MEDICAL ASSISTING

Administrative and Clinical Procedures with Anatomy and Physiology

SIXTH EDITION

MEDICAL ASSISTING

Administrative and Clinical Procedures with Anatomy and Physiology

Kathryn A. Booth, RN-BSN, RMA (AMT), RPT, CPhT, MS
Total Care Programming, Inc.
Palm Coast, Florida

Leesa G. Whicker, BA, CMA (AAMA)
Central Piedmont Community College
Charlotte, North Carolina

Terri D. Wyman, CPC, CMRS
Baystate Wing Hospital
Palmer, Massachusetts

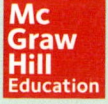

Mc
Graw
Hill
Education

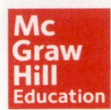

MEDICAL ASSISTING: ADMINISTRATIVE AND CLINICAL PROCEDURES WITH ANATOMY AND PHYSIOLOGY, SIXTH EDITION

Published by McGraw-Hill Education, 2 Penn Plaza, New York, NY 10121. Copyright © 2017 by McGraw-Hill Education. All rights reserved. Printed in the United States of America. Previous editions © 2014, 2011, and 2009. No part of this publication may be reproduced or distributed in any form or by any means, or stored in a database or retrieval system, without the prior written consent of McGraw-Hill Education, including, but not limited to, in any network or other electronic storage or transmission, or broadcast for distance learning.

Some ancillaries, including electronic and print components, may not be available to customers outside the United States.

This book is printed on acid-free paper.

3 4 5 6 7 8 9 0 LWI 21 20 19

ISBN   978-1-259-19774-1
MHID   1-259-19774-3

Senior Vice President, Products & Markets: *Kurt L. Strand*
Vice President, General Manager, Products & Markets: *Marty Lange*
Vice President, Content Design & Delivery: *Kimberly Meriwether David*
Managing Director: *Chad Grall*
Executive Brand Manager: *William Lawrensen*
Director, Product Development: *Rose Koos*
Senior Product Developer: *Christine Scheid*
Product Developer: *Michelle Gaseor*
Executive Marketing Manager: *Harper Christopher*
Digital Product Analyst: *Katherine Ward*
Director, Content Design & Delivery: *Linda Avenarius*
Program Manager: *Angela R. FitzPatrick*
Content Project Managers: *April R. Southwood/Brent dela Cruz*

Buyer: *Jennifer Pickel*
Design: *Srdjan Savanovic*
Content Licensing Specialists: *Lori Hancock/Lorraine Buczek*
Cover Image: *Lung:* © *Nucleus Medical Media; Taking the temperature:* © *M. Constantini/PhotoAlto;* Schedule Practice Fusion: © *Practice Fusion; Urine testing canister with rainbow squares:* © McGraw-Hill Education; *Desk:* © *MuzzyLane;* Gloved hands: © McGraw-Hill Education/Mark A. Dierker, photographer
Compositor: *SPi Global*
Printer: *LSC Communications*

All credits appearing on page or at the end of the book are considered to be an extension of the copyright page.

Library of Congress Cataloging-in-Publication Data

Booth, Kathryn A., 1957-
   Medical assisting : administrative and clinical procedures with anatomy and physiology.–Sixth edition / Kathyn A. Booth, RN-BSN, RMA(AMT), RPT, CPhT, MS, Total Care Programming, Palm Coast, Florida, Leesa G. Whicker, BA, CMA(AAMA), Central Piedmont Community College, Troy, North Carolina, Terri D. Wyman, CPC, CMRS, Wing Memorial Hospital, Monson, Massachusetts.
       pages cm
   ISBN 978-1-259-19774-1 (alk. paper)
   1. Medical assistants.   2. Clinical competence.   3. Medical offices–Management.   I. Whicker, Leesa.
   II. Wyman, Terri D.   III. Title.
   R728.8.M4 2017
   610.73'7092--dc23
                                                                                          2015032229

WARNING NOTICE: The clinical procedures, medicines, dosages, and other matters described in this publication are based upon research of current literature and consultation with knowledgeable persons in the field. The procedures and matters described in this text reflect currently accepted clinical practice. However, this information cannot and should not be relied upon as necessarily applicable to a given individual's case. Accordingly, each person must be separately diagnosed to discern the patient's unique circumstances. Likewise, the manufacturer's package insert for current drug product information should be consulted before administering any drug. Publisher disclaims all liability for any inaccuracies, omissions, misuse, or misunderstanding of the information contained in this publication. Publisher cautions that this publication is not intended as a substitute for the professional judgment of trained medical personnel.

The Internet addresses listed in the text were accurate at the time of publication. The inclusion of a website does not indicate an endorsement by the authors or McGraw-Hill Education, and McGraw-Hill Education does not guarantee the accuracy of the information presented at these sites.

mheducation.com/highered

Kathryn A. Booth, RN-BSN, RMA (AMT), RPT, CPhT, MS is a registered nurse (RN) with a master's degree in education as well as certifications in phlebotomy, pharmacy tech, and medical assisting. She is an author, an educator, and a consultant for Total Care Programming, Inc. She has over 30 years of teaching, nursing, and healthcare experience that spans five states. As an educator, Kathy has been awarded the teacher of the year in three states where she taught various health sciences, including medical assisting in both a classroom and an online capacity. Kathy serves on the AMT Examinations, Qualifications, and Standards committee, as well as the advisory board for two educational institutions. She stays current through working at various practice settings as well as obtaining and maintaining certifications. Her larger goal is to develop up-to-date, dynamic healthcare educational materials to assist her and other educators and to promote healthcare professions. In addition, Kathy enjoys presenting innovative new learning solutions for the changing healthcare and educational landscape to her fellow professionals nationwide.

Leesa G. Whicker, BA, CMA (AAMA) is a Certified Medical Assistant with a BA in art with a concentration in art history. She is an educator with more than 20 years of experience in the classroom. With 35 years of experience in the healthcare field as a medical assistant, a research specialist in molecular pathogenesis and infectious disease, and a medical assisting program director and instructor, she brings a broad background of knowledge and experience to the classroom. As a curriculum expert, she has served on several committees, including the Writing Team for the Common Course Library for the North Carolina Community College System and the Curriculum Committee at Central Piedmont Community College. She remains an active member of the Curriculum Committee. Leesa was among the first instructors to develop online courses and remains active in online curriculum development. She has presented Methods of Active and Collaborative learning on the national level. Her passion is finding novel and varied ways to reach the ever-changing learning styles of today's students. She currently teaches at Central Piedmont Community College in Charlotte, North Carolina.

Terri D. Wyman, AS, CPC, CMRS has 35 years of experience in the healthcare field, first as a CMA specializing in hematology/oncology and homecare and then in the medical billing and coding field. At the suggestion of a coworker, she began her career in education as instructor and program director for both medical assisting and medical billing and coding programs for several technical schools in New England. Currently, Terri is the financial applications analyst at Baystate Wing Hospital, where her love of teaching continues in the hospital setting. She is active with her local AAPC chapter and is on the National Advisory Board for the American Medical Billing Association (AMBA). She provides continuing education opportunities for AMBA members by writing numerous billing and coding programs and speaking at their national conferences on medical coding topics, including ICD-10. In the rapidly changing world of healthcare billing and coding, she is excited to continue sharing the language of billing and coding with instructors, students, and career professionals. Terri sends special thanks to Dale for his unending support and to Francis Stein, MD, whose patience with a new medical assistant years ago showed her the joy of learning and education.

Brief Contents

Contents

CHAPTER 7

Safety and Patient Reception 109

CHAPTER 8

Office Equipment and Supplies 138

CHAPTER 9

Examination and Treatment Areas 175

UNIT THREE

Communication

CHAPTER 10

Written and Electronic Communication 190

CHAPTER 57

Emergency Preparedness *1231*

CHAPTER 58

Preparing for the World of Work *1262*

APPENDICES

Procedures

Digital Exercises and Activities

Skills Video

Practice Medical Office

Today's medical assistants juggle many tasks in the medical office. McGraw-Hill is committed to helping prepare students to succeed in their educational program and to be successful in their chosen field. Most textbooks begin with a preface and a long list of features and supplements for both instructors and their students. While keeping with this tried-and-true format, it is our intention to give you a snapshot of some of the exciting solutions available with the sixth edition of *Medical Assisting: Administrative and Clinical Procedures with Anatomy and Physiology* for your Medical Assisting course. Instructors across the country have told us how much preparation it takes to teach medical assisting—they juggle as much, maybe more, than their students. To help, we have added more detailed information on how to organize and utilize the features as well as a breakdown of Learning Outcomes and activities that correspond in the Instructor Resources portion of Connect.

The Content—a Note from the Authors

The sixth edition of *Medical Assisting: Administrative and Clinical Procedures with Anatomy and Physiology* has many exciting and noteworthy updates. With insightful feedback from our users and reviewers, we set out to create a one-of-a-kind, dynamic, practical, realistic, *and* comprehensive set of tools for individuals preparing to become medical assistants.

When you begin the book, you will find it is not just about rote memorization of concepts. *Medical Assisting* immerses you in the world of BWW Associates Clinic, where you learn as you confront new workplace challenges in each chapter. All elements of the book—from the case studies in each chapter and the Soft Skills Success exercises to the Practice Fusion® EHR screenshots and other visuals—immerse the student in a realistic learning environment. Case studies are built around a set of patients who regularly visit BWW Associates Clinic, and you will get to know these patients as well as the employees of BWW Associates Clinic as you move through the chapters. You will also work with most of the patients of BWW Associates when using the Medical Assisting ACTIVSim™ 2.0 program.

Within this framework, we have strived to provide the most up-to-date information about all aspects of the medical assisting profession, with a focus on consistency, authenticity, and accuracy. Along with thousands of minor tweaks and updates, *Medical Assisting,* sixth edition, incorporates the following:

- Dozens of BWW EHR documentation/progress note examples in both clinical and administrative chapters

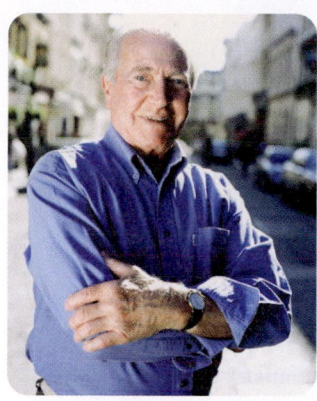

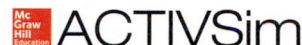

- Soft Skills Success exercises, added to the Chapter Review, test employability skills and link students to related modules in Practice Medical Office, the simulation game.
- More than 25 EHR screenshots of Practice Fusion® software, showcasing basic EHR skills in the context of the BWW Medical Associates Clinic.
- Infection control is now covered in two separate, more comprehensive chapters, with basic infection control in Chapter 7 and advanced infection control practices in Chapter 35.
- Case studies enhanced by the inclusion of more detailed clinical information and by linking the case studies and new Soft Skills Success activities where applicable.
- Revised coverage of ICD coding to focus primarily on ICD-10-CM, including detailed 1500 claim form instructions utilizing the 5010 updates to make the form compliant with ICD-10 requirements.
- Content updates, including important topics such as EHR/practice management systems, Meaningful Use, the medical assistant as a patient navigator, Globally Harmonized System (GHS), assisting in a chemical disaster, OSHA-required training, healthcare-associated infections, and other infection control practices.

A more detailed list of chapter changes is covered in the next section.

Key Chapter-by-Chapter Changes

The following chapter-by-chapter list includes the essential changes and updates made to the book. A full list of changes is available in the transition guide provided in the Instructor Resources on Connect.

Chapter 1	The medical assistant as a patient navigator, scope of practice vs. standard of care
Chapter 2	Affordable Care Act and Patient Centered Medical Care Home
Chapter 3	Professional use of personal electronic devices and social media, customer service as professionalism
Chapter 4	Difference between empathy and sympathy; introduced documentation and respecting culture differences
Chapter 5	Genetic Information Nondiscrimination Act; updated FDA regulatory functions, including the Comprehensive Drug Abuse Prevention and Control Act
Chapter 6	Changed title and content to *Infection Control Fundamentals;* transmission-based precautions and OSHA education and training requirements for ambulatory care
Chapter 7	Changed title to *Safety and Patient Reception;* medical office safety plan, Globally Harmonized System of Classification and Labeling Chemicals (GHS), and Safety Data Sheets (SDS)
Chapter 8	Computer networks and encryption, monitoring of professional e-mails, computer security
Chapter 9	ADA Amendments Act of 2008, mixing 10% bleach solution
Chapter 10	Changed title to *Written and Electronic Communication;* delivery notification, invoice vs. statement, using "rules" for e-mail management
Chapter 11	Records release rules, changed the terminology from chart to health record
Chapter 12	Meaningful Use, expanded coverage of shared data, general guidelines for using an EHR program, practice management systems
Chapter 13	Previous edition Chapter 15; now includes Retaining Files in the Office section, updated content related to filing to reflect modern office standards
Chapter 14	Previous edition Chapter 13; added automated voice response information, active listening, wireless headsets, electronic telephone messaging. Deleted information on patient courtesy phone
Chapter 15	Previous edition Chapter 14; defined modeling vs. return demonstration; sample e-newsletter, patient information form, and physician information figures added
Chapter 16	Electronic scheduler, examples of wave scheduling and modified wave scheduling
Chapter 17	Precertification, patient-centered medical homes (PCMH) concept, Medicare tax and salary requirement updates, Insurance 1500

	claim form updated to 5010 standards with new instructions
Chapter 18	Updated codes primarily to ICD-10-CM, added key terms combination codes and laterality
Chapter 19	Changed title to *Procedural Coding,* updated to 2015 codes throughout
Chapter 20	Merged chapters 20 and 21, new title *Patient Collections and Financial Management;* new sections, including In-Office Transactions, Payments After the Patient Visit, and Returned Checks, new terms added: *accounts receivable (A/R), accounts payable (A/P)*
Chapter 21	Previous edition Chapter 22; defined microvilli, added key terms word root, prefix, and suffix
Chapter 22	Previous edition Chapter 23; added acne to pathophysiology section, changed follicle description
Chapter 23	Previous edition Chapter 24; added new table The Spinal Column; defined ossification, joint junctions, and dislocation; added joint replacements and fractures to content
Chapter 24	Previous edition Chapter 25; new figures of muscle types, botulism, and tetanus
Chapter 25	Previous edition Chapter 26; new image of heart valves; added coronary circulation section
Chapter 26	Previous edition Chapter 27; added key terms *hemoglobin (Hgb), hematocrit (Hct), albumins*
Chapter 27	Previous edition Chapter 28; new table to summarize lymphatic organs, new figure of thymus and spleen; key terms *lymph node, spleen, thymus,* and *tonsils;* added celiac disease
Chapter 28	Previous edition Chapter 29; added nasal conchae parts and purposes; added parts of the pharynx
Chapter 29	Previous edition Chapter 30; new figures of Schawnn cells, movement of nerve impulse, gray and white matter and central canals
Chapter 30	Previous edition Chapter 31; new term *metabolic wastes*
Chapter 31	Previous edition Chapter 32; APGAR information with new table
Chapter 32	Previous edition Chapter 33; minor revisions to improve clarity
Chapter 33	Previous edition Chapter 34; minor revisions to improve clarity
Chapter 34	Previous edition Chapter 35; new figure of refractions, gustatory cortex
Chapter 35	New chapter *Infection Control Practices;* new content, including healthcare-associated infections, injection safety, respiratory hygiene/cough etiquette, infection control related to medical equipment, surgical site infections (SSIs), and CDC reporting requirements for infectious diseases

Chapter 36	Updated descriptions of mirroring, verbalizing, and restatement
Chapter 37	Clarified the role of pain assessment; updated image of radial pulse; key terms *hyperventilation, dyspnea,* and *rhonchi* added
Chapter 38	Improved figures of patient positions; added key term *body mechanics*
Chapter 39	Revised pelvic exam section; added better explanation of preeclampsia
Chapter 40	Added pediatric dietary guidelines table, PKU, *growth chart* as key term; new vaccine information and catch-up schedule, amblyopia added; added asthma to pathophysiology section
Chapter 41	New figure of kyphosis; added osteomalacia and sleep apnea to Table 41-1; sleep disorder feature; added adaptations and assistive devices information
Chapter 42	Added chondrosarcomas to Table 42-1; updated several images; added chemical and nuclear stress tests information
Chapter 43	Revised types of vision test and included contrast sensitivity and functional acuity tests; new figure with anatomy of the ear; added Weber and Rhine hearing tests with images
Chapter 44	Added key term *abscess;* added information about loading and unloading scalpel, suture materials, and transport bags
Chapter 45	Revised content about microscope, CLIA Certificate of Waiver, and calibration and control samples
Chapter 46	Revised content related to viruses and disease, replaced multiple images

Chapter 47	Added urine transfer straws and urine culture and sensitivity
Chapter 48	Reorganized information for clarity and added new learning outcome, new information about ESR, performing blood collection, added requisition form to chapter
Chapter 49	Updated content and photos to include MUSE Cardiology Information system; new key terms *rhythm strip, artifact,* and *peak expriatory flow rate (PEFR)*
Chapter 50	New image of stereotactic breast biopsy; added DXA section
Chapter 51	Updated information on vaccines, recordkeeping, and Rx, new key terms *adverse effects* and *side effects*
Chapter 52	Revised image of metric steps; updated images and revised the formula method explanation
Chapter 53	New images of calibrated spoons and oral syringes; additional information about needle selection
Chapter 54	New images of crutch gates to improve understanding
Chapter 55	New images of nutrients; added celiac and non-celiac gluten sensitivity, allergy treatments, preventing obesity
Chapter 56	Replenishing petty cash; new key terms, including *FICA, gross earnings, ulitization review, quality assurance, risk management, diversity*
Chapter 57	Multiple sections revised for improved understanding of content; added information about cystic duct blockage
Chapter 58	Revised information on resume types to improve understanding

A Guided Tour

Learning Outcomes, Key Terms, and Textbook Organization

Every learning outcome in *Medical Assisting,* sixth edition, is aligned with a level I heading. McGraw-Hill has made it even easier for students and instructors to find, learn, and review critical information. The chapter organization of the sixth edition is organized to promote learning based on what a medical assistant does in practice. The chapters build on one another to ensure student understanding of the many tasks they will be expected to perform. The chapters can be easily grouped together to create larger topics or units for the students to learn. For ease of understanding, content can be organized as follows:

- Unit One Medical Assisting as a Career—Chapters 1 to 5
- Unit Two Safety and the Environment—Chapters 6 to 9
- Unit Three Communication—Chapters 10 to 14
- Unit Four Administrative Practices—Chapters 15 to 20
- Unit Five Applied Anatomy and Physiology—Chapters 21 to 34
- Unit Six Infection Control and Clinical Practices—Chapters 35 to 44
- Unit Seven Assisting with Diagnostics—Chapters 45 to 50
- Unit Eight Assisting in Therapeutics—Chapters 51 to 55
- Unit Nine Medical Assisting Practice—Chapters 56 to 58

Key terms are called out at the beginning of each chapter and are set in bold throughout the text to further promote the mastery of learning outcomes.

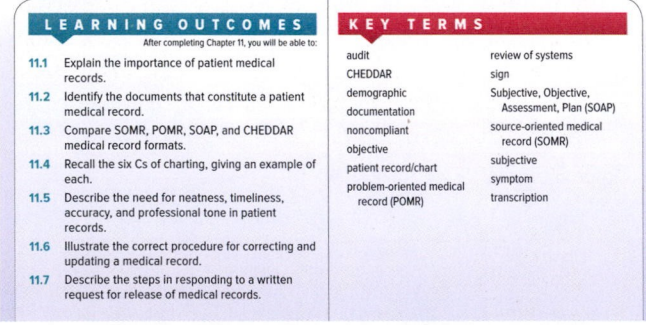

Content Correlations

Medical Assisting, sixth edition, also provides a correlation structure that will enhance its usefulness to both students and instructors. We have been careful to ensure that the text and supplements provide coverage of topics crucial to all of the following:

- CAAHEP (Commission on Accreditation of Allied Health Education Programs) Standards and Guidelines for Medical Assisting Education Programs

- ABHES (Accrediting Bureau of Health Education Schools) Competencies and Curriculum
- AAMA (American Association of Medical Assistants) CMA (Certified Medical Assistant) Occupational Analysis
- AMT (American Medical Technologists) RMA (Registered Medical Assistant) Task List
- AMT CMAS (Certified Medical Assistant Specialist) Competencies and Examination Specifications
- NHA (National Healthcareer Association) Certified Clinical Medical Assistant (CCMA)
- NHA (National Healthcareer Association) Certified Medical Administrative Assistant (CMAAA)
- CMA (AAMA) Certification Examination Content Outline
- NCCT (National Center for Competency Testing) NCMA (National Certified Medical Assistant) Detailed Test Plan
- CAHIIM (Commission on Accreditation for Health Informatics and Information Management Education)

Correlations to these are included with the instructor resources located on Connect (see later pages for information about Connect™). In addition, CAAHEP requires that all medical assistants be proficient in the 71 entry-level areas of competence when they begin medical assisting work. ABHES requires proficiency in the competences and curriculum content at a minimum. The opening pages of each chapter provide a list of the areas of competence that are covered within the chapter.

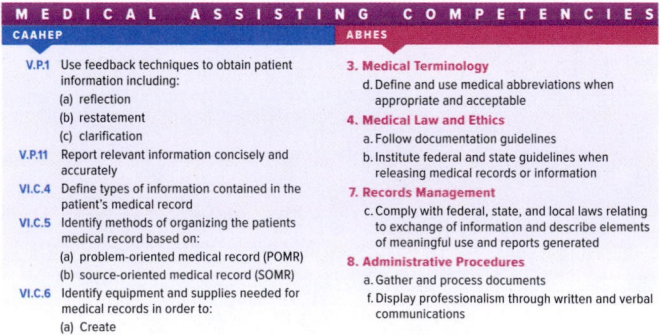

You will also find that each procedure is correlated to the ABHES and CAAHEP competencies within the workbook on the procedure sheets. These sheets can be easily pulled out of the workbook and placed in the student file to document proficiency.

Chapter Features

Each chapter opens with material that includes the Case Study, the learning outcomes, a list of key terms, the ABHES and CAAHEP medical assisting competencies covered in the chapter, and an introduction. Since the learning outcomes represent each of the level I headings in the chapter, they serve as the chapter outline. Chapters are organized into topics that move from the general to the specific. Updated color photographs, anatomical and technical drawings, tables, charts, and text features help educate the student about various aspects of medical assisting. The text features include the following:

- **Case Studies** are provided at the beginning of all chapters. They represent situations similar to those that the medical assistant may encounter in daily practice. The case studies include pictures of each of the patients who come to BWW Associates for care. Students will work with these patients in the ACTIVSim 2.0 program. Students are encouraged to consider the case study as they read each chapter. Case Study Questions in the end-of-chapter review check students' understanding and application of chapter content.

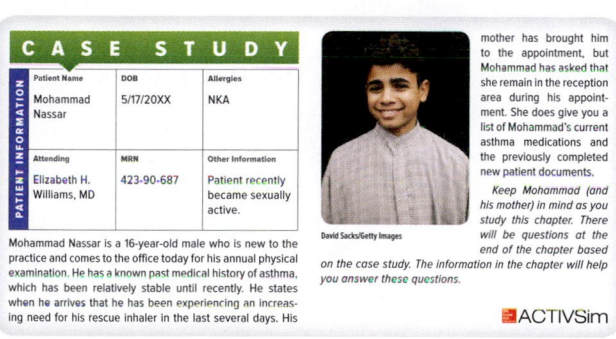

CASE STUDY

PATIENT INFORMATION	Patient Name	DOB	Allergies
	Mohammad Nassar	5/17/20XX	NKA
	Attending	MRN	Other Information
	Elizabeth H. Williams, MD	423-90-687	Patient recently became sexually active.

Mohammad Nassar is a 16-year-old male who is new to the practice and comes to the office today for his annual physical examination. He has a known past medical history of asthma, which has been relatively stable until recently. He states when he arrives that he has been experiencing an increasing need for his rescue inhaler in the last several days. His

mother has brought him to the appointment, but Mohammad has asked that she remain in the reception area during his appointment. She does give you a list of Mohammad's current asthma medications and the previously completed new patient documents.

Keep Mohammad (and his mother) in mind as you study this chapter. There will be questions at the end of the chapter based on the case study. The information in the chapter will help you answer these questions.

David Sacks/Getty Images

ACTIVSim

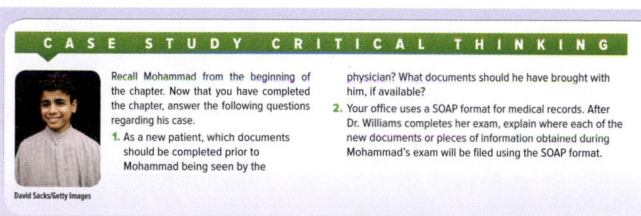

CASE STUDY CRITICAL THINKING

Recall Mohammad from the beginning of the chapter. Now that you have completed the chapter, answer the following questions regarding his case.

1. As a new patient, which documents should be completed prior to Mohammad being seen by the

physician? What documents should he have brought with him, if available?

2. Your office uses a SOAP format for medical records. After Dr. Williams completes her exam, explain where each of the new documents or pieces of information obtained during Mohammad's exam will be filed using the SOAP format.

David Sacks/Getty Images

- **Procedures** give step-by-step instructions on how to perform specific administrative or clinical tasks that a medical assistant will be required to perform. The procedures are referenced within the content when discussed. Each of the procedures is found at the end of the chapter. New figures are included with many of the procedures. In the workbook, the tearable procedure sheets that mirror the exact procedures in the book allow for easy practice and assessment. Critical procedures can also be studied in skills video exercises on Connect.

PROCEDURE 11-1 Preparing a New Patient Paper Medical Record

WORK // DOC

Procedure Goal: To assemble a new patient paper medical record

OSHA Guidelines: This procedure does not involve exposure to blood, body fluids, or tissue.

Materials: File folder, labels as appropriate (alphabet, numbers, dates, insurance, allergies, etc.), forms (patient registration, medical history, advance directives, physician progress notes, laboratory forms), and a hole punch

Method:

1. Carefully create a chart label according to practice policy. This label may include the patient's last name followed by the first name, or it may be a medical record number for those offices that utilize numeric or alphanumeric filing.
   RATIONALE: *The label must be correct to avoid filing errors.*

2. Place the chart label on the right edge of the folder, extending the label the length of the tab on the folder.

3. Place the date label on the top edge of the folder, updating the date according to practice policy. (The date is usually updated annually, if the patient has come into the office within the last year.)
   RATIONALE: *This makes it easy to identify current patient records for retrieval and identify records for purging if the patient has not been seen for a specified amount of time (often, 3 years).*

4. If alpha or numeric filing labels are utilized, place a patient name label on the chart according to practice policy.

5. Punch holes in the appropriate forms for placement within the patient's medical record.

6. Place all the forms in appropriate sections of the patient's medical record.
   RATIONALE: *Consistency in document placement assures that items can be found quickly when required.*

- **Points on Practice** feature boxes provide guidelines on keeping the medical office running smoothly and efficiently.
- **Educating the Patient** feature boxes focus on ways to instruct patients about caring for themselves outside the medical office.
- **Caution: Handle with Care** feature boxes cover the precautions to be taken in certain situations or when performing certain tasks.

CAUTION: HANDLE WITH CARE

Maintaining Standards of Cleanliness in the Reception Area

Cleanliness is (and should be) one of a medical office's hallmarks. Not only is cleanliness required in the examination and testing rooms, it is also expected in the patient reception area. A messy patient reception area reflects badly on the practice. Patients may think, "If they don't care about this, what else do they not care about?" Maintaining standards of cleanliness helps ensure that the reception area is presentable and inviting at all times.

As a medical assistant, you may be involved—along with the physician, office manager, and other staff members—in setting the office's cleanliness standards. Standards are general guidelines. In addition to setting standards, you will need to specify the tasks required to meet each standard. You also may want to create a checklist of the tasks required to meet all of these standards.

The following list outlines standards you may want to consider. Specific housekeeping tasks for meeting those standards are included in parentheses.

1. Keep everything in its place. (Complete a daily visual check for out-of-place items. Return all magazines to racks. Push chairs back into place.)

2. Dispose of all trash. (Empty trash cans. Pick up trash on the floor or on furniture.)

3. Prevent dust and dirt from accumulating on surfaces. (Wipe or dust furniture, lamps, and artificial plants. Polish doorknobs. Clean mirrors, wall hangings, and pictures.)

4. Spot-clean areas that become dirty. (Remove scuffmarks. Clean upholstery stains.)

5. Disinfect areas of the reception area if they have been exposed to body fluids. (Immediately clean and disinfect all soiled areas.)

6. Handle items with care. (Take precautions when carrying potentially messy or breakable items. Do not carry too much at once.)

After the standards have been established, type and post them in a prominent place for the office staff (but not the patients) to see. The cleaning activities checklist may be posted, but the person responsible for cleaning the office also should keep a copy. It is everyone's duty to keep the office looking clean and presentable.

A schedule of specific daily and weekly cleaning activities also should be posted. Less frequent housekeeping duties, like laundering drapes, shampooing the carpet, and cleaning windows and blinds, can be noted in a tickler file so that they will be performed on a regular basis.

It is always a good idea to have a second staff member responsible for periodically working with the medical assistant on housekeeping responsibilities. That person also may be responsible for handling cleaning duties when the medical assistant is away from the office.

- **Pathophysiology** is featured in each of the chapters on anatomy and physiology. These sections provide students with details of the most common diseases and disorders of each body system and include information on the causes, common signs and symptoms, treatment, and, where possible, the prevention of each disease.

PATHOPHYSIOLOGY

LO 23.11

Common Diseases and Disorders of the Skeletal System

Arthritis is a general term meaning "joint inflammation." Although there are more than 100 types of arthritis, we will discuss the two most common types: osteoarthritis and rheumatoid arthritis.

OSTEOARTHRITIS, also known as *degenerative joint disease (DJD),* is the most common type of joint disorder, affecting nearly everyone to some degree by the age of 70. DJD primarily affects the weight-bearing joints of the hips and knees, and the cartilage between the bones and the bones themselves begin to break down.

Causes. Research points to inflammatory processes or metabolic disorders as the etiology of DJD.

Signs and Symptoms. These include joint stiffness, aching, and pain, especially with weather changes. There is often fluid around the joint and grating noises with joint movement.

Treatment. Anti-inflammatory drugs, including aspirin and nonsteroidal anti-inflammatory drugs (NSAIDs) like naproxen and Feldene®, may be used. Intra-articular steroid injections

may be tried for severe cases. In some cases, a series of injections of hyaluronic acid–containing medications is used when other treatments do not work. These injections serve as joint fluid replacement. Some success has been found with transplanting harvested cartilage cells from the patient's healthy knee cartilage, which are then grown in the lab and reinjected into the patient's diseased joint. Surgical scraping of the joint may also be done to remove deteriorated bone fragments. As a last resort, joint replacement may be recommended.

Joint replacement prostheses can be metal, plastic, or a combination of both. The physician can surgically replace part of the joint (partial) or the entire joint (total). An example of a partial hip replacement is the Birmingham Hip Resurfacing prosthesis. In this procedure the head of the femur is replaced by an all-metal prosthesis (see Figure 23-14). One of the advantages of partial joint replacement is that it conserves more bone than conventional total joint replacement. Conserving bone is important if additional surgery is needed in the future. The surgeon will have more natural bone to work with if a revision or new prosthesis is required.

Each chapter closes with a summary of the Learning Outcomes. The summary is followed by an end-of-chapter review with questions related to the case study, as well as 10 multiple-choice exam-style questions.

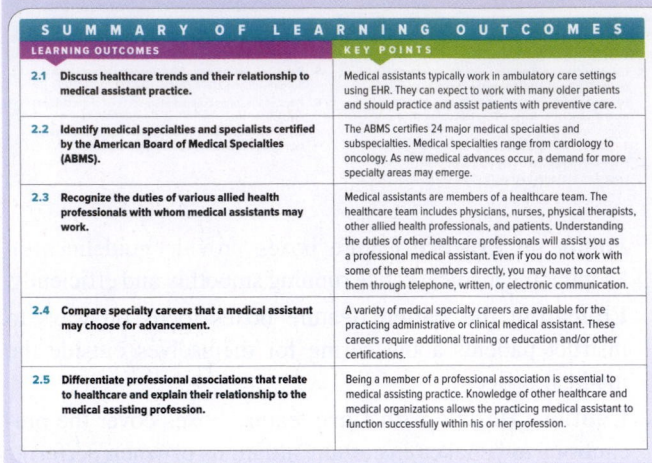

- **Medical Terminology** practice exercises have been added to all the anatomy and physiology chapters.

- **Soft Skills Success** practice scenarios emphasize employ-ability skills and critical thinking in complex situations. These new exercise features are included in most non-A&P chapters and are correlated to Practice Medical Office where applicable.

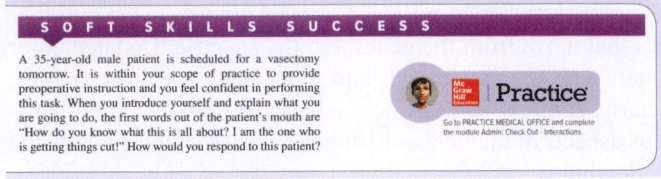

The book also includes a glossary and three appendices for use as reference tools. The glossary lists all the words presented as key terms in each chapter, along with a pronunciation guide and the definition of each term. The appendices present a list of common medical terminology, including prefixes, root words, and suffixes, as well as medical abbreviations and symbols. A Diseases and Disorders appendix provides a quick reference point for patient conditions that the student may encounter.

Digital Materials for *Medical Assisting*

For the sixth edition, we enhanced the integration between the textbook and our digital study materials and expanded our offerings to better cover all aspects of medical assisting. Links between the textbook and the key study resources are highlighted by eye-catching icons divided by resource type. Digital study resources with icons include ACTIVSim™ 2.0, BodyANIMAT3D, Practice Fusion® EHR exercises, skills videos, and Practice Medical Office.

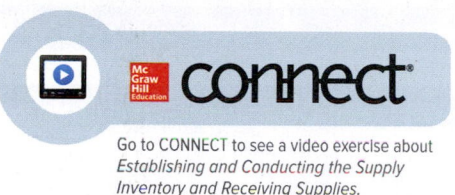

Go to CONNECT to see a video exercise about *Establishing and Conducting the Supply Inventory and Receiving Supplies.*

These different types of icons are then used to call out specific activities and exercises by name. For example, above you can see an icon for Connect skills videos (the resource) about Establishing and Conducting Supply Inventory and Receiving Supplies (the exercise name).

McGraw-Hill Connect® Medical Assisting

A number of our key resources for *Medical Assisting*, 6e—including BodyANIMAT3D activities, skills video exercises, and Practice Fusion® electronic health records simulations—are part of our Connect offering for Medical Assisting.

Here is more on what you can expect to find in Connect for *Medical Assisting*, 6e specifically:

- Pre- and Post- Tests
- End-of-Chapter Exercises
- Interactive Exercises
- Administrative and Clinical Skills Video Exercises*
- BodyANIMAT3D Exercises*
- UPDATED! EHR Exercises *
  - Utilizing both video and images, students will practice proper usage of a simulated EHR environment using Practice Fusion, the #1 cloud-based electronic health record platform. www.practicefusion.com
- NEW! Forms Exercises*
  - Utilizing common forms from a medical office, students can practice entering in the proper information from scenarios using a driver's license, an insurance form, a patient registration form, or sometimes all three. Forms include Patient Medical History, Superbill, and CMS 1500.
- NEW! Coding Exercises*
  - Utilizing scenarios developed by the authors, students can practice identifying and inputting the proper ICD-10 codes.
- NEW! Medical Terminology Practice*
  - A refresher area for the body systems chapters with Word Part exercises on select terms as well as audio terms with associated spelling practice.
- A completely revised and updated Test Bank (also available through the Instructor Resources)

*in applicable chapters

As part of Connect for Medical Assisting, we also offer SmartBook's adaptive reading experience, which is powered by LearnSmart, the most widely used adaptive learning resource.

For more information on Connect—the teaching and learning platform used with all McGraw-Hill Education products—and SmartBook look for the section *Connect, Required=Results.*

Simulations and Games for Medical Assisting

We offer two separate medical assisting study products for purchase to supplement Connect—ACTIVSim and Practice Medical Office—both of which are fully incorporated into the *Medical Assisting*, 6e learning experience.

ACTIVSim 2.0 Medical Assisting Clinical Simulator is made up of two parts: 10 Patient Case Clinical Simulators and 15 Clinical Skills Simulators. The Patient Case Clinical Simulators introduce students to nonacute medical assisting patient case scenarios, procedure simulators and quick e-learning exercises. A large portion of core clinical competencies can be simulated on virtual patients, where the learner can interact with a patient and practice the different tasks that a medical assistant performs in physicians' offices. The focus of ACTIVSim is on vital signs and obtaining patient data, including a chart feature, so that the learner can document vital signs and make notes about observations that the medical assistant can brief the doctor about. For seamless training, these patients are also used in the textbook case studies. ACTIVSim gives extensive, individualized feedback, providing students with a realistic clinical experience.

For a demo of ACTIVSim, please go to www.mhhe.com/activsim, click on Courses in the top menu, then on Health Professions in the list provided, where you'll find Medical Assisting and the option to "Try a Patient Module." An instructor's manual for ACTIVSim, updated to the sixth edition, is available in your Instructor Resources on Connect.

In **Practice Medical Office (PMO),** the student takes on the role of a new Medical Assistant in a 3D, immersive game focused on teaching the six key skills important to working in a medical office—professionalism, soft skills, office procedures, application of medical knowledge, and application of privacy and liability regulation. Practice Medical Office features twelve engaging and challenging modules representing the functional areas of a medical practice: administrative check-in interactions, clinical interactions, and administrative check-out interactions. As the players progress through each module, they will be faced with realistic situations and learning events that will test their mastery of critical job readiness skills, in a fun, engaging learning experience. PMO is accessible through a widget in Connect for *Medical Assisting*, 6e.

For a demo of Practice Medical Office, please go to http://www.mhpractice.com/products/Practice_Medical_Office and click on "Play the Demo." An instructor's manual for PMO, correlated to ABHES and CAAHEP standards by learning event, is available in your Instructor Resources on Connect.

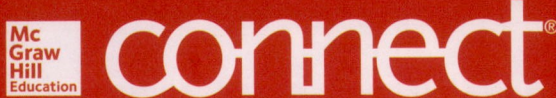

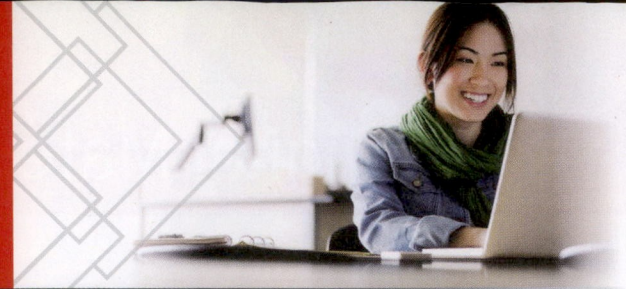

Required=Results

McGraw-Hill Connect®
Learn Without Limits

Connect is a teaching and learning platform that is proven to deliver better results for students and instructors.

Connect empowers students by continually adapting to deliver precisely what they need, when they need it, and how they need it, so your class time is more engaging and effective.

Course outcomes improve with Connect.

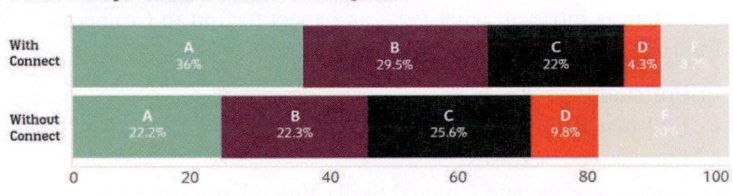

	With Connect	Without Connect
Exam Scores	80.4%	74.7%
Pass Rates	83.7%	72.9%
Attendance Rates	92.5%	74.5%
Retention Rates	87.5%	71.1%

Using **Connect** improves passing rates by **10.8%** and retention by **16.4%**.

88% of instructors who use **Connect** require it; instructor satisfaction **increases** by 38% when **Connect** is required.

Analytics

Connect Insight®

Connect Insight is Connect's new one-of-a-kind visual analytics dashboard—now available for both instructors and students—that provides at-a-glance information regarding student performance, which is immediately actionable. By presenting assignment, assessment, and topical performance results together with a time metric that is easily visible for aggregate or individual results, Connect Insight gives the user the ability to take a just-in-time approach to teaching and learning, which was never before available. Connect Insight presents data that empowers students and helps instructors improve class performance in a way that is efficient and effective.

Connect helps students achieve better grades

	A	B	C	D	F
With Connect	36%	29.5%	22%	4.3%	
Without Connect	22.2%	22.3%	25.6%	9.8%	

Based on McGraw-Hill Education Connect Effectiveness Study 2013

Students can view their results for any **Connect** course.

Mobile

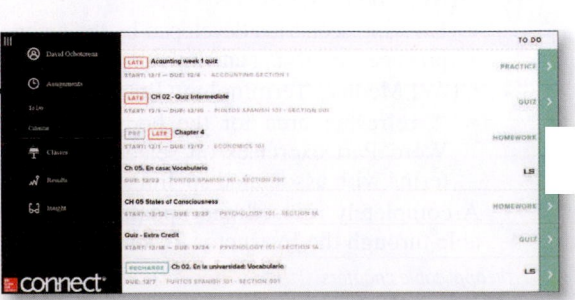

Connect's new, intuitive mobile interface gives students and instructors flexible and convenient, anytime–anywhere access to all components of the Connect platform.

Adaptive

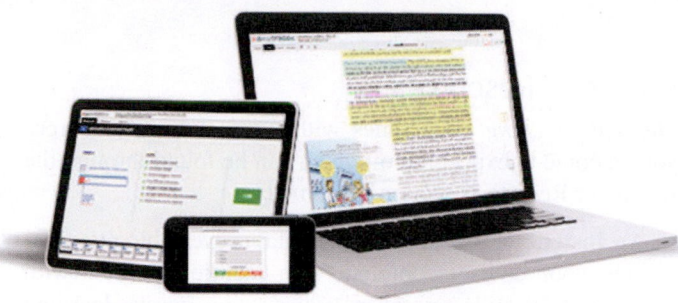

THE FIRST AND ONLY **ADAPTIVE READING EXPERIENCE** DESIGNED TO TRANSFORM THE WAY STUDENTS READ

> More students earn **A's** and **B's** when they use McGraw-Hill Education **Adaptive** products.

SmartBook®

Proven to help students improve grades and study more efficiently, SmartBook contains the same content within the print book, but actively tailors that content to the needs of the individual. SmartBook's adaptive technology provides precise, personalized instruction on what the student should do next, guiding the student to master and remember key concepts, targeting gaps in knowledge and offering customized feedback, and driving the student toward comprehension and retention of the subject matter. Available on smartphones and tablets, SmartBook puts learning at the student's fingertips—anywhere, anytime.

> Over **4 billion questions** have been answered, making McGraw-Hill Education products more intelligent, reliable, and precise.

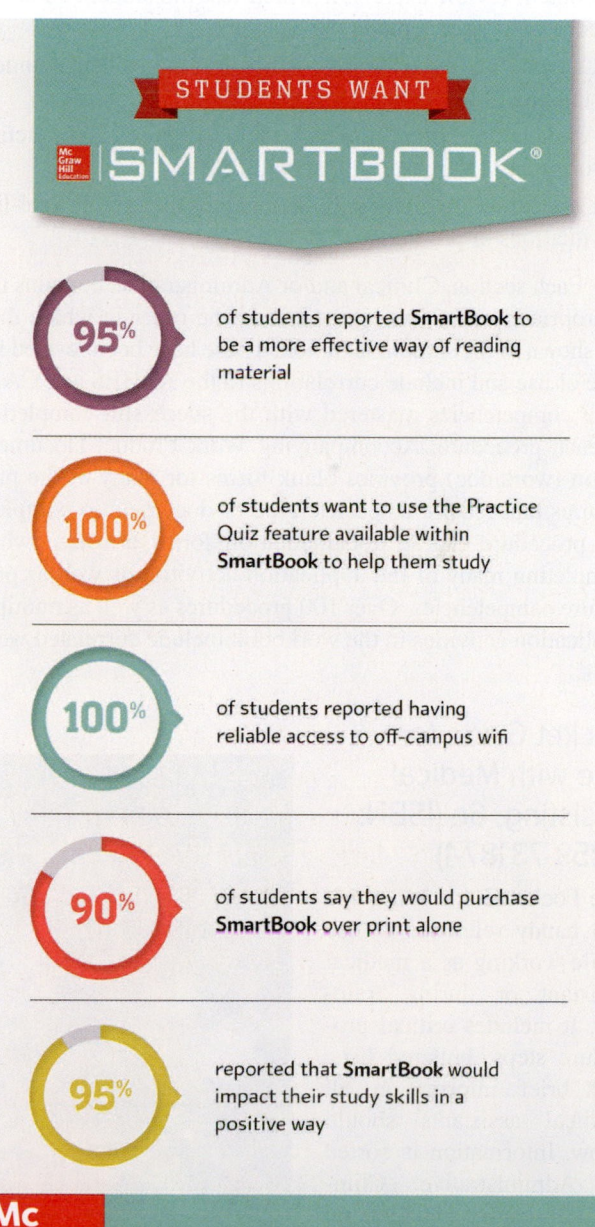

STUDENTS WANT

Mc Graw Hill Education **SMARTBOOK**®

95% of students reported **SmartBook** to be a more effective way of reading material

100% of students want to use the Practice Quiz feature available within **SmartBook** to help them study

100% of students reported having reliable access to off-campus wifi

90% of students say they would purchase **SmartBook** over print alone

95% reported that **SmartBook** would impact their study skills in a positive way

Mc Graw Hill Education

*Findings based on a 2015 focus group survey at Pellissippi State Community College administered by McGraw-Hill Education

Additional Supplementary Materials

Student Workbook for Use with Medical Assisting, 6e–in print and full color (ISBN: 1-259-73190-1)

The Student Workbook provides an opportunity for the student to review and practice the material and skills presented in the textbook. Divided into parts and presented by chapter, the first part provides the following:

- Vocabulary review exercises, which test knowledge of key terms in the chapter
- Content review exercises, which test the student's knowledge of key concepts in the chapter
- Critical thinking exercises, which test the student's understanding of key concepts in the chapter
- Application exercises, which include figures and practice forms and test mastery of specific skills
- Case studies, which apply the chapter material to real-life situations or problems

Each section, Clinical and/or Administrative, contains the appropriate procedures, presented in the order in which they are shown in the student textbook. These have been revised for ease of use and include correlations to the ABHES and CAAHEP competencies mastered with the successful completion of each procedure. Accompanying Work Product Documentation (work/doc) provides blank forms for many of the procedures that require a specific type of document to complete the procedure. These documentation forms are used when completing many of the application activities as well as procedure competencies. Over 100 procedures as well as multiple application activities in the workbook include correlated work docs.

Pocket Guide for Use with Medical Assisting, 6e (ISBN: 1-259-73187-1)

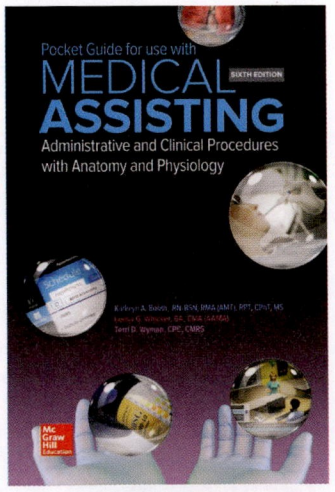

The Pocket Guide is a quick and handy reference to use while working as a medical assistant or during training. It includes critical procedure steps, bulleted lists, and brief information all medical assistants should know. Information is sorted by Administrative, Clinical, Laboratory, and General content.

Instructor Resources

Medical Assisting also comes with the instructor resources you've come to expect, all of which can be found through the Instructor Resources section in Connect.

- An **Instructor's Manual** that contains everything to organize your course, complete with lecture outlines (with PowerPoint slide references), discussion points, learning activities, and case studies. Also included are the answer keys to the book and workbook.
- **Correlation Guides** map the standards of many accreditation bureaus, including The Accrediting Bureau of Health Education Schools (ABHES) Medical Assisting competencies and curriculum; The Commission on Accreditation of Allied Health Education Programs (CAAHEP) Standards and Guidelines for Medical Assisting Education Programs competencies; American Association of Medical Assistants (AAMA) Occupational Analysis; The Association of Medical Technologists (AMT) Registered Medical Assistant (RMA) Certified Exam Topics; The National Healthcareer Association (NHA) Medical Assisting Duty/Task List; the Commission for Accreditation on Health Informatics and Information Management Education (CAHIIM); and The Secretary's Commission on Achieving Necessary Skills (SCANS) areas of competence, as well as others.
- **PowerPoint Presentations** have been fully updated to include the latest figures and content and to mirror the design of the book. Teaching notes offer suggestions—in addition to those in the Instructor's Manual—to keep your class running smoothly. We have also taken steps to make our PowerPoints more accessible, including adding alt tags for images and tables and ensuring that our slides are organized to be easily read by screen readers
- An **Asset Map** breaks down all of the resources available through the book and Connect by chapter and by learning outcome, to help you identify *what* you want to include in your course and *where* to find it.
- A **Testbank**, completely revised, with over 5,000 questions, complete with tags for learning outcomes; ABHES and CAAHEP; and Bloom's taxonomy and others to organize or modify questions to meet your course needs.
- A **Transition Guide** to help users of earlier editions make the leap to this new edition, with thorough details outlined by the authors about changes big and small.

Check out the instructor resources area on Connect for additional resources, including an image library, sample syllabi, printable procedure checklists and work documents, and more!

Acknowledgments

The task of putting together a textbook and all of its supplements, both written and digital, takes a vast amount of cumulative effort and coordination among multiple individuals and companies. To acknowledge each of them here individually would take far too long. However, we would like start by acknowledging McGraw-Hill and all of the individuals that are listed on page iv in the front of this book for their continued assistance, encouragement, and support. A special thanks for those who are so close to this edition, including Michelle, Chipper, April, Katie, Bill, Srdj, Lori, and Lorraine. Without McGraw-Hill and its valued employees, there would be no need for this acknowledgment to be written.

We would also like to distinguish some individuals who worked tirelessly and directly with us, ensuring a completely improved product: Jodie Bernard, for helping us continue the work of updating all of the figures for this edition, to keep them current, accurate, and visually appealing; Florida State University College of Medicine, Family Medicine Residency Program at Lee Memorial Health System in Fort Myers, Fort Myers Eye Associates, and Pima Heart of Arizona (specifically, David I. Lapan, MD, Claudia Rasnake, MD, and Sharlene Villanueva), for welcoming us into their institutions, allowing us to shoot more current procedural photos, and assisting us along the way. Thanks also to Jody James for picking up the pieces on numerous aspects of the project. Her attention to detail and willingness to help with whatever we needed for this edition have provided us the ability to focus on updating and reorganizing the essential content to make the 6e the best edition ever. We humbly thank each and everyone involved with this *Medical Assisting,* sixth edition.

Leesa and Terri would like to give a special thanks to Kathy Booth. Without her tireless work, team spirit and dedication to this project we would not be able to "keep the balls in the air." Her grasp of the big picture and her constant happy nature are an inspiration to us both. It is a pleasure and an honor to work with her.

Contributors and Reviewers

We, along with McGraw-Hill, would like to thank the reviewers and contributors for their assistance in developing content, offering suggestions, and shaping this revision. We appreciate you. Many of the additions, improvements, and changes are due directly to and because of their feedback. We appreciate their insight and commitment to helping us provide information that is relevant and valuable to medical assisting students.

Reviewers (Book, Workbook, LearnSmart or ActivSim)

Nick Davis, *Southern Careers Institute*
Karlene Jaggan, BIT, PN, NRCAHA *Centura College*
Shauna Phillips, RMA, CCMA, AHI *Fortis College – Phoenix*
David Martinez, MHSA, RMA *Vista College*
Kristynna Foster, MA, LVN *Charter College*
Wendy Schmerse, CPC-A, CMRS *Southern California Health Institute*
Henry Gomez, MD *ASA College*
Rebecca Ventura, RN, MSN, RMA *Davenport University – Saginaw*
Stephanie Bernard, MBA, CMA *Sanford-Brown College*
Kristy Royea, MBA, BS, CMA (AAMA), EMT-B *Mildred Elley College—Albany*
Lisa Wright, CMA (AAMA), MT, SH *Bristol Community College*
Barbara Marchelletta, CMA (AAMA), RHIT, CPC, CPT, AHI *Beal College*
Marion Odom, RMA, NCMA, CPCT, CPT, CEKG *Illinois School of Health Careers*

Melinda Wray, MA, CMA (AAMA), RMA *ECPI University*
Gerry Gordon, BA, CPC, CPB *Daytona College*
Kathleen McCall, MLT (ASCP), NCMA *DCI Career Institute*
Laura Melendez, BS, RMA, RT, BMO *Keiser University*
Adrian Rios, EMT, RMA, NCMA, MA, CPT-1 *Newbridge College*
Marlene Schmidt, MT (ASCP), DVM *Bryant & Stratton College*
Marilyn Dalton, BS, RHIT, CCS-P, CPMSM *Northeast Alabama Community College*
Mary Marks *Mitchell Community College*
Angela LeuVoy, AASMA, CMA, CBCS, CPT *Fortis College*
Luis Cedeno, BS, LPN, CPI *Miami Dade College*
Joshua Farquharson *San Joaquin Valley College – Visalia*
Marta Lopez, MD, RMA, BMO *Miami Dade College – Medical Campus*
Michelle Crissman, JD, MS, RN, CMA (AAMA) *Colorado Technical University*

Carrie Hammond, CMA (AAMA), RPT, AAS *Eagle Gate College – Murray*
Jennifer A. Leach, CCMA-NHA, BS, M.Ed *McCann School of Business and Technology*
Jean Mosley, BS, AAS, AAS, CMA (AAMA) *Surry Community College*
Jehad Ouri, CMA(AAMA) *Ohio Business College – Sheffield Village*
Kaye Bathe, CMA, BSAH *Tri-County Technical College*
Karmon Kingsley, CMA (AAMA), BS *Cleveland State Community College*
Melinda Hughes-Parnell, MSN, RN *Northwest Louisiana Technical College – Minden*
Stacey Wolfe, CMA *Community Care College*
Leeann Yurchenko, CMA (AAMA), RMA, CPC *Stautzenberger College – South*
Petra York, BS, CMA (AAMA), CPT, CET, CMAA, AHI, CPhT *Western Tech*
Lori Andrews, MSEd, RN, CMA (AAMA) *Ivy Tech Community College – Indianapolis*

Cherika de Jesus, CMA *National American University*

Leon Deutsch, MA Ed., RMA *Keiser University*

Joann Fisher, CMA (AAMA) *Elmira Business Institute (Retired)*

Rachel Houston, CMA (AAMA), AS *Cabarrus College of Health Sciences*

Beth Laurenz, BMA, BS, AAS, CMA (AAMA) *Valley View Medical Training Center*

Lynnae Lockett, RN, RMA, CMRS, MSN *Bryant & Stratton College*

Pamela McNutt, MA, RMA *National American University*

Michael Melvin, RPh, BS Pharmacy *Southern Crescent Technical College – Griffin*

Helen Mills, RN, MSN, RMA, LXMO, AHI *Keiser University*

Joanitt Montano, MD *Blue Cliff College*

Robyn Moore-Ball, RMA, AHI *Everest College – Bedford Park*

Jennifer Morrill, CMA (AAMA), RMA *North Central Michigan College*

Kim Munson, MA, CMA (AAMA), RMA (AMT) *International College of Business*

Debra Paul, BA, CMA (AAMA) *Ivy Tech Community College*

Kathleen Michael J. Perrine, MHA, RMA, NCMA, EMT *National American University*

Donna Riley, CMA (NCCT), AAS *Elmira Business Institute*

Bruno Salazar-Perea, RMA, MD *Kaplan University*

Jennifer Spencer, CMA (AAMA) *Elmira Business Institute*

Christina Steele, BS, AAGS, RMA *Dorsey Business School*

Joseph H. Balatbat, MD, RMA, RPT, CPhT, AHI *Swedish Institute College of Health Sciences*

Patti Finney, CMA (AAMA) *Ridley Lowell Business and Technical Institute*

Marissa M. Fordunski *Plaza College*

Rosemarie Scaringella, CBCS, CMAAC *Hunter Business College—Levittown*

Dawn Surridge, CMA (AAMA), AS, CPI (NCCT), CPT (NCCT) *Ridley Lowell Business and Technical Institute*

Telcida C. Dolcine, BBA, EMT-B, RMA, RPT *New York Methodist Hospital – Center for Allied Health Education*

Constantine Hatzis, MD *Mildred Elley—NYC Metro Campus*

Muhammad Khan *St. Paul's School of Nursing—Queens*

Jodi Anderson, LVN *Newbridge College*

Sixth Edition Page Proof Accuracy Checking Panel

Stephanie Bernard, BMA, CMA *Sanford-Brown College*

Kristynna M. Yateman-Foster *Charter College*

Sharon W. Breeding *Bluegrass Community and Technical College*

Carrie Mack *Premier Education Group / Branford Hall*

Tracy G. Crawford *Hinds Community College*

Melinda Wray, MA, CMA (AAMA), RMA *ECPI University*

Gerry Gordon BA, CPC, CPB *Daytona College*

Jennifer Spencer CMA (AAMA) *Elmira Business Institute*

Kristiana D. Routh, RMA *Institute of Medical and Business Careers*

Carrie Hammond, CMA (AAMA), RPT, AAS *Eagle Gate College – Murray*

Carole Zeglin, MS, BS, MT, RMA *Westmoreland County Community College*

Laura Melendez, BS, RMA, RT, BMO *Keiser University*

Angela M.B. Oliva, BSHA, CMRS, CCMA *ICDC College and OSC Computer Training*

Henry Gomez, MD *ASA College*

Debra Glover, RN, BSN *Goodwin College*

Subject Matter Expert Summit Attendees

Denise Garrow-Pruitt, Ed.D. *Middlesex Community College*

Carrie Mack *Premier Education Group/ Branford Hall*

Angela M.B. Oliva, BSHA, CMRS, CCMA *ICDC College and OSC Computer Training*

Jocelyn Lewis, PT, DPT, MS *Community College of Philadelphia*

Lorna J. Cassano, MSPT, BA *Arcadia University and Bucks County Community College*

Kevin Chakos, PharmD *American National University*

Kerry Miller, CMA, EMT-B *Globe University*

Lori Andrews, MSEd, RN, CMA (AAMA) *Ivy Tech Community College – Indianapolis*

Judith Karls, RN, BSN, MSE *Madison Area Technical College*

Mirella G. Pardee MSN, MA, RN *University of Toledo*

LearnSmart Contributors

Danielle Wilken, Ed.D, MT (ASCP) *Goodwin College*

Tammy Vannatter, BHSA, CMA (AAMA), RMA, CPC *Baker College*

Connect Practice Fusion Electronic Health Record Exercise Contributor

Amy Ensign, BHSA, CMA (AAMA), RMA (AMT) *Baker College of Clinton Township*

Connect Forms Exercise Contributor

Kerry Miller, CMA, EMT-B *Globe University*

Practice Medical Office Contributors

Suzee G. Gay, LPN

Sue Coleman, LPN, AS, RMA (AMT) *American National University*

Mario Cesar Villegas, MD *Southwest University at El Paso*

David J Holden, CMA (AAMA), RN, MSN *Bryant & Stratton College*

Dr. Marta Lopez, MD, RMA, BMO *Miami Dade College- Medical Campus*

Danielle Wilken, Ed.D, MT (ASCP) *Goodwin College*

William Hoover II, MD *Bunker Hill Community College*

Lori Andrews, MSEd, RN, CMA (AAMA) *Ivy Tech Community College – Indianapolis*

Daria M Garcia, AAS, RMA, NCMA *Kaplan College*

Helen Mills, RN, MSN, RMA, AHI, LXMO *Keiser University*

Dr. Barbara Worley, BS, DPM, RMA (AMT) *King's College*

ActivSim Instructor's Manual Contributor

Danielle Wilken, Ed.D, MT (ASCP) *Goodwin College*

PowerPoint Contributor

Yvonne Alles BS, MBA, DHA, STAR *Davenport University*

Introduction to Medical Assisting

CASE STUDY

Employee Name	Position	Credentials
Sandro Peso	Student	In Training

Supervisor	Date of Hire	Other Information
Malik Katahri, CMM	10/11/20XX	Assigned to Dr. Paul F. Buckwalter

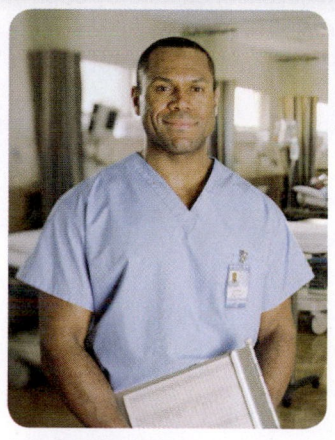

© Ryan McVay/Getty Images RF

Sandro Peso is a 33-year-old father of four who lost his job at a local factory. He is a medical assistant-in-training and is currently working at BWW Associates. He will be working in the administrative, clinical, and laboratory sections of the office. He wants to decide which area he likes best and where he might like to work when he finishes his training. It will not be long until he graduates and needs to take the test to become credentialed. He is nervous about the exam but really wants to do well to get the best job he can to help support his family.

Keep Mr. Peso in mind as you study this chapter. There will be questions at the end of the chapter based on the case study. The information in the chapter will help you answer these questions.

LEARNING OUTCOMES

After completing Chapter 1, you will be able to:

1.1 Recognize the duties and responsibilities of a medical assistant.

1.2 Distinguish various organizations related to the medical assisting profession.

1.3 Explain the need for and importance of the medical assistant credentials.

1.4 Identify the training needed to become a professional medical assistant.

1.5 Discuss professional development as it relates to medical assisting education.

KEY TERMS

accreditation

Accrediting Bureau of Health Education Schools (ABHES)

American Association of Medical Assistants (AAMA)

American Medical Technologists (AMT)

certification

Certified Medical Assistant (CMA)

Clinical Laboratory Improvement Amendments of 1988 (CLIA '88)

Commission on Accreditation of Allied Health Education Programs (CAAHEP)

continuing education

cross-training

Health Insurance Portability and Accountability Act (HIPAA)

licensed practitioner

multiskilled healthcare professional (MSHP)

Occupational Safety and Health Administration (OSHA)

patient navigator

professional development

Registered Medical Assistant (RMA)

registration

résumé

scope of practice

standard of care

MEDICAL ASSISTING COMPETENCIES

CAAHEP

V.C.12 Define patient navigator

V.C.13 Describe the role of the medical assistant as a patient navigator

X.C.1 Differentiate between the scope of practice and standards of care for medical assistants

X.C.5 Discuss licensure and certification as they apply to healthcare providers

X.P.1 Locate a state's legal scope of practice for medical assistants

ABHES

1. General Orientation

  a. Describe the current employment outlook for the medical assistant

  c. Describe medical assistant credentialing requirements and the process to obtain the credential. Comprehend the importance of credentialing

  d. List the general responsibilities & skills of the medical assistant

4. Medical Law and Ethics

  f. Comply with federal, state, and local health laws and regulations as they relate to healthcare settings

    (1) Define scope of practice for the medical assistant within the state that the medical assistant is employed

    (2) Describe what procedures can and cannot be delegated to the medical assistant and by whom within various employment settings

11. Career Development

  b. Demonstrate professional behavior

▶ Introduction

Healthcare is changing at a rapid rate. Advanced technology, implementation of cost-effective medicine, and the aging population are all factors that have caused growth in the healthcare services industry. As the healthcare services industry expands, the US Department of Labor projects that medical assisting will grow 29% between 2012 and 2022, which is much faster than the average for all occupations. The growth in the number of physicians' group practices and other healthcare practices that use support personnel will in turn continue to drive up demand for medical assistants. Medical assisting is the perfect complement to the changing healthcare industry.

Medical assistants have the training to perform a variety of duties, which qualify them to fill many different job openings in the healthcare industry. This chapter provides an introduction to the medical assisting profession. It presents a general description of your future duties, credentials, and needed training. Some basic facts about professional associations, organizations, and development related to medical assisting are also discussed. All of this will help you begin your career as a medical assistant.

▶ Responsibilities of the Medical Assistant   LO 1.1

Your specific responsibilities as a medical assistant will depend on the type, location, and size of the facility, as well as its medical specialties. General tasks performed by most medical assistants include working and communicating with patients throughout the healthcare experience. In fact, medical assistants often perform the role of **patient navigator.** They help patients find their way through the sometimes complex healthcare system, helping them overcome any barriers they may encounter to help ensure that they get the diagnosis and treatment they need in a timely manner.

Medical assistants work in an administrative, clinical, and/or laboratory capacity. As an administrative medical assistant, you may handle the payroll for the office staff (or supervise a payroll service), obtain equipment and supplies, and serve as the link between the physician or other **licensed practitioner** and representatives of pharmaceutical and medical supply companies. As a clinical medical assistant, you will be the physician's or other licensed practitioner's right arm by maintaining an efficient office, preparing and maintaining medical records, assisting the practitioner during examinations, and keeping examination rooms in order. Note that a licensed practitioner in healthcare means an individual other than a physician who is licensed or otherwise authorized by the state to provide healthcare services. Your laboratory duties as a medical assistant may include performing basic laboratory tests and maintaining laboratory equipment. In small practices, you may handle all duties. In larger practices, you may specialize in a particular duty. As you grow in your profession, advanced duties may be required. The lists of duties in Table 1-1 are provided to help you better understand what you will be doing when you practice as a medical assistant.

TABLE 1-1	Daily Duties of Medical Assistants	
Duty Type	**Entry-Level Duties**	**Advanced Duties**
General © ERproductions Ltd/Blend Images LLC RF	• Recognizing and responding effectively to verbal, nonverbal, and written communications • Explaining treatment procedures to patients • Providing patient education within scope of practice • Facilitating treatment for patients from diverse cultural backgrounds and for patients with hearing or vision impairments, or physical or mental disabilities • Acting as a patient navigator and advocate • Maintaining medical records	None
Administrative © JGI/Daniel Grill/Blend Images/Getty Images RF	• Greeting patients • Handling correspondence • Scheduling appointments • Answering telephones • Creating and maintaining patient medical records • Handling billing, bookkeeping, and insurance processing • Performing medical transcription • Arranging for hospital admissions	• Developing and conducting public outreach programs to market the licensed practitioner's professional services • Negotiating leases of equipment and supply contracts • Negotiating nonrisk and risk managed care contracts • Managing business and professional insurance • Developing and maintaining fee schedules • Participating in practice analysis • Coordinating plans for practice enhancement, expansion, consolidation, and closure • Performing as a HIPAA compliance officer • Providing personnel supervision and employment practices • Providing information systems management
Clinical © Anderson Ross/Photolibrary RF	• Assisting the licensed practitioner during examinations • Assisting with asepsis and infection control • Performing diagnostic tests, such as spirometry and ECGs • Giving injections, where allowed • Phlebotomy, including venipuncture and capillary puncture • Disposing of soiled or stained supplies • Performing first aid and cardiopulmonary resuscitation (CPR) • Preparing patients for examinations • Preparing and administering medications as directed by the licensed practitioner, and following state laws for invasive procedures • Recording vital signs and medical histories • Removing sutures or changing dressings on wounds • Sterilizing medical instruments • Instructing patients about medication and special diets, authorizing drug refills as directed by the licensed practitioner, and calling pharmacies to order prescriptions • Assisting with minor surgery • Teaching patients about special procedures before laboratory tests, surgery, X-rays, or ECGs	• Initiating an IV and administering IV medications with appropriate training, and as permitted by state law • Reporting diagnostic study results • Assisting patients in the completion of advance directives and living wills • Assisting with clinical trials
Laboratory © Adam Gault/Getty Images RF	• Performing Clinical Laboratory Improvement Amendments (CLIA)–waived tests, such as a urine pregnancy test, on the premises • Collecting, preparing, and transmitting laboratory specimens • Teaching patients to collect specific specimens properly • Arranging laboratory services • Meeting safety standards (OSHA guidelines) and fire protection mandates	• Performing as an OSHA compliance officer • Performing moderately complex laboratory testing with appropriate training and certification

You may also choose to specialize in a specific area of healthcare. For example, podiatric medical assistants make castings of feet, expose and develop X-rays, and assist podiatrists in surgery. Ophthalmic medical assistants help ophthalmologists (doctors who provide eye care) by administering diagnostic tests, measuring and recording vision, testing the functioning of eyes and eye muscles, and performing other duties. A discussion of medical specialties is found in the chapter *Healthcare and the Healthcare Team*. For specific information about medical assistant duties within medical specialty practice, review the following chapters: *Assisting in Reproductive and Urinary Specialties, Assisting in Pediatrics, Assisting in Geriatrics, Assisting in Other Medical Specialties,* and *Assisting with Eye and Ear Care.*

▶ Medical Assisting Organizations   LO 1.2

Many organizations guide the profession of medical assisting. These include professional associations such as the American Association of Medical Assistants (AAMA) and the American Medical Technologists (AMT), as well as accrediting and other organizations. As a future medical assistant, knowledge of these organizations will help you make critical decisions about your career.

Professional associations set high standards for quality and performance in a profession. They define the tasks and functions of an occupation, and they provide members with the opportunity to communicate and network with one another. Becoming a member of a professional association helps you achieve career goals and furthers the profession of medical assisting. Joining as a student is encouraged and some associations even offer discounted rates to students for a specified amount of time after graduation.

American Association of Medical Assistants

The idea for a national association of medical assistants—later to be called the **American Association of Medical Assistants (AAMA)**—was suggested at the 1955 annual state convention of the Kansas Medical Assistants Society. The next year, at an American Medical Association (AMA) meeting, the AAMA was officially created. In 1978, the US Department of Health, Education, and Welfare declared medical assisting as an allied health profession.

AAMA's Purpose The AAMA works to raise standards of medical assisting to a more professional level. It is the only professional association devoted exclusively to the medical assisting profession.

AAMA Occupational Analysis In 1996, the AAMA formed a committee whose goal was to revise and update its standards for the **accreditation** of programs that teach medical assisting. The committee's findings were published in 1997 as the "AAMA Role Delineation Study: Occupational Analysis of the Medical Assistant Profession." The study included a Role Delineation Chart that outlined the areas of competence to be mastered as an entry-level medical assistant. The Role Delineation Chart of the CMA (AAMA) was updated in 2003 to include additional competencies. In 2009, and again in 2013, it was updated and named the Occupational Analysis of the CMA (AAMA).

The Occupational Analysis provides the basis for medical assisting education and evaluation. Mastery of the areas of competence listed in the Occupational Analysis is required for all students in accredited medical assisting programs. The Occupational Analysis includes three areas of competence: administrative, clinical, and general. Each of these three areas is divided into narrower areas, for a total of 10 specific areas of competence. Within each area, a bulleted list of statements describes the medical assistant's role.

According to the AAMA, the Occupational Analysis may be used to

- Describe the field of medical assisting to other healthcare professionals.
- Identify entry-level areas of competence for medical assistants.
- Help practitioners assess their own current competence in the field.
- Aid in the development of **continuing education** programs.
- Prepare appropriate types of materials for home study.

Professional Support for CMAs (AAMA) When you become a member of the AAMA, you will have a large support group of active medical assistants. Membership benefits include

- Professional publications, such as *CMA Today*.
- A large variety of educational opportunities, such as chapter-sponsored seminars and workshops about the latest administrative, clinical, and management topics.
- Group insurance.
- Legal information.
- Local, state, and national activities that include professional networking and multiple continuing education opportunities.
- Legislative monitoring to protect your right to practice as a medical assistant.
- Access to the website at http://www.aama-ntl.org.

American Medical Technologists (AMT)

American Medical Technologists (AMT) is a nonprofit certification agency and professional membership association representing over 45,000 individuals in allied healthcare. Established in 1939, AMT began a program to register medical assistants at accredited schools in the early 1970s. The AMT provides allied health professionals with professional certification services and membership programs to enhance their professional and personal growth. Upon certification, individuals automatically become members of AMT and start to receive benefits. You will read more about the benefits of joining a professional organization later in the chapter. The AMT provides many certifications, including the Registered Medical Assistant RMA (AMT) credential and the Certified Medical Assistant Specialist CMAS (AMT) credential.

Professional Support for RMAs (AMT) The AMT offers many benefits for RMAs (AMT). These include

- Professional publications.
- Membership in the AMT Institute for Education.
- Group insurance programs—liability, health, and life.
- State chapter activities.
- Legal representation in health legislative matters.
- Annual meetings and educational seminars.
- Student membership.
- Access to the website at http://www.americanmedtech.org.

Other Medical Assisting Organizations

In addition to the AAMA, which provides the CMA credential, and the AMT, which provides the RMA and CMAS credentials, many organizations provide certification testing and medical assisting credentials. Specific information about medical assisting credentials is discussed later in this chapter.

National Healthcareer Association (NHA) This organization was established in 1989 as an information resource and network for today's active healthcare professionals. NHA provides certification and continuing education services for healthcare professionals and curriculum development for educational institutions. It offers a variety of certification exams, including Billing and Coding Specialist (CBCS), Medical Administrative Assistant (CMAA), and Clinical Medical Assistant (CCMA). Some of the NHA's programs and services include

- Certification development and implementation.
- Continuing education curriculum development and implementation.
- Program development for unions, hospitals, and schools.
- Educational, career advancement, and networking services for members.
- Registry of certified professionals.

Healthcare educators working in their various fields of study develop the National Healthcare Association certification exams. The NHA is a member of the National Organization of Competency Assurance (NOCA).

National Center for Competency Testing (NCCT) This is an independent agency that certifies the validity of competency and knowledge of the medical profession through examination. Medical assistants and medical office assistants receive the designation of National Certified Medical Assistant (NCMA) and National Certified Medical Office Assistant (NCMOA) after passing the certification examination. The NCCT avoids any allegiance to a specific organization or association.

The National Association for Health Professionals (NAHP) NAHP (http://www.nahpusa.com) offers multiple credentials for healthcare professionals. The organization, which has been in existence for 30 years, prides itself in making the process of obtaining a credential an accessible, affordable, and obtainable goal for individuals who wish to show commitment to their chosen profession. Having multiple credentials with one agency makes maintaining continuing education easier for practicing healthcare professionals. The NAHP offers many credentials, including the Medical Assistant, Phlebotomy Technician, EKG Technician, Coding Specialist, Administrative Health Assistant, Patient Care Technician, Dental Assistant, Pharmacy Technician, and Surgical Technician credentials.

With the growth of the medical assisting field, new organizations have developed to serve professionals. For example, the American Medical Certification Association (AMCA), founded in 2010, provides certification for clinical and/or administrative medical assistants. The American Registry of Medical Assistants (ARMA) is also one of many national certifying organizations, which certifies/registers medical assistants. Prospective medical assistants should be knowledgeable about the agency they will use to obtain their medical assisting credential.

▶ Medical Assistant Credentials   LO 1.3

Certification is confirmation by an organization that an individual is qualified to perform a job to professional standards. **Registration,** on the other hand, does not guarantee an individual's competence. Instead, registration is the granting of a title or license by a board that gives permission to practice in a chosen profession. Once credentialed, you earn the right to wear a pin that is obtained through the credentialing organization (Figure 1-1).

Medical assisting credentials such as certification and registration are not always required to practice as a medical assistant. However, employers today are aggressively recruiting medical assistants who are credentialed in their field. Small physician practices are being consolidated or merged into larger providers of healthcare, such as hospitals, to decrease operating expenses. Human resource directors of these larger organizations place great importance on professional credentials for their employees.

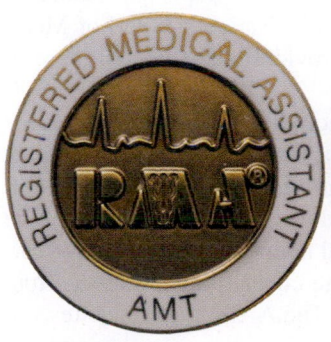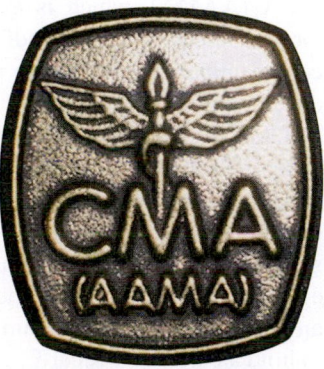

FIGURE 1-1 Wearing one of these pins indicates you have obtained a credential in medical assisting. Medical assistants registered by the American Medical Technologists must past the RMA exam to be certified and can wear the pin on the left. Members of the American Association of Medical Assistants who pass the CMA exam wear the pin on the right.
© Total Care Programming, Inc.

An accredited medical assisting program is competency based; this means that standards are set by an accrediting body for skill and proficiency in administrative and clinical tasks. Accrediting bodies are discussed later in this chapter. It is the educational institution's duty to ensure that medical assisting students learn all medical assisting competencies and that evidence is clearly documented for each student. Periodic evaluations are performed by the accrediting agencies to ensure the effectiveness of the program.

Competencies and proficiency assessments are parts of the CMA (AAMA) examination. For example, administering medications is a competency required of accredited medical assisting programs and is a component of the CMA (AAMA) examination. The CMA (AAMA) credential and the affiliation with a professional organization demonstrate competence and provide evidence of training. They also lessen the likelihood of a legal challenge to the quality of a medical assistant's work. Basically, there is less chance of malpractice if employees are credentialed through AAMA or AMT. School accreditation and credentials will be discussed in more detail later in this chapter.

State and Federal Regulations

Certain provisions of the **Occupational Safety and Health Administration (OSHA)** and the **Clinical Laboratory Improvement Amendments of 1988 (CLIA '88)** are making mandatory credentialing for medical assistants a logical step in the hiring process. OSHA and CLIA '88 regulate healthcare but presently do not require that medical assistants be credentialed. However, various components of these statutes can be met by demonstrating that medical assistants are certified. For example, some physician offices perform moderately complex laboratory testing on-site. The medical assistant can perform moderately complex tests if she or he has the appropriate training and skills.

AAMA Credential

The **Certified Medical Assistant (CMA)** credential is awarded by the Certifying Board of the AAMA. The AAMA's certification examination evaluates mastery of medical assisting competencies based on the Occupational Analysis of the CMA (AAMA), which is available at http://www.aama-ntl .org/resources/library/OA.pdf. The National Board of Medical Examiners (NBME) also provides technical assistance in developing the tests.

CMAs (AAMA) must recertify the credential every 5 years. To be recertified as a CMA (AAMA), 60 contact hours must be accumulated during the 5-year period: 10 in the administrative area, 10 in the clinical area, and 10 in the general area, with 30 additional hours in any of the three categories. In addition, 30 of these contact hours must be from an approved AAMA program. The AAMA also requires you to hold a current CPR card.

The recertification mandate requires you to learn about new medical developments through education courses or participation in an examination. Hundreds of continuing education courses are sponsored by local, state, and national AAMA groups. The AAMA also offers self-study courses through its continuing education department.

Only students who have completed medical assisting programs accredited by CAAHEP and ABHES are eligible to take the certification examination. The AAMA offers the Candidate's Guide to the Certification Examination to help applicants prepare for the examination. This guide explains the test format and test-taking strategies. It also includes a sample examination with answers and information about study references. Some schools have also incorporated test preparation reviews into their programs.

The CMA (AAMA) examination is a computerized test that may be taken any time at a designated testing site in your area. You may search the Internet for an application and test review materials. Once you have successfully passed the CMA (AAMA) examination, you have earned the right to add that credential to your name, such as Miguel A. Perez, CMA (AAMA).

AMT Credentials

The American Medical Technologists (AMT) organization credentials medical assistants as **Registered Medical Assistants (RMA)** or Certified Medical Assistant Specialists (CMAS). Although this section focuses on the RMA credential, you can find more about the CMAS credential on the AMT website at http://www.amt1.org.

Requirements for the RMA (AMT) credential include

- Graduation from a medical assistant program that is accredited by ABHES or CAAHEP, or is accredited by a regional accrediting commission, by a national accrediting organization approved by the US Department of Education, or by a formal medical services training program of the US Armed Forces.

- Alternatively, employment in the medical assisting profession for a minimum of 5 years, no more than 2 years of which may have been as an instructor in the postsecondary medical assistant program.

- Passing the AMT examination for RMA (AMT) certification.

RMAs (AMT) must accumulate 30 contact hours for continuing education units (CEUs) every 3 years if they were certified after 2006. RMAs (AMT) who were certified before this date are expected to keep abreast of all the changes and practices in their field through educational programs, workshops, or seminars. However, there are no specific continuing education requirements. Once a medical assistant has passed the AMT exam, she has earned the right to add RMA (AMT) to her name: Kaylyn R. Haddix, RMA (AMT).

The RMA (AMT) and CMA (AAMA) Examinations

The RMA (AMT) and CMA (AAMA) qualifying examinations are rigorous. Participation in an accredited program will help you learn what you need to know. The examinations cover several distinct areas of knowledge, including

- General medical knowledge, including terminology, anatomy, physiology, behavioral science, medical law, and ethics.

- Administrative knowledge, including medical records management, collections, insurance processing, and the **Health Insurance Portability and Accountability Act (HIPAA).** HIPAA is a set of government regulations that help ensure continuity and privacy of healthcare, among other things.
- Clinical knowledge, including examination room techniques, medication preparation and administration, pharmacology, and specimen collection.

Each certification examination is based on a specific content outline created by the certifying organization. You should research the Internet to gain additional information regarding any of these certifications. See Procedure 1-1, Obtaining Certification/Registration Information Through the Internet.

▶ Training Programs   LO 1.4

With continuous changes in healthcare today, the role of the medical assistant has become dynamic and wide ranging. These changes have expanded the expectations for medical assistants. The knowledge base of the modern medical assistant includes

- Administrative and clinical skills.
- Patient insurance product knowledge (specific to the workers' geographic locations).
- Compliance with healthcare-regulating organizations.
- Exceptional customer service.
- Practice management.
- Current patient treatments and education.

The medical assisting profession requires a commitment to self-directed, lifelong learning. Healthcare is changing rapidly because of new technology, new healthcare delivery systems, and new approaches to facilitating cost-efficient, high-quality healthcare. A medical assistant who can adapt to change and is continually learning will be in high demand.

Formal programs in medical assisting are offered in a variety of educational settings, including vocational-technical high schools, postsecondary vocational schools, community and junior colleges, and 4-year colleges and universities. Vocational school programs usually last 9 months to 1 year and award a certificate or diploma. Community and junior college programs are usually 2-year associate's degree programs. Training can be obtained through traditional classroom as well as online settings.

Program Accreditation

Accreditation is the process by which programs are officially authorized. The US Department of Education recognizes two national entities that accredit medical assisting educational programs:

- **Commission on Accreditation of Allied Health Education Programs (CAAHEP).** CAAHEP works directly with the Medical Assisting Educational Review Board (MAERB) of Medical Assistants Endowments to ensure that all accredited schools provide a competency-based education. CAAHEP accredits medical assisting programs in both

public and private postsecondary institutions throughout the United States that prepare individuals for entry into the medical assisting profession.
- **Accrediting Bureau of Health Education Schools (ABHES).** ABHES accredits private postsecondary institutions and programs that prepare individuals for entry into the medical assisting profession.

Accredited programs must cover the following topics:

- Anatomy and physiology
- Medical terminology
- Medical law and ethics
- Psychology
- Oral and written communications
- Laboratory procedures
- Clinical and administrative procedures

High school students may prepare for these courses by studying mathematics, health, biology, office skills, bookkeeping, and information technology. You may obtain current information about accreditation standards for medical assisting programs from the AAMA.

Medical assisting programs must also include a practicum (externship) or work experience. This applied training is for a specified length of time in an ambulatory care setting, such as a physician's office, hospital, or other healthcare facility. Additionally, the AAMA lists its minimum standards for accredited programs. This list of standards ensures that all personnel—administrators and faculty alike—are qualified to perform their jobs. These standards also ensure that financial and physical resources are available at accredited programs.

Graduation from an accredited program helps your career in three ways. First, it shows that you have completed a program that meets nationally accepted standards. Second, it provides recognition of your education by professional peers. Third, it makes you eligible for registration or certification. Students who graduate from an ABHES- or CAAHEP-accredited medical assisting program are eligible to take the CMA (AAMA) or RMA (AMT) immediately.

Work Experience

Your practicum (externship) or work experience is mandatory in accredited schools. The length of your experience will vary, depending on your particular program, so familiarize yourself with the program requirements as soon as possible. Since this is a required part of the program, no matter how good your grades are in class, if the work experience is not completed, you will not graduate from the program.

Your practicum (externship) or work experience is an extension of your classroom learning experience. You will apply skills learned in the classroom in an actual medical office or other healthcare facility. You also earn the right to include this applied training experience on your résumé under job experience, as long as you title it as "Medical Assistant Practicum, Externship, or Work Experience." The *Preparing for the World of Work* chapter will further explain your practical work experience.

▶ Professional Development LO 1.5

Professional development refers to skills and knowledge attained for both personal development and career advancement. During your training, you should strive to improve your knowledge and skills. This will help you transition into your first job with ease. You can also gain valuable knowledge and skills through volunteering prior to or in addition to work experience obtained as a student.

Once you have entered the world of work as a medical assistant, you will want to continue to develop in your profession. You can do this through additional training, **cross-training,** and other forms of continuing education.

Volunteer Programs

Volunteering is a rewarding experience. Before you even begin a medical assisting program, you can gain experience in a healthcare profession through volunteer work. As a volunteer, you will get hands-on training and learn what it is like to assist patients who are ill, disabled, or frightened.

You may volunteer as an aide in a hospital, clinic, nursing home, or doctor's office, or as a typist or filing clerk in a medical office or medical record room. Some visiting nurse associations and hospices (home-like medical settings that provide medical care and emotional support to terminally ill patients and their families) also offer volunteer opportunities. These experiences may help you decide if you want to pursue a career as a medical assistant.

The American Red Cross also offers volunteer opportunities for student medical assistants. The Red Cross needs volunteers for its disaster relief programs locally, statewide, nationally, and abroad. As part of a disaster relief team at the site of a hurricane, tornado, storm, flood, earthquake, or fire, volunteers learn first-aid and emergency triage skills. Red Cross volunteers gain valuable work experience that may help them obtain a job.

Because volunteers are not paid, it is usually easy to find work opportunities. Just because you are not paid for volunteer work, however, does not mean the experience is not useful for meeting your career goals.

Include information about any volunteer work on your **résumé**—a document that summarizes your employment and educational history. Be sure to note specific duties, responsibilities, and skills you developed during the volunteer experience. Refer to the *Preparing for the World of Work* chapter for examples of résumés.

Multiskilled Healthcare Professionals

Many hospitals and healthcare practices are embracing the idea of a **multiskilled healthcare professional (MSHP).** An MSHP is a cross-trained team member who is able to handle many different duties.

Reducing Healthcare Costs By hiring multiskilled healthcare professionals, healthcare organizations can reduce personnel costs. MSHPs can perform the functions of two or more people, so they are cost-effective employees and are in high demand.

Expanding Your Career Opportunities Career opportunities are vast if you are self-motivated and willing to learn new skills. Following are some examples of positions for medical assistants with additional experience and certifications:

- Medical office manager
- Medical biller and coder
- Medical assisting instructor (with a specified amount of experience and education)
- ECG technician
- Sterilization technician
- Patient care technician

If you are multiskilled, you will have an advantage when job hunting. Employers are eager to hire multiskilled medical assistants and may even create positions for them.

You can gain multiskill training by showing initiative and a willingness to learn every aspect of the medical facility in which you are working. When you begin working in a medical facility, establish goals regarding your career path and discuss them with your immediate supervisor. Indicate to your supervisor that you would like cross-training in every aspect of the medical facility. Begin in the department in which you are currently working and branch out to other departments once you master the skills needed for your current position. This will demonstrate a commitment to your profession and a strong work ethic. Cross-training is a valuable marketing tool to include on your résumé.

Scope of Practice

Professional development includes knowing your **scope of practice** and working within it. Medical assistants are not "licensed" healthcare professionals and most often work under a licensed healthcare provider, such as a nurse practitioner or physician. Licensed healthcare professionals may delegate certain duties to a medical assistant, providing he or she has had the appropriate training through an accredited medical assisting program or through on-the-job training provided by the medical facility or physician.

Questions often arise regarding the kinds of duties a medical assistant can perform. There is no universal answer to these questions. There is no single national definition of a medical assistant's scope of practice, so the medical assistant must research the state in which he or she works to learn about the scope of practice. You can find this information online by entering "medical assistant scope of practice" and the name of your state in any major search engine. In general, a medical assistant may not perform procedures for which he or she was not educated or trained. Examples of procedures medical assistants may not perform include administering intravenous medications (without advanced training), diagnosing patients or informing patients of a diagnosis, and giving any advice to a patient unless permitted by a facility's standard policies and procedures. The AAMA and AMT are good resources to assist you in your research. The AAMA Occupational Analysis is also a helpful reference source that identifies the procedures that medical assistants are educated to perform.

Do not confuse the terms *scope of practice* and *standard of care*. A medical assistant's scope of practice is the set of procedures that can be performed and the actions that can be taken under the terms of his or her professional license and training. **Standard of care** is a legal term that refers to the care that would ordinarily be provided by an average, prudent healthcare provider in a given situation.

Networking

Networking is building alliances—socially and professionally. It starts long before your job search. By attending professional association meetings, conferences, or other functions, medical assistants generate opportunities for employment and personal and professional growth. Networking, through continuing education conferences throughout your career, keeps the doors open to employment advancement.

PROCEDURE 1-1 Obtaining Certification/Registration Information Through the Internet

Procedure Goal: To obtain information from the Internet regarding professional credentialing

OSHA Guidelines: This procedure does not involve exposure to blood, body fluids, or tissue.

Materials: Computer with Internet access and printer

Method:

1. Open your Internet browser and use a search engine to search for the credential you would like to pursue—for example, Certified Medical Assistant or Registered Medical Assistant. If you are unsure of the credential you would like to pursue, you may just want to search for "Medical Assisting Credentials."

2. Select the site for the credential you are pursuing. Avoid sponsored links. These links are paid for and typically will not take you to the site of a credentialing organization.

3. To navigate to the home page:
   - For the CMA (AAMA) credential, enter the site http://www.aama-ntl.org.

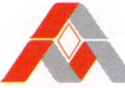

AMERICAN ASSOCIATION OF MEDICAL ASSISTANTS

Reprinted with permission from American Association of Medical Assistants.

   - For the RMA (AMT) or CMAS (AMT) credential, enter the site http://www.americanmedtech.org.

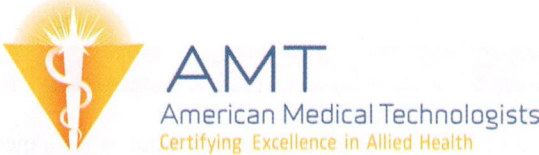

AMT American Medical Technologists
Certifying Excellence in Allied Health

Reprinted with permission from American Medical Technologists.

4. Determine the steps you must take to obtain the selected credential.
   - For CMA (AAMA), go to the drop-down menu "CMA (AAMA) Exam" and select the link "About the Exam."
   - For RMA (AMT), go to the drop-down menu "Get Certified" and select the link "Eligibility."

5. Print or write down the qualifications you must obtain.
   RATIONALE: *Maintaining a record of needed qualifications will be a reference as you pursue your chosen credential.*

6. Once you have met the qualifications, you will need to apply for the examination or certification. Download the application and the application instructions for the RMA (AMT) or the CMAS (AMT) or the candidate application and handbook for the CMA (AAMA).

7. To view or print these instructions, you may need to download Adobe Reader. You can click on a link to download Adobe Reader after you click on the "Apply Online" link for AMT or "Apply for the Exam" for AAMA.

8. Before or after you apply for the examination, you will need to prepare for the examination. Select the link "Study for the Exam" on the AAMA site or the "Prepare for Exam" link under the "Get Certified" drop-down menu on the AMT site.

9. Prepare for the exam by reviewing the content outline, obtaining additional study resources, or taking a practice exam online.

10. Print or save downloaded information in a file folder on your desktop labeled "Credentials" or another name you can recognize. To print, click the printer icon found at the bottom of the web page or click the printer icon in your browser.

11. Return to the appropriate site if you have additional questions. For the CMA (AAMA) site, you may want to check the "FAQs on CMA (AAMA) Certification" link. On the AMT site for RMA or CMAS, find the link "Take the Exam" and download the FAQs regarding the testing process.

12. Any questions you have that are not addressed on the sites can be e-mailed to the organizations. For RMA, send an e-mail to mail@americanmedtech.org. On the AAMA site for the CMA credential, click the "Contact" link on the top right-hand side of the screen and follow the instructions to send an e-mail.

LEARNING OUTCOMES	KEY POINTS
1.1 **Recognize the duties and responsibilities of a medical assistant.**	Medical assistants may have administrative, clinical, and/or laboratory duties and responsibilities. Duties range from entry-level to advanced and are listed in Table 1-1.
1.2 **Distinguish various organizations related to the medical assisting profession.**	Many organizations provide certification and support to the medical assisting profession. The AAMA and AMT are highly recognized professional associations that can help you progress in your medical assisting career.
1.3 **Explain the need for and importance of the medical assistant credentials.**	Certification and registration provide recognition of your education by peers and for advancement in your career. Medical assistants with a credential can expect more and better employment opportunities.
1.4 **Identify the training needed to become a professional medical assistant.**	Professional training for medical assistants includes formal training in a variety of educational settings. Training at a program accredited by CAAHEP or ABHES requires you to obtain work experience as part of your education.
1.5 **Discuss professional development as it relates to medical assisting education.**	*Professional development* refers to skills and knowledge attained for both personal development and career advancement. Continuing education, cross-training, and additional training help you develop within your profession. Medical assistants who network, work within their scope of practice, and are more multiskilled are highly marketable.

C A S E   S T U D Y   C R I T I C A L   T H I N K I N G

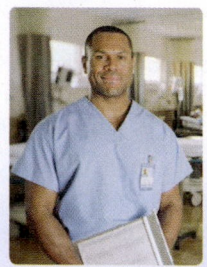

© Ryan McVay/Getty Images RF

Recall Sandro Peso from the beginning of the chapter. Now that you have completed the chapter, answer the following questions regarding his situation.

1. Describe for Sandro the skills he may perform in each of the three areas (administrative, clinical, and laboratory) of medical assisting at BWW Associates office.

2. Why should Sandro obtain a credential and membership to a professional organization?

3. How can Sandro find out what to expect on his certification test?

4. What suggestions would you give Sandro to assist him in obtaining the best job?

5. To whom will Sandro be accountable during his work at BWW Associates?

E X A M   P R E P A R A T I O N   Q U E S T I O N S

1. (LO 1.3) Two accrediting bodies for medical assisting training programs are
   a. ABHES and OSHA
   b. OSHA and AAMA
   c. ABHES and CAAHEP
   d. CAAHEP and CLIA
   e. CAAHEP and NHA

2. (LO 1.1) Entry-level administrative duties for a medical assistant include
   a. Educating patients, drawing blood, and negotiating leases
   b. Taking vital signs, performing phlebotomy, and calling in prescriptions
   c. Creating and maintaining patient medical records and billing and coding
   d. Performing ECGs, infection control, and billing and coding
   e. Checking vital signs, performing phlebotomy, and creating and maintaining patient medical records

3. (LO 1.2) The main purpose of the American Association of Medical Assistants (AAMA) is to
   a. Raise the standards of professionalism
   b. Assist with malpractice lawsuits
   c. Provide externships
   d. Support continuing education for CMAs (AAMA) and RMAs (AMT)
   e. Provide accreditation for medical assisting programs

4. (LO 1.2) You want to obtain an RMA credential. Which organization do you need to contact?
   a. NHA
   b. AAMA
   c. CAAHEP
   d. ABHES
   e. AMT

5. (LO 1.5) Which of the following is the best description of networking?
   a. Building alliances that generate opportunities
   b. Practical work experience during training
   c. Official authorization of medical assisting educational programs
   d. Training in every aspect of the medical facility
   e. Using the Internet

6. (LO 1.5) Which of the following is the *best* reason for you to become multiskilled?
   a. Reduction of healthcare costs
   b. Learning of new skills
   c. Increased employment opportunities
   d. Ability to work two jobs
   e. Recertification

7. (LO 1.2) You have become a member of the AAMA. Which of the following is most likely one of your benefits?
   a. Medical transcription
   b. Accreditation
   c. Cross-training
   d. Increased wages
   e. Group insurance

8. (LO 1.1) Which of the following would you be expected to do as an entry-level clinical medical assistant?
   a. Develop public outreach programs
   b. Be a HIPAA compliance officer
   c. Arrange laboratory services
   d. Arrange outpatient diagnostic tests
   e. Sterilize medical instruments

9. (LO 1.3) Which of the following is *least* likely the reason for the increased need to obtain a medical assisting credential?
   a. OSHA regulations
   b. An increase in malpractice
   c. An increase in organizations that require certification
   d. CLIA regulations
   e. An increase in multiskilled employees

10. (LO 1.2) Which of the following does *not* provide a certification examination for the medical assisting profession?
    a. NAHP
    b. AMT
    c. AMA
    d. NCCT
    e. NHA

Healthcare and the Healthcare Team

CASE STUDY

EMPLOYEE INFORMATION		
Employee Name Miguel A. Perez	**Position** Administrative Assistant	**Credentials** CMA (AAMA)
Supervisor Malik Katahri, CMM	**Date of Hire** 6/21/20XX	**Other Information** Wants to further his education

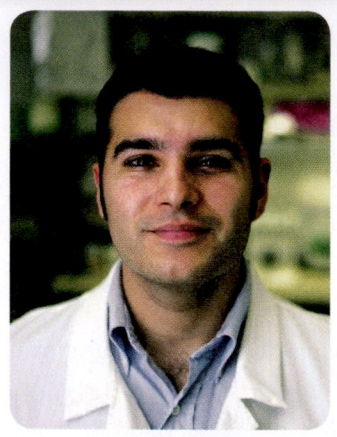
© Karen Moskowitz/Getty Images

Miguel A. Perez, CMA (AAMA), is the administrative assistant at BWW Associates. He came in early to get caught up on some important duties. He needs to schedule consults for Raja Lautu and Ken Washington, call in a medication refill for Sylvia Gonzales, and verify insurance coverage for Cindy Chen. Just as he is getting started, Kaylyn Haddix, RMA (AMT), calls from one of the exam rooms and tells him to call 911 because a patient has just gone into cardiac arrest. So much for coming in early; looks like it is going to be a busy day.

Keep Miguel in mind as you study this chapter. There will be questions at the end of the chapter based on the case study. The information in the chapter will help you answer these questions.

LEARNING OUTCOMES

After completing Chapter 2, you will be able to:

2.1 Discuss healthcare trends and their relationship to medical assistant practice.

2.2 Identify medical specialties and specialists certified by the American Board of Medical Specialties (ABMS).

2.3 Recognize the duties of various allied health professionals with whom medical assistants may work.

2.4 Compare specialty careers that a medical assistant may choose for advancement.

2.5 Differentiate professional associations that relate to healthcare and explain their relationship to the medical assisting profession.

KEY TERMS

anaphylactic shock

autopsy

biopsy

board-certified physician

electronic health records (EHR)

hormone

meridians

osteopathic manipulative medicine (OMM)

preventive care

primary care physician (PCP)

triage

wellness

whole foods

MEDICAL ASSISTING COMPETENCIES

CAAHEP	ABHES

CAAHEP

V.P.3 Use medical terminology correctly and pronounced accurately to communicate information to providers and patients

X.C.2 Compare and contrast provider and medical assistant roles in terms of standard of care

ABHES

1. **General Orientation**
   b. Compare and contrast the allied health professions and understand their relation to medical assisting
   d. List the general responsibilities of the medical assistant

3. **Medical Terminology**
   c. Apply various medical terms for each specialty

11. **Career Development**
    b. Demonstrate professional behavior

▶ Introduction

Medical assistants are an integral part of a healthcare delivery team. As such, you should recognize healthcare trends and facilities as well as the different physician specialists, allied health professionals, specialty medical assistant careers, and healthcare organizations. Medical assistants work in various roles and must be in contact with multiple other healthcare team members on an ongoing basis. For example, medical assistants are asked to call and process insurance referrals to different specialties and diagnostic departments, or they may need to contact the pharmacy to renew a prescription. A working knowledge of the different specialties and allied health professions demonstrates professionalism and competence, and it assists in developing a spirit of cooperation. Recognizing the functions of specialty careers and healthcare associations will help you perform your duties, as well as provide for advancement.

▶ Healthcare Trends   LO 2.1

Knowledge of current healthcare trends and healthcare practice settings will assist you in determining your future role as a medical assistant. Consider the following healthcare trends and how they may affect your career.

Technology

Over the last decade, the advancement of technology has affected all aspects of our life, including healthcare. Healthcare has always been affected by science and technology. For example, during the 1970s, mobile telephones seemed to be just the imaginings of science fiction. Today, a medical assistant can carry a smartphone in a pocket for easy reference and for professional communication with patients and members of the healthcare team.

Paper charts have become a thing of the past. By 2014, all healthcare facilities were required to convert to the use of **electronic health records (EHR)** in order to continue being reimbursed for Medicare and Medicaid claims (Figure 2-1). EHR allow all of a patient's data to be accessible from one location. An electronic chart provides quick access and helps prevent mistakes with medication and other medical errors. The *Electronic Health Records* chapter will provide details about how to use this essential tool.

Preventive Care and Wellness

The terms *preventive care* and *wellness* can bring to mind anything from massage therapy to *whole foods*. **Whole foods** are those that have little or no processing before they are eaten. The idea of **wellness** includes fitness. The link among exercise, diet, and good health is strong. Screening tests and drugs to prevent disease are common in **preventive care.** A healthy lifestyle goes a long way toward improving your quality of life. Physicians, insurance companies, fitness experts, and aging baby boomers all recognize the value of good health. As a medical assistant, maintaining your own health as well as guiding patients to better health practices is a must.

Aging Population

After World War II, the US economy boomed. There were plenty of jobs and people could afford to have large families. This resulted in a phenomenon known as the baby boom, which occurred from 1946 to 1964. Many of these babies are now at retirement age. In 2011, the first boomers began to receive Medicare, our national health insurance for the elderly. Because older adults require more healthcare services, medical assistants will most likely work with these patients.

Healthcare Facilities

Medical assistants may work in all types of healthcare facilities, including physicians' offices, clinics, urgent care centers, and the ambulatory or outpatient care facilities at hospitals. Two other types of healthcare facilities that commonly employ medical assistants are long-term care and hospice care. Long-term care centers provide care to people who need

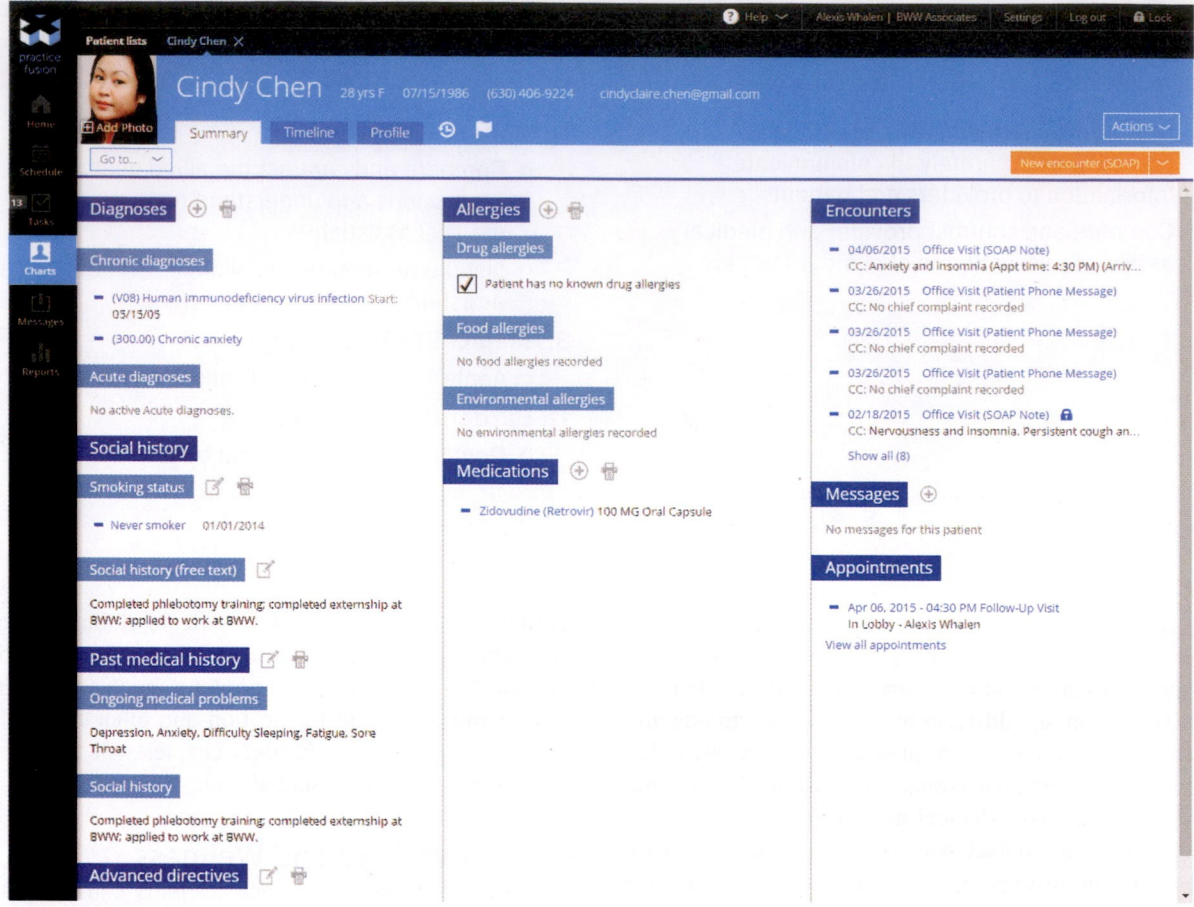

FIGURE 2-1 All healthcare employees, including medical assistants, must be able to use electronic health records.
© Practice Fusion®

nursing or other professional healthcare services on a regular basis. These patients may not need round-the-clock nursing services, but it may be unsafe for them to live alone or they may have needs their family cannot meet. Many residents in long-term care facilities are frail or elderly. They also may be disabled. Hospice is usually offered only to patients who are thought to have fewer than 6 months to live. An example of a hospice patient is a person who has terminal cancer (Figure 2-2). Anyone who has a terminal condition is eligible for this type of care.

The Affordable Care Act was passed in 2010 in an effort to lower healthcare costs and improve the quality of healthcare in the United States. With this legislation has come the creation of Patient Centered Medical Homes (PCMH), which are a potential solution to the problem of providing higher-quality care to a larger population. PCMH are meant to transform how primary care is organized and delivered and have the following functions.

- Comprehensive care. A team of care providers, including medical assistants, provides for physical and mental healthcare needs, including prevention and wellness, acute care, and chronic care. Virtual teams may also be used.
- Patient-centered care. Patients are encouraged to manage and organize their own care and are considered core members of the care team.

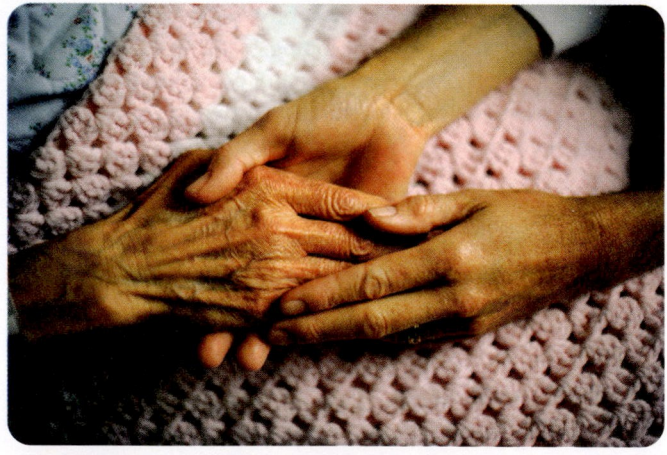

FIGURE 2-2 Hospice care provides for the needs of patients who are dying, including the need for touch.
© Royalty-Free/Corbis

- Coordinated care. Care is coordinated across healthcare services. Communication among patients, families, the PCMH, and other members of the care team is required.
- Accessible services. For all patients, it is essential to ensure shorter waiting times for urgent needs, enhanced in-person hours, around-the-clock telephone or electronic access to a member of the care team, and alternative methods of communication such as e-mail and telephone care.

- Quality and safety. Key parts of the PCMH are using evidence-based medicine and clinical decision-support tools to guide shared decision making with patients and families, engaging in performance measurement and improvement, measuring and responding to patient experiences and patient satisfaction, and practicing population health management.

With the development of PCMH, the medical assistant can expect new and expanded roles.

▶ Medical Specialties   LO 2.2

The American Board of Medical Specialties (ABMS) recognizes 24 specialties and subspecialties. The purpose of ABMS is to certify physicians in various specialties and to support their professional development. ABMS consists of 24 individual boards, one for each specialty or subspecialty. Each board is approved by both the ABMS and the American Medical Association Council on Medical Education (AMA/CME). In addition to certifying physicians, these boards develop professional and educational standards in the specialty areas.

Within each medical specialty are several subspecialties. For example, cardiology is a major specialty; pediatric cardiology is a subspecialty. As advances in the diagnosis and treatment of diseases and disorders unfold, the demand for specialized care increases and more medical specialties emerge. The education and licensing process for **board-certified physicians** is long—from 9 to 12 years—and requires multiple board tests. A medical assistant may be the "right arm" to any physician, including those described here.

Family Practice

Family practitioners (sometimes called general practitioners) are medical doctors (MDs) or doctors of osteopathy (DOs) who are generalists and treat all types of illnesses and ages of patients. Family practitioners are called **primary care physicians (PCPs)** by insurance companies. The term refers to individual doctors who oversee patients' long-term healthcare. Some people, however, have an internist or OB/GYN as their primary care physician.

A family practitioner sends a patient to a specialist when the patient has a specific condition or disease that requires advanced care. For example, a family practitioner refers a patient with a lump in her breast to an oncologist, a specialist who treats tumors, or to a general surgeon. The specialist or surgeon then does a needle biopsy of the lump to determine if it is malignant.

Working in a general practice, you will encounter patients with many different conditions and illnesses. If you work for a general practitioner, you will often be responsible for arranging patient appointments with specialists. It is therefore important for you to be familiar with the duties of each medical specialist.

Allergy

Allergists diagnose and treat physical reactions to substances such as mold, dust, fur, and pollen. An individual with allergies may also be hypersensitive to substances such as drugs, chemicals, or other elements in nature. An allergic reaction may be minor, such as a rash; serious, such as asthma; or life-threatening, such as **anaphylactic shock,** which causes swelling of the airways or nasal passages.

Anesthesiology

Anesthesiologists and anesthetists use medications that cause patients to lose sensation, or feeling, during surgery. These healthcare practitioners administer anesthetics before, during, and sometimes after surgery. They also educate patients regarding the anesthetic that will be used and its possible postoperative effects. An anesthesiologist is an MD or a DO. A certified registered nurse anesthetist (CRNA) is a registered nurse who has completed an additional program of study recognized by the American Association of Nurse Anesthetists.

Bariatrics

Bariatrics is the specialty of medicine that deals with the medical and surgical treatment of obesity. Bariatric surgery may be recommended for extremely obese patients who suffer impaired health as a result of their weight. Prior to undergoing any type of bariatric surgery, candidates must first undergo counseling and other treatment options for weight management. Therapy before and after bariatric surgery is necessary for successful weight loss and improved health.

Cardiology

Cardiologists diagnose and treat cardiovascular diseases (diseases of the heart and blood vessels). Cardiologists also read electrocardiograms (ECGs, which are sometimes referred to as EKGs) for hospital cardiology departments. They educate patients about the positive role a healthy diet and regular exercise play in preventing and controlling heart disease and recommend cardiovascular rehabilitation when needed (Figure 2-3).

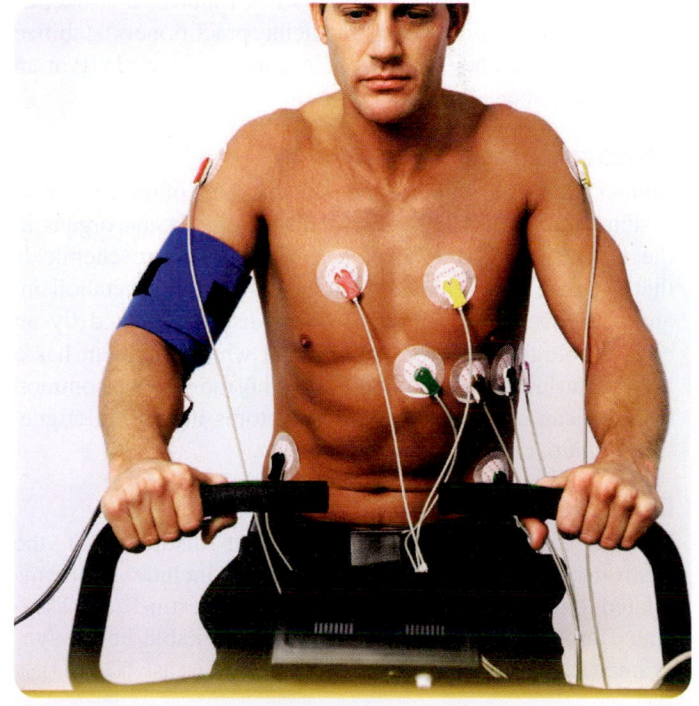

FIGURE 2-3   A cardiologist may order an exercise stress test that monitors the patient's heart while he is exercising.
© Digital Vision/Punchstock RF

Dermatology

Dermatologists diagnose and treat diseases of the skin, hair, and nails. Their patients have conditions ranging from warts and acne to skin cancer. Dermatologists treat boils, skin injuries, and infections. They also remove growths such as moles, cysts, and birthmarks; treat scars; and perform hair transplants.

Osteopathy

Doctors of osteopathy, who hold the title DO, practice a "whole-person" approach to healthcare. DOs believe that patients are more than just a sum of their body parts, and they treat the patient as a whole person instead of concentrating on specific symptoms. One key concept of osteopathy is that structure influences function. If a problem exists in one part of the body, it may affect function both in that area and in other areas.

DOs focus on the body's ability to heal itself, and they actively engage patients in the healing process. They also use **osteopathic manipulative medicine** (**OMM**), a system of hands-on techniques that help relieve pain, restore motion, and support the body's natural functions. By using OMM techniques such as muscle energy and counterstrain techniques, DOs help improve function and restore health.

Emergency Medicine

Physicians who specialize in emergency medicine work in hospital emergency rooms and outpatient emergency care centers. They diagnose and treat patients with conditions resulting from an unexpected medical crisis or accident. Common emergencies include trauma, such as gunshot wounds or serious injuries from car accidents; other injuries, such as severe cuts; and sudden illness, such as a heart attack, a stroke, or food poisoning. Emergency medicine practitioners stabilize their patients so they can then be managed by their PCP or an appropriate specialist.

Endocrinology

Endocrinologists diagnose and treat disorders of the endocrine system. The endocrine system includes glands and organs in the body that secrete hormones. **Hormones** are chemicals that regulate body functions, including growth, metabolism, and reproduction. An example of a disorder treated by an endocrinologist is hypothyroidism, in which a patient has a lower-than-normal amount of thyroid hormone. This common disorder can cause a variety of symptoms including fatigue, weight gain, dry skin, and constipation.

Gastroenterology

Gastroenterologists diagnose and treat disorders of the gastrointestinal tract. These disorders include problems related to the functioning of the stomach, intestines, and associated organs. Examples include ulcers, irritable bowel syndrome (IBS), and gastroesophageal reflux disease (GERD).

Gerontology

Gerontologists study the aging process. Geriatrics is the branch of medicine that deals with the diagnosis and treatment of problems and diseases of the older adult. A specialist in geriatrics may also be called a geriatrician. As the population of older adults increases, there is a greater need for licensed practitioners who specialize in diagnosing and treating diseases of older patients.

Gynecology

Gynecology is the branch of medicine concerned with diseases and conditions of the female genital tract, such as yeast infections, menstrual irregularities, and sexually transmitted infections (STIs). Gynecologists perform routine physical care and examination of the female reproductive system. Many gynecologists are also obstetricians.

Internal Medicine

Internists, or doctors of internal medicine, specialize in diagnosing and treating problems related to the internal organs. Some internists work with diseases and conditions related to all of the internal organs. Others choose to receive additional training that enables them to focus on 1 of 13 subspecialties. These subspecialties are adolescent medicine, allergy and immunology, cardiology, endocrinology, gastroenterology, geriatrics, hematology, infectious disease, nephrology, oncology, pulmonology, rheumatology, and sports medicine. Internists must be certified as specialists to practice in any of these areas.

Nephrology

Nephrologists study, diagnose, and manage diseases of the kidney. They may work in either a clinic or hospital setting. A medical assistant working with a nephrologist may assist in the operation of a dialysis unit for the treatment of patients with kidney failure, known as end-stage renal disease (ESRD). In a rural setting, a medical assistant might help a doctor operate a mobile dialysis unit that can be taken to the patient's home or to a medical practice that does not have this technology.

Neurology

Neurology is the branch of medical science that deals with the nervous system. Neurologists diagnose and treat disorders and diseases of the nervous system, such as strokes. The nervous system is made up of the brain, the spinal cord, and nerves that receive, interpret, and transmit messages throughout the body.

Nuclear Medicine

Nuclear medicine is a fast-growing specialty related to radiology. Nuclear medicine and radiology use radiation to diagnose and treat disease, but radiology beams radiation through the body from an outside source, whereas nuclear medicine introduces a small amount of a radioactive substance into the body and forms an image by detecting radiation as it leaves the body. The radiation that patients are exposed to is comparable to that of a diagnostic X-ray. Radiology reveals interior anatomy, whereas nuclear medicine reveals organ function and structure. Noninvasive, painless nuclear medicine procedures

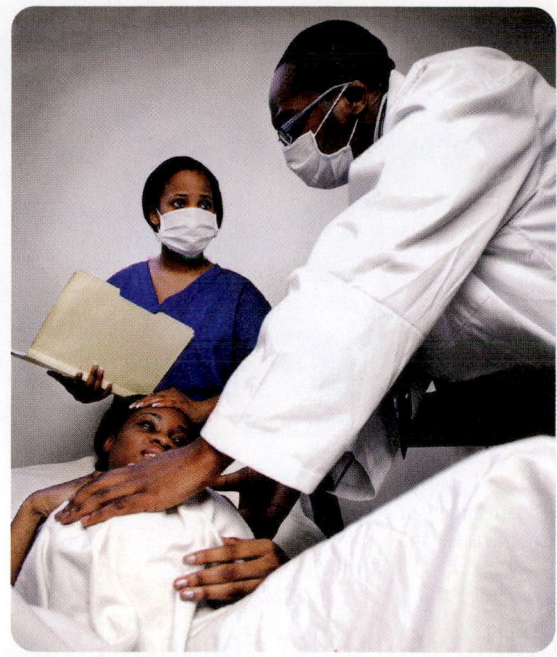

FIGURE 2-4 Obstetricians who are part of a private practice are usually connected with a specific hospital where they help their patients through labor and delivery.

© Don Thompson/Getty Images

are used to identify heart disease, assess organ function, and diagnose and treat cancer.

Obstetrics

Obstetrics involves the study of pregnancy, labor, delivery, and the period following labor, called postpartum (Figure 2-4). This field is often combined with gynecology. A physician who practices both specialties is referred to as an obstetrician/gynecologist, or OB/GYN.

Oncology

Oncologists determine whether tumors are benign or malignant and treat patients who have cancer. Treatment may involve chemotherapy, which is the administration of drugs to destroy cancer cells. Treatment may also involve radiation therapy, which kills cancer cells through the use of X-rays. Newer therapies include immune therapy, also called immunotherapy, and transplant techniques to urge the body to create healthy tissues to replace those affected by cancer. Oncologists treat both adults and children.

Ophthalmology

An ophthalmologist is an MD who diagnoses and treats diseases and disorders of the eye. This physician specialist examines patients' eyes for poor vision or disease. Other responsibilities include prescribing corrective lenses or medication, performing surgery, and providing follow-up care after surgery. The specialty of ophthalmology includes two other types of practitioners who are not MDs: optometrists and opticians. An optometrist obtains the credential

of OD (optometric doctor) and specializes in diagnosing and treating visual defects with glasses and contacts. An optician is a specialist who fills the prescriptions for glasses and contact lenses that are written by ophthalmologists and optometrists.

Orthopedics

Orthopedics is a branch of medicine that specializes in maintaining the function of the musculoskeletal system and its associated structures. An orthopedist diagnoses and treats diseases and disorders of the muscles and bones. Some orthopedists, called sports medicine specialists, concentrate on treating sports-related injuries, either exclusively for professional athletes or for nonprofessionals of all ages.

Otorhinolaryngology

Otorhinolaryngology is the study of the ear, nose, and throat. An otorhinolaryngologist diagnoses and treats diseases of these body structures. This physician specialist is also referred to as an ear, nose, and throat (ENT) specialist or otolaryngologist.

Pathology

Pathology is the study of disease. It provides the scientific foundation for all medical practice. The pathologist studies the changes a disease produces in the cells, fluids, tissues, and processes of the entire body. These samples often come from **biopsies** (samplings of cells that could be malignant or cancerous), cultures, and tissue samples. Some pathologists also perform **autopsies,** examinations of the bodies of the deceased, to determine the cause of a patient's death and to advance the clinical practice of medicine.

There are two basic types of pathologists: forensic pathologists and anatomic pathologists. Governments and police departments use forensic pathologists to determine facts about unexplained or violent crimes or deaths. Anatomic pathologists often work at hospitals in a research capacity, and they may read biopsies.

Pediatrics and Adolescent Medicine

Pediatrics is concerned with the development and care of children and adolescents from birth until 18 (in some practices, up to 21) years. A pediatrician diagnoses and treats childhood diseases and teaches parents skills to keep their children healthy.

Physical Medicine

Physical medicine specialists (physiatrists) are physicians who specialize in physical medicine and rehabilitation. They are certified by the American Board of Physical Medicine and Rehabilitation to diagnose and treat diseases and disorders such as sore shoulders and spinal cord injuries. Physiatrists offer an aggressive, nonsurgical approach to pain and injury for both adults and children.

Podiatry

Podiatry is practiced by a licensed doctor of podiatric medicine (DPM). A podiatrist studies and treats the foot and ankle. Podiatrists may diagnose, treat, prescribe medication, and perform surgery for disorders of the foot and, in some states, the ankle and leg.

Plastic Surgery

A plastic surgeon reconstructs, corrects, or improves body structures. Patients may be accident victims or disfigured due to disease or abnormal development. Plastic surgery includes facial reconstruction, facelifts, and skin grafting. Plastic surgery is also used to repair problems such as cleft lip and cleft palate, as well as disfigurement and restrictive scarring due to trauma.

Proctology

Proctology is the branch of medicine that diagnoses and treats disorders of the anus, rectum, and intestines. Proctologists treat conditions such as colitis, hemorrhoids, fistulas, tumors, and ulcers.

Radiology

Radiology is the branch of medical science that uses X-rays and radioactive substances to diagnose and treat disease. Radiologists specialize in reading X-rays. X-rays are used mostly for diagnosis—for example, to determine whether bones are broken or whether a patient has pneumonia. Radiologists often work with oncologists to apply radioactive substances to help kill cancer cells and reduce the size of malignant tumors.

Sports Medicine

Sports medicine is an interdisciplinary subspecialty of medicine that deals with the treatment and preventive care of amateur and professional athletes. Sports medicine teams consist of specialty physicians and surgeons, athletic trainers, and physical therapists. Sports medicine involves more than just treating injuries to the musculoskeletal system. Sports medicine can include an array of services, such as prevention and nutritional health.

Surgery

Surgeons use their hands and medical instruments to diagnose and correct deformities and treat external and internal injuries or disease (Figure 2-5). They work with many different specialists to surgically treat a broad range of disorders. General surgeons may, for example, perform operations as diverse as breast lumpectomy and pacemaker repair. Many surgeons specialize in a specific type of surgery, such as neurosurgery, vascular surgery, or orthopedic surgery.

Urology

A urologist diagnoses and treats diseases of the kidney, bladder, and urinary system. A urologist's patients include infants, children, and adults of all ages. Urologists also treat male reproductive diseases.

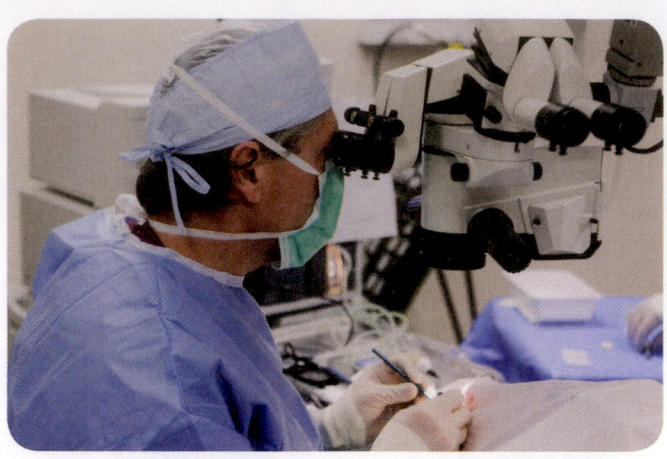

FIGURE 2-5 Most surgeons specialize in a particular type of surgery, such as heart surgery or eye surgery.
© Huntstock/Getty Images RF

▶ Working with Other Healthcare Professionals
LO 2.3

A medical assistant is a member of a healthcare team. Working as a team member is discussed in the chapter *Professionalism and Success.* That healthcare team includes doctors, nurses, specialists, and the patients themselves. Your contact with other members of the team will occur in person, electronically, or by telephone. You should recognize and understand the duties of other allied health professionals in order to be effective in your role as a medical assistant. The following is an introduction to some common allied health professionals.

Acupuncturist

Acupuncturists treat people who have pain or discomfort by inserting thin, hollow needles under the skin. The points used for insertion are selected to balance the flow of qi (pronounced chee), or life energy, in the body. The theory of acupuncture relates to traditional Chinese beliefs about how the body works. Qi is composed of two opposite forces called yin and yang. If the flow of qi is unbalanced, insufficient, or interrupted, then emotional, spiritual, mental, and physical problems will result. The acupuncturist works to balance these two forces in perfect harmony. Although there are variations in types of acupuncture—Chinese, Korean, and Japanese—all practitioners focus on many pulse points along different **meridians,** the channels through which qi flows (Figure 2-6).

Chiropractor

Chiropractors treat people using manual treatments, although they also may employ physical therapy treatments, exercise programs, nutritional advice, and lifestyle modification to help correct problems causing the pain. The manual treatments, called adjustments, realign the vertebrae in the spine and restore the function of spinal nerves. Chiropractors use diagnostic testing such as X-rays, muscle testing, and posture

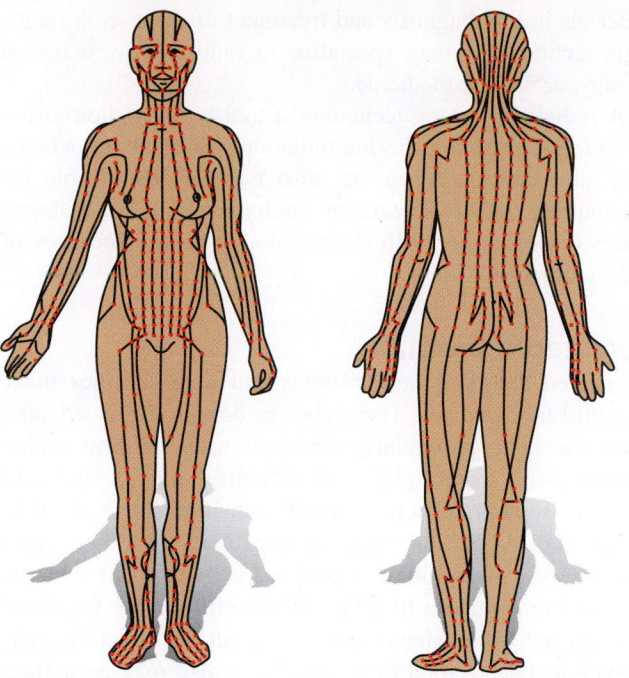

FIGURE 2-6 Meridians are pathways for the flow of qi in the body. Meridians are treated as part of traditional Chinese medicine to restore the body's harmony and wellness.

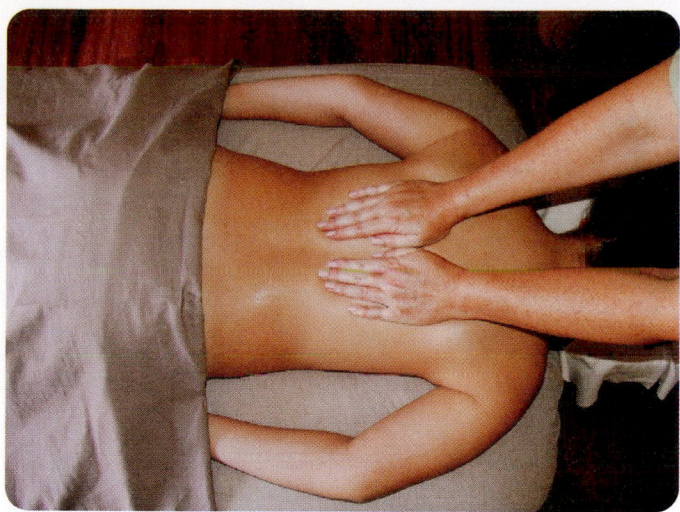

FIGURE 2-7 Massage uses kneading, pressure, stroking, and human touch to alleviate pain and promote healing through relaxation.
© McGraw-Hill Education. Shaana Pritchard, photographer

analysis to determine the location of spinal misalignments, also called subluxations. Using their findings, they develop a treatment plan, which may require several adjustments per week for several weeks or months.

Electroencephalographic Technologist

Electroencephalography (EEG) is the study and recording of the electrical activity of the brain. It is used to diagnose diseases and irregularities of the brain. The EEG technologist attaches electrodes to the patient's scalp and connects them to a recording instrument. The machine then provides a written record of the electrical activity of the patient's brain. EEG technologists work in hospital EEG laboratories, clinics, and physicians' offices.

Massage Therapist

Massage is one of the oldest methods of promoting healing. Massage therapists use pressure, kneading, stroking, vibration, and tapping to promote muscle and full-body relaxation, as well as to increase circulation and lymph flow (Figure 2-7). Increasing circulation helps remove blood and waste products from injured tissues and brings fresh blood and nutrients to the areas to speed healing. Massage is used to treat strains, bruises, muscle soreness or tightness, lower back pain, and dislocations. It also can relieve muscle spasms, restore motion and function to a body part, and decrease edema.

Medical Technology

Medical technology is an umbrella term referring to the development and design of clinical laboratory tests (such as diagnostic tests), procedures, and equipment. Two types of allied health professionals who work in medical technology are medical technologists and medical laboratory scientists.

Medical technologists (MTs) have a 4-year bachelor's degree and use complex laboratory equipment to perform clinical tests. They may be assisted by medical laboratory technicians (MLTs), who have 2-year degrees and may perform more basic tests under the supervision of an MT. MLTs and MTs perform tests in the areas of hematology, serology, blood banking, urinalysis, microbiology, and clinical chemistry.

Medical laboratory scientists examine specimens of human body tissues and fluids, analyze blood factors, and culture bacteria to identify disease-causing organisms. They also supervise and train technicians and laboratory aides. Medical laboratory scientists have 4-year degrees and may specialize in areas such as blood banking, microbiology, and chemistry.

Nuclear Medicine Technologist

A nuclear medicine technologist performs tests to oversee quality control, to prepare and administer radioactive drugs, and to operate radiation detection instruments (Figure 2-8). This allied health professional is also responsible for correctly positioning the patient, performing imaging procedures, and preparing the information for use by a physician.

Occupational Therapist

An occupational therapist works with patients who have reduced physical or mental function due to physical injuries or illnesses, psychological or developmental problems, or problems associated with the aging process. This health professional helps patients attain maximum physical and mental health by using educational, vocational, and rehabilitation therapies and activities. The occupational therapist may work in a hospital, a clinic, an extended-care facility, a rehabilitation hospital, or a government or community agency.

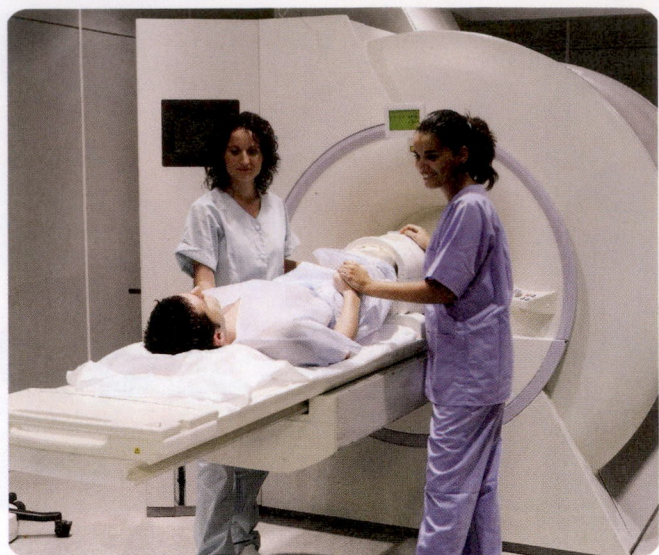

FIGURE 2-8 A nuclear medicine technologist positions the patient, performs imaging procedures, and prepares the information for use by a physician.
© Javier Larrea/age fotostock RF

Pharmacist

Pharmacists are professionals who have studied the science of drugs and who dispense medication and health supplies to the public. Pharmacists know the chemical and physical qualities of drugs and are knowledgeable about the companies that manufacture drugs.

Pharmacists inform the public about the effects of prescription and nonprescription (over-the-counter) medications. Pharmacists are employed in hospitals, clinics, and nursing homes. They also may work for government agencies, pharmaceutical companies, privately owned pharmacies, or chain store pharmacies. Some pharmacists own their own stores. Pharmacists must have 5 to 7 years of education, be registered by the state, and pass a state board examination.

Physical Therapist

A physical therapist (PT) plans and uses physical therapy programs for medically referred patients. The PT helps these patients restore function, relieve pain, and prevent disability following disease, injury, or loss of body parts. A physical therapist uses various treatment methods, which include therapy with electricity, heat, cold, ultrasound, massage, and exercise. The physical therapist also helps patients accept their disabilities.

Radiologic Technology

A radiographer (X-ray technician) assists a radiologist in taking X-ray films, which are used to diagnose broken bones, tumors, ulcers, and disease. A radiographer usually works in the radiology department of a hospital but may also use mobile X-ray equipment in a patient's room or in the operating room.

A radiologic technologist studies the theory and practice of the technical aspects of the use of X-rays and radioactive materials in the diagnosis and treatment of disease. A radiologic technologist may specialize in radiography, radiation therapy, or nuclear medicine.

A radiation therapy technologist assists the radiologist— for example, in administering radiation treatments to patients who have cancer. He or she also may be responsible for maintaining radiation treatment equipment. The technologist shares responsibility with the radiologist for the accuracy of treatment records.

Registered Dietitian

Registered dietitians help patients and their families make healthful food choices. These choices provide balanced, adequate nutrition, particularly when disease or illness makes knowing what to eat to help fight the disease difficult. Dietitians are sometimes confused with nutritionists. A dietitian has specialized training to assist ill patients with their nutritional needs; a nutritionist's goal is for those of us who are healthy to maintain a lifestyle of healthful eating. Dietitians may assist food-service directors at healthcare facilities and prepare and serve food to groups. They also may participate in food research and teach nutrition classes. Dietitians work in a variety of healthcare settings and teach at colleges and universities.

Respiratory Therapy

A respiratory therapist evaluates, treats, and cares for patients with respiratory problems. The respiratory therapist works under the supervision of a licensed practitioner and performs therapeutic procedures based on observation of the patient. Using respiratory equipment, the therapist treats patients who have asthma, emphysema, pneumonia, and bronchitis. The respiratory therapist plays an active role in newborn, pediatric, and adult intensive care units.

Respiratory therapy technicians work under the supervision of a licensed practitioner and a respiratory therapist. In addition to performing procedures such as artificial ventilation, they clean, sterilize, and maintain the respiratory equipment and document the patient's therapy in the medical record.

Nursing Aide/Assistant

Nursing aides assist in the direct care of patients under the supervision of the nursing staff. Typical functions include making beds, bathing patients, taking vital signs, serving meals, and transporting patients to and from treatment areas. Certification as a certified nursing assistant (CNA) is available and is required by many healthcare facilities, especially long-term care facilities.

Practical/Vocational Nurse

Licensed practical nurses (LPNs) and licensed vocational nurses (LVNs) are different names for the same type of nurse. Their duties involve taking and recording patient temperatures, blood pressure, pulse, and respiration rates. They also include administering some medications under supervision, dressing wounds, and applying compresses. LPNs and LVNs are not allowed, however, to perform certain other duties, such as some intravenous (IV) procedures and the administration of certain medications. LPNs/LVNs can obtain additional training to become certified in IV therapy.

Practical/vocational nurses assist registered nurses and licensed practitioners by observing patients and reporting changes in their conditions. LPNs/LVNs work in hospitals, long-term care facilities, clinics, and physicians' offices and in industrial medicine. To meet the needs of the growing aging population in this country, employment opportunities for LPNs and LVNs in long-term care settings have increased. LPNs/LVNs must graduate from an accredited school of practical (vocational) nursing (usually a 1-year program). They are also required to take a state board examination for licensure as LPNs/LVNs.

Registered Nurse

A nurse who graduates from a nursing program and passes the state board examination for licensure is considered a registered nurse (RN), indicating formal, legal recognition by the state. The RN is a professional who is responsible for planning, giving, and supervising the bedside nursing care of patients. An RN may work in an administrative capacity, assist in daily operations, oversee programs in hospital or institutional settings, or plan community health services. Registered nurses work in hospitals, long-term care facilities, public health agencies, physicians' offices, government agencies, and educational settings. They also may work in industry, providing on-site care at manufacturing facilities and other industrial workplaces.

Three types of nursing education programs qualify an individual to take a state board examination to become an RN: associate degree nurse, diploma graduate, and baccalaureate degree nurse.

Associate Degree Nurse Associate's degrees in nursing (ADNs) are offered at many junior colleges and community colleges and at some universities. These programs combine liberal arts education and nursing education. The length of the ADN program is typically 2 years.

Diploma Graduate Nurse Diploma programs are usually 3-year programs designed as cooperative programs between a community college and a participating hospital. The programs combine coursework and clinical experience in the hospital.

Baccalaureate Nurse A baccalaureate degree is awarded by a 4-year college or university program. Graduates of a 4-year nursing program are awarded a bachelor of science in nursing (BSN) degree. The curriculum includes courses in liberal arts, general education, and nursing. Graduates are prepared to function as nurse generalists and in positions that go beyond the role of hospital staff nurses. Some RNs with a BSN continue their education to earn master's or doctoral degrees.

Nurse Practitioner

A nurse practitioner (NP) is an RN who functions in an expanded nursing role. The NP usually works in an ambulatory patient care setting alongside physicians but also may work in an independent nurse practitioner practice without physicians. An independent nurse practitioner takes health histories, performs physical exams, conducts screening tests, and educates patients and families about disease prevention.

An NP who works in a physician's practice may perform some duties that a physician would, such as administering physical exams and treating common illnesses and injuries. For example, in an OB/GYN practice, the NP can perform a standard annual gynecologic exam, including taking a Pap smear or a culture to test for a yeast or bacterial infection. The nurse practitioner usually emphasizes preventive healthcare.

The NP must be an RN with at least a master's degree in nursing and must complete 4 to 12 months of an apprenticeship or formal training. With specific formal training, the student may become a pediatric nurse practitioner, an obstetric nurse practitioner (midwife), or a psychiatric nurse practitioner. Clinical medical assistants may work directly with an NP.

Physician Assistant

The physician assistant (PA) practices medicine under the laws of the specific state and the supervision of a physician. PAs provide diagnostic, therapeutic, and preventive healthcare services, as designated by the supervising physician. Physician assistants take medical histories; order laboratory and medical imaging tests; and examine, diagnose, treat, counsel, and follow up with patients. They also perform suturing, casting, and splinting for minor injuries, and some assist in surgery. PAs also prescribe certain medications. Some perform managerial duties, such as purchasing and maintaining equipment and hiring and firing personnel. The physician assistant also may take call duty for the practice and share the responsibility for afterhours call duty with the physician. A medical assistant may work directly with a physician assistant.

Speech/Language Pathologist

A speech/language pathologist treats communication disorders, such as stuttering, and associated disorders, such as hearing impairment. This health professional evaluates, diagnoses, and counsels patients who have these problems. A speech/language pathologist may work in a school, hospital, research setting, or private practice or may teach at a college or university.

▶ Specialty Career Options   LO 2.4

As a medical assistant, you have a multitude of opportunities to specialize by obtaining additional training, education, or certifications. You may determine that you prefer either the administrative or the clinical aspect of the work and move forward in your career toward that end. Tables 2-1 and 2-2 highlight some of the careers you may consider.

TABLE 2-1 Administrative Specialty Careers

Career	Duties	Organization(s)
Billing and insurance specialist	• Verifies patient insurance coverage • Processes insurance claims • Obtains fees for procedures and services performed, from both patients and insurance companies	American Medical Technologists (AMT), American Medical Billing Association (AMBA)
Certified Medical Reimbursement Specialist (CMRS)	• Facilitates the claims paying process "from patient to payment" • Plays a critical role in the healthcare provider's daily business operations, whether employed by the medical facility or self-employed as a contractor to assist the practice with its accounts receivable processes	American Medical Billing Association
Compliance officer	• Reviews and updates the office's policies and procedures manual • Creates and maintains appropriate coding and billing policies, including audit procedures • Creates, conducts, and manages compliance education programs for all staff • Establishes a process for investigating and taking action on all complaints about privacy policies and procedures • Publicizes the reporting system for all providers, staff, vendors, and business associates • Analyzes a facility's risk of releasing information incorrectly and sets policies and procedures to avoid these risks	American Health Information Management Association's Health Care Compliance Association (HCCA), American Academy of Professional Coders (AAPC)
Electronic claims professional	• Acts as the link between small and medium-sized practices and major health insurers such as Medicare • Contracts with a physician practice or healthcare facility, enters patient demographic and insurance billing information into billing software, and transmits it to the appropriate health insurance provider • Submits electronic medical (health) insurance claims to an insurance carrier	Alliance of Claims Assistance Professionals (ACAP), National Association of Claims Assistance Professionals (NACAP)
Medical biller and coder, health information coder, or medical coder	• Makes sure that all patient charges have been recorded in the billing system • Enters data such as charges into the patient accounts database • Prepares claims to send to payers such as insurance agencies • Prepares bills to send to patients • Tracks payments due from payers and patients	American Health Information Management Association (AHIMA), American Academy of Professional Coders (AAPC)
Medical transcriptionist	• Logs transcriptions of telephone calls or Internet transmissions • Sorts and distributes transcribed medical reports • Places the transcribed reports into the appropriate patient accounts in the electronic health records system	Association for Healthcare Documentation Integrity
Registered Health Information Technician (RHIT), medical record technician, medical chart specialist	• Manages patient records for a physician, group of physicians, or hospital • Ensures that all medical information is accurate and complete • Deals strictly with health information in a hospital and has no patient contact • Performs additional clerical duties such as answering the telephone in a physician's office • Checks all patient charts for completeness and accuracy	American Health Information Management Association

TABLE 2-2	Clinical Specialty Careers	
Career	**Duties**	**Organization(s)**
Anesthesiologist assistant	• Provides anesthetic care under an anesthetist's direction • Gathers patient data and assists in evaluation of patients' physical and mental status • Records planned surgical procedures, assists with patient monitoring, draws blood samples, performs blood gas analyses, and conducts pulmonary function tests	American Academy of Anesthesiologist Assistants
Cardiovascular technologist	• Performs diagnostic examinations and therapeutic interventions of the heart and/or blood vessels at the request or direction of a licensed practitioner • Uses various cardiovascular testing techniques to create a foundation of data for patient diagnosis	Cardiovascular Credentialing International
Dental assistant	• Performs many administrative and laboratory functions similar to those of a medical assistant • Serves as chairside assistant, provides instruction in oral hygiene, and prepares and sterilizes instruments	American Dental Assistant Association
Emergency medical technician (EMT)	• Works under the direction of a licensed practitioner through a radio or cellular communication network • Assesses and manages medical emergencies that occur in private and public locations • Assesses the urgency and type of condition presented, as well as the immediate medical needs, and initiates the appropriate treatment in the process known as **triage** • Records, documents, and transmits the patient's condition to the licensed practitioner, describing what has occurred	National Association of Emergency Medical Technicians
Mental health technician (psychiatric aide or counselor)	• Works with emotionally disturbed and mentally challenged patients • Assists the psychiatric team by observing behavior and providing information to help in the planning of therapy • Participates in supervising group therapy and counseling sessions	American Association of Psychiatric Technicians
Occupational therapist assistant	• Helps individuals with mental or physical disabilities reach their highest level of functioning through the teaching of fine motor skills, trades (occupations), and the arts • Prepares materials for activities, maintains tools and equipment, and documents the patient's progress	American Occupational Therapy Association
Pathologist's assistant	• May work with forensic pathologists—professionals who study the human body and diseases for legal purposes—in cooperation with government or police investigations • May prepare frozen sections of dissected body tissue • May maintain supplies, instruments, and chemicals for the anatomic pathology laboratory • Performs laboratory work (about 75% of the workday) and a variety of administrative duties	
Pharmacy technician	• Receives written or electronic prescriptions or telephone requests for prescription refills • Verifies that the information on the prescription is complete and accurate • Contacts the insurance company to verify benefits and obtain any patient copay or coinsurance requirements • Retrieves, counts, pours, weighs, measures, and, if necessary, mixes the medication for the prescription (script) • Establishes and maintains patient profiles in the pharmacy computer and prepares insurance claim submissions • Takes inventory of prescription and over-the-counter (OTC) medications • Assists in equipment maintenance and management of the pharmacy cash register	National Pharmacy Technician Association and Pharmacy Technician Certification Board
Phlebotomist	• Draws blood for diagnostic laboratory testing • Performs more advanced skills, such as drawing blood under difficult circumstances or in special situations—for example, if a blood sample is needed for an ammonia-level test, it must be drawn and stored in a particular manner phlebotomists are trained to do	National Phlebotomy Association (NPA) or American Society of Clinical Pathologists (ASCP)
Physical therapy assistant	• Assists with patient treatment by following the patient care program created by the physical therapist and licensed practitioner • Performs tests and treatment procedures, assembles or sets up equipment for therapy sessions, and observes and documents patient behavior and progress	American Physical Therapy Association
Surgical technician	• Obtains a patient's history and physical data • Discusses the data with a physician or surgeon to determine what procedures to use to treat the problem • May assist in performing diagnostic and therapeutic procedures	National Board of Surgical Technology and Surgical Assisting

▶ Healthcare Professional Associations

LO 2.5

Membership in a professional association is important for your professional development and career advancement. As discussed in the *Introduction to Medical Assisting* chapter, being part of organizations such as American Association of Medical Assistants (AAMA) and American Medical Technologists (AMT) enables you to become involved in the issues and activities relevant to your field and presents opportunities for continuing education. It is a good idea to stay informed about other healthcare associations, even those that are open to physicians only, such as the American Medical Association. Also, the physician you work for may ask you to obtain information about a particular group's activities and meetings, and by "staying in the loop," you will have better access to this information. Table 2-3 lists a few organizations that you should be familiar with.

Other organizations and professional associations help regulate healthcare. Some of the most important of these organizations are described here.

American College of Physicians

Founded in 1915, the American College of Physicians (ACP) is the largest medical specialty organization in the world. It is the only society of internists dedicated to providing education and information resources to the entire field of internal medicine and its subspecialties.

TABLE 2-3 Professional Medical Organizations

Professional Organization	Membership Requirements	Advantages of Membership
American Association of Medical Assistants (AAMA) http://www.aama-ntl.org	Interested individuals, including medical assisting students and those who practice medical assisting, may join the AAMA.	Offers flexible continuing education programs; publishes *CMA Today;* offers legal counsel, professional recognition, and various member discounts
American Association of Professional Coders (AAPC) http://www.aapc.com	Anyone interested in the coding profession may join. Student memberships are available for those currently in a coding program, as are corporate memberships for groups of six or more employees.	Training, continuing education, multiple certifications for specialties (including compliance), job board, networking, local and state chapter memberships, discounts on coding books, and educational materials
American Medical Billing Association (AMBA) http://www.ambanet.net	Interested individuals and those who want to become Certified Medical Reimbursement Specialists (CMRS) may join.	Can prepare for and take the National Medical Billing Certification Exam, also many other services such as online training, insurance, networking, and credit card processing
Association for Healthcare Documentation Integrity (AHDI) http://www.ahdionline.org	Interested individuals and those who practice medical transcription may join the AHDI.	Educates and develops medical transcriptionists as medical language specialists; offers advice and support for self-employed medical transcriptionists
American College of Physicians (ACP) http://www.acponline.org	Physicians and medical students may join.	Provides education and information resources to the field of internal medicine and its subspecialties
American Health Information Management Association (AHIMA) http://www.ahima.org	Members may be students (of approved AHIMA programs only), AHIMA-credentialed members, and noncredentialed members interested in HIM and willing to abide by the association's code of ethics.	Subscription to *Journal of AHIMA,* legislative advocacy, professional development, discounts on services and programs, job postings, members-only website, and automatic enrollment in local and/or state chapter
American Hospital Association (AHA) http://www.aha.org	Institutional healthcare providers and other individuals may join.	Provides consultant referral service and access to healthcare information resources
American Medical Association (AMA) http://www.ama-assn.org	Physicians and medical students may join.	Provides large information source; publishes *Journal of the American Medical Association* (*JAMA*); offers AMA/Net
American Medical Technologists (AMT) http://www.americanmedtech.org	Medical assistants, medical technologists, medical laboratory technicians, dental assistants, and phlebotomy technicians may join.	Offers national certification as Registered Medical Assistant (RMA); offers certification to other healthcare professionals, publications, state chapter activities, and continuing education programs
American Pharmacists Association (APhA) http:www.pharmacist.com	Pharmaceutical professionals and physicians may join.	Helps members improve skills; active in pharmacy policy development, networking, publishing, research, and public education
American Society for Clinical Pathology (ASCP) http:www.ascp.org	Any professional involved in laboratory medicine or pathology may join.	Resource for improving the quality of pathology and laboratory medicine; offers educational programs and materials; certifies technologists and technicians

American Hospital Association

The American Hospital Association (AHA) is the nation's largest network of institutional healthcare providers. These providers represent every type of hospital: rural and city hospitals, specialty and acute care facilities, free-standing hospitals, academic medical centers, and health systems and networks. The AHA works to support and promote the interests of hospitals and healthcare organizations across the country. Organizations as well as individual professionals may join the AHA. Membership benefits include use of the AHA consultant referral service, accessed, for example, by hospitals that need experts in areas not addressed by in-house personnel. Members also have access to AHA's healthcare information resources, including teleconferencing and AHA database services.

The Joint Commission

The Joint Commission (TJC) is a US-based nonprofit organization with the goal of maintaining and elevating the standards of healthcare delivery through the evaluation and accreditation of healthcare organizations. TJC employs surveyors, who are sent to healthcare organizations to evaluate their operational practices and facilities. Healthcare organizations are highly motivated to do well during a survey because accreditation by TJC is a significant factor in gaining reimbursement from Medicare and managed care organizations. In addition to hospitals, TJC evaluates and accredits ambulatory care, behavioral healthcare, home care, laboratory service, long-term care, and office-based surgery facilities.

Starting in 2003, TJC established safety requirements, known as National Patient Safety Goals, to help accredited healthcare organizations address issues of patient safety that can lead to adverse events lawsuits. The goals, found at http://www.jointcommission.org, focus on patient safety problems and how to solve them. Table 2-4 lists the requirements of the National Patient Safety Goals.

Council of Ethical and Judicial Affairs

The Council of Ethical and Judicial Affairs (CEJA) develops ethics policy for the AMA. It is composed of seven practicing physicians, a resident or fellow, and a medical student. The council prepares reports that analyze and address timely ethical issues that confront physicians and the medical profession. CEJA maintains and updates the AMA Code of Medical Ethics. This code is widely recognized as the most comprehensive ethics guide for physicians who strive to practice ethically.

American Medical Association

The American Medical Association (AMA), founded in 1847, promotes science and the art of medicine and works to improve public health. Its members include physicians from every medical specialty. As the world's largest publisher of scientific and medical information, the AMA publishes 10 monthly medical specialty journals. The AMA also accredits medical programs in the United States and Canada.

TABLE 2-4	2014 Ambulatory Care National Patient Safety Goals
The purpose of the National Patient Safety Goals is to improve patient safety. The goals focus on problems in healthcare safety and how to solve them.	
Identify Patients Correctly	• Use at least two ways to indentify patients. For example, use the patient's name *and* date of birth. This is done to make sure each patient gets the correct medicine and treatment.
	• Make sure that the correct patient gets the correct blood when they get a blood transfusion.
Use Medicines Safely	• Before a procedure, label medicines that are not labeled—for example, medicines in syringes, cups, and basins. Do this in the area where medicines and supplies are set up.
	• Take extra care with patients who take medicine to thin their blood.
	• Record and pass along correct information about a patient's medicines. Find out what medicines the patient is taking. Compare those medicines to new medicines given to the patient. Make sure the patient knows which medicines to take at home. Tell the patient it is important to bring an up-to-date list of medicines every time he or she visits a doctor.
Prevent Infection	• Use the hand cleaning guidelines from the Centers for Disease Control and Prevention or the World Health Organization. Set goals for improving hand cleaning. Use the goals to improve hand cleaning.
	• Use proven guidelines to prevent infection after surgery.
Prevent Mistakes in Surgery	• Make sure the correct surgery is done on the correct patient and at the correct place on the patient's body.
	• Mark the correct place on the patient's body where the surgery is to be done.
	• Pause before the surgery to make sure that a mistake is not being made.

Adapted from The Joint Commission 2014 National Patient Safety Goals from http://www.jointcommission.org, accessed November 28, 2014.

LEARNING OUTCOMES	KEY POINTS
2.1 **Discuss healthcare trends and their relationship to medical assistant practice.**	Medical assistants typically work in ambulatory care settings using EHR. They can expect to work with many older patients and should practice and assist patients with preventive care.
2.2 **Identify medical specialties and specialists certified by the American Board of Medical Specialties (ABMS).**	The ABMS certifies 24 major medical specialties and subspecialties. Medical specialties range from cardiology to oncology. As new medical advances occur, a demand for more specialty areas may emerge.
2.3 **Recognize the duties of various allied health professionals with whom medical assistants may work.**	Medical assistants are members of a healthcare team. The healthcare team includes physicians, nurses, physical therapists, other allied health professionals, and patients. Understanding the duties of other healthcare professionals will assist you as a professional medical assistant. Even if you do not work with some of the team members directly, you may have to contact them through telephone, written, or electronic communication.
2.4 **Compare specialty careers that a medical assistant may choose for advancement.**	A variety of medical specialty careers are available for the practicing administrative or clinical medical assistant. These careers require additional training or education and/or other certifications.
2.5 **Differentiate professional associations that relate to healthcare and explain their relationship to the medical assisting profession.**	Being a member of a professional association is essential to medical assisting practice. Knowledge of other healthcare and medical organizations allows the practicing medical assistant to function successfully within his or her profession.

CASE STUDY CRITICAL THINKING

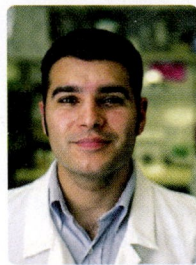

© Karen Moskowitz/Getty Images

Recall Miguel Perez, the administrative assistant from the beginning of the chapter. Now that you have completed the chapter, answer the following questions about his case.

1. What should Miguel do first, and why? What type of healthcare professional will respond to the call?

2. Raja Lautu is going to be evaluated for cancer. What type of physician will Miguel most likely be calling for this consult?

3. Ken Washington will need to have his heart evaluated. What type of physician will most likely be consulted, and what type of allied health professional will perform a special test on his heart? What is the name of the test to be performed?

4. Miguel enjoys his work as an administrative medical assistant but would like to expand his role. What specialty career would you recommend for Miguel, and why?

1. (LO 2.2) Medical specialists who deal with the medical and surgical treatment of obesity are
   a. Gastroenterologists
   b. Allergists
   c. Gynecologists
   d. Bariatric surgeons
   e. Neurologists

2. (LO 2.2) The abbreviation for a licensed doctor of podiatric medicine is
   a. DPM
   b. DVM
   c. MD
   d. OD
   e. LDPM

3. (LO 2.5) The Joint Commission (TJC) is a US-based organization that
   a. Offers continuing education for medical assistants
   b. Provides credentialing for physicians
   c. Maintains and elevates the standards of healthcare delivery through credentialing and accreditation
   d. Obtains information for medical groups
   e. Ensures the safety of employees in all facilities

4. (LO 2.4) Which of the following individuals should Miguel contact to verify Cindy Chen's insurance?
   a. Medical technologist
   b. Pharmacy technician
   c. Registered health information technician
   d. Medical billing and insurance specialist
   e. Medical transcriptionist

5. (LO 2.3) Your patient is having treatments based on qi. Which healthcare professional is most likely performing the treatments?
   a. Chiropractor
   b. Doctor of osteopathy
   c. Acupuncturist
   d. Optician
   e. Massage therapist

6. (LO 2.5) Which professional organization develops the National Patient Safety Goals?
   a. ACP
   b. AHA
   c. TJC
   d. AAMA
   e. AMA

7. (LO 2.4) Which professional would *most* likely be working outside of a healthcare facility?
   a. Occupational therapist assistant
   b. Emergency medical technician/paramedic
   c. Anesthetist's assistant
   d. Physical therapy assistant
   e. Surgical technician

8. (LO 2.3) Which healthcare team member can work independently, performing examinations and treating common illnesses?
   a. Associate degree nurse
   b. Radiologic technologist
   c. Physical therapist
   d. Medical records technologist
   e. Nurse practitioner

9. (LO 2.1) Which of the following is a trend in healthcare that has a direct effect on how medical assistants perform their job?
   a. Less hospitalized patients and more long-term care patients
   b. More hospitalized patients and fewer ambulatory care patients
   c. Lack of preventive healthcare practice and increased patient illness
   d. Increased birth rate and more contact with elderly patients
   e. Increased use of technology and EHR

10. (LO 2.1) What type of healthcare cares for patients who have terminal cancer or less than 6 months to live?
    a. Long-term care
    b. Ambulatory care
    c. Hospital care
    d. Hospice care
    e. Laboratory care

Professionalism and Success

CASE STUDY

EMPLOYEE INFORMATION		
Employee Name	**Position**	**Credentials**
Kaylyn R. Haddix	Clinical Medical Assistant	RMA (AMT)
Supervisor	**Date of Hire**	**Other information**
Malik Katahri, CMM	06/11/XX	Meeting with Malik at 1 P.M.

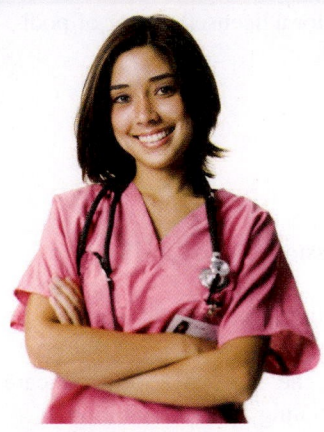
© Rubberball/Getty Images RF

Kaylyn R. Haddix does well with the "hands-on" skills and gets along fairly well with the other office personnel. However, Kaylyn has a problem with getting to work on time. She seems to show a pattern of poor planning, such as forgetting to set her alarm, losing her car keys, and neglecting to solve her various car problems when they first become apparent (brought on by skipped oil changes, worn tire treads, squeaky brakes, and a rusty muffler). The clinic suffers when Kaylyn is late because she is not ready to see the first patient upon arrival, causing patients to wait and disrupting the routines and schedules of other staff members. Following the third time she was late, Malik, the office manager, noted the problem in Kaylyn's record and informed Kaylyn that chronic tardiness could lead to termination. Although Kaylyn is sometimes afraid to ask questions, her performance is generally above average, so Malik is hoping that Kaylyn will improve.

Keep Kaylyn in mind as you study this chapter. There will be questions at the end of the chapter based on the case study. The information in the chapter will help you answer these questions.

LEARNING OUTCOMES

After completing Chapter 3, you will be able to:

3.1 Recognize the importance of professionalism in the medical assisting practice.

3.2 Explain the professional behaviors that should be exhibited by medical assistants.

3.3 Model strategies for success in medical assisting education and practice.

KEY TERMS

attitude	persistence
comprehension	prioritizing
constructive criticism	problem solving
critical thinking	punctuality
cultural diversity	self-confidence
empathy	soft skills
hard skills	teamwork
integrity	time management
organization	work ethic
patient advocacy	work quality

V.A.1 Demonstrate:
  (a) empathy
  (b) active listening
  (c) nonverbal communication

V.A.2 Demonstrate the principles of self-boundaries

V.A.3 Demonstrate respect for individual diversity including:
  (a) gender
  (b) race
  (c) religion
  (d) age
  (e) economic status
  (f) appearance

XI.P.2 Demonstrate appropriate responses to ethical issues

XI.A.1 Recognize the impact personal ethics and morals have on the delivery of healthcare

5. Psychology of Human Relations
  b. Provide support for terminally ill patients
    (1) Use empathy when communicating with terminally ill patients
  c. Intervene on behalf of patient regarding issues/concerns that may arise, i.e. insurance policy information, medical bills, physician/provider orders, etc.

11. Career Development
  b. Demonstrate professional behavior

▶ Introduction

A profession is an occupation or a career based upon specialized educational training. Professionalism is behavior that exhibits the traits or features that correspond to the standards of that profession. Professional standards vary from occupation to occupation, and some vary within the same occupation, depending on the environment. And, of course, these standards go way beyond just personal appearance, although they do include this. Imagine the difference between the professional standards required of a commercial jet pilot who logs thousands of miles despite tough weather conditions and is responsible for the lives of 200-plus passengers at any given time versus those of a hobby pilot who likes to fly his Cessna solo for a few hours on sunny weekends. Will their uniforms or dress codes be different? Is punctuality equally important in both cases? Luckily, you will not need to worry too much about airplanes as a medical assistant, but this is just one example of how professional standards may differ in a particular industry.

As discussed in *Introduction to Medical Assisting*, standards for medical assisting education and the profession are developed by professional organizations, such as the American Association of Medical Assistants (AAMA) and the American Medical Technologists (AMT). To be a professional medical assistant, not only do you need to know standards of the profession but you must also be able to exhibit appropriate personal attributes and behaviors.

Success is a favorable or desired outcome. To achieve a favorable or desired outcome from your medical assisting education and in practice, you must follow the standards and exhibit the personal behaviors established by your school and workplace. In this chapter, you will explore the professional behaviors required of a medical assistant in school and in practice, as well as the attributes and strategies needed for success in your education and career.

▶ Professionalism in Medical Assisting
LO 3.1

The mere fact that you are reading this book means you are embarking on the profession of medical assisting. To understand this profession, you should first understand what a profession consists of. A profession has two areas of competence (abilities):

1. **Hard skills**—specific technical and operational proficiencies
2. **Soft skills**—personal qualifications or behaviors that enhance an individual's interactions, job performance, and career prospects; these are sometimes called people skills (Figure 3-1)

Hard skills represent the minimum proficiencies necessary to do the job. Following are some examples of hard skills of medical assisting:

- Scheduling appointments
- Coding for insurance purposes
- Managing medical records
- Interviewing patients
- Taking vital signs
- Assisting a provider with patient examinations

These hard skills are the ones you will learn throughout this program, and your ability to perform them is readily observable. Your hard skills set is the first screen employers use to determine if you are qualified for the position.

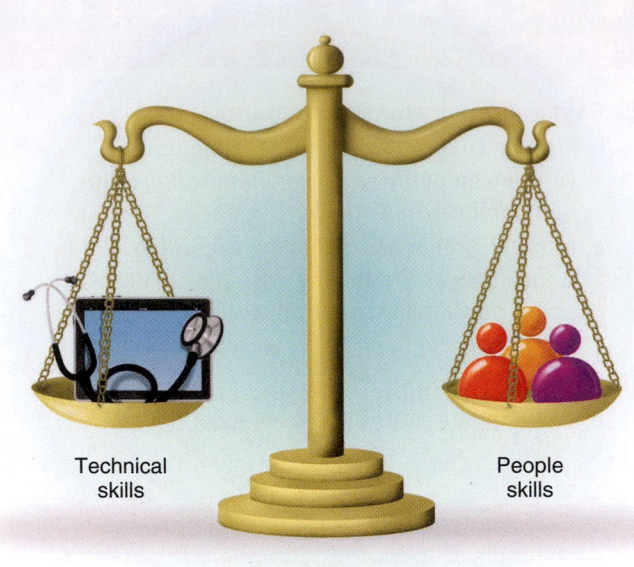

FIGURE 3-1 As a medical assistant, you need to have both technical skills (hard skills) and people skills (soft skills) and maintain a good balance between them.

Soft skills are less concrete and more difficult to observe and evaluate. These are the characteristics, attributes, or **attitudes** that people develop throughout their lives. Some examples are respect, dependability, and integrity. These personal attributes or qualities, which are sought after and significant for specific jobs, are also professional attributes or behaviors, and they tend to help define an individual's personality. Your professional behaviors together produce what is called a good **work ethic,** which is what employers seek.

A medical assisting credential and the technical skills associated with it are the reasons most graduates are hired. However, the lack of a specific soft skill or poor professional behavior is the reason for most terminations. Weakness in the soft skills is also the major reason that some students do not successfully complete their medical assisting education. So knowing how to do something is important, but behaving professionally while practicing is essential.

Much of the medical assistant's role involves dealing with other people, whether this is a patient, a patient's family member, a coworker, an insurance agent, a pharmaceutical sales representative, a laboratory staff member, or anyone else with whom you may come in contact in the workplace. Because most professional behaviors and skills are about working with other people, it only makes sense that someone going into a profession that continually deals with people should possess these behaviors and skills to do a good job. As a student and in your medical assisting career, you will experience the ongoing assessment of your professional behaviors in the following environments:

- Classroom
- Student work experience
- Hiring process

- Workplace performance evaluation
- Promotion consideration

So no matter the circumstance, your professionalism contributes to your success and should always be on the top of your list of ongoing self-improvements. For example, what if a medical assistant did not know the proper instructions to give a patient regarding a diagnostic test? She was either too shy (lacked self-confidence) to ask or chose not to ask because of a lack of time or neglect. Consequently, she gave instructions based on what she thought might be appropriate (lacked knowledge). So it is highly probable that the patient would not be adequately prepared for the test. The results of this poor decision might be

- Difficulty in performing the test on the patient.
- Cancelation of the test, wasting time and resources.
- Repetition of the test, incurring increased costs that may not be reimbursed by insurance.
- Inaccurate test results, leading to incorrect diagnosis and treatment and a poor patient outcome.
- Potential litigation (lawsuit) against the medical practice.

The issue is not that the medical assistant did not know the correct instructions but that the medical assistant did not use the correct behaviors (communication, cooperation, knowledge, persistence, work quality) to obtain and give the correct instructions. Although this scenario seems exaggerated, it has occurred. The importance of professional behaviors cannot be overemphasized.

▶ Professional Behaviors   LO 3.2

Certain behaviors distinguish medical assistants who behave professionally from those who just get by, as well as those who do not make it. Professional behaviors contribute to your overall success in life—as a medical assistant and as a human being on this planet. Let's explore essential medical assisting professional behaviors. As you read each of the following sections, take a moment to consider whether you exhibit this behavior or quality. When you have completed this section, review the sample self-evaluation document and Procedure 3-1, Self-Evaluation of Professional Behaviors, at the end of the chapter.

Comprehension

Comprehension is the ability to learn, retain, and process information. In order to function as a medical assistant, you must comprehend your role and responsibilities. This means not only to have information but also to be able to analyze that information, to know how to use it, and to retain it, no matter how infrequently you might use it. An example of comprehension is learning how to take a blood pressure, including the equipment needed, the steps in the procedure, what results to expect, how to record the results, and when to report a problem.

Persistence

Persistence is continuing in spite of difficulty—being determined and overcoming obstacles. Two other words for persistence are *perseverance* and *tenacity*. The slang is *stick-to-itiveness*. This attribute ensures that you will finish the job no matter how difficult, boring, annoying, or time-consuming it may be. One example that is not uncommon in the medical office is trying to reach a patient whose contact information is not up-to-date. The issue may be an abnormal laboratory report that requires follow-up or another vital matter. The practitioner must be able to count on you and know that you will follow through and make contact no matter how difficult it may be. The patient's well-being often depends on it.

Self-Confidence

Self-confidence means believing in oneself. It is a trait that puts people at ease. The patient, the physician, and others are more comfortable when they feel that you know what you are doing. The self-assured medical assistant is generally the one that the patient and the physician prefer to work with. However, some people are self-confident to excess, which is not a professional trait. Have you ever felt a test was easy, but when the score came back you did less than great? That is overconfidence. On the other hand, self-confidence is a professional trait that makes you desirable to be around. An overconfident person acts as if she knows everything; a self-confident person knows what she knows and what she doesn't know. Display your self-confidence by smiling, making eye contact, and remaining calm no matter what the situation.

Judgment

Judgment is evaluating a situation, reaching an appropriate conclusion, and acting accordingly. It is also referred to as **critical thinking** (Figure 3-2). Critical thinking is defined as purposeful decisions resulting from analysis and evaluation. You will examine the steps of critical thinking in the next section. Applying sound judgment in all situations—even when you are distracted, upset, or annoyed—is necessary as a medical assistant.

Knowledge

Knowledge is understanding gained through study and experience. Medical assisting is a profession that requires understanding theory (knowledge) and then applying psychomotor skills or hands-on experience. You will acquire knowledge by learning the principles and then performing the procedures. Students who do not have an understanding of the procedure and only memorize the steps may have difficulty performing when equipment varies or if a procedure is done differently (yet correctly) at the externship site. These students are often unable to function when the procedure does not go as planned. So it is best to understand the rationale for what you are doing. Avoid just memorizing steps.

Organization

Organization is planning and coordinating information and tasks in an orderly manner to efficiently complete a job in a given time frame. This attribute has many aspects, including time management and prioritizing, which will be discussed in more detail in the next section. Organization is required to know how to prioritize the issues and tasks while addressing them all in an efficient and timely manner. One example is prioritizing your work—deciding which are the most important tasks of the day and which are less important. On a day when everything seems to be "top priority," you must use your professional judgment, knowledge of office policies, and experience with providers and coworkers to determine what should be completed first, second, third, and so on.

Integrity

Integrity is adhering to the appropriate code of law and ethics and being honest and trustworthy. Ethics is a system of values that determines right or wrong behavior. Integrity involves relatively simple matters, such as not taking pens home from the workplace, to more complex matters, such as always being truthful with patients. It also deals with subjects that are punishable and illegal, such as taking cash, cheating on an exam, or falsifying a time card. Falsifying a time card is clearly dishonest, but knowingly extending breaks or lunches demonstrates a lack of integrity. Knowing that a coworker or a classmate is doing something dishonest is another area of integrity (Figure 3-3).

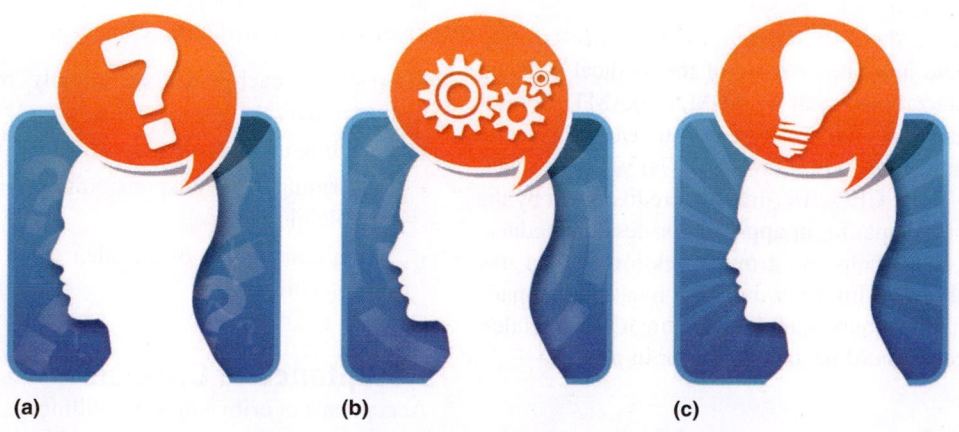

(a)   (b)   (c)

FIGURE 3-2   Using sound judgment through critical thinking requires (a) identifying a problem, (b) analyzing methods to solve it, and (c) determining an acceptable method to solve it.

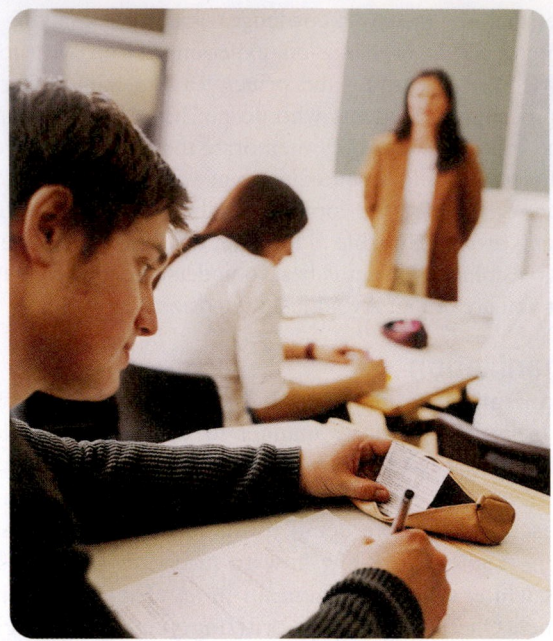

FIGURE 3-3 Being dishonest or not reporting something that you observe that is dishonest reduces your integrity and trustworthiness.
© Digital Vision RF

If you do not report your facts or suspicion of the act, you could be considered an accomplice and subject to a penalty. Besides causing harm, once a person is involved in a dishonest act or is seen as lacking integrity, it is very difficult to regain the trust of others. The *Legal and Ethical Issues* chapter provides more details about standards of integrity that involve morals, laws, and ethics.

Growth

Growth is an ongoing effort to learn and improve. Being a professional brings with it an obligation to keep up with new standards, methods, procedures, and technologies in the field. Throughout this text and your medical assisting program, you will learn current practices. However, healthcare practices change frequently. For example, electronic health records (EHR) are replacing paper health records, and the standards for cardiopulmonary resuscitation (CPR) change frequently. Growth requires staying informed.

As discussed in the *Introduction to Medical Assisting* chapter, you should join one or more of the medical assisting professional organizations, such as AAMA or AMT. Besides receiving the benefits, you are expected to earn a specific number of continuing education units (CEUs) within a specified time frame. These CEU offerings are credits given by the organization for participating in approved professional educational offerings. CEUs help you grow professionally and stay up-to-date with the latest information through taking seminars, reading articles, taking courses, and completing CEU modules, which may be accessed online, on a DVD, or in print.

Teamwork

Teamwork is working with others in the best interest of completing the job. The healthcare team, described in the *Healthcare and the Healthcare Team* chapter, is large and complex. Like any team, its members must work together and cooperate with each other in order to increase the likelihood of achieving the goal. Also, studies show that in workplaces where staff members cooperate and help each other, job satisfaction and patient (client) satisfaction are high.

In the healthcare practice, the overall goal should be providing good patient care, which is done through cooperation between team members. Everyone in the facility has an important job that depends on someone else. It is important to remember that the patient comes first and everyone is responsible for the care of that patient.

Another important aspect of teamwork and professionalism is the correct use of personal cell phones and other electronic devices while at work. Personal cell phones and other devices should never be used while you are working. Depending on the workplace policy, use of a personal cell phone or iPad may be allowed when you are on break, but otherwise you should place the device on mute or "airplane mode" and store it while you are working. In the same vein, although you may think of the computer you use at work as "yours," it belongs to your employer. Visiting social websites, such as Facebook, or checking personal e-mail or Twitter accounts should never be considered. Also, keep in mind that your work e-mail is not yours, either. Any e-mail you send from your work e-mail address reflects on your workplace and employer. Any sites you visit or e-mails you send may be tracked at any time by your employer. If you are tempted to send a "quick e-mail" to a friend or "quickly" check your Facebook account, remember, your employer and/or IT department has access to your work computer or network drive. Your employer will not ask you to work for him or her on your time; you should not be accessing personal websites and e-mail on work time.

Teamwork also requires coordination, which is the integration of activities. A typical patient may have three or more physician specialists, several prescriptions, home healthcare, routine blood work, physical therapy, hospital care, and outpatient procedures. This requires multiple appointments, insurance companies, medical claims, and other processes. These processes require all the members of the team to work together for the benefit of the patient. Frequently, coordinating these patient care activities is the role of the medical assistant and requires cooperation and coordination with everyone involved. Team dynamics consist of

- Assisting each other on a daily basis with the duties required.
- Avoiding interpersonal conflict with members of the team.
- Performing extra responsibilities without questioning or complaining.
- Being considerate of all other team members' duties and responsibilities.

Acceptance of Criticism

Acceptance of criticism is the willingness to consider feedback and suggestions to improve; it is taking responsibility for one's actions. In this context, let's focus on **constructive criticism,** which is counseling or advice that is intended to be useful with

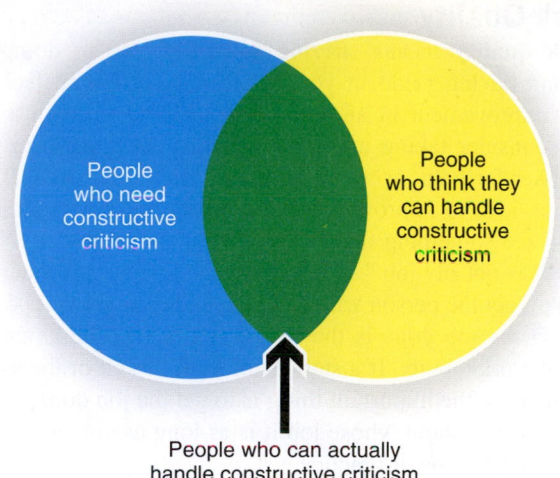

People who need constructive criticism

People who think they can handle constructive criticism

People who can actually handle constructive criticism

FIGURE 3-4 Accepting constructive criticism to improve your performance is essential to medical assisting practice. Get yourself inside the green zone.

the goal of improving something. To grow and understand the areas in which you can improve, you must be able to accept constructive criticism (Figure 3-4). This may come from medical assisting educators, classmates, physicians, coworkers, or even patients. You will be evaluated throughout your education and workplace experience. Never expect a perfect evaluation, because no one is perfect and improvements can always be made. Instead, be open to accepting criticism and suggestions and offer your own thoughts on what you can do to improve. Do not be defensive or blame others. It is not about what your classmate or coworker does; it is about you.

Relations with Others

Relations with others—the ability to get along with those around you—involves treating everyone with respect and caring even when it is difficult. This sometimes includes **empathy,** feeling and understanding another's experience without having the experience yourself. In the healthcare environment, the medical assistant works with many patients who are experiencing great loss. It may be the loss of health or function or a terminal diagnosis. Or it may be a personal loss, such as the death of a spouse. As in any other workplace, coworkers also experience losses and unfortunate events. Sometimes medical assistants are very kind to patients but do not exhibit the same behaviors with coworkers. With coworkers, they may become involved in gossip and pettiness or display impatience and rudeness.

Caring is showing concern and appropriate attention, whereas enabling, or codependency, in this context is doing for others the things that they should be doing for themselves. When you enable, you become part of the disease process. For example, a young medical assistant learned this early in her career when she became attached to a 10-year-old juvenile diabetic patient. Every time the child came into the office, the MA gave her a stuffed animal or other gift. The patient started to have more and more problems and the office visits became more frequent. An experienced medical assistant pointed out that the child was being rewarded for not managing her

illness. This exemplifies enabling. Instead of giving a gift (reward) for not managing the disease and becoming ill, the two medical assistants developed a more appropriate reward system for the patient if her diabetes was kept under control.

Professional Boundaries Having professional boundaries, or limitations, means always treating a patient as a client and not becoming involved in issues of his or her private life that do not directly relate to the healthcare. This is often difficult, especially with patients you see often and particularly enjoy, and with patients you feel you may be able to help in addition to providing care in the medical office. Generally, the guidelines for maintaining professional boundaries are

- Address the patient only by his or her last name unless first asking permission to use his or her first name (children are an exception).
- Avoid offering advice on personal matters.
- Use only tasteful, appropriate humor.
- Avoid becoming excessively friendly.
- Avoid giving or accepting money from a patient.
- Decline meeting a patient outside of the workplace unless you were acquainted prior to taking your position.

Cultural Diversity Have you heard the expression "it takes all kinds"? Professionalism involves understanding people who are different from you and respecting their right to be different. After all, from their point of view, you are the one who is different! Healthcare facilities serve patients from many countries who speak many languages. The variety of human social structures, belief systems, and strategies for adapting to situations in different parts of the world is referred to as **cultural diversity.** Showing respect to all individuals, regardless of culture, race, religion, age, gender, sexual orientation, physical challenges, special needs, lifestyle choices, or socioeconomic standing, impacts your relations with others (Figure 3-5). Being respectful does not mean that you have to agree with the lifestyles and beliefs of others. It means that you accept the idea that others have every right to be different

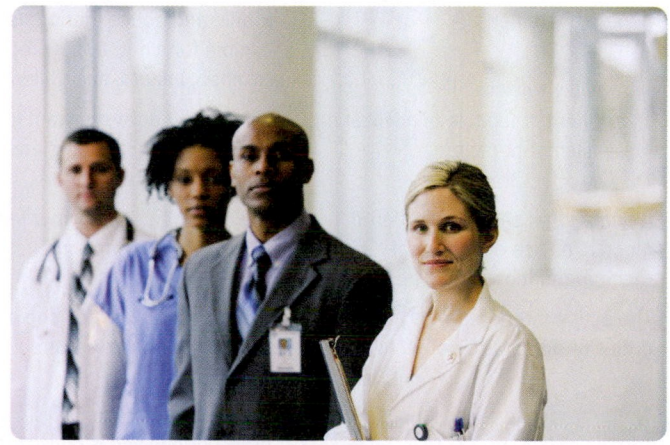

FIGURE 3-5 Respect and understanding for everyone is an essential professional behavior for the medical assistant.
© Terry Vine/Getty Images RF

from you, and as a medical assistant you treat them appropriately. The following list gives some ideas that may help you understand and respect diversity.

- Increase your awareness of diversity. Communication with patients and coworkers will help you learn about individual similarities and differences.
- Increase your awareness of your own feelings. Everyone has biases. People tend to stereotype others, and this can lead to discrimination. Examine your own biases. Are they realistic?
- Look at individuals. As you learn about people as individuals, any group stereotypes you have often begin to break down.

Patient Advocacy As a medical assistant, you may be in a position to speak or act on behalf of the patient or the patient's family. This is called **patient advocacy.** Understanding your scope of practice, as well as being professional in your relations with others and being a good communicator, will help you be an effective advocate for the patient. Be sure you have all the facts before you act, and include your supervisor or licensed practitioner as needed. Table 3-1 provides some examples of patient advocacy decisions.

Work Quality

Work quality means striving for excellence in doing the job and having pride in your performance. If you feel you need improvement in an area or would like to learn a new skill, consider taking a course, asking your supervisor or a coworker for help, or spending more time in that area. If you have an idea to improve a work process, make a suggestion. If you see something that is a potential risk, report it. Never say, "It is not my job." If it is not your job, simply state that you will get the person who can help and then get that person. Getting the job done is the focus. Being flexible is another part of work quality. If a staff member is absent or the schedule changes, the important thing is to get the job done. Again, do not worry about whose job it is as long as you are staying within your scope of practice.

Another way to look at this is to believe that patients are "customers" of the practice and, as such, deserve excellent customer service. Basically, this boils down to two things: The patient comes first and the patient is satisfied. When working with a patient, give him or her your undivided attention. Happy patients return to a practice and tell their friends about their experience. Be more than simply an employee; be part of building the practice. Keeping the following skills

TABLE 3-1	Examples of Patient Advocacy	
Circumstance	**Example**	**Suggested Action**
You have concern for the individual's safety.	You suspect an elderly patient is being abused.	Discuss with licensed practitioner; follow legal requirements and office protocols for reporting suspected elder abuse.
A complex situation requiring your level of expertise.	A patient is having difficulty with an insurance claim.	Assist the patient as needed.
A potentially bad situation exists that your knowledge may help to avoid or resolve.	You are aware that a patient will not fill a prescription for an expensive drug because he cannot afford the insurance copay.	Inform the physician, who may prescribe a generic version of the drug, or, with the physician's approval, contact the drug company to obtain free or reduced medications or contact a local pharmacy that provides low-cost medications if available.
Giving extra attention is likely to benefit the patient.	You are reviewing a 1-year-old patient's profile and notice that she is probably eligible for a nutritional program called WIC (Women, Infants, and Children).	Take the time to explain the program to the mother and provide the information for her to enroll.
The patient is capable of advocating for himself or herself.	The patient does not want to tell the physician that he does not understand why he needs a proposed procedure.	Encourage the patient to talk to the physician and assure him it is not unusual for patients to not fully understand the first time information is presented.
Anything that can be considered medical advice or a medical recommendation should be avoided.	The patient is asking your telephone advice regarding his symptoms.	Avoid saying anything that involves a potential diagnosis, such as "that sounds like the flu"; follow the office protocol for scheduling an appointment.
The action interferes with your job duties or presents a potential liability.	A patient asks you to keep an eye on her children during her exam.	Suggest the patient reschedule when she can arrange childcare; if needed, provide a contact number for a facility close to the office.
There are reasonable options.	A patient forgets to fill his monthly prescriptions and is consistently asking for an emergency refill. The office policy is that refills will be processed in 3 business days. He wants you to call and remind him each month.	Suggest to the patient that many pharmacies provide a monthly automatic refill or a monthly reminder.

sharp and using them consistently will lead to excellent customer service in the medical office.

- Using proper telephone techniques
- Writing or responding to telephone messages
- Explaining procedures to patients
- Expediting insurance referral requests
- Assisting with billing issues
- Answering questions or finding answers to patient questions
- Ensuring that patients are comfortable in your office
- Creating a warm and reassuring environment

Punctuality and Attendance

Being on time—**punctuality**—and coming to work every day that you are scheduled are essential for maintaining your job. Poor attendance is a frequent reason for termination. You are expected to be at your duty station or in your classroom, ready to work at the given time. Whether you are late or absent as a result of poor planning or an emergency, it still means that either your job is not getting done or you created additional work for your teammates. Patient care is impacted when you are not present. Recall Kaylyn in the chapter-opening case study, who is at risk for termination for frequent tardiness. Do not let this be you.

Professional Appearance

A medical professional always strives to maintain a neat appearance in the workplace, and personal cleanliness is an important part of this. Your appearance is the first impression you make on your patients, coworkers, and the physicians you work with. Medical facilities are considered "conservative" work environments, and your appearance should reflect a conservative style. Listed here are a few professional guidelines to follow in the medical environment:

- Your approved uniform or other clothing should be clean, pressed crisply, fit properly, and in good repair.
- Your shoes should be comfortable, white, clean, and in good condition. Open-toed shoes should not be worn in the patient treatment areas to prevent injury or infection to yourself.
- Choose a hairstyle that is flattering and conservative. Hair should be clean and pulled back from your face and off your collar if it is long. Natural colors for hair are the most acceptable colors in a medical environment.
- Your nails should be kept at a short working length, no more than one-fourth of an inch, and of a natural color. Acrylic nails should not be worn, as they pose a risk for infection.
- Body odors, including the odor of smoke, are offensive. Even pleasant odors such as hairspray, perfumes, and lotions may trigger nausea or allergies in some patients and should be avoided.
- Jewelry should be kept to a minimum and in good taste. No more than one ring should be worn. Rings may tear through exam gloves. Ears can be pierced with one hole, and small

earrings are appropriate. Avoid dangling earrings, as patients (particularly pediatric patients) can tear these off.

- Visible tattoos, body piercings, and tongue piercings are not acceptable.

Communication

Effective communication involves careful listening, observing, speaking, and writing. Communication even involves good manners—being polite, tactful, and respectful. You must use good communication skills during every patient discussion and in every interaction you have with providers, other staff members, and other professionals with whom your practice does business.

Communication is giving and receiving accurate information. If a person is a bad communicator, it means that he or she cannot communicate or provide information that is accurate or understandable. Sometimes the patient leaves the office confused because he or she did not understand medical terms that were used and did not communicate that he or she did not understand. Sometimes the student leaves class confused because he or she did not understand the assignment and did not communicate to the instructor that he or she did not understand. In these scenarios, communication was poor from the sender, since it was not understood. It was also poor from the receiver, since lack of understanding was not communicated back to the sender. Effective communication is a two-way process, with a responsibility on both sides. It impacts every aspect of healthcare and is discussed in-depth in the *Interpersonal Communication* chapter.

▶ Strategies for Success   LO 3.3

As you move toward and through your career as a medical assistant, you should be constantly improving your professional behaviors, as discussed earlier. As a medical assistant, you must practice specific strategies to ensure your success. These strategies include critical thinking and problem solving, time management and prioritizing, and stress management. The sections that follow will discuss these strategies, provide examples, and explain how to practice them.

Critical Thinking and Problem Solving

You will develop critical thinking skills over time as you apply your knowledge about and experience with human nature, medicine, and office skills to new situations. Critical thinking skills include quickly evaluating circumstances, solving problems, and taking action. For example, you must use critical thinking skills to assess how to react to emergency situations. If you see a patient suddenly pass out in the office reception area, you must immediately see that the patient receives first aid, notify a physician, and alert the patient's family.

Critical thinking skills are used every day, and critical thinking relies on sound judgment. More specifically, critical thinking involves the ability to

- Analyze situations.
- Determine what aspects of a situation are most important.
- Reach conclusions that go beyond the obvious.

Critical thinking includes both factual problem identification and creative decision-making skills. It is the ability to see the whole picture and to reach reasonable conclusions based on the most important facts.

Problem solving can be broken down into a step-by-step approach (Figure 3-6):

- Identify the problem and define it clearly.
- Identify the potential effects of the problem.
- Clearly identify the objectives to be achieved.
- Identify as many potential solutions and strategies as possible.
- Analyze the potential solutions and strategies.
- Implement the strategy that appears to be the best solution.
- Evaluate the results and repeat the steps as needed.

Let's use the problem-solving steps to solve a patient problem. A patient approaches your desk and complains loudly that he does not have all day to wait for the doctor to see him. His appointment was at 2:00 and the time is now 2:40. The patient is obviously angry about the delay. What should you do?

Step 1. Identify and define the problem: What is wrong with the patient?

The patient is angry because the physician did not see him promptly at his appointment time.

Step 2. Identify the potential effects of the problem: What effects might the patient's anger have?

The patient is disrupting the office; the practice may lose this client.

Step 3. Identify the objectives to be achieved: What is your goal for this situation?

Your goal is to end the disruption and calm the patient.

Step 4. Identify potential solutions and strategies: What can you do to end the disruption and calm the patient?

This is the step where you may be able to come up with more than one answer. For example, you may want to (a) inform your supervisor that the patient is causing a disruption, (b) ask the physician to talk to the patient, (c) tell the patient there is nothing you can do about it, or (d) explain the situation to the patient quietly and offer to reschedule the appointment. Remember that problem solving is not an exact science. You are attempting to come up with solutions so you can determine the one that will most effectively solve the problem.

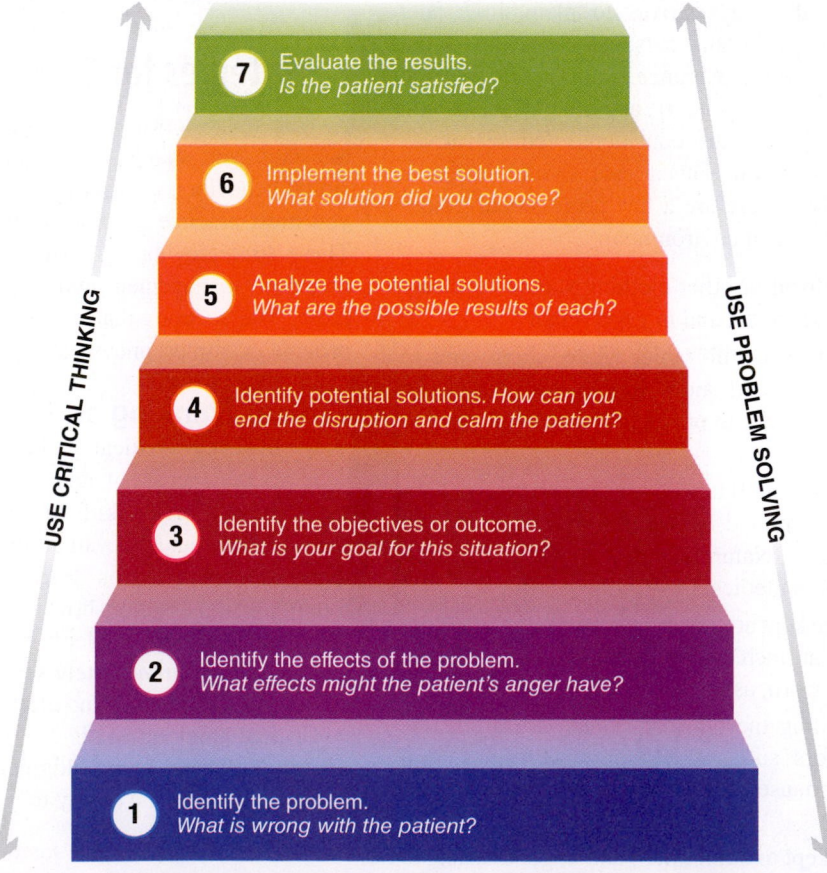

FIGURE 3-6   Use critical thinking and good judgment when following the steps of the problem-solving process.

Step 5. Analyze the potential solutions and strategies. What are the possible results from each solution?

For (a), you discover that the supervisor is busy in a room with another patient, and waiting for her to become available will allow the disruption to continue. For (b), you recall that the physician expects the office staff to take care of this type of incident. For (c), you suspect that telling the patient you cannot do anything will not make him less angry. For (d), you think that talking quietly to the patient and offering to reschedule the appointment might work.

Step 6. Implement the best solution. What solution did you choose?

You explain that an emergency earlier in the day put the physician behind schedule and offer to reschedule the patient's appointment for a more convenient time. Of course, you will need to use your judgment to provide an explanation without violating the confidentiality of the patient who had the emergency earlier.

Step 7. Evaluate the results and repeat the steps as needed. How did it go? Is the patient satisfied and calmer now? If not, try a different strategy.

This step is important because learning from experience counts. If you chose to wait for the supervisor to become available to handle the situation, and the patient stalked out of the office, saying he would not be back, you would hopefully do something different if faced with the same circumstance again. In this case, you explained the reason for the delay and offered to reschedule the patient, and he calmed down and decided to wait for the physician to see him.

Time Management and Prioritizing

Personal and professional time management skills are essential for medical assistants. **Time management** is controlling how you spend your time. People who use time management techniques routinely are the highest achievers in all walks of life, professionally and personally. Using these skills will help you function exceptionally well in the medical office, even under intense pressure. Even more importantly, you can say goodbye to the often intense stress of work overload. Setting goals and concentrating on results, not just being busy, are the main focus of time management.

Medical assistant students who are disorganized waste a great deal of time locating assignments and other materials before they get started on their work. Prepare in advance. Purchase a binder, notebook, or folders for storing your homework assignments, reminders about upcoming tests, your course syllabus, and other pertinent facts, such as your instructor's office hours and contact information and your classmates' information for study sessions. Obtain computer access with an Internet connection at home, through your school, or at the local library. Try these tips for organization:

- Study in a quiet area away from distractions.
- Find a study "buddy" who is just as committed to and focused on success as you are.

- Formal classroom courses require at least as much work time outside of class as inside it to prepare, so allow yourself enough preparation time.
- Budget your time between school and other responsibilities.
- Set aside study time by creating a study schedule.
- Set daily, weekly, or course-specific goals to accomplish the overall goal of completing your course.

The medical assistant must be organized. For example, the phone may be ringing at the same time a patient is trying to schedule a follow-up appointment, while the physician is inquiring about the results of a diagnostic report, and a coworker is asking for information about a patient's immunizations. To be an effective medical assistant, you must be able to manage your time and **prioritize** effectively. When you prioritize, you decide on the order in which tasks should be completed based on things such as the task deadline and importance. Evaluate yourself, and use the following ideas to improve your ability to manage time and prioritize.

1. Have a plan for your day. Know what needs to be done. Set your daily goals and try to meet them.
2. Take advantage of your own productivity. That is, you may work better at a particular time of day. Choose to do the most difficult tasks when you are working at your best. Remember, everybody has sluggish times, so know when yours are—maybe right after lunch or near the end of the day. Plan accordingly.
3. Avoid distractions when you can. Of course, if your job is to answer the phone, then you must do so. But if someone is just chatting or your smartphone is constantly beeping to signal text messages, this probably means you are not accomplishing what needs to be done. Personal phone calls, text messages, tweets, or other communications are not supposed to occur during your working hours. However, business electronic communication is vital. Consider setting specific times during the day to look at business e-mail so you will not have constant interruptions.
4. Evaluate yourself on a daily basis. Consider whether you accomplished your daily goal and come up with a plan to continue or do better the next day.

Stress and Burnout Professionals in the healthcare field, including medical assistants, may experience high levels of stress in their daily work environment. Stress can result from a feeling of being under pressure, or it can be a reaction to anger, frustration, or a change in your routine. Stress can increase your blood pressure, speed up your breathing and heart rate, and cause muscle tension. Stress also can cause you to behave or communicate ineffectively. For example, if you are feeling very pressured at work, you might snap at a coworker or patient, or you might forget to give the provider an important message.

Good or Bad Stress A certain amount of stress is normal. A little bit of stress—the kind that makes you feel excited or challenged by the task at hand—can motivate you to get things done and push you toward a higher level of productivity. For example, your supervisor may ask you to learn a new procedure. Learning something new, although stressful in itself, can be an exciting challenge and a welcome change of pace. Ongoing stress, however, can be overwhelming and affect you physically. For example, it can lower your resistance to colds and increase your risk for developing heart disease, diabetes, high blood pressure, ulcers, allergies, asthma, colitis, and cancer. It also can increase your risk for certain autoimmune diseases, which cause the body's immune system to attack normal tissue.

Some stress at work is inevitable. An important goal is to learn how to manage or reduce stress. Take into account your strengths and limitations, and be realistic about how much you can handle at work and in your life outside work. Pushing yourself a certain amount can be motivating. The *Points on Practice* box lists the potential causes of stress and ways to reduce stress.

Preventing Burnout Burnout is the end result of prolonged periods of stress without relief, an energy-depleting condition that will affect your health and career. Certain personality types are more prone to burnout than others. If you are a highly driven, perfectionist-type person, you will be more susceptible to burnout. Experts often refer to such a person as a characteristic Type A personality. A more relaxed, calm individual is considered a Type B person. Type B personalities are less prone to burnout but have the potential to suffer from it, especially if they work in healthcare.

According to some experts on stress, there are five stages of burnout:

1. *The honeymoon phase.* During the honeymoon phase, your job is wonderful. You have boundless energy and enthusiasm, and all things seem possible. You love the job and the job loves you. You believe it will satisfy all your needs and desires and solve all your problems. You are delighted with your job, your coworkers, and the organization.

2. *The awakening phase.* The awakening stage starts with the realization that your initial expectations were unrealistic.

The job is not working out the way you thought it would. It does not satisfy all your needs, your coworkers and the organization are less than perfect, and rewards and recognition are scarce. As disillusionment and disappointment grow, you become confused. Something is wrong, but you cannot quite put your finger on it. Typically, you work harder to make your dreams come true. But working harder does not change anything and you become increasingly tired, bored, and frustrated. You may question your competence and ability and start losing your self-confidence.

3. *The brownout phase.* As brownout begins, your early enthusiasm and energy give way to chronic fatigue and irritability. You become indecisive and your productivity drops. Your work deteriorates. Coworkers and managers may even comment on it. You become increasingly frustrated and angry and project the blame for your difficulties onto others. You are cynical, detached, and openly critical of the organization, superiors, and coworkers. You are beset with depression, anxiety, and physical illness.

4. *The full-scale burnout phase.* Unless you interrupt the process or someone intervenes, brownout drifts remorselessly into full-scale burnout. Despair is the dominant feature of this final stage. It usually takes 3 to 4 years to get to this phase. You experience an overwhelming sense of failure and a devastating loss of self-esteem and self-confidence. You become depressed and feel lonely and empty. You talk about just quitting and getting away. You are exhausted physically and mentally and prone to physical and mental breakdowns.

5. *The phoenix phenomenon.* Just like a phoenix, you can arise from the burnout ashes. But this takes time. First, you need to rest and relax. Do not take work home. If you are like many people, the work will not get done and you will only feel guilty for being lazy. Second, be realistic in your job expectations as well as your aspirations and goals. Third, create balance in your life. Invest more of yourself in family and other personal relationships, social activities, and hobbies. Spread yourself out so that your job does not have such an overpowering influence on your self-esteem and self-confidence.

Potential Causes of Stress

Sometimes stress can be difficult to measure. Just like varying thresholds for pain, different people can tolerate different amounts of stress. One person's stress may seem a lot worse than another's. For example, who can say that the stress you may be feeling over an upcoming exam is less nerve-wracking than the stress someone else may be feeling about paying off a large credit card balance? Stress can come in many forms from many directions, but here is a list of common potential causes.

- Death of a spouse or family member
- Divorce or separation
- Hospitalization (yours or a family member's) due to injury or illness
- Marriage or reconciliation from a separation
- Loss of a job or retirement
- Sexual problems
- A new baby
- Significant change in your financial status (for better or worse)
- Job change
- Children leaving or returning home
- Significant personal success, such as a promotion at work
- Moving or remodeling your home
- Problems at work, such as your boss's retiring, that may put your job at risk
- Substantial debt, such as a mortgage or overspending on credit cards

Tips for Reducing Stress

Managing your stress levels can benefit your overall well-being, both mentally and physically, at work and at home. The following is a list of helpful, doable tips for lowering stress.

- Maintain a healthy balance in your life among work, family, and leisure activities.
- Exercise regularly.
- Eat balanced, nutritious meals and healthful snacks.
- Avoid foods high in caffeine, salt, sugar, and fat.
- Get enough sleep.
- Allow time for yourself, and plan time to relax.
- Rely on the support that family, friends, and coworkers have to offer. Do not be afraid to share your feelings.
- Try to be realistic about what you can and cannot do. Do not be afraid to admit that you cannot take on another responsibility.
- Try to set realistic goals for yourself. Remember, there are always choices, even when there appear to be none.
- Be organized. Good planning can help you manage your workload.
- Redirect excess energy constructively; clean your closet, work in the garden, volunteer, invite friends for dinner, or exercise.
- Change some of the things you have control over.
- Stay focused. Focus your full energy on one thing at a time and finish one project before starting another.
- Identify sources of conflict and try to resolve them.
- Learn and use relaxation techniques, such as deep breathing, meditation, or imagining yourself in a quiet, peaceful place. Choose what works for you.
- Maintain a healthy sense of humor, as laughter can help relieve stress. Joke with friends after work. See a funny movie.
- Try not to overreact. Ask yourself if a situation is really worth getting upset or worried about.
- Seek help from social or professional support groups, if necessary.

PROCEDURE 3-1   Self-Evaluation of Professional Behaviors   WORK // DOC

Procedure Goal: To identify necessary professional behaviors and relate them to yourself in order to improve your performance as a medical assistant

OSHA Guidelines: This procedure does not involve exposure to blood, body fluids, or tissue.

Materials: Self-Evaluation Form (Figure Procedure 3-1)

Method:

1. Read and review each professional behavior.
2. Rate yourself on each behavior, considering the level at which you exhibit them.
3. Identify at least one measure to improve yourself on each behavior, as needed.
4. Place the completed form in your portfolio and review it on an ongoing basis.
5. Reevaluate your professional behavior prior to your applied training experience (practicum).
6. Compare the two scores and identify any weaknesses.
7. Obtain feedback about your professional behaviors from your instructor, coworkers, classmates, practicum coordinator, or employer.

Behavior	Example(s)	Rate Yourself (5 = Best)					Improvements Needed
		1	2	3	4	5	
Integrity	Consistently honest; able to be trusted with the property of others; can be trusted with confidential information; completes tasks accurately						
Appearance	Clothing and uniform appropriate for circumstance; neat, clean, and well-kept appearance; good personal hygiene and grooming						
Teamwork	Places the success of the team above self-interest; does not undermine the team; helps and supports other team members; shows respect to all team members; remains flexible and open to change; communicates with others to help resolve problems						
Self-confidence	Demonstrates the ability to trust personal judgment; demonstrates an awareness of strengths and limitations; exercises good personal judgment						
Communication	Speaks clearly; writes legibly; listens actively; adjusts communication strategies to various situations						
Commitment to diversity	Consistently demonstrates respect for varied cultural backgrounds, ethnicities, religions, sexual orientations, social classes, abilities, political beliefs, and disabilities						
Punctuality and attendance	Arrives at class and work on the appointed day and time						
Acceptance of criticism	Listens when constructive criticism is given; does not become defensive with criticism; appreciates constructive criticism and incorporates suggestions into behavior as appropriate						
Organization	Coordinates more than one task at a time; keeps work area neat and orderly; anticipates future work; works efficiently and systematically						
Knowledge and comprehension	Learns new things easily; retains new information; associates theory with practice						

FIGURE Procedure 3-1 Self-evaluation of professional behaviors.

SUMMARY OF LEARNING OUTCOMES

LEARNING OUTCOME	KEY POINTS
3.1 Recognize the importance of professionalism in the medical assisting practice.	Professionalism is behavior that exhibits the traits or features corresponding to the standards of that profession. Standards are developed by professional organizations and, in some states, by governmental entities. The skills are placed in two broad categories: hard skills and soft skills. Hard skills are specific technical and operational proficiencies. Soft skills are personal attributes or behaviors that enhance an individual. Professional behaviors are needed to function at a high level in medical assisting and produce a good work ethic.

LEARNING OUTCOME	KEY POINTS
3.2 Explain the professional behaviors that should be exhibited by medical assistants.	Some essential professional behaviors include comprehension—learning, retaining, and processing information; persistence—continuing in spite of difficulty; self-confidence—believing in oneself; judgment—evaluating and determining an appropriate conclusion; organization—coordinating information and tasks in an orderly manner; integrity—adhering to law and ethics; growth—engaging in ongoing efforts to learn and improve; teamwork—working with others in the best interest of completing the job; acceptance of criticism—being willing to consider feedback and suggestions to improve; relations with others—getting along with all people in all circumstances; work quality—striving for excellence in doing the job; punctuality and attendance—showing up on appointed days and times; professional appearance—adhering to the standards and codes of dress; and communication—giving and receiving accurate information.
3.3 Model strategies for success in medical assisting education and practice.	Strategies for success as a medical assistant include cultivating your skills, such as critical thinking and problem solving, time management and prioritizing, stress management, and avoidance of burnout. Practicing effective strategies can assist you during your education and employment.

CASE STUDY CRITICAL THINKING

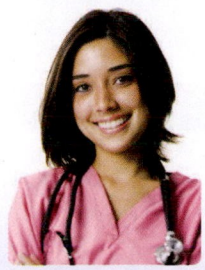

© Rubberball/Getty Images RF

Recall Kaylyn Haddix from the beginning of the chapter. Now that you have completed this chapter, answer the following questions regarding her case.

1. Why do you think Malik wants to meet with Kaylyn?
2. What professional behaviors does Kaylyn need to improve?
3. What strategies for success could Kaylyn use to prevent herself from losing her job?

EXAM PREPARATION QUESTIONS

1. (LO 3.1) The primary reason an employee is hired is usually associated with
   a. Hard skills
   b. Soft skills
   c. References
   d. Punctuality
   e. Cooperation

2. (LO 3.1) Which of the following is considered a soft skill?
   a. Communicating with a patient
   b. Measuring a patient's height
   c. Taking a telephone message
   d. Taking a patient's vital signs
   e. Scheduling an appointment

3. (LO 3.2) An indication that a person lacks integrity would be exhibited by
   a. Being rude to a coworker
   b. Coming into work late
   c. Ignoring the dress code
   d. Taking money from the cash drawer
   e. Gossiping

4. (LO 3.2) A significant part of critical thinking is
   a. Memorizing
   b. Analyzing
   c. Being tenacious
   d. Empathizing
   e. Criticizing

5. (LO 3.2) Adhering to the dress code and good personal hygiene demonstrates
   a. Persistence
   b. Growth
   c. Respect
   d. Knowledge
   e. Organization

6. (LO 3.2) If a medical assistant is not self-confident, this may lead to the patient feeling
   a. Confident
   b. Neglected
   c. Apprehensive
   d. Ignored
   e. Ill

7. (LO 3.2) An example of enabling, or codependency, would be
   a. Providing a wheelchair for a patient who is weak
   b. Helping a patient identify a community resource
   c. Scheduling a patient's next appointment
   d. Offering cookies to an obese patient
   e. Calling a taxi for a patient

8. (LO 3.2) Maintaining professional boundaries involves
   a. Showing a patient you care by being personal
   b. Being friendly but not excessively affectionate
   c. Avoiding any touch with the patient
   d. Babysitting for a patient
   e. Buying the patient lunch

9. (LO 3.3) Your coworker likes to talk about her kids and husband, usually right after lunch as you are returning to work and patients. What should you do?
   a. Talk with your coworker as much as you can, since it is important to have good relationships at work
   b. Talk with your coworker, since some personal discussions at work are OK anyway
   c. Consider telling your supervisor that your coworker talks too much and you find it disturbing
   d. Request that your supervisor ask your coworker to not talk to you so much because you cannot get your work done
   e. Realize that the time you speak with your coworker is preventing you from completing your goals, so politely explain this to your coworker

10. (LO 3.3) Once you have considered what the problem is and what effects it will have, what should you do next?
   a. Implement a solution
   b. Identify the problem
   c. Determine multiple solutions
   d. Determine the effects of the solution
   e. Evaluate your solution to determine if it works or worked

SOFT SKILLS SUCCESS

Learning the technical, or hard, skills required of a medical assistant is important. Why are the soft skills considered just as, if not more, important than these hard skills? Discuss at least four soft skills you will need as a medical assistant.

Interpersonal Communication

4

CASE STUDY

Patient Name	**DOB**	**Allergies**
Cindy Chen	7/15/19XX	NKA
Attending	**MRN**	**Other Information**
Alexis N. Whalen, MD	324-86-542	History of depression

PATIENT INFORMATION

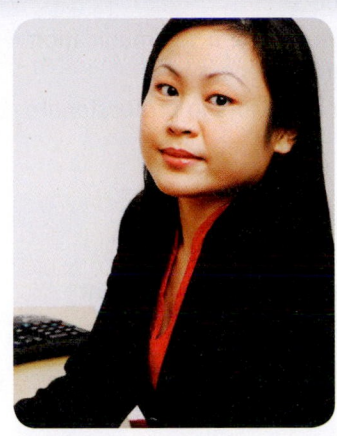

© Red Chopsticks/Getty Images RF

Cindy Chen, a 28-year-old female, arrives at your office complaining of the inability to sleep and nervousness. She tested positive for HIV in 2014, although she has been asymptomatic on antiviral drugs. Currently, she lives with her aunt and is going to school to become a phlebotomist. During her interview she asks, "Just feeling so nervous. Do you have anything you can give me until I see the doctor?"

Keep Cindy Chen in mind as you study this chapter. There will be questions at the end of the chapter based on the case study. The information in the chapter will help you answer these questions.

ACTIVSim

LEARNING OUTCOMES

After completing Chapter 4, you will be able to:

4.1 Identify elements and types of communication.

4.2 Relate communication to human behavior and needs.

4.3 Categorize positive and negative communication.

4.4 Model ways to improve listening, interpersonal skills, and assertiveness skills.

4.5 Carry out therapeutic communication skills.

4.6 Use effective communication strategies with patients in special circumstances.

4.7 Carry out positive communication with coworkers and management.

KEY TERMS

active listening

aggressive

assertive

body language

boundaries

closed posture

conflict

feedback

hierarchy

homeostasis

hospice

interpersonal skills

open posture

passive listening

personal space

rapport

V.C.1 Identify styles and types of verbal communication

V.C.2 Identify types of nonverbal communication

V.C.3 Recognize barriers to communication

V.C.4 Identify techniques for overcoming communication barriers

V.C.5 Recognize the elements of oral communication using a sender-receiver process

V.C.14 Relate the following behaviors to professional communication:

   (a) assertive

   (b) aggressive

   (c) passive

V.P.1 Use feedback techniques to obtain patient information including:

   (a) reflection

   (b) restatement

   (c) clarification

V.P.2 Respond to nonverbal communication

V.P.5 Coach patients appropriately considering:

   (a) cultural diversity

   (b) developmental life stage

   (c) communication barriers

V.A.1 Demonstrate:

   (a) empathy

   (b) active listening

   (c) nonverbal communication

V.A.3 Demonstrate respect for individual diversity including:

   (a) gender

   (b) race

   (c) religion

   (d) age

   (e) economic status

   (f) appearance

5. Psychology of Human Relations

  a. Respond appropriately to patients with abnormal behavior patterns

  b. Provide support for terminally ill patients

    (1) Use empathy when communicating with terminally ill patients

    (2) Identify common stages that terminally ill patients experience

    (3) List organizations/support groups that can assist patient and family members of patients experiencing terminal illnesses

  c. Intervene on behalf of the patient regarding issues/concerns that may arise, i.e. insurance policy information, medical bills, physician/provider orders, etc.

  d. Discuss developmental stages of life

  e. Analyze the effect of hereditary, cultural, and environmental influences on behavior

8. Administrative Procedures

  f. Display professionalism through written and verbal communications

9. Clinical Procedures

  j. Make adaptations with patients with special needs

11. Career Development

  b. Demonstrate professional behavior

▶ Introduction

Think about the last time you had a doctor's appointment. How well did the staff and physician communicate with you? Were you greeted pleasantly and invited to take a seat, or did someone thrust a clipboard at you and say, "Fill this out"? If you had a long wait in the reception area or examination room, did someone come in to explain the delay? Did you become frustrated and angry because nobody told you what was happening? The abilities to recognize human behaviors and to communicate effectively are vital to a medical assistant's success. This chapter takes a psychological approach to understanding human behavior and the challenges that influence therapeutic communication in a healthcare setting.

As the key communicator within the healthcare facility, the medical assistant must be able to communicate with each patient with professionalism and diplomacy. This includes patients from different cultures, socioeconomic backgrounds, educational levels, ages, and lifestyles. The medical assistant sets the tone for the communication circle and must be aware

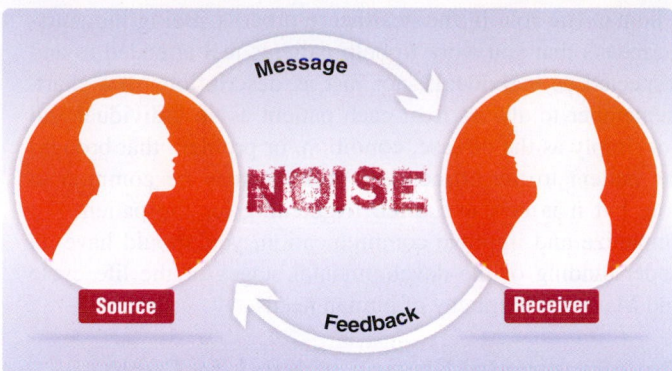

FIGURE 4-1 The process of communication involves an exchange of messages through verbal and nonverbal means.

of all the obstacles that can affect human communication. It is important that patients develop a good rapport and feel confident in the care they are receiving from your office. Developing strong communication skills in the medical office is just as important as mastering administrative and clinical tasks.

▶ Elements of Communication   LO 4.1

As you interact with patients and their families, you will be responsible for giving information and ensuring that the patient understands what you, the doctor, and other staff members have communicated. You also will be responsible for receiving information from the patient. For example, patients will describe their symptoms. They also may discuss their feelings or ask questions about a treatment or procedure. The giving and receiving of information forms the communication circle.

The Communication Circle

The communication circle involves three elements: a message, a source, and a receiver. Messages are usually verbal, written, or nonverbal. (You will explore more about nonverbal messages later in this chapter.) The source sends the message, and the receiver receives it. The communication circle is formed as the source sends a message to the receiver and the receiver responds (Figure 4-1).

Consider the following example, in which Miguel, BWW's clinical medical assistant, is speaking with Sylvia Gonzales, a patient who is having physical therapy for a back injury. Watch the communication circle at work.

| Miguel: | The physical therapist says you're making great progress and that you can start on some simple back exercises at home. I'd like to go over them with you. Then I'll give you a sheet that illustrates the exercises. How does that sound to you? |
| Sylvia Gonzales: | I'm a little nervous about doing exercises. I still have some pain when I bend over. |

| Miguel: | I understand. It's important, though, to start using those muscles again. Why don't you show me exactly where it hurts? Then we can go over proper body mechanics, such as bending down to pick something up and getting in and out of chairs, the car, and bed. Then we'll just start with one or two of the exercises and save the rest for next time, when you're feeling more ready. |
| Sylvia Gonzales: | Okay, I will try, but I only feel up to doing a little bit today. |

In this example, the medical assistant (the source) gives a verbal message about back exercises to the patient (the receiver). The patient responds by drawing attention to her pain and uneasiness about certain movements (feedback). The patient's response is also a message to the medical assistant, who responds in turn. The giving and receiving of information continues within the communication circle until the exchange is finished.

Feedback The patient's response, or **feedback,** is verbal or nonverbal evidence that the receiver got and understood the message. When you communicate information to a patient or ask a patient a question, always look for feedback. For example, if you calculate a pregnant patient's due date and tell her she's 12 weeks pregnant, look for a response. If she responds, "Oh, good, that means I'm out of danger of having a miscarriage," you may respond by saying that whereas most miscarriages occur in the first 12 weeks, some risk of miscarriage remains throughout the pregnancy. If she responds, "I thought I was 14 weeks pregnant," you need to clarify how you worked out your calculation and compare it with hers, to uncover any discrepancy. Good communication in the medical office requires patient feedback at every step.

Noise Anything that changes the message in any way or interferes with the communication process can be referred to as noise. *Noise* refers not only to sounds, such as a siren or jackhammer on the street below the medical office suite, but also to room temperature and other types of physical comfort or discomfort, such as pain, and to emotions, such as fear or sadness. If patients are feeling uncomfortable in a chilly or hot room, upset about their illness, or in great pain, they may not pay close attention to what you are saying. Conversely, if you are feeling upset about a personal problem outside work or if you are unwell or preoccupied with all the things you have on your to-do list, you may not communicate well.

As you deal with each patient, try to screen out or eliminate causes of noise. For example, before you start a conversation with a patient in an examination room, you might ask, "Are you too chilly or too warm? Is the temperature in here comfortable for you?" If there is construction going on outside the building, see if there is a less noisy inner room or office that you might use. If a patient seems nervous or upset, address those feelings before you launch into a factual discussion.

If you are feeling stressed or out of sorts, that feeling constitutes a type of noise. Try to take a "breather" between patients or a break from desk work—walk downstairs, get some fresh air, stretch your legs. Feeling dehydrated or hungry affects your communication efforts, too. Limit your caffeine and sugar intake. Drink plenty of water throughout the day. Eat a good breakfast and lunch and healthful snacks. Leave your personal problems at home.

▶ Human Behavior and Needs   LO 4.2

Medical assistants are exposed to many different personality types in addition to different illnesses. When you understand why a person is behaving in a certain way, you can adjust your communication style to adapt to that person. For example, as highly structured healthcare organizations and technological advances rapidly change the face of healthcare, many patients feel that healthcare is becoming impersonal, and consequently they may become difficult. Every time you communicate with patients, you can counteract this perception by playing

a humanistic role in the healthcare process. Being humanistic means that you work to help patients feel attended to and respected as individuals, not just as descriptions in a chart. Remember to always treat each patient as an individual and not simply as the disease, condition, or problem that brought the patient to the office. The problem may be common to you, but it is new and often frightening for the patient. To humanize and improve communication, you should have an understanding of the developmental stages of the life cycle and Maslow's hierarchy of human needs.

Developmental Stages of the Life Cycle

Understanding the stages of human growth and development will enable you to enhance your communication skills, including patient education, with patients of all age groups, cultures, and religions. Human growth includes physical, psychological, and emotional growth. Many scientists and behaviorists have studied the developmental stages of human life and have developed guidelines to assist healthcare practitioners and staff in applying effective patient communication skills. Figure 4-2 is

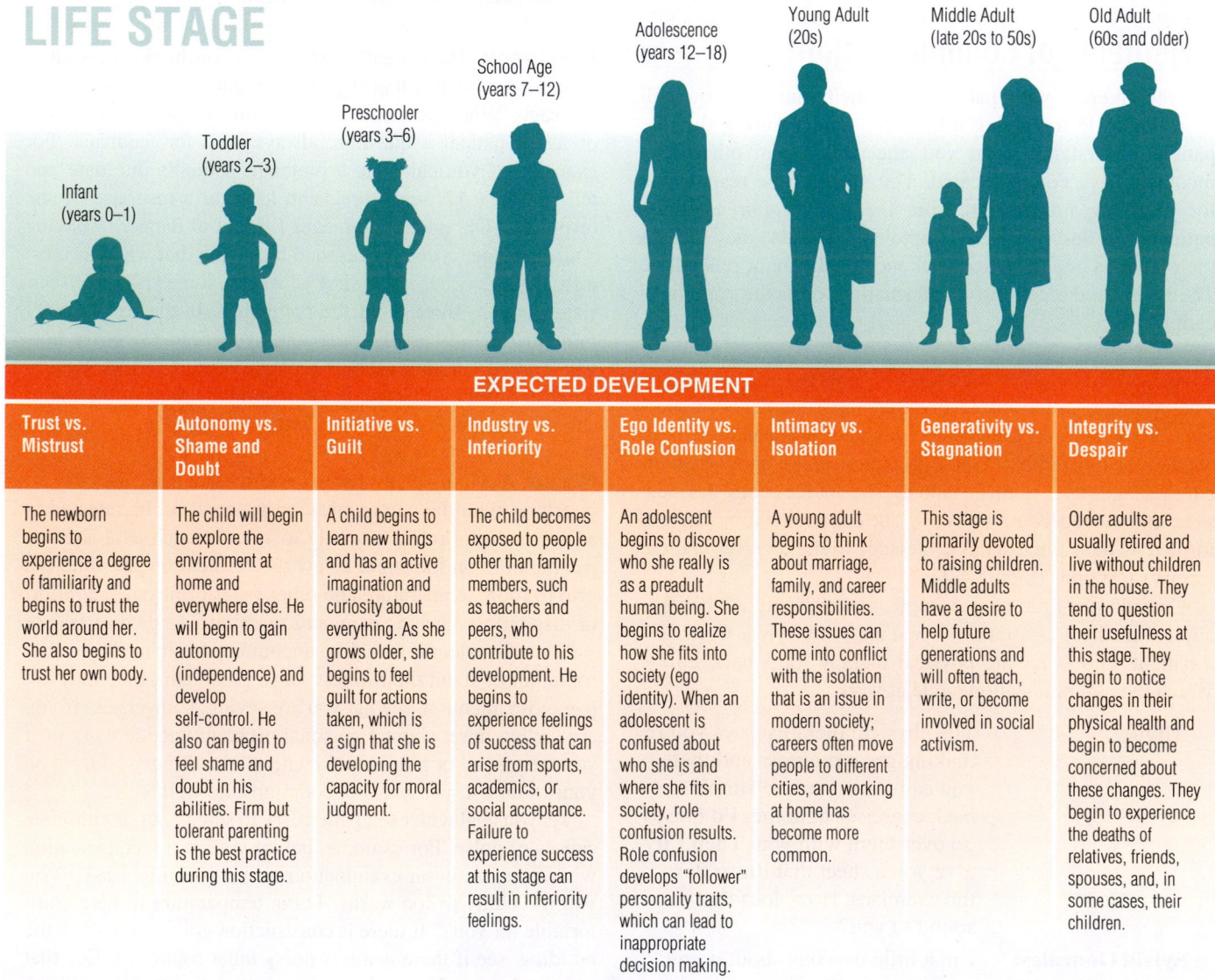

LIFE STAGE

Infant (years 0–1) · Toddler (years 2–3) · Preschooler (years 3–6) · School Age (years 7–12) · Adolescence (years 12–18) · Young Adult (20s) · Middle Adult (late 20s to 50s) · Old Adult (60s and older)

EXPECTED DEVELOPMENT

Trust vs. Mistrust	Autonomy vs. Shame and Doubt	Initiative vs. Guilt	Industry vs. Inferiority	Ego Identity vs. Role Confusion	Intimacy vs. Isolation	Generativity vs. Stagnation	Integrity vs. Despair
The newborn begins to experience a degree of familiarity and begins to trust the world around her. She also begins to trust her own body.	The child will begin to explore the environment at home and everywhere else. He will begin to gain autonomy (independence) and develop self-control. He also can begin to feel shame and doubt in his abilities. Firm but tolerant parenting is the best practice during this stage.	A child begins to learn new things and has an active imagination and curiosity about everything. As she grows older, she begins to feel guilt for actions taken, which is a sign that she is developing the capacity for moral judgment.	The child becomes exposed to people other than family members, such as teachers and peers, who contribute to his development. He begins to experience feelings of success that can arise from sports, academics, or social acceptance. Failure to experience success at this stage can result in inferiority feelings.	An adolescent begins to discover who she really is as a preadult human being. She begins to realize how she fits into society (ego identity). When an adolescent is confused about who she is and where she fits in society, role confusion results. Role confusion develops "follower" personality traits, which can lead to inappropriate decision making.	A young adult begins to think about marriage, family, and career responsibilities. These issues can come into conflict with the isolation that is an issue in modern society; careers often move people to different cities, and working at home has become more common.	This stage is primarily devoted to raising children. Middle adults have a desire to help future generations and will often teach, write, or become involved in social activism.	Older adults are usually retired and live without children in the house. They tend to question their usefulness at this stage. They begin to notice changes in their physical health and begin to become concerned about these changes. They begin to experience the deaths of relatives, friends, spouses, and, in some cases, their children.

FIGURE 4-2 Lifespan development.

an example of a lifespan development model, created by Erik Erikson (1902–1994).

Maslow's Hierarchy of Human Needs

Abraham Maslow, a well-known human behaviorist, developed a model of human behavior known as the **hierarchy** (classification) of needs (Figure 4-3). This hierarchy states that human beings are motivated by unsatisfied needs and that certain lower needs have to be satisfied before higher needs, such as self-actualization, are met. Maslow felt that people are basically trustworthy, self-protecting, and self-governing and that humans tend toward growth and love. He believed that humans are not violent by nature but are violent only when their needs are not being met.

Deficiency (Basic) Needs According to Maslow, there are general types of needs—physiological, safety, love/belonging, and esteem—that must be satisfied before a person can act unselfishly. He called these deficiency (basic) needs.

Physiological Needs Physiological needs are humans' very basic needs, such as air, water, food, sleep, and sex. When these needs are not satisfied, we may feel sickness, irritation, pain, and discomfort. These feelings motivate us to alleviate them as soon as possible to establish **homeostasis** (a state of balance, or equilibrium). Once our basic needs are met and our feelings are alleviated, we may think about other things.

Safety Needs People have the need and desire to establish stability and consistency. These basic needs are security, shelter, and a safe environment.

Love/Belonging Needs Humans have a desire to belong to groups: clubs, work groups, religious groups, families, and so on. We need to feel loved and accepted by others. Humans are like pack animals—we place great importance in belonging to society.

Esteem Needs Humans like to feel that they are important and valuable to society. There are two types of self-esteem. The first results from competence, or mastery of a task, such as completing an educational program. The second is the attention and recognition that come from others.

Self-Actualization Self-actualization is finding self-fulfillment and realizing one's potential. To reach this level, a

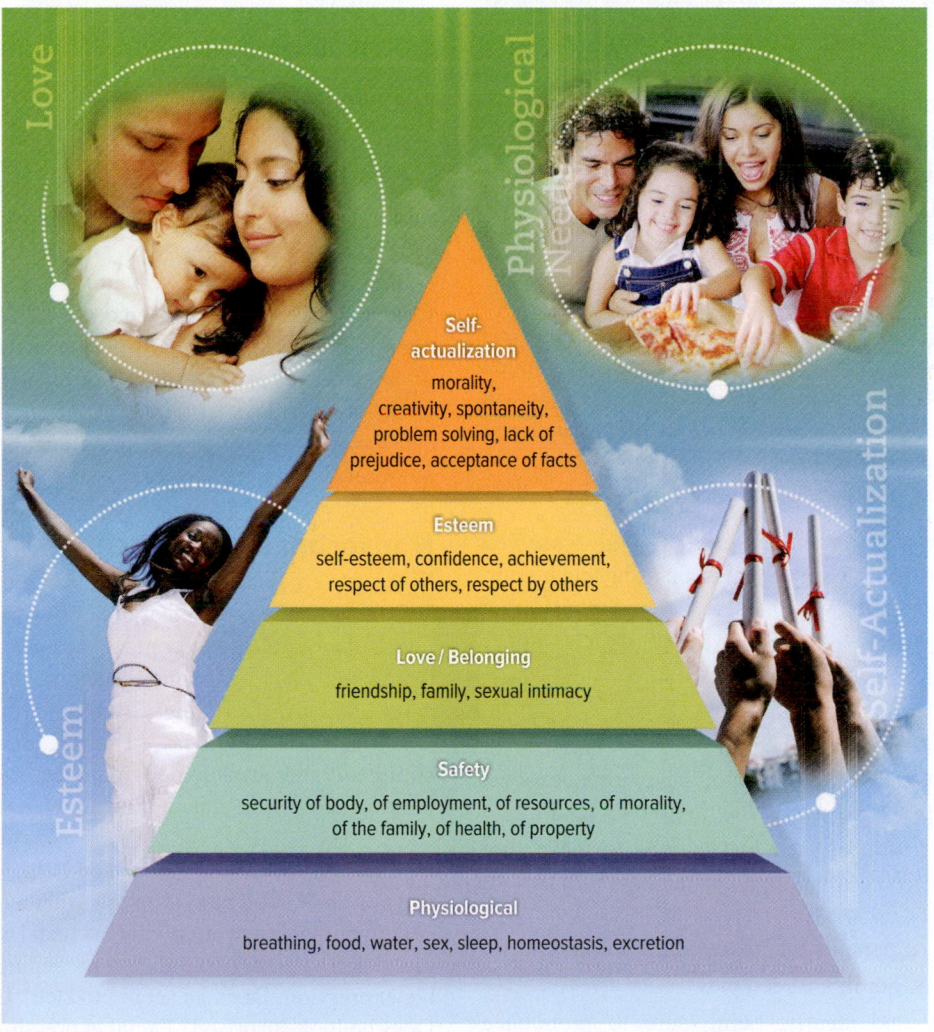

FIGURE 4-3 Maslow's hierarchy.

© Trinette Reed/Brand X Pictures/Jupiterimages RF, © BananaStock/age fotostock RF, © Gallo Images - Malcolm Dare/Getty Images RF, © baona/Getty Images RF

person utilizes many tools to maximize potential, such as education, a fulfilling career, and a balanced personal life. Self-actualized people are generally comfortable with who they are and know their strengths and weaknesses.

Considering Patients' Needs When working and communicating with patients, remember this hierarchy of human needs and observe what need a patient is deficient in. For example, if an elderly patient has recently lost her husband, she may feel lonely and deficient in the love need. You may see homeless patients who are deficient in their physiological and safety needs. You may have a young girl as a patient who is overweight and has low self-esteem. On the other hand, you may have a high-level executive as a patient who has reached self-actualization. Each of these scenarios would require a communication style adjustment in order for you to effectively communicate with these patients.

▶ Types of Communication LO 4.3

Each type of communication (verbal, nonverbal, or written) can be positive or negative. An effective communicator is familiar with these types of communication. This chapter focuses on verbal and nonverbal communication.

Positive Verbal Communication

In the medical office, communication that promotes patient comfort and well-being is essential. Treating patients brusquely or rudely is unacceptable in the healthcare setting. It is your responsibility to set the stage for positive communication.

When information—even bad news—is communicated with some positive aspect, patients are more likely to listen attentively and respond positively themselves. For example, you might explain to a patient who is about to get an injection, "This will sting, but only for a couple of seconds. When we are through, you are free to go." You would not just say, "This is going to hurt."

Other examples of positive communication are

- Being friendly, warm, and attentive ("It's good to see you again, Mrs. Armstrong. I know you're on your lunch hour, so let's get started right away.").
- Verbalizing concern for patients ("Are you comfortable?" "I understand it hurts when I do this; I'll be gentle." "This paperwork won't take long at all.").
- Encouraging patients to ask questions ("I hope I've explained the procedure well. Do you have any questions, or are there any parts you would like to go over again?").
- Asking patients to repeat your instructions to make sure they understand ("Will you explain to me how you plan to take your medicine?").
- Looking directly at patients when you speak to them.
- Smiling (naturally, not in a forced way).
- Speaking slowly and clearly, being sure to pronounce words correctly.
- Listening carefully.

Negative Verbal Communication

Most people do not purposely try to communicate negatively. Some people, however, may not realize that their communication style has a negative impact on others. Look for and ask for feedback to help you curb negative communication habits. Ask yourself, "Do the physicians and my other coworkers seem glad to speak with me? Are they open and responsive to me? Do patients seem at ease with me, or are they very quiet, turned off, or distant?" (Note that some patients may respond this way because of the way they feel, not because of the way you are communicating with them.) Here are some examples of negative communication (verbal and nonverbal):

- Mumbling
- Speaking brusquely or sharply
- Avoiding eye contact
- Interrupting patients as they are speaking
- Rushing through explanations or instructions
- Treating patients impersonally
- Making patients feel they are taking up too much of your time or asking too many questions
- Forgetting common courtesies, such as saying please and thank you
- Showing boredom

A good way to avoid negative communication is to open your eyes and ears to others in service-oriented workplace settings.

The next time you buy something at a store, call a company for information over the phone, or eat at a restaurant, take note of the way the staff treat you. Do they answer your questions courteously? Do they give you the information you ask for? Do they make you feel welcome? What specifically makes their communication style positive or negative? You expect good customer service, and so do your patients, as discussed in the chapter *Professionalism and Success*. Remember, you can always improve your communication skills, and learning by observing others is a great start.

Nonverbal Communication

Whereas verbal communication is communication that is spoken, nonverbal communication, or **body language,** consists of facial expressions, eye contact, posture, touch, and attention to personal space. In many instances, people's body language conveys their true feelings, even when their words say otherwise. A patient might say, "I'm OK about that," but if she is sitting with her arms folded tightly across her chest and avoids looking at you, she may not mean what she says.

Facial Expression Your face is the most expressive part of your body. You can often tell whether someone has understood your message simply by his facial expression. For example, when you are explaining a procedure to a patient, look at his expression. Does he seem puzzled? Is his brow wrinkled? Does he look surprised? Facial expressions can give you clues about how to tailor your communication efforts. They also serve as a form of feedback. As stated previously, your facial expressions are just as important as your words. Remain open and interested in what the patient is saying. Never look bored or impatient with a patient.

Eye Contact Eye contact is an important part of positive communication. Look directly at patients when speaking to them. Looking away or down communicates that you are not interested in the person or that you are avoiding her for some reason. Be aware of cultural differences. For example, in some cultures, it is common to avoid eye contact out of respect for someone who is considered a superior. Thus, children may be taught not to look adults in the eye.

Posture The way you hold or move your head, arms, hands, and the rest of your body can project strong nonverbal messages. During communication, posture can usually be described as open or closed.

Open Posture A feeling of receptiveness and friendliness can be conveyed with an **open posture.** In this position, your arms lie comfortably at your sides or in your lap. You face the other person, and you may lean forward in your chair. This demonstrates that you are listening and are interested in what the other person has to say. Open posture is a form of positive communication.

Closed Posture A **closed posture** conveys the opposite of open posture—a feeling of not being totally receptive to what is being said. It also can signal that someone is angry or upset. A person in a closed posture may hold his arms rigidly or fold them across his chest.

He may lean back in his chair, away from the other person. He may turn away to avoid eye contact. He may even slouch— a kind of closed posture that can convey fatigue or lack of caring. Watch for patients with closed postures that may indicate tension or pain. Avoid closed postures yourself; they have a negative effect on your communication efforts.

Touch Touch is a powerful form of nonverbal communication. A touch on the arm or a hug can be a means of saying hello, sharing condolences, or expressing congratulations. Family background, culture, age, and gender all influence people's perception of touch. Some people may welcome a touch or think nothing of it. Others may view touching as an invasion of their privacy. In general, in the medical setting, a touch on the shoulder, forearm, or back of the hand to express interest or concern is acceptable.

Personal Space When communicating with others, it is important to be aware of the concept of personal space. **Personal space** is an area that surrounds an individual. By not intruding on patients' personal space, you show respect for their feelings of privacy. In most social situations, it is common for people to stand 4 to 12 feet away from each other. For personal conversation, you would typically stand between 1 and 4 feet away from a person. Some patients may feel uncomfortable and become anxious when you stand or sit close to them. Others prefer the reassurance of having people close to them when they speak. Watch patients carefully. If they lean back

when you lean forward or if they fold their arms or turn their head away, you may be invading their personal space. If they lean or step toward you, they may be seeking to close up the personal space.

▶ Improving Your Communication Skills LO 4.4

Sharpening your communication skills should be an ongoing effort and will help you become a more effective communicator. Among the skills involved in daily communication are listening skills, interpersonal skills, and assertiveness skills.

Listening Skills

Listening involves both hearing and interpreting a message. Listening requires you to pay close attention not only to what is being said but also to nonverbal cues communicated through body language.

Listening can be passive or active. **Passive listening** is simply hearing what someone has to say without the need for a reply. An example is listening to a news program on the radio; the communication is mainly one-way. **Active listening,** on the other hand, involves two-way communication. You are actively involved in the process, offering feedback or asking questions. As seen in Figure 4-4, active listening takes place, for example, when you interview a patient for her medical history. Active listening is an essential skill in the medical office.

Ways to improve your listening skills include

- Prepare to listen. Position yourself at the same level (sitting, standing) as the person who is speaking and assume an open posture.
- Relax and listen attentively. Do not simply pretend to listen to what is being said.
- Maintain eye contact and appropriate personal space.

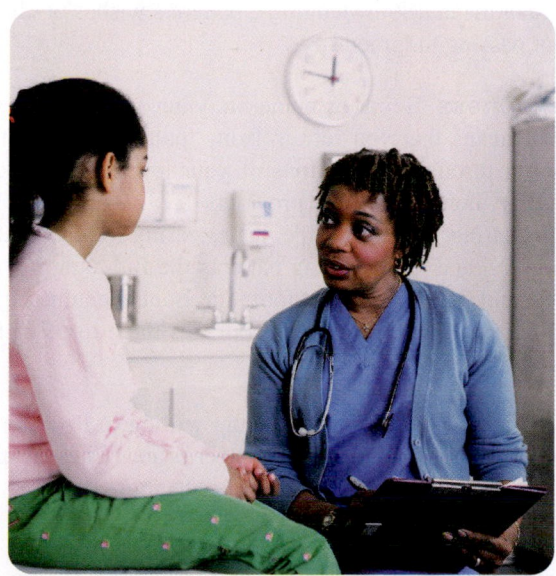

FIGURE 4-4 Active listening requires two-way communication and positive body language.
© Sean Justice/Getty Images

- Think before you respond.
- Provide feedback. Restate the speaker's message in your own words to show that you understand.
- If you do not understand something that was said, ask the person to repeat it.

Interpersonal Skills

When you interact with people, you use **interpersonal skills.** When you make a patient feel at ease by being warm and friendly, you are demonstrating good interpersonal skills. In addition to warmth and friendliness, valuable interpersonal skills include empathy, respect, genuineness, openness, consideration, and sensitivity.

Warmth and Friendliness A friendly but professional approach, a pleasant greeting, and a smile get you off to a good start when communicating with patients. When your approach is sincere, patients will be more relaxed and open.

Empathy The process of identifying with someone else's feelings is empathy. When you are empathetic, you are sensitive to the other person's feelings and problems. When you are sympathetic, you feel sorry *for* or feel pity *for* the person and his or her circumstances, but you don't really understand them. When you are empathetic, you are feeling *with* the person, putting yourself in his or her shoes. For example, if a patient is experiencing a migraine headache and you have never had one, you can still let her know you are trying to imagine, or relate to, her situation. In other words, you can acknowledge the severity of her pain and show support and care. If you were sympathetic to the patient's migraine, you would feel sorry that she did not feel well, but you would not try to put yourself in her shoes (or head) to understand how she is feeling.

Respect Showing respect can mean using a title of courtesy such as "Mr." or "Mrs." when communicating with patients. It also can mean acknowledging a patient's wishes or choices without passing judgment.

Genuineness Being genuine in your interactions with patients means that you refrain from "putting on an act" or just going through the motions of your job. Patients like to know that their healthcare providers are real people. In a medical setting, being genuine means caring for each patient on an individual basis, giving patients the full attention they deserve, and showing respect for them. Being genuine in your communication with patients encourages them to place trust in you and in what you say.

Openness Openness means being willing to listen to and consider others' viewpoints and concerns and being receptive to their needs. An open individual is accepting of others and not biased for or against them.

Consideration and Sensitivity You should always try to show consideration toward patients and act in a thoughtful, kind way. You must be sensitive to their individual concerns, fears, and needs.

Assertiveness Skills

As a professional, you need to be assertive—to be firm and to stand by your principles while still showing respect for others. Being assertive means trusting your instincts, feelings, and opinions (not in terms of diagnosing, which only the licensed practitioner can do, but in terms of basic communication with patients) and acting on them. For example, when you see that a patient looks uneasy, speak up. You might say, "You look concerned. How can I help you feel more comfortable?" versus asking the patient, "What is the matter with you?" Being assertive is different from being aggressive. When people are **aggressive,** they try to impose their position on others or try to manipulate them. Aggressive people are bossy and can be quarrelsome. They do not appear to take into consideration others' feelings, needs, thoughts, ideas, and opinions before they act or speak. To be **assertive,** you must be open, honest, and direct. Be aware of your body position: An open posture conveys the proper message. When you communicate, speak confidently and use "I" statements such as "I feel . . ." or "I think . . ."

Developing your assertiveness skills increases your sense of self-worth and your confidence as a professional. Being assertive will also help you prevent conflicts or resolve them more peacefully and increase your leadership ability. People look up to and respect professionals who are assertive in the workplace. See Table 4-1 for a comparison of nonassertive, assertive, aggressive, and nonassertive aggressive behaviors.

▶ Therapeutic Communication Skills LO 4.5

Therapeutic communication is the ability to communicate with patients in terms they can understand. At the same time, it helps patients to feel at ease with what you are saying. It is also the ability to communicate with other team members in technical terms that are appropriate in a healthcare setting. Therapeutic communication techniques can improve communication with patients. This communication must remain within your scope of practice, as discussed in the *Points on Practice* box. Therapeutic communication involves the following skills:

- *Being silent.* Silence allows the patient time to think without pressure.
- *Accepting.* This skill gives the patient an indication of reception. It shows that you have heard the patient and follow the patient's thought pattern. Some indicators of acceptance include nodding; saying "Yes," "I follow what you said," and other such phrases; and body language.
- *Giving recognition.* Show patients that you are aware of them by stating their name in a greeting or by noticing positive changes. With this skill, you are recognizing the patient as a person or an individual.
- *Offering self.* Make yourself available to the needs of the patient.
- *Giving a broad opening.* Allow the patient to take the initiative in introducing the topic. Ask open-ended questions such as "Is there something you'd like to talk about?" or "Where would you like to begin?"

TABLE 4-1 A Comparison of Nonassertive, Assertive, Aggressive, and Nonassertive Aggressive Behaviors

	Nonassertive Behavior	Assertive Behavior	Aggressive Behavior	Nonassertive Aggressive Behavior (NAG)
Characteristics of the Behavior	Emotionally dishonest, indirect, self-denying; allows others to choose for self; does not achieve desired goal	Emotionally honest, direct, self-enhancing, expressive; chooses for self; may achieve goal	Emotionally honest, direct, self-enhancing at the expense of another, expressive; chooses for others; may achieve goal at expense of others	Emotionally dishonest, indirect, self-denying; chooses for others; may achieve goal at expense of others
Your Feelings	Hurt, anxious, possibly angry later	Confident, self-respecting	Righteous, superior, derogative at the time and possibly guilty later	Defiance, anger, self-denying; sometimes anxious, possibly guilty later
The Other Person's Feelings Toward You	Irritated, pity, lack of respect	Generally respected	Angry, resentful	Angry, resentful, irritated, disgusted
The Other Person's Feelings About Himself/Herself	Guilty or superior	Valued, respected	Hurt, embarrassed, defensive	Hurt, guilty or superior, humiliated

- *Offering general leads.* Give the patient encouragement to continue by making comments such as "Go on" or "And then?"

- *Making observations.* Make your perceptions known to the patient. Say things like "You appear tense today" or "Are you uncomfortable when you . . . ?" By calling patients' attention to what is happening to them, you encourage them to notice it for themselves so that they can describe it to you.

- *Encouraging communication.* Ask patients to verbalize what they perceive. Make statements such as "Tell me when you feel anxious" or "What is happening?" Patients should feel free to describe their perceptions to you, and you must try to see things as they seem to the patients.

- *Mirroring.* Restate what the patient has said to demonstrate that you understand.

- *Reflecting.* Encourage patients to think through and answer their own questions. A reflecting dialogue may go like this:

  Patient: Do you think I should tell the doctor?

  Medical Assistant: Do you think you should?

  By reflecting patients' questions or statements back to them, you are helping patients feel that their opinions about their health are of value.

- *Focusing.* Focusing encourages the patient to stay on the topic.

- *Exploring.* Encourage patients to express themselves in more depth. Try to get as much detail as possible about a patient's complaint, but avoid probing and prying if the patient does not wish to discuss it.

- *Clarifying.* Ask patients to explain themselves more clearly if they provide information that is vague or not meaningful.

- *Summarizing.* This skill involves organizing and summing up the important points of the discussion. It gives the patient an awareness of the progress made toward greater understanding.

Ineffective Therapeutic Communication

Often, people think they are communicating thoroughly, but they are not. Here are some roadblocks that can interfere with your communication style:

- *Reassuring.* This type of communication indicates to the patient that there is no need for anxiety or worry. By doing this, you devalue the patient's feelings and give false hope if the outcome is not positive. The communication error here is a lack of understanding and empathy.

- *Giving approval.* This is usually done by overtly approving of a patient's behavior. This may lead the patient to strive for praise rather than progress.

- *Disapproving.* Overtly disapproving of a patient's behavior implies that you have the right to pass judgment on the patient's thoughts and actions. Find an alternate attitude when dealing with patients. Adopting a moralistic attitude may take your attention away from the patient's needs and instead direct it toward your own feelings.

- *Agreeing/disagreeing.* Overtly agreeing or disagreeing with thoughts, perceptions, and ideas of patients is not an effective way to communicate. When you agree with patients, they will have the perception that they are right because you agree with them or because you share their opinion. Opinions and conclusions should be the patient's, not yours. When disagreeing with patients, you become the opposition to them instead of their caregiver. Never place yourself in an argumentative situation regarding a patient's opinions.

- *Advising.* If you tell the patient what you think should be done, you place yourself outside your scope of practice. You cannot advise patients.

- *Probing.* This means discussing a topic that the patient has no desire to discuss.

- *Defending.* Protecting yourself, the institution, and others from verbal attack is classified as defending. If you become defensive, the patient may feel the need to discontinue communication.

- *Requesting an explanation.* This communication pattern involves asking patients to provide reasons for their behavior. Patients may not know why they behave in a certain manner. "Why" questions may have an intimidating effect on some patients.
- *Minimizing feelings.* Never judge or make light of a patient's discomfort. You need to be able to perceive what is taking place from the patient's point of view, not your own.
- *Making stereotyped comments.* This type of communication involves using meaningless clichés—such as "It's for your own good"—when communicating with patients. These types of comments are given in an automatic, mechanical way as a substitute for a more reasonable and thoughtful explanation.

Defense Mechanisms

When working with patients, it is important to observe their communication behaviors. Patients often develop unconscious defense mechanisms, or coping strategies, to protect themselves from anxiety, guilt, and shame. The following are some common defense mechanisms that a patient may display when communicating with the doctor, medical assistant, or other healthcare team members. These mechanisms may be adaptive (have the ability to change or adjust) or nonadaptive (not have the ability to change or adjust).

- *Compensation:* Overemphasizing a trait to make up for a perceived or actual failing
- *Denial:* An unconscious attempt to reject unacceptable feelings, needs, thoughts, wishes, or external reality factors
- *Displacement:* The unconscious transfer of unacceptable thoughts, feelings, or desires from the self to a more acceptable external substitute
- *Dissociation:* Disconnecting emotional significance from specific ideas or events
- *Identification:* Mimicking the behavior of another to cope with feelings of inadequacy
- *Introjection:* Adopting the unacceptable thoughts or feelings of others

- *Projection:* Projecting onto another person one's own feelings, as if they had originated in the other person
- *Rationalization:* Justifying unacceptable behavior, thoughts, and feelings into tolerable behaviors
- *Regression:* Unconsciously returning to more infantile behaviors or thoughts
- *Repression:* Putting unpleasant thoughts, feelings, or events out of one's mind
- *Substitution:* Unconsciously replacing an unreachable or unacceptable goal with another, more acceptable one

▶ Communicating in Special Circumstances   LO 4.6

If you make an effort to develop good interpersonal skills, most patients will not be difficult to communicate with. You will, however, encounter patients in special circumstances that can inhibit communication, such as when they are anxious or angry. Patients from different cultures may pose challenges to communication. Others may have some type of impairment or disability that makes communication difficult. Patients with terminal illnesses also may present communication difficulties. Learning about these patients' special needs and polishing your own communication skills will help you become an effective communicator in any number of situations.

The Anxious Patient

It is not uncommon for patients to be anxious in a medical office or other healthcare setting. This reaction is commonly known as the white-coat syndrome. In some cases, the anxiety even raises the patient's blood pressure. There can be many reasons for anxiety. A patient can become anxious because she is ill and does not know what is wrong with her—she may fear the worst. A patient may have recently been diagnosed with an illness that he knows nothing about, which may necessitate a severe lifestyle change. Fear of bad news or fear that some procedure is going to be painful can create anxiety. Regardless of what is causing it, anxiety can interfere with the communication process. For example, because of anxiety, a patient may not pay attention to what you are saying.

Some patients—particularly children—may be unable to verbalize their feelings of fear and anxiety. Watch for signs of anxiety, including a tense appearance, increased blood pressure and rates of breathing and pulse, sweaty palms, reported problems with sleep or appetite, irritability, and agitation. Procedure 4-1, at the end of this chapter, will help you communicate with anxious patients.

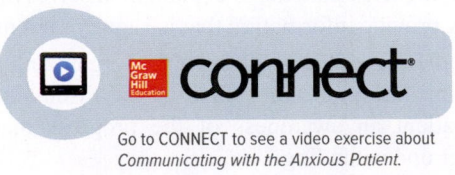

Go to CONNECT to see a video exercise about *Communicating with the Anxious Patient.*

The Angry Patient

In a medical setting, anger may occur for many reasons. It may be a mask for fear about an illness or the outcome of surgery. Anger may come from a patient's feeling of being treated unfairly or without compassion, or it may stem from a patient's resentment about being ill or injured. Anger may also be a reaction to frustration, rejection, disappointment, feelings of loss of control or self-esteem, or an invasion of privacy.

As a medical assistant, you will encounter angry patients and will need to help them express their anger constructively, for the sake of their health. At the same time, you must learn not to take expressions of anger personally; you may just be the unlucky target. The goal with angry patients is to help them refocus emotional energy toward solving the problem. Procedure 4-2, at the end of this chapter, will help you communicate with angry patients. Remember to document the facts of each encounter and its outcome in the patient's medical record (see the progress note example from Cindy Chen's chart below).

Patients of Other Cultures

Our beliefs, attitudes, values, use of language, and world views are unique to us, but they are also shaped by our cultural background. Each culture and ethnic group has its own behaviors, traditions, and values. Rather than viewing these differences as communication barriers, strive to understand them (Figure 4-5). For example, many medical facilities are located in heavily populated ethnic locations, and it is important that the medical staff understand the differences among patient cultures. A medical assistant who is employed in a medical facility in which the majority of patients are Latino should learn as much as possible about the specific Latin culture in that area in order to provide good customer service.

It is necessary to understand the difference between stereotyping and generalizing. *Stereotyping* is a negative statement about the specific traits of a group that is applied unfairly to an entire population. A *generalization* is a statement about common trends within a group, but it is understood that further investigation is needed to determine if the trend applies to an individual.

Remember, the beliefs of other cultures are neither superior nor inferior to your own. They are simply different. Never allow yourself to make value judgments or to stereotype a patient, a culture, or an ethnic group. Each patient is an individual in her own right and deserves your respect and undivided attention.

Cultural Differences Patients' cultural backgrounds have an effect on their attitudes, perceptions, behaviors, and expectations toward health and illness. The following are examples of cultural differences. More information can be found online at the National Institutes of Health website, http://sis.nlm.nih.gov/outreach/multicultural.html.

PROGRESS NOTE

Patient Name: Cindy Chen

This 28 y/o female came to office for follow up. Stated she was very nervous and requested "something to help calm me down, before I see the doctor." Became quite agitated when told Dr. Whalen would prescribe meds if needed. Encouraged her to tell me why she thought she was nervous and we talked about her schooling, exams, and her fear that her HIV status could make it difficult for her to find a position as a phlebotomist. She calmed down a bit, finally stating, "This feeling comes and goes. It is just a 'bad day.' Thank you for letting me talk." Informed Dr. Whalen of conversation.

Date: 9/1/XX

Author: K. Haddix

Done | Close

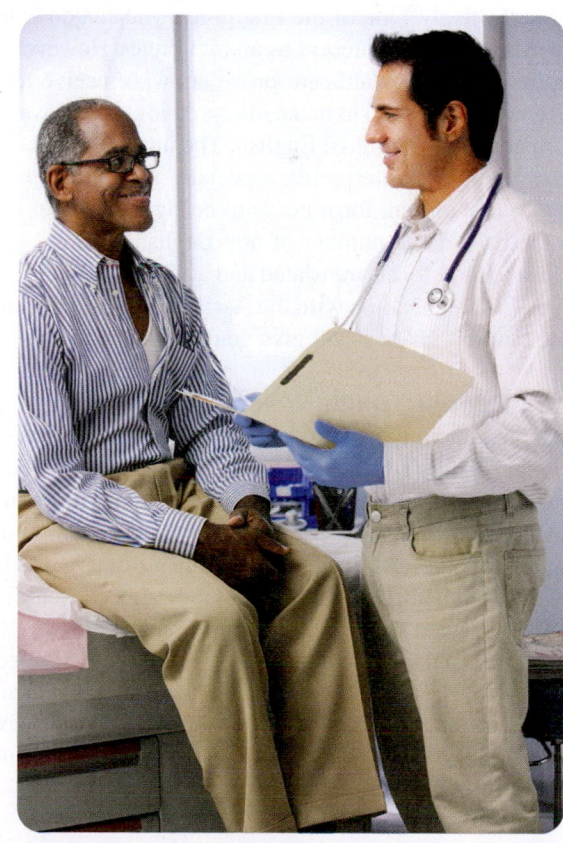

FIGURE 4-5 Knowing how to communicate across cultures is an essential skill of medical assistants.
© stockbroker/123RF

- Many cultures believe that some illnesses are caused by a change in the "vital energy" or hot and cold forces in the body.
- Certain cultures may differ in the way they perceive and report symptoms. Some may express pain very emotionally because their culture may feel that suppressing pain is harmful. In contrast, people from other cultures may not admit that they are in pain, thinking that acknowledging pain is a sign of weakness.
- Patients of certain ethnic or cultural groups often consult other types of healers before seeing a doctor. They are likely to have different expectations of treatment from each.
- Patients from other cultures may be wary of certain treatments because these treatments are so different from what they are accustomed to. This is especially true of some of the medical procedures and interventions considered to be state-of-the-art, such as laser surgery or diabetes management.
- In some cultures, it may not be appropriate to suggest making a will for dying patients or patients with terminal illnesses; this is the cultural equivalent of wishing death on a patient.
- Some cultures do not look those worthy of respect, such as healthcare workers, in the eye. If a patient does not look you in the eye when answering questions, it could be that in his culture he is not hiding anything but rather is showing you great respect.

Language Barriers Patients who cannot speak or understand English may have difficulty expressing their needs or feelings effectively. One of the first things you can do is use a family member who is present as an interpreter. However, federal policies require healthcare providers who receive federal funds (that is, Medicare) to make interpretive services available to their patients with limited English. The interpreter should be a medically trained interpreter, especially for patients having surgery or if a consent form needs to be signed. If your medical office has a large number of non-English speakers, it is a good idea to have forms translated and available for use. Procedure 4-3, Communicating with the Assistance of an Interpreter, at the end of this chapter will give you practice with this skill.

Limited Reading Skills You will find that some of your patients are functionally illiterate. They may try to hide this by saying, "I didn't bring my glasses with me" or "This is too much to read right now." Be polite, review the information with them, and ask if they have any questions. Send the information home and have them further discuss it with a family member before requesting that they sign consent forms or forms that need to be signed before having surgery. Several vendors publish patient education materials on a specific readability level. It is recommended that patient education brochures not exceed fourth- to eighth-grade reading levels. Visual media can be provided through valid Internet resources that will improve communication as well.

Cultural Competence Your cultural competence relates to your ability to respond to the cultural and language needs of the patients you encounter. Consider the following techniques to improve your communication with patients of various cultures.

- If possible, learn and use a few phrases of greeting and introduction in the patient's native language. This conveys respect and demonstrates your willingness to learn about their culture.
- Use an interpreter whenever needed to assist with communication. Look at the patient, not the interpreter, during communication.
- Be aware of nonverbal communication and respond. For example, look for signs of pain such as a grimace.
- Avoid saying "You must . . ." Instead, teach patients their options and let them decide—for example, "Some people in this situation would . . ."
- Always give the reason or purpose for a treatment or prescription.
- Make sure patients understand by having them explain it themselves.

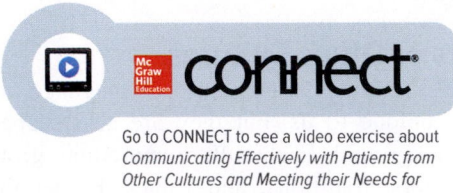

Go to CONNECT to see a video exercise about *Communicating Effectively with Patients from Other Cultures and Meeting their Needs for Privacy.*

The Patient Who Is Mentally or Emotionally Disturbed

There may be times when you will need to communicate with patients who are mentally or emotionally disturbed. When dealing with this type of patient, you need to determine what level of communication the patient can understand. Keep these suggestions in mind to improve communication.

- It is important to remain calm if the patient becomes agitated or confused.
- Avoid raising your voice or appearing impatient.
- If you do not understand what the patient said, ask him to repeat what he said.

Terminally Ill Patients

Terminally ill patients are often under extreme stress and can be a challenge to treat. It is important that healthcare professionals respect the rights of terminal patients and treat them with dignity. It is also important that you communicate with the family and offer support and empathy as their loved one accepts her condition. You also should provide information on **hospice,** which is an area of medicine that works with terminally ill patients and their families. Hospice workers often go to the home of the terminally ill patient or work with patients in facilities. Hospice care is usually staffed with RNs and other healthcare providers who have specialized training in issues related to death and dying. They work with the family and patient in the beginning, assisting with medications, comfort care, and emotional support. If the patient dies at home, they may make arrangements with the funeral home and coroner.

Elisabeth Kübler-Ross, a world-renowned authority in the areas of death and dying, developed a model that describes the behavior patients will experience on learning their condition. This is called the stages of dying or stages of grief (Figure 4-6). This model is widely used in work with terminally ill patients.

Patients' Families and Friends

Family members or friends sometimes accompany a patient to the office. These individuals can provide important emotional support to the patient. Always ask patients if they want a family member or friend to accompany them to the examination room, however. Do not just assume their preference. Acknowledge family members and friends, and communicate with them as you do with patients. They should be kept informed of the patient's progress, whenever possible, to avoid unnecessary anxiety on their part. You must always protect patient confidentiality, however. Too often, healthcare workers think that it is acceptable to discuss patient cases in detail with family members, even without the patient's consent.

The Patient with AIDS and the Patient Who Is HIV-Positive

Patients with acquired immunodeficiency syndrome (AIDS) and patients who have the human immunodeficiency virus (HIV), the virus that causes AIDS, may face social stigma or blame themselves. These patients often feel guilty, angry, and depressed.

To communicate effectively with these patients, you need accurate information about the disease and the risks involved. Take the initiative to educate yourself about AIDS and HIV. Patients will have many questions. Part of your role as a good communicator will be to answer as many questions as you can. If a patient asks a question you cannot answer, tell the patient's provider so he can respond quickly.

Remember, HIV is not transmitted through casual or common physical contact, such as brushing by a person in a crowded hall or shaking hands. It is transferred only through body fluids. Patients with AIDS and those who are HIV-positive need to know you are not afraid to be near them, to touch them, or to talk to them. Like any patient whose body is being

Kübler-Ross's stages of dying include five stages, which usually—but not always—progress in the following order:

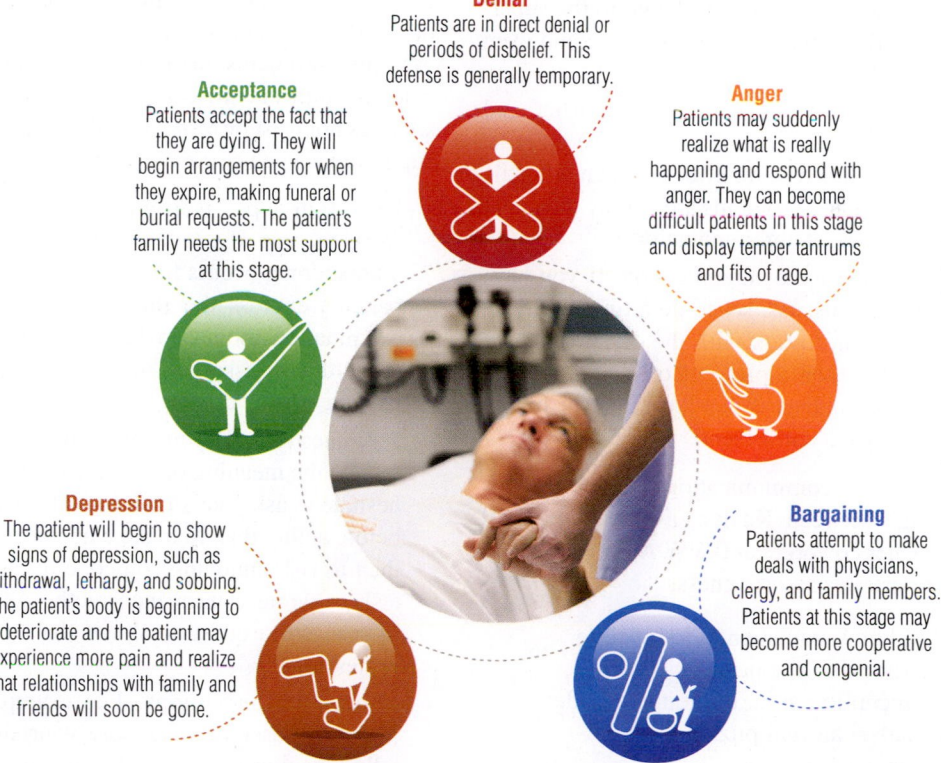

Denial
Patients are in direct denial or periods of disbelief. This defense is generally temporary.

Anger
Patients may suddenly realize what is really happening and respond with anger. They can become difficult patients in this stage and display temper tantrums and fits of rage.

Acceptance
Patients accept the fact that they are dying. They will begin arrangements for when they expire, making funeral or burial requests. The patient's family needs the most support at this stage.

Bargaining
Patients attempt to make deals with physicians, clergy, and family members. Patients at this stage may become more cooperative and congenial.

Depression
The patient will begin to show signs of depression, such as withdrawal, lethargy, and sobbing. The patient's body is beginning to deteriorate and the patient may experience more pain and realize that relationships with family and friends will soon be gone.

Even though these stages have been generalized to dying, many experts have applied them to the grieving process as well. For example, after a stroke, a patient may go through the process of grieving his loss of body function.

FIGURE 4-6 Kübler-Ross's stages of dying.
© ERproductions Ltd/Blend Images LLC RF

ravaged by a serious illness, these patients need human contact (verbal and physical) and they need to be treated with dignity.

▶ Communicating with Coworkers   LO 4.7

The quality of the communication you have with coworkers greatly influences the development of a positive or negative work climate and a team approach to patient care. In turn, the workplace atmosphere ultimately affects your communication with patients.

Positive Communication with Coworkers

In your interactions with coworkers, use the same skills and qualities that you use to communicate with patients. Have respect and empathy; be caring, thoughtful, and genuine; and use active listening skills. These skills will help you develop **rapport,** which is a harmonious, positive relationship, with your coworkers. Following are some rules for communication in the medical office.

- Use proper channels of communication. For example, if you are having problems getting along with a coworker, try first to work it out with her. Do not go over her head and complain to her supervisor. Your coworker may not have realized the effect of her behavior and may wish to correct it without involving her supervisor. If you go to the supervisor right away, working relationships can become even more strained.

- Have the proper attitude. You can avoid conflict and resolve most problems if you maintain a positive attitude. A friendly approach is much more effective than a hostile approach. Remember, many problems are simply the result of misinformation or lack of communication.

- Plan an appropriate time for communication. If you have something important to discuss, schedule a time to do so. For example, if you want to talk with the office manager about renewing the lease on a piece of office equipment, tell him you would like to discuss that topic and ask him to let you know a time that is convenient.

As an example of good communication with coworkers, consider this exchange between Kaylyn, a clinical medical assistant, and Miguel, her coworker at BWW Associates. Note the way Kaylyn demonstrates assertiveness.

Kaylyn:	I know you spent a lot of time choosing the new toys for the reception area. I love the wooden safari animal puzzles.
Miguel:	Thanks. I think the children really enjoy themselves now.
Kaylyn:	I wanted to mention to you, though, that I'm concerned about the toy tea set with miniature cupcakes and sandwiches. Anything that's smaller than a golf ball is a choking hazard to infants and toddlers.
Miguel:	I don't think the little ones pay much attention to the tea set. It's mostly for older kids.
Kaylyn:	Yes, but I'm still afraid that a baby could put one of those pieces in his mouth. What if we put up a little shelf in the play area that is low enough for kids 4 years old or more to reach but high enough to be out of reach of the babies? We could put the tea set on it in a clear plastic box and any other toys with small parts.
Miguel:	I see your point. Sounds like a good idea to me.

Kaylyn started with a statement that acknowledged the coworker's situation and feelings. Then she stated her own opinion. When her coworker disagreed, she repeated her concern, describing what could happen if the situation remained unchanged. Then, she made a constructive suggestion for solving the problem without hurting the coworker's feelings. As you interact with coworkers, be sensitive to the timing of your conversations, the manner in which you present your ideas and thoughts, and your coworkers' feelings.

Communicating with Management

Positive or negative communication can affect the quality of your relationships with your supervisor or manager. For example, problems arise when communication about job responsibilities is unclear or when you feel that your supervisor does not trust or respect you, or vice versa. Consider these suggestions when communicating with your direct supervisor:

- Keep your supervisor informed. If the office copier is not working properly, talk to your supervisor about it before a breakdown occurs that will hold everyone up. If several patients express the same types of complaint about the examination rooms, make sure the right people are told. If the doctor asks you to call a patient and you reach the patient, tell the doctor.

- Ask questions. If you are unsure about an administrative task or the meaning of a medical term, for example, do not hesitate to ask your supervisor. It is better to ask a question before acting than to make a mistake. It is also better to ask than to risk annoying someone because you carried out a task or wrote a term incorrectly. Asking your supervisor or manager a question shows that you respect him or her professionally.

- Minimize interruptions. For example, before launching into a discussion, make sure your supervisor has time to talk. Opening with "Can I interrupt you for a moment, or should I come back?" or "Do you have a minute to talk?" goes a long way toward establishing good communication. It is also better to go to your supervisor when you have several questions to ask rather than to interrupt her repeatedly.

- Show initiative. Any manager or supervisor will greatly appreciate this quality. For example, if you think you can come up with a more efficient way to get the office newsletter written and distributed, write out a plan and show it to your supervisor. He is likely to welcome any ideas that improve office efficiency or patient satisfaction.

Dealing with Conflict

Conflict, or friction, in the workplace can result from opposition of opinions or ideas or even from a difference in personalities. Conflict can arise when the lines of communication break down or when a misunderstanding occurs. Conflict also can result from preconceived notions about people or from lack of mutual respect or trust between a staff member and management. Whatever the cause, conflict is counterproductive to the efficiency of an office.

Following these suggestions can help prevent conflict in the office and improve communication among coworkers.

- Do not "feed into" other people's negative attitudes. For example, if a coworker is criticizing one of the doctors, change the subject or walk away.
- Try your best at all times to be personable and supportive of coworkers. For example, everyone has bad days. If a coworker is having a bad day, offer to pitch in and help or to run out and get her lunch if she is too busy to go out.
- Refrain from judging or stereotyping others (women are bad at math, men do not know how to communicate, and so on). Coworkers should show respect for one another and try to be tolerant and nonjudgmental.

- Do not gossip. You are there to work. Act professionally at all times.
- Do not jump to conclusions. For example, if you get a memo about a change in your schedule that disturbs you, take your concern to your supervisor. She may be able to be flexible on certain points. You do not know until you ask.

Setting Boundaries in the Healthcare Environment

As a medical assistant, your professional behavior is extremely important. In many instances, when dealing with patients, physicians, and other staff members, you must set **boundaries,** whether physical or psychological. This will limit undesirable behavior.

If a patient, physician, or staff member is acting inappropriately toward you, you must take immediate action. Do not let the situation "fester." You must act tactfully, assertively, and diplomatically. Let the aggressor know that his actions or language is inappropriate, and that you are not obligated in any way to accept such behavior. If none of your efforts help stop the unacceptable behavior, report the behavior to your immediate supervisor so she can assist you in identifying a solution. If the aggressor is your immediate supervisor, follow the office policy and procedure. Make yourself aware of policy and procedures ahead of time by reading the policy and procedure manual, which will be discussed in the *Practice Management* chapter.

PROCEDURE 4-1 Communicating with the Anxious Patient

WORK // DOC

Procedure Goal: To use communication and interpersonal skills to calm an anxious patient

OSHA Guidelines: This procedure does not involve exposure to blood, body fluids, or tissue.

Materials: Progress note

Method:

1. Identify signs of anxiety in the patient.
2. Acknowledge the patient's anxiety. (Ignoring a patient's anxiety often makes it worse.)
   RATIONALE: *Good therapeutic communication techniques can help reduce patient anxiety.*
3. Identify possible sources of anxiety, such as fear of a procedure or test result, along with supportive resources available to the patient, such as family members and friends.
   RATIONALE: *Understanding the source of anxiety in a patient and identifying the supportive resources available can help you communicate with the patient more effectively.*
4. Do what you can to alleviate the patient's physical discomfort. For example, find a calm, quiet place for the

patient to wait, a comfortable chair, a drink of water, or access to the bathroom.

5. Allow ample personal space for conversation. Note: You would normally allow a 1- to 4-foot distance between yourself and the patient. Adjust this space as necessary.
6. Create a climate of warmth, acceptance, and trust.
   a. Recognize and control your own anxiety. Your air of calm can decrease the patient's anxiety.
   b. Provide reassurance by demonstrating genuine care, respect, and empathy.
   c. Act confidently and dependably, maintaining truthfulness and confidentiality at all times.
7. Using the appropriate communication skills, have the patient describe the experience that is causing anxiety, her thoughts about it, and her feelings. Proceeding in this order allows the patient to describe what is causing the anxiety and to clarify her thoughts and feelings about it.
   a. Maintain an open posture.
   b. Maintain eye contact, if culturally appropriate.

c. Use active listening skills.

d. Listen without interrupting.

RATIONALE: *The use of open-ended questioning will result in more information about the patient's feelings of anxiety.*

8. Do not belittle the patient's thoughts and feelings. This can cause a breakdown in communication, increase anxiety, and make the patient feel isolated.

9. Be empathic to the patient's concerns.

10. Help the patient recognize and cope with the anxiety.

a. Provide information to the patient. Patients are often fearful of the unknown.

b. Suggest coping behaviors, such as deep breathing or other relaxation exercises.

RATIONALE: *Helping them understand their disease or the procedure they are about to undergo will help decrease their anxiety.*

11. Notify the doctor of the patient's concerns.

RATIONALE: *The physician must be aware of all aspects of the patient's health, including anxiety, to allow for optimal patient care. Part of your job as a medical assistant is to act as a liaison between the patient and the physician.*

12. Document your encounter with the patient.

PROCEDURE 4-2 Communicating with the Angry Patient WORK // DOC

Procedure Goal: To use communication and interpersonal skills to calm an angry patient

OSHA Guidelines: This procedure does not involve exposure to blood, body fluids, or tissue.

Materials: Progress note

Method:

1. Recognize anger and its causes. Anger is easy to recognize in most people, but it can be subtle in others. Patients who speak in a tense tone, are stubborn, or appear to ignore your attempts at communication may be angry.

2. Remain calm and continue to demonstrate genuineness and respect. Communicate that you respect and care about the patient's feelings.

3. Focus on the patient's physical and medical needs.

4. Maintain adequate personal space. Place yourself on the same level as the patient. If the patient is standing, encourage him to sit down. Maintain an open posture and eye contact but avoid staring.

RATIONALE: *Open posture and eye contact show the patient you are receptive to listening. Staring at the patient may make the person angrier.*

5. Listen attentively and with an open mind to what the patient is saying. Avoid the feeling that you need to defend yourself or to give reasons the patient should not be angry.

RATIONALE: *Most patients' anger will lessen if they know someone is really listening to them and showing an interest in their emotions and needs.*

6. Encourage patients to be specific in describing the cause of their anger, their thoughts about it, and their feelings. Be empathic and acknowledge the patient's feelings and perceptions. Follow through with any promises you make concerning correction of a problem, but avoid totally agreeing or disagreeing with the patient. State what you can and cannot do for the patient.

7. Present your point of view calmly and firmly to help the patient better understand the situation. If patients are receptive to your viewpoint, their perspective may change for the better.

8. Avoid a breakdown in communication. Allow the patient to voice anger. Trying to outtalk the patient or overexplain will only annoy and irritate him. If needed, suggest that the patient spend a few moments alone to gather his thoughts or to cool off before continuing any type of communication.

9. If you feel threatened by a patient's anger or if it looks as if the patient's anger may become violent, leave the room and seek assistance from one of the physicians or other members of the office staff.

10. Document any actual threats in the patient's chart.

PROCEDURE 4-3 Communicating with the Assistance of an Interpreter WORK // DOC

Procedure Goal: To demonstrate techniques to effectively communicate with a non-English-speaking patient through an interpreter

OSHA Guidelines: This procedure does not involve exposure to blood, body fluids, or tissue.

Materials:
Pen, forms, progress note, or computer and appropriate pictures and other visual aids if available

Method:

1. Identify the patient by name and ask if you pronounced the name correctly. Be sure to smile, even if you are feeling slightly awkward or unsure of yourself.

RATIONALE: *A smile is a form of nonverbal communication that will help the patient feel more comfortable.*

2. Introduce yourself, with your title, to the patient and the interpreter.

3. Ask the interpreter to spell his full name and provide you with identification, such as his agency's identification or a business card. Retain his business card to file in the patient's medical record. If he does not have a business card, obtain contact information, which also will be filed in the patient's medical record.

   RATIONALE: *Healthcare facilities are required to provide an interpreter, and this information must be documented.*

4. Do not take it personally if the patient appears abrupt or even rude; this behavior may be considered appropriate in the patient's culture. For example, in some cultures, male patients may not deal with a female staff member, and that should be respected if possible. Ascertain from the interpreter if there is a problem.

5. Inquire of the interpreter if the patient speaks or understands any English and if there are any communication traditions or other customs that you should be aware of. For example, traditional Navajo people consider it rude to have direct eye contact.

6. Provide a quiet, comfortable area.

7. Speak directly to the patient, and speak slowly if the patient has any understanding of English.

RATIONALE: *Eye contact and other forms of nonverbal communication are important to convey and receive information.*

8. If forms are to be completed, instruct the interpreter to translate with appropriate intervals and give opportunities for the patient to ask questions to ensure understanding. For example, If the patient is providing general consent for treatment or permission to send information and receive payment directly from the insurance company, have one area translated at a time. Instruct the interpreter to ask if there are questions at each portion.

9. If the patient and interpreter are discussing an issue in depth or appear to be leaving you out of the conversation, ask the translator what is being said.

10. Provide the same information, services, and courtesies that you would to a native English speaker. If possible, provide written information in the patient's native language.

11. Document what you would ordinarily document; note on all forms that "translation was done by" and include the name, credential, and agency of the interpreter, as well as the date and time.

SUMMARY OF LEARNING OUTCOMES	
LEARNING OUTCOMES	**KEY POINTS**
4.1 Identify elements and types of communication.	The communication circle involves a message being sent, a source, and a receiver that responds. Feedback is the response to a message, and noise is anything that may interfere with or change the message.
4.2 Relate communication to human behavior and needs.	Understanding human behavior and needs, and their correlation with professional relationships, is necessary to practicing as a medical assistant. Understanding the various stages of human life assists you in your communication skills with patients.
4.3 Categorize positive and negative communication.	Communication that promotes comfort and well-being is considered positive communication. Negative communication can be a turnoff. Medical assistants may not be aware of some of the signs of negative communication they display. Lack of eye contact with patients, except in specific cultures, or speaking sharply to a patient is considered negative communication. To help you avoid this type of communication, ask yourself, "Does this make me feel good?" or "Do I feel welcome?"
4.4 Model ways to improve listening, interpersonal skills, and assertiveness skills.	Listening and other interpersonal skills can be improved by becoming more involved in the communication process by offering feedback or asking questions of the patient. Assertive medical assistants trust their instincts. They respect their self-worth, while still making the patient feel comfortable and important. Aggressive medical assistants try to impose their positions through manipulation techniques.

LEARNING OUTCOMES	KEY POINTS
4.5 **Carry out therapeutic communication skills.**	Therapeutic communication is the ability to communicate with patients in terms that they can understand and, at the same time, feel at ease and comfortable in what you are saying. Positive therapeutic skills can enhance communication. Be aware of negative therapeutic skills that can disrupt the communication. Recognize defense mechanisims in patients and note whether the patient is using them to cope or is not able to cope.
4.6 **Use effective communication strategies with patients in special circumstances.**	Learning about the special needs of patients and polishing your communication skills will help you become an effective communicator. This will help you handle diversity in the workplace, handle anxious and annoyed patients, and deal with patients who have language barriers.
4.7 **Carry out positive communication with coworkers and management.**	The quality of communication you have with your coworkers and your supervisor greatly influences the development of a positive or negative work climate. Use proper channels of communication. Be open-minded. Keep supervisors informed of office problems as they arise and show initiative in your work habits.

CASE STUDY CRITICAL THINKING

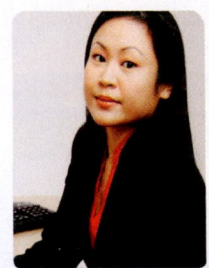

© Red Chopsticks/Getty Images RF

Recall Cindy Chen from the beginning of the chapter. Now that you have completed the chapter, answer the following questions regarding her case.

1. Cindy Chen is nervous. What techniques could you use to improve your communication with her?

2. What should you do regarding Cindy Chen's HIV-positive health status?

3. How would you best answer Ms. Chen's question "Do you have anything you can give me until I see the doctor?"

4. Ms. Chen becomes agitated when you answer her question. What should you do?

EXAM PREPARATION QUESTIONS

1. (LO 4.1) The main elements in the communication circle are
   a. A message (verbal and nonverbal), a source, and a receiver
   b. A message and a receiver
   c. A receiver, a response, a sender, and a source
   d. A source, feedback, and a receiver (verbal and nonverbal)
   e. A message, a receiver, and a response

2. (LO 4.7) Good relationships with coworkers would not include
   a. Professionalism
   b. Stress
   c. Cooperation
   d. Gossip
   e. Integrity

3. (LO 4.3) Which is an example of negative communication?
   a. Speaking sharply to the patient
   b. Listening carefully
   c. Being friendly and warm
   d. Looking directly at the patient
   e. Keeping quiet when appropriate

4. (LO 4.1) Which of the following is an example of positive communication?
   a. Treating patients impersonally
   b. Looking directly at patients when you speak to them
   c. Speaking brusquely or sharply
   d. Showing boredom
   e. Forgetting common courtesies, such as saying please and thank you

5. (LO 4.4) The ability to identify with someone else's feelings is called
   a. Sympathy
   b. Feedback
   c. Empathy
   d. Respect
   e. Assertiveness

6. (LO 4.3) Poor communication could lead to all of the following *except*
   a. Patient satisfaction
   b. Errors in billing
   c. Inefficient care
   d. Malpractice
   e. Anxiety

7. (LO 4.3) Personal space in a healthcare environment is approximately
   a. 7–18 feet
   b. 1–4 feet
   c. 3–6 feet
   d. 4–12 feet
   e. 3–10 feet

8. (LO 4.3) You want to convey an open posture while communicating with a patient. What should you do?
   a. Fold your arms and lean forward while looking into the patient's eyes
   b. Lean back gently while facing the patient
   c. Lean forward in your chair facing the patient
   d. Lean forward and avoid eye contact with the patient
   e. Extend your arms while leaning forward toward the patient

9. (LO 4.6) Your patient has been diagnosed with a terminal illness and makes the following comment: "If you could help me make it to my grandson's graduation next month before I get too sick, that would be perfect." Which of Kübler-Ross's stages of dying is this patient exhibiting?
   a. Denial
   b. Bargaining
   c. Depression
   d. Acceptance
   e. Anger

10. (LO 4.6) Which of the following is a proper technique for demonstrating cultural competence?
    a. Avoid giving the reason or purpose for a treatment or prescription, since they will not understand
    b. Do not speak in the patients' native language, because it may make them uncomfortable
    c. Look at the interpreter during communication to ensure he or she is making the correct statement
    d. Avoid saying, "You must . . ."; instead, teach patients their options and let them decide—for example, "Some people in this situation would . . ."
    e. Ignore nonverbal communication, since it is difficult to interpret

S O F T   S K I L L S   S U C C E S S

Hunter Glaspell, a 67-year-old male patient, calls BWW Medical Associates, stating his ear has been bothering him for days and the pain is getting worse. It is Monday afternoon at 4 P.M. The schedule is packed, and he wants to come in right away. When you offer him an appointment at 9 A.M. tomorrow, he becomes verbally abusive, screaming that he is in pain now. How will you handle this situation?

Mc Graw Hill Education | **Practice**

Go to PRACTICE MEDICAL OFFICE and complete Admin: Check In–Interactions.

Legal and Ethical Issues

CASE STUDY

Patient Name	DOB	Allergies
Cindy Chen	7/15/XX	NKA

Attending	MRN	Other Information
Alexis N. Whalen, MD	324-86-542	Finishes school in 6 months

PATIENT INFORMATION

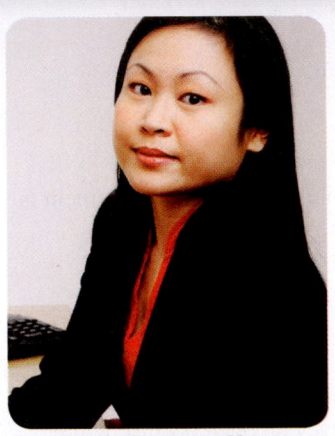

© Red Chopsticks/Getty Images RF

Cindy Chen, a 28-year-old female complaining of inability to sleep and nervousness, arrives at the office. She tested positive for HIV in 2014, although she has been asymptomatic on antiviral drugs. Currently, she lives with her aunt and is going to school to become a phlebotomist. As you are preparing to bring Cindy in from the reception area, the externship student, who is new to the office, states that she is afraid to work with you when caring for Cindy because she is afraid she might get AIDS if she works closely with her.

Keep Cindy in mind as you study the chapter. There will be questions at the end of the chapter based on the case study. The inorfmation in the chapter will help you answer these questions.

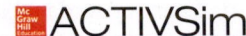 ACTIVSim

LEARNING OUTCOMES

After completing Chapter 5, you will be able to:

5.1 Differentiate between laws and ethics.

5.2 Identify the responsibilities of the patient and physician in a physician-patient contract, including the components for informed consent that must be understood by the patient.

5.3 Describe the four Ds of negligence required to prove malpractice and explain the four Cs of malpractice prevention.

5.4 Relate the term *credentialing* and explain the importance of the FDA and DEA to administrative procedures performed by medical assistants.

5.5 Summarize the purpose of the following federal healthcare regulations: HCQIA, False Claims Act, OSHA, and HIPAA.

5.6 Identify the six principles for preventing improper release of information from the medical office.

5.7 Discuss the importance of ethics in the medical office.

5.8 Explain the differences among the practice management models.

KEY TERMS

abandonment
assault
battery
bioethics
breach of contract
civil law
consent
contract
criminal law
deposition
durable power of attorney

ethics
expressed contract
felony
fraud
implied contract
law
locum tenens
minors
misdemeanor
negligence
tort

VIII.C.5	Differentiate between fraud and abuse
X.C.1	Differentiate between scope of practice and standards of care for medical assistants
X.C.4	Summarize the Patient Bill of Rights
X.C.6	Compare criminal and civil law as they apply to the practicing medical assistant
X.C.7	Define: (a) negligence (b) malpractice (c) statute of limitations (d) Good Samaritan Act(s) (e) Uniform Anatomical Gift Act (f) living will/advanced directives (g) medical durable power of attorney (h) Patient Self Determination Act (PSDA)
X.C.10	Identify: (b) Genetic Information Nondiscrimination Act of 2008 (GINA)
X.C.11	Describe the process in compliance reporting: (c) conflicts of interest
X.C.13	Define the following medical legal terms: (a) informed consent (b) implied consent (c) expressed consent (d) patient incompetence (e) emancipated minor (f) mature minor (g) subpoena duces tecum (h) respondeat superior (i) res ipsa loquitur (j) locum tenens (k) defendant-plaintiff (l) deposition (m) arbitration-mediation
XI.C.1	Define: (a) ethics (b) morals
XI.C.2	Differentiate between personal and professional ethics
XI.P.1	Develop a plan for separation of personal and professional ethics
XI.A.1	Recognize the impact personal ethics and morals have on the delivery of healthcare

4. Medical Law and Ethics

b. Institute federal and state guidelines when releasing medical records or information

c. Follow established policies when initiating or terminating medical treatment

d. Understand the importance of maintaining liability coverage once employed in the industry

e. Perform risk management procedures

f. Comply with federal, state, and local health laws and regulations as they apply to healthcare settings

▶ Introduction

Medical law plays an important role in medical facility procedures and the quality of patient care. Our modern society can be a litigious one, meaning people are inclined to sue when results or outcomes are not acceptable to them. This is particularly true with healthcare practitioners, healthcare facilities, and manufacturers of medical equipment and products. Patients, their relatives, and others expect favorable medical outcomes and often sue when these outcomes do not meet expectations. As a result, it is important for all medical professionals to understand medical law, ethics, and the Health

Insurance Portability and Accountability Act (HIPAA), which began in 1996 and has expanded since that time.

As a medical assistant, having a basic knowledge of medical law and ethics can help you gain perspective in the following three areas:

1. *The rights, responsibilities, and concerns of healthcare consumers.* Healthcare professionals need to be concerned about how law and ethics impact their respective professions and they must understand how legal and ethical issues affect patients. As medical technology advances and the use of computers increases, patients know more about their healthcare options and their rights as consumers, and more about the responsibilities of healthcare practitioners to their patients.

2. *The legal and ethical issues facing society, patients, and healthcare professionals as the world changes.* Every day new technologies emerge with solutions to biological and medical issues. These solutions often include social issues involving decisions about controversial topics like reproductive rights, fetal stem cell research, and confidentiality with sensitive medical records.

3. *The impact of rising costs on the laws and ethics of healthcare delivery.* Rising costs—of both healthcare insurance and medical treatment in general—can lead to questions concerning access to healthcare services and the allocation of medical treatment. For example, should everyone, regardless of age, race, or lifestyle, have the same access to scarce medical commodities like transplant organs and very expensive medications?

Because medical treatment and decisions surrounding healthcare today have become so increasingly complex, it is important to be knowledgeable about, and aware of, the ethical issues and the laws that govern patient care. As a medical assistant and an important member of the healthcare team, always keep in mind that any health or financial information you obtain regarding a patient (past or present) is protected. It may be shared only with the patient's express permission, except in a few very specific instances, which will be discussed in this chapter.

▶ Laws and Ethics   LO 5.1

In order to understand medical law and ethics, it is helpful to know the difference between law and ethics. A **law** is defined as a rule of conduct or action prescribed or formally recognized as binding or enforced by a controlling authority, such as local, state, and federal governments. **Ethics** is a standard of behavior based on concepts of right and wrong. Ethical behavior goes beyond the legal consideration in any given situation. *Moral values*—formed through the influence of family, culture, and society—serve as a basis for ethical conduct. Ethics will be discussed in further detail later in the chapter.

Classifications of Law

While a crime is any offense committed or omitted in violation of a public law, two types of law pertain to healthcare practitioners: criminal law and civil law. Whether the case is criminal or civil, there are always two sides, the plaintiff and the defendant. The party making the charge or claim is known as the *plaintiff*. The party against whom the charge or claim is made is the *defendant*.

Criminal Law **Criminal law** involves crimes against the state. When a state or federal law is violated, the government brings criminal charges against the alleged offender—for example, *Ohio v. John Doe.* Criminal laws prohibit such crimes as murder, arson, rape, and burglary. A criminal act may be classified as a felony or a misdemeanor. A **felony** is a crime punishable by death or by imprisonment in a state or federal prison for more than 1 year. Some examples of a felony include abuse (child, elder, or domestic violence), manslaughter, fraud, attempted murder, and practicing medicine without a license.

Misdemeanors are less serious crimes than felonies and are punishable by fines or imprisonment in a facility other than a federal prison for 1 year or less. Some examples of misdemeanors are thefts under a certain dollar amount, attempted burglary, and disturbing the peace.

Civil Law **Civil law** involves crimes against the person. Under civil law, a person can sue another person, a business, or the government. Court judgments in civil cases often require the payment of a sum of money to the injured party. Civil law includes a general category of law known as torts. A **tort** is broadly defined as a civil wrong committed against a person or property that causes physical injury or damage to someone's property or that deprives someone of his or her personal liberty and freedom. Torts may be intentional (willful) or unintentional (accidental).

Intentional Torts When one person intentionally harms another, the law allows the injured party to seek a remedy in a civil suit. The injured party can be financially compensated for any harm done by the person guilty of committing the tort. If the conduct is judged to be malicious, punitive damages may also be awarded. Examples of intentional torts include the following:

- **Assault** is the open threat of bodily harm to another, or acting in such a way as to put another in the "reasonable apprehension of bodily harm." In the medical office, if a patient were to feel threatened in any way, assault could be charged.

- **Battery** is an action that causes bodily harm to another. It is broadly defined as any bodily contact made without permission. In healthcare delivery, battery may be charged for any unauthorized touching of a patient, including such actions as suturing a wound, administering an injection, or performing a physical examination. For this reason, having a written record of a patient's informed consent is essential for all invasive medical procedures. Informed consent is discussed later in this chapter.

- *Defamation* is the act of damaging a person's reputation by making public statements that are both false and malicious.

The full term for these actions is *defamation of character*. Defamation can take the form of slander and/or libel. *Slander* is speaking damaging words intended to negatively influence others against an individual in a manner that jeopardizes his or her reputation or means of livelihood. If a patient hears members of the staff speaking about him in an unprofessional manner, or talking about his diagnosis with staff members without a "need to know," it could be considered slanderous. *Libel* is publishing in print damaging words, pictures, or signed statements that will injure the reputation of another.

- False imprisonment is the intentional, unlawful restraint or confinement of one person by another. Preventing a patient from leaving the facility might be seen as false imprisonment.

- *Healthcare fraud* and *abuse* are closely related intentional torts. **Fraud** is an intentional deception or misrepresentation of services that an individual knows to be false and that could result in an unauthorized reimbursement to a practice. An example of healthcare fraud would be billing for a procedure that is not performed. *Abuse* describes incidents or practices inconsistent with accepted and sound medical, business, or fiscal practices. Billing for unnecessary medical services is an example of healthcare abuse.

- Invasion of privacy is the interference with a person's right to keep personal matters private. Entering an exam room without knocking can be considered an invasion of privacy. The improper use of or a breach of confidentiality of medical records may be seen as an invasion of privacy.

Unintentional Torts The most common torts within the healthcare delivery system are those committed unintentionally. Unintentional torts are acts that are not intended to cause harm but are committed unreasonably or with a disregard for the consequences. In legal terms, such acts constitute negligence. **Negligence** is charged when a healthcare practitioner fails to exercise ordinary care and the patient is injured. Medical negligence is more commonly known as malpractice, which will be discussed in more detail later in this chapter.

Contracts

A **contract** is a voluntary agreement between two parties in which specific promises are made for a consideration. The elements of a contract are important to healthcare practitioners because healthcare delivery takes place under various types of contracts. To be legally binding, four elements must be present in a contract:

1. *Agreement.* One party makes an offer and another party accepts it. Certain conditions pertain to the offer:
   - It can relate to the present or the future.
   - It must be communicated.
   - It must be made in good faith and not under duress or as a joke.

- It must be clear enough to be understood by both parties.
- It must define what both parties will do if the offer is accepted.

For example, a physician offers a service to the public by obtaining a license to practice medicine and opening a business. Patients accept the physician's offer by scheduling appointments, submitting to physical examinations, and allowing the physician to prescribe or perform medical treatment. The contract is complete when the physician's fee is paid.

2. *Consideration.* Something of value is bargained for as part of the agreement. The physician's consideration is providing service; the patient's consideration is payment of the physician's fee.

3. *Legal subject matter.* Contracts are not valid and enforceable in court unless they are for legal services or purposes. For example, a contract entered into by a patient to pay for the services of a physician in private practice would be *void* (not legally enforceable) if the physician were not licensed to practice medicine. **Breach of contract** may be charged if either party fails to comply with the terms of a legally valid contract.

4. *Contractual capacity.* Parties who enter into the agreement must be capable of fully understanding all its terms and conditions. For example, a mentally incompetent individual or a person under the influence of drugs or alcohol cannot enter into a contract. In this context, *incompetent patients* are those who have mental conditions that make them incapable of understanding the concepts and meaning of a contract.

Types of Contracts The two main types of contracts are expressed contracts and implied contracts. An **expressed contract** is clearly stated in written or spoken words. A payment contract is an example of an expressed contract. **Implied contracts** are those in which the conduct of the parties, rather than expressed words, indicates acceptance and creates the contract. A patient who rolls up a sleeve and offers an arm for an injection is creating an implied contract.

Employment Contract Some medical practices—usually larger practices and hospitals—use employment contracts for their employees. This type of contract could include any or all of the following elements:

- A description of your duties and your employer's duties
- Plans for handling major changes in job responsibilities
- Salary, bonuses, and other forms of compensation
- Benefits, like vacation time, sick days, life insurance, and participation in pension plans
- Grievance procedures
- Exceptional situations under which the contract may be terminated by either you or your employer
- Termination procedures and compensation
- Special provisions, like job sharing, medical examinations, or liability coverage

If you are offered an employment contract, study it closely. Consider any local laws that apply. It is wise to have a lawyer or business adviser review the contract prior to signing it.

▶ The Physician-Patient Contract   LO 5.2

A physician has the right, after forming a contract or agreeing to accept a patient under his or her care, to make reasonable limitations (such as expecting the patient to follow through on the agreed-upon treatment plan) on the contractual relationship. The physician is under no legal obligations to treat patients who may wish to exceed those limitations (for example, expecting the physician to accept patient phone calls at home). Under the physician-patient contract, both parties have certain rights and responsibilities.

Physician Rights and Responsibilities

A physician has the right to

- Set up a practice within the boundaries of his or her license to practice medicine.
- Set up an office where he or she chooses and to establish office hours.
- Specialize.
- Decide which services he or she will provide and how those services will be provided.

Within an implied contract, the physician is not expected, or bound, to

- Treat every patient seeking care. A physician is free to use his or her discretion to form contracts within his or her practice, with one exception: If a physician is providing care to patients in a hospital emergency room or free clinic, then the physician must treat every patient who comes for treatment.
- Restore the patient to his or her original state of health.
- Make a correct diagnosis in every case.
- Guarantee the successful result of any treatment or operation. In fact, guarantees of "cures" may constitute fraud on the part of the physician.

Under an implied contract with the patient, the physician does have the responsibility (obligation) to

- Use due care, skill, judgment, and diligence in treating patients, with the same care, skill, judgment, and diligence that peers of the same medical specialty use.
- Stay informed of the best (and current) methods of diagnosis and treatment.
- Perform to the best of his or her ability, whether or not he or she is to receive a fee.
- Furnish complete information and instructions to the patient about diagnoses, options, methods of treatment, and fees for services.

Medical Assistants and Liability All competent adults are liable (legally responsible) for their actions, in both their personal lives and their professional careers. As a medical assistant, it is important to know and understand your scope of practice within the state where you are working. As healthcare providers, medical assistants have general liability in the duties they perform, as well as toward the facility in which they work. By understanding the standard of care and the duty of care, you, as the office medical assistant, can function ethically and legally within the scope of practice for your profession. Medical assistants are held to the "reasonable person standard," which means to carry out your professional and interpersonal relationships without causing harm. This also means that you are held to a higher standard, both inside and *outside* of the office and both during and *outside* of office hours.

Patient Rights and Responsibilities

Each patient has the right to see the physician of the individual's choosing, although some managed care plans limit the physician choices to those that are "in-network." Patients also have the right to terminate a physician's services if they wish. Most states have adopted a version of the American Hospital Association's *patient care partnership* (formerly called the Patient's Bill of Rights). The patient care partnership is a list of standards that patients can expect in healthcare. The Joint Commission (TJC) requires hospitals to post a copy of these standards, and most managed care organizations require contracted physicians to post them. Figure 5-1 is an example of a typical patient care partnership list for a medical office. The brochure given to the patient would go into each point in more detail.

Patient Responsibilities Patients are also part of the medical team involved in their treatment. Under an implied contract, patients have the responsibility to

- Follow any instructions given by the licensed practitioner and cooperate as much as possible.
- Give all relevant information to the licensed practitioner in order to reach a correct diagnosis. If a patient fails to inform a licensed practitioner of any medical conditions he or she has and an incorrect diagnosis is made, the licensed practitioner is not liable.
- Follow the licensed practitioner's orders for treatment.
- Pay the fees charged for services provided.

Consent means that the patient has given permission, either expressed or implied, for the licensed practitioner to examine him or her, to perform tests that aid in reaching a diagnosis, or to treat a known or found medical condition. *Expressed consent* is consent the patient gives in words. When the patient makes an appointment to be examined by a licensed practitioner, the patient has given *implied consent* to the examination and any (simple) diagnostic testing procedures needed for treatment.

Informed consent involves the patient's right to receive all information relative to his or her condition and to make a decision regarding treatment based upon that knowledge. The "doctrine of informed consent" is the legal basis for informed

BWW

BWW Medical Associates, PC
305 Main Street, Port Snead YZ 12345-9876
Tel: 555-654-3210, Fax: 555-987-6543
Web: BWWAssociates.com

Paul F. Buckwalter, MD
Alexis N. Whalen, MD
Elizabeth H. Williams, MD

Patient Care Partnership
Understanding Expectations, Rights, and Responsibilities

Welcome to our medical practice. As our patient, you have the right to certain expectations, including

1. High-quality medical care.

2. A clean and safe environment for your medical care.

3. Informed involvement in your medical care.

4. Protection of your privacy.

5. Assistance obtaining referrals and appointments with outside providers.

6. Help with billing and insurance claim issues.

You will receive a brochure outlining the details of these rights for your records. If you have any questions, comments, concerns, or suggestions regarding the information within the brochure or regarding your care with us, please let us know. We are always interested in improving your patient care experience with us.

FIGURE 5-1   Example of a patient care partnership list.

consent (or informed refusal of treatment) and is usually outlined in a state's medical practice acts. Informed consent implies that the patient understands

- Proposed treatment modes.
- Why the treatment is necessary.
- The risks involved in the proposed treatment.
- Available alternative modes of treatment.
- The risks of alternative treatments.
- The risks involved if treatment is refused.

Adult patients who are of sound mind are usually able to give informed consent. Courts have ruled that emancipated minors (those under age 18, not living at home, and self-supporting) understand as a competent adult would and therefore are able to make decisions on their own. Mature minors—although defined differently by each state—are generally minors who, depending on their medical condition, are considered capable of making their own medical decisions and do not require a guardian's consent for certain procedures like contraception, sexually transmitted infection (STI) treatment, and drug or alcohol addictions. Keep in mind, however, that although mature minors may consent to treatment, they

may not legally be allowed to enter into a financial contract for payment. The physician or business manager should make decisions regarding payment issues surrounding treatment of mature minors.

Patients who cannot give informed consent include the following:

- **Minors** or persons under the age of majority, but excluding married minors
- The mentally incompetent
- Those who speak a foreign language—interpreters may be necessary

Informed consent is a vital part of the practice of medicine. Physicians are often sued for negligence because of the failure to adequately inform patients of adverse surgical complications, drug reactions, and alternative treatment modes.

Terminating the Physician-Patient Contract

There are times when a physician feels it is necessary to terminate care of a patient. Terminating care is sometimes called withdrawing from a case and must be undertaken very carefully to avoid charges of abandonment. The following are some typical reasons a physician may choose to withdraw from a case:

- The patient refuses to follow the physician's instructions.
- The patient's family members complain incessantly to or about the physician.
- A personality conflict develops between the physician and the patient that cannot be reasonably resolved.
- The patient habitually does not pay for or fails to make satisfactory arrangements to pay for medical services. A physician may stop treatment of such a patient and end the physician-patient relationship only if adequate notice is given to the patient.
- The patient fails to keep scheduled appointments. To protect the physician from charges of abandonment, all missed and canceled appointments should be noted in the patient's chart.

A physician who terminates care of a patient must do so in a formal, legal manner, following these four steps.

1. Write a letter to the patient, expressing the reason for withdrawing from the case and recommending that the patient seek medical care from another physician as soon as possible. Thirty days is the usual norm allowed for finding another physician. Figure 5-2 shows an example of a letter terminating patient care.
2. Send the letter by certified mail with a return receipt requested. This will provide evidence that the patient received the notification by providing a signature on the return receipt.
3. Place a copy of the letter (and the return receipt, when received) in the patient's medical record.
4. Summarize in the patient record the physician's reason for terminating care and the actions taken to inform the patient.

Just as a physician may choose to end the physician-patient contract, a patient also may choose to end this contract at any time. Often, the ending of the contract on the patient's part is much less formal; he may simply stop coming to appointments. If a patient suddenly stops coming to appointments, as a medical assistant, you should always attempt

BWW

BWW Medical Associates, PC
305 Main Street, Port Snead YZ 12345-9876
Tel: 555-654-3210, Fax: 555-987-6543
Web: BWWAssociates.com

Paul F. Buckwalter, MD
Alexis N. Whalen, MD
Elizabeth H. Williams, MD

December 12, 20XX

Jack Smallwood
20 Cedarview Court
Funton YZ 13254-0987

Dear Mr. Smallwood:

This letter is to inform you of my intent to discontinue providing medical care to you due to habitual and continued noncompliance with your treatment plan. My records indicate that you have missed several appointments and have not complied with ordered testing. In order to allow you sufficient time to establish yourself with another physician, this discontinuation will go into effect 30 days from the date of this letter. My office will be happy to forward your medical records to the physician of your choice.

If you require assistance in locating a new physician, please contact your insurance plan or the Port Snead Medical Society at 1-800-666-9898.

Sincerely,

Paul F. Buckwalter, MD

Paul F. Buckwalter, MD

FIGURE 5-2 Sample letter of withdrawal of medical care.

to reach the patient to ascertain the reason the patient has stopped coming to the office. If the patient expresses dissatisfaction with the care he has received, inform the physician as soon as possible and document the call in the patient's medical record. You will have a look at patient dissatisfaction and its connection with malpractice claims a little later in this chapter.

Standard of Care

As a medical assistant, you are expected to fulfill the standards of the medical assisting profession by practicing appropriate legal concepts for your profession. According to the AAMA, medical assistants should uphold legal concepts in the following ways:

- Maintain confidentiality
- Practice within the scope of training and capabilities
- Prepare and maintain medical records
- Document accurately
- Use appropriate guidelines when releasing information
- Follow legal guidelines and maintain awareness of healthcare legislation and regulations
- Maintain and dispose of regulated substances in compliance with government guidelines
- Follow established risk management and safety procedures
- Meet the requirements for professional credentialing

Some state laws dictate what medical assistants may or may not do. For instance, in some states it is illegal for medical assistants to give injections to patients. No states consider it legal for medical assistants to diagnose a condition, prescribe treatment, or allow a patient to believe that the medical assistant is a nurse. In addition to what is stated by law, you and the physician must establish your scope of practice—the procedures that are appropriate for you to perform while working under the physician's supervision. Once that scope of practice is agreed upon, you must continue to stay within that scope of practice unless the scope is updated or changed by mutual agreement. For instance, your scope of practice may change if laws change in your state or if you receive additional training, increasing your skill and/or credential level, which allows an increase in responsibilities for your position.

Closing a Medical Practice

Distressful economic circumstances may cause a medical practice to terminate and close its services to its patients. If this becomes necessary, make sure the medical staff and all physicians do the following:

- Comply with all HIPAA laws for maintaining confidentiality
- Write letters to all patients, giving them knowledge that your practice will be closing (Figure 5-3)
- Give patients an option of choosing another physician, or make referrals. If the patient chooses another physician to take over his care, get written consent for his charts to be transferred to that physician properly.

- Keep all files in a secured location for the maximum amount of time files should be saved if contact with patients cannot be made. You will have to choose a vendor that stores files; make sure you choose a reputable vendor.
- Shred files if necessary; again, be sure to choose reputable vendors
- Stay up-to-date on any HIPAA laws that will affect the practice

▶ Preventing Malpractice Claims   LO 5.3

Malpractice litigation not only adds to the cost of healthcare but also, takes a psychological toll on both patients and healthcare practitioners. Both sides would probably agree that prevention is preferable to litigation. Healthcare practitioners who use reasonable care in preventing professional liability (malpractice) claims are less likely to be faced with defending themselves against these claims.

Risk management is the act or practice of controlling risk. This process includes identifying and tracking risk areas, developing risk improvement plans as part of risk handling, monitoring risks, and performing risk assessments to determine how risks have changed. Proper documentation, patient satisfaction, appropriate behavior, proper medical procedures, and safeguards against exposure assist with decreasing the risk of malpractice lawsuits brought against the medical facility, physicians, and their staff.

Medical Negligence

Malpractice claims are lawsuits by patients against physicians for errors in diagnosis or treatment. Medical *negligence* cases are those in which a person believes that a medical professional did not perform an essential action or performed an improper one, thus harming the patient.

The following are some examples of malpractice:

- *Postoperative complications.* For example, a patient starts to show signs of internal bleeding in the recovery room. The incision is reopened and it is discovered that the surgeon did not complete closure (cauterization) of all the severed capillaries at the operation site.
- *Res ipsa loquitur.* This Latin term means "the thing speaks for itself" and refers to a case in which the doctor's fault is completely obvious—for example, a case in which a surgeon accidentally leaves a surgical instrument inside the patient.

The following are examples of medical negligence:

- *Abandonment.* A healthcare professional who stops care without providing an equally qualified substitute can be charged with **abandonment.** For example, a labor and delivery nurse is helping a woman in labor. The nurse's shift ends, but all the other nurses are busy and her replacement is late for work. Leaving the woman would constitute abandonment. A healthcare practitioner who intends to be away from her practice for an extended period of time may hire a **locum tenens,** literally "place holder." For example, a physician taking maternity leave may hire another qualified physician to temporarily take her place. The substitute physician will

BWW Medical Associates, PC
305 Main Street, Port Snead YZ 12345-9876
Tel: 555-654-3210, Fax: 555-987-6543
Web: BWWAssociates.com

Paul F. Buckwalter, MD
Alexis N. Whalen, MD
Elizabeth H. Williams, MD

May 23, 20XX

Ms. Gisele Monahan
234 Cutter Lane
Port Snead, YZ 12345-6789

RE: Closing of Medical Practice

Dear Ms. Monahan:

I regret to inform you that our medical practice will be closing on July 30, 20XX. The practice has been purchased by the Vaughn Group, 2345 Williamsburg Court, Port Snead, YZ 12345-6789.

If you wish to use this group of medical practitioners, please sign the enclosed authorization to release medical records form so that your files may be forwarded to them promptly.

Should you choose another physician, please send me a written request with your signature, authorizing the release of your medical records to the physician of your choice. Should we not hear from you prior to the practice closing date, all records will be stored at the Vaughn Group location for retrieval at a future date.

It has been my pleasure to provide your medical care.

Sincerely,

Alexis N. Whalen, MD

Alexis N. Whalen, MD

Enc: Authorization to Release Information

FIGURE 5-3 Sample letter notifying patient of medical practice closure.

act as the practicing physician's agent; therefore, abandonment is not an issue.

- *Delayed treatment.* A patient shows symptoms of some illness or disorder, but the doctor decides, for whatever reason, to delay treatment. If the delay is the direct cause of patient harm, the patient may have a negligence case.

The following legal terms are sometimes used to classify medical negligence cases:

- *Malfeasance* refers to an unlawful act or misconduct.
- *Misfeasance* refers to a lawful act that is done incorrectly.
- *Nonfeasance* refers to failure to perform an act that is one's required duty or that is required by law.

The Four Ds of Negligence The American Medical Association (AMA) lists the following "four Ds of negligence":

1. *Duty.* Patients must show that a physician-patient relationship existed in which the physician owed the patient a duty.
2. *Derelict.* Patients must show that the physician failed to comply with the standards of the profession. For example, a gynecologist has routinely taken Pap smears of a patient and then, for whatever reason, does not do so. If

the patient then shows evidence of cervical cancer, the physician could be said to have been derelict.

3. *Direct cause.* Patients must show that any damages were a direct cause of a physician's breach of duty. For example, if a patient fell on the sidewalk and damaged her cast, she could not prove that the cast was damaged because it was incorrectly or poorly applied by her physician. It would be clear that the damage to the cast resulted from the fall. If, however, the patient's leg healed incorrectly because of the way the cast had been applied, she might have a case.

4. *Damages.* Patients must prove that they suffered injury.

To go forward with a malpractice suit, a patient must be prepared to prove all four Ds of negligence.

Malpractice and Civil Law Malpractice (medical negligence) lawsuits are part of civil law, coming under the heading of torts. Recall that a tort is the intentional or unintentional breach of an obligation that causes harm or injury. A *breach of contract* is the failure of one of the parties to adhere to the terms of the contract.

In the case of medical care contracts, which are often implied contracts, either the provider or the patient can breach the contract. The provider can breach the contract by not maintaining patient confidentiality or by not providing adequate medical care (negligence). The patient can breach the contract by not showing up for appointments or by not following the physician's plan of care.

Settling Malpractice Suits Malpractice suits often require a trial in a court of law. Sometimes, however, they are settled through arbitration or mediation. *Arbitration* is a process in which the opposing sides choose a person or persons outside the court system, often with special knowledge in the field, to hear and decide the dispute. Arbitration is generally binding—that is, the parties agreeing to settle through arbitration must follow the solution arrived at by the arbitrator. Mediation is similar to arbitration in that the goal is to settle the case. The mediator does not judge the case but simply seeks a reasonable solution that both parties can agree upon. Mediation is generally nonbinding. (Your local or state medical society has information about the policy on arbitration or mediation for your state.) If injury, failure to provide reasonable care, or abandonment of the patient is proven to have occurred, the doctor must pay damages (a financial award) to the injured party.

If the physician you work with becomes involved in a lawsuit, you should be familiar with subpoenas and depositions. A *subpoena* is a written court order addressed to a specific person, requiring that person's presence in court on a specific date at a specific time. If you were directly involved in the patient case or have knowledge of the events that precipitated the lawsuit, you might be subpoenaed to provide testimony under penalty, known as *subpoena testificandum.* Another important term to know is *subpoena duces tecum,* which is a court order to produce specific, requested documents required at a certain place and time to enter into court records. If you are in charge of patient records at the practice, you will be required to locate, assemble,

photocopy, and arrange for delivery of the requested records or be charged with contempt of court if you do not comply. Prior to appearing in court, a healthcare practitioner may be asked to give a deposition, either as a defendant or an expert witness. The **deposition** is a sworn statement regarding the facts of the case and is used to prepare the case for trial.

Law of Agency According to the law of agency, an employee is considered to be acting as a doctor's agent (on the doctor's behalf) while performing professional tasks. The Latin term *respondeat superior*, or "let the master answer," is sometimes used to refer to this relationship. For example, the medical assistant's word is as binding as if it were uttered by the doctor (so you should never promise a patient a cure). With the law of agency, the doctor is responsible, or *liable*, for the negligence of employees. A negligent employee, however, may also be sued directly because individuals are legally responsible for their own actions. So a patient can sue both the doctor and the involved employee for negligence. The employer, or the employer's insurance company, also can sue the employee. Most likely, in a case of negligence, the doctor would be sued (because you as an employee are acting on the doctor's behalf), and you are usually covered by the doctor's malpractice insurance. Some medical assistants (usually clinical MAs) choose to obtain malpractice insurance. Obtaining personal malpractice insurance is a professional decision that depends on the type of work or facility in which you are employed. The American Association of Medical Assistants (AAMA) offers medical assisting malpractice insurance through various insurance companies at reduced rates.

Courtroom Conduct Most healthcare providers will never have to appear in court, but should you be asked to appear, the following suggestions may prove helpful:

- Attend court proceedings as required. Failure to appear in court could result in charges of contempt of court or in the case being forfeited.

- Do not be late for scheduled hearings.

- Bring required documents to court and present them only when requested to do so.

- Before testifying, refresh your memory concerning all the facts observed about the matter in question, like dates, times, words spoken, and circumstances.

- Speak slowly, clearly, and professionally. Do not use medical terms. Do not lose your temper or attempt to be humorous.

- Answer all questions in a straightforward manner, even if the answers appear to help the opposing side.

- Answer only the question asked, no more and no less.

- Appear well groomed, and wear clean, conservative clothing.

Professional Liability Coverage Professional liability coverage, also known as malpractice insurance, is specialty coverage to protect the physician and staff against financial losses due to lawsuits filed against them by their clients or others. This coverage protects the physician if she is found to be negligent in her actions, and it protects the physician and her staff members if it is determined that any member is negligent in his or her actions. Professional liability coverage, however, comes at an extremely high cost to the practice. Society in general, and patients in particular, have extremely high expectations of physicians and of the medical community. Malpractice lawsuits have become quite commonplace. You have likely seen billboards advertising lawyers who offer assistance to patients who are unhappy with the medical care they have received.

It is no surprise, then, that malpractice insurance can be one of the most expensive accounts payable for the office. Depending on the type of specialty and the area of the country in which the physician practices, costs for an internist can be as low as $4,000 per year in Minnesota (which has some of the lowest malpractice rates in the country) to a high of $50,000 annually (in 2011) in Florida, which has some of the highest rates in the country. OB/GYNs, who have some of the highest rates of any specialty, can expect to pay anywhere from $15,000 in Minnesota to $80,000–$200,000 per year in Florida for coverage.

Reasons Patients Sue

The following reasons were researched by interviewing families and patients who have sued healthcare practitioners:

1. *Unrealistic expectations.* With modern advancements in medical technology, patients often expect perfection in medical outcomes. They may feel betrayed by the healthcare system when a medical outcome is not what was expected.

2. *Poor rapport and poor communication.* Patients usually do not sue healthcare practitioners whom they like and trust. Healthcare providers who do not return telephone calls or are otherwise unavailable to a patient's family members may be perceived as arrogant, cold, or uncaring. When such perceptions exist, patients and family members are more likely to sue if something goes wrong.

3. *Greed and our litigious society.* Financial gain is seldom the reason for medical malpractice, but in some cases it may be an influencing factor. Malpractice attorneys sometimes make it very easy for patients to retain their services, such as contingency arrangements.

4. *Poor quality of care.* Poor quality means that a patient is truly not receiving quality care. Poor quality in "perception" means that the patient believes he or she is not receiving quality care, even if it is not true. Either situation can lead to a malpractice lawsuit.

Statute of Limitations Statutes of limitations are laws that set the deadline or maximum period of time within which a lawsuit or claim may be filed. The most common length of time is 2 years. The deadlines may vary depending on the circumstances and the type of case or claim. The periods of time also vary from state to state and depend on whether the lawsuit or claim is filed in federal or state court. The lawsuit or claim is barred or disqualified if it is not filed before the statutory deadline. Under certain circumstances, a statute of limitations will be extended beyond its deadline. The following are examples for a civil claim for professional malpractice:

- *Medical:* 1 to 4 years from the act or occurrence of injury, or 6 months to 3 years from discovery; certain circumstances will extend the statute, including if the party is a minor, when a foreign object is involved, or in cases of fraud

- *Legal:* 1 to 3 years from date of discovery, or a maximum of 2 to 5 years from the date of the wrongful act

Four Cs of Medical Malpractice Prevention

1. *Caring.* As a healthcare professional, caring about your patients and colleagues is your most important asset. Showing patients that you care about them may result in an improvement in their medical condition and, if you are sincere, decreases the likelihood that patients will feel the need to sue if treatment has unsatisfactory results or if adverse events occur.

2. *Communication.* If you communicate in a professional manner and clearly ask for confirmation that you have been understood, you will earn respect and trust from your patients and other members of the allied health team.

3. *Competence.* Be competent in your skills and job knowledge by maintaining and updating your knowledge and skills frequently through continuing education.

4. *Charting.* Documentation is proof of competence. Make sure that all current reports and consultations have been reviewed by the physician and are evident in the chart. Chart every conversation or interaction you have with a patient.

How Effective Communication Can Help Prevent Lawsuits Patients who see the medical office as a friendly place are generally less likely to sue. Physicians, medical assistants, and other medical office staff who have pleasant personalities and are competent in their jobs will have less risk of being sued. Medical assistants can help by

- Developing good listening skills and nonverbal communication techniques so that patients feel the time spent with them is not rushed.

- Setting aside a certain time during the day for returning patient phone calls.

- Checking to be sure that all patients or their authorized representatives sign informed consent forms (after all questions and concerns have been addressed) before they undergo medical or surgical procedures.

- Avoiding statements that could be construed as an admission of fault on the part of the physician or other medical staff.

- Using tact, good judgment, and professional ability in handling patients.

- Making every effort to reach an understanding about fees with the patient before treatment so that billing does not become a point of contention.

▶ Administrative Procedures and the Law   LO 5.4

Many of your administrative duties as a medical assistant are related to legal requirements and fall under the heading of risk management. When correct policies and procedures are followed, the risk of lawsuits decreases, but if a lawsuit is brought against the physician, the same policies and procedures will be the physician's best defense. Keep in mind that everything you do and do not do reflects not only on you but also on the physician and the practice. Always follow office policies and procedures and follow your "best practices" at all times to do your part to avoid lawsuits.

Paperwork for insurance billing, patient consent forms for surgical procedures, and correspondence (such as a physician's letter of withdrawal from a case) must be handled correctly to meet legal standards. Documentation of appropriate and accurate entries in a patient's medical record not only provides proof of continuity of care but is legally important, should the physician ever require the record for a legal case involving the patient. You also may maintain the physician's appointment book—also considered a legal document—especially for tracking missed or canceled appointments. You will explore this aspect of medical assisting in the *Schedule Management* chapter.

In your role as a medical assistant, you also may be responsible for handling certain state reporting requirements. Items that must be reported include births; certain communicable diseases such as acquired immunodeficiency syndrome (AIDS) and STIs; drug abuse; suspected child abuse or abuse of the elderly; injuries caused by violence, such as knife and gunshot wounds; and deaths. Reports are sent to various state departments, depending on the content of the report. For example, suspected child and elder abuse cases are reported to the state department of social services. Addressing these state requirements is called the physician's public duty.

Phone calls also must be handled with an awareness of legal issues. For example, if the physician asks you to contact a patient by phone and you call the patient at work, you should not identify yourself or the physician by name to someone else without the patient's permission. You can say, for example, "Please tell Mrs. Arnot that her doctor's office is calling." If you do not take this precaution, the physician can be sued for invasion of privacy. You must abide by similar guidelines if you are responsible for making follow-up calls to a patient after a procedure or an office visit and when leaving messages on answering machines or on voicemail where someone other than the person you are attempting to reach may pick them up.

Documentation

Patient records are often used as evidence in professional medical liability cases, and improper documentation can contribute to the loss of a case. Physicians should keep records that clearly show exactly what treatment was performed and when it was done. It is important that physicians be able to demonstrate that nothing was neglected and that the care given fully met the standards demanded by law. One cliché to remember is "If it is not recorded, then it was not done." (On the same note, if it is recorded, it is assumed that it was done.) Pay attention to spelling in charts and keep a medical dictionary handy if you are not sure of a spelling. Today's healthcare environment requires complete documentation of actions taken and actions not taken. Medical staff members should pay particular attention to the following situations.

Referrals Make sure the patient understands whether you will be making the appointment with the referring physician, whether the specialty physician's staff will be calling to make the appointment with the patient, or whether the patient must call to set up the appointment. Document in the chart that the patient was referred, to whom, and how the appointment is to be made. If the date and time of the appointment are known, document this information also. Follow up with the specialist to verify that the appointment was kept. If a paper referral is necessary, make sure a hard copy is placed in the patient's chart. If the referral is made electronically, note the referral number in the patient's chart. Note whether reports of the consultation were received in your office, and document any further care the patient is to receive from the specialty physician.

Missed Appointments At the end of the day, a designated person in the medical office should document the charts of those patients who missed or canceled appointments without rescheduling. Charts should be dated and documented "No Call/No Show" or "Canceled/Not Rescheduled." The appointment book is also considered a legal document; make sure that all missed appointments are documented in the appointment book or within the electronic scheduling system. The treating physician should review these records and note whether follow-up is indicated.

Dismissals To avoid charges of abandonment, the physician must formally withdraw from a case. Be sure that a letter of withdrawal or dismissal has been filed in the patient's records (refer to Figure 5-2). All mailing confirmations should be filed in the record, such as the return receipt from certified mail.

All Other Patient Contact Patient records should include reports of all tests, procedures, and medications prescribed, including prescription refills. Make sure all necessary informed consent papers have been signed and filed in the chart. Make entries into the chart of all telephone conversations with the patient. Correct documentation requires the initials or signature of the person making the notation on the patient's chart as well as the date and time.

Medical Record Correction Errors made when making an entry in a medical record or errors discovered later can be corrected, but corrections must be made in a certain manner so that if the medical records are ever used in a medical malpractice lawsuit, it will not appear that they were falsified. So when deleting information, never black it out, never use correction fluid to cover it up, and never in any other way erase or obliterate the original wording. Draw a line through the original information so that it is still legible. Write or type in the correct information above or below the original line or in the margin. The *Medical Records and Documentation* chapter describes the proper procedure for correcting paper chart errors, and the *Electronic Health Records* chapter discusses the procedure for electronic health records.

Ownership of the Patient Record Patient medical records are considered the property of the owners of the facility where they were created. A physician in a private practice owns his or her charts or records, while records in a hospital or clinic belong to the facility. It is important to remember that although the facility in which the records were created owns the records, the patient owns the information they contain. Upon signing a release, patients may usually obtain access to or copies of their medical records, depending upon state law. Under HIPAA, patients who ask to see or copy their medical records must be accommodated with a few exceptions, such as with mental health records. If the physician decides it may be harmful to the patient to see the contents of the medical record and denies access, the physician is protected under the *doctrine of professional discretion.*

Retention and Storage of the Patient Record As a protection against legal litigation, records should be kept until the applicable statute of limitations period has elapsed, which is generally 7 years. In some cases, the medical records for minor patients must be kept for a specified length of time after they reach legal age. Some states have enacted statutes for the retention of medical records. Because the federal False Claims Act requires that financial records be kept for 10 years and medical records are often required to back up financial records, many legal experts suggest that medical records also should be kept for a minimum of 10 years. Most physicians retain records indefinitely to provide evidence in medical professional liability suits or for tax purposes. The medical record may provide the patient's medical history for future medical treatment. The chapter *Managing Medical Records* will go into more detail on this subject.

Credentialing *Credentialing* is used by various organizations, including insurance carriers, to ensure that healthcare providers are appropriately qualified to provide services and meet all the necessary requirements to do so. The qualifications are determined and approved by unbiased physician peer review groups. Specific criteria vary according to the physician or provider specialty and the provider's scope of practice. Physicians are broken into two types according to medical licensure—MD (medical doctor) or DO (doctor of osteopathy)— and then further broken down according to specialty.

As the office medical assistant, you may be responsible for credentialing any new providers joining the practice. In general, insurance companies require their doctors to hold and maintain the proper credentials. In order for a physician to participate with an insurance carrier such as Medicare, he must have the necessary professional credentials and go through the Medicare credentialing process, or he will not be allowed to bill Medicare for services provided to Medicare beneficiaries.

Medicare has three forms for credentialing:

1. Form 855B is used to establish or change a practice group number.
2. Form 855I is used to establish or reestablish a physician's individual number. In addition to completing this 29-page application, the physician also must provide his or her medical school diploma, individual NPI (national provider identifier), current license number, any board certifications for specialties, work history for at least 5 years, statement of any limitations, history of loss of licensure or felony convictions, history of loss or limitations of privileges or disciplinary actions, and outside verification of information provided.
3. Form 855R is used to link individual provider numbers to group practice numbers.

These forms are not complicated, but they are time-consuming. More information about Medicare's credentialing process can be found on the CMS website at http://www.cms.gov/manuals/downloads. In addition to the paper-based forms, CMS has established the Internet-based Provider Enrollment Chain and Ownership System (PECOS). This system allows physicians, nonphysician practitioners, and provider and supplier organizations to enroll, make a change in their Medicare enrollment, view their Medicare enrollment information on file with Medicare, or check on the status of a Medicare enrollment application via the Internet. Regardless of the application method used, once the Medicare credential is received, many other insurance plans will follow suit with credentialing or linking so the provider can also bill them for services provided. If a separate credentialing process is required, it is generally much less complicated than that required by Medicare.

The Food and Drug Administration Regulatory Function

The Food and Drug Administration (FDA) requires that drug manufacturers perform clinical tests on new drugs before humans use these drugs. These tests include toxicity tests in laboratory animals, followed by clinical studies (frequently called clinical trials). Venipuncture is performed and blood is drawn from controlled groups of volunteers. See Figure 5-4. Some volunteers are patients; others are healthy subjects.

Clinical tests are designed to consider the ratio of benefits to the risk of adverse side effects. If the clinical tests prove that the drug is safe and effective, the FDA approves it for marketing. The manufacturer must continue to demonstrate the drug's safety and efficacy (therapeutic value) and must submit reports whenever it discovers unexpected adverse reactions. The FDA can withdraw a drug from the market at any time if evidence suggests that it is no longer safe or effective.

During the clinical trials, the pharmaceutical (drug) company studies all aspects of the pharmacology of the new drug. When the company seeks approval from the FDA, it must document the pharmacodynamics, pharmacokinetics, safety (how many and what kind of adverse effects), and efficacy of the drug. In addition, it must present data regarding the effective dose—the amount of drug given at one time.

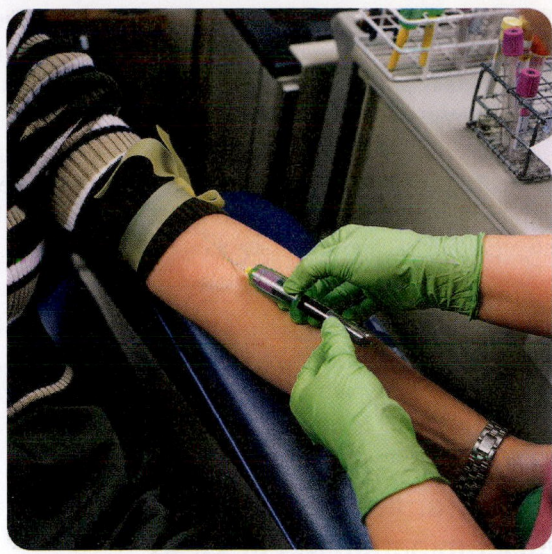

FIGURE 5-4 Blood tests provide baseline data on volunteers at the start of clinical drug trials.
© liquidlibrary/PictureQuest RF

After the FDA approves a drug, it continues its regulatory function to protect patients and consumers. These regulatory functions are discussed in detail in the chapter *Principles of Pharmacology* and include the following:

- Review of new indications proposals (applications from companies for new uses for a drug)
- Drug manufacturing—ensuring the proper identity, strength, purity, and quality of each drug
- Over-the-counter (nonprescription) drugs—approving drugs for use without supervision by a healthcare practitioner
- Prescription drugs—monitoring safety, use, and availability of drugs prescribed by healthcare practitioners
- Pregnancy categories—risk categories established by the FDA based upon the degree to which available information has ruled out risk to the fetus or breastfed infant.
- Controlled substances—regulation of drugs or drug products that are potentially dangerous or addictive
- The Comprehensive Drug Abuse Prevention and Control Act, also known as the Controlled Substances Act (CSA)—federal law established to strengthen regulation of potentially dangerous or addictive drugs by
  - Creating the Drug Enforcement Administration (DEA)
  - Designating five schedules for drugs based on the degree of potential the substance has for abuse or non-therapeutic use
  - Requiring doctors who administer, dispense, or prescribe any controlled substance to register with the DEA

Legal Documents and the Patient

You need to be aware of several legal documents that are typically completed by a patient prior to major surgery or hospitalization, including the advance medical directive, the durable power of attorney, and the uniform donor card. The Patient Self-Determination Act (PSDA), implemented in 1991, was designed to encourage patients and healthcare professionals to discuss end-of-life issues. According to the PSDA, certain healthcare facilities that are Medicare and Medicaid providers are required to ask each patient, age 18 or older, if he or she has an advance directive. Facilities are also required to inform patients of their policies regarding recognizing advance directives. They must discuss the patients' healthcare decision-making rights under state law regarding end-of-life issues. Contact your state's Public Health Department website for additional information.

Advance Medical Directive This is a legal document addressed to the patient's family and healthcare providers stating what type of treatment the patient wishes or does not wish to receive if she becomes terminally ill, unconscious, or permanently comatose (sometimes referred to as being in a persistent vegetative state). For example, an advance directive typically states whether a patient wishes to be put on life-sustaining equipment if she becomes permanently comatose. Some directives contain DNR (do not resuscitate) orders. These orders mean the patient does not wish medical personnel to try to resuscitate her if her heart stops beating. The directive is signed when the patient is mentally and physically competent to do so. It also must be signed by two witnesses. Advance medical directives are a means of helping families of terminally ill patients deal with the inevitable outcome of the illness. Having these advance directives in place can lower stress levels, as difficult decisions have already been made, and may help limit unnecessary medical costs.

Medical practices can help patients develop an advance medical directive, sometimes in conjunction with organizations that make available preprinted living will forms. The Partnership for Caring (based in Washington, DC) is one such organization.

Durable Power of Attorney Patients who have an advance medical directive are asked to name, in the second document, called a **durable power of attorney** (also known as a healthcare proxy), someone who will make decisions regarding medical care on their behalf if they are unable to do so. It is important that the person named in the durable power of attorney knows the patient's wishes ahead of time, so in the event that he is required to make medical decisions, he can be confident he is carrying out the patient's wishes.

The Uniform Donor Card In 1968, the Uniform Anatomical Gift Act was passed, setting forth guidelines for all states to follow in complying with a person's wish to make a gift of one or more organs (or the whole body) upon death. An anatomical gift is typically designated for medical research, organ transplants, or placement in a tissue bank. The uniform donor card is a legal document that states one's wish to make such a gift. People often carry the uniform donor card in their wallets. Many medical practices offer the service of helping their patients obtain and complete a uniform donor card. In some states, the Department of Motor Vehicles makes the process simple by asking you at the time you renew your driver's license if you would like to be an organ donor, with a card being issued to you at that time and a notation made on the driver's license that you are an organ donor. The patient's family should be aware of this wish to be an organ donor so that it is carried out upon the patient's death.

▶ Federal Legislation Affecting Healthcare

LO 5.5

Congress has passed legislation intended to improve the quality of healthcare in the United States, reduce fraud, and ensure that insurance providers will not discriminate against patients. The most significant healthcare laws passed in recent years are the Health Care Quality Improvement Act of 1986, the False Claims Act, the Genetic Information Nondiscrimination Act of 2008, and the Health Insurance Portability and Accountability Act of 1996. In addition, the Occupational Safety and Health Administration regulations are vital to the practice of healthcare and the safety of its practitioners, and these, too, are reviewed and often updated by the administration.

Health Care Quality Improvement Act of 1986

The Health Care Quality Improvement Act of 1986 (HCQIA) is a federal statute passed to improve the quality of medical care nationwide. Congress created HCQIA after discovering an increasing occurrence of medical malpractice and a need to improve the quality of medical care. The act requires professional peer review in certain cases, limits damages to professional reviewers, and protects from liability those who provide information to professional review bodies. One of the most important provisions of the HCQIA was the establishment of the National Practitioner Data Bank, designed to improve the quality of medical care nationwide by encouraging effective professional peer review of physicians. Information that must be reported to the National Practitioner Data Bank includes medical malpractice payments, adverse licensure actions, adverse clinical privilege actions, and adverse professional membership actions. This data bank is a resource to assist state licensing boards, hospitals, and other healthcare entities in investigating the qualifications of physicians and other healthcare practitioners.

False Claims Act

The False Claims Act is a federal law that allows individuals to bring civil actions on behalf of the US government for false claims made to the federal government, under a provision of the law call *qui tam* (from Latin, meaning to bring an action for the king and for one's self). The law was enacted because of the rising cost of healthcare, fraud, and abuse within the healthcare industry. As a result, laws have been passed to control three types of illegal conduct:

1. *False billing claims.* Fraudulently billing for services not performed is prohibited.

2. *Kickbacks.* Giving financial incentives to a healthcare provider for referring patients or for recommending services or products is prohibited under the federal Anti-Kickback Law and by state laws.

3. *Self-referrals.* Referring patients to any service or facility where the healthcare provider has financial interests is prohibited by the Federal Ethics in Patient Referral Act and other federal and state laws.

Violations of laws against healthcare fraud and abuse can result in imprisonment and fines, the loss of professional licensure, the loss of healthcare facility staff privileges, and exclusion from participating in federal healthcare programs such as Medicare and Medicaid.

Genetic Information Nondiscrimination Act of 2008

The Genetic Information Nondiscrimination Act of 2008 (GINA) was enacted by Congress to protect the rights of individuals from discrimination based on their genetic information. Protected genetic information includes the following:

- An individual's genetic test information
- Genetic test information of an individual's family member
- Information about a disease or disorder that has occurred in an individual's family member

This act prohibits insurance carriers and employers from using genetic information as a basis for denying insurance coverage or employment. Title I of GINA states that insurance carriers may not use genetic information to determine an individual's eligibility, coverage, underwriting, or premium cost. Health insurers may not require individuals to have genetic testing in order to obtain insurance coverage. Insurers also may not use previous genetic testing results to determine enrollment or coverage. Title II of GINA states that employers also are restricted from requiring genetic testing or using previous genetic testing results to determine eligibility for employment.

Occupational Safety and Health Administration

The Occupational Safety and Health Administration (OSHA), a division of the US Department of Labor, has created federal laws to protect healthcare workers from health hazards on the job. Medical personnel may accidentally contract a dangerous or even fatal disease by coming into contact with the body fluids of a patient contaminated with a virus. Medical assistants also may be exposed to toxic substances in the office. OSHA regulations describe the precautions a medical office must take with clothing, housekeeping, recordkeeping, and training to minimize the risk of disease or injury.

Some of the most important OSHA regulations are those for controlling workers' exposure to infectious disease. These regulations are set forth in the OSHA Bloodborne Pathogens Protection Standard of 1991. A pathogen is any microorganism that causes disease. Microorganisms are microscopic living bodies, such as viruses or bacteria, that may be present in a patient's blood or other body fluids (saliva or semen).

Of particular concern to medical workers are the human immunodeficiency virus (HIV), which causes AIDS, and the hepatitis B virus (HBV). AIDS damages the body's immune system and thus its ability to fight disease. Historically, AIDS has almost always been fatal, but better antiviral drugs have been more and more successful in keeping the virus under control. HBV is a highly contagious disease that is potentially fatal. It causes inflammation of the liver and may cause liver failure. Every year, about 8,700 healthcare workers become HBV-infected from patient-related or body substance exposures at work, and about 200 die from the disease.

OSHA requires that medical professionals in medical practices follow what are called Standard Precautions. These were developed by the Centers for Disease Control and Prevention (CDC) to prevent medical professionals from exposing themselves and others to bloodborne pathogens. Exposure can occur, for example, through skin that has been broken from a needle puncture or other wound and through mucous membranes, such as those in the nose and throat. If these areas come into contact with a patient's (or coworker's) blood or body fluids, a virus could be transferred from one person to another. The chapter *Infection Control Fundamentals* discusses OSHA and Standard Precautions in more detail.

Health Insurance Portability and Accountability Act

On August 21, 1996, the US Congress passed the Health Insurance Portability and Accountability Act (HIPAA). The primary goals of the act were to improve the portability and continuity of healthcare coverage in group and individual markets; to combat waste, fraud, and abuse in healthcare insurance and healthcare delivery; to promote the use of medical savings accounts; to improve access to long-term care services and coverage; and to simplify the administration of health insurance.

The primary purposes of HIPAA are to

- Improve the efficiency and effectiveness of healthcare delivery by creating a national framework for health privacy protection that builds on efforts by states, health systems, individual organizations, and individuals.

- Protect and enhance the rights of patients by providing them access to their health information and controlling the inappropriate use or disclosure of that information.

- Improve the quality of healthcare by restoring trust in the healthcare system among consumers, healthcare professionals, and the multitude of organizations and individuals committed to the delivery of care.

HIPAA is divided into two main sections of law: Title I, which addresses healthcare portability, and Title II, which covers the prevention of healthcare fraud and abuse, administrative simplification, and medical liability reform. Although in this text you will study Titles I and II in more detail, you also should be aware of three other titles included in HIPAA regulations: Title III—tax-related health provisions governing medical savings accounts; Title IV—application and enforcement of group health insurance requirements; and Title V—revenue off set governing tax deductions for employers providing company-owned life insurance premiums.

Title I: Healthcare Portability The issue of portability deals with protecting healthcare coverage for employees who change jobs, allowing them to carry their existing plans with them to new jobs. HIPAA provides the following protections for employees and their families:

- Increases workers' ability to get healthcare coverage when starting a new job

- Reduces workers' probability of losing existing healthcare coverage

- Helps workers maintain continuous healthcare coverage when changing jobs

- Helps workers purchase health insurance on their own if they lose coverage under an employer's group plan and have no other healthcare coverage available

The specific protections of this title include the following:

- Limits the use of exclusions for preexisting conditions

- Prohibits group plans from discriminating by denying coverage or charging extra for coverage based on an individual's or a family member's past or present poor health

- Guarantees certain small employers, as well as certain individuals who lose job-related coverage, the right to purchase health insurance

- Guarantees, in most cases, that employers or individuals who purchase health insurance can renew the coverage regardless of any health conditions of individuals covered under the insurance policy

Title II: Prevention of Healthcare Fraud and Abuse, Administrative Simplification, and Medical Liability Reform The HIPAA Standards for Privacy of Individually Identifiable Health Information (IIHI) provided the first comprehensive federal protection for the privacy of both IIHI and personal, or protected, health information. The *HIPAA Privacy Rule* is designed to provide strong privacy protections that do not interfere with patient access to healthcare or the quality of healthcare delivery. The privacy rule is intended to

- Give patients more control over their health information.

- Set boundaries on the use and release of healthcare records.

- Establish appropriate safeguards that healthcare providers and others must achieve to protect the privacy of health information.

- Hold violators accountable, with civil and criminal penalties that can be imposed if they violate patients' privacy rights.

- Strike a balance when public responsibility supports disclosure of some forms of data—for example, to protect public health.

Before the HIPAA Privacy Rule, the personal information transferred among healthcare providers and third-party payers fell under a patchwork of federal and state laws. This meant that unless forbidden by state or local law, IIHI could be distributed, for reasons that had nothing to do with a patient's medical treatment or healthcare reimbursement, to other agencies. For example, patient information held by a health plan could be passed on to a lender, who could then deny the patient's application for a home mortgage or a credit card; or it could be given to an employer, who could use it in personnel decisions—all without patient knowledge or consent. HIPAA stopped that.

Individually identifiable health information includes

- Patient name, address, phone numbers, and e-mail address.
- Patient dates (birth, death, admission, discharge, etc.).
- Social Security number.
- Medical record numbers.
- Health plan beneficiary numbers.
- Account numbers.
- Certificate or license numbers.
- Vehicle identifiers and serial numbers, including license plate numbers.
- Device identifiers and serial numbers.
- Web Universal Resource Locators (URLs) and Internet Protocol (IP) addresses.

The core of the HIPAA Privacy Rule is the protection, use, and disclosure of *protected health information (PHI)*. Protected health information means individually identifiable health information that is transmitted or maintained by electronic or other media, such as computer storage devices. The Privacy Rule protects all PHI held or transmitted by a covered entity, which includes healthcare providers, health plans, and healthcare clearinghouses. Other covered entities include employers, life insurers, schools or universities, and public health authorities. PHI can come in any form or medium, such as electronic, paper, or oral, including verbal communications among staff members, patients, and other providers. The Privacy Rule covers the following PHI:

- The past, present, or future physical or mental health or condition of an individual
- Healthcare that is provided to an individual
- Billing or payments made for healthcare provided

Information that is not individually identifiable or is unable to be tied to the identity of a particular patient is not subject to the Privacy Rule.

Use and *disclosure* are the two fundamental concepts in the HIPAA Privacy Rule. It is important to understand the differences between these terms. *Use* limits the sharing of information within a covered entity. Performing any of the following actions to PHI by employees or other members of an organization's workforce means the information is being used:

- Sharing
- Employing
- Applying

- Utilizing
- Examining
- Analyzing

Disclosure restricts the sharing of information outside the entity holding the information. Performing any of the following actions so that information is transmitted outside the entity constitutes disclosure:

- Releasing
- Transferring
- Providing access to
- Divulging in any manner

Managing and Storing Patient Information Because of HIPAA, medical facilities have undergone many changes to the way they manage and store patient information. Many facilities now contract consultants that specialize in HIPAA, and large facilities, such as hospitals, often employ a compliance officer. Patients must be given the opportunity to read the office privacy practices and receive a copy of them, signing an acknowledgment that they have received them. Should the patient refuse to sign the acknowledgment, the refusal should be documented in the medical record to prove *due diligence* and a "good faith effort" by the office to provide the patient with the privacy practices. The Privacy Rule requires the provider to perform activities including

- Notifying patients of their privacy rights and how their information is used.
- Adopting and implementing privacy procedures for its practice, hospital, or plan.
- Training employees so that they understand the privacy procedures.
- Designating an individual responsible for seeing that the privacy procedures are adopted and followed.
- Securing patient records containing IIHI so that they are not readily available to those who do not need them.

Patient Notification Since the HIPAA Privacy Rule's effective date, medical facilities have made major changes in how they inform patients of their HIPAA compliance. You may have noticed, as a patient yourself, the forms and information packets that are now provided by your healthcare providers. The first step in informing patients of HIPAA compliance is the communication of patient rights, conveyed through a document called Notice of Privacy Practices (NPP). This notice must

- Be written in plain, simple language.
- Include a header that reads. "This notice describes how medical information about you may be used and disclosed and how you can get access to this information. Please review carefully."
- Describe the covered entity's uses and disclosures of PHI.
- Describe an individual's rights under the Privacy Rule.
- Describe the covered entity's duties.

- Describe how to register complaints concerning suspected privacy violations.
- Specify a point of contact.
- Specify an effective date.
- State that the entity reserves the right to change its privacy practices.

See Figure 5-5 for an example of a HIPAA Notice of Privacy Practices. Procedure 5-1, found at the end of this chapter, outlines the steps in obtaining a signature for receipt of the NPP.

In addition to understanding the office obligations under HIPAA, remember, it has also given patients an increased understanding about their right to privacy regarding their health information. These rights include the following:

- The right to access, copy, and inspect their healthcare information
- The right to request an amendment to their healthcare information
- The right to obtain an accounting of certain disclosures of their healthcare information

BWW

BWW Medical Associates, PC
305 Main Street, Port Snead YZ 12345-9876
Tel: 555-654-3210, Fax: 555-987-6543
Web: BWWAssociates.com

Paul F. Buckwalter, MD
Alexis N. Whalen, MD
Elizabeth H. Williams, MD

Notice of Privacy Practices

I understand that BWW Medical Associates, PC creates and maintains medical records describing my health history, symptoms, examinations, test results, diagnoses, treatments, and plans for my future care and/or treatment. I further understand that this information may be used for any of the following:

1. Plan and document my care and treatment
2. Communicate with health professionals involved in my care and treatment
3. Verify insurance coverage for planned procedures and/or treatments for the applicable diagnoses
4. Application of any medical or surgical procedures and diagnoses (codes) to my medical insurance claim forms as application for payment of services rendered
5. Assessment of quality of care and utilization review of the healthcare professionals providing my care

Additionally, it has been explained to me that

1. A complete description of the use and disclosure of this information is included in the *Notice of Information of Privacy Practices,* which has been provided to me.
2. I have had a right to review this information prior to signing this consent.
3. BWW Medical Associates, PC has the right to change this notice and their practices.
4. Any revision of this notice will be mailed to me at the address I provided to them prior to its implementation.
5. I may object to the use of my health information for specific purposes.
6. I may request restrictions as to the manner my information may be used or disclosed in order to carry out treatment, payment, or health information.
7. I understand that it is not required that my requested restrictions be honored.
8. I may revoke this consent in writing, except for those disclosures which may have taken place prior to the receipt of my revocation.

At the time of the document signing, I request the following restrictions to disclosure or use of my health information: _____

_____

_____   _____
Printed Name of Patient or Legal Guardian   Signature of Parent or Legal Guardian

_____   _____
Printed Name of Witness/Title   Signature of Witness/Title

Date: _____

FIGURE 5-5   Example of a Notice of Privacy Practices and acknowledgment.

- The right to alternate means of receiving communications from providers
- The right to complain about alleged violations of the regulations and the provider's own information policies

Figure 5-6 gives an example of a typical privacy violation complaint form, which the office should keep on hand in case a patient feels his privacy rights have been violated. As the medical assistant, you may need to help the patient complete this form. Procedure 5-2 at the end of this chapter provides practice in assisting with this form.

Sharing Patient Information When sharing patient information, HIPAA will allow the provider to use healthcare information for *treatment, payment, and operations (TPO)*:

- *Treatment.* Providers are allowed to share information in order to provide care to patients.
- *Payment.* Providers are allowed to share information in order to receive payment for the treatment provided.
- *Operations.* Providers are allowed to share information to conduct normal business activities, such as quality improvement.

BWW

BWW Medical Associates, PC
305 Main Street, Port Snead YZ 12345-9876
Tel: 555-654-3210, Fax: 555-987-6543
Web: BWWAssociates.com

Paul F. Buckwalter, MD
Alexis N. Whalen, MD
Elizabeth H. Williams, MD

Privacy Violation Complaint

As per our Privacy Policies and Procedures, we are providing this form for individuals who feel they have a complaint regarding how their protected health information was handled by our office. You have the right to make a complaint and we may take no retaliatory actions against you because of it. We will respond to this complaint within 30 days of its receipt.

Patient Name: _____

Address: _____

DOB: _____ Date of Complaint: _____

Phone: Home _____ Cell _____ Work _____

Best time to reach you: _____

Reason for the complaint (please be as specific as possible, attaching additional documentation as necessary): _____

_____

_____

_____

_____

_____   _____
Signature   Date

Office Use Only

Received by: _____ Date _____

Follow-up Started on (date): _____

FIGURE 5-6 Sample of a Privacy Violation Complaint form.

If the use of patient information does not fall under TPO, then written authorization must be obtained before sharing information with anyone (Figure 5-7). Some of the core elements of an authorization form are

- Specific and meaningful descriptions of the authorized information.
- Persons authorized to use or disclose protected health information.
- Purpose of the requested information.

- Statement of the patient's right to revoke the authorization.
- Signature of the patient and date signed.

Procedure 5-3 at the end of the chapter outlines the steps to be taken to obtain an authorization to release PHI.

HIPAA Security Rule In February 2003, the final regulations were issued regarding the administrative, physical, and technical safeguards to protect the confidentiality, integrity, and availability of health information covered by HIPAA.

BWW

BWW Medical Associates, PC
305 Main Street, Port Snead YZ 12345-9876
Tel: 555-654-3210, Fax: 555-987-6543
Web: BWWAssociates.com

Paul F. Buckwalter, MD
Alexis N. Whalen, MD
Elizabeth H. Williams, MD

Authorization to Release Health Information

I, _____ , residing at

_____ and DOB of

_____ , give permission to (name of practice) _____

to release to _____ of BWW Medical Associates, PC the

following information: _____

_____

_____

Reason for the Request: _____

_____

Signature of Patient or Legal Guardian _____

Printed Name of Patient or Legal Guardian _____

If Guardian, Relationship to Patient _____

This authorization will expire on _____

YOU MAY REFUSE TO SIGN THIS AUTHORIZATION. You may revoke this authorization at any time by notifying BWW Medical Associates, PC in writing. Revocation will have no effect on actions taken prior to receipt of any revocation. Any disclosure of information carries the potential for unauthorized redisclosure and the information may not be protected by federal confidentiality rules.

FIGURE 5-7   An example of an Authorization to Release Health Information form.

The *Security Rule* specifies how patient information is protected on computer networks, the Internet, disks, and other storage media and extranets. However, the rapidly increasing computer use in healthcare has created new dangers for confidentiality breaches. The Security Rule mandates that

- A security officer must be assigned the responsibility for the medical facility's security.
- All staff, including management, must receive security awareness training.
- Medical facilities must implement audit controls to record and examine staff who have logged into information systems that contain PHI.
- Organizations must limit physical access to medical facilities that contain electronic PHI.
- Organizations must conduct risk analyses to determine information security risks and vulnerabilities.
- Organizations must establish policies and procedures that allow access to electronic PHI on a need-to-know basis.

Computers are not the only concern regarding workplace security. The facility layout can pose a possible violation if not designed correctly. All facilities must take measures to reduce the identity of patient information. Some examples of facility design that can help reduce a confidentiality breach include the security of patient medical records (including charts), the reception area, the clinical station (or patient care area), and the location of fax machines.

- *Chart security.* When paper health records are used, patient charts and the information contained within them can be kept confidential by following these rules:
  1. Charts that contain a patient's name or other identifiers cannot be in view at the front reception area or nurse's station. Some offices have placed charts in plain jackets to prevent information from being seen.
  2. Charts must be stored out of view of a public area to prevent unauthorized individuals from seeing them.
  3. Charts should be placed on the filing shelves without the patient name showing.
  4. Charts should be locked when not in use. Many facilities have purchased filing equipment that can be locked and unlocked without limiting the availability of patient information.
  5. Every staff member who uses patient information must be logged and a confidentiality statement signed. Signatures of staff should be on file with the office.
- *Reception area security.* To be compliant with security rules, the following steps should be taken to secure the reception area:
  1. Log off or lock your computer or terminal, shutting off the monitor when leaving your terminal or computer.
  2. The computer must be placed in an area where patients and unauthorized personnel cannot see the screen.
  3. Many facilities are purchasing flat screen monitors to prevent visibility of the screen.
  4. Patient sign-in sheets may be used but must not include

the reason or nature of the patient visit. Likewise, patient names may be called out as long as no reference to the reason for the visit is made.
  5. Call centers and reception area phone conversations must be kept confidential. Many offices put the administrative office behind sliding glass windows to allow for privacy when on the phone with other patients or offices, so that people in the reception area cannot hear phone conversations.

- *Patient care area security.* All healthcare personnel should follow these guidelines to protect PHI in patient care areas:
  1. Log off or lock computer terminals, turning off the monitor when leaving the computer station.
  2. When placing charts in exam room racks or shelves, the name of the patient or other identifiers must be concealed from view.
  3. When discussing a patient with the physician or another staff member, make sure your voice is lowered and that all doors to the exam rooms are closed. Avoid discussing patient conditions in heavy traffic areas.
  4. When discussing a condition with a patient, make sure that you are in a private room or area where no one can hear you.
  5. Avoid discussing patients in lunchrooms, hallways, or any other place in a medical facility where someone can overhear you.
- *Fax security.* As a vital link among healthcare providers, insurance plans, and others, much information is exchanged over the fax machine in a medical office, particularly if the office is paper-based and does not have access to electronic communication. Private health information can be exchanged via faxes sent to covered entities, but PHI must still be safeguarded as much as possible by taking the following precautions:
  1. Use a fax cover page. State clearly on the fax cover sheet that confidential and protected health information is included. Further state that the information included is to be protected and must not be shared or disclosed without the appropriate authorizations from the patient.
  2. Keep the fax machine in an area that is not accessible by individuals who are not authorized to view PHI.
  3. Faxes received containing PHI must be stored promptly in a protected, secure area.
  4. Always confirm the accuracy of fax numbers to minimize the possibility of faxes being sent to the wrong person. Call recipients to confirm the fax was received.
  5. Program the fax machine to print a confirmation for all faxes sent, and staple the confirmation sheet to each document sent.
  6. Train all staff members to understand the importance of safeguarding PHI sent or received via fax.
- *Copier security.* Medical assistants should follow these guidelines to protect PHI at the copier:
  1. Do not leave confidential documents anywhere on or near the copier where others can read the information.

2. Shred copies containing PHI when no longer needed—do not discard copies in a trash container.

3. If a paper jam occurs, after removing the paper causing the jam, shred it if PHI is contained within the document.

- *Printer security.* To maintain the confidentiality of printed materials, follow these guidelines:

    1. Do not print confidential material on a printer shared by other departments or in an area where others can read the material.

    2. Do not leave the printer unattended while printing confidential material.

    3. Before leaving the printing area, make sure all computer disks, CDs, DVDs, or "jump drives" containing confidential information and all printed material have been collected.

    4. Be certain that the print job is sent to the correct printer location.

    5. Shred any discarded printouts—do not throw them in a trash container.

Violations and Penalties Each staff member is responsible for adhering to HIPAA privacy and security regulations to ensure that PHI is secure and confidential. If PHI is abused or confidentiality is breached, the medical facility can incur substantial penalties or even the incarceration of staff. Violations of HIPAA law can result in both civil and criminal penalties.

- *Civil penalties* for HIPAA privacy violations can be up to $100 for each offense, with an annual cap of $25,000 for repeated violations of the same requirement.

- *Criminal penalties* for the knowing, wrongful misuse of individually identifiable health information can result in penalties ranging from $50,000 to $250,000 in fines and between 1 and 10 years in prison.

Administrative Simplification The main key to the set of rules established for HIPAA administrative simplification is standardizing patient information throughout the healthcare system with a set of transaction standards and code sets. The codes and formats used for the exchange of medical data are referred to as *electronic transaction records.* Regulated transaction information receives a transaction set identifier. For example, a healthcare claim would receive an identifier of ASC X12N 837 version 5010—a standard transaction code given to any facility that submits an electronic healthcare claim to an insurance company.

Standardized code sets are used for encoding data elements. The following books are used for the standardized code sets for all healthcare facilities:

- *ICD-9-CM/ICD-10-CM.* This book is used to identify diseases and conditions. The transition to the ICD-10 version is planned for October 2015.

- *CPT 4.* This book is used to identify physician services or procedures.

- *HCPCS.* This book is used to identify health-related services and procedures, such as pharmaceuticals or hearing and vision services, that are not included in the CPT manual.

▶ Confidentiality Issues and Mandatory Disclosure   LO 5.6

Related to law, ethics, and quality care is the issue of when a healthcare worker, including a medical assistant, can disclose information and when it must be kept confidential. The incidents that doctors are legally required to report to the state were outlined earlier in the chapter. A doctor can be charged with criminal action for not following state and federal laws.

Ethics and professional judgment are always important. Consider the question of whether to contact the partners of a patient who has a sexually transmitted infection (STI) and whether to keep the patient's name from those people. The law says that the physician must instruct patients on how to notify possibly affected third parties and give them referrals to get the proper assistance. If the patient refuses to inform involved outside parties, then the doctor's office may offer to notify current and former partners. The *Caution: Handle with Care* section addresses this issue.

In general, the patient's ethical right to confidentiality and privacy is protected by law. Only the patient can waive the right to confidentiality. A physician cannot publicize a patient case in journal articles or invite other health professionals to observe a case without the patient's written consent. Most states also prohibit a doctor from testifying in court about a patient without the patient's approval. When a patient sues a physician, however, the patient automatically gives up the right to confidentiality.

The following are six principles for preventing improper release of information from the medical office.

1. When in doubt about whether to release information, it is better not to release it.

2. It is the patient's right, not the physician's, to keep patient information confidential. If the patient wants to disclose the information, it is unethical for the physician not to do so.

3. All patients should be treated with the same degree of confidentiality, whatever the healthcare professional's personal opinion of the patient might be.

4. You should be aware of all applicable laws and of the regulations of agencies such as public health departments.

5. When it is necessary to break confidentiality and when there is a conflict between ethics and confidentiality, discuss it with the patient. If the law does not dictate what to do in the situation, the attending physician should make the judgment based on the urgency of the situation and any danger that might be posed to the patient or others.

6. Get written approval from the patient before releasing information. For common situations, the patient should sign a standard release-of-records form.

Notifying Those at Risk for Sexually Transmitted Infection

Few things are more difficult for a patient with an STI than telling current and former partners about the diagnosis. In fact, some patients elect not to do so. When patients refuse to alert their partners, the medical office can offer to make those contacts. Often that responsibility lies with the medical assistant.

You are most likely to encounter such a situation if you are a medical assistant working in a family practice, an OB/GYN practice, or a clinic. So becoming familiar with all facets of the situation—from ensuring patient confidentiality to handling potentially difficult confrontations—will help you best serve the patient.

The first step is to get the appropriate information from the patient who has contracted the STI. Because the patient may be sensitive about revealing former and current partners, help him feel more comfortable. First, spend some time talking about the STI. How much does the patient know about it? Educate him about implications, including the probable short- and long-term effects of the infection. Explain how the STI is transmitted. Alert the patient as to precautions to take so he will not continue to transmit the infection to others. Help the patient understand why it is important for people who may have contracted the infection from him to be told they may have it.

Then, offer to contact the patient's former and current partners. Fully explain each step in the notification process, assuring the patient that his name will not be revealed under any circumstances. Answer any questions and address any concerns about the notification process. If the patient is still reluctant to provide information, give him some time to think about it away from the office and follow up periodically with a phone call.

Once the patient agrees to reveal names, write down the names and other information, and preferably phone numbers. To make sure you have correct information, read it back to the patient, spelling each person's name in turn and reciting the phone number or address. Write down the phonetic pronunciations of any difficult names. Tell the patient when you will make the notifications.

You now are ready to contact these individuals. Professionals who work with STI patients recommend the following guidelines for contacting current and former partners to alert them about potential exposure to an STI. Note that these guidelines are applicable only to STIs other than AIDS. Determine how you will contact each individual: in writing, in person, or by phone.

1. If you use US mail, mark the outside of the addressed envelope "Personal." On a note inside, simply ask the person to call you at the medical office. Do not put the topic of the call in writing.

2. If you make the contact in person, ask where you can talk privately. Even if the person appears to be alone, others may still be able to overhear the conversation.

3. If you use the phone, identify yourself and your office and ask for the specific individual. Do not reveal the nature of your call to anyone but that person. If pressed, tell the person who answers the phone that you are calling regarding a personal matter.

Once on the phone or alone with the person, confirm that you are talking to the correct person. Mention that you wish to talk about a highly personal matter and ask if it is a good time to continue the discussion. If not, arrange for a more appropriate time. Inform the individual that she has come in contact with someone who has an STI and recommend that she visit a doctor's office or clinic to be tested for the infection.

Be prepared for a variety of reactions, from surprise to anger. Respond calmly and coolly. Expect to respond to questions and statements such as

- Who gave you my name?
- Do I have the disease?
- Am I really at risk? I haven't had intercourse recently (or) I've only had intercourse with my spouse.
- I feel fine. I just went to my doctor recently.

Let the person know that you cannot reveal the name of the partner because the information is strictly confidential. Assure the person that you will not reveal her name to anyone, either. Explain that exposure to the disease does not mean a person has contracted it. Encourage the person to get tested to know for sure.

Tell the person that she is still at risk, even if she hasn't had intercourse recently or has had it only with a spouse. Let the person know that someone with whom she came in close contact at some point has contracted the disease. Even if the person says, "I feel fine," she may still have the infection. Again, stress the importance of getting tested.

Provide your name and phone number for contact about further questions. Recommend local offices and clinics for testing, and provide phone numbers. If the person will come to your office, offer to make the appointment.

Finally, document the results of your call. Log in the original patient's file the date that you completed notification. Include any pertinent details about the notification. Alert the patient when all people on the list have been notified.

The AMA has several standard forms for authorization of disclosure and includes disclosure clauses in many other forms. For example, the consent-to-surgery form includes a clause about consenting to picture taking and observation during the surgery. When using a standard form, cross out anything that does not apply in that situation. Medical practices often develop their own customized forms.

▶ Ethics

Medical ethics is a vital part of medical practice and following an ethical code is an important part of your job. Ethics deals with general principles of right and wrong, as opposed to requirements of law. A professional is expected to act in ways that reflect society's ideas of right and wrong, even if such behavior is not enforced by law. Often, however, the law is based on ethical considerations.

Bioethics: Social Issues

Bioethics deals with issues that arise related to medical advances. For many people, bioethical issues are particularly sensitive and highly personal issues. This may be true for you on a personal level as well. Remember that, as a medical assistant, you must remain nonjudgmental at all times regarding patient healthcare dilemmas and decisions. Here are three examples of bioethical issues.

1. A treatment for Parkinson's disease was developed that uses fetal tissue. Some women, upon learning about this treatment, might get pregnant just to have an abortion and sell the fetal tissue. Is this ethical?

2. If a couple cannot have a baby because of a medical condition of the mother, using a surrogate mother is an option some couples choose. The surrogate mother is artificially inseminated with the sperm of the husband and carries the baby to term. The couple then raises the child. Ethically speaking, who is the real mother, the woman who bears the child or the woman who raises the child? If the surrogate mother wants to keep the baby after it is born, does she have a right to do so?

3. When a liver transplant is needed by both a famous patient who has had a history of alcohol abuse and a woman who is a recipient of public assistance, what criteria are considered when determining who receives the organ? Who makes the decision? Ethically, treating physicians should not make the decision of allocating limited medical resources. Such decisions should consider only the likelihood of benefit, the urgency of need, and the amount of resources required for successful treatment. Nonmedical criteria such as ability to pay, age, social worth, perceived obstacles to treatment, patient's contribution to illness, or the past use of resources should not be considered.

Practicing appropriate professional ethics has a positive impact on your reputation and the success of your employer's business. As a result, many medical organizations have created guidelines for the acceptable and preferred manners and behaviors, or etiquette, of medical assistants and physicians.

The principles of medical ethics have developed over time. The Hippocratic oath, in which medical students pledge to practice medicine ethically, was developed in ancient Greece (see http://www.nlm.nih.gov/hmd/greek/greek_oath.html). It is still used today and is one of the original bases of modern medical ethics. Hippocrates, the 4th century B.C. Greek physician commonly called the "father of medicine," is traditionally considered the author of this oath, but its authorship is actually unknown.

Among the promises of the Hippocratic oath are to use the form of treatment believed to be best for the patient, to refrain from harmful actions, and to keep a patient's private information confidential.

The AMA defines ethical behavior for doctors in *Code of Medical Ethics: Current Opinions with Annotations* ([Use of 174 words from the American Medical Association's Code of Medical Ethics: Current Opinions and Annotation, found within the 2015 CPT Professional Edition. © American Medical Association [1995–2015].] All rights reserved.) Medical assistants as well as doctors need to be aware of these principles, some of which are included in italics here and explained as follows:

A physician shall be dedicated to providing competent medical service with compassion and respect for human dignity.

This means that medical professionals will respect all aspects of the patient as a person, including intellect and emotions. The doctor must decide what treatment would result in the best, most dignified quality of life for the patient, and the doctor must respect a patient's choice to forgo treatment.

A physician shall deal honestly with patients and colleagues and strive to expose those physicians deficient in character or competence or who engage in fraud or deception.

Medical professionals, including medical assistants, should respect colleagues, but they also must respect and protect the profession and public welfare enough to report colleagues who are breaking the law, acting unethically, or unable to perform competently. Dilemmas may arise where one suspects, but is not able to prove, for instance, that a coworker has a substance abuse problem or another problem that is affecting performance. Ignoring such a situation in medical practice could cost someone's life as well as lead to lawsuits.

In terms of billing, a doctor should bill only for direct services, not for indirect ones such as referrals. The doctor also should not bill for services that do not really pertain to the practice of medicine, such as dispensing drugs.

It is also unethical for the doctor to influence the patient about where to fill prescriptions or obtain other medical services when the doctor has a personal financial interest in any of the choices. For example, it can be considered a conflict of interest if a physician has ownership in a surgical center and refers patients to the center without disclosing this financial interest to the patient.

A physician shall respect the law and also recognize a responsibility to seek changes in requirements that are contrary to the patient's best interests.

Several legal or employer requirements have come under scrutiny as being contrary to a patient's best interests. Among them are discharging patients from the hospital after a certain time limit for certain procedures, which may be too soon for many patients. Insurance company payment policies have sometimes been criticized as unfair. So have health maintenance organization (HMO) financial policies that conflict with a doctor's treatment preference.

A physician shall respect the rights of patients, of colleagues, and of other health professionals and shall safeguard patient confidences within the constraints of law.

As previously mentioned, the Patient Care Partnership: Understanding Expectations, Rights and Responsibilities, originally established by the American Hospital Association in 1973 and revised in 1992, lists ethical principles protecting the patient. Some states have even passed this code of ethics into law. Among a patient's rights are the right to information about alternative treatments, the right to refuse to participate in research projects, and the right to privacy.

A physician shall continue to study; apply and advance scientific knowledge; make relevant information available to patients, colleagues, and the public; obtain consultation; and use the talents of other health professionals when indicated.

Keeping up with the latest advancements in medicine is crucial for providing high-quality, ethical care. Most states require doctors to accumulate continuing education units to maintain a license to practice. These units are earned by means of educational activities such as courses and scientific meetings. As discussed in *The Profession of Medical Assisting* chapter, medical assistants who are certified by the AAMA or AMT have similar requirements by the sponsoring certification board to earn CEUs to maintain their credentialed status.

A physician shall, in the provision of appropriate patient care, except in emergencies, be free to choose whom to serve, with whom to associate, and the environment in which to provide medical services.

Ethically, doctors can set their hours, decide what kind of medicine to practice and where, decide whom to accept as a patient, and take time off as long as a qualified substitute performs their duties. Doctors may decline to accept new patients because of a full workload. In an emergency, however, a doctor is ethically obligated to care for a patient, even if the patient is not of the doctor's choosing. The doctor should not abandon that patient until another physician is available.

A physician shall recognize a responsibility to participate in activities contributing to an improved community.

This ethical obligation also holds true for the allied health professions. In addition to knowing the physician's codes of ethics, medical assistants should follow the code of ethics for their certifying body, be it the AAMA or the AMT. See the *Points on Practice* box for the AAMA's Code of Ethics and Figure 5-8 for the AMT's Standards of Practice.

▶ Legal Medical Practice Models LO 5.8

There are five basic types of medical practice:

- Sole proprietorship
- Partnership
- Group practice
- Professional corporation
- Clinics

Laws governing the types of practice vary, but medical office personnel should be aware of the laws that apply to their employers' practice management models.

Sole Proprietorship

This type of practice is often referred to as a "solo practice." In this type of practice, a physician practicing alone assumes all the benefits for and liabilities of the business. Sole proprietorship practice management is no longer a popular option, as a result of the increased expenses and decreased insurance reimbursements. So more physicians are joining group practices or professional corporations.

Partnership

When two or more physicians decide to practice together, they may form a partnership based on a legal contract that specifies the rights, obligations, and responsibilities of each partner. One advantage of partnerships is sharing the workload, expenses, profits, and assets. A disadvantage is that each partner has equal liability for acts of misconduct, losses, and deficits of the practice, unless specified otherwise in the contract.

Group Practice

Group practice is a medical practice model in which three or more licensed physicians share the collective income, expenses, facilities, equipment, records, and personnel for the practice. Physicians in group practice may be engaged in the same specialty, calling themselves, for example, Associates in Cardiology, or several physicians may offer similar specialties, such as OB/GYN and pediatrics.

POINTS ON PRACTICE
AAMA Code of Ethics

The Code of Ethics of the AAMA shall set forth principles of ethical and moral conduct as they relate to the medical profession and the particular practice of medical assisting.

Members of the AAMA dedicated to the conscientious pursuit of their profession, and thus desiring to merit the high regard of the entire medical profession and the respect of the general public which they serve, do pledge themselves to strive always to:

A. Render service with full respect for the dignity of humanity;

B. Respect confidential information obtained through employment, unless legally authorized or required by responsible performance of duty to divulge such information;

C. Uphold the honor and high principles of the profession and accept its disciplines;

D. Seek to continually improve the knowledge and skills of medical assistants for the benefit of patients and professional colleagues; and

E. Participate in additional service activities aimed toward improving the health and well-being of the community.

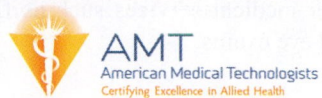

AMT Standards of Practice

The American Medical Technologists is dedicated to encouraging, establishing and maintaining the highest standards, traditions, and principles of the disciplines which constitute the allied health professions of the certification agency and the Registry.

Members of the Registry and all individuals certified by AMT recognize their professional and ethical responsibilities, not only to their patients, but also to society, to other health care professionals, and to themselves.

The AMT Board of Directors has adopted the following Standards of Practice which define the essence of competent, honorable and ethical behavior for an AMT-certified allied health care professional. Reported violations of these Standards will be referred to the Judiciary Committee and may result in revocation of the individual's certification or other disciplinary sanctions.

I.   While engaged in the Arts and Sciences that constitute the practice of their profession, AMT professionals shall be dedicated to the provision of competent and compassionate service and shall always meet or exceed the applicable standard of care.

II.   The AMT professional shall place the health and welfare of the patient above all else.

III.   When performing clinical duties and procedures, the AMT professional shall act within the lawful limits of any applicable scope of practice, and when so required shall act under and in accordance with appropriate supervision by an attending physician, dentist, or other licensed practitioner.

IV.   The AMT professional shall always respect the rights of patients and of fellow health care providers, shall comply with all applicable laws and regulations governing the privacy and confidentiality of protected healthcare information, and shall safeguard patient confidences unless legally authorized or compelled to divulge protected healthcare information to an authorized individual, law enforcement officer, or other legal or governmental entity.

V.   AMT professionals shall strive to increase their technical knowledge, shall continue to learn, and shall continue to apply and share scientific advances in their fields of professional specialization.

VI.   The AMT professional shall respect the law and pledges to avoid dishonest, unethical or illegal practices, breaches of fiduciary duty, or abuses of the position of trust into which the professional has been placed as a certified healthcare professional.

VII.   AMT professionals understand that they shall not make or offer a diagnosis or dispense medical advice unless they are duly licensed practitioners or unless specifically authorized to do so by an attending licensed practitioner acting in accordance with applicable law.

VIII.   The AMT professional shall observe and value the judgment of the attending physician, dentist, or other attending licensed practitioner, provided that so doing does not clearly constitute a violation of law or pose an immediate threat to the welfare of the patient.

IX.   AMT professionals recognize that they are responsible for any personal wrongdoing, and that they have an obligation to report to the proper authorities any knowledge of professional abuse or unlawful behavior by any party involved in the patient's diagnosis, care and treatment.

X.   The AMT professional pledges to uphold personal honor and integrity and to cooperate in protecting and advancing, by every lawful means, the interests of the American Medical Technologists and its Members.

(Revised by the AMT Board of Directors July 7, 2013)

10700 W. Higgins Road, Suite 150 | Rosemont, Illinois 60018 | (847) 823-5169 | www.americanmedtech.org

FIGURE 5-8   AMT Standards of Practice.

AMT Standards of Practice: Reprinted with permission from American Medical Technologists.

Professional Corporations

A corporation is a body formed and authorized by state law to act as a single entity. Physicians who form corporations are shareholders and employees of the organization. Forming a corporation has financial and tax advantages, and the fringe benefits for employees may be greater than in a sole proprietorship or partnership.

In forming a corporation, the incorporators and owners have limited liability in lawsuits. Some medical practices are managed by for-profit corporations that are formed by outside business interests or subsidiary corporations organized by hospitals. Physicians are hired as salaried employees with bonus options. The management corporation provides the facility, office personnel, employee benefits, human resource services, and operating expenses.

Clinics

Patients can be admitted to clinics for special circumstances and research. In many cases, clinics are hard to distinguish from large medical facilities.

Clinics are broad in their range of specialties and subspecialties, and many have sophisticated medical equipment and renowned medical practitioners. Clinics may be housed inside of a hospital or be free-standing. Urgent care centers, also known as walk-in clinics, exist so that patients have the option of being seen without an appointment.

In-store clinics are becoming more prevalent. Housed in large major chain stores and sometimes in chain pharmacies, they offer smaller medical services such as flu shots, other vaccinations, and eye exams.

Employment Law

Many medical assistants find themselves promoted into supervisory and managerial positions. Knowledge of employment and labor laws like those involving civil rights, sexual harassment, employment of persons with disabilities, fair labor laws, and family medical leave are important to all employees, but particularly so for those who oversee other employees. Labor and employment laws are covered in detail in the *Practice Management* chapter.

PROCEDURE 5-1 Obtaining Signature for Notice of Privacy Practices and Acknowledgment

WORK // DOC

Procedure Goal: To follow HIPAA guidelines and obtain the patient's signature that he or she has received and understands the office privacy policies

OSHA Guidelines: This procedure does not involve exposure to blood, body fluids, or tissue.

Materials: Preprinted Notice of Privacy Practices and Acknowledgment (see Figure 5-5), pens, and a copy machine

Method:

1. Explain to the patient the office privacy policy regarding protected health information.
   RATIONALE: *Some patients understand the spoken word more easily than the written word.*

2. Ask the patient to read the policy carefully and to feel free to ask any questions he may have regarding the policy. Answer any questions that arise.

   RATIONALE: *Patients must have a thorough understanding in order to acknowledge receipt of the privacy policy.*

3. When the patient's questions have been answered, witness the patient (or guardian) sign and print his name. Note any restrictions placed on the document.
   RATIONALE: *Restrictions must be noted so inadvertent release of information does not occur.*

4. Print your name and sign the document as witness, including your title.

5. Date the document when all signatures have been completed.

6. Make a copy of the document to file in the patient medical record and give the original to the patient.
   RATIONALE: *It is important that copies of all signed documents are in the patient's record in case of any legal proceedings that arise.*

PROCEDURE 5-2 Completing a Privacy Violation Complaint Form

WORK // DOC

Procedure Goal: To assist the patient in completing a Privacy Violation Complaint form if she feels her PHI has been compromised.

OSHA Guidelines: This procedure does not involve exposure to blood, body fluids, or tissue.

Materials: Privacy Violation Complaint form (see Figure 5-6), pens, private room to complete form, and a copy machine

Method:

1. Explain to the patient that all formal complaints must be made in writing.

   RATIONALE: *This provides legal documentation in case it is ever needed in court.*

2. Ask the patient if she feels assistance will be needed completing the form. If not, the patient may complete the form on her own. Answer any questions she may have regarding completion of the form.

3. When the patient completes the form, read it carefully, making sure it is complete and legible and the information regarding the breach of privacy is clear.

   RATIONALE: *In order to address the alleged breach, a thorough understanding of the complaint is needed.*

4. If the patient requires that any copies be made for documentation backing the claim, make the copies, returning any originals to the patient.
5. Make sure the patient signs and dates the complaint.
6. As the person receiving the complaint, sign the document as indicated and date it.

7. Explain to the patient that the office will respond to the complaint within 30 days of today's receipt.
8. Make a copy of the document for the patient and keep the original for the office files.
   RATIONALE: *Copies of all legal documents must be kept on file.*

PROCEDURE 5-3 Obtaining Authorization to Release Health Information

WORK // DOC

Procedure Goal: To follow HIPAA guidelines when obtaining the patient's protected health information without violating confidentiality regulations

OSHA Guidelines: This procedure does not involve exposure to blood, body fluids, or tissue.

Materials: Preprinted Authorization to Release Health Information form (see Figure 5-7), pens, and a copy machine

Method:

1. Explain to the patient the need for the requested medical information.
   RATIONALE: *In order for the consent to be valid, the patient must understand the need for the release of information.*
2. Obtain the name and address of the practice to which the authorization is to be mailed.
3. Fill in the patient's name, address, and DOB as required.
4. Enter the physician's or practitioner's name from your practice who is requesting the PHI.
5. Enter the information that is being requested.
   RATIONALE: *Only the required information may be requested and released to the practice.*

6. Complete the reason for request, explaining why the patient is requesting the information be sent to your office.
   RATIONALE: *To comply with HIPAA guidelines, a reason for the record release is necessary.*
7. Enter an expiration date for the authorization, giving a reasonable amount of time for the request to be fulfilled.
8. Prior to signing the release, go over with the patient the information contained within the release, answering any questions that arise. Be sure the patient understands the request may be withdrawn (in writing) at any time.
9. Witness the patient (or guardian) signature and date; if necessary, be sure the guardian relationship area is completed.
10. Sign and date the document as witness, including your title.
11. Make a copy of the document to file in the patient medical record and, if requested, give a copy to the patient.
    RATIONALE: *The release is a legal document and must be kept with the patient medical record.*
12. Make a notation in the medical record of the document signing and note the date the authorization is mailed.
    RATIONALE: *If the records are not received in a timely manner, the office will need to be contacted.*

SUMMARY OF LEARNING OUTCOMES

LEARNING OUTCOMES	KEY POINTS
5.1 **Differentiate between laws and ethics.**	A law is a rule of conduct or action prescribed or formally recognized as binding or enforced by local, state, or federal government. Ethics are standards of behavior or concepts of right or wrong beyond what the legal consideration is in any given situation.
5.2 **Identify the responsibilities of the patient and physician in a physician-patient contract, including the components for informed consent that must be understood by the patient.**	Physician responsibilities in a physician-patient contract include using due care, skill, judgment, and diligence in treating the patient; staying informed of the current diagnosis and treatment; performing to the best of the physician's ability; and providing complete information and instructions to the patient. Regarding informed consent, the physician must provide the following information: proposed treatment modes; why the treatment is necessary; risks of the proposed treatment; alternative treatments available; risks of the alternatives; and the risks if all treatment is refused.

LEARNING OUTCOMES	KEY POINTS
	Patient responsibilities in a physician-patient contract include following instructions given by the provider and cooperating as much as possible; giving relevant information to the provider; following physician instructions for treatment; and paying fees for services provided.
5.3 Describe the four Ds of negligence required to prove malpractice and explain the four Cs of malpractice prevention.	The four Ds of malpractice are duty—it must be proven that a physician-patient relationship exists; derelict—it must be proven that the physician failed to comply with standards of the profession; direct cause—it must be proven that any damages were directly caused by the physician's breach of duty; and damages—it must be proven that the patient suffered an injury. The four Cs of medical malpractice prevention are caring—the most important asset; communication—which earns respect and trust; competence—which proves abilities by maintaining and updating knowledge; and charting—which documents all aspects of patient interaction.
5.4 Relate the term credentialing and explain the importance of the FDA and DEA to administrative procedures performed by medical assistants.	The term *credentialing* refers to the approval process a healthcare provider must go through to be allowed to bill Medicare and other insurance carriers for providing medical services to patients under their insurance plans. Often, the medical assistant is in charge of submitting the required paperwork and documentation for the provider to gain this approval. The Food and Drug Administration (FDA) approves drugs for use on humans. It also regulates whether drugs are prescription-based or accessible OTC. The Drug Enforcement Agency (DEA) is responsible for controlling and overseeing the prescribing of controlled substances. Physicians must obtain and renew their license with the DEA in order to prescribe controlled substances.
5.5 Summarize the purpose of the following federal healthcare regulations: HCQIA, False Claims Act, OSHA, and HIPAA.	Congress enacted HCQIA in 1996 because it found that there was an increasing occurrence of medical malpractice and a need to improve the quality of medical care. The False Claims Act allows individuals to bring civil *qui tam* actions on behalf of the US government for false claims made to the federal government. OSHA created federal laws to protect healthcare workers from health hazards on the job. Title I of HIPAA was created so that employees could still have access to health insurance coverage when leaving employment for any reason. Title II was created to protect patients' individually identifiable personal information as well as their personal health information. It also allows patients access to their medical information on request and allows them to limit the sharing of that information. Additionally, patients on written request must be allowed to see a record of how their PHI has been shared and with whom.
5.6 Identify the six principles for preventing improper release of information from the medical office.	The six rules for preventing improper release of information include the following: (1) When in doubt about whether to release information, it is better not to release it. (2) It is the patient's right, not the physician's, to keep patient information confidential. (3) All patients should be treated with the same degree of confidentiality. (4) Be aware of all applicable laws and of the regulations of agencies involved with confidentiality. (5) When it is necessary to break confidentiality and when there is a conflict between ethics and confidentiality, discuss it with the patient. The physician may need to make the final decision. (6) Get written approval from the patient before releasing information.

LEARNING OUTCOMES	KEY POINTS
5.7 Discuss the importance of ethics in the medical office.	Ethics reflects the general principles of right and wrong. A professional, particularly a medical professional, is expected to follow especially high ethical standards.
5.8 Explain the differences among the practice management models.	There are five basic types of practice management models: (1) sole proprietorship (one physician), (2) partnership (two or more physicians), (3) group practice (three or more physicians), (4) professional corporation (a body formed and authorized by state law to act as a single entity; physicians are stakeholders and employees of the organization), and (5) clinics.

CASE STUDY CRITICAL THINKING

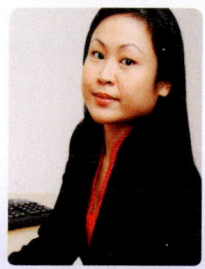

© Red Chopsticks/Getty Images RF

Recall Cindy Chen from the beginning of the chapter. Now that you have completed the chapter, answer the following questions regarding her case.

1. How will you respond to the extern's concerns?
2. Once Cindy becomes a phlebotomist, how should the information regarding her HIV-positive status be handled? Will the situation change if she develops AIDS?

EXAM PREPARATION QUESTIONS

1. (LO 5.1) A standard of behavior with a concept of right and wrong beyond the legal considerations is called
   a. Civil law
   b. Moral values
   c. Medical ethics
   d. Etiquette
   e. Ethics

2. (LO 5.1) The two types of law that pertain to healthcare professionals are
   a. Contract law and agency law
   b. Civil law and criminal law
   c. Civil law and medical law
   d. Litigation and malpractice
   e. Contract law and medical negligence

3. (LO 5.2) The physician's responsibility within the physician-patient contract includes all of the following *except*
   a. Setting up a practice within the boundaries of his or her license to practice medicine
   b. Setting up an office where he or she chooses and establishes office hours
   c. Determining whether to specialize
   d. Deciding which services to provide and how those services will be provided
   e. Treating every patient seeking care

4. (LO 5.3) Cases in which a person believes that a medical professional did not perform an essential action or performed an improper one, thus harming the patient, may result in
   a. Charges of slander
   b. Charges of medical negligence
   c. Charges of abandonment
   d. Charges of defamation
   e. Charges of fraud

5. (LO 5.3) Under the _____, words uttered to a patient by the medical assistant can be said to be the responsibility of the employer-physician.
   a. Law of agency
   b. Employee contract
   c. Civil law
   d. Criminal law
   e. Ethical considerations

6. (LO 5.4) The process used by various organizations, including insurance carriers, to ensure that healthcare providers are appropriately qualified to provide services and meet all the necessary requirements to do so is called
   a. Arbitration
   b. *Qui tam*
   c. Credentialing
   d. Subpoena
   e. Tort

7. (LO 5.5) Which of the federal acts was passed by Congress to improve the quality of medical care nationwide?
   a. HIPAA Title I
   b. HIPAA Title II
   c. OSHA
   d. HCQIA
   e. False Claims Act

8. (LO 5.6) Incidents and diseases, although normally considered confidential, that must be reported to federal, state, or local agencies come under the heading of
   a. Medical ethics
   b. HIPAA security rule
   c. STIs and AIDS
   d. Mandatory disclosure
   e. Civil law

9. (LO 5.7) Issues relating to medical advances come under the heading of
   a. Ethics
   b. Bioethics
   c. Religious freedoms
   d. Misfeasance
   e. Malfeasance

10. (LO 5.8) Which practice model provides the most legal protection for the physicians who form the practice?
   a. Sole proprietorship
   b. Partnership
   c. Group practice
   d. Professional corporation
   e. Clinics

SOFT SKILLS SUCCESS

You are a medical assistant at the family practice office of Dr. Janice Parrish. Elizabeth James and her daughter Anne have been patients at the practice for 10 years. Anne is 20 years old. Elizabeth is in the office for a blood pressure check. While you are taking her blood pressure, she tells you that Anne was in to see Dr. Parrish last week. She also says that she thinks Anne has been acting strangely and asks you if her daughter is pregnant. How would you respond to Elizabeth? What can you legally tell Elizabeth about her daughter?

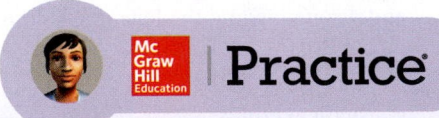

Go to PRACTICE MEDICAL OFFICE and complete the module Admin: Check In–Privacy and Liability.

Infection Control Fundamentals

6

CASE STUDY

PATIENT INFORMATION

Patient Name	DOB	Allergies
Shenya Jones	11/3/19XX	Cinnamon, peanuts
Attending	**MRN**	**Other Information**
Elizabeth Williams, MD	124-86-564	Wound C&S sent to Laboratory Services

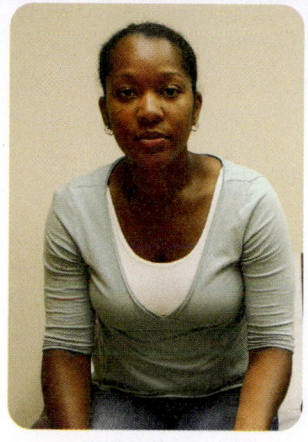

© McGraw-Hill Education

Shenya Jones, a 34-year-old female, arrives at the office with a swelling and a red pustule on her face. She states the problem started 2 days ago as a small pimple near her nose. It became irritated, then became extremely swollen and painful overnight. Now this morning there was yellow drainage noted at the site and the swelling has increased. The area of drainage is approximately 1 cm in diameter. The upper lip, side of the face, and nose are all swollen. She rates the pain in her face as 7 out of 10. The physician thinks the condition may be impetigo or methicillin-resistant *Staphylococcus aureus* (MRSA), a type of skin infection that is resistant to the common antibiotics used to treat it. Dr. Williams will culture the wound to find out what type of microorganisms are present and what specific antibiotics could be used to treat the infection.

Keep Shenya in mind as you study this chapter. There will be questions at the end of the chapter based on the case study. The information in the chapter will help you answer these questions.

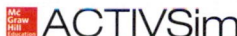

LEARNING OUTCOMES

After completing Chapter 6, you will be able to:

6.1 Identify OSHA's role in protecting healthcare workers.

6.2 Illustrate the cycle of infection and how to break it.

6.3 Summarize the Bloodborne Pathogens Standard and universal precautions as described in the rules and regulations of the Occupational Safety and Health Administration (OSHA).

6.4 Describe how transmission-based precautions supplement standard precautions.

6.5 Summarize OSHA's education and training requirements for ambulatory care settings.

KEY TERMS

alcohol-based hand disinfectants (AHD)

asepsis

carrier

endogenous infection

engineered safety devices

exogenous infection

fomite

general duty clause

healthcare-associated infections (HAI)

pathogen

reservoir host

standard precautions

susceptible host

transmission-based precautions

vector

work practice controls

MEDICAL ASSISTING COMPETENCIES

CAAHEP

III.C.2 Describe the infection cycle including:
(a) the infectious cycle
(b) reservoir
(c) susceptible host
(d) means of transmission
(e) portals of entry
(f) portals of exit

III.C.3 Define the following as practiced within an ambulatory care setting:
(a) medical asepsis
(b) surgical asepsis

III.C.4 Identify methods of controlling the growth of microorganisms

III.C.5 Define the principles of standard precautions

III.C.6 Define personal protective equipment (PPE) for:
(a) all body fluids, secretions, and excretions
(b) blood
(c) non-intact skin
(d) mucous membranes

III.C.7 Identify Center for Disease Control (CDC) regulations that impact healthcare practices

III.P.1 Participate in bloodborne pathogen training

III.P.2 Select appropriate barrier/personal protective equipment (PPE)

III.P.3 Perform handwashing

ABHES

4. Medical Law and Ethics
f. Comply with federal, state, and local health laws and regulations as they relate to healthcare settings

9. Clinical Procedures
a. Practice standard precautions and perform disinfection/sterilization techniques

10. Medical Laboratory Procedures
c. Dispose of biohazardous materials

▶ Introduction

From whooping cough in California to Ebola in West Africa, it is hard to open a newspaper or newsfeed without reading about an outbreak of disease. Despite all the medical advances of the modern world, humans continue to contract infectious diseases. As a medical assistant, you play an important role in stopping the spread of infections. In this chapter, you will be introduced to the fundamentals of infection control, including OSHA's role in protecting healthcare workers, the cycle of infection, OSHA Bloodborne Pathogens Standard, standard precautions, transmission-based precautions, and OSHA-required education and training for healthcare workers.

▶ Occupational Safety and Health Administration   LO 6.1

The Occupational Safety and Health Administration's (OSHA) mission is to "assure safe and healthful working conditions for working men and women by setting and enforcing standards and by providing training, outreach, education and assistance." Healthcare workers face safety challenges specific to caring for the sick and injured. For this reason, the Centers for Disease Control and Prevention (CDC) works closely with OSHA to ensure that these workers have documented best practices to follow. The CDC makes recommendations and guidelines regarding specific health and safety practices, and OSHA makes and enforces regulations based on these recommendations and guidelines. Copies of these guidelines can be obtained from many sources, including local OSHA offices; the CDC in Atlanta, Georgia; many industrial organizations throughout the country; and the Internet.

If a specific standard exists, its guidelines must be followed; however, if no specific standard has been developed, the **general duty clause** takes effect. This clause requires an employer to maintain a workplace free from hazards that are recognized as likely to cause death or serious injury. For example, all employers are expected to ensure that all exits are clear of obstacles and unlocked when the building is occupied. If an employer blocks a fire exit, a fire breaks out, and employees are injured because they are unable to safely leave the building, the employer has violated the general duty clause.

Employer Responsibilities

Employers have a legal responsibility to provide a safe working environment. In order to fulfill this responsibility, employers must

- Ensure that the workplace is free from serious recognized hazards and comply with Occupational Safety and Health rules and regulations.
- Inspect workplace conditions, confirming they conform to OSHA standards.
- Provide safe and properly maintained equipment.
- Maintain operating procedures and communicate new and updated procedures to employees.
- Provide accessible safety training to all workers.

Employee Responsibilities

Healthcare workers must follow regulations related to workplace safety, including chemical exposure, fire safety, electrical safety, and ergonomics and physical safety (see the chapter *Safety and Patient Reception*). In order to protect yourself, your coworkers, and your patients, you must follow the procedures, guidelines, and regulations outlined in your facility's infection control plan. Before you can understand the elements of an infection control plan, you must first understand how infections are transmitted.

▶ The Cycle of Infection   LO 6.2

As a medical assistant, your role in helping to create and maintain a safe and healthy environment for both patients and employees is key. This role includes understanding how infections occur and are transmitted in the population and practicing all necessary infection control precautions. To understand how infections are spread, you need to understand the cycle of infection.

Five elements make up the cycle of infection (Figure 6-1) These five parts must all be present for infection to occur:

1. Reservoir host
2. Means of exit
3. Means of transmission
4. Means of entrance
5. Susceptible host

Reservoir host

The infection cycle begins when the **pathogen** invades the reservoir host. The **reservoir host** is an animal, an insect, or a human whose body is capable of sustaining the growth of a pathogen. Many pathogens require a reservoir host to provide nutrition and a place to multiply.

The presence of the pathogen in the reservoir host may cause an infection in the host. At times, however, the host avoids full infection. A human **carrier** is a reservoir host who is unaware of the presence of the pathogen and so spreads the disease. The carrier exhibits no symptoms of infection. A human host also may have a subclinical case, which is a

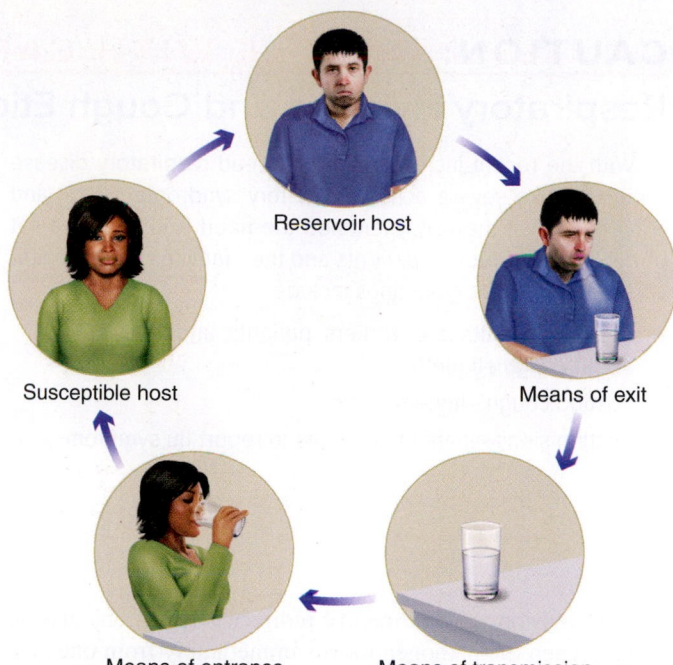

FIGURE 6-1   The cycle of infection must be broken at some point to prevent the spread of disease caused by pathogens.

manifestation of the infection that is so slight that it is unnoticeable. The host experiences only some of the symptoms of the infection or milder symptoms than in a full case. A wide range of diseases can be manifested subclinically.

An infection in the reservoir host may be either endogenous or exogenous. An **endogenous infection** is one in which an abnormality or a malfunction in routine body processes has caused normally beneficial or harmless microorganisms to become pathogenic. A bladder infection caused by *Escherichia coli* bacteria (commonly known as *E. coli*) is an endogenous infection. *E. coli* are beneficial bacteria normally found in the intestinal tract, but when introduced into the bladder via the urethra, *E. coli* can cause a bladder infection. An **exogenous infection** is one that is caused by the introduction of a pathogen from outside the body. A wound infection that occurs as the result of a healthcare worker transferring staph bacteria from her hands to a surgical site is an example of an exogenous infection.

Means of Exit

The next step in the cycle of infection is the pathogen's exiting from the reservoir host. Common routes of exit include

- Through the nose, mouth, eyes, or ears.
- In feces or urine.
- In semen, vaginal fluid, or other discharge through the reproductive tract.
- In blood or blood products from open wounds.

Means of Transmission

To reproduce after it has exited from the reservoir host, the pathogen must spread to another host by some means of transmission, either direct or indirect. Direct transmission occurs when the pathogen moves immediately from one host to another (through contact with the infected person or with the discharges of the infected person, such as saliva or blood).

Indirect transmission is possible only if the pathogen is capable of existing independently of the reservoir host. In this case, the pathogen survives until a new host encounters it and the pathogen takes up residence in that new host.

Airborne Transmission Pathogens can be transmitted to a new host through the air. For example, microorganisms may enter the respiratory tract of a new host by inhalation. Respiratory diseases such as influenza, or flu, are often transmitted this way.

Pathogens may be inhaled from a variety of sources, such as soil particles or secretion droplets from a sneeze or cough. When people inhale contaminated soil particles, fungal diseases may be contracted. If contaminated droplets are inhaled, diseases including influenza, chickenpox, and tuberculosis may be contracted. Because pathogens can spread relatively rapidly through airborne transmission, they may cause large epidemics among susceptible people. See the feature *Caution: Handle with Care* for more information on respiratory hygiene and cough etiquette.

Bloodborne Transmission Pathogens also can enter a new host through contact with blood or blood products. Bloodborne pathogens may be transmitted in a variety of ways:

- Indirectly—when pathogens are transferred through blood transfusions, needlesticks, or improperly sterilized dental equipment
- Directly—when the contaminated blood of one person comes into contact with another person's broken skin or mucous membrane, or when a pregnant woman transmits a disease to her fetus across the placenta

Transmission During Pregnancy or Birth If a mother becomes infected during her pregnancy, she can pass on pathogens to the fetus. An infection may be transmitted while the fetus is in the mother's uterus, which may result in damage to the fetus. This transmission is a form of bloodborne transmission.

Some bloodborne infections that produce only mild symptoms in the mother may be devastating to the fetus (for example, rubella). Other infections, such as herpes, gonorrhea, syphilis, or streptococcal infections, may infect the baby during passage through the birth canal. An infection that is present in a child at the time of birth is said to be congenital.

Foodborne Transmission A new host may be exposed to pathogens by ingesting contaminated food or liquids. Food can become contaminated when it is handled by an infected person who has poor hygiene habits, such as a customer at a self-service salad bar who did not wash his hands. The amount of contamination needed in a food to make someone ill varies. People who produce less stomach acid may become infected with a smaller dose of pathogens than those with higher acid production because stomach acid kills many microorganisms. An example of a pathogen transmitted by ingestion is a strain of *E. coli,* which can cause severe food poisoning.

Vector-Borne Transmission A living organism that carries microorganisms from an infected person to another person is known as a **vector.** The most common carriers are insects such as fleas, flies, mosquitoes, and ticks.

- Fleas carry the organism responsible for plague. Though the number of cases in the United States is very low, plague has been identified as a possible bioterrorism agent.
- Common houseflies carry pathogens from garbage and feces on their bodies and feet. When they land on food, they mechanically transfer these microorganisms to the food.
- Mosquitoes are carriers of several diseases of importance in the United States. They carry the organisms responsible for West Nile virus and malaria.

- Ticks carry the microorganisms responsible for Lyme disease and Rocky Mountain spotted fever.

Transmission by Touching Direct or indirect contact through touch is another method of transmitting infection. Direct transmission occurs through contact with an infected person's mucous membranes. Sexually transmitted infections are spread through the direct contact of one mucous membrane with another (in the penis, vagina, urethra, mouth, or anus) during sexual activity.

Indirect transmission occurs through contact with **fomites.** A fomite is any inanimate reservoir of pathogenic microorganisms. Examples of fomites include drinking glasses, doorknobs, shopping cart handles, pencils, and almost any surface or object that can temporarily hold microorganisms. So any object that can be contaminated by an infected person and then can transmit the infective agent to a susceptible host is considered a fomite.

Means of Entrance

Just as the pathogen needs a means of exit from the reservoir host, it also needs a means of entrance into the new host. Pathogens can enter a new host through any cavity lined with mucous membrane, such as the mouth, nose, throat, vagina, or rectum. They also can enter through the ears, eyes, intestinal tract, urinary tract, reproductive tract, or breaks in the skin. Most pathogens can take advantage of any means of exit and entry. For example, the droplets from an infected child's sneeze can land on a toy in a common play area. The next child to pick up the toy can transfer the infected droplets to her own nose, spreading the infection.

Susceptible Host

A final requirement must be met for the infection cycle to remain intact. The person into whom the pathogen has been transmitted must be an individual who has little or no immunity to infection by that organism. This individual is called a **susceptible host.**

Susceptibility is determined by a variety of factors—some related to the host, some to the pathogen, and some to the environment. Factors related to the host include the following:

- Age
- Genetic predisposition to certain illnesses
- Nutritional status
- Other disease processes
- Stress levels
- Hygiene habits
- General health

Factors related to the pathogen include the number and concentration of pathogens, the strength (virulence) of the pathogen, and the point of entry. Environmental factors, such as the host's living conditions and exposure to hazardous substances, also affect susceptibility.

Once a new host has been infected, the cycle can continue. This host becomes the reservoir host and eventually transmits the pathogen to yet another host.

Environmental Factors in Disease Transmission

The climate, food, water, animals, insects, and people in a community may greatly influence the types and courses of infection that exist there. In a highly dense population, the infection rate may be higher than in a low-density population because pathogens spread more quickly from person to person when people are in closer proximity. Proximity is one reason for the increase in respiratory disease during seasons when people are indoors for long periods.

Animals can also play a role in infection, as infections related to pathogens are found in domestic and wild animals. Unpasteurized milk from an infected cow may cause disease. Some pathogens can infect both animals and people. Butchers, hunters, and people in occupations dealing with animals may be at greater risk than other individuals for infection by those pathogens.

The environment affects the incidence of diseases carried by insects. Whether a potentially disease-carrying insect is in a certain area depends on whether that area has the appropriate climate and environment the insect needs to live. For instance, ticks may carry Rocky Mountain spotted fever or Lyme disease.

Economic and political factors also influence the pattern of infection transmission. They help determine the cleanliness of an area, the availability of medical care, and people's knowledge about preventing infection. Other factors that influence infection transmission include the availability of transportation, urbanization, population growth rates, and sexual behavior.

Breaking the Cycle

The principles of **asepsis** must be applied to break the cycle of infection and its spread. Asepsis is the condition in which pathogens are absent or controlled. For example, killing all microorganisms by sterilizing a suture removal kit and reducing the number of microorganisms on your hands by thoroughly washing them are types of aseptic practice. In medical settings, where many people are hosts to pathogens and many others are susceptible, asepsis can break the cycle by preventing the transmission of pathogens.

Specific measures to help break the cycle of infection include

- Maintaining strict housekeeping standards to reduce the number of pathogens present.
- Adhering to government guidelines to protect against diseases caused by pathogens.
- Educating patients in hygiene, health promotion, and disease prevention.

Hand Hygiene

Transmission by touching is the most common means of transmitting pathogens. The single most important aseptic procedure for a medical assistant is proper hand hygiene. The two most common methods of hand hygiene in the medical office are handwashing with plain or antimicrobial soap and water and hand disinfection with alcohol-based hand disinfectants (AHD). Consistent hand hygiene using appropriate methods protects the patient, your coworkers, and you from healthcare-associated infections.

Handwashing Aseptic handwashing removes accumulated dirt and microorganisms that could cause infection under the right conditions. Procedure 6-1 describes how to perform aseptic handwashing. In most cases, plain soap and water are adequate. There is some evidence that overuse of antimicrobial soap leads to antibiotic-resistant pathogens. For this reason, only use antimicrobial soap after assisting with exams and procedures where body fluids are present.

Alcohol-Based Hand Rubs An alternative to handwashing is the use of **alcohol-based hand disinfectants (AHD).** These are gels, foams, or liquids that have an alcohol content of 60% to 95%. AHD are the preferred method of routine decontamination and may be safely used in most situations; however, conditions in which they should not be used include

- When hands are visibly dirty or contaminated.
- Before and after eating.
- After using the bathroom.
- If you suspect you have come in contact with spore-forming bacteria.

A number of factors can affect the effectiveness of AHD:

- The type of alcohol used
- The concentration of alcohol
- Whether the hands are wet when the product is applied
- The contact time
- The amount used

If your hands feel dry before the recommended amount of time has passed, you most likely did not use enough. You should reapply the AHD using a larger amount. Procedure 6-2 describes the proper use of an alcohol-based hand disinfectant.

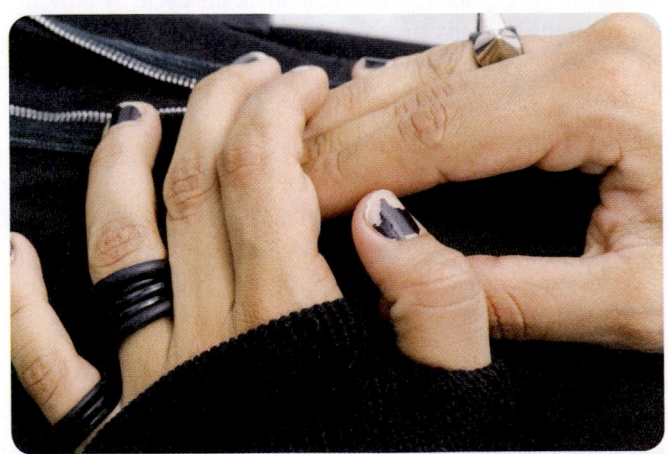

FIGURE 6-2 Chipped nail polish has a much higher bacteria count than natural, unpolished nails.
© Medioimages/Photodisc/Getty Images RF

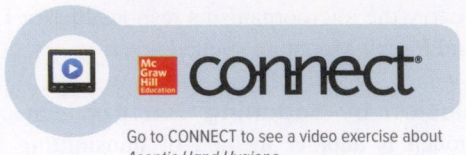
Fingernail Length Fingernails are a haven for pathogens. There is ample documentation that a large number of bacteria and some types of yeast can be cultured from underneath and around the nail, especially right next to the border of the skin and the nail. The CDC recommends that natural nail length be less than 1/4 inch.

Nail Polish and Artificial Nails The use of nail polish and artificial nails is discouraged in healthcare workers, as there is enough evidence that nail polish and artificial nails harbor pathogens. Although freshly applied nail polish has not been shown to contain increased numbers of bacteria and more research is needed, polish that is chipped has a much higher bacteria count than natural, unpolished or freshly polished nails (Figure 6-2). Healthcare workers who wear artificial nails or extensions have more gram-negative bacteria on their fingers than healthcare workers with natural nails. These increases are seen both before and after handwashing. The CDC recommends that healthcare workers not wear artificial nails or extensions when working with high-risk patients. The World Health Organization (WHO) recommends that healthcare workers not wear artificial nails when working with any patients.

▶ OSHA Bloodborne Pathogens Standard and Universal Precautions   LO 6.3

You must know the laws that require basic practices of infection control, also called infection prevention, in a medical office and how to apply these laws in your office. Federal regulations related to infection control and asepsis were developed by the Department of Labor's Occupational Safety and Health Administration and described in the OSHA Bloodborne Pathogens Standard of 1991. These laws protect healthcare workers from health hazards on the job, particularly from accidentally acquiring infections. They also help protect patients and any other people who come into the medical office.

OSHA Bloodborne Pathogens Standard

To ensure that biohazardous materials do not endanger people or the environment, laws set forth in the OSHA Bloodborne Pathogens Standard of 1991 dictate how you must handle infectious or potentially infectious waste generated during medical or surgical procedures. According to these rules, any potentially infectious waste materials must be appropriately discarded or held for processing in biohazardous waste containers. These wastes include the following:

- Blood products
- Body fluids
- Human tissues
- Cultures

- Vaccines (special preparations administered to produce immunity)
- Table paper, linen, towels, and gauze containing body fluids
- Used scalpels, needles, sutures with needles attached, and other sharp instruments (known as sharps)
- Specula
- Inoculating loops
- Used gloves, disposable instruments, cotton swabs, and disposable applicators

Many medical offices use only disposable paper gowns, drapes, coverings, and towels. Some offices, however, use cloth linens, which must be laundered. Certain rules apply to the laundering of cloth linens that are soiled with potentially infectious materials.

Medical offices use outside, licensed waste management services approved by the Environmental Protection Agency (EPA) to dispose of medical waste. A waste management service can provide instructions for preparing items before they are taken away.

The disposition and handling of contaminated sharps are of special concern because these instruments can easily puncture the skin and expose you to extremely dangerous viruses. Used sharps must never be bent, broken, recapped, or otherwise tampered with. After use, place them in a rigid, leakproof, puncture-resistant biohazardous waste container for sharps. Procedure 6-3 demonstrates the correct method for using a biohazardous sharps container. Disposable and reusable sharps are kept in separate containers. Metal basins containing disinfectant are often used to store reusable sharps until they can be processed. The outside waste management company may supply containers for the disposable items, sterilize them on its premises, and discard them in the city trash dump or incinerate them. See the *Caution: Handle with Care* section for a discussion of the guidelines you must follow when disposing of biohazardous waste and potentially infectious laundry waste.

OSHA's laws for hazardous waste disposal, as well as other OSHA regulations about measures to prevent the spread of infection, provide a margin of safety, ensuring that medical facilities meet at least the minimal criteria for asepsis. These laws include requirements for training personnel, keeping records, housekeeping, wearing protective gear, and other measures.

Although federal laws exist, individual states have some discretion in applying them. You should become familiar with the laws in your state to ensure that you are helping your medical office comply. Any outside cleaning service used by the office also should be made aware of these standards. Penalties for failing to comply with regulations can be severe (see Table 6-1).

To be in compliance with the Bloodborne Pathogens Standard, an employer must meet these requirements:

- A written OSHA Exposure Control Plan must be created and updated annually or whenever procedures that require exposure to potentially contaminated material are added or changed. The plan must be available to all employees and to authorized OSHA authorities.
- Training must be provided to all employees describing the documentation mandated by the standard. This

TABLE 6-1	Infectious Waste Disposal: Penalties for Not Following Regulations, as Set Forth by OSHA	
Type of Violation	**Characteristics of Violation**	**Penalties for Violation**
Other than serious violation	Direct relationship to job safety and health but would probably not result in death or serious physical harm	Fine of up to $7,000 (discretionary)
Serious violation	Substantial probability that death or serious physical harm could result; employer knew, or should have know, of the hazard	Fine of up to $7,000 (mandatory)
Willful violation	Violation committed intentionally and knowingly	Fine of up to $70,000 with a $5,000 minimum; if violation resulted in death of employee, additional fine and/or up to 6 months' imprisonment
Repeated violation	Substantially similar (but not the same) violation found upon re-inspection; not applicable if initial citation is under contest	Fine of up to $70,000
Failure to correct prior violation	Initial violation not corrected	Fine of up to $7,000 for each day the violation continues past the date it was supposed to stop

documentation includes the symptoms, methods of transmission, and epidemiology of infectious diseases caused by bloodborne pathogens. Employees must also be instructed in the use of personal protective equipment, universal precautions, and engineering controls designed to prevent exposure. Procedures to follow in the event of exposure or emergency situations also must be part of the training. New employee training is required before the worker can perform a task that might pose a risk of occupational exposure and then on a yearly basis. Additional training is required when a new task or procedure is introduced that may change the employees' occupational exposure risk.

- The employer must make the hepatitis B vaccine available at no charge to all employees who are at risk for occupational exposure. Employees must either receive the vaccination or decline it in writing. The employer must maintain documentation of vaccinations and refusals. Employees who initially decline the vaccine are free to reverse their decision at any point during their employment.

Universal Precautions

OSHA requires medical professionals to follow specific "universal blood and body fluid precautions" as set forth by the

Proper Use of Biohazardous Waste Containers and Handling of Infectious Laundry Waste

Biohazardous waste containers are available in a variety of designs. Frequently, more than one design is used in the clinical setting. These containers are often provided by outside sterilization and waste management companies. Examples of biohazardous waste containers include

- Bags or containers that are red or have a biohazardous waste label (for any material contaminated with blood or body fluids, such as used dressings or gloves).
- Boxes with biohazardous waste labels (sometimes lined with red bags and used for disposable gowns, examination table covers, and similar items that may be contaminated with blood or body fluids).
- Rigid, leakproof, and puncture-proof sharps containers that are red or have a biohazardous waste label (for lancets, needles, and other sharp objects).

Every biohazardous waste container has a lid that you must replace immediately after use. In addition, you may not over-fill the container, and you must replace it when it is two-thirds full. All biohazardous waste containers must have a fluorescent orange or orange-red label with the biohazard symbol and the word *BIOHAZARD* in a contrasting color (Figure 6-3). Red bags or red containers may be substituted for containers with biohazardous waste labels.

You must follow these guidelines when handling biohazardous waste:

- Always wear gloves.
- Place biohazardous waste in the appropriate biohazardous waste container immediately or as soon as possible.
- Keep biohazardous waste containers close to the place where the waste material is generated.
- Keep the containers closed when not in use, close them before removing them from the area of use, and keep them upright to avoid any spills.
- If outside contamination of the primary container occurs, place that container in a secondary container to prevent leakage during handling, processing, storage, and transport.
- Drop—do not push—intact contaminated needles into the biohazardous waste container for sharps (Figure 6-4).
- To avoid accidental puncture wounds, never break off, recap, reuse, or handle needles after use.
- If there is a danger of biohazardous waste puncturing the primary container, place that container in a secondary container.
- Do not open, empty, or clean reusable sharps containers by hand.
- When they are two-thirds full, discard disposable sharps containers in large biohazardous waste containers.

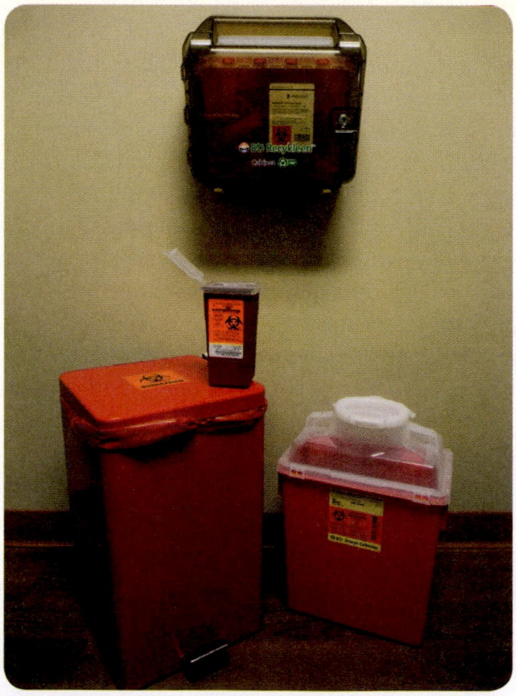

FIGURE 6-3 All biohazardous sharps containers must be rigid, leak-proof, and labeled with the biohazard symbol.
© McGraw-Hill Education. David Moyer, photographer

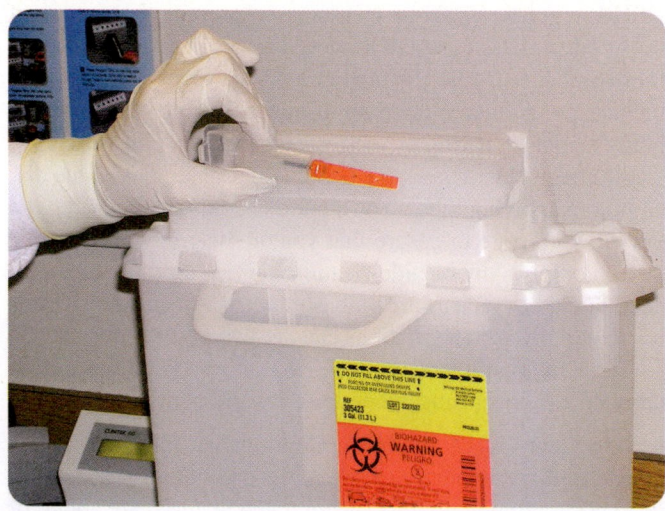

FIGURE 6-4 A sharps disposal container is a receptacle for used needles, lancets, specimen slides, transfer pipettes, and other disposable pointed or edged instruments, supplies, and equipment.
© Leesa Whicker

Spills of hazardous chemicals or biohazardous materials can happen anywhere in the office. Immediately clean up spills or splashes of potentially contaminated material. Depending on the material, you may need to use special hazardous waste control products. Be sure to dry the area if appropriate, or clearly indicate that the area is still wet. When cleaning up spills, take the following measures:

- Place material in a biohazardous waste bag.
- Ensure that the bag is leakproof on the sides and bottom and can be closed tightly.
- Place the plastic bag in a cardboard box also marked with the biohazard symbol.

The outside waste management agency will pick up the box for incineration before disposing of it in a public landfill. Procedure 6-4 demonstrates the proper disposing of biohazardous waste.

Potentially infectious laundry waste also must be handled in a specific manner. OSHA has issued these regulations for handling this type of waste:

- Place contaminated laundry in a red laundry bag that is marked with the biohazard symbol, or recognizable to facility employees as contaminated material to be handled using standard precautions.
- Pack any laundry to be transported so that it does not leak in transit.
- Have the laundry washed in a designated area onsite or at a professional laundry facility.

Any laundry service the medical office uses should abide by all OSHA regulations. For example, anyone handling laundry must wear gloves and handle contaminated materials as little as possible.

Department of Health and Human Services' Centers for Disease Control and Prevention. These universal precautions prevent healthcare workers from exposing themselves and others to infections. Following universal precautions means assuming that all blood and body fluids are infected with bloodborne pathogens. universal precautions apply to the following:

- Blood and blood products
- Human tissue
- Semen and vaginal secretions
- Saliva from dental procedures
- Cerebrospinal, synovial, pleural, peritoneal, pericardial, and amniotic fluids, which bathe various internal structures in the body
- Other body fluids, if visibly contaminated with blood or of questionable origin in the body

Breast milk, although not on the list of fluids covered by universal precautions, is generally treated as such because it has been shown that mothers can pass along the human immunodeficiency virus (HIV) to their infants through breast milk.

Healthcare facilities now use **standard precautions,** which are a combination of universal precautions and rules to reduce the risk of disease transmission by means of moist body substances (known as Body Substance Isolation [BSI] guidelines). Standard precautions apply to the following:

- Blood
- All body fluids, secretions, and excretions except sweat
- Non-intact skin
- Mucous membranes

Standard precautions are used in healthcare facilities for the care of all patients. They are an important measure for preventing the transmission of disease in the healthcare setting.

As mentioned earlier, some types of pathogens can be transmitted when the host's infected blood comes in contact with another person's skin. Skin that has been broken from a needle puncture or other wound and mucous membranes, such as those lining the nose and throat, are the areas that need the most protection. If a patient's (or coworker's) blood or body fluids come in contact with such areas, pathogens can be transferred from the patient's body to that of the medical worker.

OSHA outlines the routine safeguards to take when performing each medical procedure or task, depending on that task's level of risk. The degree of risk is determined by how much exposure to potentially infectious substances you are likely to encounter. When a procedure is explained, particular icons will be used to represent each of the OSHA guidelines. Figure 6-5 shows these icons.

OSHA divides tasks into the following three categories.

1. Category I tasks are those that expose a worker to blood, body fluids, or tissues or tasks that have a chance of spills or splashes. These tasks always require specific protective measures.
2. Category II tasks do not usually involve risk of exposure. Because they may involve exposure in certain situations, however, OSHA requires that precautions be taken.

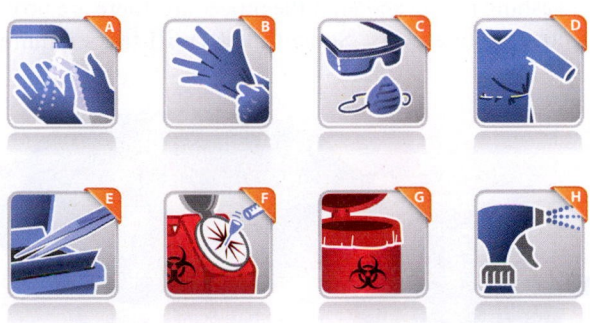

FIGURE 6-5 These icons will appear at the beginning of each Procedure to let you know which OSHA guidelines you should follow. They represent (A) handwashing, (B) gloves, (C) mask and protective eyewear or face shield, (D) laboratory coat or gown, (E) reusable sharps container, (F) sharps disposal, (G) biohazardous waste container, and (H) disinfection.

3. Category III tasks do not require any special protection. These tasks, such as taking a patient's blood pressure, involve no exposure to blood, body fluids, or tissues. (Observe patients for open wounds before you touch them to perform such tasks.)

Category I Tasks A Category I task you might perform is assisting with a minor surgical procedure in the office, such as the removal of a cyst. This procedure requires that you wash your hands before and after the procedure and that you wear protective gloves, a mask and protective eyewear or a face shield, and protective clothing. After the procedure, you must follow the guidelines for dealing with disposable and nondisposable sharp equipment and decontaminating work surfaces.

Category II Tasks A Category II task you might perform is giving mouth-to-mouth resuscitation to a patient. Because blood is usually not visible in such situations, the task is not classified as Category I. Gloves are still recommended, however, although you may not have time to get them in an emergency. Because you will be exposed to saliva in such a procedure, OSHA recommends using disposable airway equipment and resuscitation bags (shown in Figure 6-6), which medical offices are required to supply.

OSHA recommends taking these precautions to decrease the risk of transmitting infectious diseases through mouth-to-mouth resuscitation. Of particular concern to healthcare workers are HIV, which causes AIDS, and the hepatitis B virus (HBV).

AIDS damages the body's ability to fight disease and is ultimately fatal in most instances. Hepatitis B is a highly contagious and potentially fatal disease that causes inflammation of the liver and sometimes liver failure. Healthcare workers become infected with these viruses at work every year. Hepatitis B infection occurs far more frequently on the job than does HIV infection.

Category III Tasks A Category III procedure you may perform is giving a patient medicated nose drops. This task involves tilting the patient's head and holding the dropper above the patient's nostril. Although you must perform aseptic handwashing before and after the procedure, there are no other protective requirements. Some Category III tasks require no

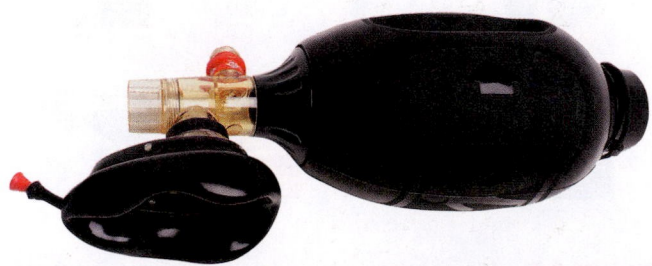

FIGURE 6-6 Resuscitation bags are used when a person requires mouth-to-mouth resuscitation. You must use one of these bags or another barrier device when performing mouth-to-mouth resuscitation.
© Stockbyte/Getty Images RF

precautions. Examples of these tasks are instructing a patient in how to use a heating pad and how to take care of a cast for a broken leg.

Written Exposure Plan

In order to reduce the risk of bloodborne pathogen exposure, OSHA requires that every medical facility have a written exposure control plan (ECP). Employees who are at risk of bloodborne exposure must have access to the ECP. This plan must be reviewed with new employees at the onset of employment and with all employees on an annual basis. A written copy of the plan must be made available if an employee requests it. The ECP must include the following:

- Determination of employee exposure
- Implementation of exposure control methods, including universal precautions, engineering and work practice controls, personal protective equipment, and housekeeping
- Hepatitis B vaccination
- Postexposure evaluation and follow-up
- Communication of hazards to employees and hazard training
- Recordkeeping
- Procedures for evaluating circumstances surrounding exposure incidents

Exposure Incidents

The OSHA Bloodborne Pathogens Standard also specifies what to do in case of an exposure incident. An exposure incident is one in which a worker, despite all precautions, has reason to believe that he has come in contact with a substance that may transmit infection. Contact may occur when a medical worker accidentally sticks himself with a used needle. A puncture exposure incident is the most common kind of exposure.

The basic rules covering exposure incidents apply to all serious infections, such as HBV and HIV. The rules covering HBV also include vaccination.

When an exposure incident occurs, the physician or employer must be notified immediately. This prompt action is extremely important because quick and proper treatment can help prevent the development of many diseases, such as hepatitis B. Timely action also can prevent the worker from exposing other people to a potentially acquired infection. Reporting the incident helps to prevent the same type of accident from happening again.

After such an exposure, the employer must offer the exposed employee a free medical evaluation. The employer must refer the employee to a licensed healthcare provider who can counsel the employee about what happened as well as about how to prevent the spread of any potential infection. The healthcare provider also takes a blood sample and prescribes appropriate treatment. If the employee does not want to participate in the medical evaluation and treatment, he has the right to refuse it. If this occurs, the employee's refusal should be documented.

If an employee who has not received the HBV vaccination and is not known to be immune is exposed to any infected person, especially someone who is HBV-positive or at high risk, it is recommended that the employee be tested for HBV and receive the vaccination if necessary. This vaccination may prevent infection. When the source person's HBV status is unknown and the person does not wish to be tested, the employee should be tested. If the source person agrees to be tested, the law requires that the employee be informed of the test results. The employee may agree to give blood but not to be tested. In such a case, the blood sample must be kept for 90 days in case the employee later develops symptoms of HBV or HIV infection and decides to be tested then.

The healthcare provider who performs the postexposure evaluation must give the employer a written report stating whether HBV vaccination was recommended and received and that the employee was informed of the results of any blood tests. Any additional information must be kept confidential.

Other OSHA Requirements

OSHA also requires that all healthcare workers who have occupational exposure to blood or other potentially infectious materials have the opportunity to receive the HBV vaccine, free of charge, as needed throughout employment. Within 10 days of a medical worker's starting a job, the doctor or employer is required to offer the worker the opportunity to receive this vaccination. The vaccine is recommended for all healthcare workers *unless*

- They have received it in the past;
- A blood test shows them to be immune to the virus; and/or
- There are medical reasons for which the vaccine is contraindicated.

In most cases, the employee is permitted to decline the vaccination if she signs a form accepting all the conditions. (A few employers require HBV vaccination as a condition for employment.) Even if the healthcare worker declines the vaccination when beginning employment, she still has the opportunity to receive the free vaccine and any necessary booster shots throughout her employment.

Needlestick Safety and Prevention Act In response to the Needlestick Safety and Prevention Act, which was signed into law in November 2000, OSHA revised the Bloodborne Pathogens Standard. The additional provisions to the standard are

- Healthcare employers must evaluate new safety-engineered control devices on an annual basis and implement the use of devices that reasonably reduce the risk of needlestick injuries.
- Healthcare facilities must maintain a detailed log of sharps injuries incurred from contaminated sharps.
- Healthcare employers must solicit input from employees involved in direct patient care to identify, evaluate, and implement engineering and **work practice controls** (controlling injuries by altering the way a task is performed).

In an effort to reduce needlestick injuries, the National Institute for Occupational Safety and Health (NIOSH) has specific recommendations for employers and employees regarding **engineered safety devices,** devices specifically designed to isolate or remove the hazard, and work practice controls. NIOSH recommendations for employers include the following:

Engineering Controls
- Eliminate the use of needles where safe and effective alternatives are available.
- Implement the use of engineered safety devices and evaluate their use on a regular basis.

Needlestick Prevention Programs
- Analyze sharps injuries to identify hazard trends in the workplace.
- Ensure employees are properly trained in the proper use and disposal of sharps.
- Adapt work practices that involve sharps to make them safer.
- Make safety awareness in the workplace a priority.
- Have established procedures for reporting all needlestick injuries.
- Evaluate prevention procedures and provide feedback to employees.

NIOSH recommendations for employees include the following:

- Avoid using needles if a safe alternative exists.
- Paticipate in choosing engineered safety devices.
- Use the engineered safety devices provided by your employer.
- Do not recap needles if possible.
- Before beginning a procedure, make sure you have a means of safe sharps disposal close by and ready for use.
- Dispose of used needles promptly and appropriately.
- Promptly report all sharps-related injuries.
- Advise your employer if you see sharps hazards in the workplace.
- Participate in bloodborne pathogen training.

▶ Transmission-Based Precautions   LO 6.4

In addition to strict adherence to standard precautions, there may be situations that require an additional level of precaution you must take in order to protect yourself, the facility staff, and other patients from exposure to infectious disease. For this reason, the CDC has developed guidelines known as **transmission-based precautions.** These guidelines are meant as a supplement to standard precautions when caring for patients with suspected or confirmed infection.

Transmission-based precautions include three categories:

- Contact precautions
- Droplet precautions
- Airborne precautions

Contact Precautions

Contact transmission is transmission by touching and is the most common means of spreading infectious diseases. The two subgroups of contact transmission are direct and indirect. As you learned earlier in the chapter, direct contact involves the spread of microorganisms from person to person by touching without an intermediate object. Microorganisms are spread indirectly by touching contaminated surfaces and objects.

Applying Contact Precautions You must use contact precautions with patients who have any of the following conditions or diseases:

- Stool incontinence/severe, uncontrolled diarrhea
- Draining wounds
- Uncontrolled secretions
- Decubitus ulcers (pressure sores)
- Ostomy tubes
- Generalized rash

Contact precautions include

- Washing your hands before and after touching the patient.
- Wearing gloves.
- Wearing a gown if considerable contact is expected.
- Washing hands after removing gloves.
- Disinfecting the exam room with EPA-registered disinfectant.

Droplet Precautions

Transmission of microorganisms by contact with secretions from the nose, throat, airways, lungs, and digestive tract is known as droplet contact. Droplets from coughs and sneezes can carry up to 3 feet from the source (Figure 6-7). Follow droplet precautions when assisting with patients suspected of having influenza, pertussis (whooping cough), mumps, respiratory syncytial virus, norovirus, and *Neisseria meningitides* (a bacterium that causes meningitis).

Applying Droplet Precautions Patients suspected of being infected with a pathogen transmitted by droplets should be placed in an exam room as quickly as possible. If you do not have an open exam room, ask the patient to put on a facemask and place the patient as far away from other patients as possible. When caring for a patient with influenza or other droplet-transmitted infection, put on a mask before entering the room. If the patient is coughing or sneezing uncontrollably and substantial spraying of respiratory droplets is expected, you should also wear gloves, a gown, and goggles or a face shield. Wash your hands before and after touching the patient or contacting respiratory secretions. Ask the patient to wear a mask when leaving the exam room and instruct her in respiratory hygiene and cough etiquette. Always clean and disinfect the exam room before allowing the next patient to enter.

Airborne Precautions

Some microorganisms are able to float in the air for substantial distances. For this reason, special airborne precautions must be taken if a patient is suspected of being infected with any known pathogen capable of being transmitted through the airborne route. The most common pathogens transmitted by the airborne route include tuberculosis, measles, chickenpox, and in some cases herpes zoster (shingles).

Applying Airborne Precautions Because airborne pathogens float in the air, anyone in the vicinity of an infected patient can easily be exposed. For this reason, it is important to isolate the patient as soon as possible. Have the patient enter through a different entrance than other patients, avoiding the reception area. Place the patient in a special airborne infection isolation room (AIIR), if one is available. If this type of room is not available, you should give the patient a facemask, close the door to the exam room, instruct the patient to keep the mask on, and change it if it becomes wet. The healthcare practitioner treating the patient will most likely transfer the patient to a facility equipped with special isolation rooms and fit-tested respirators. While caring for a patient with a suspected airborne pathogen, be sure to perform hand hygiene before and after patient contact and wear a mask, gloves, and a gown. Have the patient wear a mask at all times. After the patient leaves the room, keep the room empty for at least an hour, depending on the ventilation rate of the room. If you must enter the room before the prescribed time, you must use respiratory protection.

▶ OSHA-Required Education and Training

LO 6.5

In order for healthcare personnel to adhere to infection control policies and procedures, they must be properly trained. This training must be comprehensive and ongoing, and the trainers must have documented and demonstrated competency related to the task. Employers are required to provide infection control training at the onset of employment and then on a regular basis (usually yearly) or when a policy or procedure changes or there is a change in circumstances, such as an outbreak of influenza. Training should include the scientific rationale for infection control procedures. Understanding the rationale

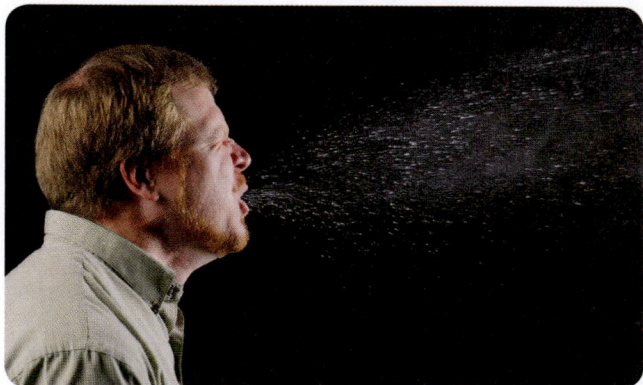

FIGURE 6-7 Uncovered coughs and sneezes can spread droplets for several feet.
James Gathany/CDC

helps healthcare workers perform the procedures correctly and alter them safely to specific situations when necessary. Anyone working in a healthcare facility who could be reasonably expected to come in contact with an infectious agent must be trained. This includes any contract worker from an outside agency, such as students participating in on-site training, housekeeping personnel, and equipment maintenance personnel who repair and maintain clinical equipment. This training must include

- Proper PPE selection and use.
- Job-specific infection prevention.

Improvement in adherence to infection control procedures and subsequent reduction in **healthcare-associated infections (HAI)** has been documented. Research shows that periodic assessment and feedback regarding healthcare workers' adherence to infection control practices in addition to education results in better adherence to those practices. Reduction in the transmission of infectious disease requires that not only healthcare workers understand how to break the chain of infection but also patients and their families. Patients and family members should be given information on standard precautions, respiratory hygiene, cough etiquette, and the importance of vaccination.

PROCEDURE 6-1 Aseptic Handwashing

Procedure Goal: To remove dirt and microorganisms from under the fingernails and from the surface of the skin, hair follicles, and oil glands of the hands

OSHA Guidelines: This procedure does not involve exposure to blood, body fluids, or tissues.

Materials: Liquid soap, disposable brush or nail cleaner, and paper towels

Method:

1. Remove all jewelry (plain wedding bands may be left on and scrubbed).
2. Turn on the faucets using a paper towel and adjust the water temperature to moderately warm. (Sinks with knee-operated faucet controls prevent contact of the surface with the hands.)

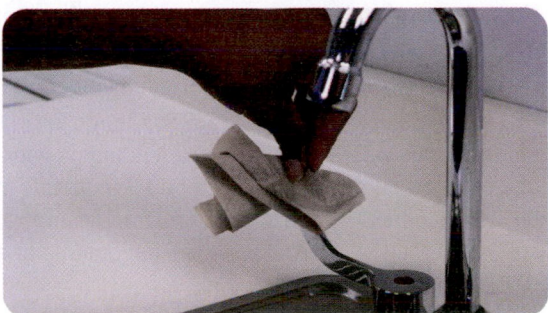

FIGURE Procedure 6-1 Step 2 Using a paper towel to turn on the faucet reduces the possibility of cross contamination.
© McGraw-Hill Education

3. Wet your hands and apply the recommended amount of liquid soap. Use a clean, dry paper towel to activate soap pump. Liquid soap, especially when dispensed with a foot pump, is preferable to bar soap.
   RATIONALE: *There is less available area for dirt to accumulate on a liquid soap dispenser than on bar soap, and there is a smaller chance of dropping the soap dispenser into the sink or onto the floor.*

4. Work the soap into a lather, making sure that all surface areas of both hands are lathered. Rub vigorously in a circular motion for 2 minutes. Keep your hands lower than your forearms so that dirty water flows into the sink instead of back onto your arms. Your fingertips should be pointing down. Interlace your fingers to clean between them, and use the palm of one hand to clean the back of the other. It is important that you wash every surface of your hands.
   RATIONALE: *Microorganisms are found on every surface of the hand and, if not washed away, can be transferred to the patient.*

5. Use a single-use disposable nailbrush or plastic, single-use nail cleaner under running water to dislodge dirt around your nails and cuticles.
   RATIONALE: *Microorganisms under the nails are not directly subjected to the running water and must be dislodged so that they can be washed away.*

6. Rinse your hands well, keeping your hands lower than your forearms and not touching the sink or faucets.

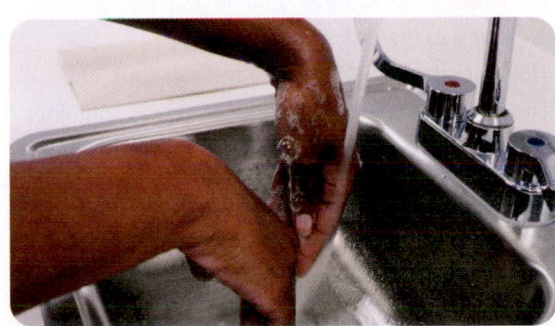

FIGURE Procedure 6-1 Step 6 Keep your hands lower than your forearms and avoid touching the sink when rinsing after an aseptic handwash.
© McGraw-Hill Education

7. With the water still running, dry your hands thoroughly with clean, dry paper towels.
8. Turn off the faucets using a clean, dry paper towel. Discard the towels.

PROCEDURE 6-2 Using an Alcohol-Based Hand Disinfectant

Procedure Goal: To use an alcohol-based hand-cleansing substance to reduce pathogens on the hand surfaces and prevent recontamination

OSHA Guidelines: This procedure does not involve exposure to blood, body fluids, or tissue.

Materials: 60% to 95% alcohol-based foam, gel, or liquid rub

Method:

1. Remove all jewelry (plain wedding bands may be left on).
2. Pump the recommended amount of AHD onto the palm of the hand.

   RATIONALE: *You must use enough AHD to cover all surfaces of the hands and there must be enough so that it does not dry too quickly.*

3. Rub the hands together vigorously, ensuring the alcohol comes in contact with all surfaces, including backs of hands, between fingers, and fingernails.

   RATIONALE: *Microorganisms are found on every surface of the hand and, if not washed away, can be transferred to the patient.*

4. Continue to rub the solution in a rotary fashion until it is evaporated and the hands are dry (10–15 seconds). Do not wave hands to hasten drying.

   RATIONALE: *Once they evaporate, AHD have no effect on pathogens.*

PROCEDURE 6-3 Using a Biohazardous Sharps Container

Procedure Goal: To ensure safe use of a sharps disposal unit

OSHA Guidelines:

Materials: Approved sharps container and gloves

Method:

1. Wash your hands and put on gloves.
2. Ensure that biohazardous waste containers are close to the place where the waste material is generated.

   RATIONALE: *To avoid accidental puncture wounds or exposure to biohazardous waste*

3. Hold the article by the unpointed, or blunt, end.
4. Drop the object directly into an approved container. (If you are using an evacuation system, do not unscrew the needle. Drop the entire system with the needle attached and the safety device engaged into the receptacle.) The container should be puncture-proof, with rigid sides and a tight-fitting lid.

   RATIONALE: *To avoid needlestick injuries*

5. Place sharps in an appropriate biohazardous waste container immediately or as soon as possible.
6. Keep containers closed when not in use. Close them before removing them from the area or use and keep them upright to avoid spills.
7. Place the container in a secondary container if the outside of the primary container becomes contaminated.
8. Drop—do not push—intact contaminated needles into the biohazardous waste container for sharps.

   RATIONALE: *To avoid accidental puncture wounds*

9. Never break off, recap, reuse, or handle needles after use.

   RATIONALE: *To avoid accidental puncture wounds*

10. Do not open, empty, or clean sharps containers.
11. Discard sharps containers that are two-thirds full in large biohazardous waste containers. Depending on your office's procedures, the container and its contents may be sterilized before further disposal, or they may be collected by an authorized waste management agency.
12. Remove the gloves and wash your hands.

PROCEDURE 6-4 Disposing of Biohazardous Waste

Procedure Goal: To correctly dispose of contaminated waste products, including sharps and contaminated cleaning and paper products

OSHA Guidelines:

Materials: Biohazardous waste containers, gloves, and waste materials

Method:

1. Wash your hands and put on gloves.
2. Carefully deposit the biohazardous materials in a properly marked biohazardous waste container. A standard biohazardous waste container has an inner plastic liner (either red or orange and marked with the biohazard symbol) and a puncture-proof outer shell (also marked with the biohazard symbol).

3. Never "dump" the contents of one biohazardous waste container into another.
   RATIONALE: *Doing so puts you at risk of exposure to biohazardous materials.*
4. If the container is full, secure the inner liner and place it in the appropriate area for biohazardous waste.
   RATIONALE: *Biohazardous waste must be held in an area separate from regular waste and trash.*
5. Remove the gloves and wash your hands.

SUMMARY OF LEARNING OUTCOMES

LEARNING OUTCOMES	KEY POINTS
6.1 Identify OSHA's role in protecting healthcare workers.	The US Department of Labor created OSHA to protect the employees' safety in the workplace. Through the creation and enforcement of standards such as the Bloodborne Pathogens Standard, Hazard Communication, and the Needlestick Safety and Prevention Act, OSHA serves to protect healthcare workers from hazards.
6.2 Illustrate the cycle of infection and how to break it.	In order for an infection to occur, these five elements must be in place: a reservoir host, a means of exit, a means of transmission, a means of entrance, and a susceptible host. The most effective means of breaking the cycle of infection is by using aseptic techniques. These include maintaining strict housekeeping standards, adhering to government health guidelines, and educating patients in hygiene, health promotion, and disease prevention.
6.3 Summarize the Bloodborne Pathogens Standard and universal precautions as described in the rules and regulations of the Occupational Safety and Health Administration (OSHA).	Laws set forth in the OSHA Bloodborne Pathogens Standard of 1991 dictate how you must handle infectious or potentially infectious waste generated during medical or surgical procedures. According to these rules, any potentially infectious waste materials must be discarded or held for processing in biohazardous waste containers.
6.4 Describe how transmission-based precautions supplement standard precautions.	Transmission-based precautions are meant to supplement standard precautions by adding an additional level of precautions. These include contact precautions, droplet precautions, and airborne precautions.
6.5 Summarize OSHA's education and training requirements for ambulatory care settings.	All ambulatory care settings must train employees and contract workers in the proper selection and use of PPE and job-specific infection prevention. This training must be done when the worker is hired and on a regular basis after that. In addition, patients and their families should be given information about preventing the spread of infection.

CASE STUDY CRITICAL THINKING

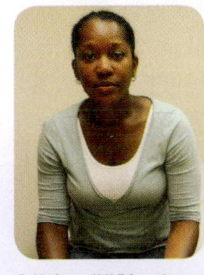

© McGraw-Hill Education

Recall Shenya Jones from the beginning of the chapter. Now that you have completed the chapter, answer the following questions regarding her case.

1. What aseptic technique practices would be most important with this patient?
2. Whom do these aseptic technique practices protect?
3. Why is it important that Dr. Williams do a wound culture?

1. (LO 6.1) The general duty clause requires
   a. That every employee perform every duty in the office
   b. An employer to maintain a safe workplace
   c. That each employee follow OSHA regulations
   d. That safety plan duties be well defined
   e. That healthcare workers not wear artificial nails when working with any patients

2. (LO 6.2) A bladder infection caused by *Escherichia coli* would be considered what type of infection?
   a. Vector-borne
   b. Exogenous
   c. Opportunistic
   d. Endogenous
   e. Foodborne

3. (LO 6.4) A set of guidelines set forth by the CDC that are meant to supplement standard precautions are known as
   a. Transmission-based precautions
   b. Training guidelines
   c. Respiratory hygiene
   d. OSHA supplemental procedures
   e. NIOSH recommendations

4. (LO 6.4) Droplet precautions pertain to someone who has which of the following?
   a. Ostomy tube
   b. Stool incontinence
   c. Draining wound
   d. Generalized rash
   e. Influenza infection

5. (LO 6.2) Which of the following is the *most* common means of transmitting pathogens?
   a. Ingesting food
   b. Sneezing
   c. Coughing
   d. Sexual contact
   e. Touching

6. (LO 6.2) Which of the following would be considered a fomite?
   a. Mosquito
   b. Pencil
   c. Sneeze
   d. *E. coli*
   e. Mucus

7. (LO 6.5) OSHA requires that all workers have initial training in PPE selection and
   a. Respirator use
   b. Job-specific infection prevention
   c. Sharps control
   d. Microbiology
   e. Equipment handling

8. (LO 6.3) Exposure to which of the following would be considered an exposure incident?
   a. Influenza
   b. Mumps
   c. HPV
   d. HIV
   e. Scabies

9. (LO 6.3) Which of the following would be considered a Category II task?
   a. Performing oral surgery
   b. Performing CPR
   c. Taking vital signs
   d. Measuring height
   e. Controlling bleeding

10. (LO 6.3) Means of controlling injuries by altering the way a task is performed is known as
    a. Universal precautions
    b. Engineering controls
    c. Personal protection
    d. Work practice controls
    e. Safety plan controls

S O F T   S K I L L S   S U C C E S S

You are a new graduate of a medical assisting program and have just been hired by an internal medicine practice with seven practitioners. This is a very busy office and you are excited to be working in the clinical area. Since you are new to the practice, you will shadow with Mary Benton, RMA. This morning is particularly busy and you have seen several patients with suspected influenza. After the morning patient session, Mary approaches you and says that you could save time by not washing your hands so much. She tells you that, if you are wearing gloves, you don't have to wash your hands after you take them off. How do you respond to Mary, and what action should you take?

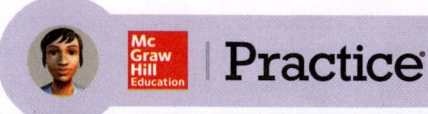

Go to PRACTICE MEDICAL OFFICE and complete Admin: Check In - Office Operations.

Safety and Patient Reception

CASE STUDY

	Patient Name	DOB	Allergies
PATIENT INFORMATION	Peter Smith	3/28/19XX	NKA
	Attending Paul F. Buckwalter, MD	**MRN** 428-69-544	**Other Information** Mrs. Smith requests to speak privately with MD.

Peter Smith is a 73-year-old male with mild Type 2 diabetes. When he called to schedule today's appointment, he stated that he was feeling very anxious and fatigued and that he was having difficulty eating and sleeping. He arrives at the reception desk today, appearing "flat" in affect. After

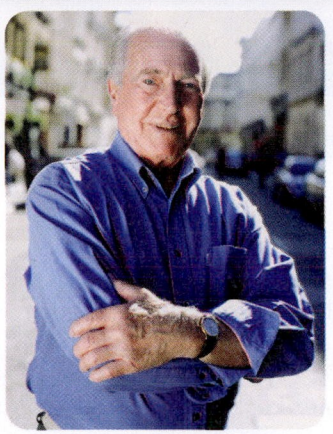

© Image Source/Getty Images RF

he signs in, his wife whispers to you, "I want to talk with the doctor about him, before he sees the doctor." Once Mr. Smith sits down, you notice him lean over and try to pick up a magazine from a table. His chair tips onto two legs while he continues to try to reach the magazine.

Keep Mr. Smith in mind as you study the chapter. There will be questions at the end of the chapter based on the case study. The information in the chapter will help you answer these questions.

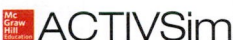

LEARNING OUTCOMES

After completing Chapter 7, you will be able to:

7.1 Describe the components of a medical office safety plan.

7.2 Summarize OSHA's Hazard Communication Standard.

7.3 Describe basic safety precautions you should take to reduce electrical hazards.

7.4 Illustrate the necessary steps in a comprehensive fire safety plan.

7.5 Summarize proper methods for handling and storing chemicals used in a medical office.

7.6 Explain the principles of good ergonomic practice and physical safety in the medical office.

7.7 Articulate the cause of most injuries to medical office workers and the four body areas where they occur.

7.8 List the design items to be considered when setting up an office reception area.

7.9 Summarize the housekeeping tasks required to keep the reception area neat and clean.

7.10 Relate how the Americans with Disabilities and Older American Acts have helped to make physical access to the medical office easier for all patients.

7.11 Describe the functions of the front office staff, including patient registration and accepting payments from patients.

7.12 Implement policies and procedures for opening and closing the office.

Americans with Disabilities Act (ADA)

color family

contagious

ergonomics

Globally Harmonized System of Classification and Labeling of Chemicals (GHS)

Hazard Communication Standard (HCS)

hazard label

infectious waste

Older Americans Act of 1965

Safety Data Sheets (SDS)

MEDICAL ASSISTING COMPETENCIES

CAAHEP

X.C.4	Summarize the Patient Bill of Rights
XII.C.1	Identify:
	(a) safety signs
	(b) symbols
	(c) labels
XII.C.2	Identify safety techniques that can be used in responding to accidental exposure to:
	(a) blood
	(b) other body fluids
	(c) needle sticks
	(d) chemicals
XII.C.3	Discuss fire safety issues in an ambulatory healthcare environment
XII.C.4	Describe fundamental principles for evacuation of a healthcare setting
XII.C.5	Describe the purpose of Safety Data Sheets (SDS) in a healthcare setting
XII.C.6	Discuss protocols for disposal of biological chemical materials
XII.C.7	Identify principles of:
	(a) body mechanics
	(b) ergonomics
XII.P.1	Comply with:
	(a) safety signs
	(b) symbols
	(c) labels
XII.P.2	Demonstrate proper use of:
	(a) eyewash equipment
	(b) fire extinguishers
	(c) sharps disposal containers
XII.P.3	Use proper body mechanics
XII.P.5	Evaluate the work environment to identify unsafe working conditions

ABHES

4. MEDICAL LAW AND ETHICS

b. Institute federal and state guidelines when releasing medical records or information

f. Comply with federal, state, and local health laws and regulations as they relate to healthcare settings

5. PSYCHOLOGY OF HUMAN RELATIONS

c. Intervene on behalf of the patient regarding issues/concerns that may arise, i.e. insurance policy information, medical bills, physician/provider orders, etc.

9. CLINICAL PROCEDURES

a. Practice standard precautions and perform disinfection/sterilization techniques

g. Recognize and respond to medical office emergencies

j. Make adaptations with patients with special needs

10. MEDICAL LABORATORY PROCEDURES

c. Dispose of biohazardous materials

▶ Introduction

In general, the medical office is divided into two broad, functional categories: The "back office" is the clinical area where patient care takes place and the "front office," including the reception area, is where business and nonclinical tasks take place. Whether you are working in the clinical area or the administrative area, safety should be foremost in your mind. Patients and staff members can fall or cut themselves and be exposed to numerous safety hazards. As a medical assistant, you have an important responsibility to remove or correct the hazards—physical, chemical, and biohazardous—that might cause injury to patients, healthcare practitioners, or staff members. In addition to safety, it is important to create an atmosphere that reflects on the quality of care patients can expect to receive. A carefully designed, well-maintained, and safe patient reception area ensures a pleasant and comfortable experience for patients while they wait to receive medical care and sets the stage for a successful interaction between the patient and the entire medical staff.

In this chapter, you will learn basic safety, including the components of a safety plan, OSHA Hazard Communication, and electrical, fire, and chemical safety. You will also be introduced to the many considerations related to the design and furnishings for the reception area of the medical office. The type of practice and the patient population's special needs are major influences, so you will explore the Americans with Disabilities and the Older Americans Acts. The roles of reception staff and what they need to accomplish in these roles will also be covered.

▶ The Medical Office Safety Plan — LO 7.1

Minimizing risk to patients, physicians, and staff by creating a safe environment in the medical office is essential. Both the administrative and clinical areas in an office environment contain many potential hazards. Having an established, routinely updated safety plan is a good first step in hazard awareness. Awareness and understanding of potential dangers facilitate the removal or correction of these hazards.

Every medical office must have a comprehensive written safety plan that is easily accessible to all employees and updated annually. Every employee is responsible for becoming familiar with and following the safety plan's policies and procedures. This plan must contain but is not limited to the following:

- OSHA Hazard Communication
- Electrical safety
- Fire safety
- Emergency action plan
- Chemical safety
- Bloodborne pathogen exposure
- Personal protective equipment
- Needlestick prevention

▶ OSHA Hazard Communication Standard — LO 7.2

OSHA's **Hazard Communication Standard (HCS)** was originally designed to keep workers safe by requiring that all workers have the right to know what chemicals they were exposed to during the course of their job. In 2012, the standard was updated with the intention that workers have a right not only to know but also to understand the dangers of any chemicals to which they may be exposed. To this end, the HSC has been aligned with the United Nations **Globally Harmonized System of Classification and Labeling of Chemicals (GHS).** The update includes changes to the information sheets that accompany each chemical, the **Safety Data Sheets** (formerly called Material Safety Data Sheets), and to the **hazard labels** required for each chemical container. Chemical

manufacturers and importers are now required to determine the hazards of the chemicals they produce. This includes the health and physical hazards and classification of chemical mixtures. This update will improve the consistency of chemical hazard information by standardizing the way it is communicated, thus improving chemical safety in the workplace.

The new standard requires each employer to:

- Train all employees on the revised standard.
- Have a written communication program.
- Provide employees with easy access to Safety Data Sheets for any chemical used in the facility.
- Keep a master list of hazardous chemicals in the facility.
- Ensure that any chemical kept in a secondary container be properly labeled.

Safety Data Sheets

Safety Data Sheets (SDS) are information sheets for every hazardous chemical. The format of these sheets has been standardized so that workers can quickly find information about hazardous chemicals in case of an accident or emergency. All Safety Data Sheets contain 16 sections. General information about the chemical is contained in sections 1–8, and additional, more technical information is found in sections 9–16.

The mandatory contents of each SDS include the following sections:

1. Identification—including the chemical, its intended uses, and contact information of the supplier
2. Hazard(s) Identification—the chemical's hazard, including the hazard classification (for example, "flammable"); a signal word, hazard statement, pictogram, and precautionary statement
3. Composition/Information on Ingredients—all ingredients contained in the product
4. First-Aid Measures—the initial care that should be rendered after exposure, including routes of exposure, symptoms, and special treatments if needed
5. Fire-Fighting Measures—proper extinguishing equipment, specific hazards resulting from the chemical during a fire, and necessary special protective equipment
6. Accidental Release Measures—action that should be taken in case of spills, leaks, or releases, including containment and cleanup
7. Handling and Storage—handling and hygiene practices and storage requirements, including incompatible chemicals and ventilation requirements
8. Exposure Controls/Personal Protections—exposure limits, required engineering controls, and PPE necessary to reduce exposure
9. Physical and Chemical Properties—appearance, odor, pH, melting and boiling points, flash point, and solubility
10. Stability and Reactivity—reactivity data, stability under normal conditions, and other information regarding hazardous reactions
11. Toxicological Information—likely routes, effects from exposure, and symptoms

The nonmandatory contents of each SDS include the following sections:

12. Ecological Information—environmental impact if the chemical is released

13. Disposal Considerations—may include appropriate disposal, recycling, or reclamation of the chemical or its package

14. Transport Information—may include guidance for shipping by air, land, or sea

15. Regulatory Information—any regulations not found elsewhere on the SDS

16. Other Information—may include when the SDS was prepared or revised and changes made in the revision

Labels

As part of the alignment with the GHS, all labels on hazardous chemicals must provide quick and simple graphic information about the chemical. Figure 7-1 is a sample of the revised hazardous chemical label. All hazardous chemical labels must include the following:

- Manufacturer's name and address
- Product identifier (name, batch number, and so on)
- Signal words (Danger, Warning, and so on)
- Hazard Statement
- Precautionary Statement (prevention, response, storage, and disposal)
- Pictograms (must be banded in red) (Figure 7-2 illustrates the OSHA-approved pictograms required on hazard labels)

Biohazard Labels In addition to containers with hazardous chemicals, all containers used to store waste products, blood, blood products, or other specimens that may be contaminated with bloodborne pathogens are considered biohazardous. They must be clearly marked with the biohazard symbol, as shown in Figure 7-3. The biohazard symbol label must be bright orange-red and clearly lettered so that no one can mistake the meaning of the warning. Labels should be securely attached to containers.

In addition to individual biohazard labels that identify particular containers, warning signs must be posted in the laboratory itself. These signs, such as the one shown in Figure 7-4, identify the presence of biohazardous material and list important safeguards to follow.

▶ Electrical Safety
LO 7.3

Because the equipment used in the medical office can make the office especially vulnerable to electrical hazards, it is critical that you know how to respond to an electrical accident. In addition to familiarizing yourself with the location of circuit breakers and emergency power shutoffs, practice these safeguards, which reduce electrical hazards:

- Avoid using extension cords. If they must be used, be sure the circuit is not overloaded. Tape extension cords to the floor to avoid tripping.

- Frayed electrical wires, overloaded outlets, and improperly grounded plugs present a danger of electric shock and fire. Contact a licensed electrician to remedy these problems. Repair or replace equipment that has a broken or frayed cord.

- Dry your hands before working with electrical devices.

- Do not position electrical devices near sinks, faucets, or other sources of water. Be sure electrical cords do not run through water.

OXI252
(disodiumflammy)
CAS #: 111-11-11xx

Danger
May cause fire or explosion; strong oxidizer
Causes severe skin burns and eye damage

Keep away from heat. Keep away from clothing and other combustible materials. Take any precaution to avoid mixing with combustibles. Wear protective neoprene gloves, safety goggles and face shield with chin guard. Wear fire/flame resistant clothing. Do not breathe dust or mists. Wash arms, hands and face thoroughly after handling. Store locked up. Dispose of contents and container in accordance with local, state and federal regulations.

First aid:
IF ON SKIN (or hair) or clothing[6]: Rinse immediately contaminated clothing and skin with plenty of water before removing clothes. Wash contaminated clothing before reuse.
IF IN EYES: Rinse cautiously with water for several minutes. Remove contact lenses, if present and easy to do. Continue rinsing.
IF INHALED: Remove person to fresh air and keep comfortable for breathing.
IF SWALLOWED: Rinse mouth. Do NOT induce vomiting.
Immediately call poison center.
Specific Treatment: Treat with doctor-prescribed burn cream.
Fire:
In case of fire: Use water spray. In case of major fire and large quantities: Evacuate area. Fight fire remotely due to the risk of explosion.

Great Chemical Company, 55 Main Street, Anywhere, CT 064XX   Telephone (888) 777-8888

FIGURE 7-1 The revised hazardous chemical label gives quick, simple, and graphic information about the chemical.

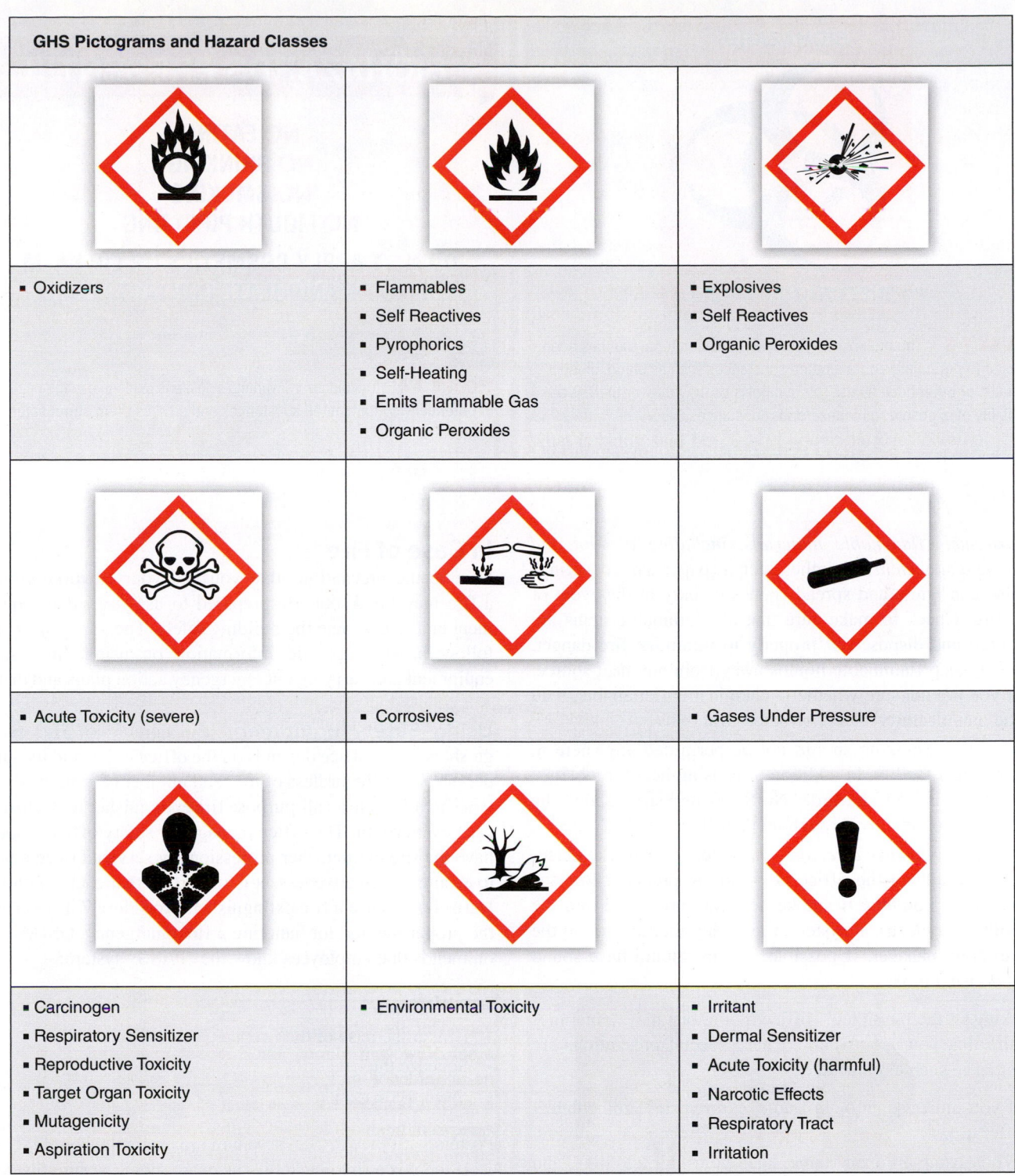

GHS Pictograms and Hazard Classes

■ Oxidizers	■ Flammables ■ Self Reactives ■ Pyrophorics ■ Self-Heating ■ Emits Flammable Gas ■ Organic Peroxides	■ Explosives ■ Self Reactives ■ Organic Peroxides
■ Acute Toxicity (severe)	■ Corrosives	■ Gases Under Pressure
■ Carcinogen ■ Respiratory Sensitizer ■ Reproductive Toxicity ■ Target Organ Toxicity ■ Mutagenicity ■ Aspiration Toxicity	■ Environmental Toxicity	■ Irritant ■ Dermal Sensitizer ■ Acute Toxicity (harmful) ■ Narcotic Effects ■ Respiratory Tract ■ Irritation

FIGURE 7-2 Pictograms are required on every hazardous chemical label and give graphic information about the chemical or chemicals inside the container.

▶ Fire Safety
LO 7.4

Fire is a safety hazard anywhere, but it is especially likely where there is sophisticated, high-voltage medical equipment such as an X-ray machine. Any electrical instrument in the exam room, however, is a potential fire hazard. Other potentially hazardous items are gas tanks and flammable chemicals. As discussed in this section, you should practice fire safety by

taking action to prevent it and knowing what action to take in the event of a fire.

Fire Prevention
Be aware of anything that might cause a fire in the exam room, examples of which are outlined in the following bullets. If you cannot correct the situation yourself, report the hazard to your supervisor.

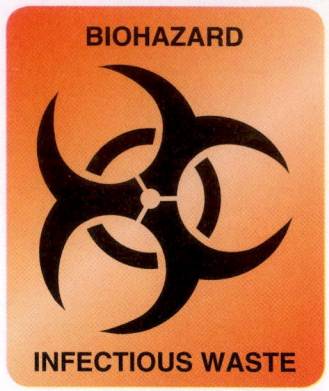

BIOHAZARD

INFECTIOUS WASTE

FIGURE 7-3 The biohazard symbol identifies material that has been exposed to potentially contaminated substances such as blood, blood products, or other body fluids. This symbol is used wherever there is a possibility of exposure to biohazardous substances.

BIOHAZARDS PRESENT!!!

NO EATING
NO DRINKING
NO SMOKING
NO MOUTH PIPETTING
DO NOT APPLY COSMETICS OR LIP BALM
DO NOT MANIPULATE CONTACT LENSES

FIGURE 7-4 The biohazard warning sign alerts personnel to the presence of potentially contaminated substances and advises them about safety guidelines.

- *Extremely flammable materials, including alcohol and some disinfectants.* Supplies such as paper table coverings also can ignite and spread flames quickly in the event of a fire. Check to make sure that all flammable items are stored and disposed of properly to minimize fire danger. Also, keep flammable liquids away from any heat source. If you are not sure whether a chemical is flammable, read the manufacturer's label or Safety Data Sheet.
- *Smoking.* Smoking should not be permitted anywhere in a medical facility. In addition to causing health problems, smoking is a fire hazard. "No Smoking" signs should be posted prominently throughout the office.
- *Inoperative smoke detectors.* Make sure that smoke detectors throughout the office are working properly. Replace batteries promptly. If smoke detectors are wired into the building's electrical system, report any malfunction to the building manager. If possible, alarms should have sound and visual modes.

Working in the physician's office laboratory may sometimes require that you use a flame. These special precautions are essential in such circumstances:

- If you must use an open flame, extinguish it immediately after use.
- When using an open flame, keep your hair, clothing, and jewelry away from the flame source.
- If you must use a chemical in a procedure that requires an open flame, double-check the SDS to identify the fire risk level for that chemical. If necessary, take a fire extinguisher to the area in which you will be working.
- Never lean over an open flame.
- Never leave an open flame unattended.
- Turn off gas valves immediately after use. If you must use an open flame in the vicinity of a gas valve, always double-check to be sure the gas is off. Make sure there is adequate ventilation.

In Case of Fire

Despite the precautions that you and your coworkers take, a fire may break out. Be prepared to use fire safety equipment and to evacuate the building safely. The paragraphs that follow provide specific information on using fire safety equipment and carrying out emergency action plans and drills.

Using Safety Equipment The number of fire extinguishers in the office depends on the office's size and its number of rooms. Regardless of the total number of extinguishers, you should locate an all-purpose fire extinguisher in or close to each exam room. The office manager or safety officer should have the fire extinguisher professionally serviced once a year to ensure its effectiveness. It is important that each employee learns how to use a fire extinguisher. Procedure 7-1 describes the proper method for handling a fire emergency. OSHA recommends that employees know the "PASS" system:

- Pull the pin.
- Aim at the base of the fire.
- Squeeze the trigger.
- Sweep side to side.

Posters with the "PASS" acronym are available from OSHA.

If there is a fire blanket in the exam room, be sure that you know how to use it and that it is stored for easy access in an emergency. To use a fire blanket to smother burning clothing, wrap the victim in the blanket and roll him on the floor. You also can contact your local fire department for more information about fire safety training.

Emergency Action Plans and Drills

Every employee must be prepared to take appropriate action during a fire emergency. An emergency action plan that outlines the employees' responsibilities is needed in order to reduce panic in an emergency and to reduce the likelihood of

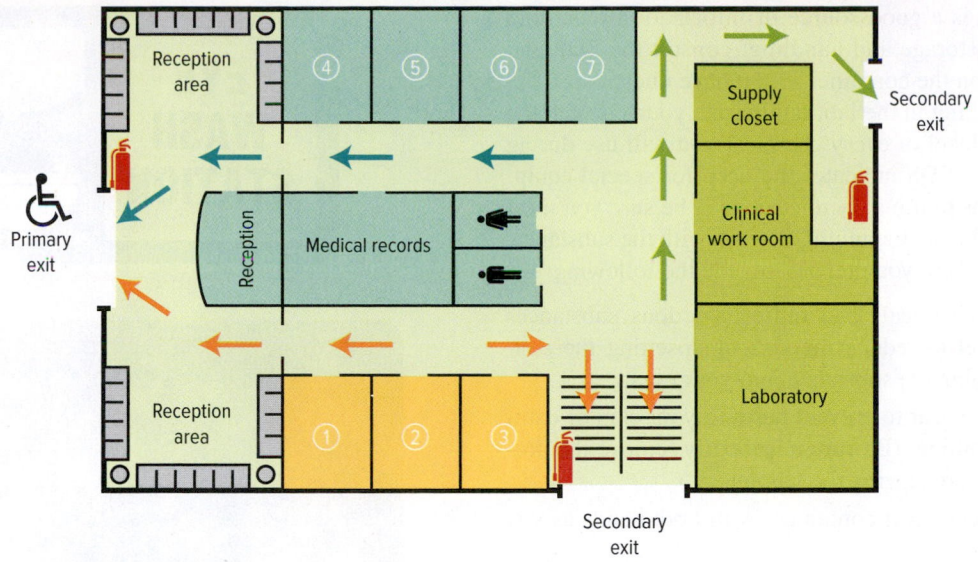

FIGURE 7-5 An evacuation route is clearly outlined on a map and posted throughout the office.

severe bodily injury. Participation in periodic fire drills is an essential part of this plan. The other important components of an effective emergency action plan are outlined in the paragraphs that follow.

Name of the person or persons responsible for reporting the fire and overseeing the entire operation. Ideally, two people are responsible for this task—a primary and a secondary. In the event the person with primary responsibility is out of the office, the person who is second on the list takes primary responsibility for reporting and overseeing.

Building evacuation routes. Maps of the office floor plan should be located throughout the office and marked with the current location and nearest exit. The route between the current location and the nearest exit should be highlighted or outlined on the map. See Figure 7-5. All exits should have a well-lit and easy-to-see exit sign. Halls leading to the exit should have emergency lighting so they remain lit in the event of a power failure. Halls also should be clutter free at all times. Exit routes should be large enough to accommodate all evacuees, including those with disabilities.

Evacuation procedure. Several employees should be responsible for ensuring that patients and staff are appropriately evacuated from the building. Patients in exam and procedure rooms may have special needs. Large medical practices may need to create different zones within the office. Each zone should have two individuals in charge of that specific area. Zones in the patient reception areas might be handled differently than zones in the clinical areas. Those responsible for evacuation should be the last to leave and should perform a quick search of bathrooms, break rooms, and other areas to ensure everyone has left the building. Two employees should be responsible for removing the book containing the SDS and handing it over to the first responders at the scene. Having designated areas outside the building to assemble the evacuees makes accounting for employees and patients easier.

A plan for accounting for all employees and patients after the evacuation is completed. Conduct a head count or roll call of all employees. To account for patients in the office, use the check-in roster. Give the name of any missing employee or patient to the person in charge. Quick action is a matter of life or death if someone is trapped in the building during a fire emergency.

Emergency action plan drills. Practice the emergency action plan on a regular basis and conduct unannounced drills so that each individual better understands her role. Having an emergency action plan drill allows for evaluation and refinement of the plan. You don't want to find out your plan doesn't work in the middle of a true emergency.

Local emergency contacts. Dialing 911 is the most common way to report an emergency; there may be other internal numbers if your facility is large. A list of fire and EMS numbers should be readily available at all times and updated regularly. The contact list also should include the name and number of the person (such as the office manager or the safety officer) who may have additional information regarding individual employee duties.

Developing and maintaining a relationship with local emergency authorities is vital. Trained fire personnel can often identify hidden workplace hazards and advise you in correcting them. Most local fire departments will come to your office and assess for fire hazards at your request.

▶ Chemical Safety   LO 7.5

A number of chemicals are used in a physician's office, and although most of these are found in the clinical lab area, they may be delivered to your office through the administrative office. If you are responsible for accepting a shipment containing chemicals, you must handle the package appropriately and make sure it is delivered to the proper person in the office. If laboratory personnel are not present when the order arrives, you must make certain that the chemical is properly stored. The SDS is a good source of information regarding proper chemical storage and handling; consult the SDS and the packing slip on the container if you have questions.

If you are working in the lab, familiarize yourself with the SDS and hazard label of every chemical you will use during a procedure. If the SDS indicates the need for special equipment or conditions to use a chemical safely, be sure you meet the requirements before beginning to work with the substance. General precautions as you prepare include the following:

- Store caustic chemicals and other hazardous substances below eye level to reduce the risk of upsetting the container and spilling the substance into your eyes.

- Wear protective gear to prevent harm to your skin or damage to your clothing. (Be sure to properly remove the protective gear before leaving the laboratory.)

- Always carry chemical containers with both hands as you gather supplies.

- Make sure you work in a properly ventilated area.

When you are ready to begin work, adhere to these guidelines:

- If you must smell the chemicals you are using, do not hold them directly under your nose. Instead, hold them a few inches away and fan air across them and toward your nose.

- Work inside a fume hood if the chemical vapor is hazardous.

- Wear a personal ventilation device when working with certain chemicals, as specified by the SDS.

- Never combine chemicals in ways not specifically required in test procedures.

- Mouth pipetting is prohibited at all times.

- If you are combining acids with other substances, always add the acid to the other substance. Adding substances to the acid increases the risk of splashing.

- If you encounter a spill of an unknown chemical substance, do not pour any other chemicals on it. Clean it up following strict hazardous waste control procedures. Never touch an unknown substance with your bare hands.

If there is an eyewash station in your lab, OSHA recommends that you know where it is and be able to find it with limited or no vision. See Figure 7-6. All employees who may incur splashes or splatters should be trained in its use. The eyewash station should be checked monthly to make sure it is working properly. Procedure 7-2 demonstrates the proper use of an eyewash station.

▶ Ergonomics and Physical Safety   LO 7.6

The medical office is a busy place, and it is sometimes easy to ignore basic safe practice when rapidly faced with multiple tasks. However, unsafe practice can have long-lasting effects on your health and quality of life. Protecting yourself from ergonomic and physical hazards ultimately reduces office costs by limiting unnecessary sick time. A safe employee is a valuable employee.

Ergonomics
Scientists study the way people work; this study is known as **ergonomics.** People who perform repetitive tasks often

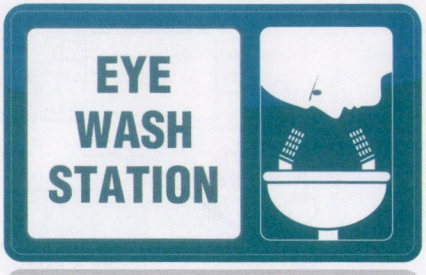

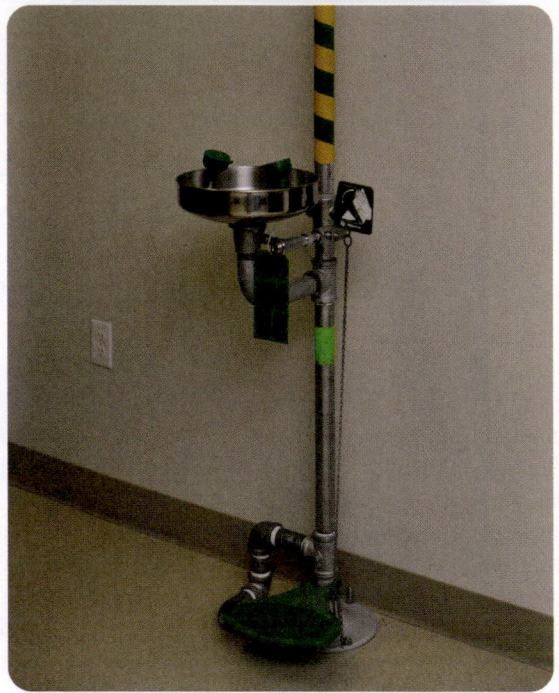

FIGURE 7-6   Eyewash station.
© Aaron Roeth Photography

develop work-related musculoskeletal disorders. Workplace injuries also may be the result of poor posture while performing a task such as leaning over to lift a patient from a wheelchair instead of bending your knees or positioning your arms too far above the computer keyboard when keying information. Good ergonomic practice (sometimes called body mechanics) is designed to reduce the likelihood of injury at work. The CDC's National Institute for Occupational Safety and Health (NIOSH) has specific recommendations for reducing work-related musculoskeletal injuries:

- Do not overextend your reach when attempting to grasp supplies. Use only approved equipment, such as stepladders or stools, to reach high shelves. Do not climb onto chairs, desks, or tables to reach anything.

- When lifting an object, squat close to the object. Keep your back straight but not rigid. Lift the item by pushing up with your legs, not by pulling with your back. Hold the load firmly with both hands, close to your body. If necessary, put on a back-support belt before attempting to move heavy loads.

- When transferring a patient, always bend at the knees to lift and ask for assistance if you are not sure you can lift or move the patient by yourself. When performing the transfer, move the patient's wheelchair as close to the exam table as possible to reduce the distance the patient must be moved. Lock the wheels of the wheelchair. Remove the wheelchair footrests if possible. Have the patient help as much as possible. If a transfer device is available, use it. Transfer devices include gait belts, sliding boards, pivot discs, and sling-type transfer equipment.

- Adjust your seat to the correct position to prevent back strain.
- If you are using a computer, take frequent breaks to reduce eyestrain and hand cramping.

Your employer has the responsibility to provide a safe work environment, including equipment designed to reduce injury and workstations that adjust to the worker. Many employers offer training seminars for reducing work-related injuries. It is your responsibility to follow safe practice when using equipment or performing tasks where there is a possibility of work-related injury.

Physical Safety

There are many ways to ensure physical safety in the medical office. You must understand and apply all the appropriate safeguards. Because accidents can happen, however, post emergency numbers in multiple locations throughout the office. Once each quarter, make sure the numbers are accurate and up-to-date.

Some safeguards come under the heading of common sense, meaning their application requires no special knowledge. These include:

- Walk, do not run, in the office.
- Prevent falls by wiping or mopping up spills immediately.
- Clear the floor of dropped objects.
- If the floor is carpeted, make sure there are no snags or tears that could cause someone to trip and fall.
- Spilled medications, chemicals, and other substances pose a threat to young children, who may ingest anything they find on the floor. Destroy and dispose of medications that are accidentally dropped on the floor.
- Be careful when carrying objects through the facility, especially when approaching blind corners.
- Close all cabinets, closet doors, desks, and worktable drawers.
- Routinely inspect the furniture in the exam room and reception area. Make sure there are no rough edges or sharp corners on the examining table, countertop, chairs, or other furniture.
- Electrical cords and medical and office equipment cables should run along the walls and be taped or fastened down securely.
- Never use damaged equipment or supplies, such as cracked or chipped glassware.

If you are asked to work in the laboratory, being aware of the laboratory environment will help you protect your health and well-being. Other safeguards to practice in the laboratory include

- Do not eat or drink in the laboratory, and do not store food there. Never use laboratory supplies, such as beakers or flasks, for eating or drinking.

- Do not put anything in your mouth while working in the laboratory. (Some people have a habit of chewing on the end of their pencils, for example.)
- Do not apply makeup or lip balm or insert contact lenses in the laboratory.
- Familiarize yourself with the location of the first-aid kit. If you are responsible for the kit in your area, check it weekly to make sure it is adequately stocked with supplies and that expiration dates on medications have not passed. See Figure 7-7.
- Familiarize yourself with the location and operation of the emergency eyewash and shower stations.

Additionally, in your efforts to promote safe practice in the laboratory, always wear appropriate protective gear and clothing. Use heat-resistant mitts or gloves to prevent burns. Wear sturdy, low-heeled, closed-toe shoes with rubber soles to prevent injury if you drop or spill something and to avoid slipping. Do not wear dangling jewelry or loose clothing that could get caught in laboratory equipment. Keep hair pulled back or covered for the same reason.

When you work with laboratory equipment, always follow manufacturers' guidelines. For example, wait for centrifuges to stop spinning before you open them.

Many laboratory materials and supplies require special handling and precautions, which include:

- Do not attempt to grasp bottles, jars, or other containers if your hands or the containers are wet.
- Close containers immediately after use.
- Clean up spills immediately.
- Clean up broken glass with a broom. Do not handle the debris. If the material is biohazardous, use tongs or forceps to pick up the glass. Package the pieces in a sturdy container with a label identifying the contents.

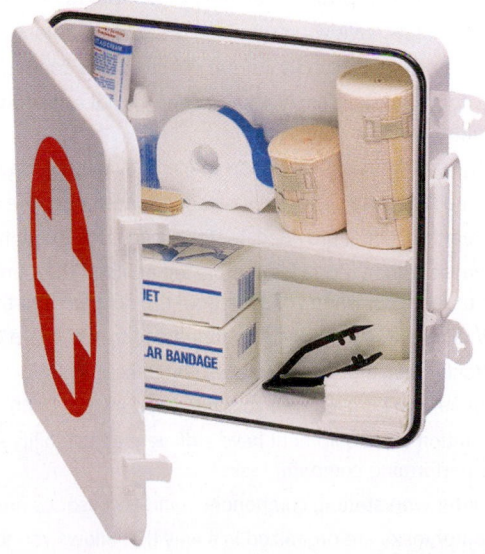

FIGURE 7-7 First-aid kit.
© Comstock/Alamy RF

▶ Preventing Injury in the Front Office

In addition to taking care of patients, medical assistants also must be aware of their environment in the medical office and how it affects their ability to perform the job effectively.

The medical office environment's many work functions require many physical tasks. Examples are using the computer, carrying and unpacking boxes, filling copy machine trays, and helping patients with impairments. The associated movements are often performed using repetitive motions, like typing, lifting, bending, stooping, and sitting.

The most common office-related injuries are those occurring to office workers, including medical assistants, who spend much of their workday seated at a computer station. Common injuries or conditions involve the forearm, wrist, hand, and back. Table 7-1 contains ergonomic excerpts from an OSHA computer station checklist to use in prevention of these common injuries.

The ideal medical office environment is an efficient, safe, and caring place for patients, visitors, and staff. You will find the *Caution: Handle with Care* feature helpful in preventing carpal tunnel syndrome (CTS), as well as identifying the symptoms and treatments for CTS, should it occur.

TABLE 7-1   OSHA Computer Workstations Checklist

1. Head and neck to be upright, or in-line with the torso (not bent down/back).
2. Head, neck, and trunk to face forward (not twisted).
3. Trunk to be perpendicular to floor (may lean back into backrest but not forward).
4. Shoulders and upper arms to be in-line with the torso, generally about perpendicular to the floor and relaxed (not elevated or stretched forward).
5. Upper arms and elbows to be close to the body (not extended outward).
6. Forearms, wrists, and hands to be straight and in-line (forearm at about 90 degrees to the upper arm).
7. Wrists and hands to be straight (not bent up/down or sideways toward the little finger).
8. Thighs to be parallel to the floor and lower legs to be perpendicular to floor (thighs may be slightly elevated above knees).
9. Feet rest flat on the floor or are supported by a stable footrest.
10. Backrest provides support for your lower back (lumbar area).
11. Seat width and depth accommodate the specific user (seat pan not too big/small).
12. Seat front does not press against the back of your knees and lower legs (seat pan not too long).
13. Seat has cushioning and is rounded with a "waterfall" front (no sharp edge).
14. Armrests, if used, support both forearms while you perform computer tasks and they do not interfere with movement.
15. Keyboard/input device platform(s) is stable and large enough to hold a keyboard and an input device.
16. Input device (mouse or trackball) is located right next to your keyboard so it can be operated without reaching.
17. Input device is easy to activate and the shape/size fits your hand (not too big/small).
18. Wrists and hands do not rest on sharp or hard edges.
19. Top of the screen is at or below eye level so you can read it without bending your head or neck down/back.
20. User with bifocals/trifocals can read the screen without bending the head or neck backward.
21. Monitor distance allows you to read the screen without leaning your head, neck, or trunk forward/backward.
22. Monitor position is directly in front of you so you don't have to twist your head or neck.
23. Glare (for example, from windows, lights) is not reflected on your screen, which can cause you to assume an awkward posture to clearly see information on your screen.
24. Thighs have sufficient clearance space between the top of the thighs and your computer table/keyboard platform (thighs are not trapped).
25. Legs and feet have sufficient clearance space under the work surface so you are able to get close enough to the keyboard/input device.
26. Document holder, if provided, is stable and large enough to hold documents.
27. Document holder, if provided, is placed at about the same height and distance as the monitor screen so there is little head movement, or need to re-focus, when you look from the document to the screen.
28. Wrist/palm rest, if provided, is padded and free of sharp or square edges that push on your wrists.
29. Wrist/palm rest, if provided, allows you to keep your forearms, wrists, and hands straight and in-line when using the keyboard/input device.
30. Telephone can be used with your head upright (not bent) and your shoulders relaxed (not elevated) if you do computer tasks at the same time.
31. Workstation and equipment have sufficient adjustability so you are in a safe working posture and can make occasional changes in posture while performing computer tasks.
32. Computer workstation, components, and accessories are maintained in serviceable condition and function properly.
33. Computer tasks are organized in a way that allows you to vary tasks with other work activities, or to take micro-breaks or recovery pauses while at the computer workstation.

Source: http://www.osha.gov/SLTC/etools/computerworkstations/checklist.html (2012).

CAUTION: HANDLE WITH CARE

Carpal Tunnel Syndrome

As the number of computers used in the home and workplace has escalated in recent years, the number of cases of carpal tunnel syndrome also has risen dramatically. Carpal tunnel syndrome is a hand disorder often associated with computer use. The term for this condition comes from the name for a canal (the carpal tunnel) located in the wrist. Several tendons pass through this tunnel, allowing the hand to open and close.

Carpal tunnel syndrome results from repetitive motion, such as keyboarding, for hours at a time. This motion may cause swelling to develop around the tendons and carpal tunnel. The swelling compresses the nerve. The people most likely to develop this disorder are workers whose jobs require them to perform repetitive hand and finger motions.

Symptoms
The symptoms associated with carpal tunnel syndrome include

- Tingling or burning in the hands or fingers.
- Weakness or numbness in the hands or fingers.
- Hands that go to sleep frequently.
- Difficulty opening or closing the hands.
- Pain that stems from the wrist and travels up the arm.

Tips for Prevention
If you use a keyboard for extended periods, you should practice proper techniques, as outlined in the following bullets, to prevent carpal tunnel syndrome (Figure 7-8).

- While seated, hold your arms relaxed at your sides. Make sure your keyboard is positioned slightly higher than your elbows. As you input, keep your elbows at your sides, and relax your shoulders.
- Use only your fingers to press keys and do not use more pressure than necessary. Use a wrist rest and keep your wrists relaxed and straight.
- When you need to strike difficult-to-reach keys, move your whole hand rather than stretching your fingers. When you

need to press two keys at the same time, such as "Control" and "F1," use two hands.
- Try to break up long periods of keyboard work with other tasks that do not require computer use.

Tips for Relieving Symptoms
If you have carpal tunnel syndrome symptoms, try these suggestions for relief:

- Elevate your arms.
- Wear a splint on the hand and forearm.
- Discuss your symptoms with a physician, who may prescribe medication.

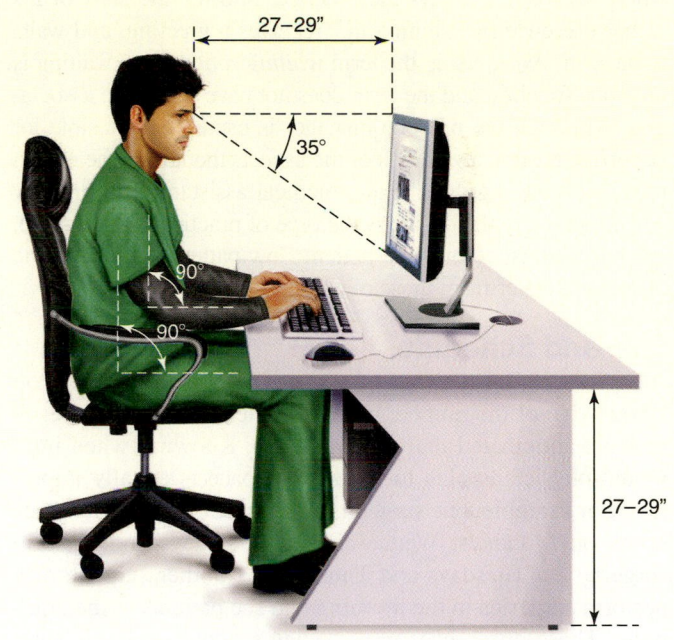

FIGURE 7-8 Maintaining proper posture and hand position helps avoid straining of the neck, back, arms, and eyes when using a computer.

Special Safety Precautions Some patients, such as children and people with disabilities, may be particularly susceptible to accidents in your office. You need to take special precautions to ensure their safety.

Children Follow these precautions when assisting children:

- Keep sharp instruments out of the reach of children.
- Store toxic items in high cabinets.
- Keep all medications and objects out of the reach of young children because children are likely to pick up items and put them in their mouths and could choke or be poisoned.
- Keep children's toys and books in the reception area or exam room picked up and stored safely when not in use.

- Toys should be washable and made of safe materials.
- Sanitize toys that children put in their mouths daily; sanitize other toys weekly.
- If well children and sick children use the same reception area or exam room, sanitize and disinfect toys after sick children play with them.
- Periodically check toys for sharp edges that might cause cuts.
- Ensure toys do not have small parts or pieces that could cause choking if swallowed.

Patients with Physical Disabilities Patients with disabilities are more likely than other patients to fall. Some patients may use walkers or canes for support, whereas others may simply be unsteady on their feet. Follow these recommendations when assisting patients with physical disabilities:

- Provide assistance as needed with disrobing prior to an exam or redressing afterward.
- Never leave severely disabled patients alone in an exam room. Check office policies for guidelines regarding appropriate chaperones for patients with disabilities.

In addition, keep in mind that patients with vision impairments may have difficulty seeing obstacles, stairs, and other potential hazards. Safe flooring and handrails in the reception area, bathroom, hallways, and exam room help ensure the safety of patients with impaired mobility or vision.

▶ Design of the Reception Area   LO 7.8

The word *reception* means the place or event where one is greeted. In the medical office, *reception* describes the area where the patient enters the practice, informs the staff of his or her presence by "signing in," receives a greeting, and waits to be seen. Avoid using the term *waiting room,* since waiting is only one function and the term does not have a positive association. Although the practice manager is usually responsible for the office design, awareness of the aspects that affect the design is valuable knowledge for any medical assistant. The primary consideration in the design is the type of practice. For example, the furnishings, colors, and patient flow patterns of a pediatric office will differ from those of an internal medicine office.

Size and Schedule

After identifying the type of practice, size is the next factor. Knowledge of the number of practitioners and the number of patients anticipated daily is important. Knowing when individual physicians plan to utilize the space is equally important. For example, one surgeon in the practice may have office hours on Mondays, Wednesdays, and Fridays and perform surgeries on Tuesdays and Thursdays. Another surgeon may perform surgeries in the morning and see patients in the afternoon. These differences in physician scheduling allow better utilization of space and relative ease in planning for the reception size. Other offices may have staggered hours where one physician will see patients between 7:00 a.m. and 3:00 p.m. and another physician in the practice will see patients from 11:00 a.m. to 7:00 p.m. This is challenging, since more space is needed during the 4 overlap hours than the remainder of the day. Dealing with overlapping office hours and other time and space issues is often part of the medical assistant's role.

Utilization of Space

Utilization of space differs by type of practice. For example, an orthopedic office or geriatric office where a significant number of patients will need room for wheelchairs and walkers requires more open space for mobility and devices than does a cardiologist's office. There may be the false assumption that pediatric offices need a smaller reception area, since the patients are smaller, but this is incorrect for a few reasons. First, a caregiver always accompanies the pediatric patient. Second, children require play space. Third, pediatric offices may need separate "well child" and "sick child" areas in an attempt to avoid cross-contamination from sick to well patients.

Overcrowding in a reception area is undesirable for patient comfort and for the potential of disease transmission. The reception area, which allows the patient to sit while waiting to be seen, is usually separated from the functional areas of the practice by a high counter and a sliding window (Figure 7-9). These areas should be HIPAA-compliant so the patient at the counter cannot overhear staff talking to or about other patients and cannot view an open computer screen or paper record.

Décor

Colors and fabrics are the primary elements that make up a room's décor. Colors can be used throughout the room—on walls, furniture, carpeting, and other items. Fabrics are used primarily on furniture and draperies.

When using several colors, it is important to decorate in color families to avoid a jarring, unprofessional look. A **color family** is a group of colors that work well together. In general, colors fall within two basic areas: cool and warm. Using all cool colors—such as white, blue, and mauve—creates a more harmonious impression in the reception area than mixing cool colors with warm ones such as red, orange, and hot pink. When choosing the color family, consider the mood you want to create, as studies demonstrate that the use of color affects mood. For example,

- Red increases heart rate and blood pressure.
- Blue causes the body to produce calming chemicals.
- Green is easy on the eyes and relaxing.
- Light browns are warm and inviting.
- Black and dark browns are associated with power and depression.
- White is related to cleanliness and purity.

Traditionally, the pediatric office incorporates primary colors for a lively atmosphere (although the use of red should

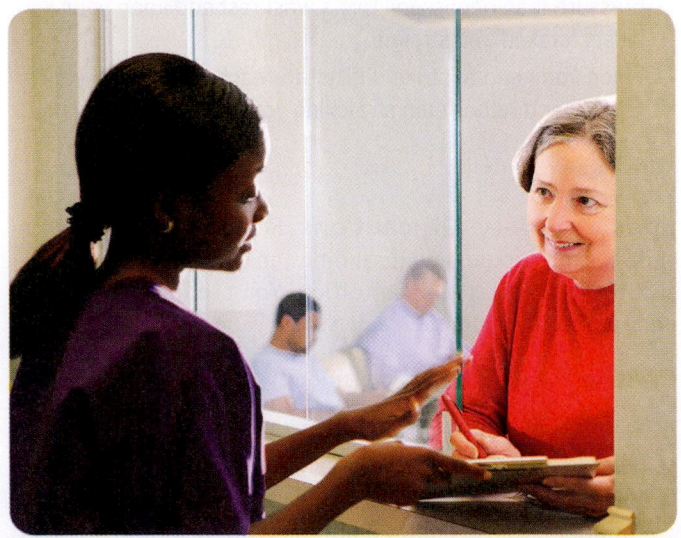

FIGURE 7-9 The receptionist's desk and window are part of every patient reception area and allow for privacy during patient check-in.
© Thinkstock Images/Getty Images RF

be limited). Obstetric offices are often decorated in pastels; geriatric offices often use soft colors in beige tones. Other offices tend to use popular decorator color palettes like earth tones and jewel tones (Figure 7-10). Colors may also reflect the cultural preferences of the dominant patient population. You might also want to consider the effect of color when choosing your scrubs or other office attire.

Fabrics, too, add to the atmosphere in the room. Heavy fabrics like velvet or brocade are more formal, whereas lightweight or sheer fabrics create a soft, delicate appearance. Patterns on fabrics or wallpaper can immediately change the mood of the room. No matter what the design, fabrics should be easy to clean and maintain.

Many medical offices are carpeted for greater appeal and improved noise reduction. Carpeting, available in a variety of colors and patterns, also provides a comfortable cushion when people walk through the office. Carpeting should be easy to clean and durable enough to handle a large volume of patient traffic. Scatter rugs, which can cause injuries if someone slips on or trips over them, should be avoided.

Furnishings

Chairs should be comfortable but have a straight back to allow the patient to get up easily, especially in obstetric, geriatric, and orthopedic offices. Many attractive stain-resistant cloth fabrics are available for medical use. Choose chairs and tables with rounded—not sharp—corners to avoid injuries.

Arranging Furniture The furniture arrangement can make the office seem comfortable or uncomfortable. If furniture is too close together, patients do not have sufficient space to move around easily or to stretch their legs. They may feel cramped. To ensure that patients have adequate room, a good rule of thumb is to allow 12 square feet of space per person. By this measurement, a 120-square-foot room (10 feet by 12 feet) can accommodate 10 people comfortably.

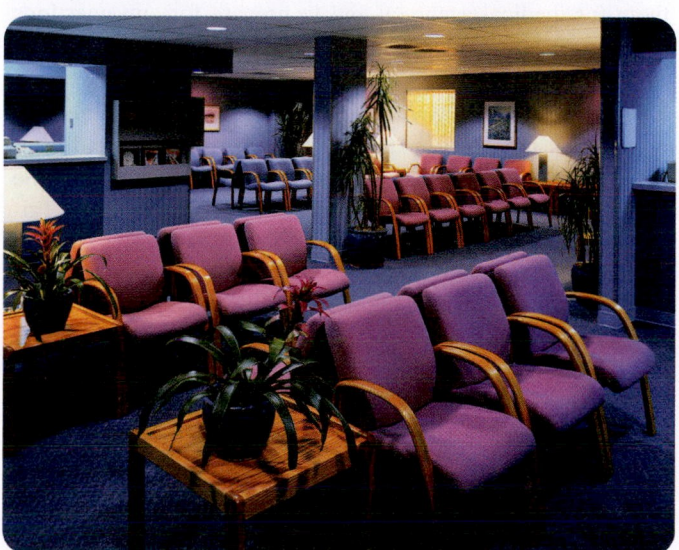

FIGURE 7-10 Decorator colors and furniture groupings make for a comfortable reception area.
© John Connell/Corbis RF

The furniture arrangement should allow maximum floor space. Patients should be able to stretch out their legs when seated and to walk around the reception area if they wish. Placing chairs against the wall usually produces the greatest amount of floor area. Additional seating in the middle of the room can be placed back-to-back to conserve space. Seats should be grouped so that families or friends can sit together. Remember to reserve room for patients in wheelchairs and to allow enough space for wheelchairs with extended leg supports. Also, keep in mind that some patients value their privacy; placing single chairs or small groups of chairs in corners of the room offers patients some measure of privacy, if needed.

Specialty Items Accessories or specialty items can make the reception area more comfortable and inviting. The following are additional items to be considered when selecting or modifying medical office furnishings:

- Artificial plants and floral arrangements are preferred due to allergies, poisons, and the potential for microbes associated with living plants; these should be kept dust-free.

- Aquariums are popular and soothing but require upkeep. Some offices employ a service to care for the aquarium; others have virtual aquariums.

- Heavy objects like large aquariums should be built into a wall if possible or securely fastened and stabilized to avoid injury. Likewise, large pictures, shelving, and bookcases should be securely fastened to walls.

- Toys and toy pieces should be easily and frequently disinfected and be larger than would fit into a small child's mouth. Balls and other throwing toys are dangerous in the medical environment.

Although specialty pieces can enhance the room's décor, they should be kept to a minimum. Too many pieces can create a cluttered look. Try to select specialty items that will be pleasing or helpful to patients. A clock is one example. Another useful item is a coat rack, which helps prevent clutter by providing a place for coats, umbrellas, and briefcases. Avoid accessories like scented candles or potpourri that may be offensive to some people or cause allergic reactions.

Other Considerations

Lighting Most medical offices use fairly bright lighting in the reception area, allowing patients to see their surroundings easily. Subdued lighting, like that sometimes used in restaurants, could be hazardous, as it may cause patients to trip over or bump into hard-to-see objects. In addition, bright lighting is essential for reading—a common activity in the patient reception area. Bright lighting also conveys an impression of cleanliness. Be aware, however, that extremely bright light can be harsh on the eyes and create an annoying glare.

Room Temperature Patients will be uncomfortable if the reception area is too hot or too cold. In an uncomfortable setting, waiting time can seem much longer than it really is, so maintaining an average, comfortable temperature is important.

To ensure a comfortable versus an uncomfortable temperature, keep the thermostat at a temperature that feels comfortable to you and to the office staff. You might periodically survey patients to see if they are comfortable and adjust the setting accordingly. Many elderly people feel cold because of lowered metabolisms. You may want to increase the temperature setting for a geriatric practice or if the office sees a large number of elderly patients. The room temperature in the reception area may be a bit cooler than in the examination rooms, where patients may be required to disrobe.

Music Many medical offices pipe soothing background music through speakers to the reception area as well as elsewhere in the office. Because the music is meant to calm patients, it should be chosen accordingly. Classical music, light jazz, and soft rock are appropriate choices, whereas heavy metal and rap music are not. Some offices use prepared compact discs. Others tune in to an "easy listening" local (or satellite) radio station.

Educational/Entertainment Materials

Practice-appropriate educational and entertainment materials are more likely to be read by patients if the materials are placed on tables close to the seating. While wall and countertop racks are appropriate and conserve space, keep some materials on tables for easier access by the elderly and differently abled (Figure 7-11). Magazines, newspapers, and other reading material also may be present. The publications should be relatively current and reflect the interests and languages of the populations served. Materials should be neatly arranged, tasteful, and not torn or dirty. Avoid tabloids. Some

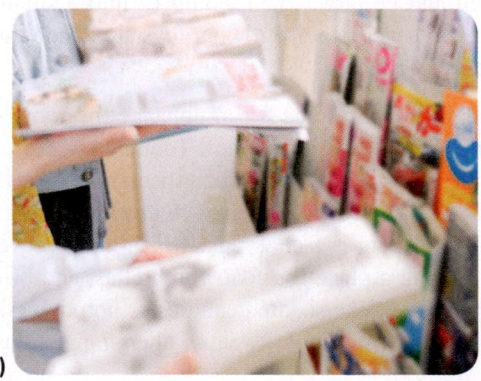

(a)

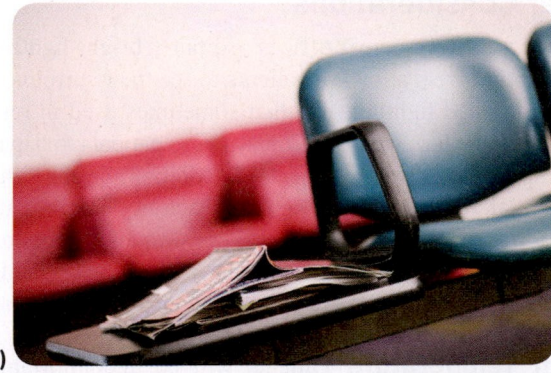

(b)

FIGURE 7-11 (a) Magazine racks save space, but do not forget to have (b) some reading material on tables for elderly or differently abled patients.
© Fuse/Getty Images RF, © Indeed/Getty Images RF

large-print editions should be available for elderly and other sight-impaired patients.

Magazines and Books Choosing the right mix of reading material to interest all patients is a challenge. You probably have been in offices that have wonderful selections, and in an equal number of offices that do not. Try to have varied types of reading material to accommodate your patients' broad range of interests. If your office sees teen and younger patients, be sure to include reading material for their interests, too.

You or someone on the office staff should be sure to screen publications for medical content so that you can alert physicians to articles that might stimulate patient questions. Make sure magazines are current. There is nothing worse than having a patient reception area full of outdated or worn magazines.

Patient Information Packet Many offices today compile a patient information packet to inform new patients about the practice. The packet can be designed in many ways, from a simple flyer to a formal folder with pockets to hold individual sheets of information. Topics covered in the packet can range from billing and insurance processing policies to biographical information on each physician in a group practice. The *Patient Education* chapter will discuss how to develop the contents of a patient information packet.

Medical Information Medical brochures are another type of reading material commonly found in the reception area. Patients may be interested in information that pertains to their general health or to specific conditions, particularly those that are treated by your physicians. Brochures on a variety of topics are available to medical offices either free of charge or for a nominal fee. These brochures are usually produced by nonprofit associations that specialize in a disease or condition (such as the American Cancer Society) and by pharmaceutical companies.

Before displaying pamphlets and brochures in the reception area, both you and the physicians may want to review them for medical accuracy and to prepare for any questions patients may have.

Bulletin Board Many reception areas contain bulletin boards that highlight area support group meetings and offer other current information. To encourage patients to look at the bulletin board, change the format and content frequently. Tailor items on the bulletin board to patient interests. Other, more general items for display on any physician's bulletin board might include the following:

- Office policies and procedures for patients such as no smoking or eating in the patient reception area, late or missed appointment policies, and patient payment information
- Government reports on drug and nutrition information
- Pamphlets or flyers from nonprofit healthcare organizations such as the American Heart Association and requests from the American Red Cross or local blood bank for blood donors
- Flyers on upcoming health fairs, including blood pressure or other health screening opportunities

- Newspaper or magazine articles on interesting medical issues pertinent to the practice specialties
- Community notices for food drives or similar charity events
- Current information about practice staff and their accomplishments

Finally, the bulletin board is an ideal place to display the office brochure. Put some extra copies of the brochure in an open envelope tacked to the bulletin board to encourage patients to take one home. To keep the bulletin board up to date, all time-sensitive materials, such as notices about a class or seminar, should be removed as soon as the date of the scheduled event has passed (Figure 7-12).

Television and Videos

Although reading remains the traditional pastime in patient reception areas, watching television and DVDs is a common activity in physician offices across the country. Many patient reception areas now include a television, which can be tuned to regular or satellite news or entertainment stations or can play preselected videos. Physicians may provide informative healthcare videos of general interest to their patients or videos that meet the more specific interests of the practice. Videos are helpful for patients with limited reading ability and can be helpful if customized for non-English speakers.

Accommodating Children

A pediatric reception area caters to a unique age group of patients. To accommodate this specialized clientele, in addition to regular chairs, child-size chairs may also be available. Playhouses or play furniture, such as small tables, are also appropriate choices. The use of bright colors and storybook characters can also help to make the décor appealing to young children. It is important to make the setting feel familiar and comfortable. The reception desk may stock rolls of stickers or other inexpensive prizes to give to young patients after they have seen the doctor. As mentioned earlier, many pediatric offices have found it helpful to include two reception areas—one for well visits and one for children who are potentially **contagious**—to separate the sick children from those who are well.

Because children—even sick ones—do not usually like to sit still for long periods, you may want to consider including toys, games, videos, and books in the pediatric reception area. If this reception area separates sick children from well children, the "well" side may include more active entertainment, like an indoor slide or playhouse, while the "sick" side may provide quieter games and activities, like books and puzzles.

Choose toys carefully. You do not want children—even well ones—to be too active in the reception area because they might disrupt other patients and their families. Avoid balls, jump ropes, and other toys meant for outside use. Puzzles and blocks are good choices because they encourage quieter play. All toys should be easy to clean (a bleach-water solution or nonaerosol disinfectant can be used) and, for safety and health reasons, should not include stuffed animals. Stuffed animals are not appropriate because they are difficult to keep clean and can be a source of infection. Their small parts can also pose a choking hazard. You might informally ask parents and children if they like the play items or if they would prefer other types of toys. Procedure 7-3 explains how to set up a pediatric reception area.

▶ The Importance of Cleanliness   LO 7.9

No matter how tastefully it is decorated, the reception area will be unappealing if it is not clean. Patients expect a physician's office to maintain a high standard of cleanliness. The perception is that a messy or dirty reception area or patient bathroom reflects a practice that does not meet minimum standards for cleanliness. A practice with a spotless, attractive reception area reassures patients that they have chosen a practice with high standards of cleanliness. Another reminder of these high standards is the availability of alcohol-based hand rubs for patient use in the reception area (as well as in patient treatment areas) with directions for their use.

Housekeeping

Keeping the patient reception area neat and clean usually falls within the medical assistant's duties. In most cases, you will be responsible for supervising the work of a professional cleaning service. In a small medical office, you may be required to clean the area yourself, using appropriate antibacterial agents and a vacuum. Cleaning should occur daily, with emergency cleanups as needed.

Because professional services generally clean in the evening after business hours, you will probably not be present while the housekeeping staff is working. You may be asked to provide feedback to the cleaning company, however. It also may be your responsibility to outline the tasks you expect workers to complete, including any special requests.

One way of communicating with the cleaning staff is to create a Cleaning Communications Notebook. Arrange with the cleaning staff to leave the notebook open every evening in the same place. Date all entries. Write short, concise directions about any special requests for cleaning. Describe the nature of any stain so the service can best treat it. Sign each entry.

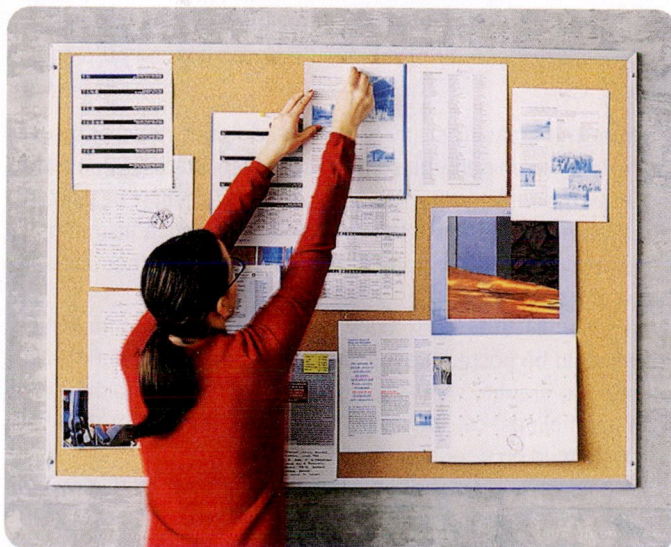

FIGURE 7-12 Keep the office bulletin board neat, current, and uncluttered so the information remains of interest to the patients.
© Rob Melnychuk/Getty Images RF

Be sure to comment when something is done especially well. Like all of us, your cleaning staff likes to hear when they have done a particularly nice job.

Tasks Although housekeeping tasks vary from office to office, basic routines are applicable to areas like the patient reception room. The *Caution: Handle with Care* section gives more information about maintaining a clean reception area.

Whether or not the office employs a professional cleaning service, you or another staff member will need to check for cleanliness throughout the day. As patients spend time in the office, items may become soiled or be moved out of place. Taking time between patient appointments or at midday to spot-clean small areas that no longer appear "spotless" and to neaten items will help keep the patient reception area pleasing to the eye.

Equipment If you, and not a professional service, are responsible for cleaning, the person in charge of the office budget will approve the purchase of cleaning equipment and supplies. Examples of cleaning equipment include handheld and upright vacuums, mops, and brooms. Supplies include trash bags, cleaning solutions, cleaning rags, and buckets. It is a good idea to have some basic cleaning materials on hand in case an emergency cleanup job is needed during office hours. Always wear gloves when doing cleaning of any kind and use OSHA guidelines for safety. Be sure to also obtain the SDS for any cleaning materials stored in the office and insert the sheets in the office SDS binder.

Removing Odors

Odors are particularly offensive in a medical office because people who are sick are often affected more severely by strong odors. Because patients are in the office for a scheduled appointment, they cannot suddenly leave to escape the odor. Some odors that may occasionally be present in a medical practice include those of urine, feces, vomit, body odors, and laboratory chemicals. A good ventilating system with charcoal filters can help minimize odors. If the system has temporary high-speed blowers, they can be activated as well. Disinfectant sprays and deodorizing sprays also may help, but deodorizers should be used sparingly, as more and more people are developing allergies to many of the scents used to mask odors.

One odor that can be prevented is smoke. Display "Thank You for Not Smoking" signs prominently in the patient reception area. Many offices, particularly those located in large buildings or attached to hospitals, are "nonsmoking zones." Smokers who visit these offices must leave not only the office but the grounds, too, if they insist on smoking. This common rule is simply because not only does smoking produce an offensive odor, it also may affect the health of other patients in the reception area. People with asthma or other breathing disorders, or who are feeling unwell for any reason, are

CAUTION: HANDLE WITH CARE

Maintaining Standards of Cleanliness in the Reception Area

Cleanliness is (and should be) one of a medical office's hallmarks. Not only is cleanliness required in the examination and testing rooms, it is also expected in the patient reception area. A messy patient reception area reflects badly on the practice. Patients may think, "If they don't care about this, what else do they not care about?" Maintaining standards of cleanliness helps ensure that the reception area is presentable and inviting at all times.

As a medical assistant, you may be involved—along with the physician, office manager, and other staff members—in setting the office's cleanliness standards. Standards are general guidelines. In addition to setting standards, you will need to specify the tasks required to meet each standard. You also may want to create a checklist of the tasks required to meet all of these standards.

The following list outlines standards you may want to consider. Specific housekeeping tasks for meeting those standards are included in parentheses.

1. Keep everything in its place. (Complete a daily visual check for out-of-place items. Return all magazines to racks. Push chairs back into place.)

2. Dispose of all trash. (Empty trash cans. Pick up trash on the floor or on furniture.)

3. Prevent dust and dirt from accumulating on surfaces. (Wipe or dust furniture, lamps, and artificial plants. Polish doorknobs. Clean mirrors, wall hangings, and pictures.)

4. Spot-clean areas that become dirty. (Remove scuffmarks. Clean upholstery stains.)

5. Disinfect areas of the reception area if they have been exposed to body fluids. (Immediately clean and disinfect all soiled areas.)

6. Handle items with care. (Take precautions when carrying potentially messy or breakable items. Do not carry too much at once.)

After the standards have been established, type and post them in a prominent place for the office staff (but not the patients) to see. The cleaning activities checklist may be posted, but the person responsible for cleaning the office also should keep a copy. It is everyone's duty to keep the office looking clean and presentable.

A schedule of specific daily and weekly cleaning activities also should be posted. Less frequent housekeeping duties, like laundering drapes, shampooing the carpet, and cleaning windows and blinds, can be noted in a tickler file so that they will be performed on a regular basis.

It is always a good idea to have a second staff member responsible for periodically working with the medical assistant on housekeeping responsibilities. That person also may be responsible for handling cleaning duties when the medical assistant is away from the office.

particularly sensitive to smoke and strong odors. It is up to the healthcare facility and its employees to protect their health while in the medical office and its grounds.

Infectious Waste

There may be times when you will need to clean up infectious waste. **Infectious waste,** also known as biohazardous waste, is waste that can be dangerous to those who handle it or to the environment. Infectious waste includes human waste, human tissue, and body fluids such as blood and urine. It also includes any potentially hazardous waste generated in the treatment of patients, such as needles, scalpels, cultures of human cells, and dressings.

Although infectious waste is not commonly generated in the patient reception area, it can happen—for example, when a patient vomits or bleeds on the rug or on furniture. If that situation should occur, you must clean up the waste promptly. Remember, infectious waste must be handled in accordance with federal law and following OSHA guidelines. Your office may choose to purchase commercially prepared hazardous waste kits for use in cleaning up spills. After cleaning infectious waste from the patient reception area, deposit it in a biohazard container. Disinfect the site to eliminate possible contamination of other patients. Refer to the chapter *Infection Control Fundamentals* to review OSHA guidelines and standard precautions.

▶ Office Access for All LO 7.10

The path patients must take to get from the parking area or street to the office and then back out again is called the office access. Some offices have easier access than others, but ease of access is important to your patients, particularly those who are older or differently abled (see Figure 7-13).

Parking Arrangements

Although some patients walk to the medical office or take public transportation, the majority of patients will probably travel by their personal vehicles. Patients who drive to the office need a place to park.

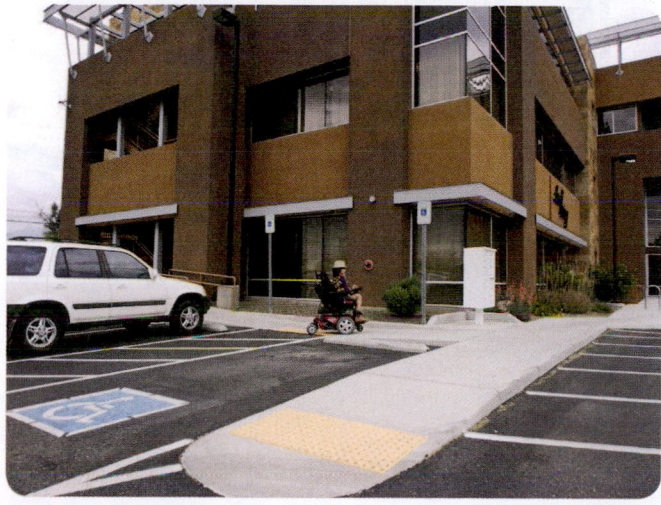

FIGURE 7-13 All patients should have access to ample parking and easy access to the office.

© McGraw-Hill Education. David Moyer, photographer

The office can offer either on-street parking or a parking lot or parking garage. On-street parking requires patients to fend for themselves. They may have to put money into parking meters, and parking spaces may be difficult to find. Both the money required and the potential problems in finding parking spots limit the ease with which patients can gain access to the office.

On the other hand, a free parking lot or parking garage improves office access. Parking lots and garages should be well lit for safety. The number of spaces needed depends on the number of patients scheduled for a specified time period and the average amount of time they spend in the facility. If patients generally spend an hour at the facility and 10 patients are scheduled per hour, then you will need no fewer than 10 parking spaces. Keep in mind that you will need to account for patients who spend more time in the office, and you will need a parking space for each staff member. Periodically reevaluate the office's parking needs because they may change over time. All offices must also provide handicapped parking spaces for patients. Visit http://www.adaptiveaccess.com/handicap_parking.php for more information on handicapped parking. You will read more about patients with special needs later in the chapter.

Entrances

The entrance to the office should be clearly marked so that patients can find the office easily. The name of the practice and of the physician(s) should be on the door or beside the door. Just outside the doorway should be a doormat to help control the amount of dirt tracked into the office. If the office door opens directly to the outside, people inside will feel a sudden change in temperature each time the door is opened in hot or cold weather. A foyer or double-door arrangement helps minimize the weather's effects by keeping the office at a consistent, comfortable temperature. All doorways must be wide enough to accommodate patients using wheelchairs and walkers. Hallways should be well lit and without obstructions.

Safety and Security

Safety and security are important concerns in any public building, and they are especially important for a medical office. To ensure both patient and staff safety, including protection from hazardous wiring or poorly lit hallways, there are guidelines for businesses, some of which pertain to the patient reception area. The medical office also must be secure from burglary.

Building Exits Make sure you and the office staff members are familiar with *all* building exits. As you learned earlier in the chapter, it may be necessary to leave the office quickly, as during a fire, flood, or other emergency. Refer to the instructions in Emergency Action Plans and Drills, discussed earlier, for more information about office exits and evacuating the office.

Security Systems No matter where the medical office is located, a security alarm system is a wise investment, even if security personnel patrol the office building. A security alarm system offers valuable protection for the confidential patient information housed in a medical office. After the alarm system is installed, all office staff members should thoroughly familiarize themselves with it. They should be able to arm and disarm it easily and know what to do if it is accidentally activated. Each staff member should have her or his own individually assigned security access code. This number is required to authorize locking or unlocking the system. Like a credit card, bank, or other security PIN (personal identification number), it should never be shared.

Considerations for Patients with Special Needs

Some patients who come into the medical office will be disabled; that is, they were born with or have acquired a condition that limits or changes their abilities. A more positive way to refer to these patients who are differently abled is the use of the term *special needs*. For example, people who are paralyzed from the waist down have special needs; so do people who are visually impaired. This does not mean that these people cannot perform the same tasks that other people can; they may simply need special accommodations to do so. With some forethought and planning, the office can appropriately accommodate special needs patients. Ensuring wheelchair access through doors and hallways, as mentioned earlier, is just one way. Using ramps instead of steps, as shown in Figure 7-14, allows easier access not only for wheelchair users but also for others who have limited mobility. Allowing additional space in the reception area for wheelchairs, walkers, crutches, and guide dogs accommodates several types of special needs patients. Procedure 7-4, found at the end of the chapter, explains how to organize the patient reception area to meet the special needs of patients who are physically challenged. For more information on meeting the needs of the differently abled, visit the Adaptive Access website at http://www.adaptiveaccess.com/index.php.

Americans with Disabilities Act Individuals with special needs are often singled out for their differences and are sometimes discriminated against. For example, if a company building does not have access ramps for wheelchairs, workers in wheelchairs cannot qualify for jobs there. This would violate the **Americans with Disabilities Act (ADA),** which prevents discrimination based solely on a person's physical or mental disability.

Passed in 1990, this federal act is sometimes referred to as the civil rights act for people with disabilities, since it forbids discrimination based on physical or mental disabilities. The intent of the ADA is to provide equal access and reasonable accommodation in several important areas, including employment, facilities, sports, and education. The two sections involving medical practices are employment (discussed in the *Practice Management* chapter) and facilities. The following are required and reasonable facility accommodations:

- Handicapped parking
- Wheelchair ramps
- Wheelchair-accessible doors, halls, and bathrooms
- Handrails in halls and bathrooms
- Handicapped bathrooms including toilets, sinks, and room for a wheelchair to turn
- Braille elevator floor indicators
- Large-print patient forms
- Devices to communicate with the hearing impaired, as discussed in the *Telephone Techniques* chapter

Service Animals A service animal may accompany a patient with special needs (Figure 7-15) into a medical office or facility. The dog is the most common service animal, but cats, monkeys, and even miniature ponies are in use. Service animals wear a special vest that identifies them and they should have a certification. Remember that these animals are not pets and should not be distracted while "on duty." Service animals are well behaved and calm unless their charge appears to be threatened.

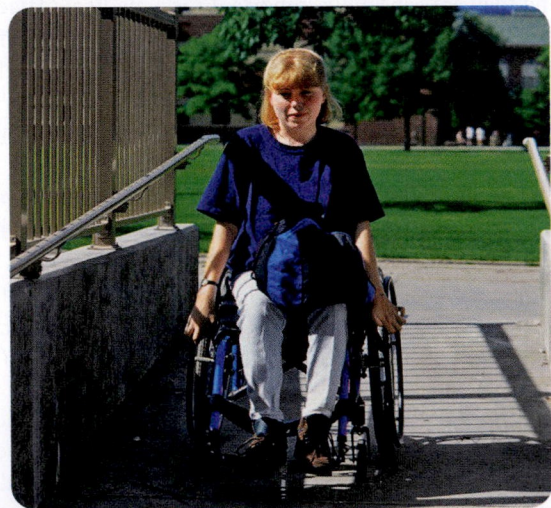

FIGURE 7-14 Ramps allow people using wheelchairs and other assistive devices easier access to the office.
© Patrick Clark/Getty Images RF

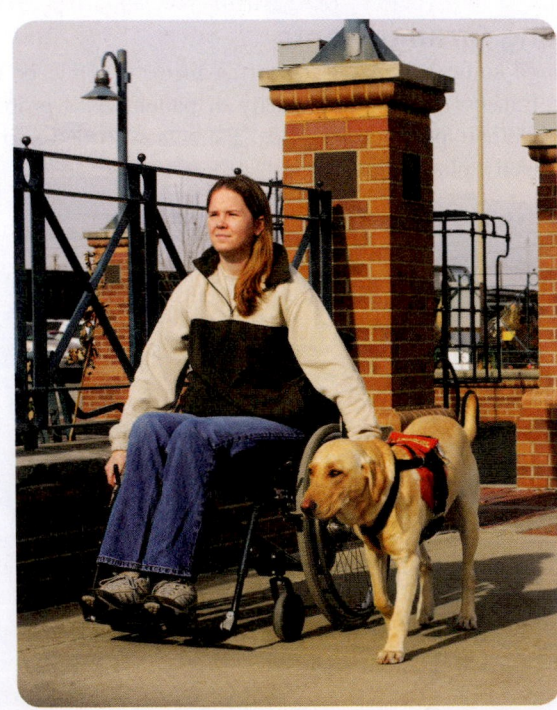

FIGURE 7-15 Service animals should not be disturbed or distracted when working.
© Don Farrall/Getty Images RF

Vision and Hearing Impairments Although they should, there are still many offices that do not make special accommodations for patients with vision or hearing impairments. As a medical assistant, you can do your part in the office by posting prominent signs in the reception area with information that patients need to know. A staff member should offer to assist patients with hearing or vision impairments as needed from the reception area to the examination room when it is their turn to see the doctor.

Patients who are hearing impaired may request the presence of a certified sign language interpreter to assist in communicating with the medical staff. If requested, federal law requires that the office provide and pay for this interpreter.

It is also helpful, but not required by law, to provide a device, also known as a telecommunications device for the deaf (TDD), for hearing-impaired patients. This specially designed telephone, formerly called a TTY (teletypewriter), looks very much like a laptop computer with a cradle for the receiver of a traditional telephone. The receiver is placed in the cradle and the hearing-impaired patient can then type the communication on the keyboard. The message can be received by another TDD or relayed through a specialty relay service.

Some states offer a relay service for patients with hearing impairments or speech disabilities. When an individual accesses this service through the TDD, the service then places the call using voice. It is important to understand that a relay service could call a medical office to make an appointment for a patient. The medical assistant needs to be careful to respond appropriately and not mistake the call as an unwanted marketing call. You will read about TDD in more detail in the *Telephone Techniques* chapter.

Preparing the Reception Area for a Child with Autism

In a medical office, you will most likely have patients who have an autism spectrum disorder (ASD). Individuals with ASD have difficulty with communication and social interactions. Children with ASD are often affected by changes in routine or schedule and new environments and may have severe reactions to sensory overload from loud noises or bright lights. For this reason, patients with ASD may need special accommodations when visiting a medical facility. As a medical assistant, you can make the visit to the healthcare facility easier by

- Scheduling the appointment first thing in the morning or last in the afternoon.
- Reducing the number of other patients and staff the patient encounters.
- Keeping the lights in the reception area low.
- Turning the volume of music down or off in the room where a patient with ASD is located.
- Taking the patient to the exam room as soon as possible.
- Alerting the healthcare practitioner that the patient is ready.
- Using visual aids and stories to explain procedures.

Older Americans Act of 1965

The fastest-growing segment of the American population is the elderly. Like those who are differently abled, many elderly people face discrimination. One reason for the discrimination may be that with age come medical conditions and disorders that create physical limitations.

Congress passed the **Older Americans Act of 1965** to eliminate discrimination against the elderly. Among other benefits, the act guarantees elderly citizens the best possible healthcare regardless of ability to pay, an adequate retirement income, and protection against abuse, neglect, and exploitation.

What does the Older Americans Act mean for the medical office reception area? If the practice serves elderly patients, the office staff must be sensitive to their special needs. The patient reception area should be as comfortable as possible for patients with arthritis, failing eyesight, and other common ailments of the elderly. Make sure there are a few straight-backed chairs located near the front door and near the examination rooms. These chairs are easier to get into and out of than soft sofas and offer greater back support than low chairs or couches with sinking cushions. In addition, arms on chairs provide support when sitting and standing for patients who are unsteady.

Place reading materials within easy reach of the chairs so that elderly patients do not have to get up from their chairs for them. Have large-print books and magazines available, if possible, for patients with poor eyesight. You also might offer magnifying glasses for patients who like to use them. In addition, make sure that the print on all office signs is large and easy to read. As stated earlier, the patient reception area and restrooms should be well lit to help everyone, including elderly patients, see more clearly.

Special Situations Patients in a medical practice are usually a diverse group of people. Their interests, needs, and medical conditions can have an impact on the design of the reception area.

Patients from Diverse Cultural Backgrounds The United States has long been called a melting pot because of its mixture of people and cultures. Each culture lends its own special qualities, and together the cultures combine to create a unique blend of people called Americans.

You may work in a neighborhood that has a distinct culture or one in which many cultures are represented. To help patients feel comfortable, make the reception area reflect aspects of the local cultural backgrounds whenever possible. This effort will help patients feel more welcome.

Suppose, for example, that the medical office where you work serves many Latino patients. Posting signs in Spanish and English acknowledges the fact that both languages are spoken in that neighborhood. Providing reading materials, such as newspapers and magazines, in a second language—for both adults and children—is another way to show respect and interest. Decorating the office for Spanish holidays in addition to American ones demonstrates that you care about what is important to patients. Displaying artwork created by local artists and artisans is another idea.

Patients Who Are Highly Contagious Patients may have to come into the physician's office when they are highly contagious. This fact is a concern for all patients, but it is especially critical for patients who are immunocompromised. The immune system of an immunocompromised patient is not functioning at a normal level. Because these patients do not have the normal ability to fight off disease, they are at greater risk than the average person for becoming sick. Patients undergoing chemotherapy and patients with AIDS, for example, have compromised immune systems. Follow transmission-based precautions when dealing with any patient who is highly contagious.

▶ Functions of the Reception Staff LO 7.11

The person who works at the *front desk* is commonly called the receptionist. The receptionist's main function is to greet people, register them, give them direction, and answer the phone. In the past, people have taken the receptionist for granted, but truly, the receptionist is one of the most important people in the practice. Just as the reception area décor gives the patient his first impression of the office itself, it is the receptionist who gives the first impression of the office staff and sets the perception of the care the patient will receive from the medical staff. The multiple tasks the receptionist is responsible for provides the very basis for the patient's medical care and for the overall positive impression you wish to convey to your patients. It is her attitude and communication skills that create this positive (or negative) first impression. This staff member, who is frequently an administrative medical assistant, should immediately acknowledge and greet the arriving patient with a smile and pleasant voice. If the receptionist is on the phone, looking up at the patient with a smile and head nod is appropriate to acknowledge the patient and let him know she will be with him shortly. This small gesture will convey that the office staff is attentive and put the patient at ease from the start of the appointment.

Patient Registration and HIPAA

Patient registration is often referred to as patient check-in or sign-in. In many offices, upon arrival, patients are asked to "sign in" to notify staff that they are there. Two commonly used forms of check-in or sign-in are the paper version and the digital or electronic version. Both may include the arrival time, the appointment time, and the practitioner's name. As you read earlier, under HIPAA, personal health information (PHI) is considered private and confidential; however, the rules do state that sign-in sheets are allowable, as long as the reason for the visit is not included on the sign-in sheet. If the physician specialty is of a confidential nature (such as psychology or drug treatment), it is suggested that sign-in sheets not be used—by the very nature of seeing the practitioner, an "assumption" about the nature of the visit can be made.

If an electronic sign-in is utilized, two methods are approved:

- Providing a digital pad (similar to electronic debit or charge)
- Use of a computer in the reception area for patients to input information

Once the patient has signed in, the receptionist will provide him or her with appropriate forms. Returning patients may receive a copy of their information to update. Some offices will interview the patient, line-by-line, and input this information directly into the system. This method is usually more time-consuming than having the patient provide hard copy and then inputting directly from the form. Regardless of which method is used, the information given should be reviewed with the patient.

New patients receive a complete new patient registration packet that includes

- Demographic/insurance coverage form.
- Authorizations for release of information to insurance carriers, assignment of benefits, and financial responsibility.
- Notice of Privacy Practices.
- Health history.
- Information regarding the payment and other policies of the practice.

The forms must be completed and signed. The patient's or insured party's insurance card and a picture identifier, such as a driver's license, are copied or scanned. The picture identifier is one method to help reduce healthcare fraud, by preventing a friend or family member who may not have health insurance from "borrowing" another insurance card. The ID should be checked every time the patient comes into the office. You will explore medical identity theft in more detail a bit later in this chapter. From the demographic and health information provided by the patient, the medical assistant initiates a medical record or electronic health record. The record may be totally electronic or a combination of electronic health record and hard-copy financial information or electronic financial information and paper health record. The components of the medical record are covered in the *Medical Records and Documentation* and *Electronic Health Records* chapters. When all forms are completed and signed, the appropriate clinical staff member is notified that the patient is ready to be seen.

Payment

Another reception responsibility is collecting the patient's insurance copayment, which is usually done prior to the visit. The amount of the copayment, if applicable, is usually shown on the patient's insurance card. Depending on the office, acceptable payment methods are cash, check, debit cards, and charge cards. Third-party checks should never be accepted, and any personal checks should be written for the exact amount. Cash and checks are kept in a cash drawer that is locked when the reception desk is unmanned. In some offices, the patient will return to the reception area after the visit and may make any payments due at that time. All financial transactions will be discussed in depth in the chapter *Patient Collections and Financial Management*. Follow-up and referral appointments are often also scheduled at the front desk. Once all patient transactions are completed, the receptionist should extend a pleasant farewell to all patients.

Observation and Updates

Another function of the front desk staff is to be observant. As discussed earlier, some patients should not sit in the main reception area. These include patients who are

- Having chest pain (adults).
- Experiencing shortness of breath.
- Bleeding.

- Feeling faint (syncope), dizzy, light-headed.
- Vomiting.
- Experiencing an undiagnosed or contagious rash.

If a patient complains of any of these symptoms, or if you notice a change in a patient's status, immediately notify a member of the clinical staff, who will determine where to place the patient. If you are concerned about the condition of any patient, do not hesitate to ask the clinical staff for advice.

As mentioned earlier in the chapter, the receptionist (or any office staff member) should address spills, trash, and any potential hazards—such as frayed cords, broken furniture, or tears in rugs—as quickly as possible. If the reception area becomes overcrowded, "traffic control" is required. Ensure chairs are not occupied with personal items and determine if there is room in treatment areas. Keeping patients updated if appointments are running late is another important function of the front office staff . If the wait time is significant, giving patients the option of rescheduling their appointments shows respect for the patient's time.

The Identity Theft Prevention Program

In many instances, HIPAA and medical identity theft go hand in hand. The person in the practice with the dual responsibility is generally the privacy or compliance officer. A three-pronged approach for the medical office's prevention program is recommended:

1. Prevention—implementing sound electronic and other security systems maintaining HIPAA compliance
2. Detection—staff training on what to look for and electronic "red flagging" such as automatic on-screen identification of a difference in date of birth
3. Mitigation—ensuring medical records of the perpetrator and the authentic patient are not co-mingled; the medical assistant should know what to look for in suspicious behaviors and both how to report such behaviors and how to find out if suspicious behavior by the patient has been previously reported

▶ Opening and Closing the Office   LO 7.12

You are learning that efficiency in the medical office is a result of good organization and adherence to office policies and procedures. These policies include establishing set procedures for opening and closing the facility. This is generally the responsibility of the staff member in the reception area. Following a set routine and using specially designed check sheets ensure no process is overlooked. Some offices perform specific tasks when opening the office, like restocking supplies, and other offices perform these tasks at closing. Let's take a general look at both of these procedures.

Beginning the Day

The person opening the office arrives approximately 30 minutes prior to the scheduled time for office operations to begin. Safety is a consideration. Be aware of the activity outside the office door such as persons in the parking area, elevators, or hallways. If you feel uncomfortable, notify the facility's security or await the arrival of another staff member. Laboratory specimens, such as blood, obtained by staff for delivery to reference laboratories are often placed in a special container on the office door or in the vicinity. Upon arrival in the morning, ensure the specimens were picked up from the previous day. Do not completely turn your back while unlocking the door. Once inside, deactivate the security system.

The first priority is accessing the answering service or answering machine to determine if any staff member may have called in with an emergency, patients have canceled appointments, patients need a same-day appointment, or hospitals reported patients seen during the night. Convey this vital information to the correct staff member as soon as possible. Other tasks may be to turn on a fax machine or coffee machine. Some offices divide the responsibility for the administrative areas and the clinical areas. Table 7-2, provides a general guideline for opening the medical office.

TABLE 7-2	Daily Checklist for Opening the Office						
Daily Checklist for Opening BWW Medical Associates, PC				W/E_____			
		M	T	W	Th	F	S
1. Security system is disarmed.							
2. Voicemail/answering service messages are retrieved.							
3. Messages are routed and ready for callback.							
4. Computers are turned on.							
5. Appointments and insurance rosters are checked.							
6. If needed, charts are pulled and paperwork is attached.							
7. Equipment is working properly.							
8. Rooms are supplied and ready.							
9. Refrigerator temperature is checked.							
10. Emergency supplies, including O_2, are checked.							
11. Reception area is in order and patient education material is available.							
12. Lab specimens from the day before were picked up.							

TABLE 7-3	Daily Checklist for Closing the Office						
Daily Checklist for Closing BWW Medical Associates, PC					W/E _____		
		M	T	W	Th	F	S
1. Computers are logged off and shut down.							
2. Contaminated supplies/equipment are properly disposed of or tagged for cleaning/sterilization.							
3. Areas are restocked.							
4. If needed, patient charts are pulled/reviewed for next day and all test results are available.							
5. Laboratory specimens are in pick-up receptacle.							
6. All office equipment is turned off (including kitchen).							
7. Reception area is neat and organized.							
8. Calls are forwarded to voicemail/answering machine.							
9. Medical records are secured.							
10. All doors and windows are locked.							
11. Security system is armed.							

Ending the Day

Table 7-3 includes typical duties for ending the day efficiently, which is just as important as beginning the day efficiently. It completes the day's responsibilities and sets the stage for the next day.

A person closing the office that has extended or split hours may not be the same person who opened the office, so cooperation and good communication are essential between staff members. Turn off equipment, such as the coffeemaker and the fax machine, if that is the office policy. Check exam rooms to be sure supplies are well stocked for the next day and give the reception room one last "look" to be sure it is neat and presentable for the morning patients. Ensure that confidential information is not in view for any cleaning or security personnel who may enter the office after hours. Notify the answering service that the office is closing or turn on the answering machine. Ensure laboratory specimens are placed in the proper container for pick-up. Activate the security system (Figure 7-16).

Be alert when exiting the building for any unusual or suspicious activity. Refer to Procedure 7-5, Opening and Closing the Medical Office, for practice on these procedures. Following consistent policies and procedures guarantees that important tasks are not forgotten and, in this case, ensures that the office, its equipment, medications, and its private information remain safe and secure at all times.

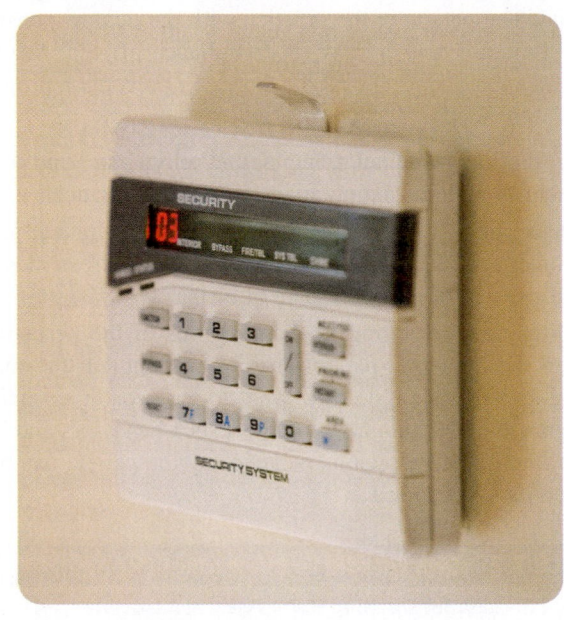

FIGURE 7-16 Arming the office security system is usually the final task to end the workday.
© 2009 Jupiterimages Corporation RF

PROCEDURE 7-1 Handling a Fire Emergency

Procedure Goal: To ensure safe use of a fire extinguisher during a fire emergency

OSHA Guidelines: This procedure does not involve exposure to blood, body fluids, or tissue.

Materials: Fully charged fire extinguisher that has been professionally serviced on a yearly basis

Method:

1. In the case of an open fire or continuous smoke, pull the fire alarm or call emergency services to alert the local fire authorities.
2. Move patients out of the area.
3. Remove the fire extinguisher from its stored location.

4. Assess the fire. If it is too large, do not attempt to extinguish the fire. Leave the building immediately and wait for the fire department to arrive.
RATIONALE: *You must determine if you can easily contain the fire so that you know whether to have everyone leave the building.*

If the Fire Cannot Be Easily Contained

5. Calmly and quickly ask each employee to follow the established fire plan.

6. Remove all patients to the outside of the building; ensure patient comfort and safety at all times.

If the Fire Is Small and Easily Contained

7. Hold the fire extinguisher upright.

8. **Pull** the safety pin on the fire extinguisher.

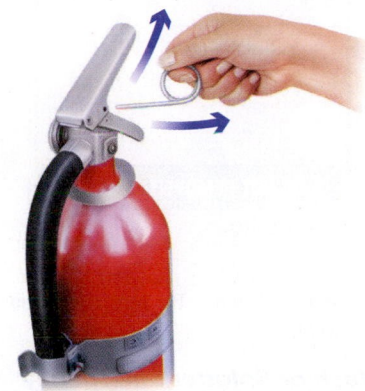

FIGURE Procedure 7-1 Step 8   To activate a fire extinguisher, pull the safety pin.

9. **Aim** at the base of the fire.

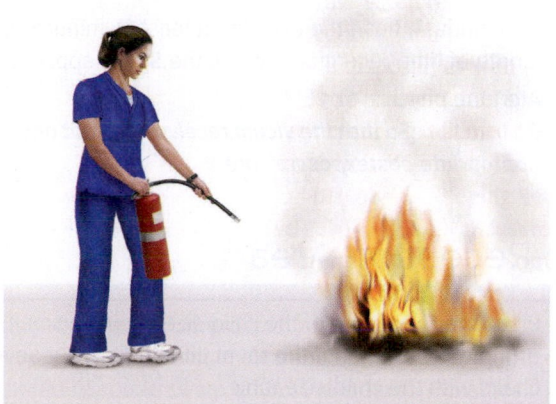

FIGURE Procedure 7-1 Step 9   You should aim at the base of the fire, not the flames. The source or fuel of the fire is at the base.

10. **Squeeze** the trigger.

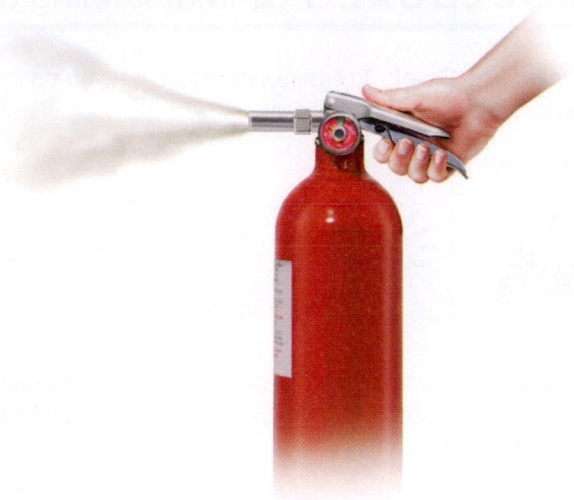

FIGURE Procedure 7-1 Step 10   Once you are aiming at the base of the fire, squeeze the lever to deliver the extinguishing agent.

11. **Sweep** side to side until the fire is out.

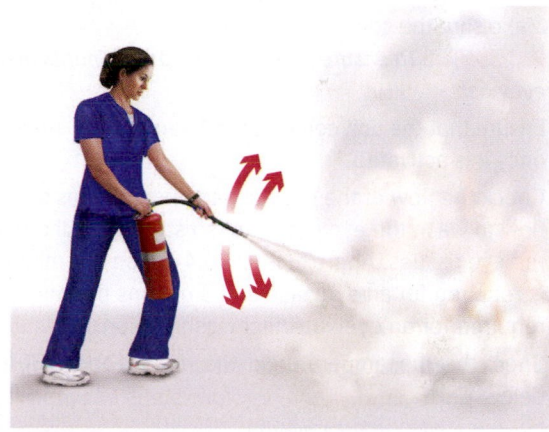

FIGURE Procedure 7-1 Step 11   Sweep back and forth at the base of the fire until it is out.

12. Do not reenter the area until the fire department assesses and clears the area.
RATIONALE: *A professional firefighter should assess the area to ascertain if there is a danger of the fire reigniting.*

PROCEDURE 7-2 Maintaining and Using an Eyewash Station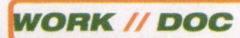

Procedure Goal: To ensure safe use of eyewash station following a splash or splatter accident

OSHA Guidelines:

Materials: Eyewash station. This may be plumbed or free-standing. Eyewash safety inspection record, gloves, moisture-proof lab coat, and goggles or face mask.

Method:

On a Weekly Basis

1. Check that the path to the eyewash station is clear and no more than 10 seconds from the hazard.
2. Ensure that the eyewash sign is easily visible.
3. Make sure the covers are in place.
   RATIONALE: *To ensure there are no contaminants on the eyewash*
4. Ensure that the unit comes on in 1 second and stays on once it is activated.
5. Check the flow of the eyewash to ensure it has sufficient flow to wash the eye but is not so strong it will damage the eye tissues. Approximately 0.4 gallon per minute is required for an eyewash and 3 gallons per minute is required for an eyewash/facewash station.
6. Check that the temperature of the water is above 60°F and below 100°F.
7. Flush the system for 1 minute.
   RATIONALE: *To remove any particulate matter such as sediment from standing water that may have collected in the water line*

8. Complete the Safety Inspection record attached to the eyewash station.

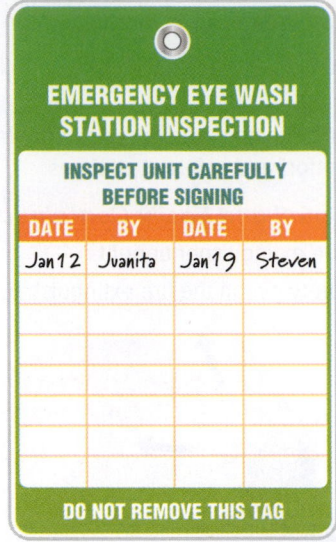

FIGURE Procedure 7-2 Step 8   The safety inspection record should be completed each week.

During a Splash or Splatter Emergency

9. Help the victim to the eyewash station.
10. Activate the system.
11. If the eyewash is a plumbed unit, have the victim lean into the eyewash, keeping her eyes continuously open. You may have to don gloves and gown and assist the victim by holding her eye or eyes open.
12. Continuously flush the eyes for at least 15 minutes or the length of time recommended on the SDS if applicable.
13. Alert the physician or EMS.
    RATIONALE: *So that the victim receives prompt and appropriate postexposure care*

PROCEDURE 7-3 Creating a Pediatric Reception Area

Procedure Goal: To create an appropriate environment for children in the patient reception area of a medical (pediatric) practice

OSHA Guidelines: This procedure does not involve exposure to blood, body fluids, or tissue.

Materials: Children's books and magazines, games, toys, nontoxic crayons and coloring books, television and DVD player, children's DVDs, child- and adult-size chairs, child-size table, bookshelf, boxes or shelves, decorative wall hangings, or educational posters (optional)

Method:

1. Place all adult-size chairs against the wall. Position some of the child-size chairs along the wall with the adult chairs.

2. Place the remainder of the child-size chairs in small groupings throughout the room. In addition, put several chairs with the child-size table.

3. Put the books, magazines, crayons, and coloring books on the bookshelf in one corner of the room near a grouping of chairs.

4. Choose toys and games carefully. Avoid toys that encourage active play, such as balls, or toys that require a large area. Make sure that all toys meet safety guidelines. Watch for loose or small (smaller than a golf ball) parts. Toys should also be easy to clean.
   RATIONALE: *Helps ensure safety in the patient reception area*

5. Place the activities for older children near one grouping of chairs and the games and toys for younger children near another grouping. Keep the toys and games in a toy box or on shelves designated for them. Consider labeling or color-coding boxes and shelves and the games and toys that belong there to encourage children to return the games and toys to the appropriate storage area.

6. Place the television and DVD player on a high shelf, if possible, or attach them to the wall near the ceiling.

Keep children's DVDs behind the reception desk, and periodically change the video in the DVD player.
RATIONALE: *Doing so helps ensure safety in the patient reception area, as DVDs and video equipment are easily damaged or destroyed by young patients. Young patients also may be harmed in trying to reach the equipment.*

7. To make the room more cheerful, decorate it with wall hangings or posters.

PROCEDURE 7-4 Creating a Reception Area Accessible to Patients with Special Needs

Procedure Goal: To arrange elements in the reception area to accommodate patients with special needs

OSHA Guidelines: This procedure does not involve exposure to blood, body fluids, or tissue.

Materials: Ramps (if needed), doorway floor coverings, chairs, bars or rails, adjustable-height tables, magazine rack, television/DVD player, large-type and Braille magazines

Method:

1. Arrange chairs to create gaps that allow substantial space along walls and near other chair groupings for wheelchairs. Keep the arrangement flexible so that chairs can be removed to allow room for additional wheelchairs if needed.
RATIONALE: *To meet all the requirements of the Americans with Disabilities Act*

2. Remove any obstacles that may interfere with the space needed for a wheelchair to swivel around completely. Also, remove scatter rugs or any carpeting that is not attached to the floor. Such carpeting can cause patients to trip and creates difficulties for wheelchair traffic.
RATIONALE: *Helps ensure safety in the patient reception area*

3. Position coffee tables at a height and location accessible to people in wheelchairs.

4. Place office reading materials, such as magazines, at a height accessible to people in wheelchairs (for example, on tables or in racks attached midway up the wall).

5. Locate the television and DVD within full view of patients sitting on chairs and in wheelchairs so that they do not have to strain their necks to watch.

6. For patients who have a vision impairment, include large-type and Braille reading materials.

7. For patients who have difficulty walking, make sure bars or rails are attached securely to walls 34 to 38 inches above the floor, to accommodate requirements set forth in the Americans with Disabilities Act. Make sure the bars are sturdy enough to provide balance for patients who need it. Bars are most important in entrances and hallways, as well as in the bathroom. Consider placing a bar near the receptionist's window for added support as patients check in.
RATIONALE: *To meet all the requirements of the Americans with Disabilities Act*

8. Eliminate sills of metal or wood along the floor in doorways. Otherwise, create a smoother travel surface for wheelchairs and pedestrians with a thin rubber covering to provide a graduated slope. Be sure that the covering is attached properly and meets safety standards.
RATIONALE: *Helps ensure safety in the patient reception area*

9. Make sure the office has ramp access.
RATIONALE: *To meet all the requirements of the Americans with Disabilities Act*

10. Solicit feedback from patients with physical disabilities about the accessibility of the patient reception area. Encourage ideas for improvements. Address any additional needs.
RATIONALE: *Doing so lets patients know that their comfort and well-being are important to you.*

PROCEDURE 7-5 Opening and Closing the Medical Office

Procedure Goal: To ensure readiness and to receive and care for patients in an efficient, organized, and safe manner

OSHA Guidelines: This procedure does not involve exposure to blood, body fluids, or tissue.

Materials: Checklist for opening and closing the office (Tables 7-2 and 7-3 may be used as samples), pen, telephone, and pad of paper

Method:

1. Using Table 7-2 , Daily Checklist for Opening the Office, as a guide, simulate the functions of opening the office. Enter the week ending date.
RATIONALE: *Using a checklist ensures no task is inadvertently skipped.*

Daily Checklist for Opening BWW Medical Associates, PC	W/E _____					
	M	T	W	Th	F	S
1. Security system is disarmed.						
2. Voicemail/answering service messages are retrieved.						
3. Messages are routed and ready for callback.						
4. Computers are turned on.						
5. Appointments and insurance rosters are checked.						
6. If needed, charts are pulled and paperwork is attached.						
7. Equipment is working properly.						
8. Rooms are supplied and ready.						
9. Refrigerator temperature is checked.						
10. Emergency supplies, including O_2, are checked.						
11. Reception area is in order and patient education material is available.						
12. Lab specimens from the day before were picked up.						

FIGURE Procedure 7-5 Step 1 Use a daily checklist when opening the office.

   a. Begin by disarming the security system.

   b. Telephone the answering service to pick up messages or set the office answering machine or voicemail system to answer calls. Document any messages and notify the appropriate person of the call.

   c. Conduct each task on the form, placing your initials in the column for the correct day of the week.

   RATIONALE: *It is important to know who performed each task in case questions arise.*

Daily Checklist for Opening BWW Medical Associates, PC	W/E 4/30/xx					
	M	T	W	Th	F	S
1. Security system is disarmed.	mk					
2. Voicemail/answering service messages are retrieved.	mk					
3. Messages are routed and ready for callback.	mk					
4. Computers are turned on.	mk					
5. Appointments and insurance rosters are checked.	mk					
6. If needed, charts are pulled and paperwork is attached.	mk					
7. Equipment is working properly.	mk					
8. Rooms are supplied and ready.	mk					
9. Refrigerator temperature is checked.	mk					
10. Emergency supplies, including O_2, are checked.	mk					
11. Reception area is in order and patient education material is available.	mk					
12. Lab specimens from the day before were picked up.	mk					

FIGURE Procedure 7-5 Step 1c Insert your initials when each task is completed under the correct day of the week.

   2. Using Table 7-3, Daily Checklist for Closing the Office, as a guide, simulate the functions of closing the office. Enter the week ending date.

     a. Begin with logging out and turning off the computers.

Daily Checklist for Closing BWW Medical Associates, PC	W/E _____					
	M	T	W	Th	F	S
1. Computers are logged off and shut down.						
2. Contaminated supplies/equipment are properly disposed of or tagged for cleaning/sterilization.						
3. Areas are restocked.						
4. If needed, patient charts are pulled/reviewed for next day and all test results are available.						
5. Laboratory specimens are in pick-up receptacle.						
6. All office equipment is turned off (including kitchen).						
7. Reception area is neat and organized.						
8. Calls are forwarded to voicemail/answering machine.						
9. Medical records are secured.						
10. All doors and windows are locked.						
11. Security system is armed.						

FIGURE Procedure 7-5 Step 2 Use a daily checklist to close the office.

   b. Use the telephone to turn on the answering machine/voicemail or notify the answering service that the office is closing.

   c. Conduct each task on the form, placing your initials in the column for the correct day of the week.

   RATIONALE: *It is important to know who performed each task in case questions arise.*

Daily Checklist for Closing BWW Medical Associates, PC	W/E 4/30/xx					
	M	T	W	Th	F	S
1. Computers are logged off and shut down.	mk					
2. Contaminated supplies/equipment are properly disposed of or tagged for cleaning/sterilization.	mk					
3. Areas are restocked.	mk					
4. If needed, patient charts are pulled/reviewed for next day and all test results are available.	mk					
5. Laboratory specimens are in pick-up receptacle.	mk					
6. All office equipment is turned off (including kitchen).	mk					
7. Reception area is neat and organized.	mk					
8. Calls are forwarded to voicemail/answering machine.	mk					
9. Medical records are secured.	mk					
10. All doors and windows are locked.	mk					
11. Security system is armed.	mk					

FIGURE Procedure 7-5 Step 2c Insert your initials when each task is completed under the appropriate day of the week.

SUMMARY OF LEARNING OUTCOMES

LEARNING OUTCOMES	KEY POINTS
7.1 Describe the components of a medical office safety plan.	The medical office safety plan should include OSHA's Hazard Communication; electrical, fire, and chemical safety; emergency action plans; bloodborne pathogen exposure plans; PPE; and needlestick prevention plans.
7.2 Summarize OSHA's Hazard Communication Standard.	The US Department of Labor created OSHA to protect the employees' safety in the workplace. Through the creation and enforcement of standards such as the Bloodborne Pathogens Standard, Hazard Communication, and the Needlestick Safety and Prevention Act, OSHA serves to protect healthcare workers from hazards.
7.3 Describe basic safety precautions you should take to reduce electrical hazards.	To reduce electrical hazards in the medical office, you should avoid using extension cords, repair or replace damaged cords, avoid overloading circuits, ensure that all plugs are grounded, dry your hands before using electrical devices, and keep electrical devices away from sinks or other sources of water.
7.4 Illustrate the necessary steps in a comprehensive fire safety plan.	A comprehensive fire safety plan must include fire prevention strategies, actions to take in the event of a fire, building evacuation routes and plans, fire drills, and local emergency contacts.
7.5 Summarize proper methods for handling and storing chemicals used in a medical office.	When using chemicals in the medical office, you should always wear protective gear, carry the container with both hands, work in a well-ventilated area, never combine chemicals unless it is specifically required in the test procedures, always add acid to water if the procedure requires that you combine chemicals, and properly clean up spills immediately.
7.6 Explain the principles of good ergonomic practice and physical safety in the medical office.	In order to protect yourself from work-related musculoskeletal disorders at work, you must follow the principles of good body mechanics. Your physical safety at work depends on understanding and applying appropriate workplace safeguards, including never running in an office, taking care when carrying objects through the facility, closing cabinets and drawers, and following appropriate safety procedures in the lab.
7.7 Articulate the cause of most injuries to medical office workers and the four body areas where they occur.	Most office-related injuries are those associated with repetitive motions, such as typing, lifting, bending, stooping, and sitting. Common injuries or conditions involve the forearm, wrist, hand, and back.
7.8 List the design items to be considered when setting up an office reception area.	The size of the space you have to work with and the schedule of the physicians seeing patients must be considered first. Utilize the space to give as much room and privacy as possible. The décor should include a color family to suit the practice type. Furnishings should be comfortable but easy to get in and out of and easy to clean. Lighting should be appropriately bright to avoid accidental falls. Accessories like wall hangings, aquariums, coat racks, and magazine racks should complement the décor but not make the room feel cluttered. Current magazines and other reading materials on multiple topics should be available to entertain and inform the patient. TV and/or informational DVDs also may be played. If the practice sees children, special accommodations to entertain them also must be made.

LEARNING OUTCOMES	KEY POINTS
7.9 Summarize the housekeeping tasks required to keep the reception area neat and clean.	Housekeeping tasks for the reception area include overseeing the professional cleaning staff (if one is employed), keeping everything in its place, disposing of trash, preventing visible dust and dirt on surfaces, spot-cleaning areas that become soiled, disinfecting areas exposed to body fluids, and handling items with care. OSHA guidelines should be followed in all aspects of keeping the office neat and clean. Standards of office cleanliness should be created and posted for all staff to see.
7.10 Relate how the Americans with Disabilities and Older American Acts have helped to make physical access to the medical office easier for all patients.	The Americans with Disabilities Act and the Older Americans Act both prevent discrimination based solely on a person's physical or mental disability or his or her age. Both of these acts mandate accessibility for the differently abled, including, but not limited to, adequate parking for vehicles with and carrying assistive devices such as wheelchairs, ramps instead of stairs, wider doorways and hallways, well-lit areas throughout the office, large-print instructions, and Braille markings for elevators and other instructions.
7.11 Describe the functions of the front office staff, including patient registration and accepting payments from patients.	The front office staff greet people, register them, give them direction, observe and report when patients should be transferred quickly to the clinical area, and answer the phone. They may also accept payment for patient visits.
7.12 Implement policies and procedures for opening and closing the office.	Maintaining specific policies and procedures for opening and closing the office ensures the necessary tasks are completed daily in a uniform manner. This results in an efficient and prepared medical office each day.

CASE STUDY CRITICAL THINKING

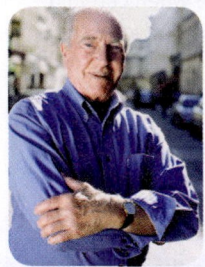

© Image Source/Getty Images RF

Recall Peter Smith from the beginning of the chapter. Now that you have completed the chapter, answer the following questions regarding his case.

1. How should you respond to Mrs. Smith's request that she be allowed to speak with Dr. Buckwalter privately?

2. Summarize your role as the "first person" Mr. Smith (and all patients) sees as he enters the office.

3. What action should you take to prevent Mr. Smith and possibly other patients from falling while trying to reach the magazines on the table?

EXAM PREPARATION QUESTIONS

1. (LO 7.8) When designing the reception area for a medical practice, the first consideration should be the
   a. Color
   b. Furnishings
   c. Patient education material
   d. Type of practice
   e. Music

2. (LO 7.2) Which of the following are the sheets that must accompany every hazardous chemical?
   a. GHS
   b. HCS
   c. SDS
   d. OSHA
   e. ADA

3. (LO 7.9) Which federal agency produces guidelines for maintaining office cleanliness and the SDS for cleaning solutions?

a. HIPAA
b. ADA
c. OSHA
d. FDA
e. DEA

4. (LO 7.10) A violation of the ADA might be not permitting

a. Smoking
b. Pharmacy refills
c. Charge cards
d. Service animals
e. Beverages in the reception area

5. (LO 7.2) OSHA requires that every facility keep a master list of hazardous chemicals in the facility. This is part of

a. Global System of Hazardous Chemicals
b. Hazmat Standard
c. DOT Safety Rule
d. Chemical Convention Rule
e. Hazard Communication Standard

6. (LO 7.7) Which injury may be caused by repetitive motions using a computer?

a. Eye strain
b. Scoliosis
c. Arthritis
d. Whiplash
e. CTS

7. (LO 7.4) PASS is an acronym for a system outlining the proper use of which of the following?

a. Fire extinguisher
b. Chemical hood
c. Gas-fed open flame
d. Alcohol-based hand disinfectant
e. Evacuation plan

8. (LO 7.2) Which of the following requires that all employees receive workplace hazard training?

a. Standard precautions
b. Emergency action plans
c. Needlestick prevention regulations
d. Hazard Communication Standard
e. Bloodborne Pathogens Standard

9. (LO 7.11) When the physician is running very late, the receptionist should

a. Inform patients they will be seen soon
b. Offer refreshments while the patients are waiting
c. Cancel appointments
d. Provide patients with the option to reschedule appointments
e. Avoid eye contact with waiting patients

10. (LO 7.6) The study of the way people work is known as

a. Economics
b. Kinesiology
c. Ergonomics
d. Posturing
e. Accommodation

S O F T   S K I L L S   S U C C E S S

You are working in the front office of a medical facility. The office is very busy; the reception area is full of patients waiting to be seen and you are currently on the phone when a man walks in and says he has to see the doctor immediately. You notice that the man is about 60 years old and appears very pale, is sweating, and is clutching his chest. What action should you take?

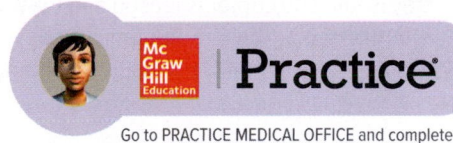

Go to PRACTICE MEDICAL OFFICE and complete the module Admin: Check In - Work Task Proficiencies.

Office Equipment and Supplies

CASE STUDY

Employee Name	Position	Credentials
Miguel A. Perez	Administrative MA	CMA (AAMA)
Supervisor	**Date of Hire**	**Other information**
Malik Katahri, CMM	6/21/20XX	15th of month: order paper & administrative supplies for office

Miguel A. Perez is the CMA (AAMA) for BWW Medical Associates, PC, a busy medical practice, and he is the first to arrive each morning. This morning, as Miguel walks through the office, turning on the lights, he notices the fire extinguisher hanging on the wall. He makes a mental note to call the maintenance company today to notify them that the expiration date on the extinguisher is this month. They will replace the old one with a new extinguisher. Miguel quickly checks the late-night pick-up specimen boxes, notes the specimens left last evening were picked up by the lab, and removes the lab reports left in the box by the lab. He switches on the copier/scanner and makes sure the paper tray is full. The copier is leased and BWW Associates is billed monthly based on the number of copies made during the month. He will call the leasing company with the number

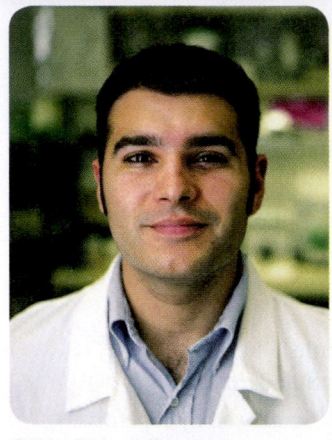

© Karen Moskowitz/Getty Images

today. He has an automatic reminder set up on his computer to do this on the 30th of each month. Next, Miguel turns on his computer and reviews his calendar and task list for the day. He has received e-mail from another practice asking about a new referral and an e-request for medical records. He prints out two computerized appointment listings for the day, placing one in the front office and one in the back office for easy reference. Because medical records in the office are computerized, he is grateful paper charts no longer need to be pulled. He takes a quick look around the administrative office to identify any items that need to be restocked, and he restocks the supply of pens and forms at the reception desk. He then scans the reception area to make sure it is neat and ready for the day.

Keep Miguel in mind as you study this chapter. There will be questions at the end of the chapter based on the case study. The information in the chapter will help you answer these questions.

LEARNING OUTCOMES

After completing Chapter 8, you will be able to:

8.1 Identify common types of computers.

8.2 Describe computer hardware components and explain the functions of each.

8.3 Describe the types of software applications commonly used in the medical office.

8.4 Summarize the options available for learning computer software programs.

8.5 Recall the steps involved in selecting new or upgrading existing office computer equipment.

8.6 Outline the basic care and maintenance required for the office computer system.

8.7 Identify several reasons security is particularly important in the computerized office.

8.8 Explain the function of other types of administrative medical office equipment.

8.9 Outline the steps to be taken in deciding whether new office equipment is needed.

8.10 Explain the difference between a maintenance contract and a service contract.

8.11 Define vital, periodic, and incidental supplies.

8.12 Outline the steps in performing a supply inventory.

8.13 List the items that should be considered when choosing a vendor for supply ordering.

central processing unit (CPU)

covered entity

database

digital subscriber line (DSL)

disbursement

disclaimer

hardware

icons

local area network (LAN)

optical character recognition (OCR)

purchase order

random-access memory (RAM)

read-only memory (ROM)

requisition

software

virtual private network (VPN)

wide-area network (WAN)

MEDICAL ASSISTING COMPETENCIES

CAAHEP

V.C.8 Discuss applications of electronic technology in professional communication

VI.C.9 Explain the purpose of routine maintenance of administrative and clinical equipment

VI.C.10 List steps involved in completing an inventory

VI.C.11 Explain the importance of a data back-up

VI.P.8 Perform routine maintenance of administrative or clinical equipment

VI.P.9 Perform an inventory with documentation

ABHES

7. Records Management

a. Perform basic keyboarding skills (i.e. Microsoft Word, etc.)

b. Utilize Electronic Medical Records (EMR) and Practice Management Systems

8. Administrative Procedures

e. Maintain inventory equipment and supplies
(1) Perform routine maintenance of administrative equipment

▶ Introduction

The modern medical office requires many different types of administrative equipment in order to function effectively and smoothly. In fact, it is fair to say that a medical office today without a computer, its related software, and other administrative equipment is like a car without gasoline. Your role as a medical assistant includes learning how to evaluate, purchase or lease, operate, and maintain this essential equipment.

Imagine how difficult it would be to function in our current culture's complex office environment without computers for claims submission, patient billing, payroll, bank deposits, and, of course, e-mail. Medical office staff also depend on copiers, scanners, and/or fax machines, adding machines, and paper shredders to accomplish daily tasks efficiently. Going hand-in-hand with this equipment are the administrative supplies like paper and toner, as well as everyday consumable supplies like pens, pencils, highlighters, staples, paper clips, and tape.

In this chapter, you will learn about the use and maintenance of many important pieces of administrative medical office equipment. You also will become proficient in the process of keeping an inventory of not only the equipment in the medical office but also the basic supplies needed to keep the office running efficiently.

▶ Computers   LO 8.1

Computer skills are essential for most career choices, and medical assisting is no exception. As a medical assistant, understanding the fundamentals of computers and their uses is a must. This knowledge will enable you to perform many office tasks with ease. The more you know about computers, the more easily you will be able to solve or avoid computer problems. In this section, we will take a closer look at computers and other electronic devices commonly used in the medical office.

Personal computers can be found in homes, offices, and schools. They are ideal for these settings because they are small, self-contained units. Because users have different needs, personal computers are available in several different types. A network is a system that links several (or even 100s) of computers together in which one of the computers commonly acts as server to store shared information such as the office database management system.

Desktop

The most common type of personal computer in the medical office, a desktop model fits easily on a desk or other flat surface. The system unit of many desktop models is housed in a tower case, which can be placed on the floor next to the desk to allow more surface area at the workstation (Figure 8-1).

Laptop and Notebook

A laptop computer is small, about the size of a magazine, and weighs only a few pounds. Laptops operate either on battery power or on an AC adapter. Using laptops and notebook computers, physicians and other healthcare professionals can instantly communicate with the medical office computer, accessing data and information from other locations. With more and more offices utilizing electronic health records, laptops and notebooks are extremely popular in offices because they are mobile and can be moved between exam rooms. Because of this mobility, offices must be very sure to use encryption software for any patient-based information that is accessible via any mobile device, including laptops.

Subnotebook and Tablet PC

Subnotebooks, which have screens measuring 14 inches or less, are smaller than laptops but larger than handheld computers. Subnotebooks are now quickly being replaced by tablet PCs. These are slate-shaped mobile computers equipped with touch screen and/or graphics table technology. This allows users to operate the computer with a stylus, a digital pen, or simply the user's finger, instead of a keyboard or mouse. Again, to protect patient information, passwords and encryption software must be utilized on any "portable" device.

Personal Digital Assistant (PDA)

PDAs are less common in medical offices and other healthcare facilities. Doctors may use them to look up medications and other reference information. They also may enter data that are transferred into a patient's chart.

Cell Phones and the Internet

Cell phone use is so widespread that imagining your life without one may be near to impossible. The days of having a landline connection in your home, complete with an actual handset and separate phone for dialing, are almost a thing of the past. Cell phones are now most often used personally and not professionally. However, for research purposes, cell phone capabilities have increased exponentially in the last several years and will continue to expand. Smartphones using Android™ technology or Apple's iPhones allow users to access the Internet and perform multiple applications in addition to simply making phone calls and sending text messages. They truly are "computers held in your hand." Cell phones will be discussed in more detail in the *Telephone Techniques* chapter.

Computers used in a medical setting usually have access to the Internet but are also frequently linked on an intranet. An intranet is a network system that connects local machines. The intranet allows information such as the office database management system to be shared locally. Database management systems contain patient-based information, and patient health information must be protected. Encryption software must be used for any patient-based information that is accessible via any mobile device, including laptops, tablets, and cell phones (Figure 8-2).

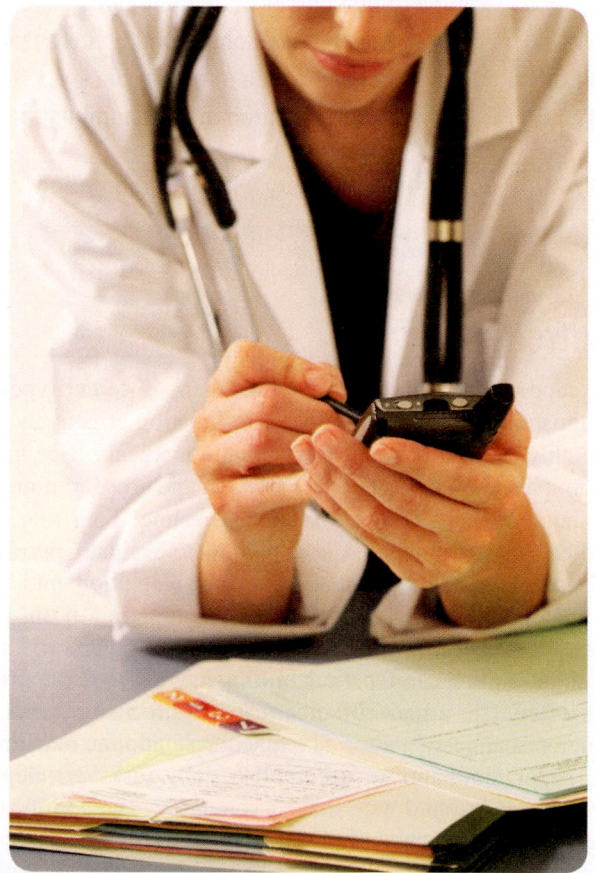

FIGURE 8-2 To protect patient health information, cell phones and other mobile devices must use encryption software when this information is accessed.

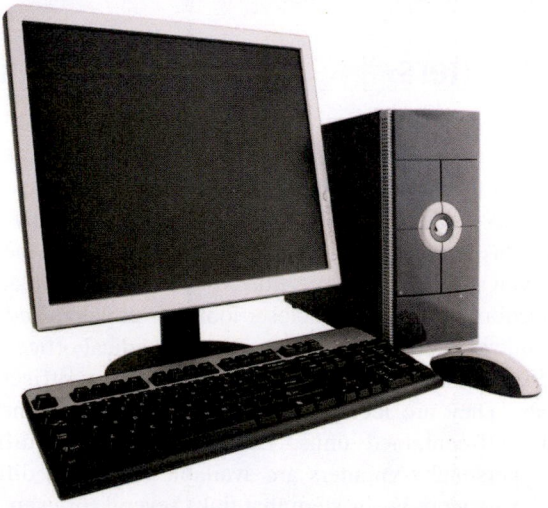

FIGURE 8-1 The desktop computer is the most common computer type in the medical office.

▶ Components of the Computer   LO 8.2

When most people talk about computer components, they are referring to the computer hardware, or its physical components, which include the monitor, keyboard, and printer. Computer hardware components are responsible for performing each of four main functions: inputting data, processing data, storing data, and outputting data. In order to work, unless the office is set up with wireless capability and wireless devices are purchased, hardware devices must be connected by a cable, such as a USB or serial cable. Let's look at the four main types of computer hardware—input devices, processing devices, storage devices, and output devices—and their respective role in the medical office.

Input Devices

For a computer to handle information like patient records, the data must first be entered, or input. Several types of input devices—keyboards, touch screens, pointing devices, modems, and scanners—may be used to enter data into the computer. After this information is entered, it can be displayed on the monitor, processed, printed, or stored.

Keyboard The keyboard is the most common input device. Most keyboards have several additional key types.

When you use the keyboard, it is important to position your hands properly to avoid injury. Refer to the *Safety and Patient Reception* chapter for more information on how to prevent and cope with carpal tunnel syndrome, a condition resulting from repetitive motion such as using a computer keyboard.

Pointing Device Many software programs require both a keyboard and a pointing device to enter information into the computer. The three common types of pointing devices are the mouse, the touch pad, and the touch screen.

- A *mouse,* the most common pointing device, has two or three buttons on top and sometimes a rolling ball on the bottom. A laser mouse detects movement through a laser and does not have a ball. As you move the mouse across a flat surface or mouse pad, you cause a light-sensing device on the bottom to move. This controls an arrow on the screen that points at the desired button or on-screen object. Then you push one of the buttons on the mouse to access a function, like opening a file.
- A *touch pad* is a form of pointing device common on laptops and notebooks. It is a small, flat device that is highly sensitive to the touch. To move the on-screen arrow, you simply slide your finger across the touch pad. To click on an item, you tap your finger on the touch pad.
- A *touch screen* is a monitor screen that is illuminated at the touch of a pen, wand, or finger. When an object is touched on the screen, the touch itself acts as a pointing device and conveys information to the computer. Touch screens are increasingly being used in clinical and hospital settings, as they are now commonly found with notebooks, iPads, and smart phones.

Modem A modem is used to transfer information from one computer to another over telephone lines. Because modems allow information to be transferred both to and from a computer, they are considered input/output devices. Modems are essential for any medical office that needs to transfer files electronically, as when submitting insurance claim forms. Modems can be internal, external, or wireless. The three standard types of modems are cable modems, digital subscriber line modems, and fax modems.

- A cable modem is a modem that operates over cable television lines to provide fast Internet access.
- **Digital subscriber line (DSL)** modems operate over telephone lines but use a different frequency than a telephone frequency. This type of modem allows computer Internet access and telephone use at the same time.
- A fax modem allows the computer to send and receive files much as a fax machine does. A fax modem is not quite as versatile as a regular fax machine, as the information being sent must first be input into the computer. In addition, without the use of a scanner, you cannot use a fax modem to send a patient record with handwritten notes on it.

Scanner A scanner is a device used to input printed matter and convert it into a readable format for the computer. Scanners are useful in the medical office because patient reports (from another doctor, hospital, or outside source) can be easily entered into the computer and, often, directly into the patient medical record. This makes it possible to move into a paperless medical system. Using a scanner is much faster than keying, or inputting the information with a keyboard. Three types of scanners are available:

- Handheld scanners are generally the least expensive but are more difficult to use and produce lower-quality results than the other two types.
- A single-sheet scanner feeds one sheet of paper through at a time and looks similar to a single-sheet printer.
- A flatbed scanner is the easiest to use and produces the highest-quality input. It works much like a small photocopier: The paper lies flat and still on a glass surface while the machine scans it. Today, most photocopiers are configured with a scanning capability and can transmit the images of scanned documents directly into computers.

Processing Devices

There are two major processing components inside the system unit, or computer cabinet: the motherboard and the central processing unit. The *motherboard* is the main circuit board that controls the other components in the system. The **central processing unit (CPU),** or microprocessor, is the primary computer chip responsible for interpreting and executing programs. The CPU is considered the most important piece of hardware in a computer system because it interprets instructions from software programs. Without a functioning CPU, the software programs will not run. Processing devices for cell phones and other mobile devices are very small electronic "chips" found inside the device.

Storage Devices

One of the computer's main tasks is to store information for later retrieval. The computer uses memory to store information either temporarily or permanently. Several types of drives are used for permanent information storage.

Memory Computers use two types of memory to store data: **random-access memory (RAM)** and **read-only memory (ROM)**. RAM is temporary, or programmable, memory. While you are working on a software program, such as Microsoft® Word, the computer is accessing RAM. In general, the more RAM that is available, the faster the computer will perform. As software programs become more sophisticated, they require more RAM.

ROM is permanent memory. The computer can read it, but you cannot make changes to it. An example of ROM is Windows® 10, a computer operating system. The purpose of ROM is to provide the basic operating instructions the computer needs to function.

Hard Disk Drive The hard disk drive is where information is stored permanently for later retrieval. Software programs and important data are usually stored on the hard disk for quick and easy access. The amount of hard disk space needed to store software programs is increasing rapidly. The more software programs you want to store, the larger the hard disk you will need.

Removable Drives Removable drives consist of CDs, jump drives, tape drives, zip drives, and DVDs.

- *CD-ROM drive.* The term *CD-ROM* stands for "compact-disc—read-only memory." CD-ROMs look like audio compact discs, but they contain software programs that often include video, sound, and other media, such as graphics, to convey information. CD-ROMs also can be used to back up information from the hard drive.
- *CD burner or recorder.* Most computers also have a CD recorder (CD-R), which allows information to be taken from one CD (or any other source) and copied to another CD.
- *External hard drive.* It is not uncommon in larger offices to use a separate computer hard drive as a backup, or to hire a company to back up the files nightly or weekly via the Internet, and store them in a separate facility.
- *Jump drive.* A jump drive—also called a flash drive, pen drive, key drive, memory key, flash key, or USB drive—is an externally attached drive that is small enough to be carried on a key chain yet holds 16 gigabytes or more of data. It provides easy portability for large bodies of data, and may be used for backup operations in a medical practice when stored off-premises. To protect any proprietary information stored on a removable drive such as a CD, DVD, or jump drive, the information should be encrypted in case the storage device is lost or stolen. Jump drives attach to the CPU via the USB ports found on the front, back, or side of the CPU device (see Figure 8-3).

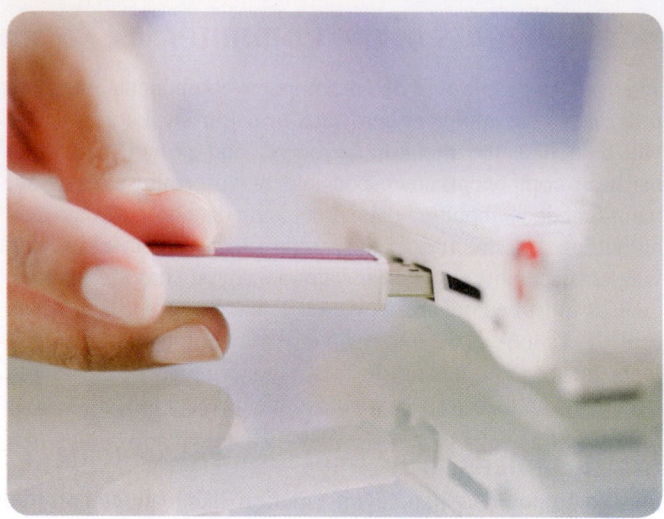

FIGURE 8-3   Plugging a jump drive into the USB port of a CPU.
© JGI/Jamie Grill/Blend Images LLC RF

- *Zip drive.* A zip drive is a high-capacity floppy disk drive developed by Iomega™. Zip disks can hold up to 750 MB of data. Zip drives are durable, are relatively inexpensive, and may be used for backing up hard disks and transporting large files.
- *DVD.* DVD (digital video disc) is optical disc storage technology. It is similar to CD technology except it is faster and can hold more information. One double-sided, dual-layer disk can store about 8 hours of high-quality video.

Output Devices

Output devices are used to display information after it has been processed. A monitor and a printer are two output devices needed in the medical office.

Monitor The monitor displays currently active information, such as a word processing document, an Internet link, or e-mail. Most healthcare facilities use LCD (liquid crystal display) monitors, which provide for better privacy than older, bulkier models because they cannot be seen from the side.

Resolution refers to the crispness of the images and is measured in dot pitch. The lower the dot pitch, the higher the resolution. For example, a monitor with a 0.26 dot pitch displays sharper images than a monitor with a 0.39 dot pitch. Using a high-resolution monitor can help you avoid eye strain.

Printer A printer produces a *hard copy*—a readable paper copy or printout of information. You will need a printer to print out correspondence, patient reports, bills, insurance claims, and other documents. Printer resolution is noted in terms of dots per inch (dpi). The higher the dpi, the better the print quality. Printer output varies, depending on the printer type and model. The two most commonly used printers are laser and ink-jet.

- Laser printers are high-resolution printers that use a technology similar to that of photocopiers. They are the fastest type of printers, produce the highest-quality output, and are now the most common type of office printer. Their cost has decreased as technology has improved.

- Ink-jet printers are nonimpact printers that form characters using a series of dots created by tiny drops of ink. Many ink-jet printers are capable of printing in both black ink and color. Because of their high-quality output and affordable prices, ink-jet printers are popular for small-office use.

Most offices have found it more economical to purchase or lease "all-in-one" devices. These function not only as the office printer but also as a fax machine, scanner, and photocopier (see Figure 8-4).

▶ Software   LO 8.3

The program, or set of instructions that tells the computer what to do, is known as its **software.** Computer software is generally divided into two categories: operating system and application software. The operating system controls the computer's operation. Application software allows you to perform specific tasks, such as scheduling appointments.

Operating System

When you turn on a computer, the operating system starts working, providing instructions that the computer needs to function. Examples of operating system software include Microsoft® Windows® 10 and Linux. Most computers come pre-installed with Windows® 7, 8, or 10.

Operating system software is sometimes referred to as the platform for the system. Most medical practices use IBM-compatible personal computers, which are very suitable for businesses that use computers primarily to manipulate words. On the other hand, advertising agencies or design firms, which are extensively involved in graphics, visual images, or desktop publishing, tend to use Apple® (Macintosh—MAC) computers.

Windows This operating system uses a graphical user interface, or GUI (pronounced "gooey"), which uses **icons,** or graphic symbols (Figure 8-5) to represent the job to be done. In this example, the "print" command is identified by a tiny illustration of a printer. When the icon is clicked, the chosen document will be printed. Most of you have been using a

GUI interface for most of your lives, using your parents' cell phones or a child's computer learning system, such as those from LeapFrog®, to play (educational) games before you even knew what else a computer could be used for.

Another important benefit of the Windows® system is that it is capable of multitasking. This means it can run two or more software programs simultaneously. For example, you might have one screen open to enter information in the patient **database** (a collection of records created and stored in the computer) at the same time as you have a word processing program open while you complete a letter for a patient who needs a letter from his primary care physician stating that he is medically cleared to return to work.

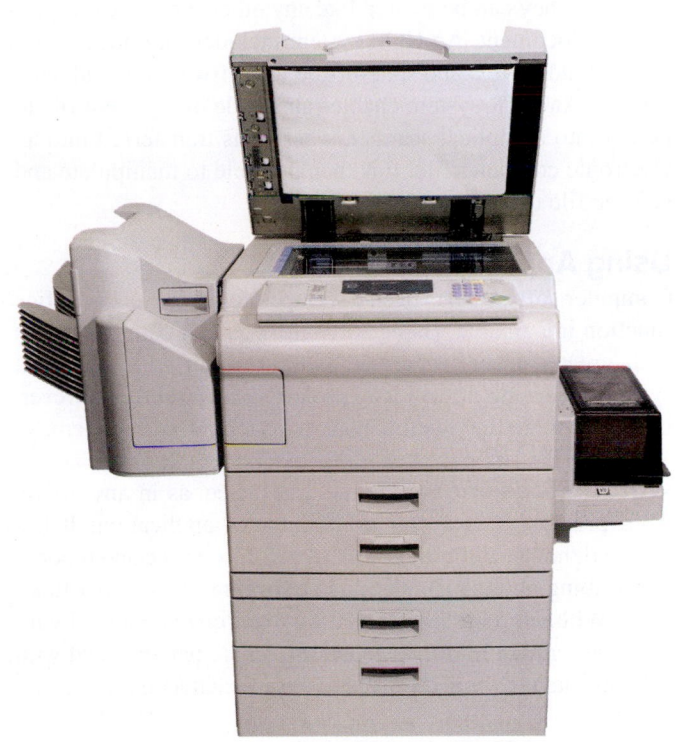

FIGURE 8-4 An all-in-one printer-scanner-fax machine can be networked to multiple computers in the office.
© Getty Images RF

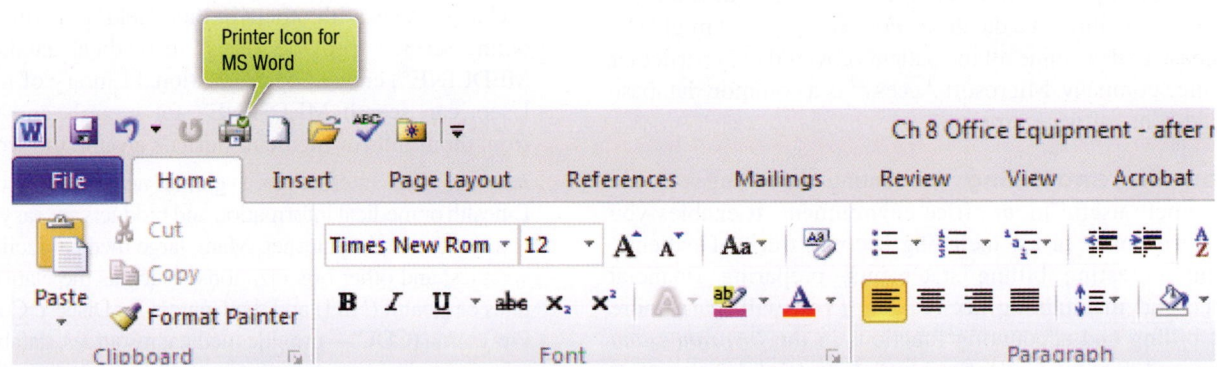

FIGURE 8-5 MS Word 2007 formatting toolbar with GUI icons, pointing out the Printer icon.

Applications

Most of the software sold in stores is application software like Microsoft® Office. Microsoft® Office includes word processing (Word), presentation software (PowerPoint), spreadsheets (Excel), database management (Access), and desktop publishing (Publisher). Medical Manager®, Medware®, Medasis, and MediSoft™ are practice management applications. These software packages are specifically designed to meet the needs of a medical practice. Standard computer practice management software packages can be purchased, and custom-made practice management software can be designed to meet the needs of a particular practice. Word processing, database, and accounting software are just a few examples of the wide variety of applications available.

Optical Character Recognition

Optical character recognition (OCR) software enables the conversion of images to text so they can be treated like any other type of word processing document. An OCR system includes an optical scanner for reading text and state-of-the-art software for analyzing images. An OCR system enables an article or a patient file to be fed into an optical scanner, where it is transferred into an electronic computer file. It is then possible to manipulate and edit the file using a word processor.

Using Application Software

Computer software has been developed for nearly every office function imaginable. Using software, you can complete tasks with greater speed, accuracy, and ease than with a manual system. Learning how to use the software correctly, however, is the key to getting the most out of your computer system.

Word Processing

In the medical office, as in any office, word processing is a common computer application. It has replaced the typewriter for writing correspondence and reports, transcribing physician notes, and performing many other functions. With word processing, a form letter can be merged with a patient mailing list to create letters that are personalized with patients' names without having to retype each letter.

Database Management

A database is a collection of records created and stored on a computer. In a medical office, databases are used to store patient records such as billing information, medical chart data, and insurance company facts. These records can be sorted and retrieved in many ways and for a variety of purposes. You may be asked to find, add to, or modify information in a database. For example, you might use a database to determine all the patients covered by a particular insurance company. Microsoft Access® is a common database management software program.

Accounting and Billing

Accounting and billing software is extremely useful in an office environment. It enables you to perform many tasks, including keeping track of patients' accounts, creating billing statements, preparing financial reports, and maintaining tax records. (You will learn more about billing and accounting functions in the *Insurance and Billing* and *Patient Collections and Financial Management* chapters.)

Appointment Scheduling

Instead of writing in an appointment book, most offices use software to schedule appointments. Some scheduling packages allow you to enter patient preferences, like day of the week and time, and then to list available appointments based on that information. If the office system is on a network, scheduling software is particularly valuable because more than one user can access the appointment schedule at a time (Figure 8-6).

Electronic Transactions

Many medical offices are now computerized and perform many transactions, such as insurance claim form submission and insurance payment posting, electronically. Procedures such as these, which formerly took minutes or hours, are now performed almost instantaneously. Instead of waiting for checks to come in the mail, credit card payments are accepted in the office and online. Insurance payments are deposited automatically into the office checking account. Instead of waiting for days for requested medical records, the office can receive them in seconds when sent securely using encrypted e-mail systems. We discuss many electronic procedures in greater detail in other chapters.

Communicating

The ability to communicate and share information with other computer users and systems is important in many medical offices. This communication may take place through e-mail, online services, and the Internet.

- *E-mail.* E-mail allows for the sending and receiving of messages almost instantly through a network. Through e-mail, it is possible to communicate with computer users in your own office, across town, or on the other side of the world. The use of e-mail in a professional context, including appropriate formats and confidentiality, is discussed in more detail in the *Written and Electronic Communication* chapter. Just a reminder, the office e-mail system is for professional use only. It is not private. Anything you send through the office e-mail system may be accessed by your supervisor and/or the office IT department. Keep office e-mail communications professional at all times.

- *Online services.* These services, known as "listserves," provide a means for healthcare professionals to communicate with one another. Most online services contain forums that offer information and discussion groups focusing on a wide range of medical topics. Healthcare workers can learn about the latest medical research and technology or exchange ideas with others in their field. In addition, some online services provide access to medical databases like MEDLINE®, created by the National Library of Medicine. Users can search MEDLINE® for records and abstracts from thousands of medical journals around the world.

- *Internet.* The Internet is a global network of computers. E-health or medical information and products are easy to access worldwide via the Internet. Many large medical facilities, universities, and other organizations—such as the National Institutes of Health (NIH) and the Centers for Disease Control and Prevention (CDC)—provide medical resources, databases, and other information on the Internet. Table 8-1 describes a few popular credible medical resources available on the Internet.

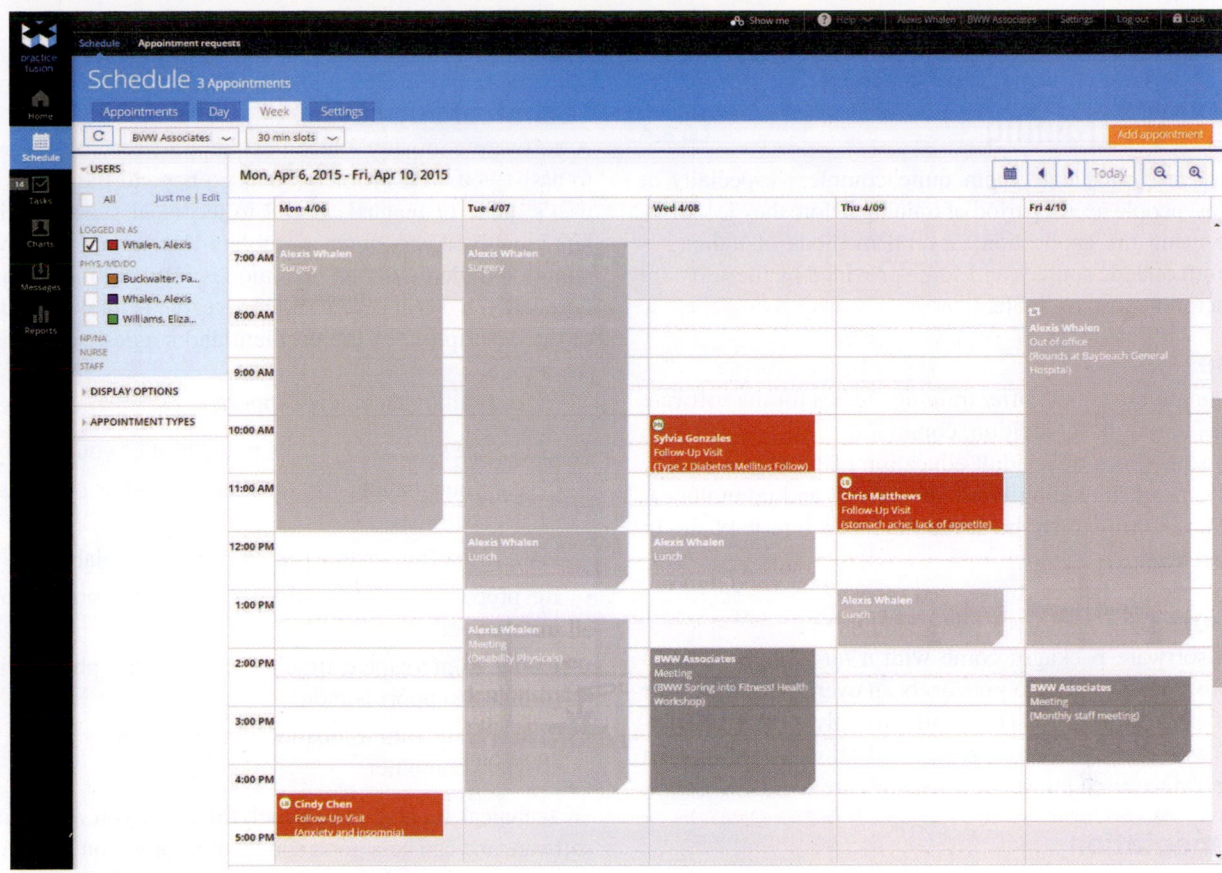

FIGURE 8-6 Practice Fusion® screen showing office appointment schedule that has been filtered to show only Alexis Whalen's schedule for the week.
© **Practice Fusion®**

TABLE 8-1	Medical Resources on the Internet	
Organization	**Web Address**	**Description**
American Medical Association	http://www.ama-assn.org	News announcements and press releases; articles from *JAMA* and other AMA journals; links to other medicine-related Internet sites
eMedicineHealth	http://www.emedicinehealth.com	Health resource center containing information about health issues and the latest treatments available
Health.gov	http://health.gov/	The Office of Disease Prevention and Health Promotion develops and coordinates high impact national disease prevention and health promotion activities, creating a healthier nation
MedlinePlus®	http://medlineplus.gov	A service of the US National Library of Medicine and NIH; site includes current health news, a medical encyclopedia, and directories for doctors, dentists, and hospitals
National Institutes of Health	http://www.nih.gov	Medical news and current events; press releases; biomedical information about health issues; scientific resources; links to Internet sites of related government agencies
National Library of Medicine	http://www.nlm.nih.gov	Internet site for world's largest biomedical library; research and developmental activities; connections to online medical information services
New England Journal of Medicine	http://content.nejm.org	Articles and abstracts; archives of past issues
WebMD Health®	http://www.webmd.com	Trustworthy, credible, and timely health information written by experts in medicine, journalism, and health communications

The Internet has also become a profitable marketing tool for medical practices. Medical websites can generate more new patients than paper advertising. Within the website, doctors can include patient education, newsletters, referring provider forms, and other patient-related information. Additionally, patients can e-mail the medical office personnel to ask questions and find out other pertinent non-PHI (protected health information).

▶ Software Training   LO 8.4

Software programs may seem quite complex, especially at first. Most people need a period of training before they feel comfortable using the application. Several methods of training—some from outside sources and some provided by the software manufacturer—are available.

Classes

Many computer vendors offer training classes for the software packages they sell. In addition, community colleges and high schools sometimes offer adult education classes for a variety of applications, including word processing and communications. These classes may be at the beginner, intermediate, or advanced level.

Tutorials

Several software packages come with a *tutorial,* which is a small program designed to give users an overall picture of the product and its functions. The tutorial usually provides a step-by-step walk-through and exercises that allow you to try out your newly acquired knowledge. (See Figure 8-7.)

Documentation

Nearly all software manufacturers provide some type of documentation with their programs. Documentation is usually in the form of written instruction manuals or online help that is accessed from within the program.

Technical Support

A software company's technical support service is designed to assist you with problems that go beyond the scope of the user's guide or manual. A call to technical support is important when you encounter a problem that cannot be solved by simple problem-solving techniques. By calling a toll-free number, you can access a knowledgeable team who will listen to the description of the problem and suggest solutions over the phone.

Before calling technical support,

- Check the system for errors to the best of your ability.
- Check your manual for answers. Ask your supervisor for assistance.
- Have the software registration number available.
- Be prepared to follow the technical support personnel's instructions.
- Allow uninterrupted time to spend on the phone with the technical support person.
- Plan to call from a location that gives ready access to the problem computer.

Technical support is also helpful when you are upgrading software and can be a good source of information regarding the latest products and their applications. Some software companies automatically notify their customers of available upgrades.

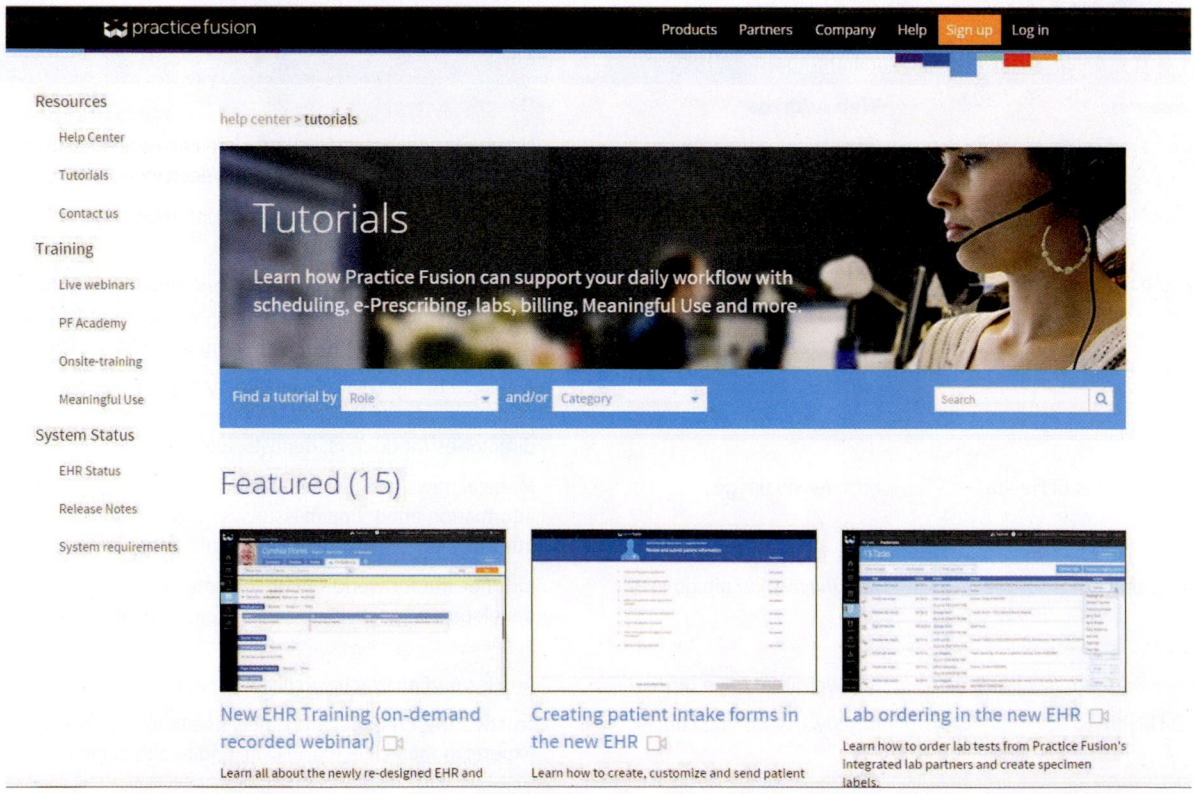

FIGURE 8-7 Practice Fusion® provides tutorials, on-demand recorded webinars, and other forms of training to help new users learn and become proficient with their system.
© Practice Fusion®

▶ Selecting Computer Equipment   LO 8.5

Most medical offices are computerized, so if the decision is made to upgrade the system, you may be a part of the decision-making process in selecting equipment. As a medical assistant who will be using the system, you may be asked for your input in selecting software, adding a network, or choosing a vendor.

The first step for helping in the selection process is to learn as much as you can about hardware and software. You can get information by taking an introductory computer class at an adult school or community college; by reading computer magazines or books; or by talking to friends, relatives, or coworkers who use computers.

Upgrading the Office System

Computer hardware is changing and improving at such a rapid pace that a system seems to become outdated almost as soon as it is purchased. In addition, more advanced software is introduced every day, and this software requires more advanced hardware in order to run, so an office system purchased only a year or two ago may need to be upgraded. Sometimes an upgrade simply requires replacement or addition of certain components. For instance, a laser printer can take the place of an ink-jet printer or portable computer devices may be added to allow healthcare providers to add information directly into the patient's medical record during the time of the visit. In other cases, such a solution is not possible or cost-effective, so an entirely new system must be purchased.

Selecting Software

Once the decision is made that a new software program, such as accounting software, is needed, research will have to be done to choose the specific software program to be purchased. To make an informed decision, you can read software reviews in computer magazines or trade publications. Check with other medical offices to get opinions on software packages. A crucial step in selecting software is to make sure the office computer system meets the minimum system requirements listed on the software box.

Adding a Network

A computer network enables users to share software programs and files and allows more than one person to work on the same patient's information at one time. While you are working on a patient's insurance claim, for example, another medical assistant might be inputting billing information. Some medical offices are virtually paperless, using a highly sophisticated network with a notebook or desktop computer in every examination room. Authorized personnel input information directly into patients' computerized records. If a doctor is in her office and a patient is waiting, a staff member at the front desk sends an e-mail message to the doctor's desktop computer (or cell phone) and a beep sounds as an alert. Networks also allow large medical facilities to communicate with employees via e-mail. For instance, an internal memo about changes in office policies may be sent by e-mail to all employees. For networks to operate, the computer must have either a network interface card or a wireless connection to the network. Networks can be run with Windows®, Novell®, or Unix® network operating systems.

Virtual Private Networks

When a group of two or more computer systems are linked together, it is known as a network system. The computers in a **local-area network (LAN)** are geographically close together (for example, in the same building). The computers in a **wide-area network (WAN)** are farther apart and are connected by telephone lines. **Virtual private networks (VPNs)** are used to connect two or more computer systems. They are also constructed using public telephone lines and use the Internet as the medium for transporting data. VPNs use encryption and other security methods to ensure that only authorized users can access the network. This type of network makes it possible for physicians to access patient records in a secure manner from a variety of locations.

Choosing a Vendor

When purchasing computer equipment, you should look for a reputable vendor who not only offers a reasonable price but also provides training, service, and technical support. A first step might be to check with personnel in other medical offices that use a computer system. Find out which dealer they use and if they are satisfied with the system, salespeople, and support. You also can ask dealers for references from medical offices that have purchased systems from them. It is a good idea to get cost estimates from at least three vendors, and it is preferable to buy all hardware components from the same vendor.

Technology Advances

Computers are evolving at such a rapid pace that it is virtually impossible to predict the changes that will take place even in the next few years. Some important new technologies, however, have already been introduced in the medical office and will be improved in the near future. Telemedicine and speech recognition technology are only two examples of new computer technologies. Undoubtedly, more will be explored and developed every year.

Telemedicine *Telemedicine* refers to the use of telecommunications to transmit video images of patient information, such as CT scans or even teleconferences involving multiple care providers. These images are already used to provide medical support to physicians caring for patients in rural areas. The use of telemedicine and advancements in computer technology allow medical practices to quickly access vast amounts of current medical information.

Speech Recognition Technology Speech recognition technology enables the computer to comprehend and interpret spoken words through the use of a specialty software program. The user simply speaks into a microphone instead of inputting information with a keyboard or a scanner. Because every human voice is different, and the English language is vast and complex, this technology is, however, difficult to perfect. As speech recognition technology becomes more advanced, more accurate, and less expensive, it will likely gain widespread acceptance. It has a great deal of potential, including the ability to virtually eliminate the need for medical assistants to transcribe physicians' notes. There are a variety of speech recognition software applications available for use.

Computer System Care and Maintenance

LO 8.6

Like a car, a computer needs routine care and maintenance to stay in sound condition; the computer user's manual outlines the steps required. Also, a good general rule is not to eat or drink near the computer. Crumbs and spilled liquids can damage the system components and storage devices.

Care for the System Unit

The system unit should be placed in a well-ventilated location, with nothing blocking the fan in the back of the cabinet. To keep the system's delicate circuitry from being damaged by an electrical power surge, you should use a power strip with a surge protector. You plug the computer into the power strip and then plug the power strip into the electrical outlet. If a power surge should occur, the surge protector will absorb the power, not the computer system. Surge protectors can also be purchased with an attached battery backup that will protect the computer during a power outage. Basic care for the system components is outlined as follows:

- *Monitor.* A screen saver automatically changes the monitor display at short intervals or constantly shows moving images on the computer monitor or screen. All Windows® operating systems come equipped with screen savers. To protect their screens, many monitors "power down" after a certain period of inactivity. If no one uses the computer for 30 minutes, for example, the monitor screen goes blank. To resume using the computer after the screen saver has been activated or the monitor has powered down, you may need to simply touch any key or move the mouse. However, if the medical office has activated the "On resume, display logon screen" feature that is standard on Windows machines you may be required to enter your login information again. Also, adding a screen cover to a monitor when it is not in use will protect the monitor.

- *Printer.* Printer maintenance generally consists of replacing the ink cartridge or toner cartridge when required. When the cartridge needs to be changed, the ink on your printouts becomes very light and colors become faded. Some integrated computer and printer systems automatically provide a "Low Ink" message on the screen when printer cartridges need replacing. The message appears when the "Print" command is given. A graph indicates the amount of ink left in the cartridge. Ink can be ordered online through a link provided with the printer program. Replacement is usually a simple process, described in the printer manual.

- *Storage devices.* Jump drives and CD-ROMs are highly sensitive devices. Even a small "injury" may cause permanent damage or make it impossible to retrieve data. To avoid problems, handle and store these devices properly. A jump drive should be protected when it is not attached to the computer. Always put the cap back on when it is not attached to the CPU or when you are transporting the drive to another location. When you handle a CD-ROM disc or pick it up, touch only the edges or the edge and the hole in the center; always be careful not to touch the flat surface of the disc. CD-ROMs should be stored in the clear plastic case (sometimes called a jewel case) in which they are packaged.

Security in the Computerized Office

LO 8.7

Although security measures are important in any office, they are especially important in a computerized medical office. Great care must be taken to safeguard confidential files, make backup copies on a regular basis, and prevent system contamination. HIPAA and HITECH laws require that privacy and security procedures be in place to prevent the misuse of health information. These procedures also must ensure confidentiality.

Safeguarding Confidential Files

Much of the information collected in a medical office is confidential. Just as with paper records, confidential information stored on the computer should be accessible only to authorized personnel. Always take care that computer screens are not visible to patients or other unauthorized personnel, and use screen savers when not use. Log off or lock your computer when leaving your desk to minimize risk of unauthorized access in your absence. Three common ways to provide security in a computerized office are to employ passwords, to encrypt sensitive information when it is being transferred electronically or stored on a "removable" storage device, and to install an activity-monitoring system.

Passwords In many hospitals and physician offices, each employee who is allowed access to computerized patient files receives a password. The employee must enter the password into the computer when using the files. Access codes or passwords only allow the user into approved areas according to the individual's job description. When you receive a password, do not divulge it to anyone else. If an employee leaves or is terminated, the user account should be deleted. When you choose a password, do not use common ones such as your birthday. This is so important that many times specific guidelines for creating a password must be followed and commonly used formats, like birthdates, will not be accepted by the password program. It is also becoming a common requirement that passwords be changed every 60–90 days and cannot repeat previous (6) passwords. Passwords should contain a variety of numbers, symbols (if accepted), and both upper- and lowercase letters.

Encryption Software Encryption software allows personal information or other PHI to be encoded in such a way that only the person with the key (password) is able to open the document in its "decoded" format.

Activity-Monitoring System In conjunction with passwords, most healthcare facilities use a computer system that monitors user activity. Whenever someone accesses computer records or an Internet site, the system automatically keeps track of the user's name and the files (or sites) that have been viewed or modified. In this way, if necessary, problems or security breaches can be traced back to specific employees.

Preventing System Contamination

Computer viruses constitute another important security issue in the computerized medical office. Viruses are programs written specifically to contaminate the hard disk by damaging or destroying data. They can be passed from computer to computer through shared, infected diskettes. Computer viruses also can be spread through infected files retrieved from online services, the Internet, e-mails, and electronic bulletin boards. Several software programs are available to detect and correct computer viruses. Most are fairly inexpensive but provide an invaluable service.

Antivirus Software and Firewalls There are literally hundreds of security vulnerabilities awaiting your computer system. You need to be concerned about everything on your computer from the operating system to the software applications. Antivirus software provides protection for your computer. It scans your system for viruses automatically and manually. If it finds a virus, it either destroys it automatically or alerts the user to respond by "cleaning" the file, thus destroying it. Antivirus software responds to spammers (persons who abuse e-mails by sending them in mass without permission), who often send malicious e-mails and files. If you do not know who sent you an e-mail, it is best not to open the file.

Firewalls (barriers to keep destructive forces away from your computer) also are called security protection. Firewalls are helpful in putting a stop to offensive Internet sites and potential computer hackers (a person who can get inside a computer legally or illegally and do anything) who are trying to gain access to your computer.

Computer Disaster Recovery Plan

When any business is dependent on computer technology for daily functioning, a computer disaster recovery plan for the business must be in place. A recovery plan offers a possible solution if the primary computer system should fail, or "crash," making all information on the hard drive unavailable. Disaster recovery planning can be developed within an organization, or it can be purchased as a software application or a service.

In a medical practice, it is important to discuss the computer disaster recovery plan with the staff so that everyone knows the part he or she will play if the computer system fails. As devices, systems, and networks become more complex, there are simply more things that can go wrong. As a result, these plans have become increasingly important and sophisticated.

Although a computer disaster recovery plan will vary from practice to practice, all plans should include these elements:

- *Minimizing damage to equipment.* Automatic warnings are built into computer systems to indicate when a fatal error has occurred. Warnings also provide direction to help prevent information loss and minimize damage to the computer equipment.

- *Retrieving information.* As stated earlier in the chapter, it is essential to routinely back up the office files using either an automated or manual backup system. An example of an automated system is a second computer, networked to the first, to which information is regularly backed up in the event the primary computer system fails. With this type of backup, the operation of the office can continue while the primary system is repaired or replaced. An example of a manual electronic backup system is copying files to CDs and keeping these backups off site. An example of a paper backup system, which is less useful, is a handwritten list of patients and the procedures performed each day.

How often backups are made varies among medical offices; your supervisor will tell you the policy for your office. If the office staff is responsible for performing the backup, remember that storing the backups properly is just as important as making them. Backup files should not be stored near the original files. Ideally, they should be kept outside the medical office—perhaps at a storage site or lock box—for security in case of fire, burglary, or other office catastrophe. Backup systems are also vital. If the main system fails, the backup system will allow all the information to be retrieved and not permanently lost.

- *Guarding protected health information.* Even during an office emergency, like a computer failure, healthcare professionals are still required to carefully protect the privacy of patient records. If an electronic or manual backup system is implemented, safeguards to protect patient information must still be observed.

▶ Administrative Medical Office Equipment
LO 8.8

Using automated equipment enables you to perform a task more easily and quickly than doing it manually. For example, adding numbers on a calculator is a much faster process than doing it on paper. Many of the administrative tasks in a medical practice can be accomplished with the help of automated equipment, allowing you more time to perform other tasks.

Facsimile Machines

Although computerized offices most often use scanners and e-mail for critical communications, alternate methods must be used when e-mail is not accepted by the recipient of the information. A facsimile (fax) machine can be an efficient way to accomplish this. A fax machine scans each page of a document, translates it into electronic impulses, and transmits those impulses over the telephone line. When another fax machine receives the impulses, they are converted into an exact copy of the original document.

A fax machine in a medical office should have its own telephone line. A separate line ensures that transmission of incoming and outgoing faxes will not be interrupted and that the machine will not tie up a needed telephone line when sending or receiving information. Always keep in mind that faxed material may include protected health information.

For this reason, fax machines should never be placed in patient examination rooms or reception areas where unauthorized persons may be able to view incoming or outgoing documents. Only staff members with a "need to know" should have access to faxed and other confidential information. Because of the confidential nature of many faxes, all faxes should also be sent with a fax cover sheet that contains a **disclaimer.** This disclaimer should state that the material within the fax is intended only for the person to whom it is being sent and if the fax is received in error, to inform the sender and destroy the fax immediately (see Figure 8-8).

Benefits of Faxing A fax machine can send an exact copy of a document to a recipient within minutes. The cost for sending a fax is the same as for making a telephone call to that location.

In addition, many fax machines have a copier function and can be used as an extra copy machine. The telephone for the fax also may be used as an extra extension for outgoing calls, if needed. Procedure 8-1, found at the end of the chapter, details the correct steps for using a fax machine.

Receiving a Fax Faxes can be received 24 hours a day if the fax machine is turned on and has an adequate paper supply

BWW

BWW Medical Associates, PC
305 Main Street, Port Snead YZ 12345-9876
Tel: 555-654-3210, Fax: 555-987-6543
Web: BWWAssociates.com

Paul F. Buckwalter, MD
Alexis N. Whalen, MD
Elizabeth H. Williams, MD

FACSIMILE COVER SHEET

Date: _____

To: _____   From: _____

Fax #: _____   Fax #: _____

# of pages (including this cover sheet): _____

Message:

_____

_____

_____

_____

_____

_____

_____

The information contained in this transmission is privileged and confidential, intended only for the use of the individual or entity named above. If the reader of this message is not the intended recipient, you are hereby notified that any dissemination, distribution, or copying of this communication is strictly prohibited. If you have received this transmission in error, do not read. Please immediately respond to the sender that you have received this communication in error and then destroy or delete it. Thank you.

FIGURE 8-8 Example of a facsimile (fax) cover sheet.

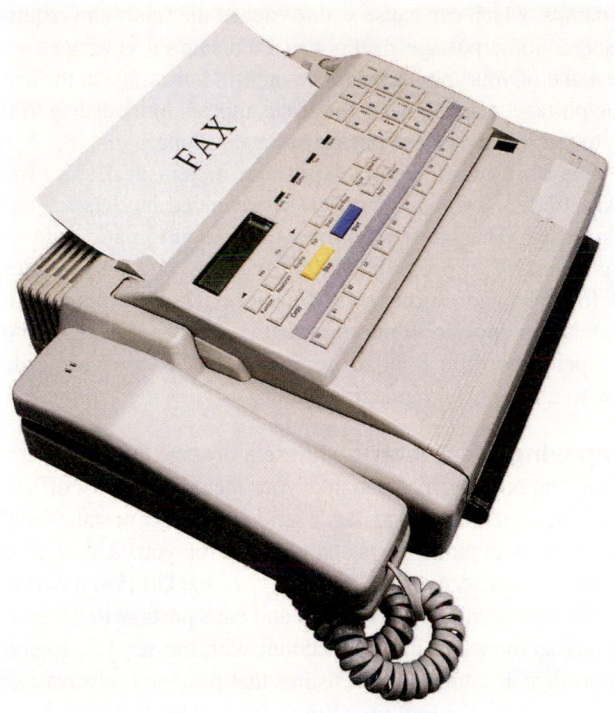

FIGURE 8-9 Typical office facsimile (fax) machine.
© Comstock Images/Alamy RF

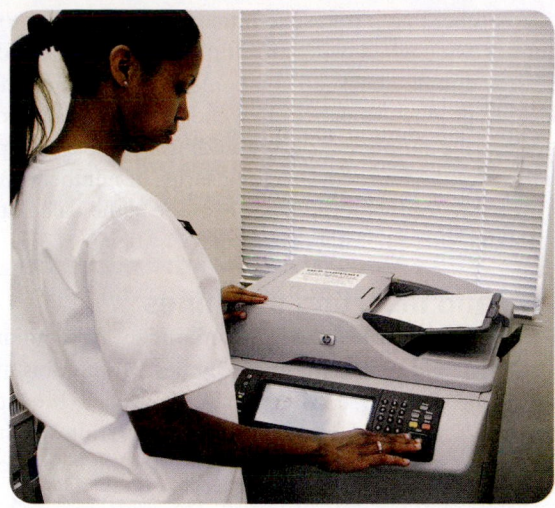

FIGURE 8-10 The office copier produces hard copies of documents.
© Total Care Programming, Inc.

(Figure 8-9). Today's fax machines have memories and can store and receive documents. If the fax machine is not already sending or receiving a fax, the fax telephone rings, or the machine buzzes briefly, signaling the start of a transmission. The transmission begins shortly thereafter, with the machine printing out the document as it is sent. When the document is completed, the machine may print a transmission report that includes the number of pages, the date and time, and the originating fax number.

Typewriters

Although typewriters are used very little in a medical practice, they may still be used to complete medical forms brought in by patients or sent from an insurance company if the office does not use electronic billing software. These forms can be completed more clearly when the information is typed instead of handwritten.

Most modern medical practices have eliminated typewriters altogether and, instead, use computers with word processing software and scanners to create and manipulate word documents.

Photocopiers

A photocopier, also called a copier or copy machine, instantly reproduces office correspondence, forms, bills, patient records, and other documents. A photocopier works by taking a picture of the document it is to reproduce and printing it on plain paper using a heat process. Photocopiers use either liquid or dry toner (a form of ink). Various kinds of paper can be used in the machine, including office stationery and colored paper. Many photocopiers accept different sizes of paper, from the standard 8 × 11 inch paper to 8 × 14 inch legal paper and even larger.

Photocopiers come in many models with varying features and speeds—from desktop machines for limited use to industrial models for continual heavy use. All styles are available through purchase or lease. Procedure 8-2, found at the end of the chapter, describes the correct method for using a photocopier machine.

Special Features In addition to the copier/scanner/fax combination machines, most copiers offer a wide range of special features. They may collate (assemble sets of multiple pages in order) and staple pages, punch holes, enlarge or reduce images, and produce double-sided copies (print on both sides of the page). Some also can adjust contrast and even track the cost of a job via a specific code input into the machine. Some photocopiers produce black-and-white copies as well as color copies. Some copiers can make transparencies (text and images printed on clear acetate), which physicians often use for presentations. Many copiers can also be networked to computers and act as both printers and copiers (see Figure 8-10).

One of the more useful features of photocopiers is the "Help" function. Selecting this function displays directions in plain English that explain how to fix a paper jam or deal with other routine copier problems. Some copiers are even programmed to indicate that service is needed.

Adding Machines and Calculators

For handling tasks such as patient billing, bank deposits, and payroll, many medical practices depend on adding machines and calculators. The difference between the two types of machines is minimal. Adding machines typically plug into an outlet and produce a paper tape on which calculations are printed. Calculators are more often battery or solar powered, with memory to store figures. Calculators are portable and usually do not produce a paper tape.

Routine Calculations Both adding machines and calculators are sufficient for most routine office calculations, such as basic arithmetic functions like addition, subtraction, multiplication, and division. More contemporary models perform such specialized functions as computing percentages and storing data. Some are even computerized.

Do remember that it is easy to hit an incorrect key or to key in a number twice when using an adding machine or a calculator. Always double-check all mathematical computations. If the machine produces a paper tape, check the numbers on the tape against the numbers you are adding. The paper tape is especially useful when adding a long series of numbers. Without a printed record, you must perform the same calculations again to make sure the total is correct.

Folding and Inserting Machines

Letter-folding equipment can help minimize the amount of time staff spends preparing large volumes of outgoing mail. Letter folders are also used for creating folded brochures. A medical practice may use folding and inserting machines for a variety of items, including invoices, newsletters, checks, statements, letters, and flyers.

Lower-end folding equipment requires letters to be fed manually. The speed of this machine is limited to the speed an individual can feed in letters, which is typically about 200 pieces per hour. An automatic feeder is required for faster folding. You will learn more about fold types and folding machines in the *Written and Electronic Communication* chapter.

Postage Meters

Every medical office uses the US Postal Service. Patient bills, routine correspondence, purchase orders, and payments are just some of the items typically sent by mail. The *Medical Records and Documentation* chapter will also provide additional information on mailing correspondence.

Although some medical offices use stamps, most use a postage meter. A postage meter is a machine that applies postage to an envelope or package, eliminating the need for postage stamps (Figure 8-11). A postage meter often has two parts: the meter, which belongs to the post office, and the mailing machine, which the practice can own. The meter actually applies the postage and the mailing machine (if available) seals the envelope.

Benefits of Using a Postage Meter Using a postage meter instead of purchasing stamps saves frequent trips to the post office. It also saves money for the office by providing the exact amount of postage needed for each item, instead of using a combination

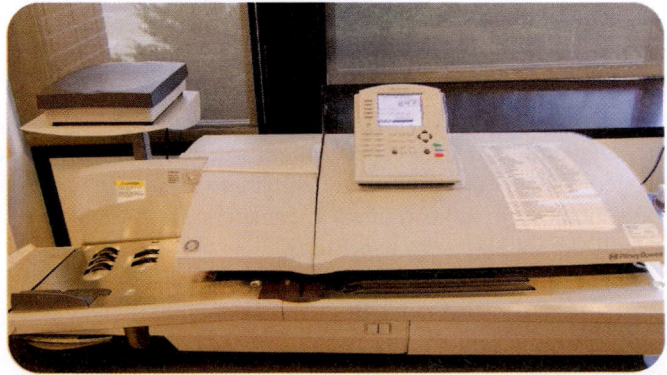

FIGURE 8-11 The postage meter is a convenient and cost-efficient way to apply postage to correspondence and packages.
© McGraw-Hill Education. Mark Dierker, photographer

of stamps, which can cause you to exceed the minimum required postage. Some postage meters can even imprint envelopes with the name of your medical practice or with a message at the same time postage is applied. The message appears immediately to the left of the postal mark, at the top of the envelope.

There are many types of postage meters available, from basic models for a small office to advanced models for large businesses. The latest machines include automatic date setting, memory to program a large mailing, and display alerts for low postage or the need for ribbon replacement. Some models can apply postage to parcels without the use of labels or tape. Procedure 8-3, at the end of this chapter, describes how to use a postage meter.

Prepaying for Postage To use a postage meter, you must prepay the postage. You can take your meter to the post office to add postage, use a postage meter service, or order postage online. A service maintains the postal account for you. Although the money in each account is the property of the US Postal Service, the provider manages the account and adds postage to the meter, as long as money is in your account with the service. Keeping the postage account current ensures that postage is always available and all mail is sent on a timely basis. This task may be one of your responsibilities. On any meter, you can check the amount of postage used and the amount remaining with the touch of a button. On some models, the meter must have $10 or more for the machine to apply postage to an envelope or package.

Postal Scales

Besides the postage meter, a medical practice also needs a postal scale. Postal scales are a good investment because they show both the weight and the amount of postage required. Some postage meters include an electronic scale. If you need a postal scale but one is not available, you can use any scale that weighs in ounces. When using a simple scale, you can then translate the weight into the correct postage by using a current postal rate chart, available from the US Postal Service, which cuts down on mail being returned for inadequate postage.

Dictation-Transcription Equipment

Healthcare professionals are seldom known for their beautiful handwriting. For offices that do not have electronic medical records, handwritten notes can be difficult, if not impossible, to read. Medical assistants, although not professional medical transcriptionists, may be asked to transcribe recorded words into written text. Using dictation-transcription equipment is the most efficient way to complete this task. *Dictation* is another word for speaking; *transcription* is another word for writing. Together, they mean to transform spoken words into written form. Should transcription be included in your job description, you will need training on using this specialized office equipment.

Check Writers

Medical practice personnel need to write checks to pay for equipment, supplies, and payroll. This common office procedure can be automated by using a check writer, which is a machine that imprints checks. Procedure 8-4, located at the end of this chapter, details the correct steps for operating a check-writing machine.

The safety advantage of using such a machine is that the name of the payee (the person receiving the check) and the amount of the check, once imprinted, cannot be altered. Numerous check-writing software packages can assist you, including QuickBooks, Checksoft, and VersaCheck.

Paper Shredders

Paper shredders cut documents into tiny pieces to make them unreadable. They are quite common in medical practices, as they allow protection of protected health information that is no longer required by the office. A paper shredder, like the one shown in Figure 8-12, is often used when confidential documents, such as patient records, need to be destroyed. The most common type of shredder cuts paper into ribbonlike strips, which differ in width, depending on the model. Other shredders cut the paper in two directions, forming small pieces. Some paper shredders offer additional options, such as an electronic eye that automatically starts the machine when paper is inserted and stops when it is done. Other features available are paper jam detection, automatic reverse, and automatic shutdown when the machine gets too hot.

How to Shred Materials A paper shredder is ready to use when it is turned on. To shred a document, insert it into the feed tray at the top of the shredder. The machine feeds the

paper through hundreds of knifelike cutters, instantaneously shredding the paper. A basket attached beneath the shredder catches the bits of paper. Different models can accommodate different amounts of paper through the cutters. Shredder baskets must be emptied periodically to allow room for additional shredded paper. Some shredders even signal when the basket

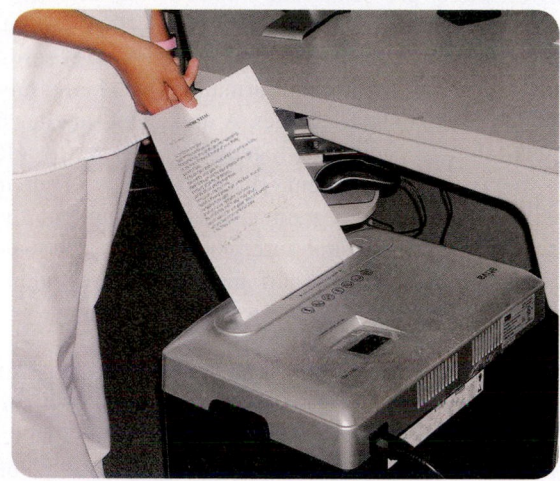

FIGURE 8-12 Using a paper shredder protects patient PHI when it is no longer needed.
© Total Care Programming, Inc.

POINTS ON PRACTICE

Recycling in the Medical Office, Hospital, Laboratory, or Clinic

You may easily incorporate recycling procedures into the daily routine of a medical office, hospital, laboratory, or clinic. Recycling may be required by state law. Some states levy large fines for noncompliance with recycling regulations. Purchase paper products that can be recycled, or those made of postconsumer recycled materials, and take care in disposing of them. Care should be taken to ensure HIPAA compliance when recycling paper. Shredding is the most effective way to comply with HIPAA regulations.

There are two essential aspects of recycling: disposal and purchasing. To create a complete recycling program, ensure that materials are disposed of properly and that purchased products have been made from recycled materials. Your town's recycling center provides guidelines for packaging recycled materials and for a pickup schedule as well as containers for recyclable materials and a list of paper materials that can and cannot be recycled. Follow regulations from OSHA and your office policy for disposal of biohazardous materials and other medical wastes. As discussed in the *Infection Control Fundamentals* chapter, these are disposed of in designed protective containers.

When purchasing items for recycling, look for the universal recycling symbol, which has three chasing arrows (Figure 8-13).

This symbol could mean that the product or package is made up of recycled materials or that the product or package is recyclable. Unless the package is made of 100% recycled materials, the law requires the package to display how much. Watch out

for claims that do not mean anything. Claims that a product or service is "environmentally friendly," "environmentally safe," "environmentally preferable," or "eco-safe" or labels that contain environmental seals are unhelpful. These phrases alone do not provide the specific information you need to compare products, packaging, or services on their environmental merits. If you want to go "green," look for claims that give some substance and additional information that explains why the product is environmentally friendly or has earned a special seal. For more about recycling, check the website of the Federal Trade Commission (http://www.ftc.gov) or the Environmental Protection Agency (http://epa.gov).

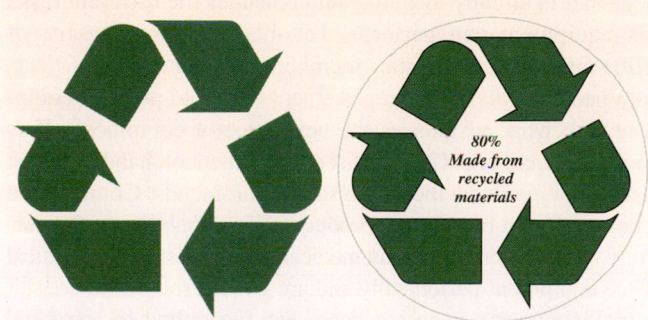

80%
Made from recycled materials

FIGURE 8-13 Check products for this symbol to determine if they are environmentally friendly.

is full. Avoid wearing loose-fitting clothing while operating a shredder to prevent an accident or personal injury.

When to Shred Materials Medical practices need to eliminate old patient records and other sensitive materials. These items cannot simply be thrown into the trash because of confidentiality problems. The shredder is an effective disposal solution. If records have incorrect information that has been corrected on subsequent documents, the old records are shredded to prevent incorrect information from being mistakenly placed in the patient's folder. A document that has been shredded cannot be put back together, so do not decide on your own to shred a document. The physician or office manager will set guidelines regarding when a document should be shredded. If you are not sure whether to shred a document, check with a senior staff member before beginning the process.

Shredding Vendors Many medical practices contract with a shredding company to come into the practice to remove and then shred designated materials. Using another company for this task does not relieve the medical practice of the responsibility for the confidential materials. The healthcare provider is still considered the **covered entity** and must comply with HIPAA law. It is important to contract only with companies that also abide by HIPAA confidentiality statutes.

▶ Purchasing Decisions for Office Equipment

LO 8.9

As the office medical assistant, in addition to your possible role in making purchasing decisions for computer equipment, you also may be involved in helping to select the most appropriate office equipment. You may be asked to investigate whether the practice needs a new photocopier or whether hiring a shredding company makes sense for the office. To make a sound decision about whether the office will benefit from such a purchase, you will need to conduct thorough research, documenting your findings for further discussion.

Evaluating Office Needs

The first step in evaluating the equipment needs of a healthcare office is the research process. Make note of the equipment that is already available and consider the different tasks this equipment can perform. To obtain a complete list of office needs, ask other staff members for their ideas.

When considering the replacement of an old piece of equipment, ask what advantages the new piece of equipment offers over the current one. Create a list of equipment on hand and a list of any new products the office staff recommends. Compare the benefits offered by the new product to the capability of the currently used equipment. Many medical magazines review medical office equipment periodically and are good resources to consult in making your purchasing decisions. Go online to shop and compare products, features, and prices. Discuss with the office manager the budget for the equipment under consideration. Consider calling a supplier for more detailed information.

Contacting Suppliers Put together a list of the features you would like in your piece of equipment. Then contact suppliers who sell models that offer those features. You can call or e-mail the manufacturer directly to find out the name of a local vendor. Many manufacturers prepare brochures giving information about their products. Request that this information be sent to you.

Go online or look in the Yellow Pages for office supply stores and other companies that sell office equipment. Obtain product and pricing information on each model. For certain equipment, such as photocopiers, a sales representative will come to your office to demonstrate and discuss the product.

Evaluating Warranty Options Most products come with a warranty, which is a contract that guarantees free service and parts replacement for a certain period, usually 1 year. Warranties are valid only for specified service and repairs. They usually do not cover accidents, vandalism, acts of God (such as damage caused by floods or earthquakes), or mistreatment of the machine. In most cases, warranty repairs must be made at an authorized service center.

If you want more coverage than the warranty allows, consider buying an extended warranty. Extended warranties increase the amount of time that equipment is covered. For expensive equipment or parts, the additional cost of an extended warranty may be justified.

After you purchase a product, you must fill out the warranty card and mail it to the manufacturer. File the receipt in a safe place in the office where it can easily be retrieved.

Preparing a Recommendation After you have obtained all the information, you are ready to evaluate it. To compare and contrast the different models, construct a chart. Place the product model names in columns across the top. Down the left side, list factors that will influence the purchase decision: cost, warranty options (including the length of the warranty and the price of an extended warranty), special features, and delivery time. Then fill in the information. This chart will provide an easy-to-use summary of your research. Finally, analyze the list and choose the product that will best meet the office's needs. Meet with the physician or office manager to discuss your recommendation.

Leasing Versus Buying Equipment

Once the product has been selected, there is one more decision to make: whether to lease or buy it. When buying a product, the purchaser becomes the owner. Owners are free to do with the product anything they choose, which may include selling it to someone else.

For most large pieces of office equipment, like photocopiers, there is also an option to *lease* the equipment. Leasing, or renting, usually involves an initial charge and a monthly fee. On average, the initial charge is equal to about two monthly payments. The ownership of a leased piece of equipment is retained by the leasing company.

Lease Agreement A lease is for a specified time, after which time the equipment is returned to the seller per the lease agreement (Figure 8-14). Some leases allow purchase of

Metropolitan Office Systems

Lease Agreement

Customer (Location)

BWW Medical Associates, PC
Full Legal Name (Please Print)

Address
305 Main Street

Port Snead _____ YZ _____ 12345-9876
City | County | State | Zip

Billing Contact

Dealer:

Customer (Billing address, if different)

Full Legal Name (Please Print)

Address

City | County | State | Zip

Phone

Quantity	Description: Make, Model, and Serial Number	Quantity	Description: Make, Model, and Serial Number
1	FT 6655 Copier AA3365430358		
1	Sorter A337502010902		
1	Document Feeder A338506		
1	RT314 Large-capacity Tray		

Minimum Lease Term:	Payment Due:	Amount of Monthly Payment with Sales, Use, and Property Tax:	Advance Payment of $965.56 (Tax Included) by Check #	Documentation Fee
	_X_ Monthly		_____ First Month's Rent	
	_____ Quarterly		_X_ First and Last	
	_____ Annually		_____ Security Deposit (Without Tax)	
60 Months	_____ Other: $455.46	$482.78	_____ Other _____	$ _0_

FIGURE 8-14 Read all lease agreements carefully before signing.

the equipment at the end of the rental period for an additional payment. The details of the purchase option are covered in the lease agreement.

Advantages and Disadvantages of Leasing When you lease a product, your office does not own it, but you have several advantages.

1. Leasing allows purchasers to keep more of their money. The initial cost of obtaining the machine is a fraction of the full cost of purchasing it. So the remainder of the money can earn interest in the bank or be used for other expenses. Leasing is advantageous when you do not have enough money to buy the equipment but need the services it provides. In addition, leasing allows businesses to update equipment every few years at the end of each lease period. Updating may not be as affordable if you buy equipment.

2. Often the company that leases the product is also responsible for servicing it.

3. In most cases, businesses are able to take lease payments as a tax deduction each year.

But leasing is not always the best solution—you will not own the equipment, so the office will not gain any equity for the money it is spending on it. It is important to weigh the advantages of leasing against the advantages of buying equipment for your medical practice.

Whether you decide to lease or buy, always ask whether the price is firm or if there is room for negotiation. Many available discounted rates are not extended to a customer simply because the customer did not ask. Although some equipment prices are nonnegotiable, terms can sometimes be negotiated on more expensive pieces of equipment. Companies that lease office equipment are often flexible in determining the monthly payment. For example, equipment companies may accept smaller payments in the beginning of the rental or purchase agreement period and require larger payments near the end.

In a competitive market, some suppliers may match their competitors' prices. When purchasing several pieces of equipment at the same time, a supplier may be able to offer some savings on the total cost of the purchase or provide some service, such as free delivery, or an extension on the service contract.

▶ Maintaining Office Equipment LO 8.10

Office equipment (as with computers) must be regularly maintained to provide optimum service. Daily or weekly maintenance, such as cleaning the glass on the photocopier or replacing toner, can be performed by the office staff.

However, more extensive maintenance should be done by the equipment supplier. Consult the equipment manual for details about the care of each piece of equipment.

Equipment Manuals

The best source of information about maintaining a piece of equipment is the manual that comes with it. This booklet gives basic information about the equipment, including how to set it up, how it works, special features, and problems you may encounter. The information in an equipment manual is extremely valuable. If the manual is lost, call the manufacturer or research the Internet to obtain another one. Equipment manuals should be stored where they can be retrieved easily. Some large pieces of office equipment provide racks or slots on the side of the equipment for manual storage.

It is helpful to write the following information on the inside front cover of the equipment manual upon initial setup. If there is a problem with the equipment that requires a maintenance call, this valuable information will be quick and easy to retrieve.

- The date of purchase or lease
- The serial number of the equipment
- The phone number of the company contracted to repair the equipment

Maintenance and Service Contracts

Equipment suppliers provide standard maintenance contracts when office equipment is purchased. A maintenance contract specifies when the equipment will be cleaned, checked for worn parts, and repaired. A standard maintenance contract may include regular checkups as well as emergency repairs.

In addition, some suppliers offer a service contract, which covers services that are not included under the standard maintenance agreement, such as emergency repairs. In some cases, service contracts are combined with maintenance contracts in one document.

Make sure to keep track of all maintenance performed on your equipment. Many offices have a maintenance log, where staff members record the date and purpose of each service call. This log is helpful in identifying whether equipment should be replaced because of the need for frequent servicing.

Troubleshooting

Before calling the service supplier for service on any piece of equipment that appears to be malfunctioning, steps should be taken to determine if you can correct the problem yourself. This process is called "troubleshooting." Resolving the problem can save you the cost of a service call that may not be covered by the standard agreement.

The first step in troubleshooting is to eliminate possible simple causes of a problem. For example, if the equipment is powered by electricity, make sure that it is plugged into a functioning outlet and that it is turned on. Are all doors and other openings in their correct positions? Are all machine connections firmly in place? If you cannot discover a simple cause for the problem, it is time to test the machine to determine what it is failing to do. In the case of a malfunctioning photocopier, for example, try making a copy and note the response. Write down any error messages the machine provides.

Next, consult the equipment manual. Many manuals devote a section to troubleshooting. If you cannot find the solution after reading the manual, call the manufacturer or the place of purchase for additional assistance. Be prepared to explain the steps you have already taken toward resolving the problem.

Backup Systems

Earlier in the chapter, you read about the importance of having a backup system for the office's computer system(s) and the information contained within it. It is also important to have a "backup plan" in case of other equipment failure. Occasionally, more than one piece of equipment can be affected by a single problem. For example, if the electricity goes off, all electrical equipment will go out at once. To avoid losing important information and records, it is important to have backup systems in place.

Telephones The use of cell phones in addition to traditional phones offers a backup to communication in the event that phone service is interrupted. Cell phones are also helpful during emergency weather conditions.

Electricity An emergency generator may supply emergency power for lighting in key hallways and exam rooms. Interior rooms and halls can quickly become very dark and hazardous when the electricity is unexpectedly cut off.

Battery Power Battery power backup is a key component of security and warning system backups. Audio warning signals sound when it is time to replace the batteries in smoke and security detectors. All batteries should routinely be replaced every six months.

Fire Extinguishers Fire extinguishers need to be serviced or replaced once a year to ensure maximum performance. The office may choose to contract with a local company to provide this annual maintenance evaluation.

Equipment Inventory

Office equipment, such as photocopiers, scanners, telephone systems, examination tables, ECG machines, lab equipment, and even reflex hammers and thermometers, is part of the medical office's assets. As such, they must be maintained and inventoried on the practice assets and liabilities balance sheet.

Traditionally, medical office equipment inventory was done manually using a master inventory such as that shown in Figure 8-15. Information kept in the master inventory log often consisted of the following items:

- Name of the equipment, including the brand name
- Brief description of the equipment
- Model number and registration number
- Date of purchase
- Place of purchase, including contact information
- Estimated life of the product
- Product warranty
- Maintenance and service contracts

EQUIPMENT INVENTORY

ITEM	PURCHASE DATE	PURCHASE PRICE
1. TotalOffice oak desk	07/25/13	$500.00
2. TotalOffice rolling desk chair	02/19/13	$225.00
3. TotalOffice 4-drawer file cabinet	12/21/11	$150.00
4. TotalOffice 2-drawer file cabinet	08/05/11	$100.00
5. HYtech Quad-core computer	03/10/15	$1150.00
6. HYtech 17-inch LED monitor	03/10/15	$200.00

FIGURE 8-15 Traditional equipment inventory, including the name and quantity of each equipment type.

With many medical offices now computerized, inventory control is no longer a manual process for these offices. Most practice management software programs for the medical office include some form of inventory control management. The information contained within the software may be the same as that in a manual system, but updates and changes are now computerized. Depending on the size of the office, bar codes, similar to those used in retail establishments, may be affixed to equipment to assist with tracking. If your office is computerized but does not run a full practice management program, there are also separate inventory control software packages available, such as Fishbowl and Intellitrack. Remember, when considering any software program, make purchasing decisions based not only on whether the program will suit the practice today but also whether it will be able to grow and expand with the practice tomorrow.

▶ Maintaining Medical Office Supplies

LO 8.11

Purchasing and maintaining the office supplies and equipment in a medical office is an essential skill in managing the office. You may be responsible for evaluating and recommending equipment and supplies, taking inventory of equipment and supplies, and negotiating prices with suppliers. When managing office supplies, your goal is to achieve efficiency, which is the ability to produce the desired result with the least effort, expense, and waste (Figure 8-16). Factors such as environmental friendliness—particularly with paper products—should be considered as well. For more information, see the feature *Points on Practice* feature on recycling supplies.

The word *supply* refers to an expendable item, or an item that is used and then must be restocked, like examination table paper. Ideally, office supplies are stored on labeled shelves.

Determining Responsibility for Organizing Supplies

The medical assistant is often responsible for organizing office supplies. In a small practice, one medical assistant may be able to handle this responsibility alone, but a practice with several physicians may require more help to manage supplies. When

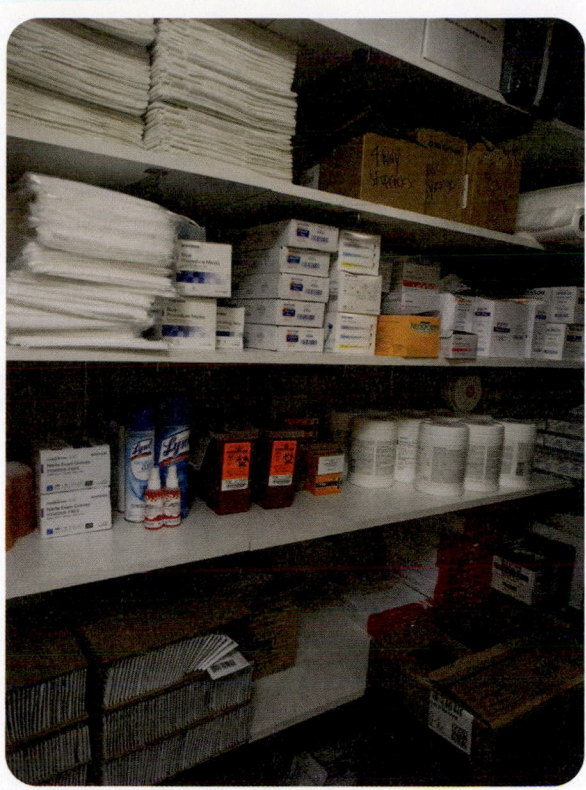

FIGURE 8-16 Keeping an up-to-date, organized inventory of supplies is crucial to a well-run office.
© McGraw-Hill Education. David Moyer, photographer

two medical assistants handle this responsibility, one is often assigned to handle administrative items and the other to handle clinical (medical) supplies. In a very large practice, a third assistant might handle computer, copier, and fax supplies.

Categorizing Supplies

Most medical office supplies fall into two main categories: administrative and clinical. Examples of administrative supplies include items that are used in the office portion of the practice, such as stationery, insurance forms, pens, pencils, and clipboards. Clinical supplies are medically related and include alcohol swabs, tongue depressors, disposable tips for otoscopes, and disposable sheaths for thermometers.

General supplies are used by both patients and staff. Examples of general supplies include paper towels, liquid hypoallergenic soap, and facial and toilet tissue.

The Supply List As discussed earlier, if the office is computerized, it is likely that both the equipment and supply inventories are computerized. To assist with inventory management, many of these systems use a bar code or other method to allow usage be tracked. By scanning the bar code as a box of supplies is opened or used, the inventory amount is adjusted accordingly within the computer system. By monitoring these numbers, you will know when specific supplies require ordering to ensure that you never run out of crucial supplies.

Regardless of how the office supply inventory is maintained, a master supply list will need to be created and maintained. One helpful way to track administrative, clinical, and general supplies is to subcategorize them in accordance with their importance within the practice. Many offices use three categories for this purpose: vital, incidental, and periodic use. The placement of supplies within each subcategory may vary depending upon the type of practice. For instance, an office specializing in pediatrics may consider the clinical supply of topical skin freeze as a vital supply for their young patients, but a cardiac office may consider it incidental. Table 8-2 lists some common supplies by their main category of administrative, clinical, or general. Think about the type of practice you might like to work in and what subcategory (vital, incidental, or periodic) these supplies might fall into.

Vital Supplies These items are absolutely essential for the practice's functioning. They include paper examination table covers and prescription pads. Without these items, the physicians and other licensed practitioners would be unable to work in a clean examination environment or to readily prescribe medication for patients during office visits. Another type of vital supply is an item that requires a special

TABLE 8-2	Typical Supplies in a Medical Office

Administrative Supplies

Appointment books, daybooks (still used in noncomputerized offices)	Insurance manuals
Back-to-school/back-to-work slips	Local welfare department forms
Clipboards	Patient education materials
Computer supplies	Pens, pencils, erasers
Copy and facsimile (fax) machine papers	Prescription pads
File folders, coding tabs	Rubber bands, paper clips
HIPAA forms (Notice of Privacy Practices, authorization forms, disclosure logs, request to inspect/copy medical records forms, request for amendment forms, acknowledgment of request for amendment forms)	Registration forms
	Social Security forms
	Stamps
History and physical examination sheets/cards	Stationery, appointment cards, bookkeeping supplies (ledgers, statements, billing forms), letterhead, second sheets, envelopes, business cards, notebooks, notepads, telephone memo pads
Insurance forms, disability, HMO and other third-party payers, life insurance examination forms, VA and W/C forms	

Clinical Supplies

Alcohol swabs	Safety pins
Applicators	Silver nitrate sticks
Bandaging materials: adhesive tape, gauze pads, gauze sponges, elastic bandages, adhesive bandages, roller bandages (gauze and elastic)	Suture removal kits
	Sutures
Cloth or paper gowns and drapes	Examination table covers
Cotton, cotton swabs	Tongue depressors
Culture tubes	Topical skin freeze
50% dextrose solution	Urinalysis test strips
Disposable sheaths for thermometers	Urine containers (sterile and nonsterile)
Disposable tips for otoscopes	Injectable medications: diazepam (Valium), diphenhydramine hydrochloride (Benadryl), epinephrine (Adrenaline), furosemide (Lasix), isoproterenol (Isuprel), lidocaine (Xylocaine: 1%, 2%, and plain), meperidine hydrochloride (Demerol), morphine, phenobarbital, sodium bicarbonate, sterile saline, sterile water
Gloves: sterile and nonsterile examination	
Hemoccult test kits	
Iodine or Betadine pads	
Lancets	
Lubricating jelly	Other medications, chemicals, solutions, ointments, lotions, and disinfectants, as needed
Microscope slides and fixative	
Needles, syringes	
Nitroglycerine tablets	

General Supplies

Liquid hypoallergenic soap	Tampons and sanitary pads
Paper cups	Tissues: facial and toilet
Paper towels	

order, such as a printed form. Special orders take time to obtain, so they must be ordered well before supplies run low.

Incidental Supplies These supplies are needed in the office but do not threaten the office's efficiency if the supply runs low. Incidental supplies include staples and rubber bands, which can be purchased at a local stationery store.

Periodic Supplies These supplies require ordering only occasionally. For example, if your office uses appointment books, you will order them only once or twice a year, probably in small numbers. The urgency of ordering some periodic items can depend on the size of the office. A multiphysician office, for example, would require more copy paper than a single-physician office. Another example of a periodic item might be holiday cards to send to the physician's colleagues and patients.

Storing Office Supplies

Storing office supplies requires good organizational skills and attention to detail. Many people in an office use these supplies, so the items should be stored neatly and in an orderly way. In addition, it is important to store supplies safely to prevent loss or theft, damage, or deterioration.

Location In a small medical office, supplies are generally kept near the areas where they are used. For example, administrative supplies are usually stored behind or adjacent to the reception area, while clinical supplies are stored near the examination rooms. If the practice has a laboratory, pertinent supplies are stored in or near the laboratory. Offices with separate supply rooms offer more storage space.

Small medical offices may not have ample storage space, so it may be tempting to store boxes on the floor behind the air-conditioning unit, stacked up close to the ceiling, or in potentially hazardous locations, such as near a heat source. However, it is essential that supplies be stored according to the guidelines described by The Joint Commission (TJC).

Items may not be stored on the floor; instead, they must be raised off the floor, as on a crate or shelf, to avoid contamination by water. Items stored close to the ceiling are considered a fire hazard. TJC standards require that supplies stored on the top shelf of a closet or storage area be at least 18 inches below the ceiling.

Avoid storing any boxes or supplies near a water heater, air-conditioning unit, heater, or stove. Many expendable items and their packaging are combustible and can quickly become a fire hazard. Air-conditioning units may drip water on the floor. If boxes of expensive forms are stored nearby, they can quickly become ruined as water seeps unnoticed into the packaging.

Storage Cabinets Each storage cabinet should be labeled with a list of its contents. Keep all stock of one item together.

Finding supplies is easier if you keep small items at eye level. Put large, bulky goods, like reams of stationery, on lower shelves. Label boxes and containers clearly so that all employees can readily find what they need and so that the inventory process is easier.

As you initially arrange items on storage shelves, label the shelves. Reserve enough space to completely stock each item. Do not put anything but the appropriate item in each

designated space. This easy system allows for a quick review when you reorder supplies, particularly if your office is using a manual inventory system.

To reduce the risk of errors on reorders, keep each item's original label attached to it. Cover the label with clear tape, if necessary. If you must replace a worn label, do it immediately when needed, making sure the new label has the same detailed information as the old one. Bottles with pouring spouts should be labeled on the side opposite the spout to prevent the liquid from dripping onto the label. Use a laundry marking pen to label linens with the name of your office. Linen services usually premark linens with the name of the company or the practice.

Many items have a shelf life after which they are no longer usable. By not overordering and by rotating supplies—using older ones first—your office will be able to use items during their shelf life. This is true not only for perishable items like medications but also for linens and paper, which can deteriorate.

Store all items based on their expiration date, so always check the dates on new items as well as those already in inventory. The oldest items should be stored in the front and the newer items stored in the rear of the cabinet. Be sure to rotate the inventory every time you add new stock, placing items with the longest expiration date at the back of the shelf. Because items can sometimes expire before they are used, be sure to check every item for the expiration date before use. Discard all expired items carefully and appropriately according to TJC and OSHA standards.

Administrative Supplies In addition to such expendable items as pens, pencils, and paper clips, paper products are important to a medical office. In general, paper products should be stored flat in their original boxes or wrappings to prevent pages from bending or curling. Information booklets may be stored upright to save space. Envelopes and other paper goods with gummed surfaces must be kept dry to prevent them from sticking together.

Clinical Supplies The rules of good housekeeping and asepsis creating the germ-free environment discussed in the *Infection Control Fundamentals* chapter apply not only to the daily office environment that is visible to patients, physicians, and office staff, but also to storage areas for clinical supplies. These areas must be kept clean and protected from damage and exposure to the elements.

All dressings and most bandaging materials must be kept sterile, including gauze that may be used to bandage an open wound. Elastic rolled bandages, which do not touch open wounds, must be clean but not necessarily sterile.

Chemicals, drugs, and solutions should be kept in a cool, dark place because light and heat cause some substances to deteriorate. Refer to the Safety Data Sheet (SDS) provided by each manufacturer for proper storage instructions. The importance of SDS is discussed in detail in the *Infection Control Fundamentals* chapter, but here are some basic guidelines:

- Store all liquids in their original containers. Line cabinets with plastic-coated shelf paper and wipe it frequently with a damp cloth. Do not store liquids above dry supplies.

- Store all poisons and narcotics separately from each other and from all other products.

- Narcotics must be stored securely out of sight in a locked cabinet.

- Never store strong acids near alkaline solutions or flammable items near sources of heat. Solutions that will be stored for a considerable length of time should have a small amount of space at the top of the bottle to allow for heat expansion.

- Some liquids should be stored in the refrigerator.

- Again, check each item for specific storage instructions. If storage space is limited, consider eliminating some items—especially bulky ones that are rarely used or items that a patient can purchase at surgical supply stores.

- Clinical refrigerators may be needed to store certain clinical supplies that require refrigeration. Never store food items and clinical items in the same refrigerator. A clinical refrigerator must be kept at a constant temperature to properly maintain the chemical integrity of lab supplies. Monitoring and recording the date and temperature of the clinical refrigerator should be completed once a week or per office protocol. Refer to each SDS for storage details on each substance.

▶ Taking a Supply Inventory   LO 8.12

As you discovered earlier, the responsibility of maintaining office supplies often falls to the medical assistant. It is a job that requires careful planning, attention to detail, and basic math skills. Accurate inventory activity ensures that the office never runs out of much-needed supplies.

Understanding Your Responsibilities

Generally, you will be responsible for overseeing the flow of supplies bought and used, calculating the budget for supplies, selecting supplies and vendors, following correct purchasing and payment procedures, and storing the goods properly.

All efficient offices will have a process for everyone within the practice to record their supply needs. The process may be as simple as a notebook stored at the front desk or a supply list positioned in a key location. As a supply need in the office is noted, it can be recorded on the supply list by anyone for the next order. Then, the medical assistant who is compiling the order should check all the inventory cards, reorder reminder cards, and supply lists, if using a manual system, before ordering.

If a computerized system is used, you will check the computerized sheet for usage as well as the office "wish list" before ordering supplies that are either low or needed but not currently purchased regularly for the office.

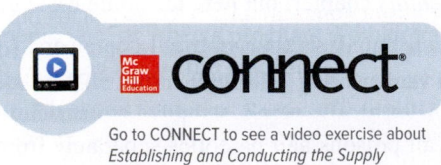

Go to CONNECT to see a video exercise about *Establishing and Conducting the Supply Inventory and Receiving Supplies.*

The Inventory Filing System

To oversee the flow of inventory efficiently, you will need a filing system. See Procedure 8-5 at the end of this chapter for a step-by-step overview of a manual inventory process. For computerized systems, the process will vary depending upon the system you are using, but the basic concept remains the same. The manual system consists of several elements:

- The list of supplies (discussed earlier in the chapter)
- An itemized inventory
- An inventory card or record page for each item
- A list of the names and addresses of current vendors
- A file of current catalogs from vendors (including some vendors not currently used, for comparison shopping)
- A wish list of brands or items that the office does not currently use but may want to try in the future
- Files for *invoices,* or bills from vendors, and completed order forms
- Reorder reminder cards to indicate when an in-stock item should be reordered
- Color-coded, removable, self-adhesive flags to indicate "Need to Order" or "On Order"
- An inventory and ordering schedule
- Order forms for each vendor (may be multicopy forms, fax forms, electronic forms, or e-mail forms)

The Inventory Card or Record Page The inventory card or record page for each item or category of items may be a 4 × 6 inch index card, a page in a loose-leaf binder, or a spreadsheet stored in the computer system (Figure 8-17). These methods make it easy to group together the items that need to be ordered at any given time. Records help you monitor how quickly items are used and how much should be ordered each time.

Of course, some information may change. As you become more proficient at monitoring inventory or as the practice grows or diminishes in size, you may find that quantities, vendors, or reorder quantities need to be adjusted. With the help of the doctor or office manager, you will be able to determine the ideal quantity of each item to have on hand, depending on the size of the practice, the available storage space, and the ordering schedule.

Be sure to check the storage areas regularly, preferably at specific times, and to count the items on hand. When the supply of an item begins to run low, you (or another staff member) should flag the inventory card or record page to indicate the need to reorder it at the next regular ordering time.

Color-coded, removable, self-adhesive flags on the inventory card or record page are an efficient way to track inventory. A red flag, for example, might indicate that a supply needs to be ordered. A yellow flag might be substituted when the item has been ordered.

Reorder Reminder Cards Reorder reminder cards (Figure 8-18) are usually brightly colored cards inserted directly into stock on the supply shelf to indicate when it is time to reorder an item. For example, if you have determined that four boxes of staples is a sufficient quantity to keep on hand and

(ITEM NAME) _Exam Table Paper 21"_

ORDER QUANTITY _____12_____   REORDER POINT _____4_____

ORDER	QTY	REC'D	UNIT COST	PRICE	PREPAID	ON ACCT.	ORDER	QTY	REC'D	UNIT COST	PRICE	PREPAID	ON ACCT.
1/4	12	1/8	$12.25	$147.00	Check 1214	X							
2/5	12	2/9	$12.25	$147.00	Check 2110	X							

INVENTORY COUNT

	JAN.	FEB.	MAR.	APR.	MAY	JUNE	JULY	AUG.	SEPT.	OCT.	NOV.	DEC.
DATE _____	7	10										
DATE _____												

ORDER SOURCE   UNIT PRICE

Smith Physician's Supply Co. _____   12 - $147.00 _____

493 Carlton Avenue _____   36 - $441.00 _____

South Union, NJ 07422 _____   _____

908-899-6123   Contact: Martin Kohn _____   _____

FIGURE 8-17 An inventory card may be manually created or computer generated.

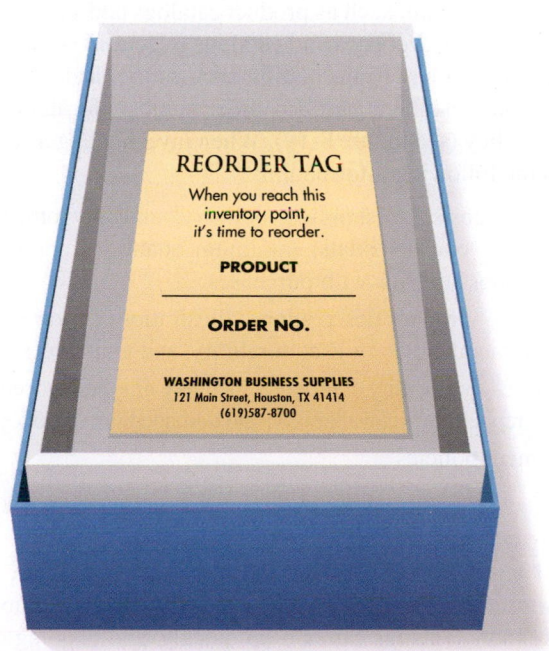

REORDER TAG

When you reach this
inventory point,
it's time to reorder.

PRODUCT
_____

ORDER NO.
_____

WASHINGTON BUSINESS SUPPLIES
121 Main Street, Houston, TX 41414
(619)587-8700

FIGURE 8-18 Reorder reminder cards are typically brightly colored cards inserted within the current supply stock, reminding you when it is time to reorder the item.

your office supply orders are filled in 2 business days, you might place the reorder reminder card between the third and fourth boxes of staples. The reorder quantity on the inventory card or record page for staples would indicate "four boxes."

The reorder reminder cards also remind other staff members to tell you when an item is in short supply. In some offices, the medical assistant labels the reminder card with the supply item's name and bar code number, such as "staples 002345." This method allows any staff member to pull the card when the last box of staples before the reminder card is taken from the supply shelf. The staff member can then place the card in a "To Be Ordered" envelope. Some offices can reorder simply by scanning the bar code. Staff members in some offices request supplies by writing them in an order book or on an order list.

Scheduling Inventory and Ordering

Establish a regular schedule for counting the office supplies, such as taking inventory every 1 or 2 weeks. Estimating when you will probably need to reorder a particular item—and putting that date on your calendar or in your appointment book—is also helpful. You and the physician can determine how often storage areas should be checked.

Established Ordering Times You should have established ordering times, such as the same day each week or month, after inventory is taken. For example, you might take inventory the first Tuesday of every month and order supplies the first Thursday of every month.

A regular schedule for taking inventory and ordering helps all staff members remember when they must give their requests to you. Although you may need to adjust the ordering time occasionally, try to stick to the schedule to avoid the expense and inconvenience of rush orders.

When to Order Ahead of Schedule When you take inventory and the spare supply of an item has not been reached but is close to the placement of the reorder reminder card, you must decide whether you should reorder then or wait until the next regular ordering time. You will probably find it is more efficient to go ahead and order rather than wait. Ordering early assures you that the supply will not be depleted before the next regular ordering time. Make sure you consider your storage capacity, as this could limit your purchases.

Ordering ahead of schedule can be especially important if there is a large demand for a particular product and manufacturers' production levels have not caught up with that demand. This situation can occur if there has been an outbreak of a particular flu or virus, or if the Food and Drug Administration has determined that a certain product is harmful, resulting in higher demand for an alternative product.

Unanticipated Shortage of a Supply Item If the supply of an item reaches the reorder reminder card, and there is still a long time before the next regular ordering time, place the order immediately so that you do not risk running out of the item.

To help you oversee inventory effectively, finish one container before opening a new one. Keep all stock of the same item in one place, as the need to count inventory of an item in more than one location or container increases the likelihood of errors. If an item is kept in more than one location, as in the case of multiple exam rooms, inventory is best maintained per room.

As a medical assistant, you want to be sure that there are always sufficient quantities of supplies to keep the office running efficiently. It is unwise to stock spare supplies in too great a quantity, however, because the administrative budget is not likely to support such expenditures. In addition, spare quantities of supplies can be a storage problem.

▶ Ordering Supplies   LO 8.13

Ordering supplies requires a procedure to deal with vendors and to order and check supplies. You can avoid common purchasing mistakes by understanding the most efficient way to order supplies for your office.

Locating and Evaluating Supply Vendors

A vendor will most likely already be in place when you join a practice. You should, however, be aware of competitors' prices, services, and other incentives intended to attract your office as a customer. Sometimes the incentives, such as bonus supplies with certain purchases, can represent sizable savings. Remember also that your time has a dollar value to the practice and services that save you time are worth comparing when evaluating vendors.

Obtaining recommendations from other medical offices is a good way to locate reputable office-supply dealers who sell items at reasonable prices. Reputable vendors fulfill orders accurately with quality items, deliver products in good condition, and charge fair prices. Keep in mind when evaluating vendors that the physician may have preferences for certain trade names or vendors.

Gathering Competitive Prices The costs of maintaining a medical practice are continually rising. Saving money on supplies through careful purchasing strategies is one way to help your physician/employer reduce spending. The medical assistant is often largely responsible for comparison pricing, ordering, and establishing and maintaining relationships with vendors. Your awareness of the most up-to-date information about vendors and supplies is valuable to your physician/employer. Discuss prices with the physician, who in turn may want to discuss them with an accountant.

Setting Up a Supply Budget The average medical practice spends 4% to 6% of its annual gross income on administrative, clinical, and general supplies. If an office is spending more than 6%, it may be time to reevaluate the office spending practices. Remember, though, that any budget is only a guide. A budget is meant to serve your office, not the reverse. You and your physician/employer may need to adjust the supply budget based on prices and discounts available from vendors.

Comparing Vendors To collect competitive data from vendors, check their website or contact them by telephone or in writing to request catalogs and other forms of product information. If you are not in charge of routing mail, make sure that supply-related mail, such as product catalogs and sale notices, is routed to you. Websites and catalogs (electronic or printed) usually include basic information such as the dealer's name, address, and telephone number; order numbers for items; and vendor policy (see Figure 8-19). When investigating a vendor, obtain the following information:

- Prices—costs for supplies, delivery, and any other services; special discounts; minimum quantities applicable; and bonus supplies with purchases
- Quality—product descriptions, illustrations, trade names, recommendations for use, durability, and guarantees
- Service—availability of products, delivery time and procedures, sales representative availability, and damaged goods policy
- Payment policies

Competitive Pricing and Quality

Part of your responsibility in managing office supplies is to stay informed about the pricing and quality of competitors to your vendors. Savings can add up quickly, and ongoing comparison pricing can save the practice hundreds of dollars a year.

Unit Pricing Because many medical items come in a variety of package sizes, you need to be aware of how much the

ORDERING INFORMATION

BY PHONE

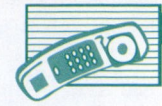

Call our toll-free number: (800) BIBBERO (800-242-2376) Monday through Friday, 6:00 a.m. – 5:00 p.m. (PT)

BY WEB

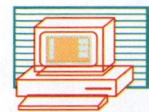

www.bibbero.com

BY MAIL

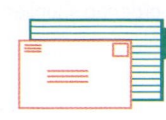

Complete order form and mail to: Bibbero Systems, Inc. 1300 N. McDowell Blvd. Petaluma, CA 94954-1180

BY FAX

Complete enclosed order form and transmit via fax to: (800) 242-9330. Our fax line is open 24 hours a day.

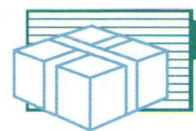

SHIPPING POLICY

Most in-stock items normally ship the same day (exclusive of file cabinets, file storage, office accessories and furnishings).

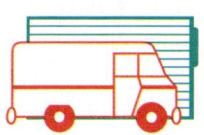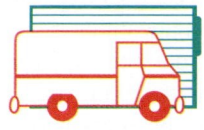

FREE DELIVERY

Free delivery on pre-paid orders totaling $300.00 or more, shipping within the Continental US.

BIBBero **SYSTEMS, INC.®**

Thank you for reviewing our catalog. We are confident that you will be pleased with both our products and our service. If you are in a hurry for product or samples, CALL us toll-free at (800) BIBBERO, FAX us at (800) 242-9330, or visit our website. Our Customer Service Department is always happy to assist you.

If ordering by mail or fax, fill out the enclosed order form located at the back of this catalog. Either return it in the enclosed postage-paid envelope or fax it to us.

For items requiring custom imprinting, please include the following information, either typed or hand printed: name, specialty, address, city/state/zip, telephone number, and state license number (when required).

Don't see what you are looking for in our catalog? Submit a sample or provide specifications for any folder, divider, patient registration form, clinical form, health history questionnaire, etc., and we will promptly provide you with a quote. We can print single or multiple part forms, custom imprint folders, and manufacture a wide range of chart dividers.

Please Note: All custom printed orders are subject to an overrun or underrun variance of 10%.

Most orders for in-stock items received by 2:00 p.m. (PT) are normally shipped the same day (excluding cabinets, file storage, office accessories and furnishings). Out-of-stock items are automatically backordered. Personalized stationery items normally ship in 5–7 working days, after proof approval. Custom printed orders normally leave our plant within 7–10 working days, after proof approval. If certain items require an extended ship time, such as those listed above, delivery time will be quoted when order is received.

Custom printing or personalization on a rush basis is available on most products for an additional charge.

Some combined stock and custom printed items can be shipped together if requested in advance. All orders are shipped via the most economical, expeditious method to your locale. Items ordered together may not ship from the same locations or be received at the same time.

Common carriers are used for large volume orders. Overnight, 2nd and 3rd Day delivery services are available upon request.

All orders prepaid by check, Visa, MasterCard or American Express totaling $300.00 or more will be shipped freight free via surface transport within the Continental US. This offer excludes file cabinets, file storage, office accessories and furnishings and special order items. We regret that the high cost of shipping outside the contiguous 48 states prohibits us from extending our freight free policy; however, we will use the most economical shipping methods available to your location.

TERMS

Full payment is due upon receipt of merchandise. Accounts are considered overdue after thirty (30) days and are subject to a 1% monthly service charge. A service charge of $10.00 will be applied to all returned checks. For information regarding special financial arrangements, please contact our Credit Department at (800) 242-2376.

GUARANTEE!

Your satisfaction Guaranteed!

We guarantee our stock products. If you wish to return something, call to obtain a return authorization number and return shipment instructions. Most of our stock items can be returned within 60 days of purchase for full credit, exchange or a refund of your purchase price, with prior return authorization. After 60 days, your return is subject to a 20% restocking charge. Call our Customer Service Department at (800) 242-2376 for your return authorization number. Dymo® Products can be returned within 30 days of receipt with prior return authorization. Opened or unpackaged items are subject to a 15% or $15.00 restocking charge, whichever is greater. For disposable products located in our Clinical Supplies section, opened packages are subject to a 15% restocking charge with prior return authorization. Personalized items, custom printed items, custom manufactured or special order items, file cabinets, high density filing systems and opened and unlocked software are not returnable.

Items damaged in transit will be replaced as quickly as possible. Note any visible damage to the cartons on the bill of lading or delivery receipt and keep the original packaging in case items within are damaged.

Please Note: Self-adhesive products have a limited shelf life. Store in a cool, dry place.

Please Note: All custom printed orders are subject to an overrun or underrun variance of 10%.

We accept Visa, MasterCard and American Express for all your purchases.

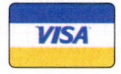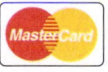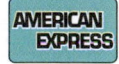

FIGURE 8-19 Examine supply catalogs and websites closely to obtain the best value for the office.
Reprinted with permission from Bibbero Systems, Inc., An InHealth Company, Petaluma, CA (800) 242-2376, www.bibbero.com.

office is actually paying per item. To calculate an item's unit price, divide the total price of the package by the quantity, or number, of items. For example, if a package of 12 pens costs $12, the unit price, or price per pen, is $1 ($12 divided by 12 pens). If another vendor provides the same type of pen in a package of 18 for $17.10, the unit price is 95 cents ($17.10 divided by 18 pens). The second set of pens is the better buy.

Unit prices are generally lower at larger quantities. So it makes sense to place one large order for a nonperishable item to cover the office until the next ordering time. Generally, however, you should not order more than a year's supply of any one item, particularly if the item is custom printed. Addresses, insurance codes, or additions to medical staff can change. When placing quantity discount orders, always consider the following factors:

- Whether the supply can be used within a reasonable time
- The possibility of spoilage or deterioration
- The amount of storage space in the office
- Whether the doctor will continue to use the item

Avoid overspending by not ordering more of an item than is reasonable or necessary.

Rush Orders Unexpected rush orders usually cost the office more money than regularly scheduled orders. (In some cases, a vendor may not charge extra to a steady customer, but these cases would be exceptions.) To avoid rush orders, be aware of approximately how long the vendor takes to deliver an order. You can obtain this information from the vendor policy and by keeping accurate records of your own experience with deliveries.

Mail-Order Companies Using large, established mail-order companies often saves money for the medical office, but there may be less control over orders and a greater potential for hidden costs. The neighborhood pharmacy may also offer discounts, but ordering from wholesalers or directly from the manufacturer is usually more economical. See the *Points on Practice* feature for helpful information about cost-efficient ordering by telephone, by fax, or through an online service.

Purchasing Groups Purchasing groups are groups of practices that order supplies together to obtain a quantity discount. For example, several medical offices associated with a nearby hospital may order through the hospital. In return for this convenience, the physicians pay dues and guarantee the vendors a certain amount of business. Some programs require members to spend a certain percentage of their supply budget through the group. Groups also may require that members not disclose the group's prices to other physicians. Large medical practices that participate in these groups usually save an average of 20% on supplies. The savings are not usually significant for small offices.

Group Buying Pools If a medical office wants to use local vendors instead of, or in addition to, a purchasing group or if it is too small to benefit from a purchasing group, it can still pool resources with other area offices to qualify for quantity discounts. Even if the offices are ordering different items, discounts are based on the total order and savings can range from 10% to 20%. Under this arrangement, the offices must usually take responsibility for distributing the items among

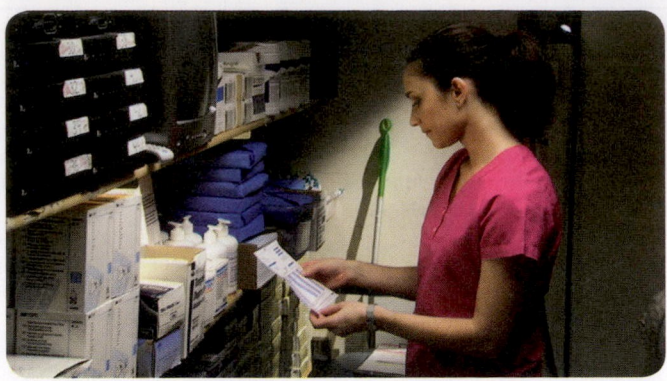

FIGURE 8-20 Jointly ordering supplies with other practices can cut down on costs for everyone.
© McGraw-Hill Education

themselves. A buying pool is convenient for medical practices that are in the same building or office complex (Figure 8-20).

Cost Controls Medical practices are increasingly interested in saving money and controlling costs in general. Physician reimbursement is constantly being reevaluated. As a result, more than ever, physicians are interested in controlling the operating costs of their practices. Managing expenses within the practice is a very important responsibility for the medical assistant. What may seem to be just a small reduction in cost to the practice can actually result in a substantial reduction to office expenses over the course of a year. As a medical assistant, it is your job to constantly look for ways to reduce costs within the practice without sacrificing quality.

Benefits of Using Local Vendors

There are many potential vendors, including local dealers, mail-order companies, and nearby pharmacies. Try to establish good credit and business relationships with reputable local vendors. Although these companies usually charge a little more than mail-order companies, spending most of the office's supply budget through one favored local dealer often results in discounts, special service in the event of an emergency, and information about upcoming sales and specials. Local dealers also may offer more personal assistance—perhaps even a salesperson's help with taking inventory—to compete with larger vendors whose business is based primarily on catalog sales. The extra service may be worth the higher cost.

Buying from local vendors also can provide a public relations benefit for physicians; it means keeping business in the community. However, specialty items may need to be ordered from other vendors. For example, letterhead should be ordered from a reliable printer, whether that printer is located in the community or out of state.

Payment Schedules

Another factor that affects the cost of supplies is the payment schedule. Many vendors do not charge for handling if an order is prepaid. Others offer a discount for enclosing a check with an order. Some delay billing for 30 to 90 days, allowing the practice to keep the money in the bank, collecting interest for a longer period.

Ordering by Telephone, Fax, or Online

You may occasionally purchase office supplies at a local office supply store, but usually you will order them without even leaving your office. Three common ways to do so are by telephone, by fax machine, and through an online service. The following tips are included to help you make sure that every order—no matter which option you choose—is successfully placed.

Ordering by Telephone

1. Clear communication is a must when ordering by telephone. Speak slowly and enunciate your words carefully to make sure you are understood. It is also a good idea to spell each word of the practice name and the address to ensure proper delivery. Use expressions like "S as in Sam, P as in people" to clarify your spelling.

2. Ask the representative taking your order to repeat the order. Check that every item is included with the appropriate price, quantity, style, and color.

3. Confirm the expected delivery date so that you will know if something is late. Also confirm how payment will be made, to prevent unexpected delays.

4. Record the name and telephone number of the person who takes the order in case there is a problem with the order. Get an order number (or confirmation number) in case you have to call back with a question or a change in your order.

5. If possible, avoid placing telephone orders on Mondays and Fridays, when call volume is typically high.

Ordering by Fax

1. When ordering by fax, use the form provided by the vendor if one is available. This form uses the format to which the supply company is accustomed and will speed your order's processing.

2. Type your order, or write it neatly and legibly, to prevent miscommunication. Fill out the form completely. Make sure you indicate quantities, descriptions, and prices (including shipping) for each item you order.

3. Proofread your order before you send it. Checking the accuracy of the order now will save time later.

4. Follow up by telephone to make sure your order was received and understood, and to confirm the delivery date and payment requirements.

Ordering Online

1. Ordering online requires a computer and a modem connection to the Internet or to an online service. Before ordering online, make sure you are fully familiar with the equipment and the process, or have your supervisor or the supply company's sales representative oversee your initial orders.

2. Type your name and address accurately.

3. If pictures of supplies are not available online, consult the company's printed catalog or CD-ROM catalog. If you do not have access to a catalog, read the online text descriptions carefully, checking trade names and specifications, to select the appropriate merchandise (Figure 8-21). If you have questions, call the supply company.

4. When you have completed the selections, the online service will display your order for you to confirm. Check that all the information is accurate, including your name, address, and telephone number.

5. If you have an account with the company, you may type in your account number to place the order. Otherwise, you may wish to arrange to make payment on delivery. If you prefer to pay by credit card, first make sure that the company is reputable and that it uses a security system that prevents your number from being read by anyone unauthorized to do so.

If, despite your best efforts, your order is processed incorrectly, take appropriate action immediately. Although ordering by telephone, by fax, or online is convenient, it still requires additional time to package items that must be returned.

By law, orders that you place must be fulfilled within a reasonable time. The Federal Trade Commission (FTC) monitors purchases by telephone, fax, and online services to protect consumers. The FTC requires supply companies to provide merchandise within 30 days or to give you the option of canceling the order and receiving a full refund.

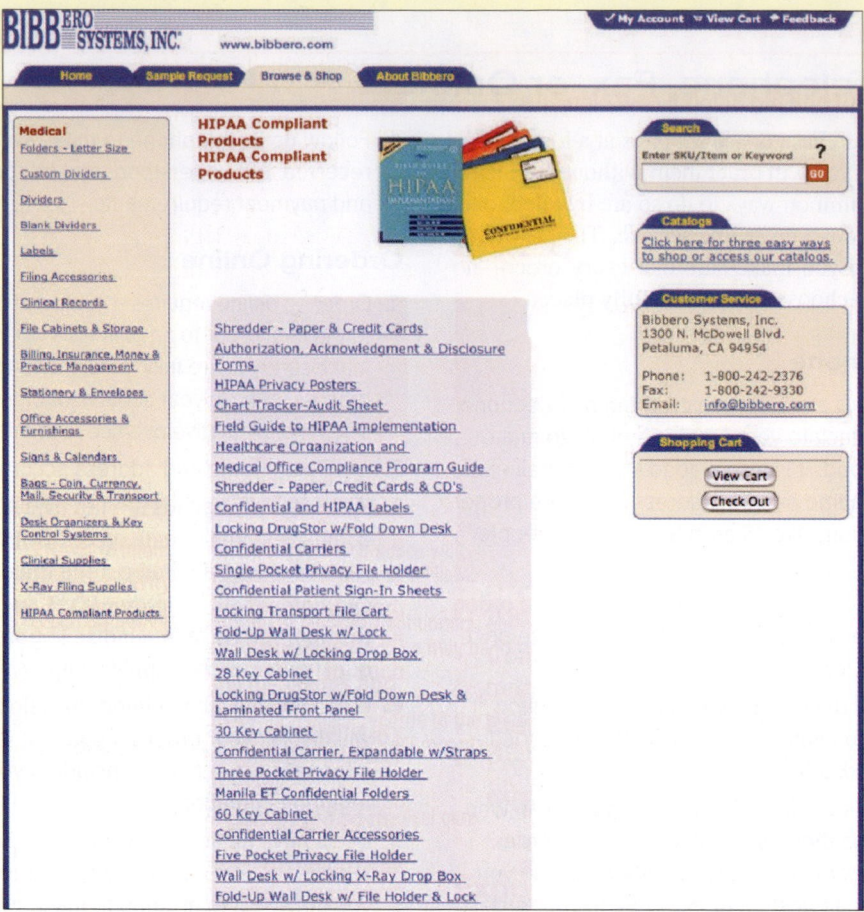

FIGURE 8-21 Read online information just as carefully as you read a printed catalog.
Reprinted with permission from Bibbero Systems, Inc., An InHealth Company, Petaluma, CA (800) 242–2376, www.bibbero.com.

The vendor's invoice usually describes payment terms. Two examples of payment terms are

- "Net 30": This means you have 30 days in which to pay the total amount.
- "1% 10 Days Net 30": This means that you will get a savings of 1% of the total price by paying within 10 days.

Copies of all bills and order forms for supplies should be kept on file for at least 7 years in case the practice is audited by the Internal Revenue Service (IRS).

Ordering Procedures

Ordering procedures for supplies vary from office to office but always involve these tasks: completing paperwork, checking orders received, correcting errors in shipments, and making payment.

Order Forms Before ordering merchandise, you should inquire about a vendor's ordering options, discuss them with the physician or practice manager, and determine which method is best for the office. Many vendors now have ordering capability through telephone, fax, e-mail, and online as well as traditional written order forms. Always be sure to keep a copy of each order you submit.

Before you place an order, gather all the necessary information, such as correct names of items, item numbers, and order and account numbers. This information helps to ensure the order's accuracy. Immediately after placing the order, note all order information on the inventory card or record page for that item.

Purchase Requisitions You will need to follow any special ordering procedures established in your medical office. The specific procedures and the medical assistant's level of authority vary from one office to another. Sometimes placing an order requires a **requisition** (a formal request from a staff member or doctor), which is given to the medical assistant who does the actual ordering. The physician's or practice manager's approval may be necessary for large purchases—for example, for orders that total more than $300. Recurring orders may not require the doctor's approval, but you may need to get approval before ordering a new brand or quantities of a particular item over a certain amount.

In a group practice where physicians or licensed practitioners order different items and several staffers are in charge of ordering, procedures for ordering can be complicated. One common way to simplify matters is to use a **purchase order**—a form that authorizes a purchase for the practice. Figure 8-22 shows a sample purchase order. Purchase orders are usually preprinted with consecutive numbers. The medical assistant submits approved purchase orders to the vendor for fulfillment. This method is most often used for expensive items, such as office equipment, but some large practices also use purchase orders for supplies.

Checking Orders Received When the shipment of supplies arrives, record on the inventory card or record page the date received and the quantity of each item. Check the shipment against the order form to make sure the correct items—in the correct sizes, styles, packaging, and quantity—have been delivered.

Then check the contents against the packing slip (a description of the package contents) enclosed in the package. This checking takes time, but catching even one error is worth the time taken. If several people on a staff have ordering responsibility, they can share the task. The employee should write on the package slip the date items were received; check off each item as you verify and initial.

Correcting Errors Any errors in a shipment should be reported immediately to the vendor so that the records can be corrected, missing supplies can be delivered, or incorrect supply orders can be canceled. When you call to report errors, be sure you have all the paperwork in front of you. You will need the invoice number, order date, name of the person who placed the order, name of the person who took the order, and a list of questions or a description of the problem. If a catalog

was used in ordering, have it open to the appropriate page. Always record the name and title of the person you speak with when reporting the error.

Invoices Typically, the vendor sends an invoice to the medical office, either accompanying the merchandise or separately. This invoice also should be checked carefully against the original order and the packing slip. It is a good idea to staple the order list, packing list, and a copy of the invoice together for the office records to verify all items were received. See Figure 8-23. Be sure to check the arithmetic, too. Then sign or stamp the invoice to confirm that the order was received. If an item you order is temporarily out of stock, the vendor usually sends an invoice stamped "Back Ordered." Later, when the item is back in stock, the vendor will ship it to your office.

It is also a good habit to record the check number, date, and amount of payment on the invoice. You, the physician, or the practice manager may initial it. By keeping a copy of the paid invoice with the attached order slip and packing slip in the office records, it will be easy to track the items included within each invoice. This step makes verifying payments easier and decreases the chance of inadvertently paying an invoice twice.

Disbursements An invoice is paid with a **disbursement** (payment of funds) to a vendor. Disbursements may be made in cash or by business credit card, check, or money order.

PURCHASE ORDER #2532

Submitted by: _____
Order Number: _____
Date Ordered: _____
Date Required: _____

SHIP TO: BWW Medical Associates, PC
305 Main Street
Port Snead, YZ 12345-9876

PHONE: 555-654-3210

NO	ITEM	DESCRIPTION/MODEL	COLOR	SIZE	QUANTITY	PRICE EACH	TOTAL
1							
2							
3							
4							
5							
6							
7							
8							
						TOTAL	

Approved: _____   Date: _____

FIGURE 8-22 Typical purchase order form.

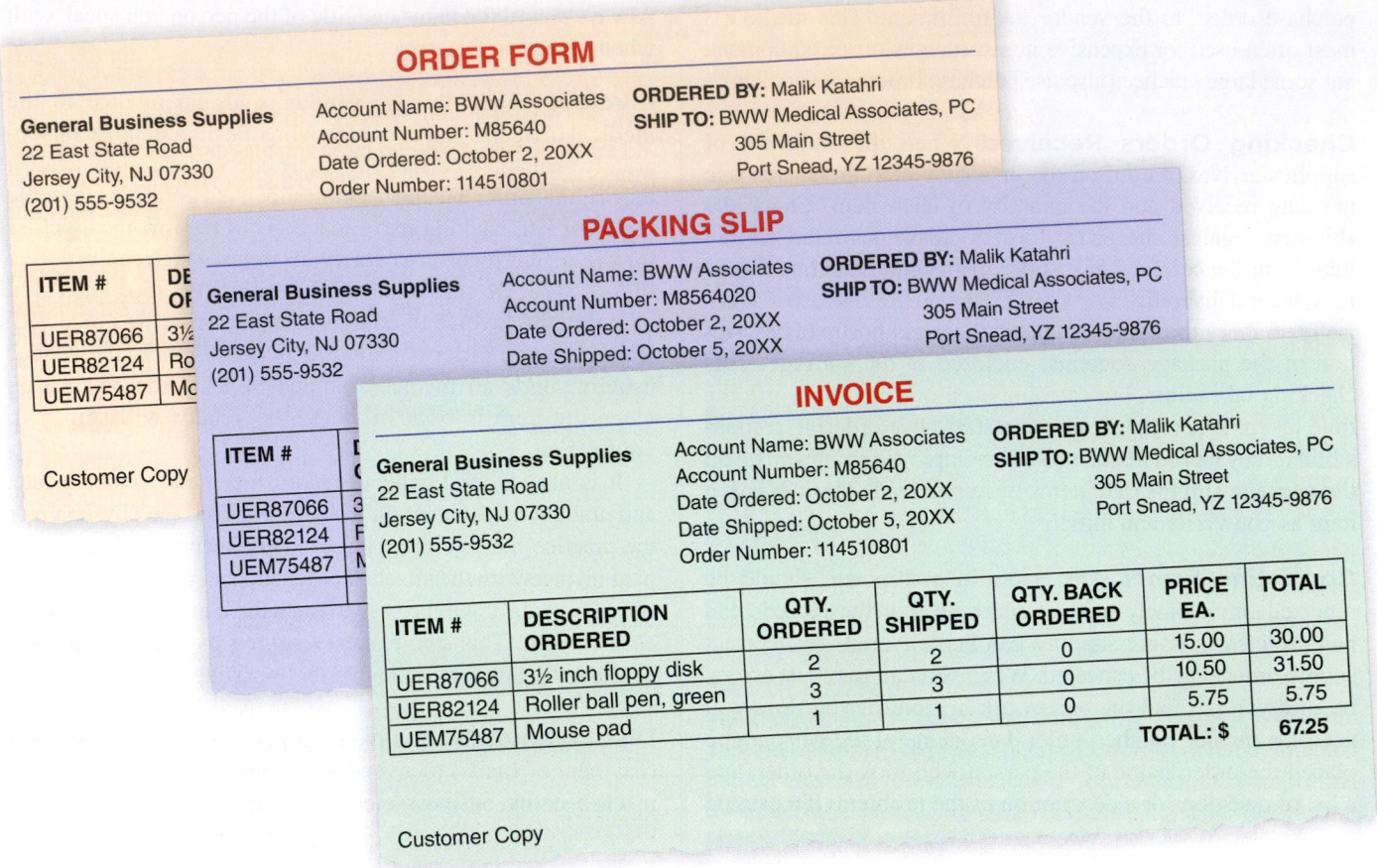

ORDER FORM

General Business Supplies
22 East State Road
Jersey City, NJ 07330
(201) 555-9532

Account Name: BWW Associates
Account Number: M85640
Date Ordered: October 2, 20XX
Order Number: 114510801

ORDERED BY: Malik Katahri
SHIP TO: BWW Medical Associates, PC
305 Main Street
Port Snead, YZ 12345-9876

ITEM #	DESCRIPTION ORDERED
UER87066	3½
UER82124	Ro
UEM75487	Mo

Customer Copy

PACKING SLIP

General Business Supplies
22 East State Road
Jersey City, NJ 07330
(201) 555-9532

Account Name: BWW Associates
Account Number: M8564020
Date Ordered: October 2, 20XX
Date Shipped: October 5, 20XX

ORDERED BY: Malik Katahri
SHIP TO: BWW Medical Associates, PC
305 Main Street
Port Snead, YZ 12345-9876

ITEM #	
UER87066	3
UER82124	R
UEM75487	M

INVOICE

General Business Supplies
22 East State Road
Jersey City, NJ 07330
(201) 555-9532

Account Name: BWW Associates
Account Number: M85640
Date Ordered: October 2, 20XX
Date Shipped: October 5, 20XX
Order Number: 114510801

ORDERED BY: Malik Katahri
SHIP TO: BWW Medical Associates, PC
305 Main Street
Port Snead, YZ 12345-9876

ITEM #	DESCRIPTION ORDERED	QTY. ORDERED	QTY. SHIPPED	QTY. BACK ORDERED	PRICE EA.	TOTAL
UER87066	3½ inch floppy disk	2	2	0	15.00	30.00
UER82124	Roller ball pen, green	3	3	0	10.50	31.50
UEM75487	Mouse pad	1	1	0	5.75	5.75
					TOTAL: $	67.25

Customer Copy

FIGURE 8-23   Check the original order form, the packing slip, and the invoice to verify that all items ordered were received.

Usually, you will write a check to the vendor and have the authorized individual sign it. Be sure to provide the original order, packing slip, and invoice. On the front of the check, record the invoice number. Finally, mail the check to the vendor with the vendor's copy of the invoice. File the office copy of the invoice, along with the original order and the packing slip, according to your inventory filing system.

On the rare occasion you make a cash disbursement, obtain a receipt to keep on file. If you are the one responsible for maintaining the practice's financial records and presenting them to the accountant, you also may be responsible for recording the payment information in the office's accounting books.

Avoiding Common Purchasing Mistakes

Even the most watchful professional can make purchasing mistakes. The best you can do is to educate yourself about common mistakes and try to avoid them. For example, be aware of the possibility of dishonest telephone or e-mail solicitations. The solicitor may claim to be a sales representative for the manufacturer of the office photocopier, offering bargains on paper or toner. It is typical, when a scam is involved, that advance payments will be required and you are instructed to send payment to a PO box, instead of to a physical address. Once you do, it is likely that the bargain will never be shipped to your office.

The best way to deal with these solicitations is to tell the caller that your office does not purchase supplies by telephone. If a telephone offer appears to be legitimate and to offer substantial savings, ask for the name and telephone number of the firm so that you can return the call at a more convenient time. This will give you time to verify the number with the telephone company and check the firm's name with the Better Business Bureau. If the solicitation is by e-mail, do not reply to the e-mail, but contact the company via its own website or by phone to verify the information.

Another disreputable tactic some vendors use is bait and switch, meaning the price of one item is lowered to attract the customer, but that item is always "sold out" and the customer is encouraged to buy a more expensive one. A vendor may also mislead you by raising the price of an item you have been ordering without informing you. Always confirm the current price, check invoices as they come in, and record everything in the item's file. Having your inventory card or record page open while ordering will prompt you to notice and question price changes. If there is an honest error, a reputable firm will readily and courteously correct it.

Problems also can be avoided by carefully supervising a new vendor's sales representative until a comfortable, professional rapport has been established. Discuss your inventory system with representatives, and ask them questions about their procedures.

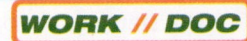

Procedure Goal: To correctly prepare and send a fax document, while following all HIPAA guidelines to guard patient confidentiality

OSHA Guidelines: This procedure does not involve exposure to blood, body fluids, or tissue.

Materials: Fax machine, fax line, cover sheet with statement of disclaimer, area code and phone number of fax recipient, document to be faxed, telephone line, and telephone

Method:

1. Prepare a *cover sheet,* which provides information about the transmission. Cover sheets can vary in appearance but usually include the name, telephone number, and fax number of the sender and the receiver; the number of pages being transmitted; and the date of the transmission. Preprinted cover sheets also can be used.
   RATIONALE: *The fax should clearly identify where it originated and to whom it is being sent. If another recipient receives the fax in error, he will know whom to notify regarding the error.*

2. All cover sheets must carry a disclaimer statement to guard the patient's privacy. A *disclaimer* is a statement of denial of legal liability. A disclaimer should be included on the cover sheet and may read something like this:

   > *This fax contains confidential or proprietary information that may be legally privileged. It is intended only for the named recipient(s). If an addressing or transmission error has misdirected the fax, please notify the author by replying to this message. If you are not the named recipient, you are not authorized to use, disclose, distribute, copy, print, or rely on this fax and should immediately shred it.*

   RATIONALE: *This step helps guard the patient's privacy.*

3. Place all pages of the document, including the cover sheet, either facedown or faceup in the fax machine's sending tray, depending on the directions stamped on the sending tray.

4. If the pages are placed facedown, write the area code and fax number on the back of the last page.

5. Dial the receiving fax machine's telephone number using either the telephone attached to the fax machine or the numbers on the fax keyboard. Include the area code for long-distance calls.

6. When using a fax telephone, listen for a high-pitched tone. Then press the "Send" or "Start" button and hang up the telephone. This step completes the call circuit in older-model fax machines. Your fax is now being sent. Newer fax machines do not require this step.
   RATIONALE: *This step completes the call circuit in older-model fax machines.*

7. If you use the fax keyboard, press the "Send" or "Start" button after dialing the telephone number. This button will start the call.

8. Watch for the fax machine to make a connection. Often a green light appears as the document feeds through the machine.

9. If the fax machine is not able to make a connection, as when the receiving fax line is busy, it may have a feature that automatically redials the number every few minutes for a specified number of attempts.

10. When a fax has been successfully sent, most fax machines print a confirmation message. When a fax has not been sent, the machine either prints an error message or indicates on the screen that the transmission was unsuccessful.
    RATIONALE: *This message confirms to the sender that the fax has been sent or indicates that the fax needs to be sent again.*

11. Attach the confirmation or error message to the documents faxed. File appropriately.
    RATIONALE: *This step ensures thorough documentation related to the fax.*

12. If required by office policy, the sender should call the recipient to confirm the fax was received.

PROCEDURE 8-2 Using a Photocopier Machine

Procedure Goal: To produce copies of documents

OSHA Guidelines: This procedure does not involve exposure to blood, body fluids, or tissue.

Materials: Copier machine, copy paper, and documents to be copied

Method:

1. Make sure the machine is turned on and warmed up. It will display a signal when it is ready for copying.

2. Assemble and prepare your materials, removing paper clips, staples, and self-adhesive flags.

RATIONALE: *This step helps avoid loose items getting caught in the copier and provides for optimum efficiency.*

3. Place the document to be copied in the automatic feeder tray as directed, or upside-down directly on the glass. The feeder tray can accommodate many pages; you may place only one page at a time on the glass. Automatic feeding is a faster process, and you should use it when you wish to collate or staple packets. Page-by-page copying is best if you need to copy a single sheet or to enlarge or reduce the image. To use any special features, such as making double-sided copies

or stapling the copies, press a designated button on the machine.

4. Set the machine for the desired paper size.
   RATIONALE: *The copier will select the paper size automatically if the size is not selected. This could result in a waste of paper.*

5. Key in the number of copies you want to make and press the "Start" button. The copies are made automatically.

6. Press the "Clear" or "Reset" button when your job is finished.
   RATIONALE: *The machine is now ready for the next user and will not perform unwanted functions on the next document.*

7. If the copier becomes jammed, follow the directions on the machine to locate the problem (for example, there may be multiple pieces of paper stuck inside the printer) and dislodge the jammed paper. Most copy machines will show a diagram of the printer and the location of the problem.

PROCEDURE 8-3 Using a Postage Meter

Procedure Goal: To correctly apply postage to an envelope or package for mailing, according to US Postal Service guidelines

OSHA Guidelines: This procedure does not involve exposure to blood, body fluids, or tissue.

Materials: Postage meter, addressed envelope or package, and postal scale

Method:

1. Check that there is postage available in the postage meter.
   RATIONALE: *For the postage meter to function, there must be money in your postal account. Contact the company that manages your account or your local post office for more information.*

2. Verify the day's date.
   RATIONALE: *US Postal Service guidelines prohibit mailing envelopes and packages that are postmarked with an incorrect date.*

3. Check that the postage meter is plugged in and switched on before you proceed.

4. Locate the area where the meter registers the date. Many machines have a lid that can be flipped up, with rows of numbers underneath. Months are represented numerically, with the number "1" indicating the month of January, "2" indicating February, and so on. Check that the date is correct. If it is incorrect, change the numbers to the correct date.

5. Make sure all materials have been included in the envelope or package. Weigh the envelope or package on a postal scale. Standard business envelopes weighing up to 1 oz require the minimum postage (the equivalent of

one first-class stamp). Oversize envelopes and packages require additional postage. A postal scale will indicate the required postage.

6. Key in the postage amount on the meter and press the button that enters the amount. For amounts over $1, press the "$" sign or the "Enter" button twice.
   RATIONALE: *This feature verifies large amounts, catching errors in case you mistakenly press too many keys.*

7. Check that the amount you typed is the correct amount. Envelopes and packages with too little postage will be returned by the US Postal Service. Sending an envelope or package with too much postage is wasteful to the practice.

8. While applying postage to an envelope, hold it flat and right side up (in order to read the address). Seal the envelope (unless the meter seals it for you). Locate the plate or area where the envelope slides through. This feature is usually near the bottom of the meter. Place the envelope on the left side and give it a gentle push toward the right. Some models hold the envelope in a stationary position. (If the meter seals the envelope for you, it is especially important that you insert it correctly to allow for sealing.) The meter will grab the envelope and pull it through quickly.

9. For packages, create a postage label to affix to the package. Follow the same procedure for a label as for an envelope. Affix the postmarked label on the package in the upper-right corner.

10. Check that the printed postmark has the correct date and amount and that everything written or stamped on the envelope or package is legible.

PROCEDURE 8-4 Using a Check-Writing Machine

Procedure Goal: To produce a check using a check-writing machine

OSHA Guidelines: This procedure does not involve exposure to blood, body fluids, or tissue.

Materials: Check-writing machine, blank checks, office checkbook, or accounting system

Method:

1. Assemble all equipment.

2. Turn on the check-writing machine.

3. Place a blank check or a sheet of blank checks into the machine.

4. Key in the date, the payee's name, and the payment amount. The check-writing machine imprints the check

with this information, perforating it with the payee's name. The perforations are little holes in the paper that prevent anyone from changing the name on the check.

5. Turn off the check-writing machine.

6. A doctor or another authorized person then signs the check.
RATIONALE: *The check is not valid without the proper signature.*

7. To complete the process, record the check in the office checkbook or accounting system.
RATIONALE: *To maintain accurate records, all financial transactions must be promptly and accurately recorded.*

PROCEDURE 8-5 Step-by-Step Overview of Inventory Procedures

Procedure Goal: To set up an effective inventory program for a medical office

OSHA Guidelines: This procedure does not involve exposure to blood, body fluids, or tissue.

Materials: Pen, paper, file folders, vendor catalogs, index cards or loose-leaf binder and blank pages, reorder reminder cards, and vendor order forms

Method:

1. Discuss and define with your physician/employer the extent of your responsibility in managing supplies. Know whether the physician's approval or supervision is required for certain procedures, whether any systems have already been established, and if the physician has any preference for a particular vendor or trade-name item. If your medical practice is large, determine which medical assistant is responsible for each aspect of supply management.

2. Know what administrative and clinical supplies should be stocked in your office. Create a formal supply list of vital, incidental, and periodic items and keep a copy in the office's procedures manual.

3. Start a file containing a list of current vendors with copies of their catalogs.

4. Create a wish list of brands or products the office does not currently use but might like to try. Inform other staff members of the list so that they can make entries.

5. Make a file for supply invoices and completed order forms. (Keep these documents on file for at least 3 years.)
RATIONALE: *Keep completed documents for future reference as well as for legal protection, if needed.*

6. Devise an inventory system of index cards, loose-leaf pages, or a computer spreadsheet for each item. List the following data for each item on its card:
   - Date and quantity of each order
   - Name and contact information for the vendor and sales representative
   - Date each shipment was received
   - Total cost and unit cost, or price per piece for the item
   - Payment method used
   - Results of periodic counts of the item
   - Quantity expected to cover the office for a given period of time

   - Reorder quantity (the quantity remaining on the shelf that indicates when reorder should be made)

7. Have a system for flagging items that need to be ordered and those that are already on order. For example, mark their cards or pages with a self-adhesive tab or note. Make or buy reorder reminder cards to put into the stock of each item at the reorder quantity level.
RATIONALE: *Having a system in place makes your job easier and will make it easier for anyone else taking over the task at a later date.*

8. Establish with the physician a regular inventory-taking schedule. Every 1 to 2 weeks is usually sufficient. As a backup system for remembering to check stock and reorder, estimate the times for these activities. Mark them on your calendar or create a tickler file on your computer.
RATIONALE: *A regular schedule means inventory and ordering will not be forgotten.*

9. Order at the same times each week or month, after inventory is taken. However, if there is an unexpected shortage of an item and more than a week or so remains before the regular ordering time, place the order immediately.

10. Fill in the vendor's order form (or type a letter of request). Order by telephone, by fax, by e-mail, or online. Online ordering will expedite the order. Follow procedures that have been approved by the physician or office manager. When placing an order, have all the necessary information at hand, including the correct name of the item and the order and account numbers. Record the order information in the inventory file for that item. Be sure to obtain from the vendor an estimated arrival time for the order and mark that date and order number on your calendar.

11. When ordering online, save the website to "Favorites" for easy, one-click future access. Select the website and establish an account with the company. To establish an account, you will need to give information about your office practice, including the name of the practice, the contact name, the address, the phone number, an e-mail address, and a payment source. Ask about adding the practice to any special contact lists for promotional materials and discounts.

12. When you receive the shipment, record the date and the amount received on the item's inventory card or record page. Check the shipment against the original order and

the packing slip inside the package to ensure that the right items, sizes, styles, packaging, and amounts have arrived. Initial each item on the packing slip as a record that the correct item and amount were received. If there is any error, immediately call or e-mail the vendor, with the catalog page and the inventory card or record page at hand.

RATIONALE: *Items should be unpacked and checked immediately so that if a problem is discovered, it will be relatively easy to prove that the error or problem is with the shipment and not caused by office personnel.*

13. Check the invoice carefully against the original order and the packing slip, making sure that the amount of the bill matches the items listed on the invoice and the packing list, and ensure that the bill has not already been paid. Sign or stamp the invoice to show that the order was received.

14. Write a check to the vendor to be signed by the physician. (Check-writing procedures are described in the *Patient Collections and Financial Management* chapter.) Be sure to show the physician the original order, packing slip, and invoice. Record the check number, date, and amount of payment on the invoice and initial it or have the physician do so. Write the invoice number on the front of the check.

RATIONALE: *Writing the invoice number on the check will ensure that the payment is posted to the correct account. Writing the check number and date on the invoice will be useful for future reference if there is a payment dispute.*

15. Mail the check and the vendor's copy of the invoice to the vendor within 30 days and file the office copy of the invoice with the original order and packing slip.

SUMMARY OF LEARNING OUTCOMES

LEARNING OUTCOMES	KEY POINTS
8.1 Identify common types of computers.	Common types of computers include desktop computers, laptops, notebooks, subnotebooks, tablets, PDAs, and some types of cell phones.
8.2 Describe computer hardware components and explain the functions of each.	Computer hardware components include the monitor, which allows information contained in the system to be seen; the keyboard, which allows for inputting of information; and the printer, which produces hard copies of information.
8.3 Describe the types of software applications commonly used in the medical office.	Software components include both the operating system that controls the computer and applications that run on the operating system. Software applications commonly used in the medical office include operating system software such as Microsoft Windows and Linux. Application software commonly used in medical offices includes word processing, database management, spreadsheets, practice management, electronic transfer, scheduling, and desktop publishing.
8.4 Summarize the options available for learning computer software programs.	Options available for learning computer software programs include classes, tutorials, manuals, documentation, and online learning with online software "Help" features.
8.5 Recall the steps involved in selecting new or upgrading existing office computer equipment.	Learn as much as you can about the hardware and software being considered. Consider the office needs now and in the future. What is the existing hardware and/or software capable of and can it meet the needs now and in the future? Will an upgrade suffice, or will new equipment or software save the office money in the long run? These are the most important considerations.
8.6 Outline the basic care and maintenance required for the office computer system.	The system unit should be placed in a well-ventilated location and a power strip with a surge protector should be used to protect the circuitry. Use screen savers and power-down capabilities when the system is not in use. Protect storage devices with appropriate covers when not in use. Never eat or drink near computers. Follow maintenance directions provided with all equipment.

LEARNING OUTCOMES	KEY POINTS
8.7 Identify several reasons security is particularly important in the computerized office.	Great care must be taken to safeguard confidential files, make backup copies on a regular basis, and prevent system contamination. HIPAA laws require that privacy and security procedures are in place to prevent the misuse of health information. These procedures also must ensure confidentiality.
8.8 Explain the function of other types of administrative medical office equipment.	Other administrative medical office equipment includes faxes to send information; photocopiers to copy information; typewriters, adding machines, and calculators to perform business functions; folding/inserting machines and postage meters to efficiently prepare mail; dictation-transcription machines for clear medical records; check writers to assist with accounts payable; and paper shredders for confidentiality.
8.9 Outline the steps to be taken in deciding whether new office equipment is needed.	The first step in evaluating the equipment needs of a healthcare office is the research process. Consider office needs and ask about advantages of new equipment versus existing equipment, comparing the benefits of each. Compare products, features, and prices, calling the suppliers for more information as needed. Do not forget to review the warranties.
8.10 Explain the difference between a maintenance contract and a service contract.	A maintenance contract specifies when the equipment will be cleaned, checked for worn parts, and repaired. A standard maintenance contract may include regular checkups as well as emergency repairs. A service contract may cover emergency repairs not covered under standard maintenance.
8.11 Define vital, periodic, and incidental supplies.	Vital supplies are items that are absolutely essential for the practice's functioning. Incidental supplies are needed in the office but do not threaten the office's efficiency if the supply runs low. Periodic supplies are those supplies that require ordering only occasionally, like appointment books.
8.12 Outline the steps in performing a supply inventory.	Review Procedure 8-5 for an outline on performing a supply inventory.
8.13 List the items that should be considered when choosing a vendor for supply ordering.	Obtaining recommendations from other medical offices is a good way to locate reputable office-supply dealers who sell items at reasonable prices. Reputable vendors fulfill orders accurately with quality items, deliver products in good condition, and charge fair prices. Compare vendors on price, quality, timeliness, and how they handle customer problems and complaints.

CASE STUDY CRITICAL THINKING

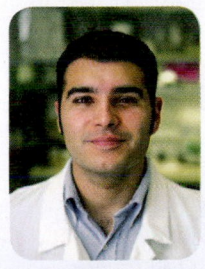

© Karen Moskowitz/Getty Images

Recall Miguel from the beginning of the chapter. Now that you have completed the chapter, answer the following questions regarding his case.

1. Why is it important that Miguel keep track of the usage of the various types of administrative equipment and supplies used by BWW Medical Associates?

2. Why is it important for Miguel to stay current with communications coming into the office via fax and e-mail?

3. Miguel has a reminder on his calendar to order paper and administrative supplies on the 15th of the month. Will he be ordering all the supplies on the inventory list? Why or why not?

4. If Miguel does not order all the supplies, how will he know which ones should be ordered?

1. (LO 8.2) Which of the following items is *not* a pointing device?
   a. Mouse
   b. Trackball
   c. Touch pad
   d. Touch screen
   e. Keyboard

2. (LO 8.1) Which of the following are considered personal computers?
   a. Desktops
   b. Laptops
   c. PDAs
   d. All of these
   e. None of these

3. (LO 8.2) Which of the following is the smallest (in physical size) storage drive?
   a. Zip drive
   b. Jump drive
   c. CD-ROM
   d. DVD-ROM
   e. Diskette

4. (LO 8.3) Which software program would be most helpful if you wanted to produce a report on your patients with a family history of breast cancer?
   a. Database management
   b. Spreadsheet
   c. Communication
   d. Appointment scheduling
   e. Word processing

5. (LO 8.2) Many copiers are now capable of multiple tasks. Which of the following is *not* one of those tasks?
   a. Copying
   b. Faxing
   c. Calculations
   d. Scanning
   e. Collating

6. (LO 8.8) Which of the following is a financial reason for considering a postage meter?
   a. It saves on trips to the post office
   b. It cuts down on the different types of stamps needed in the office
   c. Calculating postage for larger articles, including packages, is easier
   d. It saves money by calculating and printing the exact postage needed
   e. All of these

7. (LO 8.8) What is the most important reason to have paper-shredding capabilities for the medical office?
   a. Decreases waste by cutting paper into small strips
   b. Destroys "mistakes" made in a medical record
   c. Destroys unneeded documents containing PHI
   d. Increases readily available packing material
   e. Destroys records of patients who leave the practice

8. (LO 8.11) When managing office supplies, the goal is to achieve
   a. Efficiency
   b. Organization
   c. Resourcefulness
   d. Independence
   e. All of these

9. (LO 8.11) Expendable items are those that are
   a. Able to be thrown away
   b. Used and must be restocked
   c. Used indefinitely
   d. Restored and reused
   e. Vital to the running of the office

10. (LO 8.11) Examples of clinical supplies are
    a. Needles, syringes, and lubricating jelly
    b. Paper cups and toilet tissue
    c. Rubber bands, stamps, and file folders
    d. Patient education materials and insurance forms
    e. Paper drapes and HIPAA forms

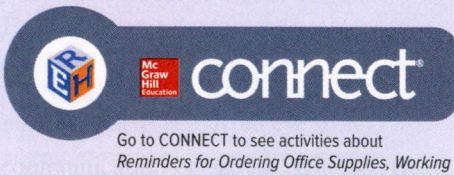

Go to CONNECT to see activities about *Reminders for Ordering Office Supplies, Working with the Task Feature,* and *Task Sequencing.*

SOFT SKILLS SUCCESS

You are in charge of ordering the administrative supplies for your office. One of your coworkers consistently uses the last ream of copy paper without letting you know. Consequently, the office frequently incurs a "rush charge" on its copy paper order. How will you deal with this situation?

Go to PRACTICE MEDICAL OFFICE and complete the module Admin: Check In - Office Operations.

Examination and Treatment Areas

CASE STUDY

PATIENT INFORMATION	**Patient Name** Shenya Jones	**DOB** 11/3/19XX	**Allergies** Peanuts and cinnamon
	Attending Elizabeth H. Williams, MD	**MRN** 124-86-564	**Other Information** CA-MRSA. Patient information brochure given to patient.

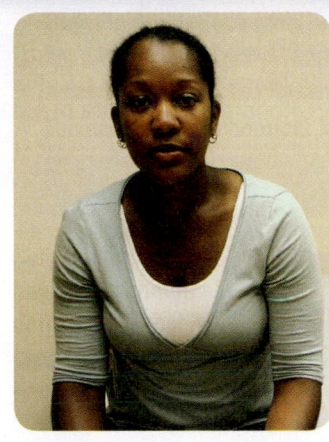

Shenya Jones, 34-year-old female, arrives at the office with swelling and a red pustule on her face. She states that the problem started 2 days ago as a small pimple near her nose. It became irritated, and then extremely swollen and painful overnight. This morning, she noticed yellow drainage at the lesion site and the swelling has increased. The area of drainage is approximately 1 cm in diameter. Her upper lip, side of the face, and nose are all swollen. The examination and treatment areas need to be prepared before you bring her to the back office.

Keep Shenya in mind as you study this chapter. There will be questions at the end of the chapter based on the case study. The information in the chapter will help you answer these questions.

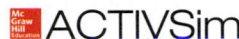

LEARNING OUTCOMES

After completing Chapter 9, you will be able to:

9.1 Describe the layout and features of a typical examination room.

9.2 Differentiate between sanitization and disinfection.

9.3 List steps to prevent the spread of infection in the exam and treatment rooms.

9.4 Describe the importance of temperature, lighting, and ventilation in the exam room.

9.5 Identify instruments and supplies used in a general physical exam and tell how to arrange and prepare them.

KEY TERMS

accessibility

ADA Amendments Act of 2008 (ADAAA)

consumable

disinfection

fixative

general physical examination

lubricant

occult blood

sanitization

spores

sterilization

III.C.4 Identify methods of controlling the growth of microorganisms

III.P.10 Demonstrate proper disposal of biohazardous material
(a) sharps
(b) regulated wastes

X.C.10 Identify:
(c) Americans with Disabilities Act Amendments Act (ADAAA)

XII.P.5 Evaluate the work environment to identify unsafe working conditions

9. Clinical Procedures
 a. Practice standard precautions and perform disinfection/sterilization techniques

10. Medical Laboratory Procedures
 c. Dispose of biohazardous materials

▶ Introduction

The care and maintenance of the medical office's examination and treatment areas are duties of the medical assistant. Preventing accidents by following physical safety guidelines discussed in the *Safety and Patient Reception* chapter are just the beginning of such duties. The medical assistant must perform specific tasks to prepare and maintain the rooms, equipment, and supplies. These tasks include knowing the equipment and supplies and practicing infection control at all times.

▶ The Exam Room   LO 9.1

The exam room is the area where the physician observes the patient, listens to the patient's description of symptoms, performs a general physical exam, and dispenses treatment. A physician performs a **general physical examination** to confirm a patient's health or diagnose a medical problem. Figure 9-1 shows a typical exam room.

Number and Size of Rooms

The number of exam rooms in a medical office depends on the number of healthcare practitioners who work there and on each practitioner's patient load. Ideally, each practitioner in a medical office has at least two exam rooms for her or his exclusive use. A minimum of two rooms per practitioner

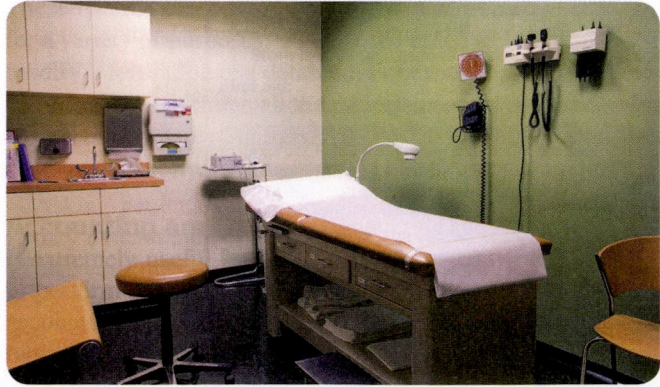

FIGURE 9-1 You are responsible for making sure the exam room is clean and orderly.
© Mark Harmel/Getty Images

enables the medical assistant to prepare one room while the practitioner examines a patient in the other room.

The customary size for an exam room is 8 × 12 feet—large enough to accommodate the practitioner, the patient, and one assistant comfortably yet small enough that instruments and supplies will be within easy reach. Doors and interior walls should be soundproofed to ensure privacy for patients. Some exam rooms have dressing cubicles in one corner, while others have screens behind which the patient may disrobe. Regardless of a room's layout, you should provide privacy for patients whenever they need to disrobe and put on gowns.

A rack for the patient's medical records may hang on the wall directly outside the exam room or on the outside of the door. As offices transition to electronic health records, many rooms now have computer stations. A light or other device like colored tabs on the wall or door may be used to signal that the room is occupied.

Furnishings

Furnishings should be arranged for efficiency, physician convenience, and patient comfort. The examining table is the exam room's key piece of equipment and should be positioned in the center of the room or extending out from the wall. This arrangement allows the physician and an assistant to attend to the patient on at least three sides. The examining table usually contains a pullout step for the patient to use when getting onto the table. It also may contain drawers for storing instruments and table coverings. Examining tables are usually adjustable to enable the patient to assume the various positions the physical exam may require. The physician will probably tell you beforehand if you need to adjust the table in a particular way. Most exam rooms also have a sink, a countertop, and a writing surface large enough to spread out the patient's records or access to a computer and electronic health records. Shelves, cupboards, and drawers store routine supplies like dressings, adhesive tape, and bandages. The exam room also may include the following items:

- One or more chairs for the patient and family member
- A rolling stool for the physician
- A weight scale with height bar (there may not be a scale in every room)
- A metal wastebasket with a lid

- Biohazardous waste containers for disposal of biohazardous materials (biological agents that can spread disease to living things)
- Puncture-proof containers for disposal of biohazardous sharps
- A high-intensity lamp
- Wall brackets for hanging instruments such as a blood pressure cuff

Special Features

The Americans with Disabilities Act of 1990 (ADA) requires that businesses, services, and public transportation provide "reasonable accommodations" for individuals with disabilities. To comply with this act, at least one exam room in a medical office must have features that make the area accessible to patients who use wheelchairs or who have visual or other types of physical impairments. **Accessibility** refers to the ease with which people can move in and out of a space.

The ADA accessibility guidelines require the following:

- A doorway at least 36 inches (915 mm) wide to allow a person in a wheelchair to pass through
- A clearance space in rooms and hallways that is 60 inches (1525 mm) in diameter to allow a person in a wheelchair to make a 180-degree turn
- Stable, firm, slip-resistant flooring
- Door-opening hardware that can be grasped with one hand and does not require the twisting of the wrist to use
- Door closers adjusted to allow time for a person in a wheelchair to enter or exit through the door
- Grab bars in the lavatory

In 2008, an amendment to the ADA, the **ADA Amendments Act of 2008 (ADAAA),** was enacted. This amendment broadens the definition of disability, making it easier for individuals who seek ADA protection to establish that they have a disability. Broadening the definition of disability made it easier for individuals with impairments or disabilities such as cancer, diabetes, and epilepsy to prove their disability and seek the protection of the ADA. Congress adopted a set of "rules of construction" to use when determining if an individual is "substantially limited." These rules include the following:

- The term *substantially limits* requires a lower degree of functional limitation than the previous standard
- The term *substantially limits* must be construed broadly
- Determining an individual's disability should not require extensive analysis
- An impairment that is episodic or in remission is considered a disability if its return would substantially limit a major life activity

▶ Sanitization and Disinfection   LO 9.2

Examination and treatment areas must be kept clean to control pathogens and to prevent the spread of infection. As discussed in the chapter *Infection Control Fundamentals,* we must apply the principles of asepsis to break the chain of infection. Two techniques used on equipment and surfaces that help maintain asepsis are sanitization and disinfection. Sanitization and disinfection are both cleaning processes that reduce pathogens. In general, sanitization is the physical act of cleaning; disinfection is the destruction of most pathogens.

Sanitization

Sanitization is the scrubbing of instruments and equipment with special brushes and detergent to remove blood, mucus, and other contaminants or media where pathogens can grow. Sanitization is used to clean items that touch only healthy, intact skin. For other equipment, sanitization is the first step before disinfection and sterilization. Examples of instruments and equipment that you can sanitize and reuse without further disinfection or sterilization include the following:

- Blood pressure cuff
- Ophthalmoscope (an instrument containing a mirror and lenses used to examine the interior of the eye)
- Otoscope (an instrument used for inspecting the ear)
- Penlight
- Reflex hammer
- Stethoscope
- Tape measure
- Tuning fork

Collecting Instruments for Sanitization Sanitize instruments as soon as possible after use. If you cannot sanitize them immediately, place them in a sink or container filled with water and a neutral-pH detergent solution so that blood and tissue will not dry on the instrument.

In a surgical setting, use a special receptacle of disinfectant solution for collecting contaminated instruments. In an examination setting, place instruments in a sink or a covered container that can be transported to a sink. Take care when placing instruments in sinks or basins, as you can damage pieces of equipment if you drop them carelessly into a receptacle. Nicks or scratches can affect their function and can provide opportunities for bacterial contamination.

When you are ready to begin the sanitization procedure, put on properly fitting, intact utility gloves. They are the barrier between your skin and any infectious material on the instruments and equipment to be cleaned. When you work with instruments that may be contaminated with blood, body fluids, or tissue, you may want the additional protection of a mask, eye protection, or protective clothing.

Separate the sharp instruments from all other equipment (Figure 9-2). This reduces the risk of blunting sharp edges or points, damaging other equipment, and injuring yourself.

Scrubbing Instruments and Equipment Begin by draining the disinfectant or detergent solution in which the equipment was soaking. Rinse each piece of equipment in hot, running water and handle only one item at a time (by its handles where applicable). Scrub each item using hot, soapy water and a small plastic scrub brush. Never use metal brushes or steel wool, which can scratch and damage instruments. Pay

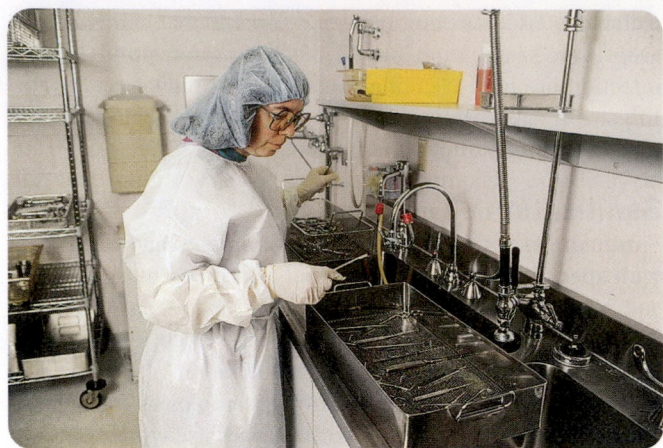

FIGURE 9-2 When working with instruments and equipment, separate pointed or sharp-edged instruments from all others.
© Cliff Moore

careful attention to hinges, ratchets, and other nooks and crannies where contaminated material may collect (Figure 9-3). Use different-sized brushes to clean all areas of each item, along with a low-sudsing, neutral-pH detergent specially formulated to dissolve blood and blood products for medical instruments and equipment. Equipment and instrument manufacturers provide guidelines for sanitizing various types of products. For example, stainless steel items must be sanitized differently than chrome-plated instruments. Follow manufacturers' guidelines when working with their products.

After scrubbing all surfaces and removing all visible stains and residue, rinse instruments individually and place each one on a clean towel. Roll the instrument in the towel to remove moisture, dry it thoroughly, and examine it closely to be sure it is operating correctly. Check that all moving parts operate smoothly and that surfaces are free from nicks, scratches, and other imperfections. Instruments that need only to be sanitized can be returned to trays or bins for storage. Wrap items that require disinfection and **sterilization** (complete destruction of

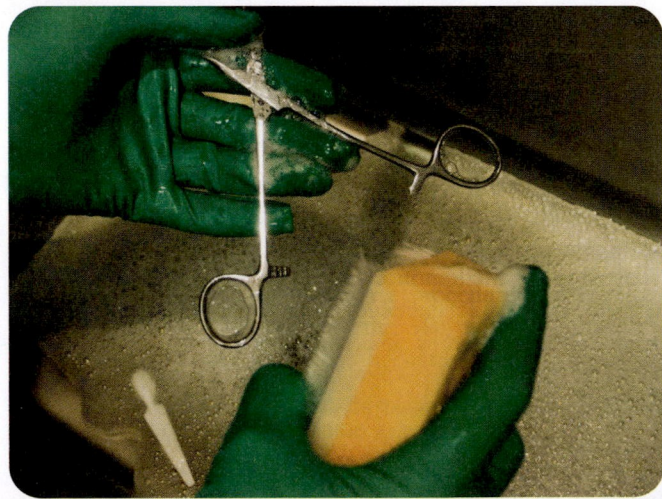

FIGURE 9-3 Clean all areas of an instrument, using a brush for hard-to-reach surfaces.
© McGraw-Hill Education. David Moyer, photographer

all living organisms) in a clean covering and set them aside for those processes. The process of sterilization is discussed in the chapter *Assisting with Minor Surgery.*

Rubber and Plastic Products To sanitize rubber and plastic products, you may need to soak them only for a short period or not at all. Be sure to follow manufacturers' guidelines, as some rubber and plastic products fade or discolor if left in a detergent solution.

Ultrasonic Cleaning Delicate instruments and those with moving parts should be sanitized using ultrasonic cleaners. Ultrasonic cleaning involves placing instruments in a special bath. The cleaner generates sound waves through a cleaning solution, loosening contaminants. Ultrasonic cleaning is safe for even very fragile instruments. Follow the manufacturer's guidelines and Procedure 9-1, Performing Sanitization with an Ultrasonic Cleaner, at the end of this chapter, when performing ultrasonic cleaning.

Disinfection

Sanitization is often only the beginning of the microorganism elimination process. After sanitization, some instruments and equipment require only disinfection before being used again. Disinfection of other items, however, is merely the second step in infection control, performed before the sterilization process.

Disinfection is a process that destroys most, but not all, microorganisms. Bacterial **spores** (thick-walled, reproductive bodies capable of resisting harsh conditions) and certain viruses have been known to survive disinfection with strong chemicals and boiling water. It is essential to understand this limitation of disinfection when you work with instruments and equipment. To destroy microorganisms, a disinfectant solution must reach every surface of an instrument. You must wear gloves when handling instruments during disinfection procedures, because instruments requiring disinfection are considered to be contaminated.

Disinfection is usually sufficient for instruments that do not penetrate a patient's skin or that come in contact only with a patient's mucous membranes or other surfaces not considered sterile. Instruments and equipment that you can disinfect and reuse without sterilization include the following:

- Enamelware
- Endotracheal tubes (tubes used to establish an artificial airway through the nose, mouth, or direct tracheal route)
- Glassware
- Laryngoscopes (tubes equipped with lighting used to examine the interior of the larynx through the mouth)
- Nasal specula (instruments used to enlarge the opening of the nose to permit viewing)

Note that you must sterilize any instrument or piece of equipment before another use, including those just listed, if there is visible contamination with blood or blood products, even if disinfection is commonly considered sufficient. Sterilization is the only reliable measure you can take to eliminate bloodborne pathogens.

Using Disinfectants Disinfectants are cleaning products—used primarily on inanimate materials—applied to instruments and equipment to reduce or eliminate infectious organisms. In contrast, cleaning products used on human tissues as anti-infection agents are called *antiseptics.*

There are no clear visual indications that an item has been properly and completely disinfected. To ensure the optimum effectiveness of disinfectants, follow manufacturers' guidelines carefully when using them. Other factors also may have an impact on a disinfectant's effectiveness. For example, if the disinfectant solution has been used many times, it may not be as powerful as a fresh solution. When wet items are put in the disinfectant bath, the surface moisture may dilute the solution. Traces of the soap used in the sanitization process can alter the chemical makeup of the disinfectant, making it nonlethal to pathogens. Evaporation also can alter the solution's chemical makeup.

Choosing the Correct Disinfectant Manufacturers' guidelines are the most accurate and up-to-date sources of information about the type of disinfectant to use on a given product. Generally, disinfect instruments and equipment by using one or more of the following agents:

- Germicidal soap products
- Alcohol
- Chlorine and chlorine products
- Formaldehyde
- Glutaraldehyde
- Hydrogen peroxide
- Iodine and iodine compounds
- Acid products

Each of these disinfectants has advantages and disadvantages. Before using any disinfectant product or procedure, it is important to understand some general guidelines about disinfectant use as well as specific concerns with each approach. Review Table 9-1 for more details about example disinfectants. Keep in mind that guidelines for the selection and use of disinfectants

---

TABLE 9-1 Disinfectants

Product	Description	Example Uses	Advantages/Disadvantages
Germicidal soap products	The germ-killing additive may increase effectiveness.	Items that do not come in contact with a patient's mucous membranes	The scrubbing and rinsing steps are most important.
Alcohol (70% isopropyl)	Used to clean instruments and equipment that would be damaged by immersion in soap and water or other disinfectant solutions	• Oral and rectal thermometers • Scissors • Stethoscopes	Corrosive product that can cause damage to instruments with long-term use and to skin when used excessively
Chlorine and chlorine compounds (bleach)	Effective in a 10% bleach solution	• Used to disinfect surfaces and soak rubber equipment before sanitization • Decontamination of blood spills	Ventilation may be necessary because the fumes should not be inhaled for a prolonged period.
Formaldehyde	• Used as a preservative in a 10% solution • Used as a germicidal and sporicidal agent in a 5% solution • Must be used at room temperature because its effectiveness is reduced in cooler environments	• Preservation of anatomic specimens • Sterilization of surgical instruments	• Irritating fumes and pungent odor • Corrosive and an irritant to body tissue • Rinse clean items thoroughly with distilled or sterile water before using on patients.
Glutaraldehyde (Cidex®, Cidex Plus®, and Glutarex®)	• Used in chemical sterilization processes and as a high-level disinfectant • Immersing instruments or equipment in a bath of glutaraldehyde for 10 to 30 minutes is sufficient for disinfection	Respiratory therapy and spirometry equipment	Any chemical used in this "cold disinfection" method must be rated as a sterilant and registered with the EPA.
Hydrogen peroxide	Available in a 3% solution	• Soft contact lenses • Spot-disinfection of fabrics	Must be stored in a dark container
Iodine and iodine compounds	• 2% or greater solutions used as disinfectants • Weaker than 2% solutions used as antiseptics	• Skin antiseptic • Disinfection of blood culture bottles	• Somewhat corrosive • Effectiveness is limited by the presence of blood products, mucus, or soap.
Acid products	Includes phenol (carbolic acid)	• Laboratory surfaces • Used as pre-cleaner before sterilization	Extremely corrosive and toxic to tissue and should be used with care

can change and that some products may have become available since this writing. Review new products carefully to be sure they are approved by the Food and Drug Administration (FDA) and the Environmental Protection Agency (EPA).

Handling Disinfected Supplies After disinfecting equipment, handle it with care to prevent contaminating any surface that may later come in contact with a patient. Use sterile transfer forceps, or sterilizing forceps, to remove items from whatever disinfection unit is used. Always wear gloves to handle disinfected items and make sure you store disinfected equipment in a clean, moisture-free environment.

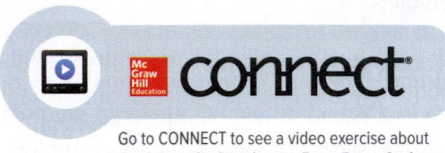

Go to CONNECT to see a video exercise about *Guidelines for Disinfecting Exam Room Surfaces.*

▶ Preparation of the Exam and Treatment Areas LO 9.3

A medical assistant must maintain the examination and treatment areas. The treatment room is basically an exam room that includes additional equipment and supplies and is used for procedures like suturing a wound or excising an abscess. Medical offices may or may not have a special treatment room. All areas of the medical office should be clean and well organized. A clean exam and treatment area is extremely important in preventing the spread of infectious diseases to patients and healthcare workers.

Infection Control

People with a variety of contagious diseases visit medical offices every day. The potential for the spread of infection is thus higher in medical offices than in most other places. For that reason, you must be especially careful to follow infection control procedures at work. You can safeguard the health of staff members and patients by

- Making hand hygiene a priority.
- Keeping the examining table clean.
- Disinfecting all work surfaces.

Hand Hygiene Clean hands are the first step in preventing infection transmission in the exam room and treatment area. Follow the steps for aseptic handwashing and the use of alcohol-based hand cleaners as outlined in the procedures in the *Infection Control Fundamentals* chapter. Review Table 9-2 for hand hygiene guidelines. After performing hand hygiene, use a clean paper towel to handle faucets or doorknobs to help you avoid contaminating your clean hands with microorganisms.

Examining Table The disposable paper that covers the examining table provides a barrier to infection during an exam. Always change the covering after each use (Figure 9-4). Your office might use precut lengths, or you might need to tear off a piece from a roll of paper.

Cover pillows with fresh paper. Also, provide tissues or special wipes for patients who need to wipe away excess

TABLE 9-2	Hand Hygiene

Recommended Practices

- Wash your hands at the beginning of the workday.
- Wash your hands with soap and water whenever they are visibly contaminated with blood or other body fluids.
- If your hands are not visibly contaminated, you should use an alcohol-based hand rub.
- Wash your hands at the end of the workday before leaving the facility.

Indications for Hand Hygiene

- Before putting on and after removing gloves
- Between patient contacts
- Between different procedures on the same patient
- After touching blood, other body fluids, secretions, excretions, and contaminated objects
- After restroom visits, eating, combing hair, handling money, and any other time hands get contaminated
- After contact with a patient's skin
- After contact with wound dressings (bandages)
- After contact with inanimate objects near a patient
- Before eating, applying cosmetics, or manipulating contact lenses
- Before and after handling clean or sterile supplies
- After blowing your nose, sneezing, or coughing
- After touching soiled items such as exam table coverings or clothing

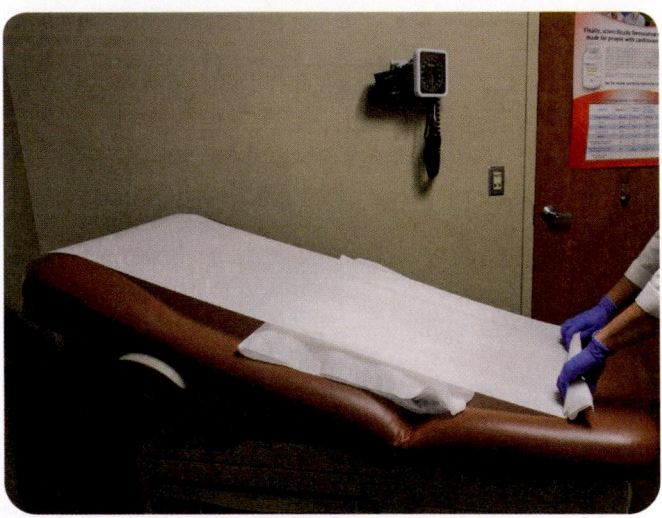

FIGURE 9-4 When you remove the cover from the examining table, roll it up tightly and quickly. Then dispose of it immediately.
© McGraw-Hill Education. David Moyer, photographer

lubricant (a water-soluble gel used during an exam of the rectum or vaginal cavity) after certain procedures.

When you remove the used covering from the examining table, roll it up quickly and carefully with the contaminated side on the inside. You should have a small, tight bundle of paper when you finish. Crumpling the paper haphazardly or shaking it in the air stirs up dust and microorganisms and can spread infection.

Dispose of used paper coverings soiled by body fluids, especially blood, in a biohazardous waste container. (Refer to the *Infection Control Fundamentals* chapter for specific guidelines for disposing of hazardous items.) Used coverings with no visible fluids may be disposed of according to the procedures established by your office. Place soiled linen cloths and pillowcases in biohazard-labeled bags to be sent to a laundry for cleaning.

Surfaces You are responsible for disinfecting work surfaces in the exam room, including the examining table, sink, and countertop. As discussed earlier, disinfection involves exposing all parts of a surface to a disinfectant like a 10% solution of household bleach in water or a product approved by the EPA. The EPA's mission is to protect human health and the environment. See *Points on Practice* for more information about mixing bleach solutions.

Surfaces must be disinfected at the following times:

- After an exam or a treatment during which surfaces have become visibly contaminated with tissue, blood, or other body fluids
- Immediately following accidental blood or other body fluid spills or splatter
- At the end of your work shift

Routinely clean and disinfect the patient lavatory toilet and sink, and inspect and disinfect reusable receptacles like wastebaskets. In most offices, these tasks are performed once a day. Follow the schedule established by your office. Procedure 9-2 at the end of this chapter describes how to disinfect work surfaces, floors, and equipment in the exam room. Replace protective coverings on equipment or surfaces that were exposed to blood, other body fluids, or tissue during the exam.

Storage During the exam, you may need to collect biohazardous specimens, like blood or urine, from the patient for testing. These specimens must be handled and stored properly because they have the potential to be biohazards. Exposure that can spread disease may occur through the following routes:

- Inhalation (breathing)
- Ingestion (swallowing)
- Transcutaneous absorption (absorption through a cut or crack in the skin)

Occupational Safety and Health Administration (OSHA) regulations require storing biohazardous materials separately from food and beverages. Do not place food and beverages in refrigerators, freezers, or cabinets where blood or other potentially infectious materials are present or put specimens in a refrigerator otherwise used to store food and beverages.

It is dangerous to put food or beverages in the laboratory refrigerator for several reasons. If a biohazardous substance is not clearly labeled and you are in a hurry, you might accidentally ingest it. There is always the possibility that containers of biohazardous substances might leak or spill or that residue from the hazardous material might not have been thoroughly cleaned from the outside of containers. This residue could contaminate food or beverages.

OSHA regulations also require that a warning label containing the biohazard symbol be clearly and securely posted on the outside of refrigerators, freezers, and cabinets where biohazardous materials are stored. The government also recommends keeping the laboratory refrigerator and the refrigerator for the employees' personal use in separate rooms. These measures help prevent employees from accidentally putting food and beverages in the wrong place.

OSHA regulations prohibit medical personnel from doing any of the following activities in a room where potentially infectious materials are present:

- Eating
- Drinking
- Smoking
- Chewing gum
- Applying cosmetics
- Handling contact lenses
- Chewing pencils or pens
- Rubbing eyes

These work practice controls, like all OSHA regulations, represent safeguards to protect workers against the health hazards of bloodborne pathogens.

POINTS ON PRACTICE
Mixing a 10% Bleach Solution

Bleach solutions are the most commonly used disinfectant in the medical office. Hard surfaces, such as countertops and floors, and softer surfaces, such as exam beds and chairs are all disinfected using 10% bleach solutions. Bleach, when mixed and handled appropriately, is known to kill or inactivate many of the most common bacteria, viruses, and fungi, including HIV, influenza A, *E. coli,* staphylococci, and candida.

In order for bleach solutions to be effective, they must be mixed at the correct concentrations. They also must be mixed fresh every day. If you have bleach solution left over at the end of the day, discard the solution and mix a fresh batch the next morning. Mixing bleach solutions is inexpensive and simple.

Mix in a Well-Ventilated Area
To make 100 mL of a 10% bleach solution, use a graduated measuring device, such as a beaker, and carefully measure

- 10 mL bleach (5.25–6.15% household bleach with no fragrance added)
- 90 mL water (tap or distilled water)

Pour the bleach directly into a spray bottle. Add the water and place the lid tightly back on the spray bottle. Gently swirl to mix the contents, being careful not to spill.

Refrigerator Temperature Control

Health inspectors visit medical facilities periodically to check that health and safety standards are being upheld. One of the first things they check is the temperature of refrigerators. To prevent spoilage or deterioration of testing kits, blood specimens, and other stored materials, the laboratory refrigerator temperature should be maintained between 36°F and 46°F (2°C and 8°C). Keep a thermometer in the refrigerator to monitor the temperature. See Figure 9-5.

Similar guidelines apply to the refrigerator in the employee area. Food spoils quickly in a refrigerator if the temperature is not low enough. The temperature of the food refrigerator should be maintained between 32°F and 40°F (0°C and 4.4°C). In addition to monitoring the temperature, make sure food is not stored in the refrigerator too long. All food containers, including brown bags containing lunches, should be dated and thrown out when their freshness has expired. You can prevent bacteria growth by wiping up food spills immediately and cleaning the interior and exterior of the refrigerator routinely.

Follow office procedures for the routine cleaning of both laboratory and food refrigerators and for the proper temperature maintenance of refrigerated contents while the refrigerator interiors are cleaned. Specimens, for example, must be kept at a specific temperature at all times. For documentation purposes, keep a log of dates when the laboratory refrigerator is cleaned.

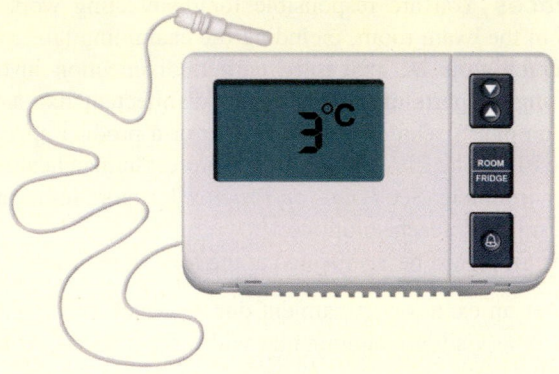

FIGURE 9-5 A temperature monitor is used to maintain a temperature within the refrigerator that prevents spoilage and deterioration of laboratory and food items.

Testing kit and specimen storage often involves refrigeration as a means of preservation. Adequate preservation requires maintaining careful temperature control in a refrigerator. Read the *Caution: Handle with Care:* Refrigerator Temperature Control section for more information on preventing spoilage by controlling refrigerator temperature.

Putting the Room in Order

After ensuring that the examining table is clean, all surfaces are properly disinfected, and all necessary items are stored, take time to straighten the exam room and put things in order. A neatly arranged room boosts patient confidence and supports the impression of a well-run office. It also contributes to the physical safety of patients and staff. Tasks include the following:

- Putting the rolling stool in its place
- Pushing in the examining-table step
- Returning supplies to containers
- Securing sample medications and solutions, prescription pads if used, and other items that may have been left in the room

▶ Room Temperature, Lighting, and Ventilation
LO 9.4

No patient wants to sit in an unkempt exam room. Nor do patients feel comfortable in a cold, dimly lit, or stuffy room. Adjusting the temperature, lighting, and ventilation is part of keeping the exam room in good order and fit for use.

Room Temperature

Because patients may be wearing only a thin paper gown or drape while in the exam room, you must be sure the exam room is warm enough. Set the thermostat to maintain the temperature at approximately 72°F and make sure there are no draft s from windows or doors. Patients often feel anxious while waiting for the physician; a warm room can help them relax.

Lighting

Good lighting is required to make accurate diagnoses, to correctly carry out medical procedures, and to read orders and instructions. A well-lit room also helps prevent accidents. Adjust room lights and blinds or drapes as necessary in preparation for an exam. If there is an exam lamp with a movable arm, be sure the arm is positioned appropriately. Replace all burned-out lightbulbs as soon as possible.

Ventilation

The air in the exam area should smell fresh and clean. Periodically, you may have to deal with offensive odors from urine, vomitus, body odors, or laboratory chemicals. First you must eliminate the source of the odor, especially if the source is potentially infectious or toxic. Then you can take steps to remove the odor.

Some exam rooms have a ventilation system with an odor-absorbing filter. If the rooms in your office do not, you may be able to turn on a high-speed blower to vent room air to the outside. In some cases, an open window and a fan may be sufficient to freshen the air. Remember to check the room temperature after using fresh-air approaches to odor control.

If necessary, you can temporarily mask unpleasant odors with a room deodorizer or spray. Some sprays also help kill germs. Be careful that the room deodorizer you choose does not have a strong odor.

▶ Medical Instruments and Supplies LO 9.5

Physicians require various instruments and supplies to perform an exam or procedure. Instruments are tools or implements physicians use for particular purposes. Disposable instruments are often referred to as supplies. You must maintain all instruments and supplies needed in the exam room. This responsibility involves the following three tasks:

- Ordering and stocking all supplies needed for exams and treatment procedures
- Keeping the instruments sanitized, disinfected, or sterilized (as appropriate) and in working order
- Ensuring all instruments and supplies are placed where the physician can easily reach them

Instruments Used in a General Physical Exam

Many of the instruments physicians use are made of reusable fine-grade stainless steel. Some of these instruments may have disposable parts. Physicians also use a number of disposable instruments, like curettes and needles, because these instruments are both convenient and sanitary. Place any such items contaminated with blood or other body fluids in biohazardous waste containers.

These commonly used instruments are shown in Figure 9-6:

- An *anoscope* is used to open the anus for an exam. Although not always used for the general physical examination, a stool specimen is usually obtained in order to check for blood.
- An *examination light* provides an additional source of light during the exam. It is usually on a flexible arm to permit light to be directed to the area being examined.
- A *laryngeal mirror* reflects the inside of the mouth and throat for exam purposes.
- A *nasal speculum* is used to enlarge the opening of the nose to permit viewing. This type of speculum may consist of a reusable handle with a disposable speculum tip, or it may be a disposable one-piece unit.
- An *ophthalmoscope* is a lighted instrument used to examine the inner structures of the eye.
- An *otoscope* is used to examine the ear canal and the tympanic membrane. The otoscope consists of a light source, a magnifying lens, and an ear speculum. An otoscope also may be used to examine the nostrils and the anterior sinuses. Like a nasal speculum, an otoscope may have disposable tips.

- A *penlight* is a small flashlight used when additional light is necessary in a small area. It also may be used to check pupil response in the eye.
- A *reflex hammer*—used to check a patient's reflexes—has a hard rubber triangular head.
- A *sphygmomanometer,* or blood pressure cuff, is a piece of equipment used to measure blood pressure.
- A *stethoscope* is used to listen to body sounds. It is described in more detail in the *Vital Signs and Measurements* chapter.
- A *tape measure* is a long, narrow strip of fabric, marked off in inches and sometimes in centimeters, used to measure size or development of an area or part of the body.
- A *thermometer* is used to measure body temperature.
- A *tuning fork* tests patients' hearing.
- A *vaginal speculum* is used to enlarge the vagina to make the vagina and the cervix accessible for visual exam and specimen collection. This instrument is used only for a female when an examination and testing of the female reproductive system are done.

Inspecting and Maintaining Instruments Prior to the exam, make sure all instruments are sanitized, disinfected, or sterilized (as appropriate) and in good working order. For example, test the otoscope and ophthalmoscope to make sure the lights work. Place all rechargeable batteries in a battery charger when the instruments are not in use.

Medical instruments are expensive and are designed to work in precise ways. Read the manufacturers' directions so you are familiar with the care and maintenance of various instruments. Routinely check instruments for chipping and rusting, and report to the physician any instruments that need repair or replacement.

Arranging Instruments The physician must be able to find and reach instruments easily during an exam. You can assist by placing instruments in the same place for every exam or by arranging them in the order the physician will use them.

Physicians usually begin a general physical exam by examining the patient's head and face and working down the body. They may want instruments placed in that order. Other physicians may have individual preferences about how they want instruments arranged. In any case, make certain you know each physician's preferences.

With the exception of the stethoscope, which most physicians carry with them, instruments are kept in one of three places during an exam:

- Mounted on the wall (sphygmomanometer, some otoscopes and ophthalmoscopes)
- Set out on the countertop (penlight, reflex hammer, tape measure, tuning fork, thermometer, some otoscopes and ophthalmoscopes)
- Set on a clean (or sterile, if appropriate) towel or tray (anoscope, laryngeal mirror, nasal speculum, vaginal speculum)

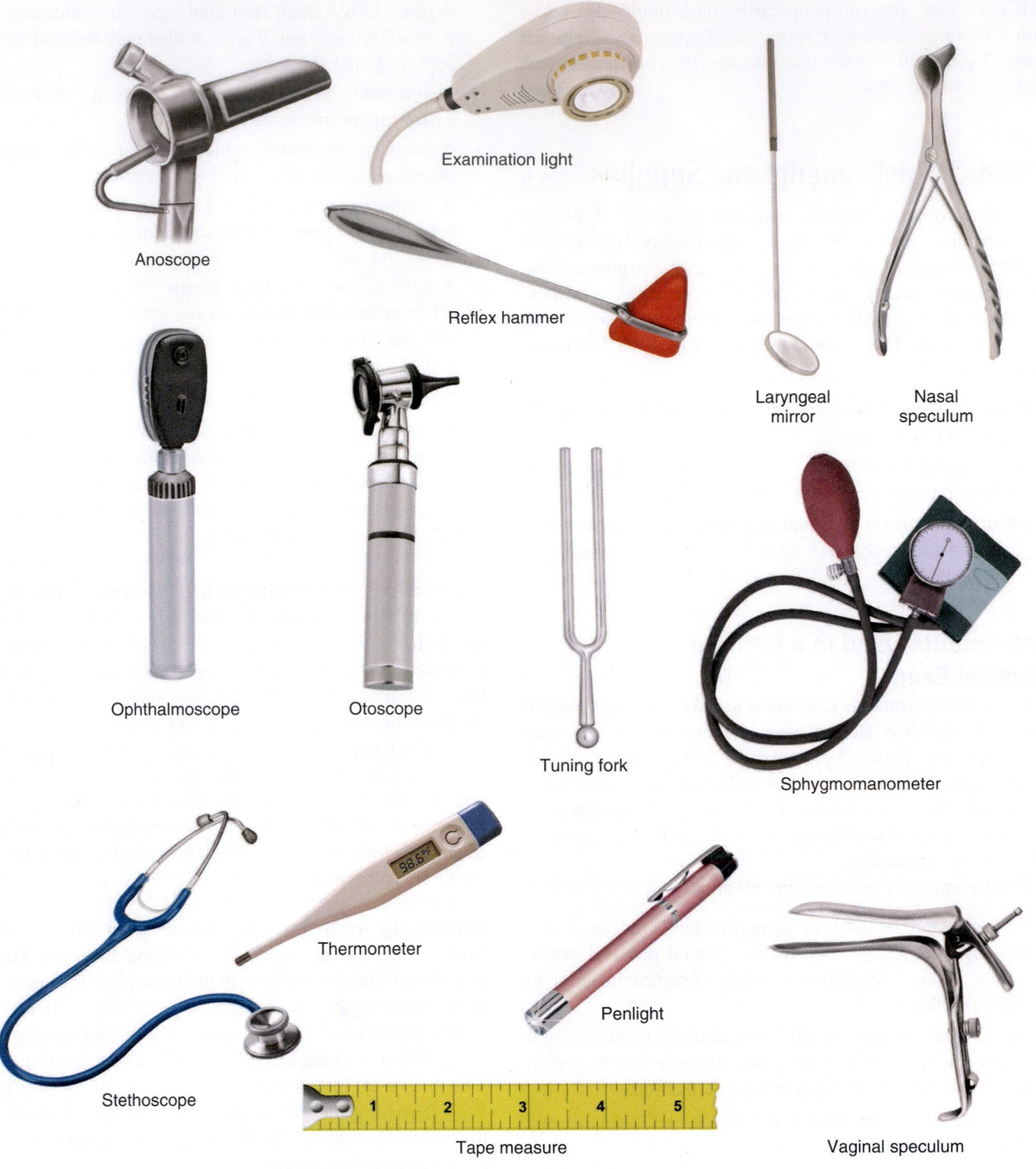

FIGURE 9-6 These instruments may be used in a general physical exam.

Preparing Instruments You must prepare some instruments before they can be used. For example, you may need to warm a vaginal speculum by holding it under warm water just prior to the exam. You might warm the mirrored end of the laryngeal mirror with water or over an alcohol lamp. You also can spray it with a special spray that prevents fogging. Any time you will be handling instruments, you must first wash your hands. If the instruments are sterile, you also must wear sterile gloves.

Cleaning Instruments After the exam, put used instruments in a container and take them to the cleaning area. Always handle instruments carefully because mishandling can alter their precision. Dispose of supplies in the appropriate containers and use approved procedures for sanitizing, disinfecting, and sterilizing reusable instruments and equipment. Refer to Table 9-3 for general guidelines on cleaning instruments.

TABLE 9-3 General Guidelines for Cleaning Instruments

Process	Guidelines*	Instruments
Sanitization	• Use detergent, or as indicated by the manufacturer. • Applies to instruments that do not touch the patient or that touch only intact skin • Disinfect these instruments after sanitization if they have come in contact with blood or other body fluids.	• Ophthalmoscope • Otoscope • Penlight • Reflex hammer • Sphygmomanometer • Stethoscope • Tape measure • Tuning fork
Disinfection	• Use only EPA-approved chemical or a 10% bleach solution to kill infectious agents outside the body. • Applies to instruments that touch intact mucous membranes but do not penetrate the patient's body surfaces	• Laryngeal mirror • Nasal speculum
Sterilization	• Use an autoclave or approved method to kill all microorganisms. • Applies to instruments that penetrate the skin or contact normally sterile areas of the body	• Anoscope • Curette • Needle (reusable) • Syringe (reusable) • Vaginal speculum

* Keep in mind, these guidelines are general. Each office may have its own methods and schedule for cleaning instruments, depending on the office's specialty.

Supplies for a General Physical Exam

Supplies for a general physical exam may be either disposable or consumable. Figure 9-7 shows various types of supplies.

Disposable supplies are items that are used once and discarded. These include the following:

- Cervical scraper (a plastic or wooden scraper used to obtain samples of cervical secretions used for female exams only)

- Cervical brush or broom (specialized collection devices often used in conjunction with a cervical scraper to obtain cervical secretions)
- Cotton balls
- Cotton-tipped applicators
- Curettes
- Disposable needles
- Disposable syringes
- Gauze, dressings, and bandages
- Glass slides
- Gloves, both sterile and exam (nonsterile) types
- Paper tissues
- Prepared paper slides used to test the stool for the presence of **occult blood** (blood not visible to the naked eye)
- Specimen containers
- Tongue depressors

Consumable supplies are items that can be emptied or used up in an exam. These items include the following:

- **Fixative** (a chemical spray used for preserving a specimen obtained from the body for pathologic exam)
- Isopropyl alcohol (for cleansing skin)
- Lubricant

As they do with instruments, physicians may have a preferred arrangement of supplies for the general physical exam. Figure 9-8 shows a typical arrangement of instruments. Certain supplies, like needles, medications, and prescription blanks, if used, should be kept in a locked cabinet away from patient access.

Storing Supplies You can use the cabinets and drawers in the exam room to store nonperishable supplies. Store every item in its own place so you can find it quickly. Consider color-coding or labeling drawers and cabinets so you can easily locate items. Store supplies that come in various sizes, like bandages, according to size and routinely straighten and clean the insides of all exam room cabinets and drawers.

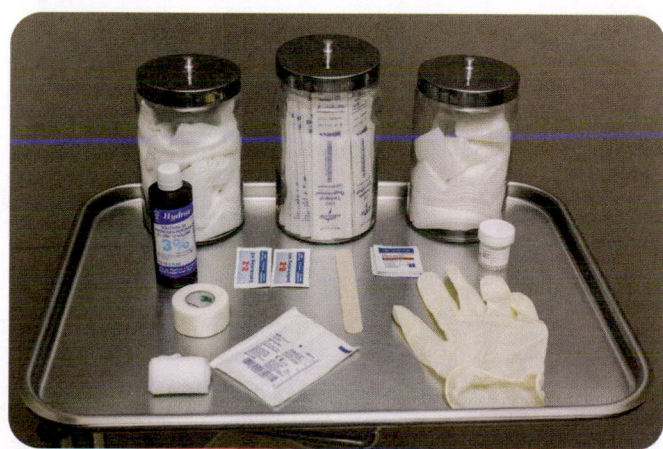

FIGURE 9-7 These supplies may be used in a general physical exam.
© McGraw-Hill Education. Aaron Roeth, photographer

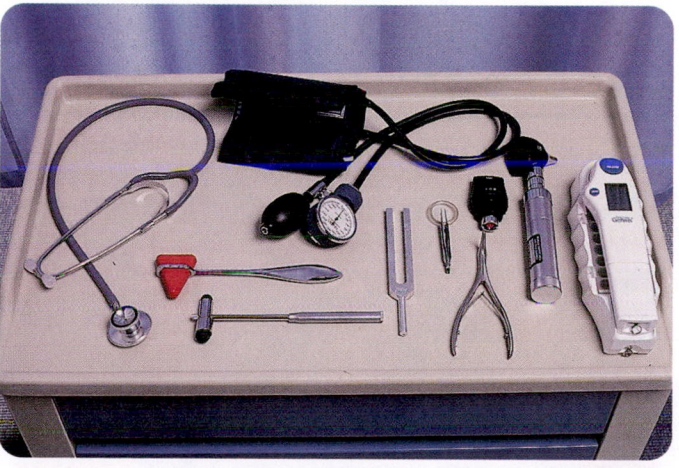

FIGURE 9-8 Arrange the instruments for a general physical exam so that they are convenient for the doctor.
© David Kelly Crow

Restocking Supplies To be sure you have a sufficient quantity of items on hand, order new supplies well in advance of needing them. A good guideline to follow is to order a new supply when the first half of a box, tube, or bottle has been used up. A recordkeeping system will help you determine which supplies you need to restock most frequently and how long it takes for new supplies to arrive. Keep track of the following information in order to develop such a system:

- The types of supplies your office uses
- The quantities of each type of supply used in a given amount of time, such as a month
- The frequency with which you must reorder particular supplies
- The names of various suppliers, along with the amount of time it takes to receive your orders

PROCEDURE 9-1 Performing Sanitization with an Ultrasonic Cleaner

Procedure Goal: To decontaminate items safely and effectively using an ultrasonic cleaner

OSHA Guidelines:

Materials: Ultrasonic cleaner, contaminated items and instruments, ultrasonic cleaning fluid, and manufacturer's directions

Method:

1. Review the manufacturer's directions for safe operation of the ultrasonic cleaner.
2. Fill the container of the ultrasonic cleaner with water. Look for the fill line on the machine. In some cases, you may use distilled water.
3. Add the directed amount of ultrasonic cleaning fluid. Typically, only a small amount of fluid is used. Check the directions.
4. Plug in and turn on the ultrasonic cleaner. Some cleaners require a warm-up period. Check the instructions.
5. Separate instruments and equipment made of different metals.
   RATIONALE: *Different metals may fuse together during the cleaning process, making them useless.*

6. Separate instruments with sharp points.
   RATIONALE: *To avoid injury*
7. Open hinges on instruments and equipment.
   RATIONALE: *Contaminated materials can become trapped between two surfaces.*
8. Place instruments and equipment in the ultrasonic cleaner, but do not overfill.
9. Close the lid, turn on the machine or timer, and wait for the cycle to be completed.
10. Rinse each instrument or piece of equipment in cool, running water and then distilled or demineralized water as policy dictates.
    RATIONALE: *Ultrasonic cleaning fluid may cause damage to instruments or equipment.*
11. Dry each instrument or piece of equipment.
12. Prepare each item for storage or further disinfection or sterilization.
13. Replace ultrasonic cleaning solution according to office policy and manufacturers' guidelines.
    RATIONALE: *Cleaning solution can be used for several cleaning baths but must be replaced as needed to maintain effectiveness.*

PROCEDURE 9-2 Guidelines for Disinfecting Exam Room Surfaces

Procedure Goal: To reduce the risk of exposure to potentially infectious microorganisms in the exam room

OSHA Guidelines:

   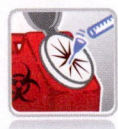

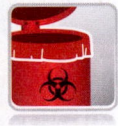

Materials: Utility gloves, disinfectant (10% bleach solution or EPA-approved disinfecting product), paper towels, dustpan and brush, tongs, forceps, and a clean sponge or heavy rag

Method:

1. Wash your hands and don utility gloves.
2. Remove any visible soil from exam room surfaces with disposable paper towels or a rag.
   RATIONALE: *Removing visible soil first allows for better penetration of the disinfectant.*
3. Thoroughly wipe all surfaces with the disinfectant.

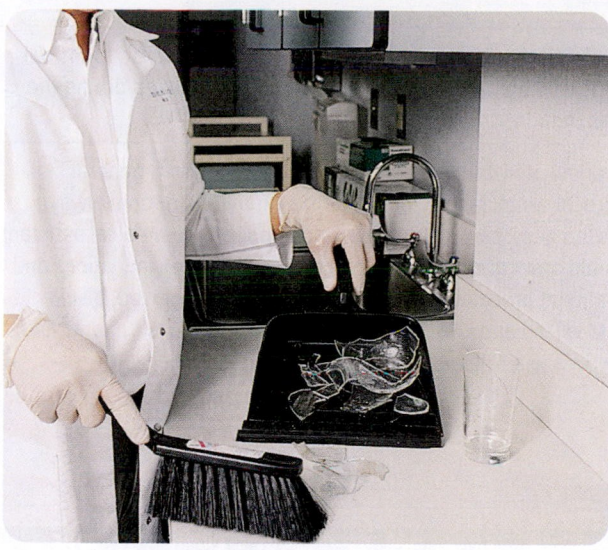

FIGURE Procedure 9-2 Step 4 Because broken glass may be contaminated, never pick it up directly with your hands. Use a brush and dustpan, tongs, or forceps to clean it up.
© Cliff Moore

4. In the event of an accident involving a broken glass container, use tongs, a dustpan and brush, or forceps to pick up shattered glass, which may be contaminated.
   RATIONALE: *Using your fingers to pick up broken glass puts you at risk for exposure to bloodborne pathogens.*

5. Remove and replace protective coverings, like plastic wrap or aluminum foil, on equipment if the equipment or the coverings have become contaminated. After removing the coverings, disinfect the equipment and allow it to air-dry. (Follow office procedures for the routine changing of protective coverings.)

6. When you finish cleaning, dispose of the paper towels or rags in a biohazardous waste receptacle. (This step is especially important if you are cleaning surfaces contaminated with blood, other body fluids, or tissue.)

7. Remove the gloves and wash your hands.

8. If you keep a container of 10% bleach solution on hand for disinfection purposes, replace the solution daily to ensure its disinfecting potency.

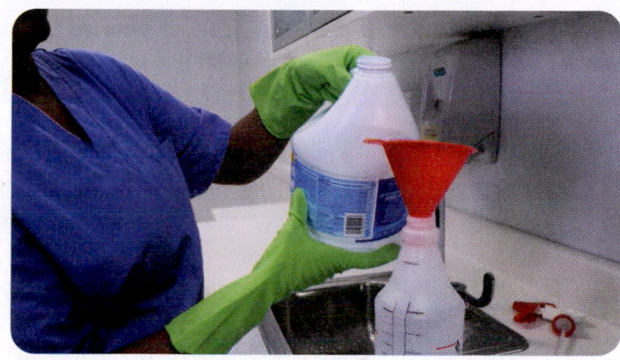

FIGURE Procedure 9-2 Step 8 Replace the bleach solution each day to ensure its disinfecting potency.
© McGraw-Hill Education

SUMMARY OF LEARNING OUTCOMES

LEARNING OUTCOMES	KEY POINTS
9.1 Describe the layout and features of a typical examination room.	A typical examination room is about 8 × 12 feet, large enough to accommodate the physician, the patient, and one assistant. Instruments and equipment in the room should be easily accessible.
9.2 Differentiate between sanitization and disinfection.	Sanitization is the scrubbing of instruments and equipment with special brushes and detergent to remove blood, mucus, and other contaminants or media where pathogens can grow. Disinfection uses special cleaning products applied to instruments and equipment to reduce or eliminate infectious organisms.
9.3 List steps to prevent the spread of infection in the exam and treatment rooms.	Steps involved in preventing the spread of infection in the examination room include covering the examination table with a paper cover and changing the cover between each patient. It is also important to disinfect all surfaces that come in contact with blood or other body fluids after each patient and at the beginning and end of the day.

9.4	**Describe the importance of temperature, lighting, and ventilation in the exam room.**	A comfortably warm, well-lit, and properly ventilated room will help the patient feel comfortable and more relaxed during the examination.
9.5	**Identify instruments and supplies used in a general physical exam and tell how to arrange and prepare them.**	A variety of instruments and supplies are used in a general physical examination. To ensure the examination room always has the necessary instruments and supplies, the medical assistant should order and stock all supplies needed for examinations and treatment procedures; keep the instruments sanitized, disinfected, or sterilized and in working order; and place all instruments and supplies where the physician can easily reach them.

CASE STUDY CRITICAL THINKING

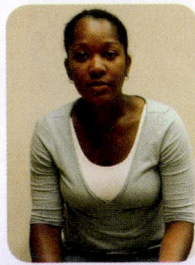

© McGraw-Hill Education

Recall Shenya from the beginning of the chapter. Now that you have completed the chapter, answer the following questions regarding her case.

1. What needs to be done before Shenya is brought back into the exam room?

2. Shenya is diagnosed with community-acquired MRSA (a highly contagious microorganism).

What measures should you take to ensure there is no transfer of infection?

3. After Shenya's examination, you will need to use an ultrasonic cleaner for sanitization. Describe how you would proceed and what source you would use if you had questions about the cleaner you are using.

EXAM PREPARATION QUESTIONS

1. (LO 9.1) Door-opening hardware required by the ADA can be grasped with one hand and
   a. Can be locked securely
   b. Is marked with reflective tape
   c. Does not require twisting the wrist to open
   d. Does not catch completely
   e. Opens automatically

2. (LO 9.5) Which of the following is a disposable supply?
   a. Glass slides
   b. Lubricant
   c. Fixative
   d. Isopropyl alcohol
   e. Nasal speculum

3. (LO 9.2) Which of the following may be sanitized and reused without further disinfection or sterilization?
   a. Curette
   b. Otoscope
   c. Laryngeal mirror
   d. Anoscope
   e. Vaginal speculum

4. (LO 9.1) Which of the following would you be *least* likely to find in an examination room?
   a. High-intensity lamp
   b. Medications
   c. Biohazardous sharps container
   d. Rolling stool
   e. Metal wastebasket with lid

5. (LO 9.2) Which disinfectant would *least* likely be corrosive or require ventilation when in use?
   a. Alcohol
   b. Bleach
   c. Hydrogen peroxide
   d. Formaldehyde
   e. Iodine

6. (LO 9.3) In which of the following situations would alcohol-based hand cleaner most likely be acceptable for use?
   a. After cleaning up a blood spill
   b. After changing the paper on the exam table
   c. After assisting with suturing
   d. After your break
   e. After helping a patient in the restroom

7. (LO 9.3) How often should you discard a 10% bleach solution?
   a. Monthly
   b. Weekly
   c. Daily
   d. Hourly
   e. Bleach solution is stable; do not discard it

8. (LO 9.4) A patient vomits in exam room 2. Which of the following would be your best course of action?
   a. Immediately call the housekeeping department to clean it up
   b. Spray the room with deodorizer and leave it empty for at least 15 minutes
   c. Clean up the vomit and then open the window or spray a room deodorizer
   d. Clean up the vomit, then turn off the ventilation system so the odor does not permeate the entire office
   e. Turn on the ventilation system and spray deodorizer

9. (LO 9.5) What instrument is used to look inside the ear?
   a. Ophthalmoscope
   b. Anoscope
   c. Nasal speculum
   d. Vaginal speculum
   e. Otoscope

10. (LO 9.5) Which of the following consumable supplies is used to preserve a specimen obtained during an exam?
    a. Lubricant
    b. Alcohol
    c. Hydrogen peroxide
    d. Fixative
    e. Bleach

SOFT SKILLS SUCCESS

Recall Shenya from the case study at the beginning of the chapter. Dr. Williams has finished seeing Shenya and asks you to help her with a patient having a mole removal in the procedure room. Dr. Williams is on a tight schedule because she needs to get to the hospital to see another patient. You know that the room in which Shenya was seen previously still needs to be disinfected and restocked, so you ask Michelle, another medical assistant in the office, to clean the room for you. You explain that Dr. Williams has asked you to assist with a mole removal. Michelle tells you that she does not want to clean the room because Shenya has MRSA and she doesn't want to get it. She also states that since the room is your responsibility she doesn't think that she should have to clean the room. How should you respond to Michelle?

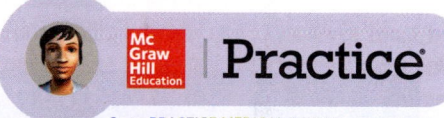

Go to PRACTICE MEDICAL OFFICE and complete the module Clinical - Office Operations.

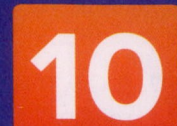

CASE STUDY

PATIENT INFORMATION		
Patient Name Valarie Ramirez	**DOB** 8/4/19XX	**Allergies** Penicillin
Attending Paul F. Buckwalter, MD	**MRN** 829-78-462	**Other Information** Past HX: AB x1

Valarie Ramirez, a 33-year-old female, arrives at the clinic with complaints of "a cold that won't go away." She states that she has had body aches, a cough, and fever for at least 3 days and feels like she is getting worse rather than better. When asked, she states that she did not get a flu shot this year. After a physical exam, Dr. Buckwalter orders a CBC

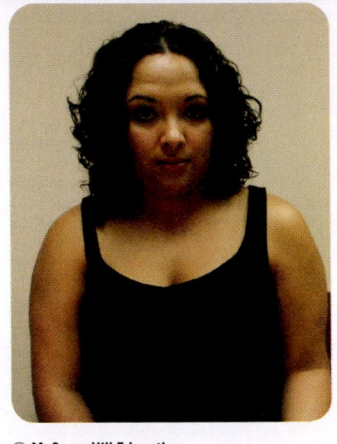

© McGraw-Hill Education

and chest X-ray and gives her a prescription for antibiotics. Dr. Buckwalter will be in touch with her when the lab and X-ray results are in. As she leaves, Valarie asks that you contact her by e-mail about her lab and X-ray results. She states that although she trusts Dr. Buckwalter, she finds him "gruff" and "unsympathetic" and would rather receive her results in this manner.

Keep Valarie in mind as you study this chapter. There will be questions at the end of the chapter based on the case study. The information in the chapter will help you answer these questions.

ACTIVSim

LEARNING OUTCOMES

After completing Chapter 10, you will be able to:

10.1 Explain why well-written documents are important to the image of the medical practice.

10.2 Describe the types of document supplies that will be used in a medical office.

10.3 Outline the general guidelines to effective writing.

10.4 List and explain the purpose of different types of documents used in a medical office.

10.5 Explain why it is important to have a signed written consent from the patient for e-mail communications.

10.6 Describe the tasks involved in editing and proofreading a document.

10.7 Outline the steps for preparing a completed letter for mailing.

10.8 Explain the differences among the types of mail services offered by the USPS.

10.9 Describe the steps involved in processing incoming mail.

KEY TERMS

annotate

body

clarity

complimentary closing

concise

editing

full-block letter style

inside address

invoice

modified-block letter style

optical character reader (OCR)

proofreading

salutation

signature block

simplified letter style

statement

subject line

template

CAAHEP	ABHES
V.C.7 Recognize elements of fundamental writing skills	**7. Records Management**
V.C.8 Discuss applications of electronic technology in professional communication	a. Perform basic keyboarding skills, i.e. Microsoft Word, etc.
V.P.8 Compose professional correspondence utilizing electronic technology	b. Utilize Electronic Medical Records (EMR) and Practice Management Systems
	c. Comply with federal, state, and local laws relating to exchange of information and describe elements of meaningful use and reports generated
	8. Administrative Procedures
	a. Gather and process documents
	f. Display professionalism through written and verbal communications

▶ Introduction

Communication skills—verbal, nonverbal, and written—are important in nearly every profession. Consider, just for a moment, the way you communicate verbally, nonverbally, and in writing, and what this may say about you to your audience. Now, consider what your communication skills may say to others about the office where you work as a medical assistant. Written documents—whether they are produced in the traditional paper format or in an electronic format—are tangible demonstrations of the office staff's ability to communicate and conduct business.

The community as a whole may often evaluate an entire medical practice by the work of one employee. When a letter, form, or document is carelessly prepared and sent into the community, the practitioner may be judged as "careless." However, when a letter or other business correspondence is constructed in a neat, concise, and well-organized fashion, the practitioner is often judged to be organized and competent. The skill demonstrated in the creation of a simple business document reflects on the medical skills of the practitioner and the practice. So it is fair to say that professional image is conveyed in all written correspondence.

Because written documents also serve as legal records, all paper and electronic documents must be prepared with great care and attention to detail. The medical assistant's administrative role includes the creation of consistently accurate and clear documents.

In this chapter, you will learn how to write effectively. You will develop skills in composing business documents using different writing styles and formats. You will also learn how to professionally manage all forms of correspondence commonly used in an ambulatory care setting.

▶ Professionalism and Document Preparation
LO 10.1

As in any business, correspondence from healthcare professionals to patients and colleagues must be handled carefully, with appropriate attention to content and presentation. By learning how to create, send, and receive correspondence and other types of documents, you can ensure positive, effective communication between your office and others. Well-written, neatly prepared correspondence is one of the most important means of communicating a professional image for the medical office (Figure 10-1).

▶ Selecting Document Supplies
LO 10.2

The first step in preparing professional-looking documents is choosing the right supplies. Many offices already have most of these supplies on hand. However, you may be responsible for selecting and ordering such supplies. You may need to make decisions about letterhead paper, envelopes, labels, invoices, and statements.

Letterhead Paper

Letterhead refers to formal business stationery on which the physician (or practice) name and address are printed at the top, along with the names of all the associates in the practice. In most cases, the office phone and fax numbers are listed along with the office website information and an e-mail address. Letterhead is used for all professional, written correspondence coming from the office, but it is important to note that letterhead is used only for the first page of a letter. If a letter is more than one page, all the additional pages are printed on plain paper (the same color and bond as the letterhead).

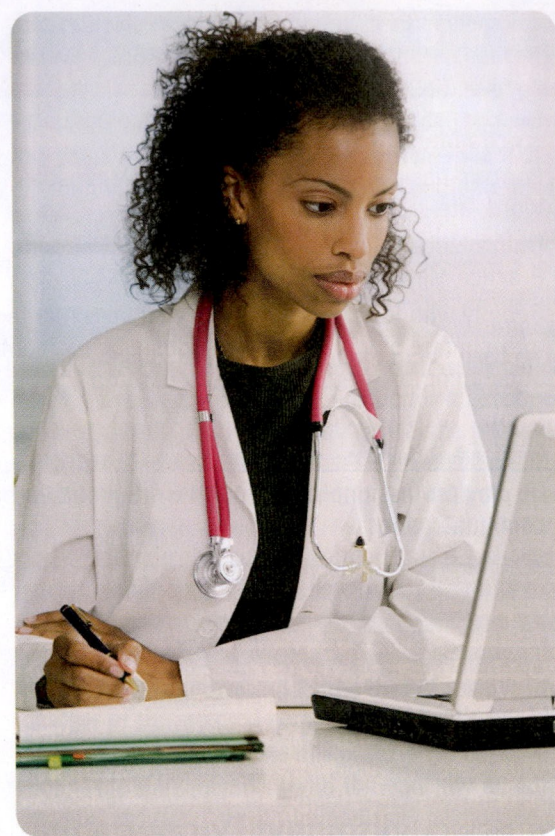

FIGURE 10-1   Well-written correspondence is vital to the professional reputation of a medical practice.
© Image Source/Getty Images RF

Letterhead paper can be cotton fiber bond (sometimes called rag bond) or sulfite bond. Cotton bond, which is usually more expensive than other paper types, contains a watermark—an impression or pattern that can be seen when the paper is held up to the light—that indicates that the paper is of high quality. The most popular cotton bond used for letterhead is 25% cotton because it is economical, but all higher grades can be used. Sulfite bond paper begins as wood pulp, which is treated with peroxide or hypochlorite to bleach it a paler color. Further chemical processes give sulfite paper a brilliant white appearance, making it a favorite for producing photographs. Businesses, including medical practices, use sulfite paper for portfolios, folders, and other items that need an attractive and durable paper.

The two most common letterhead paper sizes are standard and legal. Standard, or letter-size, paper is 8½ × 11 inches and is used for most general business documents. Legal size is 8½ × 14 inches and, as the name indicates, is used for legal and especially lengthy documents.

Formal invitations or announcements, like those announcing an office opening, may be engraved or embossed. Embossing is a process in which the letters are pressed into the paper and often set in black, gold, or silver.

Envelopes

Envelopes are used for correspondence, invoices, and statements. Typically, business letterhead and matching envelopes are printed together on higher-quality paper. Although the letterhead format for statements and invoices may be the same, these documents and their envelopes are usually printed on a lower-quality paper.

Familiarize yourself with the many types of envelopes used in the medical office.

- The most common envelope size used for correspondence is the No. 10 envelope (also called business size). It measures 4½ × 9½ inches.
- Envelopes used for invoices and statements can range from No. 6 (3⅝ × 6½ inches) to No. 10. These envelopes usually have a transparent window that allows the address on the invoice or statement to show through, saving time and reducing the potential for errors involved in retyping the address.
- Smaller payment return envelopes—preaddressed to the physician's office—are often included along with the statement, for the patient's convenience.
- Tan Kraft envelopes, or clasp envelopes, are available in many sizes and are used to send large or bulky documents.
- Padded envelopes are used to send documents or materials, like slides, that may be damaged in the normal course of mail handling.
- The stock and quality of the envelope should always match the stationery. An office typically has two grades of envelopes with a return address. One is a less expensive stock and quality of paper with a return address printed in black, used for everyday documents like insurance inquiries. The second is a higher-quality, more expensive paper with a return address printed in colors that match the office letterhead, which is used for professional correspondence.
- Data mailers are produced by a computer and are used by larger businesses and hospitals for batch mailings of items like paychecks, appointment reminders, and some invoices. The envelopes are opened by tearing off perforated sides, peeling the envelope apart, or utilizing a pull tab.

Labels

Address labels, printed from a computerized mailing list, can make the process of addressing envelopes for bulk mailings much speedier. For example, you may have to send a notice of a change in office hours or a quarterly office newsletter to a large number of patients in a practice.

You may choose to set up a system for frequently used labels. Many practices write insurance inquiries and other business letters to the same addresses repeatedly. For fast and easy access, it is helpful to print out labels of the same address a full page at a time. Pages of labels can then be stored in alphabetized folders near the transcription desk. Excel databases can also be set up to print labels and to insert names and addresses in standardized formats known as **templates.**

Invoices and Statements

Several types of invoices and statements are currently used. An **invoice** lists a product or service rendered and is used when billing for that product or service. A **statement** is a summary of total amounts owed, including outstanding charges as well as payments received. Patient statements include items such as services rendered, payments received, and outstanding balances. There are different types of statements: preprinted statements, computer-generated statements, and superbills (encounter forms)—discussed in the *Patient Collections and Financial Management* chapter.

▶ Effective Writing LO 10.3

Written communication is much like holding a conversation in person. The recipient will form a fairly quick impression of the practitioner or the office based on the appearance of the document and the way the message in the document makes the recipient feel, be it a letter, patient instructions, or even an e-mail. All written communication must be clear and well written, and it must politely and concisely convey the appropriate information to the recipient. To create effective, professional correspondence that reflects well on the practice, be sure that you use clear and **concise** language, the active voice, and an appropriate style. Following are some general guidelines to help you write more effectively.

- Before you write, know the type of person to whom you are writing. Consider him to be your audience. Is the letter to a physician, a patient, a vendor, or fellow staff members? Decide if the tone should be formal or more relaxed.

- Know the purpose of the letter before you begin and make sure your letter accurately conveys that purpose.

- Be concise. Use short sentences. Be brief. Be specific.

- Do not use unnecessary words. Use the simplest way to say what you mean.

- Show **clarity** in your writing; state your message so that it can be understood easily.

- Use the active voice whenever possible. Voice shows whether the subject of a sentence is acting or is being acted upon. Here is an example of the active voice:

"Dr. Huang is seeing 18 patients today."

Here is an example of the same sentence, written in the passive voice:

"Eighteen patients will be seen by Dr. Huang today."

Note that the active voice is more direct and livelier to read.

- Use the passive voice, however, to soften the impact of negative news:

"Your account will be turned over to a collection agency if we do not receive payment promptly."

It would sound harsher to say

"We will turn over your account to a collection agency if we do not receive payment promptly."

- Always be polite and courteous.

- Always check spelling and the accuracy of dates and monetary figures.

- Always check your grammar. Do not use slang.

- Avoid leaving "widows and orphans" or dangling words and phrases. These are words and short phrases at the end or beginning of paragraphs that are left to sit alone at the top or bottom of a page or column or separated from the rest of the thought. Do not start a paragraph at the bottom of a page if the rest of the sentence must be continued on the next page.

Grammar

Although seldom a popular topic in today's text-messaging culture, excellent grammar is essential for every medical assistant who composes professional documents. Let's look at Table 10-1 for a quick review of the parts of speech.

The basic rules of writing should be followed when composing professional documents. Table 10-2 summarizes these rules.

Because certain information in an office is used repeatedly, commonly used paragraphs and even entire letter templates are often used in many practices. These templates, or bodies of text,

TABLE 10-1	The Parts of Speech	
Part of Speech	**Description**	**Example**
Nouns	Nouns describe a person, place, thing, concept, thought, or idea. *Proper nouns* describe specific persons, places, or things.	Massachusetts, town, assistant, Dr. Whalen, freedom, kindness
Pronouns	Pronouns replace nouns by referring back to them.	He, she, it, they, him, her, us, them, theirs, you, yours, ours, mine
Verbs	Action verbs describe movement. Linking verbs express a condition or state. Linking verbs also express the senses.	Walk, type, speak, laugh Is, are, am, be, being, was Hear, smell, taste, touch, feel
Adjectives	Adjectives describe nouns and pronouns or explain which one, how many, or what kind. Adjectives also include *articles* which introduce nouns.	Playful, talented, medical, tasty; numbers are also commonly used as adjectives; common articles include the, a, and an.
Adverbs	Adverbs describe verbs, adjectives, or other adverbs and explain when, where, how, and to what extent.	Extremely, always, frequently, truly, positively
Prepositions	Prepositions are connecting words demonstrating a relationship between nouns, pronouns, or other words.	at, by, from, on, to, in, of, into, with
Conjunctions	Conjunctions join words or phrases together.	and, or, nor, but
Interjections	Interjections show strong feeling or emotion. They are often followed by an exclamation point or a comma if used in professional writing.	Help! Ouch! Call 911!

TABLE 10-2	Basic Rules of Writing
Word Division	Divide • According to pronunciation. • Compound words between the two words from which they derive. • Hyphenated compound words at the hyphen. • After a prefix. • Before a suffix. • Between two consonants that appear between vowels. • Before –ing unless the last consonant is doubled; in that case, divide before the second consonant. Do not divide • Suffixes like –sion, –tial, and –gion. • A word so that only one letter is left on a line. • A word so that only part of a word stands alone on the last line of a paragraph.
Capitalization	Capitalize • All proper names. • All titles, positions, or indications of family relation when preceding a proper name or in place of a proper noun (not when used alone or with possessive pronouns or articles). • Days of the week, months, and holidays. • Names of organizations and membership designations. • Racial, religious, and political designations. • Adjectives, nouns, and verbs that are derived from proper nouns (including currently copyrighted trade names). • Specific addresses and geographic locations. • Sums of money written in legal or business documents. • Titles, headings of books, magazines, and newspapers.

Plurals	• Add *s* or *es* to most singular nouns (plural forms of most medical terms do not follow this rule).
	• With medical terms ending in *is,* drop the *is* and add *es:*
	    metastasis/metastases
	    epiphysis/epiphyses
	• With terms ending in *um,* drop the *um* and add *a:*
	    diverticulum/diverticula
	    atrium/atria
	• With terms ending in *us,* drop the *us* and add *i:*
	    calculus/calculi
	    bronchus/bronchi
	(Two exceptions to this are virus/viruses and sinus/sinuses.)
	• With terms ending in *a,* keep the *a* and add *e:*
	    vertebra/vertebrae

Possessives	To show ownership or relation to another noun • For singular nouns, add an apostrophe and an *s.* • For plural nouns that do not end in an *s,* add an apostrophe and an *s.* • For plural nouns that end in an *s,* just add an apostrophe.
Numbers	Use numerals • In general writing, when the number is 11 or greater. • With abbreviations and symbols. • When discussing laboratory results or statistics. • When referring to specific sums of money. • When using a series of numbers in a sentence. Tips • Use commas when numerals have more than three digits. • Do not use commas when referring to account numbers, or policy numbers. • Use a hyphen or an en dash with numerals to indicate a range. An en dash is typed using CTRL plus the hyphen key on the number pad.

are saved in the computer for quick and easy repeated access. With very few keystrokes, the material can be selected and displayed almost immediately. Then, minor changes specific to the requirements of the document or letter can be made. When making changes to a template, make sure to read the document carefully once you have completed your work to ensure that all necessary changes have been made. Be sure to save your changes to a different file name, not to the actual template document.

It is also helpful to use the cut, copy, and paste features in word processing software to quickly piece together a document that uses sentences or paragraphs from other documents. Large and small bodies of text can easily be moved or copied from document to document, instead of rekeying information. These features help save time for the medical assistant.

▶ Medical Office Documents and Correspondence · LO 10.4

As a medical assistant, you will be responsible for preparing routine documents and correspondence at the physician's request. You may transcribe some documents from the doctor's dictation and compose others from notes.

The purpose of most patient correspondence is to explain, clarify, or give instructions or other information. Correspondence includes

- Letters of referral.
- Letters about scheduling, canceling, or rescheduling appointments.
- Patient reports for insurance companies.
- Instructions for examinations or laboratory tests.
- Answers to insurance or billing questions.
- Cover letters or form letters to order supplies, equipment, or magazine subscriptions.

Parts of a Business Letter

Figure 10-2 illustrates the parts of a typical business letter. Format details may vary from office to office, but the parts of a business letter are generally the same in most offices. Specific characteristics of the parts included in a typical business letter are discussed here.

Letterhead The letterhead is the preprinted portion of formal business stationery.

Dateline The dateline consists of the month, day, and year. It should begin about three lines below the preprinted letterhead text on approximately line 15. The month should always be spelled out, and there should be a comma after the day.

Delivery Notation Type any special or urgent delivery method, such as CERTIFIED MAIL, REGISTERED MAIL, or SPECIAL DELIVERY, two lines below the dateline.

Inside Address The **inside address** contains all the necessary information for the letter's correct delivery. The inside address spells out the name and address of the person to whom the letter is being sent. In general, you should

- Key, or type, the inside address on the left margin, two to four spaces down from the date. It should be two, three, or four lines in length.
- Include a *courtesy title* (Dr., Mr., Mrs., and so on) and the intended recipient's full name. Note: If Dr. is used, do not put MD after the name. For example, either of these forms is acceptable: Dr. John Smith; John Smith, MD. This form is *not* acceptable: Dr. John Smith, MD. Generally, the John Smith, MD format is used for the inside address and the Dear Dr. Smith format is used for the salutation.
- Include the intended receiver's title on the same line with the name, separated by a comma, or on the line below it.
- Include the company name, if applicable.
- Use numerals for the street address, except the single numbers one through nine, which should be spelled out—for example, Two Markham Place.
- Spell out numerical names of streets if they are numbers less than ten.
- Spell out the words *Street, Drive,* and so on.
- Include the full city name; do not abbreviate.
- Use the two-letter state abbreviation recommended by the US Postal Service (USPS). These abbreviations are easily found online by searching for "USPS state abbreviations."
- Leave one space between the state and the zip code; include the zip + 4 code, if known.

Attention Line An attention line is used when a letter is addressed to a company but sent to the attention of a particular individual. If you do not know the individual's name, call the company directly to inquire about the appropriate contact person's name. A colon between the word *Attention* and the person's name is optional. Place the attention line two lines below the inside address (if used).

Salutation When addressing a person by name, use a **salutation**—a written greeting such as "Dear"—followed by Mr., Mrs., or Ms. and the person's last name. The salutation should be keyed at the left margin on the second line below the inside address. A colon should follow. When you do not know the name, it is becoming common practice to use the business title or department in the salutation, as in "Dear Sir:" or "Dear Laboratory Director:" or "Dear Claims Representative:." This also avoids confusion if you do not know the gender of a person with a name such as Pat or Chris.

Subject Line A **subject line** is sometimes used to bring the subject of the letter to the reader's attention. The subject line is not required, but, if it is used, it should be keyed on the second line below the salutation. The subject line may be flush with the left margin, indented five spaces, or centered on the page. The subject line should be limited to two or three words and should be keyed in all capital letters to capture the reader's attention. Some offices use "RE:" (short for *regarding*) instead of the word *Subject*.

Letterhead

BWW
BWW Medical Associates, PC
305 Main Street, Port Snead YZ 12345-9876
Tel: 555-654-3210, Fax: 555-987-6543
Web: BWWAssociates.com

Paul F. Buckwalter, MD
Alexis N. Whalen, MD
Elizabeth H. Williams, MD

Dateline

November 14, 20XX

Delivery Notation

CERTIFIED MAIL

Inside Address

Mr. Hunter Boyd
4080 Magnolia Point Drive
Port, Snead YZ 12345

Salutation

Dear Mr. Boyd:

Subject Line

SUBJECT: RESCHEDULING OF APPOINTMENT

Body

Unfortunately, Dr. Buckwalter will not be in the office on December 5, 20XX, and we must reschedule your appointment for that date. Please call our office at your earliest convenience to arrange for a new appointment date and time.

Your health is of great concern to us and we apologize for any inconvenience this rescheduled appointment may cause you.

Complimentary Closing

Sincerely,

Signature Block

Malik Katahri, cmm

Malik Katahri
Office Manager

Identification Line

MK: mp

Notations

Enc: Appointment calendar

C: Miguel A. Perez, Scheduling Coordinator

FIGURE 10-2 Knowing the parts of a typical business letter enables medical assistants to create written documents that reflect well on the office.

Body The **body** of the letter begins two lines below the salutation or subject line. The text is single-spaced with double-spacing between paragraphs.

If the body contains a list, set the list apart from the rest of the text. Leave an extra line of space above and below the list. For each item in the list, indent 5 to 10 spaces from each margin. Single-space within items, but leave an extra line between items. A bulleted list has a small, solid, round circle before each item.

Complimentary Closing The **complimentary closing** is placed two lines below the last line of the body. Capitalize only the first word of the closing. "Sincerely" is a common closing. "Very truly yours" and "Best regards" are also acceptable closings in business correspondence. A comma is placed after the complimentary closing.

Signature Block The **signature block** contains the writer's name on the first line and the writer's business title on the second line. The block is aligned with the complimentary closing and typed three to four lines below it, to allow space for the signature.

Identification Line The letter writer's initials followed by a colon or slash and the typist's initials are sometimes included in the letter. These initials called the *identification line* may also be referred to as *reference initials*. This line is typed flush left, two lines below the signature block.

Notations Notations at the bottom of the letter may include an identification of any items enclosed with the letter (enclosures) and the names or initials of other people to whom a copy of the letter is being sent (Figure 10-2). Examples of enclosures include office brochures, appointment cards, and forms that the patient should complete. If the letter includes enclosures, type "Enc," "Encl," or "Encs" (for more than one enclosure) flush left, one or two lines below the identification line (if used). Check your office style to determine whether to use punctuation. Then list the items that are being enclosed with the letter. When noting copies sent to other recipients, use a separate line two lines below the enclosure line (if used) and begin the line with "C:" or "c:". Follow this with the names and titles, or in some cases the initials, of people who will receive copies of the letter.

Letter Format
Follow these general formatting guidelines for all letters.

- The margin is the space around the edges of a form or letter that is left blank. The standard setting for margins in business correspondence is 1 inch (left and right margins) for 8½-inch-wide paper.
- Roughly vertically center the letter on the page according to the length of the letter. For shorter letters, you can use wider margins and start the address farther down the page. For longer letters, use standard margins but start higher up on the page.
- Single-space the body of the letter. Double-space between paragraphs or parts of the letter.
- Use short sentences (no more than 20 words on average).
- Include at least two or three sentences in each paragraph.
- Avoid long paragraphs; use paragraphs of fewer than 10 lines.

As stated previously in the discussion on supplies, for multipage letters, use letterhead for the first page and matching plain bond paper for the subsequent pages. Use a 1-inch margin at the top and include a heading with the addressee name, date, and page number on all subsequent pages. The text of the letter should continue about three lines below the heading.

Letter Styles
Four common letter styles are used for different purposes. Your office is likely to have a preferred style in place. Let's take a look at each of these styles individually.

Full-Block Style The **full-block letter style,** also called block style, is typed with all lines flush left. Figure 10-3 shows an example of the block letter style. This style may include a

subject line two lines below the salutation. Block-style letters are quick and easy to write because all lines begin at the left margin. Block style is one of the most common formats used in the medical office.

Modified-Block Style The **modified-block letter style** is similar to full block but differs in that the dateline, complimentary closing, and signature block are aligned and begin at the center, or slightly to the right of the center, of the page (Figure 10-4). This type of letter has a traditional, balanced appearance.

Modified-Block Style with Indented Paragraphs This style is almost identical to the modified-block style except that the paragraphs are indented ½ inch (Figure 10-5).

Simplified Style The **simplified letter style** is a modification of the full-block style. Figure 10-6 shows an example of the simplified letter style. The salutation is omitted, eliminating the need for a courtesy title. A subject line in all-capital letters is placed between the address and the body of the letter. The subject line summarizes the letter's main point but does not actually use the word *subject*. All text is typed flush left. The complimentary closing is omitted, and the sender's name and title are typed in capital letters in a single line at the end of the letter. This letter style is both easy to read and quick to type. In most medical office situations, however, the simplified letter style may be too informal.

Punctuation Styles
Two different punctuation styles are used in correspondence: open punctuation and mixed punctuation. Once you have selected a style, be sure that you remain consistent and true to the chosen style throughout the letter.

Open Punctuation This style uses no punctuation after the following items when they appear in a letter:

- The word *Attention* in the attention line
- The salutation
- The complimentary closing
- The signature block
- The enclosure and copy notations

Mixed Punctuation This style includes the following punctuation marks used in specific instances:

- A colon after *Attention* in the attention line
- A colon after the salutation
- A comma after the complimentary closing
- A colon or period after the enclosure notation
- A colon after the copy notation

Now that you have a basic understanding of letter styles and formats, including punctuation styles, Procedure 10-1 at the end of the chapter outlines the steps for creating a professional business letter using word processing software.

BWW

BWW Medical Associates, PC
305 Main Street, Port Snead YZ 12345-9876
Tel: 555-654-3210, Fax: 555-987-6543
Web: BWWAssociates.com

Paul F. Buckwalter, MD
Alexis N. Whalen, MD
Elizabeth H. Williams, MD

May 28, 20XX

Mr. Shawn Collins
234 Deerfield Drive
Port Snead YZ 12345

Dear Mr. Collins:

Congratulations! Your lab results have come back and, overall, your screenings are great. However, we are a bit concerned about your cholesterol screening result, which is 225. Generally, we like to see our patients with levels under 200.

Please call our office to schedule an appointment with Kaylyn, our clinical medical assistant, to obtain information on diet and exercise programs to help you try to lower your cholesterol number naturally. At that time, she will make an appointment for you to return for a second screening in six months. Also, please check out our website at BWWAssociates.com for delicious low-fat/low-sodium recipe ideas that are easy to prepare and great for the whole family.

As always, if you have any questions at any time, please call the office.

Sincerely,

Elizabeth H. Williams MD

Elizabeth H. Williams, MD

EHW/mp

FIGURE 10-3   Example of a block-style letter with mixed punctuation. Note that all lines begin at the left margin.

Interoffice Memoranda (Memos)

Interoffice memoranda (memos) are periodically used by medical offices, clinics, and hospitals. Most word processing software has templates for formatting interoffice memos. Memos generally facilitate informal written communication within an office.

The heading for a memo generally consists of the following components, followed by a colon:

TO:

FROM:

DATE:

SUBJECT:

Traditionally, headings were written in all caps, but some templates and offices now use mixed case for the heading. Figure 10-7 reveals what a typical office memo looks like. Refer to Procedure 10-2 at the end of the chapter to review the steps for creating an interoffice memo.

In many large practices, printed memos have been replaced by "e-mail blasts" to reach all employees simultaneously. You will explore e-mail and other electronic communications next.

▶ Written Communication Using Electronic Format   LO 10.5

It is no secret that electronic communication has taken the United States by storm. Can you answer *yes* to more than two of the followings statements?

- I have multiple personal e-mail accounts.
- I have at least one social media and/or business networking media account and use it daily.
- I use a cell phone for texting.
- I "tweet" at least once a day.

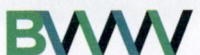

BWW Medical Associates, PC
305 Main Street, Port Snead YZ 12345-9876
Tel: 555-654-3210, Fax: 555-987-6543
Web: BWWAssociates.com

Paul F. Buckwalter, MD
Alexis N. Whalen, MD
Elizabeth H. Williams, MD

May 28, 20XX

Mr. Shawn Collins
234 Deerfield Drive
Port Snead YZ 12345

Dear Mr. Collins:

Congratulations! Your lab results have come back and, overall, your screenings are great. However, we are a bit concerned about your cholesterol screening result, which is 225. Generally, we like to see our patients with levels under 200.

Please call our office to schedule an appointment with Kaylyn, our clinical medical assistant, to obtain information on diet and exercise programs to help you try to lower your cholesterol number naturally. At that time, she will make an appointment for you to return for a second screening in six months. Also, please check out our website at BWWAssociates.com for delicious low-fat/low-sodium recipe ideas that are easy to prepare and great for the whole family.

As always, if you have any questions at any time, please call the office.

Sincerely,

Elizabeth H. Williams MD

Elizabeth H. Williams, MD

EHW/mp

FIGURE 10-4 Example of a modified-block style letter with mixed punctuation. Note that the dateline, complimentary closing, and signature block begin slightly to the right of center.

- I use other forms of electronic communication.
- I use online banking and pay my bills online.

  Now, answer the following questions, true or false.

- I have mailed a letter to someone in the past 2 weeks.
- I pay my bills by writing a check and mailing it.

Electronic communication is the preferred method of communication for many people. For the newest generation, many would rather communicate via text message or on social media than by phone or instead of in-person, face-to-face contact. For this reason, professional, grammatically correct writing (in both electronic and paper format) is largely unused by an increasingly large segment of the population. This cannot hold true for electronic communications coming from a medical office, however. Here, the information is simply too important and must be presented clearly, concisely, and professionally at all times, regardless of the format.

Electronic Media and E-mail to Patients

According to HIPAA law, transmissions that are physically moved from one location to another using magnetic tape, disk, compact disk, or any other portable computer drive are considered electronic media. When used to transport patient information, the portable device and the information it contains must be handled in the same confidential manner as patient paper records. All patient information, regardless of the form, is protected by HIPAA law and is to be guarded by the healthcare provider. The same holds true for e-mail transmissions to and from patients. One word of caution regarding e-mail communications with patients: E-mail is not considered a secure method of communication. As with cell phone communication, information can be *intercepted* and so received by someone who was not the intended recipient. Before undertaking e-mail communication with a patient, be sure to have a signed written consent for e-mail

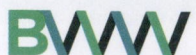

BWW Medical Associates, PC
305 Main Street, Port Snead YZ 12345-9876
Tel: 555-654-3210, Fax: 555-987-6543
Web: BWWAssociates.com

Paul F. Buckwalter, MD
Alexis N. Whalen, MD
Elizabeth H. Williams, MD

May 28, 20XX

Mr. Shawn Collins
234 Deerfield Drive
Port Snead YZ 12345

Dear Mr. Collins:

Congratulations! Your lab results have come back and, overall, your screenings are great. However, we are a bit concerned about your cholesterol screening result, which is 225. Generally, we like to see our patients with levels under 200.

Please call our office to schedule an appointment with Kaylyn, our clinical medical assistant, to obtain information on diet and exercise programs to help you try to lower your cholesterol number naturally. At that time, she will make an appointment for you to return for a second screening in six months. Also, please check out our website at BWWAssociates.com for delicious low-fat/low-sodium recipe ideas that are easy to prepare and great for the whole family.

As always, if you have any questions at any time, please call the office.

Sincerely,

Elizabeth H. Williams MD

Elizabeth H. Williams, MD

EHW/mp

FIGURE 10-5 Example of a modified-block style letter with indented paragraphs and mixed punctuation. Except for the indented paragraphs, it is identical to the modified-block style.

communication on file. Figure 10-8 gives an example of an e-mail consent form.

Once the signed consent is on file, the patient chooses the provider she wishes to communicate with. Depending on the office, by choosing a specific provider, the patient often also agrees to receive e-mail communication from members of that physician's staff, including, but not limited to, nurses, medical assistants, and administrative personnel. The office electronic health record, or EHR, program makes this communication easier in many larger offices. Many EHR programs include an e-mail component and/or a "patient portal" for patients to send and receive communications from the office, as well as pay their medical bills. The beauty of these types of programs is that the patient's e-mail address becomes part of her medical record and is then readily accessible to medical staff members who have access to the patient's chart. Figure 10-9 gives an example of a typical e-mail screen from an EHR program.

Procedure 10-3, found at the end of this chapter, outlines the steps for creating a professional e-mail message. In addition to e-mail messages, many EHR programs also contain templates for completion of electronic letters in often-used formats. Procedure 10-4 at the end of the chapter gives a basic outline of how one of these programs works. If your office uses patient e-mail or a patient portal, don't forget to verify the patient's e-mail address at each visit at the same time you re-verify other demographic information.

Interoffice E-mail

As more and more offices—medical and nonmedical—increase their e-mail use, e-mail and Internet etiquette and rules have become increasingly more important. For example, most offices with Internet access now have written policies regarding e-mail, spelling out the "dos" and "don'ts" concerning use of the practice's e-mail system. The American Medical

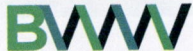

BWW Medical Associates, PC
305 Main Street, Port Snead YZ 12345-9876
Tel: 555-654-3210, Fax: 555-987-6543
Web: BWWAssociates.com

Paul F. Buckwalter, MD
Alexis N. Whalen, MD
Elizabeth H. Williams, MD

May 28, 20XX

Mr. Shawn Collins
234 Deerfield Drive
Port Snead YZ 12345

LAB RESULTS

Congratulations! Your lab results have come back and, overall, your screenings are great. However, we are a bit concerned about your cholesterol screening result, which is 225. Generally, we like to see our patients with levels under 200.

Please call our office to schedule an appointment with Kaylyn, our clinical medical assistant, to obtain information on diet and exercise programs to help you try to lower your cholesterol number naturally. At that time, she will make an appointment for you to return for a second screening in six months. Also, please check out our website at BWWAssociates.com for delicious low-fat/low-sodium recipe ideas that are easy to prepare and great for the whole family.

As always, if you have any questions at any time, please call the office.

Elizabeth H. Williams MD

Elizabeth H. Williams, MD

FIGURE 10-6   The simplified letter is considered by some to be the most readable style for correspondence.

INTEROFFICE MEMO

TO: All Staff
FROM: Malik Katahri, Office Manager
DATE: December 14, 20XX
RE: Patient PHI

It has come to my attention that a computer screen was left on while it contained patient protected health information. Worse yet, the computer is in a location where patients and visitors could view it. This is unacceptable.

We all must be very aware of what we are doing at all times and shut off computer screens, even if we are leaving the computer "just for a minute." Better yet, log off the computer prior to leaving the station. Remember, patient information is to be revealed only on a "business need-to-know basis" and it should NEVER be revealed because someone was temporarily distracted.

FIGURE 10-7   Typical office memorandum format.

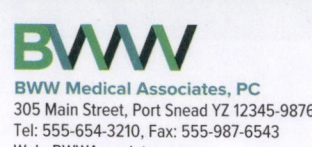

BWW Medical Associates, PC
305 Main Street, Port Snead YZ 12345-9876
Tel: 555-654-3210, Fax: 555-987-6543
Web: BWWAssociates.com

Paul F. Buckwalter, MD
Alexis N. Whalen, MD
Elizabeth H. Williams, MD

Consent to Use E-mail Communication

BWW Medical Associates pledges to use all reasonable measures to protect the private health information of our patients. This includes any information that may be transmitted to or from our office via e-mail. We cannot, however, guarantee the security or confidentiality of information shared via e-mail and we will not accept any liability for disclosure of confidential information that is not caused by professional misconduct on the part of a member of our office team. In order to honor your request to use e-mail communication, we require written consent regarding the following conditions:

- All e-mail messages to or from the patient regarding diagnosis or treatment of a medical condition will become part of the patient's permanent health record. As with any part of the health record, authorized office personnel, including billing and coding professionals in our office, will have access to the information contained within the e-mail message.

- We will forward no e-mail messages, nor the information contained within them, to any third parties, including insurance carriers, without the patient's express written consent, unless otherwise authorized or required by law.

- Because we cannot guarantee that e-mail messages will be received or read within any particular time frame, e-mail is not to be used for transmitting any time-sensitive material or information. E-mail is also not to be used for transmitting information regarding any medical emergency.

- It remains the patient's responsibility to schedule and keep any medically necessary appointments.

I have read and understand the outlined risks associated with e-mail communication between BWW Medical Associates and me. I agree to the conditions and instructions listed above, as well as to any further instructions or limitations BWW Medical Associates may impose regarding e-mail communications. All of my questions have been answered and I understand I may withdraw this consent, in writing, at any time.

_____   _____
Patient Signature   Date

_____   _____
Patient Name   Patient E-mail Address

FIGURE 10-8 E-mail consent form.

Informatics Association and Health E-mail (a nonprofit physician outreach program) are two professional organizations that have established policies relating to e-mail. Larger offices with information systems (IS) departments even audit e-mail and Internet usage. Always remember that when you are using the office computer system, no Internet site you access, and no e-mail that you send or receive, is private; it belongs to the office and the practice owners have the right to monitor and even limit the access you have to the computer system. A good rule of thumb to follow regarding any e-mail you send from your office computer is "Would I be OK with my supervisor seeing this e-mail?" If the answer is not an emphatic "Yes," do not send it.

Managing E-mail

E-mail management, while helpful on a personal level, is imperative on a professional level. Most offices limit the amount of storage each user has, so it is important to manage the documents you send, receive, keep, and delete, so that documents and e-mails that may be needed later are not inadvertently "lost in the system." The following management tools will help you manage your Inbox and your saved e-mails.

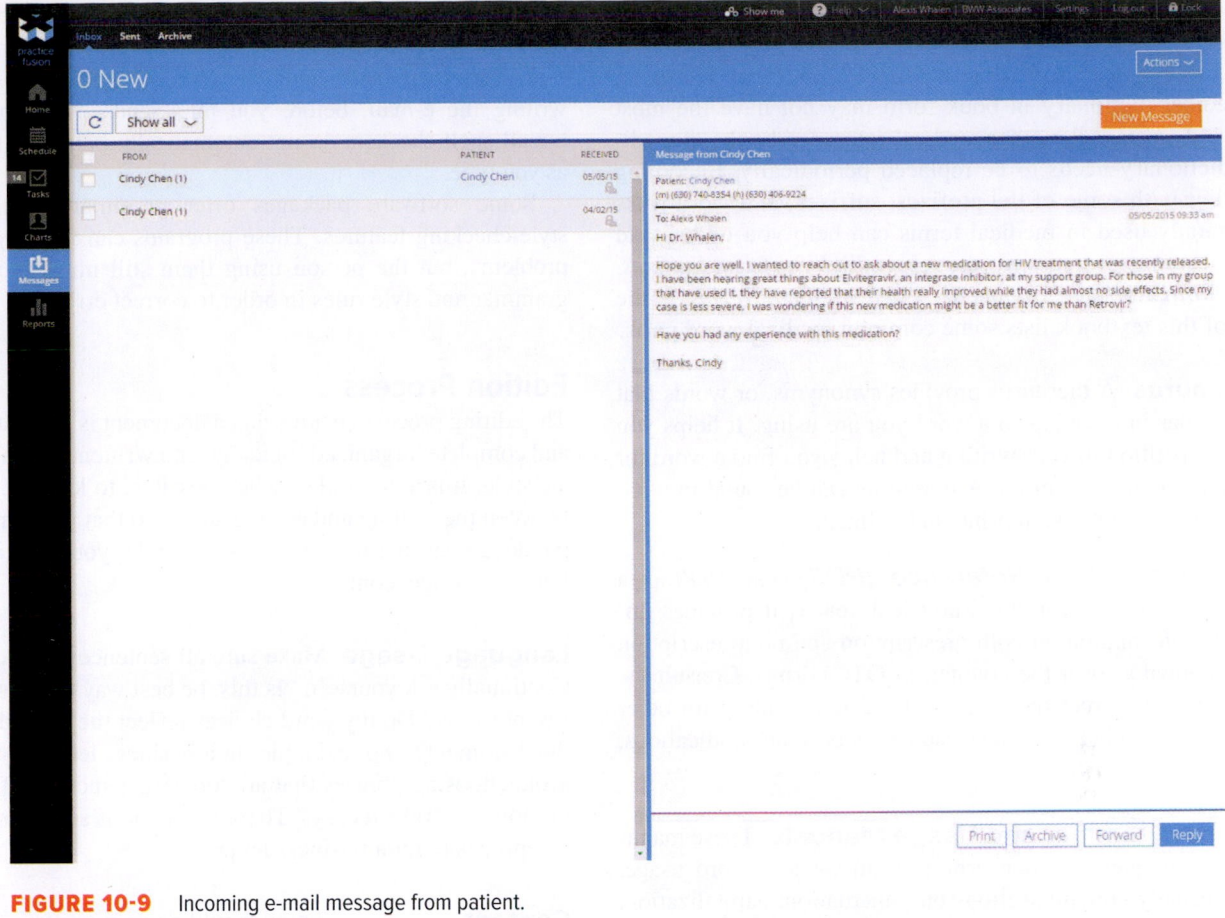

FIGURE 10-9 Incoming e-mail message from patient.

© Practice Fusion®

- Check your office e-mail regularly, emptying any unwanted e-mails.
- Do not open unidentifiable e-mails, even if they appear to be sent from someone you trust.

If there is no subject line topic, contact the sender by simply hitting reply (without opening the contents) to see if that person actually sent it or if it is SPAM (unwanted, potentially virus-carrying e-mail) that may damage your computer, or, worse, the entire office system. The office should have up-to-date antivirus software running, but always be very cautious of unsolicited e-mails.

- Set up subfolders for e-mails that have to be kept for an indefinite period of time.
- Set time limits for deleting or retaining messages.
- Save all e-mail responses that contain protected health information (PHI).
- Take advantage of the e-mail system's file management programs by setting up "rules" to automatically move certain e-mails (such as from patients or other physician offices) to folders you have set up as "high priority," so that these important messages are not accidentally "lost" or "forgotten." Check these high-priority folders several times during the day.

▶ Editing and Proofreading   LO 10.6

Editing and proofreading take place after you create the first draft of any document, on paper or in electronic format. **Editing** involves checking a document for factual accuracy, logical flow, conciseness, clarity, and tone. **Proofreading** involves checking a document for grammatical, spelling, and formatting errors. When possible, ask another person to proofread your work as well. *Never* skip over the very important steps of editing and proofreading!

Tools for Editing and Proofreading

Reference books can help you prepare letters that appear professional. Keep the following tools available.

Dictionary An up-to-date dictionary gives you more than just definitions of words. A dictionary tells you how to spell, divide, and pronounce a word and what part of speech it is, such as a noun or an adjective. A dictionary can be accessed on the Internet or in book form.

Medical Dictionary It is nearly impossible for even the most experienced healthcare professional to be familiar with every medical term and its correct spelling. So a medical dictionary will serve as a handy reference for terms with which you are unfamiliar or about which you would like more information. Like a regular dictionary, a medical dictionary can also be accessed on the Internet or in book form. However, a medical dictionary in book form may not have the most updated terms. Like other medical reference books, a medical dictionary needs to be replaced periodically. Becoming familiar with some of the prefixes, suffixes, and word roots commonly used in medical terms can help you understand the meanings of many words. Appendix I *Prefixes, Suffixes, and Word Roots in Commonly Used Medical Terms* at the end of this textbook lists some common medical word parts.

Thesaurus A thesaurus provides synonyms, or words that are similar in meaning to a word you are using. It helps you avoid repetition in your writing and helps you find a word for an idea you have in mind. A thesaurus can be found in word processing programs, in print, and online.

Physicians' Desk Reference (PDR) The *PDR* is a dictionary of medications. Published yearly, it provides up-to-date information on both prescription and nonprescription (also known as over-the-counter, or OTC) drugs. Consult the *PDR* for the correct spelling of a particular drug or for other information about its usage, side effects, contraindications, and other information.

English Grammar and Usage Manuals These manuals answer questions concerning grammar and word usage. They usually contain sections on punctuation, capitalization, and other details of written communication.

Word Processing Spell-Checkers Most word processing programs used in medical offices have built-in spell-checkers. There are also programs designed specifically to check spelling in medical documents. These spell-checkers include most common medical terms that would not be found in a regular software program. Always keep in mind that spell-checkers should not be relied on as the only means of checking a document, as they may not detect all spelling errors. Spell-checkers will not find correctly spelled words that are used incorrectly, and this type of mistake will reflect negatively on the practice. For example, if you type the word *form* instead of *from,* most spell-checkers will not recognize this as incorrect because *form* is also a correctly spelled word. Although, if the grammar setting is active in Word, it can catch incorrect grammar in some cases but like spell-checkers, should not be relied upon.

Spell-checkers do pick up many spelling errors and often give suggestions for correct spellings. If you indicate the choice you meant to input, the program automatically replaces the misspelled word. You may be able to add words—like medical terms—that are not currently recognized by the spell-checker in your computer. A word of caution is important here! Before you add the word to the computer's dictionary, be sure to look up the exact spelling in a medical dictionary. The computer will recognize only the spelling you add. If you place the *wrong* spelling in the computer, your spell-checker will not correct it.

When you type e-mails, take special care to use correct grammar and punctuation. Spell-checkers are available in most e-mail programs and should be used once you have finished writing the e-mail, before you hit "Send." Note that some e-mail spell-checkers do not automatically point out mistakes as you type.

Some software packages offer grammar-checking and style-checking features. These programs can identify certain problems, but the person using them still must know basic grammar and style rules in order to correct errors.

Edition Process

The editing process ensures that a document is accurate, clear, and complete; organized logically; and written in an appropriate style. It is a good idea, when possible, to leave some time between the writing and editing stages so that you can look at the document in a fresh light. As you edit, you must examine language usage, content, and style.

Language Usage Make sure all sentences are complete. Continually ask yourself, "Is this the best way to convey what I want to say? Do my word choices reflect the overall tone of the document?" For example, in a business letter, you would avoid choosing phrases that are too casual such as "Thanks a million" or "Take it easy." These expressions are informal and inappropriate for a business letter.

Content A business letter should contain all the necessary information the writer intends to convey. If you are editing someone else's letter and something appears to be missing, check with the writer. She or he may have omitted information by mistake.

The content of a letter should follow a logical thought pattern. Place related thoughts and ideas in paragraphs, with one paragraph for each thought or idea. A paragraph should include the message you want to convey and any supporting information. When you start a new thought, start a new paragraph as well. Create a clear, concise letter by

- Stating the purpose of the letter in the first sentence.
- Discussing one topic at a time.
- Changing paragraphs when you change topics or ideas.
- Listing events in chronological order.
- Sticking to the subject.
- Selecting words carefully.
- Reading over what you have written before printing.

Style Use a writing style that is appropriate to the reader. A letter written to a patient is likely to require a different style than one written to a physician. Consider medical terms, for example. In writing to a patient to confirm her surgery date, you might say, "The surgery to remove your gallbladder is scheduled for Friday, May 8, at 7 a.m." However, when confirming the same surgery with the physician, you would state, "Mrs. Stark's cholecystectomy is scheduled for Friday, May 8, at 7 a.m."

Proofreading

Proofreading involves thoroughly checking a document for errors in formatting, data, and grammar. Ideally, after you proofread the document, also have a coworker proofread your work. Someone else will often notice errors that you may have missed. The three types of errors that can occur when preparing a document are formatting, data, and mechanical.

Formatting Errors These errors involve the positioning of the various parts of a letter. They may include errors in indenting, line length, or line spacing. To avoid these errors, take the following two steps:

1. Scan the letter to make sure that the indentions are consistent, that the spacing is correct, and that the text is centered from left to right and top to bottom.

2. Follow the office style consistently throughout the document.

Data Errors Data errors involve mistyping monetary or other figures, like the balance on a patient statement. Mistyped monetary figures can have huge repercussions for the office, the insurance company, and the patient. Other figures, such as test results, must also be absolutely accurate. For example, look again at the first paragraph in Figure 10-6. If the medical assistant had accidentally typed "299" instead of "200" for the second figure, the sentence would not make sense. Be sure to verify the accuracy of all figures by checking them twice or by having a coworker check them.

Mechanical Errors Mechanical errors are errors in spelling, grammar, punctuation, spacing between words, and division of words. Make sure that your word processing spell-checker includes a medical terminology dictionary; otherwise, medical terms may be overlooked. Mechanical errors also include reversing words or characters, typing them twice, or omitting them altogether. Here are some tips to help you avoid mechanical errors.

- Learn basic grammar rules (refer to Tables 10-1 and 10-2). When in doubt, refer to a grammar handbook or reference manual.
- Learn basic spelling, punctuation, and word division rules. When in doubt, be sure to check a manual on English usage. Review Table 10-2, which outlines some basic rules concerning the mechanics of writing. Table 10-3 lists some of the most commonly misspelled medical terms and other words.
- Check carefully for transposed (misplaced) characters or words.
- Avoid dividing words at the end of a line. Most word processing programs automatically wrap words to the next line, so if you are writing on a computer, word division should not present a problem.

▶ Preparing Outgoing Mail   LO 10.7

After you have created, edited, and proofread a letter, you need to prepare it for mailing. This preparation includes having the letter signed, preparing the envelope, and folding and inserting the letter into the envelope. Your letter will then be ready for postage to be calculated and affixed.

Signing Letters

After your letter is complete—it has been proofread and the envelope and enclosures have been prepared—it is ready for signing. Some physicians authorize other staff members to sign for them. If you have been authorized to sign letters, you should sign the doctor's name and place your initials after the doctor's signature.

If the physician prefers to sign all letters, you should place the letter on her desk in a file folder marked "For Your Signature." If the letter is of an urgent nature, give it to the doctor as soon as possible. Otherwise, you can collect several letters in the folder and present the entire group for signing at one time. However, all prepared work should be given to the physician at the end of the day. Make sure that all enclosures are included with the letter and that they remain with the letter when it is returned to you with the physician's signature.

Using a Letter-Folding and Inserting Machine

Large offices and hospitals often have letter-folding equipment, which can help minimize the amount of time staff spends preparing large volumes of outgoing mail. Letter folders are also used for creating folded brochures. In addition to folding letters, a medical practice may use folding and inserting machines for a variety of items, including invoices, newsletters, checks, statements, letters, and flyers.

Lower-end folding equipment requires letters to be fed manually. The speed of this machine is limited to the speed at which an individual can feed in letters, which is typically about 200 pieces per hour. An automatic feeder is required for faster folding. Letter-folding machines can make many different types of folds—for example, standard business letter folds (c-fold), accordion folds (z-fold), single folds, right-angle folds, brochure or gate folds, and other folds (Figure 10-10). Most machines can fold more than one sheet of paper together but do not allow stapled pages to be fed and folded.

Many special features are available that may help the processing of mail and brochures. Batch counters and stackers help to prevent a letter-folding machine from folding more sheets than desired. A jogger helps align stacks of paper and dissipates or removes static electricity. Some machines are better designed for certain types of paper, like glossy or carbonless paper. Inserters are used to insert a folded document into an envelope.

Manually Folding a Letter

A business letter is folded twice into horizontal thirds to fit easily into a prepared standard business envelope. Be sure to include any enclosures that have been noted within the letter at the time it is being folded. See Figure 10-11 for more

TABLE 10-3 Commonly Misspelled Medical Terms and Other Words

Medical Terms

abscess	diluent	larynx	pleurisy
aerobic	dissect	leukemia	pneumonia
anergic	eosinophil	leukocyte	polyp
anesthetic	epididymis	malaise	prescription
aneurysm	epistaxis	menstruation	prophylaxis
anteflexion	erythema	metastasis	prostate
arrhythmia	eustachian	muscle	prosthesis
asepsis	fissure	neuron	pruritus
asthma	flexure	nosocomial	psoriasis
auricle	fomites	occlusion	psychiatrist
benign	glaucoma	ophthalmology	pyrexia
bilirubin	glomerular	oscilloscope	respiration
bronchial	gonorrhea	osseous	rheumatism
calcaneus	hemocytometer	palliative	roentgenology
capillary	hemorrhage	parasite	serous
cervical	hemorrhoids	parenteral	specimen
chancre	homeostasis	parietal	sphincter
choroid	humerus	paroxysm	sphygmomanometer
chromosome	ileum	pericardium	squamous
cirrhosis	ilium	perineum	staphylococcus
clavicle	infarction	peristalsis	surgeon
curettage	inoculate	peritoneum	vaccine
cyanosis	intussusception	pharynx	vein
defibrillator	ischemia	pituitary	venereal
desiccation	ischium	plantar	wheal

Other Words

absence	apparatus	changeable	definite
accept	apparent	characteristic	dependent
accessible	appearance	cigarette	description
accommodate	appropriate	circumference	desirable
accumulate	approximate	clientele	development
achieve	argument	committee	dilemma
acquire	assistance	comparative	disappear
adequate	associate	complement	disappoint
advantageous	auxiliary	compliment	disapprove
affect	balloon	concede	disastrous
aggravate	bankruptcy	conscientious	discreet
all right	believe	conscious	discrete
a lot	benefited	controversy	discrimination
already	brochure	corroborate	dissatisfied
altogether	bulletin	counsel	dissipate
analysis	business	courtesy	earnest
analyze	category	defendant	ecstasy

(continued)

TABLE 10-3 Commonly Misspelled Medical Terms and Other Words

effect	it's	pleasant	secretary
eligible	labeled	possession	seize
embarrass	laboratory	precede	separate
emphasis	led	precedent	similar
entrepreneur	leisure	predictable	sizable
envelope	liable	predominant	stationary
environment	liaison	prejudice	stationery
exceed	license	preparation	stomach
except	liquefy	prerogative	subpoena
exercise	maintenance	prevalent	succeed
exhibit	maneuver	principal	suddenness
exhilaration	miscellaneous	principle	supersede
existence	misspelled	privilege	surprise
fantasy	necessary	procedure	tariff
fascinate	noticeable	proceed	technique
February	occasion	professor	temperament
fluorescent	occurrence	pronunciation	temperature
forty	offense	psychiatry	thorough
grammar	oscillate	psychology	transferred
grievance	paid	pursue	truly
guarantee	pamphlet	questionnaire	tyrannize
handkerchief	panicky	rearrange	unnecessary
height	paradigm	recede	until
humorous	parallel	receive	vacillate
hygiene	paralyze	recommend	vacuum
incidentally	pastime	referral	vegetable
indispensable	persevere	relieve	vicious
inimitable	persistent	repetition	warrant
insistent	personal	rescind	Wednesday
irrelevant	personnel	résumé	weird
irresistible	persuade	rhythm	
irritable	phenomenon	ridiculous	
its	plagiarism	schedule	

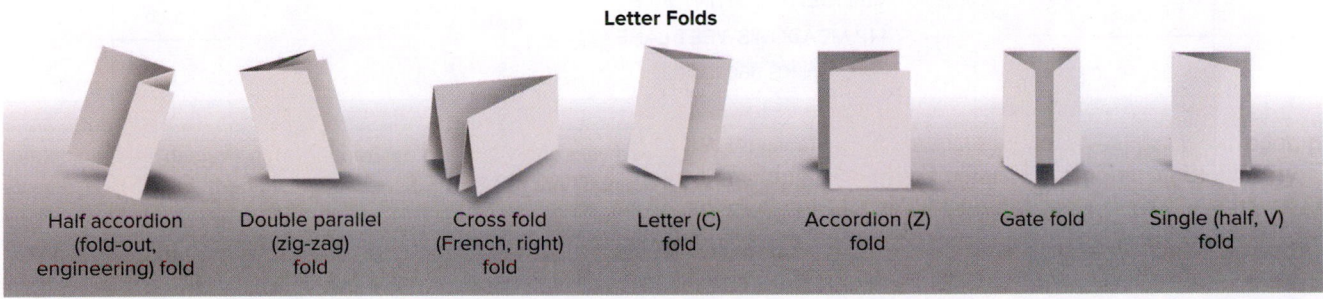

Letter Folds

Half accordion (fold-out, engineering) fold   Double parallel (zig-zag) fold   Cross fold (French, right) fold   Letter (C) fold   Accordion (Z) fold   Gate fold   Single (half, V) fold

FIGURE 10-10 Examples of different folds available with folding machines.

detailed instructions on how to manually fold and insert a business letter into an envelope.

Letters and invoices must be folded neatly before they are inserted into the envelopes. The proper way to fold a document depends on the type of envelope into which the letter will fit.

- With a small envelope, fold the enclosure in half length-wise and insert it.

- With a regular, business-size envelope, fold the letter in thirds. Fold the bottom third up first, then the top third down, and insert the letter.

- With a window envelope, use an accordion fold. Fold the bottom third up. Then, fold the top third back so the address appears in the window, and insert the enclosure.

Preparing the Envelope

To ensure the quickest delivery of mail, the USPS has issued several guidelines for preparing envelopes. The USPS uses electronic **optical character readers (OCRs)** to help speed mail processing. OCRs read the last two lines of an address and sort the mail accordingly. To take advantage of this technology, envelopes must be no smaller than 3½ × 5 inches and no larger than 6 × 11½ inches. They must be addressed in a specific format that can be read by the OCR, following USPS guidelines for addressing envelopes.

Address Placement The address must be placed in a certain location on the envelope for reading by the OCR (Figure 10-12). The area the OCR can read has the following characteristics:

How to Fold a Standard Letter

A business letter is folded twice into horizontal thirds and placed into an envelope. This ensures a little privacy in the letter. The letter is also easy to unfold after opening the envelope. The following diagram shows how a letter is normally folded. This type of fold is used regardless of letter style.

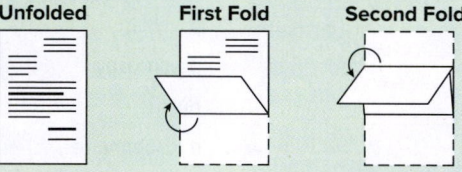

Unfolded   **First Fold**   **Second Fold**

Make a second horizontal crease one-third from the top of the letter where the bottom of the letter had been folded to. Tuck the bottom into this crease and fold the top over it. The letter will be folded into thirds. It will fit any standard envelope.

If you are folding the letter so the address faces out the envelope window, fold the letter toward the back instead of the front to create a z-fold. The letter address will appear through the envelope window, but the letter will still be folded in thirds.

FIGURE 10-11   Correct folding of a business letter.

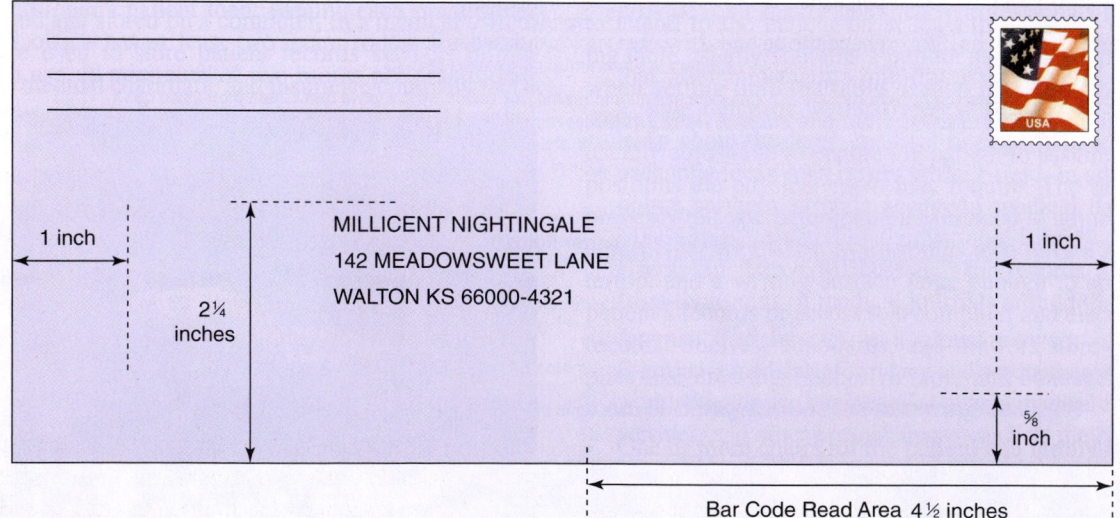

MILLICENT NIGHTINGALE
142 MEADOWSWEET LANE
WALTON KS 66000-4321

1 inch

2¼ inches

1 inch

⅝ inch

Bar Code Read Area 4½ inches

FIGURE 10-12   Correct address format and placement to allow processing by USPS electronic equipment.

- It is bordered by a 1-inch margin on both the left and right sides of the envelope.
- It has a ⅝-inch margin on the bottom. The top of the city-state-zip code line (the last line in the address block) must be no higher than 2 inches from the bottom edge of the envelope.
- An area 4½ inches wide in the bottom right corner of the envelope should be left clear. The OCR reads the address and prints a bar code that corresponds to the zip code in this area.

Two Delivery Addresses Some locations have two delivery addresses, a post office box and a street address. The mail is delivered to the address that appears directly above the city-state-zip (Figure 10-13). If the two addresses have different zip codes, the zip must be the one of the actual delivery point.

Address Format When you enter an address, follow these formatting guidelines:

- Enter the address. The OCR cannot read handwriting or fancy script fonts. Use a plain font, such as Tahoma, Times New Roman, Courier New, or Arial Black.
- Single-space the lines and use the block format. Use only one or two spaces between numbers and words in the address. Do not punctuate, because punctuation is difficult for scanners to read.
- Use only USPS-approved abbreviations for location designations, as presented in Table 10-4.
- Put the addressee's name on the first line of the address block, the department (if any) on the second line, and the company name on the third line. If the letter is to go to someone's attention at a company, per USPS OCR guidelines, put "Attention:" and the person's name on the first line, followed by the company name on the second line before the address begins.
- The line above the city, state, and zip code should contain the street address or post office box number. Include suite or apartment numbers on the same line as the street address.
- The last line of the address must include the city, state, and zip code. Use the zip + 4 code whenever possible.
- Include the hyphen in the zip + 4 code, for example, 08520-6142.
- Obtain current zip codes by logging on to the USPS website at http://zip4.usps.com.
- Insert any delivery notations (such as SPECIAL DELIVERY, CERTIFIED, or REGISTERED) two lines below the postage in all-capital letters. This information should appear outside the area the OCR can read.
- Enter any handling instructions (such as PERSONAL or CONFIDENTIAL) three lines below the return address. This information should also be outside the area the OCR can read.
- Letters going to foreign countries should have the name of the country on the last line of the address block in all-capital letters.

Monagan Medical Management Associates
2345 W Williams Street
PO Box 7654 [mail would be delivered here]
Ellenwood GA 30987

Monagan Medical Management Associates
PO Box 7654
2345 W Williams Street [mail would be delivered here]
Ellenwood GA 30987

FIGURE 10-13 When both street address and PO box are listed, delivery is dependent upon the information on line 3, or directly above the city-state-zip.

TABLE 10-4 USPS Abbreviations

Word	Abbreviation	Word	Abbreviation
Avenue	AVE	Junction	JCT
Boulevard	BLVD	Lane	LN
Center	CTR	North	N
Circle	CIR	Parkway	PKY
Corner	COR	Place	PL
Court	CT	Plaza	PLZ
Drive	DR	South	S
East	E	Street	ST
Expressway	EXPY	West	W
Highway	HWY		

Some letters may be appropriate for interoffice or company mail systems. These letters are usually placed in a large envelope with multiple address lines. The envelope can be reused many times by crossing out the previous name and address and using the next line. Place interoffice mail in a specially designated area or basket for pickup. Be sure not to mix it with outgoing mail.

▶ Mailing Options   LO 10.8

Not too long ago, there was one option for delivering correspondence or documents from one location to the other—the US Post Office. Today, aside from electronic delivery options, there are multiple ways to deliver correspondence and documents from one location to the other. Let's explore some of these options.

Mailing Equipment and Supplies

The proper equipment and supplies will help you handle the mail efficiently and cost effectively. In addition to letterhead, blank stationery for multipage letters, and envelopes described earlier in the chapter, you will need some standard supplies. The USPS provides forms, labels, and packaging for items that need special attention, like airmail, Priority Mail®, Priority Mail Express™ certified mail, or registered mail. Private delivery companies, like United Parcel Service (UPS) and Federal Express (FedEx), also provide shipping supplies to their customers.

Airmail Supplies In the past, any piece of mail that was transported by air was designated as airmail. Today, nearly all first-class mail outside a local area is routinely sent by air. However, airmail services are still available for some packages and for most mail going to foreign countries.

If you are sending an item by airmail, attach special airmail stickers, available from the post office, on all sides. (The word *AIRMAIL* can also be neatly written on all sides.) Special airmail envelopes for letters can be purchased from the USPS.

Envelopes for Overnight Delivery Services For correspondence or packages that must be delivered by the next day, a number of overnight delivery services are available through the USPS and private companies. Most companies require the use of their own envelopes and mailing materials. Make sure you keep adequate supplies on hand.

Postal Rates, Scales, and Meters Postal rates and regulations change periodically, and every medical office should have a copy of the latest guidelines—available from the USPS. The *Office Equipment and Supplies* chapter describes postal scales and meters.

Posting Mail

As stated previously, before you begin posting mail, make sure the envelope or package is complete with all noted enclosures and materials included. After inserting the document(s) in the appropriate envelope (or package in the appropriate container), apply the proper postage and place the postmarked envelope or package in the area of your office designated for mail pickup.

US Postal Service Delivery

The USPS offers a variety of domestic and international delivery services for letters and packages. As a result of a comprehensive USPS Transformation Plan in 2002, many new services were added to the post office to compete with other mail and package delivery services. Following are some of the services you will most likely use in the medical office setting.

Regular Mail Service Regular mail delivery includes several classes of mail as well as other designations like Priority Mail® and Priority Mail Express™. The class or designation determines how quickly a piece of mail is delivered.

First-Class Mail Most correspondence generated in a medical office—letters, postcards, and invoices—is sent by first-class mail. Items must weigh 11 ounces or less to be considered first-class. (An item over 11 ounces that requires quick delivery must be sent by Priority Mail®, which is discussed later in this section.) The cost of mailing a first-class item is based on its weight. The standard rate is for items 1 ounce or

less that are no larger than 6⅛ inches high, 11½ inches wide, and ¼ inch thick. Additional postage is required for items that are heavier or larger. Postage for postcards is less than the letter rate. First-class mail is forwarded at no extra cost.

Media Mail (Third-Class Mail) Media mail is also known as book rate mail. Like second-class mail, it is not often used in medical offices. Media mail is used for the mailing of books, catalogs, and other printed material that weighs less than 70 pounds. The "media" must be educational print material. CDs and digital USB drives cannot be sent by media mail, even if they contain educational material.

Parcel Post This type of mail was formerly called Parcel Post or Fourth-Class Mail. It is used for items that weigh at least 1 pound but not more than 70 pounds and have a combined length and width of not more than 130 inches. Standard post is used for items that do not require speedy delivery. Rates are based on weight and distance. There is a special fourth-class rate for mailing books, manuscripts, and some types of medical information.

Priority Mail® Priority class is useful for heavier items that require quicker delivery than is available for Standard Post. Any first-class item that weighs up to 70 pounds requires Priority Mail® service. Although the rate for Priority Mail® varies with the item's weight and the distance it must travel, the USPS offers a flat rate for all material that can fit into its special Priority Mail® envelopes and boxes, regardless of weight (up to 70 pounds). The USPS guarantees delivery of Priority Mail® items in 1 to 3 business days. Most Priority Mail® is tracked using the USPS Tracking system.

Priority Mail Express™ This is the quickest USPS service. With some exceptions, Priority Mail Express™ guarantees overnight delivery. Priority Mail Express™ deliveries are made 365 days a year. Rates vary, depending on the weight and the specific service. A special flat-rate envelope is also available. Items sent by Priority Mail Express™ are automatically insured against loss or damage. You can drop off packages at the post office or arrange for pickup service.

Special Postal Services The USPS offers a variety of special mail delivery services in addition to the regular classes of mail. These services may require an additional fee above and beyond postage costs.

Online Postage Postage can now be purchased online by using USPS-approved software. Pitney Bowes has software called ShipStream™; however, you may search the Internet for other USPS-approved software. The USPS website, http://www.USPS.com also sells postage online as well as other shipping and mailing supplies.

Certified Mail Certified mail offers a guarantee that the item has been received. The item is marked as certified mail and requires the postal carrier to obtain a signature on delivery (Figure 10-14). The signature card is then returned to the sender. The card should be added to the patient's file. When

Back side of signature card

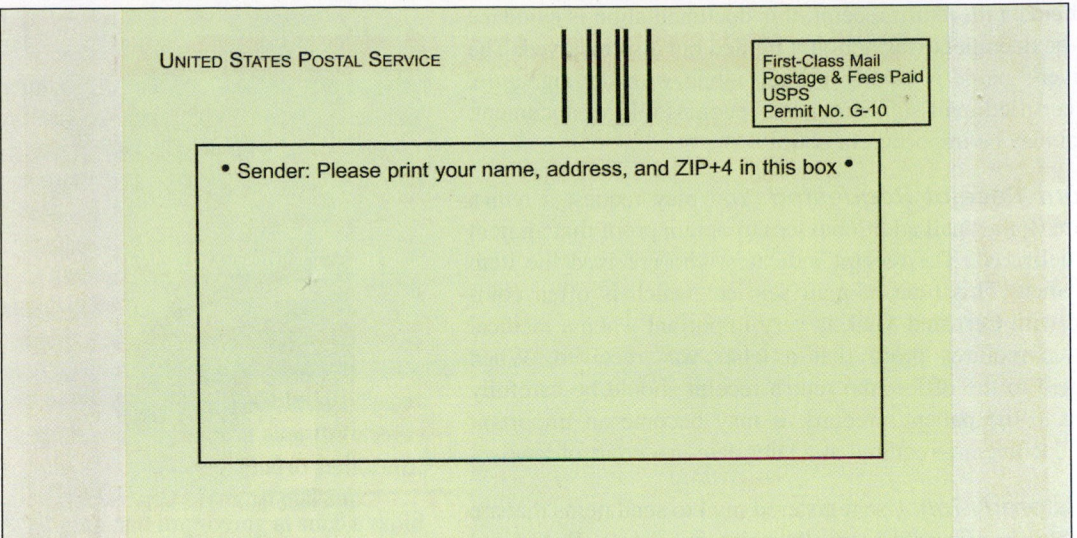

UNITED STATES POSTAL SERVICE

First-Class Mail
Postage & Fees Paid
USPS
Permit No. G-10

• Sender: Please print your name, address, and ZIP+4 in this box •

Front side of signature card

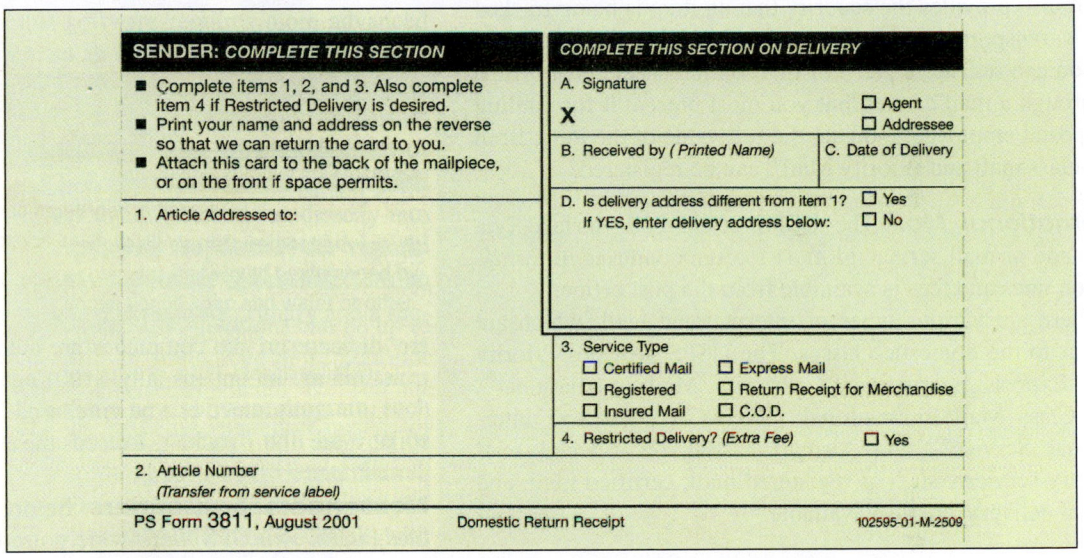

SENDER: *COMPLETE THIS SECTION*

- Complete items 1, 2, and 3. Also complete item 4 if Restricted Delivery is desired.
- Print your name and address on the reverse so that we can return the card to you.
- Attach this card to the back of the mailpiece, or on the front if space permits.

1. Article Addressed to:

2. Article Number
(Transfer from service label)

PS Form 3811, August 2001   Domestic Return Receipt   102595-01-M-2509

COMPLETE THIS SECTION ON DELIVERY

A. Signature
X
☐ Agent
☐ Addressee

B. Received by (*Printed Name*)   C. Date of Delivery

D. Is delivery address different from item 1?   ☐ Yes
If YES, enter delivery address below: ☐ No

3. Service Type
☐ Certified Mail   ☐ Express Mail
☐ Registered   ☐ Return Receipt for Merchandise
☐ Insured Mail   ☐ C.O.D.

4. Restricted Delivery? (*Extra Fee*)   ☐ Yes

Certified mail receipt

U.S. Postal Service
CERTIFIED MAIL RECEIPT
(Domestic Mail Only; No Insurance Coverage Provided)

CERTIFIED MAIL

7001 1140 0000 7637 2652

OFFICIAL USE

Postage $
Certified Fee
Return Receipt Fee
(Endorsement Required)
Restricted Delivery Fee
(Endorsement Required)
Total Postage & Fees $

Postmark
Here

Sent To

Street, Apt. No.;
or PO Box No.

City, State, ZIP+ 4

PS Form 3800, January 2001   See Reverse for Instructions

FIGURE 10-14   Certified mail with return receipt guarantees receipt of correspondence or package sent to the addressee.

combined with return receipt, this documentation is evidence that the document was not only mailed but also received. The receiver's name is clearly printed along with the signature. The certified mail signature card becomes a legal document, which may be important in court.

Return Receipt Requested You may request a return receipt (for a small additional fee) to obtain proof that an item was delivered. The receipt indicates who received the item and when. This type of mail service, which is often combined with Certified Mail, is very important when a medical practice requires proof that a letter was received. When returned to the office, the return receipt should be carefully added to the patient's record. It may become an important legal document—required at a later date in a court of law.

Registered Mail Use registered mail to send items that are valuable, irreplaceable, or otherwise important. Registered mail provides the sender with evidence of mailing and delivery. It also provides the security that an item is being tracked as it is transported through the postal system.

You can register a piece of mail online, at the post office, or through a mail carrier, but you must present it for mailing to a postal employee. Indicate the full value of the item. Both first-class mail and Priority Mail® can be registered.

International Mail The USPS offers both surface (via ship) and airmail service to most foreign countries. Information on rates and fees is available from the post office.

There are various types of international mail, which are similar to the domestic classes. The USPS provides Priority Mail Express International®, Priority Mail International®, First-Class Mail International®, First-Class Package International Service®, and Airmail M-Bags™. Special mail delivery services, such as registered mail, certified mail, and special delivery, are also available.

Tracing Mail If a piece of registered, certified, or tracked mail does not reach its destination by the expected time, you can ask the post office to trace it (Figure 10-15). You will need to present your original receipt for the item. You can also trace mail on the Internet through a UPC symbol that is scanned at the post office.

Other Delivery Services

In addition to the USPS, other companies provide mail and package delivery services around the globe. UPS, FedEx, and DHL are three of the largest and most popular of these companies; DHL is the newest of the three.

All three services deliver packages and provide overnight letter and express services. Packages can be dropped off at drop-off locations or at drop boxes (often located near post offices), or they can be picked up at your office. Locations of both can be found online or in the phone book. Fees depend on the service(s) provided, such as ground or air, and may vary among companies. Each company also offers express delivery services with rates varying according to weight, time of delivery, and whether you use office pickup or drop the package off at one of the company's local branches. Packages sent using

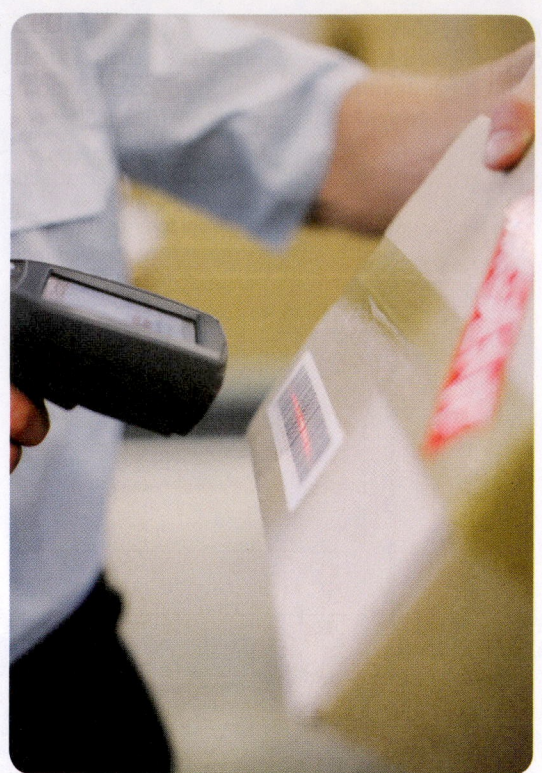

FIGURE 10-15 Items sent by registered or certified mail can be traced by the USPS if delivery is not made as expected.
© Paul Bradbury/Getty Images RF

any of these private companies are automatically insured for a minimum amount (usually $100) against theft or damage. Additional insurance can be purchased from these companies if the value of the package exceeds the standard limit.

Messengers or Couriers Before e-mail and options like FedEx and UPS were widely used, local messenger or courier services were popular for deliveries made within a local area. Except for interoffice couriers that are still used by some large organizations—like hospitals with multiple satellite locations—fewer courier services are now available for hire. Such courier services are listed in the telephone book's Yellow Pages or can be researched online.

▶ Processing Incoming Mail   LO 10.9

Mail is an important connection between the office and other professionals and patients. An office often has an established procedure for handling the mail. It is best to set aside a specific time of the day to process all the incoming mail at once rather than trying to do a little bit at a time. Although it sounds simple, processing mail involves more than merely opening envelopes. In general, it involves the following steps: sorting, opening, recording, annotating, and distributing.

Sorting and Opening

The first step in processing mail is to sort it. Always sort the mail in an uncluttered area to avoid mixing it with other paperwork. As you sort, place any personal or confidential mail aside. Unless you have special permission, never open personal mail addressed to another person. Instead, carefully place it on the addressee's desk, unopened. Sort the remaining mail according to priority. Follow a regular sorting procedure each time to avoid missing any steps. Procedure 10-5, found at the end of this chapter, outlines suggested steps for sorting, opening, and prioritizing the mail. In general, any item arriving by courier, special delivery, overnight mail, or certified or registered mail would be considered a high-priority item, but as always, sort the mail according to the procedure outlined in the office policies and procedures manual.

Recording

Keep a log of each day's mail. This daily record lists the mail received and indicates follow-up correspondence and the date correspondence is completed. This method helps in tracing items and keeping track of correspondence.

Annotating

Because you will be reading much of the incoming mail, you also may be encouraged to **annotate** it. To annotate means to underline or highlight key points of the letter or to write reminders, comments, or suggested actions in the margins or on self-adhesive notes. An example of annotating is including "please sign here" next to where a signature should be. Annotating may involve pulling a patient's chart or any previously received, related correspondence from a file and attaching it to the letter.

Distributing

Once you have reviewed the mail and made any necessary annotations, sort the letters into separate batches for distribution. These batches might include correspondence that requires the physician's attention, payments to be directed to the billing supervisor, and correspondence that requires your attention. Each batch should be presented to the appropriate person in a file folder and arranged with the highest-priority items on top. You may be given specific instructions on how to distribute magazines, newspapers, and advertising circulars.

Handling Drug and Product Samples

Many physicians receive a number of drug and product samples in the mail. Handling procedures vary from office to office. Samples of nonprescription products, like hand creams or cough drops, may be placed in the patient treatment area for patient distribution, as directed by the physician.

The physician may ask that you put samples of any new prescription drugs in his private office for him to evaluate. Store all other drug samples in a locked cabinet reserved solely for such samples. Sort and label the samples by category, such as antibiotics, sedatives, painkillers, and so on. Never give samples to patients or use them yourself unless directed by the physician. If the physician directs you to give samples to a patient, make sure to write this information in the patient's chart and date the entry.

When a box of samples is outdated, you should properly dispose of them, following all state and DEA regulations. You will most likely use the disposal company that handles your biomedical waste to dispose of unused, outdated sample medications. Flushing samples down the sink or toilet is no longer allowed, as this can pollute the environment. Samples should never be placed in the trash where unauthorized individuals could take the medications. Your local pharmacy may also have a program for disposing of outdated medications.

PROCEDURE 10-1 Creating a Professional Letter   WORK // DOC

Procedure Goal: To follow standard procedure for constructing a business letter

OSHA Guidelines: This procedure does not involve exposure to blood, body fluids, or tissue.

Materials: Computer with appropriate word processing software, letterhead paper, dictionaries or other professional tools

Method:

1. Format the letter according to the standard office procedure. Use the same punctuation and style throughout.
   RATIONALE: *Consistency in format creates a professional-looking document.*

2. Start the dateline three lines below the last line of the printed letterhead. (Note: Depending on the letter's length, it is acceptable to start between two and six lines below the letterhead.)
   RATIONALE: *The letter should be centered both vertically and horizontally on the page for visual appeal.*

3. Two lines below the dateline, enter any special mailing instructions (such as REGISTERED MAIL, CERTIFIED MAIL, and so on).

4. Three lines below any special instructions, begin the inside address. Insert the addressee's courtesy title (Mr., Mrs., Ms.) and full name on the first line. If a professional title is given (MD, RN, PhD), this title is placed after the addressee's name instead of a courtesy title.
   RATIONALE: *A professional title is used when available in professional correspondence. Never use both a courtesy title and a professional title at the same time.*

5. Enter the addressee's business title, if applicable, on the second line with the company name on the third line. The street address is entered on the fourth line, including the apartment or suite number. The city, state, and zip code appear on the fifth line. Use the standard two-letter abbreviation for the state, followed by one space and the zip code.

6. Two lines below the inside address, insert the salutation, using the appropriate courtesy title (Mr., Mrs., Ms., Dr.) prior to the addressee's last name.
   RATIONALE: *The salutation uses a courtesy title. Do not include the professional title or the addressee's first name in the salutation.*

7. Two lines below the salutation, enter the subject line, if applicable.

8. Two lines below the subject line, begin the body of the letter. Single-space between lines. Double-space between paragraphs.

9. Two lines below the body of the letter, enter the complimentary closing.

10. Leave three blank lines (return four times) and begin the signature block. (Enough space must be left to allow for the signature.) Enter the sender's name on the first line and type the sender's title on the second line.
   RATIONALE: *Adequate space must be left for the signature. If the signer has a long signature, more than three blank lines may be left. Entering the name allows the addressee to understand who sent the letter if the sender's signature is not legible.*

11. Two lines below the sender's title is the identification line. Insert the sender's initials in all capitals and your initials in lowercase letters, separating the two sets of initials with a colon or a forward slash.

12. One or two lines below the identification line, add the enclosure notation, if applicable.

13. Two lines below the enclosure notation, insert the copy notation, if applicable.

14. Edit the letter.
   RATIONALE: *Make appropriate changes to clarify the meaning of the letter.*

15. Proofread and spell-check the letter.
   RATIONALE: *Every letter must be read again to ensure there are no errors.*

PROCEDURE 10-2 Writing an Interoffice Memo

Procedure Goal: To follow standard procedure for writing an interoffice memo

OSHA Guidelines: This procedure does not involve exposure to blood, body fluids, or tissue.

Materials: Computer with appropriate word processing software, plain paper, dictionaries or other professional references as needed

Method:

1. Gather all necessary materials and documents needed to compose the memo.

2. Decide whether the memo will be created "freehand" or with an existing template.
   RATIONALE: *If a template is to be used, it must be pulled up using the appropriate computer or EHR software prior to composing the document.*

3. If using a template, fill in the headings as listed with the appropriate information. If the memo is being created freehand, use the headings DATE:, TO:, FROM:, and RE: or SUBJECT:. Fill in each heading with the appropriate information.

4. Double- or triple-space after the memo headings or, if using a template, move to the body area of the memo and begin entering the information to be included in the memo.

5. Single-space the information within the memo and double-space between paragraphs. Use either the block or the indented paragraph format, depending on office policy.

6. Spell-check and proofread the document carefully, correcting errors as necessary.
   RATIONALE: *All professional documents must be perfect to reflect well on the writer and the office.*

PROCEDURE 10-3 Composing a Professional E-mail Message

Procedure Goal: To follow standard procedure for writing a professional e-mail message

OSHA Guidelines: This procedure does not involve exposure to blood, body fluids, or tissue.

Materials: Computer with e-mail (Internet) capabilities, dictionary or other professional references as needed

Method

1. Verify that the patient's medical record contains a signed "Consent to Use E-mail" form, allowing communication by this method.
   RATIONALE: *Because e-mail is not a secure form of communication, the office must have written approval to use this form of communication with the patient.*

2. Use a classic, easy-to-read font such as Times New Roman or Arial at 12–14 pt. Use black text only.
   RATIONALE: *Larger, crisp fonts are easy to read. Black text lends a professional appearance.*

3. If responding to a patient e-mail, open the e-mail and choose "Reply." If composing a new message, choose "New" to open a new e-mail document. Carefully enter the patient's e-mail address.
   RATIONALE: *It is imperative that the correct person receives the e-mail.*

4. Add the e-mail address to the office address book for easy reference, if it is not saved in the office EHR program.

5. If answering a patient e-mail, you may keep the subject line from the original message. If you are writing a new e-mail, enter a descriptive subject line.
   RATIONALE: *The subject line gives the receiver an idea of what the e-mail pertains to.*

6. Insert a salutation, using the patient's surname as you would with an ordinary letter.

7. Compose the body of the message, aligning the information with the left margin.

8. Double-space at the end of the message and enter your name, including a signature line with the practice information, and a phone number.
   RATIONALE: *It is important that the patient can easily reach you by methods other than e-mail if needed. Including the office information and phone number makes this easier for the patient.*

9. Spell-check and proofread the message carefully for any errors.
   RATIONALE: *Even though e-mail is considered less formal, you still represent the office, and the document must be professional in tone and free of errors.*

10. Click "Send" and wait for the message informing you the message has been sent.

11. If the message is returned as undeliverable, verify that the e-mail address was entered correctly. If necessary, correct the address and attempt delivery again.

12. If the message is returned a second time as undeliverable, contact the patient by phone or an alternate communication method to be sure that he or she receives the required information.

PROCEDURE 10-4 Composing an Electronic Patient Letter

Procedure Goal: To create and send an electronic letter to a patient using EHR software

OSHA Guidelines: This procedure does not involve exposure to blood, body fluids, or tissue.

Materials: EHR software program with letter templates, information necessary to compose the letter, dictionary or other professional references as needed

Method:
1. After verifying that there is a signed "Consent to Use E-mail" in the patient's record, access the *New* menu in the appropriate screen of the software program. Choose *New Letter Template.*

2. In the *RE:* window, insert the subject line, such as "Welcome to BWW Medical Associates, PC."
   RATIONALE: *The name gives the recipient an idea of what is included in the e-mail message.*

3. In the Text box, enter the body of the letter. Begin the letter with an introductory statement, such as "Welcome to BWW Medical Associates, and thank you for choosing us for your healthcare needs. We look forward to working with you."
   Enter all pertinent information required for the letter. If continuing a "welcome to the practice" letter, be sure to include the practice name, address, phone numbers, and website information, as well as names of the medical staff, office personnel, and office hours.

4. When you complete the letter, give the template an easily identifiable name, such as *Welcome New Patient Letter.*
   RATIONALE: *This makes it easy for all users to identify each template.*

5. Enter the appropriate patient's medical record. Select the *New* menu and choose the letter template you just created. Because you are in the patient's medical record, most software programs will automatically enter the patient's address in the inside address section of the letter. The standard greeting and closure also should be inserted from the medical record. Check to be sure the information listed is correct.
   RATIONALE: *Even though this is an electronic letter, the professional format remains the same as a written letter mailed to the patient. All information must be correct.*

6. Add a signature to the letter's signature block by using the "Sign" icon within the EHR program. Choose the correct provider/staff member from the drop-down list and verify that the correct signature is inserted.

7. If the signed "Consent to use E-mail" is in the patient's chart, the letter may be sent by clicking "Send." If the consent is not signed, print the letter and send it to the patient via USPS.
   RATIONALE: *Without a signed consent, e-mail is not an approved communication between the patient and medical office.*

8. Be sure to click "Save" or "Done" depending on the EHR software used, so that the template is saved for future use.

PROCEDURE 10-5 Sorting and Opening Mail

Procedure Goal: To follow a standard procedure for sorting, opening, and processing incoming office mail

OSHA Guidelines: This procedure does not involve exposure to blood, body fluids, or tissue.

Materials: Letter opener, date and time stamp (manual or automatic), stapler, paper clips, and adhesive notes

Method:
1. Check the address on each letter or package to be sure that it has been delivered to the correct location.

2. Sort the mail into piles according to priority and type of mail. Your system may include the following:
   - Top priority. This pile will contain any items that were sent for overnight delivery, in addition to items sent by registered or certified mail delivery. (Faxes and e-mail messages are also top priority.)
   - Second priority. This pile will include personal or confidential mail.
   - Third priority. This pile will contain all first-class mail, airmail, and Priority Mail® items. These items should be divided into payments received, insurance forms, reports, and other correspondence.
   - Fourth priority. This pile will consist of packages.
   - Fifth priority. This pile will contain magazines and newspapers.
   - Sixth priority. The last pile will include advertisements and catalogs.

3. Set aside all letters labeled "Personal" or "Confidential." Unless you have permission to open these letters, only the addressee should open them.

4. Arrange all the envelopes with the flaps facing up and away from you.

5. Tap the lower edge of the envelope to shift the contents to the bottom. This step helps to prevent cutting any of the contents when you open the envelope.

6. Open all the envelopes.
   RATIONALE: *It is more efficient to open all the envelopes first and then remove the contents.*

7. Remove and unfold the contents, making sure that nothing remains in the envelope.

8. Review each document and check the sender's name and address.
   - If the letter has no return address, save the envelope, or cut the address off the envelope, and tape it to the letter.
   - Check to see if the address matches the one on the envelope. If there is a difference, staple the envelope to the letter and make a note to verify the correct address with the sender.

9. Compare the enclosure notation on the letter with the actual enclosures to make sure that all items are included. Make a note to contact the sender if anything is missing.

10. Clip together each letter and its enclosures.

11. Check the date of the letter. If there is a significant delay between the date of the letter and the postmark, keep the envelope.
    RATIONALE: *It may be necessary to refer to the postmark in legal matters or cases of collection.*

12. If all contents appear to be in order, you can discard the envelope.

13. Review all bills and statements.
    - Make sure the amount enclosed is the same as the amount listed on the statement.
    - Make a note of any discrepancies.

14. Stamp each piece of correspondence with the date (and sometimes the time) to record its receipt. If possible, stamp each item in the same location, such as the upper-right corner.
    RATIONALE: *It may be necessary to refer to the date in legal matters or in cases of collection.*

SUMMARY OF LEARNING OUTCOMES

LEARNING OUTCOMES	KEY POINTS
10.1 Explain why well-written documents are important to the image of the medical practice.	Well-written, neatly prepared documents are one of the most important means of communicating a professional image for the medical practice.
10.2 Describe the types of document supplies that will be used in a medical office.	Document supplies used in a medical office include letterhead and matching plain bond paper; matching envelopes for professional correspondence; lesser bond envelopes of varying sizes for other types of correspondence; padded envelopes and data mailers; and labels and statements.
10.3 Outline the general guidelines to effective writing.	Know the type of person to whom you are writing. Know the purpose of the letter and be concise, brief, and specific in meeting that purpose, using clarity in the writing. Use active voice whenever possible, being polite and courteous. Check spelling, grammar, and accuracy. Avoid leaving "widows and orphans."
10.4 List and explain the purpose of different types of documents used in a medical office.	The different types of documents and correspondence used in a medical office include letters of referral; letters about scheduling, canceling, or rescheduling appointments; patient reports for

LEARNING OUTCOMES	KEY POINTS
	insurance companies; instructions for examinations or laboratory tests; answers to insurance or billing questions; and cover letters or form letters to order supplies, equipment, or magazine subscriptions. Also, internal documents like memos may be used to provide staff information.
10.5 Explain why it is important to have a signed written consent from the patient for e-mail communications.	All patient information, regardless of the form, is protected by HIPAA law and is to be guarded by the healthcare provider. E-mail is not considered a secure method of communication because information can be intercepted and received by someone who is not the intended recipient. Before undertaking e-mail communication with a patient, a signed written consent for e-mail communication must be on file.
10.6 Describe the tasks involved in editing and proofreading a document.	Editing involves checking a document for factual accuracy, logical flow, conciseness, clarity, and tone. Proofreading involves checking a document for grammatical, spelling, and formatting errors.
10.7 Outline the steps for preparing a completed letter for mailing.	After you have created, edited, and proofread a letter, it must be prepared for mailing. This preparation includes having the letter signed, preparing the envelope, and folding and inserting the letter into the envelope. Be sure to include any enclosures noted in the letter when folding it for insertion into the envelope.
10.8 Explain the differences among the types of mail services offered by the USPS.	The mail delivery options offered by the USPS include certified mail, return receipt requested, registered mail Priority Mail®, Priority Mail Express®, and delivery confirmation.
10.9 Describe the steps involved in processing incoming mail.	The steps involved in processing incoming mail include sorting and opening, recording, annotating, and distributing.

CASE STUDY CRITICAL THINKING

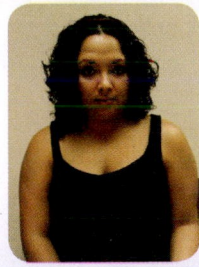

© McGraw-Hill Education

Recall Valarie from the beginning of the chapter. Now that you have completed the chapter, answer the following questions regarding her case.

1. Valarie's lab results and chest X-ray come back showing no acute pathology. You are to compose a letter to her per Dr. Buckwalter stating her results are normal and she should call the office for a flu shot when she feels better.

2. You have a "Consent to Use E-mail Communication" on file for this patient. Draft a short e-mail to her about her lab and chest X-ray results, requesting she contact the office by phone or e-mail to set up an appointment to receive a flu shot.

EXAM PREPARATION QUESTIONS

1. (LO 10.4) The _____ is the space around the edges of a form or letter that is left blank.
   a. Dateline
   b. Courtesy title
   c. Letterhead
   d. Margin
   e. Indentation

2. (LO 10.4) The complimentary closing is placed how many lines below the last line of the body?
   a. 2
   b. 6
   c. 4
   d. 3
   e. 5

3. (LO 10.8) What type of USPS mail service should be utilized to verify that the patient has received the document?
   a. Registered
   b. Certified
   c. Standard Post
   d. Certified with return receipt
   e. Media mail

4. (LO 10.6) Which of the following is spelled correctly?
   a. Professor
   b. Proffessur
   c. Profesur
   d. Profesor
   e. Proffesor

5. (LO 10.3) Which of the following is an example of a linking verb?
   a. Ran
   b. Review
   c. Be
   d. Try
   e. Type

6. (LO 10.9) Marking incoming mail to note important points for the recipient is called
   a. Opening
   b. Sorting
   c. Recording
   d. Annotating
   e. Distributing

7. (LO 10.4) Which letter format places the date, complimentary close, and signature block just to the right of center?
   a. Block
   b. Modified block
   c. Modified block with indented paragraphs
   d. Simplified
   e. Memo

8. (LO 10.5) Why is written consent required before using e-mail to communicate with a patient?
   a. The patient may not have a computer
   b. You must be sure you have a current e-mail address
   c. Parents may restrict e-mail use for their teenagers
   d. If the patient is not expecting e-mail from the office, it may be considered SPAM
   e. E-mail is not a secure form of communication

9. (LO 10.4) Which document format is traditionally used for interoffice communication?
   a. Simplified letter
   b. Block letter
   c. Modified-block letter
   d. Memo
   e. All of these

10. (LO 10.1) Better bond paper embossed with the practice name, address, and phone number is called
    a. Bonded
    b. Letterhead
    c. Envelope
    d. Label
    e. Lettering

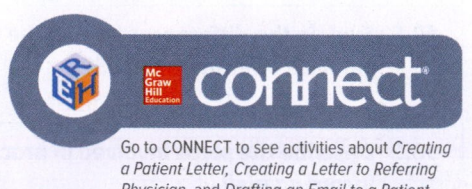

Go to CONNECT to see activities about *Creating a Patient Letter*, *Creating a Letter to Referring Physician*, and *Drafting an Email to a Patient.*

S O F T   S K I L L S   S U C C E S S

Recall Valarie from the case study at the beginning of the chapter. At the end of her appointment, Valarie asked to receive her test results by e-mail because she finds Dr. Buckwalter "gruff" and "unsympathetic" even though she trusts him.

1. What will you need from Valarie to honor her request to receive communications by e-mail?

2. How should you handle Valarie's comment about Dr. Buckwalter being "gruff and unsympathetic"?

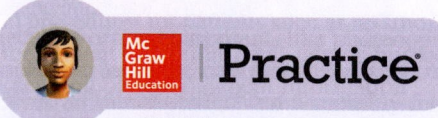

Go to PRACTICE MEDICAL OFFICE and complete the module Admin: Check In - Privacy and Liability.

Medical Records and Documentation

CASE STUDY

PATIENT INFORMATION

Patient Name	DOB	Allergies
Mohammad Nassar	5/17/20XX	NKA
Attending	**MRN**	**Other Information**
Elizabeth H. Williams, MD	423-90-687	Patient recently became sexually active.

Mohammad Nassar is a 16-year-old male who is new to the practice and comes to the office today for his annual physical examination. He has a known past medical history of asthma, which has been relatively stable until recently. He states when he arrives that he has been experiencing an increasing need for his rescue inhaler in the last several days. His

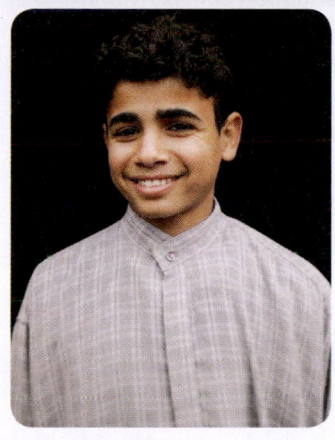

© David Sacks/Getty Images

mother has brought him to the appointment, but Mohammad has asked that she remain in the reception area during his appointment. She does give you a list of Mohammad's current asthma medications and the previously completed new patient documents.

Keep Mohammad (and his mother) in mind as you study this chapter. There will be questions at the end of the chapter based on the case study. The information in the chapter will help you answer these questions.

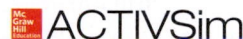

LEARNING OUTCOMES

After completing Chapter 11, you will be able to:

11.1 Explain the importance of patient medical records.

11.2 Identify the documents that constitute a patient medical record.

11.3 Compare SOMR, POMR, SOAP, and CHEDDAR medical record formats.

11.4 Recall the six Cs of charting, giving an example of each.

11.5 Describe the need for neatness, timeliness, accuracy, and professional tone in patient records.

11.6 Illustrate the correct procedure for correcting and updating a medical record.

11.7 Describe the steps in responding to a written request for release of medical records.

KEY TERMS

audit

CHEDDAR

demographic

documentation

noncompliant

objective

patient record/chart

problem-oriented medical record (POMR)

review of systems

sign

Subjective, Objective, Assessment, Plan (SOAP)

source-oriented medical record (SOMR)

subjective

symptom

transcription

V.P.1 Use feedback techniques to obtain patient information including:

    (a) reflection

    (b) restatement

    (c) clarification

V.P.11 Report relevant information concisely and accurately

VI.C.4 Define types of information contained in the patient's medical record

VI.C.5 Identify methods of organizing the patients medical record based on:

    (a) problem-oriented medical record (POMR)

    (b) source-oriented medical record (SOMR)

VI.C.6 Identify equipment and supplies needed for medical records in order to:

    (a) Create

    (b) Maintain

    (c) Store

VI.C.7 Describe filing indexing rules

VI.P.3 Create a patient's medical record

X.C.3 Describe the components of the Health Information Portability and Accountability Act (HIPAA)

X.P.2 Apply HIPAA rules in regards to:

    (a) privacy

    (b) release of information

X.P.3 Document patient care accurately in the medical record

X.A.2 Protect the integrity of the medical record

3. Medical Terminology

    d. Define and use medical abbreviations when appropriate and acceptable

4. Medical Law and Ethics

    a. Follow documentation guidelines

    b. Institute federal and state guidelines when releasing medical records or information

7. Records Management

    c. Comply with federal, state, and local laws relating to exchange of information and describe elements of meaningful use and reports generated

8. Administrative Procedures

    a. Gather and process documents

    f. Display professionalism through written and verbal communications

▶ Introduction

In your career as a medical assistant, a major part of your role will be documenting and maintaining patient health (or medical) records. These records detail the evaluation, management, and treatment given to the patient. Patient records are critical to the patient's care. Without accurate and complete patient records, medical care can easily be compromised with the potential for (unintentional) harm to the patient.

Patient health records have many sections that describe individual facets of every patient, including

- Personal information or data.
- Physical and mental conditions.
- Medical history.
- Current medical care.
- Future medical care if the patient is referred to other physicians or for further testing.

In this chapter, you will learn how to carefully manage patient records with the understanding that if the medical care is not documented, in a legal sense, the medical care did not occur at all.

▶ The Importance of Medical Records
LO 11.1

Patient medical (or health) **records,** also known as **charts,** contain important information about a patient's medical history and present condition. Patient records serve dual roles as communication tools and legal documents. They also play a role in patient and staff education and may be used for quality control and research. Patient records come in paper or electronic format. Adopting electronic health records in lieu of the traditional paper format is extremely common. This chapter will focus on the paper record format and the next chapter,

Electronic Health Records, will focus on the electronic format. Regardless of which format is used, the medical record is initiated by the medical assistant or another staff member and is consistently updated whenever the patient has contact with the office. As stated in the *Legal and Ethical Issues* chapter, it is important to remember that although the medical facility owns the physical record (electronic or paper), the patient owns the information contained within that record as his personal health information. So the patient has control over who may access that information.

The patient health record provides physicians and other medical care providers with all the important information, observations, and opinions recorded about a patient. The healthcare professional can read the complete patient medical history and information about previous treatments and outcomes. With the patient's permission, the information in the records also can be sent to other physicians or healthcare specialists if the patient needs further treatment, changes healthcare providers, or moves to a new location. The information recorded in the medical record provides a "map" or plan to follow for the continuity of patient care. It also serves as supporting documentation for billing and coding purposes, and as a legal document, it is admissible in a court of law. All medical records should include the following general information about the patient:

- Address and phone number
- Occupation
- Medical history
- Current complaint or condition
- Healthcare needs
- Medical treatment plan or services received
- Radiology and laboratory reports (when performed)
- Response to care

Standard paper patient records are usually assembled for new patients well before their actual use. The medical assistant is responsible for making sure adequate patient records are prepared and available to meet the practice's needs.

Legal Guidelines for Patient Records

In addition to being essential documents for patient care management and treatment, patient records are also important for legal reasons. As a general rule, if information is not documented, no one can prove that an event or a procedure took place. Medical records are used in lawsuits and malpractice cases to support a patient's claim of malpractice against a provider, as well as to support the provider in defense against a claim. As stated in the *Legal and Ethical Issues* chapter, legally, medical records must be retained for 7 years (for pediatric records, 7 years from the age of majority, which in most states is age 18). Remember, however, that because the Federal False Claims Act requires patient financial records to be kept for 10 years, many legal experts suggest that medical records also be kept for 10 years. This is because the medical record backs up the information within the financial record.

All medical care, evaluations, and instructions the provider gives to the patient must be documented. **Documentation** is the process of recording information in the medical record. Because every patient chart is a legal document, every entry must be clear, accurate, legible, dated, and signed. In offices that utilize paper records, some require records to be written in blue ink, so that it is easy to recognize whether the record is an original or a copy. Before making any entry, always consider how the patient record would present if it were called into a court of law for review. Never insert an opinion in a patient medical record. For instance, you would not write in a medical record "The patient appears to be drunk." Instead, "The patient's balance is unsteady and there appears to be the smell of alcohol on his breath." would be appropriate. If you are unsure how to document a situation appropriately, speak to the physician or your supervisor for appropriate guidance. In this case, you might wish to relay your observations to the physician and allow her to make the appropriate documentation.

As discussed in the *Legal and Ethical Issues* chapter, it is also very important to document when a patient is noncompliant. **Noncompliant** is the medical term used to describe a patient who does not follow the medical advice he or she receives. After a clear record has been made of the directions given to a patient for optimum health, it is essential to record the level of patient compliance. For example, after you have instructed a patient on how to collect a 24-hour urine specimen, you would write in her chart "Patient stated she understood all directions regarding collection of 24-hour urine specimen. Written instructions also given to patient." If it is determined that a patient did *not* follow the medical instructions or advice, it is then essential to chart this as well. The physician may wish to withdraw from the care of a patient because of the patient's noncompliance. However, without proper and accurate documentation of the patient's noncompliance, the physician may not be able to withdraw care without becoming legally liable. Additionally, documented noncompliance can be used in the physician's defense in a malpractice suit if it can be proven that, due to patient noncompliance, the physician was not solely responsible for inadequate medical care or results. Please refer to the *Legal and Ethical Issues* chapter for further details on noncompliance and proper steps for withdrawal from patient care.

Standards for Records

Records that are complete, accurate, and well documented can be convincing evidence that a practitioner provided appropriate care. On the other hand, altered, incomplete, inaccurate, or illegible records may imply that the care provided by the practitioner is below standard.

It is important to understand that the licensed practitioners in a practice are not the only people who document (or chart) in the practice medical records. However, it is equally important to remember that under *respondeat superior* (see the *Legal and Ethical Issues* chapter), if an employee of the practice charts inappropriately or inaccurately in a patient's medical record, in a court of law, the practitioner will also be held responsible for that action. For instance, if a medical assistant documents an erroneously high glucose level and the patient is given too much insulin based on that result and then ends up in insulin shock, the practitioner will be held responsible. All records, both medical and financial, are the physician's responsibility. As the office medical assistant, you are responsible to the patient and the practitioner for both the medical and administrative procedures you perform and the accurate recording of those procedures.

Additional Uses of Patient Records

Patient records serve as ongoing references about individual patients' medical care. They also provide valuable information for patient education, quality of treatment, and research.

Patient Education Patient health records can be used to educate patients about their own conditions and treatment plans. The healthcare provider can point out how test results have changed or how the patient's general health has improved or worsened. The provider can also emphasize the importance of following treatment instructions. The medical assistant may also use some of this information to educate the patient about his condition or its management. Records can also be used to educate the healthcare staff about unusual medical conditions, patient progress, or treatment plan results.

Quality of Care Patient medical records are frequently used to evaluate the quality of care and treatment a facility or specific physician provides. Auditing groups, such as peer review organizations or The Joint Commission (TJC), may review medical records to monitor whether the care provided and the fees charged meet accepted standards. Records also provide statistics for healthcare analysis and future healthcare plans and policy decisions.

Research Medical records also play an important role in medical research. For example, a medical research team may be testing a new antihypertensive drug with volunteers who fit a certain medical category—perhaps men between the ages of 45 and 54 who have high blood pressure. Carefully kept records are valuable sources of data about patient responses, behavior, symptoms, side effects, and outcomes.

Information in charts may spur researchers to begin a study. For example, the records may show that 80% of all patients taking a particular heart medication experience dizziness. Researchers can investigate why this reaction might be happening.

▶ Contents of Patient Medical Records   LO 11.2

As the office medical assistant, you will fill out a record for each new patient who comes to the office. Although each medical office has its own forms and physical chart type, in general, all medical records must contain certain standard information. This standard chart information covers a variety of carefully detailed notes and facts about a patient, from his medical history to the physician's diagnosis and comments on follow-up care. Let's look at each form in more detail here.

Patient Registration Form

When a new patient makes an appointment with the office, certain basic **demographic** information—specific information required of a population—must be obtained: in this case, the basic information required of all patients seen in the medical practice. Very often, the first document a new patient completes is the registration form. Depending on practice policy, the registration form may be mailed to the patient prior to the first visit with the expectation that the patient will complete it prior to the visit and bring it with her at the time of her first appointment. Some facilities have patients complete their registration online before their first appointment. Other offices ask the patient to arrive for the first appointment 15–20 minutes early and complete the registration form at that time. Although the format may vary from office to office, the information requested in the registration form itself is fairly uniform and generally includes

- Date of current (first) visit.
- Patient's legal name and physical address (PO box may be listed as the mailing address, but the physical address is also required).
- Phone numbers including area code (home, cell, work). E-mail address also may be requested, but written permission must be received prior to e-mailing the patient.
- Patient's date of birth (DOB), sex, marital status, and Social Security number.
- Medical insurance information, employer name/address, and patient occupation.
- Emergency contact name, relationship, and phone number.
- Primary care physician (if specialty office) and referral source.

The completed registration form (with front and back copies of the patient's insurance card) is the base document for each patient's financial record. Patient financial and medical records are separated into two distinct records and are filed separately. Because of the importance of this "base" demographic document, review it carefully when the patient returns it to you to be sure it is filled out completely and properly. Each time the patient returns to the office, query the patient whether her address, phone, or insurance information, and/or e-mail address (if the patient has an e-mail consent form on file) have changed since her last visit, so that the office information is always current. Figure 11-1 is an example of a patient registration form.

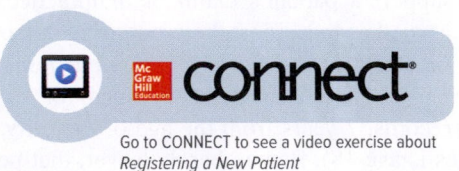

Go to CONNECT to see a video exercise about *Registering a New Patient*

Patient Medical History

The medical history form, the second part of the registration process, contains the patient's past medical history (including illnesses, surgeries, known allergies, and current medications), family medical history, and social and occupational

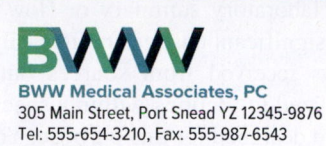

BWW Medical Associates, PC
305 Main Street, Port Snead YZ 12345-9876
Tel: 555-654-3210, Fax: 555-987-6543
Web: BWWAssociates.com

Paul F. Buckwalter, MD
Alexis N. Whalen, MD
Elizabeth H. Williams, MD

Patient Registration

Patient Information

Name: _____   Today's date: _____

Address: _____

City: _____   State: _____   Zip code: _____

Telephone (Home): _____ (Work): _____ (Cell): _____

Birthdate: _____   Age: _____   Sex: M F   Marital status: M S W D

Social Security number: _____   Employer: _____   Occupation: _____

Primary physician: _____

Referred by: _____

Person to contact in emergency: _____

Emergency telephone: _____

Special needs: _____

Responsible Party

Party responsible for payment: Self   Spouse   Parent   Other

Name (If other than self): _____

Address: _____

City: _____   State: _____   Zip code: _____

Primary Insurance

Primary medical insurance: _____

Insured party: Self   Spouse   Parent   Other

ID#/Social Security no.: _____   Group/Plan no.: _____

Name (If other than self): _____

Address: _____

City: _____   State: _____   Zip code: _____

Secondary Insurance

Secondary medical insurance: _____

Insured party: Self   Spouse   Parent   Other

ID#/Social Security no.: _____   Group/Plan no.: _____

Name (If other than self): _____

Address: _____

City: _____   State: _____   Zip code: _____

FIGURE 11-1   Typical patient registration form.

history (including diet, exercise, smoking, and use of alcohol or drugs). Usually, the history form also includes a section for the patient to describe the history of the condition or complaint that is the reason for her visit. This section is known as the *history of present illness,* or *HPI.* Medicare and managed care plans now require that the patient's complaint be entered into the medical record. This primary problem is also known as the *chief complaint,* and it should be recorded in the medical records using the patient's own words, if at all possible.

The patient medical history form—similar to the patient registration form—serves as the base document for the patient's medical record. Because of this, it should contain as much information about the patient's medical history as possible. In some offices, the medical assistant reviews the medical history form with the patient to make sure it is complete. If this task is part of your job, be sure to perform this initial interview in a private location (Figure 11-2). Make sure there are no blanks and, if you are assisting the patient with filling

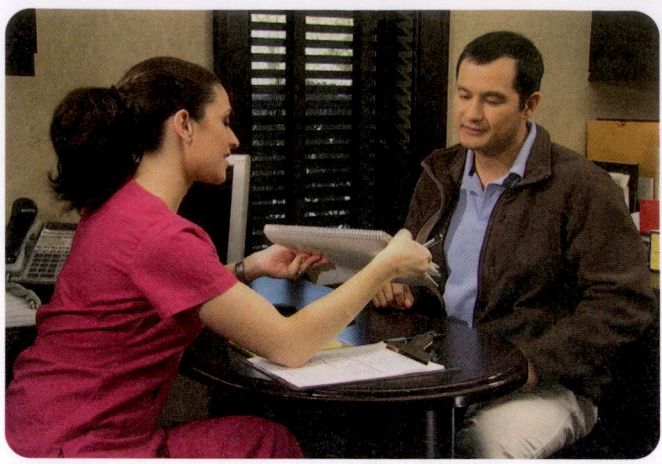

FIGURE 11-2 Perform the initial patient interview in a private location.
© McGraw-Hill Education

out the document, be sure to use his own words as much as possible. For example, when asking the patient about alcohol consumption, you might document "Patient states that . . . ," filling in the blanks using the exact words of the patient. When the interview is completed, be sure to ask the patient, "Is there anything else you would like me to share with the physician for you?" Be sure to document any positive responses. If the patient brought any medical documents with him from previous healthcare providers, including lab, X-ray, or test results, be sure to attach them to the patient's medical record for the physician's review.

In most offices, the physician will use the medical history form as the "springboard" for a discussion with the patient as to the reason for her appointment, and to get to know a little bit about each new patient. See Figure 11-3.

Physical Examination Form

Many times, a form is used to record the patient **review of systems,** often abbreviated ROS, and the results of a general physical examination. The review of systems is an "inventory" of the body obtained by the healthcare provider through a series of questions. The purpose of this review is to identify any signs or symptoms the patient is experiencing that reveal information about an illness or condition. As an "oral examination," the ROS should not be confused with the actual physical exam. The use of a physical examination form ensures consistency in the examination format and minimizes the risk of "forgotten documentation." In most offices, the physician will perform both the ROS and the physical examination, but as the medical assistant, you may perform and document the patient's vital signs (temperature, pulse, BP, respiration, and height and weight) on the physical examination form for the physician. Figure 11-4 shows a typical ROS and physical examination form.

Results of Laboratory and Other Tests

Test results include findings from tests performed in the office and those received from other physicians, hospitals,

independent laboratories, or other outside sources. Some offices use a laboratory summary or flow sheet to help the doctor detect significant changes more easily.

Test results received from sources outside the practice are best organized in sections within a specific section of the medical record designed for this purpose. You will learn more about arranging information within the medical chart a bit later in the chapter.

Documents from Other Sources

Incoming records from other sources also must be entered and stored in the patient's medical record. If a patient has requested documents from another physician or hospital to be sent to your office, a copy of the patient's written request authorizing the release of these records to your office from its original source also must be included in the medical record.

Diagnosis and Treatment Plan

The patient's diagnosis must be recorded in the medical record, along with the physician's proposed treatment plan. The treatment plan may include treatment options, the final treatment plan, instructions to the patient, and any medications prescribed. The licensed practitioner (MD, DO, PA, NP) also may include any specific comments or impressions regarding the patient and his care on record. All of this information is recorded for every patient visit in documents known as progress notes (Figure 11-5).

Operative Reports, Follow-up Visits, and Telephone Calls

Continuation of the record lasts as long as the patient is under the practitioner's care. All procedures, surgeries, follow-up care, notes, phone calls, and other patient contacts by the office staff should be recorded in the patient's medical record. Multiple progress notes may be added to the medical record as needed. A discussion on charting methods will follow later in the chapter. Depending on office policy, phone calls and between-visit contacts may be inserted in the record in chronological order, or a log of telephone contacts may be kept separately in the patient record.

Hospital Discharge Summaries

The hospital discharge summary generally includes information that summarizes the reason the patient entered the hospital; tests, procedures, and operations performed in the hospital; medications administered to the patient; and the disposition (outcome) of the case. Elements of the summary may include the following:

- Date of admission
- History of present illness (HPI)
- Date of discharge
- Admitting diagnosis
- Surgeries, procedures, or hospital course (treatment obtained in the hospital)
- Complications (if any)

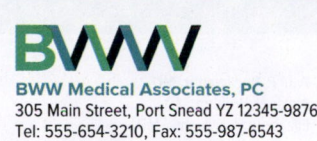

BWW Medical Associates, PC
305 Main Street, Port Snead YZ 12345-9876
Tel: 555-654-3210, Fax: 555-987-6543
Web: BWWAssociates.com

Paul F. Buckwalter, MD
Alexis N. Whalen, MD
Elizabeth H. Williams, MD

Patient Medical History

Name: _____ Age: _____ Sex: _____ MS: S M W D

Address: _____

Occupation: _____

Reason for visit: _____

History of present illness: _____

Allergies: _____

Current medications: _____

Cigarettes _____ Alcohol _____ Drugs _____

Past medical history:
Surgeries and dates: _____

Illnesses/Immunizations:

Chickenpox _____ Measles _____ Rubella _____ Mumps _____ DTP _____ TD _____ Polio _____

Whooping cough _____ Flu _____ Pneumonia _____ Hepatitis B _____

Other _____

Females: Age first period _____ LMP _____ # pregnancies _____ # children _____

Family history:

Relationship	Age If Alive	Medical Issues	Age at Death	Cause of Death
Mother				
Father				
Brothers				
Sisters				

Have you or an immediate family member (mother, father, sister, brother, grandparent) been diagnosed with:

Cancer _____ Location _____ Whom _____ Hypertension _____

Thyroid disorder _____ Heart disease _____ GI disorder _____ Blood disorder _____

Depression _____ Nervous disorder _____ Asthma _____ Migraines _____

FIGURE 11-3 Example of a patient medical history form.

- Patient instructions for follow-up care after hospital discharge
- Discharging physician's signature

Consent Forms

As discussed in the *Legal and Ethical Issues* chapter, signed informed consents must be obtained when any procedure is being performed on a patient. An example of such a form is shown in Figure 11-6. In order for any consent to be considered "informed," the patient must understand the treatment offered and the possible outcomes or side effects of the treatment. The patient also should be informed of the possible outcome if the patient receives no treatment, as well as be informed of any alternative treatments and possible risks. Once the patient signs the consent form, he may withdraw consent at

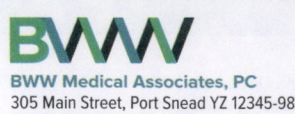

BWW Medical Associates, PC
305 Main Street, Port Snead YZ 12345-9876
Tel: 555-654-3210, Fax: 555-987-6543
Web: BWWAssociates.com

Paul F. Buckwalter, MD
Alexis N. Whalen, MD
Elizabeth H. Williams, MD

Review of Systems and Physical Examination
ROS

HEENT _____

CV _____

Resp _____

GI _____

GU _____

MS _____

Integ _____

Neuro _____

Psych _____

Endo _____

Allergic/Immuno _____

Physical Examination

T _____ P _____ BP _____ R _____ HT _____ WT _____

Appearance _____ Skin _____ Mucous membrane _____

Eyes _____ Vision _____ Pupils _____ Fundus _____

Ears _____ Nose _____ Throat _____

Chest _____ Breasts _____

Heart _____

Lungs _____

Abdomen _____

Genitalia _____

Rectum _____

Pelvic _____

Extremities _____ Pulses _____

Lymph nodes _____ Neck _____ Axilla _____ Inguinal _____ Abd _____

Neuro _____

FIGURE 11-4 Review of systems and physical examination form.

any time prior to the treatment being carried out. Signatures on informed consent documents must be witnessed; medical assistants, as members of the office medical team, are allowed to act as witnesses for such documents.

Correspondence with or About the Patient

All written correspondence from the patient or from other providers, laboratories, or independent healthcare agencies must be kept in the patient's medical record. Each piece of

correspondence should be marked or stamped with the date the medical office received the document.

Information Received by Fax

Some information—like laboratory results, practitioner comments, or correspondence—may be received by fax or even secure (encrypted) e-mail transmission if the information is required rapidly. If possible, request that an original of any faxed document be mailed to the office as a final record.

PROGRESS NOTES

Patient Name *Sylvia Gonzales*   **Date of Birth** *9/1/XX*   **MRN** *341-73-792*

Prob. No. or Letter	Date	Subjective	Objective	Assess	Plans
1	11/11/XX	*Patient states, "I have had a fever and a sore throat for the past two days"*			
			Vital signs: T 101.1 P 96 R 24 BP 124/76 Weight: 155 Height: 5' 7"		
			General: patient seems alert. HEENT: sclera clear. Pharynx red with pus pockets noted. Heart: regular w/o murmur Lungs: clear to auscultation and percussion. Abdomen: negative for tenderness		
				Strep throat	
					1. prescription for Amoxicillin, 1 tsp q8h for 10 days
					2. schedule appointment for three weeks from today's date for repeat testing

Alexis N. Whalen, MD (Attending Physician)

Kaylyn R. Haddix, RMA (AMT)

Date: November 11, 20XX

FIGURE 11-5 Typical progress note using SOAP format.

E-mails may be printed out and inserted into the patient medical record. When doing so, be sure they are printed so that the sender information and date/time are included in the printout.

Dating and Initialing You must be careful not only to date everything you put into the patient chart but also to initial each entry. This system makes it easy to identify who in the practice is responsible for each entry. In many practices, the practitioner initials or stamps reports before they are filed to prove that patient's licensed provider saw them prior to filing.

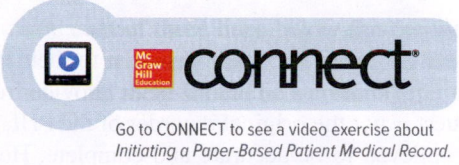

Go to CONNECT to see a video exercise about *Initiating a Paper-Based Patient Medical Record.*

Maintaining Confidentiality

As always, every patient's personal health information, whether coming into the office or being transmitted to or from another location, is covered by the HIPAA privacy and Security Rule and must be kept confidential. As per HIPAA, patients have the following specific rights regarding their protected health information (PHI) and their medical records:

1. *The right to notice of privacy practices.* Because it is unlikely that your patients will be reading federal laws, the law states that it is your responsibility to give them a copy of the laws that protect them concerning their PHI. Patients must receive a written notice of privacy practices on their first visit to a healthcare provider. They should sign a form stating they have received this information. This signed form must be carefully filed in the patient's medical record.

2. *The right to limit or request restriction on their PHI and its use and disclosure.* This means that patients can limit how your office uses their medical information and how much of that information is shared. For example, a patient with a history of sexually transmitted infection may not wish to have that information released to the orthopedic physician who is setting his broken arm. It is not necessary. In general, only the minimal amount of patient information should be released to meet the current needs of the patient. This is called the "Need to Know" general rule.

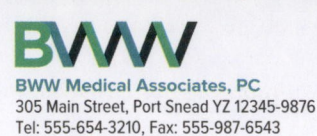

BWW Medical Associates, PC
305 Main Street, Port Snead YZ 12345-9876
Tel: 555-654-3210, Fax: 555-987-6543
Web: BWWAssociates.com

Paul F. Buckwalter, MD
Alexis N. Whalen, MD
Elizabeth H. Williams, MD

**CONSENT TO OPERATION, ADMINISTRATION OF ANESTHETICS,
AND RENDERING OF OTHER MEDICAL SERVICE**

Patient: _____ DOB: _____

1. I authorize and direct _____ with the associates and assistants
of his/her choice to perform upon myself the following procedure:

_____

_____

_____

If any unforeseen conditions arise in the course of this procedure or in the post-procedure period, calling on their judgment for other procedures or surgery, I further request and authorize them to do whatever is deemed advisable for my health and well-being.

2. The risks and alternative aspects of autologous blood transfusions (receiving my own blood donated prior to surgery), designated blood transfusions (donated in advance by family/friends for my use), or homologous blood transfusions (from the general donor population) have been explained to me. I understand autologous and designated transfusions can be accommodated only for nonemergency surgeries.

6. I certify that I understand the above consent to surgery and that the explanations referred to have been made to me.

Signature _____ Date: _____

Witness _____ Date: _____

FIGURE 11-6 An informed consent form must be completed and signed by the patient prior to any procedure being performed.

Always read record release requests carefully. Only the information requested and/or the date range required for that information should be released, nothing more.

3. *The right to confidential communications.* This means that patients can request to receive PHI in a manner other than during a medical appointment. For example, your patients may request that you call them at a variety of numbers, including home, work, or cell phone number. The patient does not have to explain the request. The law says you must make a reasonable effort to communicate with the patient in a confidential manner as the patient requests.

4. *The right to inspect and obtain a copy of their PHI.* This means that patients have a right to request and receive a copy of their own medical records. There are a few exceptions to this rule; however, in general, the medical assistant receives and processes all patient requests for medical records. It is important to always follow the protocols established in your office for medical record copying. It is considered an acceptable practice to act on a request within 30 days of the request and to charge a reasonable fee to cover the expense for copying supplies and labor.

5. *The right to request an amendment to their PHI.* Patients have the right to request an amendment to their PHI. The request may be denied if the healthcare provider receiving the request is not the original recorder of the PHI, or if the PHI is believed to be accurate and complete. Healthcare providers have the right to require that a request to amend a record be made in writing. All requests for amendment and response must be carefully documented and filed in the medical chart.

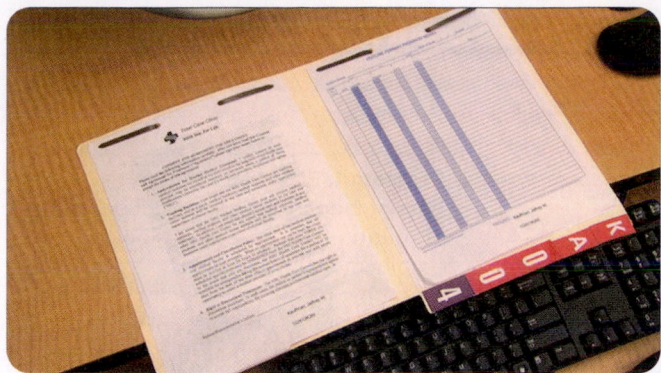

FIGURE 11-7 A newly assembled paper patient medical record.
© McGraw-Hill Education

6. *The right to know if their PHI has been disclosed and why.* For example, PHI is disclosed when a specialist or other doctor is seen. Practitioners are required to keep a written record of every disclosure made of a patient's PHI. A written record of any request by the patient for this information and the response of the healthcare provider must also be kept. This information is usually filed in the patient's medical record. When making a disclosure of information, always record the date of the disclosure, the name and address of the person receiving the PHI, a brief summary of the information released, and the purpose of the disclosure.

The HIPAA Privacy and Security Rule as it relates to all aspects of patient care, including the care and protection of patient medical records, is covered in detail in the *Legal and Ethical Issues* chapter. Now that you have learned about the forms that may be found in a medical record, Procedure 11-1, found at the end of the chapter, will outline how to assemble a new patient paper medical record. See Figure 11-7.

▶ Types of Medical Records LO 11.3

The process of documenting information in medical records can be accomplished using several formats. You should be familiar with the approaches to documenting patient information and learn to be comfortable using each approach. The most common methods are the source-oriented and problem-oriented medical records.

Source-Oriented Medical Records

In the **source-oriented medical record (SOMR)** approach, patient information is arranged within the medical record according to who supplied the data. The SOMR (sometimes called the conventional method) includes areas for data from the patient, treating physician, specialist, laboratory, hospital, or other locations to document in the record. If a specific form is used to attach these documents to the medical record, it often contains a space for patient remarks, followed by a section for the physician's comments. Often, in a SOMR, one side of the record (often the left side) is used for the practitioner's notes, which are listed in reverse chronological order. The other side of the chart contains records from the other listed sources, with like sources grouped together in reverse chronological order.

The practitioner's notes describe all problems and treatments on the same form in simple chronological order. For example, a patient's broken wrist would be recorded on the same form as her stomach ulcer. Although easy to initiate and maintain, this system presents some difficulty in tracking the progress of a specific ailment. For instance, in order for anyone to find information on the patient's stomach ulcer, the approximate time frame of the diagnosis would need to be known so that the chronological record can be searched. Another downfall of this type of record can occur if the patient has a recurrence of a problem. Because of the chronological nature of the record, if the patient develops a second stomach ulcer 2–3 years down the road, the first episode and the second one will be filed in separate locations, causing more searching to locate the related "past medical history."

Problem-Oriented Medical Records

One way to overcome the disadvantages of the source-oriented approach is to use the **problem-oriented medical record (POMR)** system. This approach, developed by Lawrence L. Weed, MD, makes it easier for the physician to keep track of a patient's progress. The information in a POMR includes the following items: database; problem list; educational, diagnostic, and treatment plan; and progress notes. Let's take a look at each of these components in a bit more detail.

Database The database includes a record of the patient's past medical history; information gained in the initial interview with the patient (for example, "Patient unemployed for the second time in past 12 months"); all findings and results from the physical examinations (such as "Pulse 105 bpm, BP 210/80"); and any tests, X-rays, and other procedure results.

Problem List Each condition or diagnosis a patient has is listed separately and given its own number, including the date of onset. Each "problem" is then identified by its number throughout the record. Work-related, social, or family problems that may be affecting the patient's health also may be listed in this problem list. For instance, the problem list for the example patient who is unemployed might include "Severe stomach pain, worse at night and after eating, has begun since the patient became unemployed for the second time."

You can alert the doctor to the fact that the patient has lost two jobs within 1 year. Such radical life changes can often provoke strong physical (and psychological) reactions. In this patient's case, the elevated blood pressure may be related to the job losses, and stress may be causing the stomach pain.

When you document problems, be careful to distinguish between signs and symptoms. **Signs** are **objective,** or external, factors—like blood pressure, rashes, or swelling— that can be seen or felt by the doctor or measured by an instrument. **Symptoms** are **subjective,** or internal, conditions felt by the patient—like pain, headache, or nausea—but are not necessarily apparent in a physical examination. Together, signs and symptoms help clarify a patient's problem and can help lead to a diagnosis.

Educational, Diagnostic, and Treatment Plan Each problem should have a detailed educational, diagnostic, and treatment summary in the record. The summary contains diagnostic workups, treatment plans, and instructions for the patient. Following are two examples. For the first problem, the summary areas are marked. Can you identify the areas of the second problem?

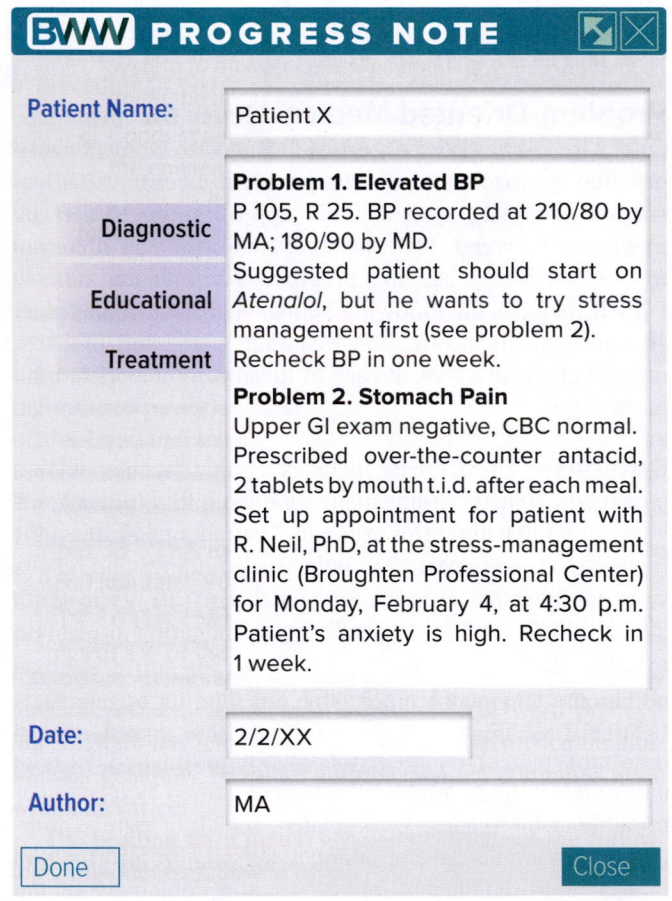

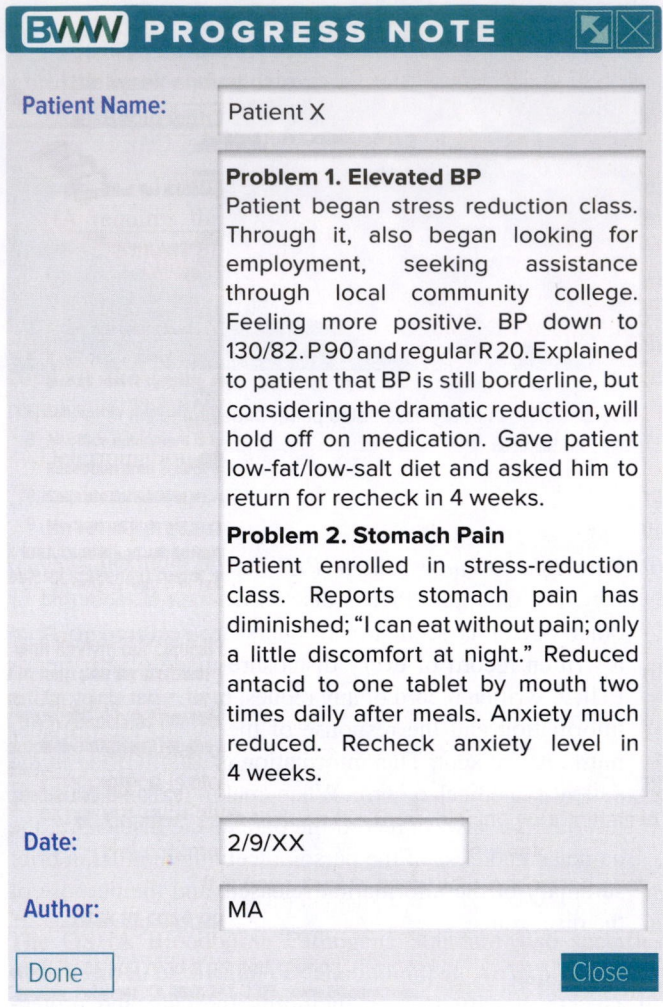

Progress Notes Progress notes are entered for each problem listed in the initial record. The documentation always includes—in chronological order—the patient's condition, complaints, problems, treatment, and responses to care. Using the same two problems, here are two examples.

SOAP Documentation

Many medical offices using the POMR format also emphasize the **Subjective, Objective, Assessment, and Plan (SOAP)** approach to documentation, which provides an orderly series of steps for dealing with any medical case. Information is documented in the record in the following order.

1. **S:** Subjective data come from the patient; the patient describes his or her signs and symptoms and supplies any other opinions or comments about the current problem.

2. **O:** Objective data come from the physician, examinations, and test results.

3. **A:** Assessment is the diagnosis or impression of a patient's problem.

4. **P:** Plan of action includes treatment options, chosen treatment, medications, tests, consultations, patient education, and follow-up.

Regardless of whether your office keeps SOMR or POMR charts, the SOAP format for documentation can still be used. It is a popular documentation model because it allows each type of data to be located within each documented note easily, instead of searching the entire entry. Figures 11-5 and 11-8 show examples of the SOAP note format using a preprinted form. The shaded columns noting where the subjective, objective, assessment, and plan information are to begin makes finding specific information easier for the user.

Note that in Figure 11-8, abbreviations such as RLQ (right lower quadrant), F (Fahrenheit), BP (blood pressure), and T (temperature) are used. If you choose to use abbreviations when charting in a medical record, use only approved medical abbreviations. To reduce confusion in medical records, abbreviations are being used less often, except for those that are very clear in meaning. Currently, The Joint Commission (TJC) does not produce an approved list of abbreviations, but it does state that the following should NOT be used when charting:

- The symbols ">" and "<"
- All abbreviations for medication names
- Apothecary units
- The symbols "@"
- The abbreviation "cc"
- The abbreviation "μg"

Before charting in the office medical record, check the policies and procedures manual to see if your office has specific abbreviations that are not to be used in patient medical records. The purpose of the patient medical record is to document information so that all who have access to the information clearly know what is being documented. If you are questioning if an abbreviation may be misunderstood, it is better to write out the word for the sake of clarity. See Appendix II *Abbreviations and Symbols Commonly Used in Medical Notations* at the end of the book for a list of the common abbreviations used in medical records.

CHEDDAR Format

The **CHEDDAR** format of medical records documentation takes the SOAP format further, breaking it down into smaller components. CHEDDAR stands for

1. **C:** Chief complaint, presenting problems, subjective statements.
2. **H:** History; past medical, family, and social histories as well as the history of presenting problem (HPI) and any other contributing information.
3. **E:** Examination, including extent of body systems examined.
4. **D:** Details of problem and complaints.
5. **D:** Drugs and dosage—for example, a list of current medications, including dosage and frequency.
6. **A:** Assessment of the diagnostic process and the impression (diagnosis) made by the practitioner.
7. **R:** Return visit information or referral, if applicable.

Figure 11-9 shows you an example of a medical record note using the CHEDDAR format.

PROGRESS NOTES

Patient Name: Mohammad Nassar   Date of Birth: 05/17/XX   MRN: 423-90-687

Prob. No. or Letter	Date	Subjective	Objective	Assess	Plans
1	6/16/XX	Patient complaining of pain in RLQ. Has been running fever between 100.5 F and 101.3F since Sunday morning. Has queasy feeling in stomach and has been unable to eat since yesterday morning.	BP 125/76. T 101.2F. Abdominal exam reveals rebound tenderness and tenderness in RLQ	Appendicitis	1. Immediate admission 2. Emergency appendectomy

Elizabeth H. Williams MD

FIGURE 11-8 Example of SOAP note using preprinted form.

Documentation and the 6 Cs of Charting

LO 11.4

Now that you have an understanding of the basic formats used in documentation, or "charting," let's discuss the types of information that will require your new expertise.

Updating Medical Forms

You have already learned that you may be asked to assist new patients with completion of the patient registration and medical history forms. You also will be updating these forms as inevitable changes take place in the lives of your patients—new addresses, changes in marital status, the birth or adoption of a child, and changes in insurance coverage. All of these changes require updates to the patient registration information. In order to make such changes in a paper record, generally you retrieve the chart from the files and cross out the old information, using one line with a note stating the information has changed. You then add the date and your initials. Depending on the extent of the change, the new information may simply be written by hand as near as possible to the original location or, more likely, a note is made to see the "updated" registration sheet. On the new sheet, the current date will be given, the updated information will be neatly typed into the required spaces, and the new registration sheet will be inserted into the appropriate location of the medical record.

Documenting Test Results

Every time a patient has an X-ray or a lab test, or a letter arrives from a specialist about the patient, it must be inserted into the medical record. Be sure to follow the office policy in placing these items in the same location in each medical record and always in reverse chronological order—which means the most current result will always be on top. If your office uses a lab flow sheet, you also may be required to record the results on a separate test summary sheet in the chart. When doing so, be extremely careful to record the results accurately and in the correct location—the patient's health and treatment will depend upon it.

PROGRESS NOTES

Patient Name _Sylvia Gonzales_   **Date of Birth** _9/1/XX_   **MRN** _341-73-792_

Prob. No. or Letter	Date	C H E D D A R
1	11/11/XX	Patient states, "I have had a fever and a sore throat for the past two days"
		Patient was healthy and well until two days ago when she noted the onset of fever and sore throat. Past history includes strep pharyngitis.
		Vital signs: T 101.1 P 96 R 24 BP 124/76 Weight: 155 Height: 5' 7"
		General: patient seems alert. HEENT: sclera clear. Pharynx red with pus pockets noted. Heart: regular w/o murmur Lungs: clear to auscultation and percussion. Abdomen: negative for tenderness.
		Other than sore throat and fever with noted temperature elevation, patient has no other complaints.
		Patient takes no daily medication except for a multi-vit. She is given an Rx for Amoxicillin 250 mg 1 tab q8h for 10 days.
		Strep Pharyngitis.
		Schedule follow-up appointment for three weeks from today for repeat throat culture.

Elizabeth H. Williams MD (Attending Physician)

Myra A. Perez, CMA

Date: November 11, 20XX

Form OMB-1243

FIGURE 11-9 Typical chart note using the CHEDDAR format.

Examination Preparation and Vital Signs

As the office medical assistant, you will often prepare each patient for his or her examination. You will record vital signs, any medication(s) the patient is currently taking, and any responses to treatment. Before you leave a patient, always remember to ask, "Is there anything else you would like the doctor to know?" The patient may be more comfortable sharing further information with you than with the doctor. You will document the vital signs, medication information, and any treatment response in the medical record. If the patient does make any additional comments, document these as well and remember to use the patient's own words if at all possible. Refer to Figure 11-10 for a sample chart note.

Follow-Up

After you record the initial interview, any background information, vital signs, and subjective information (chief complaint), the physician will decide what entries will be made regarding examination, diagnosis, treatment options and plans, including comments or observations about each case. You will then maintain the patient record by performing some or all of the following duties:

- Transcribe notes the doctor dictates about the patient's progress, follow-up visits, procedures, current status, and other necessary information. Transcription does not occur in all practices using paper records because a transcription service is often responsible for this task.

- Post laboratory or examination results in the medical record or on the summary sheet

- Record telephone calls from the patient and calls that the doctor or other office staff members make to the patient

- Telephone calls can be an important part of good follow-up care. Calls must be dated and the content of the conversations must be documented (Figure 11-11).

- You must initial the entry. Even if the doctor did not reach the patient, the call should be recorded and dated. State whether the doctor got an answer, left a message on an answering machine or with a person, and so on. Legally, if an item is not in the record, it did not happen.

- Record any medical instructions or discharge instructions the doctor gives to the patient

- At the physician's request, counsel or educate the patient regarding the treatment regimen or home care procedures the patient must follow. This information must be entered into the record, dated, and initialed. For patient convenience, many offices have preprinted instruction sheets for patients to refer to once they arrive home.

The Six Cs of Charting

To maintain accurate patient records, always keep these six Cs in mind when filling out and maintaining charts: *C*lient's (patient's) words, *C*larity, *C*ompleteness, *C*onciseness, *C*hronological order, and *C*onfidentiality.

1. *Client's words.* Be careful to record the patient's exact words rather than your interpretation of them. For instance, if a client says, "My right knee feels like it's thick or full of fluid," write that down. Do not rephrase the sentence to say, "Client says he's got fluid on the knee." Often the patient's exact words, no matter how odd they may sound, provide important clues for the physician in making a diagnosis.

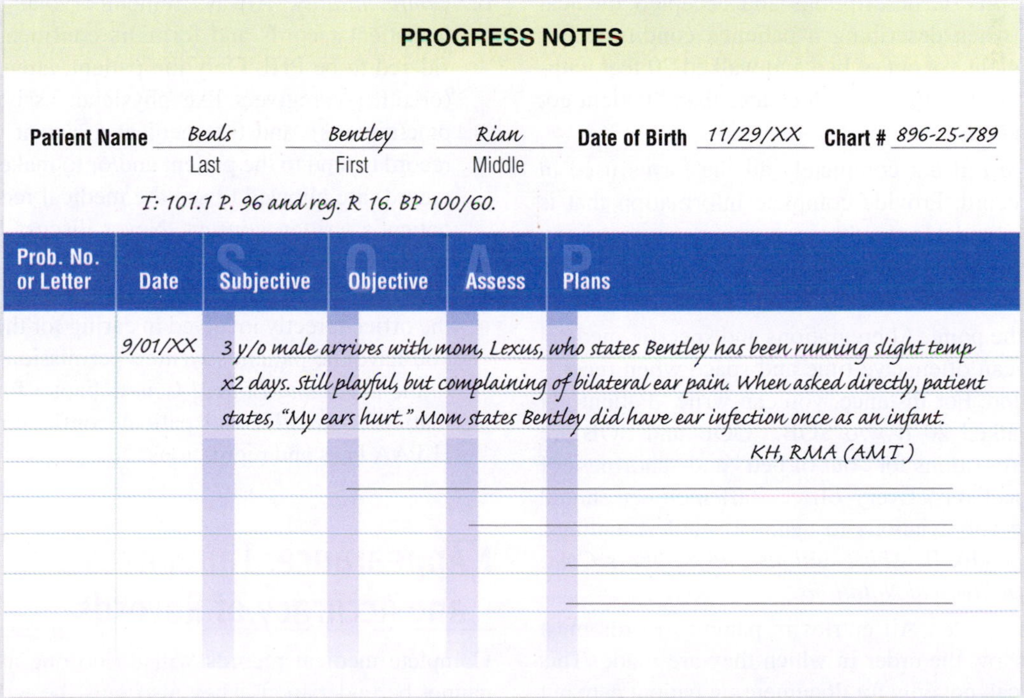

PROGRESS NOTES

Patient Name: Beals (Last) Bentley (First) Rian (Middle)   Date of Birth: 11/29/XX   Chart #: 896-25-789

T: 101.1 P. 96 and reg. R 16. BP 100/60.

Prob. No. or Letter	Date	Subjective	Objective	Assess	Plans
	9/01/XX	3 y/o male arrives with mom, Lexus, who states Bentley has been running slight temp x2 days. Still playful, but complaining of bilateral ear pain. When asked directly, patient states, "My ears hurt." Mom states Bentley did have ear infection once as an infant. KH, RMA (AMT)			

FIGURE 11-10   Chart note update started by medical assistant in preparation for patient examination.

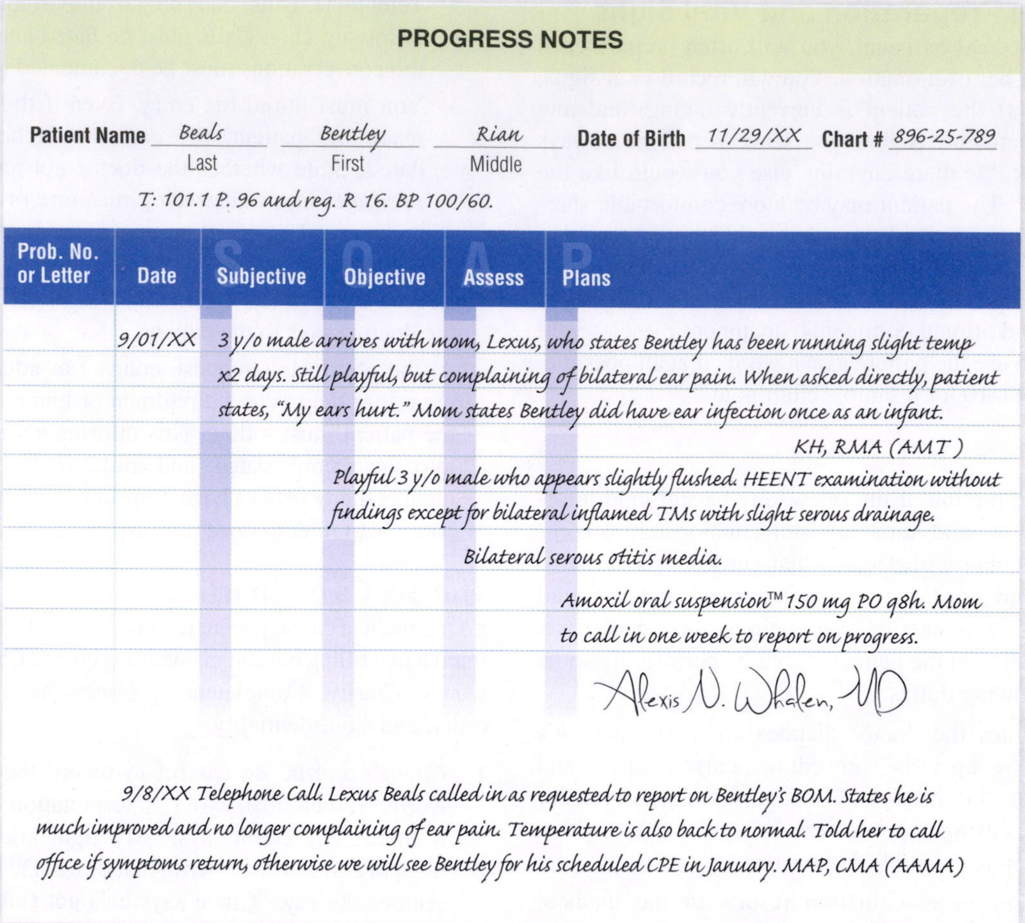

PROGRESS NOTES

Patient Name	Beals	Bentley	Rian	Date of Birth 11/29/XX	Chart # 896-25-789
	Last	First	Middle		

T: 101.1 P. 96 and reg. R 16. BP 100/60.

Prob. No. or Letter	Date	Subjective	Objective	Assess	Plans
	9/01/XX	3 y/o male arrives with mom, Lexus, who states Bentley has been running slight temp x2 days. Still playful, but complaining of bilateral ear pain. When asked directly, patient states, "My ears hurt." Mom states Bentley did have ear infection once as an infant.			
		KH, RMA (AMT)			
			Playful 3 y/o male who appears slightly flushed. HEENT examination without findings except for bilateral inflamed TMs with slight serous drainage.		
				Bilateral serous otitis media.	
					Amoxil oral suspension™ 150 mg PO q8h. Mom to call in one week to report on progress.
					Alexis N. Whalen, MD

9/8/XX Telephone Call. Lexus Beals called in as requested to report on Bentley's BOM. States he is much improved and no longer complaining of ear pain. Temperature is also back to normal. Told her to call office if symptoms return, otherwise we will see Bentley for his scheduled CPE in January. MAP, CMA (AAMA)

FIGURE 11-11 Completed chart note including telephone call from patient in follow-up.

2. *Clarity*. Use precise descriptions and accepted medical terminology when describing a patient's condition. For instance, "Patient got out of bed and walked 20 feet without shortness of breath" is much clearer than "Patient got out of bed and felt fine."

3. *Completeness*. Fill out completely all the forms used in the patient record. Provide complete information that is readily understandable to others whenever you make any notation in the patient chart.

4. *Conciseness*. While striving for clarity, also be concise, or brief and to the point. Abbreviations and specific medical terminology can often save time and space when recording information. For instance, you can write "Patient got OOB and walked 20 ft w/o SOB." OOB and SOB are standard abbreviations for "out of bed" and "shortness of breath," respectively. Every office staff member should use the same abbreviations to avoid misunderstandings. Refer to Appendix II, *Abbreviations and Symbols Commonly Used in Medical Notations*.

5. *Chronological order*. All entries in patient records must be dated to show the order in which they are made. This factor is critical, not only for documenting patient care but also in case there is a legal question about the type and date of medical services.

6. *Confidentiality*. Always remember that the information in patient records and forms is confidential and is considered to be PHI. Only the patient, attending physicians (or other caregivers like physician assistants and nurse practitioners), and the medical assistant (who needs the record to tend to the patient and/or to make entries into the record) are allowed to see the medical record without the patient's written consent. Never discuss the information in a patient record, forward it to another office, fax the information, or share it with anyone except the people in the office directly involved in caring for the patient, unless you have the patient's written permission to do so. Refer to the *Legal and Ethical Issues* chapter for detailed information about PHI and patient confidentiality, including HIPAA laws and regulations.

▶ **Appearance, Timeliness, and Accuracy of Records** LO 11.5

Complete medical records will do no one any good if they cannot be understood. They also must be written neatly and legibly; contain up-to-date information; and present an accurate, professional record of a patient's case.

Neatness and Legibility

A medical record is useless if it is difficult (or impossible) to read. Make sure that every word and number in the record is clear and legible. For this reason, if an office uses paper medical records, the records are usually transcribed. Let's look at the transcription process.

Medical Transcription Your knowledge of abbreviations, medical terminology, and medical coding will be invaluable if you are asked to transcribe a physician's notes or dictation. **Transcription** means transforming spoken notes into accurate written form. These written notes are then entered into the patient medical record. As with all parts of the medical record, they are part of the patient's continuing (and confidential) case history and often include findings, treatment stages, prognoses, and final outcomes. Always date and initial all transcription pages. With the advent of voice recognition software, transcription can be done pretty much automatically by the computer, which will type based on the words spoken by the physician. These notes still need to be proofread carefully, until the software recognizes the physician's voice and accent and its dictionary contains the words—particularly medical terms—used most often by the physician.

Regardless of how the transcription occurs, transcribed material will contain the six Cs and, as such, should be accurate and complete, using appropriate grammar, correct spelling, and accurate medical abbreviations and terminology. As always, when dealing with abbreviations, if there is any doubt as to the meaning or use of an abbreviation, use the standard rule of thumb in healthcare: "When in doubt, spell it out." Use the medical dictionary and the medical computer spell-check function to verify the spelling or meaning of words. Ask the physician only if you cannot find something in a reference source. In order to be efficient, above-average typing or word processing speed and accuracy are also important.

Keep a library of medical, secretarial, and transcription reference books and medical terminology texts near the transcription workstation. Abbreviations can save time, but you should use only those that are accepted as standard. Reference books will help you find the correct word quickly and easily and help you apply proper grammar, style, and usage to the copy.

Handwritten Notes If handwritten entries are used in the medical record, follow these tips to keep charts neat and easy to read.

- Use a good-quality pen that will not smudge or smear.
- If the records will be copied, AHIMA suggests black ink, although blue is acceptable as well, so that copies of the original are easily readable. Some medical offices prefer blue ink because blue ink used in the original record will copy as black, distinguishing the blue original from the black copy and reducing the possibility of error. Blue ink is also more difficult to match, so any additions are easy to spot. This cuts down on fraudulent entries.
- Use highlighting pens to call attention to specific items like allergies. Be aware, however, that unless the office has a color copier, most colored ink will photocopy black or gray.

Because highlighting-pen marks may not be visible on a photocopy, many offices use brightly colored stickers to list allergies within and on the medical record.

- Make sure all handwriting is legible. Take time to write names, numbers, and abbreviations clearly.
- Make any corrections to the chart by following Procedure 11-2, Correcting Paper Medical Records.

Timeliness

Medical records should be kept up-to-date and be readily available when any healthcare professional needs to see them. Follow these guidelines to ensure that information on a patient can be readily located in the medical record when it is needed.

- Record all exam and test results as soon as they are available.
- If you forget to enter a result into the record when it is received, record both the original date of receipt and the date the report was entered into the record.
- To document telephone calls, record the date and time of the call, who initiated it, the information discussed, and any conclusions or results. Depending on office policy, the call may be recorded directly into the record or a note may be made referring the reader to a separate telephone log, kept elsewhere within the medical record.
- Establish a procedure for retrieving a file quickly in case of emergency. Should the patient be in a serious accident, for example, the emergency doctor will need the patient's pertinent medical history immediately.

Accuracy

The physician must be able to trust the accuracy of the information in the medical records. Make an accuracy check of all data entered within the medical record a priority. To ensure accurate data, follow these guidelines.

- Never guess at or assume knowledge of names, procedures, medications, findings, or any other information about which there is some question. Always check all the information carefully. Make the extra effort to ask questions of the physician or senior staff member to verify information if there is any doubt as to its accuracy.
- Double-check the accuracy of findings and instructions recorded in the chart. Have all numbers been copied accurately? Are instructions for taking medication clear and complete?
- Make sure the latest information has been entered into the chart (and in the appropriate location) so that the physician has an accurate picture of the patient's current condition.

Professional Attitude and Tone

Part of creating timely and accurate records is maintaining a professional tone in your writing when recording information. As stated earlier, whenever possible, record information from the patient using his own words, particularly when recording the chief complaint (the reason for the visit). Also record the practitioner's observations and comments and any laboratory or test results. Never record your personal, subjective comments, judgments, opinions, or speculations about a patient's words, problems, or test results. You may call attention to a particular problem or observation, for example, by attaching a note to the chart, but do not make such comments a permanent part of the patient's medical record.

Correcting and Updating Medical Records

LO 11.6

In legal terms, medical records are regarded as having been created in "due course." All information in the medical record should be entered at the time of a patient's visit and not days, weeks, or months later. Information corrected or added some time after a patient's visit can be regarded as "convenient" and may damage the physician's position in a lawsuit. Untimely medical record submissions also can jeopardize a patient's care. For instance, if a medication is given to a patient but not charted appropriately in a timely fashion, the patient could inadvertently be given another dosage of the same medication, potentially causing an overdose.

Using Care with Corrections

If changes to the medical record are not done correctly, the record can become a legal problem for the physician and the practice. A physician may be able to more easily explain poor or incomplete documentation than to explain a chart where the original documentation appears to have been altered. Always be extremely careful to follow the appropriate procedures for correcting patient records.

Mistakes in medical records are not uncommon. The best defense is to correct the mistake immediately or as soon as possible after the original entry was made. To correct any mistake in a medical record, carefully draw a single line through the error, making sure that the original entry is still legible. Write or type the corrected information above or below the original entry or even in the margin, as close as possible to the original entry. If there is not enough room near the error to make the full correction, make a notation near the error as to where in the chart the correction may be found. When making the correction, note the date and reason for the correction and initial the completed correction. If at all possible, have another staff member witness the correction and initial it as witness. See Figure 11-12.

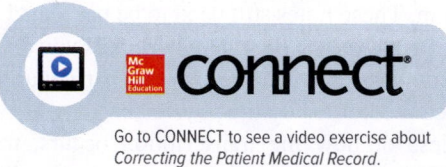

Go to CONNECT to see a video exercise about *Correcting the Patient Medical Record.*

PROGRESS NOTES

Patient Name	Beals	Bentley	Rian	Date of Birth 11/29/XX	Chart # 986-25-789
	Last	First	Middle		

T: 101.1 P. 96 and reg. R 16. BP 100/60.

Prob. No. or Letter	Date	Subjective	Objective	Assess	Plans
	9/01/XX	This 3 y/o male arrives with mom, Lexus, who states Bentley has been running slight temp x2 days. Still playful, but complaining of bilateral ear pain. When asked directly, patient states, "My ears hurt." Mom states Bentley did have ear infection once as an infant.			
					KH, RMA/AMT
		Playful 3 y/o male who appears slightly flushed. HEENT examination without findings except for bilateral inflamed TMs with slight serous drainage.			
			Bilateral serous otitis media.		
				Amoxicillin 250 mg b.i.d. x 7 days, Mom to call in one week to report on progress.	

Alexis N. Whalen, MD

9/8/XX Telephone Call. Lexus Beals called in as requested to report on Bentley's BOM. States he is much improved and no longer complaining of ear pain. Temperature is also back to normal. Told her to call office if symptoms return, otherwise we will see Bentley for his scheduled CPE in ~~January~~. MAP, CMA (AAMA) Date Error please see below

9/9/XX Correction to documentation of 9/8/XX. Patient's scheduled CPE is in June, not January as previously recorded. MAP, CMA (AAMA)

FIGURE 11-12 Example of a corrected medical record.

Updating Patient Records

All additions to a patient's record—test results, observations, diagnoses, procedures—should be done so there can be no interpretation of deception on the physician's part. In a note accompanying the material, the physician should explain why the information is being added to the record. The material may simply be the physician's recollections or observations regarding a patient visit that occurred in the past. Each item added to the record must be dated and initialed. As the office medical assistant, you may be asked to act as a third-party witness of these additions to paper records.

Most hospitals, clinics, and larger medical practices have detailed guidelines for late entries and corrections to patient charts. You must follow these guidelines carefully to avoid potential legal problems. See Procedure 11-3 at the end of this chapter for a list of steps for adding information to a paper patient record. Throughout the textbook, you will find procedures requiring you to document (chart) the procedure you just learned. This will allow you to continue to practice the charting techniques you have learned in this chapter—feel free to refer back here at any time to refresh your memory on proper techniques.

▶ Responding to Release of Records Request
LO 11.7

As you learned in the *Legal and Ethical Issues* chapter, all physical medical records, including X-rays, test results, and medical notes created by the physician, are considered the property of the practice. Although the information belongs to the patient, the law may require the physician to release the record, as in the case of a patient with a contagious disease or when a court subpoenas the records. Under no circumstances should you release patient information to insurance companies over the telephone. This information should be released in writing only after the patient has signed a written release statement. Under HIPAA, release of information over the telephone will likely be problematic.

Additionally, any request to release medical records should be approved by the physician. As stated earlier in the discussion on PHI, only the information requested should be released. Be sure to check for date ranges listed on the release as well as for specifics as to the exact information being requested. Be sure to release only the specific information requested, within any time frame restrictions outlined.

Procedures for Releasing Records

Physicians often receive requests from lawyers, other physicians, insurance companies, government agencies, and the patients themselves for copies of all or part of their medical records. Follow these steps for releasing medical information.

1. Obtain a signed and newly dated release from the patient authorizing the *transfer* of specific information—from his or her medical record to another party outside the physician's office. Please note that *verbal consent in person or over the telephone is not considered a valid authorization.* The signed and dated authorization should be filed in the patient's medical record. Refer to Figure 5-7 in the *Legal and Ethical Issues* chapter for an example of an authorization to release (transfer) health information form.

2. Make photocopies of the requested original material. Copy and send only those portions of the record covered by the release and usually only records originating from your facility. Unless the patient specifically requests that you do so, you should not release records that were obtained from other sources, such as consultations or tests done in a hospital. Do not send original documents. (If a record will be used in a court case, however, you must submit the original unless the judge specifies that a photocopy is acceptable.) In the past, originals of X-rays were often required because copies could not be made, but often today CDs can be made of X-rays and even MRIs and CT scans that will often be acceptable to the person requesting the records. If you must send the originals, the recipient should be asked to sign a statement of responsibility for the original records until they are returned to the office. Document in the patient's medical record who has possession of the original documents, the date the recipient received the originals, and the date they are returned. Do request that the recipient return the original documents as soon as possible. Remember to follow up with the recipient until the originals have been returned and placed in the patient's file.

3. Call the recipient to confirm that all materials were received. Avoid faxing confidential records. Unless the recipient has a locked and password-protected fax mailbox, there is no way to tell who will have access to documents sent by fax.

Special Cases It may not always be immediately clear who has the right to sign the authorization to release medical records form. When a couple divorces, for example, both parents are still considered legal guardians of their children, and either one can sign a release form authorizing transfer of medical records. If a patient dies, the patient's next of kin or legally authorized representative, such as the executor of the estate, may see the records or authorize their release to a third party. When you are in doubt regarding who is authorized to sign, *always* ask your supervisor before releasing confidential, protected health information.

Confidentiality

When children reach age 18, most states consider them adults with the right to privacy. No one, not even their parents, may see their medical records without the child's written consent. States extend this right to privacy to emancipated minors who are under the age of 18 and living on their own or are married, a parent, or in the armed services. Confidentiality is often extended to minors seeking care for STIs, birth control, and drug or alcohol counseling. In these instances, the minor is considered a "mature minor" and her treatment cannot be discussed with her parents without her permission, even though the parents may still be held responsible for payment of such treatment through insurance or self-payment unless the patient pays for treatment at the time of service. Refer to the information regarding minors and their access to medical care in the *Legal and Ethical Issues* chapter for more detailed information.

The main legal and ethical principle to keep in mind is that you must protect each patient's right to privacy at all times.

Auditing Medical Records

The auditing of medical records is a great housekeeping tool. To **audit** a record means to examine and review a group of patient records for completeness and accuracy—particularly as related to their ability to back up the charges sent to health insurance carriers for reimbursement. There are two types of audits: internal and external. The medical assistant, and generally the medical office manager and others who handle medical records for a medical office, should periodically perform audits to verify that the medical documentation meets required minimum standards. Many medical offices are now hiring compliance specialists to do internal auditing of their charts.

Internal Audits The medical staff can perform internal audits. Records are chosen randomly. Audits should be done both before billing is submitted (*prospective*) and after billing

BWW

Internal Medical Record Audit Form

Patient name: _____ Date of service: _____

Provider Name: _____ Supervising Physician (if needed): _____

ICD codes: _____

CPT codes: _____

Review the medical record for the following elements:

	Yes	No
1. Was the medical record for this service found?	☐	☐
2. If a paper record is used, is it legible?	☐	☐
3. If provider is not a physician, is the note written or co-signed by the supervising physician?	☐	☐
4. Does the date of service billed agree with the date of the medical record?	☐	☐
5. Does the documentation support the ICD codes billed?	☐	☐
6. Does the documentation support CPT codes billed?	☐	☐
7. Does the documentation support the level of service billed? (See below for evaluation criteria).	☐	☐

Level of service audit

History (To assign a given level, all three elements must be met or exceeded.)

History of present illness (HPI)	Review of systems (ROS)	Past, family and/or social history (PFSH)	Type of history
Brief	N/A	N/A	Problem-focused
Brief	Problem pertinent	N/A	Expanded PF
Extended	Extended	Pertinent	Detailed
Extended	Complete	Complete	Comprehensive

Physical exam (See CPT Guidelines for body area and organ system definitions)

Problem focused	Expanded PF	Detailed	Comprehensive
Limited to affected area or body system	Exam of affected area or body system & exam of related areas	Extended exam of affected area or body system & exam of related areas	General multi-system exam or complete exam of one organ system

Medical decision making (To assign given level, two of the three elements must be met or exceeded.)

Number of diagnoses or management options	Amount and/or complexity of data to be reviewed	Risk of complications and/or morbidity or mortality	Type of decision making
Minimal	Minimal or none	Minimal	Straight forward
Limited	Limited	Low	Low complexity
Multiple	Moderate	Moderate	Moderate complexity
Extensive	Extensive	High	High complexity

Time-based codes

If more than 50 percent of the face-to-face time with the patient was spent in counseling or coordination of care, indicate the total time. Counseling/coordination of care time:_____ minutes. Total face-to-face time:_____ minutes

CPT code:_____

FIGURE 11-13 Medical record audit tool.

is submitted (*retrospective*). The audit schedule of how often audits should be performed should be determined by the medical office, based on the findings of the audits themselves. Many offices perform biannual audits, while others prefer quarterly audits. If an office finds that many charts are "failing" the internal audits, medical staff training should take place and internal audits performed more frequently until the medical records meet the required standards. A sample chart review form created by Ronald Bradshaw, MD, CPA, can be found at http:// www.aafp.org/fpm/2000/0400/fpm20000400p28-rt1.pdf. See Figure 11-13 for a copy of this medical record audit tool.

External Audits Government entities (such as Medicare and Medicaid), managed care organizations (MCOs), and private insurance carriers perform external audits. The number of government (and private) audits has increased greatly in the past decade, as federal programs and private payers seek to recover possible overpayments. External auditors may want to investigate the medical records further by interviewing the staff members, patients, and all physicians who participated in the patient's care. If the medical record does not back up the charges sent to the payer, the provider (practitioner and office) may be found guilty of fraudulent billing practices. At the very least, the charges considered as fraudulently obtained will need to be returned to the payer and/or to the patient. If federal programs like Medicare and Medicaid are involved, more severe penalties may be incurred, including large financial penalties, loss of the ability to participate in federal programs, jail, and loss of the physician's medical license. More about medical billing and fraudulent practices will be discussed in the chapters on insurance, coding, and billing.

PROCEDURE 11-1 Preparing a New Patient Paper Medical Record

WORK // DOC

Procedure Goal: To assemble a new patient paper medical record

OSHA Guidelines: This procedure does not involve exposure to blood, body fluids, or tissue.

Materials: File folder, labels as appropriate (alphabet, numbers, dates, insurance, allergies, etc.), forms (patient registration, medical history, advance directives, physician progress notes, laboratory forms), and a hole punch

Method:

1. Carefully create a chart label according to practice policy. This label may include the patient's last name followed by the first name, or it may be a medical record number for those offices that utilize numeric or alphanumeric filing.
   RATIONALE: *The label must be correct to avoid filing errors.*

2. Place the chart label on the right edge of the folder, extending the label the length of the tab on the folder.

3. Place the date label on the top edge of the folder, updating the date according to practice policy. (The date is usually updated annually, if the patient has come into the office within the last year.)
   RATIONALE: *This makes it easy to identify current patient records for retrieval and identify records for purging if the patient has not been seen for a specified amount of time (often, 3 years).*

4. If alpha or numeric filing labels are utilized, place a patient name label on the chart according to practice policy.

5. Punch holes in the appropriate forms for placement within the patient's medical record.

6. Place all the forms in appropriate sections of the patient's medical record.
   RATIONALE: *Consistency in document placement assures that items can be found quickly when required.*

PROCEDURE 11-2 Correcting Paper Medical Records

Procedure Goal: To follow standard procedures for correcting a paper medical record

OSHA Guidelines: This procedure does not involve exposure to blood, body fluids, or tissue.

Materials: Patient file, other pertinent documents that contain the information to be used in making corrections (for example,

transcribed notes, telephone notes, physician's comments, correspondence), and a good ballpoint pen

Method:

1. Corrections and additions should be made so the original information remains readable, so there can be no suggestion of intent to conceal information. Draw a single line through the information to be replaced.

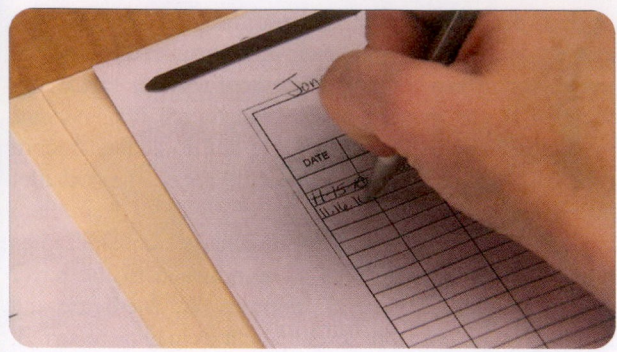

FIGURE Procedure 11-2 Step 1 Corrections should be made using a single line through the error so it can still be read.
© McGraw-Hill Education

RATIONALE: *The single line ensures that the original entry can still be seen, avoiding future potential charges of a "cover-up."*

2. Write or type in the correct information above or below the original line or in the margin. The location in the chart for the new information should be clear. If a separate sheet of paper or another document is required for the correction or addition, clearly note in the record "See attached document A" or use similar wording to indicate where the corrected information can be found.
   RATIONALE: *It is important that information within the chart may be readily found at all times to allow for excellent patient care.*

3. Place a note near the correction or addition stating why it was made (for example, "error, wrong date; error, interrupted by phone call"). Make sure you initial and date the correction. This indication can be a brief note in the margin or an attachment to the record. Do not make any changes or additions in a record without noting the reason for them.
   RATIONALE: *By noting the reason as well as the correction, you clearly indicate that the correction is intentional and necessary.*

4. Enter the date and time, and initial the correction or addition.
   RATIONALE: *No correction to a medical chart is complete or acceptable without these elements.*

5. If possible, have another staff member or the physician witness and initial the correction to the record when you make it.

PROCEDURE 11-3 Entering (Adding) Information into a Paper Medical Record

Procedure Goal: To document continuity of care by creating a complete, accurate, timely record of the medical care provided to a patient in your medical facility

OSHA Guidelines: This procedure does not involve exposure to blood, body fluids, or tissue.

Materials: Patient medical record, pertinent documents (test results, X-ray results, telephone notes, correspondence, etc.), blue ballpoint pen, notebook, keyboard, and transcription equipment

Method:

1. Verify that you have the correct chart for the documents to be filed. Carefully check the patient's name, DOB, and medical record number (if available) as verification.
   RATIONALE: *The patient's medical record is a legal document. You must be certain that documentation takes place in the correct medical record.*

2. Transcribe any dictated notes as soon as possible and enter them into the patient record. If notes are handwritten, be sure they are filed in the correct location within the medical record.
   RATIONALE: *Records must be kept up-to-date to maintain patient continuity of care.*

3. Spell out the names of disorders, diseases, medications, and other terms the first time you enter them into the patient record, followed by the appropriate abbreviation—for example, "congestive heart failure (CHF)." Thereafter, you may use the abbreviation alone.

   RATIONALE: *Follow the six Cs of documentation, one of which is clarity. There can be no confusion due to the use of abbreviations.*

4. Enter only what the doctor has dictated. Do *not* add your own comments, observations, or evaluations. Use self-adhesive flags or other means to call the doctor's attention to something you have noticed that may be helpful to the patient's case. Date and initial each entry.
   RATIONALE: *As a legal document, there is no place for personal comments or observations as part of the permanent patient medical record.*

5. Follow office procedure to record routine or special laboratory, X-ray, or other test results. These results may be posted in a particular section of the file or on a separate test summary form. If you use the summary form, make a note in the file that the results were received and recorded. Place the original report in the patient's file if required to do so by office policy. Date and initial each entry. File all correspondence and hospital records in the appropriate area of each chart, using reverse chronological order so that the most recent record is on top. Be sure that each document is initialed or stamped by the physician as having been seen, prior to filing it in the patient's chart.
   RATIONALE: *In order for the record to be useful for any medical professional using it, all documents must be filed using a consistent, easily understandable method such as POMR.*

6. Make a note in the record of all telephone calls to and from the patient. Date and initial the entries. These entries also may include the doctor's comments, observations, changes in the patient's medication, new instructions to the patient, and so on. If calls are recorded in a separate telephone log, note in the patient's record the time and date of the call and refer to the log. It is particularly important to record such calls when the patient resists or refuses treatment, skips appointments, or has not made follow-up appointments.

   RATIONALE: *As a legal representation of the patient's medical care, it is equally important to log the patient's response and responsibility toward his own medical care, plan, and treatment.*

7. Make notations in the medical record of any immunizations and vaccines that have been given to the patient. Notations should be posted in the patient's immunization record inside the medical chart. Input them into your state's public health database as well. Immunization records are kept indefinitely as a permanent part of the patient's medical history.

8. Read over the entries for omissions or mistakes. Ask the doctor to answer any questions you have.

   RATIONALE: *It is imperative that all parts of the medical record contain the six Cs of medical charting and are free of errors and omissions.*

9. Make sure that you have dated and initialed each entry.

10. Be sure that all documents are included in the file and within the appropriate location so they can be found easily when needed.

11. Return the patient's medical record to its appropriate location in the filing system as soon as possible.

   RATIONALE: *If the medical record is perfectly maintained but cannot be found, it does neither the physician nor the patient any good.*

SUMMARY OF LEARNING OUTCOMES

LEARNING OUTCOMES	KEY POINTS
11.1 Explain the importance of patient medical records.	Medical records are legal documents that give a complete, concise, chronological history of a patient's past medical history, current medical issues, treatment plan, and treatment outcome. Additionally, they act as a communication tool between care providers. The patient medical record provides physicians and other healthcare providers with all the important information, observations, and opinions that have been recorded about a patient.
11.2 Identify the documents that constitute a patient medical record.	The records that constitute the patient medical record include, but are not limited to, the following: patient registration form, medical history form, physical exam form, laboratory and other test results, records from physicians or hospitals, physician diagnosis and treatment plan, operative reports, hospital discharge summaries, follow-up notes, records of telephone calls, signed informed consents, and correspondence with or about the patient.
11.3 Compare SOMR, POMR, SOAP, and CHEDDAR medical record formats.	SOMR files documents in the medical record in strict chronological order. POMR files the same documents according to numbered problems found on the patient problem list. SOAP notes organize medical record documentation according to subjective, objective, assessment, and plan. The CHEDDAR format breaks down this information even further into chief complaint, history, exam, details, drugs, assessment, and return visit plan.
11.4 Recall the 6 Cs of charting, giving an example of each.	The six Cs of charting are client's words, clarity, completeness, conciseness, chronological order, and confidentiality.
11.5 Describe the need for neatness, timeliness, accuracy, and professional tone in patient records.	Neatness, legibility, accuracy, and professional tone are musts in maintaining medical records. Remember that patient medical records are legal documents. They must be kept up-to-date and should be easy to read. Make sure you project a professional tone when recording information. Always check for accuracy and never guess at information. Personal thoughts and observations should never be a permanent part of the patient medical record.

LEARNING OUTCOMES	KEY POINTS
11.6 Illustrate the correct procedure for correcting and updating a medical record.	The proper way to make corrections in a medical record is to draw a single line through the error so that the original entry is still legible. Make the correction as close as possible to the original entry, noting the reason for the correction, and initial the correction. Any additions to a medical record also should be made as soon as the need for the addition is noted, and the reason for the addition or change should be clearly documented.
11.7 Describe the steps in responding to a written request for release of medical records.	In order to release any confidential medical information, express written permission from the patient must be received. Unless it is impossible to do so, copies should be made and the originals should remain in the office. If originals must be released, a statement of responsibility should be signed by the receiver and should be noted in the patient's chart. Follow-up should take place until the original records are returned to the office and to the patient's record. Only release records that are expressly requested and authorized by the patient.

CASE STUDY CRITICAL THINKING

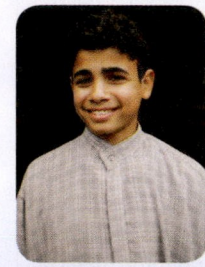

Recall Mohammad from the beginning of the chapter. Now that you have completed the chapter, answer the following questions regarding his case.

1. As a new patient, which documents should be completed prior to Mohammad being seen by the physician? What documents should he have brought with him, if available?

2. Your office uses a SOAP format for medical records. After Dr. Williams completes her exam, explain where each of the new documents or pieces of information obtained during Mohammad's exam will be filed using the SOAP format.

EXAM PREPARATION QUESTIONS

1. (LO 11.1) The process of recording information in a patient's medical record is called
   a. Auditing
   b. SOAP
   c. CHEDDAR
   d. Documentation
   e. Demographics

2. (LO 11.1) Which of the following are possible uses for patient medical records?
   a. Research
   b. Quality of care (quality control)
   c. Patient education
   d. Quality of care (quality control) and patient education only
   e. Research, quality of care (quality control), and patient education

3. (LO 11.2) Which document serves as the "base" for the patient medical record?
   a. The registration form
   b. The patient medical history form
   c. The physical examination form
   d. The patient demographic form
   e. The patient review of systems

4. (LO 11.2) Which of the following documents from other sources frequently become part of a patient's medical record?
   a. X-rays, CT scan, and MRI results
   b. Lab results from private labs or hospitals
   c. Hospital discharge summaries
   d. Hospital operative notes
   e. All of these

5. (LO 11.3) Which filing system uses the patient problem list as the source for filing within the patient medical record?
   a. POMR
   b. SOMR
   c. SOAP
   d. CHEDDAR
   e. All of these

6. (LO 11.3) Which of the following patient details would be filed under "O" using the SOAP documentation method?
   a. "I have the flu"
   b. Nausea
   c. BP 160/92
   d. Influenza
   e. Rest, fluids, ibuprofen; f/u in 5 days by phone

7. (LO 11.4) Which of the six Cs means "getting to the point"?
   a. Clarity
   b. Completeness
   c. Chronological
   d. Confidentiality
   e. Conciseness

8. (LO 11.5) In order to "trust" the information in the medical record, documentation must be _____ at all times.
   a. Timely
   b. Chronological
   c. Transcribed
   d. Accurate
   e. Professional in tone

9. (LO 11.6) Which of the following is necessary when correcting or making additions to a paper medical record?
   a. Draw a single line through the error
   b. Make the correction as close as possible to the original entry
   c. Note the reason for the correction
   d. Sign and date the correction
   e. All of these and, if possible, a witness should initial entry

10. (LO 11.7) Why are internal chart audits advisable for every medical office?
   a. To verify that the medical record "backs up" the charges being billed
   b. To give staff members practice reading physician handwriting
   c. To assure that all members of the staff are current with all patient medical issues
   d. To be sure that all possible charges are being submitted to the insurance carrier
   e. None of these

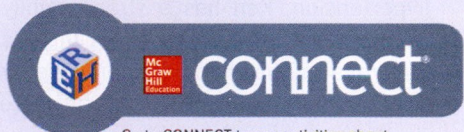

Go to CONNECT to see activities about *Updating a Patient's Chart* and *Updating Patient Demographics*.

Recall Mohammad from the case study at the beginning of the chapter.

1. Mohammad's mother brought the completed new patient forms to the office for this appointment. During Mohammad's pre-exam interview, it becomes obvious that there are some inconsistencies between what his Mother entered in the social and sexual history areas and what he is now telling you. How should this be handled?

2. Mohammad's mother asked to be invited to the post-exam discussion with Dr. Williams and Mohammad. He is OK with this as long as his "private" information is not shared with his mother. As a minor of 16, can he make this decision? (Refer to the chapter *Legal and Ethical Issues* as needed.)

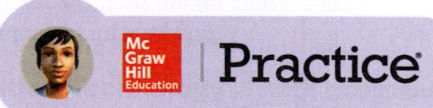

Go to PRACTICE MEDICAL OFFICE and complete the module Admin: Check In – Privacy and Liability.

Electronic Health Records

CASE STUDY

PATIENT INFORMATION

Patient Name	DOB	Allergies
Ken Washington	12/1/19XX	Sulfa
Attending	**MRN**	**Other information**
Paul F. Buckwalter, MD	891-12-743	Takes OTC Excedrin® for headaches

Ken Washington is a 61-year-old who arrives for his routine follow-up visit. Although he has not been diagnosed with hypertension, Ken has a strong family history of hypertension. He is concerned about this history and mentions today that he has had occasional weakness in his left arm and he feels that he has had an increase in headaches

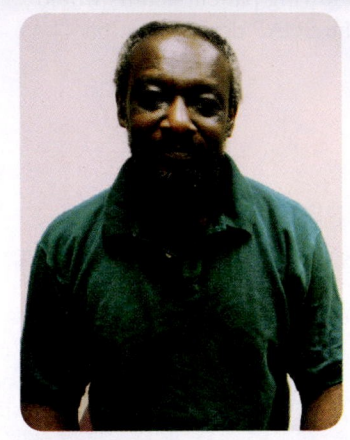

© McGraw-Hill Education

recently, which are readily addressed by OTC Excedrin®. While you are checking him in, you notice him looking at the computer monitor on your desk. The monitor is displaying the screen saver for the new EHR program recently installed at the office. He asks, "What is EHR?"

Keep Mr. Washington in mind as you study the chapter. There will be questions at the end of the chapter based on the case study. The information in the chapter will help you answer these questions.

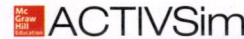

LEARNING OUTCOMES

After completing Chapter 12, you will be able to:

12.1 List four medical mistakes that will be greatly decreased through the use of EHR.

12.2 Differentiate among electronic medical records, electronic health records, and personal health records.

12.3 Explain the concept of meaningful use, identifying at least two of its goals.

12.4 Contrast the advantages and disadvantages of electronic health records.

12.5 Illustrate the steps in creating a new patient record and correcting an existing record using EHR software.

12.6 Describe some of the capabilities of EHR software programs.

12.7 Explain how you might alleviate a patient's security fears surrounding the use of EHR.

KEY TERMS

customized

electronic health record (EHR)

electronic medical record (EMR)

face page

face sheet

HITECH

meaningful use

personal health record (PHR)

Practice Management System

MEDICAL ASSISTING COMPETENCIES

CAAHEP

VI.C.8	Differentiate between electronic medical records (EMR) and a practice management system
VI.C.12	Explain meaningful use as is applies to EMR
VI.P.3	Create a patient's medical record
VI.P.4	Organize a patient's medical record
VI.P.6	Utilize an EMR
VI.P.7	Input patient data utilizing a Practice Management System
X.C.10	Identify: (a) Health Information Technology for Economic and Clinical Health (HITECH) Act
X.C.3	Describe components of the Health Information Portability and Accountability Act (HIPAA)
X.P.3	Document patient care accurately in the medical record

ABHES

7. Records Management

  a. Perform basic keyboarding skills (i.e. Microsoft Word, etc.)

  b. Utilize Electronic Medical Records (EMR) and Practice Management Systems

  c. Comply with federal, state, and local laws relating to exchange of information and describe elements of meaningful use and reports generated

8. Administrative Procedures

  a. Gather and process documents

  f. Display professionalism through written and verbal communications

11. Career Development

  b. Demonstrate professional behavior

▶ Introduction

Has your primary care physician (PCP) ever referred you to a specialist and, in the specialist's office, you spent the first 15 minutes filling out a medical history form so the medical staff had "the same medical history" that they have on file at your PCP's office? Have you ever been asked about any medication allergies or your surgical history and you just could not remember the name of the new drug you developed an allergy to or the year you had your appendix removed? Now, imagine that before you even arrive at the office, the medical staff already has that information at their fingertips, thanks to their new electronic health record (EHR) system. All you need to do is review the information with the specialist to verify that everything is correct to the best of your knowledge. Welcome to the world of electronic health records (EHR).

▶ A Brief History of Electronic Medical Records   LO 12.1

In the early 1990s, it became apparent that paper medical records could no longer meet patients' or healthcare providers' needs. The increasing need for coordination of care (consider how many physicians you see), rising healthcare costs (15% of the US gross national product), and the rather alarming increase in medical errors fueled this realization. Medical errors are the eighth leading cause of patient death in the United States. Most of these errors can be traced to communication problems, including

- Lost or misfiled paper records.
- Mishandled or "forgotten" patient messages.
- Inaccurate or unreadable information in a paper medical record.
- Mislabeled or unreadable laboratory or prescription orders.

Because of this, President George W. Bush signed an executive order in August 2006 to promote the overall efficiency and quality of healthcare in America. At the base of this order was promotion of the electronic health record, with a goal of most Americans having access to electronic health records by 2014. In many areas of the country, particularly in urban areas, this goal has been met and electronic medical records are now the rule rather than the exception. The overall goal of this order was to decrease medical errors through record legibility and record uniformity, and to increase information available among patients, medical providers, and the insurance carriers who pay for that care. Meeting this overall goal would help to control the rising cost of healthcare to both the patient and the insurance carriers, including government-funded programs like Medicare and Medicaid. Although implementation can be expensive, the electronic record (see Figure 12-1) is quickly becoming the licensed practitioner's most important business and legal record.

▶ Electronic Records   LO 12.2

The terms *electronic medical record* and *electronic health record* are seemingly used interchangeably, but they are defined differently by the National Alliance for Health Information Technology (NAHIT). The **electronic medical record (EMR)** is an electronic record of health-related information for an individual patient that is created, compiled, and managed by providers and staff members located within a *single* healthcare organization. If that same

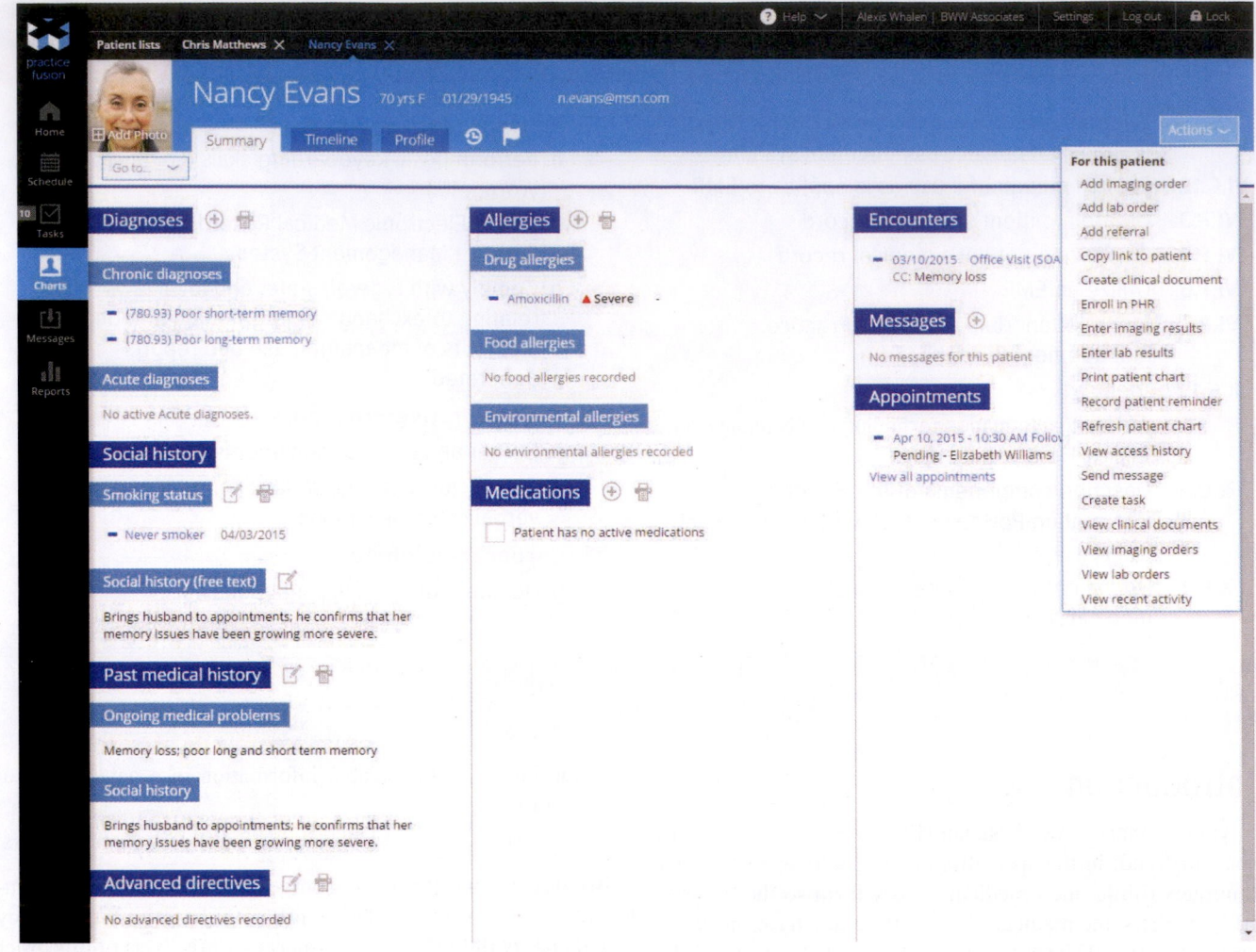

FIGURE 12-1 A face page from the Practice Fusion® Practice Management System provides an overview of Nancy Evans.
© Practice Fusion®

information on an individual patient is created, managed, and gathered in a manner that conforms to nationally recognized *interoperability standards,* so that it can be utilized by members of more than one healthcare organization, it is known as an **electronic health record (EHR).** These EHR are the federal government's ultimate goal. Because any provider with an interoperable EHR system will have access to a patient's information—no matter where the information originated—there will be increased patient continuity of care, reduction in medical errors, and, ultimately, decreased healthcare costs.

One of the offshoots of EHR that is less understood by both physicians and patients is the **personal health record (PHR).** A personal health record is basically an electronic version of the comprehensive medical history and record of a patient's lifelong health that is collected and maintained by the individual patient. This record may then be shared with providers at the patient's discretion. See Table 12-1, which outlines the basic differences between PHR and EHR.

In this era of employers, government, and insurance plans asking patients to take a much more active role in their healthcare, the PHR is a natural response to this need. PHR may be stored and maintained on secure Internet sites where the information may be efficiently managed by the patient and shared with providers as the patient wishes. Keep in mind that no matter what form a patient record takes, protected health information (PHI) is involved. As covered by HIPAA laws, PHI cannot be disclosed without patient express written permission unless allowed by federal or state statute. Refer to the *Medical Records and Documentation* chapter for more detailed information regarding HIPAA and PHI.

Because of governmental concerns surrounding data breaches possible with EHR, the American Recovery and Reinvestment Act (ARRA) became law in 2009. Part of this law includes the Health Information Technology for Economics and Clinical Health or HITECH. **HITECH** has been described as "HIPAA on steroids" because in it the Department of Health and Human Services (DHHS) greatly expands HIPAA coverage through increased compliance regulations, increased privacy regulations, and strengthened enforcement penalties relating to patient health records in EHR and Practice Management Systems. Always remember that PHI is protected, regardless of the format in which it is maintained. PHI cannot be shared with anyone without a "business need to know," unless the patient gives express written permission to share the information with that individual.

TABLE 12-1 Basic Differences Between Electronic Health Records and Personal Health Records

Description	EHR	PHR
Record ownership/management	EHR files are owned and managed by providers or facilities.	PHR files are owned and updated by the individual.
Legal document?	EHR are legal documents regulated by state and federal laws.	PHR are not legal records and have no legal regulations.
Information access	EHR access is controlled by the provider with patient authorization.	PHR access is controlled by the patient.
Providers involved	In general, EHR contain information related to treatment by one provider.	PHR contain treatment information from multiple providers.
Data entry	EHR data are entered by providers or their staff.	PHR data are entered by the patient.
Information users	EHR is used by the medical office or facility.	PHR is used by the individual patient.

▶ Meaningful Use and the EHR LO 12.3

It is impossible today to work in the healthcare industry and not hear the term **meaningful use** tossed out when speaking of electronic health records. Health IT.gov (http://healthit.gov) defines meaningful use in this way:

Meaningful use is using certified electronic health record (EHR) technology to:

- Improve quality, safety, efficiency, and reduce health disparities
- Engage patients and family
- Improve care coordination, and population and public health
- Maintain privacy and security of patient health information

It is believed that compliance with EHR programs, which support the healthcare reform tenets of the Affordable Care Act (ACT) and follow government interoperability mandates for these programs, will eventually result in better patient care, which in turn will produce the following outcomes:

- Better clinical outcomes
- Improved population health outcomes
- Increased transparency and efficiency
- Empowered individuals
- More robust research data on health systems

Let's look at each one of the hoped-for outcomes in more detail to see why EHR are considered a "core" of medical care today and in the future.

Better clinical outcomes occur when medical record documentation is clear, concise, and complete; it is easy to see what treatments work best for a patient's situation. When that documentation can be shared (PHI being omitted) with other qualified practitioners and researchers, better clinical outcomes for more patients will become possible.

Improved population health outcomes will be a natural progression from the shared knowledge of better individual outcomes. As clinicians and researchers better understand what makes us ill, the prevention and treatment of illnesses for affected populations will result.

Increased transparency and efficiency will result from the accessibility of shared records, and the results of treatment plans will be shared among practitioners, causing efficiency in the process. There will be less "reinventing of the wheel"

as more and more information is available for all practitioners regarding treatment protocols.

Empowered individuals will result from knowledgeable patients and families. *Shared data* means that patients will have access to the "track records of licensed practitioners" to allow them to choose the best provider for their needs, answers to questions such as these: Where is the best facility for treating breast cancer or leukemia? Who is most successful in helping patients and families with alcohol and substance abuse issues? Where is the most research being done on current health issues facing single parents or adult caregivers of elderly parents? All of these questions can be answered through the sharing of electronic health information. By sharing information with patients regarding their risk factors, illness, and treatment options, practitioners are engaging patients in medical decisions. Patients who are engaged partners in their care are more likely to adhere to the agreed-upon care plan when they understand the reasoning behind what they are being asked to do. Likewise, when caregivers listen to their patients, the results are more positive for the patient experience, regardless of the ultimate treatment outcome.

At the time of this writing, the government initiative through the Centers for Medicare and Medicaid Services (CMS) had recently delayed the end date for Stage 2 of its EHR implementation program to 2016. Stage 1 focused on data capture and sharing of information; Stage 2 focuses on advanced clinical processes; and Stage 3, which is still to be finalized, is due for implementation in 2017 and will focus on improved outcomes. Stage 3 will use the following criteria for this focus:

- Improving quality, safety, and efficiency, leading to improved health outcomes
- Decision support for national high-priority conditions
- Patient access to self-management tools
- Access to comprehensive patient data through patient-centered health information exchange (HIE)
- Improving population health

As Stage 3 for the EHR initiative is still in process at this time, users and participants of EHR programs will have to wait and see exactly what criteria they will have to meet in order to obtain these governmental objectives. Figure 12-2 shows a typical "dashboard" in an EHR program allowing providers to track their progress in meeting the attestation measures required during each reporting period.

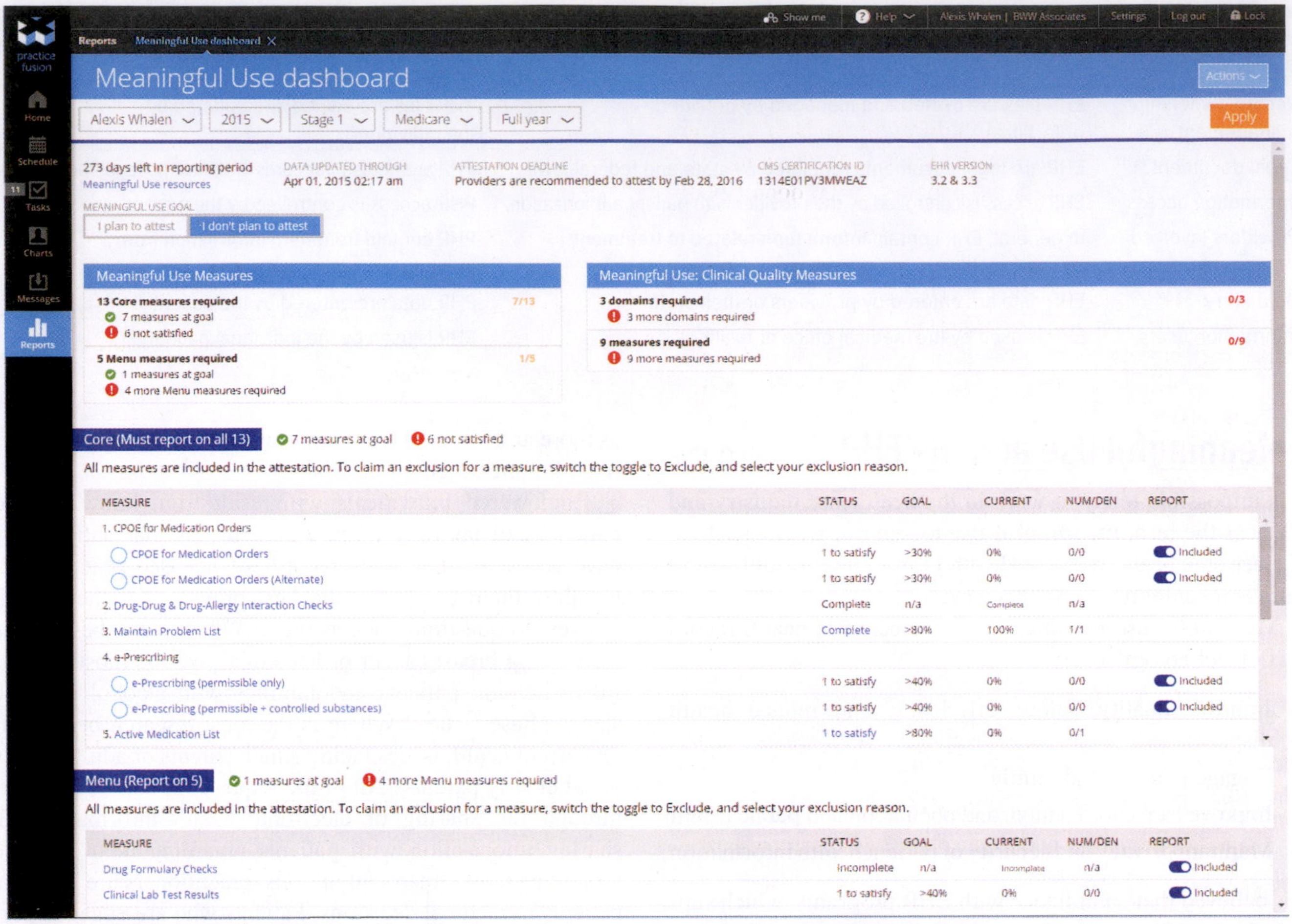

FIGURE 12-2 Built into Practice Fusion's® EHR software is a reporting system that allows you to check your practice's progress toward achieving the various stages of meaningful use.
© Practice Fusion®

▶ Advantages and Disadvantages of EHR Programs

LO 12.4

The government and proponents of EHR programs talk about all the advantages, but there are those who are reluctant to implement EHR. Let's take a look at the pros and cons of EHR programs.

Advantages of EHR Programs

Some of the advantages of EHR programs are

- Fewer lost medical records (charts do not require pulling or refiling).
- Eliminated (or reduced) transcription costs.
- Increased readability/legibility of charts.
- Ease of chart access for multiple users.
- Chart availability outside of office hours.
- Increased access to patient education materials.
- Decreased duplication of test orders.
- More efficient transfer of records.
- More efficient billing processes using electronic billing methods.
- Greatly decreased storage needs.

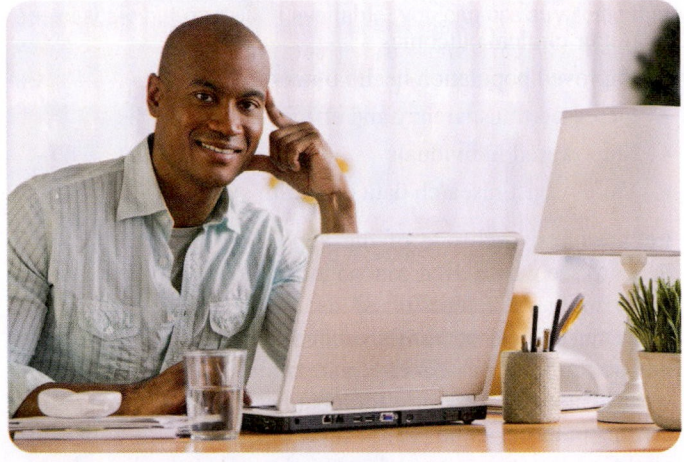

FIGURE 12-3 Electronic health records and a laptop computer with Internet access provide practitioners with easy record access no matter where they are.
© JGI/Blend Images LLC RF

In addition to these advantages, a fully functioning EHR program presents other advantages. If a practitioner is at home and needs to access a patient's record, he can access the EHR program from any computer (using his secure access code and password) at any time, review or update the file, and save it to the central computer. See Figure 12-3.

Computerized records also can be used in teleconferences, where people in different locations can look at the same record on their computer screens at the same time. Computer access to patient records is also helpful for healthcare providers with satellite offices in different cities or different parts of a city, and access may be used by a physician who is covering a practice while the patient's usual doctor is out of town.

Disadvantages of EHR Programs

Cost is the primary reason most providers give for not implementing electronic records in their offices. The estimated cost to establish an EHR program is $44,000 per full-time provider (FTP), with an estimated maintenance cost of $8,500 per year per FTP. Some practices do not have the initial financial outlay available, or feel the time needed to recoup the initial cost to implement the program does not justify the initial financial outlay. Aside from financial concerns, other reasons for not implementing electronic health records include

- Staff training requirements.
- Possible need for a full-time or part-time IT staff member.
- Possible damage to the system and to software and/or required upgrades.
- Existing programs do not fit the needs of the practice.

▶ Working with an Electronic Health Record   LO 12.5

By now, you are beginning to understand some of the EHR advantages. As a medical assistant concerned with patient care and patient confidentiality, you should also understand that the basic rules for working with a medical record do not change when that record is electronic instead of paper. The way you work with the record may change, but the way you treat a record does not. You may refer back to the chapter *Written and Electronic Communication* regarding the basic rules of working with a patient medical record.

General Guidelines for Using an EHR Program

As a medical assistant working with electronic records, you should keep the following in mind:

- Become familiar with the software and hardware used at your facility. Make sure you are not focused on the computer when you are with a patient. Becoming comfortable with the system you are using will help you to focus on the patient. If necessary, take notes and enter them into the computer when the patient is not present until you become comfortable.
- Retrieve the patient record carefully, just as you would with a paper record. Make sure you have identified the patient with at least two identifiers such as the name, date of birth, and/or medical record number.

- Keep your password information secure. Change your password on a regular basis or as directed by the healthcare facility.
- Secure the computer that maintains the electronic records and keep a backup of electronic files.
- Check your entries carefully before hitting the enter button. An EHR is a legal document just like a paper chart. What is written in the chart occurred, and what is omitted from the chart did not occur.

In addition to these guidelines, many medical record software programs use abbreviations in medical records that may or may not be used in a paper record. Common abbreviations in EHR programs include

PX for physical exam
SX for symptoms
RX for therapy, treatment, and/or prescriptions
DX for diagnosis

Additionally, because of their ability to incorporate multimedia, graphs are commonly used to track ongoing results such as BP readings, weight, recurring lab results (such as cholesterol or blood sugar), or even photos with measurements to track skin lesions. Be sure you learn and understand how to update the multimedia documents as well as how to work with the standard patient record format.

Another positive in many EHR programs is the ability to enter alerts into a patient's record to remind the practitioner if the patient is due for periodic testing such as a mammogram or colonoscopy. They can also be set up to alert the healthcare provider to abnormal test results, so that the patient can be contacted or counseled. More sophisticated programs can even document health trends, provide voice recognition, and convert notes to complete sentences.

Creating a New Patient Record Using EHR Software

Keep in mind that even though EHR programs will eventually be required to communicate with each other and they are similar in many ways, there will be differences. With practice and time, you will become an expert in your office's EHR program. All programs will have a template that will require completion for each new patient. Included in that template will be *required fields,* like the patient's name, date of birth, address, next of kin, sex, and insurance information (Figure 12-4). This information is sometimes part of a **face page,** also known as a **face sheet,** which provides an overview, or "snapshot," of patient demographic information in an EHR system. However, the way you complete these fields will vary with each software package. Procedure 12-1 at the end of this chapter outlines the basic procedure for creating a new patient record using an EHR program.

Correcting an Electronic Health Record

As you learned in the previous chapter, when correcting a paper medical record, you neatly draw a line through the error and make the correction as close to the original entry as possible. Obviously, once information is saved in an electronic

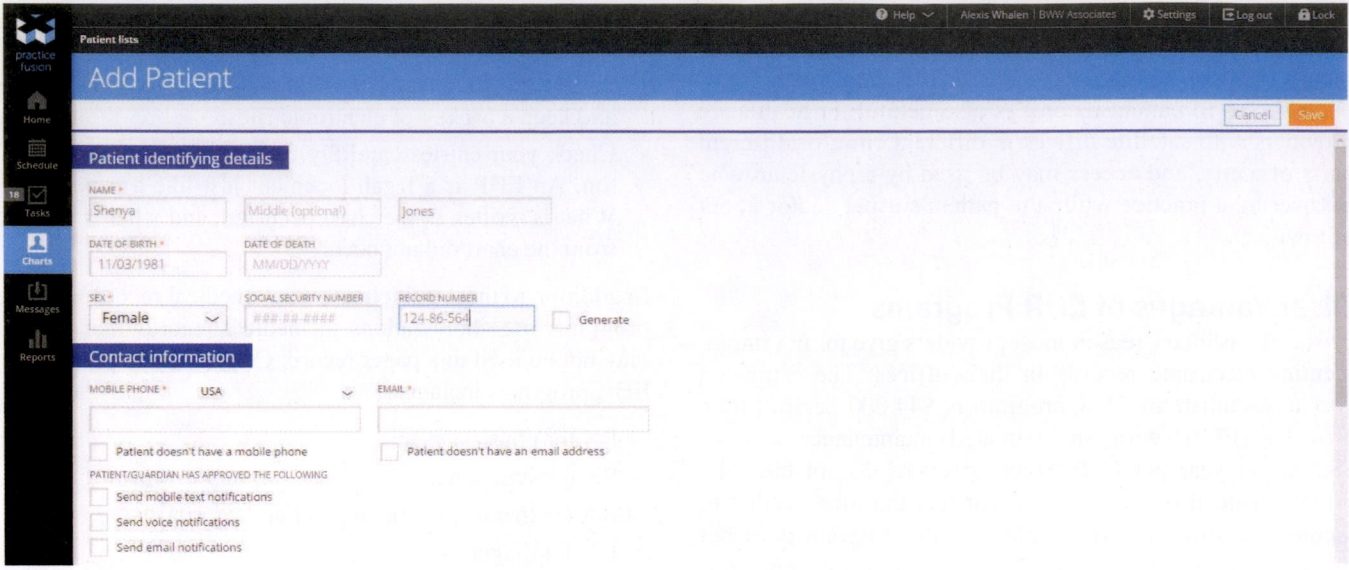

FIGURE 12-4 Screen shot from Practice Fusion®, showing Shenya Jones being added as a patient.
© Practice Fusion®

format, a line cannot be drawn through it. In fact, because electronic medical records are legal documents, once information has been saved, it cannot be changed in any way (which is why you want to double-check your work prior to clicking "save"). When an error or omission is found in an electronic record, an addendum to the omitted or incorrect information is made as soon as possible once the error or omission is noted. If an error is noted in a previous entry, many programs allow a note to be inserted at the original entry, telling the user to look at a further entry in the record for the corrected information. Procedure 12-2, found at the end of this chapter, outlines basic steps to make an addendum using an EHR program.

▶ Other Functions of EHR Programs
LO 12.6

In addition to the obvious advantages of electronic health records, all interoperable EHR programs have numerous other capabilities. When EHR programs have numerous capabilities, in addition to creating and storing medical records, they are often referred to as **Practice Management Systems.** Let's look at some of the common options for practice management and EHR programs.

Tickler Files

As stated earlier, many electronic health record programs have the capability to act as tickler files (files that need periodic attention). For example, they can alert staff members about patients who are due for yearly checkups and patients who require follow-up care. Some hospitals have begun to use electronically scanned images of patient thumbprints or photos to keep track of records. This also assists with patient security by identifying the patient at the time of each visit, which can cut down on insurance fraud. This system saves time and helps maintain patient record security. (Review the

Office Equipment and Supplies chapter for more information on computer use in the medical practice.)

Specialty Specific

Once you become accustomed to reading a medical record and documenting in it, you will begin to notice there are similarities in many of the records within any specific specialty. Cardiologists use certain terms like *cardiomegaly, congestive heart failure, echocardiogram,* and *hypertension* in many of their medical records. On the other hand, an OB/GYN would seldom use those terms, but you would see terms and abbreviations like *LMP, gravida, para,* and *C-section* in these records. Similarly, when dictating or documenting a physical exam or writing up an operative summary, physicians, like all of us, are creatures of habit and frequently use the same phrases time and time again. Recognizing this, EHR software programs may be **customized** to suit a specific specialty and style of a physician's office. Often, templates or "checkoffs" are available, so with a few simple clicks of the mouse, the physician may add entire sentences or phrases, instead of typing the same information repetitively—saving time and cutting down on errors.

Electronic Schedulers

When working with a paper appointment book, only one user at a time may make appointments. If a staff member is using the appointment book and a patient calls about an appointment, the patient on the phone must wait for the appointment book to be free before she can be assisted. Ever forget the date of an appointment? In a traditional paper book, the scheduler must go page by page in order to find the forgotten appointment—inefficient at best! Electronic schedulers (Figure 12-5) have several advantages over the traditional appointment book. Multiple users may use them at any time. Depending on the software package you are using, if you need to find a patient's appointment, you can search by the patient's name or even look up the patient's record and the date of the

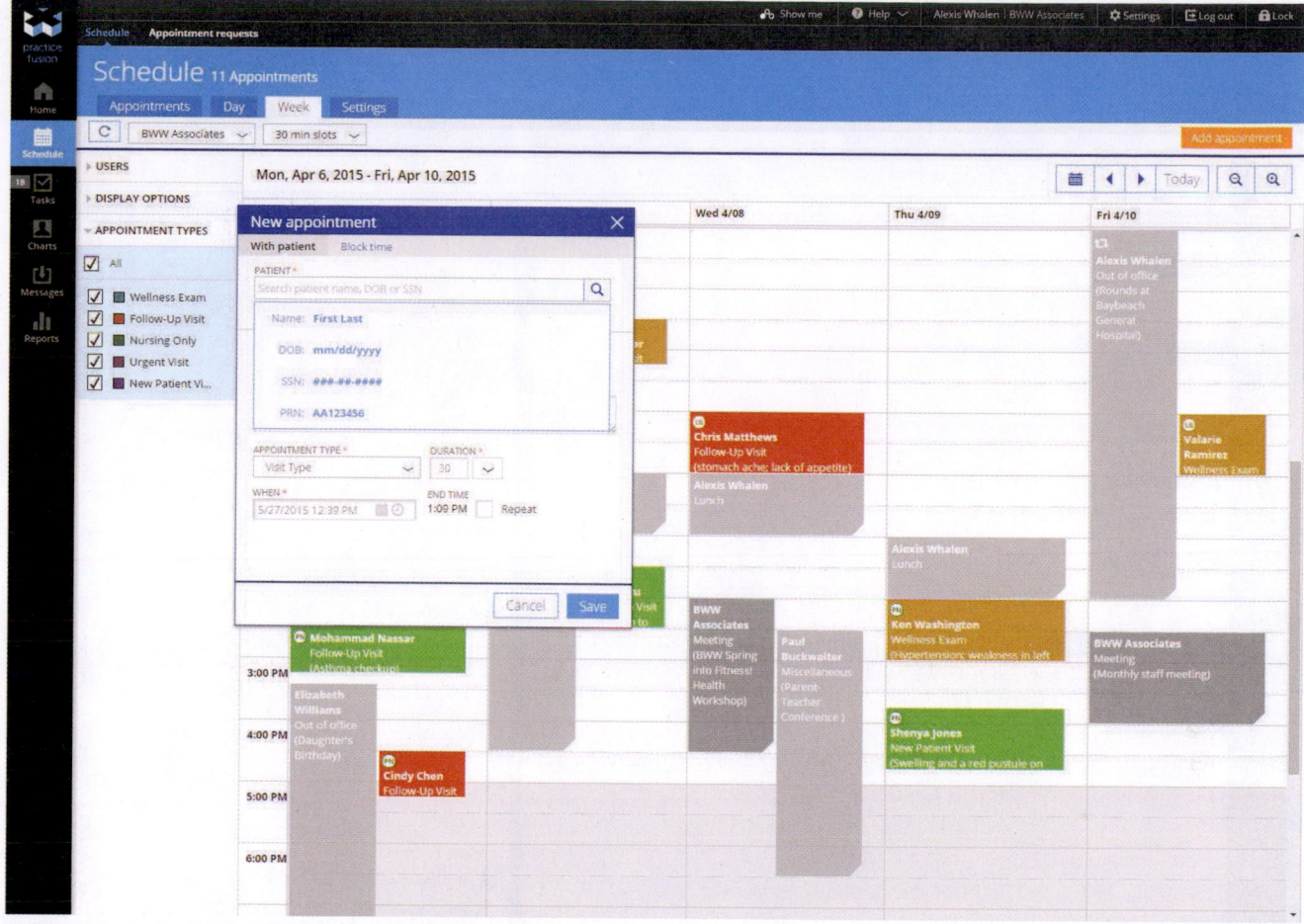

FIGURE 12-5 Electronic scheduler program in Practice Fusion®.
© Practice Fusion®

next appointment in the record. In addition to these tasks, electronic schedulers can keep a listing of patients who want an earlier appointment if one becomes available and allow you to search for appointments by time frame needed or by appointment type needed (like a complete physical or a BP check).

One disadvantage of electronic schedulers is the fact that if the computer is down, appointments cannot be made and the day's schedule is not accessible. So it is always a good idea to print out a copy of each day's schedule at the beginning of the day. Some offices also keep a backup appointment book handy in case of power failure. Some EHR scheduler programs also include appointment reminder and confirmation programs to automatically remind patients of their appointments. These programs then give patients the option to either confirm attendance or change the appointment by phone or online. Procedure 12-3 outlines the steps in creating an electronic scheduler appointment matrix. Procedure 12-4 outlines the process for booking a patient appointment using an electronic scheduler.

Eligibility Verification and Referral Management

It is always wise—before performing any procedure—to verify the patient's insurance coverage. Many Practice Management programs make this process easier by assisting with online insurance verification. In addition to verifying coverage, most programs also allow for capturing the patient's demographic information at the same time.

Many managed care programs require the patient's PCP to provide any specialist with a referral before the specialist can see the patient and before most procedures can be performed. Most EHR software programs not only allow the physicians to readily share information about the patient via the software package but also allow for electronic transmission of referrals among the PCP, the specialist, and the insurance plan involved. In addition, the number of visits allowed by the referral, the time frame involved, and the number of visits left on any given day can be tracked within the patient's medical record.

Billing and Coding Software

Many Practice Management Systems and EHR programs include billing and coding software, allowing for electronic coding of medical records, and electronic claims submission to insurance carriers. Depending on the software program being used, the procedure and diagnosis codes may be automatically chosen by the software program based on the medical record or may be coded and inserted manually by the office medical coder (Figure 12-6). Alerts to the system may be added, so if a charge does not match a diagnosis code, a flag is produced. An example would be a patient is seen for a skin biopsy, but the only diagnosis for the visit is hypertension.

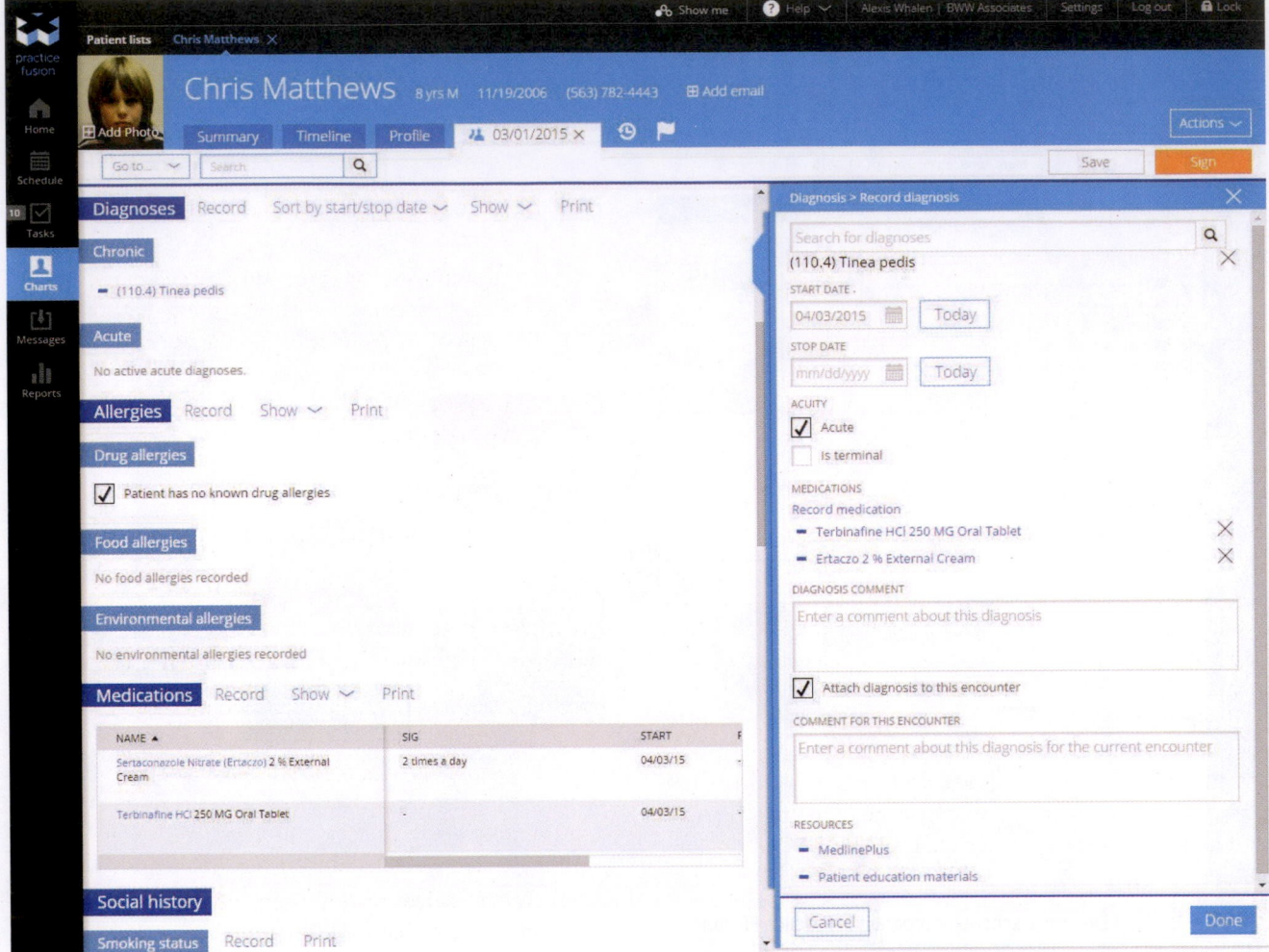

FIGURE 12-6 Practice Fusion® screen shot of office visit details for Chris Matthews, including diagnoses addition fields.
© Practice Fusion®

Because hypertension is not a reason to do a skin biopsy, an alert would appear stating the diagnosis does not meet medical necessity guidelines. Even if an electronic coding program is being used, an experienced coder should perform random internal coding audits several times a year to ensure that coding is being performed correctly. Once coding is completed, the electronic claim is submitted to the insurance carrier.

Once the insurance carrier has paid the claim, most programs also include a patient billing component so the administrative staff can produce a billing statement for the patient. This statement lists the total amount of the charges, the amount paid by the insurance plan, deductibles, and the co-payment or coinsurance balance due from the patient. You will learn more about medical billing and coding in the chapters covering these subjects later in this text.

Report Generators

Most EHR programs also include a report generator, also known as a report writer. This part of the EHR program extracts information from one or more of the patient files and presents that information in a specific format to be used for other purposes. Multiple files are accessed that meet certain conditions. Reports can be used for things such as

research or billing and accounting. Report formats may be preset or you can create your own report to reuse when needed. The types of reports that may be produced include:

- Patient demographics
- Office accounts receivable (A/R) and accounts payable (A/P)
- Office statistics (including the number of individual procedures done during a specified time frame)
- Revenue generated by specific procedures
- Other tracking mechanisms to assist the office business manager in tracking both profitable and nonprofitable procedures for the practice
- Patient and insurance carrier aging reports (reports of unpaid invoices arranged according to how long ago the invoices were generated) to see who is or who is not paying the office claims and statements promptly

Electronic Prescriptions

To encourage the use of electronic prescribing and EHR programs, Medicare and Medicaid offered e-prescribing incentives, and now virtually all EHR programs include prescription writers. These programs allow entry of prescriptions, which may be transmitted directly to the pharmacy or printed and given to the patient. Lists of the most common medications (and dosages) prescribed by the physician also may be kept in the program. Because the program communicates with the patient's individual medical record, any allergies can cause a flag for an ordered prescription; possible medication interactions will do the same.

Ancillary Order Integration

Many EHR programs also include ancillary programs for labs, X-rays, and other diagnostic and therapeutic services. Orders can be submitted to the lab or ancillary office electronically at the time the patient appointment is made. Once testing is complete, the results of the test(s) are transmitted back to the office as soon as they are available, allowing for immediate upload to the patient's medical record. This greatly cuts down on patient and physician wait time for results. Additionally, results may be faxed, scanned, or e-mailed as necessary.

Patient Access

Most patients today are technically quite savvy. In fact, many prefer most communication to occur through electronic means instead of spending telephone time on hold or waiting for someone at the office to be free to make an appointment or provide routine information. Recognizing this, many EHR packages and offices provide patient portals so that a patient can access routine information and perform routine tasks, like making an appointment, accessing a child's immunization record, or even paying a balance on his or her account, online.

▶ Security and Confidentiality and EHR   LO 12.7

When medical records are kept electronically, it is essential that the facility have policies in place to ensure the security and confidentiality of records. As already discussed, all users of the EHR program will have individual access codes and passwords. The access code will allow each user access to only the areas of the record to which the user is entitled, based on his or her job description. Additionally, these access codes insert a date and time stamp within the medical record, including the user's initials, so that office administration and the patient (if requested) may know who is accessing each medical record.

The office also should have a written procedure in place to document when someone requests information from the patient file, if the patient has given permission to release that information, and when it was released. When requested by the patient, this listing must be provided as part of the HIPAA privacy and security act. Protecting the confidentiality of patient records in computer files is the greatest concern of electronic

health records. Electronic health records should be kept just as secure as paper records are kept.

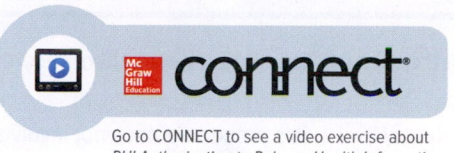

Go to CONNECT to see a video exercise about *PHI Authorization to Release Health Information.*

Remember, too, that whether you are documenting by hand or electronically, accuracy is always important. Careful key entry is essential to maintaining accurate electronic health files, to protect both the patient and the medical office. In addition, processes must be in place to back up electronic files on a regular basis to avoid accidental data loss.

Reassuring Others about EHR Confidentiality and Security

As the office medical assistant, it will often be part of your job to reassure patients and other staff members that the office EHR program and the information it contains are confidential and secure. There are several ways you can do this.

- Be knowledgeable about all the confidentiality and security aspects of the office EHR program.
- Never display negativity about the new program, even when things don't go "exactly right" when you are using it. Remember, there is a learning curve with every new process. Remain patient and interested in the process.
- Suggest the office create a pamphlet or flyer for the patients regarding the office EHR program and assist in preparing the document for the patients.
- When working in the program, show the patient his own medical record and how information is entered, maintained, and saved, including the backup process. Explain the security systems that are in place in easy-to-understand terms to reassure the patient that his medical information is accurate, safe, and secure.
- Explain the office access process to the patients, including the fact that they may view the list of people or companies (like insurance carriers) who have accessed their information, when the access took place, and why.

Overall, the benefits of electronic health records far outweigh the consequences, and with the federal government stepping in to mandate the conversion to EHR, change is inevitable. As the office medical assistant, always be willing to learn any new process, including EHR; assist others with their learning process; and help the patients understand that EHR will only improve the healthcare they receive from your office.

PROCEDURE 12-1 Creating a New Patient Record Using EHR Software

Procedure Goal: To create a new patient record using EHR software

OSHA Guidelines: This procedure does not involve exposure to blood, body fluids, or tissue.

Materials: Initial patient forms (patient information, advance directives, physician notes, referrals, and laboratory orders)

Method:

1. Open the Practice Fusion® Program and, from the Practice Dashboard, choose "Charts" from the task choices listed down the left side of the screen.

2. Click the "Add Patient" button in the upper-right corner

3. Using the initial patient forms completed by the patient, complete the patient demographic information fields one at a time. Be sure to spell the patient's name correctly.
   RATIONALE: *This is a legal record. The information must be entered correctly.*

4. Any field marked with an * is a required field. For instance, mobile phone number and e-mail address are required. If the patient does not have an e-mail address, check the box below this field stating "Patient doesn't have an email address."

   RATIONALE: *A required field is considered essential information by the practice, so the field cannot be skipped.*

5. Continue completing fields, including those for guarantor and insurance information. The guarantor will be the patient unless the patient is a minor.
   RATIONALE: *The guarantor is the person legally responsible for paying the patient's medical bills.*

6. Carefully inspect all information for accuracy and save the new patient record by clicking the "Save" button at the top right of the screen. If for any reason you do not want to save the information, click the "Cancel" button at the top right of the screen.
   RATIONALE: *This information will become part of the patient's permanent medical record. Proofread all information and verify accuracy before striking "Save."*

7. Depending on office policy, information from a hardcopy medical record may be scanned into the EHR or a manual file created to maintain it. Follow your office procedure for filing this information.
   RATIONALE: *All patient information must be readily available for healthcare providers when required for patient care.*

PROCEDURE 12-2 Making an Addition or Addendum (Correction) to an Electronic Health Record

Procedure Goal: To follow standard procedures for correcting or making an addendum to an electronic health record

OSHA Guidelines: This procedure does not involve exposure to blood, body fluids, or tissue.

Materials: Access to the patient's EHR and other pertinent documents containing the information to be used in making corrections (for example, handwritten notes, telephone notes, physician comments, correspondence, or test results)

Method:

1. Open the Practice Fusion® Program and, from the Practice Dashboard, choose "Charts" from the task choices listed down the left side of the screen.

2. From the patient roster that appears, click the patient whose record requires attention.

   RATIONALE: *Be sure to open the correct record, or another correction will be required later.*

3. From the right side of the screen, click the date for the note requiring the correction or addendum.
   RATIONALE: *Be sure to select the correct date to avoid making additional errors.*

4. Choose the area of the record requiring the changes. Make the required changes and then click the "Done" button to save the changes.
   RATIONALE: *If "Done" is not selected, the change will not be saved within the health record. The user's identity and date will automatically be stamped on the record for further reference.*

5. Back at the main screen for the patient, click "Save" at the top-right corner to finalize changes made to the record.

PROCEDURE 12-3 Creating an Appointment Matrix for an Electronic Scheduling System

Procedure Goal: Using an electronic scheduling system, to indicate the days and times when the office is not scheduling appointments

OSHA Guidelines: This procedure does not involve exposure to blood, body fluids, or tissue.

Materials: Electronic scheduling program; physician schedule of meetings, conferences, vacations, and other times of unavailability, including staff meetings and hours when patients are not seen

Method:

1. Open the Practice Fusion® Program and, from the Practice Dashboard, choose "Schedule" from the task choices listed down the left side of the screen.

2. Choose the calendar icon at the top-right corner of the screen and from the calendar that appears, select the month and day requiring the change.

3. Click "Add Appointment." From the options that appear, choose "Block Time."

RATIONALE: *When creating the matrix, this choice allows you to put in a reason without choosing patient information.*

4. Using the drop-down arrows, complete information for the following fields: When (date), Duration (amount of time), and Repeat (or never).

5. The next field is Reason. Use the drop-down menu to specify why patients will not be seen in this time frame. The choices are lunch, meeting, miscellaneous, out of office, surgery, and vacation. This is a required field.
   RATIONALE: *The reason that the time will not be used for patients will appear in the schedule for future reference.*

6. In the Description field, enter a short description regarding the reason patients will not be seen. This will be viewed by anyone looking at the schedule.

7. If any notes are needed about this blocked time, they may be added to the Notes area.

8. When all information is completed, click the "Done" button at the lower-right corner of the block time fields to save the information to the scheduler.

PROCEDURE 12-4 Scheduling a Patient Appointment Using an Electronic Scheduler

Procedure Goal: Utilizing the previously created matrix, to book patient appointments, applying the correct amount of time for each appointment

OSHA Guidelines: This procedure does not involve exposure to blood, body fluids, or tissue.

Materials: Electronic scheduler and template outlining time frames for patient appointment types

Method:

1. Establish the type of appointment required by the patients, particularly noting if the appointment is for a new patient or an established patient.
   RATIONALE: *In general, new patient appointments take longer time frames than do existing patient appointments.*

2. If needed, consult the office template for the amount of time required for the patient appointment. Keep in mind the reason for the appointment, as that may affect timing.
   RATIONALE: *If a patient is required to be fasting, for example, the appointment should be made earlier in the day and not in the afternoon.*

3. When possible, schedule appointments earlier in the day first, and then move to later time frames. Do ask if the patient has a preferred time frame and, if possible, honor the request.

4. Open the Practice Fusion® Program and, from the Practice Dashboard, choose "Schedule" from the task choices listed down the left side of the screen.

5. Click "Add Appointment." From the options that appear, choose "Patient" and enter the first few letters of the patient's last name.
   RATIONALE: *This allows you to enter the name of a new patient, or once you enter a few letters of an existing patient, choose the correct patient from the drop-down list.*

6. Enter the chief complaint given by the patient and choose the required "visit type" from the drop-down menu. Enter the length of the visit from the drop-down menu in the next field.
   RATIONALE: *The visit type is required to give the provider an idea of the type of visit scheduled.*

7. If the appointment is to be a repeated one, check the "Repeat" box and complete the fields that appear to specify when and how often the patient will be seen.
   RATIONALE: *This makes it easier to complete multiple appointments for a patient at one time.*

8. When all information is completed, click the "Save" button at the lower-right corner of the screen to save the appointment and enter it into the schedule.

LEARNING OUTCOMES	KEY POINTS
12.1 **List four medical mistakes that will be greatly decreased through the use of EHR.**	Medical mistakes that will be greatly decreased or eliminated with EHR include lost or misfiled paper records, mishandled or "forgotten" patient messages, inaccurate or unreadable information in a paper medical record, and mislabeled or unreadable laboratory or prescription orders.
12.2 **Differentiate among electronic medical records, electronic health records, and personal health records.**	The electronic medical record is an electronic record of health-related information for an individual patient that is created, compiled, and managed by providers and staff members located within a *single* healthcare organization. An electronic health record is created, managed, and gathered in a manner that conforms to nationally recognized *interoperability standards,* so that members of more than one healthcare organization can utilize it. A personal health record is an electronic version of the comprehensive medical history and record of a patient's lifelong health that is collected and maintained by the individual patient.
12.3 **Explain the concept of meaningful use, identifying at least two of its goals.**	*Meaningful use* describes EHR as improving quality, safety, and efficiency, reducing health disparities. It engages the patient and family as well as improves coordination of care for population and public health. Maintenance of privacy and security of PHI are also required. The goals include better clinical outcomes, improved population health outcomes, increased transparency and efficiency, empowered individuals, and more robust research data on health systems.
12.4 **Contrast the advantages and disadvantages of electronic health records.**	Advantages of EHR include fewer lost medical records, elimination of transcription costs, increased readability/legibility of charts, ease of chart access for multiple users, chart availability outside of office hours, increased access to patient education materials, decreased duplication of medical tests, more efficient records transfer, more efficient billing processes using electronic billing methods, and decreased need for storage space. Disadvantages include cost, need for training, possible need for F/T or P/T IT personnel, and need for computer hardware/software upgrades or changes.
12.5 **Illustrate the steps in creating a new patient record and correcting an existing record using EHR software.**	The same rules apply for EHR as for paper-based medical records when initiating or documenting in a patient's electronic health record. Follow the basic steps in Procedure 12-1 for setting up a new patient EHR and 12-2 for correcting or making an addition in an existing patient's electronic health record.
12.6 **Describe some of the capabilities of EHR software programs.**	Aside from housing patient electronic health records, many EHR programs also can perform the following functions: tickler files, specialty-specific software, electronic scheduler, eligibility verification and referral management, billing and coding capabilities, report generation, electronic prescriptions and ancillary order integration, and a patient access portal.
12.7 **Explain how you might alleviate a patient's security fears surrounding the use of EHR.**	Be knowledgeable on all aspects of the office EHR program and never display a negative attitude about it. Assist in preparing written information for the patients regarding the EHR program, including how the patient's medical information will remain confidential and secure. When the patient is in the office, offer to show the patient his EHR, and explain how information is added, entered, maintained, and kept secure. Understand and be able to explain the backup process for the EHR program. Understand the office access policy as it pertains to HIPAA, and explain it to the patients.

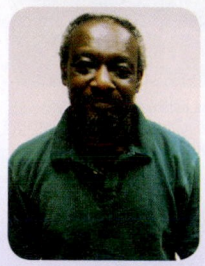

© McGraw-Hill Education

Recall Ken Washington from the beginning of the chapter. Now that you have completed the chapter, answer the following questions regarding his case.

1. How will you explain the benefits of using electronic health records to Ken Washington?

2. The screen Ken Washington has seen displays only the screen saver for the new EHR program. What precautions should be taken to ensure that patients do not see another patient's information on the computer monitor?

3. The practice you for work for wants to review all of the patients who have similar problems as Ken Washington. What function of the EHR program would you use, and what problems would you search for?

EXAM PREPARATION QUESTIONS

1. (LO 12.1) Medical errors in the United States are calculated to be the _____ leading cause of patient death.
   a. 2nd
   b. 4th
   c. 6th
   d. 8th
   e. 10th

2. (LO 12.2) Patient electronic health information created in a format meeting *interoperability standards* is defined as being in a(n)_____ format.
   a. EMR
   b. EHR
   c. PHR
   d. EMR or EHR
   e. None of these

3. (LO 12.2) An individual's lifelong health record is a(n)
   a. EMR
   b. EHR
   c. PHR
   d. Any of these
   e. None of these

4. (LO 12.3) What is the ultimate goal of EHR implementation and meaningful use?
   a. Ability to read practitioner notes
   b. Replacement of transcriptionists
   c. Selling of more Practice Management Systems
   d. Better patient care
   e. Better care of at-risk populations

5. (LO 12.3) Part of meaningful use is to empower patients and families. How is that to happen?
   a. Patients should be given reading material
   b. Providers should make sure patients understand all their options
   c. Patients should be given websites to look up information
   d. Patients should be given material and providers should make sure patients understand all of their options
   e. All of these

6. (LO 12.5) Many EHR programs use the term _____ for a correction made to an electronic health record.
   a. Deletion
   b. Error
   c. Addendum
   d. Omission
   e. Correction

7. (LO 12.6) Which of the following functions of the EHR program will be most helpful to the administration when reviewing the financial health of the practice?
   a. Report generator
   b. Tickler file
   c. Billing/coding
   d. Electronic scheduler
   e. Specialty-specific programs

8. (LO 12.6) Which of the functions of the EHR program would be most helpful to the staff who schedules appointments for patients with specialists?
   a. Billing coding
   b. Specialty-specific programs
   c. Ancillary order integration
   d. Electronic prescriptions
   e. Insurance verification

9. (LO 12.7) Which item maintains each user's ability to work in certain areas of a patient's electronic health record?
   a. Password
   b. Access code
   c. Confidentiality
   d. HIPAA
   e. None of these

10. (LO 12.8) Which of the following will *not* reassure patients about the privacy and security of the office EHR system?

   a. Showing the patient how information is entered in his or her medical record

   b. Being knowledgeable about the security of the office EHR system

   c. Sharing "computer frustrations" with the patient

   d. Explaining how the backup system for the EHR program works

   e. Assisting in the creation of a pamphlet for the patients regarding the new office EHR system

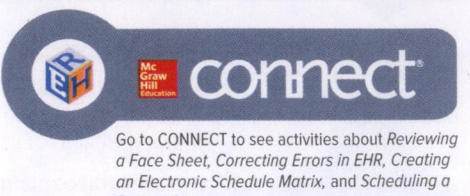

Go to CONNECT to see activities about *Reviewing a Face Sheet, Correcting Errors in EHR, Creating an Electronic Schedule Matrix,* and *Scheduling a Patient Appointment.*

S O F T   S K I L L S   S U C C E S S

Recall Ken Washington from the case study at the beginning of the chapter.

1. You have just assured Ken Washington that his medical information will be safe on the office's new EHR system. As he is checking out, the administrative assistant, who had been looking up something in his record for the physician, leaves her station momentarily, just as Ken walks by. He sees his record up on the screen and is upset. What should you say to Ken?

2. As a follow-up to the incident that occurred with Ken Washington, you have been asked to create a poster for the lounge to help remind the providers and staff on a regular basis of policies related to the use of the new EHR. What things should you include?

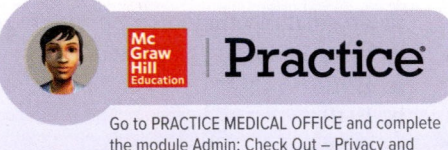

Go to PRACTICE MEDICAL OFFICE and complete the module Admin: Check Out – Privacy and Liability.

Managing Medical Records

CASE STUDY

EMPLOYEE INFORMATION

Employee Name	Position	Credentials
Malik Katahri	Office Manager	CMM

Supervisor	Date of Hire	Other Information
BWW Physicians	04/20/20XX	Meetings with EHR vendors with week

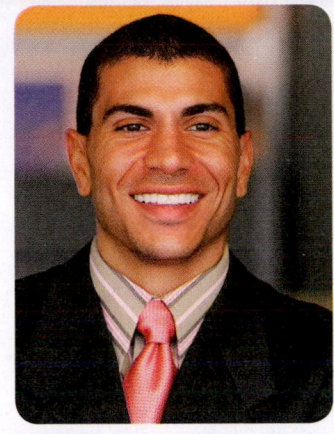

Malik Katahri is the office manager for BWW Medical Associates, PC. The number of patients the office sees is growing at an amazing rate and although good for the practice, it is taxing the current alphabetic filing system. Malik and the office staff have been discussing the pros and cons of converting to a numeric filing system or possibly doing away with paper records totally and moving toward a more progressive EHR program. The physicians are reluctant to commit to an EHR program related to the financial outlay and staff training time required.

Keep Malik in mind as you study this chapter. There will be questions at the end of the chapter based on the case study. The information in the chapter will help you answer these questions.

LEARNING OUTCOMES

After completing Chapter 13, you will be able to:

13.1 Identify the common equipment used to file and store paper medical records.

13.2 Outline the security and safety measures that should be employed when working with paper medical records.

13.3 List the common filing supplies used in the medical office.

13.4 Contrast the methods used for various filing systems and how color-coding can assist with the filing systems.

13.5 Recall the steps in the filing process.

13.6 Compare active, inactive, and closed files and how to set up a records retention program for the office.

KEY TERMS

active file

alphabetic filing system

closed file

coding

compactible file

cross-referenced

file guide

inactive file

indexing

indexing rules

indirect filing system

inspecting (conditioning)

lateral file

middle digit

numeric filing system

out guide

records management system

releasing

retention schedule

reverse chronological order

sequential order

terminal digit

tickler file

unit

vertical file

VI.C.6 Identify equipment and supplies needed for medical records in order to:
  (a) Create
  (b) Maintain
  (c) Store
VI.C.7 Describe filing indexing rules
VI.P.5 File patient medical records
X.A.2 Protect the integrity of the medical record
XII.P.3 Use proper body mechanics

8. Administrative Procedures
  a. Gather and process documents
  f. Display professionalism through written and verbal communications
11. Career Development
  b. Demonstrate professional behavior

▶ Introduction

One important administrative function of the medical assistant is the careful management of the patient medical records. The information contained in these records is the most valuable information in a medical office. For a practice using paper medical records to operate smoothly and efficiently, it is critical that these records be organized in a way that makes them easily retrievable. Maintaining a well-organized, easy-to-use **records management system** (the way patient records are created, filed, and maintained) is essential to providing good patient care.

You learned about management of EHR in the *Electronic Health Records* chapter. In this chapter, you will explore the various options for handling large volumes of paper medical records and learn how to develop an organized approach to maintaining these critical files. As you read, watch for helpful tips to locate and access patient records quickly and efficiently.

▶ Filing Equipment   LO 13.1

Filing equipment generally refers to the place where records, or files, are housed. Although there are various types of equipment, two of the most common options are shelves and cabinets. The choice of whether to use filing shelves or filing cabinets is often made according to space considerations and personal preference. Most offices already have a filing system in place before you are hired, but you may be involved in filing decisions if the practice grows or opens a satellite office. When making any equipment decision, keep in mind that any choice must take into consideration space constraints and the needs of a growing practice. To protect PHI contained within the files, the equipment must be fireproof and secure.

Filing Shelves

Filing shelves resemble traditional shelves, as shown in Figure 13-1. Many shelf systems have doors that slide from side to side or slide out from above the files. These doors can be locked for security. Filing shelves are often long, sometimes

extending the full length and height of an office wall or room, which allows several people to work in the file area at the same time.

Filing Cabinets

Filing cabinets are sturdy pieces of office furniture, usually made of wood or metal. They contain a series of drawers in which files are hung. They come in two styles:

- **Vertical files,** which are taller with narrow drawers that are approximately the width of a standard file folder
- **Lateral files,** also known as horizontal files, which have wider drawers that are usually split into three or four sections, allowing more files to be stored in each drawer (see Figure 13-2)

The drawback of each of these file cabinets is the fact that for safety reasons, only one drawer may be pulled out at a time (so the file does not fall over on the user), which means only one person at a time can access the file cabinet. For more information on patient and staff safety in all aspects of the medical office, refer to the chapter *Safety and Patient Reception.*

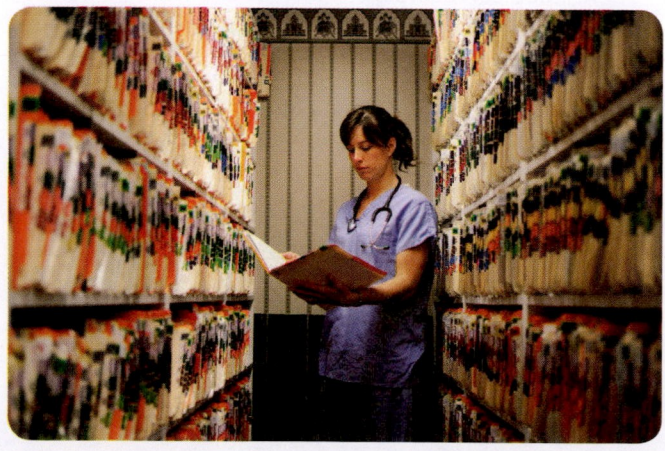

FIGURE 13-1 Medical records kept on shelves are easily accessible and can be kept secured in a separate room.
© Digital Vision/Getty Images RF

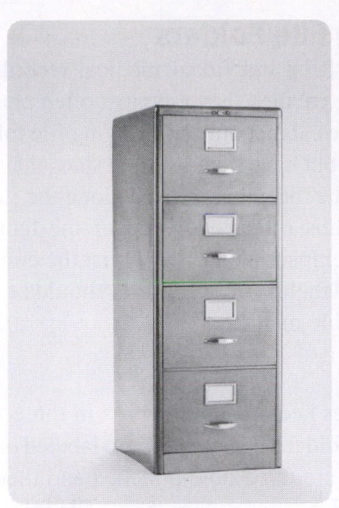

(a) Vertical files

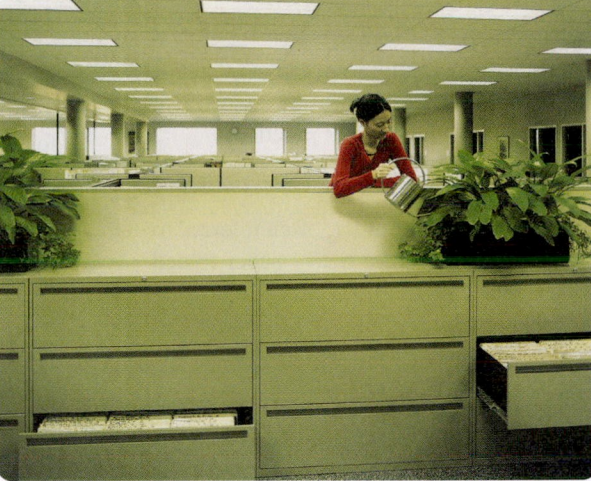

(b) Lateral files

FIGURE 13-2 (a) Example of vertical file cabinet. (b) Lateral file cabinet.
© Image Source RF; © Exactostock/SuperStock RF

Compactible Files

Many offices have limited space in which to house filing cabinets or shelves. These offices may choose to use a variation of shelf filing called **compactible files.** Compactible files are kept on rolling shelves that slide along permanent tracks in the floor.

When not in use, these files can be stored close together—even one on top of another—to conserve space. When needed, they can be rolled out into an open area so that the staff can easily use them. Compactible files can be moved manually or automatically with the touch of a button.

Rotary Circular Files

Rotary circular files are another option to consider when space is limited. These files are stored in a circular fashion, similar to a revolving door, and are accessed by rotating the files. They also can be operated either manually or electronically.

Labeling Filing Equipment

Regardless of which type of filing equipment your office uses, files should be clearly labeled on the outside of the drawer so that you do not have to open doors or drawers to know the contents. When labeling storage boxes (such as may be used for inactive records), use a permanent marker to clearly label the contents of the box. Writing directly on the box removes any possibility of a label falling off a box while in storage. If the contents may one day be destroyed, the destroy date should also be included in the labeling. For example, the label may read as follows:

Medical Records Last Names A–D. Date Last Seen 01/01/XX-06/30/XX. Destroy date: 12/31/XX

Record retention schedules will be discussed later in the chapter.

▶ Security and Safety Measures   LO 13.2

All filing systems must be secured under HIPAA privacy and security regulations. HIPAA states that there must be a "reasonable safeguard" to protect health information from any disclosure, whether intentional or unintentional. Using locking, fireproof filing cabinets to store patient records is an important element of this requirement. *Never* place patient records in an unsecured filing system. Additionally, both staff and patients must be safe when using and being around the office filing system.

Medical Record Security

Today's filing cabinets come with a lock and key. Cabinets that are not in a separate room should be locked every night when the office is being closed for the day. To protect filing shelves in a separate room, you can lock the file room. Security of the keys to that room then becomes an important issue. The number of staff members who have keys to that room should be limited— perhaps to just the healthcare providers and the office manager. When the office manager comes into the office each morning, she can unlock the files. Because the files remain open during the day, it is important to make sure they are not placed in areas where unauthorized people can obtain access to them. Posting a sign on the file room door stating "Authorized Personnel Only" helps ensure that files remain secure. To ensure office security after hours, some practices install alarm systems.

Keys and locks bring a measure of security only when they are *used.* Do not become lazy and neglect to lock filing cabinets and file rooms when leaving the office for the day. Security survey teams will always ask to see the keys to any locked door or cabinet and ask the staff to demonstrate that they work. Within a medical office, conducting regular security drills at the same time that fire drills are held will aid staff in staying sharp and aware of security risks.

▶ Filing Supplies

Once you have chosen your filing equipment, the next step is selecting filing supplies. Figure 13-3 features an assortment of filing supplies commonly used by medical practices.

File Folders

The most basic filing supply is the file folder, often referred to as a manila folder. This folder is made of heavy paper folded in half to form a pocket that can hold papers. File folders come in two sizes: letter size, which is 8½ × 11 inches, and legal size, which is 8½ × 14 inches.

Tabs The tapered, rectangular or rounded extension at the top or side of the folder is called the tab. Tabs may extend the full length of the folder, as with straight-cut folders, but more often they are cut to extend partway across a folder.

Using folders with a variety of tab locations makes it easier to read the names on the tabs. The most common type of folder for medical charts is the third-cut folder. Tabs are one-third the width of the folder and appear at the left side, center, or right side.

Labels Labels are often used on the folder tabs to identify the individual folder's contents. You can write directly on the tab area, but it is critical that each label be printed very clearly, so it is more desirable to print the chart label. This method is consistently easier to read and lends a more professional appearance. Printed labels can easily be created using a label template available with most word processing software programs, like Microsoft Word.

No matter what filing system your office uses, it is important to be consistent in preparing file labels. If all the files are labeled with the patient's last name, followed by the patient's first name and middle initial (for example, Brown, Emma L.), each label must then follow this format. It is important that the patients' names are always spelled correctly, whether on the chart label or within the record itself.

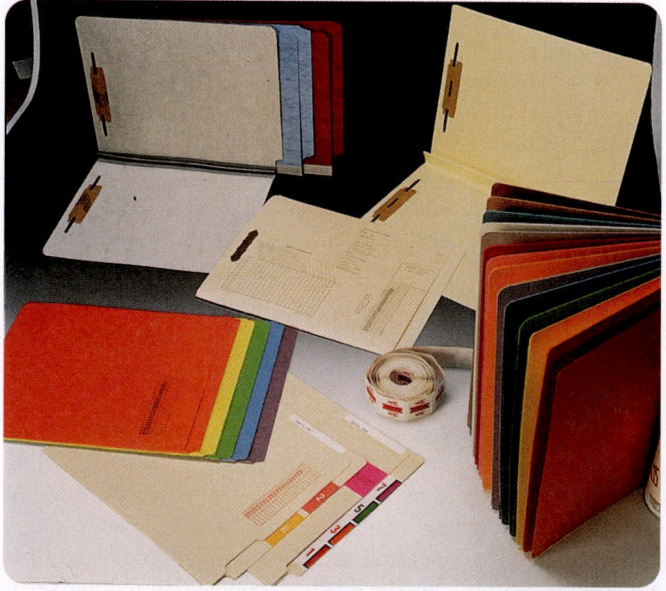

FIGURE 13-3 Medical offices use a wide assortment of filing supplies.
Courtesy Bibbero Systems, Inc.

Hanging File Folders

In order to keep individual medical records neatly organized within a file cabinet, they are most often placed in hanging file folders in the cabinet drawer. Hanging file folders resemble regular folders but have hooks on the sides that allow the folder to hang from the metal bars placed along the sides of the drawer.

Plastic tabs inserted on top of the hanging filed folders contain label inserts that clearly list the contents of the folder. As with all labeling, these inserts should be prepared in a consistent, legible manner.

Binders

Some offices keep patient records in three-ring binders rather than in file folders. The binders are labeled on the outside spine. Documents are three-hole-punched and then placed inside the binder. Binders are stronger than a file folder but require more storage space and so may not be functional for most medical offices. Inactive patient records can be transferred to a file folder for off-site storage. The binder can then be used again. Binders are especially effective for practices that see patients repeatedly, resulting in very large medical records.

File Guides

To identify a group of file folders in a file drawer, you may use **file guides,** which are heavy cardboard or plastic inserts to separate the contents so individual files can be found easily. For example, if a drawer contains the files for patients whose last names begin with the letters A through C, the guides might separate A from B and B from C.

Out Guides

Another filing supply is an **out guide.** An out guide is a marker made of stiff material. It is used as a placeholder when a file has been removed from the filing system. Many out guides include a clear pocket that can hold the name of the file that belongs in that place or the name of the individual who took the file, and its return due date. Other out guides contain a lined sheet of paper where you can write who has the chart and the date it was taken on the out guide, and then cross it out when the file is returned. Out guides can be used for both shelf and cabinet filing.

Although out guides are not essential, they are extremely helpful in ensuring that files are returned to their proper places. Out guides also save time, as they make it obvious when a file is missing and where it is to be returned. Out guides work best when the entire staff, including the practitioners, makes a dedicated effort to use the system.

File Sorters

File sorters are large, accordion-style folders with tabs in which records can be stored temporarily, until the patient records can be returned to their proper placement in the cabinet or shelf. Other file sorters may also sit on a desk and have multiple slots for temporary placement of patient records.

▶ Filing Systems

A filing system is the method by which files are organized. A variety of filing systems may be used, but every system places patient records in some sort of **sequential order**—one after another in a pattern, or sequence, that can be predicted. Always follow the office filing system exactly, as any deviation can result in lost or misplaced records. Never make any changes in the filing system without first consulting all members of the practice.

Alphabetic Filing System

One of the most common and easiest filing systems for maintaining patient files in sequential order is the **alphabetic filing system.** In the alphabetic filing system, files are arranged in alphabetic order. Each patient's medical record is labeled with the patient's last name, followed by the first name and the middle initial (if any). Let's look at this example, consisting of four patient names, filed alphabetically:

Williams, Louis R.
Wilson, Michelle A.
Wilson, T. Andrew.
Wilson, Thomas A.

The specific rules to follow when filing personal names alphabetically are called **indexing rules** (Table 13-1). These rules

TABLE 13-1 Indexing Rules for Alphabetic Filing of Personal Names

In alphabetizing, treat each part of a patient's name as a separate unit and look at the units in this order: last name, first name, middle initial, and any subsequent names or initials last. Disregard punctuation. Follow the "nothing before something" rule—an initial will come before a full name spelled out.

Name	Unit 1	Unit 2	Unit 3	Unit 4
Stephen Jacobson	Jacobson	Stephen		
Stephen Brent Jacobson	Jacobson	Stephen	Brent	
B. T. Jacoby	Jacoby	B	T	
C. Bruce Hay Jacoby	Jacoby	C	Bruce	Hay
D. Jones	Jones	D		
David Jones	Jones	David		
Kwong Kow Ng*	Ng	Kwong	Kow	
Philip K. Ng	Ng	Philip	K	

Treat a prefix, such as the "O" in O'Hara, as part of the name, not as a separate unit. Ignore variations in spacing, punctuation, and capitalization. Treat prefixes—such as De La, Mac, Saint, and St.—exactly as they are spelled.

Name	Unit 1	Unit 2	Unit 3	Unit 4
A. Serafino Delacruz	Delacruz	A	Serafino	
Victor P. De La Cruz	DeLaCruz	Victor	P	
Irene J. MacKay	MacKay	Irene	J	
Walter G. Mac Kay	MacKay	Walter	G	
Kyle N. Saint Clair	SaintClair	Kyle	N	
Peter St. Clair	StClair	Peter		

Treat hyphenated names as a single unit. Disregard the hyphen.

Name	Unit 1	Unit 2	Unit 3	Unit 4
Victor Puentes-Ruiz	PuentesRuiz	Victor		
Jean-Marie Vigneau	Vigneau	JeanMarie		

A title, such as Dr. or Major, or a seniority term, such as Jr. or 3d, should be treated as the last filing unit to distinguish names that are otherwise identical.

Name	Unit 1	Unit 2	Unit 3	Unit 4
Dr. George B. Diaz	Diaz	George	B	Dr
Major George B. Diaz	Diaz	George	B	Major
George B. Diaz, MD	Diaz	George	B	MD
James R Foster Jr.	Foster	James	R	Jr
James R Foster Sr.	Foster	James	R	Sr
Sister Theresa**	Sister	Theresa		

*In the case of foreign or Asian names, when unsure of first- and last-name order, many offices cross-reference the file with a "dummy record" at the alternate location stating "see Ng, Kwong Kow."

**"Sister Theresa" and similar names, where there is no clear first or last name, are "filed as written."

Source: Adapted from William A. Sabin, *The Gregg Reference Manual, 11th ed.* (Columbus, OH: Glencoe/McGraw-Hill, 2011).

are used as guidelines for the sequencing of files based on current business practice. They define a consistent method for the ordering of filed materials. The Association of Records, Managers, and Administrators monitors and updates these suggested methods periodically. In this way, the best, most efficient management of paper records is continually being reevaluated. From time to time, individual medical practices may choose to deviate from some of these accepted practices. However, indexing rules are the norm for most medical practice filing systems.

Indexing rules define each part of a person's name or title as a **unit.** The rules then describe the order to display and manage each unit in an alphabetized system. These rules are designed to keep alphabetizing simple and consistent, but you must know the exact spelling of a patient's name to retrieve a file. You also must know the rules of indexing. Check out the *Points on Practice* feature for common indexing rules and examples of correct filing order when indexing names that are very similar.

Chronological Filing

A chronological filing system is based on dates. Chronological filing is a type of numeric arrangement that uses numeric dates as the indexing units. The most common order of units is year, month, and day, as in 16-11-06 to denote the sixth of November 2016. It is also common practice to order the most current dates first, with the files that follow in decreasing date order.

In a medical practice, filing chronologically is one method used to file documents *within* a patient's chart. The most recent files (by date) are inserted so they are on top of documents with earlier dates in the file folder. This is known as **reverse chronological order.**

Numeric Filing

A **numeric filing system** organizes files by numbers instead of by names. In this system, each patient name is assigned a number. New patients are assigned the next unused number in sequence. Then, instead of being filed by name, the files are arranged in numeric order—1, 2, 3, 4, and so on. The resulting files are sequential by the order in which patients have come to the practice.

Only the numbers are indicated on the files. Numeric filing systems were formerly used only when patient information was considered highly confidential, but now that all patient information is considered PHI, it is found in many practices. Larger practices also find alphabetic filing more cumbersome than numeric filing, which can be expanded more easily than an alphabetic filing system.

A numeric system must include a master list of patient names and their corresponding medical record numbers (MRN). Numeric systems are known as **indirect filing systems.** If the office is not computerized, to ensure confidentiality, the office manager should keep the master list in a secure place. The provider should hold a duplicate copy, which must also be kept under lock and key. To find a patient's file number using a computer system, click the "Open Patient Chart" button and enter the first few letters of the patient's last name. Then scroll through the names and find the required patient (Figure 13-4). Choose that patient (usually by highlighting the patient name) and press the "Enter" key. The computer then provides the medical record number for that patient.

Terminal digit filing is often the filing system of choice for numeric filing systems. This type of filing allows for the storage of an endless number of files with only a minimal amount of searching needed to obtain the correct files. Numbers are assigned in small groups of two or three numbers, similar to a Social Security number. Each group of numbers is then read from right to left, starting with the last unit as the primary index. Filing is done numerically, starting with the lowest number and moving to the highest. For example, all files ending in 000 are filed first. They are then followed by files ending in 001 and so on. See Table 13-2 for an example.

Middle digit filing is similar to terminal digit filing but instead uses the middle group of numbers as the primary index, followed by the left-hand number and then the right-hand one. See Table 13-3 to view the same medical record numbers filed using the middle digit system.

Numeric, terminal digit, and middle digit filing can all be used in combination with color-coding to add even more information to the filing system.

Color-Coding

Color-coding is used when there is a need to distinguish files within a filing system. For example, you may wish to find at a glance all the new patients in the office, all patients on Medicare, or all patients whose last names begin with the letters *WI.* Coding by color can help you do so quickly and easily. Color-coding may be done in a variety of ways using colored file folders, colored labels, plastic tabs, and/or stickers.

Using Classifications To make the best use of color, you must first identify the classifications that are important to your office. For example, it may be important to identify all new patients easily, or those on Medicare. Once a classification is selected, the decision must be made as to what method of coding will be used (folder, labels, or stickers). Then, a different color must be chosen to denote each classification. For example, all new patients may be kept in red folders, or plain manila folders may be used with a red sticker or red filing label attached to the charts of new patients.

An office that uses colored charts to denote specific patient demographics might look something like this: Patients under the age of 18 have blue charts; patients over the age of 65 have red charts; and patients with diabetes have green charts, with a pink sticker added for those who are on insulin. In an emergency situation, such as when a patient with diabetes passes out while in the office, the color-coding could give staff quick and vital information at a glance.

After a color-coding system is finalized, the codes should be prominently posted on a chart in the file room so that all staff members are aware of them. This chart will help to ensure that records are filed correctly. Remember, update

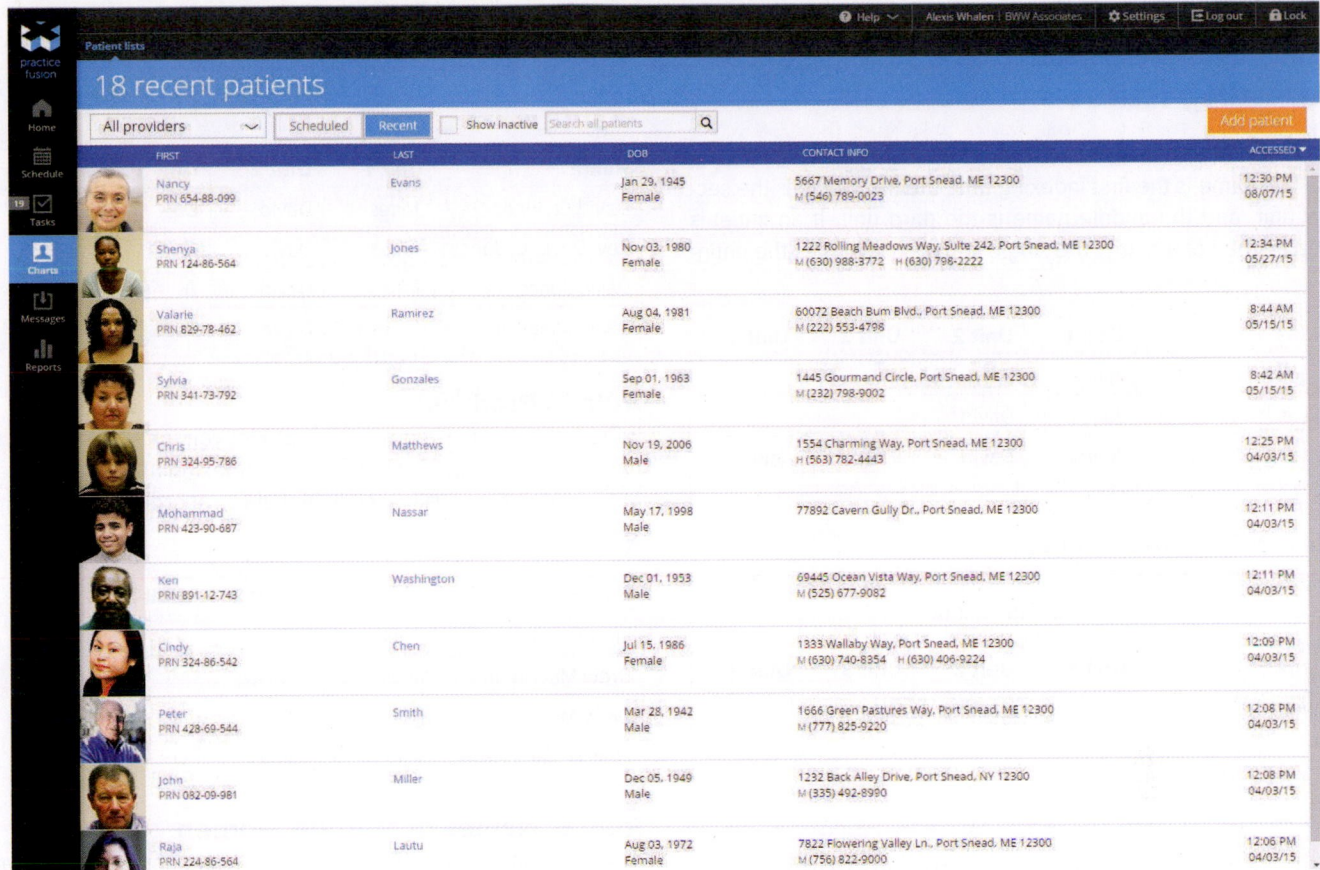

FIGURE 13-4   The recently accessed charts page in Practice Fusion®, with the "Add Patient" button in the top-right corner.

© Practice Fusion®

TABLE 13-2	MRNs Filed in Terminal Digit Order*		
Medical Record Number	Unit 1	Unit 2	Unit 3
002-25-565	565	25	002
001-25-566	566	25	001
001-24-667	667	24	001
002-24-667	667	24	002

*Showing each filing unit.

TABLE 13-3	MRNs Filed in Middle Digit Order*		
Medical Record Number	Unit 1	Unit 2	Unit 3
001-24-667	24	001	667
002-24-667	24	002	667
001-25-566	25	001	566
002-25-565	25	002	565

*Showing each filing unit.

color-coded files consistently, coding new ones and revising older ones as a patient's status changes.

Using Color in an Alphabetic Filing System
Another way to use color-coding is in conjunction with alphabetic filing systems. After files are organized alphabetically, each letter of the alphabet is assigned a color. Then the first two (or three) letters of each patient's last name are color-coded, usually with colored stickers.

The colored tabs are attached to the top of straight-edged or tabbed file folders. For example, if the letter *S* is coded as light blue and the letter *M* is coded as light green, all names starting with *SM*—like Smith—would have light blue and light green

stickers on the tabs of their medical charts. The name Snyder would be filed under a different color combination, such as light blue (for *S*) and peach (for *N*). See Figure 13-5. Because the colors will be the same in each segment of the file drawer, a color-coded system makes it easy to tell at a glance if files are filed correctly (refer back to Figure 13-1).

Using Color in a Numeric Filing System
Color can be used in a similar way with numeric systems. The numerals 1 to 9 may each be assigned a distinct color. As with the alphabetic system, color-coding helps identify numeric files that are out of place. When using color with numeric filing systems, most offices color the primary index or "key unit"

Indexing Rules

Rule 1: Individual Names

The last name is the first indexing unit, the first name is the second unit, and the middle name is the third unit. If an initial is used instead of a name, the single initial is viewed as the entire unit.

Name	Unit 1	Unit 2	Unit 3	Unit 4
D. Jones	Jones	D		
David Jones	Jones	David		
David R. James Jones	Jones	David	R	James

Rule 2: Business Names

As written (on letterhead) each word is a unit. If "The" is used as the first word, it is considered the last unit.

Name	Unit 1	Unit 2	Unit 3	Unit 4
Jones Hearing Supplies	Jones	Hearing	Supplies	
The Jones Hearing Supplies	Jones	Hearing	Supplies	The

Rule 3: Hyphenations and Abbreviations

All hyphenated names are considered to be one unit (that is, Terry-Jones, Sheila); an abbreviated name is combined to form the unit. An abbreviated name, such as Wm. for William, is filed as Wm, without the use of a period.

Name	Unit 1	Unit 2	Unit 3	Unit 4
St. Mary, William	StMary	William		
St. Mary, Wm.	StMary	Wm		
Terry-Jones, Sheila	TerryJones	Sheila		

Rule 4: Titles and Seniority Terms

Titles are normally disregarded unless they are used to distinguish between two patients with the same name. If there are patients with the same name and a title precedes the name, use it as the fourth unit. Seniority terms such as Jr. or Sr. may be indexed as the last unit. It is important to remember that if a male child has exactly the same name as his father, he is considered Jr. until his father dies. He is a III if his father and his grandfather have the same name. If II or III is used as a seniority title, the basic rule states that numbers come before letters, so David Jones III would be filed before David Jones Jr.

Name	Unit 1	Unit 2	Unit 3	Unit 4
David C. Jones	Jones	David	C	
Rev. David C. Jones	Jones	David	C	Rev
David Jones Jr.	Jones	David	Jr	
David Jones Sr.	Jones	David	Sr	

Rule 5: Prefixes

If the last name has a prefix such as Mc, Van, or de, the prefix is part of the last name. It starts the first indexing unit. The prefixes Mc and Mac are usually filed in alphabetical order as part of the last name.

Name	Unit 1	Unit 2	Unit 3	Unit 4
Elias DeLongino	DeLongino	Elias		
Drew MacDreamy	MacDreamy	Drew		
Drew McDreamy	McDreamy	Drew		
Elias D. Van Collins	VanCollins	Elias	D	

Rule 6: Names of Married Women

A woman may retain her maiden name as her last name instead of taking her husband's surname; she also may use both names and hyphenate them (see Rule 3: Hyphenations and Abbreviations). She will always keep her first and middle name as part of her original name. A married woman's name may take several forms.

Name	Unit 1	Unit 2	Unit 3	Unit 4
Mrs. David (Cynthia M.) Jones	Jones	Cynthia	M	
Mrs. Gisele Marie Jones	Jones	Gisele	Marie	
Mrs. Gisele M. Monagan-Jones	MonaganJones	Gisele	M	

Rule 7: Identical Names

If two names are identical, make sure you index them first under their names; location is next (city as the first unit, state as the second unit, street is the third unit, and street number listed lowest to highest is the fourth and final unit). This rule is used for businesses and individuals.

for each chart. If the key unit is three numbers, then all three numbers of the key unit will use a colored tab to identify each file. For example, recall our medical record numbers from Table 13-2 for terminal digit filing (see Example (a)). If #5 is blue, #6 is red, and #7 is yellow, our chart tabs for filing would look as shown in Example (b).

002-25-565
001-25-566
001-24-667
002-24-667

5	6	5
5	6	6
6	6	7
6	6	7

Example (a)   **Example (b)**

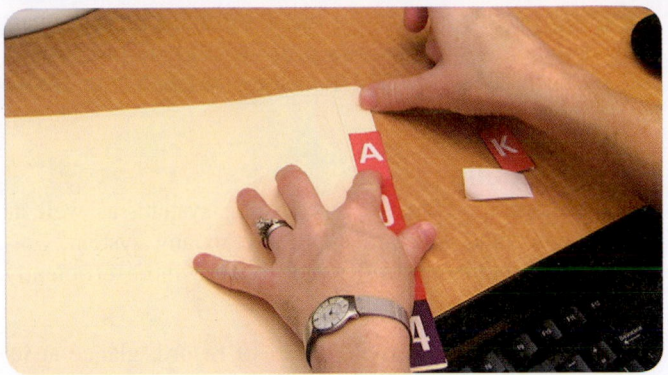

FIGURE 13-5 Colored stickers for both letters and numbers help identify charts rapidly.
© McGraw-Hill Education

Procedure 13-1, at the end of this chapter, explains how to use your knowledge of alphabetic and numeric filing and color-coding to set up a patient records system.

Supplemental Files

Occasionally, you may need to set up additional files to supplement the medical records filing system. For example, you may wish to keep some information separate from the primary file, such as older patient records or the required separate filing system for patient financial and insurance information. In these cases, you set up supplemental files, which allow you to keep this additional information about each patient without cluttering up the primary filing cabinets or making it difficult to find information.

Supplemental files are usually created using the same system as the primary files, but they are kept in a different location. Depending on frequency of use, they may be stored in a less accessible, but equally secure, area of the office. If you are keeping supplemental files, it is important to distinguish their content from that of the primary files. For example, all medical information—like patient diagnosis and treatment—will be kept in the primary files, but the financial, insurance, and billing information for each patient will be kept in a separate billing filing system. This designation will help you and other office staff members know exactly where to go to retrieve specific information.

Tickler Files

To avoid losing track of important dates, many medical practices use tickler files. A **tickler file** is a date-ordered reminder file. Think of your smartphone or home calendar; many of us record important activities and reminders, creating an informal tickler file for our personal activities. Any office activity that needs to be scheduled ahead of time can be noted and a reminder placed in the file. For example, reminders to order supplies or send patient checkup cards can be entered. When the task has been completed, the note can be crossed off the list or removed from the file and thrown away. In computerized offices, many office software packages include calendars and "tickler files" with pop-up reminders of meetings and other activities. Regardless of how it is set up, the person

involved with the activity should regularly check the tickler files at a minimum of once a week— preferably daily. This is important because tickler files only work if they are used regularly.

You can organize tickler files in a variety of ways. The common manual method, discussed in Procedure 13-2 at the end of this chapter, is to allot one file folder to each month of the year or to use a three-ring binder separated with tabs for each month. Tickler files also can be organized by day of the week or week of the month. This method is most useful if there are responsibilities that occur regularly on a certain day of the week or in a certain week within the month. If you find there are so many notes in a monthly folder that it becomes cumbersome, organizing files by the week should make this easier.

Computerized tickler files are usually in the form of a calendar. When the computer is turned on, it lists, for example, "Things to Do Today," with the tickler information posted for that date. Reminders can be set for tasks that must be completed on a regular basis—daily, weekly, or monthly—or on a one-time basis.

▶ The Filing Process   LO 13.5

Pulling and filing patient records and filing individual documents may be among your responsibilities as a medical assistant. Some practices require that records be returned to the files as soon as they are no longer in use. Other practices schedule a specific time at the end of each day to file the current day's records and pull those for the next day.

Records waiting to be filed should be placed temporarily in a file return area. To protect patient privacy, this place should be in a secure area of the office. Clear rules should designate who may handle these files and under what conditions.

The Steps in Filing

Essentially, you will be filing three types of items: new patient records, individual documents that belong in existing patient records, and patient records that are being returned to the filing system. There are five steps involved in filing: inspecting and releasing, indexing, coding, sorting, and storing.

Inspecting and Releasing **Inspecting,** sometimes called **conditioning,** is the process of making sure the item is ready for filing. Remove paper clips or other fasteners, stapling related documents together. If a document is smaller than standard size, it may be attached to a standard sheet of paper with paper or rubber cement. "Shingling" (layering) similar small documents may also be permitted to save space. If smaller documents have wording on both sides of the paper, they may also be placed in a plastic sheet protector and then filed.

Depending on office policy, either just before or immediately after conditioning, the document should be released for filing. **Releasing** usually consists of a mark or stamp on the item that indicates that the responsible licensed practitioner has seen the document and is giving permission to file it in the patient's medical record.

Indexing Another term for naming a file is **indexing.** Names should be chosen carefully, as that is how the file will be known, retrieved, and replaced. Traditionally, patient names have been used as the file names for patient records, but today this is often replaced with a numeric name or index. Most offices that use a numeric system use computer software to create new patient medical record numbers. Part of the indexing process will be to verify that the color-coding (if used) is correct and that any stickers or labels are securely fastened to the file. If colored files are used to denote patient diagnosis or insurance type, indexing is also the time to verify if any changes need to be made to the patient's file related to his or her current demographic.

Note that some files can logically be placed in more than one location. Such files should be **cross-referenced,** or filed in two or more places, with each place noted in each file. When cross-referencing a file, you may create a cross-reference form that gives the correct location to look for the file. For instance, an elderly woman might refer to herself as Mrs. John Smith. If you cannot remember her legal name, in the area where *Smith, John, Mrs.* would be located, you would place a mock folder that reads "Smith, John, Mrs., SEE Smith, Christine." You would then place the form under any heading where it is possible to look for that file. You may wish to attach it to a blank file folder, cutting the file folder in half so it consists of only one sheet, so that no documents are mistakenly filed within it.

Coding When you put an identifying mark or phrase on a document to ensure that it is placed in the correct file, that is known as **coding.** To code a document, simply write the patient's name, MRN, or the subject title of the file folder on the document. Alternatively, you can underline or highlight key words on the document itself. This step can be skipped when returning patient documents to their medical record or returning the records themselves to their properly filed location.

Sorting If you have more than one document or medical record to be filed, you must sort the files (documents) that have accumulated. Sort them in the order in which they are kept—such as alphabetically or numerically. Sorting saves you time later when you return the files to their proper places. If you will not be filing the items immediately, store them in a temporary location, like a file sorter.

Storing The final step in the filing process is to store the files in the appropriate filing equipment. Documents should be stored neatly within their file folders in the proper sequence.

Careful attention to file storage will make your job easier. Make sure the charts (folders) are in good condition. Replace them whenever they appear damaged or torn to prevent file contents from spilling out during the retrieval and filing process. If a file contains too many documents and becomes too bulky, divide it into two or more folders and label each one (for example, Glass, Ann M.—Folder 1 of 2; Glass, Ann M.—Folder 2 of 2). Also, be sure when labeling records that

consist of more than one chart that the content of each chart is clear (Folder 1 of 2, records prior to 2011; Folder 2 of 2, records from 2011 forward). Replace any labels that are no longer legible.

Filing Guidelines

There are specific rules for each filing system, as well as general guidelines that are applicable to any system. Following these guidelines will help you file more efficiently (Figure 13-6).

- Each time you pull or file a patient record, glance at its contents. You should be familiar with the typical contents and the order of a patient record folder to help avoid filing errors.

- Keep files neat. Make sure that documents fit neatly into the file folders. Papers should not extend beyond the edge of the folder. Do not place too many papers in each file folder. Folders should stay closed when laid on a flat surface.

- When inserting documents into folders already in place in the drawer, lift the folders up and out of the drawer; otherwise, this can lead to misfiling of documents. Attempting to force documents into a folder inside the drawer can damage the documents.

- Do not crowd the file drawer. Leave extra space to allow for leafing through the files and for retrieving and replacing

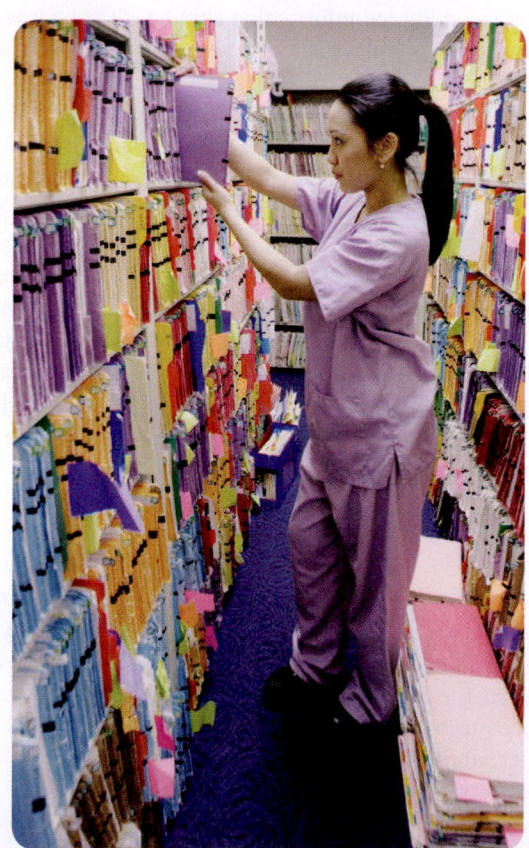

FIGURE 13-6 Filing on a regular basis keeps the task from becoming overwhelming and reduces the incidence of lost files.
© Exactostock/SuperStock RF

files easily. Where possible, use a combination of upper-case and lowercase letters to label folders. This format is easier to read than labels written completely in capital letters.

- Choose file guides with a different tab position than your folders to help them stand out. Do not place guides so close together that they hide one another. A good rule of thumb is to position guides at least 5 inches apart.
- If you are unsure whether to cross-reference a file, do it. It is better to err on the side of providing too many cross-references than too few.
- File regularly so that you are not overwhelmed with too many records or documents.
- Store only files in filing cabinets or on filing shelves.
- Do not store office equipment or supplies where files belong.
- Train all staff members who will retrieve and replace files to make sure they have a thorough understanding of the system. Update them on any changes.
- Periodically evaluate your office's filing system.

Locating Misplaced Files

Even in the best filing systems, there is a chance of temporarily misplacing or even losing a paper medical record. No matter how good a system is, errors will still be made. If a file is misplaced, here are steps you can take to try to locate it.

1. Determine the last time you or anyone else in the practice knew the file's location.
2. Go to that location and retrace the steps of the last person who handled the file. Look for the file along the way.
3. Look in the filing cabinet where the file belongs. Check neighboring files. Possibly, the file was simply put in the wrong place. Look inside other, thicker files to determine if the missing file was accidentally placed inside another file.
4. Check underneath the files in the drawer or shelf to see if the file slipped out.
5. Check the pile of items to be filed or the file sorter envelope.
6. Consider possible cross-references or similar indexes (for example, similar patient names) for the file. Check those headings to see if the file was accidentally placed there.
7. Check with other staff members to determine if they have seen the file.
8. Check to make sure the missing file was not filed under the patient's *first* name instead of the last.
9. Stand back from the file cabinet and view the *top* of the folders, looking at only the first three letters of the last names. A misfiled file will stand out.
10. If using a color-coded system, look for the color of the misfiled chart.
11. Even though files should always be kept in a secure area, occasionally individuals who are not part of the office staff, such as visiting providers may be in the area and may inadvertently pick up a file with their own materials.

If you think someone could have taken the file, call the person immediately.

12. Ask another staff person to complete steps 1 through 7 to double-check your search.
13. Straighten the office, taking care to check through all piles of information where a file could be lodged.
14. Check those charts that have been pulled for next day's appointments to see if misplaced charts have been accidentally pulled.
15. Check the provider's desk (and office).

If the misplaced file is not found within a reasonable time—24 to 48 hours—it may be considered lost. Losing a file has potentially devastating consequences, as it contains the patient's medical history, test results, and treatments. It may not be possible to duplicate the information within the file, but you can try to re-create it in a new medical record.

To do this, meet with the provider and clinical staff members to review the information needed. Record their recollections of information in the file. Note on the medical record that it is a duplicate and that the information is not official.

Consult with other offices and departments that may have records related to the file. Contact laboratories, hospitals, and other providers to request copies of documents previously included in the lost file. Place copies of those records in the new medical record, or excerpt information given to you. If the provider considers it appropriate, tell the patient whose file has been misplaced about its status and the steps you have taken to re-create it, including the offices and facilities that have been contacted to obtain information needed to re-create the medical record.

Limiting Medical Record Access

As stated earlier, the information in a patient's medical record is on a "business need to know." In computerized offices, your access ID and password will restrict the information you are allowed to see. Some offices using paper records restrict the number of people who can retrieve and return files, adding an extra measure of security to the practice. To obtain a file, staff members must fill out a requisition slip with their name, the name of the patient, and the reason for the request.

A record of who has the file is kept either in a notebook or on index cards in a card file. It also may be placed on the out guide, which is kept in the same location as the record until the record itself is returned to the filing system.

Unless required by court order, original patient medical records should not leave the practice. Photocopies can be made, if necessary. Review the *Legal and Ethical Issues* chapter regarding release of patient information.

▶ Active, Inactive, and Closed Files LO 13.6

No office has unlimited space for storage of paper records, so you need to understand the differences between active, inactive, and closed files. In your role as medical assistant, you may regularly need to transfer inactive and closed files from the office filing area to a storage area.

Active Versus Inactive Files

At any given time, there are files that you use frequently, called **active files,** and files that you use infrequently or not at all, called **inactive files.** What constitutes an active, as opposed to an inactive, file? It depends on your individual practice. In a cardiologist's office, a patient who has not been seen for a year may be considered inactive, while in a dental office, a year may simply indicate one missed appointment.

A third category of files, called **closed files,** are files of patients who have died, have moved away, or for some other reason no longer come to the office. Although closed files could be moved immediately to storage, they are usually treated in the same manner as inactive files. That is, they are kept in the office for a certain length of time to make sure that there are no requests for the information in the file.

The length of time inactive and closed files are kept or retained is 7 to 10 years. All medical records must be retained for 7 years; however, because the Federal False Claims Act requires financial records be kept for 10 years and medical records provide the medical necessity information for the billing records, many legal experts suggest also keeping medical records for 10 years (see the *Legal and Ethical Issues* chapter). Ultimately, it is the licensed practitioner who will determine when a patient file is deemed inactive or closed. You and the practitioner (or office manager) can meet regularly (once a month or once a quarter) to review these files.

Records Retention

A **retention schedule** specifies how long to keep different types of patient records in the office after files have become inactive or closed. The schedule also details when files should be moved to a storage area and how long they should be kept in storage before being destroyed. The retention schedule should be posted in the file room to make certain that all staff members are aware of it. Always be extremely careful not to destroy records prematurely, because they often cannot be re-created. Always retain a list of documents or files that have been destroyed for future reference.

For assistance in creating a retention schedule, consult the most updated and complete list of required record retention periods according to HIPAA law, which can be found on the HIPAA advisory website (http://www.hhs.gov/ocr/hipaa). Additionally, state and local retention requirements can be obtained from insurance companies, state and local agencies, and medical associations. If you do business in more than one state, follow the schedule that requires the longest retention time for materials. Remember, if your state's (retention or other) requirements are more stringent than HIPAA laws, follow your state requirements.

When counting years in a retention schedule, do not count the year in which the document was produced but begin counting with the following year. This way, documents produced near the end of a calendar year will be tracked more efficiently. Procedure 13-3 summarizes the steps for setting up a records retention program.

When records are to be eliminated, they can never simply be thrown away because of the confidential information contained within them. All medical records, as well as any document containing confidential information, must be completely destroyed by shredding.

Basic Storage Options

Before you can transfer files to storage, you need to determine how and where they will be stored. The design and layout of file storage should make even older stored files easily accessible so that they can be evaluated periodically for retention or elimination.

There are many ways to store inactive files. For example, they can be stored in their original paper state or transferred into another format, such as onto a computer disk. Files can even be electronically coded with bar codes for immediate retrieval with a computer system. Regardless of the medium chosen for storing and preserving documents, keeping related material together and retrieving it should be made as easy as possible. Inactive files contain PHI and must be kept just as secure as active files.

Paper Storage If the practice chooses to store files in their original form, they will likely be stored in boxes labeled with their contents. Choose boxes that are uniform in size so they will stack well and have lift-off lids for easy access to contents.

Although paper files are bulky to store and require roughly the same amount of space as they occupied while in the office, these files preserve the original documents. Access to these documents can be important when providing evidence of medical treatment in legal proceedings. However, if paper files start to become brittle, they should be transferred to another storage medium.

Computer Storage If storage space is limited, there are a number of paperless options for storing files, which include recordable CDs or DVDs, jump or flash drives, and external hard drives. To store records or information electronically, the office needs a computer system that can transfer documents to some type of electronic or digital format and then read them when they are retrieved from storage. (Refer to the *Office Equipment and Supplies* and the *Electronic Health Records* chapters for electronic storage options.)

The easiest way to transfer documents directly into the computer is to use a scanner, which copies a document to the computer's hard drive. This process saves countless hours of rekeying documents into the computer. Most scanners can also copy graphics and handwritten notes. The document is then labeled and saved. Documents that were originally created using the computer can also be transferred to CD, DVD, or external hard drive and then deleted from the computer system's internal hard drive. The chosen storage device is then dated and stored in labeled file boxes or other containers. The *Electronic Health Records* chapter provides more detailed information about electronic document creation and storage options.

Storage Facilities

You may wish to store files in a remote area of your office building, like an unused closet or office. Check to make sure that the area is secure, accessible, and safe for storing files (for example, do not store files where hazardous materials are stored). The practice may have to pay additional rent if the space is not within the confines of its office suite.

If there is no space in the building, consider a neighboring building, perhaps one in the same office complex. Many buildings rent space that can be used to store records. If you pursue this option, you will be responsible for managing the storage of records, including transporting them to the space, positioning them, and retrieving them as needed.

Certain storage facilities, called commercial records centers, will do some of the work for you. For a monthly fee, these centers typically house and manage stored documents. When evaluating commercial records centers, inquire about whether they will retrieve and/or deliver boxes or files and whether there is an on-site work area if someone needs to review the files at the storage location.

Maintain a separate list of files stored off-site. This list can save a wasted trip to the storage site if a needed file is not housed there. The list also provides a valuable record if files are damaged or destroyed. Remember, always update the list as new files are moved into storage and old files are taken out of storage and destroyed.

Storage Safety

No matter where you store files, you must consider the issue of safety as well as security. Beware of general storage facilities that are not specially equipped for document management. For example, these facilities may not address safety concerns by taking precautions for fire or floods—an absolute necessity for medical records. So it is wise to evaluate the storage site and to take some basic precautions.

- Choose a site with moderate temperatures year-round and adequate ventilation.
- Select waterproof storage containers that can also withstand intense heat. When possible, use metal or plastic boxes that are designated as fireproof and waterproof. Cardboard boxes, although often used for storage, are not as strong or durable. If cardboard storage boxes are used, they need to be placed on shelving well off the floor to avoid water damage.
- Choose a site equipped with a smoke alarm, a sprinkler system, and fire extinguishers.
- Select a site that is above ground and away from flood hazards. One way to find out if a site is susceptible to flooding is to inquire whether the facility has flood insurance, a requirement for sites at risk.
- Choose a site that is kept locked, is regularly patrolled, or has an alarm system, to prevent theft or vandalism.
- Remove old, brittle files as soon as possible or transfer them into another format. They can then be placed in file storage again.
- Ask for references from people at other offices who have stored files at the site. Talk to these people about what they like and dislike about the storage facility and any problems they have had in storing or retrieving documents.
- If you are storing files in another form—on computer disk or microfiche—inquire about any special precautions the site owner takes to ensure safety.

Taking the time to thoroughly research storage options ultimately saves time and effort as you manage stored files.

PROCEDURE 13-1 Creating a Filing System for Paper Medical Records

Procedure Goal: To create a filing system that keeps related materials together in a logical order and enables office staff to store and retrieve medical records efficiently

OSHA Guidelines: This procedure does not involve exposure to blood, body fluids, or tissue.

Materials: Vertical or horizontal filing cabinets with locks, tabbed file folders, labels, file guides, out guides, filing sorters

Method:

1. Evaluate which filing system is best for your office—alphabetic or numeric. Make sure the provider approves the system you choose.
   RATIONALE: *The purpose of a filing system is to provide accessibility of all medical records for the entire staff.*

2. Establish a style for labeling files and make sure that all file labels are prepared in this manner.

3. Avoid writing labels by hand. Use a keyboard, a label maker, or preprinted adhesive labels.

4. Set up a color-coding system to distinguish the files (for example, use blue for the letter *A*, red for *B*, yellow for

C, and so on). Create a chart, suitable to be hung in a professional file room, that uses the color-coding system.

5. Use file guides to divide files into sections.

6. Use out guides as placeholders to indicate which files have been taken out of the system. Include a charge-out form to be signed and dated by the person who is taking the file.
   RATIONALE: *Out guides allow for quick and easy identification of a missing file and its location.*

7. To keep files in order and to prevent them from being misplaced, use a file sorter to hold those patient records that will be returned to the files during the day or at the end of the day.

8. Develop a manual that explains the filing system to new staff members. Include guidelines on how to keep the system in good order.
   RATIONALE: *A filing system only works when all office personnel use it consistently.*

PROCEDURE 13-2 Setting Up an Office Tickler File

Procedure Goal: To create a comprehensive office tickler file designed for year-round use

OSHA Guidelines: This procedure does not involve exposure to blood, body fluids, or tissue.

Materials: 12 manila file folders or 3-ring binder with 12 separators, 12 file labels, pen or typewriter, paper

Method:

1. Write or type 12 file labels, 1 for each month of the year. Abbreviations are acceptable. Do *not* include the current calendar year, just the month.

2. Affix one label to the tab of each file folder.

3. Arrange the folders so that the current month is on the top of the pile. Months should follow in chronological order.

4. Write or type a list of upcoming responsibilities and activities. Next to each activity, indicate the date by which the activity should be completed. Leave a column after this date to indicate when the activity has been completed. Use a separate sheet of paper for each month.
   RATIONALE: *Each sheet should clearly indicate when the activity has been completed and by whom. Each sheet should be filed within the appropriate month's folder.*

5. File the notes by month in the appropriate folders.

RATIONALE: *This will create a neat and orderly way to collect tickler notes for each month.*

6. Place the folders in order, with the current month on top, in a prominent place in the office, such as in a plastic box mounted on the wall near the receptionist's desk.

7. Check the tickler file at least once a week on a specific day, like every Monday. Assign a backup person to check it in case you happen to be out of the office.

8. Complete the tickler activities on the designated days, if possible. Keep notes concerning activities in progress. Be sure to note when activities are completed and by whom.
   RATIONALE: *Keep a record of responsibilities and completed activities in case a question concerning the activity or responsibility comes up at a later date.*

9. At the end of the month, place that month's file folder at the bottom of the tickler file. If notes are remaining in that month's folder, move them to the current month's folder.
   RATIONALE: *Incomplete activities must be moved to the new month to be sure they are not overlooked.*

10. Continue to add new notes to the appropriate tickler files.
    RATIONALE: *To provide for continual update to the tickler system.*

PROCEDURE 13-3 Developing a Records Retention Program

Procedure Goal: To establish a records retention program for patient medical records that meets office needs, as well as legal and government guidelines

OSHA Guidelines: This procedure does not involve exposure to blood, body fluids, or tissue.

Materials: Updated guide for record retention as described by federal and state law (go to the HIPAA advisory website), file folders, index cards, index box, paper, pen or typewriter

Method:

1. List the types of information contained in a typical patient medical record in your office. For example, a file for an adult patient may include the patient's case history, records of hospital stays, and insurance information.

2. Research the state and federal requirements for keeping documents. Contact your appropriate state office (such as the office of the insurance commissioner) for specific state requirements, like rules for keeping records of insurance payments and the statute of limitations for initiating lawsuits. If your office does business in more than one state, be sure to research all applicable regulations. Consult with the attorney who represents your practice.

3. Compile your research results in a chart. At the top of the chart, list the different kinds of information your office keeps in patient records. Down the left side of the chart, list the headings "Federal," "State," and "Other." Then, in each box, record the corresponding information.

4. Compare all the legal and government requirements. Indicate which one is for the longest period of time.
   RATIONALE: *Retaining all records for the longest period of time required by the laws governing your organization will assure that you are in compliance with all laws.*

5. Meet with the provider (or office manager) to review the information. Working together, prepare a retention schedule. Determine how long different types of patient records should be kept in the office after a patient leaves the practice and how long records should be kept in storage. Although retention periods can vary based on the type of information kept in a file, it is often easiest to choose a retention period that covers all records. Determine how files will be destroyed when they have exceeded the retention requirements. Usually, records are destroyed by paper shredding. Purchase the appropriate equipment, or contract with a shredding company as necessary.

RATIONALE: *Shredding complies with HIPAA privacy rules regarding protected health information (PHI).*

6. Put the retention schedule in writing and post it prominently near the files. In addition, keep a copy of the schedule in a safe place in the office. Review it with the office staff.

7. Develop a system for easily identifying files under the retention system. For example, for each file deemed inactive or closed, prepare an index card or create a master list containing the following information:

   - Patient name and Social Security number
   - Contents of the file
   - Date the file was deemed inactive or closed and by whom
   - Date the file should be sent to inactive or closed file storage (the actual date will be filled in later; if more than one storage location is used, indicate the exact location to which the file was sent)
   - Date the file should be destroyed (the actual date will be filled in later)

   Have the card signed by the provider (or office manager) and by the person responsible for the files. Keep the card in an index box or another safe place. This is your authorization to destroy the file at the appropriate time.

8. Use color-coding to help identify inactive and closed files. For example, all records that become inactive in 2018 could be placed in green file folders or have a green sticker with "18" placed on them and moved to a supplemental file. Then, in January 2018, all of these files could be pulled and sent to storage.

9. One person should be responsible for checking the index cards once a month to determine which stored files should be destroyed. Before retrieving these files from storage, circulate a notice to the office staff stating which records will be destroyed. Indicate that the staff must let you know by a specific date if any of the files should be saved. You may want to keep a separate file with these notices.

10. After the deadline has passed, retrieve the files from storage. Review each file before it is destroyed. Make sure the staff members who will destroy the files are trained to use the equipment properly. Develop a sheet of instructions for destroying files. Post it prominently with the retention schedule, near the machinery used to destroy the files.

    RATIONALE: *To guard patient confidentiality and follow all HIPAA laws governing the protection of patient information.*

11. Update the index card, giving the date the file was destroyed and by whom.

12. Periodically review the retention schedule. Update it with the most current legal and governmental requirements. With the staff, evaluate whether the current schedule is meeting the needs of your office or whether files are being kept too long or destroyed prematurely. With the provider's approval, change the schedule as necessary.

SUMMARY OF LEARNING OUTCOMES

LEARNING OUTCOMES	KEY POINTS
13.1 Identify the common equipment used to file and store paper medical records.	Filing shelves, filing cabinets (horizontal and vertical), compactible files, and rotary files are all commonly used to store paper medical records. A very small office might opt to use storage bins for its medical records, but because of bulk, storage concerns, and weight and safety issues when moving the units, this method is ill advised for most practices.
13.2 Outline the security and safety measures that should be employed when working with paper medical records.	HIPAA requires that filing shelves or cabinets be fireproof and locked when the office is closed. If files are kept in a file room, the room should be locked when not in use, with only a minimal number of staff members possessing the key. Filing systems must be safe for those using them, and instructions on their proper use should be posted and understood by all staff members using them. All staff should be instructed on proper body mechanics regarding all tasks in the medical office to avoid work-related injuries.
13.3 List the common filing supplies used in the medical office.	Filing supplies used in the medical office include tabbed file folders, labels, hanging file folders, binders, tabs with inserts for labeling, file guides, out guides, and file sorters.

LEARNING OUTCOMES	KEY POINTS
13.4 Contrast the methods used for various filing systems and how color-coding can assist with the filing systems.	Alphabetic filing is the traditional filing system for medical offices. According to the filing rules found in Table 13-1 and the indexing rules in the *Points on Practice* feature, medical records are filed alphabetically using each patient's last name, first name, and middle initial as the first three filing units. Color-coding can enhance this process when each letter is assigned a different color and the first two or three letters of each patient's last name are attached to the chart using colored labels so filing errors stand out. Numeric systems are used more often because of the confidentiality they provide. These systems use a series of numbers assigned to each patient (medical record number), which are then filed by the terminal digit or middle digit format. As with alphabetic filing, color can be used in a similar way with numeric filing by assigning each number 0–9 a distinct color so that filing mistakes stand out more readily.
13.5 Recall the steps in the filing process.	The steps in the filing process include inspecting and releasing, indexing (naming), coding, sorting, and storing.
13.6 Compare active, inactive, and closed files and how to set up a records retention program for the office.	Active records are those that are used frequently. Infrequently used records are known as inactive records. Closed files are those of patients who, for whatever reason, no longer come to the office. Procedure 13-3 outlines the procedure to be used in creating an office medical records retention program.

CASE STUDY CRITICAL THINKING

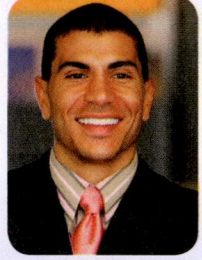

© HBSS/Corbis RF

Recall Malik Katahri from the beginning of the chapter. Now that you have completed the chapter, answer the following questions regarding his case.

1. What are some of the advantages of changing the filing system from an alphabetic system to a numeric system?

2. Would there be advantages to staying with the current system? How might you convince the physicians that electronic records would solve the filing "dilemma," making the financial outlay worthwhile? (Using information from the *Electronic Health Records* chapter may be helpful when answering this question.)

EXAM PREPARATION QUESTIONS

1. (LO 13.1) Which of the following are commonly used in medical offices as storage units for paper medical records?
   a. Filing shelves
   b. Filing cabinets
   c. Compactible files
   d. Rotary circular files
   e. All of these

2. (LO 13.2) Which of the following does not follow recommended security guidelines for medical records?
   a. Locking the records in a separate room
   b. Using locking shelves
   c. Using locking file cabinets
   d. Giving everyone in the office a key to the file room
   e. Posting a sign next to the file room stating "Authorized Personnel Only"

3. (LO 13.3) Which of the following supplies are commonly used to contain the medical record?
   a. File folders (hanging)
   b. File markers
   c. File tabs
   d. File sorters
   e. File guides

4. (LO 13.4) Which of the following lists a unit order that would never be used when filing?
   a. 1. MD   2. Po   3. Kwan   4. Quin
   b. 1. Quin   2. Kwan   3. Po   4. MD
   c. 1. Po   2. Quin   3. Kwan   4. MD
   d. 1. Po   2. Kwan   3. Quin   4. MD
   e. None of these

5. (LO 13.4) Which of the following lists the correct filing order for the names listed?
   a. Beals, Bentley Rian/Beals, Jazmyn/Beals, Kim/Beals, Lexus
   b. Johnson, B. James/Johnson, Bradley/Johnson, Bryan/Johnsen, Calvin
   c. Stark, Eleanor/Stark, Elinor/Stark-Ward, Eliner/Stark-Ward, Eleanor
   d. Whalen, Mari/Whalen, Mari L./Whalen, Mary Lou/Whalen, Mari Lou
   e. Smith, James J. II/Smith, James J. III/Smith, James J. Sr./Smith, James J. Jr.

6. (LO 13.4) Which of the following numeric sequences is correct using middle digit filing?
   a. 010   333   285 / 001   333   285 / 010   333   284 / 123   334   219
   b. 001   333   262 / 010   333   285 / 010   333   284 / 123   334   219
   c. 001   333   262 / 010   333   284 / 010   333   285 / 123   334   219
   d. 123   334   219 / 010   333   285 / 010   333   284 / 001   333   262
   e. 010   333   284 / 010   333   285 / 001   333   262 / 123   334   219

7. (LO 13.4) Which of the following numeric sequences uses terminal digit filing?
   a. 010   333   285 / 001   333   285 / 123   334   285 / 010   334   285
   b. 001   333   285 / 010   333   285 / 010   334   285 / 123   334   285
   c. 123   334   285 / 010   334   285 / 010   333   285 / 001   333   285
   d. 010   334   285 / 010   333   285 / 001   333   285 / 123   334   285
   e. 010   333   285 / 010   334   285 / 001   333   285 / 123   334   285

8. (LO 13.4) If names are absolutely identical, what is the address order that is used to choose the filing order?
   a. State, city, street name, street number
   b. City, state, street number, street name
   c. Street name, street number, city, state
   d. City, state, street name, street number
   e. Each office may choose the order that works best for them

9. (LO 13.5) The filing term that means you are *naming* the document in order to file it correctly is
   a. Inspecting
   b. Indexing
   c. Coding
   d. Sorting
   e. Storing

10. (LO 13.6) Which of the following describes the records of patients who have moved across the country?
    a. Active
    b. Inactive
    c. Closed
    d. Retained
    e. Old patients

SOFT SKILLS SUCCESS

Recall Malik Katahri, the office manager, from the case study at the beginning of the chapter.

1. One of the issues Malik has noted with internal chart audits is incomplete documentation by one practitioner. What are some of the possible consequences of incomplete or incorrect documentation?

2. How do you think Malik should handle these consequences as the office manager?

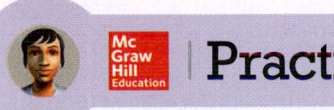

Go to PRACTICE MEDICAL OFFICE and complete the module Admin: Check Out – Work Task Proficiencies.

Telephone Techniques

EMPLOYEE INFORMATION

Employee Name	Position	Credentials
Reagan Patrick	Medical Assistant Extern	Student
Supervisor	**Date of Hire**	**Other information**
Malik Katahri	Externship Start: 9/7/20XX	Honors student. Puts a lot of pressure on herself.

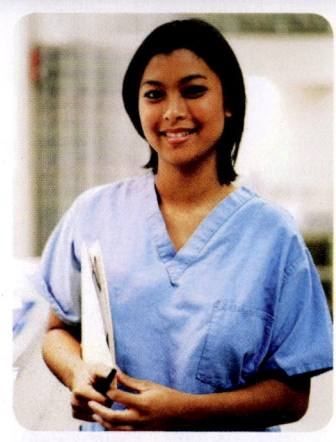
© Ablestock.com/Getty Images

Reagan Patrick has been selected by Malik Katahri and his team as their MA extern for this semester. BWW was Reagan's first choice; although excited to be working with this office, she also feels a lot of pressure to be "perfect" during this experience. She has been with them for a few days, and today she will be helping Miguel Perez, the administrative MA, with the phones and front office duties. Reagan feels she is ready but knows from the little time she has been in the office that as soon as they take the phones off the automated answering system, she is going to have to be at the top of her game as the voice of BWW Medical Associates. As the phone rings for the first time, she takes a deep breath; puts a smile on her face; and, answering on the third ring, says, "Good morning, BWW Medical Associates, this is Reagan, how may I help you?" and her morning begins.

Keep Reagan in mind as you study this chapter. There will be questions at the end of the chapter based on the case study. The information in the chapter will help you answer these questions.

LEARNING OUTCOMES

After completing Chapter 14, you will be able to:

14.1 Explain the purpose of the telecommunications equipment commonly found in the medical office.

14.2 Relate the five Cs of effective communication to telephone communication skills.

14.3 Define the following terms involved in making a good impression on the telephone: *telephone etiquette, pitch, pronunciation, enunciation,* and *tone.*

14.4 Describe how to appropriately handle the different types of calls coming into the medical practice.

14.5 Summarize the purpose of the office routing list with regard to call screening.

14.6 Carry out the procedure for taking a complete telephone message.

14.7 Outline the preparation required prior to making outgoing calls and the skills used in making the phone call.

KEY TERMS

automated voice response unit

enunciation

etiquette

interactive pager

pitch

pronunciation

telecommunications device for the deaf (TDD)

telephone triage

V.P.6 Demonstrate professional telephone techniques

V.P.7 Document telephone messages accurately

V.A.1 Demonstrate:
  (a) empathy
  (b) active listening

4. Medical Law and Ethics

  a. Follow documentation guidelines

  b. Institute federal and state guidelines when releasing medical records or information

  f. Comply with federal, state, and local health laws and regulations as they relate to healthcare settings
  (2) Describe what procedures can and cannot be delegated to the medical assistant and by whom within various employment settings

8. Administrative Procedures

  f. Display professionalism through written and verbal communications

11. Career Development

  b. Demonstrate professional behavior

▶ Introduction

Most offices have policies and procedures for routing calls that come into the office. You will learn which types of calls you may handle and which should be directed to clinical medical personnel or the physician. You will learn to triage (prioritize) calls so that emergencies are handled correctly. Of equal importance, you will learn how to take a complete telephone message, how to be prepared when placing calls, how to leave effective and HIPAA-compliant messages for patients, and how to handle difficult telephone calls, including those from angry patients with complaints and from callers who will not identify themselves.

Finally, in addition to using the telephone correctly, you will learn how other communication devices are used in the medical office, including setting up and using automated telephone menu equipment, voicemail, answering services and machines, TDDs, cell phones, and pagers.

▶ Telecommunications Equipment   LO 14.1

When thinking about telecommunications equipment in the medical office, the first item that naturally comes to mind is the office telephone system. In addition to the office telephone line(s), you will also explore how cell phones, beepers, answering machines, voicemail, and answering services play vital roles in the medical office's management.

Telephone System

The telephone is one of the most important pieces of communication equipment in the medical practice. It is not only the primary instrument patients use to communicate with the office but also the primary means of communication among providers, hospitals, laboratories, and other businesses important to the practice.

Advances in technology and the advent of the Internet are dramatically changing voice communications. Technologies like Voice over Internet Protocol (VoIP), also known as Internet Voice, allow the integration of voice and data communication through the computer and Internet service. This means that medical practices have the option of using the computer for Internet access and telephone conversations.

Multiline Phones

Few practices can function with just one or two telephone lines. Most modern medical offices have a telephone system that includes several telephones and multiple lines for incoming or outgoing calls, an intercom system, and the ability to transfer calls, leave voicemail, and put calls on hold (Figure 14-1).

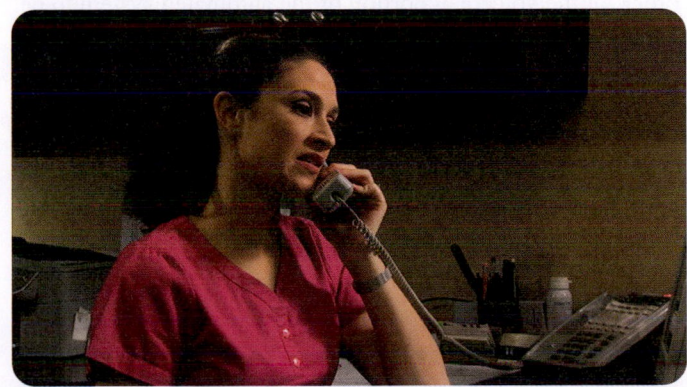

FIGURE 14-1   Most modern medical offices have multiline phones that are capable of multiple functions.
© McGraw-Hill Education

The larger the practice, the greater the demand on the phone system. Larger practices often need complex communications systems to handle all their needs.

Call Routing

The telephone system can be set up so that all incoming calls ring on all the telephones in the office, but the more common setup is that one or more "main phones" receive all calls. The receptionist then routes calls to the appropriate telephone extensions.

The **automated voice response unit** is quickly becoming a popular alternative to the traditional phone system, which requires someone to answer each call. An automated menu system answers calls for the office, separating requests into categories, so that the appropriate staff member can deal with each call efficiently. Using an automated system saves time for office personnel, because someone does not have to answer each call and then route it manually to the appropriate person or department. This allows the front office staff to complete other work without interruption.

Patients who reach an automated system hear a recorded message identifying the business. The message gives the caller a list of options from which to choose. Keep in mind that the first instruction the caller should hear is that if the call relates to a medical emergency, the caller should hang up and dial 911. After that, the caller will select an option by pressing the corresponding button on the telephone or by speaking the number of the option. The following are typical options that callers hear.

"Press or say 1 for appointments."

"Press or say 2 for prescription renewals."

"Press or say 3 for the clinical staff and triage nurse."

"Press or say 4 for the billing department."

"Press zero or say 'operator' to speak with an administrative medical assistant."

The last option is of utmost importance, so that the patient never feels lost in the system or unable to reach a "live person." Once a caller has chosen an option, the call is automatically routed to the chosen department. If no one is immediately available to answer the call, the caller may leave a message on the voicemail system, which should ask the patient to leave her name, the date and time of the call, and a brief message. In order for the voicemail portion of the automated system to be considered "successful" by the patients and other callers, it is imperative that the office staff check the system frequently (at least every hour) and return calls promptly.

Although using an automated voice response unit is efficient for the office staff, its purchase and use must be approved by the office manager and the practitioners before it is implemented. Some practitioners maintain that the patient call, as the customer and the reason for the practice, is of utmost importance above all other office tasks. If that is the belief system of the practitioner, he may be hard-pressed to feel anything other than a "live person" should be the first voice a patient hears when calling the office. Even when an automated system is in the office, always use the system per office protocol, making no changes without speaking to the office manager and licensed practitioners beforehand.

Other Automated Telephone Options

In addition to using automated voice response systems, many practices use an automated system to place routine reminder calls to patients. Medical assistants spend a great deal of time on the telephone calling patients to remind them of appointments, calling patients about no-shows, and leaving other types of messages.

Keeping in mind that some licensed practitioners believe that someone should always answer the phone, many other practitioners feel that they can make better use of staff time by automating as much of the phone system as possible. In fact, the system often pays for itself in less than a year. In addition to reminding patients of upcoming appointments, it can allow them to leave messages for staff. Automated phone systems can offer much more than just financial benefits: They can conduct patient surveys and give patients their test results through a privacy mechanism (the patient inputs his or her password). The phone system also can assist in managing referrals from the managed care organizations requiring them, and it can assist with preventive care by giving direct access to nurses or medical assistants for minor problems and concerns.

Voicemail and the Office Phone

As mentioned earlier, an automated menu often includes voicemail. If the office is closed or the person the patient is calling is on the phone or away from her desk, voicemail answers the call, and the caller can leave a message. The advantage of a voicemail system is that the caller never receives a busy signal. Another advantage is that voicemail is a more secure system, in that each person on a voicemail system has a unique password to retrieve only her messages.

Answering Machine

If the office phone system does not include voicemail, many offices use a telephone answering machine to answer calls after office hours, on weekends and holidays, and when the office is closed for any reason. A typical recorded message announces that the office is closed and states the usual business hours. In addition, the message must always indicate how the caller can reach the covering physician in the case of an emergency.

Answering Service

Instead of, or in addition to, an answering machine, many medical offices use an answering service. Unlike answering machines, answering services provide people who answer the telephone. They take messages and communicate them to the physician on call, who is responsible for handling emergencies that occur when the office is closed—at night or on weekends or holidays. Upon receiving a message from the answering service, the physician returns the patient's call and decides on the course of action.

Answering services can be used in a number of ways. The medical office may use an answering machine to record calls of a routine nature and give the number of the answering service to call in emergencies. Alternatively, the answering service may have a direct connection to the physician's office, picking up calls after a certain number of rings day or night or during specific hours. This ensures that calls do not get missed if the office is very busy and the staff cannot get to the phone.

Some answering services specialize in medical practices. These medical specialty services ask the medical practice to give specific directives for the triage of calls. Although most answering services provide satisfactory, sometimes even outstanding, service, it is good practice to check up on the service every so often by calling it during its coverage hours. This quality check ensures that the service meets office standards and expectations. Always ask any service for references before signing a contract for service.

Cellular (Cell) Phones—Personal and Business Use

Cell phones today are as common as people wearing shoes. In fact, cell phone use is so widespread that many people no longer have a land line. Instead, they depend solely on their cell phones, not only for calls but also for texting, directions, and many online applications (apps) for information and communication. Practitioners, medical practice employees, and patients may all be carrying their own cell phones into the medical office. With all that technology available at a button's touch, cell phone etiquette is a key concern. Generally, it is appropriate to turn off all personal cell phones while inside a medical office. In fact, it is not unusual for offices to have signs posted, requesting that cell phones be shut off when entering the office or at least when patients are in the treatment areas. The patients should be shown the same consideration by the practitioners and medical staff. Cell phone calls from outside the practice are usually an interruption in the communication among the practitioners, the staff, and the patient, who, as the *customer* of the practice, should have your full attention. More important, personal cell phone use should be avoided within the office, as it can interfere with other electronic equipment.

However, cell phones play an important part in the business functioning of the medical office. Licensed practitioners may use a cell phone to respond quickly to a message from staff or a hospital. Office staff may use personal cell phones in an emergency when traditional phone systems fail. Some medical practices even issue a cell phone to key employees who conduct business for the practice outside the office. In addition, patients may use their cell phones to call for a taxi after an appointment. If your medical office allows staff and patient cell phone use, make sure it is clearly noted in which areas cell phone use is permitted and, for employees, when personal cell phones may be used. In most offices, personal cell phones may be used only during break times; at other times, they must be turned off or left in vibrate mode.

Pagers (Beepers)

Physicians and other medical personnel often need to be reached when they are out of the office, so in addition to a cell phone, many also carry pagers (also known as beepers). Pagers are small electronic devices that give the user a signal to indicate that someone is trying to reach him. Although generally considered outdated technology, pagers are still used in some areas, particularly in rural areas, where cell phone signals are not as reliable.

Technology of Paging Like a cell phone, each paging device is assigned a telephone number. When the number is called, the pager picks up the signal and beeps, buzzes, or vibrates to indicate a call has been made. Most pagers have a window that displays either the caller's telephone number or a short message, so that the receiver can return the call. Pagers also can store the telephone number so that the receiver can return several calls without having to write down the numbers.

Calling a Pager Many telephone messages can wait until the physician returns to the office or calls in for messages. When a message needs to be delivered immediately, and a cell phone is not an option, paging is an efficient response. A list of pager (and cell phone) numbers for each physician in the practice should be kept in a prominent place in the office, such as by the main telephone or switchboard. Make sure you know where these numbers are kept. The paging process is as simple as making a telephone call.

1. Look up the telephone number for the pager of the practitioner you need to contact.

2. Dial the telephone number for the pager.

3. You will hear the telephone ringing and the call picked up. Listen for a high-pitched tone, which signals the connection between the telephone and the pager.

4. To operate most pagers, dial the telephone number you wish the practitioner to call, followed by the pound sign (#). (Some pager services have an operator and work much like an answering service. Give the operator a message and the operator will contact the practitioner.)

5. Listen for a beep or a series of beeps signaling that the page has been transmitted. Then hang up the phone. The practitioner should call the number at his earliest convenience.

Interactive pagers (I-pagers) are designed for two-way communication. The individual is paged in much the same way as the traditional pager. The pager can be set on "Audio" or "Vibrate" to alert the carrier that a message is coming in. However, the interactive pager screen displays a printed message and allows the physician to respond by way of a mini-keyboard.

The user can respond to the printed page by typing a return message, which is relayed back to the office in real time. The office computer and the user enter into a conversation much like e-mail or an Internet chat room. Many problems can be handled quickly and efficiently in this manner. Additionally, because the I-pager can function silently, the provider can communicate with her office while in a restaurant without disturbing others or compromising patient confidentiality.

Each interactive pager has its own wireless Internet address. The user types in the receiving party's e-mail address and creates a message on a monitor screen. The interactive pager indicates on the screen when the message has been sent, received, or read. I-pagers can communicate with other I-pagers as well, and they have broadcast capability, meaning the sender can send to more than one receiver at a time. For this reason, I-pagers can be very helpful for practices with multiple practitioners, especially where cell phone service is not always reliable.

I-pagers can also send messages to traditional telephones. The message is typed into the pager and the system "calls" the telephone number. When the telephone is answered, an electronic voice reads the message to the individual who has answered.

Telecommunications Devices for the Deaf

If your office has a significant number of patients with hearing impairments, it may be equipped with a **telecommunications device for the deaf,** known as a **TDD** (formerly known as a TTY—teletypewriter). A TDD is a specially designed telephone that looks very much like a laptop and may have a cradle for a telephone receiver (Figure 14-2). To call the office, the patient places the telephone receiver (if it has one) in the cradle and, instead of speaking, types a message using the TDD keyboard. If the office has a TDD, the message will be received in type format (similar to e-mail) on the TDD screen.

If the office does not have TDD equipment, the message may still be received through the use of a telecommunications relay service (TRS). When a patient utilizes a TRS, a specialty relay operator will receive the patient's written message through TDD equipment and then read the message to you when you answer the office phone. When a relay operator is used, the operator will identify herself as a relay operator for the patient utilizing the service. She will read the typed information from the patient. When the message is completed, she will say "go ahead" as your signal that it is your turn to reply. You will reply to the patient by speaking to the operator, and she will then enter your reply into the TDD device so that the patient can read it. You will also use the phrase *go ahead* when your message is completed.

TDD devices are becoming more common in the United States and throughout the world. Keep in mind that keying information takes longer than speaking and be patient with the process. As with text messaging, certain abbreviations are commonly used with a TDD. Table 14-1 lists some of them. Procedure 14-1, at the end of the chapter, outlines the procedure for using a TDD.

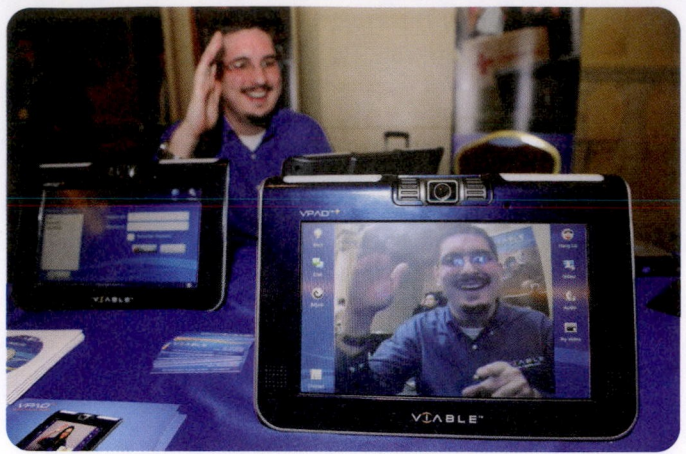

FIGURE 14-2 Telecommunications device for the deaf (TDD).
© Robyn Beck/AFP/Getty Images

TABLE 14-1	Abbreviations Commonly Used with TDD Devices
Abbreviation	**Meaning**
GA	Go ahead
SK	Stop keying
SKSK	Call complete
Q	Question
BEC	Because
U	You
UR	Your
PLS	Please
NBR	Number
TMW	Tomorrow
AM	Morning
PM	Night

▶ Effective Telephone Communication   LO 14.2

When you answer the telephone, you may be someone's first contact with the practice. The impression you leave can be either positive or negative. Your job is to ensure that it is positive.

Good telephone management leaves callers with a positive impression of you, the practitioners, and the practice. Poor telephone management can result in negative feelings, misunderstandings, and an overall unfavorable impression. The image you present over the phone should convey the message that the staff is caring, attentive, and helpful. Showing concern for each patient's welfare is a quality that patients rate highly when evaluating healthcare professionals. In addition, you must sound professional and knowledgeable when handling telephone calls. Using proper telephone management skills will help keep patients informed and ensure their satisfaction with the medical practice.

Communication Skills

Excellent communication skills are important in telephone management because they help project a positive image and thus satisfy the patient's needs and expectations. Individuals who are adept at effective communication employ the following communications skills:

- Display tact and sensitivity
- Show empathy
- Give respect
- Appear genuine
- Display openness and friendliness
- Refrain from passing judgment or stereotyping others
- Be supportive
- Ask for clarification and feedback
- Use paraphrasing to ensure that you understand what others are saying
- Be receptive to each patient's needs
- Know when to speak and when to listen

- Exhibit a willingness to consider other viewpoints and concerns

As a medical assistant, in addition to using your *active listening* skills (refer to the *Interpersonal Communication* chapter) you should also apply the five Cs of communication. Doing so will allow you to be as effective when using the telephone as you are when having a face-to-face conversation with someone. Get to know and use the five Cs of effective communication in all forms of communication:

- *Completeness.* The message must contain all necessary information.
- *Clarity.* The message must be legible and free from ambiguity.
- *Conciseness.* The message must be brief and direct.
- *Courtesy.* The message must be respectful and considerate of others.
- *Cohesiveness.* The message must be organized and logical.

Guidelines for Using the Telephone Effectively

The following guidelines will help you use the telephone effectively and professionally.

- Answer the phone promptly, by the second or third ring.
- Hold the telephone to your ear, or use a headset to hold the earpiece securely against your ear. Do not cradle the telephone with your shoulder; doing so can cause muscle strain.
- Hold the mouthpiece about an inch away from your mouth and leave one hand free to write with.
- When answering the phone, greet the caller first with the practice name, then with your name. If accepting a call routed by an automated answering system or forwarded to you by someone else, always identify yourself by name.
- Acknowledge the caller. Demonstrate your willingness to assist the caller by asking, "Ms. Jones, how may I help you?"
- Be courteous, calm, and pleasant no matter how hurried you are.
- Identify the nature of the call and devote your full attention to the caller. Do not attempt to multitask while on the phone.
- At the end of the call, allow the caller to hang up first to be sure any questions have been answered. Always say goodbye and use the caller's name.

Following HIPAA Guidelines

As you learned in the *Legal and Ethical Issues* chapter, HIPAA is the act concerned with the privacy and confidentiality of patient information, including information communicated via the telephone. Healthcare providers are allowed to disclose patient information for the purpose of treatment, payment, and health care operations (known as TPO) only. Any use of this information outside of these reasons requires a written authorization from the patient, except in emergency situations or in cases of information required by government agencies for compliance issues. As a general rule, patient information should not be revealed over the phone unless you are speaking directly to the patient or have written consent from the patient to speak to another person about his condition. Always follow your office policy and procedures manual with regard to disclosing patient information.

It is equally important to maintain patient confidentiality regarding patient appointments or their presence in the office. In the same way that you would not share patient information with anyone outside the office, you should never reveal to anyone, whether in person or on the telephone, that a patient has an appointment, is in the office, or is being treated by a member of the healthcare team. It is solely up to the patient to reveal that information.

▶ Telephone Etiquette LO 14.3

Proper telephone **etiquette** means handling all calls politely and professionally using good manners. Confidence in your role of providing quality patient care includes the ability to communicate effectively not only in person but also on the telephone. Your professionalism and caring attitude must come through the phone to the caller.

Your Telephone Voice

Customer service is critical when using the telephone. After all, your voice is representing the medical office. You must present your message effectively and professionally. Because you cannot rely on body language or facial expressions to help you communicate over the telephone, it is important to make the most of your telephone voice. Use the following tips to make your voice pleasant and effective.

- Speak directly into the receiver. Otherwise, your voice will be difficult to understand.
- Smile. The "smile" in your voice will convey your friendliness and willingness to help (Figure 14-3).

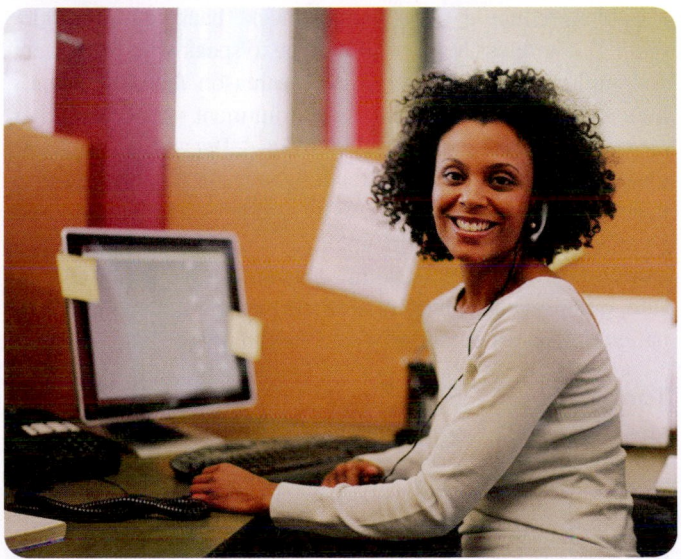

FIGURE 14-3 Smiling comes over the phone, making patients feel you want to help them.
© Thomas Barwick/Getty Images RF

- Visualize the caller and speak directly to that person.
- Convey a friendly and respectful interest in the caller.
- Be helpful and alert.
- Use language that is nontechnical and easy to understand. Never use slang.
- Speak at a natural pace, not too quickly or too slowly.
- Use a normal conversational tone.
- Try to vary your pitch while you are talking. **Pitch** is the high or low level of your speech. Varying the pitch of your voice allows you to emphasize words and makes your voice more pleasant to listen to.
- Make the caller feel important.

Pronunciation Proper **pronunciation** (saying words correctly) is one of the most important telephone skills. If you are unsure how to pronounce the name of the person on the phone, ask him to repeat it for you. This demonstrates respect for the person and shows him that he has your undivided attention. When clarifying the spelling of a name, verify letters that sound alike by repeating the letter, and include a word that begins with that letter. Examples include D as in dog, V as in Victor, and M as in Mary.

Enunciation The term **enunciation** (clear and distinct speaking) means the opposite of *mumbling*. Good enunciation helps the person you are speaking to understand you, which is especially important when you are trying to convey medical information.

Speaking clearly over the telephone is very important, because the speaker cannot be seen. Correct interpretation of the message is determined by hearing the words precisely. Activities like chewing gum, eating, or propping the phone between the ear and shoulder hinder proper enunciation. Many offices today provide the medical assistant and/or the receptionist with a wireless headset. These hands-free devices eliminate the need to hold the phone between your ear and shoulder, reducing office-related neck, back, and shoulder pain. The wireless headset allows you to speak with the patient and multitask if it is related to the reason for the patient's phone call, such as booking an appointment or accessing her electronic health record. See Figure 14-4. Because each patient deserves your undivided attention, you should not perform tasks unrelated to the caller. While using a wireless headset, always keep patient confidentiality in mind. Anything you say can be heard by people within listening range. As a general rule, do not walk around the office while on the phone with a patient unless an emergency demands that you do so.

Tone Because you are not face-to-face with the caller, the most important measurements of good telephone communication are voice quality and tone. Always speak with a positive and respectful tone.

Making a Good Impression

In a sense, your telephone duties include public relations skills. How you handle telephone calls will have an impact on the medical practice's public image.

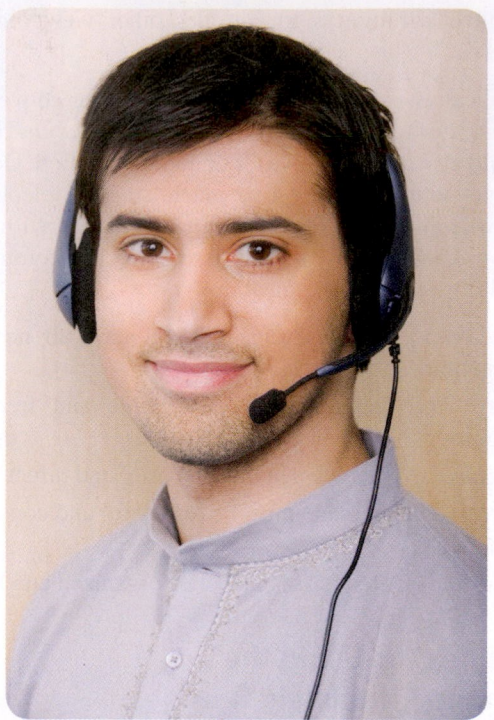

FIGURE 14-4 Using a hands-free headset allows you to speak directly into the mouthpiece, keeping your hands free to complete a task such as booking an appointment for a patient.
© Image Source RF

Exhibiting Courtesy Show common courtesy by projecting an attitude of helpfulness. Always use the person's name during the conversation and apologize for any errors or delays. When ending the conversation, be sure to ask the caller if there is anything else you can do for him and thank him before hanging up.

Giving Undivided Attention Do not try to answer the telephone while continuing to carry out another task. Before answering the phone, complete any conversations occurring in the office or excuse yourself while you answer the phone. Once you make sure that the call is not for an emergency, ask the caller if you may either put her on hold for a moment or call her back shortly. By interrupting the patient in the office briefly and giving the caller the option as to how she would like her call handled, both patients receive the undivided attention they deserve.

Putting a Call on Hold Although you should try not to put a caller on hold, there will be times when it is unavoidable. Calls may come in on another line, or a situation in the office may prevent you from devoting your full attention to the caller. Sometimes you may have to check a file or ask someone else in the office a question on behalf of the caller. Before putting a call on hold, however, always let the caller state the reason for the call. This step is essential so that you do not inadvertently put an emergency call on hold. Never answer the phone, "Dr. Buckwalter's office, please hold," and immediately put the call on hold. You must ask permission to put the caller on hold and wait for the response.

Your medical office may have a standard procedure for placing a call on hold. Typically, you will ask the caller the purpose of the call, state why you need to place the call on hold, and explain how long you expect the wait to be. Ask the caller if she would like to hold or if she would prefer you to return her call. If she requests a return call, ask her if there is a time that is best for the return call. If she decides to wait on hold and if you cannot end the task at hand quickly, return to the caller every 2 to 3 minutes, asking her if she wishes to remain on hold. An excessive wait on hold makes people feel they have been forgotten or are unimportant. Checking in with them and giving options minimizes these negative thoughts and feelings.

If you know you can return to the line shortly, put the caller on hold and complete your current task or call. If you need to answer a second call, get the second caller's name and telephone number and, unless this call includes an emergency situation, put the call on hold until you have completed the first call. You can then return to the second call. If possible, ask a coworker to assist with the second call, minimizing wait time for both callers.

Returning Patient Calls Some people do not like to hold and will request that you call them back. Obtain the caller's name and phone number, taking the time to repeat both to avoid errors. Return the call in a reasonable amount of time or as close as possible to the time requested by the caller, and give the patient your undivided attention. Be sure to apologize for the inconvenience and thank the caller for her patience.

Remembering Patient Names When patients are recognized by name, they are more likely to have positive feelings about the practice. Using a caller's name during a conversation makes the caller feel important. If you do not recognize a patient's name, it is better to ask, "Has it been some time since you've been in the office?" rather than to ask if the patient has been to the practice before.

Checking for Understanding When communicating by telephone, you do not have visual signals to convey the caller's feelings and level of understanding of the information you are discussing. If a call is long or complicated, summarize what was said to be sure that both you and the caller understand the information. Ask if the caller has any questions about what you have discussed. You may even want to have the caller repeat any instructions to make sure she understands. If a situation requires a lengthy conversation, it might be best to have the patient come in to the office or to follow up the phone call with a written summary of the discussion. Do not forget to document the call in the patient's medical record.

Communicating with Empathy Whenever information is conveyed over the telephone, feelings are also communicated. When dealing with a caller who is nervous, upset, or angry, try to show empathy (an understanding of the other person's feelings). Communicating with empathy helps the caller feel more positive about the conversation and the medical office.

Ending the Conversation It is not useful to let a conversation run on if you can effectively complete the call sooner. Before hanging up, however, take a few seconds to complete the call so that the caller feels properly cared for and satisfied. You can complete the call by summarizing the important points of the conversation and thanking the caller. Let the caller hang up first.

Occasionally, you will encounter a patient who simply will not hang up. Often these patients are merely lonely and your friendliness and helpfulness ease their loneliness. In this case, you may find that you must politely but firmly explain that another patient (or a member of the medical team) needs your assistance and you must complete the call. When you put the receiver down, never slam it—even if the caller has already hung up. Remember, all your actions reflect the medical practice's professional image. Patients in the reception area may see (and hear) you when you are talking on the telephone.

▶ Types of Incoming Calls   LO 14.4

In dealing with incoming telephone calls, you will encounter a variety of questions and requests from numerous people. Many incoming calls are from patients. You also will receive calls from various people, including attorneys, physicians, pharmaceutical sales representatives, and other salespeople.

Calls from Patients

Patients call the medical office for a variety of reasons, including rescheduling appointments and requesting prescription renewals. If you will be discussing clinical matters over the telephone, it is a good idea to pull the patient's chart. If the office uses EHR technology, this may be as simple as accessing the medical record on the computer screen. If paper records are used, you may need to ask the caller to hold for a moment while you retrieve the record. The information in the chart will often enable you to address any problems quickly. Pulling the chart also allows you to document the conversation immediately.

Always keep in mind that the physician is legally responsible for your actions, including relaying information to patients over the telephone. The office policy manual typically specifies what you may and may not discuss with patients. If you are uncertain about giving particular information to a patient, it is best to discuss the situation with the patient's practitioner or have the practitioner return the patient's call.

Appointment Scheduling Follow office procedures for making or changing appointment times over the telephone. Ask the patient to provide his name, a telephone number where he can be reached during the day, and the reason for the visit. Repeat the information back to the patient to verify all information before ending the call. (Scheduling appointments is discussed in the *Schedule Management* chapter.)

Billing Inquiries If a patient calls about a billing problem, you will need to pull the patient's billing information and possibly the medical record. With this information, you can compare the charges with the actual services performed.

If a patient claims to have been overcharged, check to see if the correct fee was charged. If you find that an error was made, apologize and tell the patient the office will send a corrected statement. Ask the patient to wait for the new statement before sending payment. If, in fact, the proper fee was charged, it may be helpful to speak to the provider before responding to the patient; she may be able to tell you if there were special circumstances regarding the visit or charge in question. Allowing the patient to pay the bill in installments is usually an acceptable option. The details on arranging for payment plans are discussed in the *Patient Collections and Financial Management* chapter.

Many offices use billing services instead of taking care of the insurance submission and monthly patient billing in the office. In that case, the patient may have called the billing service about charges and has now been referred to the office to dispute either the performance of a procedure or its cost. In this case, you may not have access to information about individual charges and may need to refer the patient to the office manager. Be aware that the patient may be upset about the bill and now is being referred to yet another person. Listen patiently to the patient and take notes regarding the complaint, remaining tactful and understanding about his concerns and possible frustration that an answer does not appear to be a simple process. No matter what your office policy is, if a patient is dissatisfied, document all appropriate comments and relay the information to the patient's practitioner and/or the office manager. If a bill has not been paid, ask if there are special circumstances affecting the patient's ability to pay. Figure 14-5 gives an example of appropriate documentation of such a call.

Requests for Laboratory or Radiology Reports If a patient calls the office requesting the results of a test, obtain the patient's chart to see if the report has been received. If it has not, suggest that the patient call back in a day or two. If the need for the result is urgent, you may call the laboratory or radiology office to obtain the results over the phone.

In some offices, you may be authorized to give laboratory results by telephone if they are normal, or negative, so the patient does not have to wait for results to be mailed or for a return phone call from the practitioner. Make a note on the patient's chart if you provide any information about test results. If a test result is abnormal, the provider will usually wish to speak with the patient. In such a case, tell the patient that the office has received the results and that the provider will call as soon as possible. Then place the patient's chart and the telephone message on the provider's desk. See Figure 14-6 for a chart note example of such a telephone call.

Questions About Medications One of the most common types of calls from patients involves questions about medications. A patient may ask about using a current prescription or may want to renew an existing one.

Prescription Renewals Calls for prescription renewals may come from the patient's pharmacy or from the patient. A pharmacist usually calls to check before dispensing refills if more than a year has passed since the original prescription was written. If the prescriber has indicated in the patient's medical record that renewals are approved, you may authorize the pharmacy to renew a prescription. In any other case, only the prescriber may authorize renewals. If the prescriber authorizes a renewal, you may be asked to telephone it in to the patient's pharmacy. Procedure 14-2 at the end of this chapter outlines the instructions for renewing a prescription by telephone. All renewals must be documented in the

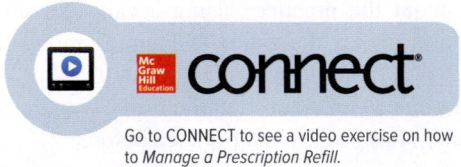

Go to CONNECT to see a video exercise on how to *Manage a Prescription Refill.*

BWW PROGRESS NOTE

Patient Name:
Shenya Jones

TC: Patient called, stating bill appears to contain an error. She was charged for a urinalysis during her last visit but states she was unable to produce a specimen for such testing. Review of medical record reveals no urinalysis was done. Patient is informed the charge will be removed from her bill. Insurance company will be notified so payment for lab can be refunded.

Date: 2/26/XX

Author: M. Katahri

Done | Close

FIGURE 14-5 Medical record documentation of a patient telephone call.

BWW PROGRESS NOTE

Patient Name:
Sylvia Gonzales

TC: Patient called inquiring about FBS result performed 5/10/XX. Reading of 130 given to patient. Per Dr. Whalen, patient is to remain on current insulin dosage.

Date: 5/12/XX

Author: M. Perez

Done | Close

FIGURE 14-6 Typical chart note documenting patient receipt of lab results by phone.

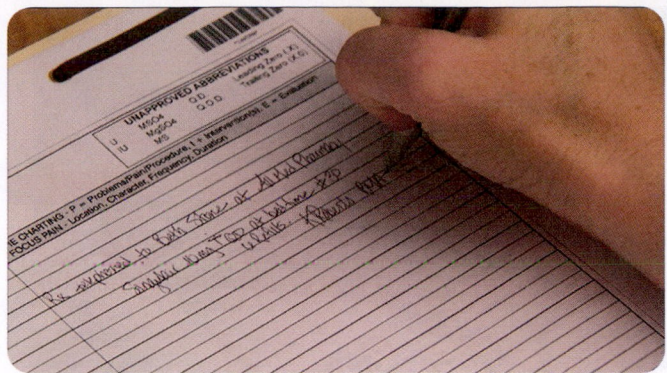

FIGURE 14-7 Documenting prescription refill.
© McGraw-Hill Education

patient's medical record, with the date and the initials of the person authorizing the renewal. See Figure 14-7.

Old Prescriptions Patients may call to ask if they can use a medication that was prescribed for a previous condition. In these instances, recommend that the patient come in for an appointment. Explain why the medication should not be used: It may be old and no longer effective, the current problem may not be the same as the previous one, the medication may not be helpful, and using the medication may mask the symptoms of the current problem, making a diagnosis (and so identifying the proper treatment) more difficult.

If the patient does not want to make an appointment, relay the information to the patient's practitioner, as he or she will probably want to speak with the patient. Again, briefly document the conversation in the patient medical record.

Progress Reports Practitioners often ask patients to call the office to let them know how a prescribed treatment is working. If a patient has a satisfactory progress report, it is not usually necessary that the patient speak to the practitioner. It is important, however, that the medical assistant relay the information to the practitioner and log the call in the patient's medical record immediately. You also may be responsible for

making routine follow-up calls to patients to verify that they are following treatment instructions. See Figure 14-8 for an example of a patient's progress report made by telephone. Figure 14-9 shows a similar patient update phone call documented using an EHR program.

Requests for Advice Sometimes patients call the office about problems or symptoms they are having. Although a patient may ask you for your medical opinion, as a medical assistant, you are not licensed to give medical advice of any kind. Explain that you are not trained to make a diagnosis or licensed to prescribe medication. Stress that the patient must see the licensed practitioner. Listen attentively to the patient. If the patient is in distress, try to schedule an appointment that day or as soon as possible.

If the patient cannot come in to the office, assure her that the practitioner will return the call or that you will call back after discussing the problem with the practitioner. Write down the patient's symptoms completely, accurately, and immediately. In many instances, the practitioner may be able to suggest simple emergency relief measures that you can relay to the patient. Occasionally, a patient will want to speak only with the practitioner, not other staff members. You must honor this request.

In some cases, the healthcare provider may feel that a patient's symptoms warrant immediate attention and will insist on seeing the patient before prescribing any treatment. If the patient refuses to come to the office, note the reason on the chart and suggest a visit to the emergency room or to a nearby medical office or urgent care center. As discussed in the *Legal and Ethical Issues* chapter, it is important to document such conversations completely in the patient's chart, including the refusal of treatment. It is always appropriate and professional to offer to take a message to have the patient's provider return the call. Figure 14-10 gives an example of such documentation.

Complaints Even when an office provides the highest-quality care, complaints still occur. When a patient calls with a complaint, such as a medication that does not appear to be

---

BWW PROGRESS NOTE

Patient Name:	Mohammad Nassar
	TC: Mohammad called in today to report that the addition of Flovent® to his medication regime is having a positive effect. He has used his rescue inhaler x2 in 3 days. Next appt in one week for recheck.
Date:	5/28/XX
Author:	K. Haddix

Done   Close

FIGURE 14-8 Patient progress note called in by telephone and documented in medical record.

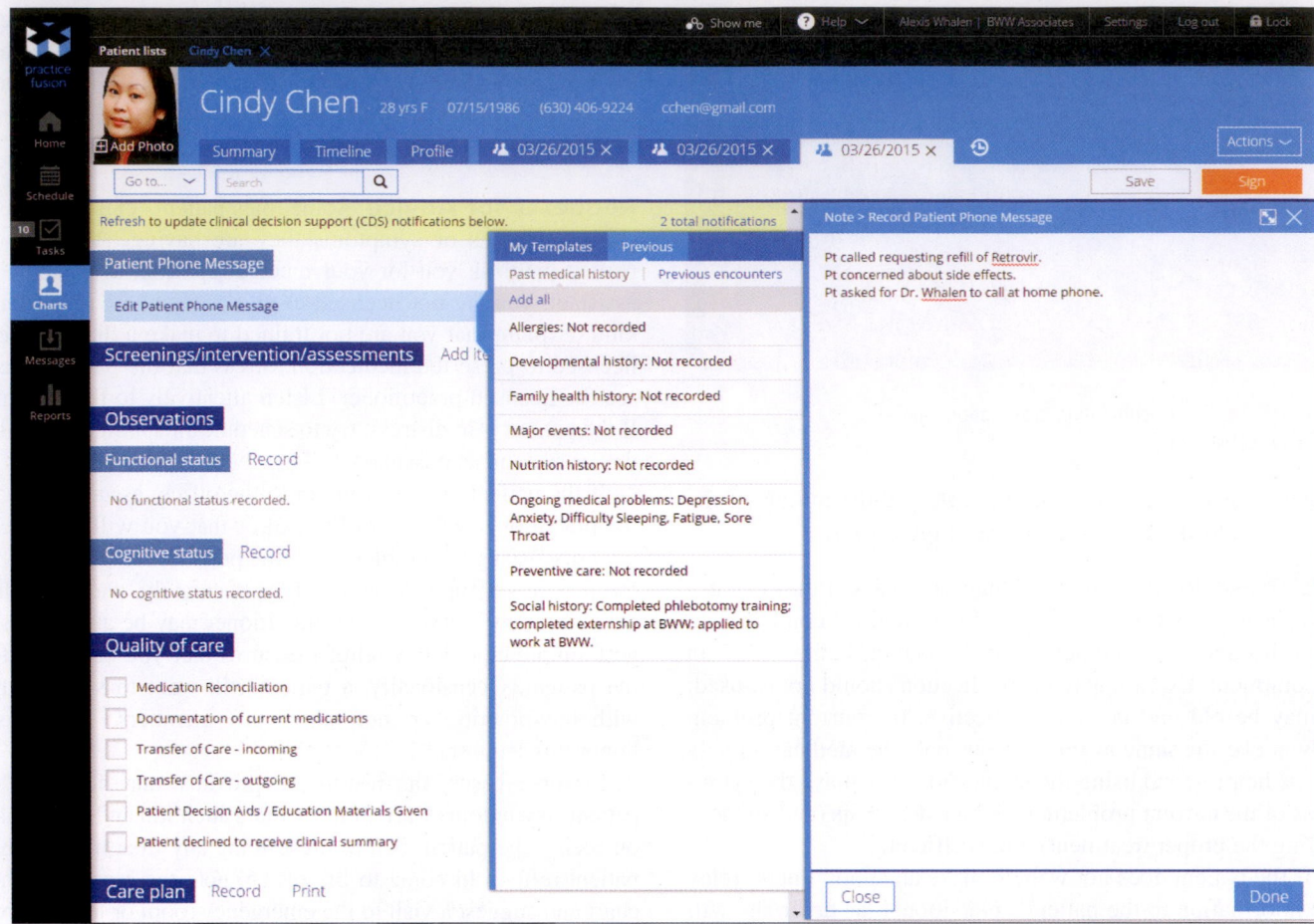

FIGURE 14-9 Telephone message from Cindy Chen documented in Practice Fusion®.

© Practice Fusion®

working, it is important to listen carefully, without interrupting. Take careful notes of all the details and read them back to the caller to ensure that you have written them down correctly. Let the caller know the person to whose attention you will bring the complaint and, if possible, when to expect a response.

Always apologize to the caller for any inconvenience the problem may have caused, even if the problem occurred through no fault of the office. Make sure the proper person receives the information about the complaint.

Sometimes a patient who calls with a complaint is angry. Responding to this type of call can be difficult and uncomfortable.

BWW PROGRESS NOTE

Patient Name: Ken Washington

TC: Patient called today stating he has had severe headaches over the last week. Advil is not helping. Requesting refill of Imitrex®, as the meds he has have expired. Dr. Buckwalter requested pt come in for BP check. Pt refused, stating he does not have time. Dr. Buckwalter informed of pt refusal. He will call pt.

Date: 3/1/XX

Author: M. Perez

Done   Close

FIGURE 14-10 Chart note documenting patient refusal of treatment request.

Your first priority is to stay calm and try to pacify the caller. Follow these guidelines when dealing with an angry caller.

- Listen carefully and acknowledge the patient's anger. By understanding the problem, you will be better able to work toward a solution.
- Remain calm and speak gently and kindly. Do not act superior or talk down to the patient. Do not interrupt the patient. Do not return the anger or blame.
- Let the patient know that you will do your best to correct the problem. This message will convey that you care.
- Take careful notes and be sure to document the call.
- Do not become defensive.
- Never make promises you cannot keep.
- Follow up promptly on the problem.
- Any time a staff member has a difficult time with a patient, it is important to inform the patient's practitioner or the office manager, even when the situation is resolved. Always inform the practitioner and/or your supervisor immediately if an angry patient threatens legal action against the office.

Other Calls

Besides calls from patients, a medical office receives many other types of calls. For example, family members and friends of patients may call providers at the office. However, the use of the office telephone is never appropriate for personal calls. Always follow office policies and procedures when handling these calls.

Remember, a patient's information is confidential. As discussed previously, HIPAA requires medical providers to obtain authorization from the patient before any information can be disclosed. This is usually in the form of a written, patient-signed authorization indicating what type of information may be given out and to whom. The following are guidelines for managing calls from attorneys, other physicians, and salespeople.

Attorneys Refer to the procedures listed in the office policies and procedures manual regarding how to handle calls from attorneys. Follow the office guidelines closely and ask the practitioner or practice manager how to proceed if you receive a call that does not fall within the guidelines. Remember, never release any patient information to an outside caller unless the patient's provider has asked you to do so.

Other Physicians Patients at your practice may be referred to surgeons, specialists, and other licensed practitioners for consultations. Consequently, you may receive calls from those providers or from their offices. Route those calls to the appropriate practitioner if the caller requests that you do so. Always remember to ask if the call is about a medical emergency. Also keep in mind that you may not give out any patient information—even to another healthcare provider—unless you have a written, signed release from the patient. The exception to this rule is information requested by practitioners to whom you have referred the patient for care. Because of the referral, there is a contract involved for continuity of care. You may release medical information specific to the care that the practitioner has been asked to provide.

Salespeople As a medical assistant, you will probably be the contact for salespeople, unless the office policy manual states that another staff member should handle this duty. On the telephone, ask the salesperson to send you information about any new products or equipment. Pharmaceutical sales representatives may want to meet with the prescribing practitioners. Forward such messages to the providers with a request to let you know when to schedule the appointment. Many prescribing practitioners see pharmaceutical sales representatives on certain days at specific times. Sometimes they limit the number of representatives they will see in one day or one week. Make sure you know your office policy and each prescriber's preferences.

POINTS ON PRACTICE
Screening Incoming Calls

Each medical office has its own policy about how to screen incoming calls before transferring them to the appropriate person. Calls come not only from patients but also from other physicians, hospital personnel, pharmacists, insurance company personnel, sales representatives, and family members and friends of patients. Here are some general tips for screening calls.

- *Find out who is calling.* A polite way to do this is to say, "May I ask who is calling?" Another option is "May I tell Dr. Williams who is calling?"
- *Ask what the call is in reference to.* When a caller asks to speak with the practitioner, you should ask the purpose of the call. Depending on the answer, you may determine that you or someone else in the office can handle the situation without disturbing the practitioner. The response may be as simple as solving a billing problem or clarifying instructions. Remember to consider the scope of practice for each member of the healthcare team when you transfer a call. Emergency calls should be transferred to the licensed practitioner right away.
- *Decide whether the call should be put through.* Although most calls are routed to the appropriate person, any callers who refuse to identify themselves should not be put through. In such a case, suggest that the caller write a letter to the practitioner and mark it "Personal."
- *Determine what to do if the matter is personal.* The practitioner may ask you to take a message in these instances. Inform the caller that the practitioner will return the call as soon as possible.

Conference Calls Periodically, providers may need to have a conference call with several individuals. For example, the physician, the nurse, and the medical assistant may need to talk with the insurance company representative at the same time. Telephone conferencing is an ideal setup in this case. All of today's telephone equipment has features for establishing and joining conference calls. In addition, offices with computerized systems now frequently use WebEx programs, such as "Go to Meeting," to allow conferencing among many participants.

▶ Managing Incoming Calls   LO 14.5

Screening Calls

Even if your office uses an automated answering unit, it is likely that part of your responsibility as the office medical assistant will be screening calls. Screening involves deciding which calls should be put through immediately and which calls are better handled by taking a message and allowing a callback at a more convenient time. The *Points on Practice* feature describes some guidelines for screening calls. The procedure will remain basically the same, whether the calls come directly to you as you answer the phone or are directed to you by a telephone answering system.

Routing Calls

Incoming phone calls can generally be separated into three distinct groups: calls dealing mainly with administrative issues; emergency calls that require immediate action by the practitioner; and calls relating to clinical issues that require the attention of the physician, physician assistant, nurse practitioner, office nurse, or clinical medical assistant. Procedure 14-3 at the end of this chapter will provide the outline for you to practice screening and routing calls.

Calls Requiring the Practitioner's Attention Certain calls will require the practitioner's personal attention:

- Emergency calls that include serious or life-threatening medical conditions, such as severe bleeding, a reaction to a drug, injuries, poisoning, suicide attempts, loss of consciousness, severe burns, or whatever your medical office deems an emergency; Table 14-2 lists symptoms and conditions that require immediate help
- Calls from other providers
- Patient requests to discuss test results, particularly abnormal results
- Reports from patients concerning unsatisfactory progress
- Requests for prescription renewals (unless previously authorized in the patient's chart)
- Personal calls

Many practitioners have a set time, such as a half hour in the late morning or at the end of the day, for returning nonemergency patient calls. If a patient prefers to discuss symptoms with his provider, you may tell the patient to expect a phone call from the provider within this set time. If the practitioner

TABLE 14-2	Symptoms and Conditions Requiring Immediate Medical Assistance*

- Allergic reactions to foods or insect stings
- Broken bones: Symptoms include being unable to move or bear weight on the injured body part; the injured part is very painful or looks misshapen
- Chemical or foreign objects in the eye
- Choking
- Drowning
- Electrical shock
- Fires, severe burns, or injuries from explosions
- Heart attack: Symptoms include chest pain or pressure; pain radiating from the chest to the arm, shoulder, neck, jaw, back, or stomach; nasuea or vomiting; sweating; weakness; shortness of breath; pale or gray skin color
- Heatstroke (sunstroke): Symptoms include confusion or loss of consciousness; flushed skin that is hot and may be moist or dry; strong, rapid pulse
- Human bites or any deep animal bites
- Hypothermia (drop in body temperature during prolonged exposure to cold): Symptoms include becoming increasingly clumsy, unreasonable, irritable, confused, and sleepy; slurred speech; slipping into a coma with slow, weak breathing and heartbeat
- Injuries to the head, neck, or back
- Lack of breathing (apnea) or difficulty breathing (dyspnea)
- Poisoning
- Pressure or pain in the abdomen that will not go away
- Severe bleeding
- Severe vomiting or bloody stools
- Shock: Symptoms include paleness; feeling faint and sweaty; weak, rapid pulse; cold, moist skin; confusion or drowsiness
- Snake bites
- Stroke: Symptoms include seizures, severe headache, slurred speech, and sudden inability or difficulty in moving a body part or one side of the body
- Unconsciousness
- Vehicle collisions

*If someone calls the office on behalf of a patient who is experiencing any of these symptoms or conditions, you may instruct the caller to dial 911 to request an ambulance. Procedure 14-4 at the end of the chapter describes the steps for handling emergency calls. If in the office, the physician should be called to the telephone immediately to offer assistance.

does not have a set time for returning phone calls, do not make a commitment as to the time of the return phone call.

In many practices, some of these calls may be handled by others on the staff, such as a nurse practitioner or physician assistant. For example, a nurse practitioner may be able to order a renewal of a regular prescription, provide advice for the care of a sprain, or answer well-baby questions or questions about the side effects of a drug.

Calls Handled by the Medical Assistant The most common calls to a medical office involve administrative and clinical issues. Depending on the practice, the office manager or someone in the billing department may handle some administrative calls. The calls handled by the medical assistant may include

- Appointments (scheduling, rescheduling, canceling).
- Questions concerning office policies, fees, and hours.
- Billing inquiries.
- Insurance questions.
- Other administrative questions.
- X-ray and laboratory reports.
- Reports from hospitals regarding a patient's progress.
- Reports from patients concerning their progress.
- Requests for referrals to other doctors.
- Requests for prescription renewals, where prior approval for refills is noted in the chart.
- Complaints from patients about administrative matters.

The Routing List Each medical office has a standard policy that documents how incoming telephone calls are to be routed and handled. A routing list, like the one shown in Figure 14-11, specifies who is responsible for the various types of calls in the office and how the calls are to be handled. For example, the routing list indicates which calls should be put through to the practitioners immediately and which ones can be returned later.

The routing list may simply identify the general title of the person responsible for handling a call. When more than one person in the office have the same title, however, the name of the individual who has that responsibility should be specified.

Telephone Triage

Depending on individual state regulations and on individual preference, some practitioners delegate part of the clinical decision making that is done over the telephone to other experienced staff members. In these instances, **telephone triage** is used to decide what action to take. The word *triage* refers to the screening and sorting of emergency incidents. Performing triage correctly is an important skill.

Using Triage Guidelines Proper office staff training is vital in providing safe, sound, and cost-effective medical care over the telephone. An increasing number of medical practices are preparing guidelines for the telephone staff to follow when patients call the office with specific medical problems or questions.

Guidelines are often written for common questions, such as how to deal with sniffles and fevers during cold and flu season or how to make a child with chickenpox more comfortable. Members of the telephone staff must realize, however, that their responsibility is to determine whether a caller needs additional medical care. They cannot diagnose or treat the patient's problem.

Office guidelines outline the specific information the telephone staff must obtain from the patient. In general, this information is the same type as that obtained during an office visit and should include the patient's age, the patient's symptoms, when the problem began, and the patient's level of anxiety about the problem.

HANDLING INCOMING TELEPHONE CALLS

	Route to doctor immediately	Take message for doctor	Route to nurse or assistant
Emergencies: bleeding, drug/allergic reaction, difficulty breathing, injury, pain, poisoning, shock, unconsciousness, incoherence or hysteria	X		
Calls from other physicians	if possible		
Patient progress report		X	
Patient request for laboratory report		X (if abnormal)	Kaylyn (if normal)
Patient questions re medication		X	
Patient questions re billing or insurance			Miguel
Patient complaints			Kaylyn
Appointments			Kaylyn
Prescription renewals or refills		X	
Office business			Miguel
Personal business		X	
Salespeople			Miguel

FIGURE 14-11 A routing list identifies the staff member responsible for each type of incoming call.

Categorizing Problems and Providing Patient Education After the patient information is obtained, the guidelines help the staff categorize the problem according to severity. The medical assistant then decides whether the problem can be handled safely with advice over the telephone, the patient needs to come in to the office, or the problem requires immediate attention at an emergency room. For instance, if a caller is having chest pains, you would be performing a type of triage by instructing her to go to the emergency room immediately, preferably by ambulance.

If a problem is deemed appropriate for telephone management, the guidelines may include recommendations for non-prescription treatment that may relieve symptoms and anxiety. This information falls under the category of patient education. Advise the caller that recommendations are based on the symptoms and are not a diagnosis. Remember, only the licensed practitioner is authorized to make a diagnosis and prescribe medication. Ask the caller to repeat any instructions you give, and tell the patient to call back within a specified time if symptoms do not improve or worsen. Be sure to document in the medical record the critical elements of the conversation that relate to the patient's health status.

▶ Taking Complete and Accurate Phone Messages · LO 14.6

Always have paper or a telephone message pad (Figure 14-12) and pen near the telephone, so that you are prepared to write down messages. Proper documentation protects the provider

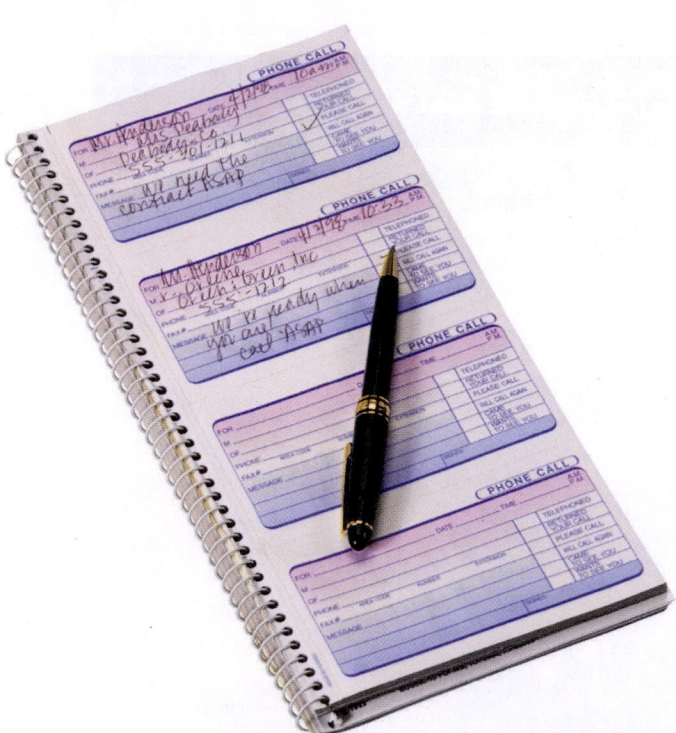

FIGURE 14-12 Using a telephone message pad ensures that no important information is omitted when the message form is filled out completely.

if the caller takes legal action. A record of telephone calls also should be included in a patient's file or electronic health record as part of a complete medical history. Because of their importance as part of the patient's legal health record, messages should never be taken on pieces of scrap paper, which are easily misplaced or accidentally discarded.

Documenting Calls

Documenting telephone calls is essential in a medical office, and several options are available to help medical assistants take a complete message every time. You can use the previously mentioned telephone message pads, a manual telephone log book, or an electronic (computerized) telephone log. Again, remember that many calls (for example, those concerning clinical problems or referrals) and the actions or decisions they lead to must be documented in patients' charts. Every entry into a patient's chart is considered a legal document, so the information must be accurate and legible.

Telephone Message Pads You can use preprinted telephone message pads, which often come in brightly colored paper, to record the following information:

- Date and time of the call
- Name of the person for whom you took the message
- Caller's name, or the patient's name if different from the caller
- Caller's telephone number (always include the area code and extension, if any)
- A description or an action to be taken, including comments like "Urgent," "Please call back," "Wants to see you," "Will call back," or "Returned your call"
- The complete message, such as "Dr. Stephenson wants to reschedule the committee meeting"
- Name or initials of the person taking the call

Figure 14-13 shows an example of a completed preprinted telephone message.

The Manual Telephone Log Some medical offices use spiral-bound, perforated message books with carbonless forms to record messages (refer to Figure 14-12). The top copy, or original, of each message is given to the appropriate person, and a copy is kept in the book for future reference in the event that the original is misplaced or accidentally destroyed.

Electronic Telephone Messaging Offices that use practice management software programs often include electronic messaging systems, which allow the telephone messages to be transmitted directly to the intended recipient's computer. These messages may be input directly into the system while on the phone with the caller instead of using the traditional message pad or telephone log that we will be discussing here. Regardless of the method used, the information to be obtained from the caller remains the same and must be complete.

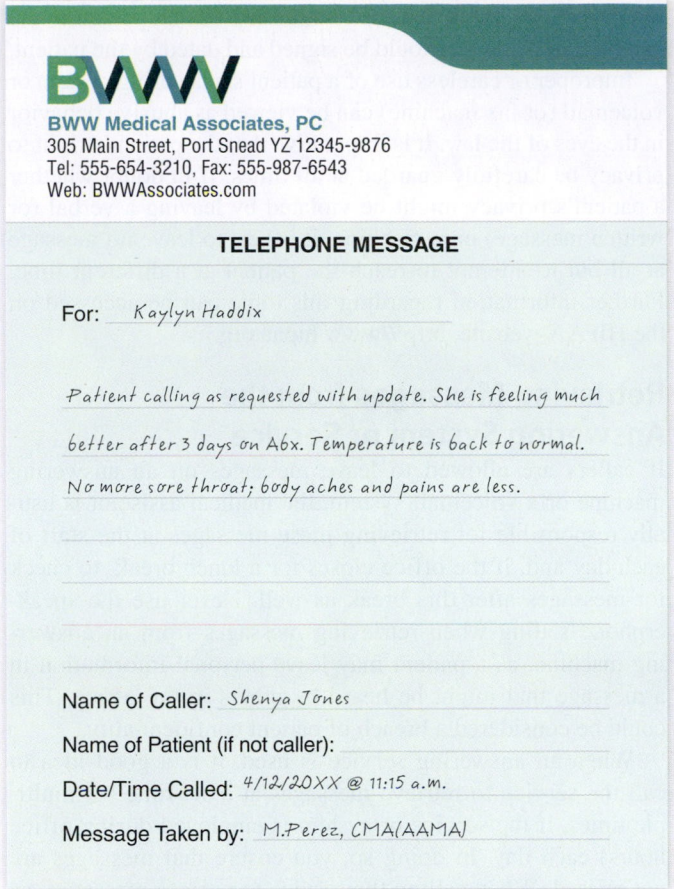

TELEPHONE MESSAGE

For: Kaylyn Haddix

Patient calling as requested with update. She is feeling much better after 3 days on Abx. Temperature is back to normal. No more sore throat; body aches and pains are less.

Name of Caller: Shenya Jones
Name of Patient (if not caller):
Date/Time Called: 4/12/20XX @ 11:15 a.m.
Message Taken by: M.Perez, CMA(AAMA)

FIGURE 14-13 It is important that messages be filled out as completely as possible.

Tips for Ensuring Accurate Messages The following suggestions will help you provide accurate documentation for incoming messages:

- Always have a pen and paper on hand. If an electronic system is used, keep the software minimized on your computer screen so you can access it quickly.
- Jot down notes as the information is given.
- Verify information, especially the spelling of patient or caller names and the correct spelling of medications.
- Obtain the patient's full name and date of birth if pulling the chart is necessary, in case there are two patients with the same name.
- Verify the correct callback number.
- When taking a phone message, never make a commitment on behalf of the intended recipient by saying, "I'll have him call you." A more appropriate response would be "I will give your message to Dr. Buckwalter."

Maintaining Patient Confidentiality

Even if you are not using a wireless headset, when you are on the phone with a patient discussing confidential information, be aware of the people around you and the volume of your voice when verifying such information. If necessary, move to a private office for such conversations so that patient confidentiality will not be inadvertently breached. When leaving paper patient messages for a practitioner containing confidential information, insert the message into a folder marked "Confidential" so it cannot readily be seen by others. If using an electronic system, each user will access the system using his or her confidential password to access all messages, allowing for maintenance of confidentiality.

▶ Placing Outgoing Calls   LO 14.7

You will often be required to place outgoing calls on behalf of the medical office. You may need to return calls, obtain information, provide patient education, pick up messages from the answering service or voicemail, or arrange patient consultations with other physicians. If you are making a long-distance call, it is important to determine the time zone and the time of day in the location you are calling before you place the call. Time zones can be determined by checking the front of the phone book, going online, or speaking with a telephone operator. For information on time zones, go to http://www.time.gov.

Locating Telephone Numbers

The medical office should have at least one telephone directory, or telephone book, for the local calling area and perhaps additional directories for surrounding areas. Use these books, an Internet phone directory such as http://www.anywho.com/ (by AT&T), the company website, or directory assistance to locate telephone numbers for outside calls. The office also may have a card file, a list, or an electronic record of commonly used telephone numbers, or these numbers may be listed in the office policies and procedures manual. If you are calling a patient, the telephone number should be in the patient's chart.

If you need to find a long-distance telephone number, many offices use the directory assistance service. You can reach this service by dialing 1-[area code]-555-1212. You also can search the Internet for free "411" services. Use directory assistance only when you have exhausted other options, however, because most long-distance carriers charge a fee each time you use the service. If you are required to call out of the country, you will need to use an international dialing code. These codes, as well as area codes and long-distance numbers, can be located through the Internet and through directory assistance. Two websites that are helpful for finding information on area codes are http://www.lincmad.com/areacodemap.html and http://www.nanpa.com.

Applying Your Telephone Skills

You can apply the telephone skills you use for answering incoming calls when placing outgoing calls. Here are additional tips for handling outgoing calls:

- Plan before you call. Have all the information you need in front of you. Plan what you will say and decide what questions to ask so you will not have to call back for additional information.
- Double-check the telephone number. If in doubt, look it up in the telephone directory. If you do dial a wrong number, be sure to apologize for the mistake.

- Allow enough time, at least a minute or about eight rings, for someone to answer the telephone. When calling patients who are elderly or physically disabled, allow additional time.
- Identify yourself. After reaching the person to whom you placed the call, give your name, and state that you are calling on behalf of the doctor or practice.
- Ask if you have called at a convenient time and whether the person has time to talk with you. If it is not a good time, ask when you should call back.
- Be ready to speak as soon as the person you called answers the telephone. Do not waste the person's time while you collect your thoughts.
- If you are calling to give information, ask if the person has a pencil and piece of paper available. Do not begin with dates, times, or instructions until the person is ready to write down the information.

Reaching Voicemail or an Answering Machine On occasion, it is important to leave a message on a patient's answering machine or voicemail. It is now required by HIPAA law that you use these pieces of equipment correctly and confidentially to guard the patient's private medical information. The goal in calling a patient's home is to speak directly to the patient or to leave a message with enough information to get the patient to call back. It is unlawful to disclose confidential patient information to anyone but the patient. HIPAA requires that you *never* leave any information if you are unsure of the phone number dialed. As a medical assistant, you cannot ensure that only the intended patient will receive any message left on an answering machine or voicemail. To guard the patient's privacy, *state only the following information:*

- The name of the individual for whom the message is intended
- The date and time of the call
- The name of your office or practice (see caution below)
- Your name as the contact person in the office (see caution below)
- The phone number of your office or practice
- The hours the office is open for a return call

A word of caution: Leave the name of the practice only if it does not reveal the purpose of the call. For instance, you would not state, "Please call Tiffany Heath from the STI Clinic." An example of an appropriate substitute is "Please call Tiffany Heath from Dr. Greene's office at 413-788-0001, Monday through Friday between 8 a.m. and 5 p.m."

Alternatively, when patients sign the Office Privacy Agreement, a release may be added inquiring if messages may be left on an answering machine or voicemail and if there are any restrictions to that permission. A second release also may be added asking if there is anyone at the home number to whom the office may speak and the relationship of that person to the patient. Each release should be signed and dated by the patient.

Improper or careless use of a patient's answering system or voicemail (or fax machine) can be viewed as abusive behavior in the eyes of the law. It is imperative that the patient's right to privacy be carefully guarded at all times. If in doubt whether a patient's privacy might be violated by leaving a verbal (or written message) on a machine, it is best to leave no message at all but to attempt to reach the patient at a different time. Further information regarding this topic can be accessed on the HIPAA website, http://www.hipaa.org.

Retrieving Messages from the Answering System or Service

If callers are allowed to leave messages on an answering machine or a voicemail system, the medical assistant is usually responsible for retrieving these messages at the start of each day and, if the office closes for a lunch break, to check for messages after this break as well. Never use the speakerphone setting when retrieving messages from an answering machine, as a patient may leave personal information in a message that might be heard by others in the office. This could be considered a breach of patient confidentiality.

When an answering service is used, it is a good idea to call the service to retrieve messages at a set time (or multiple times, if the service or system is employed during office hours) each day. In doing so, you ensure that messages are not missed. When calling the service to retrieve messages, as when taking any message, verify the information for correctness and completeness before ending the call. Procedure 14-5, located at the end of this chapter, describes how to do this.

Arranging Conference Calls

It may be necessary for you to schedule conference calls with patients, hospital personnel, or other practitioners to discuss tests or surgical results. When dealing with several people, suggest several time slots in case someone is not available at a particular time. Also keep in mind the various time zones in the country. Make sure that all the conference call participants are given the proper time in their time zone to expect the call. As mentioned earlier in this chapter, the office phone system will likely have an option allowing you to set up a conference call.

Additionally, there are services that provide "call-in conferencing." The host will provide a number and the time for you or your physician to call in as a participant, or your office may host the call. All of the participants are given a code and are asked to identify themselves as they call into the system. They will ask for an e-mail address to confirm the information, time, date, and passcodes that will be given to each individual. More information on free conference calling services can be found online. Two such services can be found at http://www.freeconference.com and http://www.freeconferencecalling.com.

PROCEDURE 14-1   Using a Telecommunications Device for the Deaf (TDD)

Procedure Goal: To properly communicate with the hearing-impaired patient using a TDD

OSHA Guidelines: This procedure does not involve exposure to blood, body fluids, or tissue.

Materials: Telephone, TDD (if available), patient chart for documentation, and a pen

Method:

Answering a Call with a TDD

1. Answer the phone as usual. If you hear a rapid clicking sound, you know you have a TDD call. You may hear no sound at all; do not hang up, as it may still be a TDD call.
   RATIONALE: *It is important to listen carefully, so as to not hang up on the patient.*

2. If you know (or believe) this is a TDD call, place your phone receiver on the TDD as directed.

3. Type your normal office greeting: "BWW Medical Associates, this is Miguel. How may I help you?"
   RATIONALE: *It is important to always identify the practice and then yourself, so the caller knows he has reached the correct party.*

4. When you complete your message, type "GA," which stands for "Go Ahead." This tells the patient you have completed your message and it is his turn to respond.

5. Give the patient time to type his response. When you see "GA" at the end of his message, it is your turn to respond.

6. When the patient receives all of the information required, he will type "Bye, SK," which stands for Good-Bye, Stop Keying.

7. If you agree the call is completed, you may also reply "Bye, SK." This will give the patient the opportunity to be the one to end the call.

8. When you receive a response of "SKSK" (Stop Keying, Stop Keying), the conversation is complete and you may hang up and turn off the TDD.
   RATIONALE: *As with a hearing/speaking patient, it is important to let the person initiating the call also be the person to end the call. This way, you know you have answered all questions and provided all needed information to the caller.*

Making a Call with a TDD

1. Turn on the TDD.

2. Dial the patient's phone number on your standard telephone and listen for the phone to ring.

3. When you hear the TDD sound, place the phone receiver on the TDD as directed.

4. After the patient types a greeting and "GA" appears on the TDD display, identify yourself and proceed with the conversation.
   RATIONALE: *It is important to identify yourself and where you are calling from when making any call.*

5. Remember to type "GA" when you complete your message so the patient knows it is his turn to respond.
   RATIONALE: *This is the only way the patient will know you have completed your communication and it is his turn to respond.*

6. Even though you were the one to initiate the call, you should still allow the patient to make the decision that the call is completed by keying "SKSK."
   RATIONALE: *You are providing a service to the patient. It is important to make sure that all information has been received and understood by him by letting him end the call.*

PROCEDURE 14-2   Renewing a Prescription by Telephone

WORK // DOC

Procedure Goal: To ensure a complete and accurate prescription is received by the patient

OSHA Guidelines: This procedure does not involve exposure to blood, body fluids, or tissue.

Materials: Telephone, appropriate phone numbers, message pad or prescription refill request form, pen, and patient chart or progress note with prescription order

Method:

1. Take the message from the call or the message system. For the prescription to be complete, you must obtain the patient's name, date of birth, phone number, pharmacy name and/or phone number, medication, and dosage.

2. Follow your facility policy regarding prescription renewals. Typically, the prescription is usually called into the pharmacy the day it is requested. An example policy may be posted at the facility and may state "Nonemergency prescription refill requests must be made during regular business hours. Please allow 24 hours for processing."

3. Communicate the policy to the patient. You should know the policy and the time when the refills will be reviewed. For example, you might state, "Dr. Williams will review the prescription between patients and it will be telephoned within 1 hour to the pharmacy. I will call you back if there is a problem."

RATIONALE: *Letting the patient know the policy demonstrates good communication skills and will result in fewer misunderstandings as to when the prescription will be available for pickup.*

4. Obtain the patient's chart or reference the electronic chart to verify you have the correct patient and that the patient is currently taking the medication. Check the patient's list of medications, which is usually part of the chart.

5. Give the prescription refill request and the chart to the physician or prescriber. Do not give a prescription refill request to the licensed practitioner without the chart or chart access information. Wait for an authorization from the practitioner before you proceed.

   RATIONALE: *All prescription refills must be authorized by the physician.*

6. Once the practitioner authorizes the prescription, prepare to call the pharmacy with the renewal information. Be certain to have the practitioner order, the patient's chart, and the refill request in front of you when you make the call. The request should include the name of the drug, the drug dosage, the frequency and mode of administration, the number of refills authorized, and the pharmacy's name and phone number. Note: You cannot call in Schedule II or III medications; these are medications that have the greatest possibility of abuse. Renewals can be called in for Schedule IV and V medications.

7. Telephone the pharmacy. Identify yourself by name, the practice name, and the practitioner's name.

   RATIONALE: *Only an identified representative from a medical practice can authorize a prescription refill.*

8. State the purpose of the call (example: "This is Miguel Perez from BWW Medical Associates. I am calling to request a prescription refill for a patient.").

9. Identify the patient. Include the patient's name, date of birth, address, and phone number.

RATIONALE: *It is essential that the correct drug be prescribed for the correct patient according to the physician's order.*

10. Identify the drug (spelling the name when necessary), the dosage, the frequency and mode of administration, and any other special instructions or changes for administration (such as "take at bedtime").

    RATIONALE: *Accuracy and complete information are essential for medication administration.*

11. State the number of refills authorized.

12. If leaving a message on a pharmacy voicemail system set up for prescribers, state your name, the name of the doctor you represent, and your phone number before you hang up.

    RATIONALE: *If the pharmacist has any questions, she must be able to reach the physician.*

13. Document the prescription renewal in the chart after the medication has been called in to the pharmacy. Include the date, the time, the name of the pharmacy, and the person taking your call. Also include the medication, dose, amount, directions, and number of refills. Sign your first initial, last name, and title. In an EHR, your credentials may be on file. Refer to Progress Note:

BWW PROGRESS NOTE		
Patient Name:	Shenya Jones	
	Rx telephoned to Beth Stone at Noname Pharmacy: Zyrtec 10 mg, one tablet daily at bedtime, #30, 6 refills	
Date:	05/03/XX	
Author:	M.A. Perez	
Done		Close

PROCEDURE 14-3 Screening and Routing Telephone Calls

WORK // DOC

Procedure Goal: To properly screen incoming telephone calls

OSHA Guidelines: This procedure does not involve exposure to blood, body fluids, or tissue.

Materials: Telephone, telephone message sheet, pen or pencil, appointment book or computerized scheduling software (computer), and office routing list

Method:
Use the office routing list to route calls appropriately.

1. Make sure all of the materials are within reach of the telephone equipment.

2. Answer the telephone promptly within two to three rings.

3. Identify the medical office and identify yourself. Make sure you know office procedure for answering the phone in your facility even if a telephone answering system is employed to route calls to you—for example, "BWW Medical Associates, this is Malik, how may I help you?"

4. If the caller does not identify himself, ask him to do so and the number he is calling from, and write down this information. Find out the reason for the call. Is it an emergency? (Refer to Table 14-2.) If so, follow office policy.

   RATIONALE: *As soon as you make certain a call is an emergency, it is important for the patient's welfare that you follow the office protocol for these situations.*

5. If you can handle the call, take care of the query. Listen carefully to what the caller has to say, paying particular attention to tone and feeling.

   RATIONALE: *If the caller's query is within your scope of practice and job description, it is up to you to take* *care of the patient's problem or request as quickly and professionally as possible.*

6. If this is a call that needs to be transferred to someone (per the routing list), tell the caller to whom and to what number you will be transferring the call. Make sure you write down the caller's name and phone number in case the call is accidentally dropped. If the other staff member does not answer promptly or is on another line, ask the caller if he would like to be transferred to the staff member's voicemail (if available) or would like to leave a message.

7. If you need to take a message, make sure you repeat the information that is given to you, especially the name of the person and his phone number. Take a complete message.
   RATIONALE: *If the message is not complete, the person receiving it may not take the appropriate action or the patient may end up needlessly being directed to multiple people.*

HANDLING INCOMING TELEPHONE CALLS

	Route to doctor immediately	Take message for doctor	Route to nurse or assistant
Emergencies: bleeding, drug/allergic reaction, difficulty breathing, injury, pain, poisoning, shock, unconsciousness, incoherence or hysteria	X		
Calls from other physicians	if possible		
Patient progress report		X	
Patient request for laboratory report		X (if abnormal)	Kaylyn (if normal)
Patient questions re medication		X	
Patient questions re billing or insurance			Miguel
Patient complaints			Kaylyn
Appointments			Kaylyn
Prescription renewals or refills		X	
Office business			Miguel
Personal business		X	
Salespeople			Miguel

FIGURE Procedure 14-3 Step 6 Use the office routing list to route calls appropriately.

PROCEDURE 14-4 Handling Emergency Calls

WORK // DOC

Procedure Goal: To determine whether a telephone call involves a medical emergency and to learn the steps to take if it is an emergency call

OSHA Guidelines: This procedure does not involve exposure to blood, body fluids, or tissue.

Materials: Office guidelines for handling emergency calls; list of symptoms and conditions requiring immediate medical attention; telephone numbers of area emergency rooms, poison control centers, and ambulance transport services; and telephone message sheets or a telephone message log

Method:

1. When someone calls the office regarding a potential emergency, remain calm.
   RATIONALE: *This attitude will help calm the caller and enable you to gather necessary information in the most efficient manner.*

2. Obtain the following information, taking accurate notes:
   a. The caller's name
   b. The caller's telephone number and the address from which the call is being made
   RATIONALE: *It may be necessary for you to put the call on hold or to hang up so you can call for medical assistance. Before you do so, however, be sure to read the information back to the caller to ensure that you have written it down correctly. If you deem the call a medical emergency, ask another medical assistant to dial 911 and give the information you have written down.*
   c. The caller's relationship to the patient (if it is not the patient who is calling)
   d. The patient's name (if the patient is not the caller)

e. The patient's age
f. A complete description of the patient's symptoms
g. If the call is about an accident, a description of how the accident or injury occurred and any other pertinent information
h. A description of how the patient is reacting to the situation
i. Treatment that has been administered

3. Read back the details of the medical problem to verify them.
   RATIONALE: *Details are necessary to determine whether or not an emergency exists and the steps you need to take next.*

4. If necessary, refer to the list of symptoms and conditions that require immediate medical attention to determine if the situation is indeed a medical emergency.

If the Situation Is a Medical Emergency

1. Put the call through to the patient's provider immediately, or handle the situation according to the established office procedures.
   RATIONALE: *Medical emergencies take precedence over all other matters.*

2. If the provider is not in the office, follow established office procedures. These may involve one or more of the following:
   a. Transferring the call to the nurse practitioner or other medical personnel, as appropriate
   b. Instructing the caller (if not the patient) to hang up and dial 911 to request an ambulance for the patient
   c. Instructing the patient to be driven to the nearest emergency room

d. Instructing the caller to telephone the nearest poison control center for advice and supplying the caller with its telephone number

e. Paging the doctor

If the Situation Is Not a Medical Emergency

1. Handle the call according to established office procedures.

2. If you are in doubt about whether the situation is a medical emergency, treat it as an emergency. You must always alert the patient's provider immediately about an emergency call, even if the patient declines to speak with the doctor.

RATIONALE: *It is better to be overly cautious than to let an emergency go untreated. The doctor should be the one to decide how to handle these situations.*

PROCEDURE 14-5   Retrieving Messages from an Answering Service or System

WORK // DOC

Procedure Goal: To follow standard procedures for retrieving messages from an answering service or system

OSHA Guidelines This procedure does not involve exposure to blood, body fluids, or tissue.

Materials: Telephone message sheets, manual telephone log, or electronic telephone log

Method

1. Set a regular schedule for calling the answering service (system) to retrieve messages.
RATIONALE: *A regular schedule ensures the procedure will not be forgotten and calls will not be missed.*

2. Call at the regularly scheduled time(s) to see if there are any messages.

3. If calling a service, identify yourself and state that you are calling to obtain messages for the practice.
RATIONALE: *Most services have a list of people at the office who are allowed to pick up messages.*

4. If calling an answering system, when the call is answered, you will enter the passcode for the office.
RATIONALE: *The passcode is given only to staff members allowed to retrieve messages.*

5. For each message, write down all pertinent information on the telephone message pad or telephone log, or key it into the electronic telephone log. Be sure to include the caller's name and telephone number, time of call, message or description of the problem, and action taken, if any.

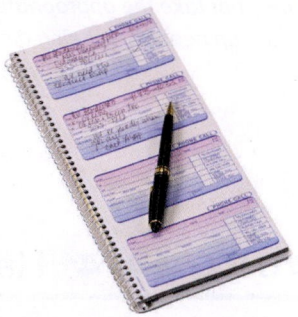

FIGURE Procedure 14-5 Step 5   Write down all pertinent information to take a complete message.
© Royalty-Free/Corbis

RATIONALE: *Always take a complete message for the convenience of the caller and the person receiving the message.*

6. If calling an answering service, repeat the information, confirming you have the correct spelling of all names and the complete, correct information.
RATIONALE: *This step ensures you have the information correct.*

7. If calling an answering system, be sure you listen carefully and replay messages if necessary to get complete information given within each message.
RATIONALE: *This step ensures you have complete and correct information.*

8. When you have retrieved all messages, route them according to office policy.

SUMMARY OF LEARNING OUTCOMES

LEARNING OUTCOMES	KEY POINTS
14.1 **Explain the purpose of the telecommunications equipment commonly found in the medical office.**	Telecommunications equipment found in the medical office includes multiline phones for incoming and outgoing calls, which may include voicemail for picking up messages; an automated voice response unit to route calls automatically to the correct person or department using a series of prompts, answered by the caller; an answering machine or answering service to pick up calls and messages when the office is extremely busy or after business hours; and cell phones and/or beepers to reach medical

	staff when they are not in the office. Additionally, a TDD may be found in the office—for communication with deaf patients.
14.2 Relate the five Cs of effective communication to telephone communication skills.	The five Cs of effective communication are important in all types of communication, and the telephone is no exception. All forms of communication are more easily understood using these principles: completeness of the message, clarity of the message, conciseness of the information, courtesy when delivering the message, and cohesiveness (logic and organization) of the message.
14.3 Define the following terms involved in making a good impression on the telephone: *telephone etiquette, pitch, pronunciation, enunciation,* **and** *tone.*	Telephone etiquette means to handle all calls professionally and politely using good manners. Pitch is the high or low level of your voice, projecting interest in what you are saying. Pronunciation is saying words correctly, and enunciation is saying them clearly. Tone projects how you are feeling; in the office, your tone should always be positive and respectful.
14.4 Describe how to appropriately handle the different types of calls coming into the medical practice.	The medical assistant may receive calls from patients, attorneys, and others. Always refer to the office policies and procedures manual regarding how to handle incoming calls appropriately. Remember, always be courteous to the caller.
14.5 Summarize the purpose of the office routing list with regard to call screening.	Screening calls categorizes the importance of the call in regard to how quickly the patient's problem or question needs to be handled. The routing list is a guideline for the entire staff to recognize which types of calls should go to each member of the medical staff, following office protocol as to the duties and scope of practice for each team member.
14.6 Carry out the procedure for taking a complete telephone message.	In addition to complete information from the caller regarding what the call is about, each complete telephone message should contain the following information: date and time of the call; name of the person for whom the message was taken; the caller's name and name of the patient (if different from the caller); the caller's telephone number with area code; a description or action to be taken; a complete and concise message; and the name or initials of the person taking the message.
14.7 Outline the preparation required prior to making outgoing calls and the skills used in making the phone call.	Prior to placing an outgoing call, be sure to have all necessary information in front of you, including the name of the person to be reached and the correct phone number. Dial the number carefully, identifying yourself when the phone is answered, asking for the person you need to reach. As always, use the five Cs of communication to complete the exchange.

CASE STUDY CRITICAL THINKING

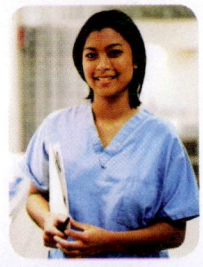

© Ablestock.com/
Getty Images

Recall Reagan Patrick from the beginning of the chapter. Now that you have completed the chapter, answer the following questions regarding her case.

1. The first phone call is easy—a routine appointment for next week, which Reagan books without a problem. The next caller states he must speak with Dr. Buckwalter immediately. How should Reagan handle this call?

2. The next call is Nancy Evans. Reagan remembers from her appointment earlier this week that Mrs. Evans has possible early-onset dementia. Mrs. Evans states she has not seen Dr. Williams in several months and wants to know why she does not "care about her anymore." While Reagan is trying to speak with Mrs. Evans, another line rings. How should Reagan handle Mrs. Evans and the ringing phone?

1. (LO 14.1) Which of the following is *not* a common function of many of today's multiline phones?
   a. Transfer options
   b. Hold
   c. Voicemail
   d. Intercom
   e. Voice recognition

2. (LO 14.1) What is the main reason pagers are not used as often in medical offices?
   a. Physicians hate carrying them
   b. Improved healthcare means fewer "emergencies"
   c. Cell phones are being used more often
   d. It is becoming harder to find signals for pagers
   e. E-mail is used more often

3. (LO 14.2) Which of the following is *not* one of the five Cs of effective communication?
   a. Compassion
   b. Clarity
   c. Conciseness
   d. Cohesiveness
   e. Completeness

4. (LO 14.2) Which of the following is an appropriate statement for answering the office telephone?
   a. "Doctor's office, Jayden speaking."
   b. "Jayden here, this is BWW Medical Associates."
   c. "BWW Medical Associates, Jayden, hold please."
   d. "BWW Medical Associates; this is Jayden. How may I help you?"
   e. All of these

5. (LO 14.3) Speaking clearly and distinctly is called
   a. Tone
   b. Enunciation
   c. Etiquette
   d. Pronunciation
   e. Clarity

6. (LO 14.4) Which of the following is *not* a common reason patients call the office?
   a. Appointment requests
   b. Billing inquiries
   c. Lab or X-ray reports
   d. Compliments to the medical staff
   e. All of these

7. (LO 14.5) Deciding how emergent a patient's problem is and how it may best be handled is a procedure known as
   a. Screening
   b. Routing
   c. Triage
   d. Paging
   e. Etiquette

8. (LO 14.5) _____ is being done when a call is transferred to an appropriate person based on the caller's request.
   a. Screening
   b. Routing
   c. Triage
   d. Paging
   e. Etiquette

9. (LO 14.6) Taking an effective message involves which of the following items?
   a. Date and time of call
   b. Whom the call is for
   c. Name and phone number of caller
   d. Message and action to be taken
   e. All of these and more

10. (LO 14.7) When placing a call to a patient with medical information, if you reach the patient's answering machine, what should you do?
    a. Leave a complete message; it is the patient's private answering machine
    b. Leave your name, the name of the practice, and your phone number so the patient can call back
    c. Leave your name and phone number, stating there is a medical issue that requires discussion
    d. Leave the practice name only if the reason for the call is not easily identifiable, your name, and your phone number; if unsure, try calling back at another time
    e. Leave your name and number with no message

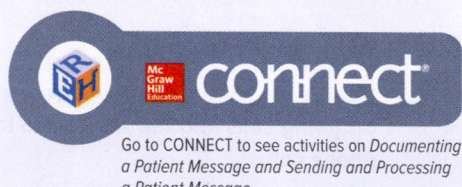

Go to CONNECT to see activities on *Documenting a Patient Message and Sending and Processing a Patient Message.*

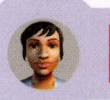

Patient Education

CASE STUDY

PATIENT INFORMATION

Patient Name	DOB	Allergies
Sylvia Gonzales	9/1/19XX	Penicillin

Attending	MRN	Other Information
Alexis N. Whalen, MD	341-73-792	04/22/XX: FBS - 152 mg/dL, A1C - 6.7% 06/18/XX: GTT - 232 mg/dL, A1C - 6.9%

A 51-year-old female, Sylvia Gonzales, is at the office for a 3-month return check for newly diagnosed Type 2 diabetes. She appears overweight and is snacking on a bag of potato

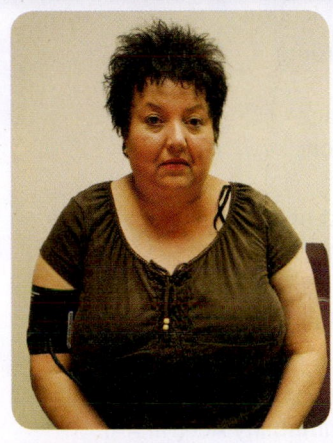

chips and chocolate milk when you take her into the exam room. She states she has taken the medication she was given for her "sugar" and she knows the doctor wants to do a special "sugar test" this time. Her medication list includes Januvia, 100 mg daily, which is a medication to help lower her blood sugar.

Keep Sylvia Gonzales in mind as you study the chapter. There will be questions at the end of the chapter based on the case study. The information in the chapter will help you answer these questions.

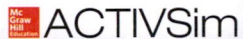

LEARNING OUTCOMES

After completing Chapter 15, you will be able to:

15.1 Identify the benefits of patient education and the medical assistant's role in providing education.

15.2 Describe factors that affect learning and teaching.

15.3 Implement teaching techniques.

15.4 Choose reliable patient education materials used in the medical office.

15.5 Explain how patient education can be used to promote good health habits.

15.6 Describe the types of information that should be included in the patient information packet.

15.7 Describe the benefits and special considerations of patient education prior to surgery.

KEY TERMS

consumer education

factual teaching

modeling

participatory teaching

philosophy

return demonstration

screening

sensory teaching

V.C.6 Define coaching a patient as it relates to:
(a) health maintenance
(b) disease prevention
(c) compliance with treatment plan
(d) community resources

V.C.8 Discuss applications of electronic technology professional communication

V.P.4 Coach patients regarding:
(a) office policies
(b) health maintenance
(c) disease prevention
(d) treatment plan

V.P.9 Develop a current list of community resources related to patients' healthcare needs

V.P.10 Facilitate referrals to community resources in the role of a patient navigator

VI.P.6 Utilize an EMR

X.C.3 Describe components of the Health Information Portability and Accountability Act (HIPAA)

X.P.3 Document patient care accurately in the medical record

2. Anatomy and Physiology
d. Apply a system of diet and nutrition
(ii) Educate patients regarding proper diet and nutrition guidelines

4. Medical Law and Ethics
f. Comply with federal, state, and local health laws and regulations as they relate to healthcare settings
(1) Define scope of practice for the medical assistant within the state that the medical assistant is employed

7. Records Management
b. Utilize Electronic Medical Records (EMR) and Practice Management Systems

8. Administrative Procedures
f. Display professionalism through written and verbal communications

9. Clinical Procedures
h. Teach self-examination, disease management, and health promotion
i. Identify community resources and Complementary and Alternative Medicine practices (CAM)
j. Make adaptations with patients with special needs

11. Career Development
b. Demonstrate professional behavior

▶ Introduction

Health education should be a lifelong pursuit for all of us. The ultimate goal of all medical professionals is to encourage and teach healthy habits and behaviors to all patients. People first have to understand what is good for them, and then they have to make a decision to follow that advice. In patient education, the medical assistant shares health information and encourages patients to make good health decisions.

In this chapter you will learn about patient education. Understanding your role and scope of practice related to patient education is necessary. Then you will develop skills in recognizing and overcoming roadblocks to education. You will become more comfortable with teaching and demonstrating procedures to others. Most importantly, you will begin to recognize the incredible responsibility of the medical assistant to correctly lead others to their highest level of health.

▶ The Educated Patient   LO 15.1

Patient education is an essential process in the medical office. It encourages patients to take an active role in their medical care. It results in better compliance with treatment programs. When patients are suffering from illness, disease, or injury, education can often help them regain their health and independence more quickly. Simply put, patient education helps patients become healthy and stay healthy. Educated patients are more likely to comply with instructions if they understand the "why" behind the instructions. Also, educated patients are more likely to be satisfied clients of the practice.

Patients benefit from education, but the medical office benefits as well. Preoperative instruction to surgical patients, for example, lessens the chance that procedures will have to be rescheduled because surgical guidelines were not followed. Educated patients will also be less likely to call the office with questions. Thus, the office staff will have to spend less time on the telephone.

Patient education takes many forms and includes a variety of techniques. It can be as simple as answering a question that comes up during a routine visit, or it can be detailed instruction regarding a procedure such as wound care. In some cases, it may involve printed materials. In others, the patient may be asked to participate by responding correctly to instructions. As a medical assistant, the amount and type of

Patient Education and Scope of Practice

A medical assistant must be competent and knowledgeable before he or she can provide patient education. If a licensed practitioner asks you to perform education, the content of that education must be approved by that practitioner. You must understand the content in order to teach it, but you should not go beyond the content you have been asked to teach. In addition, while performing education, you must not make any judgments or answer any questions that require diagnosis, assessment, or evaluation.

patient education you provide will be decided by your place of employment and scope of practice. See *Caution: Handle with Care*: Patient Education and Scope of Practice. Even if you are not providing the education, you should be aware of the patient's educational needs and ability to understand. In addition, being a role model by practicing good health behaviors is important.

▶ Learning and Teaching LO 15.2

In order to provide patient education, it is necessary to understand the process of learning. Learning is the acquiring of new knowledge, behaviors, or skills, which are also known as the *domains of learning*. Knowledge, the cognitive domain, includes the factual or practical understanding of a subject and the ability to recall it. Behavior, the affective domain, is how one approaches learning. It includes feelings, values, appreciation, enthusiasms, motivations, and attitudes. Skills, the psychomotor domain, include physical movement, coordination, and use of motor skills to complete a task. See Figure 15-1.

To better understand these domains, let's use the example of our patient, Sylvia Gonzales, who just found out she is diabetic. In order for her to be able to manage her diabetes and have the best outcome for her health, she will need to learn through all three of the domains.

- *Cognitive (knowledge):* Sylvia will need to understand the basic information about diabetes, including the effects of diet, exercise, and treatments. The information can come in many formats, as discussed later in this chapter.
- *Affective (behaviors):* Sylvia must have the desire or be motivated to make a change in order to improve her health. Once she appreciates the need, is motivated, and has a positive attitude, she will then be able to make the change. This is part of the learning process. If she does not have the desire to learn about diabetes or is not motivated to improve her health, she will not make any change. Being aware of a patient's level of motivation and

encouraging the patient are important parts of the teaching process.
- *Psychomotor (skills):* Once Sylvia has the basic knowledge and correct behavior, she will be able to learn and perform the skills necessary to improve her condition and keep her diabetes under control. This may include eating better foods, increasing exercise, and taking any medications that are prescribed.

For learning to occur, all three domains of learning must be considered during the teaching process. The patient, Sylvia, must be provided the information, she must be motivated and have a desire to learn the information, and then she must perform the skills, doing what is necessary to improve her condition.

▶ Teaching Techniques LO 15.3

Patient education can take many forms. Any instructions—verbal, written, or demonstrative—that you give to patients are types of patient education. When providing education, three types of teaching can occur: factual, sensory, and participatory. These three types of teaching correspond to the three domains of learning.

The combination of these teaching methods gives the patient an overall understanding, because it encourages learning through all three of the domains of learning.

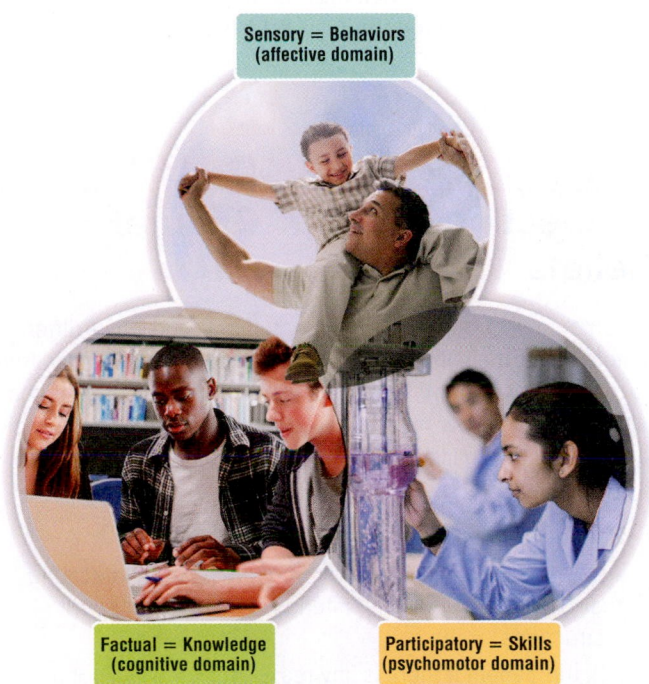

Sensory = Behaviors (affective domain)

Factual = Knowledge (cognitive domain)

Participatory = Skills (psychomotor domain)

FIGURE 15-1 Learning occurs through three domains: cognitive, affective, and psychomotor. Teaching is accomplished by factual, sensory, and participatory techniques.
(top) © Purestock/Getty Images RF; (left) © Monkey Business Images/Shutterstock; (right) © ERproductions Ltd/Blend Images LLC RF

Factual Teaching (Cognitive Domain)

Factual teaching provides detailed information about a subject. For example, when preparing a patient for surgery, you should tell the patient what will happen during the surgery, when it will happen, and why the procedure is necessary. Factual information provided to a patient before surgery can also include restrictions on diet or activity that may be necessary both before and after surgery. Factual information is usually supported with written materials so that the patient can refer to the information as needed at a later date.

Sensory Teaching (Affective Domain)

Sensory teaching provides patients with a description of the physical sensations they may have as part of the learning or the procedure involved. This learning relates to how the person is affected—that is, the affective domain. For example, prior to surgery you might need to explain how much pain or what other sensations, such as numbness or tingling, the patient may feel. All five senses may be involved: feeling, seeing, hearing, tasting, and smelling.

Participatory Teaching (Psychomotor Domain)

Participatory teaching includes demonstrations of techniques that may be necessary to show that something has been learned. For example, as part of preoperative teaching, aspects of postoperative care include cleaning the wound, changing the dressing, and applying ice packs. A new diabetic might need to be taught how to check his blood sugar. During this phase of teaching, you need to first describe the technique to the patient and then demonstrate it. By demonstrating the procedure, you are **modeling** it for the patient, or showing the patient exactly what to do. Then you should ask the patient to perform the same procedure while you watch. This practice is called **return demonstration.** The return demonstration has two purposes. First, it allows you to be sure the patient fully understands the procedure. Second, by actually performing the procedure, the patient uses motor skills and engages the psychomotor domain. Physically performing the procedure helps cement the steps in the patient's mind.

Verifying Patient Understanding

The key to the success of any educational process is verifying that patients have actually understood the information. A good way to check for understanding is to have patients explain in their own words what they have learned. This is a form of feedback. In addition, have them engage in return demonstrations.

Cultural and Educational Barriers

Some practices serve patients who cannot read well or who do not speak or understand English. It may be necessary to create educational materials written in very simple terms that present information through pictures and charts. The information also may need to be translated into one or more languages. Patients must understand the office's policies and procedures as well as any other educational information provided.

One-on-one explanations may be required for these patients. However, printed materials should still be given to these patients to take home for reference. Family members or friends may be able to read the materials for them, reinforcing what they learned in the office. When demonstrating a procedure to patients, keep in mind any physical limitations they have and adjust the procedure accordingly. Make sure patients understand the instructions by asking them to perform the procedure for you.

It is important to match the learning materials to the patient's needs and to her level of understanding. Consider the patient's cultural background, age, medical condition, emotional state, learning style, educational background, disabilities, religious background, and readiness to learn when providing new materials. Review the *Points on Practice*: Respecting Patients' Cultural Beliefs. Keep in mind that patients can refuse treatment and information. If they do, notify the doctor and document the event in the patient's chart.

▶ Patient Education Materials   LO 15.4

Patient education materials inform patients and enable and encourage them to become involved in their own medical care. Most formal types of patient education involve some printed information. They may also include visual materials, such as DVDs and Internet sites.

Printed Materials

Printed educational materials come in a variety of formats. They can be as simple as a single sheet of paper, or they can be several sheets folded or stapled together to form a booklet.

Brochures, Booklets, and Fact Sheets Many medical offices have materials available that explain procedures performed in the medical office or give information about

---

POINTS ON PRACTICE
Respecting Patients' Cultural Beliefs

Patients come from many diverse cultures and have different beliefs about the causes and treatments of illness. These differences may affect their treatment expectations, as well as their willingness to follow medical directions. Consider these simple steps when giving instructions to patients of diverse cultures:

- Speak slowly and clearly.
- Request or provide a translator as needed.
- Ask for and look for feedback from the patient, indicating that she understands and intends to follow the patient instructions.
- Ask the patient if there is any reason that she will not be able to follow the instructions.
- Address any concerns indicated by the patient, notifying the doctor if the concerns mean that the patient is not likely to follow the instructions.

specific diseases and medical conditions. For example, women who have had a cesarean section delivery may be given a fact sheet describing simple exercises they can do in bed to help regain strength in the abdominal muscles. Many educational aids are prepared by pharmaceutical companies and are provided free of charge to medical offices. Others may be written by the licensed practitioner or members of the office staff. You may be asked to help prepare some of these materials.

Electronic health record systems provide the ability to create or import informational materials for patients. Using the electronic health record system Practice Fusion®, you can quickly click a link to find up-to-date electronic information on the Internet for any diagnosis or medication you enter into the system. See Figures 15-2 and 15-3 as well as Procedure 15-1, Creating Electronic Patient Instructions, at the end of this chapter.

Whenever written materials of any kind are given to a patient, it must be noted in the patient's chart. Be sure to document exactly which brochure or leaflet was distributed. Using electronic health records, you can create and document patient receipt of pertinent information quickly and easily.

Educational Newsletters A popular patient education tool is the medical office newsletter. Newsletters contain timely, practical healthcare tips. Regular newsletters can also offer updates on office policies, information about new diagnostic tests or equipment, and news about the office staff. Newsletters are often written by the doctor or office staff. Some publishing companies and medical groups also offer newsletters that can be customized to a particular practice, using the Internet or software programs such as Microsoft® Publisher. See Figure 15-4.

Community-Assistance Directory Patients often require the assistance of health-related organizations within the community. For example, an elderly patient may need the services of a visiting nurse or a Meals on Wheels food program. Other patients may need the services of a day-care center, speech therapist, or weight clinic.

There are many community resources available in your local area that provide needed services to patients. The medical assistant should be aware of these resources and be able to navigate patients to them. The first step is to develop a community resource library by gathering a listing of local agencies. You will need the correct name, address, web address, phone number, contact person, and directions for submitting a referral for each resource listed. It may take some research on your part to locate and organize this information. Contact the community resources and request information such as brochures, newsletters, and referral applications. See

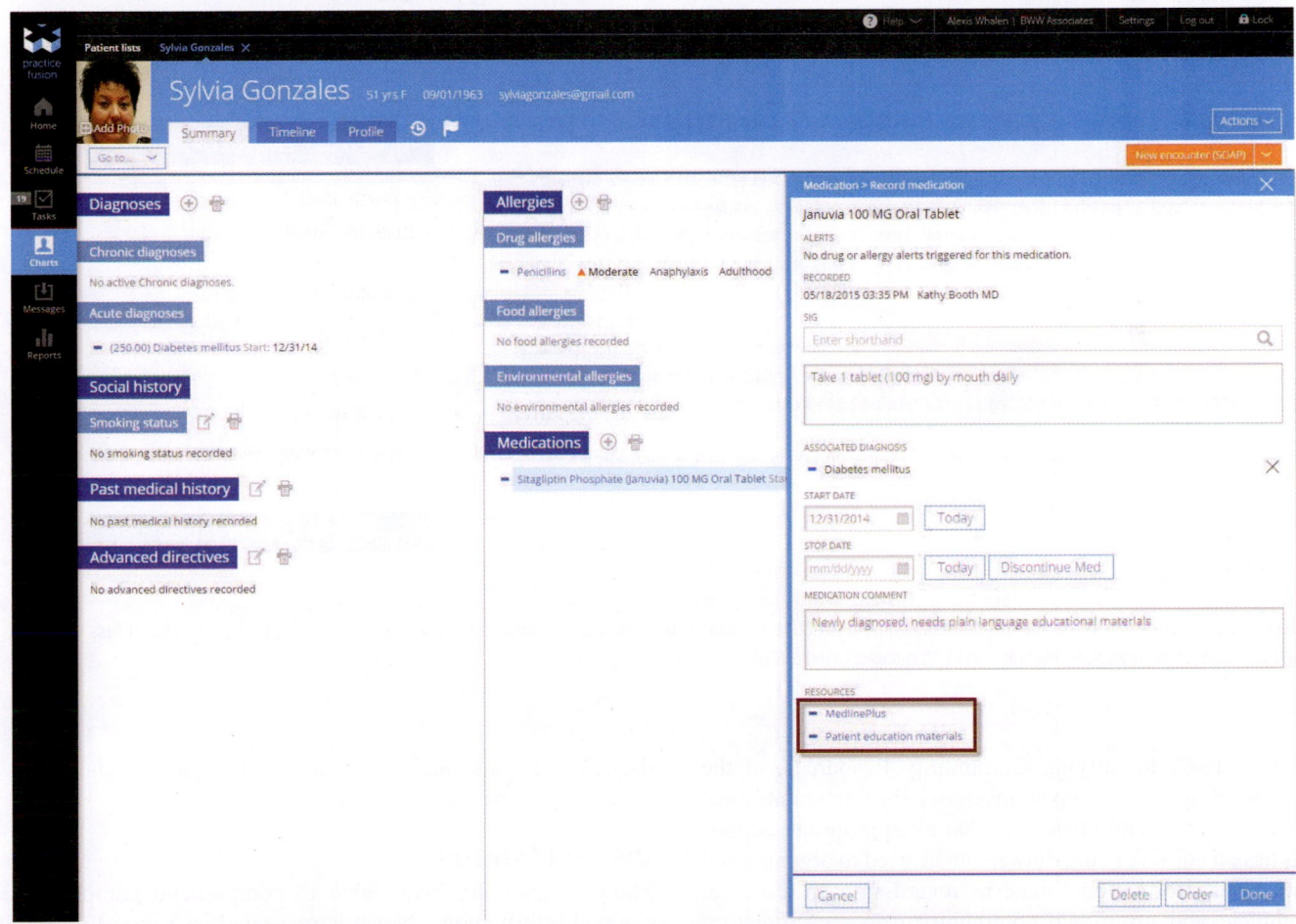

FIGURE 15-2 When you add a medication or diagnosis for a patient in Practice Fusion®, a Resources area appears with patient education materials.

© Practice Fusion®

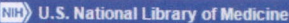
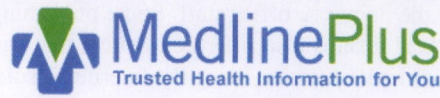
MedlinePlus
Trusted Health Information for You

Search MedlinePlus [GO]

About MedlinePlus   Site Map   FAQs   Contact Us

Health Topics   **Drugs & Supplements**   **Videos & Tools**   **Español**

Home → Health Topics → Diabetes Type 2

Diabetes Type 2
Also called: Type 2 Diabetes

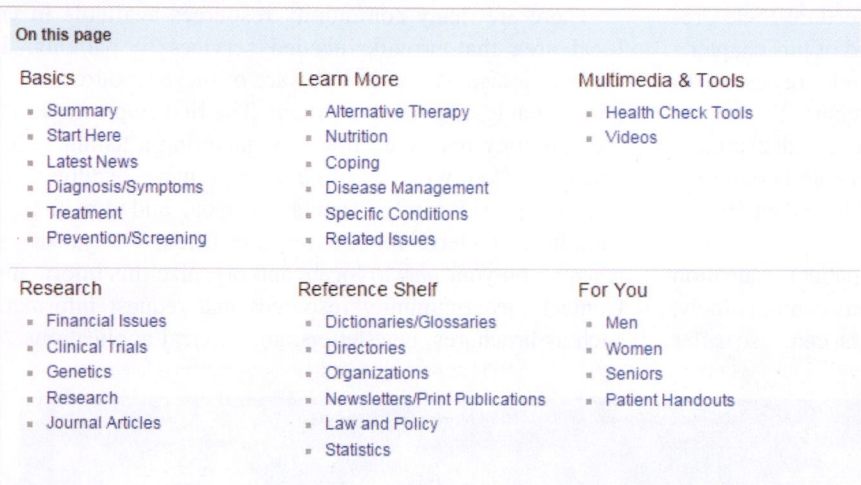

On this page

Basics
- Summary
- Start Here
- Latest News
- Diagnosis/Symptoms
- Treatment
- Prevention/Screening

Learn More
- Alternative Therapy
- Nutrition
- Coping
- Disease Management
- Specific Conditions
- Related Issues

Multimedia & Tools
- Health Check Tools
- Videos

Research
- Financial Issues
- Clinical Trials
- Genetics
- Research
- Journal Articles

Reference Shelf
- Dictionaries/Glossaries
- Directories
- Organizations
- Newsletters/Print Publications
- Law and Policy
- Statistics

For You
- Men
- Women
- Seniors
- Patient Handouts

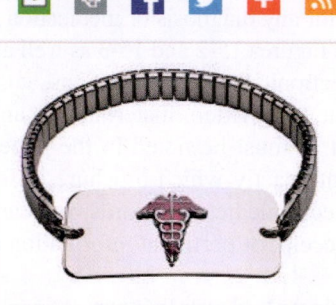

Get Diabetes Type 2 updates by email *i*

Enter email address [GO]

Summary

Diabetes means your blood glucose, or blood sugar, levels are too high. With type 2 diabetes, the more common type, your body does not make or use insulin well. Insulin is a hormone that helps glucose get into your cells to give them energy. Without insulin, too much glucose stays in your blood. Over time, high blood glucose can lead to serious problems with your heart, eyes, kidneys, nerves, and gums and teeth.

You have a higher risk of type 2 diabetes if you are older, obese, have a family history of diabetes, or do not exercise. Having prediabetes also increases your risk. Prediabetes means that your blood sugar is higher than normal but not high enough to be called diabetes.

The symptoms of type 2 diabetes appear slowly. Some people do not notice symptoms at all. The symptoms can include

- Being very thirsty
- Urinating often

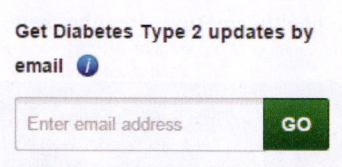

MEDICAL ENCYCLOPEDIA

A1c test

Diabetes - what to ask your doctor - type 2

Diabetes type 2 - meal planning

Giving an insulin injection

High blood sugar

Type 2 diabetes

Type 2 diabetes - self-care

Related Health Topics

Blood Sugar

FIGURE 15-3   The patient education materials link in Practice Fusion® redirects you to current, patient-oriented information on MedlinePlus.
Courtesy U.S. National Library of Medicine. Photo of bracelet: © Photodisc Collection/Getty Images RF.

Procedure 15-2, Identifying Community Resources, at the end of this chapter. Type up an inventory sheet or spreadsheet of your resources, and make sure that all appropriate departments have a copy. A filing drawer can be used to organize and maintain the informational material regarding each resource. A complete and up-to-date community resources directory prepared by the office that is accessible to staff and patients is a valuable aid for referring patients to appropriate agencies. The medical assistant provides good customer service when

they can navigate and assist in the goal of patient health and well-being using this directory.

Visual Materials

Many patients are better able to comprehend complicated medical information when it is presented in a visual format. When using visual educational materials, it is usually best to provide corresponding written materials that patients can keep for reference.

BWW Wire

Our e-newsletter is your guide to current health news, practitioner-written articles, and upcoming events for BWW Medical Associates.

BWW Staff Profile

New Year, New Electronic Health Records for All!

Over the past year, the staff of BWW prepared for the transition to a new electronic health record system. On January 1, 2015, all of our pre-existing files were officially integrated with our new Practice Fusion® EHR, and we have started primarily using electronic health records. We are excited to be able to continue to offer you the very best possible care utilizing this new system. We hope you will be patient with us as our staff get accustomed to using the new system. By January 2016, we are planning to have a patient portal system that will allow you—the patient—to access your medical records from the comfort of your home computer and to more easily request the release of your records to specialists and other providers.

Crunch Camp Challenge

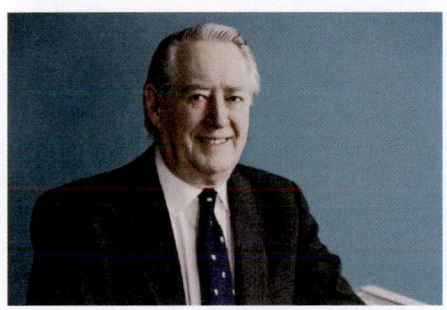

Ring in the New Year with the BWW staff as we challenge ourselves to eat healthier and exercise more. In the reception area, you'll be able to see a graph of our progress as we compete for the title of Crunch Challenge Champion and a new Vitamix blender.

Right now, Miguel is in the lead. With his marathon training regimen, he is logging an impressive number of exercise hours. Newcomer Marissa, however, is dominating the healthy eating component of the competition with her impressively varied and nutritious diet. You can log your own hours on our Crunch Camp app or at BWWAssociates.com to see if your can beat your favorite member of the BWW staff and win yourself a Vitamix blender.

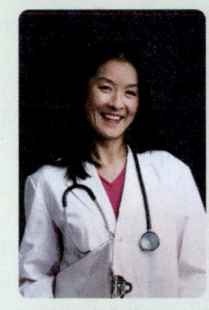
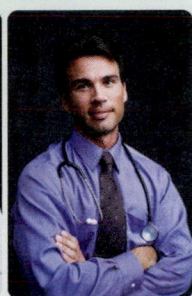

Meet Marissa T. Wang, NP and Andrew V. Utkin, PA

Starting in the New Year, BWW is happy to welcome Mrs. Wang and Mr. Utkin to our practice. Marissa started her career as a healthcare provider in the inner city, where she was a trauma nurse, before she decided to volunteer her time for a year with Doctors without Borders. She met her husband, a pharmacist, in south Sudan. Mrs. Wang just became a Nurse Practitioner, and she and her husband are expecting their first child this summer. Andrew will be splitting his time between BWW and a local non-profit clinic. Born to Ukrainian parents, Andrew spent his formative years abroad before moving to the United States for high school. He decided to enter the medical field after seeing the effects of war and the shortage of quality public healthcare.

Happy Anniversary, Dr. Buckwalter

For the past 30 years, ever since he founded BWW Medical Associates, Dr. Buckwalter has called Port Snead his home. By founding his practice, Dr. Buckwalter brought quality medical care to this underserved waterfront community. A leading citizen, Dr. Buckwalter is known for his active involvement in local government and his Scottish Terrier Jamie. Dr. Buckwalter will be retiring from practice at the end of 2015; however, we plan to make his last year one to remember!

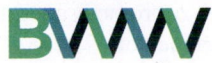
BWW Medical Associates, PC
305 Main Street, Port Snead YZ 12345-9876, Tel: 555-654-3210, Fax: 555-987-6543, Web: BWWAssociates.com

FIGURE 15-4 Practice newsletters are a great tool for patient education. They also keep patients up-to-date on practice events and advances.

DVDs DVDs are often used to educate patients about a variety of topics and to instruct them in self-care techniques. The use of DVDs is especially effective when teaching about complex subjects and procedures. Examples of helpful DVDs used in patient education include those on breast self-examination, dressing change, and infant care.

Seminars and Classes Many physicians conduct or arrange educational seminars or classes for their patients. For example, an obstetrician might offer classes in childbirth preparation for patients and their partners. Other seminars and classes may be conducted depending on the type of medical practice.

Libraries and Patient Resource Rooms Most public libraries have an assortment of books, magazines, and electronic databases pertaining to health and medical topics. Hospitals may provide patient resource rooms, which include a variety of educational materials—such as books, brochures, and DVDs—for public use. Some hospitals provide patient education materials on demand through televisions in patient rooms. A medical librarian is a healthcare team member and, if available, a good contact to assist you with obtaining and providing patient education materials.

Associations Thousands of health organizations and associations can be contacted for information about preventive healthcare and virtually every known disease or disorder. The names, addresses, telephone numbers, and websites of these organizations are provided in several directories, which are available online or at most libraries. Table 15-1 provides a sample list of patient resource organizations. Search the Internet to obtain the latest contact information for each organization.

Online Health Information The Internet is a widely used source of medical information. It will be helpful to suggest specific, reputable websites for patients to research. Website addresses should be checked for credibility before using them or referring your patients to them. See Procedure 15-3, Locating Credible Patient Education Information on the Internet, at the end of this chapter. You may need to obtain assistance and approval from the licensed practitioner, a medical librarian, or other medical staff members. Developing a list of reputable sites to suggest to patients as part of patient education is a must. After you have established the list, check the websites about every 6 months to be sure they are still active.

Once you are comfortable with the types of learning and teaching as well as the educational materials available, you should be ready to start patient education. Begin by creating a patient education plan. This plan includes identifying the education needs of the patient, creating an outline, collecting resources for teaching, carrying out the teaching, and then evaluating the effectiveness. Keep in mind that education is an ongoing process. However, the patient education plan gives you a place to start. See Procedure 15-4, Developing a Patient Education Plan, at the end of this chapter.

TABLE 15-1 Patient Resource Organizations	
Organization	**Web Address**
Alzheimer's Disease Education and Referral Center	http://www.nia.nih.gov/alzheimers
American Academy of Pediatrics	http://www.aap.org
American Cancer Society	http://www.cancer.org
American Diabetes Association	http://www.diabetes.org
Academy of Nutrition and Dietetics	http://www.eatright.org
American Heart Association	http://www.heart.org
Arthritis Foundation	http://www.arthritis.org
Asthma and Allergy Foundation of America	http://www.aafa.org
Centers for Disease Control and Prevention Department of Health and Human Services	http://www.cdc.gov
National AIDS Hotline	http://www.thebody.com
National Clearinghouse for Alcohol and Drug Information	http://www.samhsa.gov
National Health Information Center	http://www.health.gov/nhic
National Kidney Foundation	http://www.kidney.org
National Organization for Rare Disorders	http://www.rarediseases.org
President's Council on Physical Fitness and Sports Department	http://www.fitness.gov

▶ Promoting Health and Wellness Through Education · LO 15.5

Maintaining or improving your health is the best way to protect yourself against disease and illness. It is also part of being a good role model in your position as a medical assistant. **Consumer education** is geared toward the average person. It is provided in clear, everyday (nonmedical) language to help Americans become more aware of the importance of good health. As a result, many people are beginning to take greater responsibility for their own health and well-being.

There are many ways to achieve good health. You can develop healthy habits, take steps to protect yourself from injury, and take preventive measures to decrease the risk of disease or illness. Patient education in the medical office should help patients achieve these goals.

Healthy Habits

Patient education can be used to promote good health habits by teaching patients the importance of

- Good nutrition, including limiting fat intake and eating an adequate amount of fruits, vegetables, and fiber.
- Regular exercise.
- Adequate rest (7 to 8 hours of sleep a night).
- Avoiding smoking and drug use.
- Limiting alcohol consumption.

- Safe-sex practices.
- A balanced lifestyle of work and leisure activities (moderation).
- Safety practices.

Whenever possible, these guidelines should be recommended to patients of all ages. Good health should be a top priority in life. Although it is best to adopt healthy behavior before illness develops, remind patients that it is never too late to work toward improving their health.

Protection from Injury

Many accidents happen because people fail to see potential risks and do not develop plans of action. Following safety measures at home, at work, at play, and while traveling can help prevent injury. A discussion of ways to avoid accidents and injury should be part of the educational process. See the *Educating the Patient* feature Tips for Preventing Injury to help patients avoid injury at home and at work.

Another essential aspect of educating patients about injury prevention is teaching them about the proper use of medications. A prescription includes specific instructions for taking the medication. Emphasize to the patient that these instructions must be followed exactly. In addition, the patient must not change the dosage or mix medications of any kind without first checking with the physician. Patients who do not adhere to these rules run the risk of potentially dangerous side effects. Tell patients to report to the physician any unusual reactions experienced when taking medications. Patients also must be cautioned to never share their medications with anyone else, no matter how tempting it may be to "help" a family member or friend.

When providing a patient with a new prescription, always ask the patient if he has told the doctor about all the medications he is already taking, including herbs, vitamins, and over-the-counter (OTC) medications. If the patient tells you that he has not, immediately inform the physician before the patient leaves the office. Some medications taken together or with

---

EDUCATING THE PATIENT
Tips for Preventing Injury

To avoid accidents and injury, teach patients to use common sense and follow these guidelines.

At Home

- Install smoke detectors, carbon monoxide detectors, and fire extinguishers.
- Keep all medicines, chemicals, and household cleaning solutions out of the reach of children.
- Purchase products in childproof containers. Lock or attach childproof latches to all cabinets, medicine chests, and drawers that contain poisonous items.
- Keep chemicals in their original containers and store them out of children's reach.
- Install adequate lighting in rooms and hallways.
- Install railings on stairs.
- Use nonskid backing on rugs to help prevent falls, or remove rugs altogether.
- Stay with young children when they are in the bathroom.
- Do not rely on bath seats or rings as a safety device for babies and children.
- Set the water temperature on the water heater at 120° F.
- Never use appliances in the bathtub or near a sink filled with water.
- Practice good kitchen safety: Store knives and kitchen tools properly. Unplug small appliances when not in use. Wipe up spills immediately.
- When cooking, turn all handles of pots and pans inward, toward the cooking surface, to avoid spills and burns.

- Use twist-ties to shorten long electrical cords and speaker wires, or secure them with electrical tape. Avoid plugging too many electrical appliances into the same outlet.
- Exercise caution when using electrical appliances. Use outlet covers when outlets are not in use.
- To reach high places, use proper equipment, such as stepladders, not chairs.
- Use child safety gates at the top of stairwells.

At Work

- Use appropriate safety equipment and protective gear, as required.
- Lift heavy objects properly: Bend at the knees, not at the waist. As you straighten your legs, bring the object close to your body quickly. That way, strong leg muscles do the lifting, not weaker back muscles.
- Never attempt to move furniture on your own. Request that a member of the office building maintenance staff be engaged to do so.
- Use surge protectors on computer and other electronic equipment to prevent overloading outlets.
- Make sure hallways, entrance areas, work areas, offices, and parking lots are well lit.
- If your job involves desk work, practice proper posture when sitting. Do not sit for long periods of time. Get up and stretch, or walk down the hall and back.

certain foods can interfere with how well the drug works or cause side effects or adverse reactions. The physician needs to know about all drugs as well as herbal preparations and OTC medications the patient is taking.

Preventive Measures

Preventive healthcare is an area in which patient education plays a vital role. Patients need to know that they can decrease their chances of getting certain illnesses and diseases by taking preventive measures and avoiding certain behaviors. Preventive techniques can be described on three levels: *health-promoting behaviors, screening,* and *rehabilitation.*

Health-Promoting Behaviors The first level of disease and illness prevention is to form habits that lower the risk of illness or injury. Examples of these habits are given in the Healthy Habits section of this chapter. Health-promoting behaviors also include understanding the symptoms and warning signs of disease. When these signs are recognized early in the disease process, the disease can often be treated more easily and sometimes even avoided altogether.

Screening The second level of disease prevention is screening. **Screening** involves the diagnostic testing of a patient who is typically free of symptoms. Screening allows early diagnosis and treatment of certain diseases. Examples of screening tests include colonoscopy, mammography, and Pap smears for women and prostate examinations for men.

Annual screening is important to health maintenance. Although the requirements differ according to the age and condition of the patient, annual screenings usually include routine blood work, urinalysis, electrocardiogram (ECG), and a physical examination (PE).

Rehabilitation The third level of disease prevention involves the rehabilitation and management of an existing illness. At this level the disease process remains stable, but the body will probably not heal any further. The objective is to maintain functionality and avoid further disability. Examples of this level of prevention include stroke rehabilitation programs, cardiac rehabilitation, and pain management for conditions such as arthritis.

▶ The Patient Information Packet LO 15.6

When patients come to the medical practice, they need to learn not only about health and medical issues but also about the medical office itself. The patient information packet explains the medical practice and its policies. Unlike most other patient education materials, the patient information packet deals mainly with administrative matters rather than medical issues.

The patient information packet may be as simple as a one-page brochure or pamphlet. It may be a multipage brochure or a folder with multiple-page inserts. In some practices, the patient information packet is available online or through the EHR system for review or printing. See Figure 15-5.

Benefits of the Information Packet

The patient information packet is a simple, effective, and inexpensive way to improve the relationship between the office and the patients. It provides important information about the practice and the office staff. This information helps patients feel more comfortable with the qualifications of the healthcare professionals involved in their care. The packet may help clarify the roles that each office staff member has in patient care.

The information packet also informs patients of office policies and procedures. Patients will learn the doctor's office hours, how to schedule appointments, the office's payment policies, and other administrative details. This information helps limit misunderstandings about these procedures.

The patient information packet also benefits the office staff. It is both an excellent marketing tool and an aid to running the office more smoothly. Providing patients with a prepared information packet saves staff time by answering a number of potential patient inquiries. The information packet is also a good way to acquaint new office staff members with office policies.

Contents of the Information Packet Regardless of the material the information packet contains, it must be written in clear language so that patients are able to read and understand it. All materials should be written at a sixth-grade reading level to accommodate the greatest number of patients. Information should not be presented in a technical medical style. Because you may be responsible for developing portions of the information packet, you should be familiar with the contents of a typical packet.

Introduction to the Office A brief introduction welcomes the patient to the office. It may be helpful to summarize the office's philosophy of patient care. The office's **philosophy** means the system of values and principles the office has adopted in its everyday practices.

Physician's Qualifications The packet commonly includes information about the physician's professional qualifications, including where he received his medical degree and any medical specialties. It usually lists his credentials, such as board certification, and membership in professional associations. For a group practice, the information packet may contain a paragraph or a page for each physician. It may also include the qualifications of physician assistants or nurse practitioners who work in the physician's office. See Figure 15-6.

Description of the Practice The information packet should include a brief description of the practice, particularly if it is a specialty practice. Explaining the types of examinations or procedures that are commonly performed in the office as well as a list of any special services the office provides, such as physical examinations for employment, workers' compensation cases, or other occupational services, would be helpful. Be sure to make medical terms and specialties clear

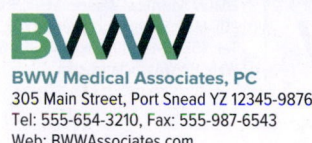

BWW Medical Associates, PC
305 Main Street, Port Snead YZ 12345-9876
Tel: 555-654-3210, Fax: 555-987-6543
Web: BWWAssociates.com

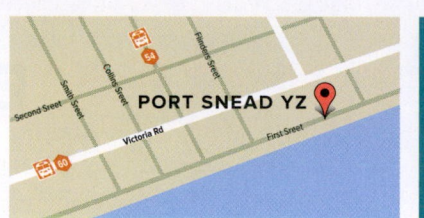

PORT SNEAD YZ

NEW PATIENT INFORMATION PACKET

PATIENT NAME: _____

DATE & TIME OF APPOINTMENT: _____

PHYSICIAN NAME: _____

Welcome to BWW Medical Associates, PC. Thank you for choosing us to assist in your healthcare needs. We have included the following information in this packet:

☐ Letter of Introduction

☐ Map to provide directions to our clinic

☐ Description of our practice, staff, and office policies

Below you will find a checklist of information to complete prior to your appointment in our office. Please fill out the entire packet and bring it in with you on your initial visit or complete it online at www.BWWAssociates.com prior to your appointment.

☐ Medical history forms

☐ Patient information sheet

☐ An authorization for release of medical information

☐ HIPAA forms

☐ Please bring all medications that you are currently taking to this appointment

☐ Please bring your insurance card(s) and a photo ID so we may make copies for your chart

☐ Please bring all radiology procedures on a CD or film to your appointment
   (CTs, PET Scan, MRIs, X-rays, etc.)

It is our desire to make your visit to BWW Medical Associates, PC as pleasant as possible. Should you have any questions, please do not hesitate to contact us at 555-654-3210 or by e-mail at patientrelations@bwwassociates.com.

FIGURE 15-5 Every clinic should have its own patient information packet for new patient orientation.

---

by avoiding the use of initials. Spell out everything the first time the reference is made and place the appropriate initials in parentheses.

Introduction to the Office Staff Many patients are not familiar with the qualifications and duties of the various members of the office staff. It is a good idea, therefore, to identify the staff positions according to their responsibilities and duties. Patients need to understand that some duties commonly thought to be a nurse's responsibilities may also be performed by a medical assistant. It may be helpful to include the professional credentials and licenses of key staff members.

Office Hours This section should list the days and hours the office is open, including holidays. In addition, patients need to know what to do if an emergency occurs outside regular office hours. Tell the patient what number to call first (for example, the answering service, 911, or the hospital emergency room) and what to do next. Include the telephone number and address of the emergency room at the hospital with which the doctor is affiliated. Assure patients that the doctor or a physician partner can be reached at all times through the answering service. Some practices have multiple offices, and the physicians rotate from office to office on a regular schedule. List all office addresses and phone numbers, along with directions to all office sites.

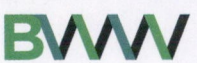

BWW Medical Associates, PC
305 Main Street, Port Snead YZ 12345-9876
Tel: 555-654-3210, Fax: 555-987-6543
Web: BWWAssociates.com

Alexis N. Whalen, MD

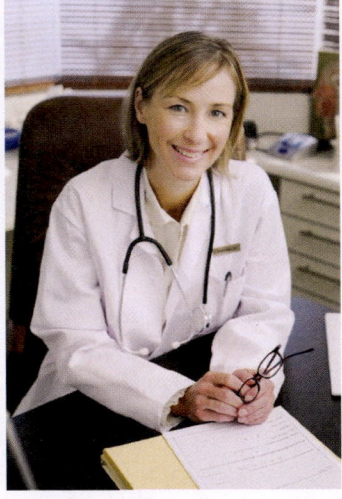

Dr. Whalen's Qualifications:

- Former Staff Pediatrician at Seattle Children's Hospital

- Board Certified OB/GYN and Pediatrician

- Residency in Family Medicine: Loyola University Chicago, Stritch School of Medicine, Chicago, IL

- Fellowship in Obstetrics & Gynecology: Stanford University, Stanford, CA

- Fellowship in Pediatrics: Seattle Children's Hospital, Seattle, WA

Dr. Whalen is a recognized expert in pediatric medicine, obstetrics, and gynecology.

Raised in Topeka, KS, Dr. Whalen completed her undergraduate studies at The University of Kansas, where she graduated first in her biochemistry class while also majoring in opera performance.

After graduation, she spent two years touring with an off-Broadway opera troop before starting medical school at Loyola University Chicago, where she went on to complete her residency in Family Medicine. During her residency, Dr. Whalen's talents for pediatrics, obstetrics, and gynecology shone, allowing her to acquire two competitive fellowships at the top research centers of Stanford and Seattle Children's Hospital.

A very well-received research study on Pediatric Cardiomyopathy earned Dr. Whalen a spot as a staff pediatrician at Seattle Children's Hospital.

While Dr. Whalen enjoyed the hustle and bustle of working at a major research hospital and the mild climate of Seattle, she and her husband decided to move back to his hometown of Port Snead five years ago.

Dr. Whalen enjoys long waterfront walks with her border collie Scout and her twin daughters Leslie and Lenore.

FIGURE 15-6   Healthcare personnel are the face of any medical practice. Providing patients with credentialing information as well as some personal information will help put new patients at ease.
© Chris Ryan/agefotostock RF

Appointment Scheduling This section of the packet should explain the procedure for scheduling and canceling appointments. You might suggest that patients can benefit by scheduling routine checkups and visits as far in advance as possible. Also note if certain times of the day are reserved for sudden or unexpected office visits.

In this section, encourage patients to be on time for appointments. Explain the problems that result from late or broken appointments. If the office charges a fee for breaking an appointment without advance notice, mention it here. Be careful to address these sensitive areas with a positive, non-threatening tone. The office's written material should simply state the office policies and the problems that can result when the policies are not followed.

Telephone Policy Providing the office's telephone policies in the information packet can help reduce the number of unnecessary calls to the office and thus save time for the office staff. Explain which procedures can be handled over the telephone and which cannot. Explain procedures such as calling in for prescription renewals or laboratory test results. If the physician returns patients' calls at a certain time of day, mention that policy in this section. Some practices bill patients for telephone calls in which medical advice is given but not for follow-up calls. For example, if a parent of a child who was vomiting uncontrollably called the physician to get immediate medical advice, the call might be billed. If the physician called to inform a patient of test results, however, the call would not be billed. It is important that patients know about these policies, particularly because many insurance plans do not cover charges for medical advice given over the phone, so the patient will be responsible for these charges.

Some offices (particularly pediatric offices) schedule a certain time of the day for patients (or parents and guardians) to call the physician for answers to their questions. This type of policy benefits both the office and the patients. The patients (or parents) have the assurance that they can speak with the physician about their concerns, and the office is spared interruptions during other times of the day.

Payment Policies Inform patients of the office's policies regarding payment and billing. State whether payment is expected at the time of a visit or whether the patient can be billed. List accepted forms of payment (for example, cash, personal checks, and credit cards). It is not common practice to mention specific fees in an information packet.

Insurance Policies List the major insurance carriers accepted by your office, or state that "most major insurance plans are accepted." Advise patients to bring proof of insurance coverage and a picture ID if this is their first visit to the office. A copy of this ID should be made and inserted in the patient's medical chart. State whether the office submits insurance claim forms directly to the insurance company or whether the patient has this responsibility. Generally, there is no charge for submission of the first insurance claim form; however, if the office charges for submission of secondary insurance forms, this should be stated. Outline the practice's policy for handling Medicare coverage, including whether the office accepts assignment on Medicare claims. If the office does not submit insurance claims directly, explain that the staff will help patients fill out insurance forms when necessary and will provide the appropriate paperwork (usually a superbill) containing dates of service and procedure and diagnosis codes for attachment to the claim form.

Patient Confidentiality Statement The information packet must include a copy of the office privacy policy. Complete information regarding the privacy policy and HIPAA regulations can be found in the *Legal and Ethical Issues* chapter. An important first step of HIPAA compliance is informing the patient of his or her rights. These rights are communicated through the Notice of Privacy Practices (NPP) (discussed in the *Legal and Ethical Issues* chapter), which must adhere to certain specifications.

The information packet also must state that no information from patient files will be released without a signed authorization from the patient. Each patient who receives a copy of the privacy notice must sign a document stating that he received the privacy notice and had the opportunity to have his questions about the notice answered. This document should remain in the patient's medical file.

Other Information The patient information packet may include the practice's policy on referrals. It may provide information about access to available community health resources or agencies. It also may include special instructions for common office procedures (for example, whether the patient needs to fast before a procedure or to avoid certain foods).

Distributing the Information Packet

For the information packet to be effective, you must make sure that new patients receive and read it. One way is to hand the packet to new patients at the time of their first office visit and briefly review the contents with them. Explain that they can find answers to many questions in the packet. Encourage patients to take the packet home, read the information, and keep it handy for future reference, but be sure to obtain the signed documentation that the patient has received and read the privacy notice for your files.

In many cases, the physician's office maintains a website where patients can view the information packet, make an appointment to see the physician, and get a map or directions to the office. The website may also allow patients to complete patient registration and consent for treatment forms online or download the forms, complete them by hand, and bring them to the office on the day of their appointment (Figure 15-7). Patients without Internet access may request to receive this information by mail, or they may be asked to arrive early for their appointment to complete the necessary forms.

▶ Patient Education Prior to Surgery

When a patient undergoes a surgical procedure, patient education is vital to a successful outcome. Although exact instructions vary according to the procedure, their purpose is to prepare the patient for the procedure and to aid the patient during the recovery period.

Providing Patient Education

Patients must receive information from the licensed practitioner (*not* the medical assistant) about the need for surgery and its nature. Educating and preparing patients for surgery may be your responsibility. You should provide support and explanations to patients. You must verify that they understand any information they have been given by other members of the healthcare team. Preoperative instruction may include discussion of postoperative care issues, such as temporary dietary restrictions or surgical wound care.

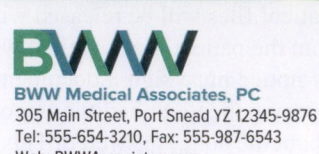

BWW Medical Associates, PC
305 Main Street, Port Snead YZ 12345-9876
Tel: 555-654-3210, Fax: 555-987-6543
Web: BWWAssociates.com

Paul F. Buckwalter, MD
Alexis N. Whalen, MD
Elizabeth H. Williams, MD

Consent for Treatment

I voluntarily give my permission to the healthcare providers of BWW Medical Associates, PC and such assistants and other healthcare providers as they may deem necessary to provide medical services to me. I understand that by signing this form, I am authorizing them to treat me for as long as I seek care from BWW Medical Associates, PC or until I withdraw my consent in writing.

_____
Signature of Patient or Guardian

_____
Printed Name of Patient or Guardian

_____
Date

_____
Relationship to Patient

Statement of Financial Responsibility/Assignment of Benefits

I acknowledge that I am legally responsible for all charges in connection with the medical care and treatment provided by BWW Medical Associates, PC and Associates. I assign and authorize payments to BWW Medical Associates, PC. I understand my insurance carrier may not approve or reimburse my medical services in full due to usual and customary rates, benefit exclusions, coverage limits, lack of authorization, or medical necessity. I understand I am responsible for fees not paid in full, co-payments, and policy deductibles and co-insurance except where my liability is limited by contract or State or Federal law.

_____
Signature of Patient or Guardian

_____
Printed Name of Patient or Guardian

_____
Date

_____
Relationship to Patient

A duplicate or faxed copy of this form is considered the same as the original document.

FIGURE 15-7 Sample patient consent for treatment form.

Determining whether patients have all the information they need before surgery is essential from both an educational and a legal standpoint. All patients who are undergoing a surgical procedure must first sign an informed consent form. This legal document provides specific information about the surgical procedure, including its purpose, the possible risks, and the expected outcome. The medical assistant may be asked to witness the patient's signature on this form. The signed informed consent form, along with documentation of all preoperative instructions, must be put in the patient's chart. (See Figure 15-8.)

Preoperative Education

Preoperative education increases patients' overall satisfaction with their care. It helps reduce patient anxiety and fear, use of pain medication, complications following surgery, and recovery time. Letting the patient know what to expect during the surgery and afterward allows the patient to emotionally educate himself about the surgical procedure. The use of effective teaching techniques is essential to ensure patient understanding. Make sure the patient has a patient instruction sheet and can repeat the expectations back to you.

It may be difficult for a patient to visualize exactly what will take place in some surgical procedures. For example, think of arthroscopy of the knee. When told that the doctor will insert a viewing instrument into the knee, patients probably have no idea of the size of this scope. As a result, they may be particularly fearful of the procedure. An anatomical model, diagram, or photo is useful to show exactly what will happen and ease patients' fears. For example, an anatomical

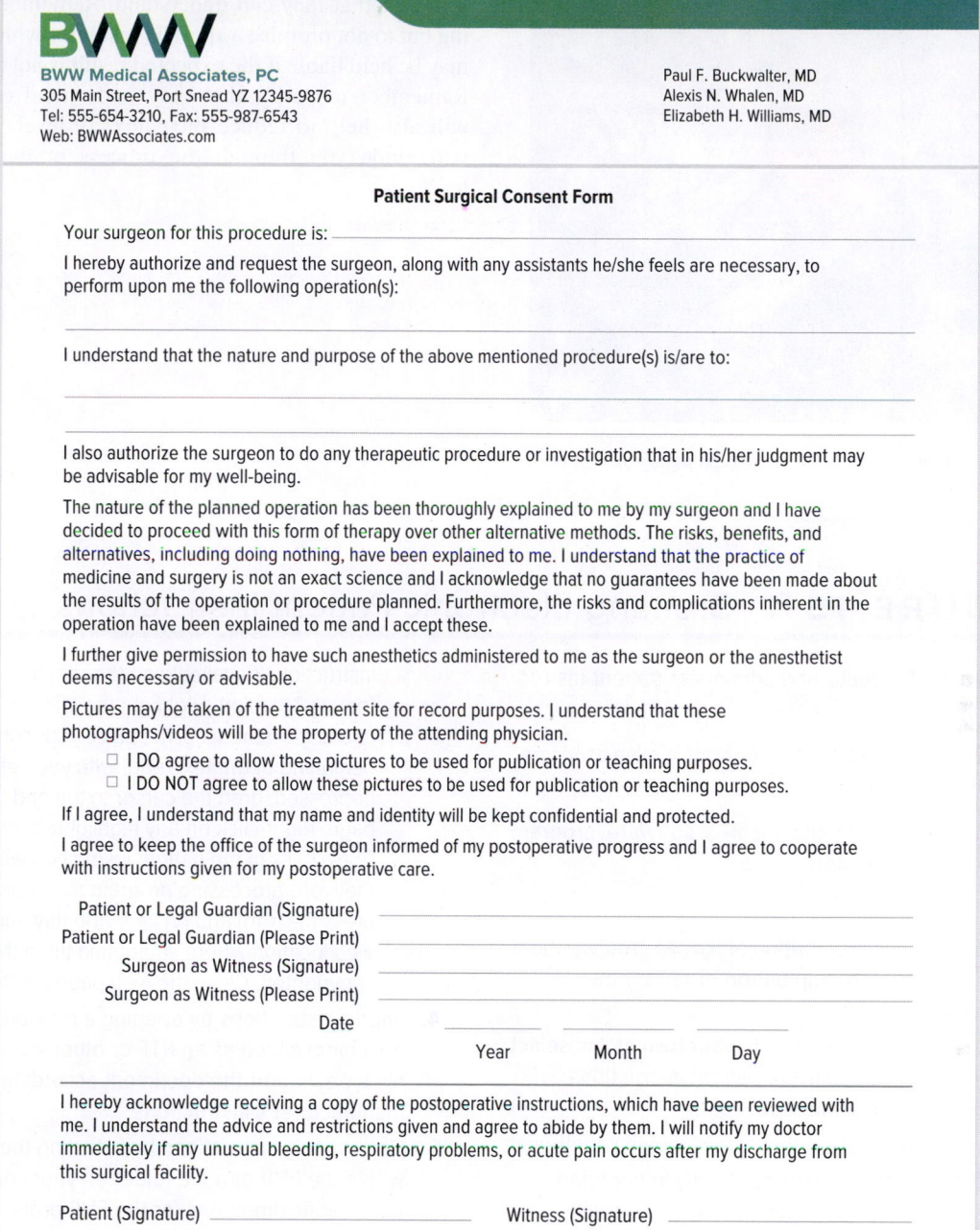

BWW

BWW Medical Associates, PC
305 Main Street, Port Snead YZ 12345-9876
Tel: 555-654-3210, Fax: 555-987-6543
Web: BWWAssociates.com

Paul F. Buckwalter, MD
Alexis N. Whalen, MD
Elizabeth H. Williams, MD

Patient Surgical Consent Form

Your surgeon for this procedure is: _____

I hereby authorize and request the surgeon, along with any assistants he/she feels are necessary, to perform upon me the following operation(s):

I understand that the nature and purpose of the above mentioned procedure(s) is/are to:

I also authorize the surgeon to do any therapeutic procedure or investigation that in his/her judgment may be advisable for my well-being.

The nature of the planned operation has been thoroughly explained to me by my surgeon and I have decided to proceed with this form of therapy over other alternative methods. The risks, benefits, and alternatives, including doing nothing, have been explained to me. I understand that the practice of medicine and surgery is not an exact science and I acknowledge that no guarantees have been made about the results of the operation or procedure planned. Furthermore, the risks and complications inherent in the operation have been explained to me and I accept these.

I further give permission to have such anesthetics administered to me as the surgeon or the anesthetist deems necessary or advisable.

Pictures may be taken of the treatment site for record purposes. I understand that these photographs/videos will be the property of the attending physician.

    ☐ I DO agree to allow these pictures to be used for publication or teaching purposes.
    ☐ I DO NOT agree to allow these pictures to be used for publication or teaching purposes.

If I agree, I understand that my name and identity will be kept confidential and protected.

I agree to keep the office of the surgeon informed of my postoperative progress and I agree to cooperate with instructions given for my postoperative care.

Patient or Legal Guardian (Signature) _____
Patient or Legal Guardian (Please Print) _____
Surgeon as Witness (Signature) _____
Surgeon as Witness (Please Print) _____
Date   _____   _____   _____
                Year   Month   Day

I hereby acknowledge receiving a copy of the postoperative instructions, which have been reviewed with me. I understand the advice and restrictions given and agree to abide by them. I will notify my doctor immediately if any unusual bleeding, respiratory problems, or acute pain occurs after my discharge from this surgical facility.

Patient (Signature) _____   Witness (Signature) _____
Patient (Please Print) _____   Witness (Please Print) _____
Date _____ _____ _____
    Year   Month   Day

FIGURE 15-8   Sample patient surgical consent form.

model may help a patient who is having surgery on his ear see how the surgical procedure will help correct his problem. (See Figure 15-9.)

Helping Relieve Patient Anxiety

When you provide preoperative education, be aware that the fear and anxiety of patients who are about to undergo a surgical procedure can adversely affect the learning process.

Consequently, allow extra time for repetition and reinforcement of material.

Always consider your choice of words carefully, stressing the positive rather than the negative whenever possible. Involving family members in the educational process is often beneficial, particularly if the patient is especially apprehensive about the surgery. Provide patients with contact information in case they have additional questions after they leave.

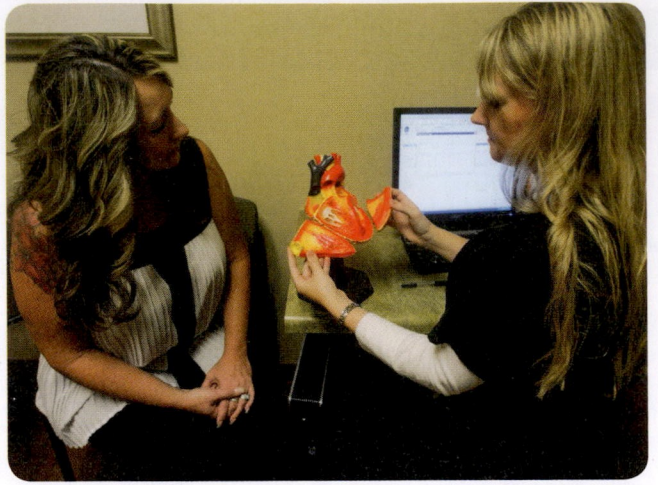

FIGURE 15-9 An anatomical model can help patients visualize what will happen during surgery.
© McGraw-Hill Education/David Moyer, photographer

Present your instructions and explanations in straightforward language that they can understand. Remember to be reassuring but to not promise a specific result for which the physician may be held liable if the expected result is not the actual result. Remember to verify that they understand everything. This will also help to reduce their anxiety level. Procedure 15-5 will guide you through the process of outpatient surgery teaching.

PROCEDURE 15-1 Creating Electronic Patient Instructions

Procedure Goal: To create and administer patient instructions electronically

OSHA Guidelines: This procedure does not involve exposure to blood, body fluids, or tissue.

Materials: An electronic health records software program that includes a patient instructions feature

Method:

1. Search the EHR to find the button or icon to create patient instructions. (Check the Help button or review the training manual.)

2. Determine if you will need to write your own or can select from a previously created list of patient instructions. Select the correct button to proceed.

3. Create new instructions by either of the following methods:

    a. Type your patient instructions directly in the open window or a word processing program. This will depend on the EHR you are using. In some cases, you may need to just click a link to go directly to previously created patient instructions.

    b. When you are within a web browser, navigate to a credible Internet site, such as MedlinePlus, for patient instruction. If available on the site, select the "printer friendly" version. Highlight the information you want to use from the website, place your cursor at the beginning of the text, and, with your left mouse button depressed, drag the cursor to the end of the instruction page. Right-click on any highlighted area and choose Copy. Click in the patient instruction window or in the word processing program and, using the keypad, press the [Ctrl] and [V] keys. Identify and credit the web location where you obtain the data if they are copyrighted. Close the web page and return to the EHR.

4. Import instructions by opening a previously created document saved as an RTF or other word processing file type. Import the document according to the manufacturer's instructions.

5. Use existing instructions by selecting them from a list within the EHR or a file folder on your computer. Check the specific directions for the EHR program you are using.

6. Record in the EHR the instructions that you provided to the patient. In most programs this occurs when you generate the instructions and they become a permanent record in the patient's chart.

PROCEDURE 15-2 Identifying Community Resources

Procedure Goal: To create a list of useful community resources for patient referrals.

OSHA Guidelines: This procedure does not involve exposure to blood, body fluids, or tissue.

Materials: Computer with Internet access, phone directory, printer

Method:

1. Determine the needs of your medical office and formulate a list of community resources. The specific needs of your

patients will help you formulate your list. Being able to help patients find outside assistance when necessary is the goal.

2. Use the Internet to research the names, addresses, web addresses, and phone numbers of local resources such as state and federal agencies, home healthcare agencies, long-term nursing facilities, mental health agencies, and local charities. Use the phone directory to help you locate local agencies such as Meals on Wheels; Alcoholics Anonymous; shelters for abused individuals; hospice care; Easter Seals; Women, Infants, and Children (WIC); and support groups for grief, obesity, and various diseases.

3. Contact each resource and request information such as business cards and brochures. Some agencies may send a representative to meet with you regarding their

services. If patients can access information easily, they are more likely to take advantage of the services available to them.

4. Compile a list of community resources with the proper name, address, phone number, e-mail address, and contact name. Include any information that may be helpful to the office.

5. Update and add to the information often, because outdated information will only frustrate you and your patients, creating even more anxiety.

6. Post the information in a location where it is readily available both in the office and on the practice's website, if available. Maintain an electronic record for easy reference.

7. Navigate patients to community resources when necessary.

PROCEDURE 15-3 Locating Credible Patient Education Information on the Internet

Procedure Goal: To determine the credibility of patient education information on the Internet

OSHA Guidelines: This procedure does not involve exposure to blood, body fluids, or tissue.

Materials: Computer with Internet access

Method:

1. Open your Internet browser and locate a search engine. Search engines vary in the way they search, so you may want to use more than one search engine for different results.

2. Search the topic. Be specific when entering the search term. For example, if you want to know about the proper diet for high cholesterol, you should type "high cholesterol diet." For different or more medical sites, try using different terms; instead of "high cholesterol" try "hyperlipidemia."

3. Select a site from the list of results and evaluate the source.

   a. Click the "about us" link to find out who developed the site. Sites should have an active link available to contact the webmaster and verify the source.

   b. Sites developed by professional organizations, educational institutions, or a branch of the federal government are generally better than those developed by an individual or a commercial company.

4. Review the "about us" page to determine the quality of the information.

   a. Review the mission statement or other detailed information about the developer.

   b. Look for information about the writers or authors of the site. Make sure they are medical professionals.

5. Check the content of the site.

   a. Avoid sites that have sensational writing or make claims that are too good to be true.

   b. Make sure the language of the information is at a level that you can understand. Avoid sites that use lots of technical jargon for patient instruction.

6. Make sure the information is current by checking the copyright or by checking with the contact information on the site. Medical information changes frequently, so check the date and avoid information over 5 years old.

7. Avoid websites that are potentially biased. For example, if the site is written by a pharmaceutical company, the site will only present information about the medication manufactured by that company. There may be alternative medications. Sites written by individuals are interesting but may be biased as well.

8. Protect your privacy. If the sites require you to register, review their privacy policy. They may be able to share your or your patient's information with other companies.

9. Once you have evaluated the site and decide to use it, you may want to have your supervisor or licensed practitioner review and approve the information you will be providing to the patient.

PROCEDURE 15-4 Developing a Patient Education Plan

Procedure Goal: To create and implement a patient teaching plan

OSHA Guidelines: This procedure does not involve exposure to blood, body fluids, or tissue.

Materials: Pen, paper, various educational aids (such as instructional pamphlets and brochures), and/or visual aids (such as posters or DVDs)

Method:

1. Identify the patient's educational needs in order to provide instruction at the patient's point of need. Consider the following:

   a. The patient's current knowledge

   b. Any misconceptions the patient may have

   c. Any obstacles to learning (loss of hearing or vision, limitations of mobility, language barriers, and so on)

   d. The patient's willingness and readiness to learn (motivation)

   e. How the patient will use the information

   RATIONALE: *Knowing what the patient already knows and understanding any special learning needs will help you tailor the instruction to the specific patient.*

2. Using the various educational aids available, develop and outline a plan that addresses all the patient's needs. Include the following areas in the outline:

   a. What you want to accomplish (your goal)

   b. How you plan to accomplish it

   c. How you will determine if the teaching was successful

   RATIONALE: *Developing an educational plan before providing the education ensures that all patient needs will be addressed.*

3. Write the plan. Try to make the information interesting for the patient.

4. Before carrying out the plan, share it with the licensed practitioner to get approval and suggestions for improvement.

5. Perform the instruction. Be sure to use more than one teaching method. For instance, if written material is being given, be sure to explain or demonstrate the material instead of simply telling the patient to read the educational materials.

6. Document the teaching in the patient's chart for continuity of care and to maintain a legal record.

   RATIONALE: *All patient education must be documented in the patient's medical chart for continuity of care and as a legal record.*

7. Revise your plan as necessary to make it even more effective. To be an effective teacher, you must evaluate the methods you use.

PROCEDURE 15-5 Outpatient Surgery Teaching

WORK // DOC

Procedure Goal: To inform a preoperative patient of the necessary guidelines to follow prior to surgery

OSHA Guidelines: This procedure does not involve exposure to blood, body fluids, or tissue.

Materials: Patient chart or progress note, surgical guidelines

Method:

1. Review the patient's chart to determine the type of surgery to be performed, and then ask the patient what procedure is being performed.

   RATIONALE: *This confirms the patient's knowledge of the procedure.*

2. Tell the patient that you will be providing both verbal and written instructions that should be followed prior to surgery.

3. Inform the patient about policies regarding makeup, jewelry, contact lenses, wigs, dentures, and so on.

4. Tell the patient to leave money and valuables at home.

5. If applicable, suggest appropriate clothing for the patient to wear for postoperative ease and comfort.

6. Explain the need for someone to drive the patient home following an outpatient surgical procedure.

   RATIONALE: *Driving after even simple surgery can be very dangerous. Surgery can be canceled if a patient does not identify a responsible driver before surgery occurs.*

7. Tell the patient the correct time to arrive at the office, surgery center, or hospital for the procedure.

8. Inform the patient of dietary restrictions. Be sure to use specific, clear instructions about what may or may not be ingested and at what time the patient must abstain from eating or drinking. Also explain these points:

   a. The reasons for the dietary restrictions

   b. The possible consequences of not following the dietary restrictions

   RATIONALE: *Surgery can be canceled if the patient has not followed dietary instructions.*

9. Ask patients who smoke to refrain from or reduce cigarette smoking during at least the 8 hours prior to the procedure. Explain to the patient that reducing smoking improves the level of oxygen in the blood during surgery.

10. Suggest that the patient shower or bathe the morning of the procedure or the evening before.

11. Instruct the patient about medications to take or avoid before surgery. For example, patients may need to stop

taking a daily aspirin or vitamin E before surgery to reduce the risk of bleeding.

RATIONALE: *Surgery can be canceled if the patient has not followed medication instructions.*

12. If necessary, clarify any information about which the patient is unclear.

13. Provide written surgical guidelines and suggest that the patient call the office if additional questions arise.

RATIONALE: *Patients may not understand or remember verbal instructions. Written instructions can be taken home and reviewed again.*

14. Document the instructions in the patient's chart for continuity of care and as a legal record. Refer to Progress Note.

RATIONALE: *All patient education must be documented in the patient's medical chart for continuity of care and as a legal record.*

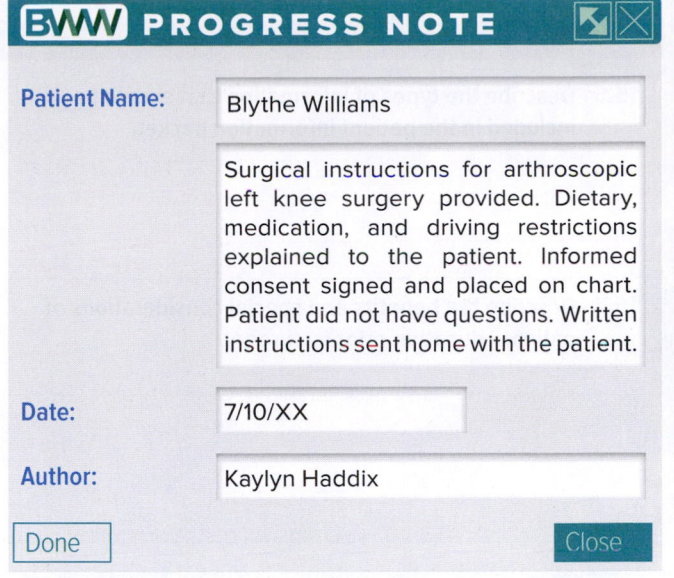

BWW PROGRESS NOTE

Patient Name: Blythe Williams

Surgical instructions for arthroscopic left knee surgery provided. Dietary, medication, and driving restrictions explained to the patient. Informed consent signed and placed on chart. Patient did not have questions. Written instructions sent home with the patient.

Date: 7/10/XX

Author: Kaylyn Haddix

Done   Close

SUMMARY OF LEARNING OUTCOMES

LEARNING OUTCOMES	KEY POINTS
15.1 Identify the benefits of patient education and the medical assistant's role in providing education.	Patients benefit from patient education because it can help them regain their health and independence more quickly. The medical office also benefits because patients will be less likely to call the office with questions and, therefore, the office staff can spend less time on the telephone. Educated patients take a more active role in their medical care.
15.2 Describe factors that affect learning and teaching.	Learning occurs in three domains: knowledge, behaviors, and skills. The patient must be able to recall the information, have the right attitude and be motivated to learn, and then implement the skills needed to demonstrate that the knowledge is retained.
15.3 Implement teaching techniques.	Teaching methods and formats are adjusted for the best possible result depending on patient need and level of understanding. The best possible education plan comes from knowing your patient and his needs and abilities, as well as the goal of the instruction. Always assess your instruction at its completion and revise the plan as needed.
15.4 Choose reliable patient education materials used in the medical office.	The types of patient education materials in medical offices include brochures, booklets, fact sheets, newsletters, DVDs, Internet sites, and community-assistance directories. Using already completed print or electronic patient instruction sheets, ensuring that Internet sources are credible, and obtaining assistance from other healthcare team members are all methods of ensuring reliability of educational materials.
15.5 Explain how patient education can be used to promote good health habits.	Patient education promotes good health by teaching patients the importance of developing healthy habits such as eating properly and exercising regularly.

LEARNING OUTCOMES	KEY POINTS
15.6 Describe the types of information that should be included in the patient information packet.	The contents of the patient's information packet should include an introduction to the medical office, the physician's qualifications, a description of the practice, an introduction to the staff, office hours, appointment scheduling, telephone policies, payment and insurance policies, a confidentiality statement, and other pertinent information.
15.7 Describe the benefits and special considerations of patient education prior to surgery.	Educating patients prior to surgery is vital to a successful outcome. Patients should learn proper procedures before surgery and sign a surgical consent.

CASE STUDY CRITICAL THINKING

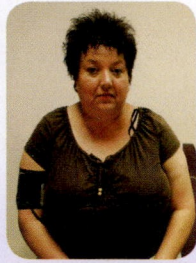

© McGraw-Hill Education

Recall Sylvia Gonzalez from the beginning of the chapter. Now that you have completed the chapter, answer the following questions regarding her case.

1. What might be important to consider when creating an educational plan for Sylvia?

2. What factors could block effective patient education?

3. Why are good listening skills an important part of teaching?

4. What do you consider behaviors that indicate you are "talking down" or behaving inappropriately to a patient?

EXAM PREPARATION QUESTIONS

1. (LO 15.6) A benefit of the patient information packet is that it
   a. Promotes better compliance with treatment programs
   b. Helps patients feel more comfortable with the qualifications of the healthcare professionals who are caring for them
   c. Can answer a treatment question that may come up during an office visit
   d. Encourages patients to help themselves achieve better health
   e. Ensures patient compliance

2. (LO 15.3) Which of the following types of teaching gives patients a description of the physical sensations they may have during the procedure?
   a. Factual
   b. Sensory
   c. Participatory
   d. Modeling
   e. Media

3. (LO 15.4) Which of the following is the *most* difficult way to create electronic patient instructions?
   a. Type the instructions directly into the open window
   b. Import the instructions from the Internet
   c. Use previously created instructions
   d. Print the instructions directly from the Internet
   e. Use preprinted instructions

4. (LO 15.1) Which of the following is the *least* likely patient benefit of patient education?
   a. Patients are less likely to call the office
   b. Patients take a more active role in their medical care
   c. Office staff are not interrupted as often by patient phone calls
   d. Patients will not need as much medication
   e. Patients are more likely to understand instructions

5. (LO 15.2) Which of the following is an example of the psychomotor learning domain?
   a. The patient is willing to read the brochure
   b. The patient performs his own blood glucose test
   c. The medical assistant tells the patient how she is going to feel during a procedure
   d. The medical assistant provides the patient with a patient information package
   e. The patient searches the Internet for information about his condition

6. (LO 15.4) When checking an Internet site for credibility, which of the following is *least* likely to be necessary?
   a. Use caution if the site uses a sensational writing style
   b. Look for the author of the information you plan to use
   c. Check the date of the document you plan to use
   d. Click links on the site to make sure they are not broken and are kept up-to-date
   e. Ensure that the site is listed on at least two search engines

7. (LO 15.6) Which of the following would *least* likely be in the patient information packet?
   a. Office policies and hours
   b. Patient instruction sheet regarding common tests done at the practice
   c. Patient instruction sheet about healthy living
   d. List of the physicians with their qualifications
   e. Patient confidentiality statement

8. (LO 15.7) What visual tool is especially helpful when performing preoperative education?
   a. Anatomical model
   b. Printed information sheet
   c. Line drawing
   d. Class or seminar
   e. Sensory teaching

9. (LO 15.5) Which of the following is a healthy habit that should be part of patient teaching?
   a. Getting adequate rest (4 to 5 hours of sleep a night)
   b. Limiting fruits, vegetables, and fiber
   c. Using cigarettes in moderation
   d. Balancing lifestyle of work and leisure activities (moderation)
   e. Exercising about 15 minutes per day

10. (LO 15.5) Your patient has a history of cardiovascular disease. Which of the following is *least* likely a screening procedure that would be done?
    a. Blood work
    b. Colonoscopy
    c. Chest X-ray
    d. ECG
    e. Cardiac rehabilitation

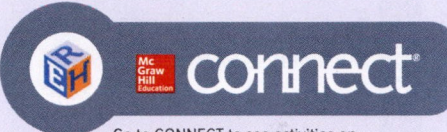

Go to CONNECT to see activities on *Administrating Patient Educational Material* and *Documenting Administration of Patient Educational Material*

SOFT SKILLS SUCCESS

A 35-year-old male patient is scheduled for a vasectomy tomorrow. It is within your scope of practice to provide preoperative instruction and you feel confident in performing this task. When you introduce yourself and explain what you are going to do, the first words out of the patient's mouth are "How do you know what this is all about? I am the one who is getting things cut!" How would you respond to this patient?

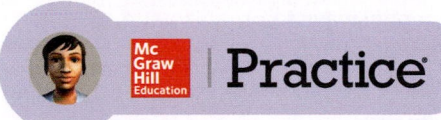

Go to PRACTICE MEDICAL OFFICE and complete the module Admin: Check Out - Interactions.

Schedule Management

CASE STUDY

PATIENT INFORMATION	Patient Name	DOB	Allergies
	John Miller	12/5/19XX	Bee stings
	Attending	MRN	Other Information
	Paul F. Buckwalter, MD	082-09-981	Hx of compliance issues w/ meds

John Miller is a 65-year-old patient with a history of hypertension, Type 2 diabetes mellitus, history of MI (myocardial infarction) 4 years ago, and a confirmed current diagnosis of CHF (congestive heart failure). He is taking glyburide 2.5 mg daily, Captopril 25 mg twice a day, and HCTZ 25 mg a day. You notice when he arrives today that he is significantly short of breath. When asked, he states, "Have been doing OK until I fell down yesterday. I was carrying a box of stuff

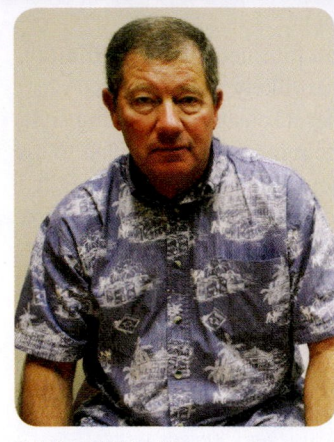

© McGraw-Hill Education

to take to the Salvation Army and lost my footing." He then shows you abrasions of his right elbow and left knee. After his examination, Dr. Buckwalter speaks to Mr. Miller's cardiologist and then asks you to book a cardiac catheterization. Mr. Miller is a Medicare patient, but he is covered under a Medicare (managed care) replacement plan instead of the traditional Medicare plan.

Keep Mr. Miller in mind as you study this chapter. There will be questions at the end of the chapter based on the case study. The information in the chapter will help you answer these questions.

McGraw-Hill Education ACTIVSim

LEARNING OUTCOMES

After completing Chapter 16, you will be able to:

16.1 Describe how the appointment book is key to the continuity of patient care.

16.2 Identify how to properly apply a matrix to an appointment book.

16.3 Compare different types of appointment scheduling systems.

16.4 Identify ways to organize and schedule patient appointments.

16.5 Model how to handle special scheduling situations.

16.6 Explain how to schedule appointments that are outside the medical office.

16.7 Implement ways to keep an accurate and efficient practitioner schedule.

KEY TERMS

advance scheduling

cluster scheduling

double-booking system

itinerary

locum tenens

matrix

minutes

modified-wave scheduling

no-show

open-hours scheduling

overbooking

time-specified scheduling

underbooking

walk-in

wave scheduling

CAAHEP

VI.C.1 Identify different types of appointment scheduling methods

VI.C.2 Identify the advantages and disadvantages of the following appointment systems:
(a) manual
(b) electronic

VI.C.3 Identify critical information required for scheduling procedures

VI.P.1 Manage appointment schedule using established priorities

VI.P.2 Schedule a patient procedure

VI.A.1 Display sensitivity when managing appointments

ABHES

7. Records Management
b. Utilize Electronic Medical Records (EMR) and Practice Management Systems

8. Administrative Procedures
d. Apply scheduling principles
(1) Schedule of in- and out-patient procedures
(2) Admission or hospital procedures

▶ Introduction

As a medical assistant, you will need to know all aspects of schedule management. This includes how to create and utilize a paper appointment book or an electronic scheduler. Electronic scheduling programs are discussed in the chapter *Electronic Health Records*. Referring back to this chapter may be necessary while learning about schedule management. In this chapter you will learn how to identify the different types of scheduling systems, how each is used, and which type of system will work best for each type of practice. You also will learn how to handle many types of scheduling situations within the medical office, including patient appointments, emergencies, pharmaceutical representatives, and the scheduling of patient appointments with other medical facilities. Legal aspects of the appointment book are discussed and proper documentation is stressed. Additional topics include appointment cards, reminder mailings, reminder calls, and recall notices for patients.

▶ The Appointment Book   LO 16.1

Time is of great value for everyone involved—the practitioner, the patient, and the office staff. Scheduling appointments in an organized fashion shows respect for everyone's time and creates an efficient patient flow. If the schedule is changed for any reason, the medical assistant must update the appointment book or scheduler and make sure that everyone involved is aware of the change. A well-managed appointment book, regardless of whether it is an actual book or an electronic format within a computer system, is key to patient continuity of care and presents the office in a positive, professional manner, ultimately keeping all parties involved on task and on time.

The office schedule depends on practitioner preferences and habits, the facilities available, and patient need. Although most patients understand that they may have to wait in the reception area before they are seen by his or her provider, few patients are willing to wait more than 20 minutes. Offices that

routinely have long waiting times can find themselves with dissatisfied patients, which can lead to other problems such as losing patients. You may find that patients will get creative in an attempt to avoid waiting. They may deliberately arrive after their scheduled appointment time to avoid waiting. Other patients may come in earlier in hopes of being seen before their scheduled appointment time. Still others may avoid the schedule entirely and walk in, expecting to be seen. All of these behaviors, if accommodated, can throw the office schedule off track. Other patients may become resentful and decide to seek medical care with a competing practice.

Even in a well-run office, however, unexpected events can disrupt the schedule. Some patients may unexpectedly require the provider to spend more time with them than was originally scheduled and patients who are ill will need to be added to the schedule, sometimes with little or no notice. Still others will forget appointments or arrive later than scheduled. For these reasons, making an office schedule flow smoothly can be a challenge. A schedule that "plans for the unexpected" combined with excellent communication between the practitioners, staff, and patients will allow a medical practice to run smoothly despite these obstacles.

Computerized Scheduling

As part of many Practice Management Systems and EHR programs discussed in the *Electronic Health Records* chapter, computerized scheduling systems are becoming more common in medical offices because they have several advantages over handwritten systems (Figure 16-1). As more practices become compliant with electronic health record regulations, the advantages seem to outweigh the disadvantages. The following are some of the advantages of computerized scheduling.

1. It enables locking out selected areas for designated purposes, such as last-minute or emergency visits.
2. It allows information to be accessed from multiple areas within the office.

3. It helps staff identify problem patients for cancellations, no-shows, and late arrivals.

4. It provides a "search" for upcoming appointments to ensure that proper follow-up care is given.

5. It provides reports on overall scheduling practices.

6. It adds color-coding as a visual aid to identify areas designated for certain types of appointments.

7. It allows searches for requested day or time availability.

Online Scheduling

The online scheduling option (e-scheduling) is gaining acceptance, but it is not recommended for all office types. Online scheduling allows patients to schedule themselves or request an appointment via the Internet. Cost and security have been the barriers to many offices; however, new security measures ensure protection of patient data online and as more programs become available, costs are also becoming more reasonable. Adding an online scheduler to the practice takes some time and requires staff training, but it can be a convenience for your patients, particularly if many of them are computer-savvy.

Before adopting an e-scheduler, assess the practice needs, survey patients regarding web access and potential for usage, and be diligent in your research about available products, particularly regarding privacy issues. One of the frontrunners in e-scheduling is Compass Scheduling, found at http://asp.compassscheduling.com

▶ Applying the Matrix   LO 16.2

Before you begin scheduling appointments, you need to prepare the appointment book or electronic scheduler. The first step is establishing the **matrix,** or basic outline of times the practitioners are and are not available to see patients. To create the matrix, block off times within the schedule during which each provider is not available to see patients. In a paper format, drawing an "X" through the unavailable time slots with a brief explanation is standard practice to avoid errors. The type of appointment book used—whether it uses 10- or 15-minute units—will determine how many "blocks" are crossed out for each designation. Electronic schedulers often use colors to designate the reason the provider is out; they may also place an "X" in the time frames selected. For example, the schedule will show when the practitioner is away for the following reasons:

- Hospital rounds
- Surgery/procedures
- Lunch
- Vacation days
- Holidays
- Personal appointments for the practitioner
- Scheduled meetings (for example, pharmaceutical company or in-service meetings)

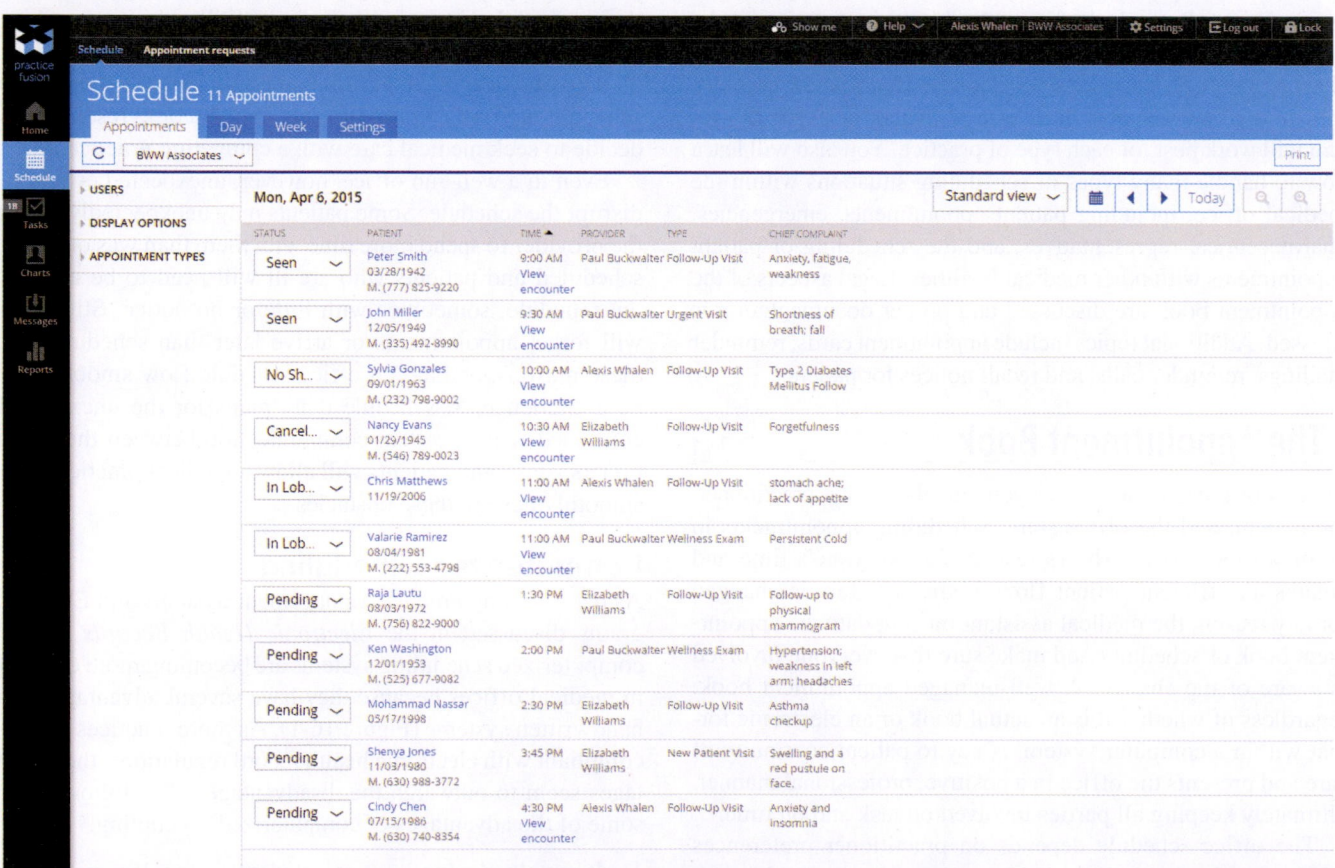

FIGURE 16-1   Screen shot from Practice Fusion® showing a day's schedule of patients, including those who did or did not show for their appointments.

© Practice Fusion®

The day's schedule is then built around the established matrix. Should the provider or office manager direct that a meeting has been canceled and patients should be seen during a time that had been blocked out, the "X" should be removed and patients scheduled as usual. Some offices prefer the "X" remain and the initials of the person approving the new schedule be added to the appointment time frame. See Figure 16-2 for an example of a matrix for a multi-practitioner office. For

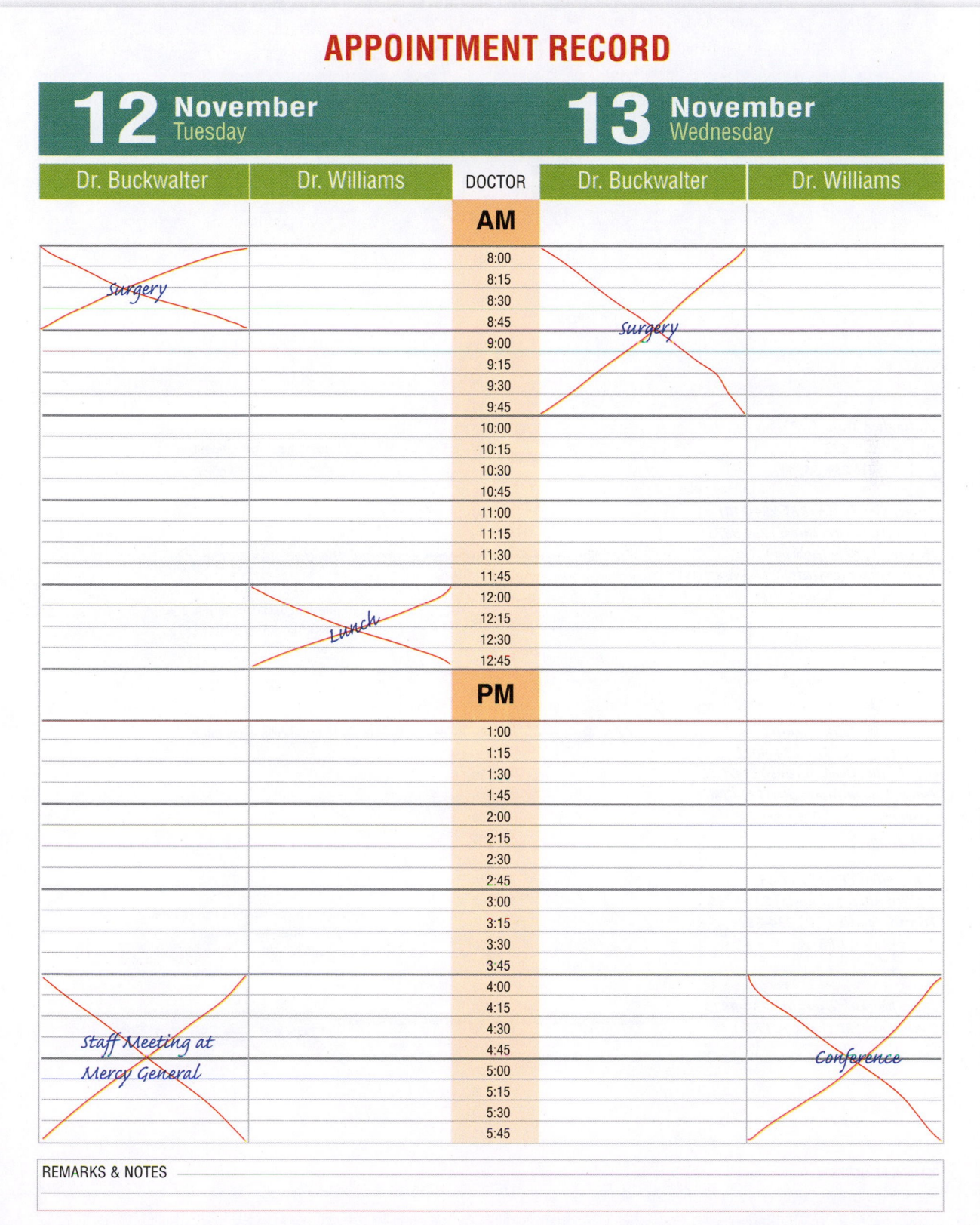

APPOINTMENT RECORD

		DOCTOR		
12 November Tuesday			**13** November Wednesday	
Dr. Buckwalter	Dr. Williams	DOCTOR	Dr. Buckwalter	Dr. Williams
		AM		
surgery (X)		8:00		
		8:15	*surgery* (X)	
		8:30		
		8:45		
		9:00		
		9:15		
		9:30		
		9:45		
		10:00		
		10:15		
		10:30		
		10:45		
		11:00		
		11:15		
		11:30		
		11:45		
	Lunch (X)	12:00		
		12:15		
		12:30		
		12:45		
		PM		
		1:00		
		1:15		
		1:30		
		1:45		
		2:00		
		2:15		
		2:30		
		2:45		
		3:00		
		3:15		
		3:30		
		3:45		
Staff Meeting at Mercy General (X)		4:00		*Conference* (X)
		4:15		
		4:30		
		4:45		
		5:00		
		5:15		
		5:30		
		5:45		

REMARKS & NOTES

FIGURE 16-2 The first step in appointment scheduling is to establish the matrix—defining when the practitioner is available to see patients.

a single-practitioner schedule with appointments in 15-minute increments, see Figure 16-3.

The same concept is true for the format of an electronic scheduler; if the matrix needs to be changed because the provider will be available to see patients, the time frame is unblocked and patients are then scheduled as usual. Figure 16-4 provides an example of an electronic scheduler. Procedure 16-1 provides the opportunity to practice completing an appointment matrix using

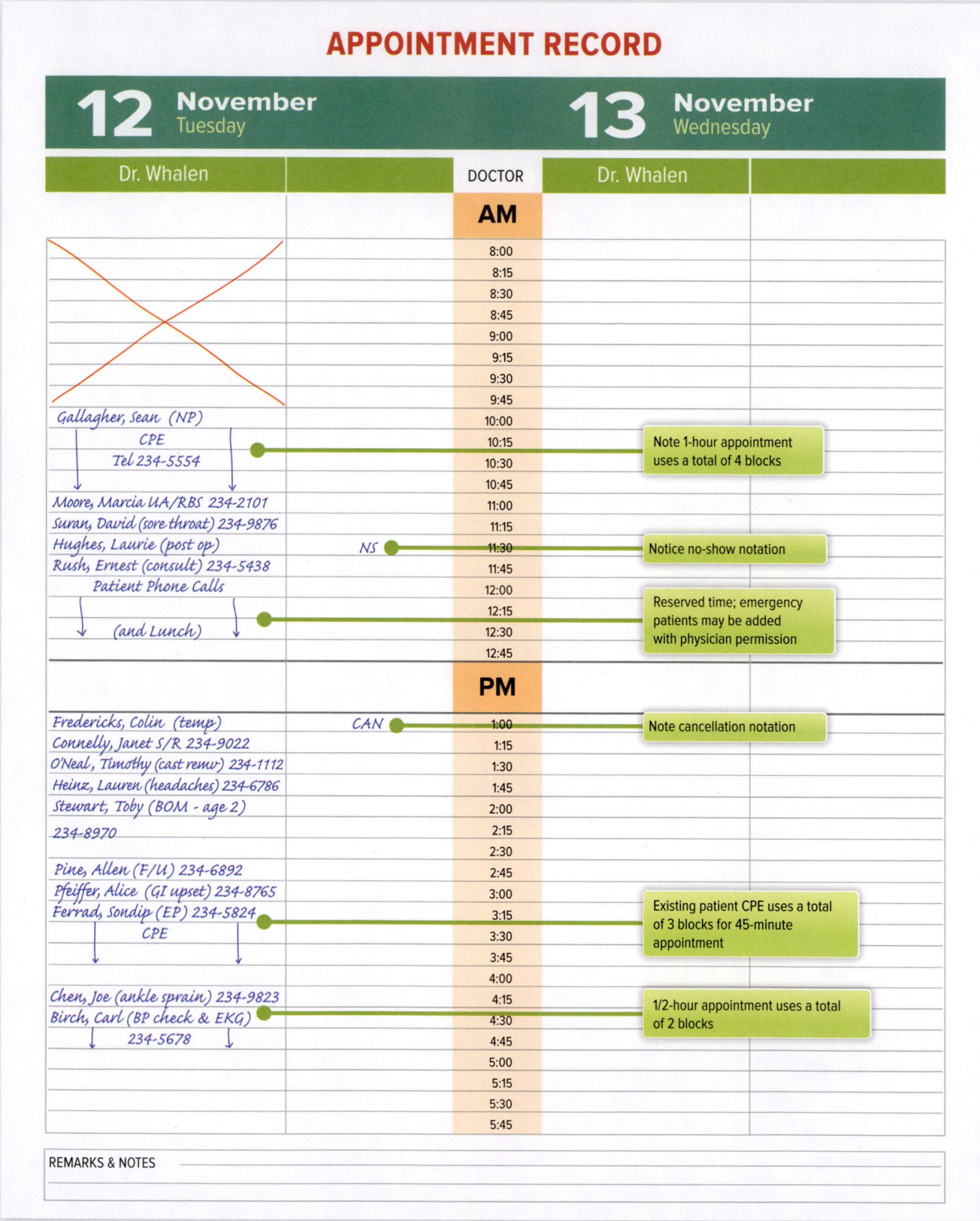

FIGURE 16-3 Single-practitioner appointment book using 15-minute appointment blocks.

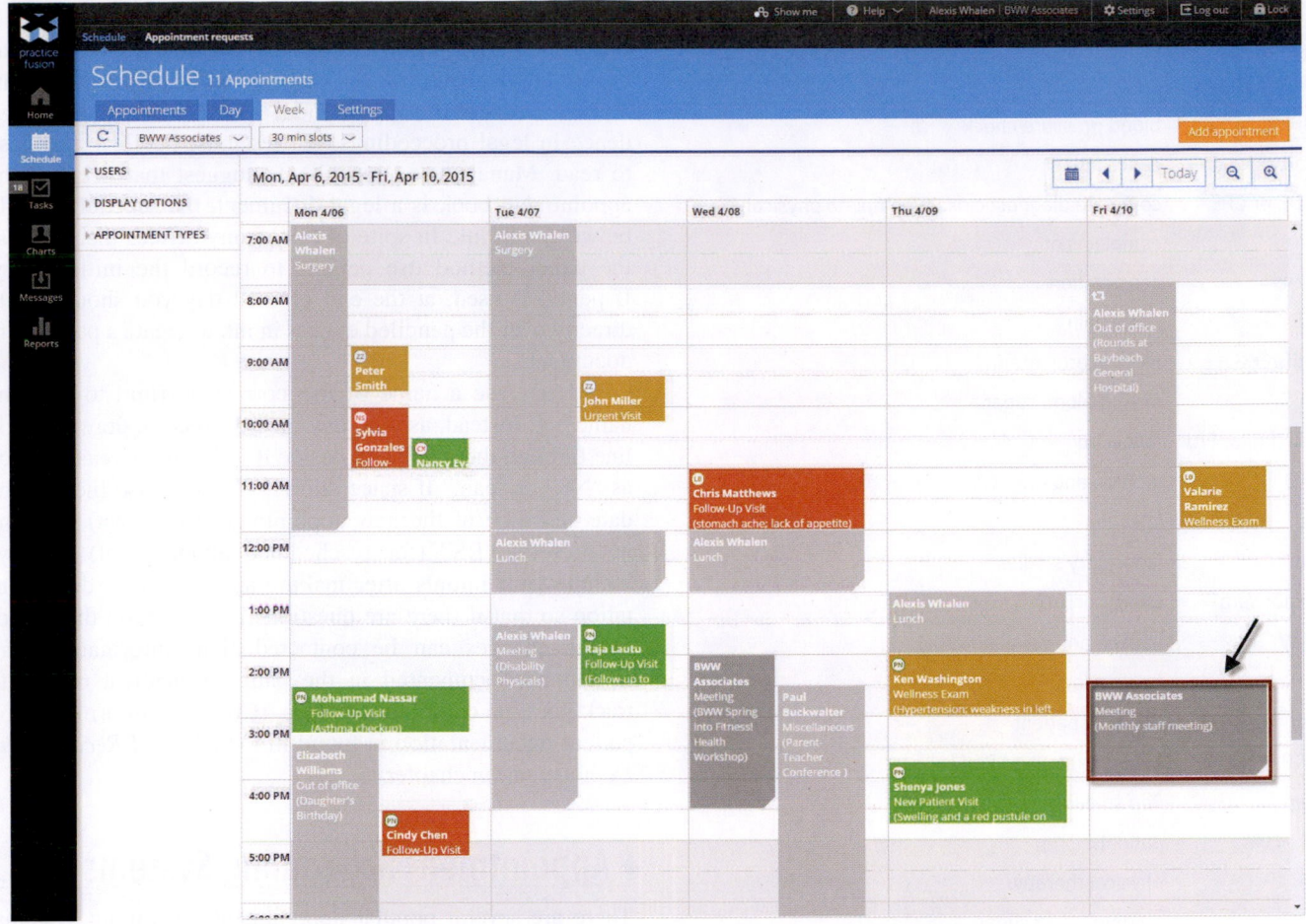

FIGURE 16-4   An example a week's schedule for BWW Medical Associates using the electronic scheduler in Practice Fusion®. Note that gray areas, like the one for the BWW Associates meeting, show times when certain practitioners are unable to see patients.

© Practice Fusion®

an appointment book. Refer to the *Electronic Health Records* chapter and Procedure 12-3 for information on creating an appointment matrix using an electronic scheduling system.

Required Patient Information

When the matrix has been established, you can begin scheduling appointments. Some practices enter the information into both traditional paper appointment books and computerized systems. Then, if the computer fails to work for some reason, the office has the book for reference. Some practitioners who have been in practice for many years are used to the appointment book method and do not want to give it up for a computerized system. Other offices are completely computerized. Per your office policy, you should obtain the following patient information in order to efficiently book a patient appointment regardless of the system used:

- Patient's full name. Obtain the correct spelling of the patient's name.
- Daytime telephone numbers. Repeat phone numbers to ensure accuracy.
- Purpose of the visit. Use a brief description and approved abbreviations when possible without disclosing the patient's diagnosis or violating HIPAA. Do not create your own abbreviations, as this can lead to errors or misunderstandings regarding the reason for the patient appointment.

Abbreviations in Appointment Scheduling

If you are the person who maintains the appointment book, you will find that certain procedures and conditions occur frequently. The use of abbreviations will depend on the office specialty. Only approved universal medical abbreviations should be used. To save space and time when entering information, use the abbreviations found in Table 16-1.

Standard Appointment Times

If you are to schedule appointments efficiently, you must have a guideline of how long visits are expected to take. Working with the provider(s) in your practice, create a list of standard appointment times. Also indicate in the list how much time to allow for tests that are commonly performed in the practice. This list, which should be kept near the appointment book or programmed into the electronic scheduling system, helps you identify which openings are appropriate for the appointment type or procedure involved. This list is intended as a guide only, as each patient visit is unique. The list will also assist you in choosing an appropriate appointment book or scheduler, as most are based on 10-, 15-, or 30-minute increments. The lengths and types of tests and procedures will depend on the practice policy and procedure manual. Table 16-2 lists the typical lengths of common office appointments and procedures.

TABLE 16-1 Common Abbreviations Used in Appointment Scheduling

Abbreviation	Description
BP	blood pressure check
can/cx	cancellation
CDE or CPE	complete diagnostic exam/complete physical exam
c/o	complains of
cons	consultation
CP	chest pain
ECG/EKG	electrocardiogram
FBS	fasting blood sugar
F/u, f/u, or F/U	follow up
I&D	incision and drainage
inj	injection
lab	laboratory studies
minor surg	minor surgery
N&V	nausea and vomiting
NP	new patient
NS	no-show patient
P&P	pelvic (exam) and Pap (smear)
Pap	Pap smear
pt	patient
PT	physical therapy
RBS	random blood sugar
re	recheck
ref	referral
RS	reschedule
Rx	prescription
Sig	sigmoidoscopy
S/R	suture removal
surg	surgery
US or U/S	ultrasound

TABLE 16-2 Typical Appointment Times for Specific Appointment Types

Appointment Type or Procedure	Time Frame Allotted
Complete physical examination (existing/new patient)	30 minutes/60 minutes
New patient visit	30–45 minutes
Follow-up appointment	5–15 minutes
Emergency office visit	15–20 minutes
Prenatal examination	15 minutes
Pelvic exam and Pap smear	15–30 minutes
Minor (in-office) surgery (e.g., mole removal)	30 minutes
Suture removal	10–20 minutes

The Appointment Book as a Legal Record

The appointment book is considered a legal record. Some experts advise keeping old appointment books for at least 3 years. Because the appointment book could be used as evidence in legal proceedings, entries must be clear and easy to read. Management consultants suggest that because the appointment book is a legal document, the schedule should be written in ink. In spite of this, many offices that still use the paper method use pencils to record the initial entry. If pencil is used, at the end of each day you should write directly over the penciled entries in ink to create a permanent document.

Never erase a name or use correction fluid to blot the name out. Instead, as with any medical record, draw a single line through the name and beside it write in the reason, such as "NS" or "can." If space allows, you may also include the date and time of the new appointment (if known) with the notation of "RS" (for rescheduled appointment). Always include your initials after making any change in documentation so that if there are questions in the future, the author of the changes can be contacted. This information also should be documented in the patient's medical record to track possible compliance issues. (Complete information on patient documentation is found in the *Medical Records and Documentation* chapter.)

▶ Appointment Scheduling Systems LO 16.3

There are several popular appointment scheduling systems. The method chosen usually depends on the type of practice and provider preferences. No matter which method your office uses, it should be regularly reviewed to see whether it is meeting its goals: a smooth flow of patients and minimal waiting time.

Open-Hours Scheduling

In the **open-hours scheduling** system, also known as the walk-in system, there are few (if any) scheduled appointments. Patients arrive at their own convenience with the understanding that they will be seen on a first-come, first-served basis. The only thing that may alter this is an emergency. Depending on how many people have arrived ahead of them, newly arriving patients may have a considerable wait. The open-hours system eliminates the problems caused by broken appointments because there are no assigned appointment times, but it increases the possibility of inefficient downtime for the practitioners and office staff, should there be no patients in the office. In addition to possible long wait times, if paper medical records are used, the medical assistant cannot retrieve patients' charts before they arrive. Although still used by emergency departments, urgent care centers, and some rural practices, most private practices have replaced this system with scheduled appointments.

Even though appointments are not booked ahead of time with an open-hours system, a matrix must still be established so that the staff will know which practitioners are available to see patients at any given time. Additionally, for legal (as well as tracking) reasons, an open-hours system still requires the use of an appointment book or electronic scheduling system to record patients as they arrive in the office.

Time-Specified Scheduling

Time-specified scheduling (also called stream scheduling) assumes a steady stream of patients all day long at regular, specified intervals. Once the matrix has been applied and provider availability has been established, it can be determined how many slots or blocks should be used for each appointment type (refer to Table 16-2). Most minor medical problems, such as sore throats, earaches, or blood pressure follow-ups, usually require only 10- to 15-minute appointment slots. More time may be required for appointments such as physical exams, which usually require 60 minutes, or new patient visits, which usually require 30 minutes. When a visit requires more time, you simply assign the patient additional back-to-back slots. Using arrows or parentheses on both sides of the appointment entry will allow you to easily see the length of existing appointments and the remaining open time slots. Refer back to Figure 16-3 for an example of a completed schedule for a single practitioner and Figure 16-4 for a multi-practitioner schedule using an electronic scheduling system.

Wave Scheduling

Wave scheduling gets its name from a "wave" at the beach. Essentially, patients are scheduled to come in "waves," or together. It works best in larger medical facilities that have enough departments and personnel to provide services to several patients at the same time. This method of scheduling is based on the reality that some patients will arrive late and that others will require more or less time than expected with the practitioner. Wave scheduling has the flexibility to allow for appointments that require more time than anticipated or for patients who miss appointments. The goal is to begin and end each hour with the overall office schedule on track. You determine the number of patients to be seen each hour by dividing the hour by the length of the average visit. If the average is 15 minutes, for example, you schedule four patients for each hour. An example of wave scheduling would be

10:00 a.m.	Mohammad Nassar	555-5683	Sore throat
10:00 a.m.	Shenya Jones	555-7322	Low back pain
10:00 a.m.	John Miller	555-4673	FU B/P
10:00 a.m.	Raja Lautu	555-2854	B12 inj

In this example, all four patients have been given appointments to see the same provider at 10 a.m. The provider will then see each patient in the order in which they arrive in the office, the goal being all four patient appointments completed by 11 a.m., when the next "wave" of four patients is scheduled to arrive. The main problem with wave scheduling is that patients may realize they have appointments at the same time as other patients. The result may be confusion and possibly annoyance or anger.

Modified-Wave Scheduling

The wave system can be modified in several ways. With **modified-wave scheduling,** as shown in Figure 16-5, patients might be scheduled in 15-minute increments. Another option is to schedule four patients to arrive at planned intervals during the first half hour, leaving the second half hour unscheduled. Appointments that are anticipated to require more time should be scheduled at the beginning of the hour. Appointments that are expected to be less time-consuming should be scheduled in 10- to 20-minute time slots. This method allows time for catching up before the next hour begins. An example of modified-wave scheduling would be

10:00 a.m.	Mohammad Nassar	555-5683	Sore throat
10:00 a.m.	Shenya Jones	555-7322	Low back pain
10:15 a.m.	(left open)		
10:30 a.m.	John Miller	555-4673	FU BP
10:30 a.m.	Raja Lautu	555-2854	B12 inj
10:45 a.m.	(left open)		

Double-Booking

With a **double-booking system,** two or more patients are purposely scheduled for the same appointment slot. Unlike the wave or modified-wave system, however, the double-booking system assumes that both patients will actually be seen within the scheduled period.

This type of system is especially useful when one patient can be managed by the nurse practitioner or physician assistant for an immunization or blood pressure check and the other patient is seen at the same time by the physician. Double-booking can also be helpful if a patient calls with a problem and needs to be seen that day but no appointments are available. You may double-book this patient with an already-scheduled patient. In such cases you should explain to the caller that he might have to wait a bit before being seen by the practitioner. To avoid these circumstances, some offices purposely leave one or two appointment slots open each morning and each afternoon to accommodate these "urgent" appointments.

Cluster Scheduling

Cluster scheduling groups similar appointments together on a specific day or for a specific block of time during the day or week (also called categorization scheduling). Cluster scheduling is often used for appointments such as blood sugar screenings, school physicals, and the like; for instance, Wednesdays after 3 p.m. might be set aside for school physicals, as it would be a more convenient time for parents. Cluster schedules are also helpful in offices where specialized equipment or services (such as physical therapy or ultrasound) are available only at certain times.

Advance Scheduling

In some specialties patients might be booked weeks or months in advance, as for annual gynecologic examinations. In such practices **advance scheduling** is used. It is still advisable to leave a few slots open each day, however, for patients who call with unexpected or unusual problems.

APPOINTMENT RECORD

12 November
Tuesday

Dr. Williams		DOCTOR		
		AM		
Auerbach, Conrad F/U	Sinclair, Monica F/U	8:00		
		8:15		
		8:30	Purdy, Marianne	Ganzalez, Hector
		8:45	↓ INJ	↓ INJ
Molini, Francesca Stomach Pain	Jacobson, Eloise LAB & ECG	9:00		
		9:15		
		9:30	Buffer	Sherbert, Philip
		9:45	↓	↓ LAB
Willis, Nina CPE	Smith, Marshall F/U	10:00		
		10:15		
		10:30	Chandler, Larry	MacDonald, Liam
		10:45	↓ GI	↓ GI
Buffer	Ward, Sylvia UTI	11:00		
		11:15		
		11:30	Campbell, Joel	Ramoson, Katrina
		11:45	↓ F/U	↓ PMS
		12:00		
		12:15		
		12:30		
		12:45		
		PM		
Gibble, Cora ECG	Bunsen, Elmer SOB	1:00		
		1:15		
		1:30	Moskowitz, Matthew	Cheng, Amy
		1:45	↓ ECG	↓ BP
Silverstein, Sidney SOB	Burns, Laura ECG & Lab	2:00		
		2:15		
		2:30	↓ Buffer ↓	↓ Osborne, Jonathan
		2:45		BP
Warren, Mary CPE	Harris, Noel CPE	3:00		
		3:15		
		3:30	McDermott, Elizabeth	Corbin, Allicia
		3:45	↓ F/U	↓ F/U
Buffer	Warner, Steve RE	4:00		
		4:15		
		4:30	Thompson, Will	Stein, Merle
		4:45	↓ Lab	↓ Emp PE
Cabrisi, Claudia US	Velone, Tina US	5:00		
		5:15		
		5:30	Tucker, Bob	Kapoor, Fatima
		5:45	↓ CONS	↓ CONS

REMARKS & NOTES _____

FIGURE 16-5 Modified-wave schedule: two patients booked each half hour.

Combination Scheduling

Some practices combine two or more scheduling methods. For example, they might use cluster scheduling for new patients and double-booking for quick follow-ups such as sore throats, hypertension, or a new medication.

▶ Organizing and Scheduling Appointments

LO 16.4

As you determine patient needs and office availability when arranging appointments, always keep in mind that you are representing the office. How you interact with patients will have either a positive or a negative impact depending on your actions and choices. Being polite and courteous while maintaining a professional manner is key. Try to be as accommodating as possible to the patient but at the same time uphold the policies and protocols of the office.

As discussed earlier in the chapter, patient status (new or existing patient) and chief complaint must be clearly identified prior to scheduling any appointment, because this will dictate the length of time the physician will spend with the patient.

New Patients

Patients who have never been seen in the practice or have not been seen by the practice in 3 or more years are considered to be new patients. A convenient decision tree to help define patients as new or existing is found in the *Procedural Coding* chapter—Figure 19-4. Appointments for new patients are most often arranged over the telephone. Be sure to obtain all the necessary information, including the correct spelling of the person's name, home address, daytime telephone number, and date of birth. The patient's insurance information as well as the full name of the guarantor (if not the patient) and his or her relationship to the patient also should be obtained at this time. With so many insurance plans available, this has become increasingly important because it is impossible for any office to accept every insurance type. Even if the insurance is accepted by the office, verification of coverage should be done prior to the patient being seen in the practice. Obtaining this information also will allow you to remind the patient that if any copayment is required by his insurance plan, the payment is expected at the time of the visit. For more information on insurance coverage and the verification process, please refer to the *Insurance and Billing* chapter.

When arranging the appointment, keep in mind that the matrix will dictate availability of some types of appointments. When scheduling an appointment for a new patient, ask the patient to arrive 15–30 minutes early to allow time for filling out the required "new patient forms," if they have not been sent to the patient prior to the appointment. Information regarding these forms may be found in the *Medical Records and Documentation* chapter. Upon arrival, the new patient also should be given the HIPAA guidelines for your office while his or her chart is being prepared for the visit.

As discussed in the *Legal and Ethical Issues* chapter, a signed receipt of the HIPAA privacy practices is now a requirement for all patients seen in the practice.

Established Patients

Established patients are those who have been seen by the practice within the last 3 years. Many times, return appointments for existing patients are made at the time they are being checked out from a current appointment. It is always good practice to ask patients returning to the reception area if they need to schedule another appointment. It is helpful for patients who are followed routinely to have appointments scheduled in a set pattern whenever possible. For instance, if a patient needs monthly B_{12} injections, scheduling the appointments for the first Tuesday of each month at 3 p.m. will be easier for the patient to remember than a different day or time each month. Scheduling patients while they are still in the office also allows you to give them an appointment card to remind them of the appointment so they can enter it in their schedule or on the "home calendar." If the patient's visit is being made by phone and is not for the immediate future, you also may ask her if she would like an appointment card mailed to her. Remember to remind existing patients, also, that any copayment is due at the time of the appointment. Procedure 16-2 at the end of the chapter outlines the procedure to utilize when booking patient appointments using a manual, paper system. Refer to the *Electronic Health Records* chapter and Procedure 12-4 for information on booking patient appointments using an electronic scheduling program.

Appointment Confirmations and Reminders

It seems today that everyone is busy with hectic schedules. It is often difficult for patients to remember their next appointment, especially if they arrange it far in advance. To help patients keep track of their appointments, you can use several types of appointment reminders.

Appointment Cards In many offices when making a return appointment at check-out, the medical assistant completes and gives the patient an appointment reminder card, like the one shown in Figure 16-6a.

To reduce the chance of error, enter the appointment in the appointment book or scheduler first; then fill out the card. Figure 16-6b shows a typical electronic scheduler screen for creating a new patient appointment. Otherwise, when the patient takes the appointment card, you have to rely on your memory when entering the appointment in the book and in a busy office this often can lead to errors. Refer to Procedure 16-3 at the end of the chapter for the steps in completing an appointment card.

Encounter Forms/Superbills As the patient leaves the office, he or she is often given paperwork to return to the front desk. This form, commonly known as the superbill or encounter form, lists services performed, diagnoses, health insurance, and demographic information regarding the

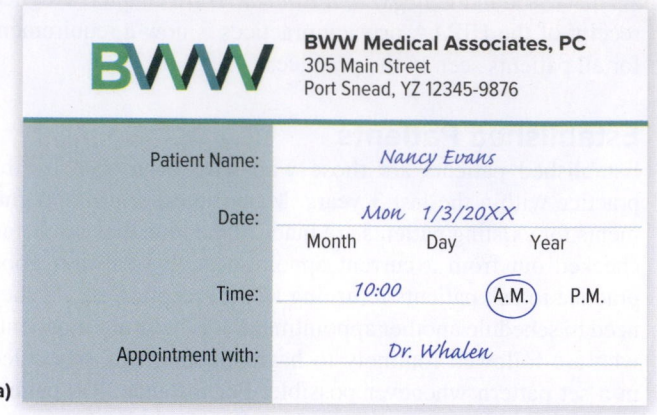

(a)

Edit patient appointment

Patient

Cindy Chen   Chart
28 yrs F   07/15/1986   M. (630) 740-8354
cindyclaire.chen@gmail.com

Appointment details

PROVIDER
Whalen, Alexis

FACILITY
BWW Associates

CHIEF COMPLAINT
Anxiety and insomnia

APPOINTMENT TYPE *
Follow-Up Visit

DURATION *
45

WHEN *
4/6/2015 4:30 PM

END TIME
5:15 PM   Repeat

(b)

Delete   Done

FIGURE 16-6   (a) Typical appointment card given to patients to remind them of upcoming appointments. (b) Screen shot of a patient appointment using Practice Fusion® program.
© Practice Fusion®

patient, as well as account balance. This *super document* also can serve as a receipt if payments are made at the time of the visit. Most superbills, like the one shown in Figure 16-7, also include an area to insert information regarding the patient's next appointment.

Reminder Mailings When making a follow-up appointment in person, ask the patient to address a postcard to himself on which you have written the next appointment's date and time. This postcard serves as a backup in case the patient loses the original appointment reminder card. Place the postcard in the tickler file under the day when it should be sent (usually a week or two before the appointment). Reminder mailings also can be sent to patients who make appointments over the telephone. In this case, of course, you must address the postcard for the tickler file yourself. Although reminder mailings are useful when appointments are made many

months in advance or for geriatric patients, they can become costly for the practice and should be limited when possible.

Confirmation Calls Depending on office policy and available time, you might also call patients 1 or 2 days before their appointments to confirm the scheduled time. This technique can be especially helpful for patients with a history of late arrivals or for **no-shows** (patients who do not call to cancel and do not come to the appointment). Writing patients' phone numbers next to their names in the appointment book makes it convenient for you to make appointment reminder calls. Procedure 16-4 at the end of the chapter outlines the steps in making appointment confirmation (or reminder) calls. Many offices that utilize electronic phone systems program the system to make reminder calls, freeing the office staff from this task. Be aware of patients who do not wish to be contacted by phone or to have messages left. Having the patient fill out a verbal contact agreement at her first visit can limit HIPAA violations. Figure 16-8 provides an example of a HIPAA-compliant verbal agreement form. If patients agree that messages may be left on voicemail or answering machines, be sure this information is added to the verbal agreement form.

Recall Notices Some offices book appointments no more than a few weeks in advance; others may not have the next year's schedule available when a patient is ready to book a return appointment. In either case, you need a way to make sure patients do not forget to call for appointments that are 6 months—or even a year—away from their last appointments.

Suppose, for example, that the practitioner tells a patient she should have an annual breast examination. How can you help her remember to call to schedule one at the appropriate time? One way is to use a system of recall notices. In a tickler file, enter the patient's name under the month when she should call the office. When the time arrives, send a form letter reminding her that she will soon be due for a breast examination and asking her to call for an appointment. Many EHR software programs offer such reminder programs as part of the software package.

E-mail Notifications With more practices trying to accommodate all patient groups, a newer approach to appointment scheduling is through the use of e-mail. Patients sign up (and sign the appropriate release to allow communication via e-mail) and are assigned passwords by the office. The patient may request an appointment via the office e-mail system (as long as it is not needed immediately). The office returns a confirmation e-mail of the scheduled appointment. When a scheduled appointment is approaching, an automatically generated notification goes out to the patient's e-mail address reminding him of the appointment. This is not suitable for all patients or all types of appointments. Some appointment types will still need to be handled by the office staff either by phone or in person because of the amount of information that needs to be relayed regarding the appointment and/or patient preparation for the appointment.

BWW Medical Associates, PC

305 Main Street, Port Snead YZ 12345-9876, Tel: 555-654-3210, Fax: 555-987-6543

☐ PRIVATE ☐ BLUECROSS ☐ IND. ☐ MEDICARE ☐ MEDI-CAL ☐ HMO ☐ PPO

PATIENT'S LAST NAME	FIRST	ACCOUNT #	BIRTHDATE / /	SEX ☐ MALE ☐ FEMALE	TODAY'S DATE / /
INSURANCE COMPANY	SUBSCRIBER		PLAN #	SUB. #	GROUP

ASSIGNMENT: I hereby assign my insurance benefits to be paid directly to the undersigned physician. I am financially responsible for non-covered services. SIGNED: (Patient, or Parent, If Minor) DATE: / /	RELEASE: I hereby authorize the physician to release to my insurance carriers any information required to process this claim. SIGNED: (Patient, or Parent, If Minor) DATE: / /

✓	DESCRIPTION	M/Care	CPT/Mod	DxRe	FEE	✓	DESCRIPTION	M/Care	CPT/Mod	DxRe	FEE	✓	DESCRIPTION	M/Care	CPT/Mod	DxRe	FEE
	OFFICE CARE						PROCEDURES						INJECTIONS/IMMUNIZATIONS				
	NEW PATIENT						Tread Mill (In Office)		93015				Tetanus		90718		
	Brief		99201				24 Hour Holter (Complete)		93224				Hypertet	J1670	90782		
	Limited		99202				Holter (setup only)		93225				Pneumococcal		90732		
	Intermediate		99203				Physician Interpret		93227				Influenza		90724		
	Extended		99204				EKG w/Interpretation		93000				TB Skin Test (PPD)		86585		
	Comprehensive		99205				EKG (Medicare)		93005				Antigen Injection-Single		95115		
							Sigmoidoscopy		45300				Multiple		95117		
	ESTABLISHED PATIENT						Sigmoidoscopy, Flexible		45330				B12 Injection	J3420	90782		
	Minimal		99211				Sigmoidos. , Flex. w/Bx.		45331				Injection, IM		90782		
	Brief		99212				Spirometry, FEV/FVC		94010				Compazine	J0780	90782		
	Limited		99213				Spirometry, Post-Dilator		94060				Demerol	J2175	90782		
	Intermediate		99214										Vistaril	J3410	90782		
	Extended		99215										Susphrine	J0170	90782		
	Comprehensive		99215				LABORATORY						Decadron	J0890	90782		
							Blood Draw Fee		36415				Estradiol	J1000	90782		
	CONSULTATION-OFFICE						Urinalysis, Chemical		81005				Testosterone	J1080	90782		
	Focused		99241				Throat Culture		87081				Lidocaine	J2000	90782		
	Expanded		99242				Occult Blood		82270				Solumedrol	J2920	90782		
	Detailed		99243				Pap Handling Charge		99000				Solucortef	J1720	90782		
	Comprehensive 1		99244				Pap Life Guard		88150-90				Hydeltra	J1690	90782		
	Comprehensive 2		99245				Gram Stain		87205				Pen Procaine	J2510	90788		
	Dr.						Hanging Drop		87210								
	Case Management		98900				Urine Drug Screen		99000				INJECTIONS - JOINT/BURSA				
													Small Joints		20600		
	Post-op Exam		99024				SUPPLIES						Intermediate		20605		
													Large Joints		20610		
													Trigger Point		20550		
													MISCELLANEOUS				

DIAGNOSIS:	ICD-9														
Abdominal Pain	789.0	Gout	274.0	C.V.A. - Acute	436.	Electrolyte Dis.	276.9	Herpes Simplex	054.9
Abscess (Site)	682.9	Asthma	493.90	Cere. Vas. Accid. (Old)	438	Fatigue	780.7	Herpes Zoster	053.9
Adverse Drug Rx	995.2	Asthmatic Bronchitis	493.90	Cerumen	380.4	Fibrocys. Br. Dis	610.1	Hydrocele	603.9
Alcohol Detox	291.8	Atrial Fib.	427.31	Chestwall Pain	786.59	Fracture (Site)	829.0	Hyperlipidemia	272.4
Alcoholism	303.90	Atrial Tachi.	427.0	Cholecystitis	575.0	Open/Close		Hypertension	401.9
Allergic Rhinitis	477	Bowel Obstruct.	560.9	Cholelithiasis	574.00	Fungal Infect. (Site)	110.8	Hyperthyroidism	242.9
Allergy	995.3	Breast Mass	611.72	COPD	492.8	Gastric Ulcer	531.90	Hypothyroidism	244.9
Alzheimer's Dis.	290.1	Bronchitis	490	Cirrhosis	571.5	Gastritis	535.0	Labyrinthitis	386.30
Anemia	285.9	Bursitis	727.3	Cong. Heart Fail.	428.9	Gastroenteritis	558.9	Lipoma (Site)	214.9
Anemia - Pernicious	281.0	Cancer, Breast (Site)	174.9	Conjunctivitis	372.30	G.I. Bleeding	578.9	Lymphoma	202.8
Angina	413.9	Metastatic (Site)	199.1	Contusion (Site)	924.9	Glomerulonephritis	583.9	Mit. Valve Prolapse	424.0
Anxiety Synd.	300.00	Colon	153.9	Costochondritis	733.99	Headache	784.0	Myocard. Infarction (Area)	410.9
Appendicitis	541	Cancer, Rectal	154.1	Depression	311.	Headache, Tension	307.81	M.I., Old	412
Arterioscl. H.D.	414.0	Lung (Site)	162.9	Dermatitis	692.9	Migraine (Type)	346.9	Myositis	729.1
Arthritis, Osteo.	715.90	Skin (Site)	173.9	Diabetes Mellitus	250.00	Hemorrhoids	455.6	Nausea/Vomiting	787.0
Rheumatoid	714.0	Card. Arrhythmia (Type)	427.9	Diabetic Ketosis	250.1	Hernia, Hiatal	553.3	Neuralgia	729.2
Osteo.	714.0	Cardiomyopathy	425.4	Diverticulitis	562.11	Inguinal	550.9	Nevus (Site)	216.9
Lupus	710.0	Cellulitis (Site)	682.9	Diverticulosis	562.10	Hepatitis	573.3	Obesity	278.0

DIAGNOSIS: (IF NOT CHECKED ABOVE)

SERVICES PERFORMED AT: ☐ Office ☐ E.R.	☐ CLAIM CONTAINS NO ORDERED REFERRING SERVICE	REFERRING PHYSICIAN & I.D. NUMBER

RETURN APPOINTMENT INFORMATION: 5 - 10 - 15 - 20 - 30 - 40 - 60 [DAYS] [WKS.] [MOS.] [PRN]	NEXT APPOINTMENT M · T · W · TH - F - S DATE / / TIME: AM PM	ACCEPT ASSIGNMENT? ☐ YES ☐ NO	DOCTOR'S SIGNATURE

INSTRUCTIONS TO PATIENT FOR FILING INSURANCE CLAIMS:	☐ CASH	TOTAL TODAY'S FEE	
1. Complete upper portion of this form, sign and date. 2. Attach this form to your own insurance company's form for direct reimbursement. **MEDICARE PATIENTS - DO NOT SEND THIS TO MEDICARE. WE WILL SUBMIT THE CLAIM FOR YOU.**	☐ CHECK # _____	OLD BALANCE	
	☐ VISA	TOTAL DUE	
	☐ MC		
	☐ CO-PAY	AMOUNT REC'D. TODAY	

FIGURE 16-7 This encounter form has an appointment block included at the bottom left.

BWW

BWW Medical Associates, PC
305 Main Street, Port Snead YZ 12345-9876
Tel: 555-654-3210, Fax: 555-987-6543
Web: BWWAssociates.com

Paul F. Buckwalter, MD
Alexis N. Whalen, MD
Elizabeth H. Williams, MD

Patient Name: _____   MRN: _____

VERBAL RELEASE OF INFORMATION

BWW Medical Associates is allowed to give verbal information or updates on your medical condition to you and your Power of Attorney for Healthcare/Legal Representative as listed in your medical record.

If you wish others, such as relatives or friends WHO ASK about your condition, to have the right to be verbally informed about your condition, please list the names of those individuals and their relationship to you.

Name: _____   Relationship: _____

Name: _____   Relationship: _____

Name: _____   Relationship: _____

Name: _____   Relationship: _____

Additionally, should verbal messages need to be relayed to me via phone when I am not available to take the call, messages may be left for me on the available voicemail or answering device at the following phone numbers:

Phone Number: _____   (Please circle)   Home   Cell   Work

Phone Number: _____   (Please circle)   Home   Cell   Work

Phone Number: _____   (Please circle)   Home   Cell   Work

- I understand that BWW Medical Associates will continue to rely on the information contained within this form as current unless I request a change in writing.

- I understand that I may revoke this verbal agreement authorization at any time.

- I understand that if I choose to revoke this authorization, I must do so in writing and present my written revocation to the Privacy Officer at BWW Medical Associates. The revocation will NOT apply to information that has already been disclosed prior to the receipt of the written revocation.

_____   _____
Signature of Patient or Guardian   Date

FIGURE 16-8   Example of verbal release of information agreement.

▶ Special Scheduling Situations   LO 16.5

In most cases scheduling is routine; however, critical thinking, creativity, and flexibility are necessary for scheduling some special cases. These special situations often involve patients, but they also may involve physicians. Here are just a few of the special situations that may arise.

Patient Scheduling Situations

On some days all patients will keep their appointments and arrive on time. On many other days, however, patients may walk in without appointments, arrive late for scheduled appointments, or miss appointments entirely. Being able to anticipate needs and being prepared for these possibilities allow you to handle them more efficiently, keeping the office schedule running smoothly.

Emergencies   Your training as a medical assistant will help you recognize the signs of an emergency. In some instances you will refer the caller to the nearest hospital emergency room or instruct the caller to call emergency medical services (EMS) for an ambulance. The procedure you will follow will depend on office policies and procedures (refer to the *Telephone Techniques* chapter). In other instances you will ask the caller to come to the office right away so you can "work" him into the schedule. It is vital that the physician see an emergency patient before patients who are already in the reception area or on the schedule. It is best to explain to waiting patients that there has been an emergency (without giving details). This announcement helps them understand and accept the delay and gives them an opportunity to reschedule their appointments if they are unable to wait. Read the *Points on Practice* feature on scheduling emergency appointments, which contains a mock emergency appointment scenario.

Referrals If your practice includes specialists, it is a common occurrence that other practitioners will refer their patients to the practice for second opinions or special consultations. A patient seeking a second opinion before deciding on surgery, often at the request of his or her insurance carrier, should be fit into the schedule as soon as possible. Other referred patients also should be seen as soon as possible, both as a professional courtesy to the referring provider and as good business practice.

Many offices maintain a listing of preferred practitioners and facilities that they would like their patients to see and use. This list should contain the physician or facility names,

specialty, address, and their phone numbers. When arranging a referral, try to give the patient two names to choose from, along with the referral phone numbers and addresses.

When choosing the referral names of either practitioners or facilities, be sure that the facility accepts the patient's insurance and that all of the paperwork required by the insurance company has been completed. Some insurance carriers require a specific paper or electronic referral (or authorization) form be filled out. Most others today utilize an area of their website as a type of point of service (POS), where the medical office enters the information into the insurance company database and an authorization is returned on the spot. Some smaller carriers may require a phone request in which the medical office speaks to a customer service representative or enters specific information into an automated voice response telephone system. Regardless of the method used, all referrals and authorizations should be documented in the patient's medical record, including the authorization number given (if applicable) by the insurance carrier, authorizing the referral.

Fasting Patients Some procedures and tests require patients to fast, or refrain from eating or drinking anything, beginning the night before. Schedule these patients as early in the day as possible to show consideration for their needs. When scheduling appointments that require the patient to fast, be sure to inform the patient of the need to fast and when the fasting should start, including the fact that the test may not be completed if the patient does not fast.

Patients with Diabetes Similar to fasting patients, patients with diabetes can use extra consideration when you schedule their appointments. In general, patients who take insulin must eat meals and snacks at regular intervals. This routine keeps their blood sugar from dropping too low—a condition that can result in confused thinking or even loss of consciousness. Therefore, you might want to avoid scheduling patients with diabetes for slots in late morning. This will help avoid the possibility of the patient waiting in the reception area during a time he should be eating a snack that is needed to keep his blood sugar levels on an even keel.

Late Arrivals If the practice has patients who are routinely late and gentle reminders to be on time have not helped, you might try booking them toward the end of the day. Even if a patient arrives late for a late-afternoon appointment, the provider will have already seen most of the day's patients and the late patient will not disrupt the schedule. Document late arrivals or missed appointments in the patient's chart. With documentation, patients who are habitually late can be called to discuss the reasons for their chronic tardiness. The goal of the discussion should be to find a solution so that patients can make their appointments on time and the schedule will run smoothly.

Walk-Ins From time to time, a patient may arrive without an appointment and still expect to see the provider. These people are called **walk-ins.** Office policies on how to handle walk-ins vary. If the person is experiencing an emergency, handle the situation as you would handle any emergency. Otherwise, you might politely explain that the doctor is fully booked for the day and offer to schedule an appointment in the usual manner. If an office PA or NP is available, suggest to the patient that this practitioner may be able to be of assistance. If, by chance, the doctor is available and willing to see the walk-in, you should still ask the person to call to schedule appointments in the future, as this is the usual policy for the practice. If your physician's office has a policy of no walk-ins, post a sign in the patient check-in area stating that patients are seen by appointment only.

Cancellations When patients call to cancel appointments, try to reschedule the appointment while they are on the telephone. If patients say they will call later to reschedule, note this information in the appointment book and thank them for the notice.

You should also write "canceled" in the appointment book, drawing a single line through the patient's name. To avoid confusion, cancel the first appointment *before* entering the patient's rescheduled appointment. Remember that the appointment book is a legal record. If you forget to cross out the name at the time of the first appointment, it may later seem that the doctor saw the patient twice. It is also important

to note the cancellation in the patient's medical record. This notation can protect the practice from possible legal action. For example, a patient whose surgical incision becomes infected cannot blame the surgeon if the patient canceled a scheduled appointment for a dressing change.

You may be able to fill slots created by cancellations by calling patients who have appointments scheduled for later in the day or week. Some patients may be willing to come in earlier than planned. When you make appointments, you can ask patients if they would be interested in coming in earlier if openings occur. Placing the names of interested patients in a tickler file or on a cancellation list can save time later.

Missed and Wrong-Day Appointments It is important for legal reasons to document a no-show in the appointment book and patient medical record. Always inform the physician of any missed appointments in case the patient's condition requires a follow-up. The provider may want you to call the patient with a polite reminder that the patient has missed an appointment and needs to reschedule. There may have been a misunderstanding about the time, or the patient may simply have forgotten the appointment. Some offices, especially ones that use computerized scheduling systems, send out form letters when patients miss appointments.

If failure to keep the appointment could endanger the patient's health, mention this possibility to the patient. The patient's provider also may wish to speak to the patient about the health issues possible due to repeated missed appointments. Some practices limit the number of times that a patient can miss, cancel, or repeatedly not show up for appointments, as this can lead to liability issues for the practitioner if the lack of follow-up leads to complications for the patient. Because of potential legal issues, it bears repeating to always document any missed or canceled appointments in the patient medical record. Refer to the *Legal and Ethical Issues* chapter to review the procedures to be followed so that providers cannot be charged with patient abandonment.

Periodically, practitioners charge for missed appointments, especially if patients habitually miss their appointments. These missed appointment charges are for missed business opportunities and not for services rendered. If your office implements this policy, make sure that you let patients know in advance before you start charging them for missed appointments. Most offices with this policy have the policy posted near the reception desk. Some offices also opt for a notation on the appointment cards that states patients will be charged for appointments that are canceled with less than 24 hours' notice.

Sometimes a patient may show up on the wrong day for her appointment. If the patient lives in the local area, rescheduling makes sense. But if the patient made special transportation arrangements or traveled from a long distance, it is good business practice to try to work the patient into the schedule for that day. If the patient provides an appointment card verifying the appointment for that day, but she is not on the schedule, the office is obligated to honor the appointment if the physician is in the office. When in doubt about the best course of action, consult with the doctor or office manager.

Practitioner Scheduling Situations

Not all scheduling problems result from patients. Sometimes practitioners disrupt the office schedule as well. They may be called away on an emergency, may be delayed at the hospital, or may simply arrive late.

Some providers are occasionally late for appointments, while others are frequently late, either when arriving in the morning or when returning from lunch or a scheduled meeting. If this situation occurs in your office, it may be handled in several ways.

Speaking to the provider directly about the problem may be helpful in resolving the situation. You also might use the staff meeting to mention that the morning or afternoon schedule often seems to get off to a late start and ask if anyone has suggestions for improving this situation. The practitioner may recognize that she is the cause of the problem and decide to resolve it.

If the practitioner does not take responsibility for the problem, however, you may need to adjust the office schedule to handle the situation. Suppose, for example, that the first patient appointment slot is at 8:30 a.m., but the practitioner habitually does not arrive until 8:35 a.m. You could simply avoid scheduling patients between 8:30 and 8:45 a.m. If a provider is often 15 minutes late returning from lunch or from meetings, you might leave open the first appointment slot after the scheduled arrival time in an attempt to avoid long wait times for patients, keeping satisfied clients.

▶ Scheduling Outside Appointments   LO 16.6

You may be responsible for arranging patient appointments outside the medical office. These appointments may include

- Consultations with or referrals to other physicians.
- Laboratory work.
- Radiology (X-ray, CT scans, MRI).
- Other diagnostic tests (EKG, stress testing)
- Hospital stays.
- Inpatient and outpatient surgeries.

Scheduling Outpatient Procedures

Always verify the patient's insurance coverage before choosing the facility or provider for the patient's referral or other service. Today, a patient's insurance coverage may dictate both where a procedure may be performed and the practitioner allowed to provide the service. A prior approval or referral from the insurance carrier also may be required. The medical assistant is often responsible for knowing not only the preferred providers and facilities for the practice providers, but also the practitioners and facilities allowed by specific insurance carriers. Obtaining referrals and prior authorizations also will often be your responsibility. (Refer to the *Insurance and Billing* chapter for more information on this topic.)

Once a facility and provider have been agreed upon by the referring practitioner, patient, and insurance carrier, document any referrals or prior authorization numbers (again, refer to the *Insurance and Billing* chapter). If the procedure is elective, ask the patient if there is a preferred date and time. If the request fits into the provider and facility schedule, try to accommodate the patient's preference, as this gesture allows the patient to have some sense of control over a situation that is likely anxiety provoking.

Before calling the surgery center, laboratory, or outpatient department required for the procedure, be sure that you have the patient's medical record; the exact name of the procedure to be performed; the approximate amount of time required (if your practitioner is performing the service); the diagnosis; and the patient's insurance information, date of birth, phone number, and home address. Give this information to the scheduler, keeping in mind the patient's preferred time frame if it can be accommodated. Once an appointment time has been agreed upon, ask the scheduler for any patient instructions, carefully documenting them to relay to the patient. If paperwork will be sent to the patient from the facility, be sure the patient also understands this.

When arrangements have been made, inform the patient orally and provide him with written instructions, asking for and answering any questions the patient may have. Be sure he understands any preprocedure instructions and the fact that if the preprocedure instructions are not followed perfectly, the procedure may need to be rescheduled or repeated. Remember to note in the patient's chart the date and time of the procedure as well as instructions provided to the patient. Procedure 16-5, found at the end of the chapter, outlines the procedure for booking an outpatient surgical appointment.

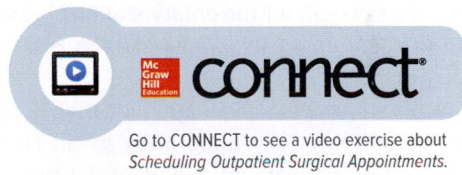

Go to CONNECT to see a video exercise about *Scheduling Outpatient Surgical Appointments.*

Reserving an Operating Room

If the surgeon in your office plans to perform surgery at a hospital, you will need to call the operating room scheduler to reserve the facility. As when booking an outpatient procedure, you will first give the preferred dates and times, the type of surgery, and the length of time the provider will need the operating room. After the day and time are set, provide the scheduler with all relevant patient information. Relay any requests from the doctor, such as the blood type and units of blood that may be needed. It also may be your responsibility to make arrangements for surgical assistants, an anesthetist, and a hospital bed for the patient following surgery. Make sure that all health insurance requirements such as referrals and prior authorizations are met and copies of forms and authorization numbers are filed appropriately. As when scheduling outpatient procedures, be sure the patient receives all necessary oral and written instructions and information regarding pre- and postsurgical care and that all questions are answered. Procedure 16-6, found at the end of the chapter, outlines the steps for booking an inpatient surgical appointment.

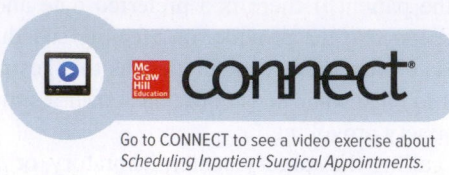

Go to CONNECT to see a video exercise about *Scheduling Inpatient Surgical Appointments.*

▶ Maintaining the Practitioner's Schedule   LO 16.7

The schedules of busy practitioners are not limited to office visits with patients. Licensed practitioners also need to attend professional meetings, travel to conferences, present speeches to colleagues, complete paperwork, and perform other duties. Your job is to help the providers in your practice make the most efficient use of their time.

One way to assist each provider with his schedule is to avoid overbooking appointments with patients. **Overbooking** (scheduling more patients than can reasonably be seen in the time allowed) creates stress for the provider and the staff and makes it difficult to maintain a timely schedule.

The opposite problem, **underbooking**—leaving large, unused gaps in the schedule—does not make the best use of the practitioner's time. Of course, you have no control over patients who cancel or do not show for appointments, but, as mentioned previously, there are ways to decrease this, such as calling patients to remind them of their appointments a day or two ahead of the scheduled appointment. If you cannot reschedule another patient for the empty slot, the provider can use the time to catch up on telephone calls to patients or to attend to other matters.

At times you will have to cancel appointments because the provider has been delayed or called away by an emergency. Apologize to waiting patients on behalf of the provider and offer them a choice. Explain that they can wait in the office (give an estimated waiting time), leave to run errands and return later, or reschedule their appointments for another day. Documentation should be noted in the patient's chart that because of an emergency in the office, the appointment had to be rescheduled by the office so the patient is not held at fault for the cancellation. Be sure to write the date of the rescheduled appointment in the chart as well. Always make sure patients who need immediate attention are seen by another provider if available, staying within office policies.

Visits Outside the Office

Some practitioners provide care outside of the office—in patient homes, in nursing homes, or during rounds within the hospital when their patients have been admitted.

House Calls Practitioners may want to check on home-bound or nonambulatory patients as part of their follow-up care.

Although not as common as it once was, house calls are a valuable service that practitioners can provide to patients who can no longer easily make it to the medical office for their appointments. Many insurance companies allow the practitioner to bill for these services with restrictions that vary depending on the plan. Supplies required for visits vary depending on the type and location of the visit, but general supplies that should be kept in a medical bag include the following:

- Blood pressure cuff
- Stethoscope
- Specimen containers
- Otoscope
- Ophthalmoscope
- Prescription pad
- Pen light
- Thermometer
- Gloves, face shield

Hospital Rounds Historically, physicians typically visited their own patients when they became hospitalized. Today, more and more hospitals are turning this responsibility over to a physician specialist known as a hospitalist. A hospitalist does not hold office hours and does not maintain a practice but only sees patients while they are hospitalized. If your office or the hospital where your physicians have privileges utilize hospitalists, they will report to the physician on the patient's progress and findings while an inpatient.

Nursing Home Visits Some practitioners check on their patients even when they are receiving around-the-clock care from a skilled nursing facility. Usually the practitioner has seen these patients for years and stays involved with their care because of the long-standing relationship or because the patient will be returning home after a rehabilitation stay and will need follow-up care.

"Mouse Calls" With all of the new technology available to them, providers are learning new ways to communicate with their patients. In their daily schedule, time is often allotted for practitioners to return phone calls, which today can also include "mouse" calls—practitioners answering e-mail inquiries from their patients. These also can be "virtual visits" covered by some insurance plans. Be sure that the appropriate releases are in the patient's file before the provider undertakes this type of communication with the patient.

Scheduling Pharmaceutical Sales Representatives

Drug manufacturers often send pharmaceutical sales representatives into medical offices with printed information about new drugs as well as free samples that can be given to patients. This is an added benefit for your patients but can be time consuming, as the representatives will want to market their products. The representatives are required to obtain signatures from the licensed practitioners in order to leave the samples behind, and for this reason, some practitioners do not want to meet with pharmaceutical representatives. Others are willing to spend a few minutes if time permits and if the products are likely to be useful to their patients. Some practitioners set aside certain times or days during the week when they will meet with pharmaceutical representatives. Many prescribers prefer that the representative leave a business card with the products represented, and if the provider is interested, she will call and arrange for an appointment at a mutually agreeable time. When a pharmaceutical representative who is unknown to you comes into the office, ask for a business card and check with the licensed practitioner or business manager before scheduling an appointment (Figure 16-9).

Making Travel Arrangements

You may be responsible for arranging transportation and lodging when practitioners attend meetings, speaking engagements, and other events out of town. You may be responsible for contacting the airlines, car rental agencies, hotels, or other services yourself, or you may use an online service such as Orbitz® or work through a travel agent. No matter which method is used to make travel arrangements, always request confirmation documents of travel and room reservations.

Before the day of departure, obtain an itinerary from the travel agent or online service, or create one yourself. An **itinerary** is a detailed travel plan, listing dates and times of flights and events, locations of meetings and lodgings, and

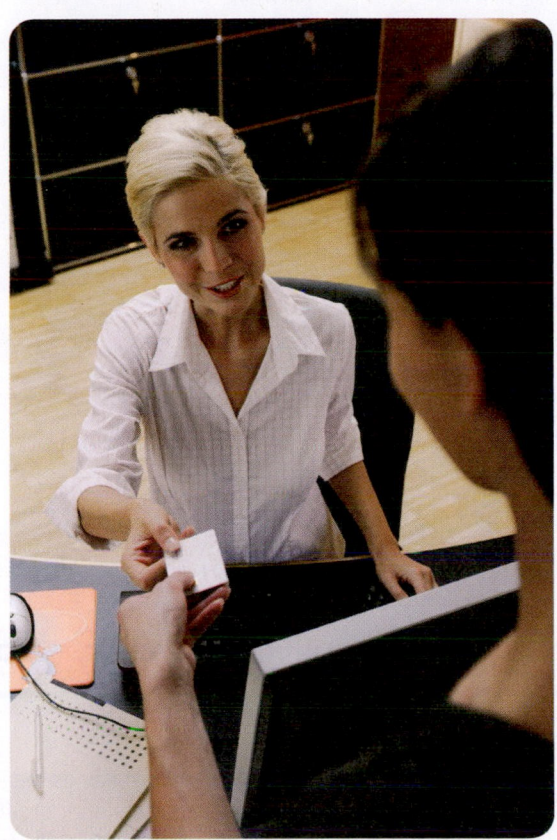

FIGURE 16-9 Pharmaceutical sales representatives who cannot see the licensed practitioners often leave a business card listing the medications from their company.
© altrendo images/Getty Images RF

telephone numbers. Give several copies to the provider and keep one for the office (Figure 16-10).

You also may be responsible for scheduling and confirming professional coverage of the practice during the physician's absence. In larger practices and more urban areas, physicians in the same or a nearby practice often provide coverage while the physician is away. This coverage may be important for legal reasons, most importantly so the physician cannot be charged with abandoning patients. If a local physician is not readily available, a **locum tenens,** or substitute physician, may be hired to see patients while the regular physician is unavailable. *Locum tenens* is Latin for "one occupying the place of another." You may have more than one *locum tenens* on call, depending on the practice. In some areas special firms provide these services and other temporary medical and nursing assistance. Before hiring a *locum tenens,* you may want to contact some of the major insurance carriers providing health insurance coverage for your patients to find out his or her credentialing and claim requirements so that the services provided by the *locum tenens* will be considered covered services.

Planning Meetings

Another of your duties may be to assist the provider in setting up meetings for professional societies or committees. To do so, you will need to know how many people are expected to attend, how long the meeting will last, and the purpose of the meeting. In addition, ask the doctor if a meal is to be served.

Some groups have a schedule of meetings planned in advance and meet in a consistent location, but if there is no established meeting place, you must choose and reserve one. Select a location with an adequately sized meeting room, sufficient parking, and, if needed, food services. Be sure also to arrange for necessary audiovisual (AV) equipment, such as a microphone, podium, or projector. Many conference centers and hotels have an on-site catering manager or conference manager to assist you with these arrangements. When the facility has been booked, mail (or e-mail) an invitation to all those expected to attend the meeting. On the invitation, provide the topic, names of the speakers, date, time, place, and admission costs or fees associated with the event if applicable.

With direction from the practitioner, you also may be responsible for creating the meeting's agenda, as discussed in more detail in the *Practice Management* chapter. After the meeting, you also may be asked to prepare the **minutes,** the report of what was discussed and decided upon at the meeting.

Scheduling Time with the Practitioner

You and the practitioner should meet on a scheduled basis to discuss any irregularities or changes in the day-to-day workings of the office. These meetings may be held between you and the provider alone or include the office manager. If items are not pressing or "private," many discussions may be included in regularly scheduled office meetings. Topics discussed may include practice finance items such as insurance premiums, taxes, and other financial matters, as well as professional licenses and renewal requirements for the medical staff. These items are discussed in further detail in the *Practice Management* chapter.

Paul F. Buckwalter, MD
Travel Itinerary

BWW Medical Associates, PC
305 Main Street, Port Snead YZ 12345-9876
Tel: 555-654-3210, Fax: 555-987-6543
Web: BWWAssociates.com

Client Information

Traveler's Name	Paul F. Buckwalter, MD
Address	560 Williamsburg Ct., Port Snead, YZ
Telephone Number	555-279-0098
Fax Number	555-987-6543
E-mail Address	
Travel Dates	May 5 – 9, 20XX

Departure Flight

Date	May 5, 20XX
Airline	United International
Flight Number	567
From	Port Snead, YZ
Departure Time	6:45 am
Departure Terminal/Gate	56C
To	Los Angeles, CA
Arrival Time	9:45 am Pacific time
Length of Flight	5 hours
Class	First Class
Seat Number	12a
Status	confirmed

Monday – May 5, 20XX

• Morning:

8:00 – 8:45	Physician Recruiter
9:00 – 10:00	Formal interview with Team, facilitated by Recruiter
10:00 – 11:00	Medical Director
11:00 – 12:00	Tour of UCLA including department with Area Manager

• Afternoon:

12:30 – 1:30	Lunch with physician(s) from another department with similar interests
2:00 – 3:00	One (1) hour with Department Chair and/or Physician Area Manager
4:00 – 6:00	One-on-one interviews with department or other physicians
	Informal time in interviewing department, as appropriate

• Evening:

7:00 – until	Dinner (or private dinner on their own)

FIGURE 16-10 Typical travel itinerary.

PROCEDURE 16-1 Creating an Appointment Matrix

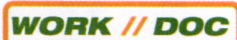

Procedure Goal: To create an appointment matrix to indicate the days and the hours the physician is not scheduling patients

OSHA Guidelines: This procedure does not involve exposure to blood, body fluids, or tissue.

Materials: Appointment record, pencil or pen; physician schedule of meetings, conferences, vacations, staff meetings, and other times of unavailability when patients are not seen

Method:

1. Using the practitioner schedule of availability as the base for the matrix, confer with the practitioner or office manager to ensure that no additional schedule changes are planned.

   RATIONALE: *The matrix should be as complete as possible to avoid the need to reschedule appointments.*

2. Indicate within each area the reason the time is being closed to appointments, such as lunch, hospital rounds, or AAMA meeting.

   RATIONALE: *Allows for all users to be aware of provider location both in and outside of the office*

3. If the office utilizes cluster scheduling for certain appointments such as physical exams and blood sugar

testing, these time frames also must be set apart. Following office policy, such as using brackets, note the appropriate appointment type to be scheduled during this time frame.

RATIONALE: *It is important for all users to know what type of appointments can be booked in each time frame.*

PROCEDURE 16-2 Scheduling Appointments

WORK // DOC

Procedure Goal: Utilizing the previously created matrix, book patient appointments applying the correct amount of time for each appointment

OSHA Guidelines: This procedure does not involve exposure to blood, body fluids, or tissue.

Materials: Appointment book and pen or pencil, or electronic scheduler (with appropriate matrix) template, outlining time frames for patient appointment types

Method:

1. Establish the type of appointment required by the patient, particularly if this is a new patient or a returning patient.

   RATIONALE: *New patients typically require a longer appointment time than do returning existing patients.*

2. If necessary, consult the template for the amount of time required for the patient appointment. Keep in mind the reason for the appointment when scheduling (for example, is the patient required to be fasting).

   RATIONALE: *Some appointments are best scheduled at certain times of the day depending on patient preparation and equipment or personnel availability.*

3. When possible, schedule appointments earlier in the day first and then move to later time frames. Do ask the patient if he or she has a preferred time frame in mind and, if at all possible, accommodate the request.

   RATIONALE: *Open appointments later in the day allow space for unexpected appointments required at a later time.*

4. When using an appointment book, enter the patient name, phone number, and reason for the appointment in the appropriate space, blocking out additional blocks of time if necessary to accommodate a longer appointment time.

5. If an electronic scheduler is used, use the search option to find the next available appointment for the time frame required for the appointment. Enter the patient name, phone number, and reason for the appointment.

6. Repeat the appointment information to the patient, giving any necessary instructions regarding preparation for the appointment, such as early arrival for blood tests. Also, this is a good time to remind patients about any copayments that will be due at the time of the appointment.

   RATIONALE: *Patients respond best when they know what is expected ahead of time.*

PROCEDURE 16-3 Completing the Patient Appointment Card

WORK // DOC

Procedure Goal: To accurately complete a patient appointment card for the patient's next visit

OSHA Guidelines: This procedure does not involve exposure to blood, body fluids, or tissue.

Materials: Appointment book or electronic scheduler, pen, and appointment card

Method:

1. After entering the patient's appointment in the appointment book or electronic scheduler, repeat the appointment date and time to the patient to verify accuracy.

2. Complete the patient appointment card, entering the appointment date and time on the card. If the practice has multiple providers, there may also be a place for the appropriate physician name to be entered, and you should do so.

   RATIONALE: *If patients see multiple providers, it is not unusual for them to forget a provider's name.*

3. Repeat appointment information to the patient one more time when giving the card to him or her, again verifying the information.

PROCEDURE 16-4 Placing Appointment Confirmation Calls

Procedure Goal: To decrease the number of no-show patients by making appointment confirmation calls 24–48 hours prior to the scheduled appointment

OSHA Guidelines: This procedure does not involve exposure to blood, body fluids, or tissue.

Materials: Office appointment book, electronic scheduler, or listing of patients scheduled to be seen tomorrow or the next day, with their home phone numbers

Method:

1. Starting with the first appointment of the day, call the patient listed.

2. If the phone is answered, ask for the patient. If you reach the patient, give your name and the name of the practice and state that you are confirming the patient's appointment for the applicable date and time.

3. Remind the patient of any special instructions regarding the appointment such as fasting, bringing in medical record or registration information, and copayments due.
   RATIONALE: *It is important that the patient come to the appointment prepared, or any testing may need to be postponed.*

4. If the patient is not available, leave your name and phone number, asking that the patient return your call.
   RATIONALE: *Unless the person answering the phone has been listed by the patient as someone to whom you may give confidential information, you must speak directly with the patient to avoid breach of patient confidentiality.*

5. If a voicemail or answering machine system is reached, follow the practice confidentiality rules of leaving only your name and phone number, asking the patient to call you back, unless you have permission from the patient to leave more explicit information on voicemail.
   RATIONALE: *Unless you have express written permission from the patient to leave a message on an answering machine or voicemail, confidentiality regulations require you not leave explicit information.*

6. Thank the patient for his or her time, stating you will see him or her at the stated date and time.

7. Allow the patient to hang up first, so if there are questions, you can answer them.
   RATIONALE: *This allows the patient to have all questions or issues addressed adequately.*

PROCEDURE 16-5 Scheduling Outpatient Surgical Appointments

WORK // DOC

Procedure Goal: To schedule an outpatient surgical procedure

OSHA Guidelines: This procedure does not involve exposure to blood, body fluids, or tissue.

Materials: Patient medical record and progress note form, calendar, telephone, pen

Method:

1. Obtain detailed information regarding the procedure to be performed from the surgeon and patient medical record. Information should include the name of procedure to be performed, the amount of time the outpatient surgical suite will be needed, and the reason (diagnosis) for the procedure.
   RATIONALE: *Without this information, you will be unable to efficiently book the required appointment.*

2. From the patient's medical record, you will need the patient's full name, DOB, allergies, current medications, address, phone number, and insurance information.
   RATIONALE: *This information will be needed by the facility booking the procedure.*

3. Place a call to the appropriate surgery center or outpatient surgical unit at the requested facility. Have the name of the surgeon, assistant, or PA (if used) available, as well as the patient's and physician's preferred dates for the procedure.

4. When the appointment scheduler answers the phone, identify yourself, the practice, and the procedure you need to schedule, as well as the preferred dates.

5. When a date for the procedure is agreed upon by the patient, give the scheduler the patient's name, address, phone number, DOB, gender, and insurance information, including the prior authorization number if needed. Also give the patient's diagnosis as required for medical necessity.
   RATIONALE: *This information will be needed by the facility for booking and billing purposes.*

6. Inquire as to any preprocedure testing that may need to be done as well as any patient preparation required prior to the procedure, including patient arrival time.
   RATIONALE: *This information will need to be relayed to the patient for adequate preparation for the procedure.*

7. Confirm the appointment date and time prior to hanging up. If necessary, book any preprocedure testing for the patient and document these appointments in the patient instructions and appropriate office form(s) and/or within the patient's medical record.
   RATIONALE: *Always document any patient-related information in the patient's medical record.*

8. Provide the patient with written instructions from the physician as well as all information obtained while

booking the appointment. The patient also should be informed that he should arrange for someone to drive him to and from this appointment.

9. Go over the written dates and instructions with the patient, asking the patient if there are any questions, answering them if possible, and, if not, asking a clinical member of the team to do so.

   RATIONALE: *It is important that the patient thoroughly understand the reason for the procedure and all preprocedure instructions to be adequately prepared for the procedure.*

10. Give a copy of instructions and information to the patient and keep a copy in the patient record. Remind the patient to feel free to call the office at any time with any questions or concerns.

    RATIONALE: *Written instructions will back up what has been relayed to the patient and serve as a reminder for the patient.*

PROCEDURE 16-6 Scheduling Inpatient Surgical Appointments

WORK // DOC

Procedure Goal: To schedule an inpatient surgical procedure

OSHA Guidelines: This procedure does not involve exposure to blood, body fluids, or tissue.

Materials: Patient medical record and progress note form, calendar, telephone, pen

Method:

1. Obtain detailed information regarding the procedure to be performed from the surgeon and patient medical record. Information should include the name of the procedure to be performed, the amount of time the inpatient surgical suite will be needed, and the reason (diagnosis) for the procedure.

   RATIONALE: *Without this information, you will be unable to efficiently book the required appointment.*

2. From the patient's medical record, you will need the patient's full name, DOB, allergies, current medications, address, phone number, and insurance information.

   RATIONALE: *This information will be needed by the facility booking the procedure.*

3. Place a call to the appropriate surgical unit at the requested hospital. Have the name of the surgeon, assistant, or PA (if used) available, as well as the patient's and physician's preferred dates for the procedure.

4. When the appointment scheduler answers the phone, identify yourself, the practice, and the procedure you need to schedule, as well as the preferred dates.

5. When a date for the procedure is agreed upon by the patient, give the scheduler the patient's name, address, phone number, DOB, gender, and insurance information, including the prior authorization number if needed. Also give the patient's diagnosis as required for medical necessity.

   RATIONALE: *This information will be needed by the facility for booking and billing purposes.*

6. Inquire as to any preprocedure testing that may need to be done as well as any patient preparation required prior to the procedure, including patient arrival time.

   RATIONALE: *This information will need to be relayed to the patient for adequate preparation for the procedure.*

7. Confirm the appointment date and time prior to hanging up. If necessary, book any preprocedure testing for the patient and document these appointments in the patient instructions and appropriate office form(s) and/or within the patient's medical record.

   RATIONALE: *Always document any patient-related information in the patient's medical record.*

8. Provide the patient with written instructions from the physician as well as all information obtained while booking the appointment. The patient also should be informed that he should arrange for someone to drive him to and from the hospital.

9. Go over the written dates and instructions with the patient, asking the patient if there are any questions, answering them if possible, and, if not, asking a clinical member of the team to do so.

   RATIONALE: *It is important that the patient thoroughly understand the reason for the procedure and all preprocedure instructions to be adequately prepared for the procedure.*

10. Give a copy of instructions and information to the patient and keep a copy in the patient record. Remind the patient to feel free to call the office at any time with any questions or concerns.

    RATIONALE: *Written instructions will back up what has been relayed to the patient and serve as a reminder for the patient.*

LEARNING OUTCOMES	KEY POINTS
16.1 **Describe how the appointment book is key to the continuity of patient care.**	The appointment book or electronic scheduler and its matrix, when used properly, allow the office staff to respect the time of both the practitioner and the patient, by keeping an efficient and timely flow of patients throughout the day.
16.2 **Identify how to properly apply a matrix to an appointment book.**	To create a matrix, in either an appointment book or an electronic scheduler, you must know the usual schedule of provider availability to see patients as well as the times the provider (or practice) will not be open to see patients. The latter times should be X'd out with a short reason given as to why the time is unavailable. Follow the instructions for the electronic scheduler to block out the appropriate time frames.
16.3 **Compare different types of appointment scheduling systems.**	The most commonly used types of scheduling systems are open-hours, time-specified, wave, modified-wave, double-booking, cluster, and advance scheduling. It is also common for offices to use any combination of these as best suits each practice.
16.4 **Identify ways to organize and schedule patient appointments.**	When organizing and scheduling patient appointments, always maintain a positive, professional image as a representative of the office. The patient's status as a new or established patient should be considered as well as patient preference whenever possible. The goal is to accommodate the patient as much as possible while maintaining an efficient office schedule. Appointments should be confirmed through appointment cards, phone calls, e-mail notification (when permitted by the patient), and mailing of recall notices.
16.5 **Model how to handle special scheduling situations.**	Handling special scheduling situations requires critical thinking skills and creativity. Scheduling situations can arise if the practitioner is running late or if a patient requires an emergency appointment. Other scheduling problems also may include a patient who does not show, arrives late, or arrives on the wrong day. Documentation of any patient-related appointment issues should be recorded in the patient's medical record for legal purposes.
16.6 **Explain how to schedule appointments that are outside the medical office.**	Outside appointments may need to be made to laboratories, for radiology services, for in- and outpatient surgeries, for hospital stays, or for other diagnostic tests. In order to efficiently book such appointments, you will require the patient's demographic and health insurance information along with the procedure or service to be performed and the reason for the service. Preferred dates and times also should be noted. If referrals or prior authorizations are required, you also may be required to obtain these so that the procedure/service is eligible for payment by the patient's insurance plan.
16.7 **Implement ways to keep an accurate and efficient practitioner schedule.**	As the office medical assistant, your duties will include maintenance of the office schedule. The practitioner's schedule should ensure an even flow of patients throughout the day. Errors or overbooking may require you to rearrange appointments as necessary and to accommodate emergency appointments with minimal interruptions to the already-established schedule. If the schedule is consistently overbooked or patient wait time becomes consistently too long, it will be your responsibility to find the cause(s) and corrections for the issues and present these to the practitioner or office manager.

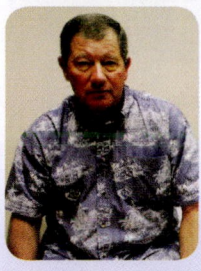

© McGraw-Hill Education

Recall John Miller from the beginning of the chapter. Now that you have completed the chapter, answer the following questions regarding his case.

1. What information will you need before you can book the cardiac catheterization?

2. Explain the process for scheduling this procedure.

1. (LO 16.1) The appointment book and its format are dependent on all of the following items *except*
   a. Practitioner preference
   b. Facilities available
   c. Patient need
   d. Practitioner habits
   e. Office location

2. (LO 16.2) When should you apply the matrix to your appointment book?
   a. On the first day of the new year
   b. When you first get it, if possible
   c. When scheduling appointments
   d. After appointments have been made
   e. At the beginning of every quarter

3. (LO 16.3) This type of scheduling groups similar appointments together on a certain day of the week or for certain times of day, which may be helpful with equipment and staffing.
   a. Time-specified
   b. Wave
   c. Open-hours
   d. Cluster
   e. Modified-wave

4. (LO 16.3) Which type of scheduling is also called *stream scheduling?*
   a. Time-specified
   b. Wave
   c. Open-hours
   d. Cluster
   e. Modified-wave

5. (LO 16.4) In terms of scheduling, the term "no-show" means
   a. The patient has passed away
   b. The patient is no longer coming to the office
   c. The patient does not call or show up for his scheduled appointment
   d. The patient comes to his appointment but then leaves before seeing the doctor
   e. The patient shows up early for his appointment

6. (LO 16.5) What is the best approach for handling the cancellation of an appointment by a patient?
   a. Send the patient a letter pointing out she canceled a necessary appointment
   b. Attempt to schedule another patient in the canceled slot
   c. Schedule other activities in those canceled slots
   d. Encourage the physician to take time off
   e. Remind the patient of the importance of follow-up care and if possible schedule her for another appointment while she is still on the phone

7. (LO 16.6) Why should the insurance company be contacted prior to scheduling an appointment outside of the office?
   a. To pay for services
   b. As a courtesy
   c. Because the test is physician ordered
   d. To give them the confirmation number
   e. To determine if the service is covered and obtain an authorization number

8. (LO 16.6) When scheduling an appointment for an abdominal CT scan, what steps should be taken?
   a. Have all information from the physician regarding the appointment and access to the patient's medical record
   b. If possible book the appointment when the patient is present to ascertain a convenient time for the patient
   c. After making the appointment, repeat the information, writing it down for the patient
   d. Give the patient oral and written instructions, answering any questions
   e. All of these

9. (LO 16.7) In what way(s) can the medical assistant assist a practitioner in managing the in-office schedule?
   a. Avoid overbooking
   b. Avoid underbooking
   c. Double-book appointments when possible
   d. Avoid overbooking and underbooking
   e. Avoid underbooking and double-booking when possible

10. (LO 16.7) All of these appointments take place outside of the medical office *except*
   a. House calls
   b. Nursing home visits
   c. Mouse calls
   d. Hospital visits
   e. ED visits

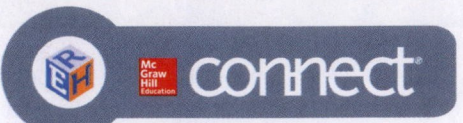

Go to CONNECT to see activities about *Scheduling an Appointment for a New Patient, Scheduling an Appointment for an Existing Patient, Blocking Appointment Times, Charting a No Show,* and *Locating an Existing Appointment.*

S O F T   S K I L L S   S U C C E S S

Recall John Miller from the case study at the beginning of the chapter.

1. Dr. Buckwalter asks you to book a cardiac catheterization for Mr. Miller. This is a day stay procedure performed at the local hospital by Mr. Miller's cardiologist. What information will you need to convey to Mr. Miller, and how will you do so?

2. Mr. Miller has a Medicare replacement plan that requires Dr. Buckwalter to obtain a prior approval for this procedure from the insurance plan. What type of information would you expect the insurance plan will need from you to issue this approval?

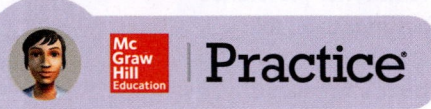

Go to PRACTICE MEDICAL OFFICE and complete the module Admin: Check Out - Work Task Proficiencies.

Insurance and Billing

CASE STUDY

Patient Name	DOB	Allergies
Sylvia Gonzales	09/01/19XX	Penicillin

Attending	MRN	Other Information
Alexis N. Whalen MD	341-73-792	HMO copay $25.00 for last visit is past due.

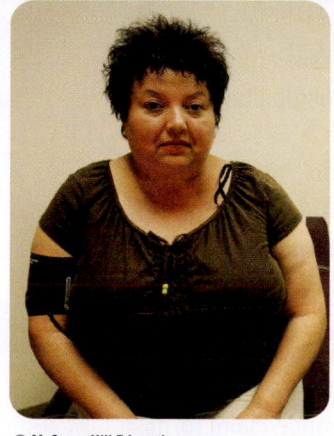

© McGraw-Hill Education

Sylvia Gonzales is a 51-year-old female with recently diagnosed Type 2 diabetes mellitus. She states that she has been faithful in taking the new medication the doctor has prescribed for her "sugar." She knows she is having a special "sugar test" done during her visit today. Her medications include Januvia 100 mg daily. Dr. Whalen has ordered a fasting blood sugar (FBS) and hemoglobin A_1C test to be done today. The FBS result is 106 and the hemoglobin A_1C result is 7.0. Mrs. Gonzales is encouraged to continue with her weight loss program through the local hospital's diabetes clinic and receives a return appointment for 3 months from now. Mrs. Gonzales has insurance through her husband, Juan (DOB 6/24/XX), as well as coverage through her own employer. Her husband's insurance is a traditional fee-for-service plan and her coverage is an HMO plan in which BWW Medical Associates participates.

Keep Sylvia Gonzales in mind as you study this chapter. There will be questions at the end of the chapter based on the case study. The information in the chapter will help you answer these questions.

McGraw-Hill Education **ACTIVSim**

LEARNING OUTCOMES

After completing Chapter 17, you will be able to:

17.1 Define the basic terms used by the insurance industry.

17.2 Compare fee-for-service plans, HMOs, and PPOs and explain the new concept of patient centered medical home.

17.3 Outline the key requirements for coverage by the Medicare, Medicaid, TRICARE, and CHAMPVA programs.

17.4 Describe allowed charge, contracted fee, capitation, and the formula for RBRVS.

17.5 Outline the tasks performed to obtain the information required to produce an insurance claim.

17.6 Produce a clean CMS-1500 health insurance claim form.

17.7 Explain the methods used to submit an insurance claim electronically.

17.8 Recall the information found on every payer's remittance advice.

KEY TERMS

allowed charge
benefits
birthday rule
capitation
clearinghouse
coinsurance
copayment
deductible
dependents
dual coverage
elective procedure
explanation of benefits (EOB)
explanation of payment (EOP)
fee-for-service

fee schedule
health maintenance organization (HMO)
patient centered medical home (PCMH)
preauthorization
precertification
preferred provider organization (PPO)
premium
remittance advice (RA)
resource-based relative value scale (RBRVS)
third-party payer
utilization review (UR)

VIII.C.1 Identify:

(a) types of third party plans

(b) information required to file a third party claim

(c) three steps for filing a third party claim

VIII.C.2 Outline managed care requirements for patient referral

VIII.C.3 Describe the processes for:

(a) verification of eligibility for services

(b) precertification

(c) preauthorization

VIII.C.4 Define a patient-centered medical home

VIII.P.1 Interpret information on an insurance card

VIII.P.2 Verify eligibility of services including documentation

VIII.P.3 Obtain precertification or preauthorization including documentation

VIII.P.4 Complete an insurance claim form

VIII.A.1 Interact professionally with third party representatives

VIII.A.2 Display tactful behavior when communicating with medical providers regarding third party requirements.

VIII.A.3 Show sensitivity when communicating with patients regarding third party requirements

X.C.8 Describe the following types of insurance

(a) liability

(b) professional (malpractice)

(c) personal injury

X.P.2 Apply HIPAA rules in regard to:

(a) privacy

(b) release of information

4. **Medical Law and Ethics**

a. Follow documentation guidelines

8. **Administrative Procedures**

a. Gather and process documents

b. Perform billing and collection procedures

(1) Payment procedures

c. Process insurance claims

(1) Differentiate between procedures of private, federal and state payers

(2) Differentiate managed care; i.e. HMO, PPO, IPA including referrals and precertification

11. **Career Development**

b. Demonstrate professional behavior

▶ Introduction

Insurance claims are a critical part of the reimbursement process. Accurate claims sent to payers ensure that medical practices receive the maximum appropriate payment for the services they provide. Patients are also concerned with their healthcare plans, asking, "How much will my insurance pay?" "How much will I owe?" "Why are this provider's fees different from my previous provider's fees?"

As the office medical assistant, you will handle questions like these every day. Not only must you correctly prepare healthcare claims, but you also will review each patient's insurance coverage, explain the provider's fees, estimate what services are covered by payers, prepare the claims to be submitted for these charges, and then understand the payment explanation

when it is returned with the payment from the payer. This chapter prepares you for these tasks by explaining the types of healthcare insurance plans available to patients today, how payers calculate their payments for services provided, and how to transmit complete and accurate claims. Finally—because, ultimately, the patient is responsible for the cost of the treatment received—you also will learn how to calculate the patient's financial responsibility for the treatment and his or her responsibility for care not covered by the insurance carrier.

▶ Basic Insurance Terminology   LO 17.1

The first step in understanding insurance is learning some basic terminology used by the insurance industry. Medical insurance, also known as health insurance, is a written contract in the form of a policy between a policyholder and a health plan (insurance carrier). The policyholder may also be called the insured, the member, or the subscriber. Under the insurance policy, the policyholder pays a **premium** (usually monthly)—the amount the policyholder pays the insurance company for the insurance coverage. In exchange, the health plan provides **benefits**—payments for medical services—for a specified time period. The policy may cover **dependents** of the policyholder, like a spouse or children. The contract also may specify a lifetime maximum benefit, which is a total sum the health plan will pay out over the patient's lifetime.

There are actually three participants under insurance contracts. The patient (policyholder) is the *first party* and the licensed practitioner who provides medical services is the *second party.* The patient often has a policy (written contract) with a health plan, the *third party,* who agrees to carry the risk of paying for those services and therefore is called a **third-party payer.**

When a patient seeks medical services and a practitioner agrees to treat the patient, the result is an implied contract between the patient and the practitioner. The patient then signs a written financial contract as the party legally responsible for paying for services. Any costs not covered by the third-party insurance company is then the responsibility of the patient.

Depending on the type of health plan, the policyholder may pay a **deductible**—a fixed dollar amount that must be paid by the insured for charges of providers, or "met," once a year in addition to the premium, before the third-party payer begins to cover medical expenses. The patient also may have to pay **coinsurance**—a fixed percentage of covered charges after the deductible is met. The coinsurance rate represents the health plan's percentage of the charge followed by the insured's percentage, such as 80-20. This means the insurance carrier pays 80% of allowed charges and the patient is responsible for the remaining 20%. If the patient belongs to a managed care health plan, like a health maintenance organization (HMO), instead of paying coinsurance the patient is responsible for a per-visit **copayment**—a fixed fee collected at the time of the visit. The patient goes to a practitioner who is a *preferred provider* for the insurance plan. The health plan pays the practitioner a set "contracted rate" agreed to by the plan and the practitioner for each service provided. The practitioner agrees to accept that payment, in addition to the patient's copayment, as payment in full for the service. Any balance on the patient's account after the copayment and insurance benefit have been received is adjusted off the patient's account, bringing the balance to zero.

Some expenses, like routine eye examinations or dental care, may not be covered under the insured's contract. These noncovered expenses are called *exclusions.* Although many insurance plans offer prescription drug benefits, be aware that such benefits often require the use of drugs listed on the plan's *formulary* (a list of approved brands). If a prescription for a nonformulary medication is written, the pharmacy or health plan case manager will usually contact the prescriber, asking if a substitution of a formulary drug can be made. If not, the patient may be responsible for a large portion, if not all, of the prescription's cost.

Many procedures and surgeries done today are "planned" procedures—that is, done at the convenience of the physician or surgeon and the patient. This type of procedure is known as an **elective procedure.** Many of these procedures are covered by third-party payers but only if certain rules prior to performance of these procedures are followed. **Precertification** is the process of confirming with an insurance company that a patient's insurance plan offers coverage for a specific procedure or service. When planning an elective procedure or service for a patient, most offices take this process one step further, by performing a preauthorization, also known as a prior authorization. A **preauthorization** is the receipt of confirmation from the patient's insurance plan that the proposed procedure or service will be considered a *covered service* because of the individual patient's specific circumstance that requires the procedure or service to be performed. If the insurance carrier agrees that the patient requires the procedure—in other words, it is *medically necessary*—the insurance carrier will issue a prior authorization number approving the need for the service or procedure. The prior authorization does not, however, mean that the insurance carrier agrees to pay for the service. This requires the next step of *predetermination,* in which the insurance carrier informs the provider of the maximum amount it will pay for the procedure to be performed. Once preauthorization is given, the documentation about the care given must "back up" the procedure codes submitted to the insurance carrier, or the charges may still be denied.

▶ Private Health Plans   LO 17.2

All insurance companies have their own rules about benefits and procedures. Most even have their own printed and/or online manuals that must be kept handy in the office for reference. Most insurance plans also have websites and toll-free numbers available for providers to answer questions. Do not be afraid to use these tools. If the first answer you receive does not sound correct, hang up and call back. You will more than likely get a different representative. Ask your question again. If you get the same answer the second time, it is more likely to be correct. Always get the name and extension number of the representative you speak with and document the call. Many companies also give you a call reference number in case a similar issue arises later. Keep all of this information with the patient's financial or insurance record for further reference. In order to refer back to the original call, you will need to give the insurance company that original reference number.

It is important for you to understand each insurance plan's rules and regulations, not only for the patient, but also so you can explain to the provider which plans require a referral or preauthorization for certain procedures. You must also understand (and explain to patients and providers) which plans require patients to utilize specific hospitals, surgical centers, or ancillary providers for labs and X-rays, in order for the services to be covered for payment.

In the United States, the majority of individuals with insurance are covered by group policies, usually through their employers. Some people (often the self-employed) have individual plans. Many others are covered under a government plan (Medicare, Medicaid, TRICARE), which will be discussed later. Still others—over 49.9 million Americans (according to the US Census Bureau figures for 2010)—have had no health insurance. The federal government through the Obama administration has changed that. On March 23, 2010, President Barack Obama signed into law a massive healthcare overhaul bill known as the Affordable Care Act, or ACA, also referred to as "Obamacare." The core of this new law, which has taken several years to fully phase in, is the extension of insurance coverage to all Americans who now lack healthcare coverage. Also included in the law are bans on the ability of private insurance carriers to impose lifetime limits on coverage, to deny coverage for preexisting conditions, and to cancel a policy when an insured person becomes ill. Parents in many circumstances can also keep their children covered under the family policy until age 26.

Although ACA has allowed many more Americans to have insurance, many plans have very high deductibles of $5,000 per year or higher. This means that although patients now have coverage, they will be liable for the cost of their care until their deductible is met. Most people who have high-deductible insurance choose the plan in order to afford the insurance, because premiums are lower. The front office staff will often be responsible for collecting the money patients owe the practice. We will talk more about patient collections in the *Patient Collections and Financial Management* chapter.

Traditionally, every insurance plan issued each of their providers an identification number, similar to the policy number given to each subscriber. Since the advent of HIPAA, although individual insurers may still issue individual ID numbers, every physician and provider who submits a claim to an insurance carrier must now use a specific provider number, known as a National Provider Identifier (NPI), from the Centers for Medicare and Medicaid Services (CMS). During the transition period, while providers obtained their NPIs, certain non-NPI numbers and two-character qualifiers (Table 17-1) were allowed. Now that all providers have an NPI, these non-NPI numbers and their identifiers are used only for certain payers who still require them.

TABLE 17-1	National Uniform Claim Committee (NUCC) Non-NPI Qualifiers
Qualifier	**Description**
0B	State License Number
1B	Blue Shield Provider Number
1C	Medicare Provider Number
1D	Medicaid Provider Number
1G	Provider UPIN Number
1H	CHAMPVA Identification Number
E1	Employer's Identification Number
G2	Provider Commercial Number
LU	Location Number
N5	Provider Plan Network Identification Number
SY	Social Security Number (may not be used for Medicare)
X5	State Industrial Accident Provider Number
ZZ	Provider Taxonomy Number

Fee Schedules and Charges

Physicians establish a list of their usual fees—charged to most of their patients most of the time under typical conditions—for procedures and services they frequently perform. These fees are listed on the office **fee schedule.** Figure 17-1 shows a sample of an office fee schedule.

Fee-for-Service and Managed Care Plans

There are two major types of health plans: traditional fee-for-service plans and managed care plans. **Fee-for-service** plans, the oldest and most expensive type, pay the practitioner a set amount for each service provided based on a fee schedule listed in the insurance policy, and the patient is responsible for the balance. The practitioner who provides the service controls the amount charged for services, but the insurance carrier controls the amount paid for each service.

Managed care organizations (MCOs) control both the financing and delivery of healthcare to policyholders. They enroll policyholders, and they also enroll licensed practitioners and other care providers to provide services for their members at reduced rates. This allows them to control all aspects of the care provided to their members, including the providers their members may see; the fees those providers may charge the MCO; and the copayment charge the provider may bill the patient. Many people who are insured through their employers are covered by some form of managed care plan.

Healthcare providers who enroll with managed care plans are called *participating providers.* They have contracts with the MCOs that stipulate not only the practitioner fees but also the credentials they must have and their responsibilities to the patients and to the MCO itself. Most MCOs also publish their participating providers' names in booklets and on their website so that policyholders can easily choose a participating provider from the list.

Managed care plans pay their participating providers in one of two ways—by either contracted fees or a fixed prepayment called **capitation.** In most plans, the primary care physician, or PCP, is reimbursed using the capitation method, which is payment of a fixed amount per patient who signs up with a particular PCP. The physician is paid a set amount per month for each patient enrolled in her practice, regardless of whether she sees that patient multiple times during the month or not at all. In addition to these capitated payments, the PCPs will be paid additional contracted fees for certain other services they provide for the patient such as labs and immunizations. In most managed care plans, specialists are paid in a negotiated fee-for-service manner. These contracted rates are usually less than those paid by private fee-for-service plans, but more than those paid by the government health plans. Providers and insurance carriers negotiate these contracts and fee schedules on a periodic basis.

As shown in Figure 17-2, more than half of all health plans are **preferred provider organizations (PPOs).** A PPO is a managed care plan that establishes a network of providers to perform services for plan members. In exchange for the PPO sending them patients, the practitioners agree to charge discounted fees. In most PPOs, plan members may also choose to receive care from providers outside the network. However, if they do, they are responsible for paying a higher percentage of the charges for

BWW Medical Associates, PC
Multi-Specialty Fee Schedule

SERVICES RENDERED	CPT	FEE	SERVICES RENDERED	CPT	FEE
Initial OV	99204	$100.00	EKG with Interp	93000	$80.00
Follow-up Visit	99214	$65.00	24-Hour Holter Monitor	93224	$300.00
LCMDM Consultation	99241	$120.00	Sigmoidoscopy	45330	$800.00
HCMDM Consultation	99245	$180.00	Spirometry	94010	$35.00
Hospital Admission	99223	$150.00	Throat Culture	87081	$25.00
Hospital Consultation	99253	$150.00	Flu Immunization	90724	$25.00
ER Visit	99284	$150.00	Pneumococcal Immunization	90732	$25.00
Hospital Visit	99232	$125.00	Allergy Injection, Single	95115	$25.00
Urinalysis w/ Micro	81000	$25.00	Allergy Injection, Multiple	95117	$60.00
Culture	87086	$45.00	Hemoccult x 3	82270	$30.00
CBC	85025	$60.00	Tetanus Injection	90718	$20.00
Venipuncture	36415	$35.00	Screening Mammography	77057	$425.00

FIGURE 17-1 The practice fee schedule shows the charge for each service provided by the practice.

Distribution of Health Plan Enrollment for Covered Workers, by Plan Type, 1988–2013

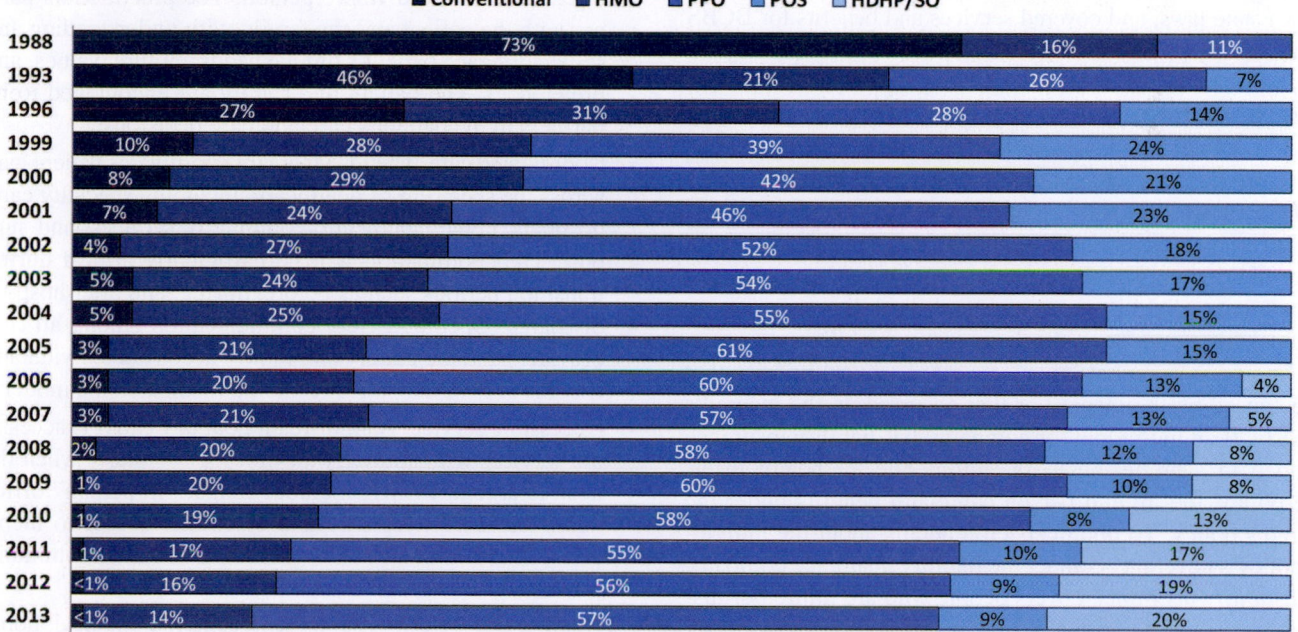

NOTE: Information was not obtained for POS plans in 1988. A portion of the change in plan type enrollment for 2005 is likely attributable to incorporating more recent Census Bureau estimates of the number of state and local government workers and removing federal workers from the weights. See the Survey Design and Methods section from the 2005 Kaiser/HRET Survey of Employer-Sponsored Health Benefits for additional information.

SOURCE: Kaiser/HRET Survey of Employer-Sponsored Health Benefits, 1999-2014; KPMG Survey of Employer-Sponsored Health Benefits, 1993, 1996; The Health Insurance Association of America (HIAA), 1988.

FIGURE 17-2 Distribution of health plan enrollment for covered workers, by plan type, 1988–2013.

these visits and may be subject to a deductible they would not be responsible for if they saw in-network providers.

Another common type of managed care system, covering 14% of those with private healthcare insurance, is a **health maintenance organization (HMO).** Physicians with HMO contracts are often paid a capitated rate, or they may be employees of the organization who are paid salaries. Patients who enroll in an HMO pay yearly premiums to maintain the insurance coverage and usually also pay a copayment, often $15 to $35, at the time of the office visit. No other fees are required for any covered service a member needs. In HMOs, patients must usually choose from a specific group of healthcare providers. If they seek services from a provider who is not in the health plan, the HMO does not pay for the care. Patients also pay for excluded services—those not included in the plan as covered services.

An important aspect of cost control used by managed care organizations is a process known as **utilization review (UR).** In this process, medical peers who have training similar to that of the practitioner providing the medical care review individual cases to be sure that all services provided were medically necessary and that there was appropriate use of medical resources. Should UR find that services were not medically necessary, payment can be denied at a loss to the practice, as the patient cannot be billed for services considered not medically necessary.

Commercial Payers

Blue Cross and Blue Shield Although many people think Blue Cross and Blue Shield (BCBS) is one large corporation, it is actually a nationwide federation of nonprofit and for-profit service organizations that provide prepaid healthcare services to BCBS subscribers. Each state's organization operates under its own state laws, and covered services and benefits for BCBS plans can vary greatly from state to state and plan to plan.

Private Commercial Carriers There are too many private commercial payers to list, and rules and regulations among the carriers vary as much as the covered services and the fees allowed for those covered services. Aetna, CIGNA, and Travelers are common commercial carriers.

In addition to health insurance, two other special types of insurance—liability insurance and disability insurance—are available to cover medical expenses. *Liability insurance,* also known as personal injury insurance, covers injuries that were caused by the insured or that occurred on the insured's property. If an individual (or company) has liability insurance included in a home, business, automobile, or health insurance policy, the injured person can claim benefits under the insured's policy. To obtain specific details about the individual policy's coverage, contact the liability insurance company.

Disability insurance covers people who are injured or disabled for nonwork reasons. It may be offered by an employer to employees at employee expense, or provided free of charge by an employer for its employees. Disability insurance may also be purchased privately by self-employed individuals. Disability insurance is not health insurance and does not cover medical expenses. When an insured person cannot work, and can provide the insurance carrier with documentation as to the medical reason he or she cannot work, the insurance company pays the insured a prearranged monthly amount to assist with the insured's normal daily expenses. There are two types of disability policies. Short-term policies offer coverage for shorter periods of time, usually 7 (consecutive) days to 6 months, and long-term disability policies may last for 1 year or more depending on policy stipulations.

Patient Centered Medical Home

Providers, insurers, patients, and US politicians continue to search for a better way to provide healthcare for all citizens. One model that has shown promise is the **patient centered medical home,** also known as *primary care medical home* (*PCMH*). The premise behind the patient centered medical home is to change the organization and delivery of primary care in America.

According to the Agency for Healthcare Research and Quality (AHRQ), the five functions and attributes of the PCMH are as outlined here.

- Comprehensive care. Comprehensive care is the goal and charge of the medical team responsible for meeting the majority of the patient's physical and mental health needs. These services include preventive care and wellness, as well as acute and chronic care. The team of providers involved might include any or all of the following practitioners: advanced practice nurses (APRN), physician assistants (PA), physicians, nurses, pharmacists, nutritionists, social workers, educators, and care coordinators. These providers may be in physical, "brick and mortar" locations or connected in a virtual fashion to link patients with providers and care within their communities.

- Patient centered. The goal of the PCMH is primary care oriented toward the whole person. The practitioners partner with the patient and the family with understanding and respect for each patient's unique needs, culture, values, and preferences. The patient and family are encouraged to be partners in the patient's care and care decisions.

- Coordinated care. The PCMH team coordinates patient care across the spectrum of healthcare, including specialty care, hospitals, home healthcare, community services, and support. The coordination will be particularly critical during transition periods such as before, during, and after hospital discharge. Open and clear communication among all care providers and the patient and family is considered vital and is at the core of the patient centered medical home model.

- Accessible service. A significant goal of PCMH is accessible services with shorter wait times, particularly when the need is urgent. PCMH includes longer "in person" office hours and 24/7 telephone and electronic access to members of the heathcare team, including alternate communication methods such as e-mail and telemedicine.

- Quality and safety. The patient centered medical home concept is committed to quality and continuous quality improvement by engaging in evidence-based medicine and clinical decision support tools to guide decision making with patients and families. The patient experience is measured and improved by gauging patient experience and satisfaction. Transparency of satisfaction is included by public sharing of safety and data improvement activities.

Many legislatures, providers, patients, and even insurers recognize that in many ways the healthcare system in the United States is "broken." Ideas and healthcare models such as the patient centered medical home is at the forefront of the movement to provide healthcare for everyone. For more information on PCMH, visit http://www.pcmh.ahrq.gov.

▶ Government Plans   LO 17.3

Government plans are generally designed to offer healthcare to retirees, low-income and disadvantaged individuals, and active or retired military personnel and their families. Some of these plans maintain many of the features of managed care plans.

Medicare

The largest federal program providing healthcare is *Medicare,* which provides health insurance for citizens aged 65 and older. Other people who are eligible for Medicare include people under the age of 65 who are dependent widows aged 50 to 65, the disabled, the blind, and workers of any age who have chronic kidney disease requiring dialysis or end-stage renal disease (ESRD) requiring transplant. Kidney donors are also eligible for Medicare. The Medicare program is managed by CMS. Two websites are available to obtain more information regarding Medicare: http://www.medicare.gov (supplies patients and beneficiaries with information) and http://www.cms.gov (includes provider and claims information for both Medicare and Medicaid). Medicare is divided into two main parts—Part A and Part B.

Part A Medicare Part A is the hospital benefit, which is billed by hospitals (or other healthcare facilities) and financed through contributions collected from the Federal Insurance Contributions Act (FICA) tax on income earned by workers and the self-employed. Currently, the FICA tax for workers is 6.2% (with the employer matching the 6.2%, for a total of 12.4%) and 12.4% for the self-employed up to a wage maximum of $110,000. You will learn more about FICA tax deductions in the *Practice Management* chapter. Medicare Part A pays most of the costs for the following individuals:

- Patients who are admitted as inpatients for up to the 90-day benefit period. A benefit period begins the day a patient is admitted to the hospital and ends when that patient has not been hospitalized or placed in a skilled nursing facility for a period of 60 continuous days after discharge.

  The 90-day benefit period is divided into two parts. The initial benefit period is 60 days; after the patient pays a deductible, hospital coverage is at 100%. After the first 60 days, the patient enters into a 30-day period called coinsurance days. During this 30-day period, the patient must pay an additional per-day payment, or coinsurance. If the hospital stay extends beyond the 30 coinsurance days, the patient may use up to 60 lifetime reserve days, which also include a per-day charge. It is important to note these 60 lifetime reserve days are not renewable. Once they are used up during the patient's lifetime, they are no longer available. If the patient is admitted to the hospital again for longer than 90

days, after the reserve days are exhausted, the patient will be responsible for all charges after the 90th day.

- A patient who has been admitted to a skilled nursing facility (SNF) after inpatient hospitalization. Coverage is for no more than 100 days in each benefit period—usually 1 calendar year.
- A patient who is receiving medical care at home
- A patient receiving hospice care either at home or in a hospice facility. Terminally ill patients with a prognosis (prediction) of 6 months or less to live are eligible for hospice care. Hospice programs provide *palliative care,* including pain relief and support for terminal patients and their family members.
- A patient who requires psychiatric treatment. Currently, Medicare covers only 190 days of psychiatric hospitalization in a patient's lifetime.
- A patient who requires respite care. In certain clearly and narrowly defined circumstances, Medicare provides for a respite, or short break, for the person who cares for a terminally ill patient at home. The terminally ill patient is moved to a care facility for the respite.

Anyone who receives Social Security benefits is automatically enrolled in Part A and does not have to pay a premium. Individuals aged 65 or older who are not eligible for Social Security benefits may enroll in Part A, but they must pay premiums for the coverage.

Part B Medicare Part B covers a portion (usually 80%) of the allowed charges for a wide range of outpatient procedures and supplies. For example, it covers licensed and credentialed provider services, outpatient hospital services, diagnostic tests, clinical laboratory services, and outpatient physical and speech therapy as long as these services are considered medically necessary. Individuals entitled to Part A benefits automatically qualify for Part B benefits. In addition, US citizens and permanent residents over the age of 65 are also eligible. Part B is a voluntary program; eligible persons may or may not take part in it. However, those desiring Part B must enroll because coverage is not automatic. The Medicare beneficiary has a 6-month time frame to apply, beginning 3 months prior to his 65th birthday until 3 months after it. If the deadline is missed, the beneficiary must wait until open enrollment, which is from January to March 31 of each year. If the Medicare B enrollment takes place more than 12 months after the initial enrollment period, there is a permanent 10% increase in the premium for each year the beneficiary was eligible to enroll but did not. Unlike Part A, Part B coverage is not premium free. Starting in 2007, the Medicare Part B premium is based on the beneficiary's income. The standard premium in 2015 of $104.90/month has not increased since 2013. This standard amount may increase or decrease depending on the individual's income, so it is important to check the CMS website yearly for accurate information. Each Medicare enrollee receives a health insurance card that lists the beneficiary's name, sex, effective dates for Part A and Part B coverage, and Medicare number. CMS assigns the Medicare number, which

TABLE 17-2 Comparison of Medicare A and B Premiums, Deductibles, and Benefits

Medicare Plan	Premium	Deductible	Benefit Period	Patient Coinsurance
Medicare A	None	Yes/per admission		
Hospitalization			Days 1–60	$0—Medicare pays 100%
			Days 61–90	$315/day
			Days 91–150 (includes 60 lifetime reserve days)	$630/day
			After 150 days	100%—no Medicare benefit
Skilled nursing facility (patient must have been hospitalized at least 3 days and be admitted to approved skilled nursing facility within 30 days of hospital discharge)			Days 1–20 Days 21–100 After 100 days	$0—Medicare pays 100% $157.50 100%—no Medicare benefit
Home healthcare (includes part time home nursing and aide services, durable medical equipment [DME], and supplies)			Unlimited, as long as Medicare criteria are met and services are *medically necessary*	$0 for home health service 20% of allowed charges for DME
Hospice services (palliative care for the terminally ill and family members)			Patient elects hospice care and physician certifies need for hospice	$0 except for outpatient medication and inpatient hospital care
Blood				First 3 pints per year
Medicare B (Outpatient Medical)	Yes	Yes/per year	January 1–December 31	20% of approved charges
Outpatient mental health				50% of approved charges
Outpatient laboratory				$0 of approved charges (Medicare pays 100%)
Home healthcare (includes part time home health nursing and aides, physical/occupational/speech therapies, DME supplies and services)				$0 for home care (Medicare covers 100%) 20% for DME
Blood				First 3 pints and 20% of approved charges
Ambulatory surgery				20% of predetermined charge after deductible

usually consists of the Social Security number followed by an alpha or alphanumeric suffix. The suffix indicates how the beneficiary is eligible for Medicare. The three most common suffixes are as follows:

- Suffix "A" is attached to the patient's own Social Security number because it was her income making eligible for Medicare.
- Suffix "B" is attached to the Social Security number of the spouse because the patient (who usually has not paid enough into the system to be eligible under his own number) is eligible because of his spouse's contributions.
- Suffix "D" is attached to the Social Security number of a spouse who is deceased. This benefit type has commonly been known as "widows' benefits."

See Table 17-2 for an overview of Medicare A and B premium, deductible, and benefit differences as of 2015.

Medicare Part C and Part D Medicare Part C, introduced in 1997, provides several plan choices for individuals called Medicare Advantage plans. These include PPOs, HMOs, private fee-for-service (PFFS) plans, special needs plans, and Medicare medical savings account (MSA) plans. The MSA plan started in 2007.

In 2003, the legislature passed the Medicare Part D prescription drug plan, and coverage began January 1, 2006. All Medicare beneficiaries can enroll in a prescription drug plan through the Medicare Prescription Drug plan, Medicare Advantage, or other Medicare plans, and through employers and unions. Figure 17-3 is the Medicare Part D coverage determination request form.

Medicare Plan Options Medicare beneficiaries can choose from a number of insurance plan options, including fee-for-service and Medicare Advantage plans consisting of different types of managed care plans.

Fee-for-Service—the Original Medicare Plan The Medicare fee-for-service plan allows the beneficiary to choose any licensed practitioner certified by Medicare. Each time the beneficiary receives outpatient services, a fee is billable. Medicare generally pays part of this fee and part is due from the beneficiary. Once the patient meets the annual deductible, if

Plan Name _____

Phone # _____

Fax # _____

Medicare Part D Coverage Determination Request Form

This form cannot be used to request:

➢ Medicare non-covered drugs, including barbiturates, benzodiazepines, fertility drugs, drugs prescribed for weight loss, weight gain or hair growth, over-the-counter drugs, or prescription vitamins (except prenatal vitamins and fluoride preparations).

➢ **Biotech or other specialty drugs for which drug-specific forms are required. [See <Part D plan website.>] OR [See links to plan websites at http://www.cms.hhs.gov/PrescriptionDrugCovGenIn/04_Formulary.asp]**

Patient Information			Prescriber Information		
Patient Name:			Prescriber Name:		
Member ID#:			NPI# (if available):		
Address:			Address:		
City:	State:		City:		State:
Home Phone:	Zip:		Office Phone #:	Office Fax #:	Zip:
Sex (circle): M F	DOB:		Contact Person:		

Diagnosis and Medical Information		
Medication:	Strength and Route of Administration:	Frequency:
☐ New Prescription OR Date Therapy Initiated:	Expected Length of Therapy:	Qty:
Height/Weight:	Drug Allergies:	Diagnosis:
Prescriber's Signature:		Date:

Rationale for Exception Request or Prior Authorization
FORM CANNOT BE PROCESSED WITHOUT REQUIRED EXPLANATION

☐ Alternate drug(s) contraindicated or previously tried, but with adverse outcome (eg, toxicity, allergy, or therapeutic failure)

➔ Specify below: (1) Drug(s) contraindicated or tried; (2) adverse outcome for each; (3) if therapeutic failure, length of therapy on each drug(s);

☐ Complex patient with one or more chronic conditions (including, for example, psychiatric condition, diabetes) is stable on current drug(s); high risk of significant adverse clinical outcome with medication change

➔ Specify below: Anticipated significant adverse clinical outcome

☐ Medical need for different dosage form and/or higher dosage

➔ Specify below: (1) Dosage form(s) and/or dosage(s) tried; (2) explain medical reason

☐ Request for formulary tier exception

➔ Specify below: (1) Formulary or preferred drugs contraindicated or tried and failed, or tried and not as effective as requested drug; (2) if therapeutic failure, length of therapy on each drug and adverse outcome; (3) if not as effective, length of therapy on each drug and outcome

☐ Other:_____ ➔ Explain below

REQUIRED EXPLANATION:_____

_____

_____

Request for Expedited Review

☐ REQUEST FOR EXPEDITED REVIEW [24 HOURS]

➔ BY CHECKING THIS BOX AND SIGNING ABOVE, I CERTIFY THAT APPLYING THE 72 HOUR STANDARD REVIEW TIME FRAME MAY SERIOUSLY JEOPARDIZE THE LIFE OR HEALTH OF THE MEMBER OR THE MEMBER'S ABILITY TO REGAIN MAXIMUM FUNCTION

Information on this form is protected health information and subject to all privacy and security regulations under HIPAA.

FIGURE 17-3   Medicare Part D coverage determination request form.

the patient sees a participating provider, Medicare pays 80% of approved charges directly to the provider and the patient is responsible for the remaining 20% and any disallowed charges. Providers who accept the Medicare-allowed charge as payment in full are known as those who "accept assignment." These providers cannot charge the patient more than this allowed charge, regardless of the original fee. A Medicare beneficiary may choose a provider who does not participate in the Medicare program and who does not accept assignment. In that case, the provider does not have to accept the Medicare allowable as payment in full and may charge the patient up to the "limiting charge"—usually defined as 115% of the nonparticipating allowable fee—as described by Medicare. This usually results in an increased out-of-pocket expense for the patient.

To help with the responsibility of the 20% coinsurance, individuals enrolled in the Original Medicare B Plan often buy additional insurance called a *Medigap* plan. While coverage of these plans varies from policy to policy, the core benefits common to all Medigap plans include coverage of the patient's Part B deductible and the 20% balance of all charges that are allowed by Medicare. However, if Medicare does not pay a claim, Medigap is not required to pay the claim, either. Although private insurance carriers offer Medigap plans, federal and state laws regulate coverage and standards. As for any insurance, the policyholder pays a monthly premium for Medigap insurance policies. A number of different options, labeled A through J, are available. Monthly premiums vary widely across the different plan levels as well as within a single plan level, depending on the insurance company selected. In 2009, CMS changed how claims were processed through Medicare contracting reform. At the forefront of these changes was the creation of Medicare Administrative Contractor (MAC) jurisdictions for claims processing. Table 17-3 outlines the jurisdictions for Medicare medical claims and the states contained within each. Durable medical equipment (DME) claims are separated from medical claims and are submitted to MACs set up specifically for DME. More information on all Medicare MACs can be found at http://www.cms.gov/Medicare/Medicare-Contracting/Medicare-Administrative-Contractors/MACJurisdictions.html.

Medicare Managed Care Plans Instead of the traditional Medicare A and B plans, many Medicare beneficiaries choose from a variety of managed care plans approved by CMS for their healthcare coverage. Medicare managed care plans charge a monthly premium and a small copayment for each office visit, but not a deductible. Like private payer managed care plans, Medicare managed care plans often require patients to select a primary care physician (PCP), who oversees and manages the patient's medical care through *referrals.* Usually, patients are also required to use a specific network of providers, hospitals, and other facilities. Some plans allow members the option of receiving services from providers outside the network, but the member's portion of the charges will be higher. Medicare MCOs offer coverage for services not reimbursed in the Original Medicare Plan, like physical examinations and immunizations.

Medicare Preferred Provider Organization Plan In the Medicare preferred provider organization (PPO) plan, patients pay less when they use doctors within a network, but they may choose to go outside the network for additional costs, such as a higher copayment or higher coinsurance. Patients do not need a PCP, and referrals are not required.

Medicare Private Fee-for-Service Plan Under a Medicare private fee-for-service plan, patients receive services from the provider they choose as long as Medicare has approved the provider or facility. This plan is operated by private insurance companies that have a contract with Medicare to provide services to Medicare beneficiaries. The private insurance company sets its own rates for services, and physicians are allowed to bill patients the amount of the charge not covered by the plan. A copayment may or may not be required.

Recovery Audit Contractor Program In 2008, CMS announced aggressive new steps to find and prevent waste, fraud, and abuse in Medicare. Since then, CMS has been working closely with beneficiaries and providers, consolidating its fraud detection efforts, strengthening its oversight of medical equipment suppliers and home health agencies, and launching the national recovery audit contractor (RAC) program. Contracts have been awarded to four permanent RACs, each of which audits one-fourth of the country. The RACs are designed to guard the Medicare Trust Fund by fighting fraud, waste, and abuse in the Medicare program. The recovery audit program's goal is to identify improper payments—overpayments or underpayments—made on claims of healthcare services provided to Medicare beneficiaries. Overpayments can occur when healthcare providers submit claims that do not meet Medicare's coding or medical necessity policies. Underpayments can occur when healthcare providers submit claims for a simple procedure but the medical record reveals that a more complicated procedure was actually performed. Healthcare providers subject to review by the RACs include hospitals, physician practices, nursing homes, home health agencies, durable medical equipment suppliers, and any other provider or supplier that bills Medicare Parts A and B. For further information, go to http://www.cms.hhs.gov and search for the recovery audit program.

TABLE 17-3	Medicare MAC Jurisdictions for Medical Claims
A/B MAC Jurisdiction Number	**States Included in Each Jurisdiction**
E	American Samoa, California, Guam, Hawaii, Nevada, and Northern Mariana Islands
F	Alaska, Idaho, Oregon, Washington, Arizona, Montana, North Dakota, South Dakota, Utah, and Wyoming
H	Colorado, New Mexico, Oklahoma, Texas, Arkansas, Louisiana, and Mississippi
5	Iowa, Kansas, Missouri, and Nebraska
6	Illinois, Minnesota, and Wisconsin
8	Indiana and Michigan
N	Florida, Puerto Rico, and US Virgin Islands
J	Alabama, Georgia, and Tennessee
11	North Carolina, South Carolina, Virginia, and West Virginia
L	Delaware, District of Columbia, Maryland, New Jersey, and Pennsylvania
K	Connecticut, New York, Maine, Massachusetts, New Hampshire, Rhode Island, and Vermont
15	Kentucky and Ohio

Medicaid

Medicaid, also run by CMS, is a health-benefit program designed for low-income, blind, or disabled patients; needy families; foster children; and children born with birth defects. Medicaid is a health cost assistance program, *not* an insurance program. The difference between an assistance program and a health insurance program is this: The government provides assistance programs to the recipient (or patient) at no charge, while the subscriber (or patient) pays for health insurance programs through premiums. The federal government provides funds to all 50 states to administer Medicaid (covering specified mandated services), and then each state adds its own funds (for additional optional services). Every state has a program to assist with medical expenses for citizens who meet its qualifications. Such programs may have different names and slightly different rules, but they provide basically the same assistance:

- Licensed, credentialed practitioner services
- Emergency services
- Laboratory services and X-rays
- Skilled nursing facility (SNF) care
- Early diagnostic screening and treatment for minors (aged 21 and younger)
- Vaccines for children

Accepting Assignment Any licensed practitioner who agrees to treat Medicaid patients also agrees to accept the established Medicaid payment for covered services as payment in full. Recall that this agreement is called accepting assignment. If the practitioner's fee is higher than the Medicaid payment, the patient cannot be billed for the difference. For services that Medicaid does *not* cover, however, the provider may bill the patient directly. Note that, as a federally funded assistance program, Medicaid is known as the *payer of last resort,* meaning that if both a private insurance plan and Medicaid cover a patient, the private plan must be billed before Medicaid. It is considered fraud to knowingly bill Medicaid if another insurance company also provides medical coverage for a patient.

Dual Coverage, or Medi/Medi Elderly or disabled patients who have Medicare and who cannot pay the difference between the charges submitted and the Medicare payment may qualify for Medicare and Medicaid. Formerly known as Medi/Medi, this is now more commonly known as **dual coverage.** In such cases, Medicare is the primary payer and Medicaid is the secondary payer. The patient with dual coverage is never billed for a balance unless a noncovered service is provided (and the patient is notified in advance in writing of this fact) or Medicare/ Medicaid states that the patient may be billed.

State Guidelines Medicaid benefits can and often do vary greatly from state to state. Eligibility is based on how much income the patient reported for the previous month. It is important to understand the Medicaid guidelines in your state

so that the Medicaid reimbursement to your office is prompt and trouble free. Here are some suggestions:

- Do not submit a claim to Medicaid without verification of Medicaid benefit eligibility. Doing so may constitute fraud. You should contact Medicaid to verify eligibility every time the patient is seen in the office.

- Ensure that the provider signs all claims, unless claims are submitted electronically (the provider's signature is kept on file). Send the completed and signed claims to the state's Medicaid-approved contractor (which pays on behalf of the state) or to the state department that administers Medicaid (for example, the state department of social services or public health). Check with your state Medicaid office if you are unsure where to send the claim.

- Unless the patient has a medical emergency, Medicaid often requires authorization before services are performed, which must be obtained from the state Medicaid office in advance. If the patient is seen on an emergency basis, it is not unusual for the Medicaid office to require that they be notified as soon as possible of any emergency treatment given to the patient. Not meeting these requirements can result in claim denial.

- Check the time limit (deadline) on claim submission with your state's Medicaid office. It can be as short as 2 months or as long as 1 year from the date of service. Claims submitted after this time limit will be denied or rejected. Any charges denied by Medicaid because they were submitted after the time limit must be adjusted from the account. The patient cannot be billed for the charges. The practice is expected to absorb the loss of income when charges are not submitted within the time frame allowed to be considered for payment.

- Treat Medicaid patients with the same professionalism and courtesy you extend to other private-pay patients. Simply because a patient qualifies for Medicaid assistance does not mean the patient is in any way inferior to those with private insurance.

TRICARE and CHAMPVA

The US government provides healthcare benefits to families of current military personnel, retired military personnel, and veterans through the TRICARE and CHAMPVA programs. TRICARE and CHAMPVA patients are most commonly seen at a military-related facility.

Run by the Defense Department, TRICARE (formerly known as Civilian Health and Medical Program for Uniformed Services, or CHAMPUS) is not a health insurance plan. Rather, it is a healthcare benefit for families of uniformed personnel and retirees from the Army, Navy, Marines, Air Force, Coast Guard, Public Health Service, and National Oceanic and Atmospheric Administration (Figure 17-4). TRICARE offers families three choices of healthcare benefits:

1. TRICARE Prime, a health maintenance organization
2. TRICARE Extra, a managed care network of healthcare providers families can use on a case-by-case basis without a required enrollment
3. TRICARE Standard, a fee-for-service plan

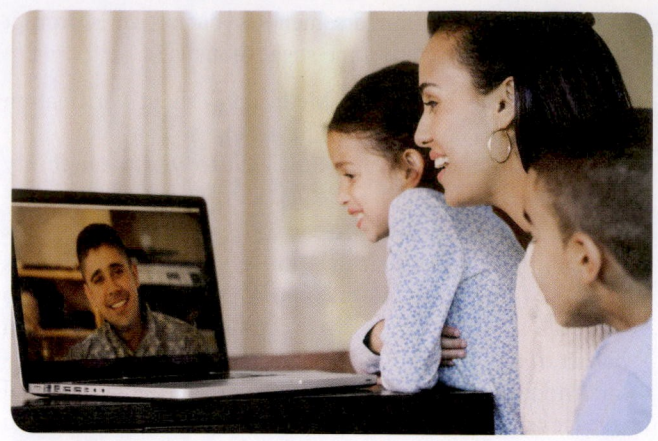

FIGURE 17-4 TRICARE covers healthcare services for family members of active military personnel as well as retirees.
© Ariel Skelley/Getty Images RF

Another program, TRICARE for Life, is aimed at Medicare-eligible military retirees and Medicare-eligible family members. TRICARE for Life offers the opportunity to receive healthcare at a military treatment facility to individuals aged 65 and older who are eligible for both Medicare and TRICARE.

Under TRICARE for Life, enrollees in TRICARE who are aged 65 and older can continue to obtain medical services at military hospitals and clinics as they did before they turned 65. As a general rule, TRICARE for Life acts as a secondary payer to Medicare; Medicare pays first and TRICARE pays the remaining out-of-pocket expenses.

CHAMPVA is the acronym for Civilian Health and Medical Program of the Veterans Administration and it covers the expenses of the families (dependent spouses and children) of veterans with total, permanent, service-connected disabilities. It also covers surviving spouses and dependent children of veterans who died in the line of duty or as a result of service-connected disabilities.

TRICARE and CHAMPVA Eligibility As with any healthcare plan, you must verify TRICARE eligibility. All TRICARE patients should have a valid identification card. To receive TRICARE benefits, eligible individuals must be enrolled in the Defense Enrollment Eligibility Reporting System (DEERS)—a computer database.

Eligibility for CHAMPVA is determined by the nearest Veterans Affairs medical center. Contact this center if any questions arise. Patients can choose the doctor they wish after CHAMPVA eligibility is confirmed.

Unlike Medicaid-participating providers who must accept all Medicaid patients once they agree to participate, TRICARE- and CHAMPVA-participating providers have the option of deciding whether to accept patients on a case-by-case basis. Make sure you know the policy of the providers in your office regarding this issue.

State Children's Health Insurance Plan

Originally enacted in 1997, the State Children's Health Insurance Plan (SCHIP) was reenacted in 2009 and is now more commonly known simply as CHIP. The plan allows states to provide health coverage to uninsured children in families whose incomes are too high to qualify for Medicaid but too low to afford private insurance. States have raised eligibility levels to provide coverage to more families. Check your state's requirements for this plan through its website.

Workers' Compensation

Workers' compensation insurance covers employment-related accidents and diseases. Federal law requires employers to purchase and maintain a certain minimum amount of workers' compensation insurance for their employees. Workers' compensation laws vary from state to state, but, in most states, this insurance includes these benefits:

- Basic medical treatment
- A weekly amount paid to the patient for a temporary disability, which compensates workers for loss of income until they can return to work
- A weekly or monthly sum paid to the patient for a permanent disability
- Rehabilitation costs to restore an employee's ability to work again
- Death benefits for survivors

Not all medical practices accept workers' compensation cases. Every procedure or treatment deemed necessary must be approved in order for payment to be made. Prior to treating a patient who states her care is related to a work-related illness or injury, call the employer to verify this information. When contacting the employer, speak to the office manager or human resources department. Be sure to get the name and extension of the person who verifies information for you. Give the verifier the patient's name and ask if the treatment is to be covered by workers' compensation. If the answer is yes, be sure to get the date of the original injury or illness and a brief description of the event causing the illness or ask the verifier if a workers' compensation case has been opened by the employer with the insurance carrier and obtain the case number. If a case has not been opened, ask the employer to report the incident. Until this report—known as the Employer's First Report of Illness or Injury—is received from the employer, the insurance carrier will not open a case, which means you will not be paid. Obtain the name, address, and phone number of the insurance carrier and carefully document this information. After completing the call to the employer and receiving permission to treat the patient, call the insurance carrier and verify that the employer has an active workers' compensation policy with them.

Records management of workers' compensation varies by state. If you see a patient privately and then she comes to you for a work-related illness or injury, be sure to keep the medical and financial records of the private care separate from the records of the care related to the workers' compensation case. Because the employer and insurer have contracted with the practitioner to provide care, they have the right to see all treatment and applicable financial records related to the workers' compensation claim without patient consent. It is up to the office to maintain the patient's confidentiality related to any care provided to her that is not related to the workers' compensation claim; keeping separate files makes it easier to do so.

Procedure 17-1, found at the end of the chapter, outlines the steps for verifying a patient's workers' compensation coverage.

▶ Payer Payment Systems   LO 17.4

As stated earlier, many traditional indemnity payers and even some MCOs base their reimbursement for medical care on fee schedules, but some payers, including Medicare, use differing formulas and processes for calculating provider payments. Let's look at some of these methods.

Medicare Payment System: RBRVS

Third-party payers set the fees they are willing to pay providers; these fees are often less than the physician's fee schedule. Most payers base their fees on the amounts Medicare allows because the Medicare method of fee setting takes into account important factors other than only the usual fees.

The payment system Medicare uses is called the **resource-based relative value scale (RBRVS).** The RBRVS establishes the relative value units for services, replacing the providers' consensus on fees (the "usual" or historical charges) with amounts based on resources (what each service really costs to provide).

An RBRVS fee has three parts and uses the formula RVU × GAF × CF. Listed below is an explanation for each part of this formula:

1. The national uniform relative value unit (RVU). The relative value of a procedure is based on three cost elements: the physician's work, the practice cost (overhead), and the cost of malpractice insurance. For example, the relative value unit for a simple office visit—say, to administer a flu shot—is much lower than the relative value for a complicated encounter, like planning a patient's treatment of uncontrolled diabetes.

2. A geographic adjustment factor (GAF). A GAF is used to adjust each relative value to reflect a geographic area's relative costs, such as office rent and utilities.

3. A nationally uniform conversion factor (CF). A uniform CF is a dollar amount used to multiply the relative values to produce a payment amount. It is used by Medicare to make adjustments according to changes in the cost-of-living index.

When RBRVS fees are used, providers receive considerably lower payments than when usual fees are used. Each part of the RBRVS—the relative values, the geographic adjustment, and the conversion factor—is updated each year by CMS. The Medicare fee schedule (MFS) is also published each year by CMS in the *Federal Register* at http://www.cms.gov/.

Payment Methods

Most third-party payers use one of three methods for reimbursing providers:

1. Allowed charges
2. Contracted fee schedule
3. Capitation

Allowed Charges Most payers set an **allowed charge**—the maximum amount the payer will pay any provider—for each procedure or service. The term *allowed charge* has many equivalent terms, including *maximum allowable fee, maximum charge, allowed amount, allowed fee,* and *allowable charge.*

The provider's usual charge is often greater than a plan's allowed charge. If the provider participates in the plan, only the allowed charge will be the basis for the payer's payment. The plan's contract with the provider governs whether the provider is permitted to bill a patient for the part of a usual charge the payer does not cover. Billing a patient for the difference between a higher usual fee and a lower allowed charge is called *balance billing.* Under most contracts, participating providers may not balance bill the patient. Instead, the provider must write off the difference between the fee charged and the allowed charge. The common term for this write-off is *adjustment.*

For example, Medicare-participating providers may not collect any amount greater than the Medicare-allowed charge. Medicare is responsible for paying 80% of this allowed charge after patients have met their annual deductible, and patients (or their secondary insurance) are responsible for the other 20%.

Here is an example of a Medicare billing. A Medicare-participating provider reports a charge of $200 for a service and the Medicare-allowed charge is $84. The provider must write off the difference between the two charges. The patient is responsible for 20% of the allowed charge, not of the provider's usual charge:

Provider's usual fee:	$200.00
Medicare-allowed charge:	$ 84.00
Medicare pays 80% of allowed charge:	$ 67.20
Patient pays 20% of allowed charge:	$ 16.80
Adjustment ($200 − $84):	$116.00

The total the provider can collect is $84.00. The provider must write off the difference between the usual fee and the allowed charge, or $116.00 in this example. Remember, in this example, it is assumed the patient has paid her annual deductible; otherwise, her coinsurance would be higher.

Contracted Fee Schedule Some payers, particularly PPOs, establish fixed fee schedules with their participating physicians. The plan's terms determine what percentage of the charges, if any, the patient owes and what percentage the payer covers. Participating providers can typically bill patients their usual charges for procedures and services not covered by the plan.

Capitation The fixed prepayment for each plan member in capitation contracts is determined by the managed care plan that initiates contracts with providers. The plan's contract with the provider lists the services and procedures covered by the capitation rate. For example, a typical contract with a primary care provider might include the following services:

- Preventive care, including well-child care, adult physical exams, gynecologic exams, eye exams, and hearing exams
- Counseling and telephone calls
- Office visits

- Medical care, including medical care services such as therapeutic injections and immunizations, allergy immunotherapy, electrocardiograms, and pulmonary function tests
- The local treatment of first-degree burns, the application of dressings, suture removal, the excision of small skin lesions, and the removal of foreign bodies or cerumen from the external ear

For instance, HMO B has a contract with Dr. Williams stating that her capitation rate is $150.00/month per patient. For each patient with HMO B who chooses Dr. Williams to be his or her PCP, Dr. Williams will receive $150/month, whether she sees each patient that month or not. When she does see a patient for, let's say an office visit and an EKG, she will receive the $150 and the patient's copay but no other reimbursement from HMO B, regardless of what her actual charges might be.

If a provider and patient decide a service is required that is not covered by the managed care plan, the provider often must notify the patient in advance that a service is not covered and state the fee for which the patient will be responsible. It is always a good idea to have the patient sign a waiver of liability—a notification in writing that he will be responsible for any noncovered charges, and the expected amount, prior to performing any such procedure.

Calculating Patient Charges

In addition to premiums, patients may be obligated to pay deductibles, copayments, coinsurance, excluded and over-limit services, and balance billing (only if allowed by the insurance plan).

All payers require patients to pay for excluded (noncovered) services. Providers generally can charge their usual fees for these services. Likewise, in managed care plans that set limits on the annual (or other period) usage of covered services, patients are responsible for usage beyond the allowed number. For example, if one preventive physical examination is permitted annually, additional preventive examinations are denied by the payer and become the patient's responsibility.

Communicating with Patients About Charges

When patients have office visits with a provider who participates in the plan under which they have coverage, like a Medicare-participating (PAR) provider, they generally sign an *assignment of benefits* statement. With this statement, the provider agrees to prepare and submit healthcare claim forms for patients, to receive payments directly from the payers, and to accept a payer's allowed charge. Patients are billed for charges that payers deny or do not pay. When patients have encounters with nonparticipating (nonPAR) providers, the procedure is usually different. To avoid the difficulty of collecting patient payments at a later date, practices may require the patient to either (1) assign benefits directly to the practice or (2) pay in full at the time of services.

Patients often call the office regarding statements they receive from the practice. For example, suppose a patient receives a bill for $100 from your practice. She calls to say that she has paid her deductible for the year, so her insurance company should have paid 80% of the charges. You call the patient's insurance company and, after confirming coverage,

learn that her deductible increased to $200 this year and she still has to pay $100 to meet her deductible. If she pays the $100 bill in full, her deductible will then be met. Alternatively, many insurance carrier websites now include a calculator that, based on the CPT (procedure) code and ICD (diagnosis) codes you enter, will calculate the payment to expect from the insurer, and the probable patient balance, as well as give you information as to the deductible amount and balance still owed by the patient. You now can call the patient to explain these facts to her.

To estimate patients' responsibility for charges, you should check with the payer to find out

- The patient's deductible amount and how much of the deductible is still owed, any coinsurance or copayment amounts that are the patient's responsibility, and whether the planned service or treatment is a covered service on the patient's plan.
- The payer's allowed charges for the services the provider anticipates providing. This will allow you to anticipate how much the payer will be paying the office for the service provided.

Patients should always be reminded of their financial obligations under their plans, including their obligation to pay charges that were denied by the insurance provider, according to practice procedures. The practice's financial policy regarding payment for services is usually either displayed on the reception area wall or included in the new patient information packet. The policy should explain what payments are required of the patient and when payment is due. For example, the policy may state the following:

- For unassigned claims: Payment for the practitioner's services is expected at the time of your appointment, unless you have made other arrangements with our practice manager.
- For assigned claims: After your insurance company processes your claim, you will be billed for any amount that is your responsibility. You are responsible for any part of the charges that are denied or not paid by the carrier. Payment for these charges is expected in full within 30 days of the statement date, unless prior arrangements have been made.
- For managed care members: Copayments must be paid prior to seeing the practitioner.

It is also good practice to notify patients in advance of the probable cost of procedures that are not going to be covered by their plan. For example, some private plans as well as Medicare do not pay for services like chiropractic care and some preventive services. Patients should be asked to sign a document known as a waiver of liability, which should specify why the service will not be covered and the cost of the procedure, *before* the service is provided.

The Advance Beneficiary Notice of Noncoverage, or ABN (CMS-R-131), is a notice given to Medicare beneficiaries to convey that Medicare is not likely to provide coverage in a specific case (Figure 17-5). "Notifiers" include physicians, providers (including institutional providers like outpatient hospitals), other licensed practitioners, and suppliers paid under Part B (including independent laboratories), and hospice providers and religious nonmedical healthcare institutions (RNHCIs) paid exclusively under Part A.

(A) Notifier(s):
(B) Patient Name: _____   **(C) Identification Number:** _____

ADVANCE BENEFICIARY NOTICE OF NONCOVERAGE (ABN)

NOTE: If Medicare doesn't pay for **(D)**_____ below, you may have to pay.

Medicare does not pay for everything, even some care that you or your health care provider have good reason to think you need. We expect Medicare may not pay for the **(D)**_____ below.

(D)_____	**(E) Reason Medicare May Not Pay:**	**(F) Estimated Cost:**

WHAT YOU NEED TO DO NOW:

- Read this notice, so you can make an informed decision about your care.
- Ask us any questions that you may have after you finish reading.
- Choose an option below about whether to receive the **(D)**_____ listed above.
   Note: If you choose Option 1 or 2, we may help you to use any other insurance that you might have, but Medicare cannot require us to do this.

(G) OPTIONS: Check only one box. We cannot choose a box for you.
❑ **OPTION 1.** I want the **(D)**_____ listed above. You may ask to be paid now, but I also want Medicare billed for an official decision on payment, which is sent to me on a Medicare Summary Notice (MSN). I understand that if Medicare doesn't pay, I am responsible for payment, but **I can appeal to Medicare** by following the directions on the MSN. If Medicare does pay, you will refund any payments I made to you, less co-pays or deductibles.
❑ **OPTION 2.** I want the **(D)**_____ listed above, but do not bill Medicare. You may ask to be paid now as I am responsible for payment. **I cannot appeal if Medicare is not billed.**
❑ **OPTION 3.** I don't want the **(D)**_____ listed above. I understand with this choice I am **not** responsible for payment, and **I cannot appeal to see if Medicare would pay.**

(H) Additional Information:

This notice gives our opinion, not an official Medicare decision. If you have other questions on this notice or Medicare billing, call **1-800-MEDICARE** (1-800-633-4227/**TTY**: 1-877-486-2048).

Signing below means that you have received and understand this notice. You also receive a copy.

(I) Signature:	**(J) Date:**

According to the Paperwork Reduction Act of 1995, no persons are required to respond to a collection of information unless it displays a valid OMB control number. The valid OMB control number for this information collection is 0938-0566. The time required to complete this information collection is estimated to average 7 minutes per response, including the time to review instructions, search existing data resources, gather the data needed, and complete and review the information collection. If you have comments concerning the accuracy of the time estimate or suggestions for improving this form, please write to: CMS, 7500 Security Boulevard, Attn: PRA Reports Clearance Officer, Baltimore, Maryland 21244-1850.

Form CMS-R-131 (03/08)   Form Approved OMB No. 0938-0566

FIGURE 17-5   Advance Beneficiary Notice of Noncoverage.
Source: Centers for Medicare and Medicaid Services.

The ABN must be verbally reviewed with the beneficiary or his or her representative and any questions raised during that review must be answered before it is signed. The ABN must be delivered far enough in advance that the beneficiary or representative has time to consider the options and make an informed choice. Employees or subcontractors of the notifier may deliver the ABN. ABNs are never required in emergency or urgent care situations. Once all blanks are completed and the form is signed, the beneficiary or representative receives a copy. In all cases, the notifier must retain the original notice on file.

The Claims Process: An Overview LO 17.5

From the time the patient enters a medical office until the time the insurer pays the practice for that office visit and associated services, several steps are carried out. In brief, the provider's office performs the following services:

- Obtains patient information
- Delivers services to the patient and determines the diagnosis and fee
- Records charges and codes, records payment from the patient, and prepares and submits the healthcare claim
- Reviews the insurer's processing of the claim, remittance advice, and payment

In offices that use electronic billing, medical assistants use the medical billing program to support administrative tasks such as:

- Gathering and recording patient information.
- Verifying patients' insurance coverage.
- Recording procedures and services performed.
- Recording applicable diagnosis and codes for each procedure performed.
- Filing insurance claims and billing patients.
- Reviewing and recording payments.

Billing programs streamline the important process of creating and following up on healthcare claims sent to payers and bills sent to patients. For example, a large medical practice with a group of providers and thousands of patients may receive a phone call from a patient who wants to know the amount owed on an account. With a billing program, the medical assistant can key the first few letters of the patient's last name and the patient's account data will appear on the screen. The outstanding balance can then be communicated to the patient. Billing programs are also used to exchange health information about the practice's patients with health plans. Using *electronic data interchange* (*EDI*), similar to the technology behind ATMs, information is sent quickly and securely between the medical practice and the insurance carrier.

Obtaining Patient Information

You will need certain information to be able to complete insurance claims and bill correctly for the patients of the medical practice where you work. This information is usually completed on a patient registration form, as discussed in the *Medical Records and Documentation* chapter.

Basic Facts When the patient first arrives, obtain or verify the following personal information:

- Patient Name (be sure to get the correct spelling of the patient's *legal* name)
- Current home address
- Current home telephone number
- Date of birth (month, day, and the four digits of the year)
- Social Security number
- Next of kin or person to contact in case of an emergency

Obtain the following insurance information:

- Current employer (may be more than one)
- Employer address and telephone number
- Insurance carrier and effective date of coverage
- Insurance group plan number
- Insurance identification number
- Name of subscriber or insured

Obtain the following release signatures:

- Patient's signature on a form authorizing release of information to the insurance carrier
- Patient's signature on a form for assignment of benefits

Eligibility for Services After verifying the patient's personal and insurance information, copy or scan the front and back of the patient's insurance card and obtain the release signatures for inclusion in the patient's financial record. Without the signed authorization to release information, you do not have legal permission to give the insurance carrier information regarding the patient's diagnosis and treatment. And without the assignment of benefits signature, the insurance carrier may send the payment for services to the patient instead of to the office. Also, verify the effective date of insurance coverage; the insurance carrier will not cover services performed before this date. To reduce possible payment problems, remember to inform the patient (in writing) before a service is performed if there is a possibility it may not be covered. By signing the waiver, the patient agrees to accept responsibility for payment, should the insurer not pay for the service. Be sure to retain the original waiver of liability in the patient's financial record and provide a copy to the patient for his records.

Obtaining Prior Authorization In today's medical office, you can often receive prior authorization for anticipated treatment(s) using the insurance carrier's website or over the phone. When calling the insurance company to request prior authorization, have the patient's insurance group number and ID number available, as well as the name, address, phone number, and date of birth for identification purposes. If the patient is covered under someone else's policy and is not the subscriber (insured), you should have the subscriber's name and birth date available and the relationship between the patient and the subscriber. You also will need the name and CPT (procedure) code of the planned procedure and the diagnosis and ICD (diagnosis) code to document medical necessity. A standard prior authorization request form is accepted by many payers for providers who do not have access to electronic technology to obtain prior authorizations. This standard form may be viewed in Figure 17-6 and is accepted by payers either via fax or US mail.

If you call the insurance carrier, ask for or select the prior authorization department. You will likely be speaking to a nurse case manager, who will take down the information regarding the planned procedure. She may give authorization over the phone; if so, carefully write down the authorization number and place it in the patient's chart for further reference. If the insurance plan website gives you the ability to obtain prior authorization online,

BWW

BWW Medical Associates, PC
305 Main Street, Port Snead YZ 12345-9876
Tel: 555-654-3210, Fax: 555-987-6543
Web: BWWAssociates.com

Prior Authorization Request Form

Instructions: Complete all applicable fields. Prior to completing this form, please confirm the patient's benefits and eligibility. Benefits for services received are subject to eligibility and plan terms and conditions in place at the time services are provided. For specific policies, please reference payers' specific websites.

URGENT REQUEST? ☐

Have you verified that pre-authorization is required? ☐ Yes ☐ No
You must verify pre-authorization by checking the pre-authroization list on the plan's website or by calling the number on the back of the member's card.

Is this request: ☐ New ☐ Authorization Extension ☐ Providing Additional Information
In case of authorization extension or providing additional information, please list pre-existing authorization number here: _____

SECTION 1: PATIENT INFORMATION

Last Name:	First Name:	MI:	DOB (MM/DD/YYYY):
PCP Name:	PCP Phone:		PCP Fax:

SECTION 2: INSURANCE INFORMATION

Insurance Name:	Member ID #:	Group #:
Insurance Address 1:	Insurance Address 2:	

City:	State:	Zip:	Phone:	Fax:

SECTION 3: PROVIDER INFORMATION

Please check one: *You are the* ☐ Requesting Provider ☐ Servicing Provider

Name:	Tax ID #:	NPI:
Address:	City:	State:	Zip:
For additional information, contact:	Phone:	Fax:

SECTION 4: PRE-AUTHORIZATION REQUEST

Anticipated Service Date:	Provider Name:
Provider Address	

City:	State:	Zip:

Service Type Requiring Authorization[1,2,3] (Check all that apply)

Ambulatory/Outpatient Services
☐ Surgery/Procedure (SDC)
☐ Infusion or Oncology Drugs

Ancillary
☐ Acupuncture
☐ Chiropractic
☐ IV/ART

Nutrition/Counseling
☐ Counseling
☐ Enteral Nutrition
☐ Infant Formula
☐ Total Parental Nutrition

Durable Medical Equipment
☐ Prosthetic Device
☐ Purchase
☐ Renal Supplies
☐ Rental

Outpatient Therapy
☐ Occupational Therapy
☐ Physical Therapy
☐ Pulmonary/Cardiac Rehab
☐ Speech Therapy

Inpatient Care Observation
☐ Acute Medical/Surgical
☐ Long Term Acute Care
☐ Acute Rehab
☐ Skilled Nursing Facility
☐ Observation

Dental
☐ Adjunctive Dental Services
☐ Endodontics
☐ Maxilliofacial
☐ Prosthetics
☐ Oral Surgery
☐ Restorative

Home Health/Hospice
☐ Home Health (Circle: SN, PT, OT, ST. HHA, MSW)
☐ Hospice
☐ Infusion Therapy
☐ Respite Care

Transportation
☐ Non-emergent Ground ☐ Non-emergent Air

☐ **Other-please specify:**

ICD Code(s) and Description(s)	CPT or HCPCS Code(s), Description(s), and Units OR # of Days	DME ONLY Line Item Cost
Primary:		$
Secondary:		$
Tertiary:		$

Please submit any clinical information with this form needed to prove medical necessity. Refer to specific guidelines of each plans medical policy.

[1] *Please attach plan specific supporting documentation.*
[2] *Note all services listed will be covered by the benefits in member's health plan product.*
[3] *This form does not replace payer specific prior authorizaton requirements.*

FIGURE 17-6 Standardized prior authorization request form from Healthcare Administrative Solutions.

you will complete the authorization form as directed, keying the required information in the fields as requested. The authorization will be given either immediately or within 24 hours, and an authorization will be sent to the office via secure e-mail or USPS. Keep this authorization in the patient's record as proof of receipt. As always, note the authorization number for insertion in block 23 of the CMS-1500 claim form when submitting the procedure for payment. Completion of the CMS-1500 claim form will be covered a bit later in the chapter. Procedure 17-2 at the end of this chapter outlines the steps for obtaining prior authorization.

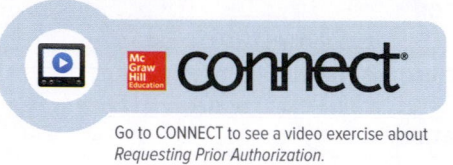

Go to CONNECT to see a video exercise about *Requesting Prior Authorization.*

Coordination of Benefits This refers to legal clauses in insurance policies that prevent payment duplication by restricting insurance company payments to no more than 100% of the covered benefits' cost. In many families, the husband and wife are both wage earners, so they and their children are frequently eligible for health insurance benefits through both employers' plans. In such cases, the two insurance companies coordinate their payments to pay up to 100% of a procedure's cost. A payment of 100% includes the policyholder's deductible and coinsurance or copayment. The *primary* plan is the policy that pays benefits first. The *secondary,* or supplemental, plan pays the deductible and coinsurance or copayment. A policyholder's primary plan is always his employer group health plan. If both a husband and wife have insurance through their employers, the husband's plan is his primary plan and the wife's insurance plan is her primary plan. To determine the primary plan for dependents who are covered by two or more medical plans, in many states, the **birthday rule** is followed. It states that the insurance policy of the policyholder whose birthday comes first in the calendar year is the primary payer for all dependents.

For example, if a husband's birthday is July 14 and his wife's birthday is June 11, following the birthday rule, the wife's insurance plan is the primary payer for their children and the husband's is the secondary payer. If a husband and wife were born on the same day, the policy that has been in effect the longest is the primary payer. Be sure to check with your state's insurance commission to see if the birthday rule applies in your state. Table 17-4 lists widely used coverage guidelines.

Delivering Services to the Patient

To ensure claims processing accuracy, any services the physician or other healthcare team members deliver to the patient in the office must be entered into the patient record, along with referrals to outside licensed practitioners.

Practitioner Services The licensed practitioner who examines the patient notes the patient's symptoms, a diagnosis, a treatment plan (including prescribed medications), and if and when the patient should return for a follow-up visit—all in the

TABLE 17-4	Guidelines for Determining Primary Insurance Coverage

- If the patient has only one policy, it is primary.
- If the patient has coverage under two plans, the plan covering the employee for the longest period of time is primary. However, if an active employee has a plan with the present employer and is still covered by a former employer's plan as a retiree or a laid-off employee, the current employer's plan is primary.
- If the patient is also covered as a dependent under another insurance policy, the patient's plan is primary.
- If an employed patient has coverage under the employer's plan and additional coverage under a government-sponsored plan, the employer's plan is primary. An example of this is a patient enrolled in a PPO through employment who is also covered by Medicare.
- If a retired patient is covered by the plan of the spouse's employer and the spouse is still employed, the spouse's plan is primary, even if the retired person has Medicare.
- If the patient is a dependent child covered by both parents' plans and the parents are not separated or divorced (or have joint custody of the child), the primary plan is determined by which parent has the first birth date in the calendar year (the birthday rule).
- If two or more plans cover the dependent children of separated or divorced parents who do not have joint custody of their children, the children's primary plan is determined in this order:
  1. The plan of the custodial parent
  2. The plan of the spouse of the custodial parent (if the parent has remarried)
  3. The plan of the parent without custody

medical record. After completing the visit, the practitioner writes the diagnosis, treatment, and sometimes the fee on an encounter form (superbill) (Figure 17-7) or charge slip (Figure 17-8) and instructs the patient to give you the superbill or charge slip before leaving. If the patient has a per-visit copayment, it is collected prior to seeing the practitioner or it is collected at the time the patient is leaving the office.

Medical Coding Today, the superbills used by most offices are preprinted with common procedures and procedure codes. If the charges are not preprinted, there is a space next to each procedure where the current charge may be inserted. For a procedure not listed on the superbill, a blank space at the bottom can be completed with the procedure name, procedure code, and charge. It is critical to verify that the procedure checked off on the form was actually completed by comparing the superbill to the medical record. This step ensures the patient is not inadvertently charged for a procedure that did not take place. Also, be sure the appropriate diagnosis codes are checked off, proving medical necessity for the procedures performed. If your office uses a charge slip instead of a superbill, you will need to translate the procedures listed on the charge slip into charge codes for the insurance carrier. This topic is covered in the *Diagnostic Coding* and *Procedural Coding* chapters.

Referrals and Authorizations for Other Services

You may be asked to secure authorization from the insurance company for additional procedures to be performed by one of

BWW Medical Associates, PC

305 Main Street, Port Snead YZ 12345-9876, Tel: 555-654-3210, Fax: 555-987-6543

☐ PRIVATE ☐ BLUECROSS ☐ IND. ☐ MEDICARE ☐ MEDI-CAL ☐ HMO ☐ PPO

PATIENT'S LAST NAME		FIRST		ACCOUNT #	BIRTHDATE / /	SEX ☐ MALE ☐ FEMALE	TODAY'S DATE / /
INSURANCE COMPANY		SUBSCRIBER			PLAN #	SUB. #	GROUP

ASSIGNMENT: I hereby assign my insurance benefits to be paid directly to the undersigned physician. I am financially responsible for non-covered services. SIGNED: (Patient, or Parent, If Minor) DATE: / /	RELEASE: I hereby authorize the physician to release to my insurance carriers any information required to process this claim. SIGNED: (Patient, or Parent, If Minor) DATE: / /

✔	DESCRIPTION	M/Care	CPT/Mod	DxRe	FEE	✔	DESCRIPTION	M/Care	CPT/Mod	DxRe	FEE	✔	DESCRIPTION	M/Care	CPT/Mod	DxRe	FEE
	OFFICE CARE						PROCEDURES						INJECTIONS/IMMUNIZATIONS				
	NEW PATIENT						Tread Mill (In Office)		93015				Tetanus/Diphtheria		90718		
	Brief		99201				24 Hour Holter (complete)		93224				MMR		90707		
	Limited		99202				Holter (setup only)		93225				Pneumococcal		90732		
	Intermediate		99203				Physician Interpret		93227				Influenza		90656		
	Extended		99204				EKG w/Interpretation		93000				TB Skin Test (PPD)		86580		
	Comprehensive		99205				EKG (tracing only)		93005				Antigen Injection-Single		95115		
							Sigmoidoscopy		45300				Multiple		95117		
	ESTABLISHED PATIENT						Sigmoidoscopy, Flexible		45330				B12 Injection	J3420	90782		
	Minimal		99211				Sigmoidos. , Flex. w/Bx.		45331				Injection, IM		90782		
	Brief		99212				Spirometry, FEV/FVC		94010				Compazine	J0780	90782		
	Limited		99213				Spirometry, Post-Dilator		94060				Demerol	J2175	90782		
	Intermediate		99214										Vistaril	J3410	90782		
	Extended		99215										Susphrine	J0170	90782		
	Comprehensive		99215				LABORATORY						Decadron	J0890	90782		
							Blood Draw Fee		36415				Estradiol	J1000	90782		
	CONSULTATION-OFFICE						Urinalysis, Chemical		81000				Testosterone	J1080	90782		
	Focused		99241				Throat Culture		87081				Lidocaine	J2000	90782		
	Expanded		99242				Occult Blood		82270				Solumedrol	J2920	90782		
	Detailed		99243				Pap Handling Charge		99000				Solucortef	J1720	90782		
	Comprehensive 1		99244				Pap Life Guard		88150-90				Hydeltra	J1690	90782		
	Comprehensive 2		99245				Gram Stain		87205								
	MCR Pts - use E/M codes						Hanging Drop		87210				INJECTIONS - JOINT/BURSA				
	Case Management		98900				Urine Drug Screen		80100				Small Joints		20600		
													Intermediate		20605		
	Post-op Exam		99024										Large Joints		20610		
							SUPPLIES						Trigger Point		20552		
													MISCELLANEOUS				

DIAGNOSIS:	ICD-9		Gout	274.0		C.V.A. - Acute	436.		Electrolyte Dis.	276.9		Herpes Simplex	054.9
Abdominal Pain	789.0		Asthma	493.90		Cere. Vas. Accid. (Old)	438		Fatigue	780.7		Herpes Zoster	053.9
Abscess (Site)	682.9		Asthmatic Bronchitis	493.90		Cerumen	380.4		Fibrocys. Br. Dis	610.1		Hydrocele	603.9
Adverse Drug Rx	995.2		Atrial Fib.	427.31		Chestwall Pain	786.59		Fracture (Site)	829.0		Hyperlipidemia	272.4
Alcohol Detox	291.8		Atrial Tachi.	427.0		Cholecystitis	575.0		Open/Close			Hypertension	401.9
Alcoholism	303.90		Bowel Obstruct.	560.9		Cholelithiasis	574.00		Fungal Infect. (Site)	110.8		Hyperthyroidism	242.9
Allergic Rhinitis	477		Breast Mass	611.72		COPD	492.8		Gastric Ulcer	531.90		Hypothyroidism	244.9
Allergy	995.3		Bronchitis	490		Cirrhosis	571.5		Gastritis	535.0		Labyrinthitis	386.30
Alzheimer's Dis.	290.1		Bursitis	727.3		Cong. Heart Fail.	428.9		Gastroenteritis	558.9		Lipoma (Site)	214.9
Anemia	285.9		Cancer, Breast (Site)	174.9		Conjunctivitis	372.30		G.I. Bleeding	578.9		Lymphoma	202.8
Anemia - Pernicious	281.0		Metastatic (Site)	199.1		Contusion (Site)	924.9		Glomerulonephritis	583.9		Mit. Valve Prolapse	424.0
Angina	413.9		Colon	153.9		Costochondritis	733.99		Headache	784.0		Myocard. Infarction (Area)	410.9
Anxiety Synd.	300.00		Cancer, Rectal	154.1		Depression	311.		Headache, Tension	307.81		M.I., Old	412
Appendicitis	541		Lung (Site)	162.9		Dermatitis	692.9		Migraine (Type)	346.9		Myositis	729.1
Arterioscl. H.D.	414.0		Skin (Site)	173.9		Diabetes Mellitus	250.00		Hemorrhoids	455.6		Nausea/Vomiting	787.0
Arthritis, Osteo.	715.90		Card. Arrhythmia (Type)	427.9		Diabetic Ketosis	250.1		Hernia, Hiatal	553.3		Neuralgia	729.2
Rheumatoid	714.0		Cardiomyopathy	425.4		Diverticulitis	562.11		Inguinal	550.9		Nevus (Site)	216.9
Lupus	710.0		Cellulitis (Site)	682.9		Diverticulosis	562.10		Hepatitis	573.3		Obesity	278.0

DIAGNOSIS: (IF NOT CHECKED ABOVE)

SERVICES PERFORMED AT: ☐ Office ☐ E.R. ☐	☐ CLAIM CONTAINS NO ORDERED REFERRING SERVICE	REFERRING PHYSICIAN & I.D. NUMBER

RETURN APPOINTMENT INFORMATION: 5 - 10 - 15 - 20 - 30 - 40 - 60 [DAYS] [WKS.] [MOS.] [PRN]	NEXT APPOINTMENT M - T - W - TH - F - S DATE / / TIME:	ACCEPT ASSIGNMENT? AM ☐ YES PM ☐ NO	DOCTOR'S SIGNATURE

INSTRUCTIONS TO PATIENT FOR FILING INSURANCE CLAIMS:	☐ CASH	TOTAL TODAY'S FEE	
1. Complete upper portion of this form, sign and date. 2. Attach this form to your own insurance company's form for direct reimbursement. **MEDICARE PATIENTS - DO NOT SEND THIS TO MEDICARE. WE WILL SUBMIT THE CLAIM FOR YOU.**	☐ CHECK # ___ ☐ VISA ☐ MC ☐ CO-PAY	OLD BALANCE / TOTAL DUE / AMOUNT REC'D. TODAY	

FIGURE 17-7 A superbill (encounter form) can be used as a charge slip and invoice and contains the information required to submit a health insurance claim.

DATE	DESCRIPTION–CODE	CHARGE	PAYMENT	CURRENT BALANCE

521-234-0001

BWW Medical Associates, PC
305 Main Street,
Port Snead, YZ 12345-9876

Tax ID No. 11-0004004

99205	Office Visit, New Patient	36425	Venipuncture	59025	NST
99215	Office Visit, Established Patient	57454	Colposcopy with Biopsy	54150	Circumcision
99213	Office Visit, Established, Brief	57511	Cryosurgery	58300	IUD Insertion
88155	Pap	58100	Endometrial Biopsy	57170	Diaphragm Fitting
84703	Urine Pregnancy Test	56600	Vulva Biopsy		

NAME _____ DX _____ No. 0005807

FIGURE 17-8 A charge slip shows the services performed for a patient and the charge for those services.

your providers at a facility outside of your office, such as a hospital or an ambulatory surgical center. If so, contact the insurance company to explain the reason for the procedure(s) and obtain an authorization number using the previously described procedures. Enter this authorization number in the billing program for inclusion on claims related to this procedure.

Frequently, you will be asked to arrange an appointment for required services, particularly if the practitioner believes they are urgently needed. For example, a physician may send a patient to a specialist's office for evaluation on the same day the patient visits your office. If the patient is a member of a managed care program, prior to making the required appointment, you will need to verify with the insurance plan that the insurance company allows the specialist requested. If so, a referral also may be needed. Depending on the insurance plan and your office capabilities, this referral, like prior authorizations, may be completed in writing or via the insurance plan's website. Without this referral, the specialist's charges may not be covered.

Patient Checkout

As stated earlier, everyone who receives services from a physician in the practice is ultimately responsible for paying the practice for those services. When the patient brings you the superbill at the end of the visit, you may do one or more of the following, depending on your practice's policy:

- Prepare and transmit a healthcare claim on behalf of the patient directly to the insurance company.
- Accept payment from the patient for the full amount. The patient will submit a claim to the insurance carrier for reimbursement. With offices increasingly submitting electronic claims, this option is becoming less common.
- Accept an insurance copayment or coinsurance from the patient and credit the account appropriately.

Specifics on the patient checkout procedure are covered in the *Patient Collections and Financial Management* chapter.

Right now, let's look at the processes involved in completing and submitting a healthcare insurance claim form.

▶ Preparing and Transmitting the Healthcare Claim LO 17.6

Healthcare claims are a critical communication between medical offices and payers on behalf of patients. Processing claims is a major task in most offices, and the numbers can be huge. For example, a 40-physician group practice with 55,000 patients served annually typically processes 1,000 claims (or more) daily!

Filing Limits In order for claims to be processed, they must be considered "clean"—free of errors. The first item the insurance carrier is going to review when receiving the claim is the date of service, as the time limit for timely filing begins on this date. Time limits for filing claims vary from company to company. For example, some insurers will not pay a claim unless it is filed within 60 or 90 days from the date of service, while others, like Medicare, allow up to a year for claim submission. In the typical medical practice, claims are transmitted within a few business days after the date of service. Many large practices file claims every day or several times a week to ensure that they never miss the filing deadline.

Electronic Claims Transmission

The electronic claim transaction is the HIPAA Healthcare Claim or Equivalent Encounter Information, commonly referred to as the "HIPAA (or 5010) claim" or simply the "837P claim" (P for physician). Its official name is *X12 837 Health Care Claim*. If you hear someone refer to a "5010 claim," he is speaking of the current format for electronic claims submission.

As of October 2003, Medicare mandated the X12 837 transaction for all Medicare claims except those from very small practices. Third-party payers may continue to accept paper transactions. Practices that elect to use paper claims must have two versions of their medical billing software: one to capture the necessary data elements for HIPAA-compliant electronic Medicare claims and another version to generate CMS-1500 paper claims. Also, under HIPAA regulations, only medical offices that do not handle any other HIPAA-related transactions may still use paper claims. Because most insurance carriers accept electronic claims and the process for submitting electronic claims has become more streamlined and cost efficient, even smaller offices are submitting electronic claims, which, in general, are paid within a week or two instead of the usual 6–8 weeks for paper claim reimbursement.

Preparing Electronic Claims The information entered on electronic claims is called data elements. Many elements, like the patient's personal and insurance information, are entered in the billing program before or at the time of the patient appointment, based on the patient registration form and on payer information and requirements. After the appointment is concluded, the claim is completed when the medical assistant keys the billing transactions—the services, charges, and payments—as detailed on the superbill (encounter form) into the billing claims software program. Once all the claims for the day are prepared, or often at a specified time each day, the software program is programmed to prepare claims for editing ("scrubbing") and transmission.

Follow these tips when entering data in medical billing programs:

- Enter data in all capital letters.
- Do not use prefixes for people's names, such as Mr., Ms., or Dr.
- Unless required by a particular insurance carrier, do not use special characters like hyphens, commas, or apostrophes.
- Use only valid data in all fields; avoid words such as "same."

The X12 837 transaction requires a lot of information, and all of it must be correct. Most billing programs or claim transmission programs automatically reformat data such as dates into the correct formats. These data elements are reported in five major sections:

1. Provider
2. Subscriber (the insured or policyholder)
3. Patient (who may be the subscriber or another person)
4. Claim details
5. Services

Not all data elements are required. Some are considered situational and are required only when a certain condition applies. When it does apply, that data element also becomes required. For example, if a claim involves pregnancy, the date of the last menstrual period is required. If the claim does not involve pregnancy, that date should not be reported.

One of the provider elements required for electronic claims is the provider *taxonomy code*—a 10-digit number representing a provider's medical specialty. Providers select the taxonomy code that most closely matches their education, license, or certification. The code is reported on claims because payment for some services is impacted by the specialty of the provider

performing them and by payers' contracts. For example, nuclear medicine is usually a higher-paid specialty than internal medicine. An internist who also has a specialty in nuclear medicine would report the nuclear medicine taxonomy code when billing for that service and use the internal medicine taxonomy code when reporting internal medicine claims.

Before the HIPAA mandate for standard transactions, some payers required additional records, like their own information sheet, when providers billed them. Some payers also used their own coding systems. The HIPAA Electronic Health Care Transactions and Code Sets (TCS) mandate means that all health plans are required to accept the standard claim submitted electronically, although the information required by each payer may vary. Be sure to follow each payer's specifications when submitting claims.

Other standard transactions also support the claim process—such as advising the office of claim status and payment—and apply to the treatment, payment, and operations (TPO) information exchanged between medical offices and health plans. Each electronic transaction has both a title and a number. Each number begins with X12—the number of the EDI format—followed by a unique number that stands for the transaction. Here are some examples of titles and numbers medical assistants may encounter while processing X12 837 healthcare claims:

Number	Title
X12 276/277	Claim status inquiry and response
X12 270/271	Eligibility inquiry and response
X12 278	Referral authorization inquiry and response
X12 835	Payment and remittance advice
X12 820	Health plan premium payments
X12 834	Enrollment in and withdrawal from a health plan

Paper Claim Completion

As stated previously, regardless of the office's billing method, the patient's demographic and billing information is usually updated at the patient's office visit and entered into the office medical billing program. Then the program is instructed to print the data on a CMS-1500 paper form (also called the CMS-1505 because of the form's 2005 update), shown in Figure 17-9. This claim may be mailed or faxed to the third-party payer.

Because of the HIPAA mandate regarding electronic claims submission, the paper claim is not as widely used as previously; however, the information it contains is very similar to the X12 837. The CMS-1500 contains 33 form locators, which are numbered blocks. Blocks 1–13 refer to the patient information and the patient and guarantor insurance coverage information. Blocks 14–33 contain information about the provider and the transaction information, including the patient's diagnoses, procedures, and charges.

The following instructions provide step-by-step guidance in completing a CMS-1500 paper form, which you can practice with Procedure 17-3, Completing the CMS-1500 Claim Form, found at the end of this chapter. Figure 17-10 is an example of a completed Medicare claim that includes a secondary payer.

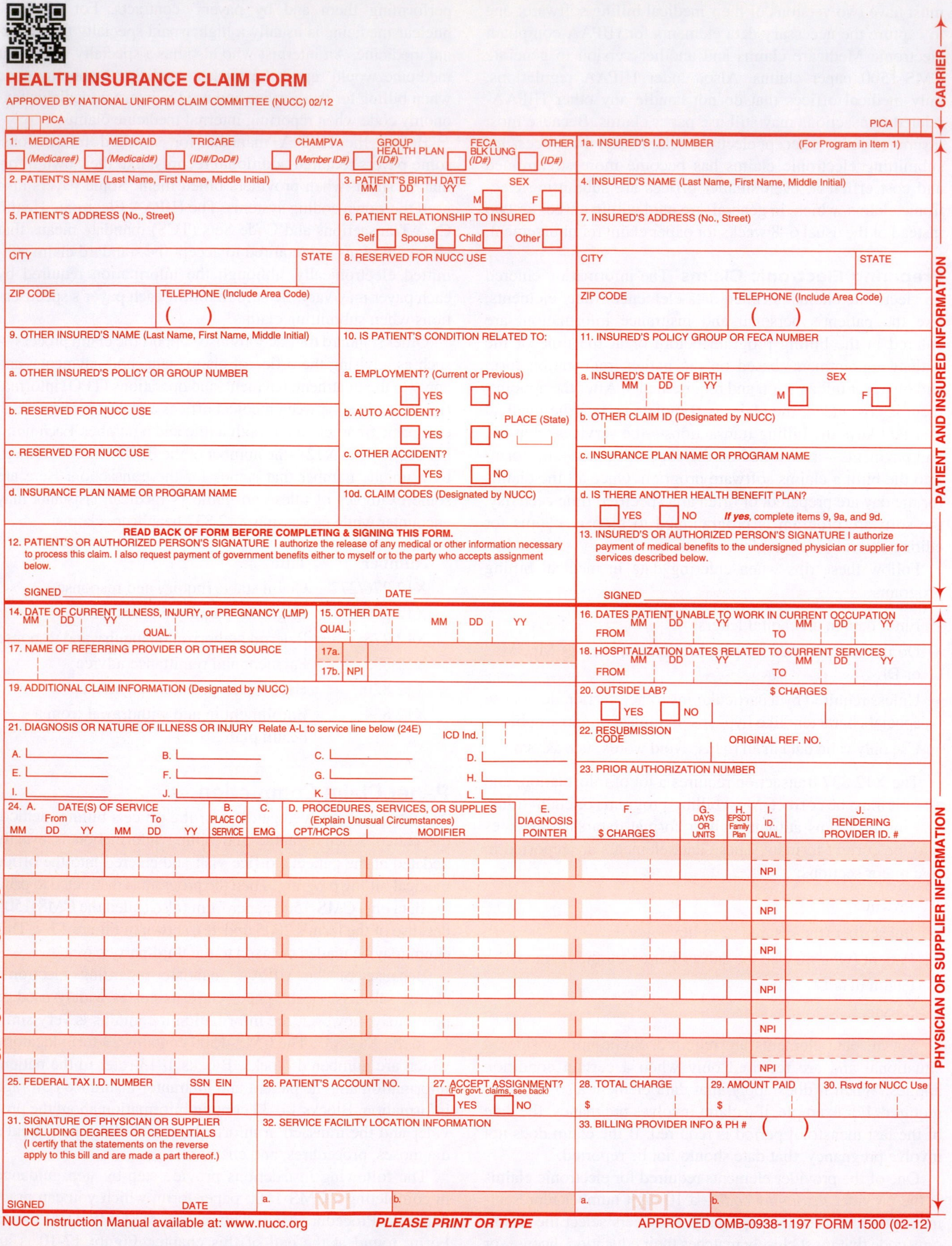

HEALTH INSURANCE CLAIM FORM

APPROVED BY NATIONAL UNIFORM CLAIM COMMITTEE (NUCC) 02/12

FIGURE 17-9 The CMS-1500 is the paper professional health insurance claim form.

HEALTH INSURANCE CLAIM FORM

APPROVED BY NATIONAL UNIFORM CLAIM COMMITTEE (NUCC) 02/12

PICA			PICA

1. MEDICARE [X] (Medicare#) **MEDICAID** [ ] (Medicaid#) **TRICARE** [ ] (ID#/DoD#) **CHAMPVA** [ ] (Member ID#) **GROUP HEALTH PLAN** [ ] (ID#) **FECA BLK LUNG** [ ] (ID#) **OTHER** [ ] (ID#)

1a. INSURED'S I.D. NUMBER (For Program in Item 1)
000112345A

2. PATIENT'S NAME (Last Name, First Name, Middle Initial)
WARD ELEANOR M

3. PATIENT'S BIRTH DATE 02 02 1929 **SEX** M [ ] F [X]

4. INSURED'S NAME (Last Name, First Name, Middle Initial)

5. PATIENT'S ADDRESS (No., Street)
305 MAIN STREET
CITY ASHFIELD **STATE** XY
ZIP CODE 12345 **TELEPHONE** (Include Area Code) ( )

6. PATIENT RELATIONSHIP TO INSURED
Self [X] Spouse [ ] Child [ ] Other [ ]

8. RESERVED FOR NUCC USE

7. INSURED'S ADDRESS (No., Street)
CITY **STATE**
ZIP CODE **TELEPHONE** (Include Area Code) ( )

9. OTHER INSURED'S NAME (Last Name, First Name, Middle Initial)
WARD ELEANOR M

a. OTHER INSURED'S POLICY OR GROUP NUMBER
XXM625743289

b. RESERVED FOR NUCC USE

c. RESERVED FOR NUCC USE

d. INSURANCE PLAN NAME OR PROGRAM NAME
MEDEX

10. IS PATIENT'S CONDITION RELATED TO:

a. EMPLOYMENT? (Current or Previous) YES [ ] NO [X]

b. AUTO ACCIDENT? YES [ ] NO [X] **PLACE** (State)

c. OTHER ACCIDENT? YES [ ] NO [X]

10d. CLAIM CODES (Designated by NUCC)

11. INSURED'S POLICY GROUP OR FECA NUMBER
NONE

a. INSURED'S DATE OF BIRTH MM DD YY **SEX** M [ ] F [ ]

b. OTHER CLAIM ID (Designated by NUCC)

c. INSURANCE PLAN NAME OR PROGRAM NAME

d. IS THERE ANOTHER HEALTH BENEFIT PLAN? YES [ ] NO [X] If yes, complete items 9, 9a, and 9d.

READ BACK OF FORM BEFORE COMPLETING & SIGNING THIS FORM.
12. PATIENT'S OR AUTHORIZED PERSON'S SIGNATURE I authorize the release of any medical or other information necessary to process this claim. I also request payment of government benefits either to myself or to the party who accepts assignment below.
SIGNED SIGNATURE ON FILE DATE

13. INSURED'S OR AUTHORIZED PERSON'S SIGNATURE I authorize payment of medical benefits to the undersigned physician or supplier for services described below.
SIGNED SIGNATURE ON FILE

14. DATE OF CURRENT ILLNESS, INJURY, or PREGNANCY (LMP) MM DD YY QUAL.

15. OTHER DATE QUAL. MM DD YY

16. DATES PATIENT UNABLE TO WORK IN CURRENT OCCUPATION FROM MM DD YY TO MM DD YY

17. NAME OF REFERRING PROVIDER OR OTHER SOURCE
DN WARNER RICHARD MD
17a.
17b. NPI 4235436543

18. HOSPITALIZATION DATES RELATED TO CURRENT SERVICES FROM MM DD YY TO MM DD YY

19. ADDITIONAL CLAIM INFORMATION (Designated by NUCC)

20. OUTSIDE LAB? YES [ ] NO [X] **$ CHARGES** 0 00

21. DIAGNOSIS OR NATURE OF ILLNESS OR INJURY Relate A-L to service line below (24E) **ICD Ind.** 0

A. J159 B. J449 C. D508 D.
E. F. G. H.
I. J. K. L.

22. RESUBMISSION CODE ORIGINAL REF. NO.

23. PRIOR AUTHORIZATION NUMBER

24. A. DATE(S) OF SERVICE From MM DD YY	To MM DD YY	B. PLACE OF SERVICE	C. EMG	D. PROCEDURES, SERVICES, OR SUPPLIES (Explain Unusual Circumstances) CPT/HCPCS	MODIFIER	E. DIAGNOSIS POINTER	F. $ CHARGES	G. DAYS OR UNITS	H. EPSDT Family Plan	I. ID. QUAL.	J. RENDERING PROVIDER ID. #
1	05 10 16	05 10 16	11		99213		A	80 00	1		NPI	1578597456
2	05 10 16	05 10 16	11		71020		A	120 00	1		NPI	1578597456
3	05 10 16	05 10 16	11		82805		B	65 00	1		NPI	1578597456
4	05 10 16	05 10 16	11		85025		C	45 00	1		NPI	1578597456
5											NPI	
6											NPI	

25. FEDERAL TAX I.D. NUMBER 222519813 SSN [ ] EIN [X]

26. PATIENT'S ACCOUNT NO. VAA00255

27. ACCEPT ASSIGNMENT? (For govt. claims, see back) YES [X] NO [ ]

28. TOTAL CHARGE $ 310 00

29. AMOUNT PAID $ 0 00

30. Rsvd for NUCC Use

31. SIGNATURE OF PHYSICIAN OR SUPPLIER INCLUDING DEGREES OR CREDENTIALS (I certify that the statements on the reverse apply to this bill and are made a part thereof.)
SIGNED Alexis N. Whalen, MD DATE 03/02/2015

32. SERVICE FACILITY LOCATION INFORMATION
a. NPI b.

33. BILLING PROVIDER INFO & PH # (555) 654-3210
BWW MEDICAL ASSOCIATES
305 MAIN STREET
PORT SNEAD XY 12345-6789
a. 1962410233 b.

NUCC Instruction Manual available at: www.nucc.org **PLEASE PRINT OR TYPE** APPROVED OMB-0938-1197 FORM 1500 (02-12)

FIGURE 17-10 Completed CMS-1500 claim form for a Medicare patient with secondary insurance coverage.

HIPAA laws are equally important when working with patient financial information and when working with patient PHI in the medical record. Remember, keep access to patient medical and financial records confidential at all times, including the information contained within a paper or electronic health or claim file.

Completing the CMS-1500 Form In this section, let's complete the CMS-1500 claim form block by block.

Here is how to complete blocks 1–13, the patient and insured's information:

Block 1 Place an X in the appropriate insurance box.

(Note: Each box is to the left of the insurance plan it represents.)

1. MEDICARE	MEDICAID	TRICARE	CHAMPVA	GROUP HEALTH PLAN	FECA BLK LUNG	OTHER
☐ (Medicare#)	☐ (Medicaid#)	☐ (ID#/DoD#)	☐ (Member ID#)	☐ (ID#)	☐ (ID#)	☐ (ID#)

Block 1a Insert the insured's ID number exactly as it appears on the insurance card.

For W/C claims enter the patient's employee ID. For property or casualty claims, enter the federal tax ID or SSN of the insured person or entity.

1a. INSURED'S I.D. NUMBER	(For Program in Item 1)

Block 2 Enter the patient's name in this order: last, first, middle initial (if used). Commas may be used to separate name components and a hyphen may be used between hyphenated last names. Do not use periods within the patient's name. If the patient is the insured, it is not necessary to complete the block, but check specific payer instructions before leaving it blank. Medicare requires this block to be completed.

2. PATIENT'S NAME (Last Name, First Name, Middle Initial)

Block 3 Enter the patient's birth date in the 8-digit format: XX/XX/XXXX. Place an X in the box representing the patient's sex.

3. PATIENT'S BIRTH DATE MM DD YY	SEX M ☐ F ☐

Block 4 Enter the insured's name in this order: last, first, middle initial (if used). For Medicare, leave blank; if TRICARE, enter the sponsor's name.

Commas may be used to separate name components and a hyphen may be used between hyphenated last names. Do not use periods within the patient's name.

4. INSURED'S NAME (Last Name, First Name, Middle Initial)

Block 5 Enter the patient's street address, city, state, and zip code. Do not use punctuation or symbols in the address fields. If the 9-digit zip code is used, include the hyphen. If the patient is the insured,

these fields may be left blank, but check individual payer guidelines before leaving them blank. Medicare requires these fields to be completed.

(Note: "Patient's Telephone" does not exist in 5010A1 [electronic claim]. The NUCC recommends that the phone not be reported.)

5. PATIENT'S ADDRESS (No., Street)	
CITY	STATE
ZIP CODE	TELEPHONE (Include Area Code) ( )

Block 6 Enter an X for the patient's relationship to the insured. If the patient is insured, use Self; if Medicare, leave blank; if TRICARE, enter the patient's relationship to the sponsor. If the patient is a dependent, but has a unique member ID number that is reported on the claim, report Self, since the patient, although a dependent, is uniquely identified by this ID number.

6. PATIENT RELATIONSHIP TO INSURED
Self ☐ Spouse ☐ Child ☐ Other ☐

Block 7 Enter the insured's street address, city, state, and zip code if the insured's name is inserted in block 4. Do not use punctuation or symbols in the address fields. If the 9-digit zip code is used, include the hyphen. For Medicare claims, leave these fields blank. For W/C claims, enter the employer's address. For property and casualty claims, enter the address for the person entered as the insured.

(Note: "Insured's Telephone" does not exist in 5010A1 [electronic claim]. The NUCC recommends that the phone not be reported.)

7. INSURED'S ADDRESS (No., Street)	
CITY	STATE
ZIP CODE	TELEPHONE (Include Area Code) ( )

Block 8 Reserved for NUCC Use (This field was previously used to report "Patient Status," which does not exist in 5010A1, so the field has been eliminated.)

8. RESERVED FOR NUCC USE

Block 9a–d *(Note: Block 9 is used for the **secondary** insurance information and block 11 is used for the **primary** insurance information. You may find it easier to complete blocks 11 and 10 first, and then come back to block 9.)*

9 If the patient has a *secondary* policy, enter the name (last, first, middle initial) of the insured

for this *secondary* policy. Commas may be used to separate name components and a hyphen may be used between hyphenated last names. Do not use periods within the patient's name.

9a Enter the *secondary* policy's group number or individual policy ID number. For a Medigap plan, enter the word "Medigap" before the ID number. No hyphens or spaces are allowed in group numbers.

9b This field was previously used to report "Other Insured's Date of Birth, Sex." The field has been eliminated because this information does not exist in 5010A1.

9c This field was previously used to report "Employer's Name or School Name." This information does not exist in 5010A1, so this field has been eliminated.

9d Enter the name of this *secondary* insurance plan. If this is a Medigap plan, enter the 9-digit CMS-assigned PAYERID.

| 9. OTHER INSURED'S NAME (Last Name, First Name, Middle Initial) |
| a. OTHER INSURED'S POLICY OR GROUP NUMBER |
| b. RESERVED FOR NUCC USE |
| c. RESERVED FOR NUCC USE |
| d. INSURANCE PLAN NAME OR PROGRAM NAME |

Block 10a–c Place an X in the correct Yes or No box in each area to indicate whether the patient's condition is related to employment, auto accident, or other accident. If auto accident is answered Yes, insert the two-letter abbreviation for the state in which the accident occurred.

(*Note: If any of these questions are answered yes, a workers' compensation, automobile, or other liability insurer may be responsible for the charges.*)

| 10. IS PATIENT'S CONDITION RELATED TO: |
| a. EMPLOYMENT? (Current or Previous)   ☐ YES   ☐ NO |
| b. AUTO ACCIDENT?   ☐ YES   ☐ NO   PLACE (State) |
| c. OTHER ACCIDENT?   ☐ YES   ☐ NO |

Block 10d Claim Codes (Designated by NUCC) When required by individual payers, condition codes approved by the NUCC may be inserted in this field. The condition codes approved for use on the 1500 claim form are available at http://www.nucc.org, under Code Sets.

| 10d. CLAIM CODES (Designated by NUCC) |

Block 11a–d (*Note: Block 11 is used for the* primary *insurance information. Many administrative assistants and billers find it easiest to complete block 11 before completing blocks 9 and 10.*)

11 Enter the policy or group number for the primary insurance plan. If Medicare is the primary payer, enter the word NONE here and leave 11a–d blank. (The word NONE tells Medicare it is the primary payer. If the word NONE is not placed here, Medicare assumes it is the secondary payer.) Do not use hyphens or spaces within a policy or group number.

11a For primary payers other than Medicare, enter the insured's date of birth (XX/XX/XXXX) and sex. If gender is unknown, leave blank.

11b Enter the "Other Claim ID" designated by the NUCC, if applicable. At this time, the only qualifier approved is "Y4," identifying any property or casualty claim number. The qualifier is entered to the left of the vertical dotted line and the claim number listed to the right of the vertical dotted line.

11c Enter the insurance plan name for the primary insurance.

11d Place an X in the appropriate box indicating whether there is a secondary payer. If Yes is chosen, blocks 9a–d will be completed; if No is chosen, blocks 9a–d will be left blank.

| 11. INSURED'S POLICY GROUP OR FECA NUMBER |
| a. INSURED'S DATE OF BIRTH   MM   DD   YY   SEX   M ☐   F ☐ |
| b. OTHER CLAIM ID (Designated by NUCC) |
| c. INSURANCE PLAN NAME OR PROGRAM NAME |
| d. IS THERE ANOTHER HEALTH BENEFIT PLAN?   ☐ YES   ☐ NO   *If yes,* complete items 9, 9a, and 9d. |

Block 12 The patient or authorized representative signs here, giving the provider permission to release his or her medical information to the insurance carrier.

Block 13 The patient or authorized representative signs here, authorizing the insurance carrier to send payment directly to the provider.

| READ BACK OF FORM BEFORE COMPLETING & SIGNING THIS FORM. |
| 12. PATIENT'S OR AUTHORIZED PERSON'S SIGNATURE I authorize the release of any medical or other information necessary to process this claim. I also request payment of government benefits either to myself or to the party who accepts assignment below.   SIGNED_____ DATE_____ | 13. INSURED'S OR AUTHORIZED PERSON'S SIGNATURE I authorize payment of medical benefits to the undersigned physician or supplier for services described below.   SIGNED_____ |

Now let's move on to blocks 14–33, the provider's information. In blocks 14-18, dates may be listed in either the 6-digit (MMDDYY) or 8-digit format, but once chosen, the format must be consistent within the claim.

Block 14 Enter the date of the current illness, injury, or pregnancy (last menstrual period [LMP]) using the 8-digit format. The qualifier entered to the right of the dotted vertical line identifies the date as LMP or other symptom:

431 Onset of Current Symptoms or Illness

484 Last Menstrual Period

14. DATE OF CURRENT ILLNESS, INJURY, or PREGNANCY (LMP)
MM | DD | YY
QUAL.

Block 15 Enter an "Other Date" related to the patient's condition or treatment. Previous pregnancies are not considered a similar illness. Leave blank if unknown. The identifying qualifier is listed first between the vertical dotted lines. Acceptable qualifiers include

454 Initial Treatment

304 Latest Visit or Consultation

453 Acute Manifestation or a Chronic Condition

439 Accident

455 Last X-ray

471 Prescription

090 Report Start

091 Report End

444 First Visit or Consultation

15. OTHER DATE
QUAL. | MM | DD | YY

Block 16 Enter the dates the patient is or was unable to work, using the chosen date format. (This information could signal a workers' compensation case if work-related.)

16. DATES PATIENT UNABLE TO WORK IN CURRENT OCCUPATION
FROM MM | DD | YY TO MM | DD | YY

Block 17 Enter the name of the referring, ordering, or supervising physician (first, middle, and last) with credential. To the left of the vertical dotted line, enter the qualifier to identify the provider:

DN—Referring Provider

DK—Ordering Provider

DQ—Supervising Provider

(*Note: Medicare will reject claims containing the provider's middle name or initial and/ or the credential. It requires neither.*)

Block 17a–b Some insurers require provider identifiers other than the NPI.

17a If required, enter the approved 2-digit qualifier from Table 17-1 with the provider identifier next to it; otherwise, leave blank. Medicare requires this field to be blank. Only the provider NPI is submitted to Medicare.

17b Enter the referring provider NPI number.

17. NAME OF REFERRING PROVIDER OR OTHER SOURCE | 17a. |
| 17b. | NPI |

Block 18 If applicable, enter the dates the patient was hospitalized during this claim, using the chosen date format for consistency.

18. HOSPITALIZATION DATES RELATED TO CURRENT SERVICES
MM | DD | YY MM | DD | YY
FROM TO

Block 19 Additional Claim Information (Designated by NUCC). To use this field, refer to the most current instructions from the public or private payer regarding use of this field and the qualifiers required. Otherwise, leave this field blank. Medicare uses this field for information related to chiropractic manipulations. See the Medicare Claims Processing Manual, Chapter 26, Section 10.4, for specific instructions for chiropractic claims. W/C programs also have very specific guidelines. Check with the individual W/C program involved for their instructions.

19. ADDITIONAL CLAIM INFORMATION (Designated by NUCC)

Block 20 If the office is billing for services provided by an outside laboratory, place an X in the Yes box and enter the amount being billed for the lab. Enter the laboratory name, address, and NPI in block 32. If only labs performed in your office are being billed, enter an X in the No box.

20. OUTSIDE LAB? $ CHARGES
YES NO

Block 21 Enter the multi-character ICD-10 codes indicating the patient diagnoses. (You will learn more about diagnosis coding in the *Diagnostic Coding* chapter.) Enter the codes in spaces A–L in descending order of importance. Do NOT use decimal points when inserting the diagnosis codes. The ICD indicator will be inserted in the upper right corner between the two vertical dotted lines, indicating which type of ICD codes is being used.

9—ICD-9 codes (replaced 10/1/15 with ICD-10 codes)

0—ICD-10 codes

21. DIAGNOSIS OR NATURE OF ILLNESS OR INJURY Relate A-L to service line below (24E) ICD Ind.
A. B. C. D.
E. F. G. H.
I. J. K. L.

Block 22 If required by the payer, enter the original reference number for claims being resubmitted. The resubmission code identifies the type of claim being submitted:

7 Replacement of prior claim

8 Void/cancel of prior claim

22. RESUBMISSION CODE ORIGINAL REF. NO.

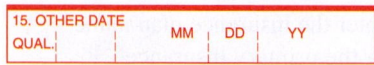

Block 23 If required, enter the prior authorization number received by the payer for the procedure performed (if prior authorization is required and not received, or if authorization is received but the number is not present on the claim, the claim will be denied). Hyphens and spaces are not allowed within an authorization number.

23. PRIOR AUTHORIZATION NUMBER

Blocks 24 A–J The six service lines here are used to enter the services provided to the patient. They are divided horizontally between shaded and nonshaded areas to accommodate supplemental information that may be required by the payer regarding the service provided. Check with individual payers regarding the use of these shaded areas. For 24I and 24J, the NPI is inserted in the nonshaded areas and the non-NPI information with its appropriate qualifier is inserted in the shaded areas. Follow individual payer requirements for use of these shaded areas. Remember that Medicare requires only that the NPI be submitted.

24A Enter the dates of service using the 6-digit format. If the service is provided on one date, enter the same date twice.

24B Enter the 2-digit place of service code from Table 17-5. Keep a listing nearby for handy reference.

24C EMG stands for emergency service indicator. If the insurer requires this information, and the service was provided on an emergency basis, enter Y for yes. If service was not provided on an

emergency basis or if the insurer does not require the information, leave blank. For Medicare, leave blank.

24D Enter the appropriate CPT or HCPCS code with modifier, one per line, to represent each service provided. (You will learn more about CPT and HCPCS coding in the *Procedural Coding* chapter.)

24E Enter the reference number A–L from block 21 to represent the diagnosis code associated with each procedure or service performed. This identifies the medical necessity for the service provided.

24F Enter the fee charged for each service provided.

24G Enter the days or units for each service provided. For instance, if the patient had three 15-minute (15 minutes = 1 unit) physical therapy treatments, enter 3. Even if the unit is one, enter the number 1.

24H EPSDT stands for Early, Periodic, Screening, Diagnosis, and Treatment. It is for Medicaid programs. If the procedure is related to EPSDT for a Medicaid patient, enter Y; otherwise, leave blank. If the program requires a reason code instead of a Y/N response, the following codes will be substituted for the Y/N response:

AV Available—Not Used (Patient refused referral.)

S2 Under Treatment (Patient currently under treatment for referred diagnostic or corrective health problem.)

ST New Service Requested (Referral to another provider for diagnostic or corrective treatment/scheduled for another appointment with screening provider for diagnostic or corrective treatment for at least one health problem identified during an initial or periodic screening service, not including dental referrals.)

NU Not Used (Used when no EPSDT patient referral was given.)

24I If the payer requires a non-NPI identifier, enter its qualifier (see Table 17-1) in the shaded area. If it is not required, leave blank. For Medicare, leave the shaded area blank.

24J If a non-NPI qualifier was entered in the shaded area, enter the appropriate non-NPI identifier in the shaded area. If it is not required, leave the shaded area blank. Enter the provider's NPI number in the nonshaded area. For Medicare, leave the shaded area blank.

TABLE 17-5	Place of Service Codes for CMS-1500 Form
Code	**Place of Service**
11	Office
12	Home
21	Inpatient Hospital
22	Outpatient Hospital
23	Emergency Department—Hospital
24	Ambulatory Surgical Center
25	Birthing Center
26	Military Treatment Facility
31	Skilled Nursing Facility
32	Nursing Facility
33	Custodial Care Facility
34	Hospice

24. A. DATE(S) OF SERVICE						B. PLACE OF SERVICE	C. EMG	D. PROCEDURES, SERVICES, OR SUPPLIES (Explain Unusual Circumstances)		E. DIAGNOSIS POINTER	F. $ CHARGES	G. DAYS OR UNITS	H. EPSDT Family Plan	I. ID. QUAL.	J. RENDERING PROVIDER ID. #
From			To					CPT/HCPCS	MODIFIER						
MM	DD	YY	MM	DD	YY										
1														NPI	
2														NPI	
3														NPI	
4														NPI	
5														NPI	
6														NPI	

Block 25 Enter the provider's Tax ID number. Place an X in the box identifying it as SSN (Social Security number) or EIN (employer identification number).

25. FEDERAL TAX I.D. NUMBER   SSN EIN
☐ ☐

Block 26 Enter the patient's account number (if used by your office). No hyphens or spaces are accepted in account numbers.

26. PATIENT'S ACCOUNT NO.

Block 27 Place an X in the Yes box to indicate the provider is accepting assignment on the claim (the check will be issued directly to the provider). Place an X in the No box to indicate the provider is not accepting assignment on the claim (the check will be issued to the patient).

27. ACCEPT ASSIGNMENT?
(For govt. claims, see back)
☐ YES   ☐ NO

Block 28 Enter the total charges for the claim by totaling charges from column 24F in lines 1–6.

Block 29 Enter any amount paid by a primary payer or patient on covered services. If this is a primary claim, leave blank. For Medicare claims, leave blank.

Block 30 Reserved for NUCC use. This block was used to enter the "Balance Due," which does not exist in 5010A1, so the field has been eliminated here.

28. TOTAL CHARGE   29. AMOUNT PAID   30. Rsvd for NUCC Use
$ $

Block 31 The physician or provider should sign and date the form here. Be sure the provider's credential is included in the signature.

31. SIGNATURE OF PHYSICIAN OR SUPPLIER
INCLUDING DEGREES OR CREDENTIALS
(I certify that the statements on the reverse
apply to this bill and are made a part thereof.)

SIGNED   DATE

Block 32 Enter the name and address of the facility providing the services if different from the billing provider. Post office boxes are not accepted for the facility or billing provider address and the zip code must consist of the full 9 digits given by the US Postal Service. No punctuation is used within the address, but a hyphen is included within the 9-digit zip code. If the billing provider and service facility provider are the same or if the service took place in the patient's home, leave block 32 blank.

32a   Enter the servicing provider's NPI.

32b   If required by the insurer, enter the servicing provider's appropriate 2-digit qualifier followed by the non-NPI identifier required. For Medicare, leave this field blank.

32. SERVICE FACILITY LOCATION INFORMATION

a.   NPI   b.

Block 33 Enter the billing provider's name, address, city, state, 9-digit zip code, and phone number. No punctuation is used within the address, but a hyphen is included within the 9-digit zip code. No PO Boxes may be used in this field.

33a   Enter the billing provider's NPI.

33b   If required by the insurer, enter the billing provider's appropriate 2-digit qualifier, followed by the non-NPI identifier required. For Medicare, leave this field blank.

33. BILLING PROVIDER INFO & PH # (   )

a.   NPI   b.

Although the basic information required to complete the CMS-1500 claim is the same for every provider and insurance plan, you will find that instructions for completing the claim form vary among insurance carriers. So follow the individual carrier's instructions carefully to obtain a clean claim with every submission. Procedure 17-3 provides an outline for completing the CMS-1500 claim.

▶ Transmitting Electronic Claims LO 17.7

Although hospitals and large practices have been using the X12 837 healthcare claims for quite some time now, smaller offices are still using paper claims for many of their claims submissions. Although even larger practices that have been using electronic claims processing consistently may be hesitant about choosing an electronic health records (EHR) software program, they will find health claims filing to be more efficient with EHR, as many of these programs can streamline the overall claims process. For example, with an EHR program, there is no need to repeatedly handwrite, key, or produce a computer-generated claim. The electronic claim template contains the instructions on placement of the information within the electronic claim. This information is pulled from the patient record automatically with a few of the medical assistant's simple keystrokes, which queue the claim for processing. At the time of transmission, all queued "clean" claims are transmitted with a few basic computer commands.

Practices handle electronic claims transmission—also called electronic media claims, or EMC—in a variety of ways. Some practices transmit claims themselves; others hire outside vendors to handle this task for them.

Three major methods are used to transmit claims electronically: direct transmission to the payer, clearinghouse use, and direct data entry.

Transmitting Claims Directly

In the direct transmission approach, medical offices and payers exchange transactions directly, using the necessary information systems—including a translator and communications technology—to conduct electronic data interchange (EDI).

Using a Clearinghouse

Many offices whose medical billing software vendors do not have translation software must use a **clearinghouse** in order to send and receive data in the correct EDI format. Clearinghouses can translate nonstandard formats into standard formats and many also "scrub" the claims "clean" prior to submission to ensure each claim meets coding and payer claim standards so the claim will be paid rapidly. Clearinghouses also apply software checks to claims they receive and transmit back reports of errors or missing information to the provider so claims can be corrected before they even reach the payer. To ensure that the standard format is compliant, the clearinghouse must receive all the required data elements from the physician, as clearinghouses are prohibited from creating or modifying data content.

Medical offices may use a clearinghouse to transmit all their claims, or they may use a combination of direct transmission and a clearinghouse. For example, they may send claims directly to Medicare, Medicaid, and a few other major commercial payers and use a clearinghouse to send claims to other, smaller payers.

Using Direct Data Entry

Some payers offer online direct data entry (DDE), which uses an Internet-based service into which employees can key the standard data elements. Although the data elements must meet the HIPAA standards requirements regarding content, EDI formatting is not required. Instead, the elements are loaded directly in the health plans' computer. One drawback is that each claim must be hand-keyed into the system each time the patient is seen, unlike the office billing software, which keeps the patient's prior information within its database.

Generating Clean Claims

Although healthcare claims, whether submitted electronically or by paper, require many data elements and are complex, it is often simple errors that prevent you from generating "clean" claims—those accepted for processing by the payer. Claims should be carefully checked for common errors (Table 17-6) before transmission or printing. Prior to submitting any insurance claim, make sure you have access to the insurance carrier's most recent claim submission manual. Following the instructions in that manual carefully will result in clean claims the majority of times.

If you receive a paper query from an insurance carrier or electronic notification of claim rejection for any reason (including those shown in Table 17-6), provide the missing or corrected information or, if required, submit a new claim with corrected information. For instance, if any facility information is missing, insert the missing information and submit a corrected claim. If a provider number is missing, obtain the correct provider number from the referring or treating physician's office and submit a corrected claim with the appropriate ID number. Do note that most errors are errors of omission and if claims are checked carefully prior to submission, most errors can be caught, resulting in clean claims the first time around.

Claims Security

Most medical offices use computer networks in which personal computers are connected to a local area network (LAN), so users can exchange and share information and hardware. The LAN is linked to remote networks like the Internet by a router that determines the best route for data (which include electronic patient data) to travel across the network. Packets of data traveling between the LAN and the Internet—like electronic claims—must usually pass through a firewall, a security

---

TABLE 17-6 Common Errors Preventing Clean Claims

- Missing or incomplete service or billing provider name, address, and identification for the services rendered, including invalid zip codes or state abbreviations
- Missing Medicare assignment indicator or benefits assignment indicator
- Missing part of the name or the identifier of the referring provider
- Missing or invalid subscriber or patient information, including misspelling of names
- Missing or invalid information regarding secondary insurance plans
- Missing payer name and/or payer identifier, required for both primary and secondary payers

device that examines information (for example, e-mails) that enters and leaves a network, determining whether to forward the information to its destination.

The HIPAA rules set standards for protecting individually identifiable protected health information (PHI) when it is maintained or transmitted electronically. Medical offices use a number of security measures to protect the confidentiality, integrity, and availability of this information, including

- Access control, passwords, and log files to keep intruders out.
- Backups (saved copies of files) to replace items after damage to the computer.
- Security policies to handle violations that do occur.

Refer to the *Legal and Ethical Issues* chapter for further information regarding all HIPAA and confidentiality standards, including those for electronic transmissions.

▶ Insurer Processing Claims and Payments

LO 17.8

The Claims Register

If claims are transmitted electronically, the billing program or the clearinghouse will create a log of transmitted claims to allow you to track the progress of the submitted charges. If your office submits paper claims, you should create and maintain a claims register like the one shown in Figure 17-11. Procedure 17-4, at the end of the chapter, outlines the steps for creating a claims register.

Your transmitted claim for payment will undergo a number of reviews by the insurer. Currently, much of the review process occurs electronically.

Review for Medical Necessity

The insurance carrier reviews each claim to determine whether the procedures provided and the accompanying diagnoses are compatible and whether the treatment is medically necessary, as explained further in the *Diagnostic Coding* and *Procedural Coding* chapters.

Review for Allowable Benefits

The claims department also compares the fees the provider has charged with the benefits provided by the patient's health insurance policy. This review determines the amount of deductible and/or coinsurance the patient owes. The amount the patient owes the practice is known as patient liability.

Payment and Remittance Advice

After reviewing and accepting the claim, the insurer pays a benefit, either to the practice or to the subscriber (patient), depending on whether an assignment of benefits was signed and on the policy of the insurance carrier. With the payment, the insurer sends a **remittance advice (RA)** or an **explanation of payment (EOP),** sometimes called an **explanation of benefits (EOB).** If the payment is made electronically, the RA will also be received electronically. In this case, the RA is known as an electronic remittance advice (ERA) or electronic explanation of benefits (EEOB). A patient who receives the payment receives an RA summary containing only his information and the practice receives a practice RA that typically contains information for multiple patients at one time. Each insurance plan has its own EOP (RA) format and you will learn those of your office's most popular payers. Because many patients may be included on each EOP (RA), you may find it easiest to use a ruler to read each line of a paper RA and check off each line as you credit each patient's account. If a secondary insurance carrier requires a copy of a patient's primary insurance EOP, remember to black out any information on the EOP that does not pertain to the patient information required by the insurance carrier, to protect the information of the other patients on the EOB. The RA or the EOP explains the medical claim. For each service submitted to an insurer, the RA or EOP form gives the following information:

- Name of the insured and identification number
- Patient name
- Claim number
- Date of service, place of service, and procedure code for service provided
- Amount billed by the practice

Patient Name	Insurance Company	Claim Filing		Insurance Response Pd, Denied, Rejct, Suspd, Info Req		Date Resubmitted	Payment		Patient Balance	Date Patient Billed
		Date	Amount		Date		Date	Amount		
Smith, Peter	Aetna	1/4/XX	182 50	Info Req	1/5/XX	1/6/XX	1/25/XX	85 25	25.12	2/2/XX

FIGURE 17-11 After submitting each claim, track it in an insurance claims register similar to this one.

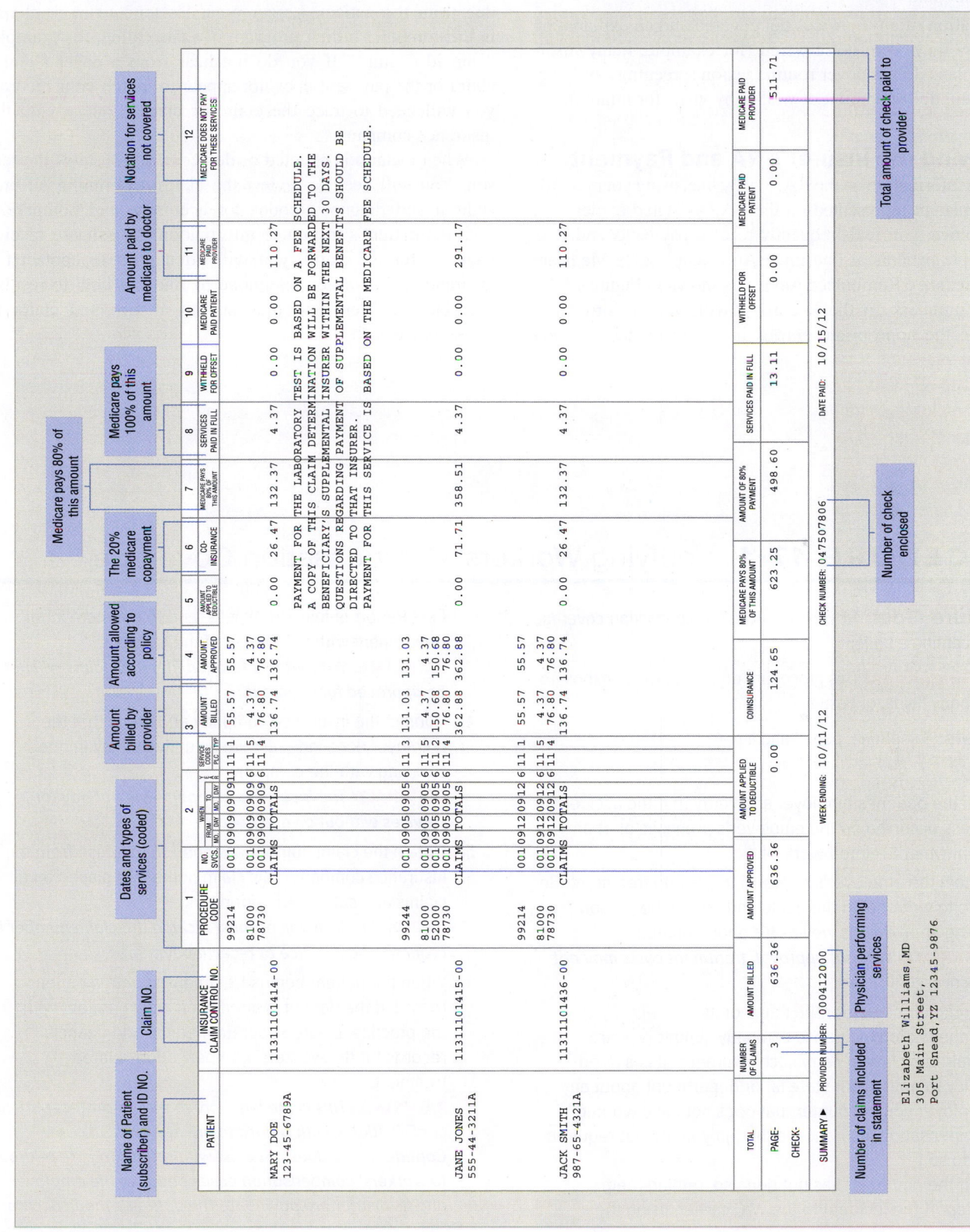

FIGURE 17-12 The payer sends a remittance advice to explain payment made to the medical practice.

- Amount allowed
- Amount of patient liability (coinsurance, copayment, deductible, or noncovered services)
- Amount paid
- A notation of any services not covered and an explanation of why they were not covered (for example, many insurance plans do not cover routine vision screenings and only a certain dollar amount of well-baby visits for infants)

Reviewing the Insurer's RA and Payment

Verify all information on the RA, line by line, using your records for each patient represented on the RA. As stated earlier, in a large practice, you will frequently receive payments and RAs for multiple patients at one time. An example of a Medicare RA, or Medicare Remittance Advice, is shown in Figure 17-12.

If all numbers on the RA agree with your records, you can make the appropriate entries in the insurance tracking log for claims paid. In a small practice, the insurance tracking log is used to track filed claims, using such information as patient name, date the claim was filed, services the claim reflects, notations about the claim results, and any balance due from the patient. Larger practices tend to track claims in the computer billing program in a file called, for example, "Unpaid Claims." If you do not hear from a payer about a claim or the payment does not appear to match your records, you will need to trace the claim or place a query with the insurance company.

When a claim is rejected or denied, the RA states the reason. You will need to review the claim, examining all procedural and diagnosis codes for accuracy, and compare it with the patient's insurance information. In order to receive payment for the claim, you will often need to contact the insurance company by telephone to find out how to resolve the claim problem and then submit a corrected claim to obtain payment.

PROCEDURE 17-1 Verifying Workers' Compensation Coverage

Procedure Goal: To verify workers' compensation coverage before accepting a patient

OSHA Guidelines: This procedure does not involve exposure to blood, body fluids, or tissue.

Materials: Telephone, paper, and a pen

Method:

1. Call the patient's employer and verify that the accident or illness occurred on the employer's premises or at an employment-related work site.

2. Obtain the employer's approval to provide treatment. Be sure to write down the name and title of the person giving approval, as well as his phone number.
   RATIONALE: *Without approval, treatment costs may not be covered.*

3. Ask the employer for the name of its workers' compensation insurance company. (Employers are required by law to carry such insurance. It is a good policy to notify your state labor department about any employer you encounter that does not have workers' compensation insurance, although you are not required to do so.)

   If the employer has not done so, remind them to report the incident to the W/C carrier, using the First Report of Injury or Illness, and to the state labor department within 24 hours of the incident.
   RATIONALE: *Without this form on file, the claims will not be approved for payment.*

4. Contact the insurance company and verify that the employer does indeed have an active policy in good standing with the company.
   RATIONALE: *The insurance company will not pay for services without a valid policy.*

5. Obtain the claim number assigned to the case from the insurance company. This claim number is placed on all claims and submitted paperwork.
   RATIONALE: *All invoices must include the claim number in order for the practice to receive payment.*

6. When the patient begins treatment, create a patient record. If the patient is already an active patient with the practice, create separate medical and financial records for the workers' compensation-related treament.
   RATIONALE: *This is the legal procedure to protect patient confidentiality with regard to private medical care. Confidentiality does not exist with regard to care related to workers' compensation cases because the employer and its insurer are paying for the patient's medical care.*

PROCEDURE 17-2 Submitting a Request for Prior Authorization

Procedure Goal: To submit a request for prior authorization

OSHA Guidelines: This procedure does not involve exposure to blood, body fluids, or tissue.

Materials: Prior authorization form, patient medical chart with planned procedure and CPT code, diagnosis and ICD code for proof of medical necessity, and patient financial record or the following information: patient name, address, DOB, subscriber name and relationship to patient if not the same, insurance policy group, and ID numbers

Method:

1. Place a call to the insurance carrier or access the website if available.

2. When you reach the nurse manager for the patient's policy, explain that you would like to obtain prior authorization for the requested procedure. She will ask a series of questions regarding the patient, procedure, and diagnosis. Answer these questions using the assembled materials from the patient's medical and financial records.
   RATIONALE: *The more information available regarding the proposed procedure and the reason for it, the easier it is to obtain prior authorization.*

3. If obtaining authorization via the insurance carrier's website, access the website utilizing your user ID and password. Enter the prior authorization area of the website and enter the required information using the assembled materials from the patient's medical and financial records.
   RATIONALE: *The more information available regarding the proposed procedure and the reason for it, the easier it is to obtain prior authorization.*

4. When prior authorization is obtained, carefully record the authorization number and the name and extension number of the person issuing the authorization (if obtained over the phone). If the authorization is obtained via a website, print out the authorization documentation.
   RATIONALE: *If authorization is received, but the authorization number is not on the claim form or is incorrect, payment may still be denied.*

5. Place the authorization number and/or documentation in the patient medical and financial record for further reference, as it will be required when submitting the patient's health insurance claim.

PROCEDURE 17-3 Completing the CMS-1500 Claim Form

Procedure Goal: To complete the CMS-1500 claim form correctly

OSHA Guidelines: This procedure does not involve exposure to blood, body fluids, or tissue.

Materials: Patient record, CMS-1500 form, NUCC Non-NPI Qualifiers and Place of Service Codes, typewriter, computer or pen, and patient ledger card or charge slip

Method:

Note: The numbers below correspond to the numbered fields on the CMS-1500.

1. Place an X in the appropriate insurance box.
   a. Insert the insured's ID number exactly as it appears on the insurance card.

2. Enter the patient's name, as it appears on the insurance card, in this order: last, first, middle initial (if used).

3. a. Enter the patient's birth date in the 8-digit format.
   b. Place an X in the box representing the patient's sex: male or female.

4. Enter the insured's name, as it appears on the insurance card, in this order: last, first, middle initial (if used).

5. Enter the patient's street address, city, state, and zip code.

6. Enter an X for the patient's relationship to the insured. If the patient is the insured, use Self.

7. Enter the insured's street address, city, state, and zip code. For Medicare claims, leave these fields blank.
   RATIONALE: *Medicare patients are always both the insured and the patient.*

8. Reserved for NUCC Use. Leave blank unless instructed otherwise by the insurer.

9. Enter the last name, first name, and middle initial of the insured (as shown on the insurance card) for this *secondary* policy covering the patient.
   RATIONALE: *This is the block for the secondary insurance. The primary insurer will want to know who carries the secondary insurance.*
   a. Enter the *secondary* policy's group number or individual policy ID number.
   b. This field is now left blank.
   c. This field is now left blank.
   d. Enter the name of this *secondary* insurance plan. If this is a Medigap plan, enter the 9-digit CMS-assigned PAYERID.
   RATIONALE: *The PAYERID tells Medicare the coverage is a Medigap plan.*

10. Place Xs in the appropriate Yes or No box in a, b, and c to indicate whether the patient's place of employment, an auto accident, or another accident caused the patient's condition. If an auto accident is responsible, for the

PLACE, enter the two-letter state postal abbreviation for the location of the accident.

RATIONALE: *If any of these boxes is marked "Yes," another insurance plan is probably liable for the charges (workers' compensation, auto insurance, or other liability plan).*

d. If a claim code is required by an individual payer, insert in this field.

11. Enter the policy or group number for the primary insurance plan. If Medicare is the primary payer, enter the word NONE here and leave 11a–d blank.

   a. Enter the insured's date of birth (XX/XX/XXXX) and sex. If gender is unknown, leave blank.

   b. Enter the "Other Claim ID" designated by the NUCC, if applicable.

   c. Enter the insurance plan name for the primary insurance.

   d. Place an X in the appropriate box indicating if there is a secondary payer or not.

   RATIONALE: *If the answer is "No," there is no other insurance coverage, and fields for block 9 will remain blank.*

12. The patient or authorized representative signs and dates the form here. If signatures are on file, this may be noted by inserting "Signature on File."

   RATIONALE: *Without a signature authorizing release of information, you do not legally have permission to submit this information to the insurance carrier.*

13. The patient or authorized representative signs here. If signatures are on file, this may be noted by inserting "Signature on File."

   RATIONALE: *Without this signature, the insurance carrier may send payment for the provider's services to the patient.*

Provider Information Section

14. Enter the date of the current illness, injury, or pregnancy (LMP) using the 8-digit format. Enter the qualifier to the right of the dotted vertical line to identify the date as LMP or other symptom.

15. If an "Other Date" related to the patient's condition or treatment is known, enter here. Leave blank for Medicare or if unknown. If completed, enter the identifying qualifier between the vertical dotted lines found just prior to this date.

   RATIONALE: *Information is used to analyze "pre-existing conditions"; Medicare does not require this information.*

16. Enter the dates the patient is or was unable to work, using the chosen date format. This information could signal a workers' compensation claim.

17. Enter the name of the referring, ordering, or supervising physician (first, middle, and last) with credential. For Medicare, omit the middle name and credential. To the left of the vertical dotted line, enter the qualifier to identify the provider.

   RATIONALE: *Medicare may reject the claim if a middle initial and/or credential is submitted.*

a. If required by the payer, enter the approved 2-digit qualifier from Table 17-1 with the provider identifier next to it; otherwise, leave blank. Medicare requires this field to be blank. Only the provider NPI is submitted to Medicare.

b. Enter the referring provider NPI number.

RATIONALE: *All payers require the provider NPI.*

18. If applicable, enter the dates the patient was hospitalized during this claim.

19. Refer to the most current instructions from the public or private payer regarding use of this field and the qualifiers required. Otherwise, leave this field blank. Medicare uses this field for information related to chiropractic manipulations.

20. Place an X in the Yes box if a laboratory test was performed outside the provider's office and enter the amount being billed for the lab for these procedures. Enter the laboratory name, address, and NPI in block 32. Place an X in the No box if the test was done in the provider's office that is billing the insurance carrier.

21. Enter the ICD codes indicating the patient diagnoses in spaces A–L in descending order of importance.

   a. Enter the ICD indicator in the upper right corner between the two vertical dotted lines indicating which type of ICD code is being used.

   RATIONALE: *All payers require the indicator to tell them whether ICD-9 or ICD-10 codes are being used. Diagnosis codes are required by payers to demonstrate medical necessity of the services provided.*

22. If required by the payer, enter the original reference number for claims being resubmitted. The resubmission code identifies the type of claim being submitted.

23. Enter the prior authorization number if required by the payer. For Medicare, leave blank.

   RATIONALE: *Payers who require prior authorizations will deny claims without them. Medicare does not require prior authorization and will reject claims with "unauthorized" information in this area.*

24. The six service lines here are used to enter the services provided to the patient. They are divided horizontally between shaded and nonshaded areas to accommodate supplemental information that may be required by the payer regarding the service provided.

   a. Enter the dates of service using the 6-digit format.

   b. Enter the 2-digit place of service code from Table 17-5.

   c. EMG stands for emergency service indicator. If the insurer requires this information, and the service was provided on an emergency basis, enter a Y for yes. If service was not provided on an emergency basis or if the insurer does not require the information, leave blank.

   d. Enter the appropriate CPT or HCPCS code with modifier, one per line, to represent each service provided.

   RATIONALE: *These codes tell the payer which service was provided to or for the patient.*

e. Enter the reference number A–L from block 21 to represent the diagnosis code associated with each procedure or service performed.

RATIONALE: *Each "pointer" identifies the medical necessity for each service provided.*

f. Enter the fee charged for each service provided.

g. Enter the days or units for each service provided.

h. If the procedure is related to EPSDT for a Medicaid patient, enter Y; otherwise, leave blank.

i. If the payer requires a non-NPI identifier, enter its qualifier in the shaded area.

j. If a non-NPI qualifier was entered in the shaded area, enter the appropriate non-NPI identifier in the shaded area. If it is not required, leave the shaded area blank. Enter the provider's NPI number in the nonshaded area. For Medicare, leave shaded area blank.

RATIONALE: *The NPI identifies the practitioner providing the service.*

25. Enter the provider's Tax ID number. Place an X in the box identifying it as SSN (Social Security Number) or EIN (Employer Identification Number).

RATIONALE: *This information is required for tax purposes.*

26. Enter the patient's account number (if used by your office).

27. Place an X in the Yes box or the No box to indicate whether the provider is accepting assignment on the claim.

RATIONALE: *This block tells the payer if you are a participating provider.*

28. Enter the total charges for the claim.

29. Enter any amount paid by a primary payer or patient on covered services. If this is a primary claim, leave blank. For Medicare claims, leave blank.

RATIONALE: *Medicare does not require this information.*

30. Block 30 is to be left blank.

31. The physician or provider should sign and date the form here.

RATIONALE: *The provider's signature confirms that he or she provided the services listed.*

32. Enter the name and address of the facility providing the services if different from the billing provider. If the billing provider and service facility provider are the same or if the service took place in the patient's home, leave block 32 blank.

a. If block 32 is completed, enter the servicing provider's NPI.

b. If block 32 is completed and if required by the insurer, enter the servicing provider's appropriate 2-digit qualifier followed by the non-NPI identifier required.

33. Enter the billing provider's name, address, city, state, 9-digit zip code, and phone number.

a. Enter the billing provider's NPI.

b. If required by the insurer, enter the billing provider's appropriate 2-digit qualifier, followed by the non-NPI identifier required.

PROCEDURE 17-4 Tracking Insurance Claims Submissions WORK // DOC

Procedure Goal: To create and use a spreadsheet to track insurance claims submissions

OSHA Guidelines: This procedure does not involve exposure to blood, body fluids, or tissue.

Materials: CMS-1500 claims prepared for submission or record of CMS-1500 claims submitted electronically; Insurance Claims Register or computer with software program such as MS Excel, allowing for the creation of a spreadsheet.

Method

1. Use the Insurance Claims Register or create a spreadsheet with the following headings: Patient Name (and/or account number); Insurance Company; Date of Submission and Amount of the Claim; Insurance Response and Date of Response; Date of Resubmission; Date of Payment; Payment Amount; Patient Balance; and Date of Patient Billing.

2. Using the list of claims submitted, complete the blanks for patient name, insurance company, date of submission, and amount of the claim.

3. When the RA (EOB) is received, complete the date and response columns, including whether the claim is paid, rejected, or denied or a request was made for more information.

RATIONALE: *This allows you to follow up in the future once correction or requested information is submitted to the insurance carrier.*

4. If resubmission is required, enter the date of resubmission.

5. If payment is received, enter the date of receipt and the amount of the payment.

RATIONALE: *This information tells you the insurance carrier has met its obligation.*

6. Record patient balance (if any) and the date the patient is billed.

RATIONALE: *You now can track the remaining balance owed by the patient.*

SUMMARY OF LEARNING OUTCOMES

LEARNING OUTCOMES	KEY POINTS
17.1 Define the basic insurance terms used by the insurance industry.	The following are terms used by insurance companies, knowledgeable medical assistants, medical billers, and coders: *premium, benefit, lifetime maximum, deductible, coinsurance, copayment, exclusions, formulary, elective procedure, precertification,* and *preauthorization.*
17.2 Compare fee-for-service plans, HMOs, and PPOs and explain the new concept of patient centered medical home.	Fee-for-service plans are traditional plans where, after a yearly deductible is met, the insurance plan pays for a percentage of the charges and the patient is responsible for the other percentage (often 80% insurance plan and 20% patient). HMOs are prepaid plans that pay the providers either by capitation or by contracted fee-for-service with patients choosing a PCP, seeing preferred providers, and paying a fixed per-visit copay. A PPO is a managed care plan that establishes a network of providers to perform services for plan members. Members may seek out-of-network care, but their costs will be higher. The patient centered medical home model is a new approach to preventive care that puts the patient and family at the center of the decision-making process using a coordinated team approach to patient care.
17.3 Outline the key requirements for coverage by the Medicare, Medicaid, TRICARE, and CHAMPVA programs.	Medicare provides health insurance for citizens aged 65 and older as well as for certain disabled workers, disabled widows of workers, and patients with long-term disability related to chronic kidney disease on dialysis and end-stage renal disease requiring transplant. Medicaid is a health benefit plan for low-income, blind, or disabled patients; needy families; foster children; and children born with birth defects. TRICARE is a healthcare benefit for families of uniformed personnel and retirees from the uniformed services. CHAMPVA covers the expenses of the families of veterans with total, permanent, service-connected disabilities as well as expenses for surviving spouses and dependent children of veterans who died in the line of duty or as a result of service-connected disabilities.
17.4 Describe allowed charge, contracted fee, capitation, and the formula for RBRVS.	An allowed charge is the maximum dollar amount an insurance carrier will base its reimbursement on—it is also the maximum amount a participating provider is allowed to collect. A contracted fee is a negotiated fee between the MCO and the provider. Capitation is a fixed prepayment paid to the PCP in most plans. RBRVS stands for resource-based relative value scale. Its formula is RVU $\times$ GAF $\times$ CF.
17.5 Outline the tasks performed to obtain the information required to produce an insurance claim.	The claims process includes obtaining patient information, delivering services to the patient and determining the diagnosis and fee, recording charges and codes, documenting payment from the patient, and preparing the healthcare claims.
17.6 Produce a clean CMS-1500 health insurance claim form.	Using the step-by-step instructions within the chapter and Procedure 17-3, and given a completed encounter form (superbill) with all necessary information, the student should produce a legible, clean, and acceptable CMS-1500 claim form.
17.7 Explain the methods used to submit an insurance claim electronically.	The three methods used to submit claims electronically are a claims submission directly to the payer's website via an electronic data interchange, the use of a clearinghouse to "scrub" and submit claims to the payer for the provider, and the use of direct data entry, or DDE.

LEARNING OUTCOMES	KEY POINTS
17.8 Recall the information found on every payer's remittance advice.	Although the format may vary from payer to payer, all RAs (EOBs) contain the following information: name of the insured and identification number; patient name; claim number, date of service, place of service, and code for the service provided; amount billed; amount allowed; amount of subscriber liability; amount paid; and a notation of any services not covered and an explanation of why they were not covered.

CASE STUDY CRITICAL THINKING

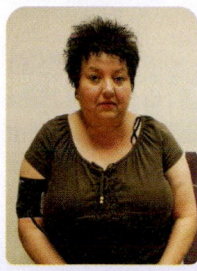

© McGraw-Hill Education

Recall Sylvia Gonzales from the beginning of the chapter. Now that you have completed the chapter, answer the following questions regarding her case.

1. Which insurance plan will be primary for Mrs. Gonzales if the state she lives in uses the birthday rule?

2. If Mr. Gonzales's insurance is primary, explain how the payment will be calculated by the insurance carrier for today's office visit and two lab tests.

3. If the HMO plan is considered primary, what will Sylvia's portion of the charges consist of?

EXAM PREPARATION QUESTIONS

1. (LO 17.1) A fixed-dollar amount the subscriber must pay, or "meet," each year before the insurer begins to cover expenses is the
   a. Copayment
   b. Deductible
   c. Premium
   d. Coinsurance
   e. Lifetime maximum

2. (LO 17.1) Depending upon the type of plan, the patient's portion of the medical charges after the insurance has paid is known as the
   a. Copayment
   b. Deductible
   c. Coinsurance
   d. Premium
   e. Copayment or coinsurance

3. (LO 17.2) Most specialists are paid by MCOs using which of the following methods?
   a. Fee-for-service
   b. Capitation
   c. Copayment
   d. Coinsurance
   e. Negotiated per-service fees

4. (LO 17.3) The national health insurance plan for Americans age 65 and older is
   a. Medicaid
   b. Medicare
   c. TRICARE
   d. CHAMPVA
   e. Workers' compensation

5. (LO 17.3) The appropriate definition for Medicaid plans is
   a. Health insurance plan
   b. Welfare
   c. Health benefit plan
   d. Liablity plan
   e. Health insurance benefit

6. (LO 17.4) RBRVS consists of which components?
   a. RVU
   b. GAF
   c. CF
   d. RVU, GAF, and CF
   e. RVU and CF only

7. (LO 17.5) Which of the following is *not* performed by the medical practice when preparing a healthcare claim for payment and reviewing the insurance payment?

   a. Submitting the employer's first report of illness or injury

   b. Obtaining patient information

   c. Delivering services to the patient and determining the diagnosis and fee

   d. Recording charges and codes, recording payment from the patient, and preparing and submitting the healthcare claim

   e. Reviewing the insurer's processing of the claim, remittance advice, and payment

8. (LO 17.6) Why is it important that each procedure on the CMS-1500 be matched with a diagnosis code?

   a. It proves the procedure was performed

   b. It keeps the coder employed

   c. It increases the reimbursement amount

   d. It proves medical necessity for the procedure

   e. It truly does not matter

9. (LO 17.7) Which of the following is the most common method for medical practices to submit electronic medical claims to third-party payers?

   a. Paper claims via US mail

   b. DDE

   c. Direct submission

   d. Clearinghouse

   e. DDE and paper claims

10. (LO 17.8) Which of the following documents provides information regarding the payer's payment (or denial) of charges received?

   a. RA

   b. EOB

   c. RA or EOB

   d. Claims register

   e. 1505

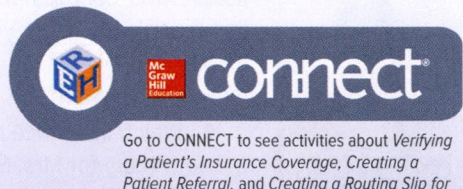

Go to CONNECT to see activities about *Verifying a Patient's Insurance Coverage*, *Creating a Patient Referral*, and *Creating a Routing Slip for Billing*.

SOFT SKILLS SUCCESS

Recall Sylvia Gonzales from the case study at the beginning of the chapter.

1. In this state, each employee's insurance plan is considered primary for him or her, which means Mrs. Gonzales's HMO is her primary payer and the $25 copay from her last visit is now past due, because she wanted this submitted to her husband's insurance. Insurance company refused coverage because of a $1,000 yearly deductible, which has not yet been met. How will you handle this?

2. What policies should be implemented now that you know that Mrs. Gonzales's secondary insurance will not cover her copayments until her high yearly deductible is met?

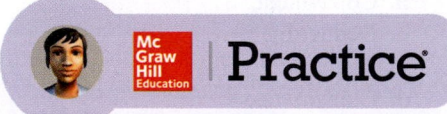

Go to PRACTICE MEDICAL OFFICE and complete the module Admin: Check In - Work Task Proficiencies.

Diagnostic Coding

CASE STUDY

	Patient Name	DOB	Allergies
PATIENT INFORMATION	Cindy Chen	7/15/19XX	NKA
	Attending	**MRN**	**Other Information**
	Alexis N. Whalen, MD	324-86-542	History of depression

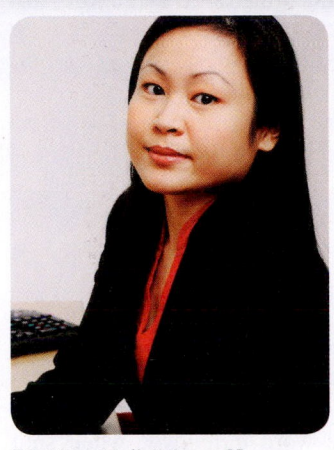

Cindy Chen, a 28-year-old female complaining of inability to sleep and nervousness, arrives at the office. She tested positive for HIV in 2014, although she has been asymptomatic on antiviral drugs. Currently, she lives with her aunt and is going to school to become a phlebotomist. During her interview, she says she thinks her nervousness may be due to upcoming exams and the recurrent sore throat and tiredness she has been experiencing in the last several months.

Keep Cindy Chen in mind as you study this chapter. There will be questions at the end of the chapter based on the case study. The information in the chapter will help you answer these questions.

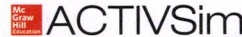

LEARNING OUTCOMES

After completing Chapter 18, you will be able to:

18.1 Recall the six ways that ICD codes are used today.

18.2 Compare ICD-9-CM and ICD-10-CM.

18.3 Describe the conventions used in ICD-10.

18.4 Outline the steps to code a diagnosis using ICD-10-CM.

18.5 Explain the purpose and usage of external cause of injury and health status codes.

18.6 Illustrate unique coding applications for neoplasms, diabetes mellitus, fractures, signs and symptoms, poisonings, and Z codes.

KEY TERMS

Alphabetic Index
category
chapters
chief complaint (CC)
combination code
conventions
cross-reference
diagnosis (Dx)
diagnosis code
etiology
International Classification of Diseases

laterality
morbidity
mortality
primary diagnosis
principal diagnosis
rubric
secondary diagnosis
subcategory
Tabular List
World Health Organization (WHO)

MEDICAL ASSISTING COMPETENCIES

CAAHEP	ABHES
IX.C.2 Describe how to use the most current diagnostic coding classification system	3. **Medical Terminology**
IX.P.2 Perform diagnostic coding	d. Define and use medical abbreviations when appropriate and acceptable
IX.P.3 Utilize medical necessity guidelines	4. **Medical Law & Ethics**
IX.A.1 Utilize tactful communication skills with medical providers to ensure accurate code selection	f. Comply with federal, state, and local health laws and regulations as they relate to healthcare settings
	8. **Administrative Procedures**
	c. Process insurance claims
	(3) Perform diagnostic and procedural coding

▶ Introduction

Patients who come to the medical office have a variety of reasons for seeking medical care. Each of those reasons results in at least one diagnosis. The word *diagnosis,* when split into its component word parts, means "the condition of complete knowledge" (*osis*—condition, *dia*—complete, *gnos*—knowledge). When submitting claims to insurance carriers to receive reimbursement for the care the patient receives, this knowledge must be converted into numeric and alphanumeric codes, known as ICD codes. ICD stands for **International Classification of Diseases.** Prior to October 1, 2015, the diagnostic coding system was known as ICD-9-CM, which stood for the ninth edition, clinical modification. The current system, for dates of service beginning October 1, 2015, is the 10th edition, so it is named ICD-10-CM.

With the passage of the Medicare Catastrophic Coverage Act of 1988, diagnosis coding became mandatory for Medicare claims (using ICD-9), and shortly thereafter, its use was also mandated for Medicaid and commercial insurance carriers. Just as you learn medical terminology to communicate with all members of the healthcare team, as a medical assistant, it is equally important to learn the *language* of coding—in this chapter, ICD-10, and in the following chapter, the language of CPT and HCPCS procedural coding. Because insurance carriers pay claims based on the codes assigned to describe the information within the medical record (not on the medical record itself), it is vital that you understand what the codes mean and how to choose the correct code based on the information found on the encounter forms and within the patient medical record.

▶ The Reasons for Diagnosis Codes LO 18.1

Patients present to healthcare providers with a description of their medical problem, called their **chief complaint (CC),** which is documented at each visit. To diagnose a patient's condition, the practitioner follows a complex decision-making process based on the patient's statements, an examination, and the practitioner's evaluation of this information. The practitioner establishes a **diagnosis (Dx)** that describes the primary condition for which a patient is receiving care. Additional conditions or symptoms that affect the patient's management are called *coexisting conditions,* or *comorbidities.* These conditions may be related or totally unrelated to the primary condition, but if they currently affect the patient's condition or treatment, they also must be noted in the chart, coded, and reported to the insurance carrier. The diagnoses listed on a healthcare claim form should prove medical necessity for the treatment provided.

The diagnosis is communicated to the third-party payer through a **diagnosis code** (or diagnostic code) on the healthcare claim. Until the transition, diagnosis codes used in the United States were found in the 9th edition of the clinical modification of the ICD reference, now replaced by the 10th edition; ICD-10. Also available on CD-ROM, the ICD code set is based on a system maintained by the **World Health Organization (WHO)** of the United Nations.

The Health Insurance Portability and Accountability Act (HIPAA) mandates ICD code use in the healthcare industry for reporting patients' diseases and conditions, or their signs and symptoms if no actual diagnosis has been assigned. The codes are updated every year on October 1, which explains why ICD-10 was effective October 1, 2015 instead of in January 2016 when the new procedural codes come out. It is important to remember that the edition of diagnosis codes being used is based on the date of service (DOS), not on the date the claim is submitted.

For instance, when completing claims on October 1, 2015, you would have used 2015 ICD-9 codes on a claim for services provided on September 30, 2015. However, for a claim reporting services provided on October 1, 2015, the new 2016 ICD-10 codes will have been used. Even though the new codes became effective in October 2015, they will be used until September 30, 2016 and so the manual is dated 2016. The edition published in October 1, 2016 will be dated 2017 and so on. The medical office must always have the current year's coding reference books and should update office forms and computer programs containing diagnosis (and procedure) codes because using outdated codes will result in denied claims.

The ICD coding system was originally created for the classification of patient **morbidity** (sickness) and **mortality** (death) statistics and to provide access for medical research, education, and administration. Today, ICD codes are increasingly important and they are used for

- Facilitation of payment for medical services.
- Evaluation of utilization patterns (patient use of healthcare facilities).
- Study of healthcare costs.
- Research regarding quality of healthcare.
- Prediction of healthcare trends.
- Planning for future healthcare needs.

Keep in mind as you learn coding that just as whatever you document in a patient's health record becomes part of his or her permanent record, so does any code you assign to the patient for receipt by the insurance carrier. It also may be part of statistical reporting for communicable diseases, pregnancies, cancer diagnosis, and so on, so it is extremely important that you understand the information in the medical record that you are coding, as well as the descriptions of the codes you are assigning.

▶ A Basic Comparison of ICD-9-CM and ICD-10-CM
LO 18.2

The ICD was originally introduced in 1893 by The International Statistical Institute as the first International List of Causes of Death, requiring physicians to better track a patient's diagnosis and medical care. The responsibility of ICD was taken over by WHO in 1948 when morbidity causes were added in the sixth edition. ICD-9, introduced in 1975, did not allow the addition of new, more precise diagnoses that have developed over the years. There were approximately 14,200 codes in the ICD-9-CM, while the ICD-10-CM contains over 68,000 codes. This allows greater specificity for diagnosis classifications and provides expansion for new codes. This is particularly important relating to *code linkage*—between ICD diagnosis codes and the CPT procedure codes to prove the *medical necessity* of a patient's procedure or treatment (refer to the *Insurance and Billing* chapter for more information). You will learn more about CPT in the *Procedural Coding* chapter. At this time, many other countries in the world have adopted at least some version of ICD-10-CM. As with any change or update in the medical office, such as the claim update from the 4010 to the 5010 format or from paper medical records to an EHR program, the transition from ICD-9 to ICD-10 presented challenges to medical offices. The medical offices were required to not only learn the new system but also accommodate both systems during an overlap period. Table 18-1 shows basic comparisons between the two systems.

Additionally, ICD-9 also included a volume for hospitals (called volume 3), which contained procedures performed primarily in the inpatient hospital setting. Because of the increase in the number of diagnoses and hospital-based procedures codes available with ICD-10, it includes a totally separate volume for hospital procedure codes, called ICD-10-PCS (Procedural Coding System). Unless you decide to expand your training to include inpatient hospital coding, it is likely you will never use the PCS coding system.

TABLE 18-1	Basic Comparisons of ICD-9-CM and ICD-10-CM Codes	
Feature	**ICD-9**	**ICD-10**
Number of codes	14,200	68,000+
Format	3–5 characters; first character may be alpha or numeric; 2–5 are numeric	3–7 characters; first character alpha (uppercase); 2 and 3 are numeric; 4–7 may be alpha or numeric
Specificity	Limited	Expanded
Laterality	None	Has laterality
Decimal point	After 3rd character; not always used	Decimal must be used after 3rd character
Placeholder	0 as 4th digit is present when 5th digit is required	"X" used as placeholder for a nonexistent digit when 6th or 7th digit is required for code specificity
Combination codes	Some	Expanded number of combination codes
External causes of morbidity and mortality, including poisonings	E codes	Instead of a separate section, external causes are included as V01–Y99 codes
Factors influencing health status	V codes	Instead of a separate section, health status codes are included as Z00–Z99 codes

TABLE 18-2   Chapter, Description, and Code Ranges for ICD-10-CM

Chapter	Description	Code Range
1	Certain infectious and parasitic diseases	A00–B99
2	Neoplasms	C00–D49
3	Diseases of the blood and blood-forming organs and certain disorders involving the immune mechanism	D50–D89
4	Endocrine, nutritional, and metabolic diseases	E00–E89
5	Mental and behavioral disorders	F01–F99
6	Diseases of the nervous system	G00–G99
7	Diseases of the eye and adnexa	H00–H59
8	Diseases of the ear and mastoid process	H60–H95
9	Diseases of the circulatory system	I00–I99
10	Diseases of the respiratory system	J00–J99
11	Diseases of the digestive system	K00–K95
12	Diseases of the skin and subcutaneous tissue	L00–L99
13	Diseases of the musculoskeletal system and connective tissue	M00–M99
14	Diseases of the genitourinary system	N00–N99
15	Pregnancy, childbirth, and the puerperium	O00–O9A
16	Certain conditions originating in the perinatal period	P00–P96
17	Congenital malformations, deformations, and chromosomal abnormalities	Q00–Q99
18	Symptoms, signs, and abnormal clinical and laboratory findings; not elsewhere classified	R00–R99
19	Injury, poisoning, and certain other consequences of external causes	S00–T88
20	External causes of morbidity	V01–Y99
21	Factors influencing health status and contact with health services	Z00–Z99

ICD-10 Information

As you can see from Table 18-1, by converting to ICD-10, we jumped from 14,200 diagnosis codes available with ICD-9 to 68,000+ possibilities with ICD-10. Because of this increase in codes, the number of chapters also increased from 17 to 21 for ICD-10.

Alphabetic and Numeric Indexes

Like ICD-9, the 10th edition of ICD contains an **Alphabetic Index** of the diseases, conditions, and related terms. When coding in ICD-10, you will begin with the Alphabetic Index, in the front of the book to look up the diagnostic term, such as *appendicitis*. Once the term is identified in the Alphabetic Index, it directs you to the lists of appropriate codes in the **Tabular** (numeric) **List.** The ICD-10 Tabular List incorporates 21 **chapters** with the alphanumeric range for each as listed in Table 18-2. A **category,** also known as a **rubric,** has 3 characters and a **subcategory** has 4 or 5 characters, with the final code consisting of up to 7 characters. The use of the ICD-10 manual and the code characters involved will become clearer as examples are provided later in the chapter. It is important to always look up a code in the Alphabetic Index first and then *verify* the code in the Tabular List because often the Tabular List contains specific information about the diagnosis often not found in the Alphabetic Index. Never code using only the Alphabetic Index. It is simply your start point. We will discuss this concept in more detail later in the chapter.

Characters and Specificity

Although there are similarities between ICD-9 and ICD-10, perhaps the most striking difference is the way the ICD-10 code looks in comparison to an ICD-9 code. The change in the look is directly related to the need to expand the specificity of many of the diagnosis codes and so a new format was required. All ICD-10 codes begin with an alpha character. The number of possible characters increased from 3–5 in ICD-9 to 3–7 in ICD-10. Again, the intent of the ICD-10 is to provide a more precise clinical picture of the patient and enhanced trending analysis. Table 18-3 provides an example of the increased specificity of the new coding system using the diagnosis of breast cancer.

TABLE 18-3 Example of Greater Specificity Available with ICD-10 vs. ICD-9

ICD-9 (limited specificity)	ICD-10 (expanded specificity)
Code: 233.0 Carcinoma in situ breast (vague as to cancer type)	Code: D05.01 Lobular carcinoma in situ of right breast
	OR
	Code: D05.11 Intraductal carcinoma in situ of right breast

TABLE 18-4 Example of ICD-10 Placeholder, Not Available in ICD-9

ICD-9-CM	ICD-10-CM
910.0 Face, neck, and scalp; abrasion or friction burn without mention of infection	S00.01 Abrasion of scalp (code noted to √X7th)
910.1 Face, neck, and scalp; abrasion or friction burn, infected	S00.01XA Abrasion of scalp, initial encounter S00.01XD Abrasion of scalp, subsequent encounter S00.01XS Abrasion of scalp, sequela

TABLE 18-5 Example of an ICD-10 Combination Code

ICD-9-CM	ICD-10-CM
995.92 Severe sepsis AND 785.52 Septic shock	R65.21 Severe sepsis with septic shock

From the example in Table 18-3, some of the limitations of ICD-9 can be clearly seen. For example, code 233.0, which consists of only 4, all-numeric characters, only tells us the patient has carcinoma in situ of the breast—it does not tell us the type of cancer, nor does it tell us which breast is affected. In order to choose the most specific code in ICD-10, which consists of 5 characters, you need to know both the type of cancer affecting the patient and which breast is affected (replacing the 5th character 1 for these ICD-10 codes with a 2 means the patient's cancer is affecting the left breast).

Placeholders

The ICD-9 did not incorporate a placeholder in anticipation of new codes. The ICD-10 uses an "X" to hold a place for future expansion of the code's specificity. An example is illustrated in Table 18-4. The diagnosis statement is *Abrasion of scalp,* which points us to code *S00.01* with a notation to "check X7th." Immediately below this code are three options, all beginning with the base code *S00.01,* followed by the placeholder of "X" followed by "A," "D," or "S."

The 7th character is used to explain the encounter determination:

- "A" designates an initial encounter.
- "D" designates a subsequent encounter.
- "S" designates sequel.

If the "X" placeholder and 7th character are not present, the code will not be accepted. Keep in mind that, these "additional characters" are not optional. You must also be careful when adding characters that you do not "drop" the "X" placeholder. For example, if you dropped the "X" placeholder in coding the initial encounter for a scalp abrasion, you would end up with S00.01A—a code that does not exist in ICD-10 and would be rejected. You must be very detail-oriented to code efficiently and accurately.

Combination Codes

A **combination code** is one in which two diagnoses are included in one code. This may be a diagnosis with an associated secondary process (known as a manifestation) or a diagnosis with an associated complication. The ICD-9-CM accommodated only a relatively small number of combination codes, often requiring the use of multiple codes to completely code a condition, illness, or injury. The ICD-10-CM contains many more combination codes, greatly cutting down on the need for multiple codes for a single diagnosis. An example of a combination code appears in Table 18-5.

In some cases, multiple codes are also used with ICD-10 coding when appropriate. One example is coding for pregnancy and prenatal visits, which often require more than one code to describe completely.

▶ An Overview of ICD-10   LO 18.3

The ICD-10-CM, as stated earlier, consists of two parts: the Tabular List, known as Volume 1, and the Alphabetic Index, known as Volume 2, found at the beginning of the manual (Figure 18-1).

The correct procedure when using the ICD reference is to look up the diagnosis description in the Alphabetic Index (Volume 2) and then verify the code given by cross-referencing it in the Tabular List (Volume 1). In order to use both indices easily, you must understand the *conventions* they use.

Conventions

A list of abbreviations, punctuation, symbols, typefaces, and instructional notes appears at the beginning of ICD-10. These items, called **conventions,** provide basic guidelines for using the code set. Here are some important conventions:

- NOS. This abbreviation means "not otherwise specified," or "unspecified." It is used when a condition is not described in enough detail to choose a more specific code. In general, codes with NOS should be avoided unless no other option is available. The provider should be asked for more specific information to help select a more specific code, if possible. Most of the NOS codes end with the number 9.

Example:

A41.9	**Sepsis, unspecified organism**
	Septicemia NOS

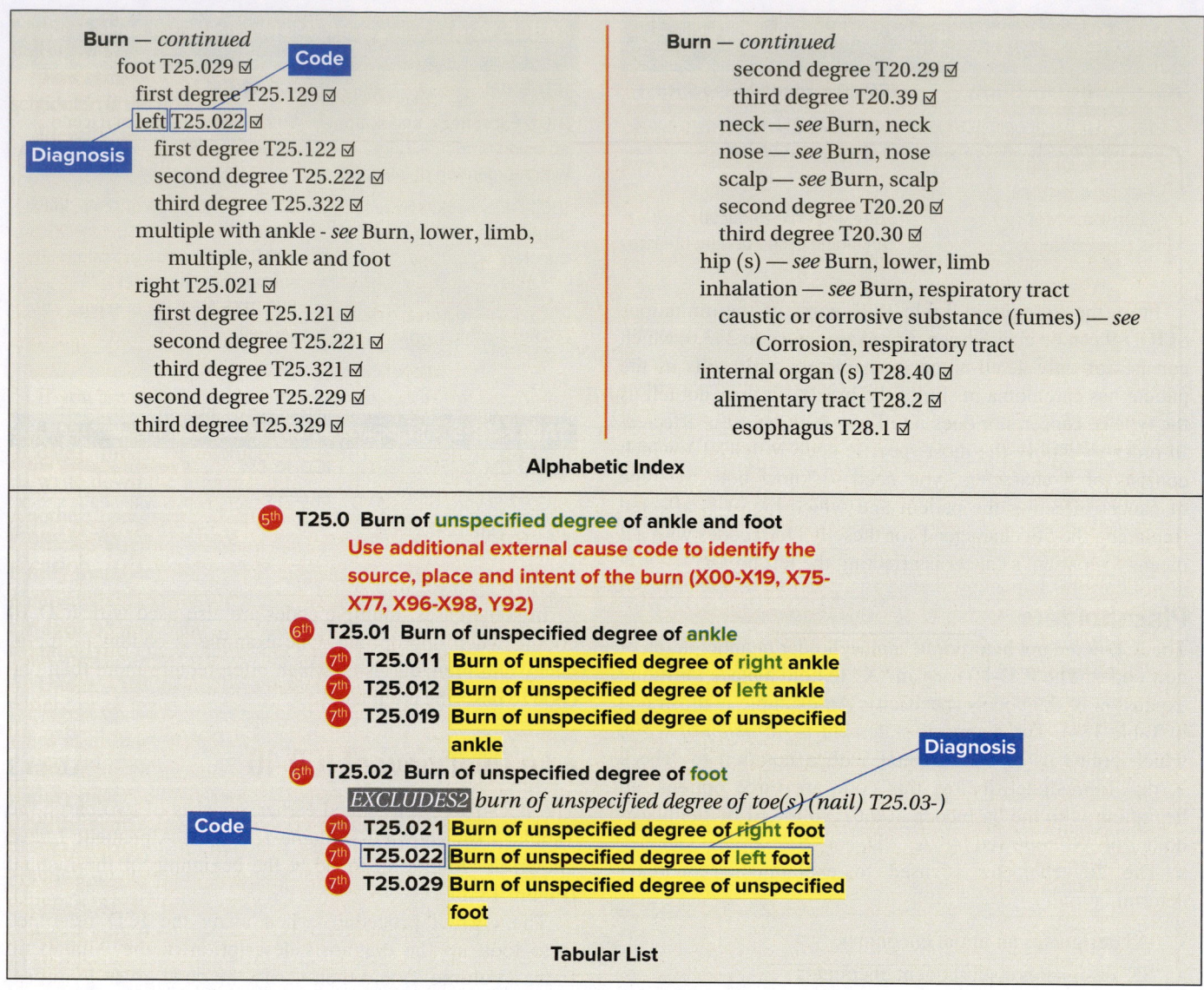

FIGURE 18-1 ICD Alphabetic Index and Tabular List.

Source: International Classification of Diseases, Tenth Revision, Clinical Modification, 2015, Complete Draft Code Set.

- NEC. This abbreviation means "not elsewhere classified." It is used when the ICD-10 does not provide a code specific enough for the patient's condition. Only use these codes when you are sure a more specific code does not exist. In general, the NEC codes end with the number 8.

Example:

E03.8	Other specified hypothyroidism

- [ ] Brackets. In the Tabular List, brackets are used around synonyms, alternative wordings, or explanations. These terms may help you pick out the correct code, but it is not mandatory that they be found in the medical record. For instance, in the example, the patient's diagnosis may include "croup," but it does not have to in order to use code J05.0.

Example:

J05.0	Acute obstructive laryngitis [croup]

- [ ] Brackets. Brackets that appear in the Alphabetic Index indicate that two codes will be required to completely code the diagnosis. The code in the bracket will be the secondary code.

Example:

Hydrothorax, filarial
(see also infestation, filiarial) B74.9 [J91.8]

- ( ) Parentheses. These are used around descriptions in the Alphabetic Index that do not affect the code—that is, nonessential or supplementary terms that may assist you in choosing the correct code.

Example:

Fleischer (-Kayser) ring (corneal pigmentation)
H18.04-

- **:** Colon. This is used in the Tabular List after an incomplete term that needs one of the terms that follow the colon to make it assignable to a given category.

Example:

I52	Other heart disorders in diseases classified elsewhere
	Code first underlying disease, such as:
	  congenital syphilis (A50.5)
	  mucopolysaccharidosis (E76.3)
	  schistosomiasis (B65.0–B65.9)
	  Diarrhea:
	  dysenteric
	  epidemic

- *INCLUDES.* This note indicates that the entries following it further define the content of a preceding entry. In this example, in the medical record, the practitioner may refer to the patient as having acute myocarditis or subacute myocarditis; the same diagnosis code will be used for both.

Example:

I40	**Acute myocarditis**
	INCLUDES *subacute myocarditis*

- *Excludes.* There are two types of Excludes notes in ICD-10. Although they both indicate that codes (diagnoses) are excluded from the code containing the note, they are used for different reasons.

- *EXCLUDES1* indicates that the code is excluded and never should be used at the same time as the code above the *EXCLUDES1* note.

Example:

I33	**Acute and subacute endocarditis**
	EXCLUDES1 *acute rheumatic endocarditis (I01.1) endocarditis NOS (I38)*

- *EXCLUDES2* means "not included here." An *Excludes2* note indicates that the condition excluded is not part of the condition represented by the code, but if documented, the patient may have both conditions at the same time. When an *EXCLUDES2* note appears under a code, it is acceptable to use both the code and the excluded code together if required by the medical record documentation. In the example, if the patient is documented as having both acute and chronic tonsillitis, it is acceptable to code both J03 and J35.0 together (in that order, because acute always precedes chronic conditions).

Example:

J03	**Acute tonsillitis**
	EXCLUDES2 Chronic tonsillitis (J35.0)

- *Use additional code.* This note indicates that an additional code should be used, if available. The additional code is always listed after the primary code.

Example:

N18.6	**End stage renal disease** Chronic kidney disease requiring chronic dialysis Use additional code to identify dialysis status (Z99.2)

- *Code first underlying disease.* This instruction appears when the category is not to be used as the primary diagnosis. These codes may not be used as the first listed code on the insurance claim form; they must always be preceded by another code for the primary diagnosis. In this example, the underlying disease such as African trypanosomiasis (B56.-) or poliovirus infection (A80.-) will be listed first, followed by the meningitis code (G02).

Example:

G02	**Meningitis in other infectious and parasitic diseases classified elsewhere** Code first underlying disease such as: African trypanosomiasis (B56.-) poliovirus infection (A80.-)

- *Code first, if applicable, any causal condition.* This note means that the code may be used as a primary diagnosis if the underlying, or "causal condition," is unknown or not applicable.

Example:

N13.8	**Other obstructive and reflux ureteropathy** Urinary tract obstruction due to specified cause Code first, if applicable, any causal condition, such as enlarged prostate (N40.1)

Two other conventions to be aware of in the Tabular List are the use of bold and italicized typeface. Bold is used for all codes and titles in the Tabular List. Italicization is used for all Exclusion notes and to identify codes that are not used to describe the primary diagnosis; they are only used as secondary diagnoses.

The Alphabetic Index includes two notations you should also be aware of:

- *See Condition.* When found in the Alphabetic Index, it is meant to refer you to a different "main term" for the condition. For instance, if you look up the term *Ankle* in the Alphabetic Index, you will be directed to *See Condition.* Ankle is not a diagnosis; it is a location. Keep in mind that the diagnosis (and its main term) is "what is wrong with the patient." The location will be used as a subterm. If the patient has a diagnosis of ankle fracture, you will look up fracture, ankle, and then type (open, closed, and so on) as the main term and condition.

Example:

Ankle—See Condition

- *See also.* If the diagnosis for the patient is cervical inflammation, the main term is *inflammation.* When you look up *inflammation, cervix* (subterm for the location of the inflammation), you are directed to *See also* "Cervicitis."

Example:

> **Inflammation**
> Cervix (uteri) (See also Cervicitis)

The direction "See Condition" is a directive; you must do so to locate the code. "See also" is a suggestion; you might find a better code for the diagnosis you are coding. In the case of "cervicitis," you will find multiple codes available depending on what is causing the cervicitis. Follow all directions in ICD-10. It will make you a better coder and, in many cases, increase the reimbursement for the provider because you are giving the insurance carrier the most specific information available for the medical necessity for the services provided. Read the coding guidelines in the beginning of the manual. Broken out by section, these guidelines give very specific instructions on how to code each of the 21 chapters of the ICD-10 manual. Read and highlight this area of the manual as you learn to code—you will be glad you did.

The Alphabetic Index

As stated earlier, when coding, the Alphabetic Index is your start point (after you read the guidelines). It contains all the medical terms necessary to locate codes in the Tabular List—including common terms that are not found in the Tabular List. The index is organized by condition. To use the Alphabetic Index, think about what is wrong (the problem) and not where the problem occurred. For example, you would find the term *wrist fracture* by looking under *fracture* (the condition) and then, below it, *wrist* (the location), rather than by looking under *wrist* to find *fracture.* In fact, if you look up the word *wrist,* you will be told "See also condition," telling you to look up the problem with the wrist.

The assignment of the correct code begins with looking up the medical term that describes the patient's condition in the Alphabetic Index. The following example illustrates the index's format. Each main term is printed in boldface type and is followed by its code number. For example, if the diagnostic statement is "the patient presents with blindness," the main term *blindness* is located in the Alphabetic Index.

> **Blindness** (acquired) (congenital) (both eyes)
> H54.0
> blast S05.8X-√
> color—See Deficiency, color vision
> concussion S05.8X-√
> cortical H47.619
>   left brain H47.612
>   right brain H47.611

Any other terms that are needed to select correct codes are printed and indented after the main term. These terms, called *subterms,* may show the cause or source of the disease or describe a particular type or body site for the main term. In this shortened example, the main term *blindness* is followed by multiple additional terms (some listed in the previous example), each indicating a different type—such as color blindness—for this medical condition. Additionally, when coding cortical blindness, note that each of its subterms, which denote the location in the brain cortex causing the color blindness, has its own code. When cross-referencing with the Tabular List, you will note that the main code of H54.0 represents blindness of both eyes. The characters after the decimal point further delineate the type, the causal location, and, in the case of cortical blindness, which side of the brain is affected.

Other helpful terms found in parentheses, known as *nonessential terms,* also may be shown. Nonessential terms are those that assist you in choosing the correct code, but it is not mandatory that they be present within the code description. In the example, any of the terms *acquired, congenital,* and *both eyes* may be in the diagnostic statement, such as "the patient presents with blindness acquired in childhood."

Cross-references of *See* or *See also* are used frequently in ICD. If the cross-reference *See* appears after a main term, you *must* look up the term that follows the word *See* in the index. The *See* reference means that the main term where you first looked is not correct; another category must be used. In the previous example regarding color blindness, to code *Color* (blindness), you are instructed to *See* the term *Deficiency, color vision* to locate the correct code. As stated earlier, the reference *See also* is a suggestion that you may find more information looking under a different term.

The Tabular List

The Tabular List for ICD-10 consists of 21 chapters of disease descriptions and codes. In addition to chapters for each body system, it also includes a chapter for injuries related to poisonings, anaphylactic reactions, and the like; a chapter for injuries related to "external causes" (known as E codes in ICD-9); and a chapter for health encounters for healthy patients (such as for physicals and well-child visits), which were known as V codes in ICD-9. Table 18-2 outlines the list of chapters in the Tabular List for ICD-10.

The Tabular List contains very specific information in numeric sequence to back up, or expand on, the information found in the Alphabetic Index. Once you find the condition you believe is needed—your "start point"—in the Alphabetic Index, then locate in the Tabular List, the code given by the Alphabetic Index to obtain the "final destination." This is the exact code, including any 5th, 6th, or 7th "optional" characters, required to give you the most specific, accurate diagnosis code available for the information you are given in the medical record.

Code Structure As stated earlier in the comparison between ICD-9 and ICD-10, I-10 diagnosis codes as they are commonly abbreviated, are made up of 3 to 7 alphanumeric characters. The system continues to use 3-character categories, known as **rubrics,** for diseases, injuries, and symptoms. Many of these categories are divided into 4- or 5-character codes known as subcategories. Many codes are then further subdivided into 6- or 7-character codes to produce the final code—for example,

> **S90 Superficial injury of ankle, foot and toes**
> **The appropriate 7th character is to be added to each code from category S90**
> **A = initial encounter**
> **D = subsequent encounter**
> **S = sequela**
> S90.0 Contusion of ankle
> S90.00 Contusion of unspecified ankle
> S90.01 Contusion of right ankle
> S90.02 Contusion of left ankle

When listed in the ICD-10, codes available using 4, 5, 6, or even 7 characters must be reported on claims because they represent the most specific diagnosis documented in the patient medical record. This is known as coding to the *highest level of specificity* and payers require it. For example, CMS rules state that a Medicare claim will be rejected when the most specific code available is not used. In the previous example, it would be incorrect to use code S90, S90.0, or even S90.00, S90.01, or S90.02 because the instructions under the rubric state that a 7th character must be added. In these examples, the most specific codes given consist of only 5 characters, so the aforementioned *placeholder* will be used in the sixth position. For an initial encounter, the final codes will look like this example:

> **S90.00XA** Contusion of unspecified ankle (initial encounter)
> **S90.01XA** Contusion of the right ankle (initial encounter)
> **S90.02XA** Contusion of the left ankle (initial encounter)

One other item to keep in mind is that although every ICD-10 code contains a decimal after the 3rd character, this decimal point is never placed on the insurance claim form. All diagnostic decimal points are omitted when completing an insurance claim form. Refer to the *Insurance and Billing* chapter for further information.

▶ Coding with ICD-10   LO 18.4

You may think that if your office uses a superbill or an EHR program to select codes, you will not need to understand coding. This is simply not true. Every diagnosis and procedure checked off on the encounter form must be verified in the medical record. EHR programs do not understand *medical necessity*—figuring out which diagnoses best explain why a specific procedure was performed. With the limited room on an encounter form, it is very possible that the most specific diagnosis code available for the patient's condition is not listed on the encounter form. It may be your responsibility to locate the "best code for the job." If the provider uses a SOAP note format when charting (see the *Medical Records and Documentation* chapter), you can locate the diagnosis in the assessment area. If a more "free-hand" approach or "narrative" style note is used, a little detective work may be needed.

The diagnosis is peptic ulcer.

Now, decide what the main term is for the condition or the diagnosis. For the diagnosis in Example #1, the main term is *ulcer*. The word *peptic* (stomach) describes the type of ulcer and is considered a subterm. Because there is an exact diagnosis, the pain and reflux will not be coded in outpatient facilities like physician offices. Inpatient facilities such as hospitals have different rules, and the symptoms would be coded.

Once you find the description, locate the code given for that description; it is usually to the right of the description or just below it. Verify the code in the Tabular List and be sure to read all instructions in this section because there are often more specific instructions in the Tabular List that will help you find the right code or affirm that you have the correct code; here are some examples.

1. For the first diagnosis of peptic ulcer (site unspecified), the code given is K27.9. When looking up the main code in the Tabular List, you will note that the rubric of K27 is *Peptic ulcer, site unspecified*. You then have the choice of adding 0–9 as the 4th character to complete the code. Since we have not been told whether the ulcer is with hemorrhage or perforation (or both), or whether the ulcer is acute or chronic, we will complete the code using the digit 9. Our completed code description will then read *Peptic ulcer, site unspecified, unspecified as acute or chronic, without hemorrhage or perforation.*

2. In Example #2, the sebaceous cyst, the code given as our start point is L72.3, which states *cyst, sebaceous (duct) (gland)*. In verifying in the Tabular List, rubric L72 includes the description of *Follicular cysts of skin and subcutaneous tissue*. Again, 4th-character options of 1–9 are given. Note that if a 4th character of 1 is chosen, then a 5th character of 1 or 2 must be added to complete the description. Because we are told the patient has a sebaceous cyst, we verify that L72.3 is defined as sebaceous cyst, and this is the code that will be used.

In both of these cases, the level of specificity of each diagnosis was increased by the addition of the "optional" 4th character, and we noted that in the second example, depending what type of cyst was diagnosed, a 5th character might be required to complete the code. As we move forward we will see more codes that include 6- and 7-character codes, as well as those utilizing the placeholder "X." As you can see, these optional characters truly are not optional at all. Finally, do not forget to look for instructions such as *Code also* and *Code first underlying condition,* as well as *Includes* and *Excludes* notes that assist you in deciding on the correct code or codes.

Additional Guidelines for ICD-10 Coding

Now that you understand that you must first look up the main term and then the subterm in the Alphabetic Index, then confirm the code in the Tabular List (a step that can never be skipped), let's look at some guidelines in more detail that will make your coding more specific and efficient.

Acute Versus Chronic Conditions An acute (including subacute for coding purposes) condition is defined as one that is of sudden onset or a more long-standing (chronic) condition that has suddenly worsened. There are times, such as with bronchitis, when the patient has both the acute form (J20.9) and the underlying chronic form (J42). When this occurs and both codes must be reported, the acute code is always listed first, followed by the code for the chronic form of the condition.

Combination Codes When a combination code is available, it must be used in place of the two single codes. An example of this is cholelithiasis (gallstones), code K80.20, with acute cholecystitis (gallbladder inflammation), code K81.9. However, because they are being diagnosed together, when you look up *cholecystitis* and see the subterm "with," you will find a direction stating "See Calculus, gallbladder, with cholecystitis." When you do so, you will note that cholelithiasis with cholecystitis, acute, is coded K80.10 with a notation to check the 5th character. You are given two options: 0 represents *Calculus of the gallbladder with chronic cholecystitis without obstruction.* 1 represents *Calculus of the gallbladder with chronic cholecystitis with obstruction.* Because there is no mention of obstruction in our diagnosis, the correct full code is K80.10. One other note on acute versus chronic conditions: If the condition is not defined as acute or chronic and the provider cannot be located to provide this detail, the assumption is that the condition is chronic. See Figure 18-2.

Multiple Coding Prior to the ICD-10 code set, there were many instances when one code did not fully describe the patient's diagnosis. With ICD-10, this happens less often, but there are still times when more than one code will be required to fully "explain" the patient's condition. This most often occurs when a disease or condition is the manifestation (result) of another condition. For instance, if a patient is diagnosed with otitis externa of the right ear, caused by impetigo, two codes will be required because the otitis is caused by the underlying condition of the impetigo. When you look up otitis externa in the Alphabetic Index, follow the subset "in (due to)," and locate impetigo, you will note code L01.00 followed

(a)
Cholecystitis K81.9
    with
        calculus, stones in
            bile duct (common) (hepatic) — *see* Calculus, bile duct,
                with cholecystitis
            cystic duct — *see* Calculus, gallbladder, with cholecystitis
            gallbladder — *see* Calculus, gallbladder, with cholecystitis
            choledocholithiasis — *see* Calculus, bile duct, with
                cholecystitis
            cholelithiasis — *see* Calculus, gallbladder, with
                cholecystitis

(b)
Calculus — *continued*
    common duct (bile) — *see* Calculus, bile duct
    conjunctiva — *see* Concretion, conjunctiva cystic N21.0
        duct — *see* Calculus, gallbladder
    dental (subgingival) (supragingival) K03.6 diverticulum
        bladder N21.0
        kidney N20.0
    epididymis N50.8
    gallbladder K80.20
        with
            bile duct calculus — *see* Calculus, gallbladder and
                bile duct
            cholecystitis K80.10
                with obstruction K80.11
                acute K80.00

(c)
🔴5th **K80.0 Calculus of gallbladder with acute cholecystitis**
    Any condition listed in K80.2 with acute cholecystitis
    K80.00 Calculus of gallbladder with acute cholecystitis without obstruction
    K80.01 Calculus of gallbladder with acute cholecystitis with obstruction
🔴5th **K80.1 Calculus of gallbladder with other cholecystitis**
→   **K80.10 Calculus of gallbladder with chronic Cholecystitis without obstruction**
        Cholelithiasis with cholecystitis NOS
    K80.11 Calculus of gallbladder with chronic cholecystitis with obstruction
    K80.12 Calculus of gallbladder with acute and chronic cholecystitis without obstruction
    K80.13 Calculus of gallbladder with acute and chronic cholecystitis with obstruction
    K80.18 Calculus of gallbladder with other cholecystitis without obstruction
    K80.19 Calculus of gallbladder with other cholecystitis with obstruction

FIGURE 18-2 (a) Alphabetic Index for cholecystitis directing you to calculus, gallbladder. (b) Alphabetic Index showing calculus wth cholecystitis (K80.10). (c) Tabular List for K80.10 verifying correct description of calculus of gallbladder with chronic cholecystitis without obstruction. **Source:** International Classification of Diseases, Tenth Revision, Clinical Modification, 2015, Complete Draft Code Set.

by a code in brackets: [H62.40]. Remember from the conventions discussed earlier in the chapter that codes in brackets must follow the primary code. See Figure 18-3a.

When verifying the code choices in the Tabular List, first look up L01.00 for impetigo. Note that you have five choices, all utilizing 5 characters for types of impetigo. Because you

(a)

Otitis — *continued*
  with effusion (*see also* Otitis, media, nonsuppurative, chronic)
→ externa H60.9☑
    abscess — *see* Abscess, ear, external
    acute (noninfective) H60.50☑
      actinic H60.51☑
      chemical H60.52☑
      contact H60.53☑
      eczematoid H60.54☑
      infective — *see* Otitis, externa, infective
      reactive H60.55☑
      specified NEC H60.59☑
    cellulitis — *see* Cellulitis, ear
    chronic H60.6☑
    diffuse — *see* Otitis, externa, infective, diffuse
    hemorrhagic — *see* Otitis, externa, infective
      hemorrhagic
→ in (due to)
    aspergillosis B44.89
    candidiasis B37.84
    erysipelas A46 [H62.40]
    herpes (simplex) virus infection B00.1
      zoster B02.8
→ impetigo L01.00 [H62.40]
    infectious disease NEC B99 ☑ [H62.4-☑]
    mycosis NEC B36.9 [H62.40]
    parasitic disease NEC B89 [H62.40]
    viral disease NEC B34.9 [H62.40]
    zoster B02.8

(b)

Diseases of the skin and subcutaneous tissue (L00-L99)

> EXCLUDES2 certain conditions originating in the perinatal
>   period (P04-P96)
>   certain infectious and parasitic diseases
>   (A00-B99)
>   complications of pregnancy, childbirth and the
>   puerperium (O00-O9A)
>   congenital malformations, deformations, and
>   chromosomal abnormalities (Q00-Q99)
>   endocrine, nutritional and metabolic diseases
>   (E00-E88)
>   lipomelonotic reticulosis (I89.8)
>   neoplasms (C00-D49)
>   symptoms, signs and abnormal clinical and
>   laboratory findings, not elsewhere classified
>   (R00-R94)
>   systemic connective tissue disorders (M30-M36)
>   viral warts (B07.-)

Infections of the skin and subcutaneous tissue (L00-L08)

> EXCLUDES2 hordeolum (H00.0)
>   infective dermatitis (L30.3)
>   local infections of skin classified in Chapter 1
>   lupus panniculitis (L93.2)
>   panniculitis NOS (M79.3)
>   panniculitis of neck and back (M54.0-)
>   Perlèche NOS (K13.0)
>   Perlèche due to candidiasis (B37.0)
>   Perlèche due to riboflavin deficiency (E53.0)
>   pyogenic granuloma (L98.0)
>   relapsing panniculitis [Weber -Christian] (M35.6)
>   viral warts (B07.-)
>   zoster (B02.-)

L00 Staphylococcal scalded skin syndrome
  Ritter's disease
  Use additional code to identify percentage of skin
  exfoliation (L49.-)
  EXCLUDES1 bullous impetigo (L01.03)
    pemphigus neonatorum (L01.03)
    toxic epidermal necrolysis [Lyell] (L51.2)

→ 4th **L01 Impetigo**
  EXCLUDES1 impetigo herpetiformis (L40.1)
  5th **L01.0 Impetigo**
    Impetigo contagiosa
    Impetigo vulgaris
→ **L01.00 Impetigo, unspecified**
    Impetigo NOS
  L01.01 Non-bullous impetigo
  L01.02 Bockhart's impetigo
    Impetigo follicularis
    Perifolliculitis NOS
    Superficial pustular perifolliculitis
  L01.03 Bullous impetigo
    Impetigo neonatorum
    Pemphigus neonatorum
  L01.09 Other impetigo
    Ulcerative impetigo
  L01.1 Impetiginization of other dermatoses

(c)

  H61.329 Acquired stenosis of external canal secondary to inflammation and infection, unspecified ear
6th **H61.39 Other acquired stenosis of external ear canal**
  H61.391 Other acquired stenosis of right external ear canal
  H61.392 Other acquired stenosis of left external ear canal
  H61.393 Other acquired stenosis of external ear canal, bilateral
  H61.399 Other acquired stenosis of external ear canal, unspecified ear
5th **H61.8 Other specified disorders of external ear**
6th **H61.81 Exostosis of external canal**
  H61.811 Exostosis of right external canal
  H61.812 Exostosis of left external canal
  H61.813 Exostosis of external canal, bilateral
  H61.819 Exostosis of external canal, unspecified ear
6th **H61.89 Other specified disorders of external ear**
  H61.891 Other specified disorders of right external ear
  H61.892 Other specified disorders of left external ear
  H61.893 Other specified disorders of external ear, bilateral
  H61.899 Other specified disorders of external ear, unspecified ear
5th **H61.9 Disorder of external ear, unspecified**
  H61.90 Disorder of external ear, unspecified, unspecified ear
  H61.91 Disorder of right external ear, unspecified
  H61.92 Disorder of left external ear, unspecified
  H61.93 Disorder of external ear, unspecified, bilateral
→ 4th **H62 Disorders of external ear in diseases classified elsewhere**
→ 5th **H62.4 Otitis externa in other diseases classified elsewhere**
  Code first underlying disease, such as:
  erysipelas (A46)
→ impetigo (L01.0)
  EXCLUDES1 otitis externa (in):
    candidiasis (B37.84)
    herpes viral [herpes simplex] (B00.1)
    herpes zoster (B02.8)
  H62.40 Otitis externa in other diseases classified elsewhere, unspecified ear
→ **H62.41 Otitis externa in other diseases classified elsewhere, right ear**
  H62.42 Otitis externa in other diseases classified elsewhere, left ear
  H62.43 Otitis externa in other diseases classified elsewhere, bilateral
5th **H62.8 Other disorders of external ear in diseases classified elsewhere**

(d)

Diagnosis: Otitis externa of right ear, due to Impetigo
  L01.00 Impetigo, unspecified
  H62.41 Otitis externa in other diseases classified elsewhere, right ear

FIGURE 18-3 (a) Alphabetic Index for otitis externa in impetigo. (b) Tabular List for impetigo, unspecified. (c) Tabular List for otitis externa in diseases classified elsewhere. (d) Final coding order for otitis externa of the right ear due to impetigo.

Source: International Classification of Diseases, Tenth Revision, Clinical Modification, 2015, Complete Draft Code Set.

have no specific information as to the type, you will choose L01.00, Impetigo, unspecified. See Figure 18-3b.

Now look up the code in brackets: H62.40. Note that under the classification of H62.4, *Otitis externa in other diseases classified elsewhere,* you are instructed to "Code first underlying disease, such as: erysipelas (A46), impetigo (L01.0)." Also note your 5th-character choices for the otitis codes: 0 = unspecified ear, 1 = right ear, 2 = left ear, and 3 = bilateral ears (Figure 18-3c).

Because your patient diagnosis is with the right ear, you will use code H62.41. As you have been instructed, the correct order for these codes will be L01.00 (Impetigo) first followed by H62.41 (Otitis externa, right ear), as shown in Figure 18-3d.

Remember that 4th, 5th, 6th, and 7th characters, when provided, are not optional and must be used when given. See Figure 18-4 for examples of each.

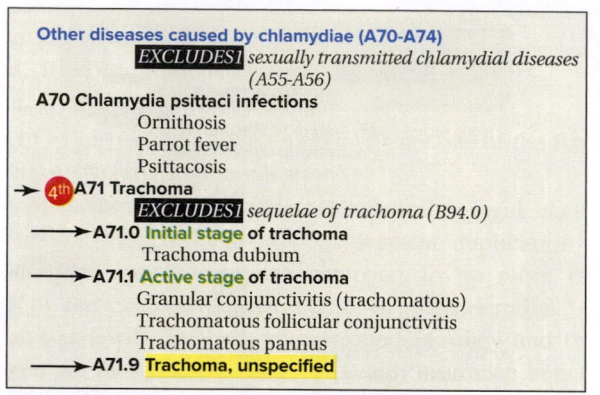

FIGURE 18-4 (a) Fourth-character categories for trachoma. (b) Fifth-character subclassifications for Other chlamydial diseases. (c) Sixth-character subclassifications for diabetes mellitus with diabetic arthropathy. (d) Seventh-character extension for injury of nerves and spinal cord at thorax level.
Source: *International Classification of Diseases, Tenth Revision, Clinical Modification, 2015, Complete Draft Code Set.*

Coding Unclear Diagnoses

Practitioners frequently do not have an exact diagnosis documented. Terms such as *probable, suspected, likely, questionable, possible,* or *rule out* flag a diagnosis as being uncertain. Outpatient coding rules require that unclear diagnoses be coded using the symptoms that led the patient to seek care, until an absolute diagnosis is made. The rules are different for inpatient coding.

Example:

> **Diagnosis:** Nonproductive cough and fever,
> Rule out bronchitis
> **Outpatient diagnosis:** Cough (R05)
> Fever (R50.9)

A similar situation occurs with "impending" or "threatened" conditions. If the condition actually occurs, code it as a confirmed diagnosis. If it did not occur, check to see if a code exists for the threatened condition, and if it exists, use it. If it does not exist, code the underlying conditions or symptoms as if the condition did not exist.

Example:

> **Diagnosis:** Hemorrhage in early pregnancy
> with threatened abortion
> **ICD:** O20. Hemorrhage in early pregnancy
> O20.0 Threatened abortion

Use code O20.0, as it describes exactly the diagnosis given. One word of caution is in order regarding diagnosis codes from ICD-10 Chapter 15, *Pregnancy, Childbirth, and the Puerperium:* Remember that ICD-10 codes always begin with a letter. The first character in this chapter is an "O," not a zero (0). Now that you have the foundation to begin using the ICD manual, Procedure 18-1 at the end of this chapter outlines the steps for locating an ICD-10-CM code.

Principal Versus Primary Diagnosis

The **principal diagnosis** is defined by the Uniform Hospital Discharge Data Set (UHDDS) as "that condition established after study to be chiefly responsible for occasioning the admission of the patient to the hospital for care." Outpatient coding does not generally use principal diagnoses; instead, it uses the **primary diagnosis,** defined as the main reason for the patient's visit. The **secondary** (or subsequent) **diagnoses** are other conditions that are also affecting the patient at the time of the visit and so are coded after the primary diagnosis.

Diagnosis-Related Groups and IP Coding

Unlike outpatient claims where payment is often based on the procedure performed, inpatient claims are paid based on a system known as *Diagnosis-related groups,* or *DRGs.* There are over 700 DRGs, which are based on four elements: principal diagnosis; other diagnoses; significant procedures performed; and the age, sex, and discharge status of the patient. As a medical assistant, you will probably never assign a DRG, but the information you give to the admitting clerk regarding the patient's condition on admission can affect the DRG assigned, so you must be thorough and accurate in the information you give regarding your patients.

▶ External Cause of Injury and Health Status Codes   LO 18.5

Earlier versions of ICD contained two "extra" chapters at the end of the Tabular List. One was the external cause chapter, known as E codes because they all began with the first character E. E codes were supplemental codes used to describe how an injury or illness occurred when caused by an accident or poisoning. The last chapter, known as V codes because they all began with the character V, were for healthcare visits classified as "Supplementary Classification of Factors Influencing Health Status and Contact with Health Services." This very long title was (and is) for codes describing patients who are not currently ill but come to the office for reasons including history of an illness (personal or family); preventive medicine (such as immunizations and physical exams); employment, school, and camp exams; well-baby care; contraception; screenings; aftercare (such as postsurgical care); carrier status; organ donor; testing for status; and so on. ICD-10 made these codes part of the Tabular List and split the external cause codes into two chapters: Chapter 19, *Injury, Poisoning, and Certain Other Consequences of External Causes.* These are the codes that answer "how" an injury or poisoning occurred. For instance, if you see a friend on crutches and he tells you he broke his ankle, naturally your question would be "How did you do that?" Whatever answer he gives you provides the information for using a code or codes from Chapter 19 to act as a secondary code(s) to the primary code describing his fractured ankle. Codes in Chapter 19 begin with the letter "S" or "T." Chapter 20 is the *External Causes of Morbidity* chapter. Chapter 20 codes begin with the letter "V," "W," "X," or "Y." External cause codes are not required by all payers but are intended to provide data for injury research and evaluation of injury prevention strategies.

Chapter 21 in ICD-10 contains the *Supplementary Classification of Factors Influencing Health Status and Contact with Health Services.* Because the codes in this chapter begin with the letter "Z," they are now sometimes referred to as "Z codes." Let's look at both of these accident and "well" visits in a bit more detail. For conciseness, we will simply call codes from this chapter health status codes.

Health Status Codes

Because the patient is basically "healthy," Z codes are generally used in the outpatient setting. Examples of common health status codes include the following:

- Z23: Encounter for vaccination (remember this is a diagnosis, not a procedure code)
- Z51.11: (Encounter for) Chemotherapy treatment

(The patient does have cancer, but the reason for the visit today is the chemotherapy administration. This will be followed by the appropriate code for the neoplasm being treated.)

- Z88.0: History (personal) of allergy to penicillin
- Z37.0: Vaginal delivery of single, live-born newborn (status of the newborn child for the mother's medical record)

Z codes are coded via the same Alphabetic Index as the other ICD-10 codes. For the preceding examples, the key terms *vaccination, encounter, history,* and *outcome of delivery* will be italicized in the Alphabetic Index. Their Tabular List for verification is located in Chapter 21 at the end of the Tabular List. Procedure 18-2 outlines the procedure for locating a Z code.

External Cause Codes

Because coding external cause (T, V, and Y) codes can be complicated, let's focus on getting acquainted with the basic concepts first. Some of the major categories of these codes include transport accidents; poisonings and adverse effects; accidental falls; accidents from fire and flames; accidents due to natural and environmental factors; late effects of accidents; assaults or self-injury; assaults or purposely inflicted injury and suicide; and self-inflicted injury. Both the Table of Drugs and Chemicals and the Alphabetic Index for external cause codes are found at the end of the main Alphabetic Index for ICD-10 codes. Now, let's discuss some specifics for the general use of these codes.

General Use of External Cause Codes
External cause codes are used with any diagnosis code from 001–V84.4, except for CMS (Medicare), which does not require these codes on its claim forms. In general, external cause codes are only used for the initial treatment for an acute illness or injury, and not for subsequent visits. The exception to this rule is treatment for acute fractures. In this case, use the external cause code for as long as acute treatment of the fracture is taking place. Use as many external cause codes as necessary to completely explain how the incident occurred. For instance, if a patient accidentally overdoses on a combination of alcohol and Valium®, at least two codes will be necessary to explain the overdose of both substances. Another example may relate to your friend with the broken ankle. Two external cause codes may be applicable. If he was at work and fell from scaffolding while painting a house, two codes would be necessary for the initial encounter—fall from scaffolding (W12.XXXA) and a place of occurrence code denoting that the accident took place at a private residence (Y92.009).

Place of occurrence codes are found under the key term of *place*. All accidents occurring while using machinery or any type of motorized vehicle (including boats, motorcycles, ATVs, and heavy machinery) require an external cause code describing the vehicle involved in the accident. Many of these codes contain a 4th character that describes the person injured, such as the driver (0), passenger (1), person outside the vehicle (3), person boarding or alighting the vehicle (4), and so on. Always use the code bringing the highest level of specificity. Many of these codes also require a 7th character describing the type of encounter for the visit.

A—initial encounter

D—subsequent encounter

S—sequela

Be careful when adding these 7th characters. Be sure to use the placeholder X as needed. For instance, with the example of your friend who fell from the scaffolding, the base code is W12 with a note to add the 7th character for the encounter. Did you notice that in order to put the A for the initial encounter in the correct location, three X placeholders were required: W12.XXXA?

Poisonings and Adverse Effects The Table of Drugs and Chemicals is located directly after the Alphabetic Index. The table consists of a row for each drug name and then six columns with the following titles: Poisoning, Accident, Therapeutic Use, Suicide Attempt, Assault, and Undetermined. Refer to the poisoning column when the medical record states "poisoning," "overdose," "wrong substance given or taken," or "intoxication." ICD-9 coding required at least two codes for poisonings, first a code describing the poisoning and then an E code to describe how the poisoning took place. ICD-10 has created combination codes for poisonings so that in many cases only one code will be required. If the patient has a secondary symptom due to the poisoning, such as vomiting, this will be coded as secondary to the poisoning code, which will be a T code from Chapter 19. The following definitions will be helpful when deciding which column to use when choosing the correct type of poisoning code using the Table of Drugs and Chemicals:

- Poisoning, Accidental (unintentional). This column is used for accidental overdose, wrong substance given or taken, drug taken by mistake, accidental drug usage, and accidents in drug usage in a medical facility.
- Poisoning, Intentional (self-harm). This column is used when the patient intentionally intended to harm him- or herself (suicide attempt).
- Poisoning, Assault. This column is used when it has been determined that the patient was intentionally harmed by or poisoned by another person with the intent to injure or kill the patient.
- Poisoning, Undetermined. These codes are to be used when the intent of the poisoning or injury cannot be determined.
- Adverse effect. This column is used when the correct substance is properly administered in the correct dosage but caused a poisoning or other adverse effect.
- Underdosing. This column is used as a *secondary* diagnosis when the patient is taking less of a medication than

is prescribed, causing or exacerbating a medical condition, which would be the primary code. If noncompliance or care is complicated because of the underdosing, these issues may also be coded.

Examples:

# 1 Diagnosis:	Hives (urticaria) due to newly diagnosed Penicillin allergy (taken as prescribed); initial encounter
ICD-10 Codes:	T36.0X5A Adverse effect of Penicillins and L50.0 Urticaria due to drugs (allergic)
# 2 Diagnosis:	Vomiting due to intentional overdose of Valium; subsequent encounter
ICD-10 Codes:	T42.4X2D Poisoning, intentional (self harm) by benzodiazpines and R11.10 Vomiting, unspecified

Burns Coding burns typically requires three codes: the degree of the burn (if there are multiple burns, they are sequenced with the highest degree first); the extent (percentage of the body burned); and the external cause code for how the burn occurred. To code burns, first use the key term *Burn,* then find the indented subterm for the burn location, and, finally, use the subclassification for the extent of the burn (1st, 2nd, or 3rd degree). Locations with multiple burn degrees are coded to the highest extent of the burn. Once that code is completed, return to the key term *Burn* and subterm *Extent.* Using the Rule of Nines, found in the Tabular List at the beginning of the T31 section, calculate the percentage of the body burned. Finally, locate the external cause code description from the Alphabetic Index for External Cause Codes and verify it in the Tabular List.

Example:

Diagnosis:	Patient presents with 1st and 2nd degree burns to right hand and wrist from boiling water; initial encounter
ICD-10 Codes:	T23.201A (1st & 2nd degree burn right hand and wrist), T31.0 (less than 10% of body surface burned) and X12.XXXA (Contact with other hot fluids)

Always remember that external cause codes are never the primary or first diagnosis listed. When used, they are listed after the primary (or secondary) diagnosis to which they relate. More than any other type of diagnosis code, external cause codes require practice to get perfect. Procedure 18-3 found at the end of the chapter outlines how to code using external cause codes.

▶ Synopsis of ICD-10 Coding Guidelines by Chapter
LO 18.6

You now have a basic idea of how to use the ICD-10 manual and locate and verify an ICD-10 code. The majority of ICD-10 codes follow the general guidelines. However, unique coding applications also exist. These include but are not limited to neoplasms, diabetes mellitus, fractures, pregnancy, external causes of morbidity and mortality, R codes (abnormal findings), poisonings, and expanded Z codes (formerly V codes). In this section we are going to take a quick look at the unique guidelines for some of the chapters in ICD-10, to allow you to better understand how to code correctly and efficiently with the ICD-10 manual.

Chapter 1: Certain Infectious and Parasitic Diseases (A00–B99)

In an outpatient setting, requesting a confirmatory serology or culture for HIV is not enough to code HIV positivity. Only a diagnostic statement such as "known HIV" or "positive HIV" is adequate from the provider. When no definitive diagnosis or manifestation of HIV is present and the patient has an inconclusive serology, code R75, inconclusive laboratory evidence of human immunodeficiency virus, should be assigned. Patients who have had a positive serology or culture and have developed an HIV-related illness should be assigned code B20 on every encounter. Patients who are HIV positive but asymptomatic in status should be assigned code Z21. This code should be assigned for all patients with the diagnostic statement of positive HIV. When a patient presents with any signs or symptoms while being seen for HIV testing, code only the signs and symptoms. If counseling is provided during the same encounter, an additional counseling code out of Z71.7 may be reported.

Chapter 2: Neoplasms (C00–D49)

Chapter 2 of ICD-10-CM deals with neoplasms. To assign a proper code, first remember that all cancers are found under the term *neoplasm* and that the documentation of the neoplasm must state whether it is benign, malignant, in situ, or of uncertain behavior. Found in the Table of Neoplasms, neplasms are listed alphabetically by anatomical location such as breast or bone. Each site may further be broken down to a certain area. In the case of a bone neoplasm, in order to code the diagnosis, you must know in which bone (rib, femur, vertebra, etc.) the neoplasm has been found. When coding malignant neoplasms, the primary site is the location where the cancer originated. The secondary, or metastatic, sites are the areas to which the cancer or malignancy has spread. Once the site and type of the neoplasm are identified, any additional instructions for coding must be observed. An additional code, such as one identifying exposures to carcinogenic (cancer-causing) substances that may be the underlying cause of the patient's cancer diagnosis, may be required. Two examples of carcinogens as underlying causes are exposure to tobacco smoke (Z77.22) and exposure to tobacco smoke in the perinatal period (P96.81).

The correct coding and sequencing of neoplasms is critical. If the treatment is directed at the primary neoplasm, that code is used as the principal (or primary) diagnosis. If the neoplasm has metastasized and the patient's treatment is for the secondary site, then the secondary neoplasm becomes the primary diagnosis. If chemotherapy, radiation therapy, or immunotherapy—although each is generally considered a procedure and not a diagnosis—is the primary reason for medical care, it is coded first (and linked to the appropriate procedure), followed by the code for the malignancy being treated.

Chapter 4: Endocrine, Nutritional, and Metabolic Diseases (E00–E89)

Chapter 4 contains the codes for diabetes mellitus. Codes for diabetes mellitus are combination codes that include the type of diabetes:

- Type 1—insulin-dependent diabetes (IDDM), sometimes referred to as juvenile diabetes
- Type 2—noninsulin-dependent diabetes (NIDDM)

In addition to the type of diabetes which must be documented as type 1 or type 2, the body system affected by diabetes and the condition affecting the anatomical structure are included. When the type of diabetes is not documented in the medical record (and the provider cannot be queried), then the patient should be assigned a code for Type 2 diabetes mellitus. In many cases one code will identify both the type of diabetes and its manifestation. For instance, if a patient with Type 2 diabetes is discovered to have retinopathy without macular edema, the code of E09.319 will completely code his condition. If, however, the patient's diabetes is caused by another underlying factor, two codes will be needed. Look at Figure 18-5. The first code will identify the underlying condition, for instance, Cushing's syndrome (E24.-) followed by the appropriate code for the type of diabetes from category E08. Do note also that the Cushing's syndrome code will require additional digits as noted in the Alphabetic Index by the dash after the decimal point.

Chapter 5: Mental and Behavioral Disorders (F01–F99)

When patients experience pain, whether acute or chronic, it should be documented if the pain is exclusively psychological. Pain that is associated with and is exclusively psychological should be assigned code F45.41, pain disorder with related psychological factors, followed by the appropriate code from the category G89.

Chapter 6: Diseases of the Nervous System (G00–G99)

The nervous system chapter in ICD-10 no longer includes the eye and ear; they have each been given an individual chapter (7 and 8); otherwise, the coding for the nervous system has changed very little since ICD-9. As stated earlier, code G89 is used for pain diagnoses. This code may be used as a first-listed diagnosis when the reason for the encounter is the treatment of the pain. If the patient is seen for a definitive diagnosis (such as cancer) and pain is also noted, then the definitive diagnosis should be listed first, followed by the most specific pain code possible. If malignant neoplasm is the underlying cause of the pain, the appropriate pain code is G89.3.

Diabetes mellitus (E08-E13)

E08 Diabetes mellitus due to underlying condition
    Code first the underlying condition, such as:
        congenital rubella (P35.0)
        Cushing's syndrome (E24.-)
        cystic fibrosis (E84.-)
        malignant neoplasm (C00-C96)
        malnutrition (E40-E46)
        pancreatitis and other diseases of the pancreas (K85-K86.-)
    Use additional code to identify any insulin use (Z79.4)
    Excludes1: drug or chemical induced diabetes mellitus (E09.-)
        gestational diabetes (O24.4-)
        neonatal diabetes mellitus (P70.2)
        postpancreatectomy diabetes mellitus (E13.-)
        postprocedural diabetes mellitus (E13.-)
        secondary diabetes mellitus NEC (E13.-)
        type 1 diabetes mellitus (E10.-)
        type 2 diabetes mellitus (E11.-)
    E08.0 Diabetes mellitus due to underlying condition with hyperosmolarity
        E08.00 Diabetes mellitus due to underlying condition with hyperosmolarity without nonketotic hyperglycemic-hyperosmolar coma (NKHHC)
    E08.01 Diabetes mellitus due to underlying condition with hyperosmolarity with coma
    E08.1 Diabetes mellitus due to underlying condition with ketoacidosis
        E08.10 Diabetes mellitus due to underlying condition with ketoacidosis without coma

FIGURE 18-5 Diabetes mellitus codes with underlying conditions using ICD-10 2016 version from CMS.gov website.
Source: 2016 version from CMS.gov website, https://www.cms.gov/Medicare/Coding/ICD10/2016-ICD-10-CM-and-GEMs.html

Chapter 9: Diseases of the Circulatory System (I00–I99)

ICD-10 uses the hypertension table in the Alphabetic Index, and the rules for coding hypertension have not changed since ICD-9. Primary hypertension, also known as essential hypertension, is coded as I10. When hypertension is caused by an underlying condition (secondary hypertension), two codes are required—the first to identify the underlying **etiology** (cause) and the second to code the hypertension. A patient who has elevated blood pressure may not necessarily have a diagnosis of hypertension. This is known as transient hypertension, and the code R03.0 should be assigned.

Chapter 10: Diseases of the Respiratory System (J00–J99)

Coding within the respiratory system is not difficult as long as you continue to follow the basic guidelines and the guidelines within the chapter. It should be noted, however, that positive laboratory documentation is not required in order to code either novel A or H1N1 influenza as a diagnosis. When the provider's documentation states "suspected or probable" novel A influenza or H1N1 influenza, codes should be assigned as if the condition existed (J09.0 category). Documentation of any another type of influenza should be assigned codes from the J10 category. Figure 18-6 shows the difference in the Tabular List between novel A influenza codes and descriptions and those for influenza due to other influenza virus. Note that manifestations of novel A and H1N1 virus are included in the code descriptions.

Chapter 13: Diseases of the Musculoskeletal System and Connective Tissue (M00–M99)

This chapter contains the categories for fractures, which are coded quite differently in ICD-10 than they were in in ICD-9. **Laterality** (which describes the side of the body affected by the diagnosis) for fractures is new and designated as follows:

- Unilateral—4th character "1"
- Laterality designated by—5th character:
  - 0—unspecified
  - 1—right
  - 2—left

Another major change in ICD-10 is the addition of a 7th character designating the type of encounter for which the patient is being seen. Coding pathological fractures due to osteoporosis includes this 7th character. Shown in Figure 18-7 are the six capital letters used for this mandatory 7th character.

For the purposes of these 7th-character extensions, the term *initial* means an active fracture that is still healing, *subsequent* defines follow-up after the active fracture care, and *sequela* refers to care after the injury has healed, but there are now different issues related to the initial injury that must be attended to. To better understand the coding concepts within this section, let's take a look at Figure 18-8 for a patient who has age-related osteoporosis with a current pathological fracture of the right shoulder. Based on the information in Figure 18-8, the code would be M80.011; however, because of the information you received on the necessary 7th characters (see Figure 18-7), you know that if the patient had a subsequent visit for the fracture as a routine checkup for a healing fracture, you would use the code M80.011D.

Chapter 14: Diseases of the Genitourinary System (N00–N99)

ICD-10 provides for four stages of chronic kidney disease (CKD). Code N18.1 is the beginning stage; N18.2, mild CKD; N18.3, moderate CKD; and N18.4, severe CKD. If end-stage renal disease (ESRD) is documented, use code N18.6. This code will be used alone, even if both chronic kidney disease and end-stage renal disease are documented. Keep in mind that kidney transplant (Z94.0—kidney transplant status) may not totally restore kidney function, so both Z94.0 and a code for chronic kidney disease, if still present, may be coded.

Chapter 15: Pregnancy, Childbirth, and the Puerperium (O00–O9A)

When coding pregnancy-related diagnoses, ICD-10 often requires a 7th character (the highest specificity for the system). With many codes, the 7th character specifies the trimester of the pregnancy in which the condition occurs. Read these descriptions carefully. If the patient is in a different trimester than the one stated, you must look for a different code. With codes describing pregnancy conditions related to multiple gestation, the 7th digit specifies the number of fetuses in utero. Maternity coding can be complicated, but thorough reading of the medical record documentation and understanding of the coding guidelines specific to this chapter will allow optimal confidence in coding.

Chapter 17: Congenital Malformations, Deformations, and Chromosomal Abnormalities (Q00–Q99)

Codes from this chapter are used exclusively when a patient's medical record documents that the diagnosis or condition is congenital or chromosomal in nature. Codes Q00–Q99 may be listed as either primary or secondary diagnoses, depending on the guidelines given within the coding instructions. Diseases and conditions in this section include hydrocephalus, spina bifida, atrial septal defect, limb malformations and deformities, cleft lip/palate, trisomy 21 (Down syndrome), and many others.

J09 Influenza due to certain identified influenza viruses

Excludes1: influenza due to other identified influenza virus (J.10.-)
influenza due to unidentified influenza virus (J11.-)
seasonal influenza due to other identified influenza virus (J10.-)
seasonal influenza due to unidentified influenza virus (J11.-)

J09.X Influenza due to identified novel influenza A virus

Avian influenza
Bird influenza
Influenza A/H5N1
Influenza of other animal origin, not bird or swine
Swine influenza virus (viruses that normally cause infections in pigs)

J09.X1 Influenza due to identified novel influenza A virus with pneumonia

Code also, if applicable, associated:
lung abscess (J85.1)
other specified type of pneumonia

J09.X2 Influenza due to identified novel influenza A virus with other respiratory manifestations

Influenza due to identified novel influenza A virus NOS
Influenza due to identified novel influenza A virus with laryngitis
Influenza due to identified novel influenza A virus with pharyngitis
Influenza due to identified novel influenza A virus with upper respiratory symptoms
Use additional code, if applicable, for associated:
pleural effusion (J91.8)
sinusitis (J01.-)

J09.X3 Influenza due to identified novel influenza A virus with gastrointestinal manifestations

Influenza due to identified novel influenza A virus gastroenteritis
'intestinal flu' [viral gastroenteritis] (A08.-)

J09.X9 Influenza due to identified novel influenza A virus with other manifestations

Influenza due to identified novel influenza A virus with encephalopathy
Influenza due to identified novel influenza A virus with myocarditis
Influenza due to identified novel influenza A virus with otitis media
Use additional code to identify manifestation

(a)

J10 Influenza due to other identified influenza virus

Excludes1: influenza due to avian influenza virus (J09.X-)
influenza due to swine flu (J09.X-)
influenza due to unidentified influenza virus (J11.-)

J10.0 Influenza due to other identified influenza virus with pneumonia

Code also: associated lung abscess, if applicable (J85.1)

J10.00 Influenza due to other identified influenza virus with unspecified type of pneumonia

J10.01 Influenza due to other identified influenza virus with the same other identified influenza viruspneumonia

J10.08 Influenza due to other identified influenza virus with other specified pneumonia

Code also: other specified type of pneumonia

J10.1 Influenza due to other identified influenza virus with other respiratory manifestations

Influenza due to other identified influenza virus NOS
Influenza due to other identified influenza virus with laryngitis
Influenza due to other identified influenza virus with pharyngitis
Influenza due to other identified influenza virus with upper respiratory symptoms
Use additional code for associated pleural effusion, if applicable (J91.8)
Use additional code for associated sinusitis, if applicable (J01.-)

J10.2 Influenza due to other identified influenza virus with gastrointestinal manifestations

Influenza due to other identified influenza virus gastroenteritis
EXCLUDES 1 'intestinal flu' [viral gastroenteritis] (A08.-)

J10.8 Influenza due to other identified influenza virus with other manifestations

J10.81 Influenza due to other identified influenza virus with encephalopathy

J10.82 Influenza due to other identified influenza virus with myocarditis

J10.83 Influenza due to other identified influenza virus with otitis media

Use additional code for any associated perforated tympanic membrane (H72.-)

J10.89 Influenza due to other identified influenza virus with other manifestations

Use additional codes to identify the manifestations

(b)

FIGURE 18-6 (a) Tabular List for influenza due to avian influenza virus and (b) Tabular List for influenza due to other influenza virus 2016 version from CMS.gov website.

Source: 2016 version from CMS.gov website, https://www.cms.gov/Medicare/Coding/ICD10/2016-ICD-10-CM-and-GEMs.html

M.80 Osteoporosis with current pathological fracture
Includes: osteoporosis with current fragility fracture
Use additional code to identify major osseous defect, if applicable (M89.7–)
Excludes1: collapsed vertebra NOS (M48.5)
pathological fracture NOS (M84.4)
wedging of vertebra NOS (M48.5)
Excludes 2: personal history of (healed) osteoporosis fracture (Z87.310)
The appropriate 7th character is to be added to each code from category M80:
A – initial encounter for fracture
D – subsequent encounter for fracture with routine healing
G – subsequent encounter for fracture with delayed healing
K – subsequent encounter for fracture with nonunion
P – subsequent encounter for fracture with malunion
S – sequela

FIGURE 18-7 Codes and the 7th characters for osteoporosis with pathological fracture 2016 version from CMS.gov website.
Source: 2016 version from CMS.gov website, https://www.cms.gov/Medicare/Coding/ICD10/2016-ICD-10-CM-and-GEMs.html

M80.01 Age-related osteoporosis with current pathological fracture
Involutional osteoporosis with current pathological fracture
Osteoporosis NOS with current pathological fracture
Postmenopausal osteoporosis with current pathological fracture
Senile osteoporosis with current pathological fracture
M80.00 Age-related osteoporosis with current pathological fracture, unspecified site
M80.01 Age-related osteoporosis with current pathological fracture, shoulder
M80.011 Age-related osteoporosis with current pathological fracture, right shoulder
M80.012 Age-related osteoporosis with current pathological fracture, left shoulder
M80.013 Age-related osteoporosis with current pathological fracture, unspecified shoulder

FIGURE 18-8 Tabular List for subclassification M80.01, Age-related osteoporosis with current pathological fracture, shoulder 2016 version from CMS.gov website.
Source: https://www.cms.gov/Medicare/Coding/ICD10/2016-ICD-10-CM-and-GEMs.html

Chapter 18: Signs, Symptoms, and Abnormal Clinical and Laboratory Findings (NEC) (R00–R99)

Chapter 18 is primarily used to code for the following types of conditions:

- Cases that do not have a more specific diagnosis after all the findings are analyzed
- Transient signs and symptoms at the initial encounter with undetermined cause
- Provisional diagnosis in a patient not returning for further care
- Cases without a definitive diagnosis referred elsewhere
- Cases in which a definitive diagnosis could not be determined
- Additional information that represents a significant but currently asymptomatic medical problem (such as an asymptomatic HIV-positive patient)

There are multiple combination codes available in this chapter. Watch for them and follow guidelines for their use. If a combination code is available, it must be used to avoid unbundling the code.

Chapter 19: Injury, Poisoning, and Certain Other Consequences of External Causes (S00–T88)

As stated earlier in the chapter, the 7th-character extension is used extensively in this chapter for poisonings. You will also note that because poisoning codes require specificity, the "X" placeholder is often found in the 5th position, the 6th character 1–6 describes how the poisoning took place, and then a 7th character A (initial), D (subsequent), or S (sequela) is used to describe the type of encounter. An illustration for the substance sulfonazide is in Table 18-6.

Note that the table does not give you the 7th-character options. This is a perfect example of why you must always verify codes in the Tabular List to obtain the entire correct code. If a 7th character is required and is not in place, the insurance carrier will not accept the code. For any of the poisoning codes for sulfonazide to be complete, the letter, A, D, or S will have to be added to the code describing the encounter as initial, subsequent, or a sequela.

Burns and Corrosions Always remember that burns are classified by three factors: depth of the burn (first-degree, second-degree, or third-degree), the extent (total body area—based on the rule of nines), and the agent (fire, thermal, or appliance). Burns that are caused by a corrosive material are coded the same as any burn with the additional code for the corrosive material being sequenced first. It is also important to note that if the same area of the body sustains multiple burn degrees, the area should be coded as the most extensive degree listed. For instance, if the left foot sustains both

TABLE 18-6   Excerpt from ICD-10 Table of Drug and Chemicals for the Substance Sulfonazide

Substance	Poisoning Accidental	Poisoning Intentional	Poisoning Assault	Poisoning Undetermined	Adverse Effect	Underdosing
Sulfonazide	T37.1X1	T37.1X2	T37.1X3	T37.1X4	T37.1X5	T37.1X6

first- and second-degree burns, code the entire foot as a second-degree burn.

Chapter 20: External Causes of Morbidity (V00–Y99)

Codes within this chapter identify who, what, when, and where an accident or injury occurred. They are used for data in determining research and prevention strategies for injuries. These codes may be used as secondary codes to describe health conditions and are applicable for categories A00–T88.9 and Z00–Z99. Figure 18-9 shows some of the categories for these secondary codes, previously referred to as E codes in ICD-9. The use of these codes should completely identify the patient's cause of injury. An example would be a sprained ankle while playing football. The cause of the injury is a fall, the activity is football, and the location is the playground at the time of injury. When assigning multiple external cause codes, the code indicating the cause or intent, or medical misadventure, is reported before the code for the place, activity, or external status codes. When reporting multiple causes of injuries, codes for child and adult abuse take priority over all other external cause codes. Read the guidelines carefully.

Chapter 21: Factors Influencing Health Status and Contact with Health Services (Z00–Z99)

As explained earlier in the chapter, the unique ICD-9 V codes (used to code for healthcare encounters other than injury or illness, such as prenatal care or administration of immunizations) were replaced by Chapter 21, *Factors Influencing Health Status and Contact with Health Services,* Z00–Z99 in ICD-10. In addition to the usual "well" visits thought of in this section, the following reasons for healthcare encounters are included in this section:

- Chemotherapy, radiation therapy, and immunotherapy
- Aftercare
- Administrative exams (such as a sports physical)

V00-X58	Accidents
V00-V99	Transport accidents
V00-V09	Pedestrian injured in transport accident
V10-V19	Pedal cycle rider injured in transport accident
V20-V29	Motorcycle rider injured in transport accident
V30-V39	Occupant of three-wheeled motor vehicle injured in transport accident
V40-V49	Car occupant injured in transport accident
V50-V59	Occupant of pick-up truck or van injured in transport accident
V60-V69	Occupant of heavy transport vehicle injured in transport accident
V70-V79	Bus occupant injured in transport accident
V80-V89	Other land transport accidents
V90-V94	Water transport accidents
V95-V97	Air and space transport accidents
V98-V99	Other and unspecified transport accidents
W00-X58	Other external causes of accidental injury
W00-W19	Slipping, tripping, stumbling and falls
W20-W49	Exposure to inanimate mechanical forces
W50-W64	Exposure to animate mechanical forces
W65-W74	Accidental non-transport drowning and submersion
W85-W99	Exposure to electric current, radiation and extreme ambient air temperature and pressure
X00-X08	Exposure to smoke, fire and flames
X10-X19	Contact with heat and hot substances
X30-X39	Exposure to forces of nature
X52-X58	Accidental exposure to other specified factors
X71-X83	Intentional self-harm
X92-Y08	Assault
Y21-Y33	Event of undetermined intent
Y35-Y38	Legal intervention, operations of war, military operations, and terrorism
Y62-Y84	Complications of medical and surgical care
Y62-Y69	Misadventures to patients during surgical and medical care
Y70-Y82	Medical devices associated with adverse incidents in diagnostic and therapeutic use
Y83-Y84	Surgical and other medical procedures as the cause of abnormal reaction of the patient, or of later complication, without mention of misadventure at the time of the procedure
Y90-Y99	Supplementary factors related to causes of morbidity classified elsewhere

FIGURE 18-9   Code range descriptions for external cause of illness or injury for ICD-10 2016 version from CMS.gov website.
Source: https://www.cms.gov/Medicare/Coding/ICD10/2016-ICD-10-CM-and-GEMs.html

- Family history if the patient may be at risk for like illness
- Personal history if the patient's habits or past illnesses or condition place him at risk

Diagnostic coding can be intimidating. Like learning anything new, take it a little bit at a time, and remember, practice does make perfect. Read all guidelines carefully. Don't be afraid to ask questions—particularly if you do not understand terminology—so that you are capable of choosing the most appropriate code. Coding takes concentration, an in-depth knowledge of anatomy, physiology, and medical terminology,

and, most importantly, an "inquiring mind" to get to the heart of the patient's diagnosis and make sure that the codes truly describe what is wrong with each patient.

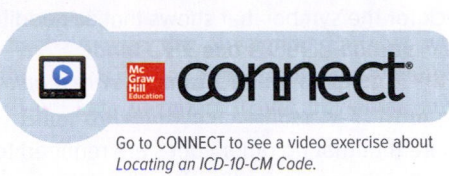

Go to CONNECT to see a video exercise about
Locating an ICD-10-CM Code.

PROCEDURE 18-1 Locating an ICD-10-CM Code

Procedure Goal: To analyze diagnoses and locate the correct ICD code

OSHA Guidelines: This procedure does not involve exposure to blood, body fluids, or tissue.

Materials: Patient record, charge slip or superbill, and ICD-10-CM manual

Method:

1. Locate the patient's diagnosis on the superbill (encounter form) or elsewhere in the patient's chart. If it is on the superbill, verify documentation in the medical chart.
   RATIONALE: *The medical record documentation must back up all diagnosis codes used for billing.*

2. Find the diagnosis in ICD-10's Alphabetic Index. Look for the condition first; then locate the indented subterms that make the condition more specific. Read all cross-references to check all the possibilities for a term, including its synonyms and any eponyms.

3. Locate the code from the Alphabetic Index in ICD-10's Tabular List.

RATIONALE: *All codes must be verified in the Tabular List to be sure the most accurate code is chosen.*

4. Read all information to find the code that corresponds to the patient's specific disease or condition. Study the list of codes and descriptions. Be sure to pick the most specific code available. Check for the symbol that shows that additional characters may be required.
   RATIONALE: *The additional characters allow for specificity. If they are given, they must be used, or the insurance carrier will not accept the code for payment.*

5. Be sure that all necessary codes are chosen to completely describe each diagnosis. Check for instructions stating that an additional code is needed. If more than one code is needed, be sure instructions are followed and the codes are listed in the correct order.
   RATIONALE: *In order to accurately code the patient's condition, all applicable codes must be chosen and recorded as instructed by the ICD manual.*

6. Carefully record the diagnosis code(s) on the insurance claim and proofread the numbers.

PROCEDURE 18-2 Locating a Health Status (Z) Code

Procedure Goal: To analyze the patient record (or encounter form) and decide whether a Z code is an appropriate diagnosis code

OSHA Guidelines: This procedure does not involve exposure to blood, body fluids, or tissue.

Materials: Patient record, charge slip or superbill, and ICD-10-CM manual

Method:

1. Locate the patient's diagnosis. This information may be found on the superbill (encounter form) or elsewhere in the patient's chart. If it is on the superbill, verify documentation in the medical chart.

RATIONALE: *All information billed to the insurance carrier must be backed up by the patient medical record.*

2. If the reason for the patient encounter relates to a physical exam, immunization, well-child visit, or other visit where there is no diagnosis or condition of illness found, a Z code will be used to code the reason for the visit (diagnosis).

3. Find the diagnosis in ICD-10's Alphabetic Index. Look for the condition first and then locate any indented subterms that make the condition more specific. Read all cross-references.
   RATIONALE: *Subterms assist in locating codes with the greatest specificity.*

4. Locate the code from the Alphabetic Index in the Z code area of ICD-10's Tabular List.

5. Read all descriptive information to find the code that corresponds to the patient's specific reason for today's visit. Be sure to pick the most specific code available. Check for the symbol that shows that any additional specificity characters are required.

    RATIONALE: *Fourth to 7th characters are required to record the most specific code available.*

6. Be sure that that no other codes are required to describe the patient's reason for the visit. Check for instructions stating that an additional code is needed. If more than one code is needed, be sure instructions are followed and the codes are listed in the correct order.

    RATIONALE: *The patient's condition must be coded so that all information about the diagnosis is included. If codes are listed in the wrong order, the insurance carrier may reject them.*

7. Carefully record the diagnosis code(s) on the insurance claim and proofread the numbers.

PROCEDURE 18-3 Locating an External Cause Code

Procedure Goal: To analyze the patient record (or encounter form) and decide whether an external cause code is required to completely code the encounter

OSHA Guidelines: This procedure does not involve exposure to blood, body fluids, or tissue.

Materials: Patient record, charge slip or superbill, and ICD-10-CM manual

Method:

1. Locate the patient's diagnosis. This information may be found on the superbill (encounter form) or elsewhere in the patient's chart. If it is on the superbill, verify documentation in the medical chart.

    RATIONALE: *All information billed to the insurance carrier must be backed up by the patient medical record.*

2. If the patient's diagnosis begs the question "How did that happen?" an external cause code is required to give the insurance carrier as much information as possible.

    RATIONALE: *Without the external cause code, the payer does not know how the injury or illness occurred.*

3. After coding the diagnosis of the condition requiring treatment, open the ICD-10 manual to the External Cause Alphabetic Index or, if necessary, use the Table of Drugs and Chemicals. Find the appropriate description in ICD-10's Alphabetic Index, looking for the condition first, and then locate any indented subterms that make the condition more specific. Read all cross-references.

    RATIONALE: *Subterms assist in locating codes with the greatest specificity.*

4. Locate the code from the Alphabetic Index in the external cause code area of ICD-10's Tabular List.

5. Read all descriptive information to find the code that corresponds to how the patient's current condition came about. Choose the most specific code available. Check for the symbol that shows that any additional characters are required; many external cause codes require these.

    RATIONALE: *Fourth to 7th characters are often required to record the most specific code available.*

6. Carefully record the diagnosis code(s) on the insurance claim and proofread the numbers.

7. External cause codes are always secondary, so be sure that the primary diagnosis code is listed first. Check for instructions stating an additional code is needed. If more than one code is needed, be sure instructions are followed and the codes are listed in the correct order.

    RATIONALE: *The coding order is important. Insurers may deny claims if codes are not placed in the appropriate order.*

LEARNING OUTCOMES	KEY POINTS
18.1 **Recall the six ways that ICD codes are used today.**	ICD codes are used to facilitate payment for medical services, evaluate utilization patterns (patient use of healthcare facilities), study healthcare costs, research quality of healthcare, predict healthcare trends, and plan for future healthcare needs.
18.2 **Compare ICD-9-CM and ICD-10-CM.**	ICD-10-CM is intended to provide a more precise clinical picture of the patient and enhanced trending analysis for data reporting. The number of codes increased from under 15,000 in ICD-9 to 68,000+ in ICD-10, and the characters changed from 3–5 numeric (with the exception of the E and V codes) to 3–7 alphanumeric. Both the 9th and 10th revisions contain the Alphabetic Index of the diseases, conditions, and related terms. The ICD-10 Tabular List consists of 21 chapters (versus ICD-9, with 17 chapters) with a corresponding range of codes. Many codes use an "X" as a placeholder for future expansion, which was not possible with ICD-9.
18.3 **Describe the conventions used in ICD-10.**	The conventions used in ICD include NOS; NEC; brackets; parentheses; colon; includes and Excludes (1 and 2) notes; instructions to use additional code, code first underlying disease, and code, if applicable, any causal condition first. Additionally, bold and italics are used in both the Alphabetic Index and Tabular List. Instructions to See condition and See also are found exclusively in the Alphabetic Index.
18.4 **Outline the steps to code a diagnosis using ICD-10-CM.**	To choose an ICD code, check the encounter form (superbill) and/or patient medical record for all applicable diagnoses. Find the key term in the Alphabetic Index and then search for any applicable subterms. Once the code has been located, verify its description in the Tabular List, again reading all applicable notations for other coding options and instructions. Document each code carefully using instructions for code sequencing on the CMS-1500 claim form.
18.5 **Explain the purpose and usage of external cause of injury and health status codes.**	Z codes are defined as Supplementary Classification of Factors Influencing Health Status and Contact with Health Services. They are used for patients who, although not ill, are seeking healthcare. They are used for exams, counseling, donors, chemotherapy encounters, and so on. The Supplementary Classification of External Causes of Injury and Poisoning are used to explain how an illness or injury came about. They are used for all types of accidents and poisonings, as well as to describe the external cause for morbidity.
18.6 **Illustrate unique coding applications for neoplasms, diabetes mellitus, fractures, signs and symptoms, poisonings, and Z codes.**	The majority of ICD-10-CM codes follow the general guidelines. However, unique coding applications do exist and chapter guidelines must be followed. These include but are not limited to the chapters on neoplasms, diabetes mellitus, fractures, signs and symptoms, poisonings, and the new Z codes.

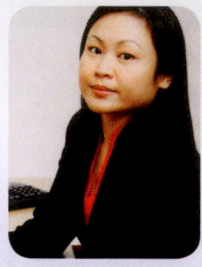

Recall Cindy Chen from the beginning of the chapter. Now that you have completed the chapter, answer the following questions regarding her case.

1. How would you code Cindy's HIV-positive status using ICD-10?

2. What other diagnosis codes would you use related to Cindy's symptoms, using the ICD-10 coding system?

3. You note in Cindy's record that she has a history of mild depression. Should this diagnosis be coded and, if so, how would this diagnosis be coded?

© Red Chopsticks/Getty Images RF

EXAM PREPARATION QUESTIONS

1. (LO 18.1) Which organization maintains and updates the ICD system?
   a. AMA
   b. AAMA
   c. WHO
   d. TJC
   e. BWW

2. (LO 18.3) The Alphabetic Index for ICD-10-CM is organized by
   a. The part of the body involved
   b. Symptoms the patient displays
   c. Codes found in the Tabular List
   d. The condition
   e. The alphabet

3. (LO 18.3) _____ provide coding guidelines for using the ICD code set.
   a. Abbreviations
   b. Certain forms of punctuation
   c. Chapter openers
   d. Notes
   e. Conventions

4. (LO 18.2) Matching a procedure with the diagnosis describing why the procedure was done is known as
   a. Reasonable doubt
   b. Medical necessity
   c. Proof of need
   d. Rationale
   e. A requirement

5. (LO 18.4) Which diagnosis gives the primary reason for a patient's outpatient visit?
   a. Primary diagnosis
   b. Principal diagnosis
   c. Secondary diagnosis
   d. Probable diagnosis
   e. Z code diagnosis

6. (LO 18.5) Which diagnosis code type can never "stand alone"?
   a. A principal diagnosis
   b. A Z code
   c. An external cause code
   d. A primary diagnosis
   e. A supplemental diagnosis

7. (LO 18.5) What is the purpose of external cause codes?
   a. To act as the primary diagnosis
   b. To describe well-child visits
   c. To describe poisonings
   d. To describe how an accident occurred
   e. To describe poisonings, accidents, and other causes of injury and morbidity

8. (LO 18.1) The primary reason for the ICD-10 update is
   a. There are more diagnoses to choose from
   b. It works better with EHR programs
   c. It provides greater specificity for diagnosis classifications
   d. It provides room for expansion for new codes
   e. It provides greater specificity and room for code expansion

9. (LO 18.3) Which coding convention is *not* new in ICD-10?
   a. Includes 1 & 2
   b. Excludes 1 & 2
   c. Default code
   d. See/See also
   e. Placeholders

10. (LO 18.6) Which ICD-10 chapter replaces the V codes found in previous versions of ICD?
    a. Chapter 21
    b. Chapter 20
    c. Chapter 10
    d. Chapter 5
    e. Chapter 1

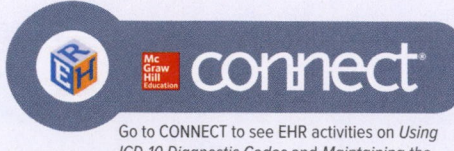

Go to CONNECT to see EHR activities on *Using ICD-10 Diagnostic Codes* and *Maintaining the ICD-10 Database*.

Recall Cindy Chen from the case study at the beginning of the chapter.

1. You receive a call from Cindy, who is quite upset. She has just received an EOB from her insurance company clearly stating a diagnosis of AIDS. Although HIV positive, she has not been diagnosed with AIDS. How will you help Cindy's immediate concern of her diagnosis?

2. In looking at Cindy's insurance claim, you see that the new coder did indeed use the diagnosis code for AIDS instead of HIV. How can this be corrected with the insurance company? What will you say to the coder regarding the need for accuracy when coding any claim?

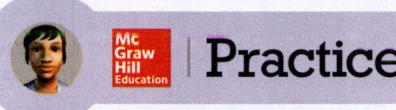

Go to PRACTICE MEDICAL OFFICE and complete the module Admin: Check Out - Office Operations.

Procedural Coding

CASE STUDY

Patient Name	DOB	Allergies
Raja Lautu	8/3/19XX	Benzalkonium Chloride, Sulfa

Attending	MRN	Other Information
Elizabeth H. Williams, MD	224-86-564	Family hx of breast CA. Nonsmoker. Occ. wine w/ meals.

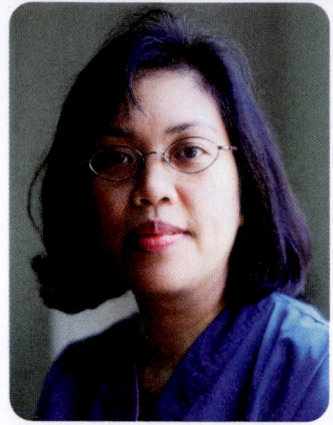

© ERproductions Ltd/Blend Images LLC RF

Raja Lautu is a 42-year-old woman who had a (screening) digital mammogram with CAD (computer-aided detection) performed recently as part of her physical examination (she is a new patient for Dr. Williams and BWW Medical Associates). When the mammogram revealed a small density in the right breast, a complete ultrasound of this breast was ordered with stereotactic breast biopsy. Considering Raja's family history reveals that both her mother and maternal aunt have had breast cancer, she is understandably nervous about this development.

Keep Raja in mind as you study this chapter. There will be questions at the end of the chapter based on the case study. The information in the chapter will help you answer these questions.

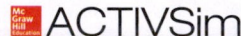

LEARNING OUTCOMES

After completing Chapter 19, you will be able to:

19.1 List the sections of the CPT manual, giving the code range for each.

19.2 Describe briefly each of the CPT's general guidelines.

19.3 List the types of E/M codes within the CPT.

19.4 List the areas included in the surgical coding section.

19.5 Locate a CPT code using the CPT manual.

19.6 Explain how to locate a HCPCS code using the HCPCS coding manual.

19.7 Explain the importance of code linkage in avoiding coding fraud.

KEY TERMS

add-on code

bundled codes

concurrent care

consultation

counseling

critical care

Current Procedural Terminology (CPT)

downcoding

E/M code

established patient

global period

HCPCS Level II codes

Healthcare Common Procedure Coding System (HCPCS)

modifier

new patient

panel

procedure code

unbundling

upcoding

M E D I C A L   A S S I S T I N G   C O M P E T E N C I E S

CAAHEP

ABHES

IX.C.1 Describe how to use the most current procedural coding system	**3. Medical Terminology** d. Define and use medical abbreviations when appropriate and acceptable
IX.C.3 Describe how to use the most current HCPCS level II coding system	**8. Administrative Procedures** c. Process insurance claims (3) Perform diagnostic and procedural coding
IX.C.4 Discuss the effects of: (a) upcoding (b) downcoding	
IX.C.5 Define medical necessity as it applies to procedural and diagnostic coding	
IX.P.1 Perform procedural coding	
IX.P.3 Utilize medical necessity guidelines	
IX.A.1 Utilize tactful communication skills with medical providers to ensure accurate code selection	

Introduction

In the previous chapter, you were introduced to diagnostic coding—the reason(s) the patient sought healthcare. In this chapter, you will explore the language of procedural coding. You will learn how to translate the medical terms for the procedures and services provided to patients into code numbers selected from standardized procedural coding systems. These codes, when placed correctly on the healthcare claims introduced in the *Insurance and Billing* chapter, explain to third-party payers the services patients received from the provider.

After you study the concepts of procedure or CPT codes, you will explore the "linking" of diagnosis codes with procedure codes to explain the *medical necessity* of each procedure or service performed. Finding the correct codes can require detective work! The reward is accurate procedure codes that, when combined with accurate and appropriate diagnosis codes, bring the maximum appropriate reimbursement to the practitioners in your medical office.

The CPT Manual   LO 19.1

After an office or clinic visit, hospital or nursing home visit, inpatient or outpatient consultation, or even a house call, each procedure and service performed on or for a patient is reported on healthcare claims using a **procedure code.** These codes represent medical procedures, such as surgery and diagnostic tests, as well as medical services, such as physical examinations to evaluate a patient's condition. Medical assistants often choose these procedure codes—based on the information provided by the practitioner on the encounter form, or from the patient medical chart or electronic health record—and use them to report medical services.

Current Procedural Terminology (CPT)

The most commonly used system of procedure codes is found in the *Current Procedural Terminology* or simply *CPT,* a reference manual published by the American Medical Association (AMA). CPT is the HIPAA-required code set that translates descriptions for physicians' and other providers' healthcare-related procedures into 5-digit codes.

Like ICD, the CPT manual is updated yearly; new codes are used for services provided beginning January 1 of each new year. In each edition, newly developed procedures are added and old ones are revised or, if obsolete, deleted. These changes are also available in an electronic file for computerized medical offices. As with ICD codes, remember that the choice of which set of codes to use is based on the date of service, not the date of the claim. If claims are submitted January 2, 2017, and the date of service was December 23, 2016, CPT codes from 2016 would be used; for services provided on January 2, 2017, the 2017 edition of the CPT codes would be used.

Medical offices should always have the current year's CPT available for reference and keep forms up to date. Like ICD codes, if current codes are not used, medical claims are often denied. Previous editions of each coding manual should be kept for at least several months after the new edition is released for use with claims for dates of service in the prior year, and for reference in case questions arise regarding previously submitted claims.

Organization of the CPT Manual

CPT codes are organized into six main sections:

Section	Range of Codes
Evaluation and Management	99201–99499
Anesthesiology	00100–01999
	99100–99140
Surgery	10021–69990
Radiology	70010–79999
Pathology and Laboratory	80047–89398
Medicine (except for anesthesia)	90281–99199
	99500–99607

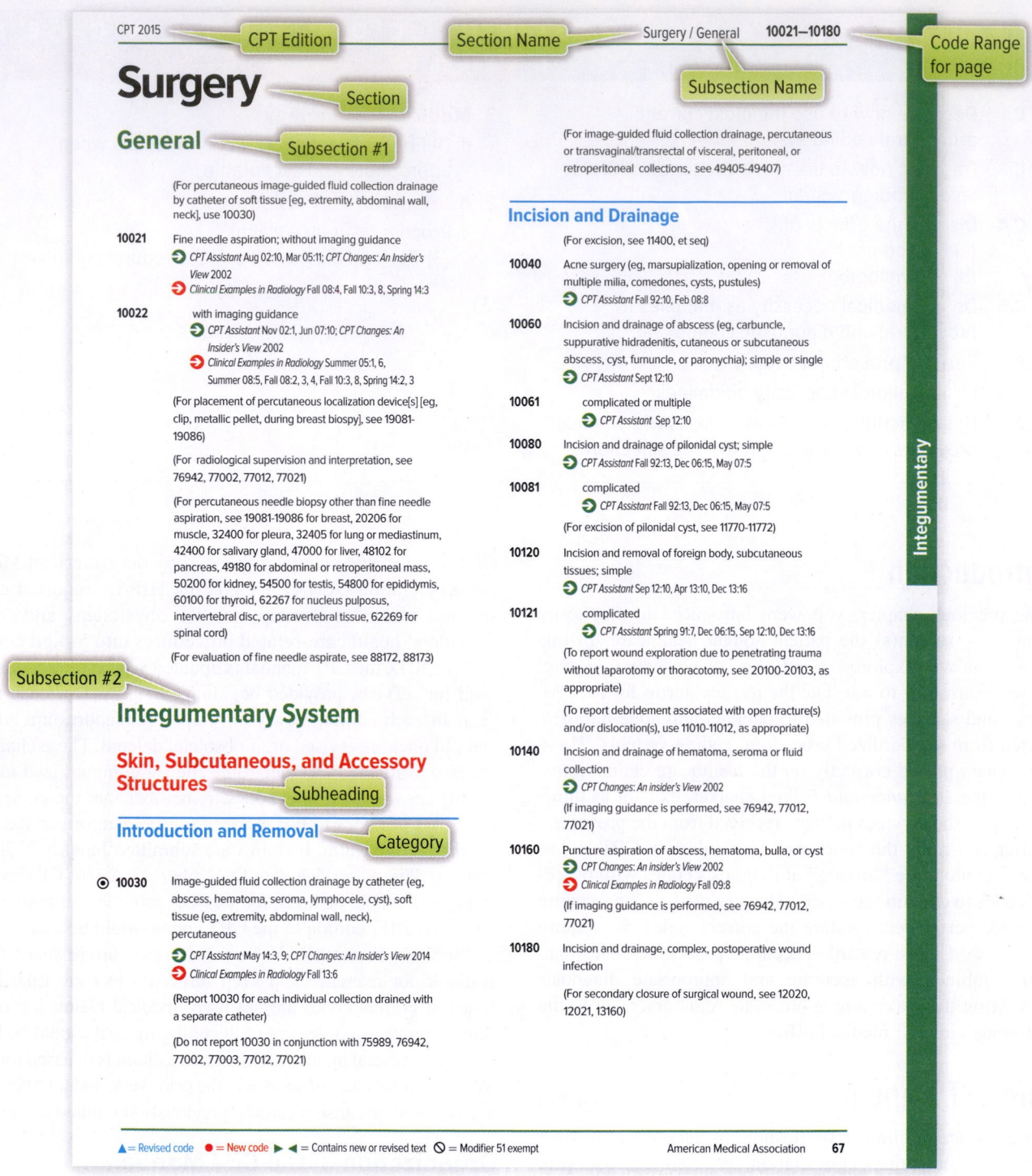

FIGURE 19-1 CPT manual page showing edition, section, subsection, subheading, and category names as well as the code range on the page.
Use of the CPT Manual page, found within the 2015 CPT Professional Edition. © American Medical Association [2014]. All rights reserved.

In looking at the section numbers, you will note that except for the Evaluation and Management section, the sections are listed in numeric order by code range. Because Evaluation and Management (E/M) codes are used so frequently, they are placed in the front of the manual for easy reference.

The Introduction to the CPT manual gives the user important general instructions for the use of CPT. In this section, you will also find helpful information regarding common prefixes, suffixes, and word roots found within the manual. CPT is also full of helpful illustrations of the human body.

A descriptive list of illustrations with the page number where each can be found is also in the Introduction. In addition, pay close attention to the guidelines found at the beginning of each section, as these provide important overall information for coding in each section. The CPT sections are divided into categories, which, in turn, are further divided into headings according to the type of test, service, or body system. Code number ranges included on a particular page are found in the upper-right corner so that a code can be located quickly after using the index (see Figure 19-1).

Note that each page also gives you other important information, including

1. **Section name.** The section is the name used by CPT to denote each chapter. In Figure 19-1, the section name is Surgery.

2. **Subsection name.** The subsection is the area within the section detailing the body system you are in. In Figure 19-1, the first subsection is General. Note that the next subsection for Surgery—Integumentary System—starts part of the way down the page.

3. **Subheading.** The subheading describes the body area for the body system you are looking at. Figure 19-2 shows the subheading of Skin, Subcutaneous, and Accessory Structures.

4. **Category.** The category describes the procedure area. In Figure 19-2, you will find the Incision and Drainage (I&D) category.

▶ General CPT Guidelines   LO 19.2

As stated earlier, each CPT section contains guidelines for that section. Now, let's discuss the general guidelines, found at the beginning of the manual and followed throughout.

CPT Code Format

CPT codes are 5-digit numeric codes. Most codes are stand-alone codes with the complete description listed next to the appropriate code. The exception to this rule is the code description containing a semicolon, which is then followed by a code with an indented description. An indented description means that you refer back to the previous code description, reading the information prior to the semicolon and adding the indented code information after the colon to complete the description. Let's look at the following example:

Example:

25500	Closed treatment of radial shaft fracture; without manipulation
25505	with manipulation

To read the full description for code 25505, read code 25500 up to the semicolon and then substitute the description for 25505 after the semicolon. Following these instructions, the full description for 25505 is *Closed treatment of radial shaft fracture; with manipulation.*

Add-on Codes

A plus sign (+) is used for **add-on codes.** These codes are used to describe procedures done in addition to a "main" procedure. For example, in Figure 19-3, you will note that code 11001 has a plus sign in front of it with a description of *each additional 10% of body surface, or part thereof (List separately in addition to code for primary procedure).*

CPT code 11001 is also an indented code, meaning it is related to the code immediately preceding it (code 11000). The description for code 11000 is *Debridement of extensive eczematous or infected skin; up to 10% of body surface.* In putting the two codes together, you would be telling the insurance carrier that up to 20% of the body surface was debrided.

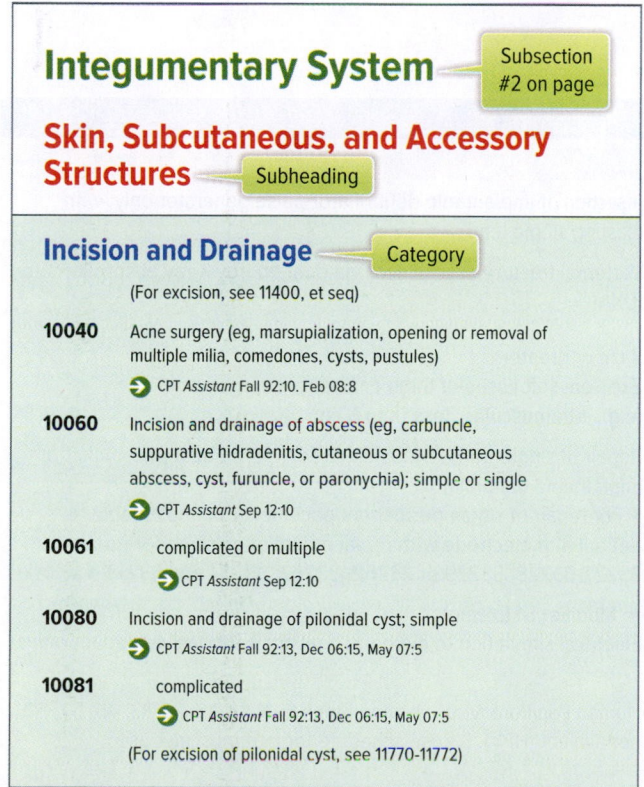

FIGURE 19-2 The Incision and Drainage category of the Integumentary System subsection.

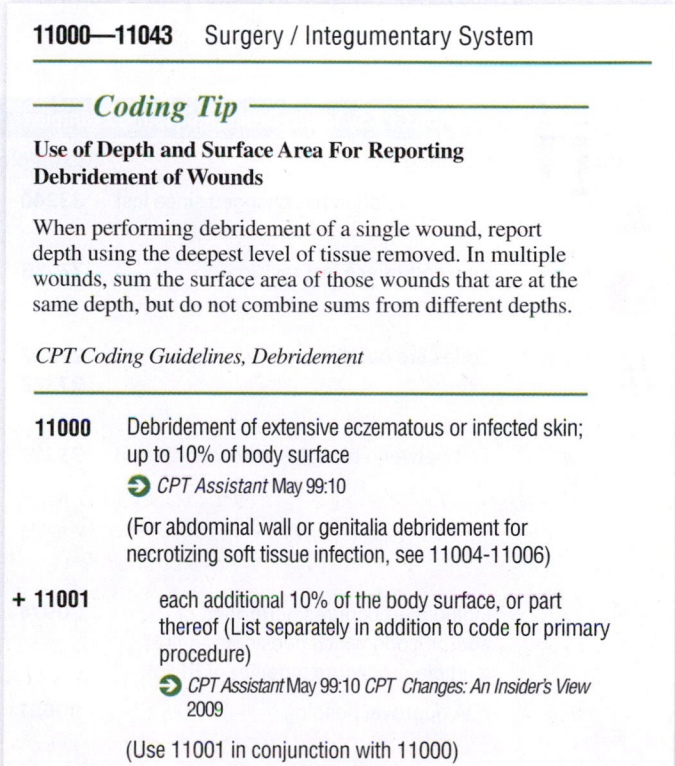

FIGURE 19-3 Add-on code 11001 for use exclusively with primary code 11000.

Example #1 shows you the correct coding when 20% of the body surface area is debrided; Example #2, when 25% (up to 30%) of the body is debrided.

Example #1: Debridement of 20% of body surface area

Code 11000	(debridement of first 10% of body surface)
	And
Code 11001	(debridement of second 10% of body surface area or part thereof)

Example #2: Debridement of 25% of body surface area

Code 11000	(debridement of first 10% of body surface)
	And
Code 11001	(debridement of second 10% of body surface area)
	And
Code 11001	(debridement for the next 5% as the description states "next 10% or part thereof")

Appendix D in the CPT manual contains a complete listing of all add-on codes in the manual. Add-on codes are never reported alone. They always follow the primary code.

As stated previously, also be alert for indented codes. For these codes, you will read the description of the "parent code" up to the semicolon and then replace the information following the semicolon with the information found in the indented code description. In Figure 19-1, codes 10022, 10061, 10081, and 10121 are all examples of indented codes.

Symbols Used in CPT

The CPT manual uses instructional symbols to give repetitive information without adding multiple pages. Refer to Table 19-1 for examples of each symbol.

- *Blue triangle.* This symbol tells the user that the code description has been revised in some way from last year. Note in Table 19-1 that code 33240 has a blue triangle next to it; this indicates that the code description has changed from the 2014 CPT manual's description. This information could be important, as the change could mean the procedure performed by the physician may now require a different code. It could also mean something as simple as the placement of a comma or semicolon has changed.
- *Red dot.* The symbol denotes a new code for this edition of the CPT. In Table 19-1, note that code 77086 is a new procedure code as of 2015 CPT.
- *The # sign.* The # (pound) sign is used to denote codes that are out of numeric sequence. Referring to Table 19-1, (indented) code 27337 "works with" code 27327. It is followed by code 27328—causing it to be out of numeric order.

Example:

#27327	Excision, tumor, soft tissue of thigh or knee area, subcutaneous; less than 3 cm
#27337	3 cm or greater
#27328	Excision, tumor, soft tissue of thigh or knee area, subfascial (eg, intramuscular); less than 5 cm

TABLE 19-1 Common CPT Symbols, Descriptions, and Examples

Symbol	Meaning	Example	
▲	Code description has changed since last revision	33240	Insertion of implantable defibrillator pulse generator only; with existing single lead
●	New code since last revision	77086	Vertebral fracture assessment via dual-energy X-ray absorptiometry (DXA)
#	Codes are out of numeric sequence	27337 27328	3 cm or greater Excision, soft tissue of thigh or knee area, subfascial (e.g., intramuscular); less than 5 cm
►◄	Text between triangles is new or revised	33218	Repair of single transvenous electrode, permanent pacemaker or implantable defibrillator ► For repair of single permanent pacemaker or implantable defibrillator electrode with replacement of pulse generator, see 33227, 33228, 33229 or 33262, 33263, 33264 and 33218 ◄
⊘	Multiple procedures performed or add-on code which does not require multiple procedure modifier of 51	20974	= Modifier 51 Exempt Electrical simulation to aid bone healing; noninvasive (nonoperative)
⚡	FDA approval pending	90651	Human Papillomavirus vaccine types 6, 11, 16. 18. 31, 33, 45, 52, 58, nonavalent (HPV), 3 dose schedule for intramuscular use
◉	Moderate (conscious) sedation is included in the procedure	44388	Colonoscopy through stoma, diagnostic, including collection of specimen(s) by brushing or washing, when performed (separate procedure)

This was done so code numbers would not be "reshuffled" every year. If the pound sign were not used and codes were to remain in numeric order, for code 27327 to have an indented code, code 27328 would have to be used. Code 27328 had previously been assigned its description. To keep all codes in numeric order, all codes from 27328 with its new description and all other codes on this page would have to be assigned new descriptions. This is a lot of work and very confusing with constantly changing code descriptions on a yearly basis. Note that each code is also found in red, in its "proper numeric place" with directions telling the coder in what code range to locate the out-of-sequenced code.

- *Triangles pointing toward each other.* Triangles pointing toward each other with text between them denote new or revised text information. Traditionally, these arrows have been green. You will also see them used for the out-of-sequence coding information. See code 33218 in Table 19-1.

  Example:

◎▲ 33218	Repair of single transvenous electrode, permanent pacemaker or implantable defibrillator
	➲*CPT Assistant* Summer 94:10, 19, Oct 96:9, Nov 99:15-16, Jun 12:3; *CPT Changes: An Insider's View* 2000, 2012, 2015
	▶ (For repair of single permanent pacemaker or implantable defibrillator electrode with replacement of pulse generator, see 33227, 33228, 33229 or 33262, 33263, 33264 and 33218) ◀

- *Circle with diagonal line.* This symbol is noted in Table 19-1 as "Modifier 51 Exempt." Modifier 51 is used when multiple procedures are performed in the same session. Modifier 51 exempt codes are those to which the multiple procedure modifier does not apply. Appendix E of the CPT manual lists the modifier 51 exempt codes. Note that modifier 51 is never appended to a designated add-on code.

- *Lightning bolt.* The lightning bolt is used to denote vaccines pending FDA approval. Appendix K in the CPT manual lists the vaccines affected by this symbol. When the vaccines are approved, these along with other current codes will be listed on the AMA site at http://www.ama-assn.org/ama/pub/physician-resources/solutions-managing-your-practice/coding-billing-insurance/cpt/about-cpt.page? and then in subsequent CPT editions.

- *Bull's-eye.* The bull's-eye symbol denotes moderate (conscious) sedation and means it is understood that conscious sedation is necessary for the procedure performed, so conscious sedation is included in the procedure; it cannot be billed separately. Many endoscopy procedures include this symbol.

  Example:

◎▲ 44388	Colonoscopy through stoma; diagnostic, including collection of specimen(s) by brushing or washing, when performed (separate procedure)
	➲*CPT Assistant* Nov 07:8, Dec 13:3; *CPT Changes: An Insider's View* 2015
	▶ (Do not report 44388 in conjunction with 44389-44408) ◀

Because this code includes sedation as part of the procedure, administered by the physician performing the procedure, there will be no separate charge for the anesthesia. The CPT manual's Appendix G lists all codes that include moderate (conscious) sedation.

Whenever you are coding, always watch carefully for these symbols. Their instructions are explicit and must be followed to ensure correct procedure coding.

Modifiers

One or more two-digit **modifiers** (up to four per procedure) may be assigned to the 5-digit main code. Modifiers are written in column 24D on the CMS-1500 Claim Form (see Figure 17-9). The use of a modifier shows that one or more special circumstances apply to the service or procedure the physician performed. For example, in the Surgery section, the modifier 62 indicates that two surgeons worked together, each performing part of a surgical procedure during an operation. Each surgeon will be paid part of the amount normally reimbursed for that procedure code. The CPT's Appendix A explains the proper use of each modifier. Some section guidelines also discuss the use of modifiers within the individual section's coding information. Table 19-2 gives a brief overview with examples of common CPT modifiers.

Category II Codes, Category III Codes, and Unlisted Procedure Codes

Category II codes are optional, supplemental tracking codes used to track healthcare performance measures, like programs and counseling to avoid tobacco use (Code 4000F or 4001F if medication is instituted to assist patient). Category III codes are "temporary" CPT codes for emerging technology, services, and procedures. An example of a category III code is 0051T Implantation of a total replacement heart system (artificial heart) with recipient cardiectomy. If available, these codes should be used instead of the *unlisted codes* found throughout the CPT manual. Category II and III codes are both found directly after the last of the Medicine codes in the CPT manual.

When no code is available to completely describe a procedure, a code for an unlisted procedure is selected. Unlisted procedure codes are used for new services or procedures that have not yet been assigned codes in CPT. When these codes are used, which is rare, a procedure or service description (usually from the medical record) is sent with the claim submission. Some payers, including Medicare and Medicaid, prefer the use of HCPCS codes (when available) instead of the unlisted procedure codes used with CPT. Check with individual payers to learn each payer's preferences. HCPCS codes will be discussed in further detail later in the chapter.

Coding Terminology

Before you begin coding, you must have a basic understanding of common terminology used throughout the CPT manual. Some of these terms are defined in the following paragraphs.

TABLE 19-2   Common CPT Modifiers

Modifier	Description	Example
22	**Increased Procedural Services.** When the work required to complete the service is much more than usually required, modifier 22 may be added to the CPT code. Medical record documentation will be required. This modifier cannot be attached to an E/M code.	Because of extreme scarring and previous surgeries, lysis of adhesions (CPT 58740) requires almost twice the normal time frame. Code 58740-22.
23	**Unusual Anesthesia.** Once in a while, a procedure that normally does not require anesthesia or anesthetic will require general anesthesia because of unusual situations.	Excision of subcutaneous tumor of neck, because of patient age of 4, requires general anesthesia. Code 11424-23.
24	**Unrelated E/M Service by the Same Physician During a Post-operative Period.** The patient may require the services of the physician for treatment of an unrelated condition during a global surgical period.	The patient is one week post-op laparoscopic cholecystectomy. During post-op check, patient states asthma appears to be in exacerbation. Code 99024 for post-op visit. Code 99213-24 for E/M visit for asthma.
25	**Significant, Separately Identifiable E/M Service by the Same Physician on the Same Day of the Procedure or Other Service.** While in the office for a specific procedure, the patient may require an E/M service above and beyond that normally provided during the usual pre- and/or post-procedure period.	Patient comes in for a previously scheduled mole removal (11401). Prior to the procedure, the physician notes that the patient's BP is elevated. When the procedure is completed, BP is still noted to be elevated. Physician makes an adjustment to the patient's antihypertensive medication and counsels diet adjustments. Code 11401. Code 99212-25.
26	**Professional Component.** Some procedures (such as radiology) contain a combination of professional and technical components. If the physician provides only the professional component, modifier 26 is added.	Screening mammography, bilateral (CPT 77057). Hospital performs the mammogram; physician provides interpretation. Code 77057-26.
TC	**Technical Component.** This is the HCPCS modifier that is the "reverse" of modifier 26. It designates the provision of the technical component only.	Screening mammography, bilateral (CPT 77057). Hospital performs the mammogram; physician provides interpretation. Hospital Code 77057-TC.
32	**Mandated Services.** Service (such as a consult) is required by the insurance carrier, government agency, or regulatory agency.	Insurance carrier requires a second opinion prior to an elective surgical procedure. Physician performs consult regarding need for surgery. Code 99242-32.
47	**Anesthesia by Surgeon.** Surgeon provides and administers anesthesia other than local anesthesia. Modifier is appended to the surgical procedure.	Procedure performed is shoulder manipulation under regional anesthesia by orthopedic surgeon. Code 23700-47.
50	**Bilateral Procedure.** Modifier is used if the procedure is not defined as bilateral but the procedure is performed on both sides of the body.	Procedure: Bilateral knee arthroscopy. Code 29870-50.
51	**Multiple Procedures.** When the same provider performs multiple procedures (other than E/M, PT, and Rehab or supply provision) in the same session, the first procedure is listed as usual, and subsequent procedures should include the addition of modifier 51.	Code 15877. Suction-assisted lipectomy; trunk. Code 15879-51. Suction-assisted lipectomy; lower extremity.
52	**Reduced Services.** Due to circumstances, service is reduced or eliminated by the physician.	Exploratory laparotomy for removal of malignant neoplasm, but cancer is widely metastasized so procedure is halted. Code 49000-52.
53	**Discontinued Procedure.** Similar to modifier 52, except in this case, the procedure is discontinued due to patient condition becoming endangered.	Patient is undergoing diagnostic colonoscopy when significant PVCs become evident and uncontrollable. Procedure is halted. Code 45330-53.
54	**Surgical Care Only.** Surgeon provides only the surgical care with other physician(s) providing pre- and post-op care.	Total abdominal hysterectomy with bilateral salpingo-oophorectomy (TAH-BSO) surgery only. Code 58150-54.

(continued)

TABLE 19-2 Common CPT Modifiers

Modifier	Description	Example
55	**Postoperative Management Only.** Physician provides postoperative care only.	Total abdominal hysterectomy with bilateral salpingo-oophorectomy (TAH-BSO) postoperative care only. Code 58150-55.
56	**Preoperative Management Only.** Physician provides preoperative care only.	Total abdominal hysterectomy with bilateral salpingo-oophorectomy (TAH-BSO) preoperative care only. Code 58150-56.
57	**Decision for Surgery.** During an E/M service, decision is made that surgery is required.	Patient in office for biopsy results. Decision is made that treatment option includes mastectomy. Code 99214-57.
58	**Staged or Related Procedure or Service by the Same Physician During the Postoperative Period.** Circumstances may include staged (planned) procedure, procedure being more extensive than originally thought, or therapy following original procedure.	Patient has breast biopsy, which has a post-op period. During this period, mastectomy is decided upon and performed. Code 19302-58.
59	**Distinct Procedural Service.** Used when the secondary procedure is identified as *different session, different procedure/surgery, different site or organ system. Separate incision/excision, separate lesion, separate injury or area of injury when injuries are extensive.* (Some Medicare codes have edits that state certain procedures cannot be performed together regardless of use of 59 modifier.)	Medical records indicate that colonoscopy with polyp removal using snare (45385) and colonoscopy with hot biopsy forceps (45384) were done in same session. Code 45385. Code 45384-59.
62	**Two Surgeons.** Modifier indicates that two surgeons performed a procedure that normally is performed by one surgeon, each performing distinct aspects of the procedure.	Two surgeons work as a team for spinal cord exploration and decompression. Code 63075-62. Code 63077-62.
66	**Surgical Team.** As with modifier 62, this modifier is used when a team of surgeons is required for a complicated procedure.	Patient requires a heart-lung transplant. Team includes cardiac surgeon, thoracic surgeon, perfusionist, and anesthesiologist. Code 33935-66.
76	**Repeat Procedure or Service by Same Physician.** Procedure is performed and complication requires repeat or related service. Used to explain this is not a duplicate service but is medically necessary.	Patient undergoes arteriovenous anastomosis (36821), but anastomosis does not hold and requires repeat procedure. Code 36821-76.
77	**Repeat Procedure by Another Physician.** As with modifier 76, a second procedure is required, but in this case, a different physician provides the service.	Patient undergoes arteriovenous anastomosis (36821), but anastomosis does not hold and requires repeat procedure; performing physician is not available. Code 36821-77.
78	**Unplanned Return to the OR by the Same Physician Following Initial Procedure for Related Procedure During the Postoperative Period.** Complications related to the initial procedure are most often the reason for the return to surgery.	Patient undergoes implantation of central venous access device (36558), which clots off later in the day, requiring declotting. Code 36593-78.
79	**Unrelated Procedure or Service by the Same Physician During the Postoperative Period.** Usually, patient undergoes a primary procedure and, for an unrelated issue, requires a second surgery or procedure during the post-op period.	Patient undergoes laparoscopic cholecystectomy (47562). Two weeks later, experiences acute appendicitis episode and undergoes emergency appendectomy. Code 44970-79.
80	**Assistant Surgeon.** Surgeon acts as assistant to primary surgeon. (A physician assistant may function in this role.)	Surgeon performs total knee replacement with assistant surgeon. Code 27447-80.
81	**Minimum Assistant Surgeon.** This modifier is used only when minimal assistance during surgery is required.	Patient undergoing 4-vessel CABG. Second physician asked to assist only in stabilizing patient during procedure. Code 33536-81. Code 33518-81.

(continued)

TABLE 19-2 Common CPT Modifiers

Modifier	Description	Example
82	**Assistant Surgeon (When Qualified Resident Surgeon Is Not Available).** This modifier is used only in teaching hospitals where resident surgeons are normally available.	Patient undergoing 4-vessel CABG. Second physician asked to assist only in stabilizing patient during procedure because the surgical resident is assisting with another procedure. Code 33536-82. Code 33518-82.
90	**Reference (Outside) Laboratory.** Modifier is used when physician is billing for services provided by an outside laboratory. (Not allowed by Medicare.)	Provider office bills for comprehensive metabolic panel performed by "Allied Labs" and then reimburses the lab. Code 80053-90.
91	**Repeat Clinical Diagnostic Laboratory Test.** This modifier is used when serial (multiple) labs are required on the same day to monitor the patient's condition.	After surgery, the patient appears to be in acute renal failure, requiring monitoring of kidney function. Code xxxxx-91.
92	**Alternative Laboratory Platform Testing.** Modifier 92 is used for disposable kit testing such as HIV testing.	Patient is tested for HIV using disposable test at hospital bedside. Code 86701-92.
99	**Multiple Modifiers.** Used when more than three modifiers are applicable to CPT code being used and the payer only accepts one modifier per code.	Medical Insurance Inc. accepts only one modifier per line, requiring modifier 99 be used and applicable modifiers be listed in block 19 of the CMS form. Procedure performed: Bilateral (50) mastectomy with assistant surgeon (80). Code 19307-99.

Note: You can see the complete listing of all modifiers in the *Current Procedural Terminology* manual, Appendix A.
Source: American Medical Association, *Current Procedural Terminology*, 2015 Professional Edition, copyright 2015.

Bundled codes consist of any code that includes more than one procedure in its description. Read code descriptions carefully, as it is unethical (and often considered fraudulent) to intentionally unbundle procedures into component codes when a bundled procedure code is available. For instance, all therapeutic procedures include diagnostic codes unless noted otherwise, so if a diagnostic knee arthroscopy (29870) is turned into a therapeutic arthroscopy (29871), only the therapeutic arthroscopy will be reported because it is understood that a diagnostic procedure must have taken place in order for the therapy to have taken place.

Concurrent care is described as similar care being provided by more than one physician. This frequently occurs when a patient is hospitalized and multiple specialists are caring for the patient. The services provided may be similar, but because of the differing specialties, the care is not considered to be duplication of services.

Critical care is provided to unstable, critically ill patients. Constant bedside attention is needed in order to code critical care, so the physician's documentation must be explicit regarding the time spent with the patient. The time need not be continuous, but the time is added together so that critical care codes chosen are based on the sum total of the critical care given during one particular date. Unlike emergency care codes, which can only be used when the patient's care is provided in an emergency department, the patient need not be in a critical care or intensive care bed in order for the codes to be used, but his condition must be critical in nature.

Consultations are patient visits or appointments provided at the request of other healthcare providers. The CPT codes for consultations include 99241–99245 for outpatient consultations and 99251–99255 for inpatient consultations. A service can only be considered a consultation if the 3Rs are present: *request* (from another practitioner), *record* (documentation) findings and recommendations, and *report* to the referring practitioner. If the consulting provider takes over the care of the patient, then he is no longer considered a consulting provider, but a treating provider. In this case, he will use standard "visit" E/M codes and no longer use consultation codes. As of January 2010, Medicare stopped accepting consultation codes; comparable inpatient and outpatient E/M service codes (such as 99201–99205 and 99211–99215 for outpatient visits) are to be used instead. Many commercial payers, following Medicare's lead, also have begun denying consultation codes, so again, it is important to know each payer's rules and regulations before submitting claims to the payers. We will discuss E/M codes and services in greater detail in just a bit.

Counseling is considered part of E/M (Evaluation and Management) services, but if a complete history and physical exam does not take place (making an E/M code inappropriate), counseling codes may be used. These codes may be used when discussing with the patient and family questions or concerns regarding one or more of the following: diagnostic results and recommendations; prognosis, risks, and benefits of options; instructions for treatment and/or follow-up; importance of compliance; risk factor reduction; and patient/family education.

Downcoding is the term used when the insurance carrier bases reimbursement on a code level lower than the one submitted by the provider. This can occur for several reasons:

- The coding system used by the insurer does not match that used by the provider. This can occur if the provider uses a HCPCS code the insurer does not recognize. Always verify the code set accepted by the payer.

- If a workers' compensation carrier bases payment on an RVS (relative value system), the carrier may convert a CPT code to the lowest-paying code within the system. Again, check with the payer as to the system in use.

- A payer requests backup documentation (medical records) on a case and finds the documentation does not "back up" the level of code used on the claim. This is by far the most common cause of downcoding in medical offices. Be sure your provider's documentation always is specific enough to back up the level of code used.

Unbundling, as stated in the bundling definition, is defined as breaking a bundled code into its component parts for higher reimbursement and is not allowed. Code 77055 is defined as mammography, unilateral. Without research, you might think a bilateral mammography would be coded by adding modifier 50, but this is not the case. Code 77056 is an indented code with the description of mammography, bilateral—this code without a modifier is used for bilateral mammography.

Upcoding refers to coding a procedure or service at a higher level than that provided to receive a higher level of reimbursement. Other terms for this process are *code creep, overcoding,* and *overbilling,* and all are fraudulent practices when done knowingly or repeatedly.

It is important to remember that insurers, particularly federally funded ones like Medicare and Medicaid, assume that if they are being billed, those doing the billing are appropriately trained to bill services following all appropriate guidelines. Ignorance is not considered an excuse when these payers are repeatedly billed excessive amounts for procedures. So it is imperative that each provider's documentation in the patient medical record is clear and concise and proves the level of service being billed actually occurred.

▶ Evaluation and Management Services

LO 19.3

To diagnose conditions and plan treatments, physicians use a wide range of time, effort, and skill for different patients and circumstances. Evaluation and management codes (**E/M codes**) are often considered the most important of all CPT codes because all physicians in any medical specialty can use them. Table 19-3 gives the E/M breakdown by type with code range.

Many E/M codes are divided based on the patient status of **new patient** versus **established patient.** This is simply because, in many cases, a practitioner will need to spend more time with a new patient, getting to know her and her history, than will be necessary with a patient who has been coming to the practice for several years and whose history is well known.

The general rule of thumb is if a patient has been seen by a practitioner of the same specialty in the same practice within 3 years, he is an existing patient. If the patient has not been seen in the practice within the last 3 years, he is considered a new patient. Figure 19-4 shows an example of a new versus established patient decision tree.

In addition to being the most important codes in the CPT manual, the E/M codes are considered by many the most difficult to code because of the many factors that must be considered when choosing an E/M Code. Let's examine the various components that must be considered when choosing an E/M code. As with any coding exercise, practice is the most important factor when learning procedure (or diagnostic) coding.

TABLE 19-3   E/M Code Breakdown with Code Ranges

E/M Type	Code Range
Office/Other Outpatient Services	New Pt 99201–99205 Est. Pt 99211–99215
Hospital Observation Services	99217–99226
Hospital Inpatient Services	99221–99239
Consultations	OutPt 99241–99245 InPt 99251–99255
Emergency Department Services	99281–99288
Critical Care Services	99291–99292
Nursing Facility Services	99304–99318
Domiciliary, Rest Home (Boarding Home), or Custodial Care Services	New Pt 99324–99328 Est. Pt 99334–99337
Domiciliary, Assisted Living Facility, or Home Care Plan Oversight Services	99339–99340
Home Services	New Pt 99341–99345 Est. Pt 99347–99350
Prolonged Services	99354–99360
Case Management Services	99363–99368
Care Plan Oversight Services	99374–99380
Preventative Medicine Services (includes counseling services)	New Pt 99381–99387 Est. Pt 99391–99397 Other 99420–99429
Non-Face-to-Face Physician Services	99441–99449
Special Evaluation and Management Services	99450–99456
Newborn Care Services	99460–99465
Inpatient Neonatal Intensive Care Services and Pediatric and Neonatal Critical Care Services	99466–99486
Care Management Services	99487–99490
Transitional Care Management Services	99495–99496
Advance Care Planning	99497–99498
Other Evaluation and Management Services	99499

Source: American Medical Association, *Current Procedural Terminology,* 2015 Professional Edition, Copyright 2015.

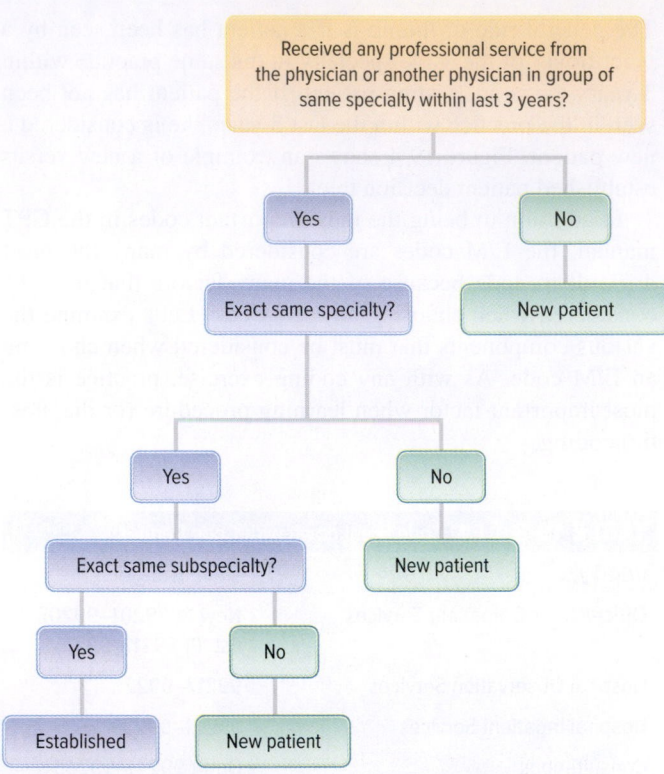

FIGURE 19-4 Decision tree for new versus established patients.

Key Factors in Determining Level of Service

The E/M section guidelines explain how to code different levels of these services. Three key factors documented in the patient's medical record help determine the level of service:

1. The extent of the patient history taken
2. The extent of the examination conducted
3. The complexity of the medical decision making

Let's look briefly at each of these key factors.

Patient History The elements of a history include the chief complaint (CC); history of present illness (HPI); review of systems (ROS); and past, family, and/or social history (PFSH). When coding, the history is described using one of the following terms:

- Problem-focused—history is limited to the chief complaint and a brief history of the present problem.

- Expanded problem-focused—history includes the chief complaint, a brief history of the current problem, and a "problem-pertinent" review of systems.

- Detailed—history still focuses on the chief complaint but includes an extensive history of the current problem and an extended review of systems and pertinent past, family, and/or social history.

- Comprehensive—the most complex of the histories; all four components of CC, HPI, ROS, and PFSH are documented.

Physical Exam The elements of the physical exam include the same terminology but relate to the level of examination performed. The physical exam has three elements:

1. The constitutional exam includes any of the following: BP sitting or lying, pulse, respirations, temperature, height, weight, and general appearance.

2. Body areas (BA) include head (including face), neck, chest (including breasts and axillae), abdomen, genitalia, groin and buttocks, back, and each extremity.

3. Organ systems (OA) include the following systems: ophthalmologic (eyes), otolaryngologic (ears, nose, throat, and mouth), cardiovascular, respiratory, GI (gastrointestinal), GU (genitourinary), musculoskeletal, integumentary (skin), neurologic, psychiatric, and hematologic/lymphatic/immunologic (blood, lymph, immunity).

Physical exam terms include the following:

- Problem-focused—exam is limited to the body area or organ system directly related to the chief complaint. (1 BA or OS)

- Expanded problem-focused—limited exam of the affected body area or organ system and any other symptomatic or related BA or OS. (2–7 limited BA or OS)

- Detailed—includes an extended exam of the affected body area and any other related, symptomatic BA or OS. (2–7 extended BA or OS)

- Comprehensive—the most extensive exam; includes either a complete single-specialty exam or a complete multisystem examination. (8 + BA or OS)

Medical Decision Making The most important key component in establishing an E/M code is the medical decision making (MDM) and it is probably the most difficult to document. It is based on the complexity of the decision making by the provider about the patient's care and diagnosis. The three elements that must be documented to establish MDM are the number of diagnoses or management options (minimal, limited, multiple, or extensive); the amount or complexity of data to be reviewed (none or minimal, limited, moderate, or extensive); and the risk of complication or death if the condition is untreated (minimal, low, moderate, or high). Here we outline the complexity levels of medical decision making:

- Straightforward MDM—there are minimal diagnosis and management options with a minimal amount or complexity of data to be reviewed and minimal risk to the patient of complication or death if the condition is left untreated.

- Low-complexity MDM—there are a limited number of diagnoses and management options with a limited amount or complexity of data to be reviewed and low risk of complication or death if the patient is not treated.

- Moderate-complexity MDM—there are multiple diagnoses and management options with a moderate amount or complexity of data to review. If not treated, the condition presents a moderate risk of complication or death to the patient.

- High-complexity MDM—the physician has extensive diagnosis and management options with an extensive amount and complexity of data for review. The patient is at high risk for complication and/or death if not treated.

Some medical assistants and billers/coders like to use a grid similar to the one in Table 19-4 to assist with the MDM decision-making process when assigning E/M codes.

Three Contributory Factors in Assigning Codes

In addition to these three key components, some E/M codes take three *contributory factors,* listed as follows, into consideration when codes are assigned:

1. Counseling. This component is only considered critical for E/M codes when counseling is the reason for the encounter and constitutes 50% or more of the total time of the visit.
2. Coordination of care. This is the time the licensed practitioner uses to coordinate patient care with other healthcare agencies like home care or nursing home care.
3. Nature of the presenting problem. This is another term for the severity of the patient's chief complaint.
   - A minimal complaint may not require the presence of a physician, but service is provided under the licensed clinician's supervision such as a BP reading or dressing change.
   - A self-limited complaint is a minor problem that will run a "known" course and is transient in nature. A problem with a good prognosis when the patient is compliant also may be considered self-limiting.
   - Low-severity complaints are those with a low risk of morbidity and mortality (death) if there is no treatment. Full recovery is expected.
   - Moderate-severity complaints have a moderate risk of morbidity and mortality if there is no treatment. Prognosis is uncertain and there is increased risk of impairment.
   - High-severity complaints are those of high to extreme risk. Risk of death is moderate to high and there is a high risk of prolonged functional impairment.

Finally, *time* is listed as a component to some codes after being incorporated in 1992 to assist with code choice. The times listed are considered averages and unless the code choice, such as with face-to-face contact codes, is based on time, time should not be considered a critical factor when choosing an E/M code. As noted in Table 19-3, the location of the service is also important because different E/M codes apply to services performed in a provider's office or other outpatient location, a hospital inpatient room, a hospital emergency department, a nursing facility, an extended-care facility, or a patient's home.

Appendix C of the CPT code manual lists medical record documentation examples of each E/M code type to assist you in choosing appropriate E/M codes for your provider.

▶ Surgical Coding   LO 19.4

Figure 19-5 illustrates an encounter form listing codes from the integumentary part of the surgical section. Many insurance carriers cover the surgical procedures found in CPT as part of a *surgical package.* Included in most surgical packages are the preoperative exam and testing; the surgical procedure itself, including local or regional anesthesia if used; and routine follow-up care for a set period of time. Payers assign a fee to each of these packaged codes that pays for all the services provided in this package. If using anesthesia other than local anesthesia, the anesthesiologist billing for her services would use an anesthesia code.

The period of time covered for follow-up care is called the **global period.** For example, the global period for repairing a tendon might be set at 15 days. A global period for major surgery like an abdominal hysterectomy might be set at 90 days. During the global period, any care provided related to the surgical procedure is included in the surgical fee and cannot be billed separately; remember, any attempt to do so is called *unbundling* and is considered fraud. As discussed earlier, if a patient is seen for an unrelated problem, the service or procedure may be billed separately using modifier 24 for E/M services, or modifier 79 for an unrelated surgical procedure taking place in a global period. After the global period ends, additional services related to the initial surgery can be reported separately for payment.

As shown in Figure 19-5, to make the coding process more efficient, most medical offices list frequently used procedures and their applicable CPT codes on superbills, or encounter forms. After seeing the patient, the provider checks off the appropriate procedures or services and the patient returns the form to the medical assistant at the front desk. The medical assistant then inputs the information into the facility computer system, if the office is computerized. If the office uses a manual system, the administrative medical assistant will put the office copy of the completed superbill in a designated area so it can be used to quickly and efficiently complete the CMS-1500 form for submission to the patient's insurance carrier. If superbills are used in the office, the office must remember to update both the ICD and CPT codes on the superbills and in any computer programs when the new codes are available

TABLE 19-4	Medical Decision-Making Elements for E/M Codes				
Elements	**Straightforward**	**Low**	**Moderate**	**High**
Number of diagnostic or management options	Minimal	Limited	Multiple	Extensive
Amount or complexity of data to be reviewed	Minimal/none	Limited	Moderate	Extensive
Risk of complication or death	Minimal	Low	Moderate	High

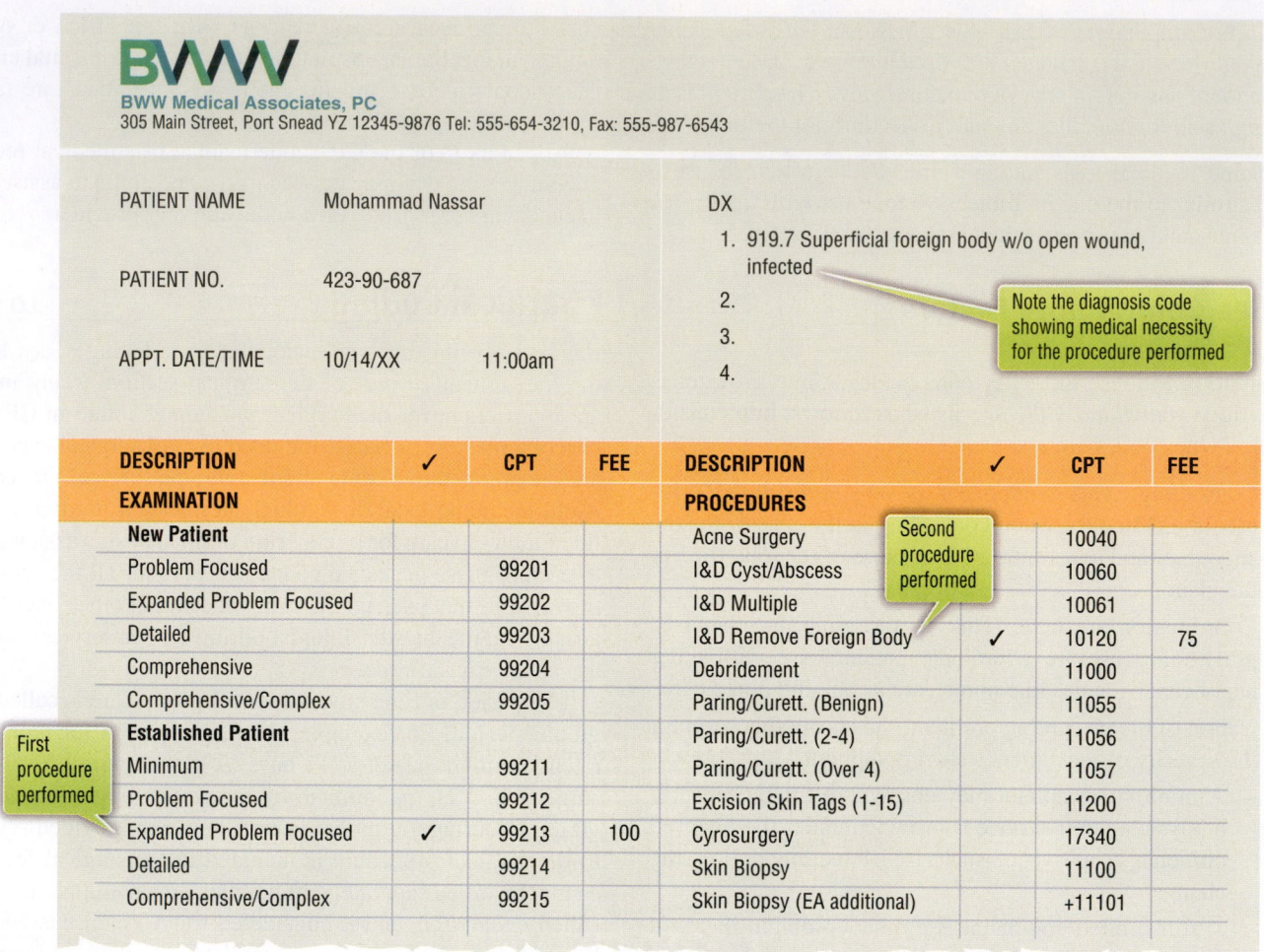

FIGURE 19-5 Superbill (encounter form) with procedures and diagnosis proving medical necessity for procedure performed.

each year (October for ICD codes and January for CPT codes). See Figure 19-6 for an example of an electronic billing report for BWW Medical Associates's EHR. This report will let you know which records have been coded with both diagnostic and procedural coding systems and are ready for billing to each patient's insurance plan.

Let's look at each subsection of the surgery chapter of the CPT manual with a brief overview of coding guidelines for each area.

Integumentary System

Integumentary subheadings are skin, subcutaneous, and accessory structures; nails; pilonidal cyst; introduction; repair (closure); destruction; and breast. These are further subdivided by the procedures done within each subheading, such as I&D, excision, paring, and biopsy benign and malignant lesions. Many codes in this section are based on size and location; choose carefully. Carefully read instructions regarding closure of any removed or repaired lesion. Simple closure is often included in the main code, so often you will code closure only if they are intermediate (layered) or complex (greater than layered). The instructions within the integumentary section give great information as to how to choose the correct closure type. Read everything carefully and follow the instructions exactly.

Musculoskeletal System

The musculoskeletal subheadings begin with general and then start with the head and work their way down to the foot and toes. You will find this to be true for the rest of the CPT manual. Codes start from the top of the body and work their way down within each section and subsection. Casts and strappings as well as endoscopy and arthroscopy are also found in this chapter. Probably the most common codes from this section include the fracture codes. Here are a couple of straightforward rules:

- A fracture treatment is closed unless stated otherwise; that is, treatment occurs without opening the skin. Open treatment means that surgery occurred to repair the fracture. Percutaneous treatment (fixation) immobilizes the fracture with hardware (pins) inserted using X-ray guidance.

- Be careful with cast and strapping codes. Fracture repair assumes cast application and includes it. Cast application and removal for fractures are coded only when the physician applying or removing the cast did not initially treat the patient's fracture.

- Last, any therapeutic procedure (like arthroscopy) includes the diagnostic procedure, so if a diagnostic procedure becomes a therapeutic (surgical) procedure, in the end, only the therapeutic procedure will be coded.

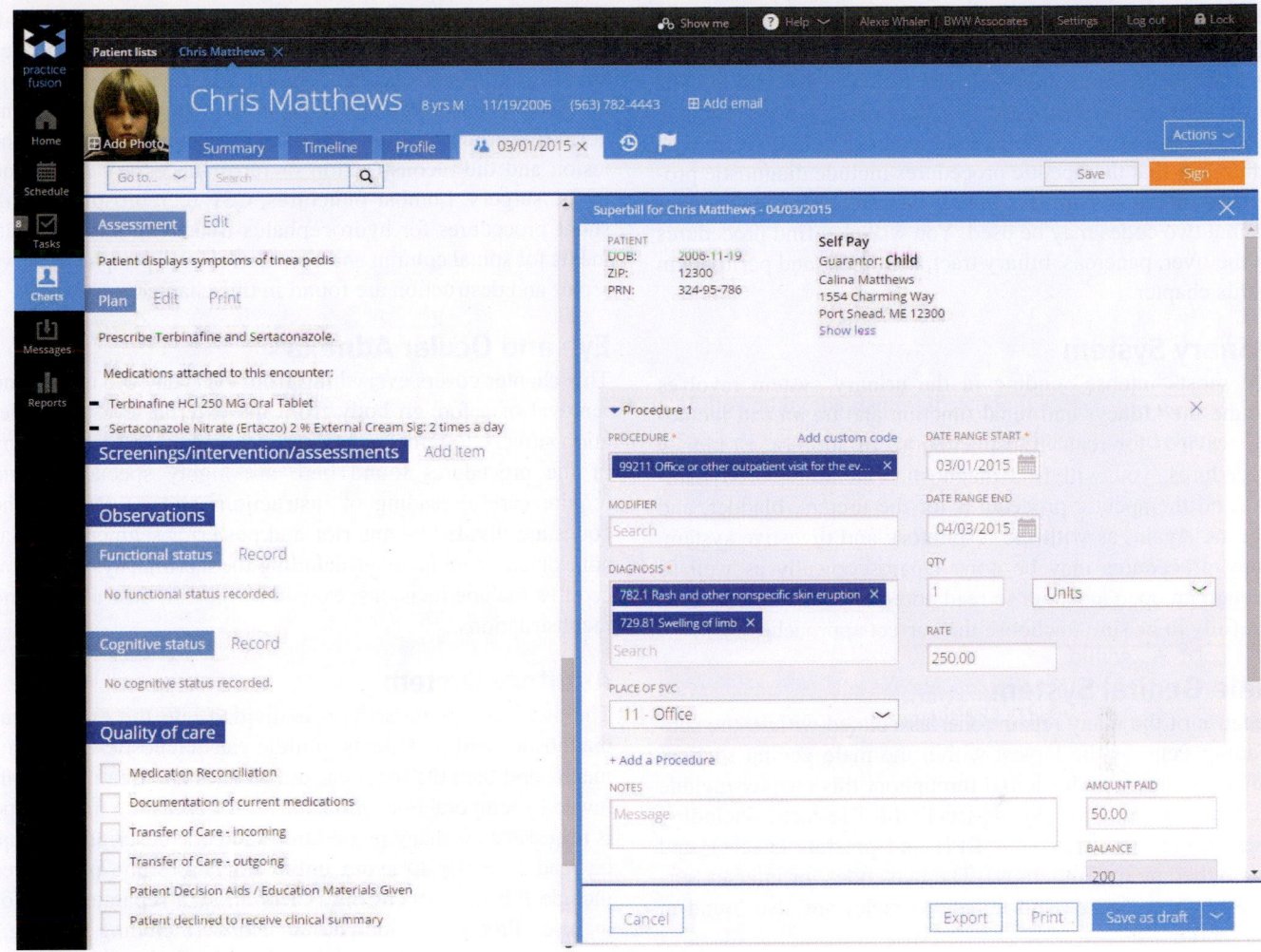

FIGURE 19-6 A Practice Fusion® superbill (encounter form) for Chris Matthews.

© Practice Fusion®

Respiratory System

The most important item to remember when coding the respiratory system is to code to the furthest extent of the procedure. For instance, many endoscopy procedures for the respiratory system begin with the nose and proceed further into the respiratory system. If the procedure results in a laryngoscopy, the scope passes through the trachea, so the code includes scoping of the trachea, which is not coded separately, as the description for code 31515 states *with or without tracheoscopy, for aspiration.* Be sure to also read information regarding the approach for the procedure. Many procedures can be done via a scope (*-scopy*) or as an open procedure using an incision (*-tomy*); these procedures are very different, so be cautious when coding similar procedures using different approaches. Be alert also for *incision* codes versus *excision* codes (removal—*ectomy*) and for the suffix *-plasty,* signifying a repair procedure like rhinoplasty. Your anatomy and terminology knowledge will be invaluable when coding.

Cardiovascular System

As you might expect, cardiology coding consists of some of the more complicated coding scenarios. Often, in order to completely code cardiovascular surgery, codes from the cardiovascular surgery section, medicine section (for nonsurgical services), and radiology section (for diagnostic or visualization assistance) will all be necessary. When coding bypass procedures, read instructions carefully. You must know not only whether veins or arteries (or both) are used in the bypass but also the correct coding sequence; the right codes in the wrong order will also hold up a claim. Injection codes will be used for diagnostic and therapeutic procedures and you will also find embolectomy and thrombectomy codes in this section. Nonsurgical cardiography procedures include ECGs, Holter monitors, and exercise tests. The echocardiography area includes all cardiac ultrasound procedures as well as vascular Doppler procedures for noncardiac vascular areas, such as the extremities. Read *everything* and make sure to code procedures completely, using as many codes as necessary.

Hemic/Lymphatic Systems and Mediastinum and Diaphragm

These two short subsections of the surgery section include procedures on the spleen, bone marrow, and lymph nodes as well as surgical procedures related to the mediastinum and diaphragm. Coding in these sections is pretty straightforward *if* you read carefully.

Digestive System

The most common procedures done in the upper digestive system are incisions and excisions followed by repairs. The lower digestive system (stomach, intestines, rectum) include these as well as endoscopies (and laparoscopies). As always, remember that therapeutic procedures include diagnostic procedures unless you are specifically instructed within the chapter that two codes may be used. You will also find procedures on the liver, pancreas, biliary tract, abdomen, and peritoneum in this chapter.

Urinary System

The most "intense" coding in the urinary system revolves around the kidneys and renal function and treatment, including services for renal transplantation. In addition to kidney procedures, you will find diagnostic (including urodynamics) and therapeutic procedures for the ureters, bladder, and urethra. Again, as with the respiratory and digestive system, many procedures may be done laparoscopically as well as through an open incision, so read notes and code descriptions carefully to be sure to choose the correct approach.

Male Genital System

Because of the many repair codes associated with it, the subheading Penis is the largest within the male genital section. Other procedure codes found throughout this chapter include excision, incision, biopsy, destruction (of lesions), including laser surgery (treatment for BPH and prostate cancer), and brachytherapy (radiotherapy). The two codes for intersex surgery (male to female and female to male) are also found in this section.

Female Genital System/ Maternity and Delivery

Medical assistants and coders use this section either extensively or almost never, as the codes found here are used almost exclusively by OB/GYN providers. This chapter is set up from "the outside in," starting with the introitus (vaginal opening) moving to the ovaries within the pelvis, with a separate subsection devoted to labor and delivery. This chapter has definitions and specialized guidelines too numerous to cover here, so if you find yourself coding for the specialty of OB/GYN, read the entire chapter carefully, taking notes and highlighting important information. Seeking the assistance of an experienced OB/GYN coder will be very helpful when you start out.

Endocrine System

Another short section, the endocrine system codes include those for procedures on the thyroid, parathyroid, thymus, adrenal glands, pancreas, and carotid body. Procedures include incisions, excisions, and laparoscopies.

Nervous System

Codes describing procedures on the brain, spinal cord, and peripheral nerves are all found in this section. Anatomic sites create the subheadings, which are subdivided by the procedure performed. Because of the complicated nature of coding procedures related to this delicate system, multiple specialized guidelines are found within this chapter. The approach again is an important consideration when coding surgery on the brain (anterior, middle, or posterior cranial fossa), as is the definitive procedure that describes the procedure done to the lesion and the reconstruction or repair necessary at the end of the surgery. Lumbar punctures, CSF (cerebrospinal fluid) shunt procedures for hydrocephalus treatment, and all treatments for spinal column and cord defects and peripheral nerve repair and destruction are found in this chapter.

Eye and Ocular Adnexa

This chapter covers everything from everyday eye exams and removal of a foreign body from the external eye to enucleation surgery to remove the contents of the eye socket. Many of the procedures found here are highly specialized and require careful reading of instructions and guidelines. The codes are divided by anterior and posterior segments, ocular adnexa, and conjunctiva (including the lacrimal system). Procedures include incisions, excisions, repairs, destruction, and reconstructions.

Auditory System

The auditory system section is divided into the external ear diagnostics and treatments, middle ear diagnostics and treatments, and then the inner ear diagnostics and treatments, followed by temporal bone procedures. An operating microscope is necessary for many procedures and code descriptions must be read carefully to avoid unbundling, as some procedures include this component but others allow a separate code for its use. Procedures include incisions (including "tubing," or tympanostomy), excisions, introductions, and repairs (tympanoplasty).

Radiology

The radiology section includes diagnostic radiology (imaging), diagnostic ultrasound, radiologic guidance, mammography, bone and joint procedures, radiation oncology, and nuclear medicine.

Many diagnostic radiology procedures use modifiers 26 (professional component only) and TC (technical component only); however, read descriptions carefully. When a code states that it includes "radiologic supervision and interpretation," as with code 77021, the code is all-inclusive and modifiers cannot be used. There are many instructions throughout this chapter leading you to correct code usage. Read all *includes* and *excludes* instructions carefully.

Laboratory Procedures

Organ or disease-oriented **panels** listed in the pathology and laboratory section of the CPT include tests frequently ordered together. An electrolyte panel, for example, includes tests for carbon dioxide, chloride, potassium, and sodium. Each element of the panel has its own procedure code. However, when the tests are performed together, the code for the panel must be used, rather than the separate procedure codes. To code a panel correctly, the provider must order each test listed within the panel and there must be a need for each of them. If a panel is appropriate but one or two laboratory tests are also ordered that are not included in the panel, code the panel and then the additional tests separately.

If each test in a panel or procedure in a surgical package is coded separately, it will cause unbundling of the panel or package. The review performed by the insurance carrier's claims department will "rebundle" the services under the appropriate code, which could delay payment. Remember—when unbundling is done intentionally or repeatedly to receive more payment than is correct, you and the practice can be investigated for fraud.

Medicine and Immunizations

Injections and infusions of immune globulins, vaccines, toxoids, and other substances require two codes—one for giving the injection and one for the particular vaccine or toxoid that is given. An E/M code is not used along with the codes for immunization unless a significant evaluation and management service is also performed (like a yearly physical exam) and documented appropriately by the doctor. Modifier 59 would be appended to the E/M code in this case, indicating the need for both procedures.

▶ Using the CPT Manual   LO 19.5

Now that you have a basic understanding of the CPT manual's format, its conventions, and its sections, including where to find section guidelines and instructions, it is time to actually use the CPT manual. Remember, when choosing E/M codes you must know whether the patient is a new or established patient and where the services took place. Use all of the information you have studied, and the chapter guidelines, to assist you in locating the correct codes.

The next step is to find the procedures and services provided by the office. As with diagnosis codes, these may be found on the superbill. However, remember to check the patient's chart to verify that documentation of the procedures and services provided exists within the medical chart (if it is not written down, it did not happen). When coding E/M codes, you may find it easiest to go directly to the E/M section in the front of the CPT manual to choose the correct code. For all other procedures, you will need to use the alphabetic listing of procedures in the back of the CPT manual.

When using the alphabetic listing of procedures, the number or number range in the index to the right of the description represents the coding possibilities for the description. If a hyphen is between two codes, this indicates a code range and each code in the range will need to be checked in the numeric index to choose the correct code. Code numbers with commas between them indicate that there is more than one possible correct location for the code required. Again, all codes will have to be checked. In some cases, the patient's medical record may show an abbreviation, an *eponym* (a person or place for which a procedure is named), or a synonym. For example, the record might state "treated for bone infection." In the CPT's index, the entry for "Infection, Bone," is followed by the instruction "See Osteomyelitis." The greater your knowledge of anatomy, physiology, and terminology, the easier it will be for you to code. Let's look at a couple of examples.

Example #1: Procedure—Dressing Change

To find the code for "dressing change," first look alphabetically in the index for that procedure. Then find the procedure code in the body of the CPT to be sure the code accurately reflects the service performed. The procedure code 15852 explains the dressing change is for "other than burns" and "under anesthesia (other than local)." (A dressing change without anesthesia would be included in an E/M code.) Per the notes in CPT, a dressing for a burn is found in procedure codes 16010–16030.

Example #2: Procedure—Excision of Vaginal Cyst

To code the excision of a vaginal cyst, you would first look under "Excision" (the main term). There is a listing for the subterm "Cyst" beneath "Excision," followed by a list of organs, regions, or structures involved. Note that each subterm is indented under the main term. Additionally, the subterms relating to cyst locations are indented even further under that subterm. This is a common occurrence in the CPT manual. Look for "Vagina" to find the code (57135). Another way to find the code is to look under "Vagina" as the main term and then find the listing for "Cyst Excision" as a subterm beneath it.

Once you decide on the appropriate CPT code(s), the next step is to check for any applicable modifiers. The use of modifiers can greatly enhance your reimbursement and can cut down on claim inquiries from the insurance carrier, but the ability to use modifiers correctly and proficiently will require practice. As discussed earlier, Appendix A of the CPT manual contains all CPT modifiers, and many of the section guidelines also contain information regarding the use of modifiers within that section. This is not an optional step. Modifier use is required if one is available for the situation.

Example #3: Procedure—Bilateral Breast Reconstruction

A bilateral breast reconstruction requires the modifier -50. Find the code for "breast reconstruction with free flap": 19364. To show the insurance carrier that the procedure was performed on both breasts, attach the -50: 19364-50. (Some insurers will require that you list the code once and then a second time with the modifier: 19364, 19364-50.) The insurance company will often pay the full charge for the first procedure and then pay the second procedure at 50%.

Once all procedures and services have been assigned a CPT code and modifier as needed, carefully enter the 5-digit code(s) and modifiers in block 24D of the CMS-1500 form, as you learned in the *Insurance and Billing* chapter. Remember that the primary procedure—often this is the most labor-intensive one or the principal reason for the patient's encounter—is listed first and is matched with the appropriate diagnosis code, often the primary diagnosis, to demonstrate medical necessity for the insurance carrier. After the principal procedure is listed, enter all other procedures provided to the patient during this date of service and match each with its appropriate diagnosis to verify its medical necessity as well.

Procedure 19-1, found at the end of this chapter, outlines the correct steps for locating a CPT code.

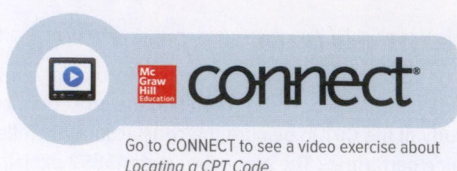

Go to CONNECT to see a video exercise about *Locating a CPT Code.*

▶ The HCPCS Coding Manual   LO 19.6

The **Healthcare Common Procedure Coding System, commonly referred to as HCPCS** (pronounced hick-picks), was developed by the Centers for Medicare and Medicaid Services (CMS) for use in coding services for Medicare patients. Today, in addition to Medicare, Medicaid and private insurance programs also accept some HCPCS codes. To avoid claim denials due to an invalid or unacceptable code, be sure to check with the insurance carrier to see if they accept HCPCS codes and, if so, which ones. The HCPCS coding system has two levels:

1. HCPCS Level I codes are more commonly known as CPT codes.
2. **HCPCS Level II codes,** issued by CMS, are called national codes and cover many supplies, such as sterile trays, drugs, injections, and DME (durable medical equipment). If CPT and HCPCS have identical descriptions, the HCPCS Level I (CPT) code should be used. However, if CPT has a generic description and HCPCS has a more specific description, HCPCS Level II should be used. Level II codes also cover services and procedures not included in the CPT. For instance CPT has one (generic) code to cover the supplies and materials used for in-office procedures (99070), whereas the HCPCS manual lists very specific codes for each item supplied.

The HCPCS codes for Level II have five characters, either numbers, letters, or a combination of both. At times, there are also two-character modifiers, either two letters or a letter with a number. These modifiers are different from the CPT modifiers but may be used with CPT codes as well as with Level II codes. For example, HCPCS modifiers may indicate social worker services (HO) or equipment rentals (KH). Appendix 2 of the HCPCS manual gives a complete list of all HCPCS modifiers.

Examples of Level II codes are listed here:

Code Number	Description
A0225-QN	Ambulance service, neonatal transport, base rate, emergency transport, one way, furnished directly by the provider of services
E0781	Ambulatory infusion pump, single or multiple channels . . .
G0008	Administration of influenza virus vaccine
G0104	Colorectal cancer screening; flexible sigmoidoscopy
Q0091	Screening Papanicolaou (Pap) smear; obtaining, preparing, and conveyance of cervical or vaginal smear to laboratory
V5298	Hearing aid, not otherwise specified

In medical offices where the HCPCS system is used, regulations issued by CMS are reviewed to determine the correct code and modifier for use on each payer's claims. Medical assistants who code with the HCPCS manual find its steps for coding mimic those of CPT, except that the Alphabetic Index is found in the front of the manual, with the alphanumeric index toward the back.

As with all coding procedures, the first step is to locate the description of the service, procedure, or item in the Alphabetic Index. Once this is located, note the code(s) or code range given and move to that area of the alphanumeric index to verify the description. Choose the code description that exactly matches the service, procedure, or item supplied as documented in the medical record. If you are coding medications supplied to the patient, you will find it easiest to locate the drug name in the Table of Drugs found in Appendix 1 of HCPCS. This table lists the unit, route of administration, and appropriate "J" code. Even though only one code is given, do not skip the step of verifying the information in the alphanumeric index.

Once all CPT and HCPCS codes are located and verified, enter them in block 24D of the CMS-1500 form if your office is not computerized. Otherwise, enter the codes in the appropriate area of the office medical billing software so that the information may be transmitted to the health insurance carrier electronically. Procedure 19-2, at the end of the chapter, outlines the steps for locating a HCPCS code. Procedure 19-3 outlines the procedure for entering CPT (HCPCS) and ICD codes into an electronic system.

▶ Coding Compliance   LO 19.7

Licensed practitioners have the ultimate responsibility for proper documentation and correct coding as well as for compliance with regulations, but many expect their medical assistants to have working knowledge of these, too. Medical assistants help ensure maximum appropriate reimbursement for reported services by submitting correct healthcare claims. These claims, and the process used to create them, must comply with the rules imposed by federal and state law and with payer requirements.

Code Linkage

As you learned in the *Insurance and Billing* chapter, clean claims are those in which each reported service is connected to a diagnosis that supports the procedure as necessary to investigate or treat the patient's condition. Insurance company representatives analyze this connection between the diagnostic and the procedural information, called code linkage, to evaluate the medical necessity of the reported charges. Correct claims also comply with many other government agency regulations.

The possible consequences of inaccurate coding and incorrect billing include the following:

- Denied claims
- Delays in processing claims and receiving payments
- Reduced payments
- Fines and other sanctions
- Loss of hospital privileges
- Exclusion from payers' programs

- Prison sentences
- Loss of the practitioner's license to practice medicine

To avoid errors, the codes on healthcare claims are checked against the medical documentation. A code review, also known as a coding audit, checks these key points:

- Are the codes appropriate to the patient's profile (age, gender, condition; new or established), and is each coded service billable?
- Is there a clear and correct link between each diagnosis and procedure?
- Have the payer's rules about the diagnosis and the procedure been followed?
- Does the documentation in the patient's medical record support the reported services?
- Do the reported services comply with all regulations?

Insurance Fraud

The majority of those involved in the delivery of healthcare are trustworthy people devoted to patients' welfare. However, some people are not. For example, according to the Department of Health and Human Services (DHHS), in 2013 alone, the federal government recovered more than $1.57 billion in judgments, settlements, and other fees in healthcare fraud cases. Fraud is an act of deception used to take advantage of another person or entity (refer to the *Legal and Ethical Issues* chapter). For example, it is fraudulent for people to misrepresent their credentials or to forge another person's signature on a check.

Claims fraud occurs when physicians or other practitioners falsely represent their services or charges to payers. For example, a provider may bill for services that were not performed (phantom billing), overcharge for services, or fail to provide complete services under a contract. A patient may exaggerate an injury to get a settlement from an insurance company or ask the medical assistant to change the date a service was actually provided so that the service is covered by a health plan policy that is no longer active.

A number of coding and billing practices are fraudulent. Investigators reviewing physicians' billings look for patterns like these:

- Reporting services that were not performed

    Example: A lab bills Medicare for a general health panel (CPT 80050) but fails to perform one of the tests in the panel.

- Reporting services at a higher level than was carried out

    Example: After a visit for a flu shot, the provider bills the encounter as an evaluation and management service plus an injection.

- Performing and billing for procedures not related to the patient's condition and therefore not medically necessary

    Example: After reading an article about Lyme disease, a patient is worried about having worked in her garden over the summer and requests a Lyme disease diagnostic test. Although no symptoms or signs have been reported, the physician orders and bills for the Lyme disease test, stating an exposure had occurred.

- Billing separately for services bundled in a single procedure code (unbundling)

    Example: When a physician orders a comprehensive metabolic panel (CPT 80053), the provider bills for the panel as well as for a quantitative glucose test, which is included in the panel.

- Reporting the same service twice

    Example: The office submits a claim the same day the patient is in the office for a urinalysis, but the patient was unable to produce a specimen. When the patient returns later in the week with the specimen, a second claim is submitted for the urinalysis.

Note that HIPAA calls for penalties for giving remuneration to anyone eligible for benefits under federal healthcare programs. The forgiveness or waiver of copayments may violate the policies of some payers; others may permit forgiveness or waiver if they are aware of the reasons for the forgiveness or waiver, such as the patient's inability to pay (be sure to have documentation of such inability to avoid charges of discrimination). Routine forgiveness or waiver of copayments or deductibles constitutes fraud when billing federal programs like Medicare or TRICARE. The practice should ensure that its policies on copayments are consistent with applicable law and with the requirements of its agreements with payers.

Compliance Plans

To avoid the risk of fraud, medical offices have a compliance plan to uncover compliance problems and correct them. A compliance plan is a process for finding, correcting, and preventing illegal medical office practices. Its goals are to

- Prevent fraud and abuse through a formal process to identify, investigate, fix, and prevent repeat violations relating to reimbursement for healthcare services provided.
- Ensure compliance with applicable federal, state, and local laws, including employment laws and environmental laws as well as antifraud laws.
- Help defend providers if they are investigated or prosecuted for fraud by showing the desire to behave compliantly and thus reduce any fines or criminal prosecution.

When a compliance plan is in place, it demonstrates to payers like Medicare that honest, ongoing attempts have been made to find and fix weak areas of compliance with regulations. The development of this written plan is led by a compliance officer and committee with the intention to (1) audit and monitor compliance with government regulations, especially in the area of coding and billing; (2) develop consistent written policies and procedures; (3) provide for ongoing staff training and communication; and (4) respond to and correct errors. Although coding and billing compliance are the compliance plan's major focus, it covers all areas of government regulation of medical practices, such as equal employment opportunity (EEO) regulations (for example, hiring and promotion policies) and OSHA regulations (for example, fire safety and handling of hazardous materials like bloodborne pathogens). For further information, go to http://www.oig.hhs.gov/fraud/docs/complianceguidance/thirdparty.pdf.

PROCEDURE 19-1 Locating a CPT Code

Procedure Goal: To locate correct CPT codes using the CPT manual

OSHA Guidelines: This procedure does not involve exposure to blood, body fluids, or tissue.

Materials: Patient record, superbill or charge slip containing procedure(s) performed, and CPT manual

Method:

1. Find the services listed on the superbill (if used) and in the patient's record.

   RATIONALE: *Only documented services and procedures may be coded for submission to the insurance carrier.*

   a. Check the patient's record to see which services were documented. For E/M procedures, note whether the patient is a new or established patient and then look for clues as to the location of the service and the extent of the history, examination, and medical decision making that were involved.

   RATIONALE: *To code E/M services correctly, all of this information is required.*

2. Look up the procedure code(s) in the Alphabetic Index of the CPT manual.

   a. Verify the code number in the Tabular List, reading all notes and guidelines for that section.

   RATIONALE: *All codes must be verified in the Tabular List; never code only from the Alphabetic Index.*

   b. If a code range is noted, look up each code in the range and choose the correct code given in the Tabular List. If the correct description is not found, start the process again. Use the same process if multiple codes are given, looking each one up in the Tabular List until you find the correct code description.

   RATIONALE: *The Tabular List gives specific information and direction not found in the Alphabetic Index.*

3. Determine appropriate modifiers.

   a. Check section guidelines and Appendix A to choose a modifier if needed to explain a situation involving the procedure being coded, such as bilateral procedure, surgical team, or a discontinued procedure.

   RATIONALE: *Modifiers give the payer specific information about the procedure, which may affect payment for that procedure.*

4. Carefully record the procedure code(s) on the healthcare claim or, if the office is computerized, enter the codes into the office billing system for placement on an electronic health claim form. Usually, the primary procedure—the one that is the primary reason for the encounter or visit—is listed first.

5. Match each procedure with its corresponding diagnosis. The primary procedure is often (but not always) matched with the primary diagnosis.

   RATIONALE: *This code-linking provides the payer with the medical necessity for each procedure—the reason the service or procedure was needed.*

PROCEDURE 19-2 Locating a HCPCS Code

Procedure Goal: To locate correct HCPCS codes using the HCPCS manual

OSHA Guidelines: This procedure does not involve exposure to blood, body fluids, or tissue.

Materials: Patient record, superbill or charge slip containing procedure(s) performed, and HCPCS manual

Method:

1. Locate the service, supplies, and equipment requiring a HCPCS code from the encounter form or from the patient's record. If an encounter form is used, verify procedure completion in the medical record.

   RATIONALE: *Only services, supplies, and equipment documented as provided may be billed to the insurance carrier.*

2. Use the Alphabetic Index in the beginning of the manual to locate the section in which the category of codes is found.

3. Find the code or code range listed, reading descriptions carefully. Do not code from the Alphabetic Index.

   RATIONALE: *The Tabular List includes further information on each code so that the correct code can be chosen.*

4. Look up the code or each code in the code range listed in the Tabular List. Read descriptions carefully.

   RATIONALE: *The Tabular List includes further information on each code so that the correct code can be chosen.*

5. Make sure the code is valid for the type of insurance the patient carries.

   RATIONALE: *If the insurance carrier does not accept HCPCS codes, the equivalent CPT code will need to be used instead of HCPCS.*

6. Enter the correct code(s) on the superbill, or encounter form, if necessary and, if the office uses a computerized billing program, in the patient's computerized record so that it can be used for billing purposes. Otherwise, place the HCPCS code in block 24D of the 1500 claim form for submission to the insurance carrier. Match each HCPCS code with the appropriate diagnosis code to demonstrate medical necessity.

   RATIONALE: *This code-linking provides the payer with the medical necessity for each procedure—the reason the service or procedure was needed.*

PROCEDURE 19-3 Entering CPT/HCPCS and ICD Codes into an EHR Program

Procedure Goal: To enter procedure and diagnosis codes into the Practice Fusion® EHR/billing program

OSHA Guidelines: This procedure does not involve exposure to blood, body fluids, or tissue.

Materials: Paper or electronic superbill, patient's medical record, and a computer with Practice Fusion® EHR program loaded

Method:

1. Log in to the Practice Fusion® EHR Program as instructed and from the Tasks on the right side of the screen, choose **Charts.**

2. Double-click the name of the patient requiring EHR update with procedural and diagnostic coding for billing to the insurance carrier.

3. From the right side of the patient's screen choose the encounter date requiring code insertion by double-clicking it.

4. Scroll down the screen to locate the Diagnosis section and click **Record.**

5. In the blank diagnosis field that appears, key the first few letters of the first diagnosis. From the available listing, reading carefully, choose the diagnosis code and description required.
   RATIONALE: *The diagnosis will become a permanent part of the patient's medical history and record; choose carefully.*

6. If a start date for the diagnosis is known, enter it in the appropriate field. If medications were given for this diagnosis, click **Medications** and they may be listed if desired. Otherwise, at the bottom of the screen, select the box next to **Attach Diagnosis to this Encounter** and click **Done.**
   RATIONALE: *The diagnosis now becomes part of the medical necessity for this visit.*

7. Repeat the process to add all diagnoses pertaining to this encounter.

8. To add all procedures and services provided during this encounter, move to the bottom of the screen and click the **Record** button next to **Superbill.**

9. In the procedure field, enter the CPT code desired.

10. Check the description for the CPT or HCPCS code entered, making sure it matches the procedure performed. If so, click the procedure and the code will be entered.
    RATIONALE: *The procedure selected will be billed to the insurance plan. It must match the medical record describing the procedures or services provided during this encounter.*

11. In the next field, add any required modifiers to the procedure code following payer guidelines.

12. In the diagnosis field, select the diagnosis from the list that has been saved for this patient; that is the reason this procedure or service was provided.
    RATIONALE: *The diagnosis provides the medical necessity or reason the service or procedure was required.*

13. Enter the number of units (or times) the service was provided on this date.

14. At the top-right corner of the screen, click **Save** after checking your work.

15. Repeat these steps for each procedure or service performed until all services are recorded and diagnosis is attached, and perform a final save.

SUMMARY OF LEARNING OUTCOMES	
LEARNING OUTCOMES	**KEY POINTS**
19.1 List the sections of the CPT manual, giving the code range for each.	The sections for the CPT manual are Evaluation and Management, Anesthesiology, Surgery, Radiology, Pathology and Laboratory, and Medicine, with code ranges from 00100 to 99602.
19.2 Describe briefly each of the CPT's general guidelines.	A CPT code is a 5-digit code representing the service provided to the patient. The CPT manual general guidelines include the following symbols, each of which represents important information about the code being described: blue triangle, red dot, # sign, triangles facing each other, circle with a diagonal through it, lightning bolt, bull's-eye, as well as add-on codes and modifiers. Always begin coding by looking up the description in the Alphabetic Index and verifying in the Tabular (numeric) List. Carefully read all guidelines and information surrounding the codes.

LEARNING OUTCOMES	KEY POINTS
19.3 List the types of E/M codes within the CPT.	The E/M code types include office and other outpatient services; hospital observation; hospital inpatient; consultations; ED services; critical care, nursing facility, domiciliary, and rest home services; domiciliary and assisted-living services; home care plan oversight; home services; prolonged services; case management; care plan oversight; preventative medicine; non-face-to-face physician services; special E/M; newborn care, neonatal ICU, and critical care services; and other E/M services.
19.4 List the areas included in the surgical coding section.	Surgical coding sections include integumentary, musculoskeletal, respiratory, cardiovascular, digestive, urinary, male and female genital systems, endocrine, nervous, eye and ear, radiology, pathology and lab, and medicine.
19.5 Locate a CPT code using the CPT manual.	Student answers will vary depending upon the information (encounter forms or mock medical records) they are given to practice coding with the CPT manual. They should be able to select an accurate code for simple, straightforward coding scenarios.
19.6 Explain how to locate a HCPCS code using the HCPCS coding manual.	Student answers will vary depending upon the information (encounter forms or mock medical records) they are given to practice coding with the HCPCS manual. They should be able to select an accurate code for simple, straightforward coding scenarios.
19.7 Explain the importance of code linkage in avoiding coding fraud.	Code linkage demonstrates the medical necessity of services provided to the patient by accurately linking each procedure code to its appropriate diagnosis. All procedures, services, and diagnoses must be documented in the patient's medical record to be used on any health insurance claim form.

CASE STUDY CRITICAL THINKING

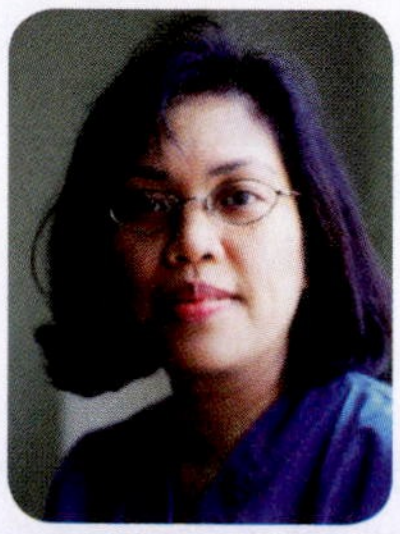

© ERproductions Ltd/Blend Images LLC RF

Recall Raja Lautu from the beginning of the chapter. Now that you have completed the chapter, answer the following questions regarding her case.

1. What is the correct CPT code for the physical examination that was performed on Raja?
2. Code the screening bilateral mammogram using both the CPT and HCPCS coding references. Which payer will require the HCPCS code instead of the CPT?
3. Using the CPT manual, code the ultrasound of the breast and the breast biopsy. Include any necessary modifiers.

1. (LO 19.1) All of the following are sections of the CPT manual *except*
   a. Anesthesiology
   b. E/M
   c. Surgery
   d. Pathology and Lab
   e. Integumentary

2. (LO 19.1) Which area gives instructions on how to code within a specific chapter?
   a. Appendix A
   b. Section notes
   c. Guidelines
   d. Modifiers
   e. Index

3. (LO 19.2) Which of the following CPT conventions indicates the code is new to the current edition?
   a. Triangle
   b. Plus sign
   c. Lightning bolt
   d. Red dot
   e. Bull's-eye

4. (LO 19.2) Which of the following CPT conventions indicates the code description is revised?
   a. Blue triangle
   b. Plus sign
   c. Lightning bolt
   d. Red dot
   e. Bull's-eye

5. (LO 19.3) The _____ codes are considered to be the most important of the CPT codes.
   a. Level II
   b. E/M
   c. Add-on
   d. Unlisted procedure
   e. Surgical

6. (LO 19.3) For reporting purposes, CPT considers a patient "new" if he or she has not received professional services within the past _____ year(s).
   a. 1
   b. 2
   c. 3
   d. 4
   e. 5

7. (LO 19.4) Which of the following are components of a surgical package?
   a. Preoperative work-up
   b. Surgery itself
   c. Usual postoperative follow-up
   d. All of these
   e. Only the surgery itself and usual post-op care

8. (LO 19.5) Which of the following is the correct code for vaginal hysterectomy (255 g) including removal of fallopian tubes and ovaries with appendectomy?
   a. 58291, 44950
   b. 58291, 44950-51
   c. 58260, 44955
   d. 58262, 44950–51
   e. 58262, 44955

9. (LO 19.6) What is the correct HCPCS code for a folding walker with wheels?
   a. E0143
   b. E0141
   c. E0149
   d. E0148
   e. E0144

10. (LO 19.7) The "key" to showing medical necessity for a procedure or service is
   a. A working compliance plan
   b. The use of appropriate ICD codes
   c. Upcoding
   d. Downcoding
   e. Accurate code linkage

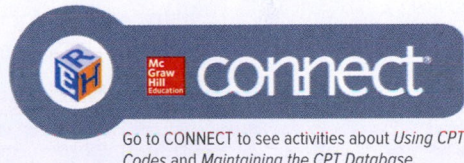

Go to CONNECT to see activities about *Using CPT Codes* and *Maintaining the CPT Database*.

Recall Raja Lautu from the case study at the beginning of the chapter.

1. Raja is very relieved when her breast biopsy comes back negative; however, she is upset that the insurance company appears to think she already has a history of breast cancer. In looking at her claim form, you see that the coder mistakenly chose a code for history of breast cancer instead of family history of breast cancer. How will you handle this?

2. Physical exam code 99396 was submitted on the same insurance claim form. Is this correct? If not, why not, and how should this be handled?

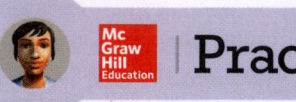

Go to PRACTICE MEDICAL OFFICE and complete the module Admin: Check Out - Work Task Proficiencies.

Patient Collections and Financial Management

CASE STUDY

PATIENT INFORMATION		
Patient Name	**DOB**	**Allergies**
Nancy Evans	1/29/19XX	Amoxicillin
Attending	**MRN**	**Other Information**
Elizabeth H. Williams, MD	654-88-099	Increasing short-term memory loss. MRI scheduled.

Nancy Evans is a 71-year-old female who has been referred to the neurologist because of a possible diagnosis of Alzheimer's disease. The charges for today total $360.00. Her husband reminds you that she has Medicare and a Medigap plan that picks up her 20% coinsurance after

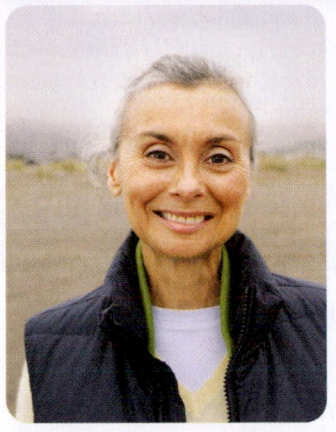

© John Lund/Sam Diephuis/Blend Images LLC RF

Medicare. You inform Mr. Evans that the office is a participating provider with Medicare. You bill Medicare and find out from the remittance advice (RA) that Nancy has $122.65 left on her deductible for this year.

Keep Nancy Evans in mind as you study this chapter. There will be questions at the end of the chapter based on the case study. The information in the chapter will help you answer these questions.

LEARNING OUTCOMES

After completing Chapter 20, you will be able to:

20.1 Summarize the importance of and how to establish good bookkeeping and banking practices.

20.2 Compare single-entry, double-entry, and write-it-once bookkeeping systems and explain accounts receivable and accounts payable.

20.3 Describe the common payment methods accepted in medical practices today.

20.4 Identify the different types of documents used as statements to bill patients and how these documents are used in cycle billing.

20.5 Compare open-book, written-contract, and single-entry accounts and the purpose of creating an accounts receivable aging.

20.6 Explain the purposes of the following credit and collections acts: ECOA, FCRA, FDCPA, and TLA.

20.7 Relate the required components of a Truth in Lending Statement to credit practices in the medical office.

20.8 Summarize two common types of problem collection accounts in the medical office.

20.9 Identify negotiable instruments and the items that must be present for a check to be negotiable.

20.10 Describe the different types of check endorsements and the steps in creating a bank deposit.

20.11 Carry out the process of reconciling the office bank statement.

20.12 List several advantages to electronic banking.

20.13 Implement setting up, classifying, and recording disbursements in a disbursements journal.

ABA number	check	limited check	skip
accounting	counter check	money order	statute of limitations
accounts payable (A/P)	credit	negotiable	third-party check
accounts receivable (A/R)	credit bureau	open-book account	tracking
age analysis	cycle billing	payee	traveler's check
bookkeeping	disclosure statement	payer	Truth in Lending Statement
cash flow statement	endorsement	power of attorney	voucher check
cashier's check	guarantor	reconciliation	write-it-once (pegboard) system
certified check	journalizing	single-entry account	written-contract account

MEDICAL ASSISTING COMPETENCIES

CAAHEP

VII.C.1 Define the following bookkeeping terms:
(a) charges
(b) payments
(c) accounts receivable
(d) accounts payable
(e) adjustments

VII.C.2 Describe banking procedures as related to the ambulatory care setting

VII.C.3 Describe precautions for accepting the following types of payments:
(a) cash
(b) check
(c) credit card
(d) debit card

VII.C.4 Describe types of adjustments made to patient accounts including:
(a) non-sufficient funds (NSF) check
(b) collection agency transaction
(c) credit balance
(d) third party

VII.C.5 Identify types of information contained in the patient's billing record

VII.C.6 Explain patient financial obligations for services rendered

VII.P.1 Perform accounts receivable procedures to patient accounts includng posting:
(a) charges
(b) payments
(c) adjustments

VII.P.2 Prepare a bank deposit

VII.P.3 Obtain accurate patient billing information

VII.P.4 Inform a patient of financial obligations for services rendered

VII.A.1 Demonstrate professionalism when discussing patient's billing record

VII.A.2 Display sensitivity when requesting payment for services rendered

ABHES

4. Medical Law and Ethics

f. Comply with federal, state, and local health laws and regulations

5. Psychology of Human Relations

c. Intervene on behalf of the patient regarding issues/concerns that may arise, i.e. insurance policy information, medical bills, physician/provider orders, etc.

8. Administrative Procedures

a. Gather and process documents

b. Perform billing and collection procedures
(1) Accounts payable and accounts receivable
(2) Post adjustments
(3) Payment procedures; i.e. credit balance, non-sufficient funds, refunds

11. Career Development

b. Demonstrate professional behavior

▶ Introduction

Often, when you ask someone why he or she entered the medical field, you will hear, "I wanted to be involved with patient care." Excellent patient care is at the heart of every medical office, but what is behind this heart? The true backbone of the practice–financial management. Without current, sound financial practices and management in place, a medical practice cannot succeed. A licensed practitioner may have a thriving practice and be loved by her patients, but without employees who understand and perform sound business and financial management procedures, the practice will fail and ultimately close. In this chapter, you will explore the practices necessary to keep a successful medical practice thriving.

▶ The Medical Practice as a Business   LO 20.1

A medical practice is a business. If it is to prosper, its income must exceed its expenses. In other words, it must produce a profit. The process of communicating the income and expenses of a business and its financial health is known as **accounting.** The practice's finances must be watched closely to be sure that expenses do not exceed income. Part of this process is the systematic recording of business transactions, known as **bookkeeping.** As the office medical assistant, recording daily business transactions may be part of your responsibility. Your records, along with other financial records, will later be analyzed by an accountant or by a more experienced medical assistant to monitor the practice's financial health. In addition to bookkeeping, banking is another key responsibility of many medical assistants. To fulfill these administrative responsibilities, you need an understanding of basic accounting systems and the procedures surrounding banking and financial management.

Importance of Accuracy

Whenever you perform bookkeeping or banking procedures, strive for 100% accuracy. Because bookkeeping records form a chain of information, an undetected error at the first link will be carried through all other links in the chain. You might compare this to a set of dominoes: If one domino is not perfectly balanced, it will affect all those that come after it, collapsing the entire bunch. Undetected errors in the medical office can result in billing a patient twice for the same visit, omitting bank deposits, or making improper payments to suppliers. These actions can result in lost money—and patients—for the practice. Establishing procedures that are consistently carried out will help ensure accuracy and help keep you from forgetting a potentially important step in the procedure.

Establishing Procedures

Here are some general suggestions to assist you in maintaining accuracy in bookkeeping and banking procedures for your medical practice:

- Be organized. Maintain the practice's bookkeeping and banking records and written procedures in a logical and organized way.

- Be consistent. Always handle the same kinds of transactions in exactly the same way. For example, endorse all checks with the same information, regardless of who wrote them or when you will be depositing them. Using a pre-printed bank stamp is helpful for consistency with this procedure.

- Use markers. Make check marks as you work to avoid losing your place if you are interrupted. For example, place a red check mark on each checkbook entry as you check it against the bank statement when you reconcile the office checkbook with the bank statement.

- Write clearly. Always use the same type and color pen and clear, easy-to-read handwriting. If more than one person performs bookkeeping and banking tasks, each person should initial her part of the procedure to identify her work. It is recommended that as few people as possible perform these tasks to minimize possible duplication or accidental "skipping" of steps because "Judy and Michaela each mistakenly thought the other had performed the bank reconciliation." You may use pencil for trial balances and worksheets, but you should use pen for final bookkeeping entries.

- Check your work. Frequently review your work to detect and correct any errors. To correct errors, draw a straight line through the incorrect figure and write the correct figure above it. Never erase errors or delete them with correction fluid or tape. As with medical records, the office financial records are legal documents and every entry, even corrected ones, needs to be readable at all times.

- Use straight columns. Keep all columns of figures straight, so that decimal points align correctly. This makes totaling of figures easier and looks neat and professional.

Using set procedures, even as more and more of these procedures become computerized, will help you organize your work, help ensure accuracy, and make you a more valuable member of the practice staff because others will trust that your work will be concise and accurate.

▶ Medical Office Accounting Methods   LO 20.2

Patient accounting methods within a medical practice may be computerized or manual, but more and more offices are turning to computerized patient accounting systems. Three types of manual accounting systems may be used by medical practices that are not computerized: single-entry, double-entry, and write-it-once (pegboard) systems. All accounting systems record income, *charges* (money owed to the practice), *disbursements* (money paid out by the practice), and other financial information. The choice of system is based on the size and complexity of the practice. Even if your office is computerized, it is important to have a basic understanding of each of these systems, as you will find that computerized systems work in the same manner. Not only that, but if the office computer system goes down for any reason, you will still need to have a mechanism to track any transactions that take place during the "computer down time."

Electronic Bookkeeping

Offices that utilize a computerized bookkeeping system enjoy several important benefits over traditional manual bookkeeping methods. With computerized bookkeeping, you save time because

- The computer performs repetitive tasks.
- The computer software automatically performs mathematical calculations.
- Built-in tax tables are available that calculate tax liabilities for you.

Many bookkeeping software programs and practice management software programs are available on the market and perform the same tasks that are performed manually. Understanding these tasks is an essential part of managing books on a computer as well as with a manual system. The practice in which you work may already have a computerized bookkeeping program in place, which you will learn as the office medical assistant. It is also a good idea to stay current on new software programs as they become available by reading computer software magazines or joining your local medical assisting organization, which often keeps members updated on new trends in the market. If you learn about a more efficient way to use the practice's current financial management software or discover a new software program that you feel might be helpful to your office, gather the pertinent information and make a recommendation to the physician or office manager regarding your proposal.

Manual Bookkeeping Systems

Traditionally, there were two types of accounting systems: single-entry and double-entry. In the single-entry system, a transaction is listed once (each) in the patient ledger, the daily log, and the checkbook. Although simple to use, this system is not self-balancing and errors may easily go undetected. In the double-entry system, all entries are listed twice, based on the accounting formula of Assets = Capital + Liabilities. An asset is anything owned by the company (or practice). Capital is the portion of the asset that is paid for, and a liability is the amount of money owed by the practice on the asset. To better understand this formula, consider the new ECG machine purchased by the practice in the following example. The cost of the machine is $15,000 and the office made a down payment of $5,000.

Example:

$$\$15,000 \text{ (Asset)} = \$5,000 \text{ (Capital)} + \$10,000 \text{ (Liability)}$$

Every month, when a payment is made, the asset amount will remain the same, but the capital amount will increase and the liability amount will decrease. However, both sides of the equation will continue to balance.

Write-It-Once, or Pegboard, System Most medical offices using a manual bookkeeping system use the **write-it-once (pegboard) system,** which contains a formula to check your work. The write-it-once system uses the same bookkeeping forms as the single- and double-entry systems, but the day sheet, also called the daily log, has pre-punched holes on the right or left side of the log. There are similar holes in the shingled (layered) charge sheets that are placed in designated areas on top of the day sheet, which has been placed on the pegboard. Each charge sheet is made with no-carbon-required (NCR) paper, so when the patient ledger card is placed between the day sheet and charge sheet and an entry is made, it appears on all three documents at the same time—hence the term "write-it-once." You will examine this system in more detail later in the chapter.

Bookkeeping Forms Regardless of the type of bookkeeping method used, all of these systems use similar forms and records to maintain the bookkeeping system. Each form is discussed in further detail in the following paragraphs.

Daily Log The daily log is also known as a general ledger, day sheet, or daily journal, depending on the practice. Regardless of the name used, it is a chronological list of each patient's charges, any payments made on the account, and any adjustments on the account (like the difference between the charge billed to the insurance carrier and the "allowed charge" that the payment is based on). See Figure 20-1. In the daily log, you record the name of each patient seen that day. Across from the name, you record the service provided (using the proper procedure codes), the fee charged, and the payment (if any) received. This process is called **journalizing.** You then post (copy) the charges, adjustments, and payments from the daily log to patient ledger cards. Using a daily or monthly cash control sheet, you record checks and cash received as well as deposits made each day.

Date: 4/15/XX							
Patient	Service	Charge	Payment	Adj	Cur Bal	Prev Bal	MD
Washington, Ken	99212, 93000	150.00	25.00		125.00	0.00	PFB
Ramirez, Valarie	99213	80.00			190.00	110.00	PFB
Lautu, Raja	99384	145.00	20.00		160.00	35.00	EHW
Chen, Cindy	99215, 36415	210.00		25.00	185.00	0.00	ANW
Matthews, Chris	99212	65.00	65.00		0.00	0.00	ANW
TOTALS		650.00	110.00	25.00	660.00	145.00	

FIGURE 20-1 The daily log is used to record all patient-based financial activity in the office for each day.

In most offices, medical assistants maintain the daily log. You can obtain the information you need to post transactions from the charge slip, which may also be called the encounter form or superbill. (Note: A charge slip is the original record of all of the doctor's charges and services performed on that day for an individual patient.) Because some charge slips include the areas for payment and next appointment information, the term *superbill* is often used. Typically, a charge slip/receipt includes duplicate (and sometimes triplicate) copies underneath to use for bookkeeping purposes—one copy for the patient, one for the medical office, and one for the business office, if that is a separate entity. Remember, you need to track charges *and* receipts for payment, for each patient, regardless of the bookkeeping method used. If the provider also performs house calls or visits to nursing homes, records of these visits must also be accounted for, so additional copies of charge slips may be sent with the provider to use when visiting these outside facilities.

As a medical assistant, it is also your job to record any night calls or other unscheduled visits in the daily log. Simply check with the provider each morning to determine if a charge slip needs to be generated to record the proper fees. If the physician has not noted the charge amount on a charge slip/receipt or record of outside visits, you may have to apply the appropriate fees according to the agreed-upon fee schedule for your office.

In addition to payments made by patients while in the office, other payments will come into the office by mail from both insurance companies and patients. These payments also must be recorded in the daily log for proper tracking of **accounts receivable (A/R).** When payment is sent from an insurance company, it is usually in the form of a check (or electronic payment) and has an explanation of benefits (EOB) or remittance advice (RA) attached, displaying the amount paid on each patient's behalf. You must post the amount indicated to each patient account and record any adjustment required according to the contract the practice has with the insurance company.

If extra columns are available, and if it is part of office policy, you also may record additional financial information in the daily log. For example, in addition to showing the total amount charged to the patient, you might show a breakdown of that total into the amounts generated by different practitioners in a group practice or by different functions of the office, such as the laboratory or X-ray department.

At the end of each day, total the charges and receipts in the daily log and post these totals to the monthly summary of charges and receipts. To double-check your totals, perform the following steps, outlined in Procedure 20-1 at the end of this chapter:

- Ensure that the day's total cash and check receipts are the same as the day's total bank deposit.
- Ensure that the sum of the day's charges for each type of service is the same as the total of the day's charges.

Patient Ledger Cards Another bookkeeping task is preparing a *patient ledger card* for each patient. This card includes the patient's name, address, home and work telephone numbers, health insurance information, Social Security number, and employer's name; the name of the guarantor (the

one who is responsible for payment of the charges, if different from the patient); and any special billing instructions. Figure 20-2 shows an example of a patient ledger card.

You will use the patient ledger card to record charges incurred by the patient, payments received, adjustments made, and the resulting balance owed to the doctor as described in Procedure 20-1. Because these cards document the financial transactions of the individual patient account, they are sometimes called *account cards.* In some practices that perform manual billing procedures, they are photocopied for use as monthly statements.

The information for the patient ledger cards comes from the daily log and includes the information found on the superbill (charge slip). It is best to complete all the cards at the end of each business day. If this is not possible, you may complete them as time permits during the next business day. To prevent duplicate or omitted postings, put a small check mark next to each entry in the daily log after you post it to the proper ledger card. Take great care when posting because errors posted on the patient's ledger card will be reflected on the patient billing statements. To ensure accuracy, add up the total charges and receipts from the ledger cards and make sure the information matches the total charges and receipts in that day's daily log.

When working with patient financial records, including patient ledger cards, keep in mind that each patient's financial records must be kept just as confidential as his or her medical record information. Regardless of whether you are working with paper financial records or using an electronic system, just as with medical information, be sure that only those staff members with a "need to know" are allowed access to any patient's financial information.

Bookkeeping Records Regardless of whether the office bookkeeping system is computerized or manual, the records kept on the office finances remain the same. Let's look at each of these records.

Accounts Receivable Each day, you must update the accounts receivable record, which shows the total owed to the practice (the amount able to be received but not yet received). Total up the items on the accounts receivable record and then total up the outstanding balances on the patient ledger cards. The two numbers should match. If they do not, recheck your work to find the cause of the discrepancy.

Accounts Payable Accounts payable (A/P) are the amounts the practice owes to vendors (the amount able to be paid but not yet paid). If your responsibilities include accounts payable, keep careful records of equipment and supplies ordered and compare orders received against the invoices. In the checkbook register, keep detailed and accurate records of accounts paid.

Record of Office Disbursements This record is a list of the amounts paid for items like medical supplies, office rent, office utilities, employee wages, postage, and equipment over a certain period of time. It shows the **payee** (the person who will receive the payment), the date, the check number, the amount paid, and the type of expense. Figure 20-3 is an example of a disbursement record.

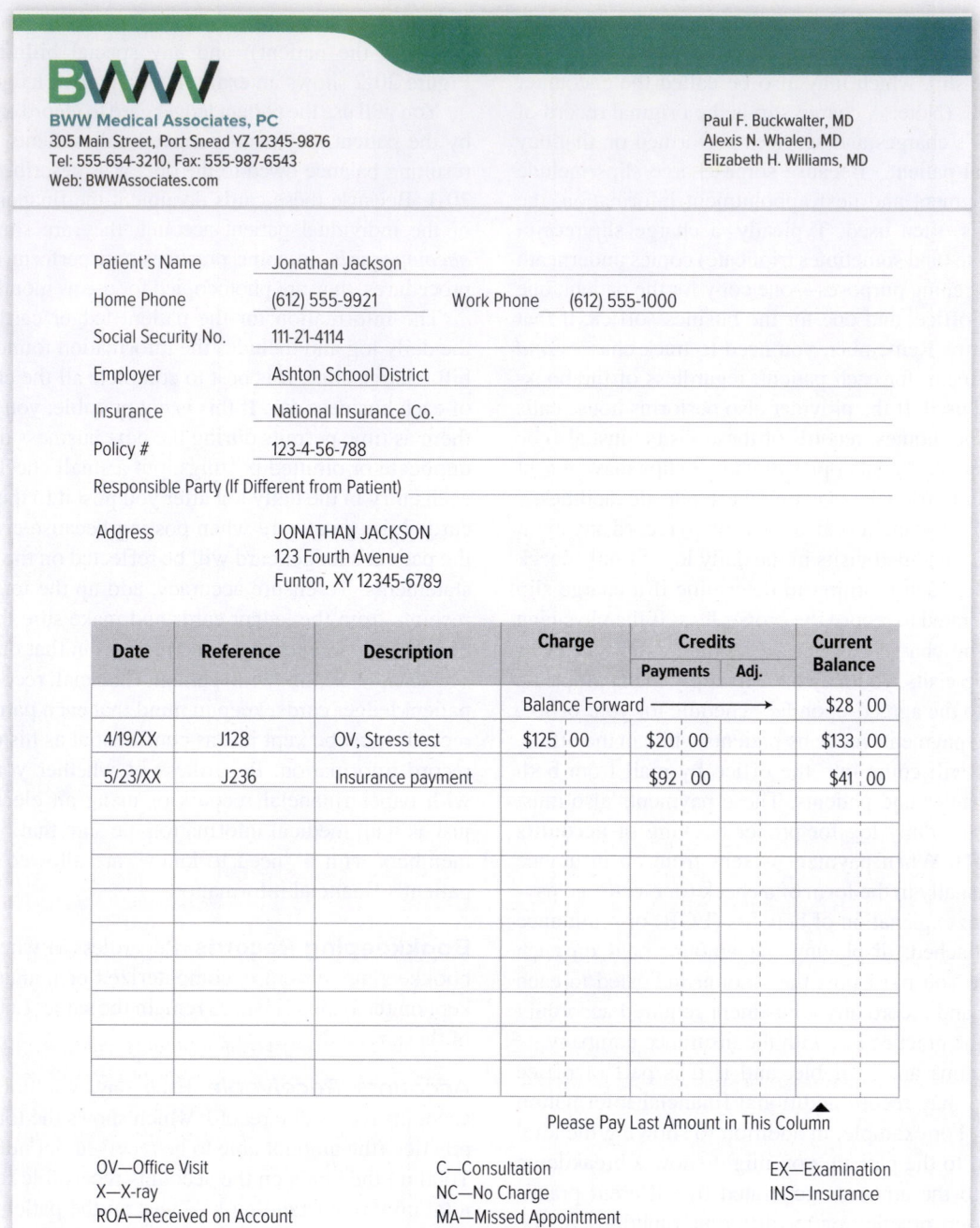

Patient's Name	Jonathan Jackson		
Home Phone	(612) 555-9921	Work Phone	(612) 555-1000
Social Security No.	111-21-4114		
Employer	Ashton School District		
Insurance	National Insurance Co.		
Policy #	123-4-56-788		
Responsible Party (If Different from Patient)			
Address	JONATHAN JACKSON 123 Fourth Avenue Funton, XY 12345-6789		

Date	Reference	Description	Charge	Credits Payments	Adj.	Current Balance
			Balance Forward ⟶			$28 00
4/19/XX	J128	OV, Stress test	$125 00	$20 00		$133 00
5/23/XX	J236	Insurance payment		$92 00		$41 00

Please Pay Last Amount in This Column ▲

OV—Office Visit	C—Consultation	EX—Examination
X—X-ray	NC—No Charge	INS—Insurance
ROA—Received on Account	MA—Missed Appointment	

FIGURE 20-2   A patient ledger card shows an individual patient's charges, adjustments, receipts, and balance due.

A checkbook register may be used to record office disbursements. As an alternative, a disbursement journal or the bottom section of the daily log may also be used to record office disbursements. For income tax purposes, this record should include only office expenses. The practitioner's personal expenses should not be listed here.

Summary of Charges, Receipts, and Disbursements

Charges, receipts, and disbursements are usually summarized at the end of each month, quarter, or year depending on your office policies and procedures (Figure 20-4). The summary is used to compare the current period's income and expenses with any previous period's income and expenses.

By analyzing summaries, a provider (or practice manager) can see which functions of the practice are profitable, the total amount charged for services, the payments received for services, the total cost of running the office, and a breakdown of expenses into various categories. Based on this information, the practice can make vital business decisions. For example, after analyzing monthly summaries, it may decide to budget expenses differently, collect payments more promptly, cut unprofitable services, or expand profitable services.

Although an accountant may prepare these reports, an experienced administrative medical assistant can prepare them. If you are asked to prepare them, follow these guidelines.

Record of Office Disbursements - April 20XX

Date	Payee	Ck. No.	Total Amount	Rent	Utilities	Postage	Lab/X-Ray	Medical Supplies	Office Supplies	Wages	Insurance	Taxes	Travel	Misc.
01	Philips' Med. Suppl.	1778	$125.00					$125.00						
01	Postage	1779	$16.85			$16.85								
02	Medi Path	1780	$32.50				$32.50							
02	Quik Service Co.	1781	$82.40						$82.40					
02	Philips' Med. Suppl.	1782	$92.00					$92.00						
02	Jean Medina	1783	$77.06							$77.06				
05	State Dept. of Rev.	1784	$189.16									$189.16		
06	General Insurance	1785	$165.92								$165.92			
07	Postage	(Cash)	$5.19			$5.19								
07	Micah Smith	(Cash)	$15.00										$15.00	
08	IRS	1786	$419.41									$419.41		
12	Quik Service Co.	1787	$124.00						$124.00					
13	City Laundry	1788	$75.00											$75.00
13	National Insurance	1789	$189.00								$189.00			
14	Broyer Assoc.	1790	$1 500.00	$1 500.00										
14	Postage	(Cash)	$12.11			$12.11								
15	City Gas Co.	1791	$125.00		$125.00									
19	Jean Medina	1792	$85.92							$85.92				
19	Postage	(Cash)	$8.95			$8.95								
21	Philips' Med. Suppl.	1793	$85.00					$85.00						
13	Medi Path	1794	$67.90				$67.90							
14	Micah Smith	(Cash)	$10.00										$10.00	
14	Elena Paxson	1795	$126.00								$126.00			
27	Postage	1796	$17.32			$17.32								
28	Johnson Assoc.	1797	$123.45				$123.45							
Total			$3770.14	$1 500.00	$125.00	$60.42	$223.85	$302.00	$206.40	$288.98	$354.92	$608.57	$25.00	$75.00

FIGURE 20-3 The office disbursements journal is a record of payments made by the office, showing who was paid, when the payment was made, and the amount paid.

- Every business day, post the total charges and receipts from the daily log to the appropriate line and column of the monthly summary.
- Each business day, also post the disbursements from the record of office disbursements to the appropriate lines and columns of the monthly summary.
- At the end of the month, total the columns on the monthly summary.
- At the end of each quarter, post the charges, receipts, and disbursements for each of the previous 3 months to the quarterly summary. Then, total each column.
- At the end of the year, post the charges, receipts, and disbursements for each of the previous 12 months (or 4 quarters) to the annual summary. Then, total each column.

Remember, the total charges and total receipts in any summary should be almost the same. They may not be identical because some bills may not have been fully collected.

▶ In-Office Transactions
LO 20.3

Once health insurance claims have been filed and the insurance pays its portion of the patient's charges, the patient will be held accountable for his portion of the fees. Billing and collections are vitally important tasks because they convert the practice's accounts receivable into income, or cash flow, from which the accounts payable can be paid. Unless billing and collections are carried out effectively, a practice might have plenty of money due in accounts receivable but not enough cash on hand to pay its accounts payable, including staff salaries.

There are methods of improving billing and collection procedures to increase income for the practice. You will need to know about standard payment, billing, and collection procedures as well as credit arrangements and common problems in collecting payment. Patients who have insurance (a third-party payer) often request that the office submit a claim to the insurance carrier and then bill them for the balance, and most offices do so. It makes good business sense, however, if a patient belongs to a managed care organization (MCO) with a known copayment for each visit that this charge should be collected at each visit. And most medical offices require this. (Refer to the *Insurance and Billing* chapter for more information.) Immediate patient payment not only brings income into the practice faster but also saves the cost of preparing and mailing statements (patient bills) and collection of past-due accounts. Many offices post a small sign at the reception desk that states, for example, "Payment is requested when services are rendered unless other arrangements are made in advance." As the medical assistant, you are responsible for collecting these payments. If the patient cannot pay all or part of the charges at the time of the visit, it may be your responsibility to bill for the practitioner's services and possibly to extend credit utilizing payment plans for larger patient-due balances.

Quarterly Summary of Charges, Receipts, and Disbursements, 20XX

	MONTH	1 CHARGES	2 RECEIPTS	3 DISBURSE-MENTS	Types of Disbursements							
					4 WAGES	5 RENT & UTILITIES	6 OFFICE EXPENSES	7 GENERAL MEDICAL	8 X-RAY/ LAB.	9 TAXES	10 PERSONAL	11 MISC.
1	Jan.	15400.00	14800.00	6218.14	3349.50	1625.00	129.86	93.45	241.86	589.02	100.00	89.45
2	Feb.	18255.00	18950.00	7050.40	3872.80	1683.08	235.00	118.72	266.00	611.20	186.60	77.00
3	Mar.	13850.00	13250.00	6530.14	3666.10	1702.85	43.85	243.11	187.02	577.00	88.11	22.10
4												
5	Subtotal	47505.00	47000.00	19798.68	10888.40	5010.93	408.71	455.28	694.88	1777.22	374.71	188.55
6												
7	Apr.											
8	May											
9	June											
10												
11	Subtotal											
12												
13	July											
14	Aug.											
15	Sept.											
16												
17	Subtotal											
18												
19	Oct.											
20	Nov.											
21	Dec.											
22												
23	Subtotal											
24												
25	Grand Total											
26												
27												
28												
29												
30												
31												
32												
33												
34												
35												
36												

FIGURE 20-4 Depending on office policy, the monthly, quarterly and/or yearly summary of office charges, receipts, and disbursements is used to summarize the office financial health.

Starting the Business Day

At the beginning of each day, place a daily log sheet on the pegboard. Then, place the stack of superbills (charge slips/receipts) on the pegs, aligning the top line of the first superbill with the daily log top line. Because the superbills are layered one over the other from top to bottom, alignment of the first will align all others. The superbills are prenumbered. This numbering promotes good cash control and theoretically prevents embezzlement. Figure 20-5 shows the setup for the pegboard system.

Patient Process

As each patient comes in to the office, place the patient's ledger card under the next available superbill, aligning the card's first blank line with the carbon strip on the superbill. Write the date, the patient's name, and the patient's previous balance on the charge slip section. The information will automatically be recorded in the daily log and on the patient ledger card. Most pegboard sheets also contain a column just to the right of the superbill where the preprinted number of the patient's superbill may be recorded on the day sheet as a checks and balances entry.

Attach the Superbill to the Patient Chart

Remove the superbill and attach it to the patient chart so that it is ready for the provider to check off both the services provided and the applicable diagnoses for the day's visit. After examining the patient, the provider checks off or fills in the appropriate charges and diagnoses on the superbill, indicates when the next appointment is needed, and gives the superbill to the patient to return to the front desk on the way out.

Patient Checkout

When the patient returns the completed superbill you again place the ledger card between the superbill and the daily log, checking to ensure proper alignment. On the superbill, enter the date, procedure (or code), charges, payments, new balance, and date and time of the next appointment (if any). As you write this information, it should be automatically transferred onto the ledger card and daily log. Finally, tear off the receipt and give it to the patient. You can now return the patient ledger card to the file.

Accepting Patient Payment

When the patient comes to you at the completion of his visit with the superbill (refer to the *Insurance and Billing* chapter), you enter the charges for the services provided (if they are not preprinted on the form) and ask for payment. There are several effective yet diplomatic ways to request payment. Two examples are "For today's visit, the total charge is $50. How

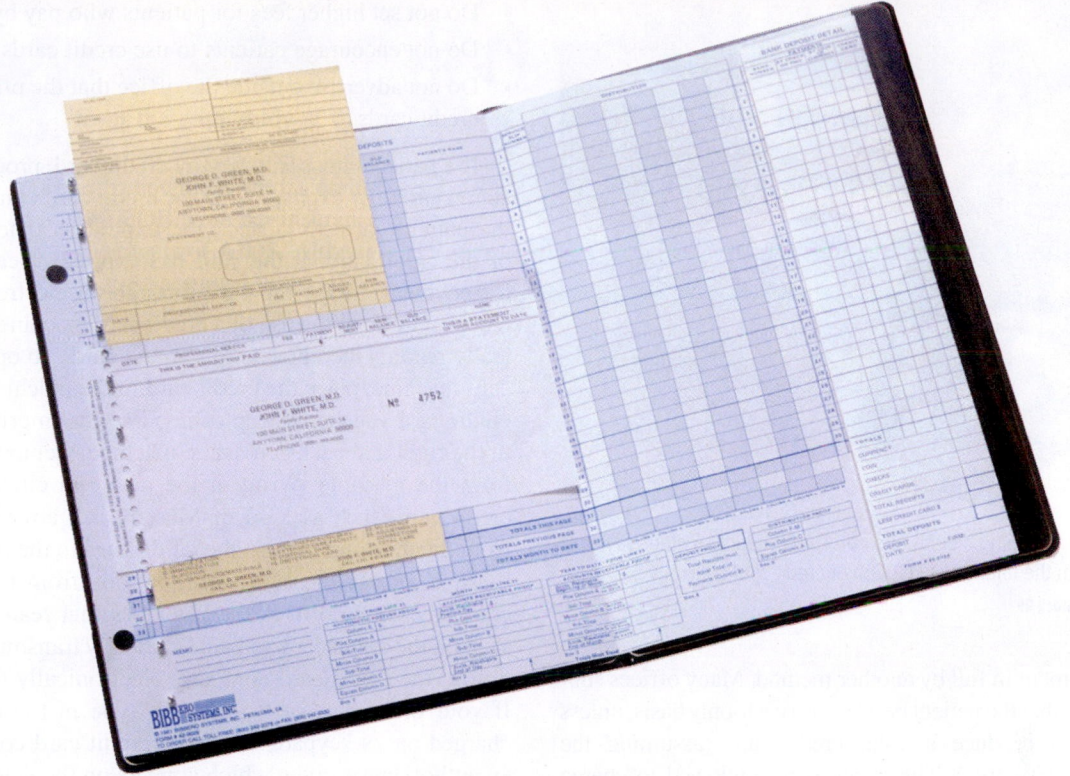

FIGURE 20-5 Using the pegboard system, shown here with a correctly aligned ledger card and superbill on the pegboard.
Courtesy of Bibbero Systems, Inc.

would you like to pay for that today?" and "The charge for your laboratory work today is $80. Would you like to pay for that now?" The first example is the preferred method because, in the second example, asking the patient if he would like to pay for the service now leaves him open to say, "No, bill me," which will slow your cash flow and cost the practice the expense of sending a billing statement. Computerized offices post the payments to the patient's account using the office billing software. Offices that use a manual, paper system often use the previously described write-it-once, or pegboard, system, which allows you to record the payment on the patient ledger card and produce a receipt for payment simultaneously.

To encourage patients to pay for treatment at the time of service, most practices accept several forms of patient payment, including cash, check, and debit and credit cards. Giving the patient these options encourages payment at the time of service.

Cash If the patient chooses to pay in cash, count the money carefully to be sure you have received the proper amount. Next, record the payment on the patient's ledger card or, with a computerized system, credit the patient's account per system instructions and give the patient a receipt.

Once the money is posted to the account, a computerized billing program gives you the option of printing a receipt you can give to the patient. If the office uses superbills, one of the copies can be given to the patient as the receipt. If your office does not use either of these methods, prepare a cash receipt manually, as shown in Figure 20-6. Be sure that whatever method is used, the office also retains a copy of the receipt. Then place the money in the cash drawer or cash box.

No. _102_		Date _10/15_ , 20XX
Received from	Nancy Evans	
	Twenty and 00/100	Dollars
For Professional Services	Account Amount	$ 20.00
	This Payment	$ 20.00
	Balance	$ 0
	Thank You!	

BWW Medical Associates, PC
305 Main Street, Port Snead YZ 12345-9876
Tel: 555-654-3210, Fax: 555-987-6543

FIGURE 20-6 A receipt such as this may be used when the patient makes a payment while in the office.

Check If your office accepts checks, always ask for proof of identity if you do not know the person writing the check, to avoid the accidental acceptance of fraudulent checks. The check should be completed fully and correctly. Many offices have a stamp with the office name on it for patient convenience and to ensure that the practice name is spelled correctly. Unless the patient has made previous arrangements, the check should be made out for the full amount owed. Verify that the check is dated for the current date and signed when accepting it. Endorse it immediately and place it with other checks for the day's deposit. If a check is returned for nonsufficient funds (NSF), notify the patient immediately,

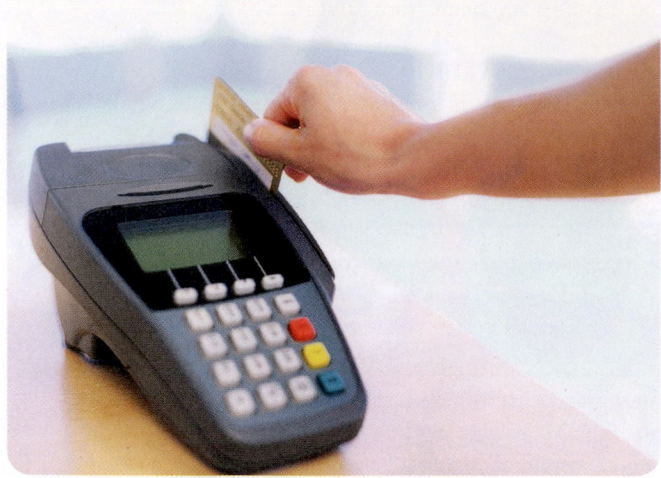

FIGURE 20-7 Swiping a debit or credit card produces instant payment authorization from the financial institution or credit card company.
© Exactostock/SuperStock RF

requesting payment in full by another method. Many offices subsequently insist that the patient be seen on a cash-only basis, unless the patient can produce a valid credit card (assuming the office takes credit cards). The office is also allowed to charge the patient an additional fee for the expense of processing the NSF check. You will learn more about this process a bit later in the chapter.

Debit Card Many patients use debit cards instead of paying by cash or check. A debit card looks like a credit card but immediately transfers the funds from the patient's bank account to the practice account. The advantage to the practice is that if there are insufficient funds in the account, the transaction will be refused and other arrangements can be made immediately. Debit cards, like credit cards, are read through electronic readers (Figure 20-7) and the patient inputs a personal identification number (PIN) verifying his or her wish that funds be transferred.

Credit Card Many medical practices accept credit cards, such as Visa or MasterCard. This payment method offers advantages for both the practice and the patient. For the practice, it provides prompt payment from the credit card company, thus increasing cash flow. It also reduces the amount of time and money spent on preparing and mailing statements, thus decreasing expenses. For the patient, it is convenient and allows a large bill to be paid in several smaller amounts, usually once a month.

Credit cards have one major disadvantage for the practice—cost. The credit card company deducts a percentage of each transaction for its collection service, usually between 1% and 5%. If a patient charges $100 in services on a credit card, for example, the practice receives only $95 to $99. The credit card company keeps the difference. Some banks are beginning to charge a similar fee for the convenience of accepting debit cards as well. A disadvantage for patients is the accrued interest charges on unpaid balances.

If the practice accepts credit card payments, the American Medical Association (AMA) suggests several guidelines.

- Do not set higher fees for patients who pay by credit card.
- Do not encourage patients to use credit cards for payment.
- Do not advertise outside the office that the practice accepts credit cards.

If a patient chooses to pay by credit card, process the transaction carefully to ensure that the credit card company charges the patient correctly. Check the expiration date on the front of the credit card. If the card has expired, it cannot be used for payment. Swipe the card through an electronic reader or record it through the use of a credit card machine that mechanically records the information on the card. To operate a credit card machine, place the credit card in the machine and place a credit card voucher on top of it. Slide the imprint arm firmly to the right and back across the machine. Remove the voucher from the machine. Write in the date and circle the type of credit card, such as Visa or MasterCard, after it is removed from the machine. Return the credit card to the patient.

Next, obtain the authorization code from the credit card company. Some offices have devices that read the magnetic strip on the credit card and automatically transmit the information to the credit card company electronically (Figure 20-7). If your office has such a device, type in the amount to be charged on its keypad. Then, the credit card company issues an authorization code, which appears on the device's screen.

If your office does not have such a device, call the credit card company for the authorization code. Give the operator the patient's credit card number and the amount of the payment. The operator then gives you the authorization code.

Write the authorization code in the box marked "Authorization" on the credit card voucher. Initial the voucher in the appropriate box. Then, fill in the services provided and the amount of the charges. Enter the total charges in the box marked "Total."

Give the receipt to the patient to sign. Compare the patient's signature on the receipt with the signature on the back of the credit card (they should be identical). Keep one copy of the receipt for the office. Give the other copy (and the credit card) to the patient.

When the payment comes in from the credit card company, they will have deducted their fee from the funds being deposited in the office account. When posting these payments to the individual patient account, you will need to adjust (write off) the amount withheld by the credit card company so that the patient is not inadvertently billed for this charge.

Online Payments Many hospitals and larger practices that accept credit and debit card payments also accept payments online through their websites or via the patient's online banking program. The payment is then directed into the office checking account with notification to the practice so that the patient's account can be credited appropriately.

Payment Responsibility

The person with financial responsibility for the patient is known as the **guarantor,** the person who "guarantees" payment. In most cases, any patient who is 18 or over is legally considered to be her own guarantor. This is true even if someone else (such as a spouse or parent) is the insured person (the person who carries the insurance for the family). As with every rule, there are some exceptions to this rule. A few are listed here.

Responsibility for Minors When a child's parents are married, either parent may consent to treatment for the minor child. Both parents are responsible for payment for the minor's treatment, although usually only one is listed on the patient's account as the guarantor. If you must send a bill for services provided to a minor child, it should be addressed to the guarantor to ensure payment. Emancipated minors are the exception to this process. If you have been shown legal proof of emancipation, any bills will be addressed to the emancipated minor; because of the emancipation process, the minor is legally responsible for her bills.

The legal and financial arrangements of a divorced couple are private. Unless you have legal documentation stating otherwise (retain a copy of this document in the patient financial record), you should assume that the parent bringing the patient to the office has consent ability and payment responsibility. Unless you have documentation otherwise, it should be made clear to the parents that payment is due at the time of the visit, regardless of which parent brings the child to the office. Refer to the *Legal and Ethical Issues* chapter for a more in-depth discussion on this topic.

Elderly Patients and Patients with Disabilities Sometimes when elderly patients or patients with disabilities are brought in for medical care, you may be asked to send the bill to another party such as an adult child. Because of HIPAA confidentiality laws, you cannot send a patient's bill to another person without first obtaining written consent to do so from the patient and the person accepting responsibility for payment. If the patient has been found to be incompetent, you should request proof of legal guardianship (keeping a copy in the patient's financial file) prior to sending a bill to the guardian.

Professional Courtesy Although much less common than in the past, a practitioner may treat some patients free of charge or for just the amount covered by the patient's insurance. This practice is known as professional courtesy. These patients often include other practitioners and their families, the practice's staff members and their families, other healthcare professionals, and clergy members. If the patient is part of a managed care organization or has Medicare, the provider must collect any copayment or deductible as part of the contracted agreement with the insurance carrier. It is considered fraud to consistently not collect copayments or deductibles if the collection of such payments is stipulated in the provider-insurer contract.

Follow the office policy regarding provision of professional courtesy. If you are unsure, check with the practitioner or office manager before making such adjustments to any patient's account.

▶ Standard Billing Procedures   LO 20.4

In today's practice, most offices receive payments from insurance carriers and then find they must bill the patient for any balance due. As the medical assistant, part of your duties may include preparing these patient billing statements. You also may have to manage related billing responsibilities, such as establishing and maintaining billing cycles.

Preparing Statements

Part of the medical assistant's job may be to prepare statements to mail to patients who do not pay when services are rendered or who make only a partial payment. Figure 20-8 shows a statement with an itemized list of services. You can obtain most of the information for the statement from the patient ledger card or from the patient's computerized account. Regardless of the format used, all statements should include the following information:

- Practice name, address, and telephone number (usually preprinted on the statement or prepared by the computer program)
- Patient's name and address
- Guarantor's name (if different from the patient)
- Balance (if any) from the previous month(s)
- Itemized list of services and charges, by date, for the current month
- Payments from the patient or insurer during the month
- Total balance due

Whatever billing procedure you use, enclose a self-addressed envelope with the statement to encourage prompt payment. Some offices have found that using a lightly colored return envelope, such as pale yellow, actually encourages faster payment because the color stands out against the usual white envelopes, jogging the patient's memory to "pay that one."

Manual Statements If the office wishes to produce manual statements, a template can be made on the computer in a format similar to Figure 20-8. Each procedure should be listed using abbreviations for common procedures, such as OV for office visit. Be sure that an explanation of the abbreviations appears on the statement, usually at the bottom. Also include the CPT codes for the procedures performed. Some statements also include the diagnosis code attached to each procedure. Using an itemized list of services provided on statements is standard practice in most medical offices, as it decreases the number of patient calls asking, "Why am I being billed?" After completing the statement, fold it in thirds and mail it in a typewritten or window business envelope.

The Patient's Ledger Card as a Statement A common alternative to typing up statements, especially in smaller, noncomputerized offices, is to photocopy the patient's ledger card and fold the photocopy so that the patient's address shows through the window in a window envelope. If your practice uses ledger cards for this purpose, be sure there are no stray marks or comments on the card and that the copy is clean and easy to read.

Computer-Generated Statements If the practice utilizes an electronic billing program, statements similar to Figure 20-8 will be produced by the program, either automatically at certain times during the month after insurance payments

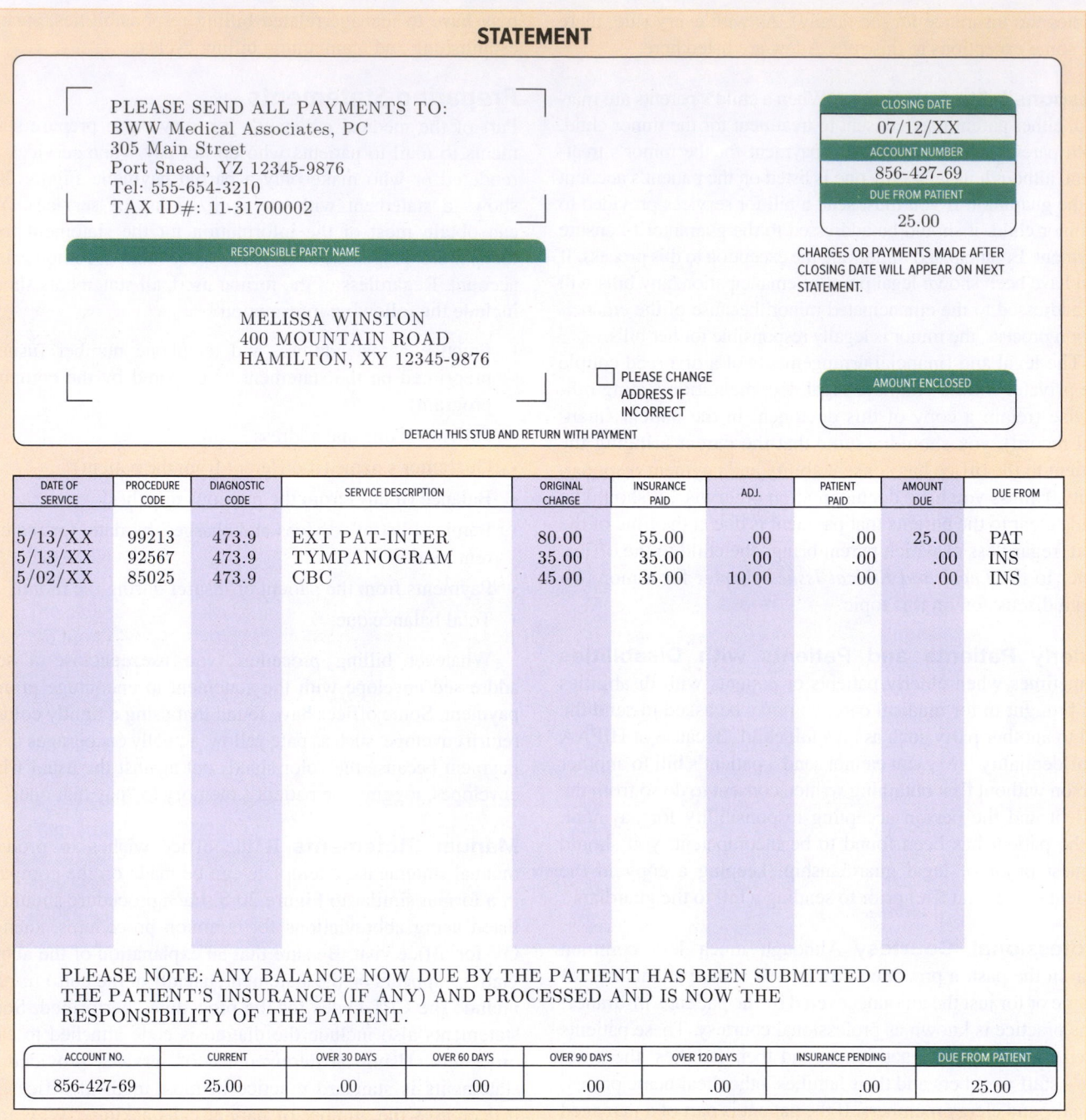

STATEMENT

PLEASE SEND ALL PAYMENTS TO:
BWW Medical Associates, PC
305 Main Street
Port Snead, YZ 12345-9876
Tel: 555-654-3210
TAX ID#: 11-31700002

CLOSING DATE
07/12/XX
ACCOUNT NUMBER
856-427-69
DUE FROM PATIENT
25.00

CHARGES OR PAYMENTS MADE AFTER CLOSING DATE WILL APPEAR ON NEXT STATEMENT.

RESPONSIBLE PARTY NAME

MELISSA WINSTON
400 MOUNTAIN ROAD
HAMILTON, XY 12345-9876

☐ PLEASE CHANGE ADDRESS IF INCORRECT

AMOUNT ENCLOSED

DETACH THIS STUB AND RETURN WITH PAYMENT

DATE OF SERVICE	PROCEDURE CODE	DIAGNOSTIC CODE	SERVICE DESCRIPTION	ORIGINAL CHARGE	INSURANCE PAID	ADJ.	PATIENT PAID	AMOUNT DUE	DUE FROM
5/13/XX	99213	473.9	EXT PAT-INTER	80.00	55.00	.00	.00	25.00	PAT
5/13/XX	92567	473.9	TYMPANOGRAM	35.00	35.00	.00	.00	.00	INS
5/02/XX	85025	473.9	CBC	45.00	35.00	10.00	.00	.00	INS

PLEASE NOTE: ANY BALANCE NOW DUE BY THE PATIENT HAS BEEN SUBMITTED TO THE PATIENT'S INSURANCE (IF ANY) AND PROCESSED AND IS NOW THE RESPONSIBILITY OF THE PATIENT.

ACCOUNT NO.	CURRENT	OVER 30 DAYS	OVER 60 DAYS	OVER 90 DAYS	OVER 120 DAYS	INSURANCE PENDING	DUE FROM PATIENT
856-427-69	25.00	.00	.00	.00	.00	.00	25.00

FIGURE 20-8 The patient billing statement should list all services and their charges, any payments made, and the amount now due.

have been made and a patient balance remains or on demand with a few keystrokes. Follow the instructions in the software procedure manual. You can then fold the printouts and mail them in window envelopes with a return payment envelope.

Using an Independent Billing Service Large practices may have both their insurance and patient billing procedures handled by an independent billing service. In addition to billing the insurance plan, the billing service may rapidly copy ledger cards or produce computer-generated statements listing the practice business office address for patients with balances due. The statements are then mailed to patients, usually with an envelope for sending payment directly to the provider's office.

Using the Superbill as a Statement

As stated earlier in the chapter, many paper-based practices still use a superbill (encounter form), which lists the charges and procedure codes (CPT) for services rendered on that day, including appropriate diagnoses and codes (ICD). As a carbonless form, when the charges and any payments are entered on the superbill, an automatic receipt and first statement are generated at the same time, saving time and money. Some offices even give the patient a return envelope if there is a balance on the account to encourage prompt payment, as this is considered the first bill received by the patient. Procedure 20-2, located at the end of the chapter, will give you practice billing with a superbill.

Managing Billing Cycles

Smaller practices send out their statements monthly, usually at the end of the month. Larger practices tend to spread the billing process out over the month in a process known as **cycle billing.** In cycle billing the accounts are split into groups and statement mailing dates are staggered.

For example, you may bill on the fifth of the month for patients whose last names begin with A through D. Then, on the tenth of the month, you may bill patients whose names begin with E through H, and so on. Using cycle billing not only staggers the workload throughout the month, but also tends to spread out the payments coming into the office, giving the office a more even cash flow.

▶ Standard Collection Procedures LO 20.5

Although many patients pay a statement within the standard 30-day period, some do not. When a patient does not pay his bill during the standard period, you need to take steps to collect the payment. For example, you may need to call or write the patient to determine the reason for nonpayment or to set up a payment arrangement.

Whether you use telephone calls, notes, or letters, there are laws, such as each state's statute of limitations, as well as professional standards and guidelines to direct your efforts in collecting overdue payments from patients.

Statute of Limitations

A **statute of limitations** is a state law that sets a time limit on when a collection suit on a past-due account can legally be filed. The time limit varies with the type of account and the state in which the debt was incurred.

Open-Book Account An account that is left open to charges that are made on an intermittent basis is known as an **open-book account.** Most of a provider's long-standing patients have this type of account. An open-book account uses the last payment date or the date of the last charge for each illness as the start date to determine the time limit for that specific debt.

Written-Contract Account As it sounds, a **written-contract account** is one in which the practitioner and patient sign an agreement regarding the treatment and the payment agreement. For this type of an account, the payment agreement often states that the patient will pay the bill in more than four installments. Some states allow longer time limits for these accounts than for open-book accounts. Written-contract accounts are regulated by the Truth in Lending Act, discussed later in this chapter.

Single-Entry Account An account consisting of only one charge is referred to as a **single-entry account.** For example, someone vacationing in your area might come in for treatment of a cold. This person's account would list only one office visit. If the vacationer did not become a regular patient, the account would be considered a single-entry account. Some states impose shorter time limits on single-entry accounts than on open-book accounts.

Using Collection Techniques

Individual practices have their own ways of approaching the task of account collections. Most begin the process with statements, then telephone calls, and finally letters.

Initial Telephone Calls When calling a patient (or sending a letter) about collections, be friendly and sympathetic. Call the patient at home unless you have specific permission to call her at work. The first phone call to the patient should occur if payment has not been received after 30–45 days. Because the patient received a receipt or superbill at the time of the visit, any statement mailed after that is essentially the second notice of payment due. The first mailed statement usually contains a message that is friendly in tone, such as "Your prompt payment is appreciated." When you call, assume that the patient forgot to pay or was temporarily unable to pay. You should ask the patient for the full amount due but have a minimum amount you would accept in mind (for instance, half). If the patient states that she cannot afford full payment, ask her what amount she feels she can send; if that amount is acceptable, obtain a date you can expect to receive the payment. If you do not receive the payment within 24 hours of the stated date, a phone call may be made and another statement sent. The message on this statement will be more urgent in tone because the patient did not respond to your phone call, and the tone of any subsequent communication will be still more urgent.

Follow-up Statements and Collection Letters Once an account is 60 days past due, it is advisable to send an initial letter of inquiry. Usually this letter still has a friendly, "we want to help" tone, giving the patient options to take care of his obligation, but makes it clear that the patient must take some sort of action. Figure 20-9 shows an example of such a letter.

If an account is 90 days past due, your collection letter can contain stronger wording. For example, it might say "Please let us know when you plan to pay the $250 past-due balance. We have sent you three monthly reminders. If you cannot pay in full now, please contact us at (number) to make payment arrangements. We want to be understanding but need your cooperation."

If an account is 120 days or more past due, you can send a final letter. It might state "Every courtesy has been extended to you in arranging for payment of your long overdue account. Unless we hear from you by (date), the account will be given to (name of collection agency) for collection." Be sure to note the cutoff date on the patient's ledger card. By law, you cannot threaten to send an account to a collection agency unless it will actually be sent on that cutoff date. Therefore, you must be sure you are ready to do so before you send such a letter. This collection letter should be mailed by certified mail with return receipt so that you have proof that the letter was sent and that the intended recipient received the letter.

If the patient does not respond with payment prior to the date stated in the letter, the practice will have no choice but to turn the account over to the office collection agency. We will discuss collection agencies later in the chapter.

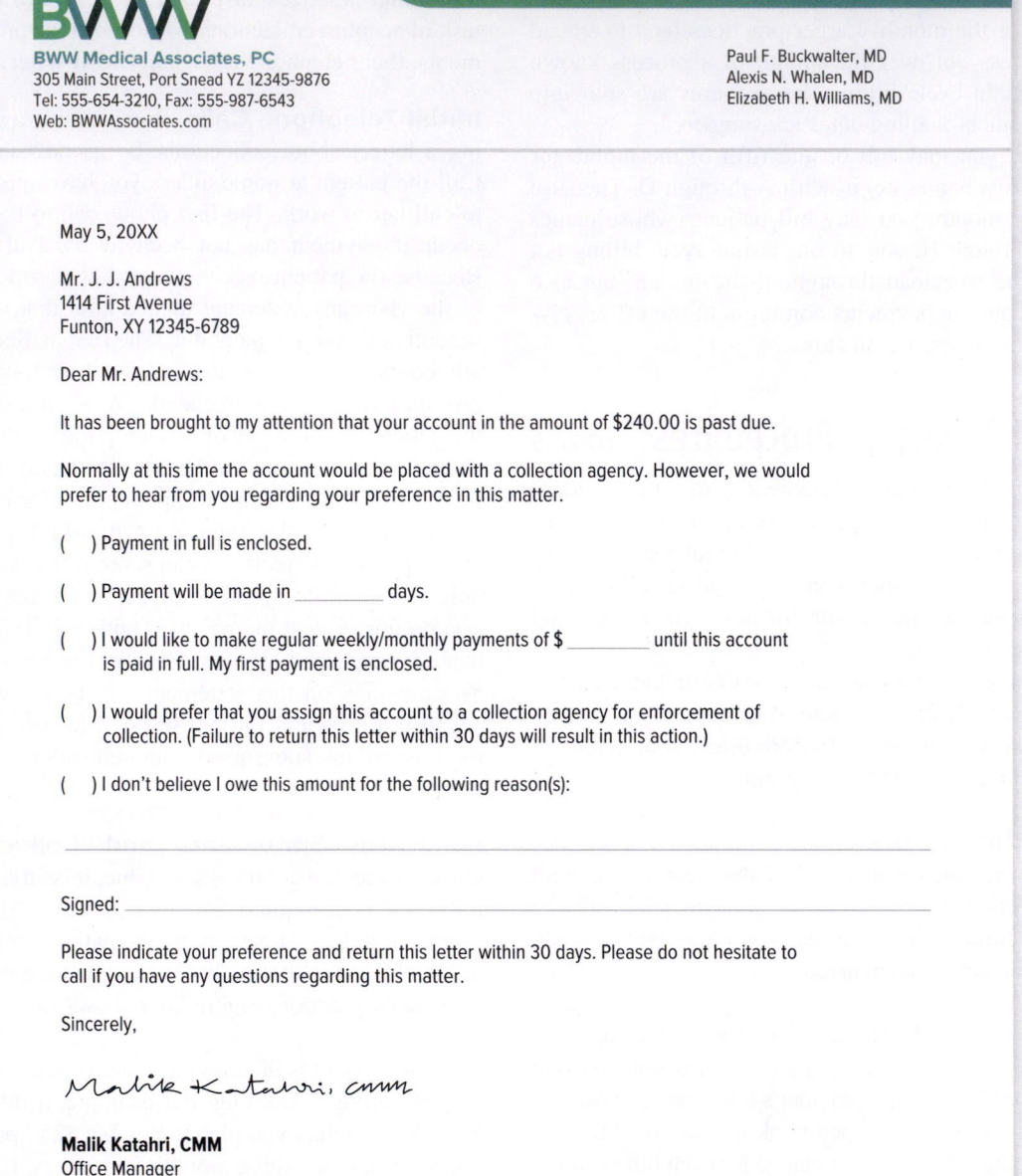

BWW

BWW Medical Associates, PC
305 Main Street, Port Snead YZ 12345-9876
Tel: 555-654-3210, Fax: 555-987-6543
Web: BWWAssociates.com

Paul F. Buckwalter, MD
Alexis N. Whalen, MD
Elizabeth H. Williams, MD

May 5, 20XX

Mr. J. J. Andrews
1414 First Avenue
Funton, XY 12345-6789

Dear Mr. Andrews:

It has been brought to my attention that your account in the amount of $240.00 is past due.

Normally at this time the account would be placed with a collection agency. However, we would prefer to hear from you regarding your preference in this matter.

(   ) Payment in full is enclosed.

(   ) Payment will be made in _____ days.

(   ) I would like to make regular weekly/monthly payments of $ _____ until this account
        is paid in full. My first payment is enclosed.

(   ) I would prefer that you assign this account to a collection agency for enforcement of
        collection. (Failure to return this letter within 30 days will result in this action.)

(   ) I don't believe I owe this amount for the following reason(s):

_____

Signed: _____

Please indicate your preference and return this letter within 30 days. Please do not hesitate to
call if you have any questions regarding this matter.

Sincerely,

Malik Katahri, CMM

Malik Katahri, CMM
Office Manager

FIGURE 20-9 Most offices use a collection letter similar to this so that the patient can simply make a choice, sign the letter, and return it to the office.

Payments After the Patient Visit

If you receive payments sometime after the patient visit, either by mail or in person, record them on the patient ledger card and day sheet, as you normally would. Record charges for practitioner visits to hospitalized patients or other out-of-office visits in the same way. If required, you can use the pegboard system to record bank deposits and petty cash disbursements in the daily log, but you will need the appropriate disbursement journal and overlapping forms.

Returned Checks

If a patient's check does not clear due to nonsufficient funds (NSF), you must adjust the account accordingly. NSF payments are first deducted from the office checking account. The patient's account is then updated with a negative payment (noted in parentheses in the payment column) for the amount of the check, adding that amount back to the patient balance. The patient may also be charged an office fee for the inconvenience of dealing with the NSF check. Any fees your office charges for NSF must be clearly stated and in plain view for patients to see. In addition, if the bank imposes a fee on the office, these bank fees also should be passed to the patient to recoup the loss for the practice and marked on the patient's ledger. Depending on office policy, the patient may now be seen on a *cash-only* basis by the practice. Procedure 20-3, at the end of this chapter, explains the procedure for posting an NSF payment.

Refunding an Overpayment (Credit Balance)

Periodically, the combination of insurance payments and patient payments exceeds the allowed charges. This is called an overpayment. Sometimes this happens when patients feel they have not met their annual deductible, they pay their balance, and then the insurance carrier also makes a payment on the patient's behalf. After posting the payments, the account balance will be a negative number, which is called a *credit balance*. When this happens, the medical office owes the patient money. In some medical offices, if this amount is small, they leave it in place so that the next scheduled visit's new charges will be applied against this amount. Procedure 20-4, at the end of this chapter, outlines the procedure for processing a credit balance.

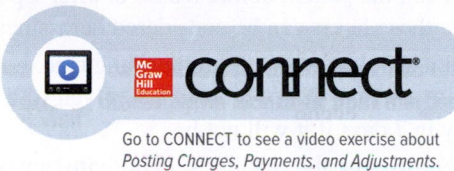

Go to CONNECT to see a video exercise about *Posting Charges, Payments, and Adjustments.*

Many times, instead of leaving a credit balance on the books, the office will need to refund the overpayment amount to the patient. This refunded amount is noted in the patient's account, bringing the balance to zero. When this happens, you will create a letter explaining how the overpayment occurred and enclose the check for the refund amount. Procedure 20-5, at the end of this chapter, outlines the steps for processing refunds to patients.

Uncollectable Accounts

In every office, despite the best collection efforts by the staff and even an outside collection agency, there will be patients who simply will not, or cannot, pay their medical bills. These accounts are known as *uncollectable*. In most offices the medical assistant and office manager or practitioner will meet monthly to discuss these accounts. When it is agreed that the money owed is never going to be collected, the practice manager or practitioner will give approval to adjust the remaining balance off the account. This practice *relieves* the A/R of these funds that will never be brought into the practice. An adjustment is made on the account for the full balance due, bringing the current balance to zero. Be sure to note the account with the name of the person giving approval for this adjustment. If it is office policy, also send the patient a registered letter informing him that he has 30 days to find a new provider because of the nonpayment of his account.

End of the Day

At the end of each day, total and check the calculations in all columns. If you find an error, correct it immediately by drawing a line through it and making a new entry on the next available writing line. Remember to make the correction on the patient ledger card and to issue a new receipt to the patient. To balance a pegboard system or patient ledger card, after adding the figures in each column, use the following formula for the column totals:

Previous balance + Today's charges − (Payments + Adjustments)
= New accounts receivable total

Preparing an Age Analysis

Age analysis is the process of classifying and reviewing past-due accounts by age from the first date of billing. A monthly age analysis, such as that shown in Figure 20-10, helps you keep on top of past-due accounts and determine which ones need follow-up. Computer billing programs will prepare an age analysis for you, but you can prepare one by hand if your office

Accounts Receivable–Age Analysis								Date: October 1, 20XX
Patient	Balance	Date of Charges	Most Recent Payment	30 Days	60 Days	90 Days	120 Days	Remarks
Black, K.	120.00	5/24	5/24			75.00	45.00	3rd Notice
Brown, R.	65.00	8/30	8/30	65.00				
Green, C.	340.00	8/25						Medicare Filed
Jones, T.	500.00	6/1	6/30		125.00	125.00	250.00	3rd Notice
Perry, S.	150.00	7/28	7/28	75.00	75.00			1st Notice
Smith, J.	375.00	6/15	7/1			375.00		2nd Notice
White, L.	200.00	6/24	7/5	20.00	30.00	150.00		2nd Notice

FIGURE 20-10 An age analysis organizes accounts by how long each has been on the A/R.

is not computerized. Offices that use ledger cards to track patient accounts often have a procedure to track how long since the last payment has been received. For instance, color-coded tags may be placed on the cards—yellow denoting 30 days past due; green, 60 days past due; red, 90 days past due; and black, 120 days past due. By pulling the ledger cards by color grouping, an age analysis can be completed easily either on graph paper or a spreadsheet. Include the patient's name, balance due, date of charges, and date of most recent payment, as well as how long each part of the balance has been "waiting" on the A/R. It also may be helpful to insert a column at the end for action the office has taken in attempting to collect this debt. Procedure 20-6, at the end of the chapter, outlines this process.

▶ Laws That Govern Credit and Collections
LO 20.6

Federal and state laws govern debt collection. Table 20-1 outlines the penalties for violating laws that regulate credit and debt.

Fair Debt Collection Practices Act of 1977

This act governs the methods that can be used to collect unpaid debts. Its goal is to eliminate abusive, deceptive, or unfair debt collection practices, such as threatening to take action that is illegal or that is not actually planned. It is this law that states that if you threaten to turn an account over to a collection agency if a payment is not made by the 15th of the month, you must actually do so.

Following are guidelines for sending letters and making calls requesting payment from patients. For further information, visit http://www.ftc.gov/bcp/edu/pubs/consumer/credit/cre27.pdf.

- Do not call the patient before 8 a.m. or after 9 p.m. Calling outside those hours can be considered harassment.
- Do not make threats or use profane language. For example, do not state that an account will be given to a collection agency in 7 days if it will not be.
- Do not discuss the patient's debt with anyone except the person responsible for payment. If the patient is

TABLE 20-1	Laws That Govern Credit and Collection Procedures	
Law	Requirements	Penalties for Breaking the Law
Equal Credit Opportunity Act (ECOA) http://www.ftc.gov/bcp/edu/pubs/consumer/credit/cre15.shtm	• Creditors may not discriminate against applicants on the basis of sex, marital status, race, national origin, religion or age. • Creditors may not discriminate because an applicant receives public assistance income or has exercised rights under the Consumer Credit Protection Act.	• If an applicant sues the practice for violating the ECOA, the practice may have to pay damages (money paid as compensation), penalties, lawyers' fees, and court costs. • If an applicant joins a class action lawsuit against the practice, the practice may have to pay damages of up to $500,000 or 1% of the practice's net worth, whichever is less. (A class action lawsuit is a lawsuit in which one or more people sue a company that wronged all of them the same way.) • If the Federal Trade Commission (FTC) receives many complaints from applicants stating that the practice violated the ECOA, the FTC may investigate and take action against the practice.
Fair Credit Reporting Act (FCRA) https://www.ftc.gov/enforcement/statutes/fair-credit-reporting-act	• This act requires credit bureaus to supply correct and complete information to businesses to use in evaluating a person's application for credit, insurance, or a job.	• If one applicant sues the practice in federal court for violating the FCRA, the practice may have to pay damages, punitive damages (money paid as punishment for intentionally breaking the law), court costs, and lawyers' fees. • If the FTC receives many complaints from applicants stating that the practice violated the FCRA, the FTC may investigate and take action against the practice.
Fair Debt Collection Practices Act (FDCPA) http://www.ftc.gov/bcp/edu/pubs/consumer/credit/cre27.pdf	• This act requires debt collectors to treat debtors fairly. It also prohibits certain collection tactics such as harassment, false statements, threats, and unfair practices.	• If one debtor sues the practice in a state or federal court for violation of the FDCPA, the practice may have to pay damages, court costs, and lawyers' fees. • If the debtor joins a class action suit against the practice, the practice may have to pay damages of up to $500,000 or 1% of the practice's net worth, whichever is less. • If the FTC receives many complaints from debtors stating that the practice violated the FDCPA, the FTC may investigate and take action against the practice.
Truth in Lending Act (TLA) http://www.occ.treas.gov/handbook/til.pdf	• This act requires creditors to provide applicants with accurate and complete credit costs and terms, clearly and obviously.	• If one applicant sues the practice in a federal court for violation of the TLA, the practice may have to pay damages, court costs, and lawyers' fees. • If the FTC receives many complaints from applicants stating that the practice violated the TLA, the FTC may investigate and take action against the practice.

represented by a lawyer, discuss the problem only with the lawyer, unless the lawyer gives you permission to talk to the patient.

- Do not use any form of deception or violence to collect a debt. For example, do not pose as a government employee or other authority figure to try to force a debtor to pay.

Telephone Consumer Protection Act (TCPA) of 1991

This act protects telephone subscribers from unwanted telephone solicitations, commonly known as telemarketing. The act prohibits autodialed calls to emergency service providers, cellular and paging numbers, and patients' hospital rooms. It prohibits prerecorded calls to homes without prior permission of the resident and it prohibits unsolicited advertising via fax machine.

These regulations do not apply to people who have an established business relationship with the telemarketing firm or people who have previously given the telemarketing firm permission to call. The law also does not apply to telemarketing calls placed by tax-exempt nonprofit organizations, such as charities.

Although most provisions of this federal law do not apply to medical practices, you should be aware of the law. One way to avoid an unknowing violation of this law is to limit your calls to patients to the hours between 8 a.m. and 9 p.m. (some states, however, have exceptions for the TCPA provisions). Do not use an automated dialing device for calls to patients regarding their accounts; always place the calls yourself.

Observing Professional Guidelines for Finance Charges and Late Charges

According to the AMA, it is appropriate to assess finance charges or late charges on past-due accounts if the patient is notified in advance. Advance notice may be given by posting a sign at the reception desk, giving the patient a pamphlet describing the practice's billing practices, and/or including a note on the statement.

The practice must adhere to federal and state guidelines that govern these charges. The practice also should use compassion and discretion when assigning charges, especially in hardship cases. Because of the nature of medical care, many offices choose not to assess finance or late charges to patient accounts.

Using Outside Collection Agencies

If in-house collection efforts do not result in payment, the practice may wish to select a collection agency to manage the account. Because collection agencies keep a percentage of any funds they collect for their clients (usually between 40% and 60% of the collected amount), the office staff should use all reasonable methods to collect unpaid balances prior to sending an account to collection. Because of the humanitarian and ethical standards of the medical profession, practitioners must be careful to avoid collection agencies that use harsh or harassing collection techniques. Getting referrals for collection agencies from other medical offices will be helpful. The American Collectors Association International

(http://www.acainternational.org) may also be of assistance when choosing a collection agency.

Once an agency is chosen and accounts are deemed eligible for referral to the agency (after the appropriate notice has been given), the following information must be supplied to the agency regarding each account:

- Full name of patient and the last known address
- Occupation and business name and address
- Name of spouse, if any
- Total amount of the debt
- Date of the last activity (payment or charge) on the account
- Description of actions taken to collect the debt
- Response(s) received to collection attempts

Once an account has been turned over to the collection agency, all communication between the patient and the office concerning her debt must cease. All inquiries must be referred to the collection agency. If a payment is received after the account has been turned over, follow the procedure outlined in the agreement with the agency—some agencies allow the office to deposit the check and send the agency its percentage, and others ask you to return the check to the patient with the request that the patient call the agency.

When you receive a payment from the collection agency, it will list the total amount collected from the patient, the amount deducted for its fee, and the amount being forwarded to the office. When posting this payment, insert the amount received from the agency in the paid column. Use the adjustment column to insert the portion of the payment that was paid to the collection agency for its services. Subtract both amounts from the patient's balance to obtain the current balance. If the payment was considered payment in full, be sure to take the full balance on the account as an adjustment to bring the patient's balance to zero. Follow your office procedure regarding this account once the payment is made. Once a patient goes to collection, some offices also send a letter of discontinuation of services due to nonpayment, giving the patient 30 days to locate a new healthcare provider. Procedure 20-7, at the end of the chapter, outlines the steps in turning an account over to a collection agency and posting a payment from the agency for a collection account.

Because the debt is now the responsibility of the collection agency, it is important to note all accounts that have been turned over to the agency. For computerized accounts, a comment may be made to the account or the patient's name and account number may be color-coded, denoting collection proceedings have begun. For practices that use ledger cards, the color-coded tabs used for aging may also be used to denote collection proceedings (often black tabs are used for this purpose).

Finally, it should always be the decision of the practice (and not the collection agency) whether to pursue legal action regarding an account or to adjust the debt off the books. All collection agencies should make a monthly report to the office, documenting the activity on the accounts they are working with. Give the collection agency a set amount of time to collect the debt, such as 60–90 days. After that time, the practice should decide how to best deal with the account if the debt has not been paid.

As stated earlier, when an account is deemed "uncollectable" by the practitioner or the office manager, the balance may be written off to "relieve" the A/R of money that will not be received.

Insuring Accounts Receivable

To protect the practice from lost income because of nonpayment, the practice may buy accounts receivable insurance. Policies can pay when a large number of patients (or one large account or insurance plan) do not pay and the practice must absorb the lost income. Some policies also protect the practice in the event that its A/R records are destroyed and the individual records may no longer be available. It will not pay to re-create the records, but it will allow for recoupment of at least some of the outstanding A/R. Accounts receivable insurance can protect the practice cash flow and help ensure that the practice will have sufficient income to cover expected expenses.

▶ Credit Arrangements   LO 20.7

Sometimes a practitioner or practice agrees to extend credit to a patient who is unable to pay immediately. This situation is common when a patient's medical bills are high. By extending **credit,** the provider gives the patient time to pay for services, which are provided on trust. If the provider knows the patient well, she may offer credit without checking the patient's credit history. However, to avoid charges of discrimination under the Equal Credit Opportunity Act (ECOA), you will normally perform a credit check prior to extending credit.

Following Laws Governing Extension of Credit

When you help the physician decide whether to grant credit to a patient, you must comply with certain laws governing extension of credit.

Equal Credit Opportunity Act The Equal Credit Opportunity Act states that credit arrangements may not be denied based on a patient's sex, race, religion, national origin, marital status, or age. Credit also cannot be denied because the patient receives public assistance or has exercised rights under the Consumer Credit Protection Act, such as disputing a credit card bill or a credit bureau report. (Credit bureau reports are discussed in further detail a bit later.)

Under ECOA, the patient has a right to know the specific reason that credit was denied. Some reasons might include having too little income or not being employed for a certain period of time. Vague reasons about not meeting minimum standards or not receiving enough points on a credit-scoring system are not acceptable. In order to comply with ECOA, a credit check is required on any patient the practice is considering for extension of credit.

Performing a Credit Check To perform a credit check, be sure you have the patient's most current information, including the patient's address, telephone number, and Social Security number, as well as the name, address, and telephone number of the patient's employer. With this information you can verify employment and generate a credit bureau report.

Employment Verification Explain to the patient that you will be calling his employer to verify employment. Many employers have a designated person to handle such calls. The patient may be able to give you that name before you call the place of employment. After calling, record the updated information on the patient's registration card, along with any credit references obtained from the patient.

Credit Bureau Report A **credit bureau** is a company that provides information about the creditworthiness of someone seeking credit. If a patient's credit history is in question, you may request a report from a credit bureau, a sample of which is shown in Figure 20-11. A credit bureau collects information about an individual's payment history on credit cards, student loans, and similar accounts. The three leading national credit bureaus are TRW Inc., Equifax Inc., and Trans Union Credit Information Company. If the practice decides not to extend credit based on the credit report, the Fair Credit Reporting Act states that you must inform the patient in writing that credit was denied based on the credit report. You also must provide the name and address of the credit bureau, but you are not required to discuss the information obtained from the report. The patient may contest the credit report and have any inaccurate information corrected. Once the information has been corrected, the provider may then decide to extend credit to the patient.

Extending Credit If the practice decides to extend credit, two common arrangements are made: the unilateral agreement and the mutual (bilateral) agreement.

Unilateral Agreement If the patient offers to pay the debt over a period of months, and the provider agrees, the patient will be billed every month for the full amount owed and should make whatever payment is possible each month. This type of arrangement is considered a unilateral agreement and is not regulated by the Truth in Lending Act.

Mutual Agreement The second option is the mutual, or bilateral, agreement between practitioner (practice) and patient. They might agree that the patient will be billed for the full amount owed each month and will pay a minimum amount each month. If the practice does not assess finance charges, and if the total number of payments is four or fewer, this type of agreement is also not covered by the Truth in Lending Act. If the practice and patient make a bilateral agreement that includes more than four payments, or if the practice assesses finance charges, the agreement is subject to the requirements of the Truth in Lending Act.

Truth in Lending Act

The Truth in Lending Act comes under Regulation Z of the Consumer Credit Protection Act. This act covers credit agreements that involve more than four payments. It requires

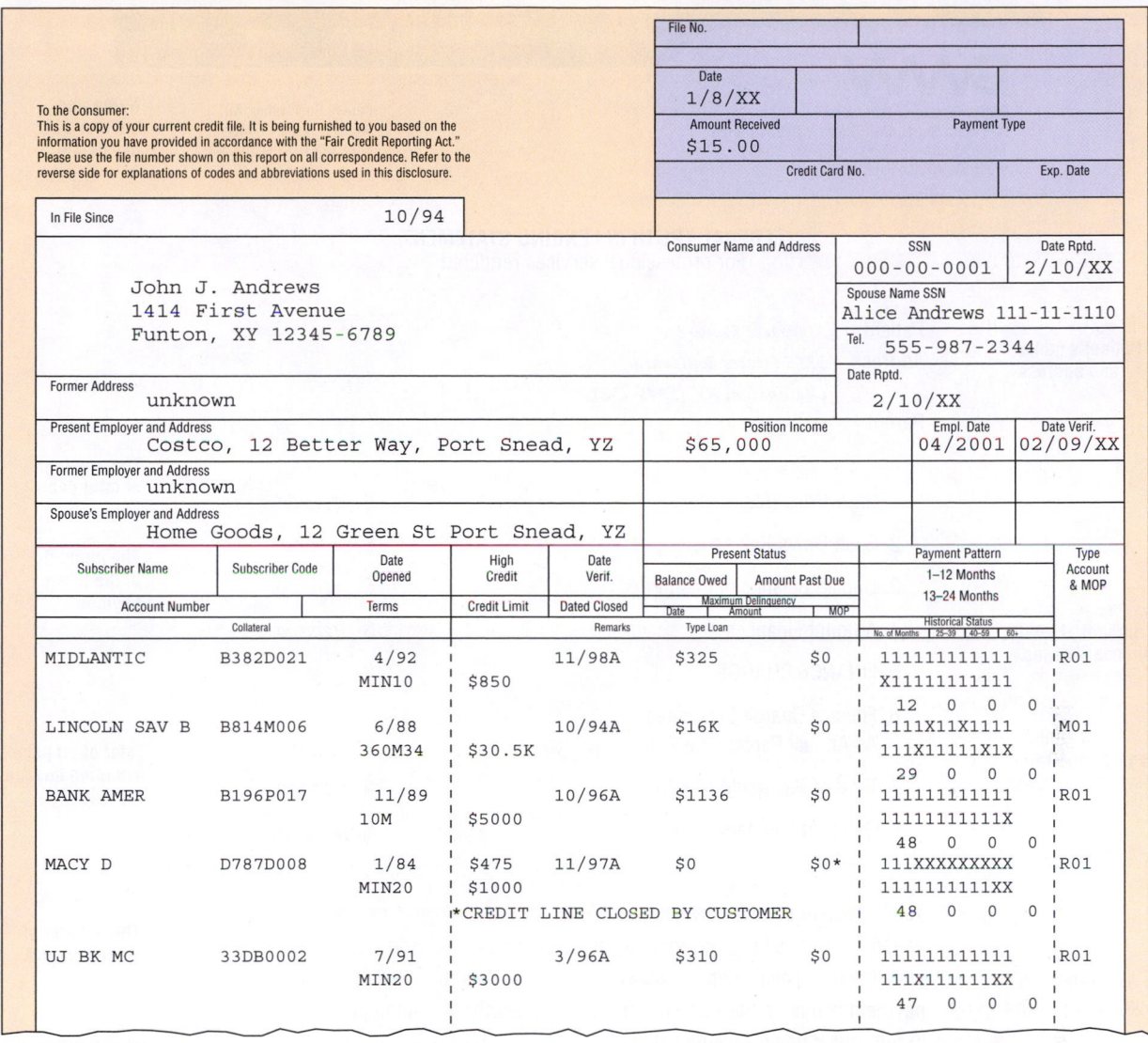

FIGURE 20-11 Credit reports can be used to help the practice decide whether to extend credit on a case-by-case basis.

the practice and patient to discuss, sign, and retain copies of a **disclosure statement** (frequently called a federal **Truth in Lending Statement**), which is a written description of the agreed terms of payment (Figure 20-12). According to the Truth in Lending Act, a disclosure statement must meet the following two requirements:

1. The agreement must be discussed with the patient when the terms are first determined. The practice and the patient must agree on the payment terms.

2. Both the practitioner (or his representative) and the patient must sign the document to indicate mutual agreement on the written terms.

Further, a disclosure statement must include the following six pieces of information:

1. The amount of total debt (the amount for which the patient is receiving credit)

2. The amount of the down payment

3. The amount of each payment (which may be weekly or monthly or for another period) and the date it is due (frequently the total number of payments to be made after the down payment is also included)

4. The due date for the final payment and the amount of the final payment if different from the other payment amounts

5. The interest rate, if interest is to be paid, expressed as an annual percentage

6. The total finance charges, if any (if interest is charged, the total amount of interest accrued during the course of the debt will be entered here)

The practice and the patient should each keep a copy of the signed disclosure agreement. Procedure 20-8, at the end of the chapter, outlines the steps in creating and completing a Truth in Lending Statement (Agreement). Under the Truth in Lending Act, the patient is billed only for the monthly amount agreed upon, not the total amount of the debt. To avoid mailing a monthly statement, some offices create

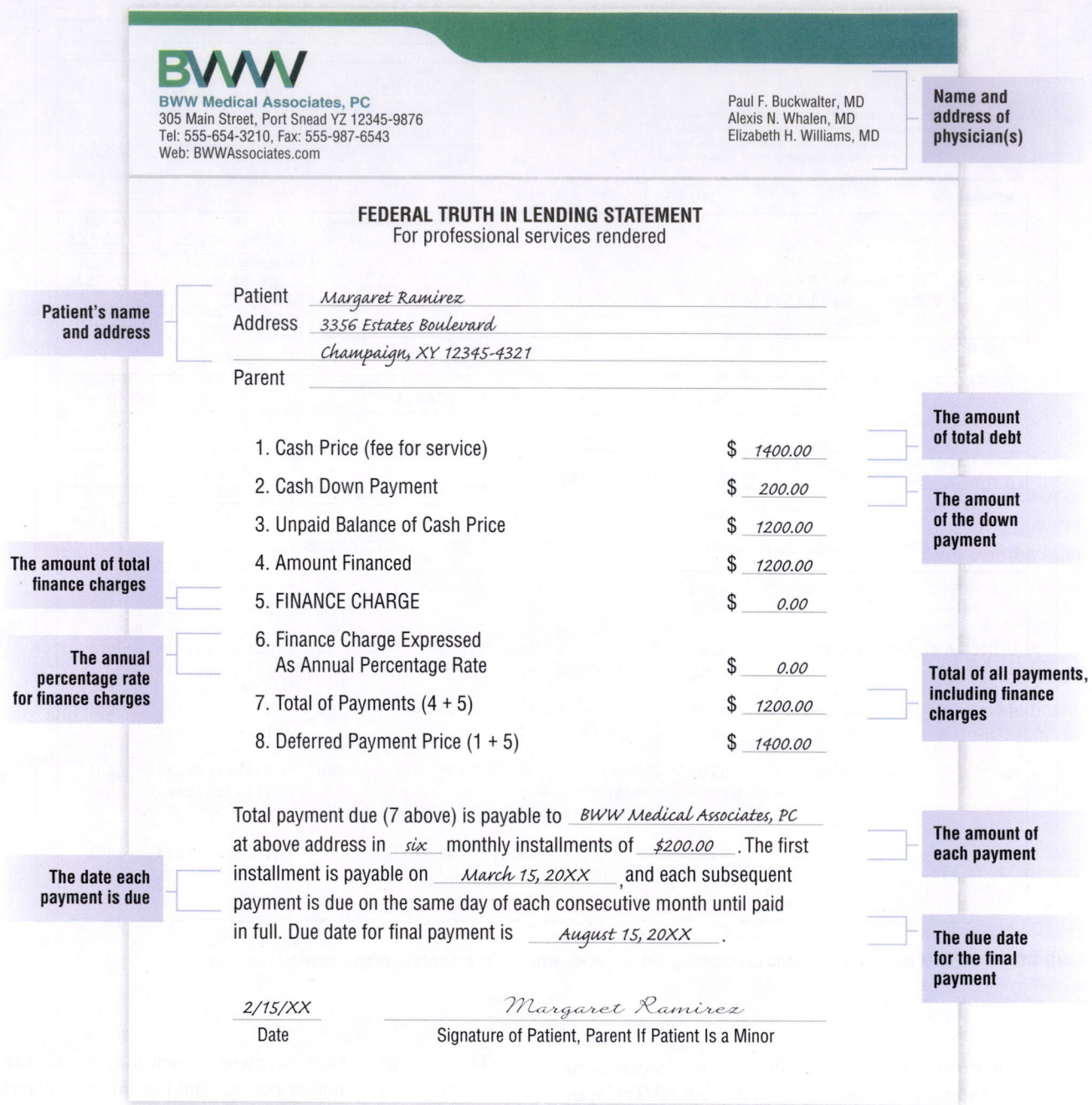

FIGURE 20-12 Typical Truth in Lending Statement completed and signed by the patient.

a master document, given to the patient at the time of the agreement signing, that outlines each month's due date and the amount due, with a running total of the new balance once the payment is made. Figure 20-13 is an example of such a document.

▶ Common Collection Problems   LO 20.8

Collection problems come in many forms, but there are two common collection problems encountered by medical practices. The first is patients who cannot pay—also called hardship cases—and the second is patients who have moved

without leaving a forwarding address and therefore have not received a statement.

Hardship Cases

A practitioner may decide to treat some patients without charge—or at a deep discount—simply because they cannot pay. These patients may be poor, uninsured, underinsured, or elderly and on a limited income. They may be patients who have suffered a severe financial loss or family tragedy. Medical ethics require practitioners to provide care to individuals who need it, regardless of their ability to pay. Nevertheless, free treatment for hardship cases is at the practitioner's discretion.

BWW

BWW Medical Associates, PC
305 Main Street, Port Snead YZ 12345-9876
Tel: 555-654-3210, Fax: 555-987-6543
Web: BWWAssociates.com

Paul F. Buckwalter, MD
Alexis N. Whalen, MD
Elizabeth H. Williams, MD

February 15, 20XX

Margaret Ramirez
3356 Estates Boulevard
Champaign, XY 12345-4321

RE: Monthly Payment Agreement

Dear Ms. Ramirez:

As outlined in the Truth and Lending Statement signed in our office today, for your convenience we have outlined below your monthly payment schedule.

Amount Financed: $1200.00

Monthly Payments: $200.00

Date of Payment	Current Balance
3/15/20XX	$1000.00
4/15/20XX	$ 800.00
5/15/20XX	$ 600.00
6/15/20XX	$ 400.00
7/15/20XX	$ 200.00
8/15/20XX	$ 0.00

If for any reason, you cannot make the agreed-upon monthly payment as outlined above, please call me immediately so a new arrangement may be made.

As always, we thank you for choosing BWW Medical Associates, PC for your healthcare needs.

Sincerely,

Malik Katahari, cmm

Malik Katahari, CMM
Office Manager

MK/map

FIGURE 20-13 Patient letter outlining the Truth in Lending Statement, including the payment dates and the amount of each payment.

Providing free care must be undertaken very carefully because, under the ECOA, if a patient is given free or reduced-fee treatment based on her inability to pay and another patient under similar circumstances is treated, she also must be extended the same financial consideration or a charge of discrimination may be levied against the provider. Some providers treat such patients for urgent problems and then refer the patients to federally funded clinics that are allowed to provide free or reduced-fee services related to their government funding.

Patient Relocation and Address Change

Sometimes a patient account remains unpaid because the patient has moved without leaving a forwarding address and has not received the statement. These patients are known as **skips.** Obviously, reaching such a patient about payment issues will provide a challenge.

Remember, you cannot discuss a debt with anyone except the person responsible for the charges. When you make a telephone call for collection, however, you may ask a third party for the patient's new address or phone number if known.

If the third party states the new address is not known, do not call again unless there is reason to believe that the third party has learned of the person's address or phone number since the first inquiry. If the patient had given permission to e-mail him, you may also try that avenue. Ask the post office for a forwarding address. If these avenues do not locate the patient, he may be labeled a skip and then referred to the office collection agency. Be sure to keep the returned statement and envelope stamped by the post office as "addressee unknown" or "no forwarding address" to prove a reasonable attempt to collect the debt.

Banking and Negotiable Instruments

LO 20.9

In addition to the financial practices outlined earlier in the chapter, your administrative responsibilities also may include handling the practice's banking. Because a practice may use traditional (manual) or electronic (computerized) banking methods, you should be familiar with both. Regardless of which method you use, remember to keep all banking materials secure because they represent the finances of the practice. For example, to prevent theft of checks, always put the checkbook in a securely locked place when it is not in use. Also, file deposit receipts promptly. If they are lost, you have no proof that a deposit was made. Lack of proof could cost the practice thousands of dollars. Because you will be responsible for office funds, it is important that protocols be in place and consistently followed. Be sure you are clear regarding the procedure to be followed and to whom within the practice you should report suspected lost or stolen funds.

Banking Tasks

Common banking tasks in the medical office practice include the following:

- Writing checks
- Accepting checks
- Endorsing checks
- Making deposits
- Reconciling bank statements
  - Recordkeeping of bank accounts
  - Balancing of individual accounts

Because many manual banking procedures revolve around the writing and receipt of checks, you must first have a thorough understanding of the terminology surrounding this common "piece of paper."

Checks

A **check** is a bank draft or order for payment (Figure 20-14). The person who writes the check is called the **payer.** By writing a check, the payer directs the bank to pay a sum of money

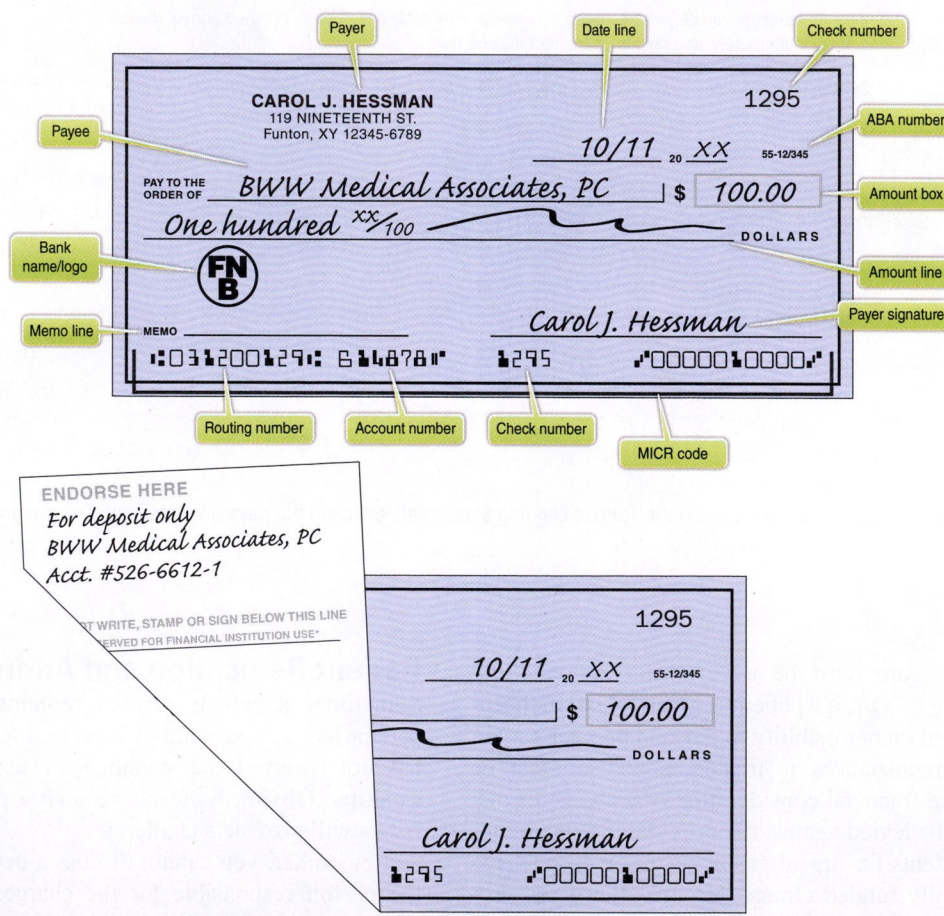

FIGURE 20-14 Parts of a check, with an example of a restrictive endorsement.

on demand to the payee. In order to be considered **negotiable** (legally transferable from one person to another), a check must

- Be written and signed by the payer or maker.
- Include the amount of money to be paid, considered a promise to pay a specified sum.
- Be made payable to the payee (the person named on the check) or bearer.
- Be made payable on demand or on a specific date.
- Include the name of the bank that is directed to make payment.

Types of Checks and Other Negotiable Papers

In addition to personal checks from patients and business checks from insurance companies and other offices, you may also receive or even use the following types of checks in the medical office.

- **Cashier's check**—a check issued from the bank's account and signed by a bank representative. It is usually purchased by individuals who do not have checking accounts or for use in purchases where large sums are required, such as a down payment for a car or house, when the payee wants a guarantee that the check will not be returned for insufficient funds.
- **Certified check**—a personal or business check that is written and signed by the payer, taken to the bank the check will be drawn on, and stamped "CERTIFIED" by the bank. This stamp means the bank has already drawn the money from the payer's account and set it aside to guarantee that the check will be paid when submitted. Many banks no longer use certified checks, having replaced them with cashier's checks.
- **Voucher check**—a business (or personal) check with a perforated stub attached for recordkeeping. Instead of using a checkbook register, before the check is written out, the stub is completed with all of the payee information for the user's records. Voucher checks come in various styles and often in a three-ring binder format.
- **Limited check**—a check that is valid for redemption during a specific time frame, often only 30–90 days and usually used for payroll. Some accounts limit the amount of checks written as well as the valid time frames.
- **Counter check**—a bank-issued check that allows the depositor to withdraw funds from his account only. It states "PAY TO THE ORDER OF MYSELF ONLY." This may be used when the provider wants to draw off of the account in the absence of his or her checkbook; a counter check is similar to a withdrawal slip.
- **Traveler's check**—a check preprinted in established denominations of $10, $20, $50, and $100. These checks must be signed at the location where they were purchased. When using a traveler's check, it must be signed in the presence of the payee, and the signatures must match in order for the traveler's check to be valid for redemption.
- **Money order**—another kind of guaranteed payment. Money orders are purchased in banks or from other vendors for a small fee, using cash. They are often used by people without checking accounts who wish to have a receipt of payment for their records.

Check Codes

The face (front) of every check contains two important items: the American Banking Association (ABA) number and the magnetic ink character recognition (MICR) code (Figure 20-14). The **ABA number** appears as a fraction, such as 60-117/310, on the upper edge of all printed checks. It identifies the geographic area and specific bank on which the check is drawn.

Found at the bottom of a check, the MICR code consists of numbers and characters printed in magnetic ink, which can be read by MICR equipment at the bank. This code, which includes the bank's routing number, the customer's account number, the check number, and an area for bank use, enables checks to be read, sorted, and recorded by computer.

Parts of a Check

The checks you encounter both personally and in your office contain many important features that should be inspected upon receipt to ensure prompt payment. Refer back to Figure 20-14 to familiarize yourself with the location of each item.

- *Payer*—account holder's legal name, usually preprinted with address and possibly other information like phone numbers and e-mail addresses
- *Date line*—date that is written in by the payer, stating that the funds are available as of this date
- *Check number*—indicates the number in a series
- *ABA number*—preprinted numbers appearing as a fraction, such as 55-12/345, identifying the geographic area and specific bank on which the check is drawn
- *Payee*—the name written on the "pay to the order of" line to whom the payer wishes the funds to be paid
- *Amount box*—box in which the check's numeric amount should be entered
- *Amount line*—line where the check's dollar amount is written out in words and the cents are usually put into a fraction over 100, followed by a line, to reduce the ability for someone to write in information. If there is a discrepancy between the amount box and the amount line, the amount line is the amount used when paying out the funds.
- *Bank information*—information that identifies the processing facility or the city and state of the account holder's branch bank that the funds are coming from; it may list the logo, address, e-mail, or any other special branch information
- *Memo line*—line that can be left blank but should be filled in to ensure that the payment is credited to the correct account. This can be done by entering any account information, which is extremely helpful when the payer is someone other than the patient, such as the spouse or parent.
- *Payer signature line*—line where the payer MUST sign the check in order for the funds to be legally drawn
- *Routing number*—9-digit portion of the MICR code that routes the check back to the issuing bank and should match the bank name and ABA fraction code number

- *Account number*—part of the MICR code that indicates the payer's account within the bank
- *Check number*—part of the MICR code that identifies and refers back to the check number at the top right of the check
- *MICR recording area*—space for bank use only to record the branch and amount of the check

Accepting Checks Before accepting any check, review it carefully. First, be sure the check has the correct date, amount, and signature and that no corrections have been made. Refer to Figure 20-14, which shows a correctly written and endorsed check. Do not accept a **third-party check** (one made out to the patient rather than to the practice) unless it is from a health insurance company. Also, do not accept a check marked "Payment in Full" unless it actually does pay the complete outstanding balance. You may accept a check signed by someone other than the payer if the person who signed the check has power of attorney. **Power of attorney** gives a person the legal right to handle financial matters for another person who is unable to do so. Frequently, power of attorney is granted to a patient's spouse, son, or daughter.

Be sure to follow your practice's policy when accepting a check. For example, if a patient is new or unfamiliar, office policy may require you to request patient identification and to compare the signature on the identification with the signature on the check. Many offices will not accept post-dated checks because they are then responsible for holding the check until the date the bank will accept the check. Policy also may require that you not accept a check for more than the amount due because cash will be due back to the patient and then if the check is returned for insufficient funds, the office will be out not only the amount of the check but also the amount of the cash given to the patient.

Checking Account Types

It is not uncommon for a practitioner to have at least three different types of checking accounts: a personal account, a business account for office expenses, and an interest-earning account. The interest-earning account will be used for paying special expenses, like property taxes and insurance premiums. As a medical assistant, most of your banking tasks will involve the business checking account. You may sometimes, however, make payments from, or transfer money to and from, the interest-earning account, as directed.

▶ Preparing a Bank Deposit LO 20.10

Endorsing Checks

Once a check has been presented for payment and received by the office, it should be inspected and then immediately endorsed, or accepted for payment. There are four principal types of **endorsement:**

- Blank endorsement. A blank endorsement consists simply of the payee's signature. Once this endorsement is made, anyone who has possession of the check may cash it, so it should only be signed when the check is being cashed or deposited immediately, not prior to arriving at the bank.
- Restrictive endorsement. A restrictive endorsement specifies how the check may be redeemed. In the case of the medical office, the endorsement is often made by a stamp and "restricts" redemption of the check to depositing it in the office checking account. Refer back to Figure 20-14 for an example of this type of endorsement.
- Special endorsement. A special endorsement may also be called a third-party endorsement, as the payee of the check signs it over to another person. For example, if an insurance check is sent to Nancy Evans, our case study patient, instead of the office, she could sign it over to the office like this:

    Pay to the order of BWW Medical Associates, PC
    Nancy Evans

    By endorsing the check in this manner, Nancy ensures that only BWW Medical Associates can redeem this check.
- Qualified endorsement. Attorneys, who may accept a check on behalf of their client but have no personal claim on the transaction, most often use qualified endorsements. In this case, the attorney might endorse the check "without recourse," which disclaims any future liability regarding this transaction.

If, after reading about the types of endorsements, you think the best type of endorsement is a restrictive endorsement, you would be correct. A restrictive endorsement prevents the check from being cashed if it is lost or stolen because the only way the check can be redeemed is by deposit into the specified account; if you do not use a restrictive endorsement for your personal checking account, do you think you might consider doing so now?

No matter what type of endorsement is chosen, always be sure to make all endorsements in ink, using a pen or rubber stamp. Place the endorsement in the 1.5-inch area indicated on the back of the check. Most personal and business checks have a number of lines or a shaded area preprinted on the checks for this purpose. (Refer to Figure 20-14.) Leave the rest of the back of the check blank for the bank's use.

Completing the Deposit Slip

After endorsing the check, post the payment to the patient ledger card and to the daily log or day sheet. Then put the check with others to be deposited. Even if your office does not make daily deposits, it is a good idea to have a deposit slip started at the beginning of the day, adding each check to the deposit slip by hand or electronically as you receive it, as shown in Figure 20-15. In this way, you will have a running list of checks (and cash) to be deposited and can compare this to the day sheet at any time to verify the amount of the payments received by the office. The account number is printed on deposit slips in MICR numbers that match those on the checks. As mentioned, these numbers enable checks and deposit slips to be read, sorted, and recorded by computer.

Banks will accept a list of deposited items on something other than the bank-provided deposit slip if the bank's deposit slip is attached. For example, if you are depositing 50 checks,

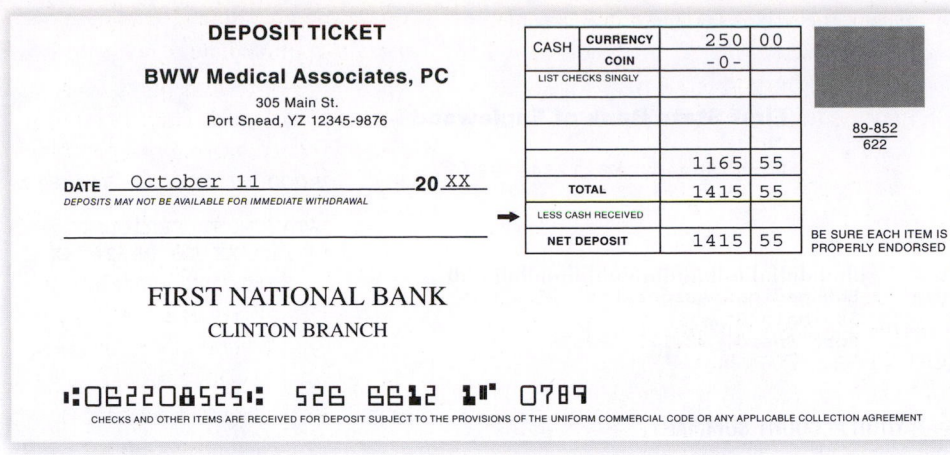

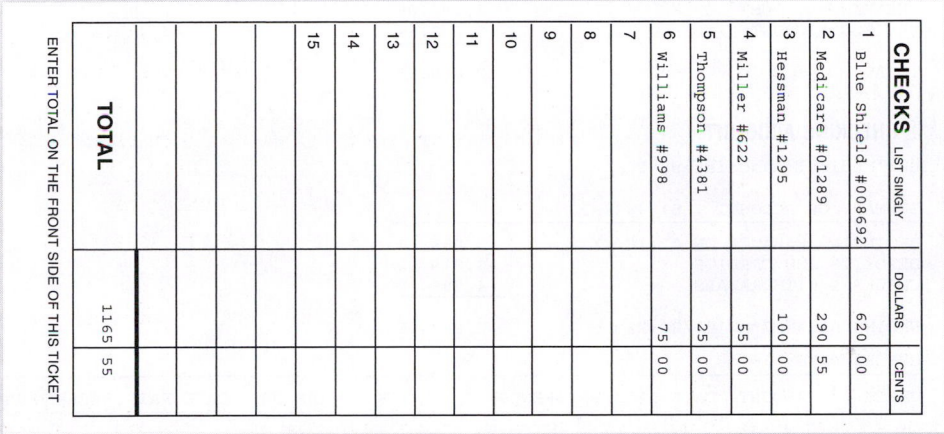

FIGURE 20-15 A correctly completed deposit slip.

you may create a computer printout listing the payers' names, check numbers, amount of each check, and total. You can then attach the printout to a deposit slip with the total written on the deposit slip. Another method is to attach a calculator or adding machine tape listing the individual check amounts and including the total amount.

Making the Deposit

Plan to deposit checks and cash into the practice's bank account in person at the bank, as described in Procedure 20-9 at the end of this chapter. Make sure you are aware of your surroundings when making deposits because of safety issues. Always obtain a deposit receipt from the bank.

Again, depending on practice size, the frequency of deposits may be limited to several days a week; however, it should be done as often as possible to reduce theft, loss, bounced checks, and inaccurate recordings.

Electronic Deposits

With the advent of electronic claims submission, many payers and offices prefer to receive their insurance payments electronically as well. Electronic funds transfers, or EFTs, may be set up between the office and many insurance carriers, greatly decreasing the amount of time it takes to receive payment from the insurance carriers via US mail. Even smaller offices

that still submit paper claims to insurance carriers may be able to receive their insurance payments electronically. The office will receive notification from the insurance carrier of any payment (deposit) sent to the office checking account along with the explanation of benefit (EOB), also known as the remittance advice (RA), explaining which patient accounts the payment pertains to. You can learn more about remittance advices, both electronic and paper, in the *Insurance and Billing* chapter.

▶ Reconciling the Bank Statement LO 20.11

Another important administrative task that often is part of the medical assistant's role is the banking task of reconciling the bank statement. **Reconciliation** involves comparing the office financial records, the checkbook or disbursements journal, with the bank records (statement) to ensure that they are consistent with each other and accurate. In most practices, this task is performed once a month when the practice receives the monthly checking account statement from the bank, either in the mail or electronically if the office utilizes the bank's electronic banking services. Figure 20-16 shows an example of a typical bank statement.

When reconciling the checkbook with the bank statement, keep in mind one thought: "the bank needs to 'know' everything I know regarding what I have paid and deposited and I,

```
First State Bank of Englewood
CN 1                                           PAGE 1
Port Snead, YZ 12345-9876
                                   ACCOUNT NO.    518-833-3

                                   STATEMENT PERIOD
                                   07/19/XX TO 08/20/XX


    |||..|.|.|.||.|.|.|.||.....||.|.|.|.|.|.||.....||.|...||.||
    BWW Medical Associates, PC
    305 Main St.
    Port Snead, YZ 12345-9876
```

YOUR ACCOUNT SUMMARY

DEPOSIT ACCOUNTS	BALANCE
CHECKING ACCOUNT	2,088.08
SAVINGS ACCOUNT	10,602.54
TOTAL	12,690.62

CHECKING ACCOUNT

BWW Medical Associates, PC

SUMMARY OF ACCOUNT   518-833-3

BEGINNING BALANCE ON 07/18/XX	3,055.24
DEPOSITS AND CREDITS	+3,819.02
CHECKS & WITHDRAWALS	−4,786.18
ENDING BALANCE ON 08/20/XX	2,088.08

CHECKS PAID: 38

CHECK	AMOUNT	DATE PAID	REFERENCE#	CHECK	AMOUNT	DATE PAID	REFERENCE#
CHECK	450.00	07/19/12	81569110	2226	181.00	08/12/12	05105878
2202	146.23	07/31/12	29521570	2227	24.74	08/19/12	06120827
2203	122.03	07/29/12	29141271	2228	140.00	08/12/12	05022086
2210*	43.00	07/29/12	07046380	2229	148.71	08/16/12	27248941
2211	60.09	08/01/12	04597911	2230	53.16	08/13/12	27852752
2214*	123.59	07/24/12	29470425	2231	50.00	08/14/12	01018325
2215	47.70	07/19/12	12357289	2232	50.00	08/13/12	05080148
2216	9.00	07/22/12	05479786	2233	15.00	08/16/12	04709533
2217	30.00	07/26/12	29841864	2234	13.95	08/19/12	06008593
2218	19.00	07/30/12	04330539	2235	123.59	08/14/12	27050650
2219	12.00	07/24/12	04037820	2236	50.00	08/13/12	05099115
2220	35.93	07/24/12	04068844	2237	50.00	08/15/12	03014667
2221	10.00	08/12/12	05091269	2238	20.00	08/16/12	04675854
2222	23.48	07/24/12	29465653	2239	47.70	08/14/12	06172997
2223	242.43	07/26/12	29804419	2240	24.74	08/19/12	06120925
2224	150.00	07/30/12	29405827	2243*	400.00	08/14/12	29652307
2225	830.00	08/07/12	02242873	2344	400.00	08/14/12	29652306

FIGURE 20-16 A typical bank statement used to reconcile the office checking account.

in comparing the bank statement to the checking account, need to be sure that I have recorded everything that the bank knows." Let's look at a simple scenario:

When the bank statement comes in, you immediately block out some quiet time to take care of the reconciliation. In comparing the deposits and payments recorded by the bank as completed, you note a $2,000 deposit made 2 days ago, which is not yet recorded, and three checks you sent out totaling $800, which also have not yet been redeemed. These items are not yet "known" by the bank. You also notice that the automatic payment of $500 for quarterly payroll taxes has not been recorded in the checkbook. The bank statement shows a balance of $10,900. The office checkbook shows a balance of $12,600.

Bank Statement		Checkbook	
Balance	10,900.00		12,600.00
(deposit)	+ 2,000.00	(autopay)	−500.00
	12,900.00		12,100.00 √
(outstanding checks)	− 800.00		
	12,100.00 √		

Once the deposit that has not cleared is added to the bank statement balance and the outstanding checks are subtracted, the new balance is $12,100. At the same time, when the auto-payment is subtracted from the checkbook balance, its balance is also $12,100. You have successfully reconciled the

BANK RECONCILIATION

CLIENT NAME: _____

MONTH OF: _____

BANK: _____ ACCOUNT NO. : _____

GENERAL LEDGER

ACCOUNT BALANCE........................

ADD DEBITS:

_____

_____

_____

_____

TOTAL DB.............

TOTAL........................

LESS CREDITS:

Checks

Auto Withdrawals

Bank Fees

_____

_____

TOTAL CR.............

BANK BALANCE PER GENERAL LEDGER..

BALANCE PER BANK STATEMENT

AS OF:

ADD DEPOSITS IN TRANSIT:

_____

_____

_____

TOTAL IN TRANSIT........................

TOTAL........................

LESS CHECKS OUTSTANDING:

(SEE LIST BELOW)

TOTAL.................

BANK BALANCE PER RECONCILIATION.................

CHECKS:

NUMBER	AMOUNT	NUMBER	NUMBER	NUMBER	AMOUNT
					TOTAL
TOTAL		TOTAL		GRAND TOTAL	

FIGURE 20-17 A typical reconciliation worksheet to aid in reconciling the checkbook to the bank statement.

bank statement. Figure 20-17 shows you an example of a reconciliation worksheet. The complete reconciliation process is explained in Procedure 20-10 at the end of the chapter.

▶ Electronic Banking   LO 20.12

Compared with traditional banking methods, electronic banking has several advantages. Electronic banking can improve productivity, cash flow, and accuracy. The use of electronic banking can also speed up many banking tasks. If your medical office uses electronic banking, your basic tasks will be the same as in an office that uses traditional banking methods. How these tasks are performed, however, may be quite different. When you use electronic banking, you are still responsible

for recording and depositing checks, just as if you were using traditional methods, but you will see these differences:

- Rather than your recording each check in a paper checkbook and determining the new balance, the computer software calculates the new balance for you.
- Rather than your reconciling the office bank statement on paper, the computer software does it automatically.
- Rather than putting the checkbook and banking forms in a securely locked place at the end of the day, you use a computer password for security.

Many medical office software programs are available today and each one has a different interface, uses different menus, and prompts you for information in different ways. However, certain general concepts apply to all. All software will allow you to record deposits, pay bills, display the checkbook (and account balances), and reconcile the bank statement. For specific information, consult the user's manual that comes with the program used by your practice. Before electing to sign up for electronic banking, check with the current bank used by the office to see what safeguards and protections it offers regarding the information the office is transferring electronically. Electronic banking can speed up processes for the office, but it is extremely important that the office remain in control of how that information is protected and who has access to the information. If the bank currently used by the office does not use appropriate safeguards for electronic banking procedures, the office may want to consider changing financial institutions.

Record Deposits

If you select "Record Deposits," a message on the computer screen prompts you to enter information about each check to be deposited that day. This information usually includes the check writer's name and the amount of the check. The check's ABA number also may be requested. After you enter this information, the computer gives you a chance to double-check it. If all the information is correct, you continue entering and checking the other checks, one at a time. You can then select a command to print a deposit slip that contains the information you have just entered. To make the deposit, place the cash and checks in a deposit bag along with the computerized deposit slip and the bank's deposit slip.

Pay Bills

The bill pay function allows you to log checks that you write into a computerized checkbook register. For each check you want to write, a message should prompt you for information, such as the payee and the amount of the check. The computer also should give you a chance to verify and correct this information before moving on to the next check or printing the checks. More and more programs, depending upon the bank the office uses, also allow for electronic bill pay. Recording these payments in the electronic (or paper) checkbook register is the same as when writing a check, except instead of recording the check number, you will record the transaction number assigned by the bank as proof the payment has been sent.

Some software programs automatically assign the next available check number to each new check you enter. To double-check that the computer-assigned check numbers match those on the actual checks, print a list of the checks you have entered and compare it with the checks before mailing them.

Display the Checkbook

The checkbook display function allows you to review the electronic checkbook register. Although you cannot change information that appears in the register—unless your software and your bank allow total electronic banking—you can print it out so you can be sure the checks have been recorded properly and you can check your latest balance.

If you select "Display Checkbook" from the "Banking" menu, the computer displays a list of all checks that have been entered into the register. Information includes check number, date, payee, and amount. Scrolling up and down reveals all the checks in the register. This area also will reveal any auto withdrawals or auto deposits that have been made up until the current date (one of the advantages of electronic banking), and the balance and current statement may be checked at any time, not just once a month when the bank statement arrives.

Balance Checkbook

The "Balance Checkbook" option electronically reconciles the monthly bank statement. After you enter the appropriate date or dates, the computer screen displays all the checks and deposits that were logged into the register in the order they were posted.

The next screen highlights each check or deposit that has not been seen on a previous bank statement. You are prompted to indicate whether that item appears on the current statement, usually using Y for yes and N for no. After the computer queries these items, it may ask you to enter any items that appear on the current bank statement but are not in the checkbook, such as service charges.

Finally, a message on the screen prompts you to enter the current account balance from the bank statement. Then, the computer reconciles the bank statement. It will alert you if the system balance does not agree with the balance on the bank statement. If the balance does not agree, recheck the information you entered for possible errors. If you have rechecked your work and a coworker has also acted as a "second set of eyes" and has verified no errors or omissions, yet the balances still do not agree, call the bank to determine if a bank error has been made.

▶ Accounts Payable and Managing Disbursements   LO 20.13

Accounts payable (A/P) are the practice expenses, and accounts receivable reflect the practice income. This section focuses on accounts payable and the process of making those payments, known as disbursements. A basic accounting principle to bear in mind is that when a practice's income exceeds its expenses, it has a profit, commonly called "being in the black." If a practice's expenses exceed its income, it has a loss, known as "being in the red."

Because of this relationship between income and expenses, most practices try to reduce expenses by controlling accounts payable. As the office medical assistant, you play an important role in helping control accounts payable in order to maximize profits.

Accounts payable fall into three main groups:

- Payments for supplies, equipment, and practice-related products and services
- Payroll, which may be the largest of the accounts payable
- Taxes owed to federal, state, and local governments and agencies

A practice's accounting system usually consists of several elements. These elements include the daily log, patient ledger cards, the checkbook, the disbursements journal, the petty cash record, and the payroll register. In this chapter, you are focusing on the first four elements. You will explore the petty cash record and payroll register in the *Practice Management* chapter.

As discussed earlier in this chapter, the daily log and patient ledger cards are used primarily for accounts receivable. The disbursements journal (as well as the petty cash record and payroll register) is used primarily in accounts payable.

Disbursements

A disbursement is any payment the practice makes for goods or services. One of the most common disbursements is payment for office supplies. Other disbursements include payments for equipment, dues, rent, taxes, salary, and utilities. No matter what type of disbursement you make on behalf of the practice, you must keep accurate records of the purchase and the payment.

Recording Disbursements You may record disbursements in a check register, in a disbursements journal, or on the bottom section of the daily log. If you use a disbursements journal, follow these steps to record disbursements:

1. When beginning a new journal page, give each column a heading to reflect the type of expense, such as utilities or rent. Procedure 20-11, at the end of this chapter, outlines how to set up a disbursements journal.

2. For each check, fill in the date, payee's name, check number, and check amount in the appropriate columns.

3. Determine the expense category of the check.

4. Record the check amount in the column for that type of business expense.

5. If you must divide a check between two or more expense columns, record the total in the check amount column. Then record the amount that applies to each type of expense in the appropriate column. The total amount listed in the check amount column must equal the sum of the amounts listed in the expense columns.

Writing Checks

Virtually all disbursements are made by check, although electronic payments are becoming more and more common. Paying by check gives the practice complete, accurate records of all financial transactions. If your office uses electronic banking, including bill pay, the transaction number given by the bank, at the time the bill is paid, should be recorded in place of the check number in the disbursements journal and checkbook for future reference.

Before writing a check, make sure the checking account balance is up-to-date and large enough to cover the check you want to write. Enter the date, check number, payee information, and reason for the payment on the check stub and then subtract the amount of each check from the previous balance,

enter the new balance, and carry that balance forward to the next stub. Do this step before writing the check so that the payment entry is not accidentally omitted from the disbursements journal. The same information holds true when electronic banking is utilized. Be sure to record the payment in the disbursements journal or online checkbook prior to sending the payment.

If you use a pegboard system for your checkbook/disbursements journal, you will automatically record the date, check number, payee, and check amount on the check register as you write out the check because of the carbonless paper that is on the back of the check itself. You must note the reason for payment and the new balance manually, however. Record that information in the appropriate spaces on the register.

If you make an error when completing a check, write VOID in ink across the front of the check in large letters so that it cannot be used again. Then file the voided check in numeric order with the returned checks.

After filling out the check properly, detach it from the checkbook and give it to the doctor to sign, along with the invoice to be paid. Mark the date, check number, and amount paid on the invoice. Make a copy of the invoice for your records. Keep these copies with supporting documents, like order forms or packing slips, in a paid-invoice file. Then, mail the check and the original invoice to the payee in a neatly hand-addressed or typewritten envelope. If you use a window envelope, be sure the payee's address shows through the window.

Recording disbursements in columns for each type of expense allows you to total and track expenses by category. **Tracking** (watching for changes) is important because it helps control expenses. Before tracking, check your calculations by performing a trial balance:

1. Total the check amount column.

2. Calculate the total for each expense column.

3. Add together all the expense column totals. The combined expense column total should match the total in the check amount column.

4. If the amounts do not match, recheck every entry until you find the error. When you find it, draw a line through it and record the correct information neatly above it or to the side.

5. When the two amounts match (or balance), carry forward all column totals to the disbursements journal for the next month. Remember to prepare summaries and perform balances at the end of every month, quarter, and year.

If your office uses an office management software package, trial balances and financial summaries are created with a few keystrokes. Remember, however, computer programs are only as good as the information entered into the programs. If you make a keystroke error when entering information, the trial balance and/or financial summary will contain errors. Always enter financial information—whether you write it by hand or key it into a computer program—with great care.

Understanding Financial Summaries

The practitioner or practice manager may periodically analyze the practice's income and expenses. Financial summaries provide an easy-to-read report on the business transactions for a given period, such as a month, quarter, or a year.

In the past, it was necessary to have an accountant to prepare financial summaries. But with more offices utilizing practice management software, creating these reports using the software package or templates is a relatively simple process once the procedure is understood. A medical assistant with a basic understanding of the information contained within financial summaries will be an asset in helping the practice to remain financially stable. Following are some of the records found in most financial statements.

Statement of Income and Expense Also called a profit-and-loss statement, a statement of income and expense highlights the practice's profitability. It shows the physician the practice's total income and then lists and subtracts all expenses.

Cash Flow Statement A **cash flow statement** shows how much cash is available to cover expenses, to invest, or to take as profit. The cash flow statement begins with the cash on hand at the beginning of the period and shows the income and disbursements made during that period. It concludes with the new amount of cash on hand at the end of the period.

Trial Balance The practitioner or practice manager may review trial balances periodically to ensure that the books balance. As described earlier in this chapter, the combined expense column total should match the total in the check amount column. If the amounts do not match, recheck every entry until you find the error and the column amounts balance.

Although not considered by many to be as "glamorous" as patient care, the medical assistant who focuses and excels in the administrative procedures for the practice—particularly its financial practices—and takes an interest in controlling expenses while maintaining quality care for patients will be an outstanding asset to any practice in the "business of medicine."

PROCEDURE 20-1 Posting Charges, Payments, and Adjustments

WORK // DOC

Procedure Goal: To post charges, payments, and adjustments to the patient account

OSHA Guidelines: This procedure does not involve exposure to blood, body fluids, or tissue.

Materials: Daily log sheets, patient ledger cards, and check register or computerized bookkeeping system; summaries of charges, receipts, and disbursements

Method:

1. Create a ledger card (patient account) for each new patient and maintain a ledger card for each existing patient. Include the following information on each ledger card:
   a. Patient name
   b. Patient address
   c. Patient home and work phone numbers
   d. Insurance carrier with policy number and guarantor information

2. Update the ledger card every time the patient incurs a charge or makes a payment. Be sure to adjust the account balance after every transaction. In a computerized system, a patient record contains the same information as a ledger card. This record also must be maintained and updated.
   RATIONALE: *The information on each patient's ledger card must match that of the daily log.*

3. Use a new log (day) sheet each day. For each patient seen that day:

   a. Record the following: patient name, the relevant charges, and any payments received.
   b. Calculate any necessary adjustments and new balances.
   c. When using a computerized system, enter the patient's name or account number, the relevant charges, along with any payments received and adjustments made in the appropriate areas. The computer program will calculate the new balances.
   RATIONALE: *Each day's transactions must be accurately and promptly recorded.*

4. Record all deposits accurately in the check register.

5. File the deposit receipt—with a detailed listing of checks, cash, and money orders deposited—for later use in reconciling the bank statement.

6. The deposit amount should match the amount of money collected by the practice for that day.
   RATIONALE: *If the receipts for the day and the deposit for the day match, you have balanced for the day.*

7. Prepare or, if using a computerized program, print a summary of charges, receipts, and disbursements every month, quarter, or year, as directed. Double-check all entries and calculations from the monthly summary before posting them to the quarterly summary. Also, double-check the entries and calculations from the quarterly summary before posting them to the yearly summary.
   RATIONALE: *Double-checking all entries ensures that mistakes are found and corrected as soon as possible.*

PROCEDURE 20-2 Using the Superbill as Bill/Receipt

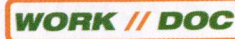

Procedure Goal: To complete a superbill accurately for use as the patient's first bill or receipt

OSHA Guidelines: This procedure does not involve exposure to blood, body fluids, or tissue.

Materials: Superbill, patient ledger card, patient information sheet, fee schedule, pen

Method:

1. From the patient ledger card and information sheet, fill in the patient data, such as name, sex, date of birth, and insurance information.

2. Fill in the date of service. If there are multiple practice locations, circle the location where the service is taking place.

3. Attach the superbill to the patient's medical record and give them both to the practitioner.
   RATIONALE: *The practitioner must have the superbill to enter the services performed during the visit.*

4. At the end of the visit, accept the completed superbill from the patient. Make sure that the practitioner has indicated the procedures performed and an appropriate diagnosis for each.
   RATIONALE: *The diagnosis ensures medical necessity for the insurance carrier to allow for payment.*

5. If the practitioner has not already recorded the charges, refer to the fee schedule for procedures that are marked. Then fill in the charges next to those procedures.
   RATIONALE: *Each procedure must have a charge for accurate billing.*

6. In the appropriate blanks, list the total charges for the visit and the previous balance (if any).

7. Calculate the subtotal.

8. Fill in the amount and type of payment (cash, check, money order, debit or credit card) made by the patient during this visit.
   RATIONALE: *This information ensures accurate posting to the patient's account.*

9. Calculate and enter the new balance.

10. If not already on file, have the patient sign the authorization-and-release section of the superbill.
    RATIONALE: *Without this signature, there is no authorization to share information with the insurance carrier, nor is there agreement for the payer to pay the service provider directly for the services provided.*

11. Keep a copy of the superbill for the practice records. Give the original to the patient along with one copy to file with the insurer.

PROCEDURE 20-3 Posting a Nonsufficient Funds (NSF) Check

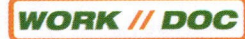

Procedure Goal: To post a nonsufficient funds (NSF) check amount and any applicable fees to the patient's account

OSHA Guidelines: This procedure does not involve exposure to blood, body fluids, or tissue.

Materials: Computer, returned check, patient ledger, calculator (optional), daily log sheet

Method:

1. Locate the patient's account on the computer, or pull the patient's ledger card for manual processes.
   RATIONALE: *You must be sure that you have the correct patient (account) to record the NSF check.*

2. Use your medical facility code for NSF check (if used). Using today's date, create a new charge log for the patient. Use the code and the description *Check returned by bank* in the description column.

3. In the payment/adjustment column, place the amount of the check in parentheses to indicate that the amount is debited as an *adjustment*. Add the amount of the returned check to the old balance and enter it in the *current balance* column.
   RATIONALE: *This negative payment/adjustment will increase the patient's amount due by the amount of the NSF check. The parentheses remind you to add the payment to the balance, instead of subtracting it as you usually would do.*

4. On the next line, also using today's date, enter the medical facility's code for the NSF charge allowed by the office. Enter the charge amount in the *charge column* and add this amount to the patient's current balance.
   RATIONALE: *The office has the right to charge the patient for the inconvenience of dealing with an NSF check.*

PROCEDURE 20-4 Processing a Payment Resulting in a Credit Balance

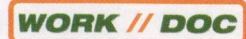 **WORK // DOC**

Procedure Goal: To process a payment that results in a credit balance on the patient's account

OSHA Guidelines: This procedure does not involve exposure to blood, body fluids, or tissue.

Materials: Daily log or day sheet, patient ledger card, computer, calculator, patient explanation of benefits (EOB) or remittance advice (RA) if applicable, and patient or insurance payment

Method:

1. Locate the patient's account in the computer, or pull the patient's ledger card for paper-based systems.
   RATIONALE: *Patient financial records are legal documents, so you must be sure to post financial information to the correct account.*

2. Post the total amount of the payment received to the patient's account by writing (or keying) the remittance amount in the paid column.

3. Subtract the payment amount from the previous balance and insert the new balance in the balance column. If the balance created is a *credit* balance, insert the figure in the current balance column within parentheses.
   RATIONALE: *Inserting figures in parentheses tells the office staff that the balance is owed by the practice (credit balance), not to the practice (debit balance).*

4. Review the account thoroughly, checking to see if any more receipts are expected on the patient's account.
   RATIONALE: *Some patients have multiple insurance plans and more than one insurance payment may be expected on the account.*

5. If a credit balance is verified, adjust the credit balance off the patient's account by issuing a refund (see Procedure 20-5).

PROCEDURE 20-5 Processing Refunds to Patients

WORK // DOC

Procedure Goal: To process a patient refund due to a credit balance

OSHA Guidelines: This procedure does not involve exposure to blood, body fluids, or tissue.

Materials: Payment (check), ledger card, computer, calculator, remittance advice (RA) or explanation of benefits (EOB) if applicable

Method:

1. Calculate and determine the amount to be refunded (from Procedure 20-4). If the amount to be refunded is determined by the EOB or RA, verify the amount listed.
   RATIONALE: *If the patient made a payment and the insurance plan directs the office to return the patient's payment, that amount must be refunded to the patient.*

2. Record the check number and amount in the disbursements journal or checkbook and write a check to the patient for the amount to be refunded.

RATIONALE: *Always record transactions in the checkbook first so that you never forget this step.*

3. Ask the practitioner or business manager to sign the check so that it can be given or mailed to the patient.

4. Post the refund as a negative payment (credit) to the patient's ledger card or to the patient's account if a computerized system is being used. Using parentheses around the figure is a common way to record the credit.

5. Make a copy of the check, retaining a copy in the patient's financial record. Give or mail the check to the patient. If the check is being mailed, be sure to verify the patient's address prior to mailing and utilize certified return receipt mail to be sure the patient receives the check.

PROCEDURE 20-6 Preparing an Age Analysis

WORK // DOC

Procedure Goal: To create and examine an age analysis of practice accounts

OSHA Guidelines: This procedure does not involve exposure to blood, body fluids, or tissue.

Materials: Computer, patient accounts, ledger cards (if a manual system is used), accounts receivable age analysis form or template (Figure 20-10), policies and procedures manual, pen

Method:

1. Using the reporting section of your billing computer program, create an age analysis report for patients and insurance companies. This also can be done manually by pulling patient ledger cards, noting balances due and dates of last payments. Use Figure 20-10 as a guide to create a spreadsheet for your findings.
   RATIONALE: *If the office billing is computerized, pulling an aging report from the system is efficient and reliable.*

2. Review the accounting report. Check the report—highlight each account for proposed actions according to your office policy.
RATIONALE: *Efforts to collect outstanding accounts become more urgent as accounts age and it becomes more difficult to collect the outstanding balance.*

3. Mark the accounts that are under 31 days as "No action to be taken at this time."
RATIONALE: *Accounts of this age are considered current.*

4. Bills that are unpaid at more than 31 days should be marked as "Contact or follow up with insurance company."
RATIONALE: *Patients frequently wait for the insurance carrier to pay its portion before they pay the patient balance.*

5. Accounts that are 31–60 days old should be marked according to your office policy. An initial phone call may be made inquiring as to payment arrangements.
RATIONALE: *The older an account becomes, the more difficult it is to collect. These accounts are at "prime time" to be collected.*

6. Accounts that are 61–90 days old should be marked according to your office policy. Make notations such as "Account Past Due." A follow-up phone call and/or more insistent statement message letter for payment may be in order.

RATIONALE: *Collecting accounts aged less than 91 days have a better success rate than those that are older.*

7. Accounts that are 91–120 days old should be marked according to your office policy. A last phone call to attempt discussing the account and more insistent collection statement/letter should be sent.

8. For accounts older than 120 days, make sure you review previous collection attempts. At this point, after discussion with the physician, a letter stating the account will be turned over to the collection agency will take place with a specific date listed in the letter. This letter should be mailed by certified, return receipt mail.
RATIONALE: *After 120 days without a payment, it is unlikely the patient will pay the bill without a more aggressive course of action.*

9. Record all actions that have been taken beside each account.
RATIONALE: *This diary provides a written record of all attempts to collect the debt.*

10. Finally, write follow-up letters to patients and document any agreements that you and the patient have discussed via telephone. Be sure to keep a copy of any correspondence mailed to the patient in the financial record.
RATIONALE: *All documentation will be necessary, should any legal action be taken regarding this debt.*

PROCEDURE 20-7 Referring an Account to a Collection Agency and Posting the Payment from the Agency

Procedure Goal: To follow the correct procedure in turning an account over to a collection agency and posting the payment from them when received

OSHA Guidelines: This procedure does not involve exposure to blood, body fluids, or tissue.

Materials: Computer, patient accounts, ledger cards (if a manual system is used), patient's financial record containing demographic information, collection agency's phone number, pen

Method:

1. Make sure all attempts that have been made to collect the debt per office policy have been documented, including the return receipt from the letter sent to the patient stating that the account would be turned over to the collection agency by a specific date (today).
RATIONALE: *To avoid charges of harassment, once a threat of collection proceedings has been made, the account must be turned over on the specified date.*

2. Verify that the following information is in the patient's financial file to be turned over to the collection agency:
- Last known phone number and address for the patient
- Employer (if any) name and phone number
- Name of spouse, if applicable
- Total amount of debt, with last payment amount and date
- If there has been no payment, the last date a service was provided
- Description of office actions to collect debt
- Any patient response to those actions

RATIONALE: *This information is required by the collection agency prior to taking over the account.*

3. Place a call to the agency, identifying yourself and the office, and explain you are calling to turn accounts over to them.

4. For each account to be turned over, supply the information listed in step 2.

5. When a payment arrives from the agency, each account will be identified with the total amount of the debt collected. The agency will also deduct its fee from this amount.
RATIONALE: *The agency will collect its fee up front from the payment received per contracted agreement with the practice.*

6. When posting the payment, post the actual amount of the payment sent to the office from the collection agency to the patient's account, not the full amount of the payment made by the patient.
RATIONALE: *The agency kept a portion of the payment as its fee; it will not be posted to the patient's account.*

7. Make an adjustment (write-off) on the patient's account in the amount kept by the agency as its fee.
RATIONALE: *You cannot add the fee charged by the collection agency to the patient's account. It is a "cost of doing business."*

8. Subtract both the payment and the adjustment from the patient's balance. If the payment is noted by the agency as being the full payment on the account, the payment and adjustment should result in a zero balance on the patient's account.

PROCEDURE 20-8 Completing a Truth in Lending Statement (Agreement)

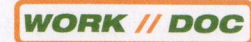

Procedure Goal: To create an accurate and complete Truth in Lending Statement

OSHA Guidelines: This procedure does not involve exposure to blood, body fluids, or tissue.

Materials: Computer, paper, patient financial record, Truth in Lending patient letter (sample), Truth in Lending Statement, name of the procedure or service to be financed, total cost of procedure or service to be financed, amount of down payment, number of payments, amount of each payment, date of month for each payment, pen

Method:

1. Create a document (or use a template) similar to that of Figure 20-12 to use as the Truth in Lending Statement.

2. Make sure the following information is included:
   - Patient name and address
   - Price for service or procedure
   - Amount of down payment received
   - Unpaid balance
   - Amount financed
   - Finance charge (if applicable)
   - Finance charge as a percentage rate (if applicable)
   - Total amount to be financed
   - Number of payments and the amount of each
   - Date payments are due, including final payment date

3. Once the template is completed, fill in the information for the patient's agreement. Make calculations carefully and check your work.
   RATIONALE: *For the Truth in Lending Statement to be valid, all information must be included and accurate.*

4. After going over the statement with the patient, have the patient sign and date the agreement.
   RATIONALE: *Without the patient's signature the agreement is not valid.*

5. Give a copy of the signed agreement to the patient and keep a copy in the patient's financial record for future reference.

6. If desired, a master document, such as that found in Figure 20-13, may be created outlining the agreement and listing the actual date and payment amount for each month of the agreement.
   RATIONALE: *This document avoids the need for mailing a monthly statement for the agreed-upon amount to the patient.*

PROCEDURE 20-9 Making a Bank Deposit

Procedure Goal: To prepare cash and checks for deposit and to deposit them properly into a bank account

OSHA Guidelines: This procedure does not involve exposure to blood, body fluids, or tissue.

Materials: Bank deposit slip and items to be deposited, such as checks, cash, and money orders

Method:

1. Divide the bills, coins, checks, and money orders into separate piles.

2. Sort the bills by denomination, from largest to smallest. Then, stack them—portrait side up—in the same direction. Total the amount of the bills and write this amount on the deposit slip on the line marked "currency" or cash.
   RATIONALE: *The bank will require bills to be sorted for ease of counting by the teller to verify deposit information.*

3. If you have enough coins to fill coin wrappers, put them in wrappers of the proper denomination. If not, count the coins and put them in the deposit bag. Total the amount of coins and write this amount on the deposit slip on the line marked "Coin."
   RATIONALE: *If there are enough coins to fill denomination wrappers, the bank will require this to be done.*

4. Review all checks and money orders to be sure they are properly endorsed with a restrictive endorsement. List each check on the deposit slip, including the check number and amount.
   RATIONALE: *Without a proper endorsement, the bank will not accept a check for deposit.*

5. List each money order on the deposit slip. Include the notation "money order" or "MO" and the name of the writer.

6. Calculate the total deposit (total of amounts for currency, coin, checks, and money orders). Write this amount on the deposit slip on the line marked "Total." If you do not use deposit slips that record a copy for the office, photocopy the deposit slip for your office records.
   RATIONALE: *Deposit slips must be kept in case there is ever a discrepancy between the office and bank records. The deposit slip is proof of deposit.*

7. Record the total amount of the deposit in the office checkbook register.

8. If you plan to make the deposit in person, place the currency, coins, checks, and money orders in a deposit bag. If you cannot make the deposit in person, put the checks and money orders in a special bank-by-mail

envelope or put all deposit items in an envelope and send it via registered mail.

RATIONALE: *If a deposit absolutely must be mailed, registered mail provides insurance for the amount of the deposit and proof of receipt by the bank.*

9. Make the deposit in person or by mail.

10. Obtain a deposit receipt from the bank. File it with the copy of the deposit slip in the office for later use when reconciling the bank statement.

PROCEDURE 20-10 Reconciling the Bank Statement   WORK // DOC

Procedure Goal: To ensure that the bank record of deposits, payments, and withdrawals agrees with the practice record of deposits, payments, and withdrawals

OSHA Guidelines: This procedure does not involve exposure to blood, body fluids, or tissue.

Materials: Previous month's bank statement, current month's bank statement, reconciliation worksheet (if not part of current bank statement), deposit receipts, red pencil, check stubs or checkbook register, returned checks or listing of checks returned

Method:

1. Check the closing balance on the previous month's statement against the opening balance on the current month's statement. The balances should match. If they do not, call the bank.

   RATIONALE: *If the ending balance from last month does not match the beginning balance of this month, there may be a problem with the bank's system.*

2. Record the closing balance from the current statement on the reconciliation worksheet (Figure 20-17). This worksheet usually appears on the back of the bank statement.

   RATIONALE: *This is the starting point for adjusting the bank balance as needed to accomplish reconciliation.*

3. Check each deposit receipt against the bank statement.

   a. Place a red check mark in the upper-right corner of each receipt recorded on the statement.

   b. Also place a check mark next to each deposit recorded in the checkbook to be sure none was skipped in this record.

4. Total the amount of deposits that do *not* appear on the statement. Add this amount to the closing balance from the bank on the reconciliation worksheet.

   RATIONALE: *These deposits are in transit, but the amount must be added to the bank balance in order for reconciliation to occur.*

5. Compare each redeemed check with the bank statement, making sure that the amount on the check agrees with the amount on the statement.

   a. Place a red check mark in the upper-right corner of each redeemed check recorded on the statement.

   b. Also, place a check mark on the check stub or check register entry.

   c. Any checks that were written but do not appear on the statement and were not returned as redeemed are considered "outstanding" checks. You can find these easily on the check stubs or checkbook register because they have no red check mark next to them.

6. List each outstanding check separately on the worksheet, including its check number and amount. Total the outstanding checks and subtract this total from the bank statement balance.

   RATIONALE: *These checks will eventually be honored by the bank. In order to balance the checkbook and bank statement, these outstanding checks must be subtracted from the bank balance. (You cannot add the amount back to your checkbook because the money will not be returned to the account.)*

7. Record the ending balance found in the office checkbook in the appropriate area of the reconciliation worksheet.

   RATIONALE: *This is the starting point for adjusting the checkbook balance as needed to accomplish reconciliation.*

8. If the statement shows that the checking account earned interest, add this amount to the checkbook balance.

   RATIONALE: *You did not know the interest amount prior to today, so now it must be added to the bank balance both in the checkbook and on the reconciliation worksheet.*

9. If the statement lists such items as service charge, check printing charge, or automatic payment, subtract them from the checkbook balance and add these charges to the checkbook register itself.

   RATIONALE: *In order to balance with the bank statement, you must now enter the information you did not know until now, both in the checkbook register and on the reconciliation worksheet.*

10. Compare the new checkbook balance with the new bank statement balance. They should match. If they do not, repeat the process, rechecking all calculations. Double-check the addition and subtraction in the checkbook register. Review the checkbook register to make sure you did not omit any items. Ensure that you carried the correct balance forward from one register page to the next. Double-check that you made the correct additions or subtractions for all interest earned and charges incurred.

11. If you have double-checked your work and the balances still do not agree, ask a coworker to check your figures. If the coworker also finds no error or omission, call the bank to determine if a bank error has been made. Contact the bank promptly because the bank may have a time limit for corrections and may consider the bank statement correct if you do not point out an error within a specified time. Check with your individual bank for its policy.

   RATIONALE: *Always ask a "fresh set of eyes" to look at the reconciliation prior to calling the bank. If anyone looks at figures for too long, it is not unusual to see "what you want to see," instead of what is really there.*

PROCEDURE 20-11 Setting Up the Disbursements Journal

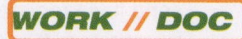

Procedure Goal: To set up the office disbursements journal

OSHA Guidelines: This procedure does not involve exposure to blood, body fluids, or tissue.

Materials: Disbursements journal (either paper or electronic), pen (if journal is in a paper format), listing of the headings required for the disbursements journal

Method:

1. Write in or key column headings for the basic information required for each check: date, payee's name, check number, and check amount.
   RATIONALE: *This information is needed for accounting purposes.*

2. Enter column headings for each type of business expense, such as utilities, payroll, and taxes.

3. Write in column headings (if space is available) for deposits and the account balance.

4. Record the data from completed checks under the appropriate column headings.
   RATIONALE: *The amount spent on each type of business expense is entered and tracked for income and expense reports. The practice manager will know exactly where money is being made or lost.*

5. Be sure to subtract payments from the balance and add deposits to it.
   RATIONALE: *This step allows for a running tally of income and expenses, including the current balance.*

SUMMARY OF LEARNING OUTCOMES

LEARNING OUTCOMES	KEY POINTS
20.1 Summarize the importance of and how to establish good bookkeeping and banking practices.	Procedures to be established to help maintain consistency in financial practices include being organized and consistent. Write clearly and use markers to keep track of your current location. Check your work frequently and correct any errors using the approved method of drawing one line through the error and correcting the information directly above that location. All entries must be kept readable at all times. Finally, keep all figure columns straight so that decimal points line up. Following through on these procedures can help ensure that your work will be concise and accurate.
20.2 Compare single-entry, double-entry, and write-it-once bookkeeping systems and explain accounts receivable and payable.	The single-entry accounting system is easy to use because each entry is written once on the patient ledger, on the daily log, and in the checkbook but contains no checks and balances for accuracy. The double-entry system is based on Assets = Capital + Liabilities. It has checks and balances but can be cumbersome and complicated. The write-it-once system is used in manual offices because it allows all transactions to be recorded in one procedure, using carbonless forms on all necessary documents. Many office management software packages are based on the write-it-once concept. *Accounts receivable* refers to the money that is owed to the practice (able to be received). *Accounts payable* refers to the money that the practice owes other vendors (able to be paid).
20.3 Describe the common payment methods accepted in medical practices today.	Common payment methods accepted by medical practices include cash, check, money orders, and debit and credit cards.
20.4 Identify the different types of documents used as statements to bill patients and how these documents are used in cycle billing.	Common statement documents include the use of superbills, typed or computer-produced itemized statements, and copies of ledger cards. In cycle billing the accounts are split in groups and statement mailing dates are staggered.

LEARNING OUTCOMES	KEY POINTS
20.5 Compare open-book, written-contract, and single-entry accounts and the purpose of creating an accounts receivable aging.	An open-book account is the account type most commonly found in a medical practice, consisting of periodic charges and payments added as needed when patients are seen in the practice. A written-contract account is used when the physician and patient sign a contract for a specific service or procedure. A single-entry account is used for patients when it is expected they will be seen only once, such as for a relative visiting the area on vacation. An age analysis is the process of classifying and reviewing past-due accounts by age from the first date of billing. It helps you keep on top of past-due accounts and determine which ones need follow-up.
20.6 Explain the purposes of the following credit and collections acts: ECOA, FCRA, FDCPA, and TLA.	The Equal Credit Opportunity Act (ECOA) prohibits discrimination based on sex, marital status, race, national origin, religion, or age. Applicants also cannot be discriminated against for receiving public assistance income or exercising their rights under the Consumer Credit Protection Act. The Fair Credit Reporting Act (FCRA) requires credit bureaus to supply correct and complete information to businesses to use in evaluating a person's application for credit, insurance, or a job. The Fair Debt Collections Practices Act (FDCPA) requires debt collectors to treat debtors fairly and prohibits certain collection tactics, including harassment, false statements, threats, and unfair practices. The Truth in Lending Act (TLA) requires creditors to provide applicants with accurate and complete credit costs and terms.
20.7 Relate the required components of a Truth in Lending Statement to credit practices in the medical office.	The Truth in Lending Statement must include the following elements: the amount of total debt, the amount of the down payment, the amount of each payment and the date due, the due date for the final payment, the interest rate (if any) expressed as an annual percentage rate, and the total finance charges (if any).
20.8 Summarize two common types of problem collection accounts in the medical office.	The two most common types of collection problems in the medical office are hardship cases, who simply cannot afford to pay their debt, and accounts known as skips, where the debtor moved and left no valid forwarding information so it is not possible to bill the patient.
20.9 Identify negotiable instruments and the items that must be present for a check to be negotiable.	A negotiable instrument is one that is legally transferable from one person to another. To be negotiable, a check must be written and signed by the payer or maker, include the amount of money to be paid, be made payable to the payee or bearer, be made payable on demand or on a specific date, and include the name of the bank that is directed to make payment.
20.10 Describe the different types of check endorsements and the steps in creating a bank deposit.	The types of check endorsements are blank, restrictive, special, and qualified. To make a bank deposit, follow the steps outlined in Procedure 20-9.
20.11 Carry out the process of reconciling the office bank statement.	Follow Procedure 20-10 to successfully reconcile a mock bank statement with a mock office checkbook.

LEARNING OUTCOMES	KEY POINTS
20.12 List several advantages to electronic banking.	The computer software calculates each new balance for you. It can reconcile the monthly bank statement automatically and, instead of locking up bank forms and the office checkbook, a computer password and security system keep the information safe and confidential.
20.13 Implement setting up, classifying, and recording disbursements in a disbursements journal.	Following Procedure 20-11, set up a mock disbursements journal consisting of several columns of expenses. Once set up, given a list of several "bills" to be paid, document the check information and record the disbursement amount in the correct column(s) of the journal.

CASE STUDY CRITICAL THINKING

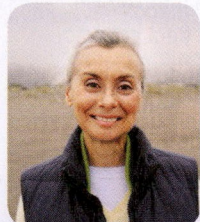

© John Lund/Sam Diephuis/Blend Images LLC RF

Recall Nancy Evans from the beginning of the chapter. Now that you have completed the chapter, answer the following questions regarding her case.

1. How much of the $360 bill for the neurology consult services will be Nancy's responsibility? (Refer to the *Insurance and Billing* chapter if necessary.)
2. What is the best way to bill Nancy for this balance?
3. Why is this way the preferred method?

EXAM PREPARATION QUESTIONS

1. (LO 20.1) Which of the following is *not* a procedure to be followed when setting up bookkeeping or banking systems?
   a. Be organized in your work area
   b. Be consistent in your procedure
   c. Use markers, jotting a red "x" as you work to avoid losing your place
   d. Write clearly in pen, using the same color of ink
   e. Check your work carefully

2. (LO 20.3) The form that contains a single patient's financial information and record of transactions is called the patient
   a. Day sheet
   b. Check
   c. Pegboard
   d. Daily log
   e. Ledger card

3. (LO 20.3) Which of the following is the preferred way to ask a patient for payment?
   a. "I need $50 for today's visit."
   b. "The total for today's visit is 50 bucks. How do you want to pay for that?"
   c. "That will be $50. What is your check number?"
   d. "Your anticipated charge for today is $50. We require payment up front."
   e. "Your charge for today's visit is $50. We take cash, check, and credit and debit cards."

4. (LO 20.4) Which of the following would *not* be acceptable for use as a patient statement?
   a. A completed superbill
   b. A handwritten statement
   c. A computer-generated statement
   d. A "clean" copy of the office ledger card
   e. A typed statement

5. (LO 20.5) What is the most important reason for running an age analysis of the patient accounts?
   a. It allows you to see "deadbeats" at a glance
   b. It allows you to track the "high dollar" accounts
   c. It tracks delinquent insurance payments
   d. It allows you to track past-due accounts so that the patients can be contacted
   e. It lets the physician know how much money is owed to the practice

6. (LO 20.6) Which of the following laws govern(s) collection policies in medical practices?
   a. ECOA
   b. FCRA
   c. FDCPA
   d. TLA
   e. ECOA, FCRA, and TLA

7. (LO 20.7) Under what conditions is a Truth in Lending Statement required?
   a. When the physician informally agrees that the patient can pay a bill in installments
   b. If a bilateral agreement of fewer than four installments is reached
   c. When the patient pays at the time of service
   d. When a finance charge is to be assessed by the practice
   e. All of these require a Truth in Lending Statement

8. (LO 20.9) Business (or personal) checks with stubs attached are known as
   a. Counter checks
   b. Voucher checks
   c. Limited checks
   d. Traveler's checks
   e. Cashier's checks

9. (LO 20.9) The best endorsement to use on a daily basis when preparing checks for the office deposit is the _____ endorsement.
   a. Blank
   b. Special
   c. Restrictive
   d. Third-party
   e. Qualified

10. (LO 20.13) A payment made by the office for goods or services purchased is known as
    a. Disbursement
    b. Accounts payable
    c. Accounts receivable
    d. Liability
    e. Capital

SOFT SKILLS SUCCESS

Recall Nancy Evans from the case study at the beginning of the chapter.

1. Even though her short-term memory is starting to be affected by her disease, Mrs. Evans is still interested and involved in her medical care and financial matters. In fact, she asks about her balance today. How can you help make sure that she does not forget important information?

2. Because Mrs. Evans asked about her balance, you give her a copy of today's encounter form. She states (correctly) that this is not the "usual bill." What will you say to her?

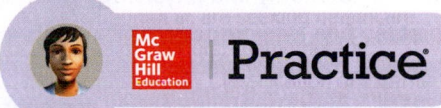

Go to PRACTICE MEDICAL OFFICE and complete the module Admin: Check Out - Work Task Proficiencies.

Organization of the Body

CASE STUDY

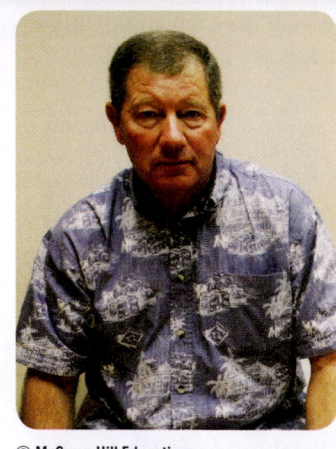

© McGraw-Hill Education

John Miller, a 65-year-old male, arrives at the clinic complaining of his shoes not fitting and feeling like he cannot take a deep breath. During the patient interview, he also states he is having intermittent pain in his chest. He has not taken his blood pressure medication for 2 weeks because he ran out of the medication and there were no refills left on his prescription. He is hoping to get this medication renewed. The licensed practitioner wants to evaluate his congestive heart failure and orders a chest X-ray. You know from your study of anatomy that the X-ray will provide an image of the structures in the thoracic cavity.

Keep John in mind as you study this chapter. There will be questions at the end of the chapter based on the case study. The information in the chapter will help you answer these questions.

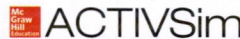

LEARNING OUTCOMES

After completing Chapter 21, you will be able to:

21.1 Explain the importance of understanding both anatomy and physiology when studying the body.

21.2 Illustrate body organization from simple to more complex levels.

21.3 Describe the locations and characteristics of the four main tissue types.

21.4 Describe the body organ systems, their general functions, and the major organs contained in each.

21.5 Use medical and anatomical terminology correctly.

21.6 Explain anatomical position and its relationship to other anatomical positions.

21.7 Identify the body cavities and the organs contained in each.

21.8 Relate a basic understanding of chemistry to its importance in studying the body.

21.9 Name the parts of a cell and their functions.

21.10 Summarize how substances move across a cell membrane.

21.11 Distinguish the stages of cell division.

21.12 Explain the uses of these genetic techniques: the polymerase chain reaction and DNA fingerprinting.

21.13 Describe the different patterns of inheritance and common genetic disorders.

21.14 Describe the causes, signs and symptoms, and treatments of various genetic diseases and disorders.

MEDICAL ASSISTING COMPETENCIES

CAAHEP

I.C.1 Describe structural organization of the human body

I.C.2 Identify body systems

I.C.3 Describe:
(a) body planes
(b) directional terms
(c) quadrants
(d) body cavities

I.C.4 List major organs in each body system

I.C.5 Identify the anatomical location of major organs in each body system

I.C.7 Describe the normal function of each body system

I.C.9 Analyze pathology for each body system including:
(a) diagnostic measures
(b) treatment modalities

V.C.9 Identify medical terms labeling the word parts

V.C.10 Define medical terms and abbreviations related to all body systems

ABHES

2. Anatomy & Physiology

a. List all body systems, their structure and functions

b. Describe common diseases, symptoms and etiologies as they apply to each system

3. Medical Terminology

a. Define and use entire basic structure of medical words and be able to accurately identify in the correct context; i.e. root, prefix, suffix, combinations, spelling, and definitions

b. Build and dissect medical terms from roots/ suffixes to understand the word element combinations that create medical terminology

c. Apply the various medical terminology for each specialty

▶ Introduction

The human body is complex in its structure and function. Think of your own body for a moment. If you were to choose just one body part—say, your eyes—consider everything about how they look, how they function, how they are connected to the rest of your face, and how your skull supports them. Consider what happens to your eyes when you smile, cry, or glimpse bright sunlight or when a misguided insect or piece of dirt makes its way into them and you have to rub one eye with your finger and you end up scratching it accidentally, causing temporarily blurred vision.

Of course, the eyes are just one example. You have your entire body to deal with. This chapter provides an overview of the human body. It introduces you to the way the body is organized from the chemical level all the way up to the organ system level. You will learn important terminology used to describe body positions and parts. You will also explore how diseases develop at the genetic and organism levels.

▶ The Study of the Body   LO 21.1

Anatomy is the scientific term for the study of body structure. For example, the heart may be described as a hollow, cone-shaped organ that is an average of 14 centimeters long and 9 centimeters wide. Understanding anatomy allows us to understand the normal positions of body structures and how to describe these positions precisely and correctly. **Physiology** is the term for the study of the function of the body's organs. For example, the physiology of the heart can be described by saying that the heart pumps blood into blood vessels to transport nutrients throughout the body. Anatomy and physiology are commonly studied together because they are intimately related. For example, the anatomy of the heart (a hollow, muscular organ) allows it to do its function (pump blood into tubular blood vessels). If the heart were not hollow, it could not allow blood to flow into it. If the heart were not muscular, it could not pump blood.

Knowledge of anatomy and physiology will help you grasp the meaning of diagnosis and procedure codes and help you understand the clinical procedures you will perform and assist with as a medical assistant. Understanding anatomy and physiology can also make it easier to see how and why certain diseases develop. Diseases develop in the body when homeostasis—the relative consistency of the body's internal environment—is not maintained. Body conditions that must remain within a stable range include body temperature, blood pressure, and the concentration of various chemicals within the blood. Individual cells must also maintain homeostasis. For example, if chemicals within a cell change the deoxyribonucleic acid (DNA), or genetic makeup of the cell, that cell can become cancerous.

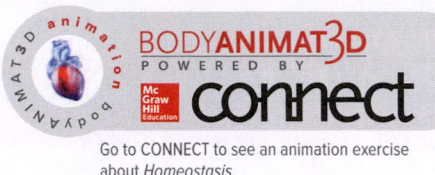

Go to CONNECT to see an animation exercise about *Homeostasis.*

▶ Structural Organization of the Body

LO 21.2

The body's structure can be divided into different levels of organization. The chemical level is the simplest level—the billions of atoms and molecules in the body. Atoms are the simplest units of all **matter,** anything that takes up space and has weight, and many are essential to life. The four most common atoms in the human body are carbon, hydrogen, oxygen, and nitrogen. **Molecules** are made up of atoms that bond together. Proteins and carbohydrates are examples of molecules that consist of hundreds of atoms.

Molecules join together to form **organelles,** which can be thought of as cell parts. Organelles combine to form cells such as leukocytes (white blood cells), erythrocytes (red blood cells), neurons (nerve cells), and adipocytes (fat cells). **Cells** are considered to be the smallest living units in the body. When similar types of cells organize together, they form **tissues.** Two or more tissue types combine to form **organs,** and organs arrange to form **organ systems.** Finally, organ systems combine to form an **organism.** Figure 21-1 illustrates the organization of the body's organ systems.

▶ Major Tissue Types

LO 21.3

Tissues are groups of cells that have similar structures and functions. The four major tissue types in the body are epithelial, connective, muscle, and nervous tissue. These are explained more fully in the following paragraphs.

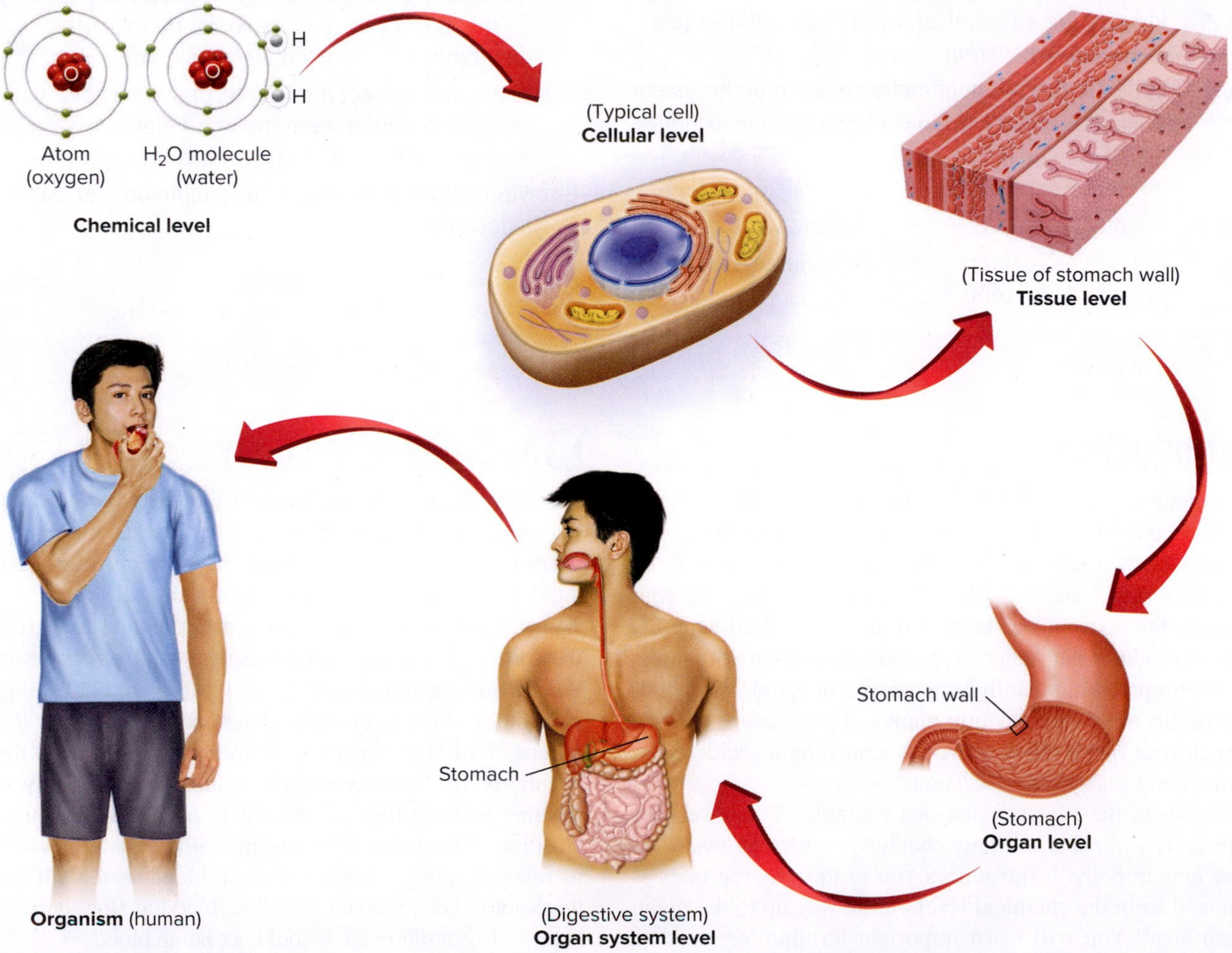

Atom
(oxygen)

H₂O molecule
(water)

Chemical level

(Typical cell)
Cellular level

(Tissue of stomach wall)
Tissue level

Stomach wall

(Stomach)
Organ level

Stomach

Organism (human)

(Digestive system)
Organ system level

FIGURE 21-1   The human body is organized in levels, beginning with the chemical level and progressing to the cellular, tissue, organ, organ system, and organism (whole body) levels.

Epithelial Tissue

When you think of epithelial tissue, think of a covering, lining, or gland. Epithelial tissue covers the body and most organs in the body. It lines the body's tubes, such as blood vessels and the esophagus, and the body's hollow organs, such as the stomach and heart. This type of tissue also lines body cavities, such as the thoracic cavity and the abdominopelvic cavity.

Glandular tissue is also classified as a type of epithelial tissue. It is composed of cells that make and secrete (give off) substances. If a gland secretes its product into a duct, as does a sweat or oil (sebaceous) gland, it is called an *exocrine gland*. If a gland secretes its product directly into surrounding tissue fluids or blood, it does not have ducts and is called an *endocrine gland*. The pancreas and thyroid are considered endocrine glands because they release their hormones directly into the bloodstream.

Epithelial tissues are avascular, which means they lack blood vessels. However, these tissues have a nerve supply and are very mitotic, meaning they divide constantly. In addition, the cells within epithelial tissues are packed together tightly. Epithelial tissues have many different functions, depending on their location in the body. For example, those covering the body protect against invading pathogens and toxins. Those that line the digestive tract secrete a variety of enzymes needed for digestion. They often possess microvilli—tiny, fingerlike projections that allow the body to absorb nutrients. Epithelial tissues lining the respiratory tract have goblet cells and cilia. The goblet cells produce mucus, which traps small particles that enter the respiratory tract. The cilia constantly push the mucus and trapped particles away from the lungs (see Figure 21-2). Epithelial cells within the kidneys act as filters to help remove waste products from the blood.

Connective Tissue

Connective tissue is the most abundant tissue in the body. The cells of connective tissue are not packed together tightly. Instead, a matrix separates the cells. Think of the matrix simply as the matter between the cells of connective tissue. The matrix may contain fibers, water, proteins, inorganic salts, and other substances. The components of the matrix vary, depending on the type of connective tissue. Connective tissue generally has a rich blood supply, except for cartilage and some dense connective tissues that contain a very poor blood supply.

Many different cell types are located in connective tissue; the most common are fibroblasts, mast cells, and macrophages. Fibroblasts are responsible for secreting collagen and making fibers. They are essential for the normal development and repair of connective tissue. Mast cells secrete substances such as heparin and histamine that promote inflammation when tissue is damaged. Macrophages are cells that destroy unwanted material, such as bacteria or toxins.

The following sections discuss the various types of connective tissue in more detail.

Blood This tissue is composed of red blood cells, white blood cells, platelets, and plasma. Plasma is the matrix of blood. Unlike other connective tissues, this matrix does not contain fibers. Blood transports substances throughout the body. Blood and its cell functions will be discussed in depth in a later chapter.

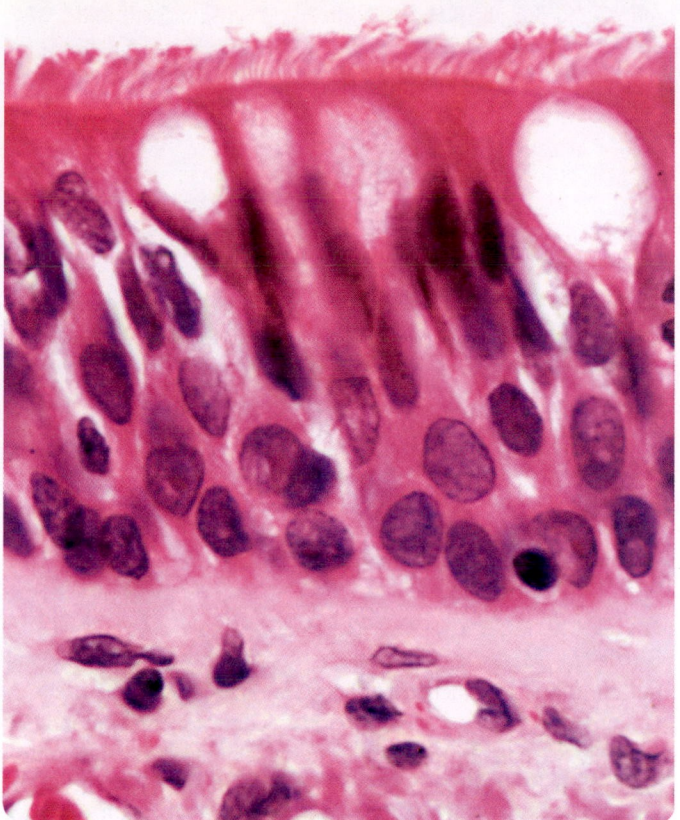

FIGURE 21-2 Epithelial tissue lining the respiratory tract.
© McGraw-Hill Education/Al Telser, photographer

Osseous (Bone) Tissue The matrix of osseous tissue contains mineral salts that make it a very hard tissue. Contrary to popular belief, bone is a living tissue—it is metabolically active.

Cartilage The matrix of cartilage is rigid, although it is not as hard as osseous tissue. Cartilage gives shape to structures such as the ears and nose. It also protects the ends of long bones and forms the discs between the vertebrae of the neck and spine.

Dense Connective Tissue The matrix of dense connective tissue is packed with tough fibers that make it a soft but very strong tissue. Ligaments, tendons, and joint capsules have large amounts of this tissue type. Ligaments connect bones to bones, tendons connect muscles to bones, and joint capsules surround moveable joints in the body. Dense connective tissue also makes up a large part of the skin's dermis. When skin is damaged, this tissue "fills in" the damaged space and forms a scar.

Adipose (Fat) Tissue Within adipose tissue, unique cells—adipocytes—store fats. This tissue type stores energy for body cells, cushions body parts and organs, and insulates the body against excessive heat or cold (see Figure 21-3).

Muscle Tissue

Muscle is a specialized type of tissue that contracts and relaxes. The three types of muscle tissue are skeletal, visceral (smooth), and cardiac.

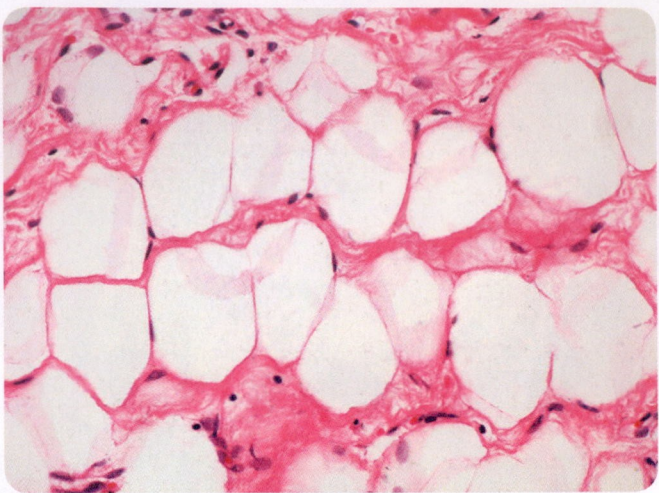

FIGURE 21-3 Adipose tissue.
© McGraw-Hill Education/Al Telser, photographer

Skeletal Muscle Tissue As its name suggests, skeletal muscle tissue is attached to the skeleton. This type of tissue is voluntary because we can consciously control its movement. For example, we can consciously decide to contract the skeletal muscles attached to our arm bones and make them move. It is also referred to as striated because the cells of this muscle tissue type have striations, or stripes, in their cytoplasm (see Figure 21-4).

Visceral Muscle Tissue This smooth muscle tissue is located in the walls of hollow organs (except the heart), the walls of blood vessels, and the dermis of skin. It is involuntary—we cannot consciously control its movement. For example, you do not consciously decide when the visceral muscle of your stomach contracts. This tissue is also called *smooth muscle* because its cells do not have striations in their cytoplasm.

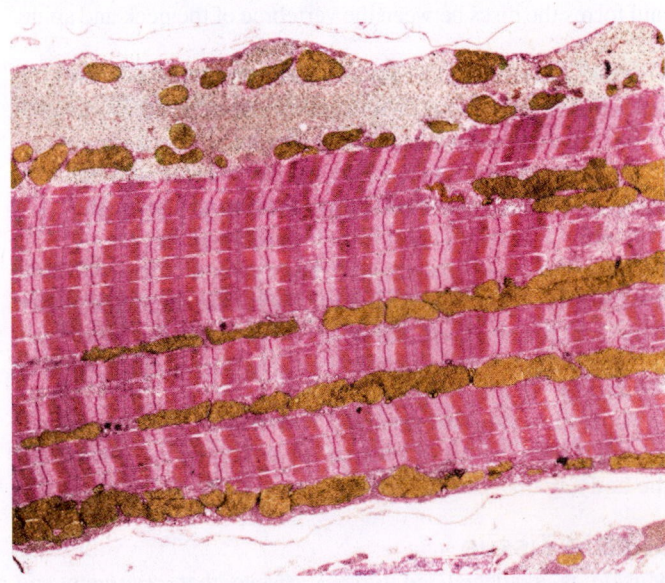

FIGURE 21-4 Skeletal muscle tissue.
© Science Photo Library RF/Getty Images

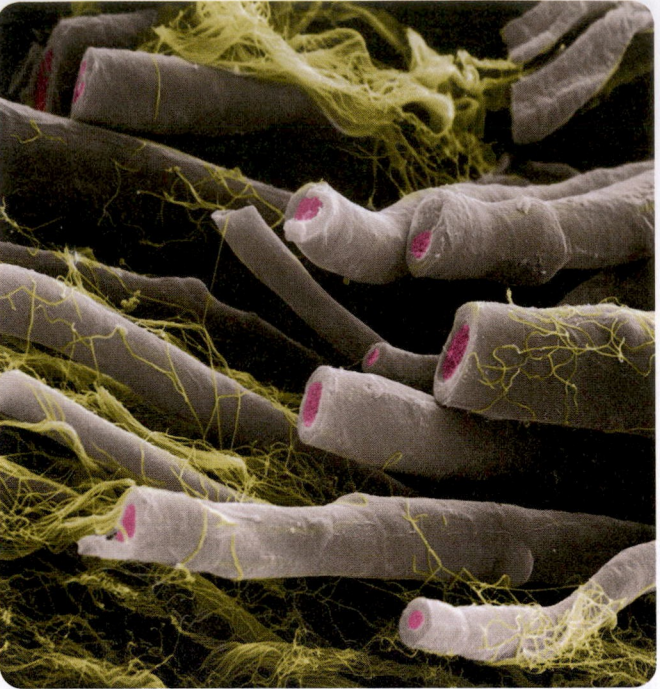

FIGURE 21-5 Nervous tissue.
© Science Photo Library RF/Getty Images

Cardiac Muscle Tissue This specialized muscle tissue is located in the wall of the heart. Like skeletal muscle tissue, cardiac muscle is striated. Like smooth muscle tissue, it is not under voluntary control; it is involuntary.

Nervous Tissue

Nervous tissue is located in the brain, spinal cord, and peripheral nerves. This tissue specializes in sending impulses, or electrical messages, to the neurons, muscles, and glands in the body (see Figure 21-5). Nervous tissue contains two types of cells: neurons and neuroglial cells. Neurons are the largest cells, and they transmit impulses. Although neuroglial cells are smaller, they are more abundant and act as support cells for the neurons. They do not transmit impulses.

▶ Body Organs and Systems   LO 21.4

Organs are structures formed by the organization of two or more different tissue types that work together to carry out specific functions. For example, the heart is made up of cardiac muscle tissue, connective tissue, and epithelial tissue. These tissues work together to carry out the heart's function—to effectively pump blood into blood vessels. Organ systems are formed when organs join together to carry out vital functions. For example, the heart and blood vessels unite to form the cardiovascular system. The organs of the cardiovascular system circulate blood throughout the body to ensure that all body cells receive enough nutrients. See Figure 21-6 for a summary of the human body's organ systems, their general functions, and the organs within each.

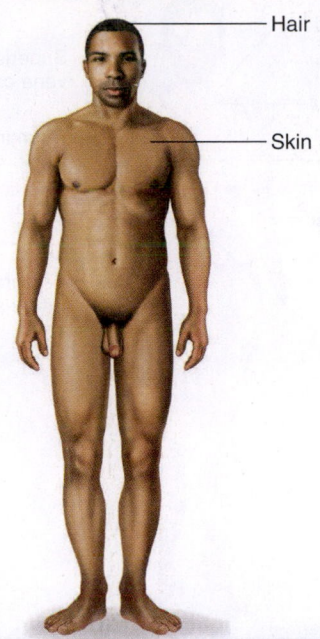

Integumentary System

Serves as a sense organ for the body, provides protection, regulates temperature, prevents water loss, and produces vitamin D precursors. Consists of skin, hair, nails, and sweat glands.

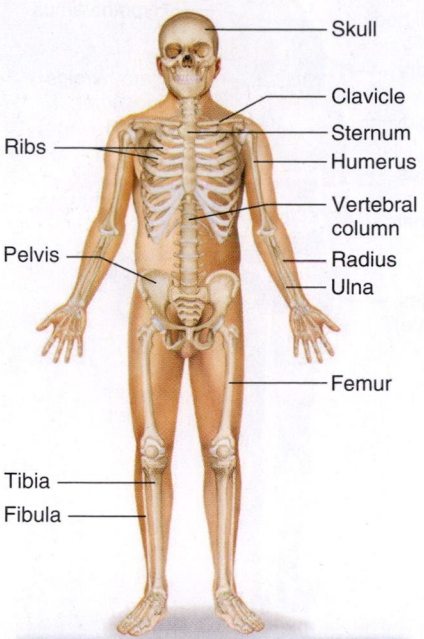

Skeletal System

Provides protection and support, allows body movements, produces blood cells, and stores minerals and fat. Consists of bones, associated cartilages, ligaments, and joints.

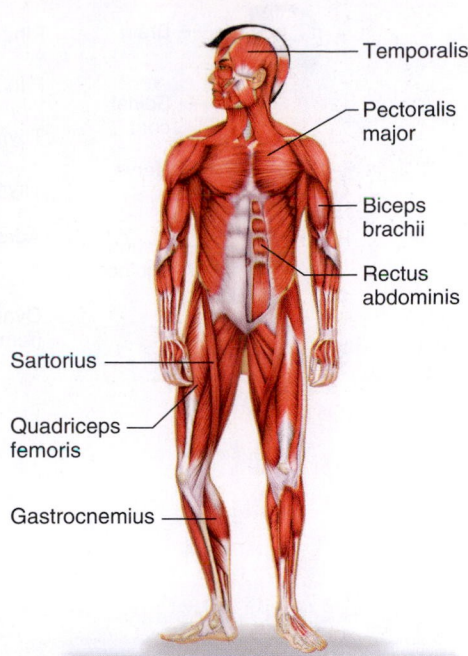

Muscular System

Produces body movements, maintains posture, and produces body heat. Consists of muscles attached to the skeleton by tendons.

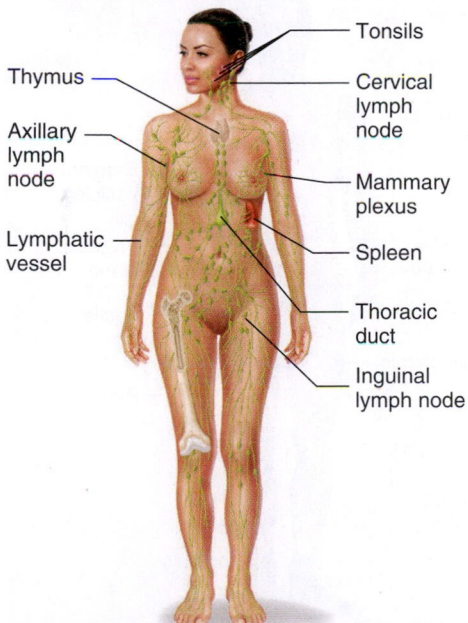

Lymphatic System

Removes foreign substances from the blood and lymph, combats disease, maintains tissue fluid balance, and absorbs fats from the digestive tract. Consists of the lymphatic vessels, lymph nodes, and other lymphatic organs.

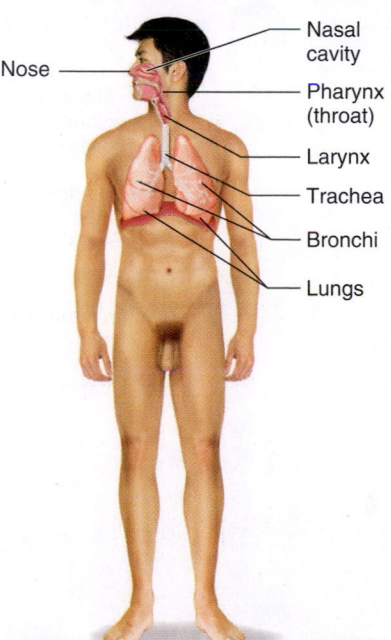

Respiratory System

Exchanges oxygen and carbon dioxide between the blood and air and regulates blood pH. Consists of the lungs and respiratory passages.

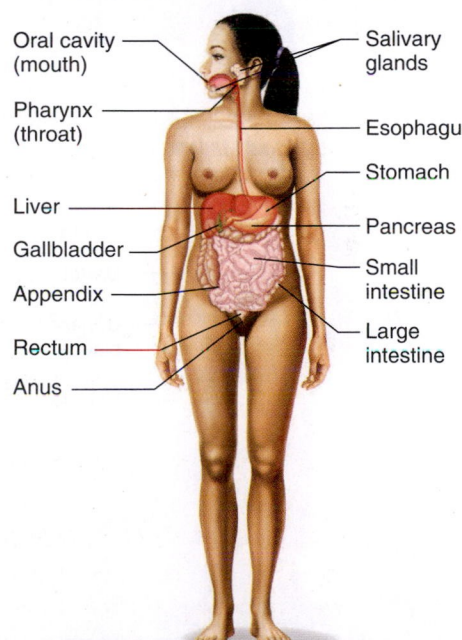

Digestive System

Performs the mechanical and chemical processes of digestion, absorption of nutrients, and elimination of wastes. Consists of the mouth, esophagus, stomach, intestines, and accessory organs.

FIGURE 21-6   Organ systems of the body.

(continued)

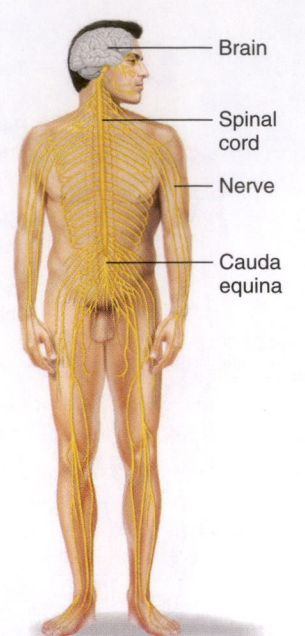

Nervous System

A major regulatory system that detects sensations and controls movements, physiologic processes, and intellectual functions. Consists of the brain, spinal cord, nerves, and sensory receptors.

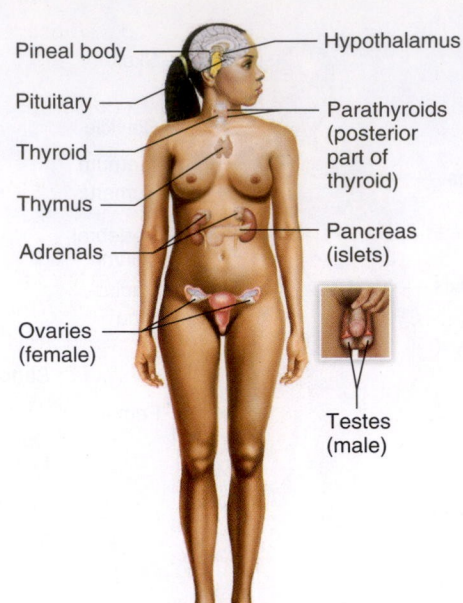

Endocrine System

A major regulatory system that influences metabolism, growth, reproduction, and many other functions. Consists of glands, such as the pituitary, that secrete hormones.

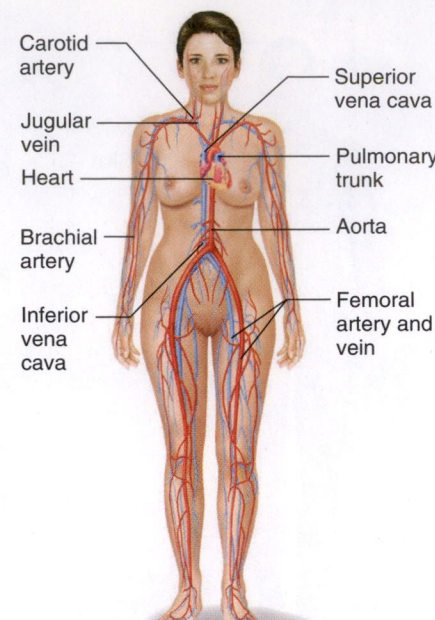

Cardiovascular System

Transports nutrients, waste products, gases, and hormones throughout the body; plays a role in the immune response and the regulation of body temperature. Consists of the heart, blood vessels, and blood.

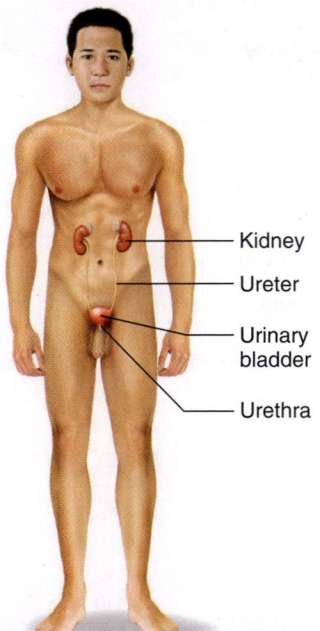

Urinary System

Removes waste products from the blood and regulates blood pH, ion balance, and water balance. Consists of the kidneys, urinary bladder, and ducts that carry urine.

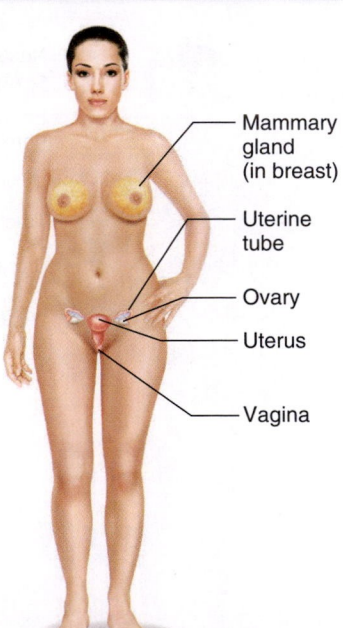

Female Reproductive System

Produces oocytes and is the site of fertilization and fetal development; produces milk for the newborn; produces hormones that influence sexual function and behaviors. Consists of the ovaries, vagina, uterus, mammary glands, and associated structures.

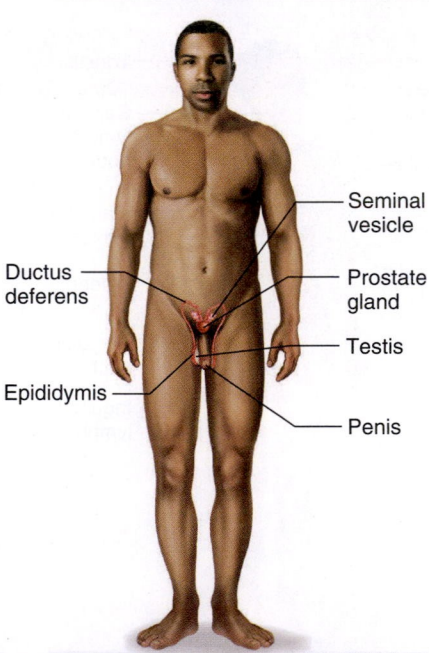

Male Reproductive System

Produces and transfers sperm cells to the female and produces hormones that influence sexual functions and behaviors. Consists of the testes, accessory structures, ducts, and penis.

FIGURE 21-6 Organ systems of the body.

► Understanding Medical Terminology

LO 21.5

Unlike the English language, in which word meanings often seem to have no rhyme or reason—like the overly used "whatever" and various difficult-to-translate modern slang—medical terminology often can be broken down into word parts that make the meaning concrete and easy to understand. All medical terms must have a **word root** that contains the base meaning for the term and a **suffix** at the end of the term that alters the word root's meaning. In the term *appendectomy,* for example, the word root *append* refers to the appendix and is combined with the suffix *-ectomy,* which means "surgical removal." So *appendectomy* means "surgical removal of the appendix." The word parts' meanings stay consistent, making it easier to learn new terms containing already understood word parts. Using your new knowledge, if you are told that the word root *hyster* means "uterus," you can easily see that *hysterectomy* means "surgical removal of the uterus."

In addition to word roots and suffixes, some terms also contain a **prefix,** which comes at the beginning of the term and, like the suffix, alters the term's meaning. Let's take the terms *premenstrual* and *postmenstrual.* In defining terms, the general rule is to start with the suffix, then add the prefix (if present), and finally the word root(s)—for example,

- The suffix *-al* means "pertaining to."
- The prefix *pre-* means "before."
- The prefix *post-* means "after."

The word root *menstru* refers to the menstrual period. Putting them together, *premenstrual* means "pertaining to *before* the menstrual period" and *postmenstrual* is "pertaining to *after* the menstrual period."

For terms in which the suffix begins with a consonant, a combining vowel—often an "o"—is used between the word root and the suffix to ease pronunciation. An example of this is the term *tracheotomy.* The word root *trache* ("windpipe") is joined to the suffix *-tomy* ("to cut into"). The letter "o" is inserted between the two to make pronunciation easier. Unlike prefixes and suffixes, combining vowels do not change the meaning of the term. Appendix I contains commonly used word roots, suffixes, and prefixes. Table 21-1 summarizes information on understanding medical terminology.

► Anatomical Terminology

LO 21.6

Anatomical terms describe the locations of body parts and various body regions. To correctly use these terms, it is assumed that the body is in the anatomical position. For example, picture yourself in the **anatomical position:** Your body is standing upright and facing forward, and your arms are at your sides with the palms of your hands facing forward. Even if patients are lying down, for consistency and correct communication when you use anatomical terms, always refer to patients as if they were in the anatomical position. Anatomical position is pictured later in this chapter.

TABLE 21-1	Understanding Medical Terminology		
Word Part	**Description**	**Term Using Word Part**	**Term Meaning**
Word root	Base meaning of the term	Colostomy	Colo = colon; -stomy = to cut (or create) a new opening colostomy: to cut a new opening for the colon
Suffix	Ending of term; alters meaning of the word root	Cardiology	Cardi = heart; -logy = knowledge of cardiology: knowledge (specialty) of the heart (with the combining vowel "o" between the two to ease pronunciation)
Prefix	Beginning of the term; alters the meaning of the word root	Tachycardia	Tachy- = rapid; cardi = heart; -ia = condition of tachycardia: condition of rapid heart (beat)
Combining vowel	Placed between word root and suffix to ease pronunciation	Cardiologist	Cardi = heart; o = combining vowel to ease pronunciation; -logist = specialist in knowledge of cardiology: specialist in the knowledge of the heart

TABLE 21-2	Directional Anatomical Terms	
Term	**Definition**	**Example**
Superior (cranial)	Above or close to the head	The thoracic cavity is superior to the abdominal cavity.
Inferior (caudal)	Below or close to the feet	The neck is inferior to the head.
Anterior (ventral)	Toward the front of the body	The nose is anterior to the ears.
Posterior (dorsal)	Toward the back of the body	The brain is posterior to the eyes.
Medial	Close to the midline of the body	The nose is medial to the ears.
Lateral	Farther away from the midline of the body	The ears are lateral to the nose.
Proximal	Close to a point of attachment or to the trunk of the body	The knee is proximal to the toes.
Distal	Farther away from a point of attachment or from the trunk of the body	The fingers are distal to the elbow.
Superficial	Close to the surface of the body	Skin is superficial to muscles.
Deep	More internal	Bones are deep to skin.

Directional Anatomical Terms

The directional anatomical terms that identify the position of body structures compared to other body structures are *superior* (*cranial*), *inferior* (*caudal*), *anterior* (*ventral*), *posterior* (*dorsal*), *medial, lateral, proximal, distal, superficial,* and *deep.* For example, the eyes are medial to the ears but lateral to the nose. See Table 21-2 and Figure 21-7 for an explanation and illustration of these important directional terms.

Anatomical Terms That Describe Body Sections

Sometimes in order to study internal body parts, it helps to imagine the body as being divided into sections. Medical professionals often use the following terms to describe how the body is divided into sections:

- A *sagittal plane* divides the body into left and right portions.
- A *midsagittal plane* runs lengthwise down the midline of the body and divides it into equal left and right halves.

- A *transverse plane* divides the body into superior (upper) and inferior (lower) portions.
- A *frontal,* or *coronal,* plane divides the body into anterior (frontal) and posterior (rear) portions.

Figure 21-8 illustrates these planes.

Anatomical Terms That Describe Body Parts

Many other anatomical terms describe different regions or parts of the body. For example, the term *brachium* refers to the arm, and the term *femoral* refers to the thigh. Figure 21-9 illustrates anatomical position in (a) and many of the common anatomical terms that describe body parts.

▶ Body Cavities and Abdominal Regions LO 21.7

Body cavities house and protect the internal organs. The largest body cavities are the dorsal cavity and the ventral cavity. The dorsal cavity is divided into the cranial cavity (which

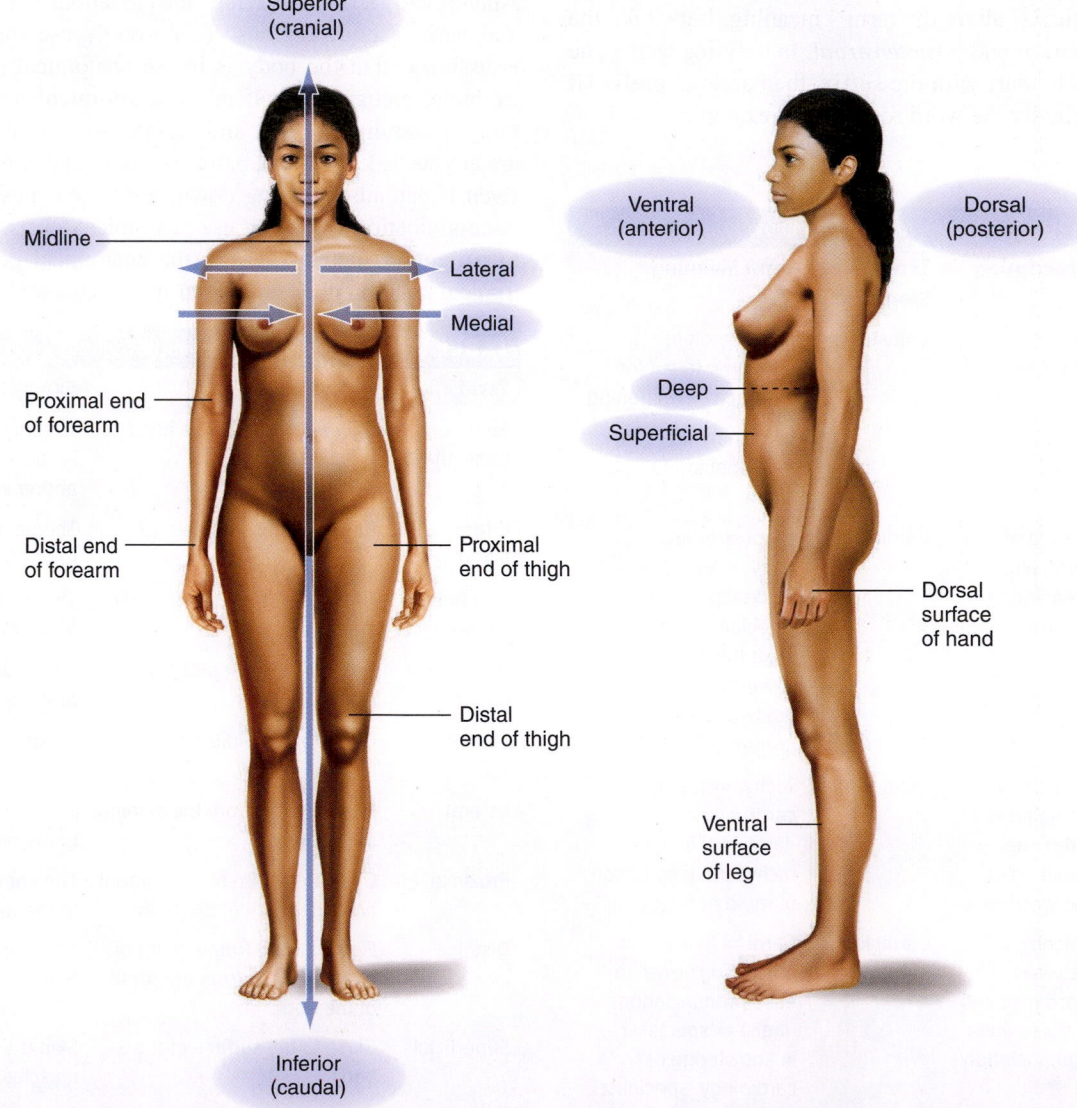

FIGURE 21-7 Directional terms provide mapping instructions for locating organs and body parts.

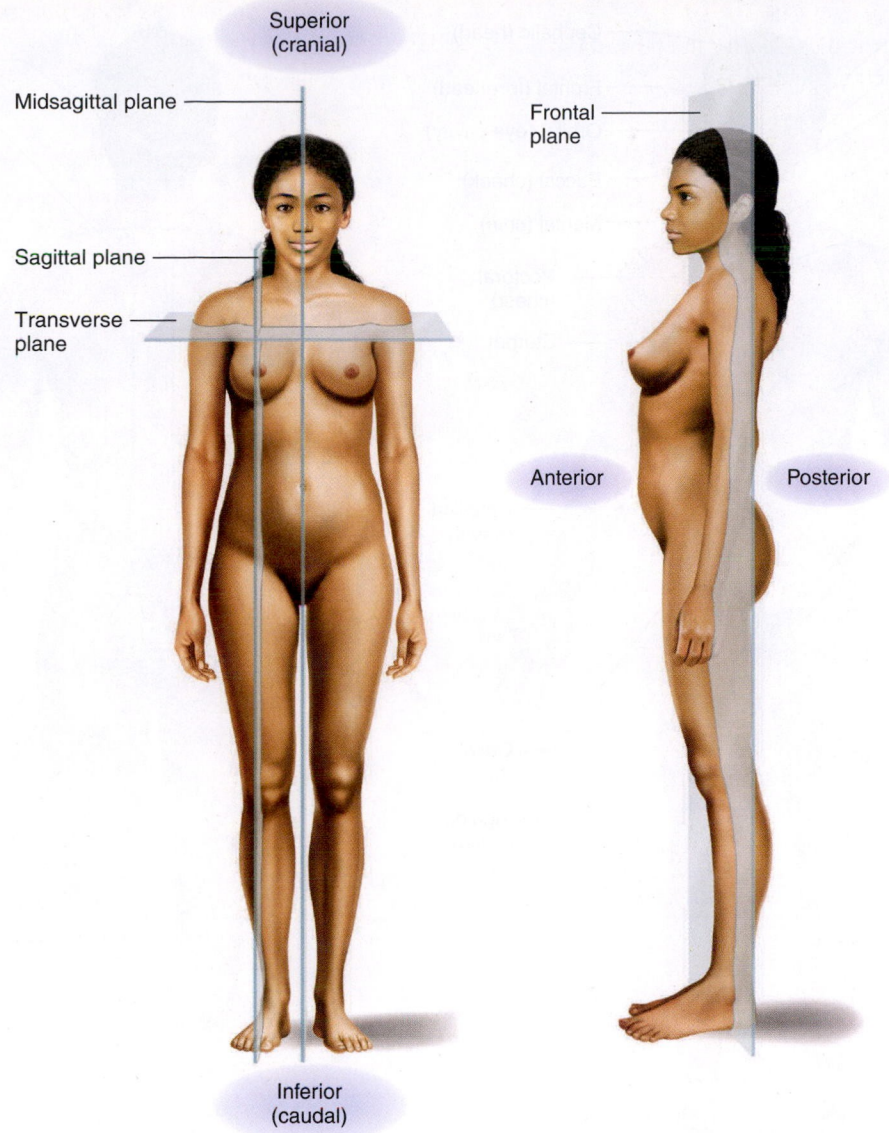

FIGURE 21-8   Spatial terms are based on imaginary cuts, or planes, through the body.

houses the brain) and the spinal cavity (which contains the spinal cord). The ventral cavity is divided into the thoracic cavity and the abdominopelvic cavity. The muscle called the *diaphragm* separates the thoracic and abdominopelvic cavities. The thoracic cavity contains the following:

- Lungs
- Heart
- Esophagus
- Trachea

The abdominopelvic cavity is divided into a superior abdominal cavity and an inferior pelvic cavity. It contains the following:

- Stomach
- Small and large intestines
- Gallbladder

- Liver
- Spleen
- Kidneys
- Pancreas

The bladder and internal reproductive organs are located in the pelvic cavity, which is depicted in Figure 21-10. The abdominal area is further divided into nine regions or four quadrants, which are illustrated in Figure 21-11.

▶ Chemistry of Life   LO 21.8

Now that you have studied how the body is organized structurally, you need to learn about its chemical structure. **Chemistry** is the study of what matter is made of and how it changes. It is important to have a basic understanding of chemistry when studying anatomy and physiology because

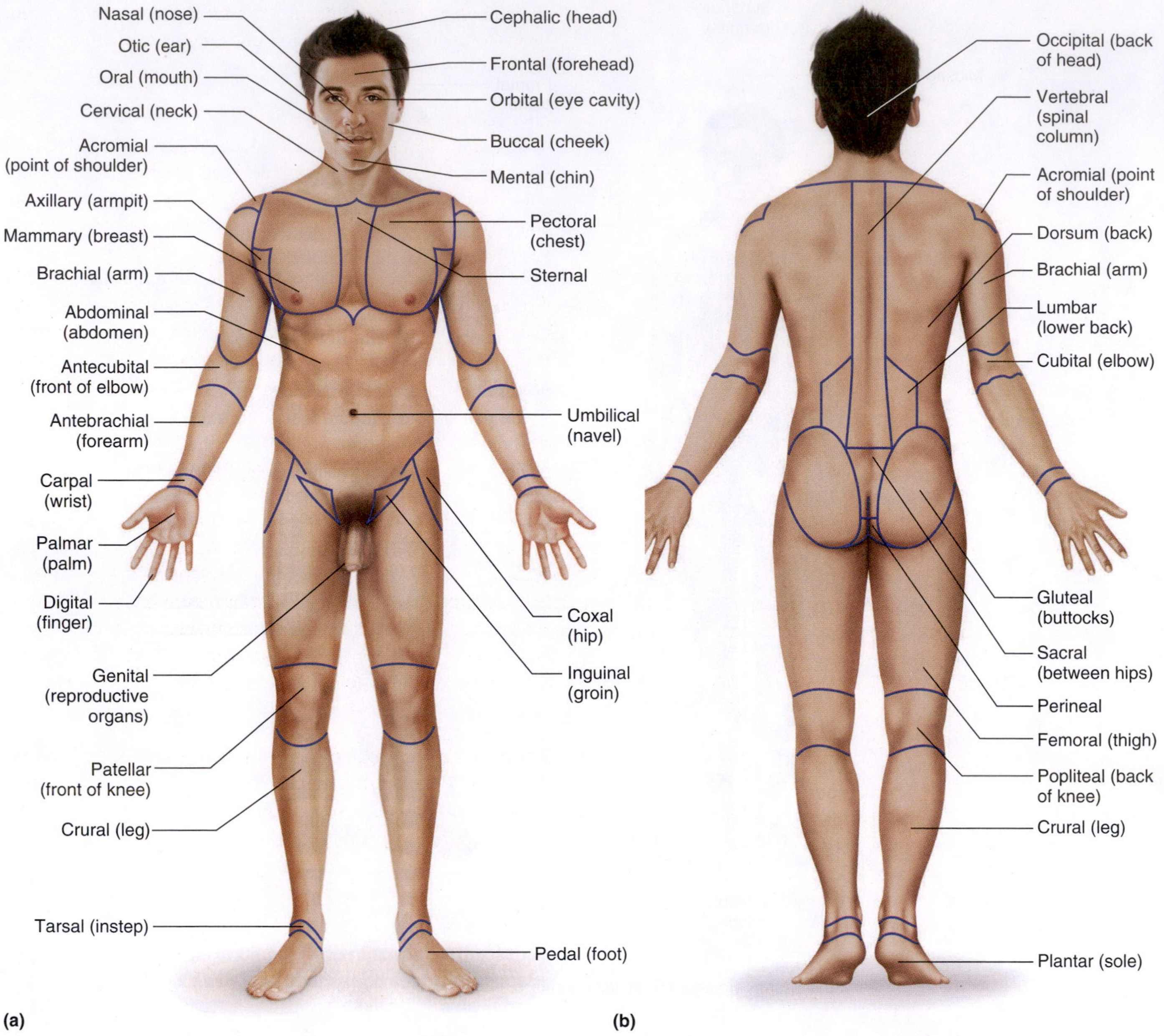

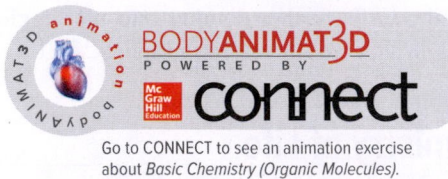

Labels (anterior view, a):
- Nasal (nose)
- Otic (ear)
- Oral (mouth)
- Cervical (neck)
- Acromial (point of shoulder)
- Axillary (armpit)
- Mammary (breast)
- Brachial (arm)
- Abdominal (abdomen)
- Antecubital (front of elbow)
- Antebrachial (forearm)
- Carpal (wrist)
- Palmar (palm)
- Digital (finger)
- Genital (reproductive organs)
- Patellar (front of knee)
- Crural (leg)
- Tarsal (instep)
- Cephalic (head)
- Frontal (forehead)
- Orbital (eye cavity)
- Buccal (cheek)
- Mental (chin)
- Pectoral (chest)
- Sternal
- Umbilical (navel)
- Coxal (hip)
- Inguinal (groin)
- Pedal (foot)

Labels (posterior view, b):
- Occipital (back of head)
- Vertebral (spinal column)
- Acromial (point of shoulder)
- Dorsum (back)
- Brachial (arm)
- Lumbar (lower back)
- Cubital (elbow)
- Gluteal (buttocks)
- Sacral (between hips)
- Perineal
- Femoral (thigh)
- Popliteal (back of knee)
- Crural (leg)
- Plantar (sole)

(a)   (b)

FIGURE 21-9 Numerous anatomical terms describe regions of the body: (a) anterior view and (b) posterior view.

body structures and functions result from chemical processes that occur within body cells and fluids.

BODY **ANIMAT3D**
POWERED BY
McGraw Hill Education **connect**

Go to CONNECT to see an animation exercise about *Basic Chemistry (Organic Molecules).*

As you learned earlier in the chapter, the chemical level is the lowest level of organization. The building blocks of every living organism are the same chemical elements that make up all matter, liquids, solids, and gases. When two or more atoms are chemically combined, a molecule is formed. A compound is formed when two or more atoms of different elements are combined. For example, a molecule of oxygen (O_2) is not a compound, because it is made up of only one element. In contrast, a water molecule is a compound, because it is made up of atoms of two different elements—two hydrogen atoms and one oxygen atom. Water is critical to both chemical and physical processes in human physiology, and it accounts for approximately two-thirds of a person's body weight.

Metabolism is the overall chemical functioning of the body. It is a series of life-sustaining processes, including the breakdown of food and its transformation into energy. The two processes of metabolism are anabolism and catabolism. In anabolism, small molecules combine to form larger ones

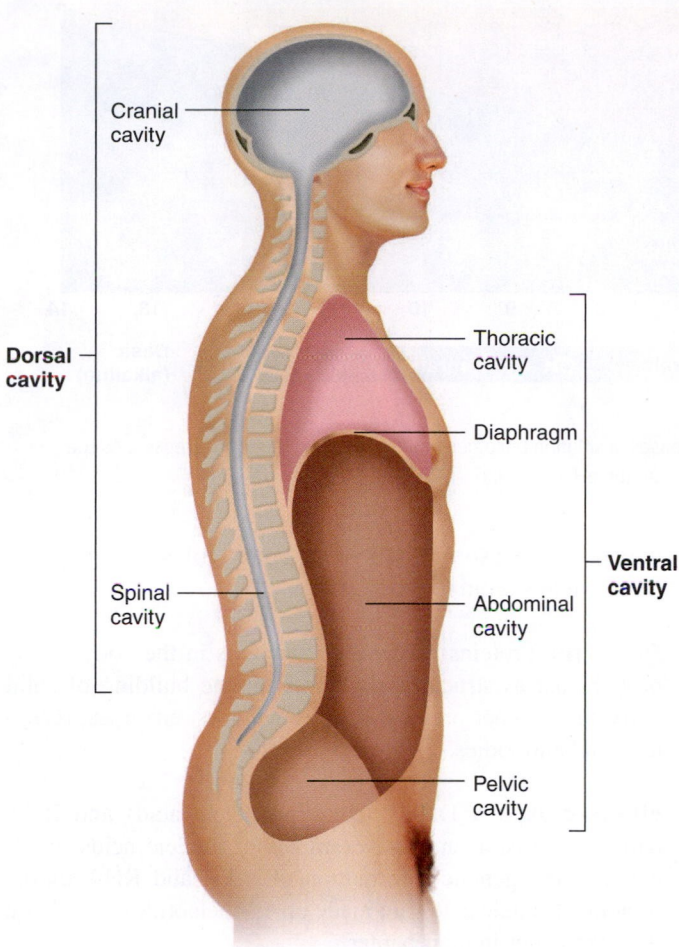

Cranial cavity

Dorsal cavity

Thoracic cavity

Diaphragm

Spinal cavity

Ventral cavity

Abdominal cavity

Pelvic cavity

FIGURE 21-10 The two main body cavities are dorsal and ventral.

(for example, when amino acids combine to form proteins). In catabolism, larger molecules are broken down into smaller ones (for example, when stored glycogen is converted to glucose molecules for energy).

Electrolytes

When put into water, some substances release **ions,** which are either positively or negatively charged particles. These substances are called **electrolytes.** For example, when you put sodium chloride (NaCl) in water, it releases two electrolytes: the sodium ion (Na) and the chloride ion (Cl). Electrolytes are critical because the movements of ions into and out of body structures regulate or trigger many physiologic states and activities in the body. For example, electrolytes are essential to fluid balance, muscle contraction, and nerve impulse conduction. Exercising makes you sweat, causing fluid and electrolyte loss. Drinking a sports drink after exercising helps you maintain fluid balance because sports drinks contain water and electrolytes such as sodium and potassium.

Acids and Bases Acids are substances that release hydrogen ions (H^+) in water. Many acids, such as lemon juice and vinegar, have a sour taste. Bases are substances that release hydroxyl ions (OH^-) in water. A basic substance may also be referred to as an alkali. Many basic substances are slippery and bitter to the taste. Laundry detergents, bleach, dish soaps, and many other household cleaning agents are examples of basic substances.

Testing Acids and Bases In the clinical setting, litmus paper, liquid pH indicator test kits, or a pH meter is often used to determine if a substance is acidic or basic. An acidic

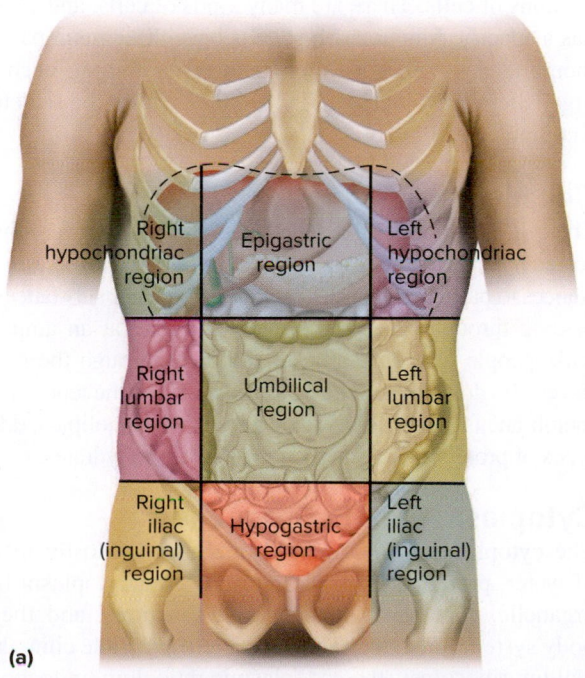

Right hypochondriac region

Epigastric region

Left hypochondriac region

Right lumbar region

Umbilical region

Left lumbar region

Right iliac (inguinal) region

Hypogastric region

Left iliac (inguinal) region

(a)

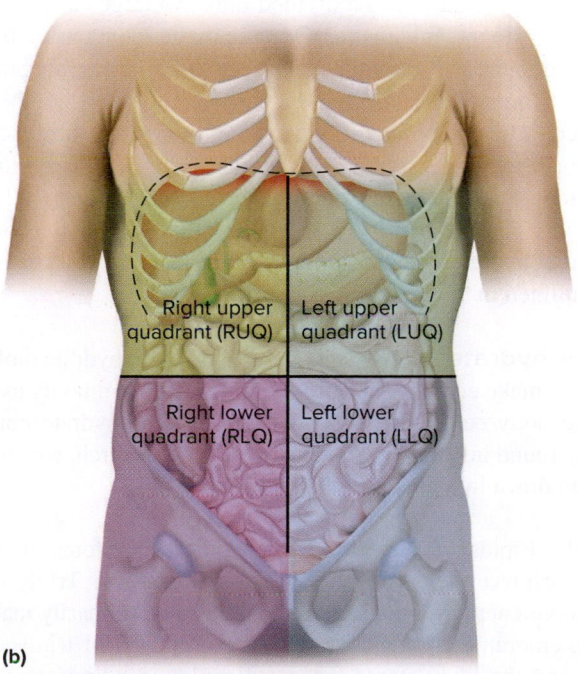

Right upper quadrant (RUQ)

Left upper quadrant (LUQ)

Right lower quadrant (RLQ)

Left lower quadrant (LLQ)

(b)

FIGURE 21-11 (a) The abdominal area divided into nine regions and (b) the abdominal area divided into four quadrants.

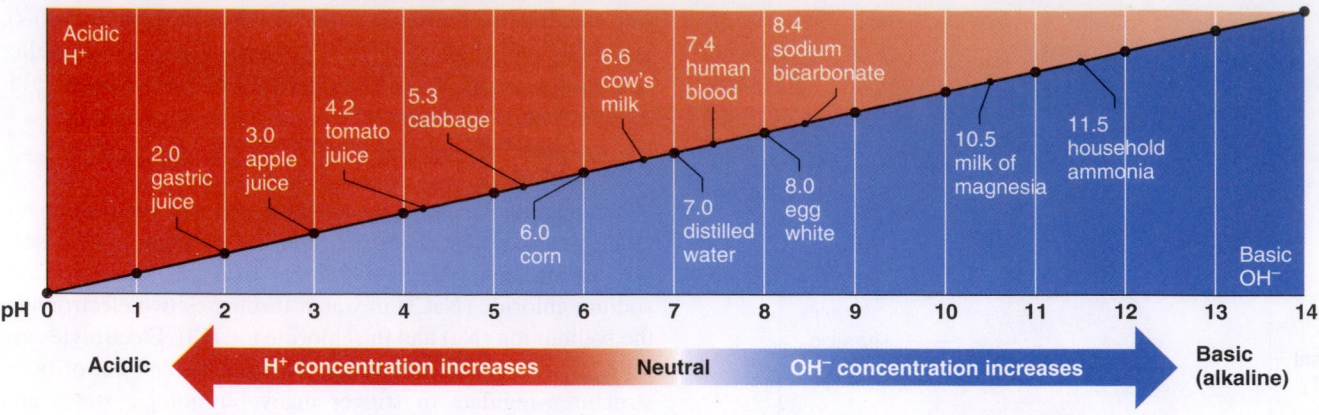

FIGURE 21-12 pH scale. As the concentration of hydrogen ions (H^+) increases, a solution becomes more acidic, and the pH decreases. As the concentration of hydroxl ions (OH^-) increases, a solution becomes more basic and the pH increases.

substance will turn blue litmus paper red, and a basic substance will turn red litmus paper blue. The pH scale runs from 0 to 14. If a solution has a pH of 7, the solution is neutral, which means it is neither acidic nor basic. If a solution has a pH less than 7, the solution is acidic. If a solution has a pH greater than 7, it is basic, or alkaline. The more acidic a solution is, the higher the concentration of hydrogen ions it contains. The pH values of some common substances are shown in Figure 21-12.

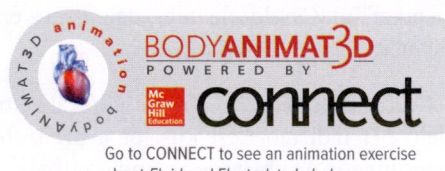

Go to CONNECT to see an animation exercise about *Fluid and Electrolyte Imbalances.*

Biochemistry

Biochemistry is the study of matter and chemical reactions in the body. Matter can be divided into two large categories: organic and inorganic matter. Organic matter contains carbon and hydrogen, and its molecules tend to be large. Inorganic matter generally does not contain carbon and hydrogen; these molecules tend to be small. Examples of inorganic substances are water, oxygen, carbon dioxide, and salts such as sodium chloride. Water is the most abundant inorganic compound in the body. The four major classes of organic matter in the body are carbohydrates, lipids, proteins, and nucleic acids. These are outlined in the following sections.

Carbohydrates Body cells depend on carbohydrate molecules to make energy. The carbohydrate most commonly used by the body cells is glucose. A type of carbohydrate commonly found in potatoes, pastas, and breads is starch, which is broken down into glucose when needed.

Lipids Lipids are fats. Three types of lipids are found in the body: triglycerides, phospholipids, and steroids. Triglycerides store energy for cells, and phospholipids primarily make cell membranes. Butter and oils are composed of triglycerides, and the body stores these molecules in adipose tissue (fat). Steroids are very large lipid molecules that make cell

membranes and some hormones. Cholesterol is an example of an essential steroid for body cells.

Proteins Proteins have many functions in the body. Many proteins act as structural materials for the building of solid body parts. Other proteins act as hormones, enzymes, receptors, and antibodies.

Nucleic Acids DNA (deoxyribonucleic acid) and RNA (ribonucleic acid) are two examples of nucleic acids. DNA contains the genetic information of cells, and RNA makes proteins. Nucleic acids are made up of nucleotides, which are discussed later in this chapter.

▶ Cell Characteristics   LO 21.9

Chemicals react to form the complex substances that make up cells, the basic unit of life. The human body is composed of millions of cells. There are many kinds of cells, and each type has a specific function. Most cells have three main parts: cell membrane, cytoplasm (liquid matrix containing each cell's organelles), and nucleus. Figure 21-13 shows the structure of a composite cell.

Cell Membrane

The cell membrane is the outer limit of a cell. It is very thin and selectively permeable, which means that it allows some substances to pass through it while preventing other substances from passing through. Think of a fence and gate at an amusement park; people who have a ticket can enter through the gate, but those who do not have a ticket are kept behind the fence. The cell membrane is composed of two layers of phospholipids, different types of proteins, cholesterol, and a few carbohydrates.

Cytoplasm and Its Organelles

The cytoplasm is the "inside" of the cell. Mostly made up of water, proteins, ions, and nutrients, the cytoplasm houses organelles that perform many cell functions, and therefore body system functions. These organelles include cilia, the flagellum, ribosomes, the endoplasmic reticulum, mitochondria, the Golgi apparatus, lysosomes, and centrioles.

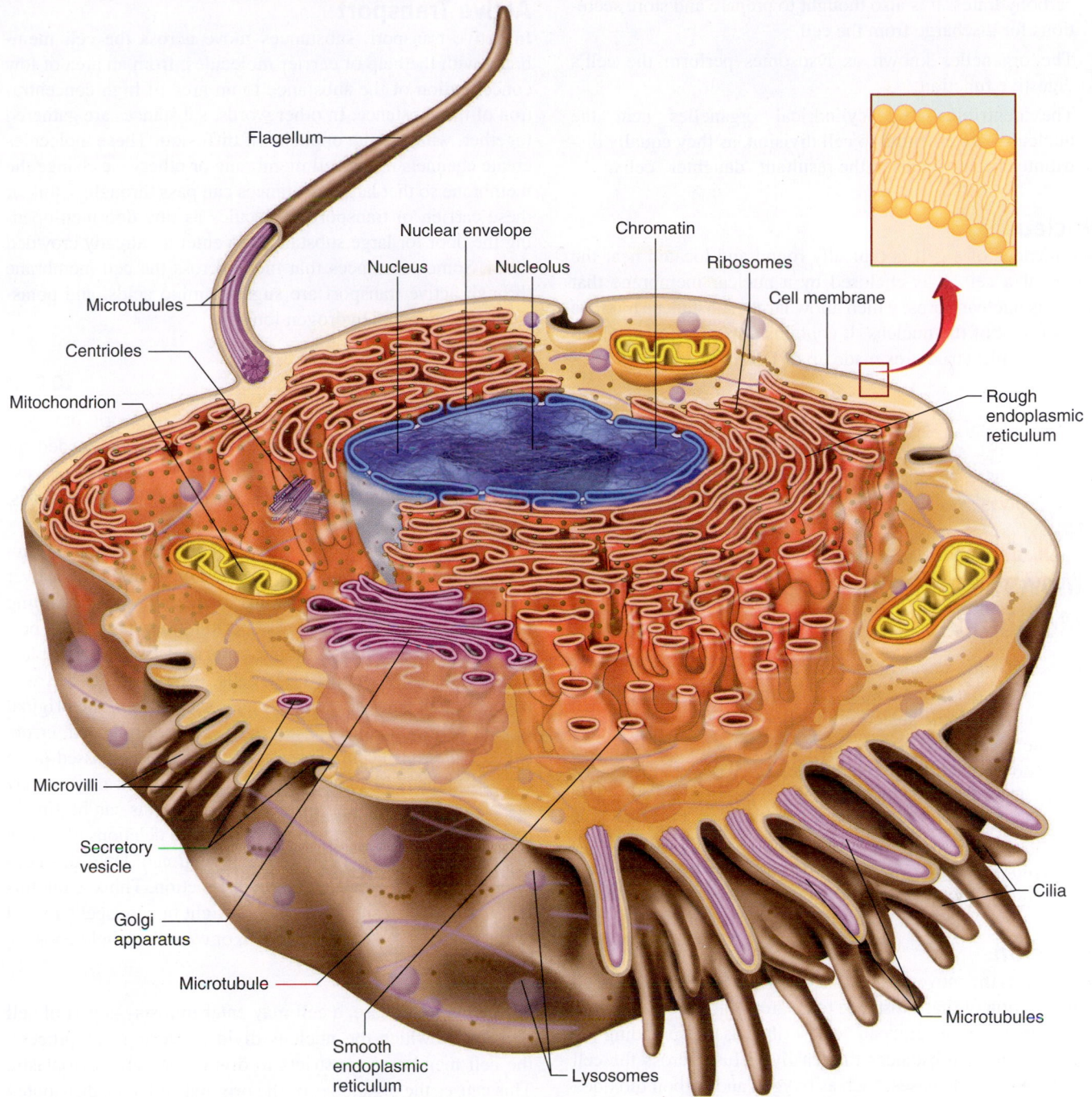

Flagellum

Microtubules

Centrioles

Mitochondrion

Nuclear envelope

Nucleus

Nucleolus

Chromatin

Ribosomes

Cell membrane

Rough
endoplasmic
reticulum

Microvilli

Secretory
vesicle

Golgi
apparatus

Microtubule

Smooth
endoplasmic
reticulum

Lysosomes

Cilia

Microtubules

FIGURE 21-13 A composite cell drawing showing the structures that are common to many cell types. Not all types of cells have all of these structures.

- Many cells contain hair-like projections on the outside of the cell membrane called *cilia*. Cilia assist with propelling matter throughout the body tracts, including the respiratory system. Cells with cilia are often found in the mucous membranes.

- A flagellum is a tail-like structure found on the human sperm cell and provides its "swimming" type of locomotion.

- Ribosomes, in conjunction with RNA molecules, are responsible for protein synthesis. Amino acids are connected together to form proteins through a specialized process involving different types of RNA molecules. The ribosome supports the protein chain as it is formed.

- The endoplasmic reticulum comes in two forms—smooth and rough. The rough endoplasmic reticulum is named for the presence of ribosomes on its surface, which give it a bumpy or rough appearance. Both types of endoplasmic reticulum form networks, or passageways, for transporting substances throughout the cytoplasm.

- Mitochondria—the centers for cell respiration—provide energy for the cell. There may be only one mitochondrion in a cell or many, depending on how much energy each cell type requires.

- The cell's Golgi apparatus is known to process and sort proteins from the ribosome and to synthesize or produce carbohydrates. It is also thought to prepare and store secretions for discharge from the cell.

- The organelles known as lysosomes perform the cell's digestive function.

- The centrioles—two cylindrical organelles near the nucleus—are essential to cell division, as they equally distribute chromosomes to the resultant "daughter" cells.

Nucleus

The nucleus of a cell is typically round and located near the center of a cell. It is enclosed by a nuclear membrane that contains nuclear pores, which allow larger substances to move into and out of the nucleus. It contains **chromosomes,** which are thread-like structures made up of DNA.

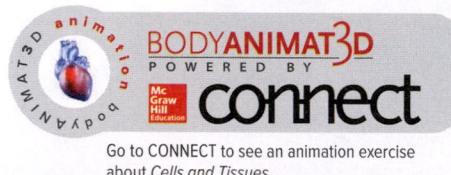

Go to CONNECT to see an animation exercise about *Cells and Tissues.*

▶ Movement Through Cell Membranes

LO 21.10

The selectively permeable cell membrane controls what moves into and out of a cell. Recall that selective permeability means there is some selection, or choice, in what substances cross the membrane. Some substances, such as oxygen and water, move across the cell membrane without the use of energy. These movements are called *passive mechanisms.* Sometimes the cell has to use energy to move a substance across its membrane in movements known as *active mechanisms.* Large molecules, such as glucose and proteins, move across the cell membrane by active transport.

Diffusion

Diffusion is the movement of a substance from an area of high concentration of that substance to an area of low concentration of the same substance; it can be described as the spreading out of a substance. Substances that easily diffuse across the cell membrane include gases, such as oxygen and carbon dioxide.

Osmosis

Osmosis is the diffusion, or movement, of water across a semi-permeable membrane, such as a cell membrane. A semipermeable membrane lets water and other solvent liquids through but nothing else. Remember, water will always try to diffuse toward the higher concentration of solutes (solids in solution).

Filtration

In filtration, some type of pressure, such as gravity or blood pressure, forces substances across a membrane that acts as a filter. Filtration separates substances in solutions. For example, you could separate sand from water by pouring the sand/water mixture through a filter. In the body, capillaries in the kidneys act as filters to separate the components of blood.

Active Transport

In active transport, substances move across the cell membrane with the help of carrier molecules, from an area of low concentration of the substance to an area of high concentration of the substance. In other words, substances are gathered together, which is the opposite of diffusion. These molecules create channels in the cell membrane or otherwise change the membrane so that large substances can pass through. Think of these carrier, or transport, molecules as tiny doormen opening the door for large substances to enter an already crowded room. Some substances that move across the cell membrane through active transport are sugars, amino acids, and potassium, calcium, and hydrogen ions.

▶ Cell Division

LO 21.11

Cells can become damaged, diseased, or worn out, and replacements must be made. Also, new cells are needed for normal growth. Cells reproduce by cell division, a process that involves splitting the nucleus, through **mitosis** or **meiosis,** and splitting the cytoplasm, called **cytokinesis.**

A cell that carries out its normal daily functions and is not dividing is said to be in *interphase.* For example, if a liver cell is in interphase, it is making liver enzymes, detoxifying blood, and processing nutrients. During interphase, a cell prepares for cell division by duplicating its DNA and cytoplasmic organelles. For most body cells, each daughter cell will have an exact copy of the DNA and organelles in the original mother cell. Sometimes when the DNA is duplicated, errors called *mutations* occur. These mutations will be passed on to the descendants (daughter cells) of that cell and may or may not affect the cells in harmful ways. Mutations can be simple changes in the DNA sequence or complete deletions of a gene or part of a gene. A **gene** is a discrete section of DNA that contains a code for a specific protein or function. Think about this book as a gene; a simple mutation might be a mispelled word or the loss of a sentence, a chapter, or even the whole book.

Mitosis

Following interphase, a cell may enter mitosis—a part of cell division in which the nucleus divides. During this process, the cell membrane constricts to divide the cell's cytoplasm. This causes the organelles of the original cell to be distributed almost evenly into the two new cells. The stages of mitosis are listed here and pictured in Figure 21-14.

- *Prophase* occurs when the centrioles that have replicated just prior to the onset of mitosis move to opposite ends of the cell. As they separate, they create spindle fibers between them.

- During *metaphase,* the chromosomes line up in the middle of the cell between the centrioles on these spindle fibers.

- During *anaphase,* the centromeres divide, pulling the chromatids (now chromosomes) toward the centrioles at opposite sides of the cell.

- The final stage is called *telophase.* As the chromosomes reach the centrioles, each with its complete set, cytokinesis, or division of the cytoplasm, takes place and mitosis is complete.

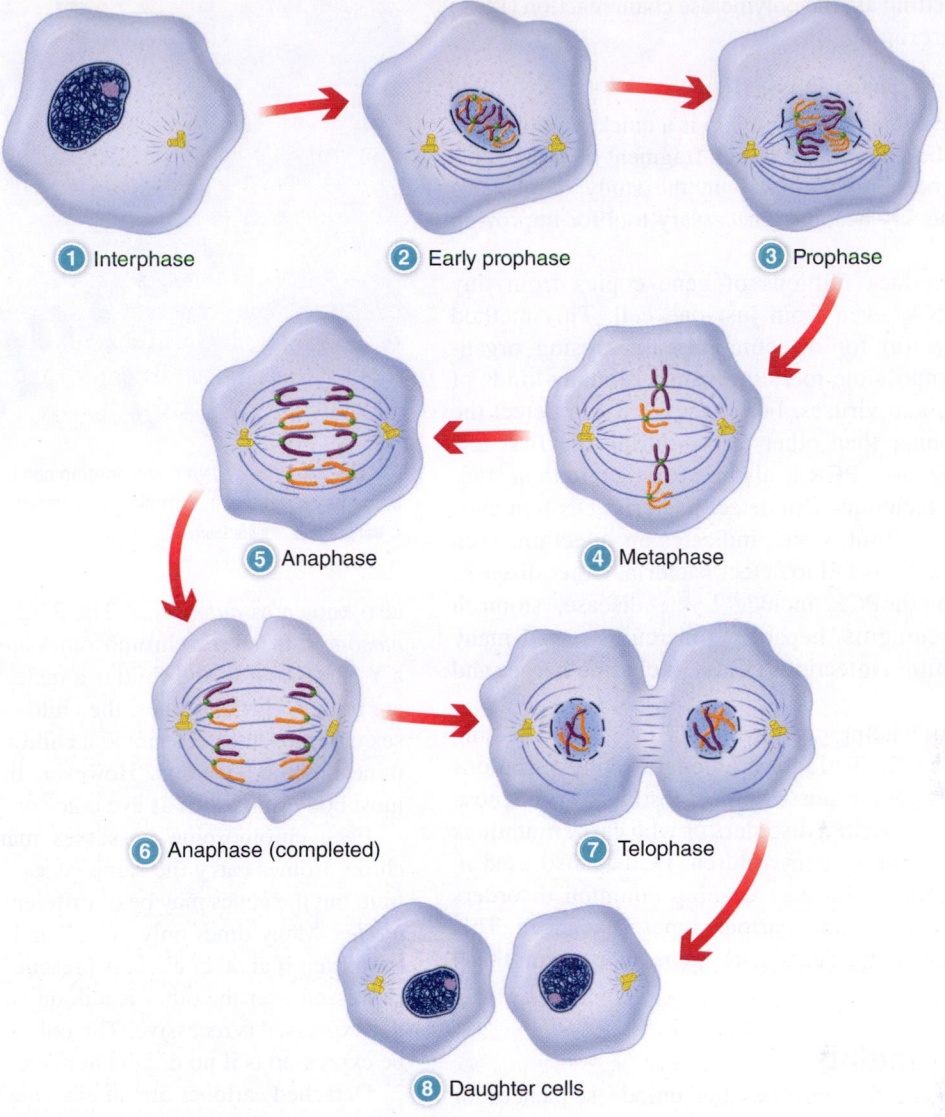

1. Interphase 2. Early prophase 3. Prophase

5. Anaphase 4. Metaphase

6. Anaphase (completed) 7. Telophase

8. Daughter cells

FIGURE 21-14   Cell mitosis.

Remember, during mitosis, the nucleus makes a complete copy of all 23 of its chromosome pairs (46 chromosomes altogether). As the cell divides, each new cell receives a complete set of chromosome pairs. The resulting cells are identical to each other.

Meiosis

Meiosis is reproductive cell division. It takes place only in the reproductive organs when the male and female sex cells are formed. During meiosis, the nucleus copies all 23 chromosome pairs, but two divisions take place. The four cells that are formed each contain only one of each chromosome pair, for a total of 23 chromosomes. This type of cell division must occur so that when the sex cells combine during fertilization, the resulting cell contains the usual number of chromosomes (46).

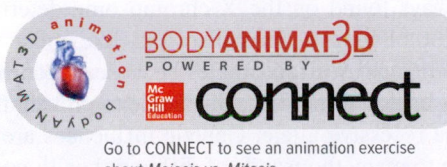

Go to CONNECT to see an animation exercise about *Meiosis vs. Mitosis.*

▶ Genetic Techniques   LO 21.12

DNA is the primary component of genes and is found in the nucleus of most cells within the body. As mentioned earlier in the chapter, a gene is a section of DNA that contains the code for a specific protein or function. Genetic techniques involve using or manipulating genes.

The chemical structure of every person's DNA is the same. The unique sequence of the *nucleotides* (groups of molecules that form the basic unit of DNA) determines an individual's characteristics. As an illustration, take the statement "my cat has blue eyes." Think of each letter as one nucleotide. If you change the letter "c" in the statement to an "r" you have an entirely different statement: "my rat has blue eyes." Many genetic differences—excessively large muscles in sheep, for instance—are caused by changes in just a few nucleotides. One DNA molecule contains hundreds or thousands of genes. Each gene occupies a particular location on the DNA molecule, making it possible to compare the same gene in a number of different samples. Two widely used genetic techniques in the clinical setting are the polymerase chain reaction (PCR) and DNA fingerprinting.

Polymerase Chain Reaction

The polymerase chain reaction (PCR) is a quick, easy method for making millions of copies of any fragment of DNA. This technique has been revolutionary in the study of genetics and has very quickly become a necessary tool for improving human health.

PCR can produce millions of gene copies from tiny amounts of DNA, even from just one cell. This method is especially useful for detecting disease-causing organisms that are impossible to culture, such as many kinds of bacteria, fungi, and viruses. For example, it can detect the AIDS virus sooner than other tests—during the first few weeks after infection. PCR is also more accurate than standard tests. The technique can detect bacterial DNA in children's middle ear fluid, which indicates an infection, even when culture methods fail to detect bacteria. Other diseases diagnosed through PCR include Lyme disease, stomach ulcers, viral meningitis, hepatitis, tuberculosis, and many sexually transmitted infections (STIs), including herpes and chlamydia.

PCR is also leading to new kinds of genetic testing because it can easily distinguish among the tiny variations in DNA that all people possess. This testing can diagnose people who have inherited disorders or who carry mutations that could be passed to their children. PCR is also used in tests that determine who may develop common disorders such as heart disease and various types of cancer. This knowledge helps individuals take steps to prevent those diseases.

DNA Fingerprinting

A DNA "fingerprint" comprises the unique sequences of nucleotides in a person's DNA and is the same for every cell, tissue, and organ of that person. Consequently, DNA fingerprinting is a reliable method for identifying and distinguishing among human beings to establish paternity and identify suspects in criminal cases (see Figure 21-15).

It is also used to diagnose genetic disorders such as cystic fibrosis, hemophilia, Huntington's disease, familial Alzheimer's, sickle cell anemia, thalassemia, and many others. Detecting genetic diseases early, or in utero, allows patients and medical staff to prepare for proper treatment. Researchers also use this information to identify DNA patterns associated with genetic diseases.

▶ Heredity and Common Genetic Disorders
LO 21.13

Heredity is the transfer of genetic traits from parent to child. When a sperm cell and an ovum (egg) unite, a cell called a *zygote* forms. The zygote has 46 chromosomes, or 23 chromosomal pairs. One half of each pair comes from the sperm, and the other half from the ovum. The first 22 pairs, which are the same size and shape, are called *homologous chromosomes,*

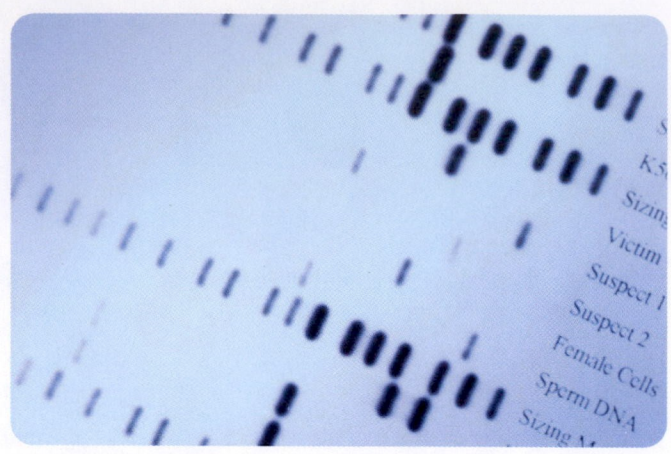

FIGURE 21-15 DNA fingerprinting can be used to establish paternity or identify a suspect in a criminal investigation.
© Martin Shields/Science Source

also known as *autosomes.* The 23rd pair are called *sex chromosomes.* If the sex chromosomes are an X chromosome and a Y chromosome, the child is a male. If the sex chromosomes are both X chromosomes, the child is a female. Although the sex chromosomes determine a child's gender, they also determine other body traits. However, the autosomes determine most body traits such as eye color or freckles.

Each chromosome possesses many genes. Homologous chromosomes carry the same genes that code for a particular trait, but the genes may be of different forms, which are called *alleles.* Many times only one allele is actually expressed as a trait, even if another allele is present. The allele that is always expressed over the other is a dominant allele. The one that is not expressed is recessive. The only way a recessive allele can be expressed is if no dominant allele is present.

Detached earlobes are an example of a trait determined by a dominant allele. If a child inherits a dominant allele for this trait from one parent but inherits the recessive allele from the other parent, the child will have detached earlobes. If the child inherits recessive alleles from both parents, then he or she will have attached earlobes. See Figure 21-16.

Most traits in the body are determined by multiple alleles. For example, hair color, height, skin tone, eye color, and body build are each determined by many different genes. *Complex inheritance* is the term that describes inherited traits that are determined by multiple genes. It explains why different children within the same family can have different characteristics.

Sex-linked traits are carried on the sex chromosomes, X and Y. The Y chromosome is much smaller than the X chromosome and does not carry many genes. So if the X chromosome carries a recessive allele, it is likely to be expressed because there is usually no corresponding allele on the Y chromosome. For example, the presence of a recessive allele that is always found on the X chromosome determines red-green color blindness. This disorder (like most sex-linked disorders) primarily affects males because the corresponding Y chromosome does not have any allele to prevent the expression of the recessive allele. Genetic influences are known to contribute to many thousands of different health conditions.

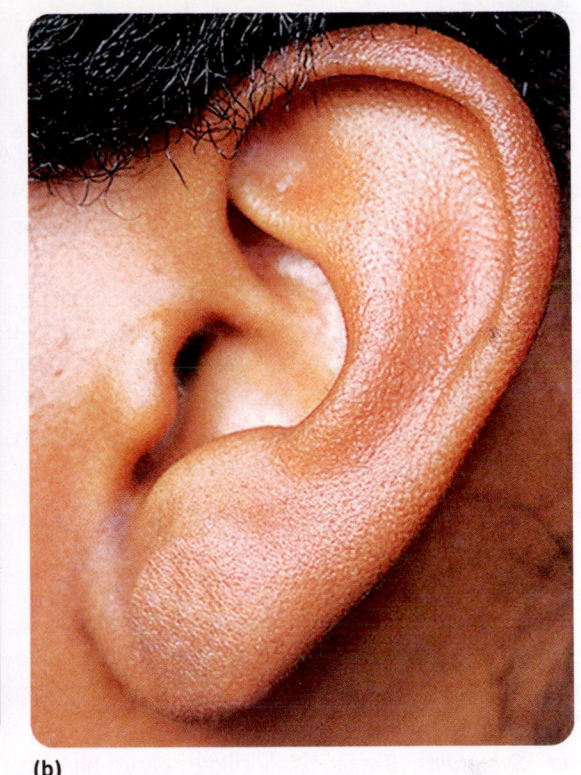

(a) (b)

FIGURE 21-16   Heredity determines whether your earlobes are (a) attached or (b) detached.
© McGraw-Hill Education/Joe DeGrandis, photographer

PATHOPHYSIOLOGY

Common Genetic Disorders

In addition to your understanding of the human body's anatomy and physiology, as a medical assistant it is very important to be able to recognize and comprehend the associated causes, characteristics, and available treatments of common genetic disorders. These genetic disorders, and their respective causes, signs and symptoms, and treatments are described here.

ALBINISM is a condition in which a person is born with little or no pigmentation in the skin, eyes, or hair. Albinism affects all races; in most cases there is no family history of it.

Causes. At least six different genes are involved with pigment production. This condition develops when a person inherits one or more faulty genes that do not produce the usual amounts of a pigment.

Signs and Symptoms. In addition to lack of pigment, people with the condition experience visual problems and sun-sensitive skin.

Treatment. Although there is no cure, treatments are available to help the symptoms. Prenatal testing for the condition is available.

CYSTIC FIBROSIS is a life-threatening disease that mainly affects the lungs and pancreas. This disease is one of the most common inherited life-threatening disorders among Caucasians in the United States.

Causes. Inheritance is autosomal recessive, so if both parents are carriers, there is a 25% chance that each child born to them will develop cystic fibrosis.

Signs and Symptoms. Patients with this disorder have increasing problems with breathing. Thick secretions eventually block passages in the airways, and these secretions may become infected.

Treatment. There is no cure, but treatments are available to help patients live with the complications associated with this disorder. Newborn babies are commonly screened for the disease because, the sooner treatment begins, the healthier the child can be. Parents are also commonly screened for the gene to determine the likelihood of having a child with cystic fibrosis.

DOWN SYNDOME, also called *trisomy 21,* is a disorder that causes intellectual disabilities and physical abnormalities.

Causes. This disorder occurs when a person has three copies of chromosome 21 instead of two. This condition can be diagnosed through prenatal tests such as amniocentesis. The risk of having a child with Down syndrome increases with the mother's age.

Signs and Symptoms. The signs of Down syndrome include a flat facial profile; a protruding tongue; oblique, slanting eyes; abundant neck skin; short, broad hands; and poor muscle tone. Heart, digestive, hearing, and visual problems are also common in people with this condition. Learning difficulties are common in Down syndrome and can range from moderate to severe.

Treatment. There is no cure, but support programs and the treatment of health problems allow many patients with Down syndrome to live a relatively normal life.

FRAGILE X SYNDROME is the most common inherited cause of learning disability. All races and ethnic groups seem to be affected equally by this syndrome.

Causes. In this disorder, one of the genes on the X chromosome is defective and makes the chromosome susceptible to breakage. This sex-linked disorder affects boys more severely than girls. It is estimated that approximately 1 in 300 females is a carrier for this disorder.

Signs and Symptoms. Mental impairment, learning disabilities, attention deficit disorder, a long face, large ears, and flat feet are some of the signs and symptoms. Fragile X syndrome can be easily diagnosed using prenatal tests such as amniocentesis.

Treatment. There is no cure, but some treatments and support groups are available to patients with this disorder.

HEMOPHILIA is a group of inheritable blood disorders. Each condition may be mild to severe.

Causes. In each type of hemophilia, an essential clotting factor is low or missing. Most types are X-linked recessive disorders; therefore, this disorder primarily affects males. Carriers of the gene can be identified with a blood test, and prenatal tests can diagnose the condition in the fetus.

Signs and Symptoms. Symptoms include easy bruising, spontaneous bleeding, and prolonged bleeding. Repeated bleeding in the joints leads to arthritis and permanent joint damage.

Treatment. Treatment includes injections of the missing clotting factors, often factor VIII.

KLINEFELTER SYNDROME is a chromosomal abnormality that affects males.

Causes. Males with this disorder have an extra X chromosome.

Signs and Symptoms. Tall stature, pear-shaped fat distribution, small testes, sparse body hair, and infertility are the most common signs and symptoms. Thyroid problems, diabetes, and osteoporosis are also common in patients with this syndrome.

Treatment. There is no cure, but treatments such as testosterone replacement therapy can decrease the risk of osteoporosis and produce more male characteristics.

PHENYLKETONURIA (PKU) develops if a person cannot synthesize the enzyme that converts phenylalanine to tyrosine. Phenylalanine is an essential amino acid, but too much of it can be harmful, so the body regularly converts it to tyrosine.

Causes. This condition is inherited as an autosomal recessive disorder.

Signs and Symptoms. If phenylalanine builds up in the blood, it can lead to irreversible damage to organs, including the brain.

Treatment. Phenylalanine is found in many proteins, so meats and other protein-rich foods must be avoided. Early detection of PKU is important to prevent developmental delays. There is no cure for PKU, but special diets allow a person to lead a normal life. Most newborns are tested for PKU, and prenatal diagnosis is available.

SUMMARY OF LEARNING OUTCOMES

LEARNING OUTCOMES	KEY POINTS
21.1 Explain the importance of understanding both anatomy and physiology when studying the body.	Knowledge of anatomy (the study of the body's structure) and physiology (the study of the body's function) is important when learning to assign diagnosis and procedure codes and perform clinical procedures. Since the structure of an organ is related to its function, it is necessary to learn both.
21.2 Illustrate body organization from simple to more complex levels.	The body organization levels from simplest to most complex are chemical, cellular, tissue, organ, organ system, and organism.
21.3 Describe the locations and characteristics of the four main tissue types.	Epithelial tissues cover body surfaces and line body cavities or are glandular tissues. Connective tissue contains a matrix between its cells. Muscle tissue is specialized tissue that contracts and relaxes; there are three types of muscle tissue. Nervous tissue sends signals to the neurons, muscles, and glands and is located in the brain, spinal cord, and nerves.
21.4 Describe the body organ systems, their general functions, and the major organs contained in each.	The body organ systems include integumentary, skeletal, muscular, lymphatic, respiratory, digestive, nervous, endocrine, cardiovascular, urinary, and reproductive systems. Each system has its particular set of organs and vessels.
21.5 Use medical and anatomical terminology correctly.	Knowledge and use of anatomical and medical terminology are important for medical personnel to communicate with each other in a consistent manner.

LEARNING OUTCOMES	KEY POINTS
21.6 **Explain anatomical position and its relationship to other anatomical positions.**	In anatomical position, the body is erect, facing forward with arms at the sides and palms facing forward. All other body positions are defined based on their relation to anatomical position.
21.7 **Identify the body cavities and the organs contained in each.**	The dorsal cavity consists of the cranial cavity, which contains the brain, and the spinal cavity, which contains the spinal cord. The ventral cavity is composed of the thoracic cavity, the abdominal cavities, and, below the abdominal cavity, the pelvic cavity. The body's organs are contained within these cavities.
21.8 **Relate a basic understanding of chemistry to its importance in studying the body.**	It is important to have a basic understanding of chemistry when studying anatomy and physiology because body structures and functions result from chemical processes that occur within body cells and fluids.
21.9 **Name the parts of a cell and their functions.**	The main components of a cell are cell membrane, cilia, flagellum (may be present), ribosomes, endoplasmic reticulum, mitochondria, Golgi apparatus, lysosomes, and centrioles. Each has its own specialized function in the life of a cell.
21.10 **Summarize how substances move across a cell membrane.**	Cells use both active and passive mechanisms to transport substances across the cell membrane. Passive mechanisms include diffusion, osmosis, and filtration. Active transport uses carrier molecules.
21.11 **Distinguish the stages of cell division.**	A cell at rest is said to be in interphase. During mitosis, prophase, metaphase, anaphase, and telophase occur. Reproductive cell division is known as meiosis and takes place only in the reproductive cells.
21.12 **Explain the uses of these genetic techniques: the polymerase chain reaction and DNA fingerprinting.**	Genetic techniques allow the identification of individuals through the unique sequences of nucleotides found within DNA. Polymerase chain reactions allow millions of copies from just a fragment of DNA. DNA fingerprinting is used in paternity testing and in identifying suspects in criminal cases.
21.13 **Describe the different patterns of inheritance and common genetic disorders.**	Dominant traits occur through alleles. If a dominant allele is received from a parent, the trait will appear in the child. Complex inheritance is more common and is determined by multiple genes given by both parents. Sex-linked traits are carried on the sex chromosomes.
21.14 **Describe the causes, signs and symptoms, and treatments of various genetic diseases and disorders.**	There are many genetic disorders including albinism, cystic fibrosis, Down syndrome, Fragile X-syndrome, hemophilia, Klinefelter syndrome, and phenylketonuria. They are caused by an abnormal chromosome from one or both parents. Treatment varies and is based upon the signs and symptoms since most of these disorders do not have a cure.

CASE STUDY CRITICAL THINKING

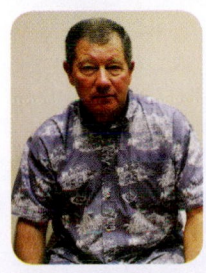

© McGraw-Hill Education

Recall John Miller from the beginning of the chapter. Now that you have completed the chapter, answer the following questions regarding his case.

1. What organs are found in the thoracic cavity?

2. What structure separates the thoracic and abdominopelvic cavities?

3. Mr. Miller's radiology report states that the X-ray views included an AP view. You ask the nurse practitioner what this means, and she states that the direction of the X-ray beam was from anterior to posterior. Describe, in lay terms, what that means.

1. (LO 21.3) Which of the following are characteristics of skeletal muscle?
   a. Smooth and voluntary
   b. Striated and involuntary
   c. Striated and voluntary
   d. Smooth and involuntary
   e. None of these

2. (LO 21.13) The clinical name for Down syndrome is
   a. Hemophilia
   b. Trisomy 21
   c. Klinefelter syndrome
   d. Fragile X syndrome
   e. Phenylketonuria

3. (LO 21.5) Which word part does not change the meaning of a medical term but aids in pronunciation?
   a. Word root
   b. Prefix
   c. Suffix
   d. Combining vowel
   e. All of these

4. (LO 21.7) Which abdominal region is named for its location under the stomach?
   a. Hypogastric
   b. Epigastric
   c. Hypochondriac
   d. Umbilical
   e. Iliac

5. (LO 21.8) Acids release which type of ion in water?
   a. Cl^-
   b. OH^-
   c. H^+
   d. Na^+
   e. K^+

6. (LO 21.9) Which of the following organelles is responsible for protein synthesis in the cell?
   a. Ribosome
   b. Nucleus
   c. Mitochondrion
   d. Golgi apparatus
   e. Centriole

7. (LO 21.6) Which plane divides the body into right and left portions?
   a. Transverse
   b. Lateral
   c. Sagittal
   d. Frontal
   e. Coronal

8. (LO 21.5) The medical term meaning "wrist" is
   a. Tarsal
   b. Palmar
   c. Radial
   d. Brachial
   e. Carpal

9. (LO 21.11) An error in DNA duplication is known as a(n)
   a. Mitosis
   b. Mutation
   c. Allele
   d. DNA fingerprint
   e. Chain reaction

10. (LO 21.6) The term meaning "close to the point of attachment" is
    a. Distal
    b. Superficial
    c. Medial
    d. Proximal
    e. Superior

M E D I C A L   T E R M I N O L O G Y   P R A C T I C E

Analyze the following medical terms, presented throughout the chapter. Using a medical dictionary (or Appendix I) place a / mark between each word part. Define each word part and then define the whole word.

EXAMPLE: **append/ectomy** = append means "appendix" + ectomy means "surgical removal"
APPENDECTOMY means "surgical removal of the appendix."

1. anterior
2. caudal
3. cranial
4. distal
5. dorsal
6. femoral
7. frontal
8. inferior
9. lateral
10. medial
11. midsagittal
12. posterior
13. proximal
14. sagittal
15. superficial
16. superior
17. transverse
18. ventral

The Integumentary System

PATIENT INFORMATION

Name	DOB	Allergies
Christopher Matthews	11/19/19XX	NKA

Attending	MRN	Other Information
Alexis N. Whalen, MD	324-95-786	Oldest child, one sister age 5, one brother age 6 mos. He is home-schooled by Mom.

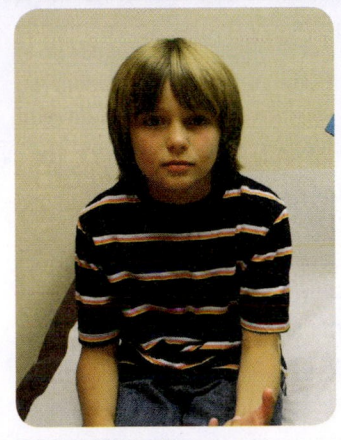

© McGraw-Hill Education

Chris is an existing patient, age 7. Dad brings him in today, stating that Chris has been complaining that his feet "hurt and itch." Dad adds as an aside that Chris has developed an "aversion" to soap and water and, even after showering, wears the same sneakers, often without socks, for days at a time. After taking both of them into the exam room and checking Chris's vital signs, you ask Chris to take off his sneakers. There is an obvious odor to his feet (and sneakers), although Chris states he showered just this morning. His feet, particularly his toes, are red, with cracking between the toes, and he is obviously uncomfortable, rubbing his bare feet together because "they itch like crazy."

Keep Chris in mind as you study this chapter. There will be questions at the end of the chapter based on the case study. The information in the chapter will help you answer these questions.

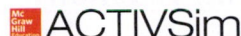

LEARNING OUTCOMES

After completing Chapter 22, you will be able to:

22.1 Describe the functions of skin.

22.2 Describe the layers of skin and the characteristics of each layer.

22.3 Explain the factors that affect skin color.

22.4 Summarize types of common skin lesions.

22.5 Describe the accessory organs of skin along with their structures and functions.

22.6 Explain the process of skin healing, including scar production.

22.7 Describe the common diseases and disorders of the skin.

KEY TERMS

alopecia
apocrine gland
arrector pili
dermis
eccrine gland
epidermis
follicle
hypodermis
keratin
keratinocyte

melanin
melanocyte
nail bed
oxygenated
sebaceous
sebum
stratum basale
stratum corneum
subcutaneous
sudoriferous

CAAHEP	ABHES

I.C.4 List major organs in each body system	**2. Anatomy & Physiology**
I.C.5 Identify the anatomical location of major organs in each body system	a. List all body systems, their structure and functions
I.C.6 Compare structure and function of the human body across the life span	b. Describe the common diseases, symptoms and etiologies as they apply to each system
I.C.7 Describe normal function of each body system	c. Identify diagnostic and treatment modalities as they relate to each body system
I.C.8 Identify common pathology related to each body system including:	**3. Medical Terminology**
(a) signs	a. Define and use entire basic structure of medical words and be able to accurately identify in the correct context, i.e. root, prefix, suffix, combinations, spelling, and definitions
(b) symptoms	
(c) etiology	
I.C.9 Analyze pathology for each body system including:	b. Build and dissect medical terms from roots/ suffixes to understand the word element combinations that create medical terminology
(a) diagnostic measures	
(b) treatment modalities	c. Apply various medical terms for each speciality
V.C.9 Identify medical terms labeling the word parts	d. Define and use medical abbreviations when appropriate and acceptable
V.C.10 Define medical terms and abbreviations related to all body systems	

▶ Introduction

The integumentary system consists of skin and its accessory organs. Skin is the body's outer covering and its largest organ. The accessory organs of skin are hair follicles, nails, and skin glands. Consider what you see of your own skin when you stand undressed facing a full-length mirror. In fact, pretty much everything you see in the reflection is either skin or its accessory organs. Your skin accounts for approximately 15% of your entire body weight.

▶ Functions of the Integumentary System

LO 22.1

People are often interested in the appearance of their skin—the color, the texture, the presence or absence of freckles, lines, wrinkles, puffiness, redness—but rarely consider its functions. The integumentary system serves many important purposes, including

- *Protection.* As long as skin is intact, it is the body's first line of defense against bacteria and viruses. It also protects underlying structures from ultraviolet (UV) radiation and dehydration.
- *Body temperature regulation.* Skin plays a major role in regulating body temperature. When a person is hot, dermal blood vessels dilate, which is why a person's skin becomes pinkish. Because the dermal blood vessels are dilated, more blood than normal passes through the skin. This is beneficial because blood carries a lot of the body's heat.

When the blood gets close to the body's surface (to skin), the heat can escape. On the other hand, if a person is cold, the dermal blood vessels constrict, preventing the heat in blood from escaping.

- *Vitamin D production.* When exposed to sunlight, the skin produces a molecule that is turned into vitamin D. The body needs vitamin D for calcium absorption.
- *Sensation.* The skin is packed with sensory receptors that can detect touch, heat, cold, and pain.
- *Excretion.* Small amounts of waste products, such as water and salts, are lost through skin when a person perspires. This is why hydration is so important when exercising or during exposure to high temperatures, as the amount of perspiration increases and higher amounts of water and salts are lost.

▶ Skin Structure

LO 22.2

The skin is a complex organ that consists of three layers. The **epidermis** (top layer) and the dermis (middle layer) sit on a third layer called the subcutaneous layer or hypodermis (see Figure 22-1).

Epidermis

The epidermis is the most superficial layer of skin. It is made up of many layers of tightly packed cells and can be divided into two major sublayers: the stratum corneum and the stratum basale.

The **stratum corneum** is the most superficial layer of the epidermis. Most of the cells in this layer are dead and very

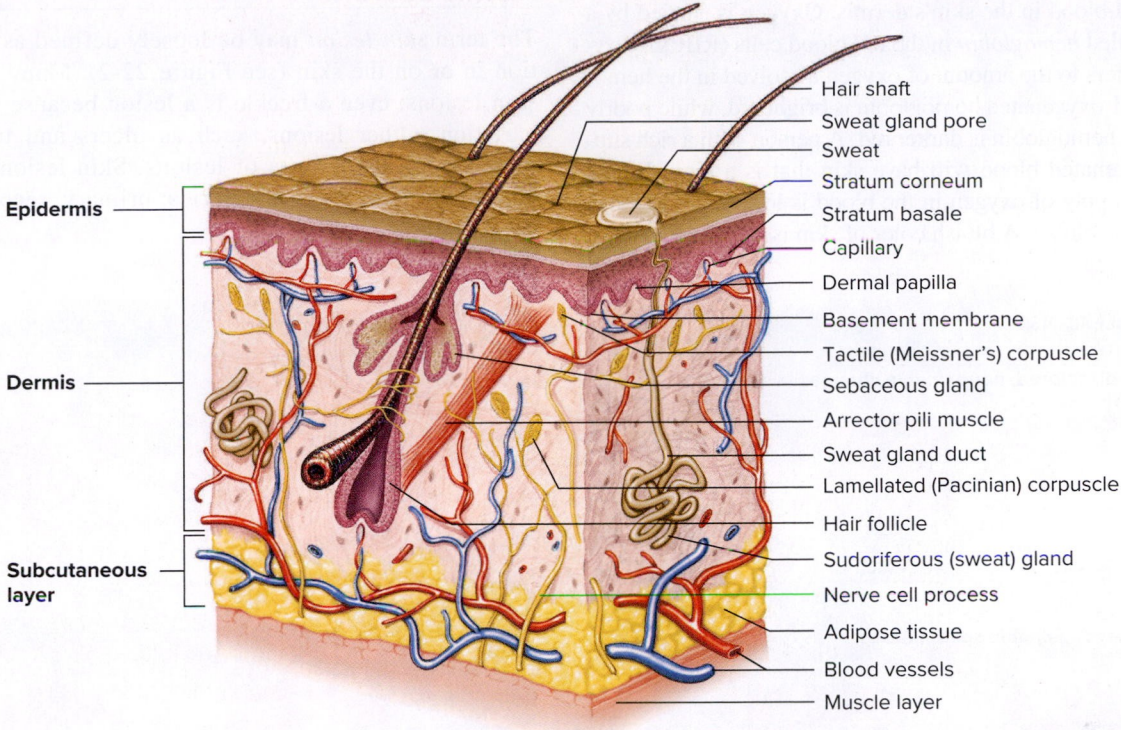

Epidermis

Dermis

Subcutaneous layer

Hair shaft
Sweat gland pore
Sweat
Stratum corneum
Stratum basale
Capillary
Dermal papilla
Basement membrane
Tactile (Meissner's) corpuscle
Sebaceous gland
Arrector pili muscle
Sweat gland duct
Lamellated (Pacinian) corpuscle
Hair follicle
Sudoriferous (sweat) gland
Nerve cell process
Adipose tissue
Blood vessels
Muscle layer

FIGURE 22-1 Section of skin.

flat. Because they have accumulated a tough protein called **keratin,** the cells in this layer stick together and form an impermeable layer for skin. Most bacteria, viruses, and water cannot penetrate the stratum corneum.

The **stratum basale,** also known as the *stratum germinativum,* is the deepest layer of the epidermis. The cells in this layer are constantly dividing (or germinating), which pushes older cells up toward the stratum corneum.

The most common cell type in the epidermis is the **keratinocyte.** This cell makes and accumulates keratin, which makes the epidermis waterproof and resistant to bacteria and viruses. Another cell type of the epidermis is the **melanocyte,** which makes the pigment **melanin.** Melanin is deposited throughout the layers of the epidermis. This pigment absorbs UV radiation from sunlight and prevents the radiation from harming structures in the skin's underlying layers.

Dermis

Lying below the epidermis is the dermis. The **dermis** is living tissue that binds the epidermal top layer to the underlying subcutaneous tissue layer. As living tissue, the dermal layer includes all major tissue types, as well as the following:

- Epithelial, connective, muscle, and nervous tissues
- Sudoriferous (sweat) glands
- Sebaceous (oil) glands
- Hair follicles
- The arrector pili muscles
- Collagen fibers, elastin fibers, nerve fibers, and many blood vessels

Subcutaneous Layer

The **subcutaneous** layer of skin, or **hypodermis,** is largely made up of adipose and loose connective tissue. This layer also contains blood vessels and nerves. The adipose, or fat, tissue acts as a storage facility. It also cushions and insulates the underlying structures and organs. The amount of adipose tissue varies from body region to body region, and from person to person.

▶ Skin Color   LO 22.3

The amount of melanin in the skin's epidermis is what most determines skin color. Melanin can range in color from yellowish to brownish. The more melanin a person has in the skin, the darker the skin color. All people have about the same number of melanocytes, regardless of skin color. What varies from person to person is how active the melanocytes are in producing melanin. For example, a person with dark skin has very active melanocytes. Sunlight, UV lamps, and X-rays stimulate melanin production. This is why your skin darkens when you go to a tanning bed or to the beach for the day. Patients undergoing radiation therapy often have tanned skin in the treatment area.

As you studied in the chapter *Organization of the Body,* your inherited characteristics come from your parents. So your skin color—meaning the activity of the melanocytes—is directly related to the genes you received from your parents. As the gene pool is varied between ethnic backgrounds, it is also varied within families, which explains the differences in skin color not only among races but also within families.

Another factor that determines skin color is the amount of **oxygenated** blood in the skin's dermis. Oxygen is carried by a pigment called *hemoglobin* in the red blood cells (RBCs). *Oxygenation* refers to the amount of oxygen dissolved in the hemoglobin. Well-oxygenated hemoglobin is bright red, while poorly oxygenated hemoglobin is darker red. A person with a rich supply of oxygenated blood will have skin that is a pinkish hue. When the supply of oxygen in the blood is low, the skin looks rather pale or bluish. A bluish color of skin is called *cyanosis*.

▶ Skin Lesions LO 22.4

The term *skin lesion* may be loosely defined as any variation in or on the skin (see Figure 22-2). Many of us have skin lesions; even a freckle is a lesion because it is a skin variation. Other lesions, such as ulcers and tumors, are more troublesome types of lesions. Skin lesions are classified into three major categories: primary, secondary, and vascular.

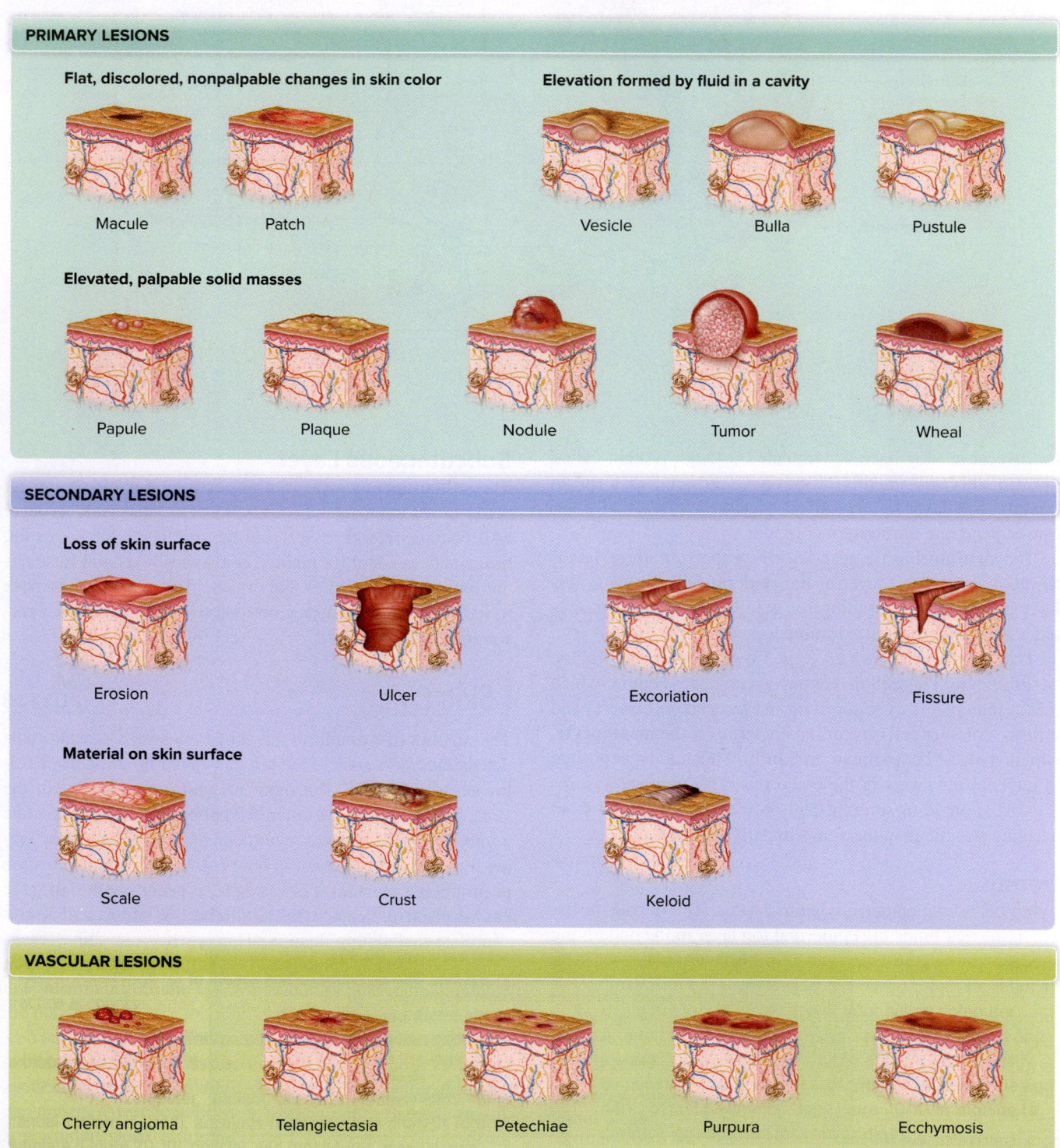

PRIMARY LESIONS

Flat, discolored, nonpalpable changes in skin color

Macule   Patch

Elevation formed by fluid in a cavity

Vesicle   Bulla   Pustule

Elevated, palpable solid masses

Papule   Plaque   Nodule   Tumor   Wheal

SECONDARY LESIONS

Loss of skin surface

Erosion   Ulcer   Excoriation   Fissure

Material on skin surface

Scale   Crust   Keloid

VASCULAR LESIONS

Cherry angioma   Telangiectasia   Petechiae   Purpura   Ecchymosis

FIGURE 22-2   Types of skin lesions.

TABLE 22-1	Common Skin Lesions and Descriptions
Lesion Name	**Description**
Bulla	A large blister or cluster of blisters
Cicatrix	A scar, usually inside a wound or tissue
Crust	Dried blood or pus on the skin
Ecchymosis	A black and blue mark, or bruise
Erosion	A shallow area of skin worn away by friction or pressure
Excoriation	A scratch; may be covered with dried blood
Fissure	A crack in the skin's surface
Keloid	An overgrowth of scar tissue
Macule	A flat skin discoloration, such as a freckle or a flat mole
Nodule	A large pimple or small node (larger than 6 cm)
Papule	An elevated mass similar to but smaller than a nodule
Petechiae	Pinpoint skin hemorrhages that result from bleeding disorders
Plaque	A small, flat, scaly area of skin
Purpura	Purple-red bruises, usually the result of clotting abnormalities
Pustule	An elevated (infected) lesion containing pus
Scale	Thin plaques of epithelial tissue on skin's surface
Tumor	A swelling of abnormal tissue growth
Ulcer	A wound that results from tissue loss
Verrucae	Another term for warts
Vesicle	A blister
Wheal	Another term for hive

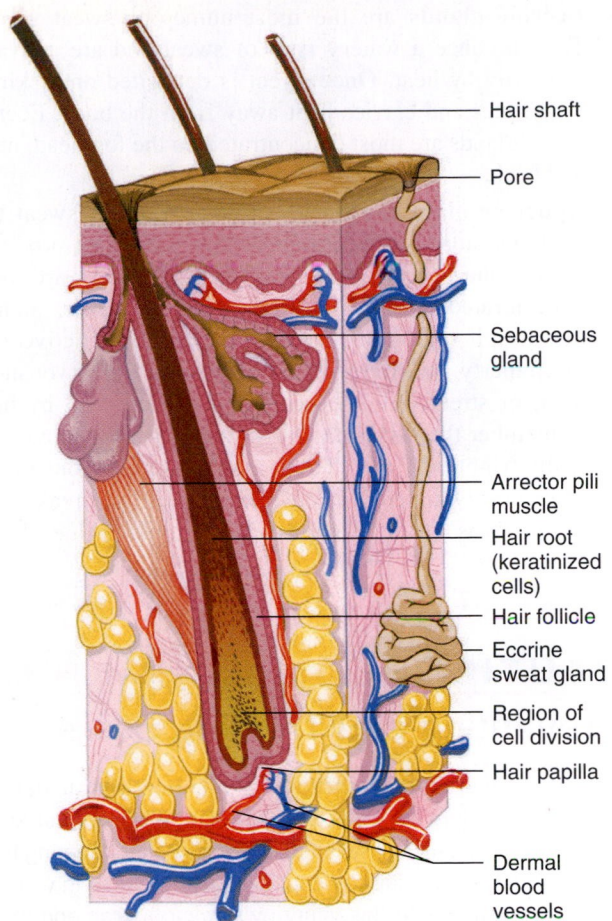

FIGURE 22-3 The hair follicle extends into the dermis.

- Primary lesions such as macules and vesicles originate from disease or body changes.
- Secondary lesions, which include ulcers and keloids, are caused by a reaction to external traumas like scratching or rubbing, the healing process, or primary lesions.
- Vascular lesions are anomalies of the blood vessels and include telangiectasias, which are small dilated blood vessels on the skin's surface, and ecchymoses, commonly called bruises.

Table 22-1 lists some of the common types of skin lesions.

▶ Accessory Organs LO 22.5

The skin's accessory organs include hair follicles, **sebaceous** (oil) glands, nails, and **sudoriferous** (sweat) glands. Technically, breasts are considered an accessory organ of the integumentary system, but because they are more closely associated with the female reproductive system, they will be discussed in *The Reproductive Systems* chapter.

Hair Follicles

Hair **follicles** are tube-like structures in the skin's dermis; they are made up of epithelial tissue. Their function is to generate

hairs (see Figure 22-3). Keratinocytes make up most of the hair follicle. As hair follicles produce new keratinocytes, old ones are pushed toward the skin's surface. The old keratinocytes stick together to produce a hair. The portion of the hair embedded in the skin is called the *root,* and the portion of the hair extending from the surface of skin is called the *shaft.*

Melanocytes are also found in hair follicles. They produce and distribute pigments to create hair color. A person develops gray hair when these melanocytes produce less pigment than normal.

When a hair follicle goes into a resting cycle, the hair falls out. Most of the time, the hair follicle will begin a growing cycle again and produce a new hair. However, sometimes hair follicles completely die, and **alopecia** (baldness) develops.

Arrector pili muscles are attached to most hair follicles. When a person is cold or nervous, these muscles pull on hair follicles and cause hairs to stand erect. These muscles also pull on fibers in the skin's dermis, causing goose bumps (see Figure 22-3).

Sudoriferous Glands

Most sudoriferous glands are located in the skin's dermis. However, their ducts open onto the skin's epidermis. There are two types of sweat glands—eccrine and apocrine.

- **Eccrine glands** are the most numerous sweat glands. They produce a watery type of sweat and are activated primarily by heat. Once sweat is deposited onto skin, it evaporates and carries heat away from the body. Eccrine sweat glands are most concentrated on the forehead, neck, and back.

- **Apocrine glands** produce a thicker type of sweat that contains more proteins than the type of sweat produced by eccrine sweat glands. Apocrine glands are most concentrated in areas of skin with coarse hair, such as the armpit and groin areas. They become active during puberty and are primarily activated by nervousness, pain, or stress, but they can also be activated by heat. Remember the last time you watched a scary movie that really frightened you? These glands were responsible for producing your cold sweat. Bacteria often break down the proteins in the sweat produced by apocrine glands.

As the proteins are digested, the bacteria release a foul-smelling waste product that is responsible for the smell of body odor.

Sebaceous Glands

Sebaceous glands—more commonly called *oil glands*—produce an oily substance called **sebum.** Sebum is secreted onto hairs to keep them soft and pliable, and it is eventually deposited onto skin to keep it soft as well. Sebum also prevents bacteria from growing on skin (see Figure 22-1).

Nails

Nails protect the ends of the fingers and toes. They are formed by epithelial cells with hard keratin, which is more permanent than the softer keratin found in your skin. For this reason, the nails must be cut because they do not slough off by themselves as your skin cells do. The portion of a nail that you can

CAUTION: HANDLE WITH CARE

Preventing and Treating Scars

One of the skin's major functions is to protect your underlying tissues from injury and infection. Whether skinning your knees as a child or cutting yourself in the kitchen while preparing food, you have most likely injured your skin at some time in your life. Your skin responds to this injury by forming a scab and then a scar. Many scars simply retract and go away in time. The size and extent of the scar depend on the following:

- *Extent of the wound.* Deep or jagged wounds may produce a larger scar.
- *Wound location.* Wounds over mobile areas like the knees and elbows often have larger scars because they are constantly under tension.

It is important that you seek medical attention for wounds that

- Bleed profusely.
- Are larger than ½ inch deep or wide.
- Are located on the face.
- Are caused by a rusty tool or nail.
- Are jagged in appearance.
- Are caused by an animal bite.
- Show signs of infection.

These basic tips may help prevent the formation of lasting scars:

- Wash wounds with mild soap and water and clean out any debris left in the wound.
- Do not use harsh soaps, hydrogen peroxide, or alcohol to clean a wound, as these can damage tissues and delay healing.
- Cover the wound to keep out bacteria, dirt, and debris to reduce the possibility of infection.

- Keep the wound moist by applying an antibiotic ointment. This keeps the bandage from sticking to the wound and may reduce the likelihood of infection.
- Do not pick or pull at a scab. This reopens the wound and may cause infection or larger scar formation.
- Use medical honey. Honey has antibacterial properties and has been found to accelerate healing. Special medical products are available for hard-to-heal wounds.

If a scar forms, numerous treatments are available:

- *Sunscreen.* Protecting a newly healed wound from UV radiation by using sunscreen with an SPF of 30 or higher helps reduce scar thickening and hyperpigmentation.
- *Silicone gel sheeting.* Studies show that covering a wound with a silicone gel sheet reduces healing time and scar formation. These sheets may be used for surgical and nonsurgical wounds.
- *Dermabrasion.* This procedure literally "sands" the surface of the skin and scar and is most often used for raised scars.
- *Surgical scar repair.* A large or hyperpigmented scar can be reduced in size by removing it surgically. Scar reduction surgical procedures include the following:
  - Z-plasty—a specialized plastic surgical technique that alters the pull on a tightened scar by lengthening it
  - Scar shaving—a technique for shaving off a raised scar
  - Scar removal—making an elliptical incision around the scar and removing it, which results in a scar that is thinner than the original scar

see is the nail body, and the portion embedded in skin is the nail root. The nail root contains active keratinocytes that constantly divide to produce nail growth. The white, half-moon-shaped area at the base of a nail is called a *lunula*. The lunula also contains very active keratinocytes. Beneath each nail is a layer called the **nail bed,** which holds the nail down to underlying skin and provides nutrients to the nail from the blood supply under the nail bed (see Figure 22-4). Extending from the nail bed beyond the fingertip is the free edge of the nail. This is the part that you cut and file so that your nails look neat and trimmed.

▶ Skin Healing   LO 22.6

When skin is injured, it becomes inflamed. Redness, swelling, localized warmth, and pain are characteristics of inflammation. An inflamed area looks red because nearby blood vessels dilate. The inflamed area also swells because the dilated blood vessels "leak" and fluids seep into spaces between cells. Inflamed areas are often painful because the excess fluid activates pain receptors. However, inflammation promotes healing because more blood travels to the area, and this extra blood carries more nutrients needed for skin repair. It also carries defensive cells to clear up the cause of inflammation.

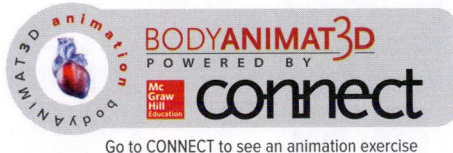

Go to CONNECT to see an animation exercise about *Inflammation*.

When structures and blood vessels of the dermis are injured, a blood clot initially forms. A scab, which is basically clotted blood and other dried tissue fluids, eventually replaces the blood clot. The scab is normally replaced by collagen fibers that bind the edges of the wound together. Collagen

fibers are whitish and serve as the major component of scars. Sometimes skin scars are replaced with new skin, but if the wound is extensive, a scar will persist. Scars can be merely a cosmetic nuisance, or they can cause problems with underlying structures. For example, a large scar over a joint can cause loss of movement in that joint. See the *Caution: Handle with Care* feature for more information on preventing and treating scars.

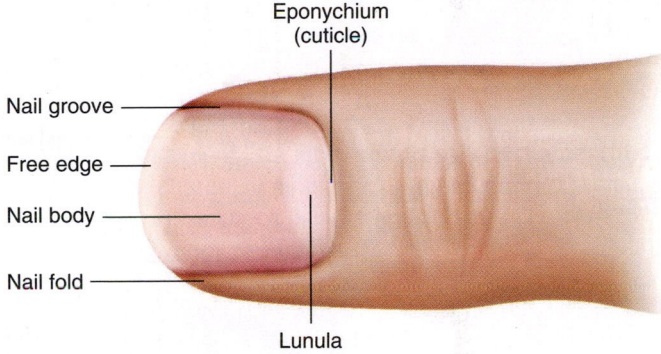

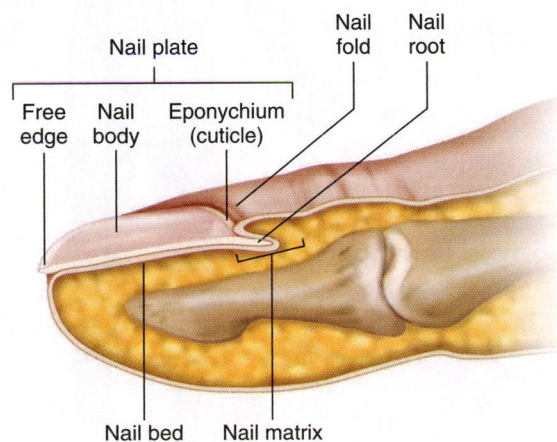

FIGURE 22-4   Anatomy of a nail.

Common Diseases and Disorders of the Skin

BURNS

Although many of the skin conditions discussed in this chapter can be extremely serious and even life-threatening (such as skin cancer), the skin is also prone to burns. In fact, burns are a leading cause of accidental death in the United States, where there are approximately 150 burn care centers devoted to this type of skin injury. Burns may be caused by heat, chemicals, electricity or radiation, as well as extreme cold or friction.

It is also important to note that an estimated 450,000 people seek medical treatment for burn injuries each year; 45,000 require hospitalization; and more than 3,500 patients die annually from burn injuries. Worldwide, more than a million people each year suffer from burn injuries that cause significant or permanent disability.

The extent of the affected body surface area and the severity (degree) of a burn are the most important factors in predicting the risk of death associated with burn injuries. The rule of nines is a quick way to estimate the extent of body surface area affected by burns. This method divides the body into 11 areas, each accounting for 9% of the total body surface. The genital area accounts for 1%. (See Figure 22-5.)

Rule of Nines. Following are the 11 body areas of the rule of nines, with their percentages:

• Head	9% (front and back, 4.5% each)
• Right arm	9% (front and back, 4.5% each)
• Left arm	9% (front and back, 4.5% each)
• Front of right leg	9%
• Front of left leg	9%
• Back of right leg	9%
• Back of left leg	9%
• Front of body	18% (both areas) trunk is two areas
• Back of body	18% (both areas) trunk is two areas
• Genital area	1%
	Total body area = 100%

Burn Severity. The severity of burns indicates the thickness of the injury (see Figure 22-6). The following terms are used to report burn severity:

- *Superficial (first-degree).* These burns involve only the epidermis and are characterized by pain, redness, and

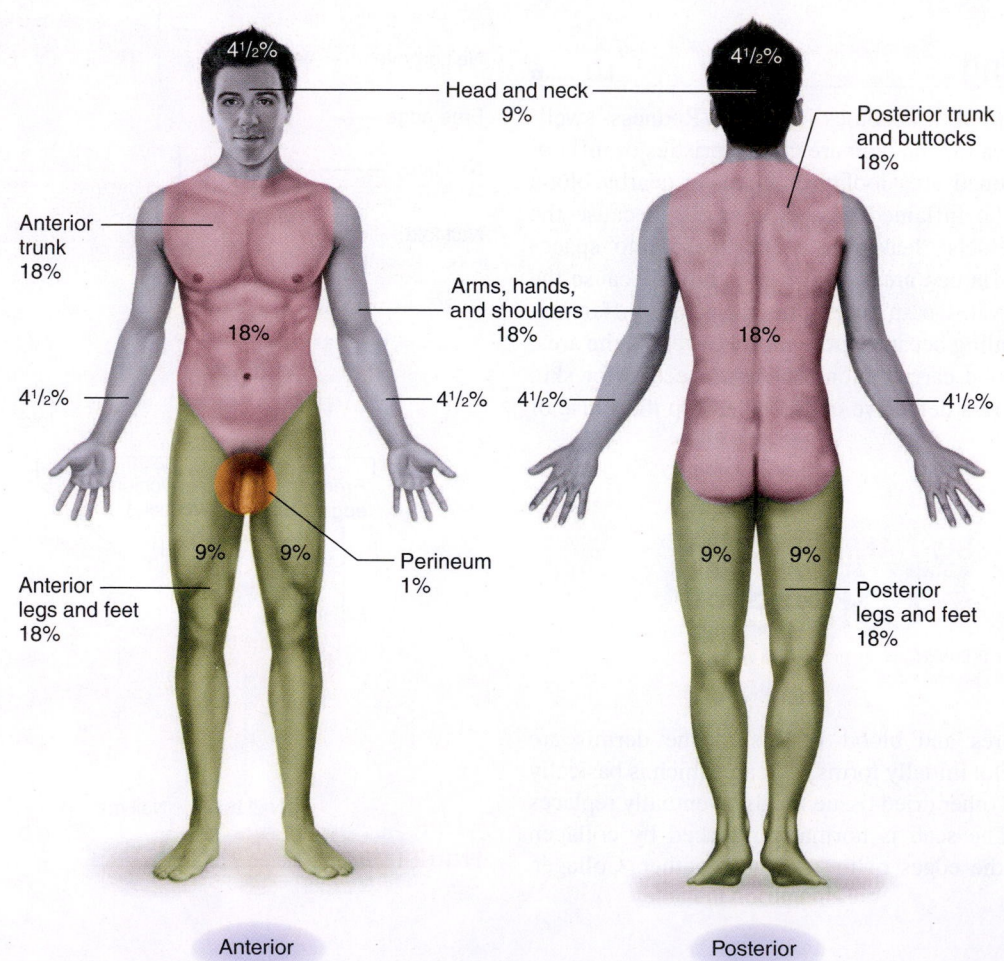

FIGURE 22-5 Using the rule of nines aids in estimating the extent of burns.

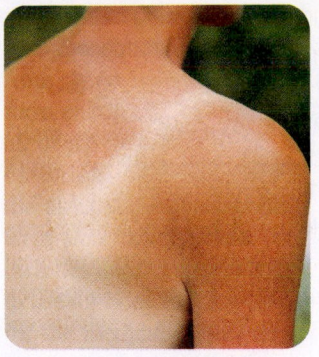

(a) First degree (superficial)

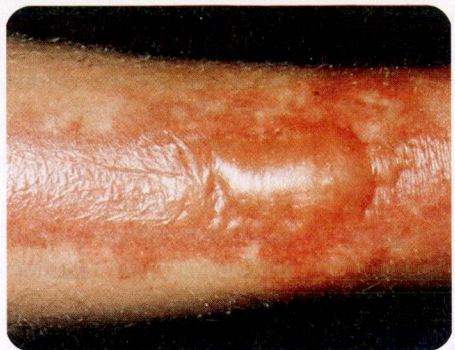

(b) Second degree (partial thickness)

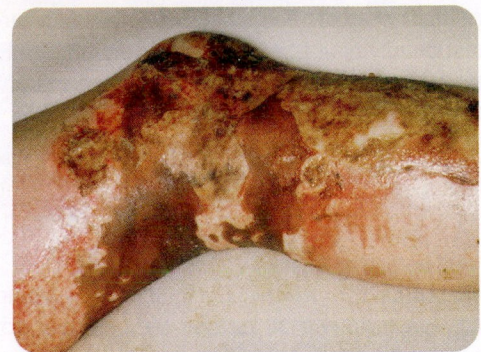

(c) Third degree (full thickness)

FIGURE 22-6   The degrees of burn severity include (a) superficial (first-degree) burns, (b) partial-thickness (second-degree) burns, and (c) full-thickness (third-degree) burns.

© Sheila Terry/Science Source; © Dr. P. Marazzi/Science Source; © John Radcliffe Hospital / Science Source

swelling. Unless they are extensive, they do not require medical attention and usually heal well.

- *Partial-thickness (second-degree).* These burns involve the epidermis and dermis. Pain, redness, swelling, and blisters characterize them. Medical staff should treat any partial-thickness burn that affects 1% or more of the body surface. A body surface area of 1% is about the size of a person's hand. Shock is likely to develop in partial-thickness burn injuries that affect 9% or more of the body surface. These burns can be life-threatening, depending on their extent.

- *Full-thickness (third-degree).* These burns involve all layers of skin and often underlying structures such as muscles and bones. The skin frequently looks black or charred, which is known as *eschar.* Full-thickness burns always require medical attention regardless of the extent or the size of the burn area.

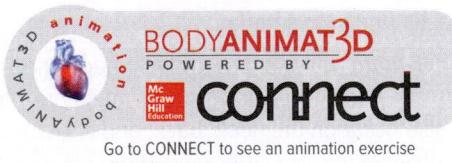

Go to CONNECT to see an animation exercise about Burns.

General Guidelines for Treating Burns.

- Anything sticking to the burn should be left in place.

- Do not apply butter, lotions, or ointments to the burn. Only use ointments prescribed by a doctor or recommended by a pharmacist.

- Cool the burn with large amounts of cool water. Avoid ice or extremely cold water.

- Cover the burn with a sterile sheet. However, do not cover burns to the face.

- Contact emergency medical personnel for serious burns.

- With burns to the mouth and throat, check the airways for swelling. Burns to the head are always more serious than burns to other body parts. They almost always require emergency medical treatment.

Skin Cancer and Common Skin Disorders

Skin is vulnerable to many disorders because it is the most exposed of all body organs. The following sections discuss skin cancer and common skin disorders.

SKIN CANCER

Skin cancer develops from cells in the skin's epidermis. It is more common in people who have light-colored skin and who have had excessive exposure to sunlight. It can occur anywhere on the body, but it is most likely to appear on skin that is readily exposed to sunlight. The two most common types of skin cancer

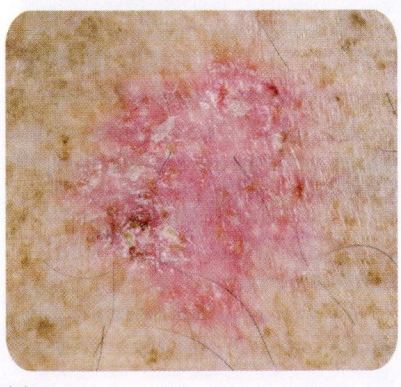

(a)

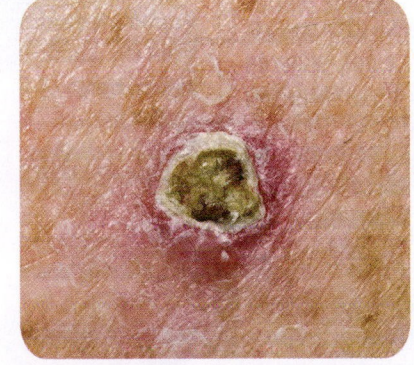

(b)

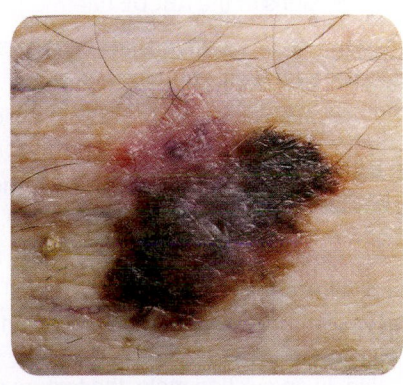

(c)

FIGURE 22-7   Types of skin cancer: (a) squamous cell carcinoma, (b) basal cell carcinoma, and (c) malignant melanoma.

© Dr. P. Marazzi / Science Source; © Dr. P. Marazzi / Science Source; © Dr. P. Marazzi / Science Source

are basal cell carcinoma and squamous cell carcinoma, but the most deadly type is malignant melanoma (see Figure 22-7). For more information on the general symptoms of cancer, refer to the feature *Educating the Patient.*

BASAL CELL CARCINOMA accounts for approximately 90% of all skin cancers in the United States. Fortunately, it progresses slowly and rarely spreads to other body parts. It is derived from cells of the stratum basale of the epidermis.

Signs and Symptoms. These include changes on the skin and a new growth or sore on the skin that does not heal. Its appearance may be waxy, smooth, red, pale, flat, or lumpy, and it may or may not bleed.

Treatment. Several forms of treatment are available:

- *Curettage and electrodessication.* In curettage, a sharp instrument is used to scoop out the cancerous lesion. Electrodessication uses electrical currents to minimize bleeding as well as to kill any remaining cancer cells.
- *Mohs surgery.* The cancerous lesion is shaved off one layer at a time. Each layer is then examined under a microscope by the surgeon until no tumor is detected in the last layer removed.
- *Cryosurgery.* Freezing is used to kill cancer cells.
- *Laser therapy.* A beam of light destroys cancer cells.

SQUAMOUS CELL CARCINOMA is much less common than basal cell carcinoma but is more likely to spread to surrounding tissues. It arises from flat cells of the epidermis and is most likely to appear on the face, lips, ears, and the backs of the hands. The signs and symptoms of and the treatments for this type of cancer are the same as for basal cell carcinoma.

MALIGNANT MELANOMA, a cancer that arises from melanocytes, is the most aggressive of the skin cancers. It is also the fastest-growing skin cancer, with rates increasing 5% to 7% per year. The lifetime risk of developing malignant melanoma is 1 in 75. It appears to be more prevalent in females, but males, when diagnosed, seem to have a poorer prognosis. Melanoma can occur anywhere on the body but most often appears on the trunk, head, and neck in men and on the arms and legs in women.

Signs and Symptoms. A mole that itches or bleeds is a common symptom. New moles may develop near it, or it may change to have any signs of the ABCDE rule:

- *Asymmetry.* The mole should not be asymmetrical. It should look equal in size from side to side.
- *Border.* The border of the mole should not be irregular. The edges should not blur into nearby normal tissue.
- *Color.* The mole should be even. It should not darken or lighten or contain a mixture of colors.
- *Diameter.* The mole should not grow larger than 6 mm, about the diameter of a pencil eraser.
- *Evolving.* The mole has been changing in size, shape, color, or appearance or growing in an area of previously normal skin. In an existing mole, the texture of the mole may change and become hard, lumpy, or scaly. Although the skin may feel different and may itch, ooze, or bleed, melanoma usually does not cause pain.

Treatment. The treatment depends on the staging of this cancer. Melanoma has five stages, including the following, from the least to the most serious:

- Stage 0. Malignancy is found only in the epidermis.
- Stage I. Malignancy has spread from the epidermis to the dermis and has a thickness of 1 to 2 millimeters.
- Stage II. Malignancy has a thickness of 2 to 4 millimeters and may be ulcerated.
- Stage III. Malignancy has spread to one or more nearby lymph nodes.
- Stage IV. Malignancy has spread to other body organs or other lymph nodes far away from the original melanoma site.

Available treatments for melanoma include the following:

- Surgery to remove the melanoma
- Lymph node biopsy to determine if the cancer has spread
- Removal of cancerous lymph nodes
- Chemotherapy for advanced stages of cancer
- Radiation therapy for advanced stages of cancer
- Immunotherapy to boost the patient's immune system

Common Skin and Hair Disorders

ACNE VULGARIS, commonly known as acne, is an inflammatory condition of the skin follicles and sebaceous glands. See Figure 22-8.

Causes. Acne often appears in adolescence as a result of a surge of sex hormones, which increases the amount of sebum the sebaceous glands produce. Excess sebum and dead skin cells clog the pores, where bacteria then accumulate, causing the pimples. These pimples may rupture or leak, and as the bacteria then infect the adjacent skin areas, they cause the characteristic skin inflammation.

Signs and Symptoms. Comedos (blackheads and whiteheads), as well as papules and pustules occur mainly on the face, but they can also occur on the neck, back, and chest.

Treatment. Patients may find the following instructions helpful in controlling their acne. Wash your face twice a day, removing all makeup and using *noncomedogenic* (non-pore-clogging)

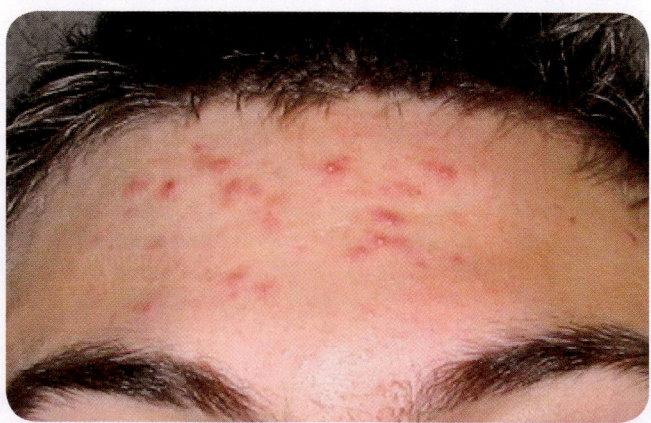

FIGURE 22-8 Acne is common during adolescence and is frequently seen on the face and back.
© McGraw-Hill Education

skin care products. Wash your hair frequently because oils from your hair can end up on your face. Always use makeup or lotions containing sunscreen, and keep your hands away from your face during the day. Seek the care of a dermatologist for severe cases of acne, as these may require oral antibiotics (tetracycline) or other prescription medications, such as retinol.

ALOPECIA is a disorder that specifically targets hair and results in hair loss.

Causes. Most of the time, alopecia is inherited. Other common causes include hormonal changes, chemotherapy, stress, burns, and fungal infections of the skin.

Signs and Symptoms. Loss or lack of hair on the scalp or other areas of the body, alopecia is more commonly called *baldness.*

Treatment. If a result of heredity, this disorder is not curable. Hair transplants and some drugs, such as Rogaine®, may slow down hair loss. Hair loss caused by other factors, such as chemotherapy, is often temporary, but the hair may grow back a different color or texture.

CELLULITIS is an inflammation of connective tissue in skin and primarily occurs on the face and legs. See Figure 22-9.

Causes. This skin disease is caused by staphylococcal and streptococcal bacteria.

Signs and Symptoms. Skin appears red and tight and is often painful. The inflammation may trigger a fever.

Treatment. Treatment includes oral and topical antibiotics. In serious cases, intravenous (IV) antibiotics and hospitalization may be required.

DERMATITIS is a general term defined as inflammation of skin or a rash. It has many causes and is a sign of many types of skin disorders. A common type of dermatitis is contact dermatitis, which results from contact with allergens or irritants. If you have ever had poison ivy, you had a type of contact dermatitis. Another common form of dermatitis is eczema.

ECZEMA is one type of chronic dermatitis that has acute phases characterized by a blistered rash that itches severely. Eczema often appears in childhood but is also commonly seen in adults.

Causes. Causes of eczema are mostly unknown, but it is thought to be a type of allergy or the result of an often unknown underlying inflammatory condition. Environmental irritants, stress, diet, and medications can exacerbate or worsen the signs and symptoms of this disease.

Signs and Symptoms. The rashes of eczema are red, scaly, and itchy.

Treatment. Treatments include topical steroids and other types of anti-inflammatory drugs. Antibiotics may be needed for any secondary infections that develop. Avoiding known factors that trigger eczema, such as stress, is also helpful.

FOLLICULITIS, sometimes called "swimmer's rash," is an inflammation of hair follicles. See Figure 22-10.

Causes. This disorder usually results from shaving or excess rubbing of skin areas. It may also be caused by bacteria and fungi, which may develop from prolonged wearing of wet swimwear or using undertreated hot tubs.

Signs and Symptoms. Follicles become red and itchy and often look like pimples.

Treatment. Treatments include regular cleansing of skin, topical antibiotics, and the use of electric razors instead of razor blades. Wearing wet swimwear for prolonged periods of time should also be avoided.

HERPES SIMPLEX types 1 and 2 are the most common types of herpes simplex.

Causes. Herpes simplex types 1 and 2 are both caused by a virus. Herpes simplex type 1 causes cold sores. It is very

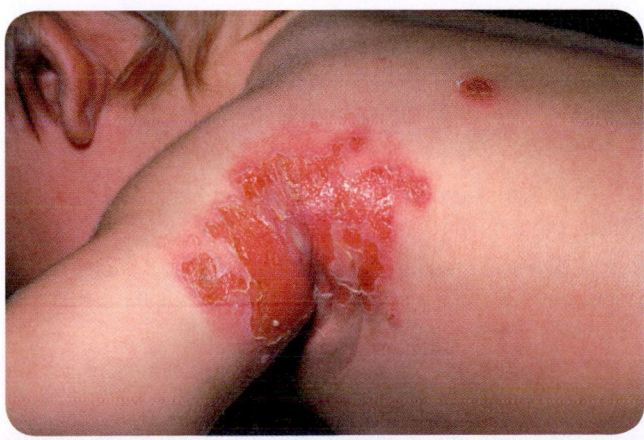

FIGURE 22-9   Cellulitis is inflammation of the skin caused by staphylococcal or streptococcal bacteria.
CDC/Allen W Mathies, MD, Califorinia EPO, Immunization Branch

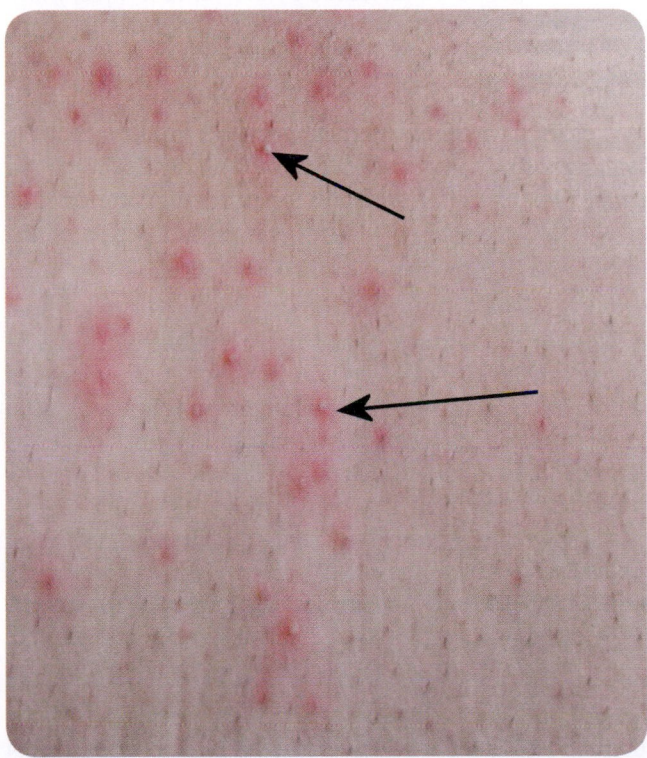

FIGURE 22-10   Folliculitis can be caused from shaving or rubbing of the skin and often looks like pimples.
© McGraw-Hill Education

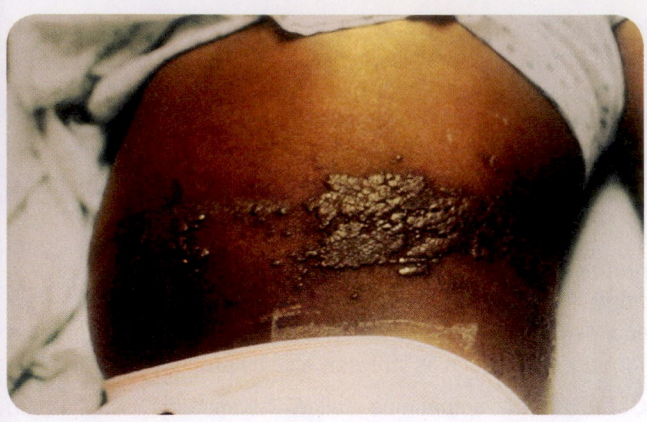

FIGURE 22-11 Herpes zoster, more commonly known as shingles, is a painful, blistering rash that follows the pathway of an affected nerve root. CDC

contagious and is spread through saliva. Herpes simplex type 2, known as *genital herpes,* is sexually transmitted.

Signs and Symptoms. Herpes simplex type 1 causes painful sores on the lips, mouth, and face. Herpes simplex type 2 normally causes painful sores on genital areas.

Treatment. There is no cure for herpes simplex, and its skin lesions usually recur throughout life. However, antiviral drugs such as acyclovir (Zovirax®) prevent frequent outbreaks. Patients should also be instructed to get adequate rest and nutrition and to control stress as much as possible.

HERPES ZOSTER is a disorder commonly known as *shingles.* See Figure 22-11.

Causes. Herpes zoster is caused by the *Varicella* virus, which also causes chickenpox. After a person has chickenpox, the virus becomes dormant in the spine's dorsal nerve root but can become active again later in life to cause shingles.

Signs and Symptoms. Herpes zoster causes a painful, blistering rash usually on one side of the body following the *dermatome*—the skin area along the pathway of the affected nerve root. Shingles usually starts as a tingling or pain on the torso or neck, followed by a rash that eventually blisters.

Treatment. Some antiviral medications, such as Zovirax®, shorten the duration of the disease, and pain medications assist with pain control. Recovery is usually complete, but recurrences of the disease do occur. Some patients suffer from the complication known as *post-herpetic pain syndrome,* where nerve pain continues even though the rash is no longer present. It is uncertain whether the chickenpox vaccine prevents herpes zoster. The vaccine Zostavax® by Merck Pharmaceuticals is a preventive alternative for patients 60 years of age and older with a history of having had chickenpox. Patients considering Zostavax® should know that it is advertised as reducing the risk of developing shingles; it does not guarantee that shingles will not occur.

IMPETIGO causes the formation of oozing skin lesions that eventually crust over. It is highly contagious for those who come in contact with the lesions or the exudates (exuded substances) from them.

Causes. This disease is caused by staphylococcal and streptococcal bacteria.

Signs and Symptoms. The skin develops itchy, oozing lesions that eventually crust over with a distinctive, honey-colored crust from the drying exudates.

Treatment. This condition is treated with antibiotics. Washing the lesions two or three times a day with soap and water will help remove the exudates and decrease the spread to other skin areas.

PEDICULOSIS is more commonly known as *lice* and comes in three forms: head lice (*Pediculosis capitis*), body lice (*Pediculosis corporis*), and pubic lice (*Pediculosis pubis*).

Causes. All forms are caused by parasitic lice and are associated with overcrowded conditions causing person-to-person contact. Pubic lice are also spread by sexual contact.

Signs and Symptoms. Skin itches and can become irritated from scratching. Head lice are also identifiable by the dandruff-like nits that cannot be shaken off.

Treatment. Prescription medications and shampoos are often necessary. For head lice, some patients find equal success with over-the-counter (OTC) treatments such as Nix®.

PSORIASIS is a common chronic, inflammatory skin condition.

Causes. This skin disorder is most likely an inherited autoimmune disorder.

Signs and Symptoms. Patients with psoriasis have recurring episodes of itching and redness with outbreaks of distinctive silvery, scaly skin lesions. Some people also have joint pain with this condition known as psoriatic arthritis.

Treatment. Mild cases are treated with anti-inflammatory drugs and therapeutic ointments such as creams with vitamins A and D, hydrocortisone creams, and retinoids. Some patients also experience relief with controlled UV ray treatments. Severe cases may require hospitalization.

RINGWORM is a fungal skin infection, commonly occurring in three forms: *Tinea corporis* (body), *Tinea capitis* (scalp), and *Tinea pedis* (feet), which is commonly known as athlete's foot. See Figure 22-12.

Causes. All forms of ringworm are caused by fungi called *dermatophytes.*

Signs and Symptoms. Flat, circular lesions that may be dry and scaly or moist and crusty are the hallmarks of ringworm. *Tinea capitis* is characterized by small papules that may cause small, patchy areas of baldness.

Treatment. Topical and oral antifungal agents are used to treat all forms of ringworm. The spread is contained by not sharing sheets, towels, and other personal care items.

ROSACEA is a skin disorder that commonly appears as facial redness, predominantly over the cheeks and nose.

Causes. Rosacea results from dilation of small facial blood vessels, but the cause of this dilation is unknown. It occurs most frequently in fair-skinned people.

Signs and Symptoms. Redness and acne-like symptoms on the face are the most common symptoms.

Treatment. Although it is not curable, rosacea is usually managed well with topical cortisone or antibiotic creams. In severe cases, electrolysis may be useful in destroying large or dilated blood vessels.

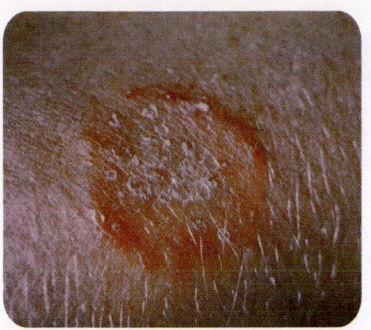

(a) *Tinea corporis* affects the body.

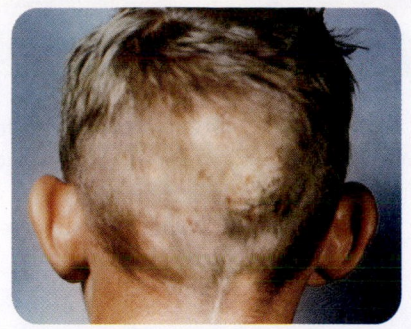

(b) *Tinea capitis* affects the scalp.

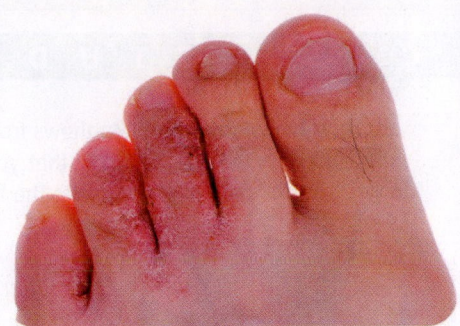

(c) *Tinea pedis* affects the feet.

FIGURE 22-12   Ringworm is a fungal infection that affects the body in three places.
CDC/Dr. Lucille K. Georg; CDC; carroteater/Getty Images RF

SCABIES is a highly contagious skin condition.

Causes. Scabies is caused by an itch mite that burrows beneath skin and lays its eggs. Sometimes the burrows of the mites can be seen and look like red pencil marks.

Signs and Symptoms. Redness and severe itching, especially at night, are usually the only symptoms of scabies.

Treatment. Most cases are easily treated with prescription medications such as Elimite™, which is left on the skin for 6 to 10 hours and followed by a bath. Antipyretic (anti-itching) or steroid creams may control the itching. Because scabies is contagious, it is wise to treat an entire family if one member is infected.

WARTS (verrucae) are harmless skin growths that can appear almost anywhere on the body surface but most commonly occur on the hands, feet, and face.

Causes. These growths are caused by a virus.

Signs and Symptoms. Warts vary greatly in appearance; they can be smooth, flat, rough, raised, dark, small, or large.

Treatment. Warts are often removed with OTC medications but can also be treated through surgery, lasers, freezing, or burning.

SUMMARY OF LEARNING OUTCOMES

LEARNING OUTCOMES	KEY POINTS
22.1 Describe the functions of skin.	The functions of skin include protection, body temperature regulation, vitamin D production, sensation, and excretion.
22.2 Describe the layers of skin and the characteristics of each layer.	The topmost layer of the skin is the epidermis. The dermis is the complex middle layer. The innermost layer attaching the skin to muscle is the subcutaneous layer.
22.3 Explain the factors that affect skin color.	The amount of melanin affects and determines skin color. The amount of oxygen-carrying hemoglobin in the blood also affects skin color.
22.4 Summarize types of common skin lesions.	Skin lesions are split among three main types: primary lesions such as macules and vesicles; secondary lesions, which include ulcers and keloids; and vascular lesions, which involve blood vessels and include telangiectasias and ecchymoses.
22.5 Describe the accessory organs of skin along with their structures and functions.	The accessory organs of skin include hair follicles, arrector pili muscles, sebaceous glands, sudoriferous glands, and keratin-filled nails.
22.6 Explain the process of skin healing, including scar production.	Injured skin becomes inflamed from dilating blood vessels that leak and cause swelling. A blood clot is formed, which is replaced by a scab, which is then replaced by collagen fibers that produce scar tissue.
22.7 Describe the common diseases and disorders of the skin.	Common diseases and disorders of the skin include acne, alopecia, cellulitis, dermatitis, eczema, folliculitis, herpes simplex, herpes zoster, impetigo, pediculosis, psoriasis, ringworm, rosacea, scabies, and warts.

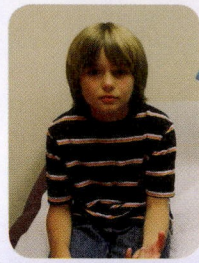

© McGraw-Hill Education

Recall Chris Matthews from the beginning of the chapter. Now that you have completed the chapter, answer the following questions regarding his case.

1. Considering the information you already have on Chris's feet and his behavior, what is the likely diagnosis?

2. What is the clinical name for this condition? During and after treatment, what are some tips you can give Chris to avoid a recurrence?

EXAM PREPARATION QUESTIONS

1. (LO 22.2) Which protein gives skin its protective quality?
   a. Melanin
   b. Vitamin D
   c. Keratin
   d. Hemoglobin
   e. Collagen

2. (LO 22.4) Which of the following lesions is a vascular lesion?
   a. Tumor
   b. Macule
   c. Ecchymosis
   d. Wheal
   e. Plaque

3. (LO 22.7) The patient has burned his left arm front and back from elbow to fingertips as well as his left chest and abdomen (approximately half of his trunk). Using the rule of nines, what percentage of his body is burned?
   a. 27%
   b. 18%
   c. 13.5%
   d. 9.5%
   e. 22.5%

4. (LO 22.5) The medical term for hair loss is
   a. Folliculitis
   b. Alopecia
   c. Pediculosis
   d. Impetigo
   e. Excoriation

5. (LO 22.4) Which medical condition is more commonly known as a *hive*?
   a. Cicatrix
   b. Vesicle
   c. Pustule
   d. Wheal
   e. Erosion

6. (LO 22.4) *Verrucae* is a medical term meaning
   a. Bruises
   b. Warts
   c. Nodules
   d. Wrinkles
   e. Moles

7. (LO 22.1) Which of the following is *not* a function of skin?
   a. Temperature regulation
   b. Protection
   c. Excretion
   d. Sensation
   e. Vitamin B production

8. (LO 22.7) Scabies is caused by
   a. Fungi
   b. Lice
   c. Mites
   d. Bed bugs
   e. Bacteria

9. (LO 22.2) The most superficial layer of the epidermis is the
   a. Stratum basale
   b. Stratum corneum
   c. Stratum germinativum
   d. Stratum dermis
   e. Stratum keratin

10. (LO 22.5) The part of the nail that holds it down to the underlying tissues and provides nutrients to the nail is the
    a. Lunula
    b. Nail bed
    c. Cuticle
    d. Free edge
    e. Nail root

Analyze the following medical terms, presented throughout the chapter. Using a medical dictionary (or Appendix I) place a / mark between each word part. Define each word part and then define the whole word.

EXAMPLE: **chemo/therapy** = chemo means "chemical" + therapy means "treatment"

CHEMOTHERAPY means "treatment with chemicals."

1. cellulitis
2. cyanosis
3. dermatitis
4. dermatome
5. epidermis

6. folliculitis
7. hemoglobin
8. hypodermis
9. keratinocyte
10. lunula

11. melanocyte
12. pediculosis
13. sebaceous
14. subcutaneous
15. sudoriferous

The Skeletal System

23

CASE STUDY

PATIENT INFORMATION		
Patient Name John Miller	**DOB** 12/5/19XX	**Allergies** Bee Stings
Attending Paul F. Buckwalter, MD	**MRN** 082-09-981	**Other Information** X-Ray Report: AP and lateral knee films show no factures. Joint alignment is normal.

John Miller is a 65-year-old patient returning to the clinic for a follow-up visit. He has a history of hypertension, diabetes Type 2, myocardial infarction (heart attack, 2008), and a recent confirmed diagnosis of congestive heart failure. He is taking glyburide, captopril, and HCTZ. When he arrives at the clinic, you notice he is walking with difficulty. He is seeing Olivia Ntombi, FNP, today as a work-in patient, since Dr. Buckwalter's schedule is fully booked. Mr. Miller states, "I was doing okay until I fell down yesterday. I was carrying

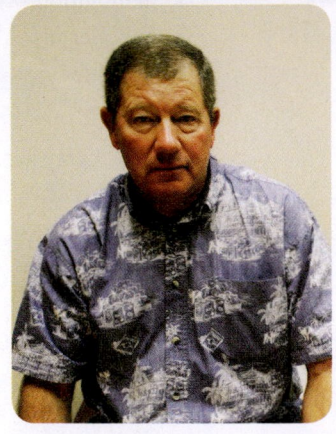
© McGraw-Hill Education

a box of stuff to take to the Salvation Army and lost my footing." The patient shows you an abrasion on his left knee and his right elbow. He says his knee is popping and very tender, and his elbow does not bend as much as it did before he fell. He is concerned that the bursitis in his knee might flare up. He also wonders why his elbow does not bend. The nurse practitioner orders X-rays of his knee and elbow.

Keep John in mind as you study this chapter. There will be questions at the end of the chapter based on the case study. The information in the chapter will help you answer these questions.

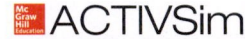

LEARNING OUTCOMES

After completing Chapter 23, you will be able to:

23.1 Describe the structure of bone tissue.

23.2 Explain the functions of bones.

23.3 Compare intramembranous and endochondral ossification.

23.4 Describe the skeletal structures and one location of each structure.

23.5 Locate the bones of the skull.

23.6 Locate the bones of the spinal column.

23.7 Locate the bones of the rib cage.

23.8 Locate the bones of the shoulders, arms, and hands.

23.9 Locate the bones of the hips, legs, and feet.

23.10 Describe the three major types of joints and give examples of each.

23.11 Describe the common diseases and disorders of the skeletal system.

KEY TERMS

appendicular

articulations

axial

clavicle

diaphysis

dislocation

epiphysis

femur

fibula

metacarpal

metatarsal

ossification

patella

pectoral girdle

pelvic girdle

radius

scapula

sternum

suture

temporal mandibular joint (TMJ)

tibia

ulna

I.C.1 Describe structural organization of the human body

I.C.6 Compare structure and function of the human body across the life span

I.C.7 Describe the normal function of each body system

I.C.8 Identify common pathology related to each body system including:
(a) signs
(b) symptoms
(c) etiology

I.C.9 Analyze pathology for each body system including:
(a) diagnostic measures
(b) treatment modalities

V.C.9 Identify medical terms labeling the word parts

V.C.10 Define both medical terms and abbreviations related to all body systems

2. Anatomy & Physiology

a. List all body systems, their structure and functions

b. Describe common diseases, symptoms and etiologies as they apply to each system

c. Identify diagnostic and treatment modalities as they relate to each body system

3. Medical Terminology

b. Build and dissect medical terms from roots/suffixes to understand the word element combinations that create medical terminology

c. Apply various medical terms for each specialty

▶ Introduction

Imagine that you are walking along a bustling city sidewalk, and someone behind you calls your name. As you pause and turn your head to see who it is, you catch a glimpse of your profile in the reflection of a coffee shop window. You stand taller than you think you are, with one leg in front of the other as if pivoting. You bring your right hand up to your forehead and quickly rub your brow, then let it drop to your side. Your friend then appears beside you and the two of you hug. Although it may seem as if your body is simply made of only the surface features you can see reflected in this window, dressed for the day in nice clothing and hugging your friend, of course, there is much more to this picture. After all, your bones are behind this picture, scattered all throughout your body to provide it with the structure and support you need for daily functioning.

In this chapter, you will learn about the bones of the body, their structure, and how the joints of the body work. The skeletal system is composed of 206 bones as well as joints and related connective tissues. Now, picture this many bones hiding within that person—*you!*—reflected earlier in the coffee shop window.

The skeleton has two major divisions—the **axial** skeleton and the **appendicular** skeleton (see Figure 23-1). These divisions differ in the following ways:

- The axial skeleton contains 80 bones, including the bones of the skull, vertebral column, and rib cage. It supports the head, neck, and trunk, and it protects the brain, spinal cord, and organs in the thorax. The hyoid bone, which anchors the tongue, is also included in the axial skeleton.

- The body's other 126 bones belong to the appendicular skeleton, which includes the bones of the arms, legs, **pectoral girdle**, and **pelvic girdle.** The pectoral girdle attaches the arms to the axial skeleton, and the pelvic girdle attaches the legs to the axial skeleton.

▶ Bone Structure   LO 23.1

Bones contain various kinds of tissues, including osseous tissue, blood vessels, and nerves. Osseous tissue can be compact or spongy (see Figure 23-2). At the microscopic level, spongy, or cancellous, bone has more spaces within it than compact bone does. Spongy bone looks a lot like a natural sea sponge with the spaces filled with *red bone marrow.* Compact bone looks solid, like granite or marble. However, the following structures within these bones can be observed with a microscope:

- *Osteons,* also known as the *Haversian system,* are elongated cylinders that run up and down the bone's long axis. Each osteon has a central canal that contains blood vessels and nerves.

- *Bone matrix,* made of inorganic salts, collagen fibers, and proteins, is the substance between bone cells. Bone cells are called *osteocytes.* The primary salt of the matrix is calcium phosphate, which makes bone matrix very hard.

- *Lamellae* are layers of bone surrounding the canals of osteons.

- *Lacunae* are holes in the matrix of bone that hold osteocytes.

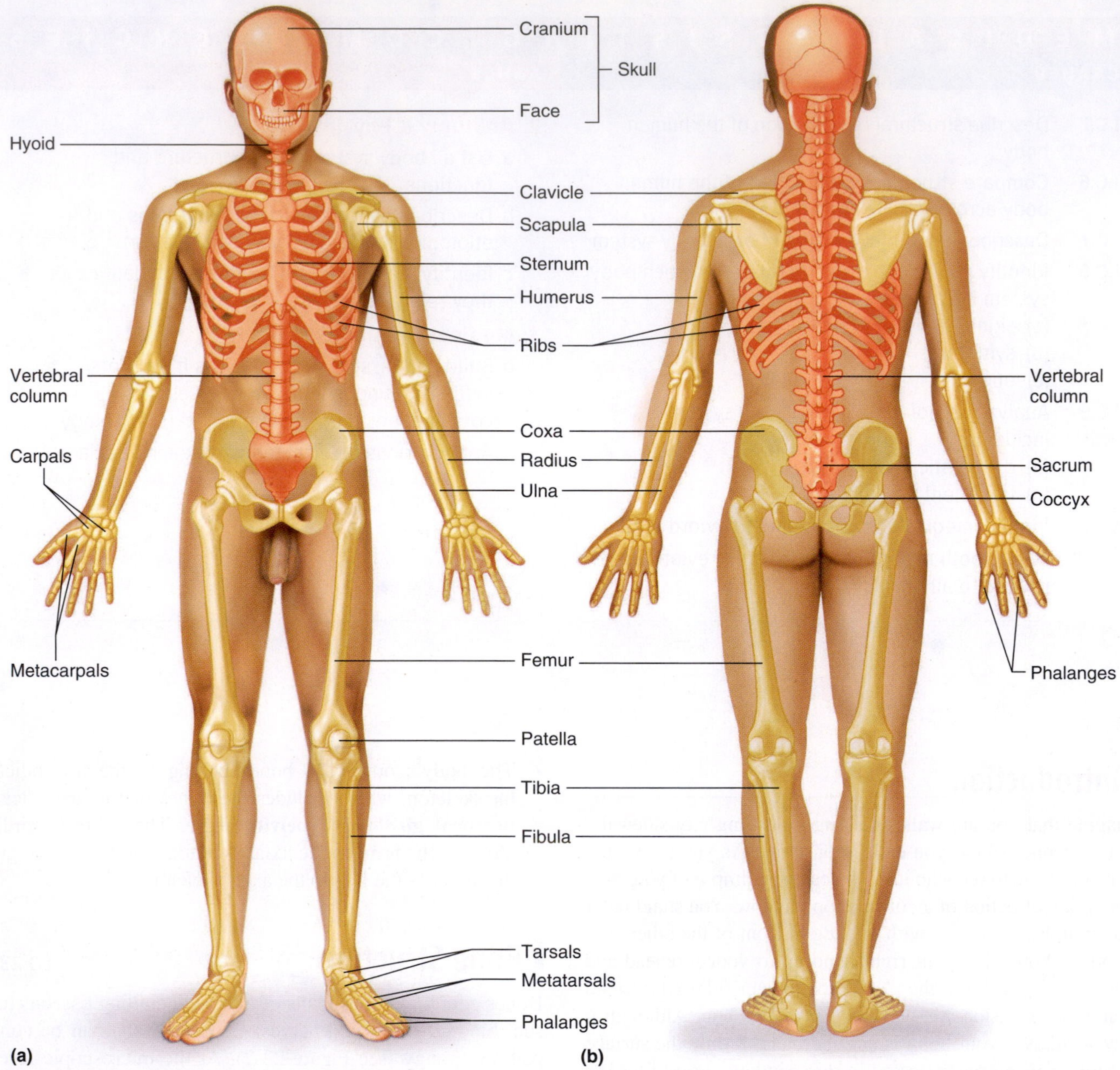

Cranium

Skull

Face

Hyoid

Clavicle

Scapula

Sternum

Humerus

Ribs

Vertebral
column

Carpals

Coxa

Radius

Ulna

Vertebral
column

Sacrum

Coccyx

Metacarpals

Femur

Phalanges

Patella

Tibia

Fibula

Tarsals

Metatarsals

Phalanges

(a)   (b)

FIGURE 23-1   Major bones of the skeleton: (a) anterior view and (b) posterior view. The axial skeleton is shown in orange and the appendicular skeleton is shown in yellow.

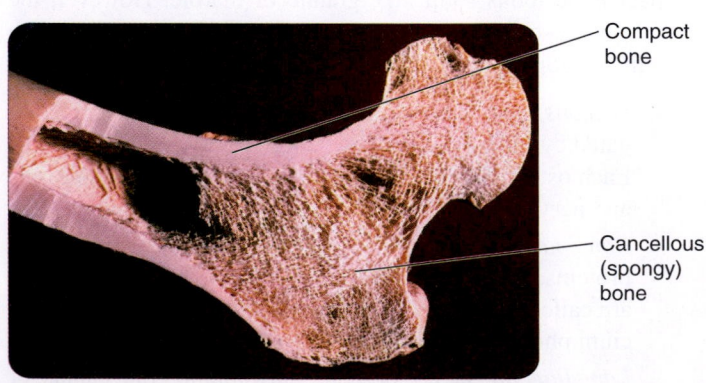

Compact
bone

Cancellous
(spongy)
bone

FIGURE 23-2   Cross section of bone showing compact and cancellous (spongy) bone tissue.

© Lester V. Bergman/Corbis

- *Canaliculi* are tiny canals that connect lacunae to each other and allow osteocytes to spread nutrients to each other.

All bones are made up of both compact and cancellous bone. They are classified according to their shape (see Figure 23-3):

- *Long bones* are located primarily in the arms and legs. Examples include the **femur** (thighbone, see Figure 23-4) and the humerus (upper arm bone). Long bones have the following parts (see Figure 23-5):

  - **Diaphysis**—the shaft of a long bone. It is tubular and consists of a thick collar of compact bone that surrounds the central medullary cavity.

  - **Epiphysis**—the expanded end of a long bone. It consists of a thin layer of compact bone surrounding cancellous bone. Long bones have an epiphysis at both ends.

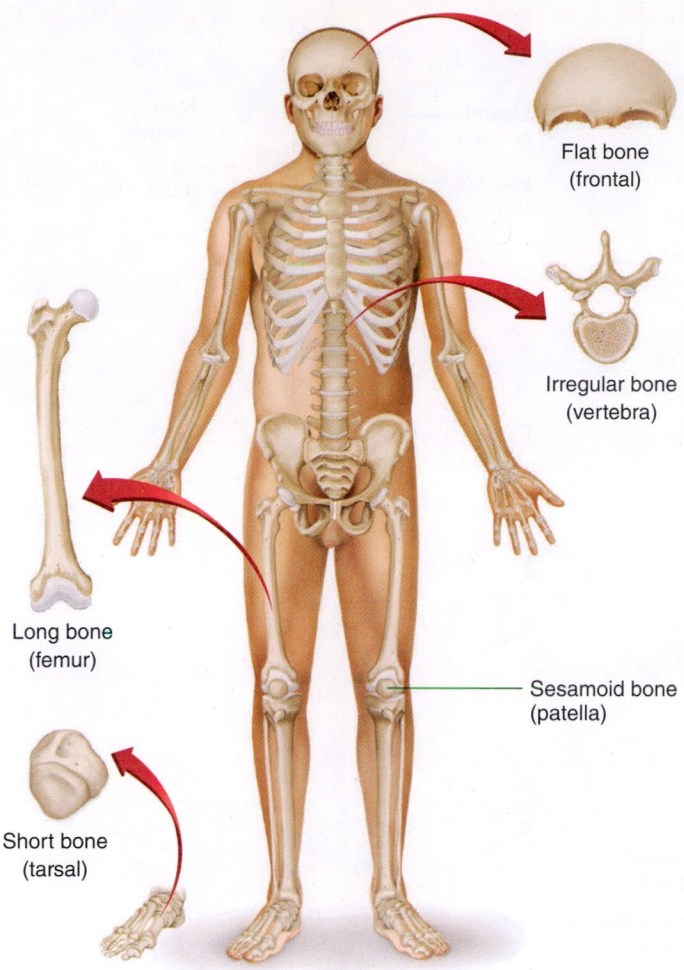

Flat bone
(frontal)

Irregular bone
(vertebra)

Long bone
(femur)

Sesamoid bone
(patella)

Short bone
(tarsal)

FIGURE 23-3 Classification of bone by shape: Five different classes of bone are recognized according to shape—long, short, flat, irregular, and sesamoid.

- *Articular cartilage*—the cartilage that covers the epiphyses of long bones. It cushions bones and absorbs stress during bone movements.
- *Medullary cavity*—the canal that runs through the center of the diaphysis. In adults, it contains *yellow bone marrow* (mostly fat).
  - *Periosteum*—a membrane that surrounds the diaphysis. It contains bone-forming cells, dense fibrous connective tissue, nerves, and blood vessels.
  - *Endosteum*—a membrane that lines the medullary cavity and the holes of cancellous bone. It contains bone-forming cells.
- *Short bones* are located in the wrists and ankles. Examples include the carpals (wrist bones) and some of the tarsals (ankle bones).
- *Flat bones* are primarily located in the skull and rib cage. Examples include the ribs and frontal bone.
- *Irregular bones* include the vertebrae and the pelvic girdle bones.
- *Sesamoid bones* are small, rounded bones usually found next to joints or embedded in a tendon. An example is the patella, or kneecap.

Gender Differences in Skeletal Structure

You may wonder how physicians, pathologists, and archeologists can tell if a skeleton is male or female. Table 23-1 outlines some of the skeletal differences between the sexes.

▶ Functions of Bones   LO 23.2

Bones have many functions. Without bones, the body would be more like a glob of jelly and not capable of very much. Bones give shape to body parts such as the head, legs, arms, and trunk. They also support and protect soft structures in the body. For example, the skull protects the brain. Bones also function in body movement because skeletal muscles attach to them, allowing you to create willful, or voluntary, movements.

The red marrow within cancellous bone produces new blood cells in a process called *hematopoiesis.* Blood cells have a limited lifespan, so they need to be replaced. Red blood cells, for example, need replacing as often as every 90 to 120 days. Your red marrow is actively making more blood cells 24 hours a day. Bones also store calcium for the body. Every cell in the body needs calcium, so the body must have a large supply readily available.

▶ Bone Growth   LO 23.3

Bones grow through a process called **ossification.** Ossification is the process of creating bone from either fibrous membranes or cartilage. These two types of ossification are called intramembranous and endochondral ossification.

In *intramembranous* ossification, bones begin as tough, fibrous membranes. Eventually, bone-forming cells called *osteoblasts* turn the membrane to bone. Except for the lower jaw bone, the bones of the skull are formed by intramembranous ossification.

In *endochondral* ossification, bones start out as cartilage models. Eventually, the osteoblasts form a bone collar around the diaphysis of the cartilage model. Think of a sculptor who first builds a framework or model of soft material before applying sculpting clay over the framework. Eventually, when the clay hardens, either through drying or firing in a kiln, there is more hard material than there is soft framework. Then bone is formed in the diaphysis of the bone. This area is called the *primary ossification center.* Later, the epiphyses turn to bone (secondary ossification centers), and the medullary cavity and spaces in cancellous bone are formed. The cells that form holes in bone are called *osteoclasts.* As long as a bone contains some cartilage between an epiphysis and the diaphysis, it can continue to grow in length. This plate of cartilage is called an *epiphyseal disk* or *growth plate.* Once the cartilage is gone, bone growth stops. For most people, bone growth stops between the ages of 18 and 25.

Even after bone growth stops, osteoclasts and osteoblasts continually remodel bone tissue. Throughout life, osteoclasts break down bone when the body needs more calcium in the blood, and osteoblasts replace the bone when there is excess calcium in the blood.

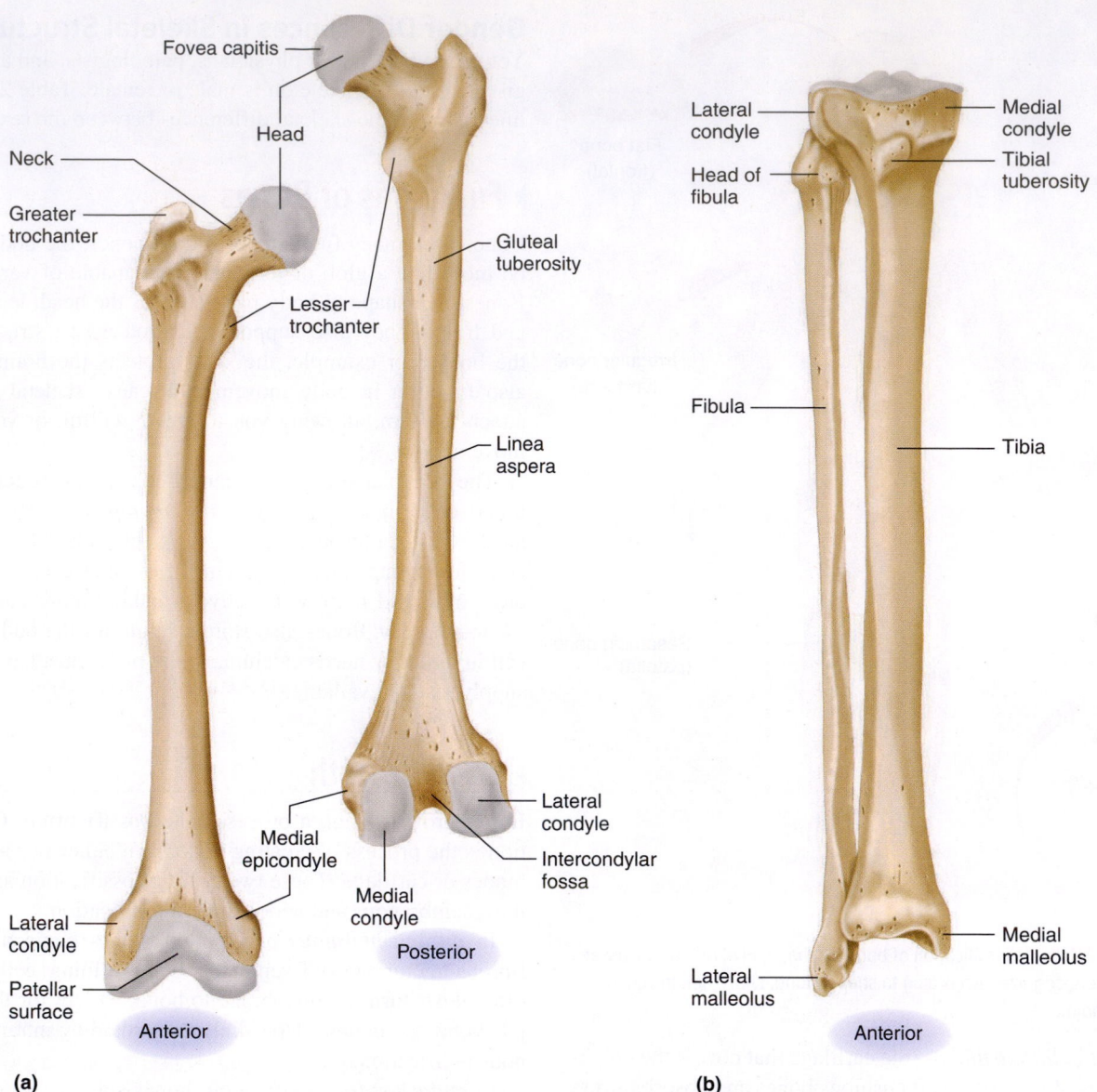

FIGURE 23-4 Bone structures: (a) bone structures of the femur and (b) bone structures of the tibia and fibula.

Building Better Bones

Many factors influence bone health, including diet, exercise, and a person's overall lifestyle. You can help patients improve or maintain their bone health by teaching them about behaviors that will support it.

Bone-Healthy Diet Good nutrition is essential for proper bone growth during childhood and the teen years. It is equally important in adulthood in order to maintain healthy bones. Bone-building nutrients are found in dairy products, broccoli, kale, spinach, salmon, sardines, egg yolks, whole grains, and fruits—especially bananas and oranges. Calcium and vitamin D are particularly important for healthy bones. Without vitamin D, the bloodstream cannot absorb calcium from the digestive tract. Without calcium, bone tissue will slowly wear away. Supplements can always be taken if a person's diet does not include adequate amounts of calcium and vitamin D.

Bone-Healthy Exercises Weight-bearing and strength-training exercises are best for bone health. When your muscles contract, they pull on your bones. This tension stimulates bones to thicken and strengthen. Lifting weights is an effective way to increase the tension on bones. Other activities such as jogging, walking briskly, or playing a sport regularly will also stimulate your bones to increase in density.

Bone-Healthy Lifestyle A person with a bone-healthy lifestyle avoids smoking and alcohol. Smoking rids the body of calcium, which is necessary for bone growth. Alcohol prevents calcium absorption in the digestive tract. Smokers are almost twice as likely to develop osteoporosis as nonsmokers.

Bone Tests

Bone density tests and bone scans are currently the most useful tools in determining bone health. Bone density tests are

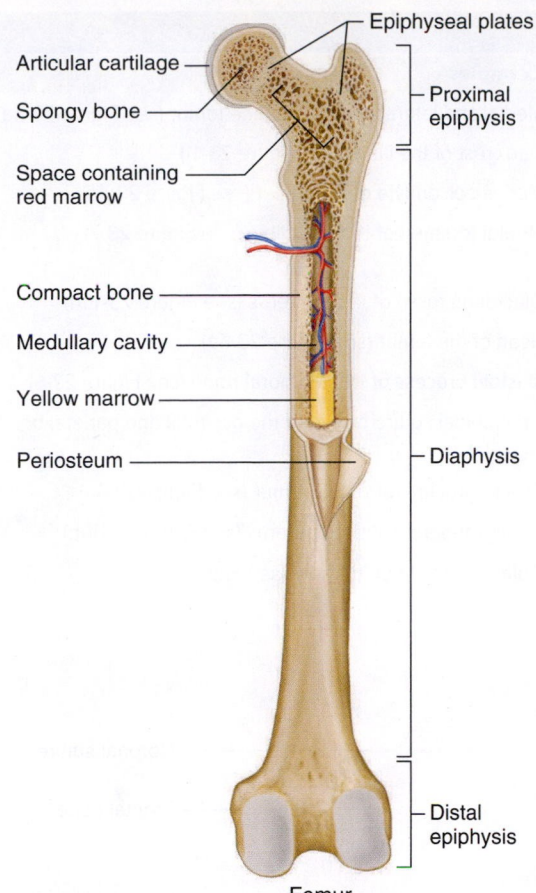

Parts of a long bone labels:
- Articular cartilage
- Spongy bone
- Space containing red marrow
- Compact bone
- Medullary cavity
- Yellow marrow
- Periosteum
- Epiphyseal plates
- Proximal epiphysis
- Diaphysis
- Distal epiphysis
- Femur

FIGURE 23-5   Parts of a long bone.

painless procedures used to determine the density of a person's bones. Because osteoporosis shows no symptoms in early stages, it is important to have these tests done when your doctor recommends them. Bone scans help diagnose the causes of bone pain, arthritis, bone infections, and bone cancers. These scans use radioactive tracers that are injected into the patient and concentrate in bone tissue.

▶ Bony Structures   LO 23.4

The skeletal bones act as your body's rigid foundation. By design, they are not perfectly smooth or perfectly rounded.

Bones have projections and processes for muscle and ligament attachment. For bones to come together at joints, or **articulations,** there are depressions and hollows. In addition, blood vessels and nerves need openings within bones for entrances and exits. Each of these structures has a specific name and design. Table 23-2 lists some of these common terms to describe skeletal structures and directs you to the appropriate figures throughout this chapter.

▶ The Skull   LO 23.5

Skull bones are divided into two types: cranial and facial bones. Cranial bones form the top, sides, and back of the skull (see Figure 23-6). Facial bones form the face (see Figure 23-7). The skull bones of an infant are not completely formed. The "soft spots" felt on an infant's skull are actually *fontanels,* which are tough membranes that connect the incompletely developed bones. These structures allow the infant's skull to be somewhat moldable to assist with delivery through the birth canal. As the fontanels close, the sutures of the skull are formed.

The major cranial bones are the following:

- The *frontal bone* forms the anterior portion of the cranium. It is also called the forehead bone.
- *Parietal bones* form most of the top and sides of the skull.
- The *occipital bone* forms the back of the skull. The large hole at the base of the occipital bone is called the *foramen magnum.* It allows the spinal cord to connect to the brain. Two bumps called occipital *condyles* are on either side of the foramen magnum. They sit on top of the first vertebra. When you nod your head, your occipital condyles are rocking back and forth on the first vertebra of the spinal column.
- Two *temporal bones* form the lower sides of the skull.
  - A canal called the *external auditory meatus* (commonly called the ear canal) runs through each temporal bone. A large bump called the *mastoid process* is located on each temporal bone just behind each ear. Major neck muscles attach to your skull at the mastoid processes.
  - A *sphenoid bone* forms part of the floor of the cranium. It is shaped like a butterfly. In the center is a deep depression called the *sella turcica.* The pituitary gland sits in this deep depression.

Part	Differences
Skull	Male skull is larger and heavier, with more conspicuous muscular attachments. Male forehead is shorter, facial area is less round, jaw is larger, and mastoid processes are more prominent than those of a female.
Pelvis	Male pelvic bones are heavier, thicker, and have more obvious muscular attachments. The obturator foramina and the acetabula are larger and closer together than those of a female.
Pelvic cavity	Male pelvic cavity is narrower in all diameters and is longer, less roomy, and more funnel-shaped. The distances between the ischial spines and between the ischial tuberosities are less than in a female.
Sacrum	Male sacrum is narrower, sacral promontory projects forward to a greater degree, and sacral curvature is bent less sharply posteriorly than in a female.
Coccyx	Male coccyx is less movable than that of a female.

TABLE 23-1   Differences Between the Male and Female Skeletons

TABLE 23-2 Terms Used to Describe Skeletal Structures

Term	Definition	Examples
Condyle	A rounded process that usually articulates with another bone	Medial and lateral condyles of the femur (see Figure 23-4a)
Crest	A narrow, ridge-like projection	Iliac crest of the ilium (see Figure 23-11)
Epicondyle	A projection situated above a condyle	Medial epicondyle of the femur (see Figure 23-4a)
Foramen	An opening through a bone that is usually a passageway for blood vessels, nerves, or ligaments	Mental foramen of the mandible (see Figure 23-7)
Fossa	A relatively deep pit or depression	Olecranon fossa of the humerus (see Figure 23-10d)
Head	An enlargement on the end of a bone	Head of the femur (see Figure 23-4a)
Process	A prominent projection on a bone	Mastoid process of the temporal bone (see Figure 23-6)
Suture	An interlocking line of union between bones	Lambdoidal suture between the occipital and parietal bones (see Figure 23-6)
Trochanter	A relatively large process	Greater trochanter of the femur (see Figure 23-4a)
Tubercle	A small, knob-like process	Greater tubercle of the humerus (see Figure 23-10b)
Tuberosity	A knob-like process usually larger than a tubercle	Tibial tuberosity of the tibia (see Figure 23-4b)

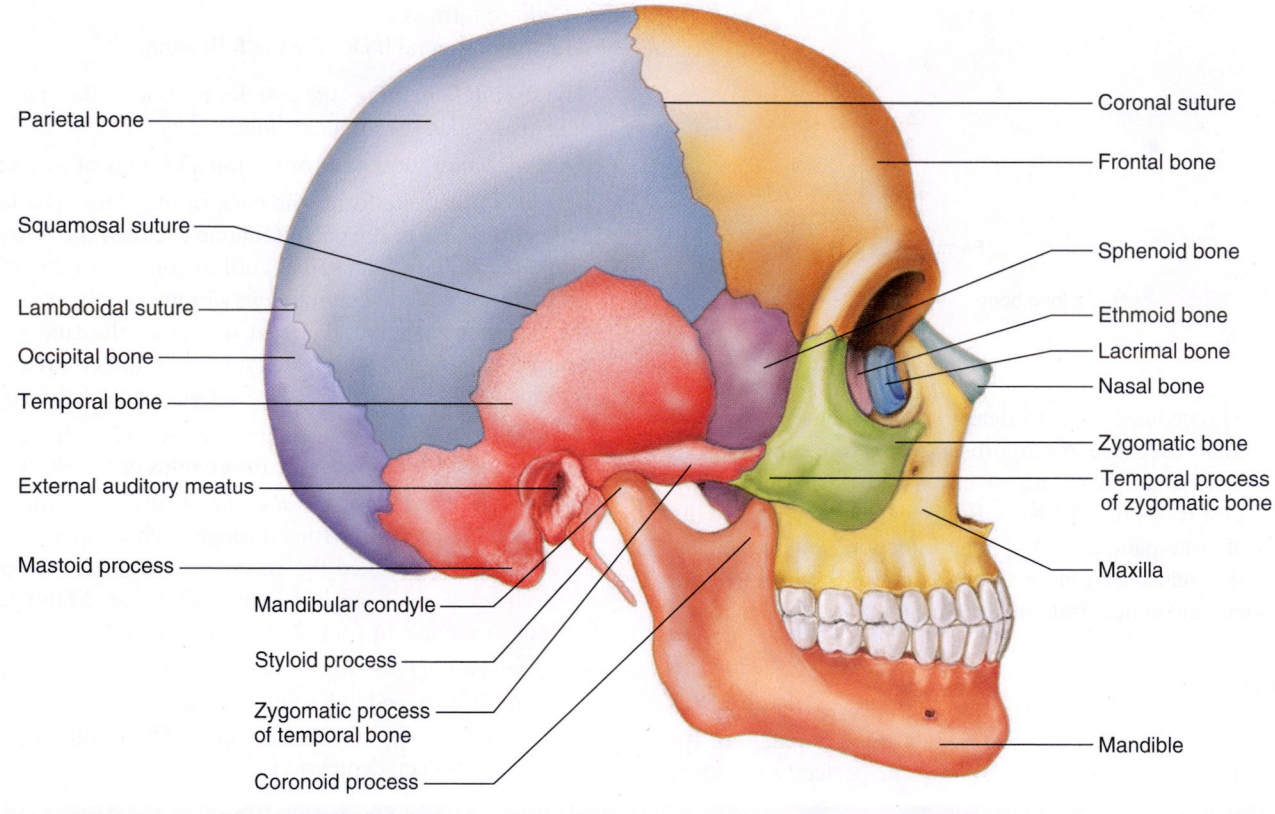

FIGURE 23-6 Lateral view of the skull.

- *Ethmoid bones* are between the sphenoid bone and the nasal bones. They also form part of the floor of the cranium.
- *Ear ossicles* are the body's smallest bones. They are the malleus, incus, and stapes and are in the middle ear cavities of the temporal bones.

The following are major facial bones:

- The *mandible* is the lower jaw bone and is the only movable bone in the skull. It attaches to the temporal bone in front of the external auditory meatus in an area known as the **temporal mandibular joint (TMJ).** The mandible anchors the lower teeth and forms the chin.
- The *maxillae* form the upper jaw bone of the facial skeleton, to which the upper teeth anchor.
- The *zygomatic bones* are the cheekbones. Several thin nasal bones fuse together to form the bridge of the nose.
- *Palatine bones* form the hard palate, which is the roof of the mouth.
- The *vomer* is a thin bone that divides the nasal cavity.

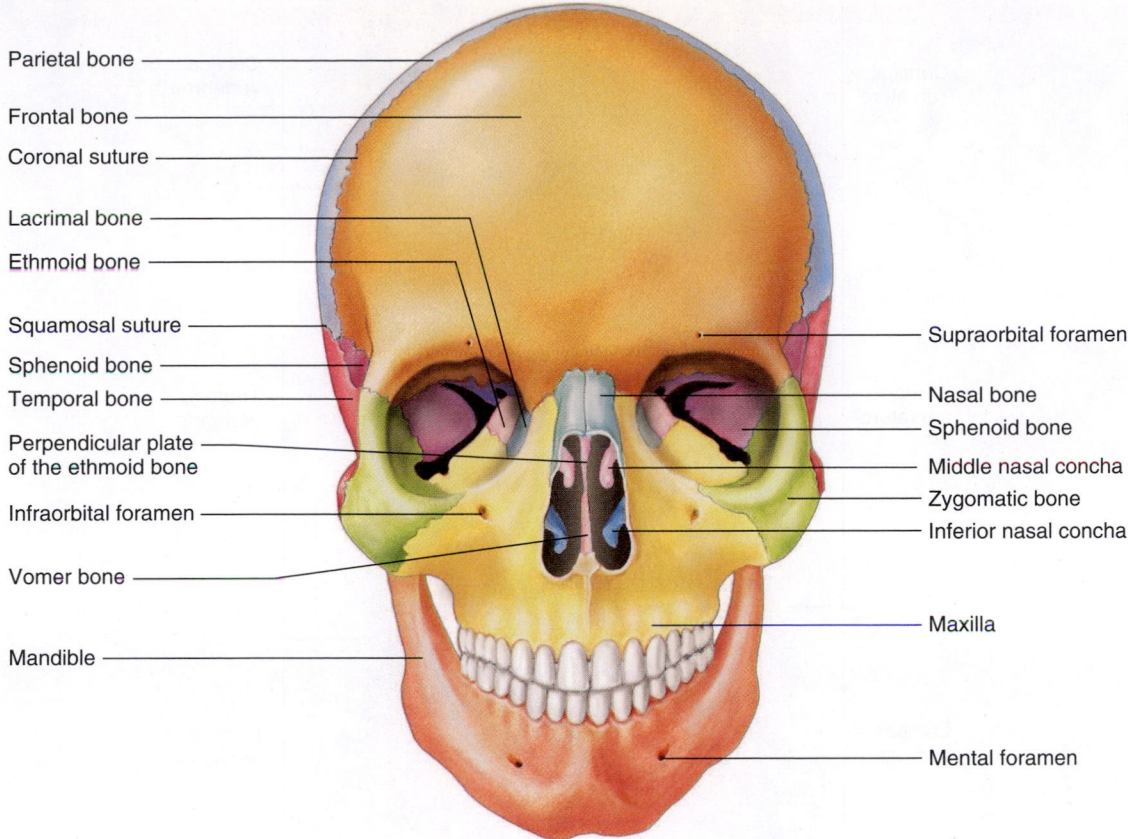

Parietal bone
Frontal bone
Coronal suture
Lacrimal bone
Ethmoid bone
Squamosal suture
Sphenoid bone
Temporal bone
Perpendicular plate of the ethmoid bone
Infraorbital foramen
Vomer bone
Mandible

Supraorbital foramen
Nasal bone
Sphenoid bone
Middle nasal concha
Zygomatic bone
Inferior nasal concha
Maxilla
Mental foramen

FIGURE 23-7   Anterior view of the skull.

▶ The Spinal Column

LO 23.6

The spinal column consists of 7 cervical vertebrae, 12 thoracic vertebrae, 5 lumbar vertebrae, a sacrum, and a coccyx (see Figure 23-8 and Table 23-3):

- *Cervical vertebrae,* which are located in the neck, are the smallest and lightest vertebrae. The first cervical vertebra is called the *atlas* and the second is called the *axis.* When you turn your head from side to side, your atlas is pivoting around your axis.
- *Thoracic vertebrae* are the posterior attachment for the 12 pairs of ribs. They have long, sharp spinous processes that you can feel when you run your finger down someone's spine.
- *Lumbar vertebrae* are very sturdy structures. They form the small of the back and bear the most weight of all the vertebrae.

TABLE 23-3	The Spinal Column	
Vertebrae Name	**Number**	**Description**
Cervical	7	Smallest and lightest
Thoracic	12	Posterior attachments for ribs
Lumbar	5	Form the small of the back
Sacrum	5	Bones are fused
Coccyx	3 to 5	Bones are fused

- The *sacrum* is a triangular-shaped bone that consists of five fused vertebrae.
- The *coccyx* (commonly called the tailbone) is a small, triangular-shaped bone made up of three to five fused vertebrae; it is considered nonessential in humans.

▶ The Rib Cage

LO 23.7

The rib cage is made of 12 pairs of ribs and the **sternum** (see Figure 23-9). The sternum—often called the breastplate—forms the front middle portion of the rib cage. The cartilaginous tip of the sternum is known as the *xiphoid process.* The sternum joins with the clavicles and most ribs. All 12 pairs of ribs are attached posteriorly to thoracic vertebrae. The ribs themselves are classified in three groups based on their anterior attachment:

- True. The first seven pairs of ribs are *true ribs.* They attach directly to the sternum through pieces of cartilage called *costal cartilage.*
- False. Rib pairs 8, 9, and 10 are called *false ribs.* They do not attach directly to the sternum by individual cartilage but instead attach to the costal cartilage of rib pair number 7.
- Floating. Rib pairs 11 and 12 are called *floating ribs* because they do not attach anteriorly to the sternum or to any other structure.

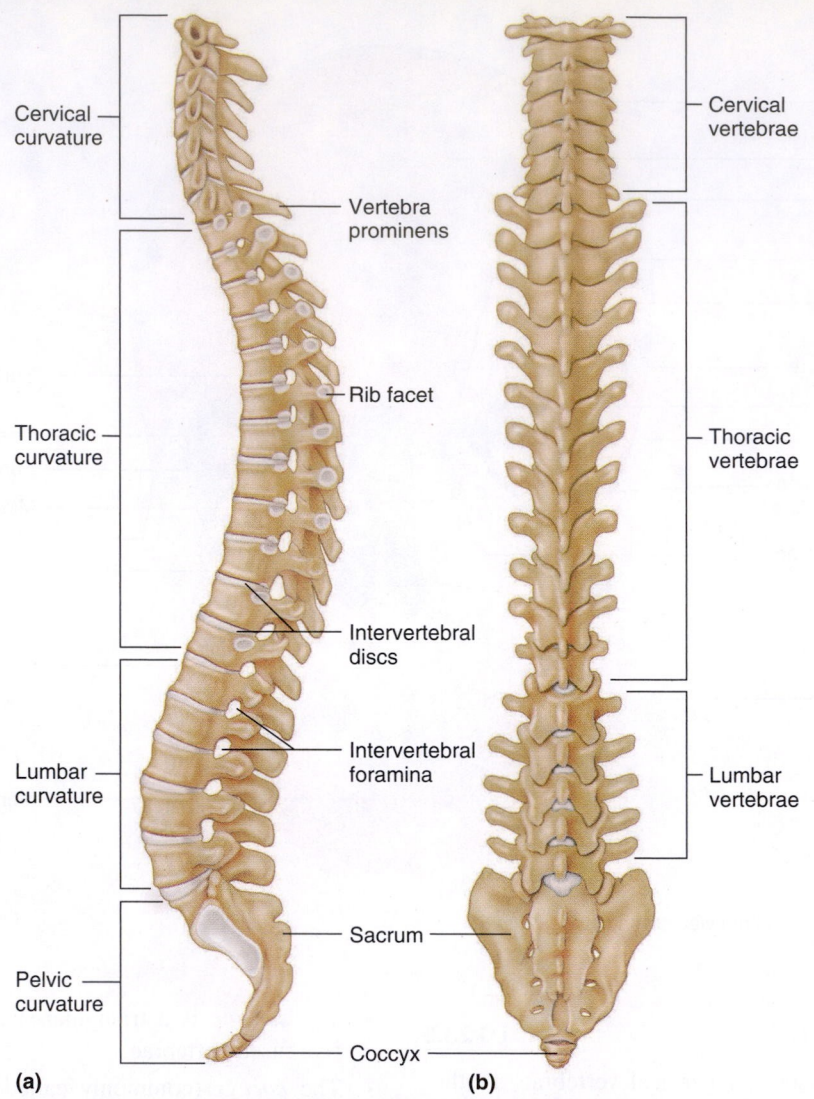

FIGURE 23-8 Vertebral column: (a) lateral view and (b) posterior view.

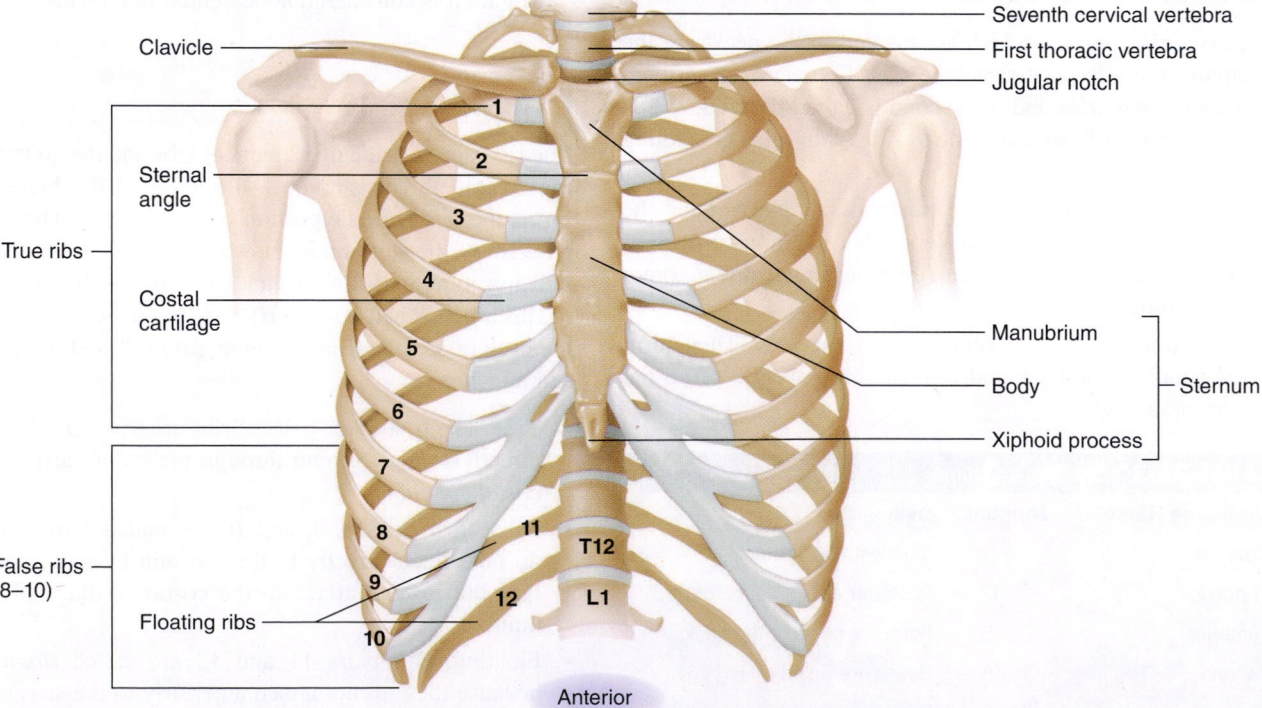

FIGURE 23-9 Thoracic rib cage showing pectoral girdle attachment of upper extremities.

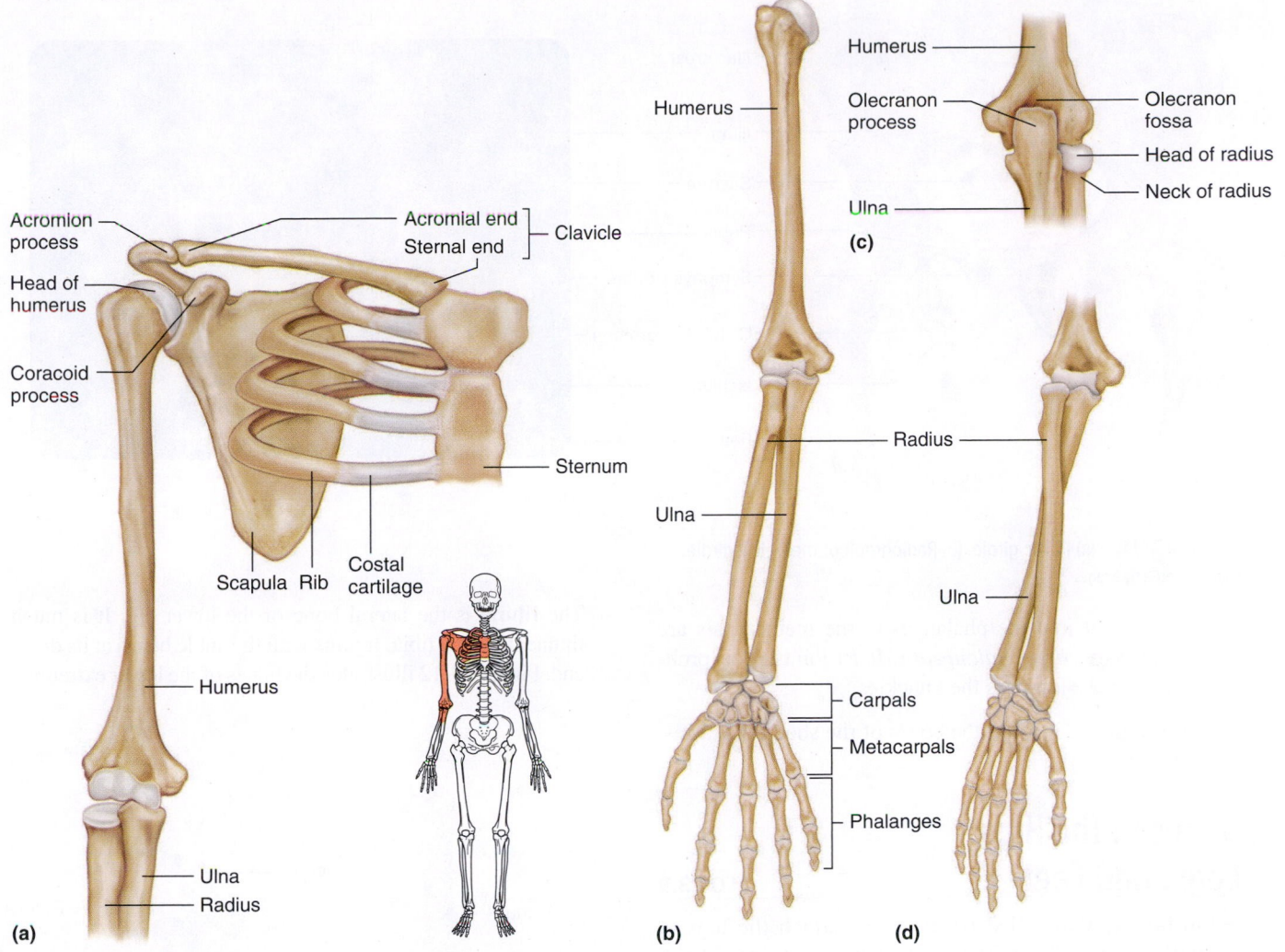

FIGURE 23-10   (a) The pectoral girdle with upper limb attached. (b) Frontal view of upper limb (palm anterior). (c) Frontal view of upper limb (palm posterior). (d) Posterior view of right elbow.

▶ Bones of the Shoulders, Arms, and Hands

LO 23.8

The bones of the shoulders make up the pectoral girdle and include the clavicles and the scapulae (see Figure 23-10). They attach the arms to the axial skeleton.

- The **clavicles,** or collar bones, are slender in shape. Each joins with the sternum and a scapula.
- **Scapulae** (or shoulder blades) are thin, triangular-shaped flat bones located on the dorsal surface of the rib cage. Each scapula joins with the head of a humerus and a clavicle.

The upper limb, or arm, bones include the humerus, radius, and ulna:

- The *humerus* is located in the upper part of the arm. Its proximal end joins with the scapula, and its distal end attaches at the radius and the ulna.

- The **radius** is the lateral bone of the forearm. It is on the same side of the arm as your thumb. Proximally, it joins with the humerus and the ulna, and distally with the carpal (wrist) bones.

- The **ulna** is the medial bone of the lower arm. The proximal end of the ulna joins with the humerus to form the elbow joint. Distally, it also joins with the radius and some of the carpal bones of the wrist.

The bones of the hand include carpals, metacarpals, and phalanges:

- *Carpals* are wrist bones. Each wrist contains eight marble-sized carpal bones.
- **Metacarpals** form the palms of the hands. Each hand has five metacarpals.
- *Phalanges* are the bones of the fingers. There are 14 phalanges in each hand—3 for each finger and 2 per thumb.
- The joints between the phalangeal bones are the proximal and distal *interphalangeal* (PIP and DIP) joints.

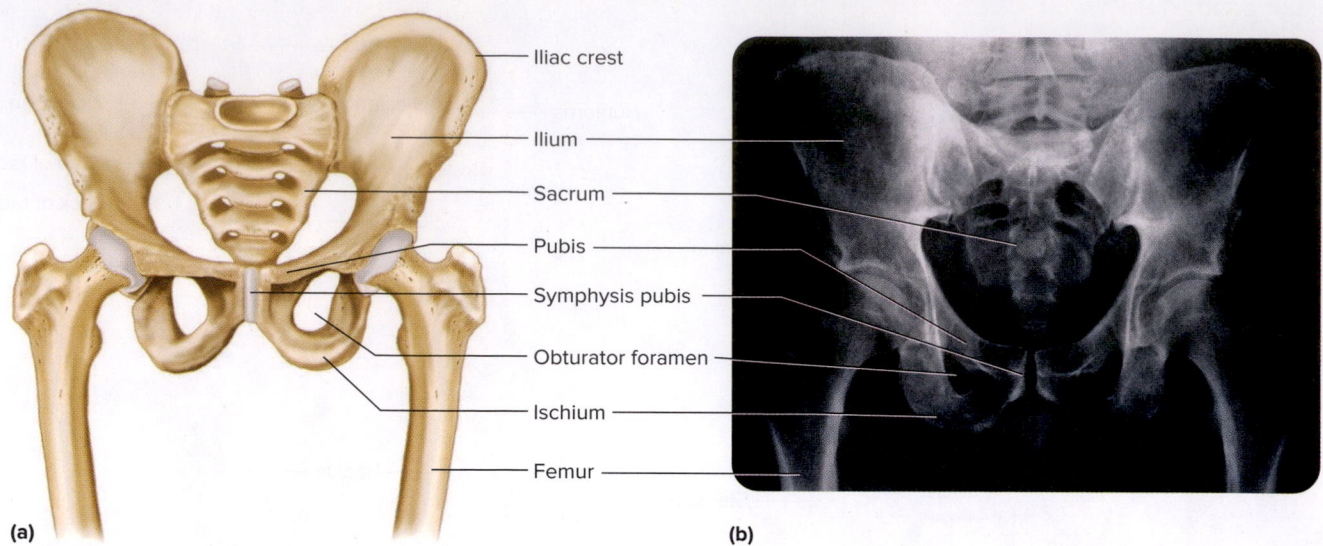

(a)   (b)

FIGURE 23-11 (a) Pelvic girdle. (b) Radiograph of the pelvic girdle.
© Sandra Baker/Getty Images

- The joints that join the phalanges to the metacarpals are called the *metacarpophalangeal (MCP)* joints. You probably know these joints as the knuckles.

    Refer to Figure 23-10 for the bones of the shoulders, arms, and hands.

▶ Bones of the Hips, Legs, and Feet

LO 23.9

The hip bones, also called *coxal* bones, attach the legs to the axial skeleton. They also protect pelvic organs. Each coxal bone has three parts: the ilium, the ischium, and the pubis.

- The *ilium* is the most superior part of a coxal bone. When you put your hands on your hips, you are touching the part of the ilium called the *iliac crest.*
- The *ischium* forms the lower part of a coxal bone and the pubis forms the front.
- The *pubis* bones of each coxal bone join together to form the *symphysis pubis,* which is also referred to as the *pelvic girdle* (see Figure 23-11).

    The bones of the lower limb, or leg, include the femur, the patella, the tibia, and the fibula.

- The femur is the thigh bone and the largest bone in the body. Its proximal end joins with the hip bone at the *acetabulum* (or hip socket). Ligaments and muscles hold it in place.
- The distal end of the femur attaches to the tibia and the **patella** (kneecap). The patella is a sesamoid bone that literally resembles a sesame seed—a small, rounded bone in front of the knee joint.
- The **tibia** (or shinbone) is the medial bone of the lower leg. Its proximal end joins with the femur and fibula, and distally to the ankle bones.

- The **fibula** is the lateral bone of the lower leg. It is much thinner than the tibia. It joins with the ankle bones at its distal end. Figure 23-12 illustrates the bones of the lower extremity.

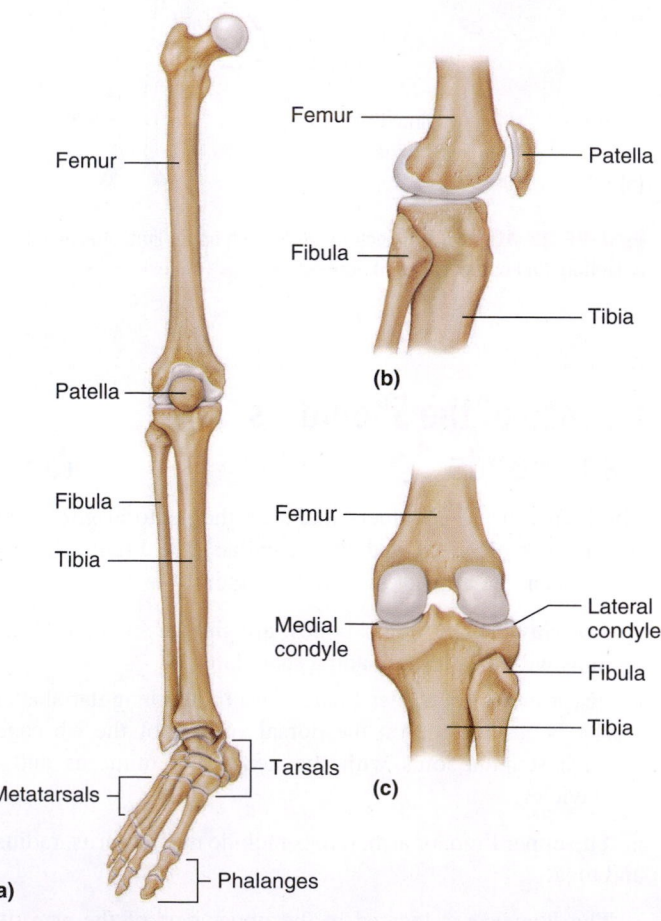

FIGURE 23-12 (a) Anterior view of the right lower limb. (b) Lateral view of the right knee. (c) Posterior view of the right knee.

The bones of the foot include the tarsals, the metatarsals, and the phalanges.

- The *tarsal* bones form the back of the foot. The *calcaneus,* or heel bone, is the largest tarsal bone. There are seven tarsal bones per foot.
- **Metatarsals** are bones that form the front of the foot. There are five metatarsals per foot.
- The bones of the toes are called *phalanges.* Each foot contains 14—2 for each big toe and 3 in all the other toes. The joints between these lower phalanges are interphalangeal joints, just like those of the fingers.
- The joints that join the toes to the foot are called *metatarsophalangeal (MTP)* joints.

▶ Joints
LO 23.10

Joints are the junctions between bones. Based on their structure, joints can be classified as fibrous, cartilaginous, or synovial.

- The bones of *fibrous joints* are connected together with short fibers. So the bones of this type of joint do not normally move against each other. Most fibrous joints are found between cranial bones and facial bones. Fibrous joints in the skull are called **sutures.**
- The bones of *cartilaginous joints* are connected together with a disc of cartilage. This type of joint is slightly movable. The joints between vertebrae are cartilaginous joints.
- The bones of *synovial joints* are covered with hyaline cartilage and are held together by a fibrous joint capsule (see

Figure 23-13). The joint capsule is lined with a synovial membrane, which secretes a slippery fluid called *synovial fluid.* This fluid allows the bones to move easily against each other. Bones are also held together through tough, cord-like structures called *ligaments.* Synovial joints are freely movable. Examples of synovial joints are the elbows, knees, shoulders, and knuckles.

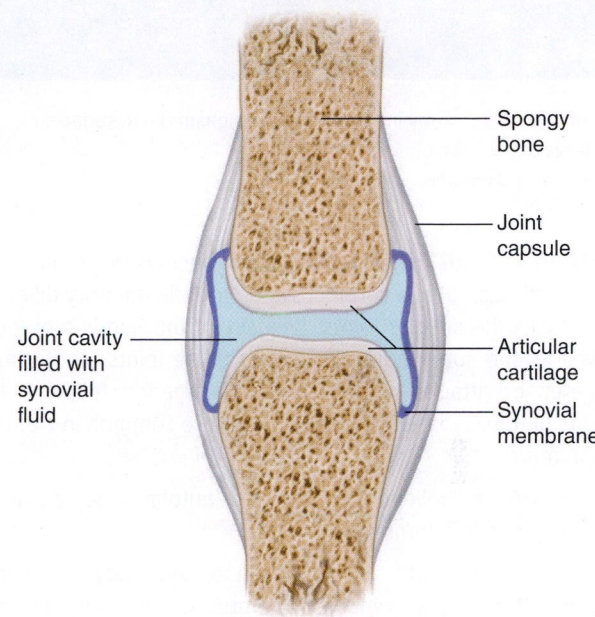

Spongy bone

Joint capsule

Joint cavity filled with synovial fluid

Articular cartilage

Synovial membrane

FIGURE 23-13 Structure of a synovial joint.

PATHOPHYSIOLOGY
LO 23.11

Common Diseases and Disorders of the Skeletal System

Arthritis is a general term meaning "joint inflammation." Although there are more than 100 types of arthritis, we will discuss the two most common types: osteoarthritis and rheumatoid arthritis.

OSTEOARTHRITIS, also known as *degenerative joint disease (DJD),* is the most common type of joint disorder, affecting nearly everyone to some degree by the age of 70. DJD primarily affects the weight-bearing joints of the hips and knees, and the cartilage between the bones and the bones themselves begin to break down.

Causes. Research points to inflammatory processes or metabolic disorders as the etiology of DJD.

Signs and Symptoms. These include joint stiffness, aching, and pain, especially with weather changes. There is often fluid around the joint and grating noises with joint movement.

Treatment. Anti-inflammatory drugs, including aspirin and nonsteroidal anti-inflammatory drugs (NSAIDs) like naproxen and Feldene®, may be used. Intra-articular steroid injections

may be tried for severe cases. In some cases, a series of injections of hyaluronic acid–containing medications is used when other treatments do not work. These injections serve as joint fluid replacement. Some success has been found with transplanting harvested cartilage cells from the patient's healthy knee cartilage, which are then grown in the lab and reinjected into the patient's diseased joint. Surgical scraping of the joint may also be done to remove deteriorated bone fragments. As a last resort, joint replacement may be recommended.

Joint replacement prostheses can be metal, plastic, or a combination of both. The physician can surgically replace part of the joint (partial) or the entire joint (total). An example of a partial hip replacement is the Birmingham Hip Resurfacing prosthesis. In this procedure the head of the femur is replaced by an all-metal prosthesis (see Figure 23-14). One of the advantages of partial joint replacement is that it conserves more bone than conventional total joint replacement. Conserving bone is important if additional surgery is needed in the future. The surgeon will have more natural bone to work with if a revision or new prosthesis is required.

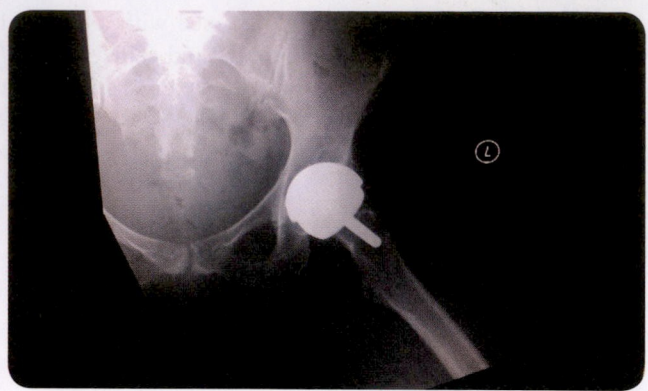

FIGURE 23-14   X-ray image of the Birmingham Hip Resurfacing prosthesis of the left hip.

© Total Care Programming, Inc.

RHEUMATOID ARTHRITIS (RA) is the second most common form of arthritis. RA is a chronic, systemic, inflammatory disease that attacks the smaller joints, typically of the hands and feet, as well as the surrounding tissues of those joints. There may be flares or attacks of pain and inflammation followed by periods of remission. RA is three times more common in women than in men.

Causes. RA is believed to be an autoimmune disease, triggering joint inflammation.

Signs and Symptoms. In this disease, the body's immune system attacks the synovial membrane, causing edema (swelling) and congestion. Tissue becomes granular and thick, eventually destroying the joint capsule and bone. Scar tissue forms, bones atrophy, and visible deformities become apparent due to the bone malalignment and immobility. Patients also have moderate to severe pain in the affected joints.

Treatment.   Treatment includes anti-inflammatory drugs, exercise, heat or cold treatments, and cortisone injections. Researchers are working with genetic techniques to block the immune system reaction. Low-impact aerobic exercise may be helpful, and some patients find warm water exercises beneficial, too.

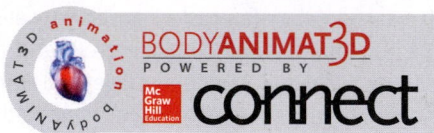

Go to CONNECT to see an animation exercise about *Osteoarthritis vs. Rheumatoid Arthritis.*

BURSITIS is inflammation of a bursa, which is a fluid-filled sac that cushions tendons. It occurs most commonly in the elbow, knee, shoulder, and hip.

Causes.   Overuse of and trauma to joints are the most common causes of this condition. Bacterial infections can also cause bursitis.

Signs and Symptoms.   These include joint pain and swelling, as well as tenderness in the structures surrounding the joint.

Treatment.   The most common treatments are bed rest, pain medications, steroid injections, aspiration of excess fluid from the bursa, and antibiotics.

EWING SARCOMA FAMILY OF TUMORS (ESFT) is a group of tumors that affect different tissue types. However, the tumors primarily affect bone.

Causes.   Causes of ESFT are not clear, but it mostly affects Caucasians between the ages of 10 and 20. The tumors are usually located in the lower extremities but may also occur in the pelvis, chest wall, upper extremities, spine, and skull.

Signs and Symptoms. Fever, pain in the tumor location, fractures, and bruises in the tumor location are the primary symptoms.

Treatment.   Treatment options include surgery, chemotherapy, radiation therapy, a bone marrow transplant, and stem cell transplant.

FRACTURES are cracks, breaks, or splintering of a bone. Fractures are categorized in several ways (Figure 23-15). Complete fractures go across the entire bone; incomplete fractures go through only part of the bone. Comminuted fractures are those in which the bone has broken into several fragments. In a greenstick fracture, the bone is bent, but only one side is fractured. Greenstick fractures occur most often in children because their bones are still soft and pliable. A fracture is closed if it does not cause a break in the skin. In open fractures, the bone breaks through the skin. A **dislocation** is the displacement of a bone end from the joint.

Causes. Fractures and dislocations are most often caused by falls, automobile accidents, and sports injuries. Fractures may also occur in people with bone disorders such as tumors, osteoporosis, and Paget's disease.

Signs and Symptoms. After an accident or a fall, the patient may have intense pain, localized swelling, bruising, bleeding, a limb or joint that is deformed or out of place, numbness, and loss of use of the limb.

Treatment. Fractures and dislocations must be realigned (put back in place) and immobilized. This is usually accomplished by casting or splinting but may require surgical placement of plates, screws, or pins. For more information about emergency treatment of fractures, refer to the *Emergency Preparedness* chapter.

GOUT, also known as *gouty arthritis,* is a type of arthritis that usually occurs more frequently with age.

Causes.   Gout is caused by deposits of uric acid crystals in the joints. People with gout cannot properly break down uric acid and remove it from their bloodstream.

Signs and Symptoms. Symptoms include sudden or chronic joint pain, commonly in the great toe, joint swelling and stiffness, and fever.

Treatment. The most common treatments are pain medications and changes to the patient's diet. Patients should eliminate from their diet certain foods that cause the formation of uric acid (meats, fish, beer, and wine). There are medications available that increase uric acid elimination by the kidneys (uricosuric agents) or decrease uric acid production (xanthine oxidase inhibitors).

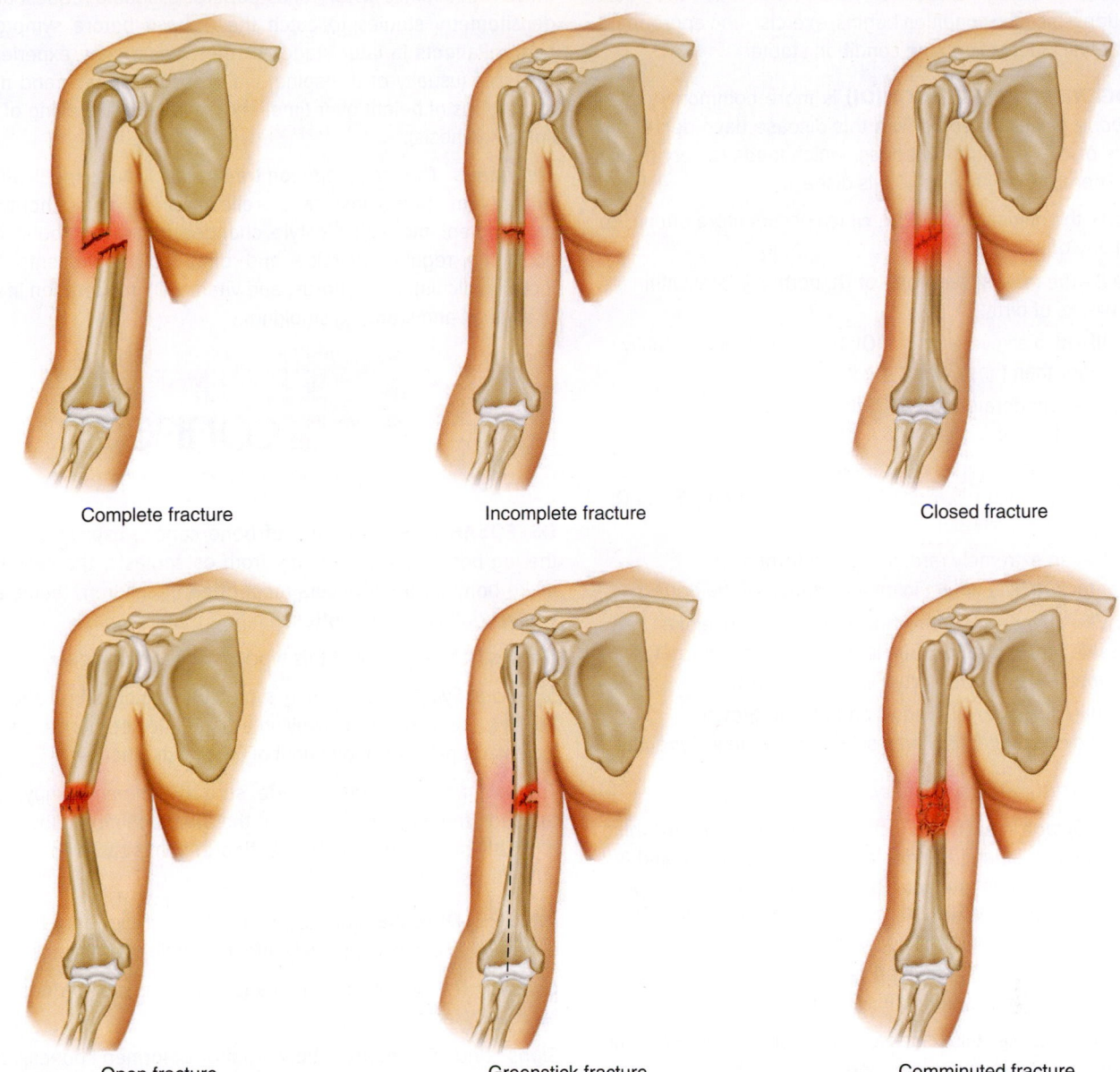

Complete fracture   Incomplete fracture   Closed fracture

Open fracture   Greenstick fracture   Comminuted fracture

FIGURE 23-15   Various types of fractures.

KYPHOSIS is an abnormal curvature of the spine, most often at the thoracic (chest) level. This condition is often referred to as humpback.

Causes. Adolescent kyphosis may result from growth retardation or improper development of the epiphyses as a result of rapid growth. Poor posture may exacerbate or worsen this condition. The adult form of kyphosis is frequently the result of aging and degenerative disc disease of the intervertebral discs and vertebral fracture from underlying osteoporosis.

Signs and Symptoms. In adolescent kyphosis, there may be no symptoms other than visible back curvature. There may be mild pain, tiredness, tenderness, or stiffness of the thoracic spine. In adult kyphosis, the upper back is rounded and there may be pain, back weakness, and fatigue.

Treatment. Childhood kyphosis can be treated with exercise, a firm mattress, and a back brace if needed until growth is completed to keep the spine in alignment. Spinal fusion or grafting may be needed in rare cases of neurological damage or disabling pain. Harrington rods may also be used to keep the vertebrae aligned.

LORDOSIS is an exaggerated inward (convex) curvature of the lumbar spine. Sometimes this condition is called swayback.

Cause. Wearing high heels is a frequent cause. The positioning of the feet with the elevated heel height causes an inward positioning of the back as a counter-balancing measure.

Signs and Symptoms. The main sign is visual inward curvature of the lower back. There may be mild pain with this exaggerated curvature.

Treatment. Avoiding excessive heel height is the best prevention. Once the condition begins, exercise and appropriate footwear will at least keep the condition stable.

OSTEOGENESIS IMPERFECTA (OI) is more commonly called *brittle-bone disease*. People with this disease have decreased amounts of collagen in their bones, which leads to very fragile bones. There are eight types of this disease:

- Type I—the mildest form of OI, which occurs more often than any of the other types
- Type II—the most severe form of OI, normally fatal within a few weeks of birth
- Type III—also a severe type of OI; however, infants usually live longer than those with Type II
- Type IV—a moderate form of OI that is usually diagnosed later in childhood
- Type V—similar to Type IV except that large callouses form around bone fractures. This type accounts for only 5% of OI cases
- Type VI—an extremely rare, moderate form of OI characterized by a defect in mineralization of the bone
- Type VII—a moderate form caused by inheritance of a recessive gene mutation. Similar to Type IV. Moderately abnormal bone growth occurs in this type of OI.
- Type VIII—similar to OI Types II and III, and growth deficiency is severe; however, sclera are white in Type VIII

Cause. The disorder is hereditary.

Signs and Symptoms. These include fractures (all types); blue sclera (types I, II, III, and IV): dental problems (types III and IV); hearing loss (type I); a triangular face (type III); abnormal spinal curves (types I, III, IV, V, and VI): very small stature (types II, III, IV, VII, and VIII); a small chest (types II and III); fractures at birth (types II and III); loose joints (type IV); muscle weakness (types I, III, and IV); and respiratory difficulties (types I, II, III, and VIII).

Treatment. Because this disease has many symptoms, the list of treatments is extensive and includes fracture repair, surgery to strengthen bones by inserting metal rods into them, dental procedures, physical therapy, braces to prevent bone deformities, wheelchairs and other supportive aids, medications, and counseling. Other surgeries may be required to treat lung and heart problems that sometimes occur with this disease.

OSTEOPOROSIS is a condition in which bones become thin (more porous) over time. It is a very common disorder in the United States and affects women more than men and Caucasians more than any other race. This condition occurs because of hypocalcemia in which bone is broken down to release calcium and is not replaced in sufficient amounts; thus, bone density decreases.

Causes. These include hormone deficiencies (estrogen in women and testosterone in men), a sedentary lifestyle, a lack of calcium and vitamin D in the diet, bone cancers, corticosteroid excess (usually as a result of endocrine diseases), smoking, excess alcohol consumption, and steroid use.

Signs and Symptoms. There are usually no symptoms in the early stages of this disease. Patients at high risk, especially those with a family history of osteoporosis, should request bone densitometry studies to catch the disease before symptoms begin. Patients in later stages of the disease may experience fractures (usually of the spine, wrists, or hips), back and neck pain, a loss of height over time, and an abnormal curving of the spine (kyphosis).

Treatment. The most common treatments include medications to prevent bone loss and relieve bone pain; hormone replacement therapy; lifestyle changes to prevent bone loss (including regular exercise and diets or supplements that include calcium, phosphorus, and vitamin D); moderation in use of alcohol; and stopping smoking.

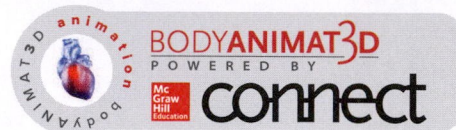

Go to CONNECT to see an animation exercise about *Osteoporosis*.

OSTEOSARCOMA is a type of bone cancer, usually affecting the leg bones, that originates from osteoblasts, the cells that make bony tissue. It occurs most often in children, teens, and young adults and more often in males than females.

Causes. The etiology of this type of cancer is unclear.

Signs and Symptoms. Primary symptoms include pain in affected bones (usually the legs), swelling around affected bones, and an increase in pain with movement of the affected bones.

Treatment. Treatments include surgery, chemotherapy, and radiation therapy. Amputation of the affected limb, followed by a prosthesis fitting, may be needed in some cases to prevent metastasis.

PAGET'S DISEASE causes bones to enlarge and become deformed and weak. It usually affects people over the age of 40.

Causes. This disease may be caused by a virus or various hereditary factors.

Signs and Symptoms. Bone pain, deformed bones, and fractures are common symptoms. Patients may experience headaches and hearing loss if the disease affects skull bones.

Treatment. Treatments include surgery to remodel bones, hip replacements, medications to prevent bone weakening, and physical therapy.

SCOLIOSIS is an abnormal, S-shaped, lateral curvature of the thoracic or lumbar spine.

Causes. This disorder can develop prenatally when vertebrae do not fuse together. It can also result from diseases that cause weakness of the muscles that hold vertebrae together. Other causes of scoliosis are unknown, but they may be genetic.

Signs and Symptoms. A patient with scoliosis usually has a spine that looks bent to one side, with one shoulder or hip appearing to be higher than the other. Patients often experience back pain.

Treatment. Treatment includes different types of back braces, surgery to correct spinal curves, and physical therapy to strengthen the muscles of the back and abdomen.

LEARNING OUTCOMES	KEY POINTS
23.1 Describe the structure of bone tissue.	Bones consist of the following substances: osteons (the Haversian system), bone matrix between osteocytes (bone cells), collagen fibers and proteins, lamellae, and canaliculi. Long bones include the femur and humerus; short bones include the carpals and tarsals; flat bones include the ribs and the frontal bone; irregular bones include the vertebrae and bones of the pelvic girdle. The diaphysis is the shaft of the long bone. The epiphysis is an end of a long bone. Articular cartilage covers the end of the long bones. The endosteum lines the medullary cavity. The periosteum is the membrane surrounding the diaphysis.
23.2 Explain the functions of bones.	Bone functions include giving shape to body parts, protecting soft structures of the body, and assisting in movement. The red bone marrow is responsible for hematopoiesis. Bones also store calcium.
23.3 Compare intramembranous and endochondral ossification.	Bones grow through two types of ossification: intramembranous ossification and endochondral ossification. The cartilage plate between the diaphysis and the epiphysis allows for growth of the long bone.
23.4 Describe the skeletal structures and one location of each structure.	Skeletal structures include the following: condyles, crests, epicondyles, foramina, fossae, heads, processes, sutures, trochanters, tubercles, and tuberosities.
23.5 Locate the bones of the skull.	The major bones of the skull are the frontal, parietal, temporal, and occipital bones. The fontanels are the membranous structures that connect the incompletely developed cranial bones. Within the skull are the mastoid processes, sphenoid, ethmoid, and ear ossicles. The facial bones include the mandible, maxillae, zygomatics, nasal and palatine bones, and vomer. Locations are shown in Figures 23-6 and 23-7.
23.6 Locate the bones of the spinal column.	The spinal column includes cervical, thoracic, and lumbar vertebrae; the sacrum; and the coccyx. Locations are shown in Figure 23-8.
23.7 Locate the bones of the rib cage.	There are 12 pairs of ribs, a sternum, and the xiphoid process. Locations are shown in Figure 23-8.
23.8 Locate the bones of the shoulders, arms, and hands.	Each upper extremity includes the clavicle, scapula, humerus, radius, ulna, carpals, metacarpals, and phalanges. Locations are shown in Figure 23-10.
23.9 Locate the bones of the hips, legs, and feet.	The bones of the hip, leg, and foot include the coxal bones, the femur, patella, tibia, fibula, metatarsals, tarsals, and phalanges. Locations are shown in Figures 23-11 and 23-12.
23.10 Describe the three major types of joints and give examples of each.	The three joint types are fibrous joints (for example, sutures of the skull), cartilaginous joints (for example, the joints between vertebrae), and synovial joints (for example, the elbow). A synovial joint consists of hyaline-covered bones held together by a fibrous joint capsule, which is lined by a synovial membrane that secretes synovial fluid. Ligaments hold the bones of these joints together.

LEARNING OUTCOMES	KEY POINTS
23.11 Describe the common diseases and disorders of the skeletal system.	There are many common diseases and disorders of the bones and the skeletal system with varied signs, symptoms, and treatments. Examples include arthritis, bursitis, EFT, fractures, gout, kyphosis, lordosis, and scoliosis, as well as osteoporosis and osteosarcoma.

CASE STUDY CRITICAL THINKING

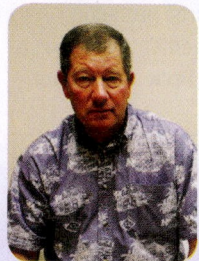

© McGraw-Hill Education

Recall John Miller from the beginning of the chapter. Now that you have completed the chapter, answer the following questions regarding his case.

1. Explain to John what bursitis is and what causes it.

2. What treatment might the family nurse practitioner prescribe for John's bursitis?

3. Why do you think John's family nurse practitioner suspects bursitis and not a fracture?

4. John's family nurse practitioner thinks that John may have bruised the sesamoid bone in front of his knee joint. What is the medical term for this bone?

5. The X-ray findings state that AP and lateral views of the knee and elbow showed no fractures. Describe the terms *AP* and *lateral*.

EXAM PREPARATION QUESTIONS

1. (LO 23.1) The tiny canals of cancellous bone that allow for the spread of nutrients are called
   a. Lamellae
   b. Lacunae
   c. Osteons
   d. Canaliculi
   e. Osteoblasts

2. (LO 23.3) Which substance is necessary for bone to absorb calcium?
   a. Vitamin C
   b. Phosporus
   c. Vitamin D
   d. Protein
   e. Carbohydrates

3. (LO 23.4) Articulation is another name for a
   a. Fossa
   b. Joint
   c. Foramen
   d. Suture
   e. Tubercle

4. (LO 23.5) Neck muscles attach to the skull via the _____ process.
   a. Mastoid
   b. Xiphoid
   c. Styloid
   d. Zygomatic
   e. Coracoid

5. (LO 23.9) The acetabulum is the
   a. Hip bone
   b. Knee joint
   c. Hip socket
   d. Shoulder bone
   e. Shoulder socket

6. (LO 23.11) A lateral curvature of the spine is known as
   a. Lordosis
   b. Kyphosis
   c. Osteoporosis
   d. Scoliosis
   e. Sarcoma

7. (LO 23.11) The medical term for brittle-bone disease is
   a. Ewing sarcoma family of tumors
   b. Osteogenesis imperfecta
   c. Rheumatoid arthritis
   d. Osteoporosis
   e. Paget's disease

8. (LO 23.1) Which of the following is the shaft of a long bone?
   a. Spine
   b. Epiphysis
   c. Crest
   d. Periosteum
   e. Diaphysis

9. (LO 23.1) The bones of the rib cage are
   a. Long bones
   b. Flat bones
   c. Irregular bones
   d. Short bones
   e. Sesamoid bones

10. (LO 23.4) Which of the following is an interlocking line of union between bones?
   a. Suture
   b. Condyle
   c. Process
   d. Articulation
   e. Fossa

MEDICAL TERMINOLOGY PRACTICE

Analyze the following medical terms, presented throughout the chapter. Using a medical dictionary (or Appendix I) place a / mark between each word part. Define each word part and then define the whole word.

EXAMPLE: **mast/oid** = mast means "breast" + oid means "resembling"
   MASTOID means "resembling a breast." (A mastoid process resembles a breast.)

1. arthritis
2. bursitis
3. scoliosis
4. costal
5. coxal
6. metacarpophalangeal
7. metatarsophalangeal
8. osteoblast
9. osteoclast
10. osteocyte
11. osteoporosis
12. osteosarcoma
13. hematopoiesis
14. interphalangeal
15. intramembranous
16. synovial
17. periosteum
18. temporal

The Muscular System

CASE STUDY

PATIENT INFORMATION			
Patient Name	**DOB**	**Allergies**	
Ken Washington	12/1/19XX	Sulfa	
Attending	**MRN**	**Other Information**	
Paul F. Buckwalter, MD	891-12-743	AFO brace ordered	

Ken F. Washington, a 61-year-old male patient, has arrived for a follow-up visit from a recent hospitalization for a stroke. Until this hospitalization, he had no major health issues. However, he now has weakness in his left arm and his speech is difficult to understand. He has left-leg weakness with foot drop, a condition characterized by an inability to raise the front part of the foot. The foot drop is causing

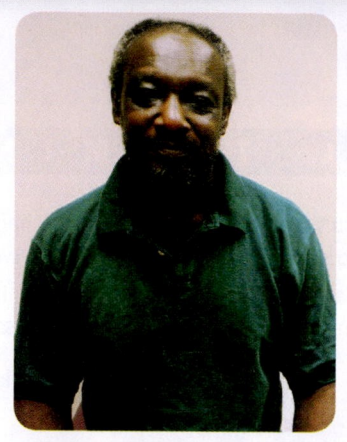

© McGraw-Hill Education

him to trip when he walks more than a few steps. The physician has ordered a physical therapy evaluation and treatment as needed. The patient has been placed on an exercise regimen for his left-arm weakness. A special ankle foot orthosis (AFO) brace has been ordered to help Ken with his foot drop.

Keep Ken in mind as you study this chapter. There will be questions at the end of the chapter based on the case study. The information in the chapter will help you answer these questions.

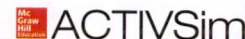

LEARNING OUTCOMES

After completing Chapter 24, you will be able to:

24.1 Describe the functions of muscle.

24.2 Compare the three types of muscle tissue, including their locations and characteristics.

24.3 Explain how muscle tissue generates energy.

24.4 Describe the structure of a skeletal muscle.

24.5 Differentiate between the terms *origin* and *insertion*.

24.6 Identify the major skeletal muscles of the body, giving the action of each.

24.7 Summarize the changes that occur to the muscular system as a person ages.

24.8 Describe the causes, signs and symptoms, and treatments of various diseases and disorders of the muscular system.

KEY TERMS

acetylcholine
acetylcholinesterase
agonist
antagonist
aponeurosis
creatine phosphate
fascicle
insertion
lactic acid
multi-unit smooth muscle

myofibrils
origin
prime mover
sarcolemma
sarcoplasm
sarcoplasmic reticulum
sphincter
striations
synergist
visceral smooth muscle

▶ Introduction

Your bones and joints do not produce movement all by themselves. Instead, your muscles—by alternating between contraction and relaxation—cause your bones and supported structures to move. The human body has more than 600 individual muscles. Although each muscle is a distinct structure, muscles act in groups to perform particular movements. In this chapter, you will explore the differences among three muscle tissue types, the structure of skeletal muscles, muscle actions, and the names of skeletal muscles.

▶ Functions of Muscle   LO 24.1

Muscle tissue is unique because it has the ability to contract. This contraction allows muscles to perform various functions. In addition to allowing the human body to move, muscles provide stability, control body openings and passages, and warm the body.

Movement

Skeletal muscles are attached to bones by tendons. Because skeletal muscles cross joints, when these muscles contract, the bones they attach to move. This allows for various body motions, like walking or waving your hand. Facial muscles are attached to the skin of the face; when they contract, different facial expressions are produced, such as smiling or frowning. Smooth muscle is found in the walls of various organs, like the stomach, intestines, and uterus. The contraction of smooth muscle in these organs produces the movement of their contents, such as the movement of food material through the intestine or the birth of a child being pushed from the mother's uterus. Cardiac muscle of the heart produces the atrial and ventricular contractions that pump blood into the blood vessels.

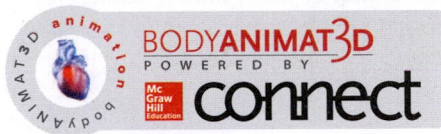

BODYANIMAT3D
POWERED BY
McGraw Hill Education
connect

Go to CONNECT to see an animation exercise about *Muscle Contraction*.

Stability

You rarely think about it, but muscles are holding your bones tightly together so that your joints remain stable. There are also very small muscles holding your vertebrae together to stabilize your spinal column.

Heat Production

When muscles contract, heat is released, which helps the body maintain a normal temperature. This is why moving your body—say, jogging in place for a few seconds—can make you warmer if you are cold.

Control of Body Openings and Passages

In addition to providing important structural support for your bones and joints, muscles also form valve-like structures called **sphincters** around various body openings and passages. These sphincters control the movement of substances into and out of these passages. For example, a urethral sphincter prevents urination until you relax it to permit urination.

▶ Muscle Cells and Tissue   LO 24.2

There are three types of muscle tissue: skeletal, smooth, and cardiac. Muscle tissue is made of muscle cells. Muscle cells, or *myocytes,* are called muscle fibers because of their long lengths. The cell membrane of a muscle fiber

TABLE 24-1   Types of Muscle Tissue

Muscle Group	Major Location	Major Function	Striated (Yes/No)	Mode of Control	Rate of Contraction	Intercalated Discs
Skeletal muscle	Attached to bones and the skin of the face	Produces body movements and facial expressions	Yes	Voluntary	Fast to contract and relax	No
Smooth muscle	Walls of hollow organs, blood vessels, and iris	Moves contents through organs; vasoconstriction	No	Involuntary	Slow to contract and relax	No
Cardiac muscle	Wall of the heart	Pumps blood through heart	Yes	Involuntary	Groups of muscle fibers contract as a unit	Yes

is called a **sarcolemma.** The cytoplasm of this cell type is called **sarcoplasm,** and the endoplasmic reticulum is called **sarcoplasmic reticulum.** Most of the sarcoplasm is filled with long structures called **myofibrils.** It is the arrangement of the actin and myosin filaments in myofibrils that produces the **striations,** or stripes, observed in skeletal and cardiac muscle cells. Muscle fibers are controlled by motor neurons that release chemical substances called *neurotransmitters,* such as acetylcholine, dopamine, and epinephrine, onto the fibers. See Figure 24-1 for an illustration of the structure of a skeletal muscle. Study Table 24-1 to review the locations and features of the three types of muscle tissue.

Skeletal Muscle

Skeletal muscle fibers respond only to the neurotransmitter **acetylcholine,** which causes skeletal muscle to contract. Once contraction has occurred, skeletal muscles release an enzyme called **acetylcholinesterase,** which breaks down acetylcholine. This allows the muscle to relax. Figure 24-2a shows a photomicrograph of skeletal muscle. These muscles are responsible for body movement, posture, and heat generation through shivering.

Smooth Muscle

There are two types of smooth muscle: multi-unit and visceral. **Multi-unit smooth muscle** is found in the iris of the

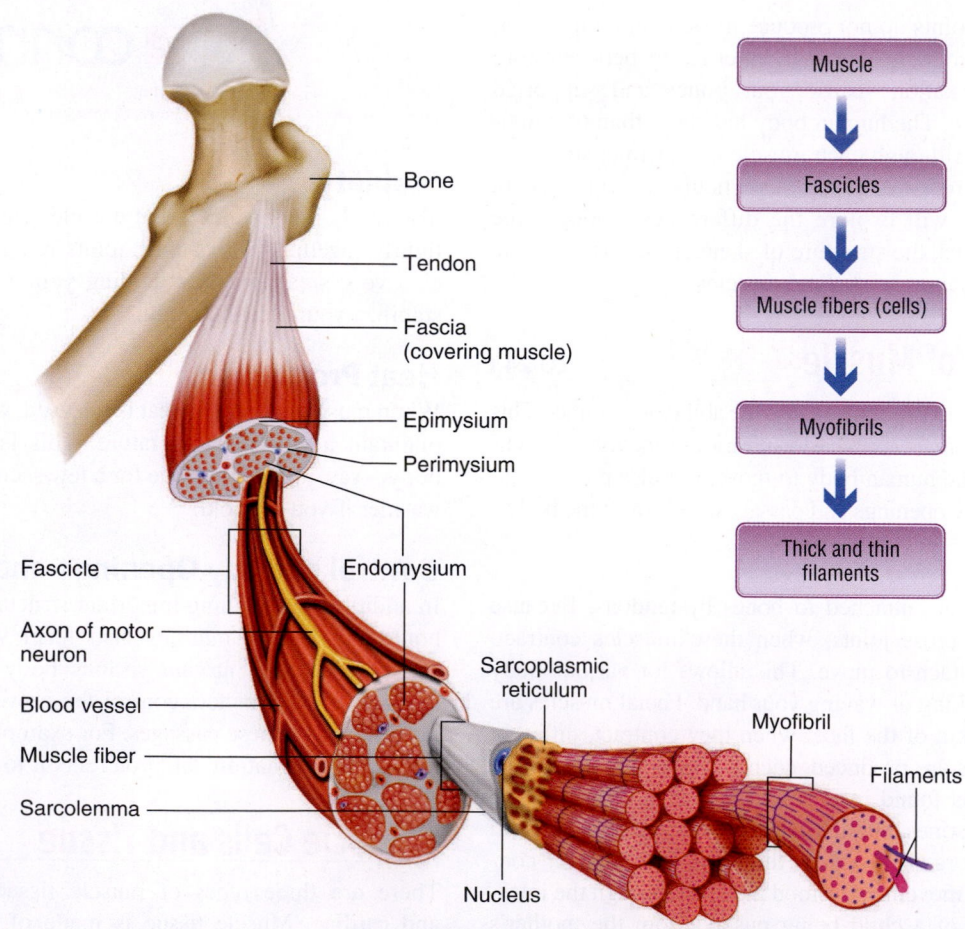

FIGURE 24-1   Structure of a skeletal muscle.

eye and the walls of blood vessels. This muscle type contracts in response to neurotransmitters and hormones. **Visceral smooth muscle** contains sheets of muscle cells that closely contact each other. It is found in the walls of hollow organs like the stomach, intestines, bladder, and uterus. Muscle fibers in visceral smooth muscle respond to neurotransmitters, but they also stimulate each other to contract, so the muscle fibers tend to contract and relax together. This type of muscle produces an action called peristalsis. *Peristalsis* is a rhythmic contraction that pushes substances through tubes of the body. For example, peristalsis in the lower two-thirds of the esophagus moves the *bolus* of food through the stomach; peristaltic muscle movements in the fallopian tubes propel the ovum (egg) through the tubes toward the uterus.

Two neurotransmitters are involved in smooth muscle contraction—acetylcholine and norepinephrine. Depending on the smooth muscle type, these neurotransmitters cause or inhibit contractions. Figure 24-2b is a photomicrograph of smooth muscle.

Cardiac Muscle

Groups of cardiac muscle are connected to each other through *intercalated discs*—discs with tunnels that physically connect the cardiac muscle cells. These discs allow the fibers in each group to contract and relax together—a design that allows the heart to work as a pump. First, the atria (holding chambers) contract and relax together; then the ventricles (pumping chambers) contract to send blood to the lungs and body, after which they relax and the cycle starts again. Cardiac muscle is also self-exciting, which means that it does not need nerve stimulation to contract. Nerves only speed up or slow down the contraction of the heart. Like smooth muscle, cardiac muscle responds to two neurotransmitters—acetylcholine and norepinephrine. Acetylcholine slows the heart rate, and norepinephrine speeds it up. Figure 24-2c is a photomicrograph of cardiac muscle.

▶ Production of Energy for Muscle   LO 24.3

Because a lot of adenosine triphosphate (ATP)—a type of chemical energy—is needed for sustained or repeated muscle contractions, a muscle cell must have multiple ways to store or make this substance. Muscle cells make this energy in three ways:

- **Creatine phosphate** production. Creatine phosphate production is a rapid way for a muscle to produce energy. When ATP is used during muscle contraction, it loses a phosphate and, therefore, energy. Imagine a desk toy that has five ball bearings suspended by strings. You create potential energy by lifting one of the ball bearings away from the others. When you release the ball bearing—breaking the bond between your fingers and the ball—the potential energy is released and the ball bearing hits the others, causing them to swing back and forth for several minutes. As with the ball bearing, energy stored in the phosphate bond is released when the bond is broken. Creatine phosphate "donates" a phosphate group, restoring energy potential.

- *Aerobic respiration*—an energy-forming biochemical process that requires oxygen—uses the body's store of glucose to

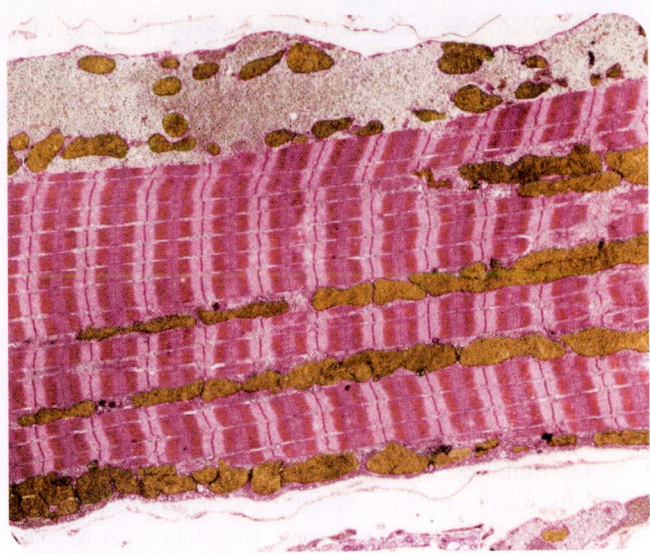

(a)

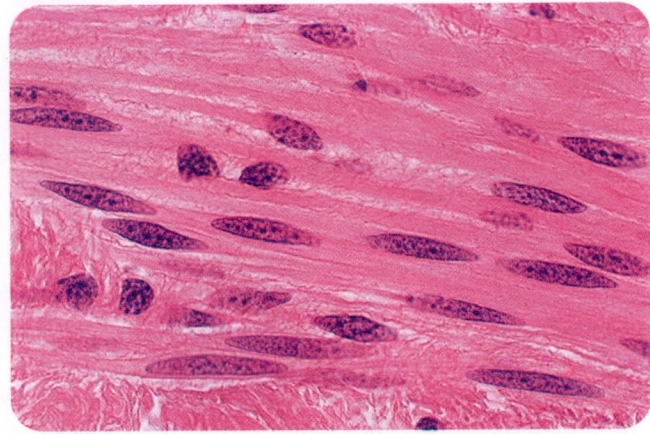

(b)

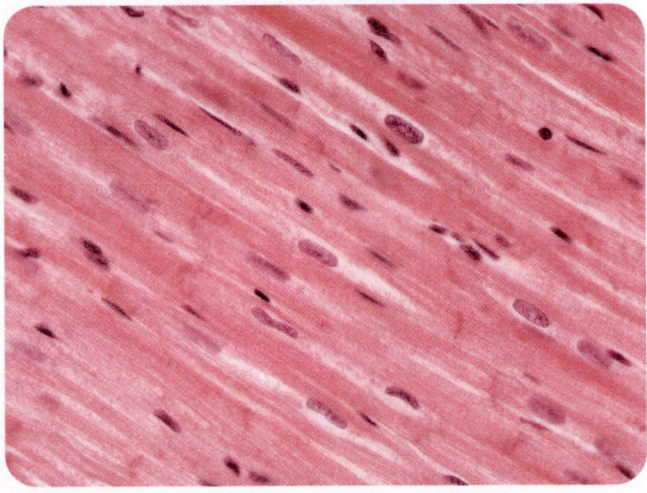

(c)

FIGURE 24-2   Photomicrographs of (a) skeletal, (b) smooth, and (c) cardiac muscle.

© Science Photo Library RF/Getty Images; © McGraw-Hill Education/Dennis Strete, photographer; © McGraw-Hill Education/Al Telser, photographer

make ATP. A cell breaks down glucose into pyruvic acid using oxygen (hence the term *aerobic*). The pyruvic acid is further converted into acetyl coenzyme A, which begins a series of reactions known as the *Krebs cycle,* or citric acid cycle. The oxygen needed for this method is stored in the muscle pigment called *myoglobin,* which also gives muscle its pinkish color.

- **Lactic acid** production occurs when a cell is low in oxygen and must convert pyruvic acid to lactic acid. This conversion produces a small amount of ATP for the cell, but because lactic acid is a waste product, it must then be released from the cell.

Oxygen Debt

Oxygen debt occurs when skeletal muscle is used strenuously for several minutes. When pyruvic acid is converted to lactic acid for energy production, the lactic acid builds up and causes muscle fatigue and soreness. The lactic acid is taken to the liver via the bloodstream to be converted back into glucose, which requires more energy. The amount of oxygen the liver cells need to make enough ATP for this conversion results in the oxygen debt. This process explains why your body still burns energy even after you are done exercising.

Muscle Fatigue

Muscle fatigue is a condition in which a muscle has lost its ability to contract. It usually develops because of an accumulation of lactic acid. It can also occur if the blood supply to a muscle is interrupted or if a motor neuron loses its ability to release acetylcholine onto muscle fibers. Cramps—painful, involuntary contractions of muscles—can accompany muscle fatigue. For this reason, if you have just finished an intense workout, it is important to replenish your electrolytes by drinking fluids and eating foods that are good sources of sodium, potassium, and calcium.

▶ Structure of Skeletal Muscles   LO 24.4

Skeletal muscles are the major organs that make up the muscular system. A skeletal muscle consists of connective tissue, skeletal muscle tissue, blood vessels, and nerves. When you see marbling in a steak, you are actually viewing connective tissue. The red portion of the steak is the muscle tissue.

The following connective tissue coverings are associated with skeletal muscles (see Figure 24-1):

- *Fascia.* Connective tissue located just below the skin that helps support and hold together muscles, bones, nerves, and blood vessels.
- *Tendon.* Tough, cord-like structure made of fibrous connective tissue that connects muscles to bones.
- **Aponeurosis.** Tough, sheet-like structure made of fibrous connective tissue. It typically attaches muscles to other muscles.
- *Epimysium.* A thin covering that is just deep to the fascia of a muscle. It surrounds the entire muscle.
- *Perimysium.* A sheath of connective tissue surrounding a group of 10 to 100 muscle fibers. This grouping of muscle fibers is called a **fascicle.**
- *Endomysium.* The connective tissue that surrounds individual muscle cells.

▶ Attachments and Actions of Skeletal Muscles   LO 24.5

In order for skeletal muscle to produce movement, it must cross a joint and have at least two attachments to bone—one to the bone proximal to the joint and the second distal to the joint. Typically, one of the bones is more movable than the other when the muscle contracts. These attachments are known as the *origin* and *insertion.* An **origin** is an attachment site for the less movable bone during muscle contraction. An **insertion** is an attachment site for the more movable bone during muscle contraction. For example, the biceps brachii (the muscle on the anterior upper arm) attaches to two places on the scapula and to one site on the radius. When the biceps brachii contracts, the radius moves and the arm bends at the elbow. So the origin of the biceps brachii is where it attaches to the scapula. The insertion site of the biceps brachii is its attachment site on the radius (see Figure 24-3).

Most of the time, body movement is not produced by only one muscle, but by a group of muscles. However, one muscle is responsible for most of the movement; this muscle is called the **prime mover** or **agonist.** Other muscles help the prime mover by stabilizing joints; these muscles are called **synergists.** An **antagonist** is a muscle that produces a movement opposite to the prime mover. When the prime mover contracts, the antagonist must relax in order to produce a smooth body movement. For example, when you bend your arm at the elbow, the prime mover (agonist) is the biceps brachii. The synergist muscles are the brachialis and brachioradialis. The antagonist is the triceps brachii because its action is to extend the arm at the elbow. While the prime mover and synergists contract, the agonist relaxes; when the antagonist contracts, the prime mover and synergists relax.

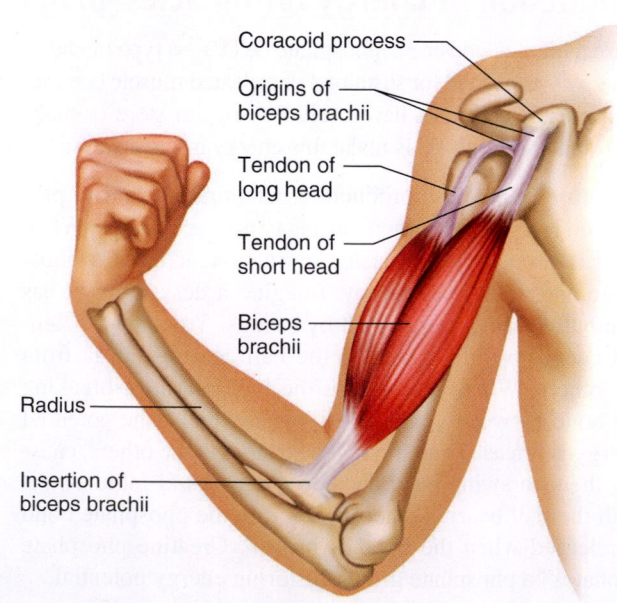

Coracoid process

Origins of biceps brachii

Tendon of long head

Tendon of short head

Biceps brachii

Radius

Insertion of biceps brachii

FIGURE 24-3   Origins and insertion of biceps brachii.

The body movements produced by skeletal muscles include the following:

- *Flexion*—bending a body part or decreasing the angle of a joint
- *Extension*—straightening a body part or increasing the angle of a joint
- *Hyperextension*—extending a body part past the normal anatomical position
- *Dorsiflexion*—pointing the toes up
- *Plantar flexion*—pointing the toes down
- *Abduction*—moving a body part away from the midline of the body
- *Adduction*—moving a body part toward the midline of the body
- *Rotation*—twisting a body part—for example, turning your head from side to side
- *Circumduction*—moving a body part in a circle—for example, moving your arm in a circular motion
- *Pronation*—turning the palm of the hand down or lying face down
- *Supination*—turning the palm of the hand up or lying face up
- *Inversion*—turning the sole of the foot medially
- *Eversion*—turning the sole of the foot laterally
- *Retraction*—moving a body part posteriorly
- *Protraction*—moving a body part anteriorly

- *Elevation*—lifting a body part—for example, elevating your shoulders as in a shrugging gesture
- *Depression*—lowering a body part—for example, lowering your shoulders

See Figures 24-4, 24-5, and 24-6 for illustrations of these types of movements. As a medical assistant, it is important to understand these movements so that you can assist with judging and measuring your patients' ability to perform range-of-motion (ROM) exercises when assessing injuries and illnesses.

▶ Major Skeletal Muscles   LO 24.6

The name of a skeletal muscle often describes it in some way. Usually, the name indicates the location, size, action, shape, or number of attachments of the muscle. For example, the pectoralis major is named for its large size (major) and its location (pectoral, or chest, region). The sternocleidomastoid is named for its attachment sites—*sterno* (sternum), *cleido* (clavicle), and *mastoid* (the mastoid process of the temporal bone, located behind the ear). As you study muscles, you will find it easier to remember them if you think about what the name describes. Figures 24-7 and 24-8 show the anterior and posterior views of superficial skeletal muscles.

Muscles of the Head
The muscles of the head include those that move the head, provide facial expression, and move the jaw. Muscles that

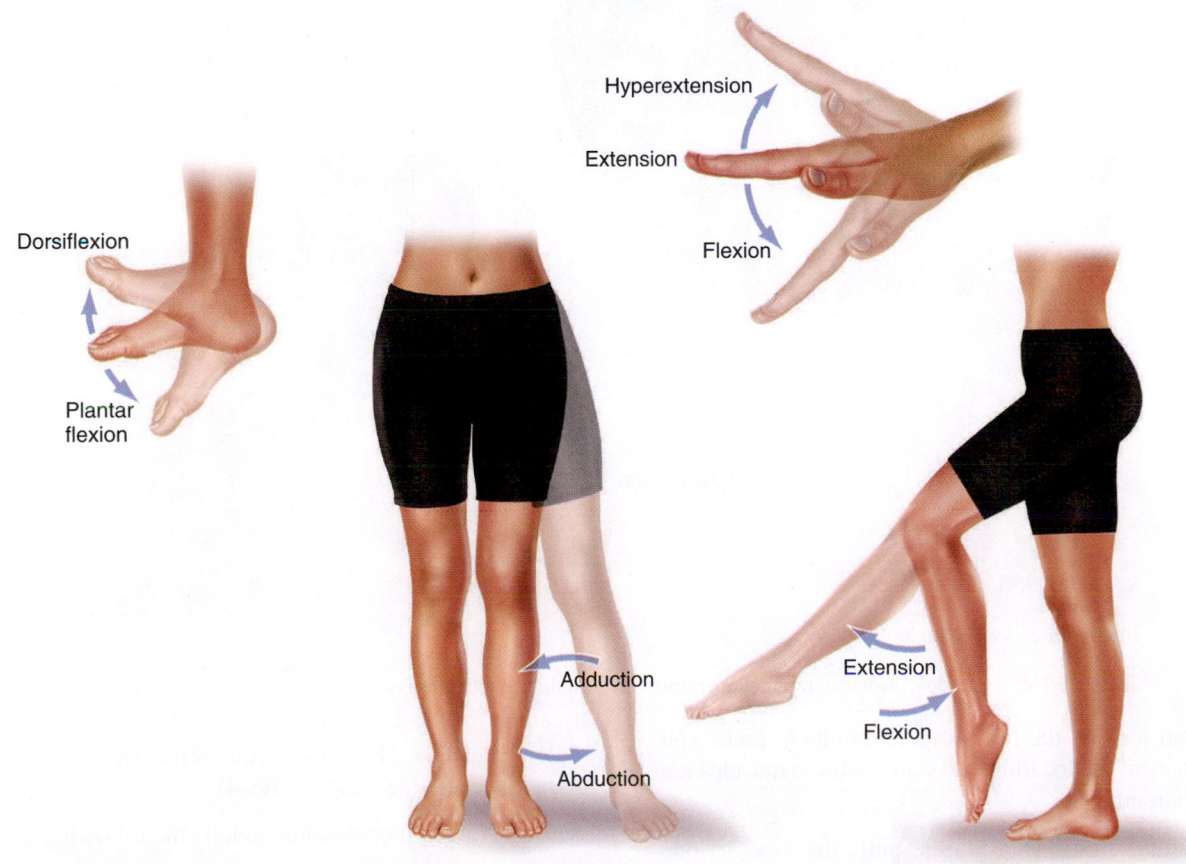

FIGURE 24-4 Adduction, abduction, dorsiflexion, plantar flexion, hyperextension, extension, and flexion.

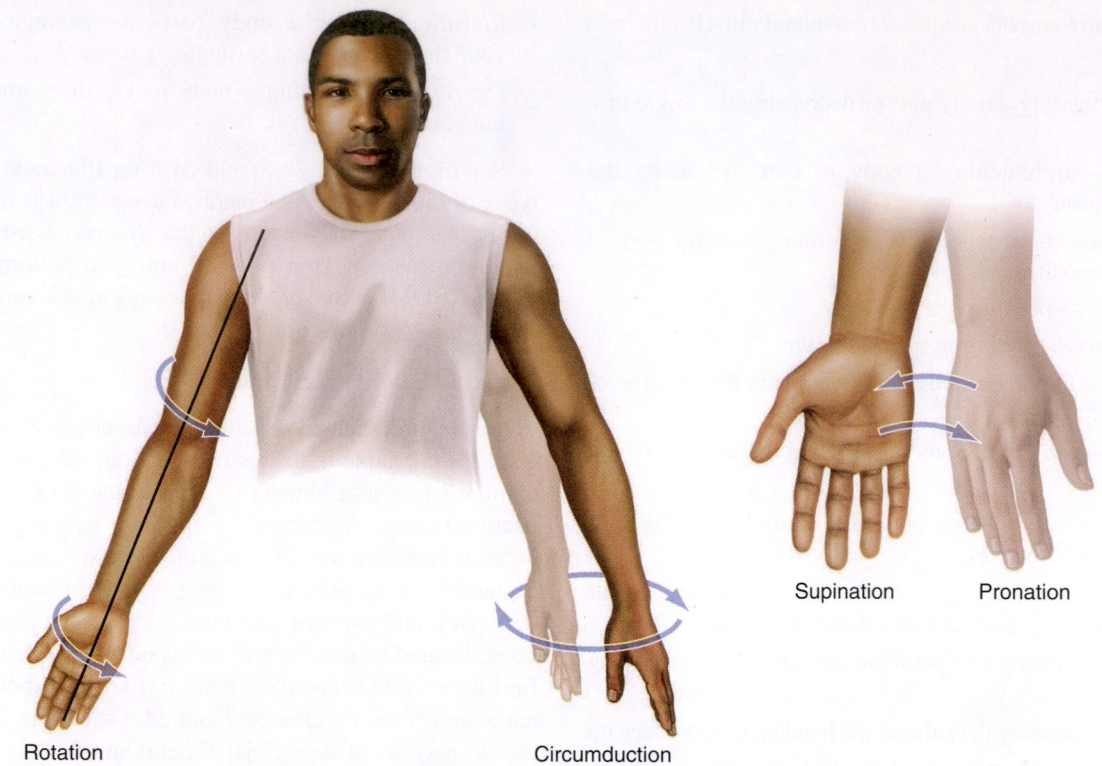

FIGURE 24-5 Rotation, circumduction, supination, and pronation.

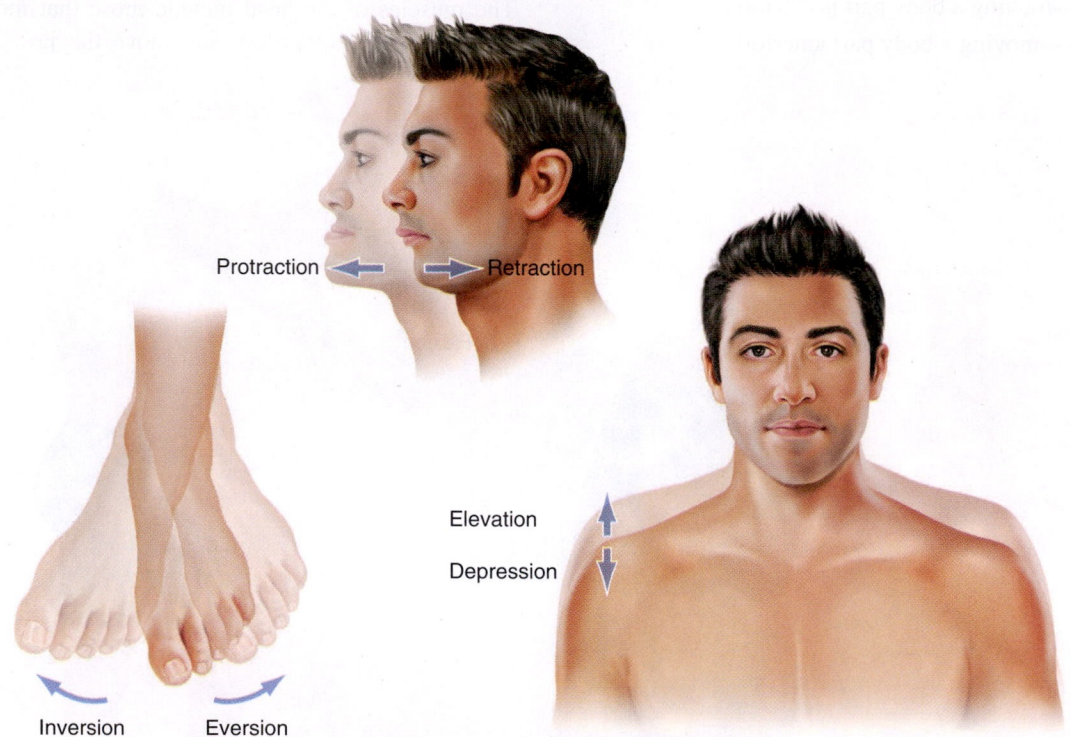

FIGURE 24-6 Eversion, inversion, protraction, retraction, elevation, and depression.

move the head include the following, and hints to assist you with remembering the locations for some of these muscles are provided in parentheses:

- Sternocleidomastoid. This muscle pulls the head to one side and pulls the head to the chest. (sterno = sternum, cleido = clavicle, mastoid = mastoid)

- Splenius capitis. This muscle rotates the head and allows it to bend to the side. (capit = head)

Muscles of facial expression include the following:

- Frontalis. This muscle raises the eyebrows. (frontal = pertaining to the front)

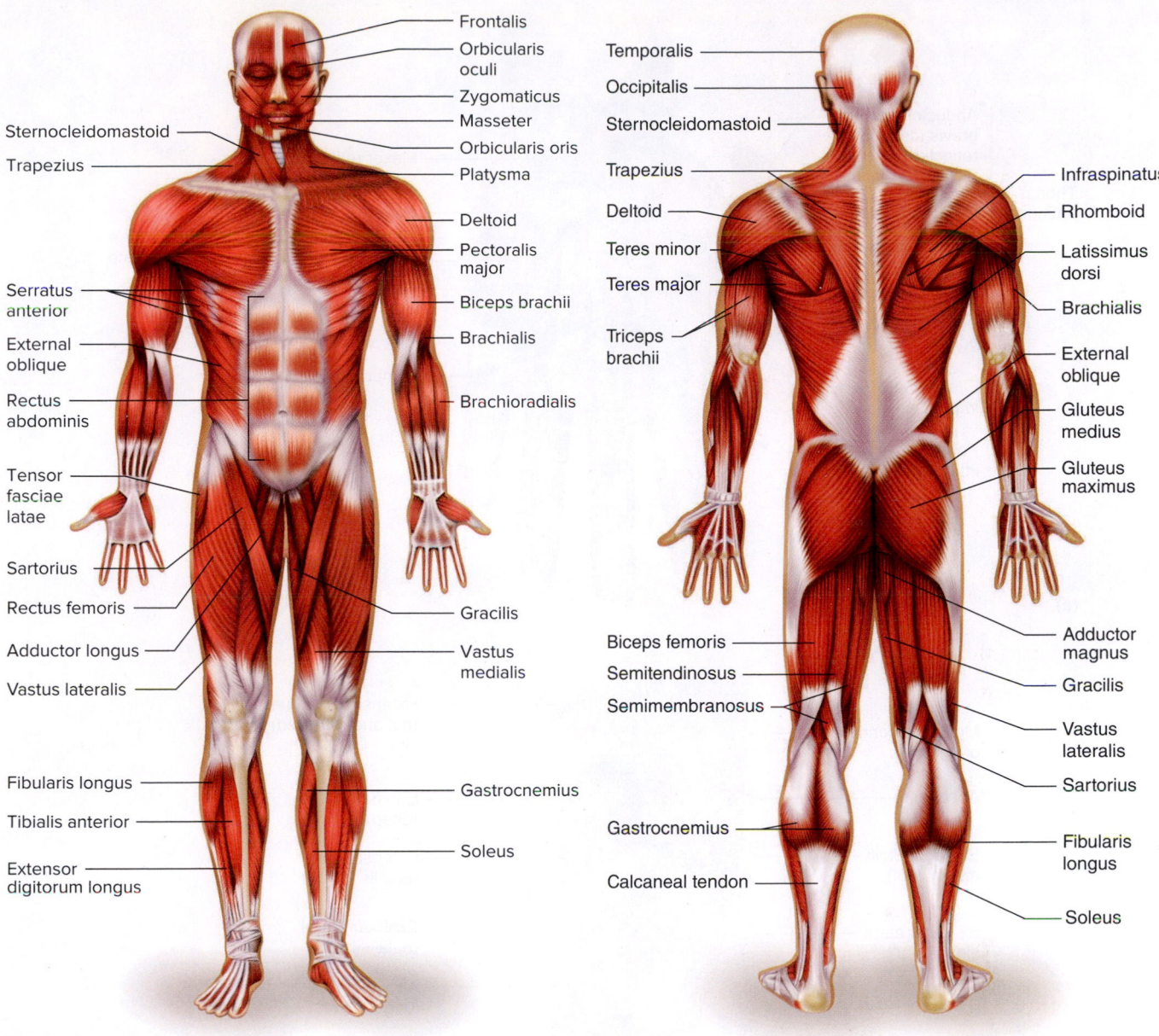

FIGURE 24-7 Anterior view of superficial skeletal muscles.

FIGURE 24-8 Posterior view of superficial skeletal muscles.

- Orbicularis oris. This muscle allows the lips to pucker. (oris = oro or mouth)
- Orbicularis oculi. This muscle allows the eyes to close. (oculi = eye)
- Zygomaticus. This muscle pulls the corners of the mouth up. (zygomat = cheekbone)
- Platysma. This muscle pulls the corners of the mouth down.

The muscles of the jaw allow for mastication (chewing) and include the following:

- Masseter and temporalis. These muscles close the jaw. (masseter as in mastication or chewing, temporo = temple)

- Internal and external pterygoids. These muscles help position the jaw.
- Sternohyomastoid. This muscle opens the jaw. (hyo = hyoid bone)

Arm Muscles

Muscles that move the arm include muscles of the arm and forearm (see Figures 24-7, 24-8, and 24-9). These muscles include

- Pectoralis major. This muscle pulls the arm across the chest; it also rotates and adducts the arms. (pectoro = chest)

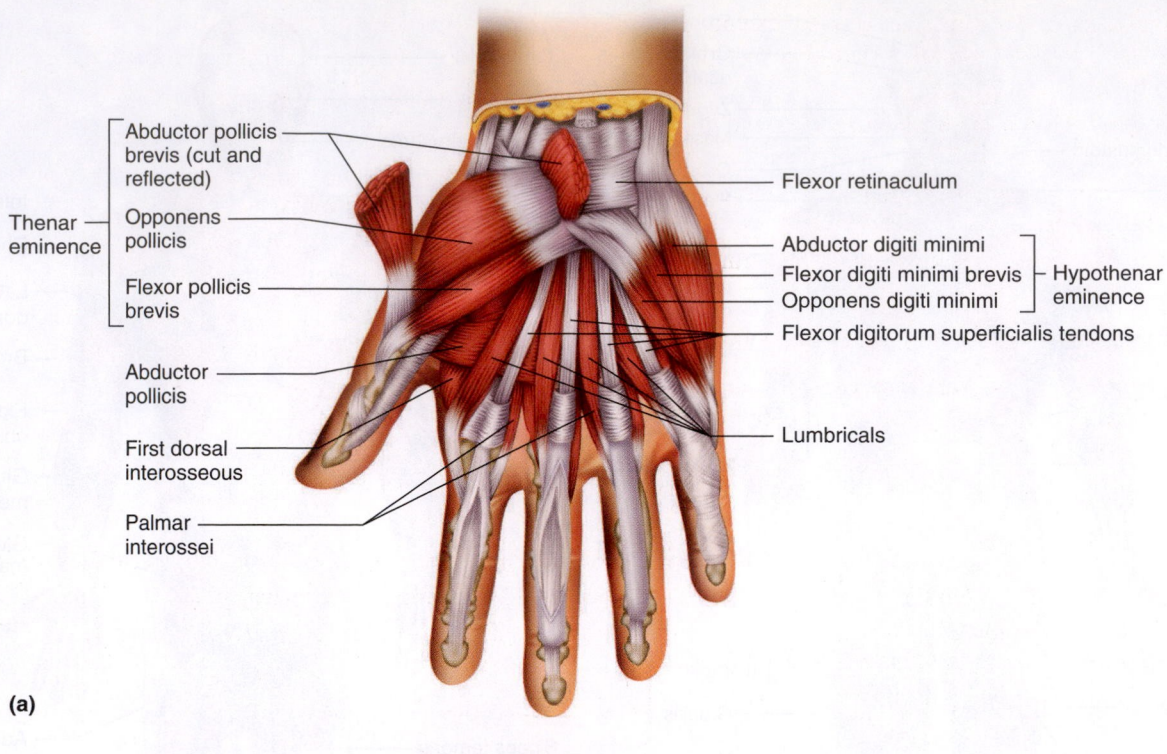

(a)

Abductor pollicis brevis (cut and reflected)

Thenar eminence

Opponens pollicis

Flexor pollicis brevis

Abductor pollicis

First dorsal interosseous

Palmar interossei

Flexor retinaculum

Abductor digiti minimi
Flexor digiti minimi brevis — Hypothenar eminence
Opponens digiti minimi

Flexor digitorum superficialis tendons

Lumbricals

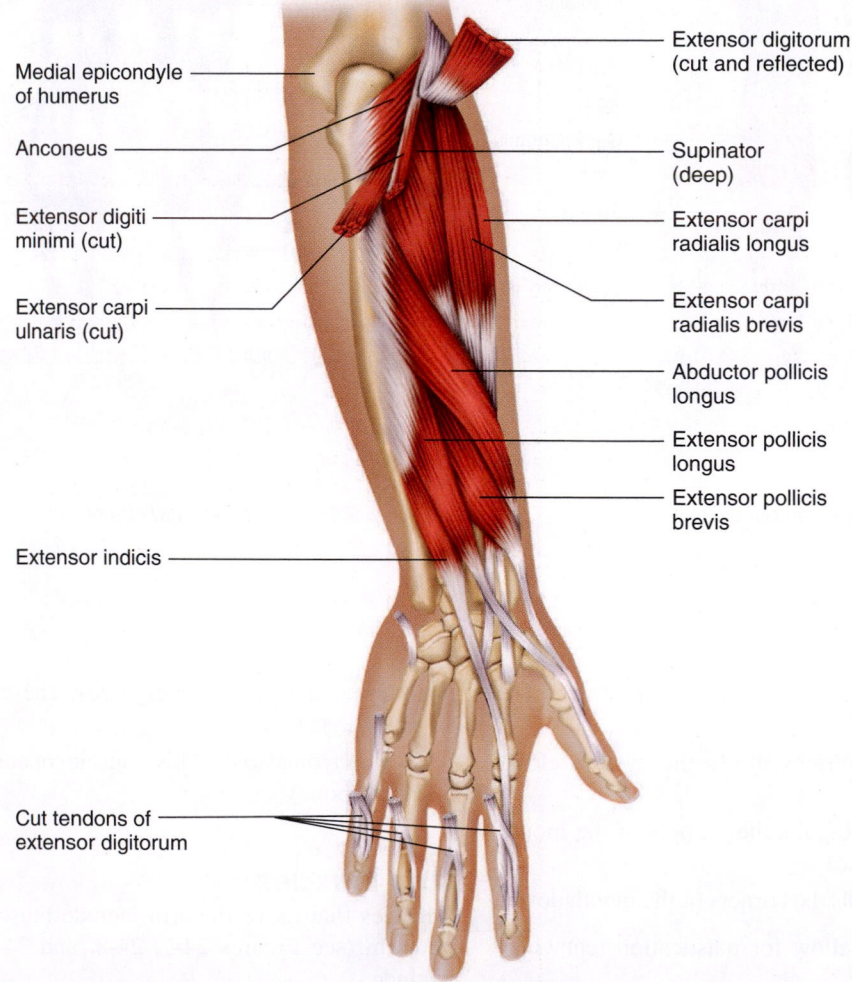

(b)

Medial epicondyle of humerus

Anconeus

Extensor digiti minimi (cut)

Extensor carpi ulnaris (cut)

Extensor indicis

Cut tendons of extensor digitorum

Extensor digitorum (cut and reflected)

Supinator (deep)

Extensor carpi radialis longus

Extensor carpi radialis brevis

Abductor pollicis longus

Extensor pollicis longus

Extensor pollicis brevis

FIGURE 24-9 Muscles of the (a) anterior hand and (b) posterior forearm.

- Latissimus dorsi. This muscle acts to extend, adduct, and rotate the arm inwardly. (latissimus = butterfly, dorsi = back)
- Deltoid. This muscle acts to abduct and extend the arm at the shoulder.
- Subscapularis. This muscle rotates the arm medially. (sub = below, scapulo = shoulder blade)
- Infraspinatus. This muscle rotates the arm laterally. (infra = below, spinat = spine)

Muscles that move the forearm include the following:

- Biceps brachii. This muscle flexes the arm at the elbow and rotates the hand laterally. (bi = two, ceps = insertion, brachii = arm)
- Brachialis. This muscle flexes the arm at the elbow. (brachii = arm)
- Brachioradialis. This muscle flexes the forearm at the elbow. (brachii = arm, radio = radius)
- Triceps brachii. This muscle extends the arm at the elbow. (tri = three, ceps = insertion, brachii = arm)
- Supinator. This muscle rotates the forearm laterally (supination). (supine = palm up)
- Pronator teres. This muscle rotates the forearm medially (pronation). (prone = palm down)

Muscles of the Wrist, Hand, and Fingers

Muscles that move the wrist, hand, and fingers can be seen in Figures 24-7, 24-8, and 24-9. These muscles include the following:

- Flexor carpi radialis and flexor carpi ulnaris. These muscles flex and abduct the wrist. (radio = radius, ulna = ulna)
- Palmaris longus. This muscle flexes the wrist.
- Flexor digitorum profundus. This muscle flexes the distal joints of the fingers but not the thumb. (digits = fingers)
- Extensor carpi radialis longus and brevis. These muscles extend the wrist and abduct the hand. (carpo = wrist, radio = radius, long = long, brev = brief or short)
- Extensor carpi ulnaris. This muscle extends the wrist. (carpo = wrist, ulna = ulna)
- Extensor digitorum. This muscle extends the fingers but not the thumb. (digit = finger)

Respiratory Muscles

The muscles of respiration—breathing—include the following:

- Diaphragm. This muscle separates the thoracic cavity from the abdominal cavity; its contraction causes inspiration—breathing in.
- External and internal intercostals. The contractions of these muscles expand and then lower the ribs during breathing. See Figure 24-10 on the next page for an illustration of the internal intercostal muscle. (inter = between, costo = rib)

Abdominal Muscles

The muscles of the abdominal wall include the following:

- External and internal obliques. These muscles compress the abdominal wall. (oblique = diagonal)
- Transverse abdominis. This muscle also compresses the abdominal wall. (transverse = across)
- Rectus abdominis. This muscle acts to flex the vertebral column and compress the abdominal wall. (rectus = erect)

See Figures 24-7, 24-8, and 24-10 for illustrations of these muscles.

Muscles of the Pectoral Girdle

The muscles that move the pectoral girdle (shoulder) include the following:

- Trapezius. This muscle raises the arms and pulls the shoulders downward. (trapezius = trapezoid)
- Pectoralis minor. This muscle pulls the scapula downward and raises the ribs. (pectoro = chest, minor = smaller)

See Figures 24-7, 24-8, and 24-10 for illustrations of these muscles.

Leg Muscles

The leg muscles include muscles of the thigh and lower leg (see Figures 24-7 and 24-8). Muscles that move the thigh include the following:

- Iliopsoas major. This muscle flexes the thigh.
- Gluteus maximus. This muscle extends the thigh.
- Gluteus medius and minimus. These muscles abduct the thighs and rotate them medially.
- Adductor longus and magnus. These muscles adduct the thighs and rotate them laterally. (adduct = toward the midline)
- Biceps femoris, semitendinosus, and semimembranosus. These three muscles are known as the *hamstring group*. They act to flex the leg at the knee and extend the leg at the thigh.
- Rectus femoris, vastus lateralis, vastus medialis, and vastus intermedius. These four muscles are known as the *quadriceps group;* they act to extend the leg at the knee.
- Sartorius. This muscle flexes the leg at the knee and thigh. It also abducts the thigh, rotating the thigh laterally but rotating the lower leg medially; it carries out the act of sitting cross-legged.

Muscles of the Ankle, Foot, and Toes

Muscles that move the ankle, foot, and toes include the following:

- Tibialis anterior. This muscle inverts the foot and points the foot up (dorsiflexion).
- Extensor digitorum longus. This muscle extends the toes and points the foot up.

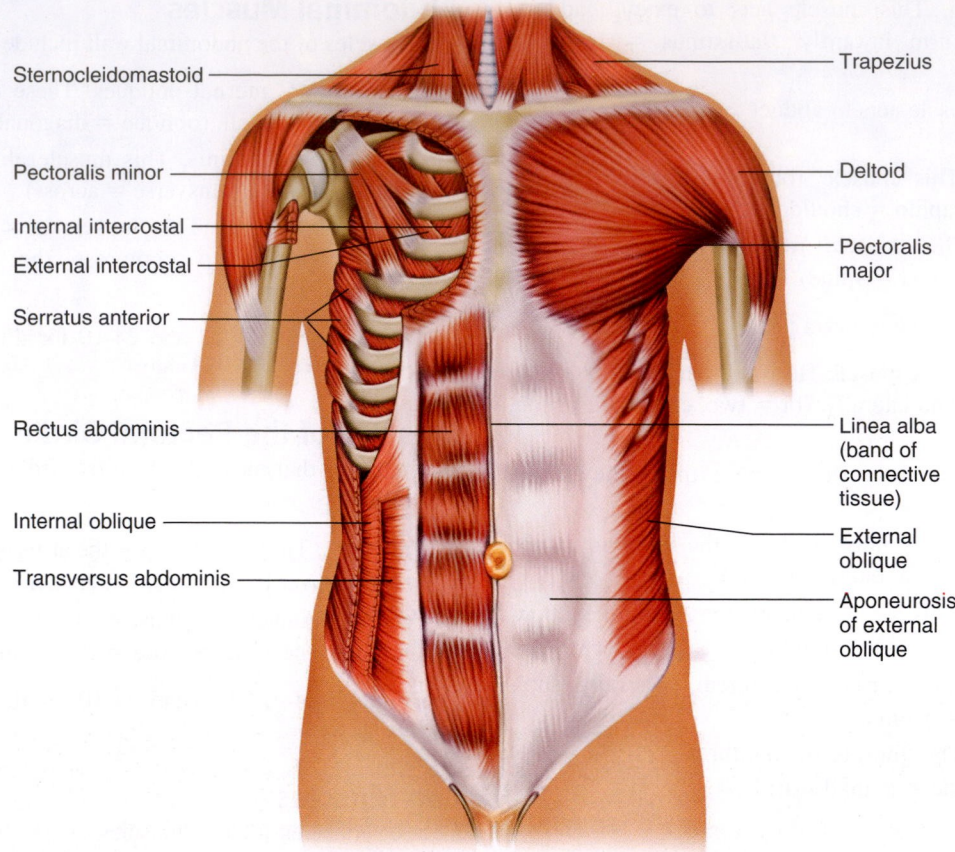

FIGURE 24-10 Muscles of the anterior chest and abdominal wall.

CAUTION: HANDLE WITH CARE

Muscle Strains and Sprains

Strains are injuries that excessively stretch muscles or tendons. Sprains are more serious injuries that consist of tears to tendons, ligaments, and/or the cartilage of joints. You can teach patients to prevent these types of injuries by doing the following:

- Warm up. Warming up muscles for just a few minutes before an intense activity raises muscle temperature. This increase in temperature prevents injuries by making muscle tissue more pliable.

- Stretch. Stretching improves muscle performance and should always be done after the warm up or after exercising. A person should never stretch further than he can hold for 10 seconds.

- Cool down. Slowing down the exercise before completely stopping prevents dizziness and fainting. If a person suddenly stops exercising, blood can pool in the legs and is prevented from reaching the brain. Cooling down also helps to remove lactic acid from muscles.

If sprains or strains do occur, immediate RICE treatment is recommended:

- R is for rest. Resting minimizes bleeding, further injury, and swelling. Sometimes a splint, sling, or crutches may be needed.

- I is for ice. Ice minimizes swelling and pain. A bag filled with crushed ice conforms better to a body part than one filled with ice cubes. A bag full of frozen peas or other small vegetables can also be used. The ice should be applied for 10 minutes and then removed for 10 minutes. This should be kept up for about an hour and repeated several times during a 48-hour period.

- C is for compression, which minimizes swelling. A bandage should be loosely wrapped around the injured area and the bag of ice. Compression should be applied and removed along with the ice.

- E is for elevation. The injured muscle should be elevated, which minimizes swelling, and elevation should be continued as long as swelling is present.

If the patient does not think his symptoms have improved in several days to a week, a physician should be contacted to rule out a more serious injury, such as a torn ligament or muscle, or even a bone fracture.

- Gastrocnemius. This muscle flexes the foot and flexes the leg at the knee. It is more commonly referred to as the calf muscle.
- Soleus. This muscle also flexes the foot.
- Flexor digitorum longus. This muscle flexes the foot and toes.

See Figures 24-7 and 24-8 for illustrations of these muscles.

▶ Aging and the Musculoskeletal System
LO 24.7

Although the aging of the skeletal system causes more obvious difficulties for patients with diseases and conditions like arthritis, fractures, and osteoporosis, muscular decline often goes hand-in-hand with these changes. Aging causes a decline in the speed and strength of muscle contractions, even though the actual endurance of muscle fibers changes very little. Elderly patients often have increasing difficulty with dexterity and gripping ability. Mobility may decrease related to the combined decline of the musculoskeletal system. The patient's diet and exercise history, as well as family history, also has a direct impact on the patient's mobility and activity level as he or she ages.

Assistive devices like railings, tub and shower seats, and gripping devices can assist patients who are experiencing difficulties. Exercise routines, particularly pool exercises like swimming and physical therapy, are often helpful in maintaining strength and mobility. Guarding against sprains and strains during exercise routines is essential. See the *Caution: Handle with Care* Muscle Sprains and Strains for more information.

PATHOPHYSIOLOGY
LO 24.8

Common Diseases and Disorders of the Muscular System

BOTULISM is usually thought of as a disease that affects the gastrointestinal tract, but it can also affect various muscle groups. This disease most commonly affects infants. Although a person can survive this disease, its effects may be long-lasting.

Causes. This is a rare but serious disorder caused by the bacterium *Clostridium botulinum,* which normally lives in soil and water. If this bacterium gets on food, it produces a toxin that can lead to a type of food poisoning. The foods most likely to contain *Clostridium botulinum* are canned vegetables, cured pork, raw fish, honey, and corn syrup. A person can also acquire this bacterium through improperly cleaned open wounds.

Signs and Symptoms. This disease causes many symptoms, including dysphagia (difficulty swallowing), paralysis, muscle weakness, nausea and vomiting, abdominal cramps, double vision, dyspnea (difficulty breathing), poor feeding and suckling in infants, the inability to urinate, the absence of reflexes, and constipation. The signs and symptoms usually appear 8 to 40 hours after the toxin is ingested. The diagnosis is usually made by either a blood test to identify the toxin or an analysis of the suspected food. See Figure 24-11.

Treatment. Treatment includes emergency hospitalization, intubation—inserting a tube into the upper airway to open airways, mechanical ventilation if respiratory muscles are impaired, intravenous fluids or nasogastric (through nose to stomach) feeding if swallowing is impaired, and the administration of an antitoxin.

Prevention Tips. You can instruct patients to prevent botulism by observing the following guidelines:

- Never give honey or corn syrup to infants.
- Sterilize home-canned food containers properly (240°F for 35 minutes).
- Do not use foods from bent or bulging cans.
- Never eat foods that smell as if they may have spoiled.
- Cook and store foods properly.

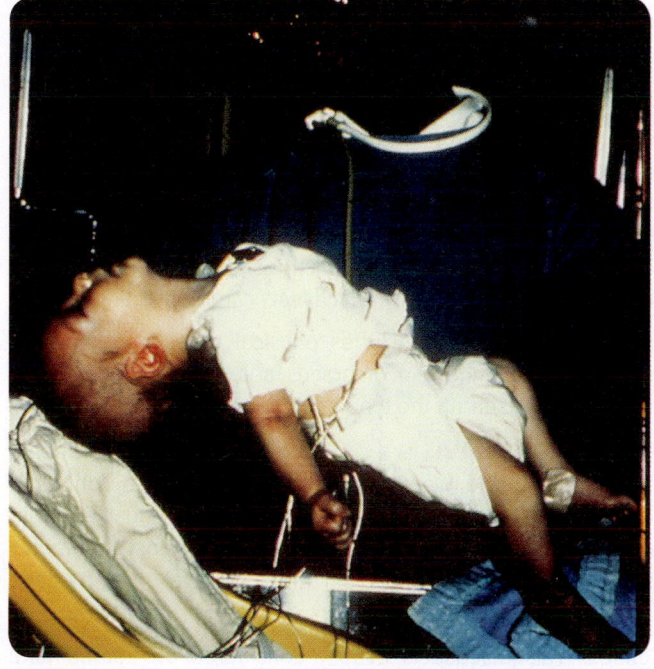

FIGURE 24-11   An infant with paralysis caused by botulism.
CDC

FIBROMYALGIA is a fairly common condition that results in chronic pain, primarily in joints, muscles, and tendons. It most ordinarily affects women between the ages of 20 and 50.

Causes. The causes of this disorder are poorly understood. Fibromyalgia may be caused or exacerbated by sleep disturbance, emotional distress, decreased blood flow to muscles, a virus, or any combination of these factors.

Signs and Symptoms. Symptoms include fatigue, tenderness in different areas of the body, sleep disturbances, and chronic facial pain. The diagnosis is usually made by ruling out other possible diseases. It is not normally diagnosed unless a person has muscle and joint pain for at least 3 months in certain body areas.

Treatment. Treatment is varied and includes antidepressants, anti-inflammatory and nerve pain medications, physical therapy, lifestyle changes to reduce stress, counseling to improve coping skills, reduction or elimination of caffeine to improve sleeping, and dietary supplements to improve nutrition.

MUSCULAR DYSTROPHY (MD) is a group of inherited disorders characterized by muscle weakness and a loss of muscle tissue. There are at least seven types of muscular dystrophy, and they are distinguished from each other by types of symptoms, the age at when symptoms appear, and the cause.

Causes. The causes of this disorder are primarily hereditary. Genetic fetal testing is available.

Signs and Symptoms. The signs and symptoms vary widely and depend on the type of muscular dystrophy. The symptoms of Duchenne muscular dystrophy—the most common and widely known type—progress steadily and are eventually fatal. Other types cause mild symptoms, and patients usually have normal life expectancies. Specific signs and symptoms include muscle weakness in various muscle groups, depending on the type of dystrophy; difficulty walking; drooling; a delayed development of motor skills; frequent falls; intellectual disability in some types; a curved spine; the formation of a claw hand or clubfoot; a loss of muscle mass; the accumulation of fat or fibrous connective tissue in muscles; and arrhythmias (irregular heart rhythms) in some types. The progression of the muscular weakness may also include eventual paralysis of the affected muscle groups. The diagnosis is primarily made through a muscle biopsy. Other tests include deoxyribonucleic acid (DNA) testing; an electromyography (EMG) test, which tests muscle weakness; or an electrocardiogram (ECG), which tests cardiac function.

Treatment. Treatment includes physical therapy to maintain muscle function, the use of braces and wheelchairs, various medications based on the type of MD, and spinal surgery.

MYASTHENIA GRAVIS is a condition in which affected people experience muscle weakness. In this autoimmune condition, a person produces antibodies that prevent muscles from receiving neurotransmitters from neurons. It most commonly affects young women and older men, especially if they have other autoimmune disorders.

Causes. This disease is usually considered an autoimmune disorder.

Signs and Symptoms. The signs and symptoms usually get better with rest and worsen with activity. They include double vision; muscle weakness; dysphagia (difficulty swallowing); difficulty talking, chewing, lifting, or walking; fatigue; drooling; and difficulty breathing. The diagnosis may be difficult, but a single-fiber EMG test is often useful. This test measures the response of a muscle fiber to nervous stimulation. Other tests include acetylcholine receptor antibody tests and the edrophonium test. In a positive edrophonium test, muscle activity increases after medication is given that blocks the breakdown of acetylcholine.

Treatment. Treatments include lifestyle changes to avoid excessive stress, adequate rest, the use of an eye patch to treat double vision, medications to improve communication between nerves and muscles, medications to suppress the immune system, plasmapheresis to remove harmful antibodies from blood, and removal of the thymus.

RHABDOMYOLYSIS is a condition in which the kidneys have been damaged in relation to serious muscle injuries.

Causes. Kidneys become damaged because of toxins released from muscle cells. When muscles are damaged, excessive amounts of the pigment myoglobin are released, which is then broken down into harmful chemicals. Muscles are most often damaged through trauma; excessive use (for example, marathon running); overdoses of cocaine, heroin, and other drugs; alcoholism; and a blockage of the blood supply to the muscles.

Signs and Symptoms. Symptoms include dark urine, muscle tenderness, muscle weakness, muscle stiffness, seizures, joint pain, and fatigue. Diagnosis includes urinalysis for the presence of myoglobin, creatine phosphokinase (CPK), and creatinine; blood is also tested for the presence of myoglobin, CPK, or high levels of potassium. CPK is an enzyme released into the blood when muscles are damaged. Creatinine is a protein released by the breakdown of muscle tissue.

Treatment. Treatment includes hydration to rapidly eliminate toxins from the kidneys, diuretics to help flush toxins from the body, medications to flush excess potassium from the body, and therapy for kidney failure.

TENDONITIS is described as the painful inflammation of a tendon as well as of the tendon-muscle attachment to a bone. The most common locations for tendonitis are the shoulder, hip, heel, and hamstrings. Tendonitis may also be associated with bursitis, the inflammation of the bursa located in synovial joints like the shoulder, elbow, and knee.

Causes. Tendonitis usually occurs after a sports-related activity that results in injury to the tendon-muscle or tendon-to-bone attachment. Other musculoskeletal disorders may also cause or exacerbate this condition.

Signs and Symptoms. These include pain at the joint or muscle attachment that results in limited range of motion (ROM) of the affected area.

Treatment. For the initial injury, using ice for the first 12 to 24 hours will minimize inflammation. After this initial time period, applying heat will help with joint and muscle pain. If calcium deposits are found in the tendon, which can be confirmed by X-ray, heat will aggravate the condition, whereas continued use of ice packs will help to relieve the discomfort. Resting the affected area and taking oral analgesics will also help control pain and reduce inflammation.

TETANUS is commonly called lockjaw. This disease has a high mortality rate, especially in infants. Immediate treatment is necessary to prevent death or long-lasting effects. However, tetanus is completely preventable through regular vaccinations.

Causes. A toxin produced by the bacterium *Clostridium tetani*, which lives naturally in soil and water, causes this disease. People most commonly acquire this bacterium through open wounds caused by objects contaminated with soil.

Signs and Symptoms. Symptoms usually appear between 5 and 10 days after infection. Muscle spasms in the jaw, neck, and facial muscles are usually the first signs. Other signs and symptoms include worsening of the muscle spasms (which spread to other body locations and may cause bone fractures), dyspnea (breathing difficulties), irritability, fever, profuse sweating, and drooling. See Figure 24-12. The diagnosis is usually based on the type of wound and the characteristic signs and symptoms of the disease. Tetanus antibody tests can also be used in diagnosis, but cultures of the wound site often produce false-negative findings.

Treatment. Administering antitoxin and antibiotics is a key treatment. Others include wound cleaning, muscle relaxants, sedation, and bed rest. The insertion of an endotracheal tube and mechanical ventilation may be needed for patients with severe breathing difficulties.

TORTICOLLIS is also known as wry neck. This disease is a cervical deformity in which the head bends toward the affected side while the chin rotates to the opposite side.

Causes. Torticollis may be acquired or congenital. It is caused by spasm or shortening of the sternocleidomastoid muscle. Breech or other difficult birth is often the cause of the congenital form as a result of the previously noted malpositioning, or from injury or scar tissue from ruptured muscle fibers before or during the birth process. The acquired form is the result of underlying disease, cervical spine injury, or chronic muscle spasms.

Signs and Symptoms. There is obvious malpositioning of the head and neck in an affected individual.

Treatment. For the congenital form, passive exercises to stretch the muscles as well as corrected head positioning during sleep (to maintain the straightening accomplished through the exercises) may be helpful. The treatment for acquired torticollis should consist of treating the underlying disease if possible. Otherwise, heat, cervical traction, a neck brace, exercise, massage, and psychotherapy to help the patient deal with the psychological and emotional effects related to the deformity are all treatment options.

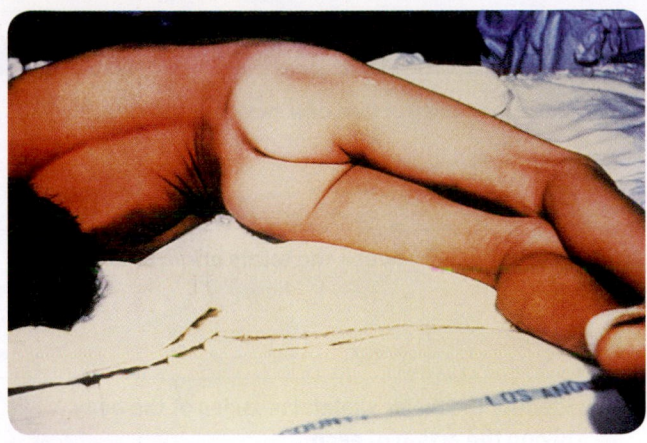

FIGURE 24-12   A patient with advanced tetanus.
CDC

TRICHINOSIS is an infection caused by parasites (worms).

Causes. This disease is caused by worms that are usually ingested by eating undercooked meat. Once ingested, the worms can leave the digestive tract and infect skeletal muscles, the heart, the lungs, and the brain. This disease is preventable by not eating wild animal meat. Proper cooking will also prevent trichinosis. There is no cure for this disease once the worms leave the digestive tract and infect other tissues.

Signs and Symptoms. Common symptoms include abdominal pain, diarrhea, muscle pain, fever, and pneumonia. In more serious cases, arrhythmias, heart failure, and encephalitis (swelling of the brain) can result. The diagnosis is usually based on the symptoms, a blood test to determine if there is an increase in eosinophils (white blood cells) in the blood, or a muscle biopsy that reveals the presence of the worms.

Treatment. Patients with this disease are treated with medications to kill worms in the digestive tract and with anti-inflammatory drugs to reduce muscle pain and swelling.

SUMMARY OF LEARNING OUTCOMES

LEARNING OUTCOMES	KEY POINTS
24.1 Describe the functions of muscle.	The functions of muscles include movement, stability, control of body openings and passages, and the production of heat. Valve-like muscular structures called sphincters control the passage of substances into and out of organs like the stomach and bladder.
24.2 Compare the three types of muscle tissue, including their locations and characteristics.	The three types of muscle tissue are striated, voluntary skeletal muscle; smooth, involuntary visceral muscle; and specialized striated and involuntary cardiac muscle.
24.3 Explain how muscle tissue generates energy.	There are three ways muscles create energy. Creatine phosphate is a rapid method for muscles to create energy; aerobic respiration uses stored glucose to produce ATP in the Krebs cycle; and lactic acid production occurs when a cell is low in oxygen and converts pyruvic acid to lactic acid.

LEARNING OUTCOMES	KEY POINTS
24.4 Describe the structure of a skeletal muscle.	Skeletal muscle is composed of connective tissue, skeletal muscle tissue, blood vessels, and nerves. The coverings of skeletal muscles include fascia, tendon, aponeurosis, epimysium, perimysium, and endomysium.
24.5 Differentiate between the terms *origin* and *insertion*.	The origin of a muscle is the attachment site of the muscle to the less movable bone during muscle contraction. The insertion of a muscle is the attachment site for the muscle to the more movable bone during muscle contraction.
24.6 Identify the major skeletal muscles of the body, giving the action of each.	The major muscles of the head are the sternocleidomastoid, splenius capitis, frontalis, orbicularis oris and oculi, zygomaticus, platysma, masseter, and temporalis. The upper extremity muscles include the pectoralis major, latissimus dorsi, deltoid, subscapularis, infraspinatus, biceps brachii, brachialis, brachioradialis, triceps brachii, supinator, pronator teres, flexor carpi radialis and ulnaris, plamaris longus, flexor digitorum profundus, extensor carpi radialis longus and brevis, extensor carpi ulnaris, and extensor digitorum. The major respiratory muscles are the diaphragm and the external and internal intercostals. The abdominal muscles include the external and internal obliques, transverse abdominis, and rectus abdominis. The pectoral girdle muscles include the trapezius and pectoralis minor. The muscles of the lower extremity include the iliopsoas major; gluteus maximus, medius, and minimus; adductor longus and magnus; biceps femoris; semitendinosus and semimembranosus; rectus femoris; vastus lateralis, medialis, and intermedius; sartorius; tibialis anterior; extensor digitorum longus; gastrocnemius; soleus; and flexor digitorum longus.
24.7 Summarize the changes that occur to the muscular system as a person ages.	The common diseases of aging include arthritis, fractures, osteoporosis, and muscular decline. Aging causes a decline in strength and speed of muscle contractions. Dexterity and gripping abilities lessen, and mobility often decreases related to skeletal and muscular decline.
24.8 Describe the causes, signs and symptoms, and treatments of various diseases and disorders of the muscular system.	There are many common diseases and disorders of the muscular system with varied signs, symptoms, and treatments. Some of these are botulism, fibromyalgia, muscular dystrophy, myasthenia gravis, rhabdomyolysis, tendonitis, tetanus, torticollis, and trichinosis.

CASE STUDY CRITICAL THINKING

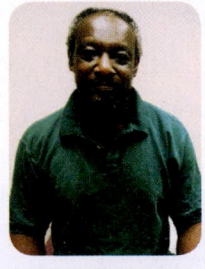

Recall Ken Washington from the beginning of the chapter. Now that you have completed the chapter, answer the following questions regarding his case.

1. Relate the benefits of exercise to the musculoskeletal system.

2. Identify the arm muscles Ken will need to strengthen.

3. The physical therapist wants Ken to strengthen the extensor digitorum longus muscle. Where is this muscle, and why does the therapist think this will help Ken's foot drop?

1. (LO 24.2) Groups of cardiac muscle are connected by
   a. Striations
   b. Multi-units
   c. Intercalated discs
   d. Fascia
   e. Myofibrils

2. (LO 24.2) Skeletal muscle responds to which of the following neurotransmitters?
   a. Epinephrine
   b. Acetylcholine
   c. Norepinephrine
   d. Dopamine
   e. Glucagon

3. (LO 24.5) Increasing the angle of a joint produces which of the following body movements?
   a. Extension
   b. Plantar flexion
   c. Flexion
   d. Hyperextension
   e. Elevation

4. (LO 24.6) Which muscle acts to abduct and extend the arm at the shoulder?
   a. Biceps brachii
   b. Gluteus maximus
   c. Triceps brachii
   d. Deltoid
   e. Brachioradialis

5. (LO 24.6) Which muscle separates the thoracic and abdominal cavities and assists in respiration?
   a. Internal/external obliques
   b. Internal/external intercostals
   c. Diaphragm
   d. Pectoralis major
   e. Serratus anterior

6. (LO 24.6) Which of the following muscles assists with mastication?
   a. Masseter
   b. Frontalis
   c. Platysma
   d. Zygomaticus
   e. Orbicularis oculi

7. (LO 24.8) The medical term for a condition known as wry neck is
   a. Tetanus
   b. Fibromyalgia
   c. Rhabdomyolysis
   d. Tendonitis
   e. Torticollis

8. (LO 24.8) Trichinosis is caused by a(n)
   a. Autoimmune disorder
   b. Parasitic worm
   c. Cervical deformity
   d. Soil bacterium
   e. Genetic mutation

9. (LO 24.5) The attachment site for the more movable bone during muscle contraction is the
   a. Origin
   b. Agonist
   c. Synergist
   d. Insertion
   e. Antagonist

10. (LO 24.5) Pointing the toes downward is known as
    a. Plantar flexion
    b. Abduction
    c. Inversion
    d. Dorsiflexion
    e. Pronation

MEDICAL TERMINOLOGY PRACTICE

Analyze the following medical terms, presented throughout the chapter. Using a medical dictionary (or Appendix I) place a / mark between each word part. Define each word part and then define the whole word.

EXAMPLE: **myo / globin** = myo means "muscle" + globin means "protein" *MYOGLOBIN* means "muscle protein."

1. abduction
2. adduction
3. circumduction
4. dorsiflexion
5. eversion
6. fibromyalgia
7. hyperextension
8. inversion
9. tendonitis
10. myocytes
11. triceps
12. rhabdomyolysis

The Cardiovascular System

CASE STUDY

PATIENT INFORMATION			
Patient Name	**DOB**	**Allergies**	
John Miller	12/5/19XX	Bee stings	
Attending	**MRN**	**Other Information**	
Paul F. Buckwalter, MD	082-09-981	Current Medications: Glyburide 2.5 mg daily, Captopril 25 mg bid, HCTZ 25 mg daily	

John Miller, a 65-year-old patient, was referred to the cardiologist's office for an evaluation. The patient has a history of hypertension and had a myocardial infarction (heart attack) 4 years ago. More recently, he was diagnosed with mild congestive heart failure (CHF). Three weeks ago, on the advice of his primary care physician, he started a light exercise program for weight loss. Following exercise he has had a radiating chest pain (angina pectoris) that stopped after rest.

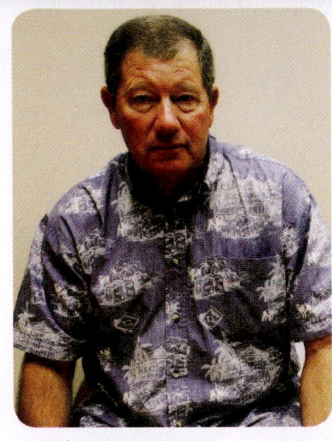
© McGraw-Hill Education

The condition has worsened in the last week. The cardiologist ordered a stress echocardiogram (a test that visualizes the heart during increasing stress). The stress echocardiogram results suggested that the chest pain may be due to coronary artery disease (CAD). The patient was scheduled for a cardiac catheterization the next morning. It was noted in the patient's chart that he smokes two packs of cigarettes per day.

Keep John in mind as you study this chapter. There will be questions at the end of the chapter based on the case study. The information in the chapter will help you answer these questions.

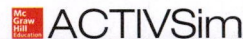
McGraw-Hill Education ACTIVSim

LEARNING OUTCOMES

After completing Chapter 25, you will be able to:

25.1 Describe the structures of the heart and the function of each.

25.2 Explain the cardiac cycle, including the cardiac conduction system.

25.3 Differentiate among the different types of blood vessels and their functions.

25.4 Compare the various types of circulation.

25.5 Explain blood pressure and tell how it is controlled.

25.6 Describe the causes, signs and symptoms, and treatments of various diseases and disorders of the cardiovascular system.

KEY TERMS

atrioventricular node (AV node)

bundle of His

cardiac output

chordae tendineae

coronary circulation

diastolic pressure

embolus

endocardium

epicardium

hepatic portal system

myocardium

pericardium

pulmonary circulation

Purkinje fibers

sinoatrial node (SA node)

stenosis

systemic circulation

systolic pressure

vasoconstriction

vasodilation

viscosity

MEDICAL ASSISTING COMPETENCIES

CAAHEP	ABHES

CAAHEP

I.C.4 List major organs in each body system

I.C.5 Identify the anatomical location of major organs in each body system

I.C.7 Describe the normal function of each body system

I.C.8 Identify common pathology related to each body system including
(a) signs
(b) symptoms
(c) etiology

I.C.9 Analyze pathology for each body system including:
(a) diagnostic measures
(b) treatment modalities

V.C.9 Identify medical terms labeling the word parts

V.C.10 Define medical terms and abbreviations related to all body systems

ABHES

2. Anatomy & Physiology
a. List all body systems, their structure and functions
b. Describe common diseases, symptoms, and etiologies as they apply to each system
c. Identify diagnostic and treatment modalities as they relate to each system

3. Medical Terminology
a. Define and use entire basic structure of medical words and be able to accurately identify in the correct context, i.e. root, prefix, suffix, combinations, spelling, and definitions
b. Build and dissect medical terms from roots/suffixes to understand the word element combinations that create medical terminology
c. Apply various medical terms for each specialty
d. Define and use medical abbreviations when appropriate and acceptable

Introduction

The cardiovascular system consists of the heart and blood vessels. It pumps blood to the lungs to pick up oxygen and to the digestive system to pick up nutrients. It then delivers the oxygen and nutrients to all of the body cells. At the same time, it picks up waste products from the body cells and transports them to the lungs, kidneys, and other organs for removal from the body.

The Heart   LO 25.1

The heart is a cone-shaped organ about the size of a loose fist. It is located within the mediastinum (central part of the chest) and extends from the level of the second rib to about the level of the sixth rib. Although many people think the heart is in the left side of the chest, it is located only slightly left of the midline of the body. The heart is bordered laterally by the lungs, posteriorly by the vertebral column, and anteriorly by the sternum. Inferiorly, the heart rests on the diaphragm.

Cardiac Membranes

The heart is enclosed by a membrane called the **pericardium,** or pericardial sac (see Figure 25-1). The pericardium has two parts. The outer part, called the *fibrous pericardium,* consists of a tough, fibrous material that helps protect the heart and anchor it in the chest. The inner part of the pericardium, which is called the *serous pericardium,* has two layers: the *parietal pericardium* and the *visceral pericardium.* The visceral pericardium is actually the outermost layer of the heart. The area

between these two layers of the pericardium is known as the pericardial cavity. It contains pericardial fluid, which reduces the friction between the membranes when the heart contracts and relaxes.

The Heart Wall

The wall of the heart (see Figure 25-2) is composed of the following three layers:

- **Epicardium.** This outermost layer is the visceral pericardium. It contains fat, which helps to cushion the heart.
- **Myocardium.** This middle layer is the thickest layer of the wall and is made primarily of cardiac muscle.
- **Endocardium.** This innermost layer is thin and very smooth. This layer contains part of the cardiac electrical conduction system, which is discussed later in this chapter.

Heart Chambers and Valves

The heart contains four hollow chambers, two on the left and two on the right (see Figure 25-3). The upper chambers of the heart are called *atria* (the singular form is *atrium*). They have thin walls and receive blood returning to the heart from the lungs and the body. The bottom chambers of the heart are the *ventricles.* The ventricles pump blood into the arteries, which send the blood to the lungs and the body. The wall that separates the left and right sides of the heart is the septum.

For the heart to function properly, the blood must move through it in only one direction. The four valves within the heart that keep blood flowing in one direction are the tricuspid and the bicuspid (mitral) valves, which are located

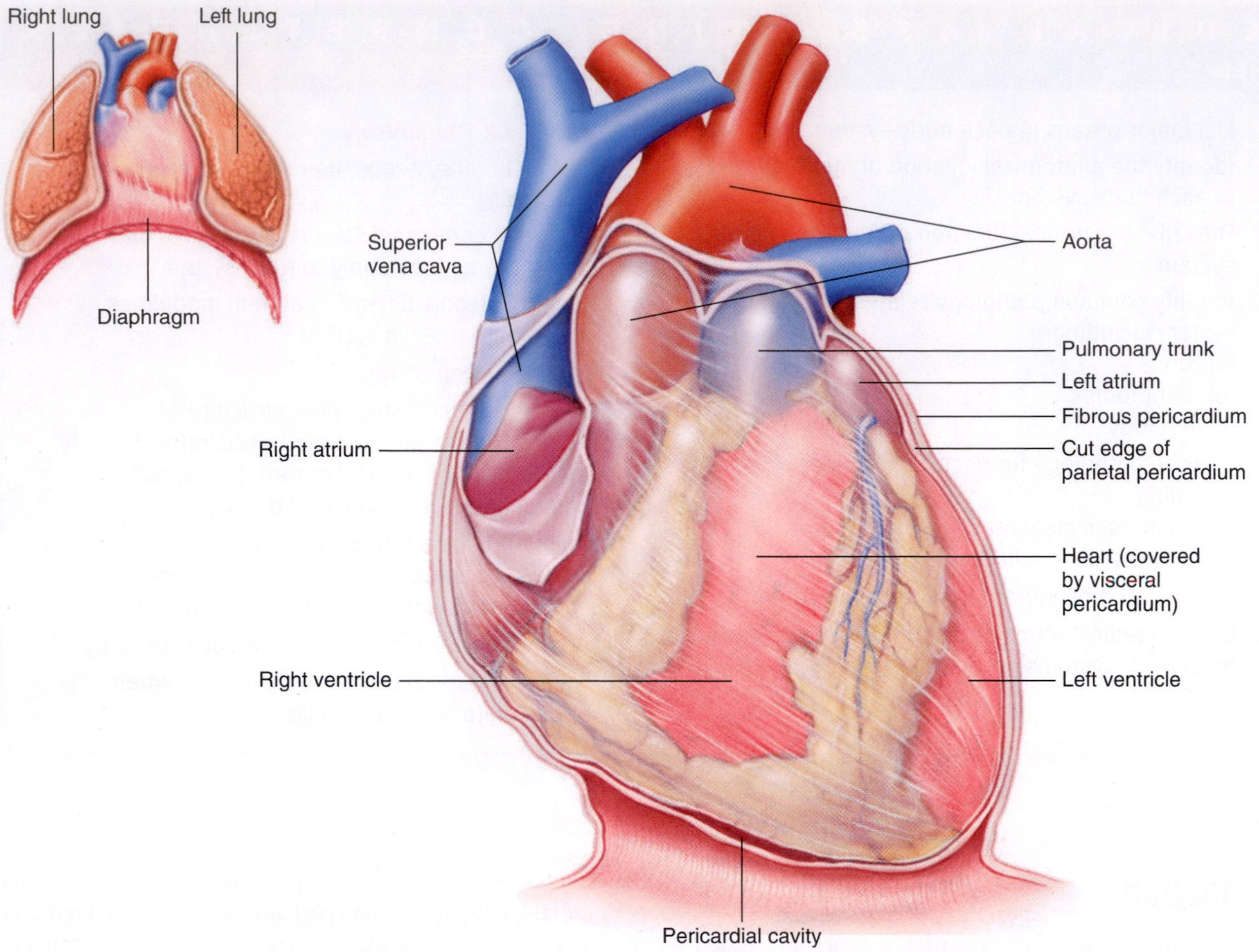

Right lung   **Left lung**

Superior vena cava

Diaphragm

Aorta

Pulmonary trunk

Left atrium

Fibrous pericardium

Cut edge of parietal pericardium

Right atrium

Heart (covered by visceral pericardium)

Right ventricle

Left ventricle

Pericardial cavity

FIGURE 25-1   Location and membranes of the heart.

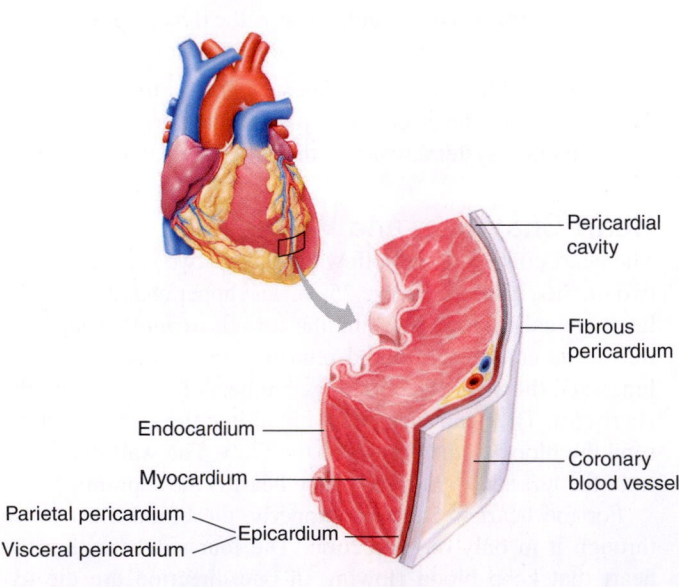

Pericardial cavity

Fibrous pericardium

Endocardium

Coronary blood vessel

Myocardium

Parietal pericardium

Visceral pericardium

Epicardium

FIGURE 25-2   Layers of the wall of the heart.

between the atria and ventricles, and the pulmonary semilunar and aortic semilunar valves, which are located between the ventricles and their arteries.

Tricuspid Valve   The *tricuspid valve* has three cusps and is located between the right atrium and the right ventricle (see Figure 25-4). It prevents blood from flowing back into the right atrium when the right ventricle contracts. This valve is also called the *right atrioventricular (AV) valve*. The cusps of this valve are anchored by cord-like structures called **chordae tendineae** to bumps of cardiac muscle called *papillary muscles*. These muscles contract when the ventricles contract, closing the valve.

Bicuspid Valve   The *bicuspid valve* has two cusps and is located between the left atrium and the left ventricle. It prevents blood from flowing back into the left atrium when the left ventricle contracts. This valve is also known as the *mitral valve* and the *left AV valve*. Like the tricuspid valve, the bicuspid valve also has chordae tendineae attached to papillary muscles.

Pulmonary Semilunar Valve   The *pulmonary semilunar valve* is located between the right ventricle and the trunk of the pulmonary arteries. It prevents blood from flowing back into the right ventricle. Because its cusps are shaped like a half moon, this valve is called a *semilunar valve*.

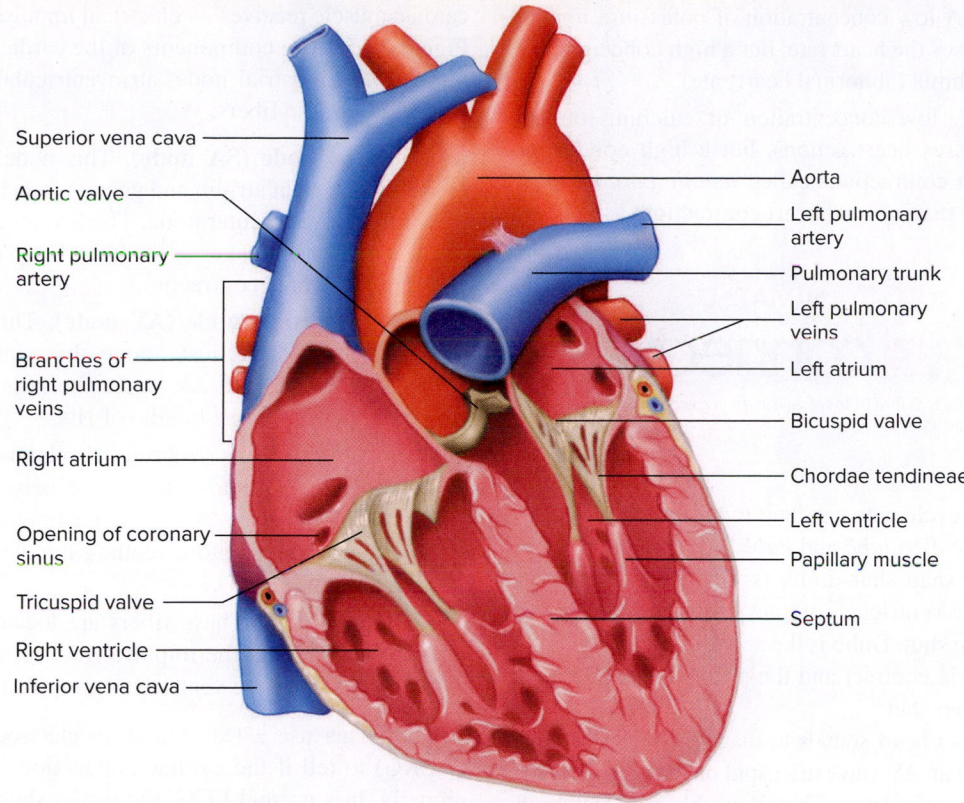

FIGURE 25-3 The chambers and valves of the heart are visible in this coronal section.

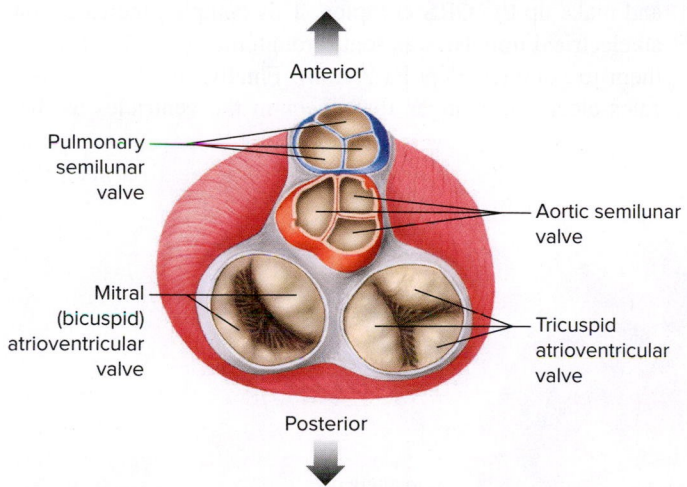

FIGURE 25-4 Valves viewed from a cross section of the heart.

Aortic Semilunar Valve The *aortic semilunar valve* is between the left ventricle and the aorta. It prevents blood from flowing back into the left ventricle and is also a semilunar valve.

▶ Cardiac Cycle LO 25.2

One heartbeat makes up one cardiac cycle. During the course of one cardiac cycle, all four heart chambers contract and then relax. The atria contract first, then the ventricles. Here are the actions that occur:

- Right atrium contracts → tricuspid valve opens → blood flows into the right ventricle.
- Left atrium contracts → bicuspid valve opens → blood flows into the left ventricle.
- Right ventricle contracts → tricuspid valve closes, pulmonary semilunar valve opens → blood is pushed into the trunk of the pulmonary artery.
- Left ventricle contracts → bicuspid valve closes, aortic semilunar valve opens → blood is pushed into the aorta.

The following factors influence the cardiac cycle:

- Exercise. Strenuous exercise increases the heart rate because skeletal muscles need more oxygen.
- Parasympathetic nerves. The parasympathetic nerve to the heart is the vagus nerve, and it generally keeps the heart rate relatively low.
- Sympathetic nerves. The sympathetic nerves increase the heart rate during times of stress. Parasympathetic and sympathetic nerves are discussed in more detail in *The Nervous System* chapter.
- Cardiac control center. This center is located in the medulla oblongata, which is part of the brainstem. When blood pressure rises, this control center sends impulses to decrease the heart rate. When blood pressure falls, it sends impulses to increase the heart rate.
- Body temperature. An increase in body temperature usually increases the heart rate. This explains the high heart rate when a person runs a fever.

- Potassium ions. A low concentration of potassium ions in the blood decreases the heart rate, but a high concentration causes a dysrhythmia (abnormal heart rate).
- Calcium ions. A low concentration of calcium ions in the blood depresses heart actions, but a high concentration causes heart contractions called *tetanic contractions,* which are longer than normal heart contractions.

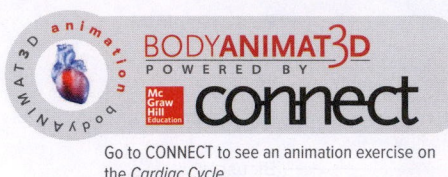

Go to CONNECT to see an animation exercise on the *Cardiac Cycle.*

Heart Sounds

During one cardiac cycle, you can hear two heart sounds. The sounds, commonly called *lubb* and *dubb,* are generated when valves in the heart snap shut. Lubb is the first heart sound and occurs when the ventricles contract and the tricuspid and bicuspid valves snap shut. Dubb is the second heart sound and occurs when the atria contract and the pulmonary and aortic semilunar valves snap shut.

Physicians listen to heart sounds to diagnose certain conditions. For example, if an AV valve (tricuspid or bicuspid) is damaged, it will not close completely. This allows blood to leak back into the atria when the ventricles contract and produces an abnormal heart sound called a *murmur.* Murmurs may indicate serious heart conditions, although many heart murmurs are harmless.

Cardiac Conduction System

The cardiac conduction system consists of a group of structures that send electrical impulses through the heart. When cardiac muscle receives an electrical impulse, it contracts (see Figure 25-5). The components of the cardiac conduction system are the sinoatrial node, atrioventricular node, bundle of His, and Purkinje fibers.

- **Sinoatrial node (SA node).** This node is located in the wall of the right atrium and generates an impulse that flows to the atrioventricular node. The SA node is also known as the natural pacemaker of the heart because it generates the heart's rhythmic contractions.
- **Atrioventricular node (AV node).** This node is located between the atria, just above the ventricles. After the impulse reaches the AV node, the atria contract and the impulse is sent to the bundle of His.
- **Bundle of His.** This structure, also known as the *atrioventricular,* or *AV, bundle,* is located between the ventricles and splits into two branches, forming the left and right *bundle branches,* before sending the electrical impulse to the Purkinje fibers.
- **Purkinje fibers.** These fibers are located in the walls of the ventricles. As the impulse flows through the Purkinje fibers, it causes the ventricles to contract.

Physicians use a test called an electrocardiogram (ECG or EKG) to tell if the cardiac conduction system is working properly. In a normal ECG, the waves shown in Figure 25-6 are produced. The first wave (P wave) indicates that an electrical impulse was sent through the atria, causing them to contract (depolarization). The Q, R, and S waves occur together and make up the QRS complex. This complex indicates that an electrical impulse was sent through the ventricles, causing them to contract (depolarization). Finally, the T wave indicates electrical changes that occur in the ventricles as they

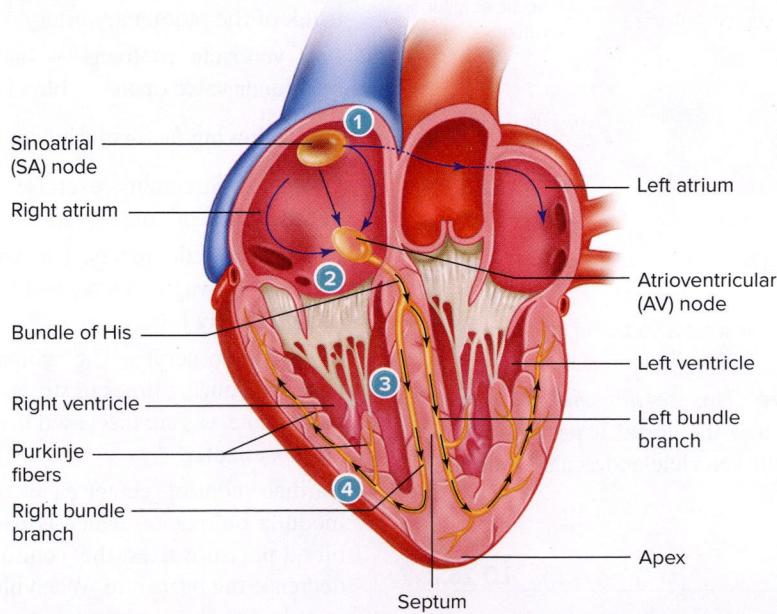

FIGURE 25-5 In the cardiac conduction system, impulses begin at the sinoatrial (SA) node and travel through the heart in the order shown here.

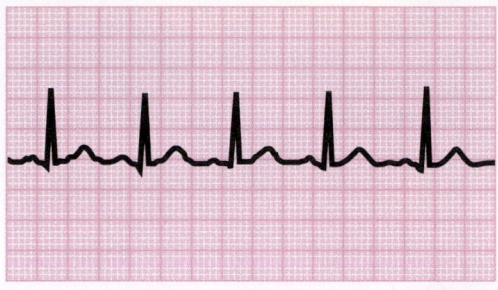

(a)

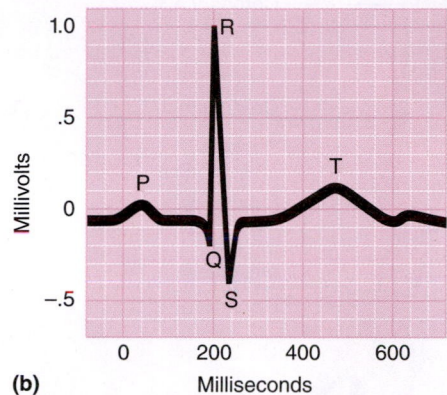

(b)

FIGURE 25-6 Electrocardiogram: (a) a normal ECG and (b) waves of a normal ECG pattern.

relax (repolarization). You will learn more about the electrical conduction system of the heart and ECGs, including how to perform them, in the chapter *Electrocardiography and Pulmonary Function Testing.*

▶ Blood Vessels   LO 25.3

Blood circulation takes place in blood vessels that form a closed pathway to carry blood from the heart to cells and back again. These vessels include arteries, arterioles, veins, venules, and capillaries.

TABLE 25-1   Major Arteries of the Body

Artery	Anatomical Location or Organ Supplied
Lingual	Tongue
Facial	Face
Occipital	Back of scalp and neck
Maxillary	Teeth, jaw, and eyelids
Ophthalmic	Eye
Axillary	Armpit area
Brachial	Upper arm
Ulnar	Forearm and hand
Radial	Forearm and hand
Intercostals	Rib area
Lumbar	Posterior abdominal wall
External iliac	Anterior abdominal wall
Common iliac	Legs, gluteal area, and pelvic organs
Femoral	Thigh
Popliteal	Posterior knee
Tibial	Lower leg and foot

Arteries and Arterioles

Arteries carry blood away from the heart and are the strongest of the blood vessels. They have a thick layer of smooth muscle that can withstand the high pressure the heart exerts on them (see Figure 25-7). This pressure is necessary to carry the blood throughout the body. Small branches of arteries are called *arterioles.*

The largest artery in the body is the aorta, which receives its blood directly from the left ventricle. The aorta branches into the coronary arteries and many other major arteries that supply blood to various parts of the body. Major arteries are summarized in Table 25-1 and illustrated in Figure 25-8. Many arteries are paired, meaning there is a left and a right artery of the same name.

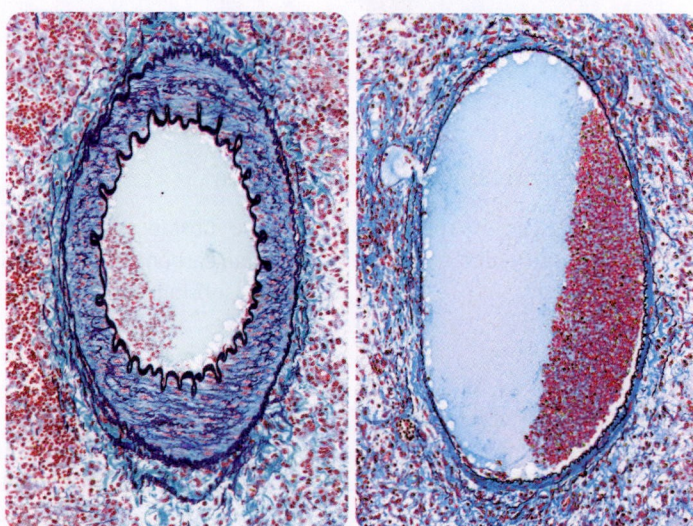

FIGURE 25-7 Arteries have much thicker walls than other blood vessels. (left) Cross section of an artery. (right) Cross section of a vein.
© Microscape/SPL/Science Source

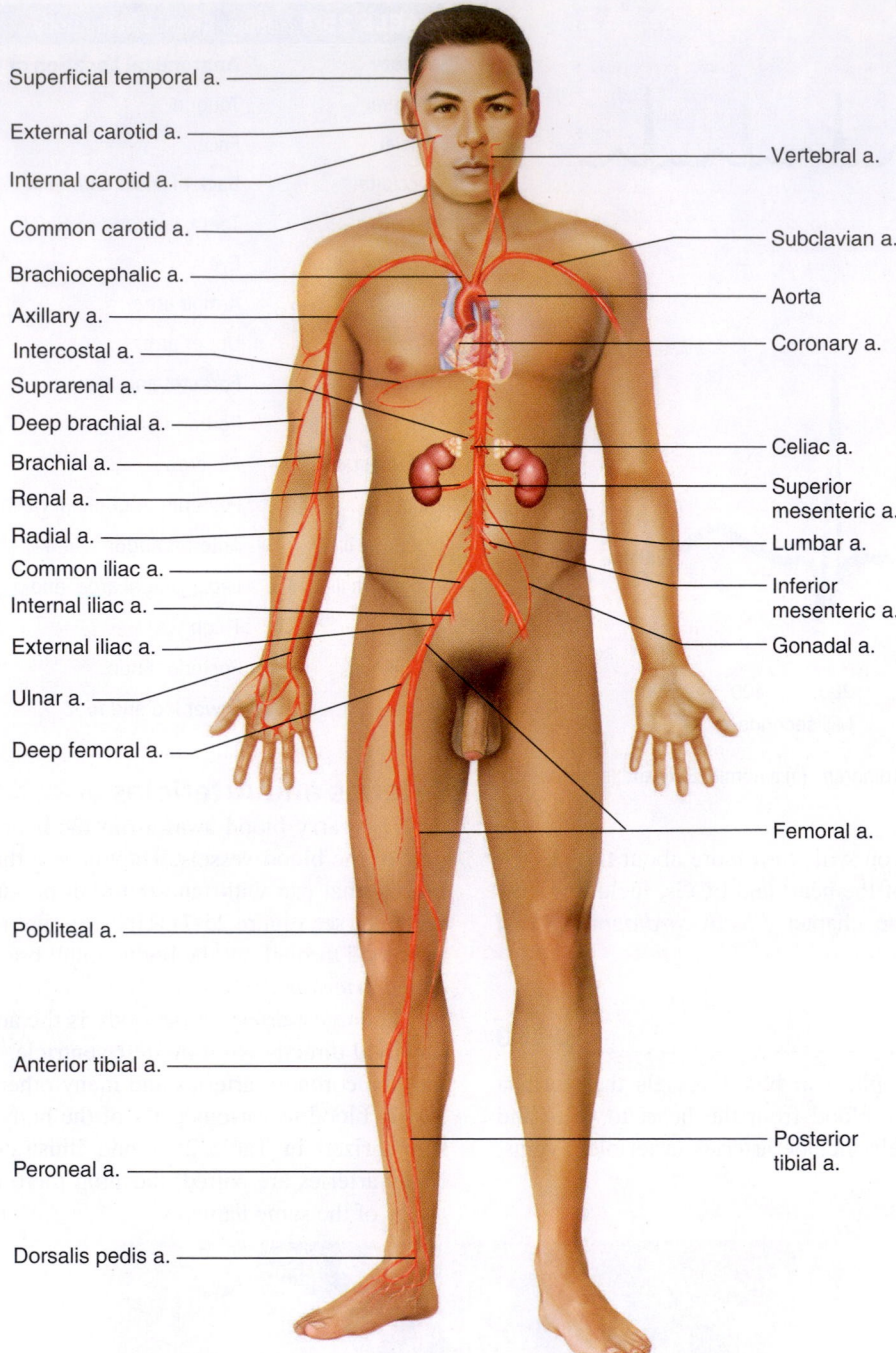

Superficial temporal a.
External carotid a.
Internal carotid a.
Common carotid a.
Brachiocephalic a.
Axillary a.
Intercostal a.
Suprarenal a.
Deep brachial a.
Brachial a.
Renal a.
Radial a.
Common iliac a.
Internal iliac a.
External iliac a.
Ulnar a.
Deep femoral a.
Popliteal a.
Anterior tibial a.
Peroneal a.
Dorsalis pedis a.

Vertebral a.
Subclavian a.
Aorta
Coronary a.
Celiac a.
Superior mesenteric a.
Lumbar a.
Inferior mesenteric a.
Gonadal a.
Femoral a.
Posterior tibial a.

FIGURE 25-8   Major arteries of the body (a. stands for *artery*).

Most arteries carry oxygenated blood. The exceptions to this are the pulmonary arteries, which carry deoxygenated blood from the heart to the lungs.

Capillaries

Capillaries are the smallest type of blood vessel. They branch off of arterioles and have walls that are only about one cell layer thick. These thin walls make the exchange of oxygen, carbon dioxide, and nutrients possible between the blood and the body cells (see Figure 25-9). In fact, capillaries are the only type of blood vessels that allow substances to move into and out of the blood. Tissues that require a lot of oxygen, such as muscle and nervous tissues, have a lot of capillaries.

The substances that move through the capillary walls include oxygen, carbon dioxide, nutrients, water, and metabolic wastes. These substances move through the walls through one of three processes: diffusion, filtration, or osmosis. These processes are described in the *Organization of the Body* chapter.

Veins and Venules

Veins are blood vessels that carry blood toward the heart. Unlike arteries, they are not under high pressure, so they do not need thick, muscular walls. Their walls are thinner than those of arteries. Because the blood in veins is not under pressure, veins have valves that prevent backflow and keep the blood moving toward the heart (see Figure 25-10).

EDUCATING THE PATIENT

Chest Pain

Chest pain, or angina, is a common reason for people to go to the emergency room or an urgent care center. Explain to patients that there are many causes of chest pain, both cardiac and noncardiac. Cardiac causes include myocardial infarction (MI, or heart attack), pericarditis, and coronary spasms. See the Pathophysiology section of this chapter for more detailed descriptions of these causes. Noncardiac causes include heartburn, panic attacks, lung conditions, broken ribs, inflammation of the gallbladder or pancreas, and even just sore muscles. However, tell patients that all chest pain should be taken seriously, because some conditions, both cardiac and noncardiac, can be life-threatening if not treated.

Skeletal muscle contractions help move the blood through veins. When the muscles contract, they squeeze the veins and blood is pushed through them, much the way toothpaste is pushed out of a tube. The sympathetic nervous system also influences the flow of blood through veins. If blood pressure becomes abnormally low, the sympathetic nervous system causes vein walls to constrict, which forces blood through the veins.

Venules are very small veins formed when capillaries merge together (see Figure 25-11). The venules then merge to form the veins.

Most veins carry deoxygenated blood. The exceptions to this are the pulmonary veins, which carry oxygenated blood from the lungs to the left ventricle of the heart. Large veins often have the same names as the arteries they run next to, but there are exceptions. For example, the veins next to the carotid arteries are the jugular veins.

Large veins empty blood into the superior vena cava and the inferior vena cava (plural: *venae cavae*), which are the largest veins in the body. The superior vena cava generally collects blood from veins above the heart, and the inferior vena cava collects blood from veins below the heart. The major veins are summarized in Table 25-2 and are illustrated in Figure 25-12.

The veins of the intestines carry blood from the digestive tract to the liver. The liver then processes nutrients in the blood and returns it to general circulation through the hepatic veins. The veins involved in this process are known as the **hepatic portal system.**

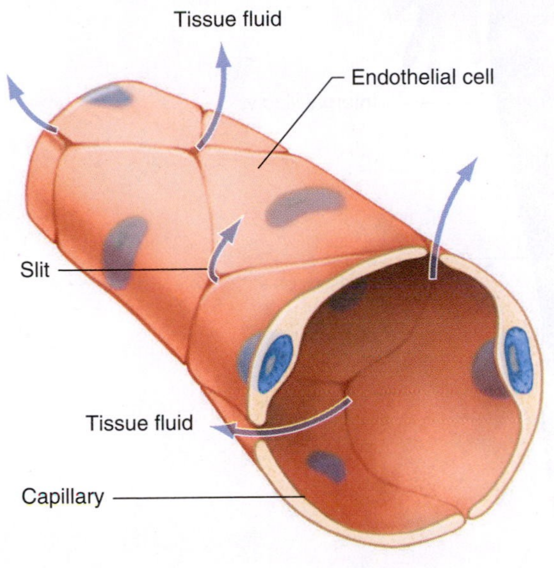

FIGURE 25-9 Structure of a capillary wall.

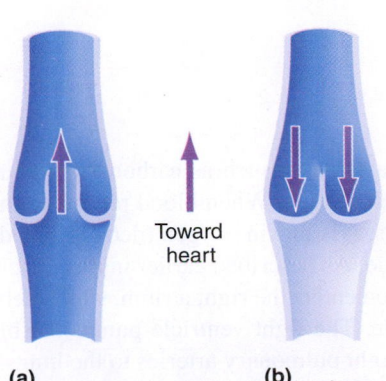

FIGURE 25-10 Venous valve: (a) valve opens when blood is flowing toward the heart and (b) valve closes to prevent blood from flowing away from the heart.

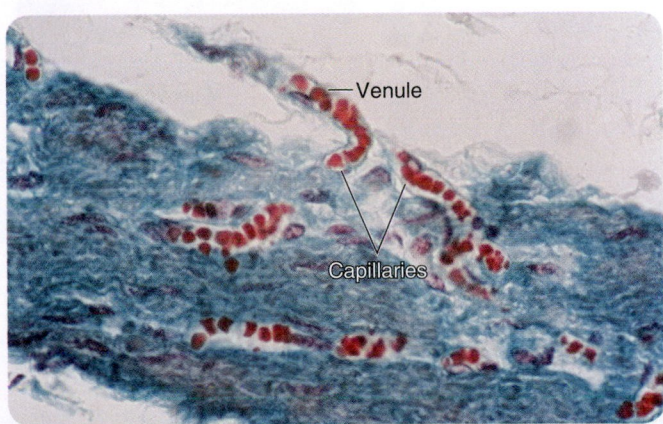

FIGURE 25-11 This light micrograph of a capillary network shows the capillaries merging to become venules.
© Biophoto Associates/Science Source

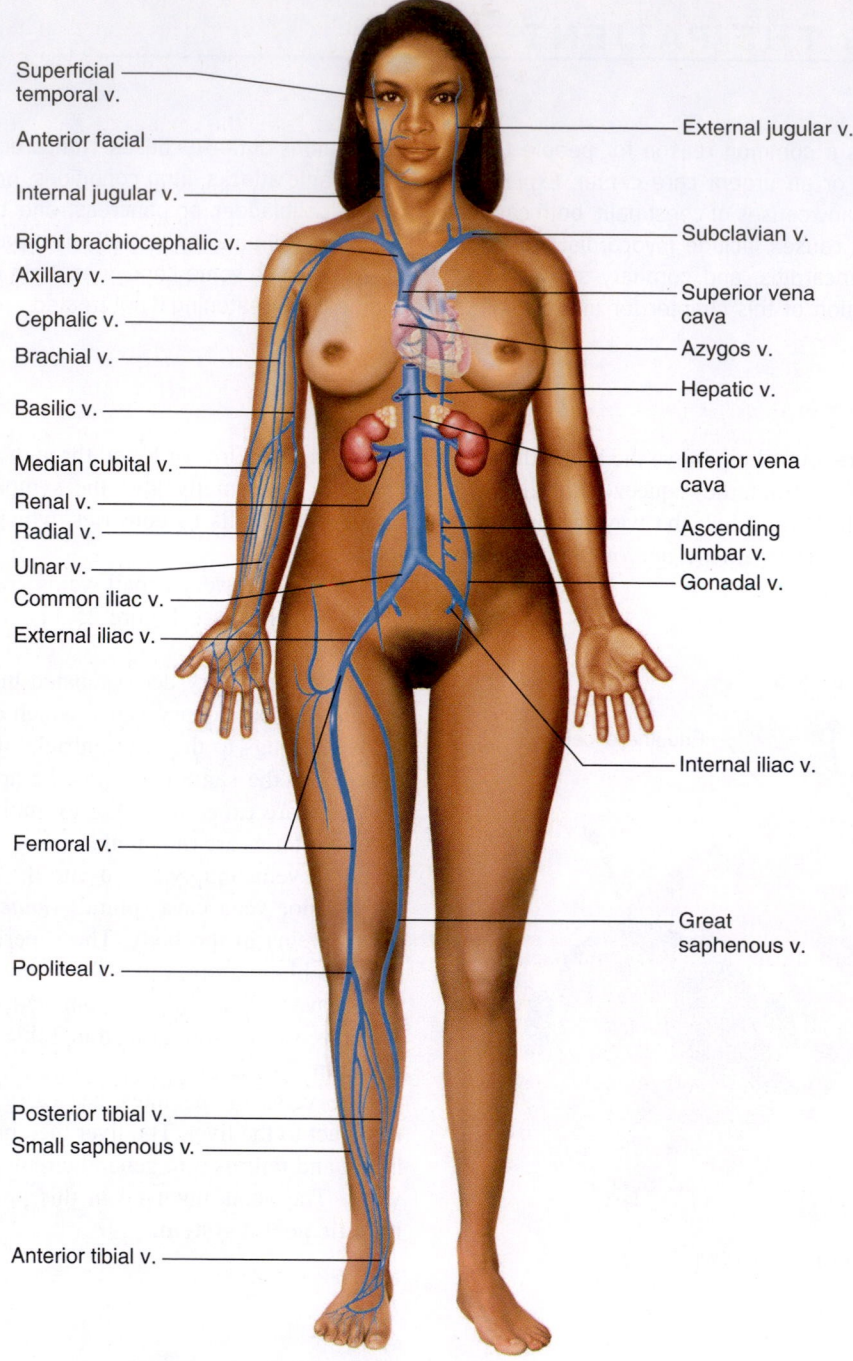

Superficial temporal v.

Anterior facial

Internal jugular v.

Right brachiocephalic v.

Axillary v.

Cephalic v.

Brachial v.

Basilic v.

Median cubital v.

Renal v.

Radial v.

Ulnar v.

Common iliac v.

External iliac v.

Femoral v.

Popliteal v.

Posterior tibial v.

Small saphenous v.

Anterior tibial v.

External jugular v.

Subclavian v.

Superior vena cava

Azygos v.

Hepatic v.

Inferior vena cava

Ascending lumbar v.

Gonadal v.

Internal iliac v.

Great saphenous v.

FIGURE 25-12 Major veins of the body (v. stands for *vein*).

▶ Circulation

LO 25.4

Blood circulates through the body through three main circuits. The *pulmonary circuit* provides oxygen, the *systemic circuit* distributes the oxygen throughout the body, and the *coronary circuit* distributes the oxygen to the heart muscle.

Pulmonary Circulation

The pulmonary circuit, or **pulmonary circulation,** is the route blood takes from the heart to the lungs and back to the heart again (see Figure 25-13). The purpose of this circuit is

to remove waste gases such as carbon dioxide and replenish the blood with oxygen. When blood returns to the heart from the body cells, it is low in oxygen (deoxygenated) and rich in carbon dioxide. As described earlier in this chapter, the deoxygenated blood enters the right atrium, which delivers it to the right ventricle. The right ventricle pumps the blood through the left and right pulmonary arteries to the lungs.

In the lungs, blood picks up oxygen and gets rid of carbon dioxide. Blood rich in oxygen and low in carbon dioxide then returns to the heart through the four pulmonary veins. The pulmonary veins empty the oxygenated blood into the left atrium.

TABLE 25-2	Major Veins of the Body
Vein	**Anatomical Location or Organ Drained**
Jugular	Head and neck
Brachiocephalic	Head and neck
Axillary	Armpit area
Brachial	Upper arm
Ulnar	Lower arm and hand
Radial	Lower arm and hand
Intercostal	Rib area
Azygos	Thorax and abdomen
Iliac	Pelvic organs, legs, and gluteal areas
Femoral	Thighs
Popliteal	Knees
Saphenous	Legs
Hepatic	Liver to the inferior vena cava
Hepatic Portal System	
Gastric	Stomach to the liver
Splenic	Spleen, pancreas, and stomach to the liver
Mesenteric	Intestines to the liver
Hepatic portal	Gastric, splenic, and mesenteric veins to the liver

Systemic Circulation

The systemic circuit, or **systemic circulation,** is the route blood takes from the heart through the body and back to the heart. The purpose of this circuit is to deliver oxygen and nutrients to the body cells. It also picks up carbon dioxide and waste products from the body cells (see Figure 25-13).

Blood that returns from the lungs and enters the left atrium is oxygen rich (oxygenated) and has a low level of carbon dioxide. It flows from the left atrium to the left ventricle, which contracts to pump the oxygenated blood into the aorta, which branches off to various arteries to deliver the blood throughout the body.

The arteries branch into the smaller arterioles, and the arterioles branch into capillaries. In the capillaries, oxygen and nutrients picked up from the digestive system move from the blood into the body cells. Carbon dioxide and metabolic wastes move from the body cells into the blood. The blood then moves through the venules and veins and is collected into the vena cava, which delivers the blood back to the right atrium of the heart, and the whole process starts over again with pulmonary circulation.

Coronary Circulation

Coronary circulation is the part of systemic circulation that supplies oxygen and nutrients to the heart and removes carbon dioxide and other wastes. The coronary arteries branch directly off the aorta immediately after the blood leaves the left atrium (see Figure 25-14). Like all other arteries, the coronary arteries branch into smaller and smaller vessels, ending in capillaries, where oxygen and nutrients move into the heart

cells and carbon dioxide and wastes move into the blood. The blood then travels through the venules and the cardiac veins, which merge to form a large vein called the *coronary sinus.* Unlike other veins, however, the coronary sinus does not empty into the vena cava. It empties directly into the right atrium.

Blockage of one or more of the coronary arteries may cause chest pain, or angina, and may lead to myocardial infarction (MI, or heart attack) if not corrected. See the *Educating the Patient* feature and the Pathophysiology section of this chapter for more information about these disorders.

▶ Blood Pressure   LO 25.5

Blood pressure is the force that blood exerts on the inner walls of blood vessels. Blood pressure is highest in arteries and lowest in veins. In the clinical setting, *blood pressure* refers to the pressure in arteries.

Arterial blood pressure rises and falls as the ventricles of the heart contract and relax. It is highest when the ventricles contract. This highest point of pressure is called the **systolic pressure** or systole. When the ventricles relax, blood pressure in arteries is at its lowest. This pressure is called the **diastolic pressure** or diastole. Blood pressure is usually reported as the systolic pressure over the diastolic pressure. For example, in the blood pressure reading 120/80, 120 denotes the systolic pressure and 80 refers to the diastolic pressure.

You can feel the surge of blood through arteries when you take a pulse. The pulse is created as the artery expands when pressure increases and then subsequently relaxes as blood pressure decreases. Common places to feel a pulse are the carotid and radial arteries.

Many factors affect blood pressure, including cardiac output, blood volume, vasoconstriction, vasodilation, and blood viscosity. **Cardiac output** is the total amount of blood the heart pumps in 1 minute. As cardiac output increases, it causes an increase in blood pressure. When cardiac output decreases, blood pressure decreases accordingly.

When a person loses a large volume of blood, his blood pressure significantly decreases. If the blood pressure falls too low, the muscular walls of the arteries can constrict to increase blood pressure. This process is known as **vasoconstriction.** If a person's blood pressure is too high, the blood vessels dilate, decreasing the blood pressure. This process is known as **vasodilation.**

The **viscosity,** or thickness, of blood also plays a part in blood pressure. Under certain circumstances, such as dehydration, the blood becomes more viscous, or thicker. The thicker blood requires more energy to move and results in higher blood pressure.

Blood pressure is controlled to a large extent by the amount of blood pumped out of the heart. The amount of blood entering the heart should be equal to the amount of blood pumped out of the heart. The heart has a way to ensure that this happens. When blood enters the left ventricle, the wall of the ventricle is stretched. The more the wall is stretched, the harder it will contract and the more blood it will pump out. This is referred to as *Starling's law of the heart.* If only a small amount

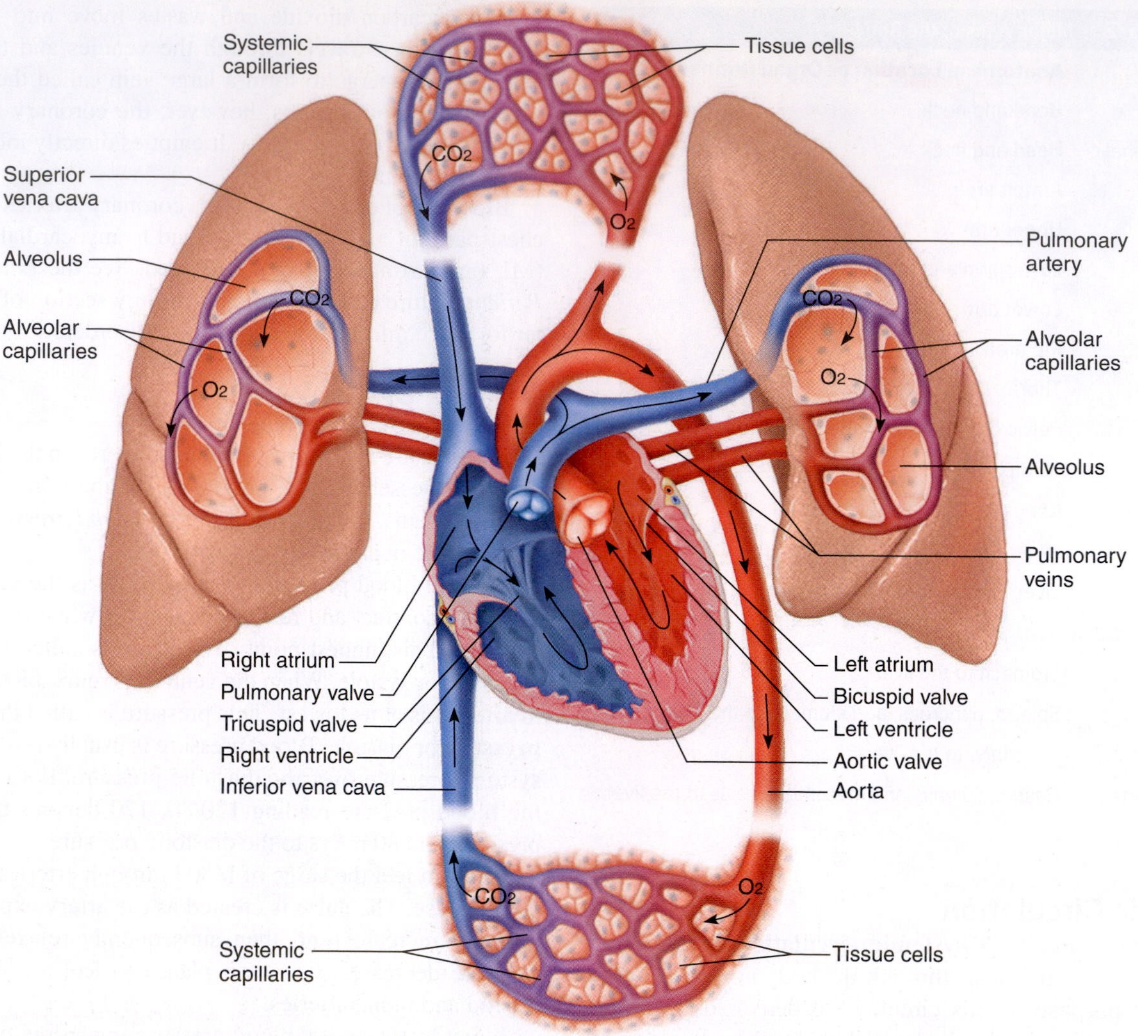

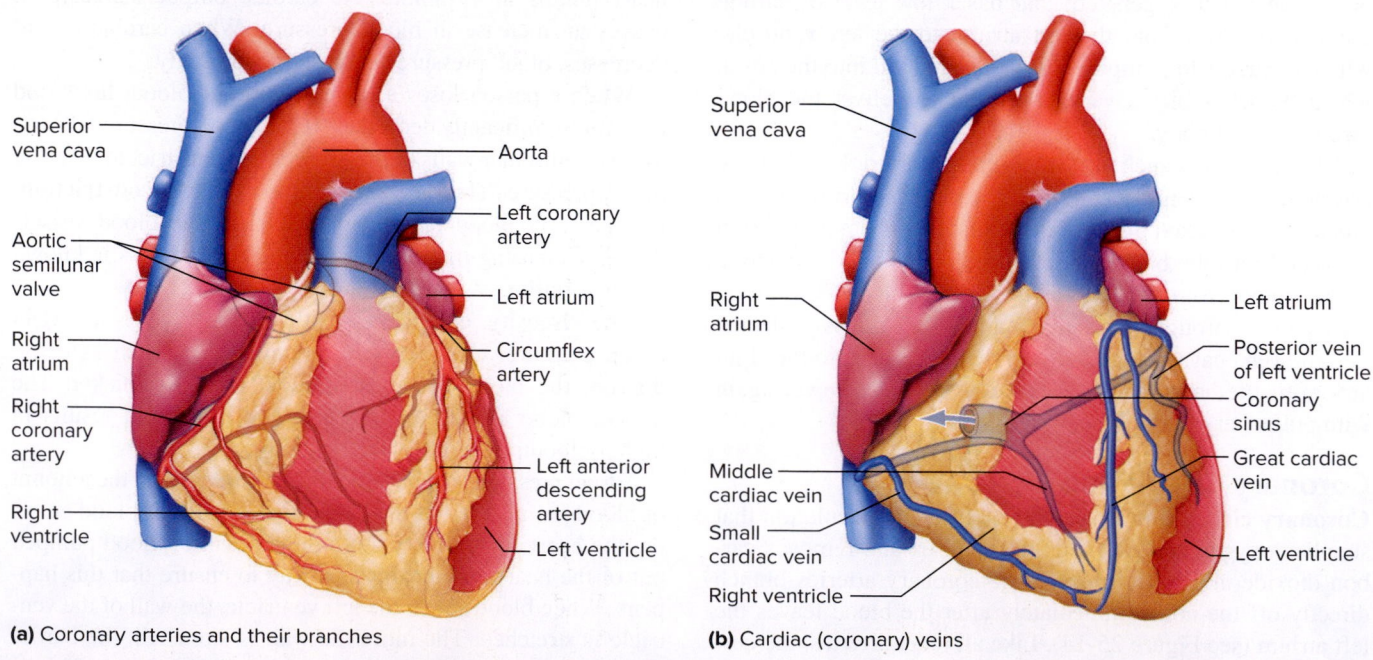

FIGURE 25-13   Pathway of blood through the heart and lungs and on to other body parts. The right side of the heart delivers blood to the lungs (pulmonary circulation), and the left side delivers blood to all other body parts (systemic circulation).

Heart diagram labels (top figure):

Systemic capillaries
Tissue cells
CO_2
Superior vena cava
Pulmonary artery
Alveolus
CO_2
O_2
Alveolar capillaries
CO_2
O_2
Alveolar capillaries
Alveolus
Pulmonary veins
Right atrium
Pulmonary valve
Tricuspid valve
Right ventricle
Inferior vena cava
Systemic capillaries
CO_2
O_2
Tissue cells
Left atrium
Bicuspid valve
Left ventricle
Aortic valve
Aorta

(a) Coronary arteries and their branches

Superior vena cava
Aorta
Aortic semilunar valve
Left coronary artery
Left atrium
Circumflex artery
Right atrium
Right coronary artery
Right ventricle
Left anterior descending artery
Left ventricle

(b) Cardiac (coronary) veins

Superior vena cava
Right atrium
Left atrium
Posterior vein of left ventricle
Coronary sinus
Great cardiac vein
Middle cardiac vein
Small cardiac vein
Right ventricle
Left ventricle

FIGURE 25-14   Coronary circulation. (a) The coronary arteries and their branches supply blood to the heart muscle. (b) The cardiac (coronary) veins collect the deoxygenated blood and deposit it into the coronary sinus, which empties into the right atrium.

of blood enters the left ventricle, it will not be stretched very much and therefore will not contract very forcefully. In this case, not much blood is pumped out of the heart.

Baroreceptors also help regulate blood pressure. Baroreceptors measure blood pressure and are located in the aorta and carotid arteries. If pressure increases in these blood vessels, this information is sent to the cardiac center in the medulla oblongata. The cardiac center then knows to decrease the heart rate, which lowers blood pressure. If pressure gets too low in the aorta, baroreceptors pick up this information and relay it to the cardiac center. The cardiac center then increases the heart rate to raise blood pressure.

PATHOPHYSIOLOGY

LO 25.6

Common Diseases and Disorders of the Cardiovascular System

HYPERTENSION, or high blood pressure, is a consistent resting blood pressure of 140/90 mm Hg or higher. It is known as the "silent killer," because it increases a person's risk of heart attack, stroke, heart failure, and kidney failure, sometimes without presenting symptoms that could warn the person of medical risk. The American Heart Association estimates that 73 million American adults have hypertension, with African Americans having a higher incidence than Caucasians.

Causes. Known causes and risk factors for hypertension include narrowing of the arteries, kidney disease, endocrine disorders, pregnancy, drug use (especially cocaine and amphetamines), sleep apnea, obesity, smoking, a high-sodium diet, excessive alcohol consumption, stress, diabetes, and various medications such as oral contraceptives and cold medicines. However, many of the causes of hypertension are unknown.

Signs and Symptoms. Hypertension often causes no symptoms at all. When symptoms are present, they include excessive sweating, muscle cramps, fatigue, frequent urination, headaches, dizziness, and an irregular heart rate.

Treatment. Hypertension cannot be cured, but it can be controlled. The first method of treatment is to treat the underlying causes, if they are known. For example, the patient may be placed on a low-sodium/low-cholesterol diet and may be encouraged to make lifestyle changes such as getting regular exercise, managing stress, and stopping smoking. The physician may also prescribe medications to slow the heart rate and/or dilate the blood vessels and diuretics to reduce blood volume.

Patient compliance is the key to successful management of hypertension. Because hypertension often has no symptoms, but the prescribed medications may have noticeable side effects, patients may stop taking the medications because they feel better when they do not take it. Be sure patients understand that taking the medication(s) is crucial to their treatment and long-term health. If they experience unacceptable side effects, they should tell the physician, because many options are available, and the physician may be able to prescribe a different medication that has fewer or less noticeable side effects.

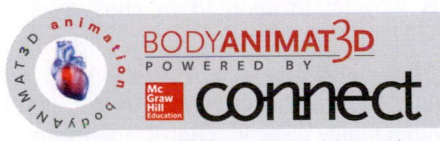

Go to CONNECT to see an animation exercise about *Hypertension.*

DYSRHYTHMIAS are abnormal heart rhythms. The heart may beat too fast (tachycardia), too slowly (bradycardia), or irregularly. The most common type of dysrhythmia is atrial fibrillation, which is a sporadic, rapid beating of the atria that may or may not affect the ventricles. The most serious type of dysrhythmia is ventricular fibrillation, in which disorganized electrical activity in the heart causes the ventricles to quiver ineffectively instead of beating. Most sudden cardiac deaths are caused by ventricular fibrillation.

Causes. Most dysrhythmias result from abnormal flow of electrical impulses through the heart. Abnormal impulse conduction has many potential causes, including electric shock, certain medications, some herbal supplements, hypertension, previous heart attack, decreased blood flow to the heart, coronary artery disease, heart valve disorders, weakening of the heart muscle (cardiomyopathy), some genetic diseases, diabetes mellitus, sleep apnea, electrolyte (potassium, sodium, and calcium) imbalances, excess alcohol consumption, and drugs such as cocaine and amphetamines.

Signs and Symptoms. Dysrhythmias may cause signs and symptoms including shortness of breath, dizziness or fainting, an unusually fast or slow heart rate, a fluttering feeling in the chest, and chest pain.

Treatment. The first goal of treatment is to correct the underlying cause of the dysrhythmia. Other treatment options include

- Vagal maneuvers to slow the heart rate. These include holding the breath, straining (bearing down as if for a bowel movement), and putting the face in cool water.
- Medications such as beta blockers and anti-dysrhythmics.
- Pacemakers.
- Radiofrequency catheter ablation. This procedure destroys a small amount of heart tissue to change the flow of the electrical impulses through the heart.
- Maze procedure; this operation forms scars in the atria to correct the flow of electrical impulses through the heart.
- Implantation of an implantable cardioverter defibrillator (ICD) to regulate the heart rhythm.
- Surgery to correct heart defects such as narrow coronary arteries.
- Electric shock (defibrillation) to reset heart rhythms.
- Cardiopulmonary resuscitation if there is no evidence of blood flow.

ANGINA is chest pain that occurs when the heart does not receive enough oxygen to carry out its job of pumping blood throughout the body. It is not immediately life threatening, but if the reason for the angina is not found and corrected, the angina may become unstable (difficult to treat and less responsive to medications). This type of angina is a warning of serious or life-threatening conditions.

Causes. Angina is caused by a narrowing of the coronary arteries. Arteries may become too narrow due to coronary spasms or as a result of coronary artery disease (atherosclerosis), in which fatty deposits accumulate in the arteries.

Signs and Symptoms. The pain of angina is usually described as a tight feeling in the chest. It is often brought about by stress or physical activity. When the stress or activity stops, the pain usually goes away.

Treatment. A doctor should monitor patients with angina regularly. Most patients with angina carry sublingual nitroglycerin with them to dilate the coronary blood vessels and relieve the pain. Treatment must also address the underlying cause of the angina to prevent more serious conditions such as a heart attack or stroke. The physician may order several tests to determine the cause of angina, such as an electrocardiogram (ECG), a stress test, blood tests, chest X-rays, cardiac catheterization, or an echocardiogram.

CORONARY ARTERY DISEASE (CAD), also called **ATHEROSCLEROSIS,** is an accumulation of fatty deposits in the arteries as a result of too much glucose in the blood. The deposits cause the arteries to become narrow, reducing the amount of blood that can flow through them. CAD affects more Americans than any other type of heart disease. The American Heart Association estimates that one in three American adults has one or more types of coronary artery disease.

Causes. This condition is usually caused by a buildup of fat, cholesterol, and calcium in the arteries. The risk factors for developing CAD include high levels of LDL (low-density lipoprotein) cholesterol in the blood, a diet high in fat and cholesterol, smoking, high blood pressure, obesity, a lack of exercise, and diabetes mellitus.

Signs and Symptoms. There are often no signs or symptoms until a heart attack occurs. The most common symptoms include angina, shortness of breath, tightness in the chest, fatigue, and swelling in the legs of feet (edema). As with most cardiac conditions, the first line of defense against CAD is prevention. CAD may be prevented or reduced by controlling high blood pressure and high cholesterol, not smoking, eating healthy foods, engaging in regular exercise, and treating any existing conditions such as diabetes or atherosclerosis.

Treatment. Existing CAD is treated using lipid-lowering agents such as Mevacor® or Lipitor®, aspirin therapy, and medications to slow a rapid heart rate. The patient can help by adopting a low-fat diet, exercising moderately, and not smoking. Severe CAD may require surgery such as coronary angioplasty or coronary artery bypass grafting (CABG) to repair, widen, or detour around narrowed coronary arteries.

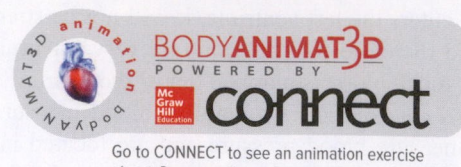

Go to CONNECT to see an animation exercise about *Coronary Artery Disease (CAD).*

A MYOCARDIAL INFARCTION (MI), commonly called a *heart attack,* is nonreversible damage to the heart caused by a lack of oxygen. Historically, MIs have been fatal, and they often still are, but with new treatments, more and more people survive them. However, the body cannot replace the damaged cardiac cells, so a heart attack can result in permanent damage to the heart.

Causes. The causes and contributing factors include blockage of coronary arteries as a result of atherosclerosis (CAD) and a blood clot that blocks the flow of blood through an artery. Drugs such as cocaine can cause coronary arteries to spasm, which may also cause an MI.

Signs and Symptoms. Common symptoms include recurring, squeezing chest pain or angina; pain in the shoulder, arm, back, teeth, or jaw; chronic pain in the upper abdomen; shortness of breath, especially on exertion; sweating (diaphoresis); dizziness or fainting; and nausea or vomiting.

Treatment. The first treatment, if possible, is chewing an aspirin at the onset of symptoms. In an unconscious patient who has no pulse and is not breathing, cardiopulmonary resuscitation (CPR) should be administered. Other immediate treatment options include the use of a defibrillator and thrombolytic medications to destroy the blood clots that block a coronary artery. It should be noted that thrombolytic drugs are effective only if begun within 3 hours of the first symptom, so time is crucial. Surgery (angioplasty or CABG) may be necessary to replace or repair blocked coronary arteries. Long-term treatment includes anticoagulant medications such as heparin and warfarin to thin the blood, and medications such as atenolol to slow the heart rate.

AN ANEURYSM is a ballooned, weakened arterial wall. The most common locations of aneurysms are the aorta and arteries in the brain, legs, intestines, and spleen. An aortic aneurysm is a bulge in the wall of the aorta. Most aortic aneurysms occur in the abdominal aorta (abdominal aortic aneurysm), but some occur in the thoracic aorta (see Figure 25-15). Most aortic aneurysms do not rupture; however, when they do, the resulting hemorrhage is a life-threatening emergency.

Causes. Most causes are unknown. One identified risk for developing an aneurysm is atherosclerosis, which is usually associated with a high-cholesterol diet. Smoking and obesity also increase the risk of atherosclerosis. Congenital conditions may cause an aneurysm—some individuals are born with weak aortic walls. A traumatic injury to the chest also may be a risk factor. The risk of developing an aneurysm can be reduced by not smoking, by losing excess weight, and by eating a low-fat, low-cholesterol diet. Periodic screening is an option for patients with a family history of aortic aneurysms.

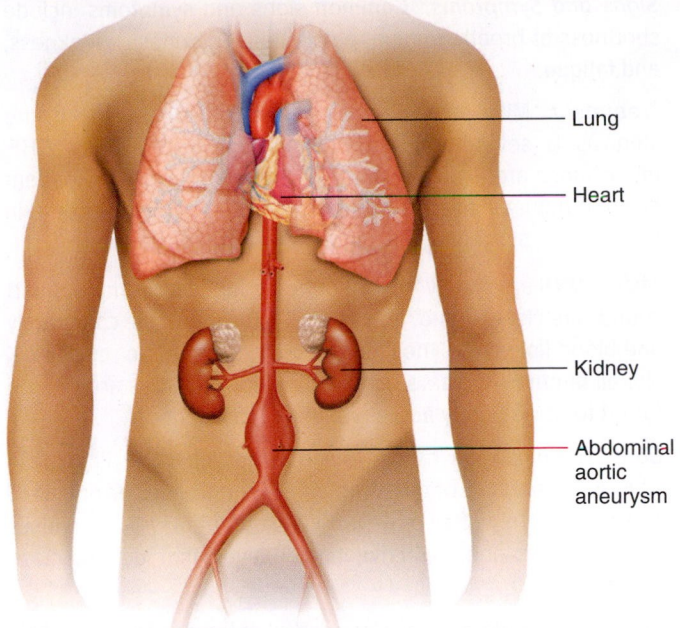

FIGURE 25-15 Abdominal aneurysms can occur without symptoms, but if they rupture they are frequently life threatening.

Signs and Symptoms. There are usually no signs or symptoms of an aneurysm, although hypertension may be present. When symptoms do exist, the most common are a pulsation in the abdomen and back pain. A sudden pain in the abdomen or back, dizziness, a fast pulse, or a loss of consciousness can be a sign that an aneurysm has ruptured.

Treatment. The primary treatment is surgery to repair the aneurysm.

ENDOCARDITIS is an inflammation of the innermost lining of the heart, including the heart valves.

Causes. Bacterial infections are the most common cause of endocarditis. Patients are more susceptible to this condition if they have abnormal heart valves.

Signs and Symptoms. Common signs and symptoms include weakness, fever, excessive sweating, general body aches, difficulty breathing, and blood in the urine.

Treatment. The treatment for this condition is intravenous antibiotics followed by oral antibiotics for up to 6 weeks.

MYOCARDITIS is an inflammation of the muscular layer of the heart. It is relatively uncommon but very serious because it leads to weakening of the heart wall.

Causes. The most common cause of myocarditis is a viral infection, but it also may be caused by exposure to certain chemicals, allergens, and bacteria.

Signs and Symptoms. Signs and symptoms include fever as well as chest pains that feel like a heart attack. Difficulty breathing, decreased urine output, fatigue, and fainting also may accompany myocarditis.

Treatment. Treatment normally includes steroids to reduce inflammation, bed rest, and a low-sodium diet.

PERICARDITIS is inflammation of the pericardium, which is the group of membranes that surround the heart.

Causes. This condition is most commonly caused by complications of viral or bacterial infections. However, heart attacks and chest injuries also can lead to pericarditis.

Signs and Symptoms. Symptoms include sharp, stabbing chest pains, especially during deep breaths. Fever, fatigue, and difficulty breathing while lying down are also common symptoms.

Treatment. Diuretics are used to remove excess fluids around the heart. If bacteria caused the pericarditis, antibiotics are used as well. In chronic cases, surgery may be required to remove part of the membranes surrounding the heart. Because pericarditis can be very painful, treatment also generally includes painkillers.

CONGESTIVE HEART FAILURE (CHF) is a slowly developing condition in which the heart weakens over time. Eventually, the heart is no longer able to pump enough blood to meet the body's needs.

Causes. There are many risk factors for this condition, including smoking, being overweight, a diet high in cholesterol, a lack of exercise, atherosclerosis, history of MI, high blood pressure, a damaged heart valve, excessive alcohol consumption, and diabetes mellitus. Congenital heart defects (those present at birth) and drugs that weaken the heart (especially cocaine, heroin, and some antineoplastic drugs for cancer) also may contribute to the development of this disorder. Patients may reduce the risk factors for CHF by controlling high blood pressure and high cholesterol, not smoking, maintaining a healthy diet, engaging in regular exercise, and treating any existing atherosclerosis or diabetes.

Signs and Symptoms. Signs and symptoms include shortness of breath; constant wheezing; prominent neck veins; fluid retention that causes swelling in the legs, feet, or abdomen; nausea; dizziness; and an irregular or rapid heartbeat. (See Figure 25-16.)

Treatment. Common treatment options include medications to slow a rapid heartbeat, diuretics to decrease edema and fluid accumulation in the lungs, and medications to reduce blood pressure. In more serious cases, surgery to repair defective heart valves or other heart defects, implantation of a cardiac pacemaker, or a heart transplant may be needed.

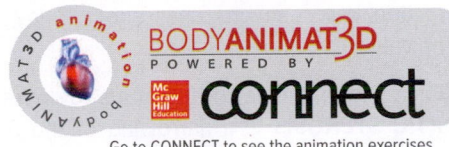

Go to CONNECT to see the animation exercises *Heart Failure Overview, Left-Side Heart Failure,* and *Right-Side Heart Failure.*

MITRAL VALVE PROLAPSE (MVP) is a condition in which the mitral valve falls into the left atrium during systole. This prevents the valve from sealing properly. In severe cases, blood may flow back into the atrium. Although most cases are mild, MVP can become worse over time. It also increases the risk of heart valve infections and endocarditis.

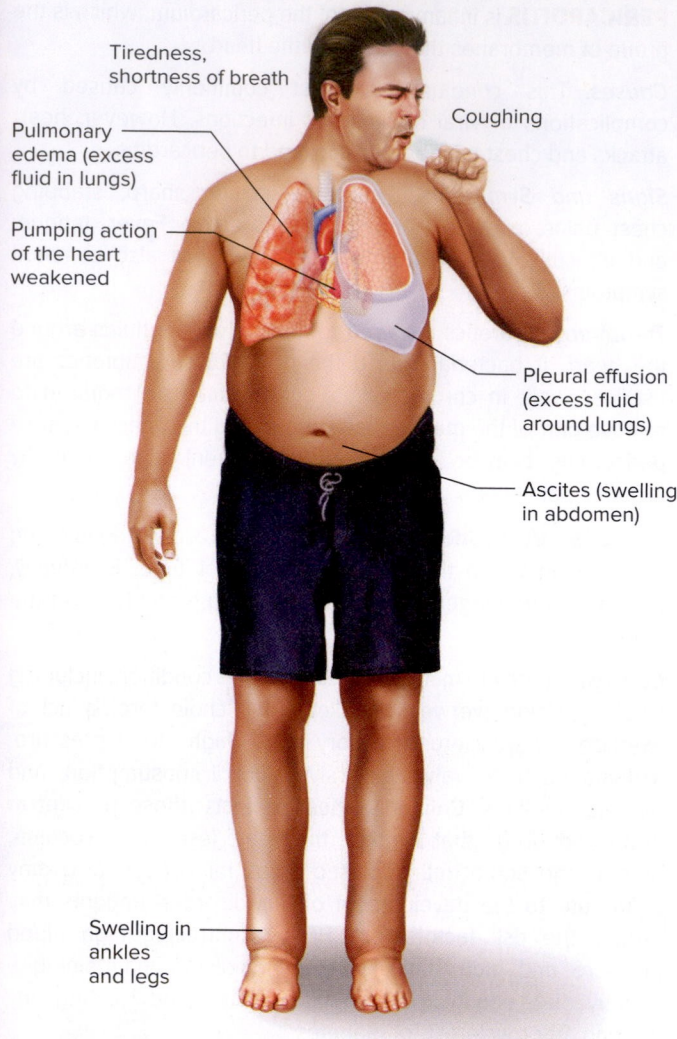

Tiredness, shortness of breath

Coughing

Pulmonary edema (excess fluid in lungs)

Pumping action of the heart weakened

Pleural effusion (excess fluid around lungs)

Ascites (swelling in abdomen)

Swelling in ankles and legs

FIGURE 25-16   When the heart muscle is damaged and weak, a patient will suffer symptoms of heart failure.

Causes. The cause of MVP is unknown in most cases. However, it may be hereditary, and it has been linked to autonomic nervous system disorders.

Signs and Symptoms. In mild cases, symptoms may not develop. In more severe cases, palpitations, shortness of breath, and chest pain may occur.

Treatment. No treatment is needed for mild cases. Medications are used to treat symptoms and to help prevent complications such as infection. In very severe cases, surgery may be required to repair the valve.

STENOSIS is an abnormal narrowing of a body passage. In the heart, **AORTIC STENOSIS** is a narrowing of the aortic valve, and **MITRAL STENOSIS** is a narrowing of the mitral valve. Stenosis causes these valves to fail to open fully. As a result, blood flow from the heart decreases and pressure inside the left ventricle increases. In severe cases, stenosis may cause heart dysrhythmias or congestive heart failure.

Causes. Aortic or mitral stenosis can be congenital or may occur later in life. Noncongenital cases are common in patients who have had rheumatic fever.

Signs and Symptoms. Common signs and symptoms include shortness of breath, angina, palpitations, dizziness, weakness, and fatigue.

Treatment. Mild stenosis may not need treatment. If the stenosis is severe enough to cause dysrhythmias or CHF, medications are used to control these disorders. If the patient has had rheumatic fever, antibiotics may also be prescribed. In some cases, surgery or valvuloplasty may be performed.

MURMURS are simply abnormal heart sounds. Normally, heart sounds are clear, strong, and smooth as valves close completely and blood flows over the lining of the heart with no resistance. Not all murmurs indicate a heart disorder. Murmurs are graded from 1 to 6; 1 is barely audible and the least serious.

Causes. Not all the causes of heart murmurs are known. In children, the failure of the foramen ovale or ductus arteriosis to close completely after birth can cause murmurs. Other causes include stress and defective heart valves that do not close completely.

Signs and Symptoms. The signs and symptoms vary considerably depending on the cause and severity of the heart murmur. Severe symptoms include weakness, pallor, edema (fluid retention), and other signs commonly associated with heart failure.

Treatment. In many cases, no treatment is required. Surgery to correct valvular defects or other heart defects may be needed in more serious cases.

THROMBOPHLEBITIS is a condition in which a blood clot blocks or partially blocks blood flow in a vein, causing inflammation, swelling, and pain. It most commonly occurs in the leg veins. The danger of thrombophlebitis is that the blood clot may break loose, becoming an **embolus** that moves through the circulatory system. The embolus can cause major problems, depending on where it lodges in the body. If it blocks a blood vessel in the lungs, it becomes a pulmonary embolism (obstruction in the lungs). If it blocks a coronary artery, it may cause a myocardial infarction (heart attack). If it blocks an artery in the brain, it may cause a cerebrovascular accident (stroke).

Causes. The causes and risk factors include prolonged inactivity, oral contraceptives, postmenopausal hormone replacement therapy (HRT), certain types of cancer, paralysis in the arms or legs, the presence of a venous catheter, a family history of thrombophlebitis, varicose veins, and trauma to veins.

Signs and Symptoms. The most common symptoms are tenderness and pain in the affected area; redness, swelling, and tenseness of the affected areas; fever; and a positive Homan's sign (pain behind the knee that is caused by a blood clot, when the foot is forceably dorsiflexed).

Treatment. This disorder is most often treated by applying heat to the affected area, wearing support stockings, and elevating the legs. Anti-inflammatory medications and anticoagulants may be prescribed. In some cases, surgery may be performed to remove the clot.

VARICOSE VEINS are twisted, dilated veins usually seen in the legs. They affect women more often than men. When varicose veins occur in the rectum, they are called *hemorrhoids*.

Causes. Varicose veins may be caused by prolonged sitting or standing, damage to valves in the veins, a loss of elasticity in the veins, obesity, pregnancy, oral contraceptives, or hormone replacement therapy. Family history also seems to play a part in the development of varicose veins. In some cases, varicose veins may be prevented or at least minimized through exercise and elevation of the legs.

Signs and Symptoms. Signs and symptoms include discomfort in the legs, discolorations around the ankles, clusters of veins, and enlarged, dark veins seen through skin.

Treatment. The treatment of varicose veins includes the following:

- Sclerotherapy, a procedure that prevents blood from flowing through varicose veins
- Laser surgery to prevent blood from flowing through affected veins
- Vein stripping, which involves removing affected veins
- Insertion of a catheter into the affected veins in order to destroy them
- Endoscopic vein surgery to close off affected veins

SUMMARY OF LEARNING OUTCOMES

LEARNING OUTCOMES	KEY POINTS
25.1 Describe the structures of the heart and the function of each.	The structures of the heart include the pericardium, epicardium, myocardium, and endocardium. The chambers of the heart consist of the atria (upper chambers) and the ventricles (lower chambers). The four valves within the heart are the tricuspid, the bicuspid, the pulmonary semilunar, and the aortic semilunar valves.
25.2 Explain the cardiac cycle, including the cardiac conduction system.	One cardiac cycle consists of one complete heartbeat. The atria contract and relax together, and the ventricles contract and relax together. As each chamber contracts, associated valves open and close to control the flow of blood through the heart. Contractions are initiated by the cardiac conduction system, which consists of the sinoatrial node, the atrioventricular node, the bundle of His, bundle branches, and Purkinje fibers.
25.3 Differentiate among the different types of blood vessels their functions.	Types of blood vessels include arteries and arterioles, which take blood from the heart to the body; veins and venules, which carry blood back from the body to the heart; and capillaries, which act as the connectors between the arterioles and venules. The largest artery in the body is the aorta. Other major arteries include lingual, facial, occipital, maxillary, ophthalmic, axillary, brachial, ulnar, radial, intercostals, lumbar, external iliac, common iliac, femoral, popliteal, and tibial. The largest veins in the body are the superior and inferior venae cavae. Other major veins are jugular, brachiocephalic, axillary, brachial, ulnar, radial, intercostals, azygos, iliac, femoral, popliteal, saphenous, hepatic, gastric, splenic, mesenteric, and hepatic portal.
25.4 Compare the various types of circulation.	Pulmonary circulation is the path the blood travels from the right side of the heart to the lungs and back to the left side of the heart. Its purpose is to oxygenate the blood and remove waste gases. Systemic circulation is the route blood takes from the left side of the heart, throughout the body, and back to the right side of the heart. Its purpose is to deliver oxygen and nutrients to body cells and to remove metabolic wastes from the cells. Coronary circulation delivers oxygenated blood to the coronary arteries and removes metabolic wastes from the heart muscle.

LEARNING OUTCOMES	KEY POINTS
25.5 Explain blood pressure and tell how it is controlled.	Blood pressure is the force exerted on the inner wall of blood vessels by blood as it flows through vessels. It is highest in arteries and lowest in veins. Clinically, blood pressure is the force of blood within the arteries. Blood pressure is largely controlled by the amount of blood pumped out of the heart, but various other events also may raise and lower blood pressure.
25.6 Describe the causes, signs and symptoms, and treatments of various diseases and disorders of the cardiovascular system.	Many different types of cardiac and blood diseases are described within this chapter. The signs, symptoms, and treatments are as varied as the diseases themselves. The last section of this chapter outlines the most common of these diseases, their signs and symptoms, and their treatments.

CASE STUDY CRITICAL THINKING

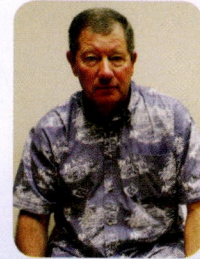

© McGraw-Hill Education

Recall John Miller from the beginning of this chapter. Now that you have completed this chapter, answer the following questions regarding his case.

1. What symptoms suggest that this patient is suffering from coronary artery disease and not some other disorder?

2. Why is it important to test the heart under stress rather than obtaining a resting echocardiogram?

3. Why is a cardiac catheterization needed in addition to the stress echocardiogram?

4. What lifestyle changes should this patient make to prevent future heart attacks?

EXAM PREPARATION QUESTIONS

1. (LO 25.1) Which heart valve is between the left atrium and left ventricle?
   a. Tricuspid
   b. Bicuspid
   c. Pulmonary semilunar
   d. Aortic semilunar
   e. Right atrioventricular

2. (LO 25.2) Which part of the cardiac conduction system receives electrical impulses from the bundle branches?
   a. AV node
   b. SA node
   c. Bundle of His
   d. Purkinje fibers
   e. Chordae tendineae

3. (LO 25.3) In which blood vessels does the exchange of oxygen and waste gases occur?
   a. Arteries
   b. Arterioles
   c. Veins
   d. Venules
   e. Capillaries

4. (LO 25.4) Which chamber of the heart receives oxygenated blood from the lungs?
   a. Left atrium
   b. Right atrium
   c. Pulmonary trunk
   d. Left ventricle
   e. Right ventricle

5. (LO 25.6) Which of the following causes of chest pain is *not* cardiac in nature?
   a. Angina
   b. Pericarditis
   c. Heartburn
   d. Myocardial infarction
   e. Coronary spasms

6. (LO 25.5) The amount of pressure in the arteries when the ventricles contract is called
   a. Cardiac output
   b. Vasodilation
   c. Vasoconstriction
   d. Diastole
   e. Systole

7. (LO 25.1) The layer of the heart wall that is made mostly of cardiac muscle that allows the heart to contract and relax is the
   a. Pericardial space
   b. Myocardium
   c. Epicardium
   d. Visceral pericardium
   e. Endocardium

8. (LO 25.6) A condition in which a blood clot and inflammation develop in a vein is
   a. Mitral stenosis
   b. Varicose veins
   c. Thrombophlebitis
   d. Myocardial infarction
   e. Pericarditis

9. (LO 25.3) The largest veins in the body are the
   a. Hepatic portal veins
   b. Jugular veins
   c. Venae cavae
   d. Pulmonary veins
   e. Femoral veins

10. (LO 25.5) The total amount of blood pumped out of the heart in 1 minute is known as the
   a. Cardiac output
   b. Systolic pressure
   c. Systemic circulation
   d. Coronary sinus
   e. Diastolic pressure

MEDICAL TERMINOLOGY PRACTICE

Analyze the following medical terms, presented throughout the chapter. Using a medical dictionary (or Appendix I) place a / mark between each word part. Define each word part and then define the whole word.

EXAMPLE: **vaso / spasm** = vaso means "vessel" + spasm means "cramp or twitching"
VASOSPASM means "twitching or cramping of a vessel."

1. atherosclerosis
2. atrioventricular
3. baroreceptor
4. echocardiogram
5. electrocardiogram
6. intercostal
7. myocardium
8. pericarditis
9. stenosis
10. thrombophlebitis
11. vasoconstriction
12. ventricular

The Blood

CASE STUDY

Patient Name	DOB	Allergies		
Cindy Chen	7/15/19XX	NKA		
Attending	**MRN**	**Other Information**		
Alexis N. Whalen, MD	324-86-542	CD4 (T-cell) count: 480 cells/mm^3 CBC 　RBC: 3.9 million/mm^3 　Hgb: 12.1 g/dL 　Hct: 39% 　MCV: 98 fL 　Platelets: 90,000 　WBC: 4,100		

PATIENT INFORMATION

Cindy Chen is a 28-year-old Asian female complaining of inability to sleep and nervousness. She tested positive for HIV in 2014 and has been taking the antiviral drug Retrovir® as prescribed by her physician. She currently lives with her aunt

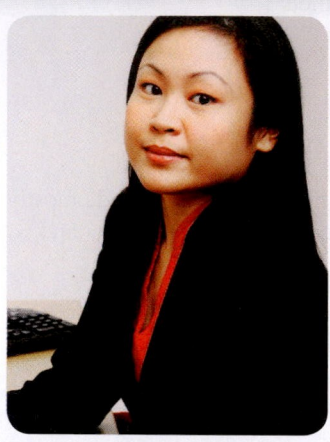

and is going to school for phlebotomy. When looking at her chart, you notice that she has lost 20 pounds in the last 3 months. When she was in for a checkup a week ago, Dr. Whalen ordered a series of blood tests, including helper T-cell tests and CBC with platelet count. She is in the office today to discuss the results of the tests.

Keep Cindy in mind as you study the chapter. There will be questions at the end of the chapter based on the case study. The information in the chapter will help you answer these questions.

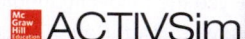

LEARNING OUTCOMES

After completing Chapter 26, you will be able to:

26.1 Describe the components of blood, giving the function of each component listed.

26.2 Explain how bleeding is controlled.

26.3 Differentiate among blood types A, B, AB, and O related to their compatibility.

26.4 Explain the difference between Rh-positive blood and Rh-negative blood.

26.5 Describe the causes, signs and symptoms, and treatments of various diseases and disorders of the blood.

KEY TERMS

agglutination
agranulocyte
albumins
basophil
coagulation
eosinophil
erythrocyte
erythropoietin
fibrinogen
globulins
granulocyte

hematocrit (Hct)
hemoglobin (Hgb)
hemostasis
leukocyte
lymphocyte
monocyte
neutrophil
platelets
serum
thrombocytes
thrombus

▶ Introduction

Your blood is a type of connective tissue that is made up of multiple parts, including red and white blood cells, cell fragments called platelets, and plasma (the fluid part of the blood). The average-sized adult body contains approximately 4 to 6 liters of blood, or approximately 8% of the total body weight. Blood volume varies from person to person depending on the person's size, the amount of adipose tissue in the body, and the concentrations of certain ions in the blood. In general, partly because of their smaller size, females generally have less blood volume than males.

Blood performs many essential functions. It carries oxygen, nutrients, and hormones to cells throughout the body, and it carries carbon dioxide and other wastes away from the body cells. It also helps regulate body temperature.

▶ Components of Blood   LO 26.1

Red Blood Cells

Red blood cells (RBCs), also called **erythrocytes,** are biconcave-shaped cells, similar to a doughnut with a depression where the hole should be. RBCs are small enough to pass through capillaries (see Figure 26-1).

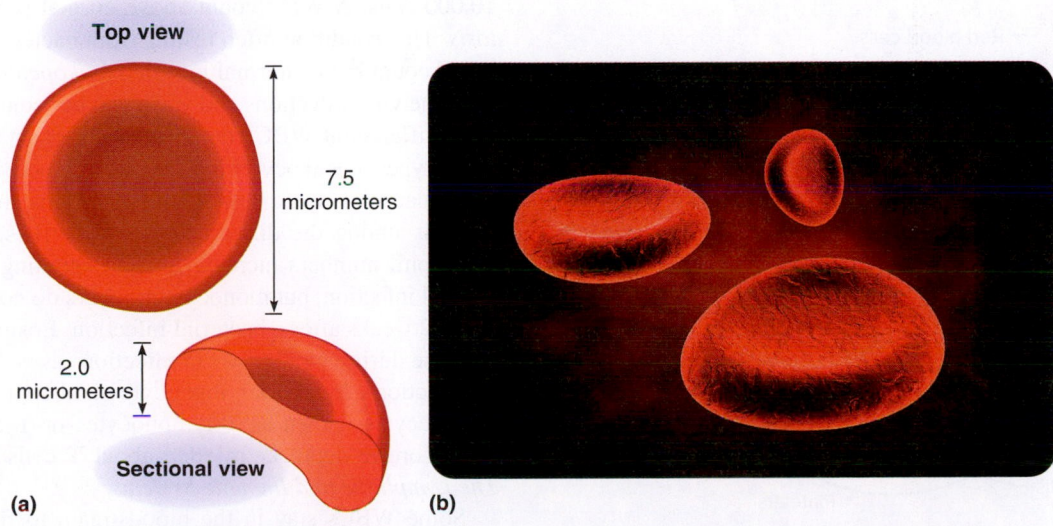

Top view

7.5 micrometers

2.0 micrometers

Sectional view

(a)   (b)

FIGURE 26-1   Red blood cells: (a) biconcave shape of red blood cells and (b) scanning electron micrograph of red blood cells.
© Cre8tive Studios/Alamy RF

The percentage of red blood cells in a sample of blood is called the **hematocrit (Hct).** A healthy person normally has a hematocrit level of about 45%. Almost 99% of the "formed elements," or cells in blood, are red blood cells; white blood cells and platelets make up only about 1%. The rest of blood (approximately 55%) is plasma (see Figure 26-2).

Mature RBCs do not contain nuclei. They do, however, contain a pigment called **hemoglobin (Hgb).** The function of hemoglobin is to carry oxygen from the lungs to the body tissues, and to carry carbon dioxide from the tissues to the lungs for release from the body. Hemoglobin that carries oxygen is called *oxyhemoglobin* and is bright red; hemoglobin that is not carrying oxygen is called *deoxyhemoglobin* and is a darker red. Often, because the deoxyhemoglobin is now carrying carbon dioxide, it is referred to as *carboxyhemoglobin.*

An RBC count consists of the number of red blood cells in 1 cubic millimeter (roughly 20 drops) of blood. A normal RBC count varies among laboratories, but a typical normal count is between 4.2 and 5.4 million RBC/cubic milliliter (mm^3) for adult males and between 3.6 million and 5.0 million RBC/mm^3 for adult females. Because the function of an RBC is to transport oxygen throughout the body, a low count reflects a decreased ability to carry oxygen, causing a condition known as *anemia.* Likewise, if the RBC count is adequate but the amount of hemoglobin within the red blood cells is decreased, thus impairing the ability to carry adequate oxygen, anemia may also be diagnosed.

During fetal development, RBCs are made in the yolk sac, the liver, and the spleen. However, once a baby is born, most blood cells are produced in red bone marrow by cells called *hemocytoblasts.* The average lifespan of an RBC is only about 120 days, so red bone marrow is constantly making new cells. The hormone **erythropoietin,** produced by the kidneys, stimulates the red bone marrow and is responsible for regulating the production of RBCs. The kidneys release erythropoietin when oxygen concentrations in the blood get low.

Iron is necessary to make hemoglobin. In addition to iron, vitamin B_{12} and folic acid (vitamin B_9) are two dietary factors that affect RBC production. These vitamins are necessary for DNA synthesis, so red bone marrow, like all actively dividing tissue, is affected when DNA cannot be produced. As stated earlier, too few RBCs or too little hemoglobin can result in one of the many types of anemia, which will be discussed in more detail in the Pathophysiology: Common Diseases and Disorders of the Blood System section of this chapter.

As RBCs age, macrophages in the liver and spleen destroy them. When an RBC is destroyed, a pigment called *biliverdin* is released from the cell. The liver usually converts biliverdin into an orange-colored pigment called *bilirubin.* Bilirubin is used to make bile, which is needed for the digestion of fats. However, when there is too much bilirubin, it builds up in the bloodstream. This causes the individual's skin and the sclera of the eyes to appear yellow-orange in color, a condition known as *jaundice* (or *icterus*).

White Blood Cells

White blood cells (WBCs), commonly called **leukocytes,** are divided into two categories: granulocytes and agranulocytes. **Granulocytes** have granules (small particles) in their cytoplasm and include neutrophils, eosinophils, and basophils. **Agranulocytes** do not have granules in their cytoplasm and include monocytes and lymphocytes. The types of WBCs and their characteristics are described in Table 26-1.

A WBC count is the number of WBCs in 1 cubic millimeter of blood. This count is normally between 5,000 and 10,000 cells. A WBC count above normal is called *leukocytosis.* This condition often results from bacterial infections. A WBC count below normal is called *leukopenia* and is caused by some viral infections and various other conditions.

A differential WBC count lists the percentages of the different types of leukocytes in a sample of blood. This is a useful test because certain diseases and conditions change the usual balance among the different types of WBCs. For example, neutrophil numbers increase at the beginning of a bacterial or viral infection, but monocyte numbers do not increase until about 2 weeks after a bacterial infection. Eosinophil numbers increase during viral or worm infections as well as with allergic reactions. In AIDS, lymphocyte numbers fall, particularly lymphocytes known as T lymphocytes or T cells. You will gain more in-depth knowledge about T cells in the chapter *The Lymphatic and Immune Systems.*

Some WBCs stay in the bloodstream to fight infections, whereas others leave the bloodstream by squeezing through blood vessel walls to reach other tissues. This squeezing of a

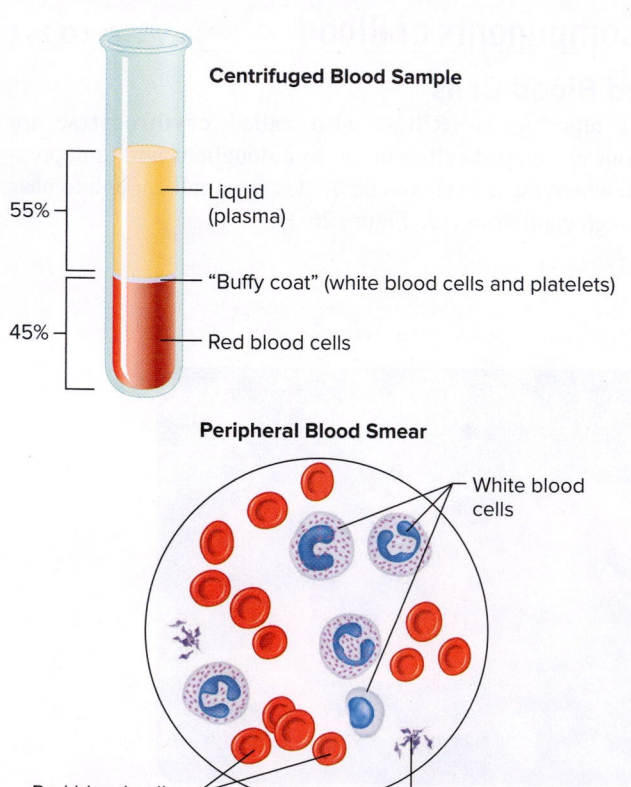

FIGURE 26-2 Centrifuged blood sample and peripheral blood smear slide seen through a microscope showing blood components.

TABLE 26-1 Types of White Blood Cells

Cell Type	Description	Adult Normal Range % of Total WBC Count	Function
Granulocytes (Polymorphonuclear)			
 © Ed Reschke	**Neutrophils** have distinct nuclei with 3 or 4 lobes. They show neutral staining: tan, lavender, or pink.	60–70%	Aid in immune system defense; release pyrogens (chemicals produced by leukocytes to cause fever); phagocytize (engulf) bacteria; use lysosomal enzymes to destroy bacteria; level increases during infection and inflammation
 © Ed Reschke	**Eosinophils** have a bilobed nucleus and cytoplasmic granules that stain orange-red.	1–4%	Assist with inflammatory responses; secrete chemicals that destroy certain parasites; level increases with allergies and parasitic infection
 © Ed Reschke	**Basophils** have a bilobed nucleus and cytoplasmic granules that stain deep blue.	0–1%	Assist with inflammatory response by releasing histamine; release heparin (anticoagulant) and produce a vasodilator; count increases with chronic inflammation and during healing from infection
Agranulocytes (Mononuclear)			
 © Ed Reschke	**Monocytes** have large, kidney-shaped nuclei.	2–6%	Are the largest WBCs; become macrophages; phagocytize dying cells, microorganisms, and foreign substances; levels increase during chronic infections, such as tuberculosis (TB)
 © Ed Reschke	**Lymphocytes** have round nuclei and a minimum amount of cytoplasm. Lymphocytes may be B cells, T cells, or natural killer (NK) cells.	20–30%	B-cell lymphocytes assist the immune system by producing antibodies; T-cell lymphocytes assist the immune system through interactions with other leukocytes; NK cells quickly respond to stressed cells; lymphocyte levels increase during viral infections; see the chapter *The Lymphatic and Immune Sytems*

cell through a blood vessel wall, which is called *diapedesis,* is shown in Figure 26-3.

Blood Platelets

Platelets are fragments of cells that are found in the bloodstream (refer back to Figure 26-2). Platelets are also called **thrombocytes** (thrombo = clot; cyte = cell) and are important in the blood-clotting process. Platelets come from cells called *megakaryocytes* found in red bone marrow. A normal platelet count is between 150,000 and 450,000 platelets per microliter of blood.

Blood Plasma

Plasma is the liquid portion of blood. It is mostly water but also contains a mixture of proteins, nutrients, gases, electrolytes, and waste products. The three major types of proteins in plasma are

- **Albumins**—the smallest plasma proteins; they pull water into the bloodstream to help maintain blood pressure.
- **Globulins**—transport lipids and some fat-soluble vitamins in plasma; some globulins become antibodies.
- **Fibrinogen**—an important protein for the blood-clotting process.

The term **serum** refers to the fluid that is left when all clotting factors are removed from plasma. You will learn more about serum in the *Processing and Testing Blood Specimens* chapter.

Nutrients in plasma are absorbed from the gastrointestinal tract and include amino acids, glucose, nucleotides, and lipids. Because lipids are not water soluble and because plasma is mostly water, lipids must combine with molecules called *lipoproteins* to be transported. The different types of lipoproteins are chylomicrons, very low-density lipoproteins (VLDL), low-density lipoproteins (LDL), and high-density lipoproteins (HDL). You will learn more about lipids and their effect on the body in the *Nutrition and Health* chapter.

The gases dissolved in plasma include oxygen, carbon dioxide, and nitrogen. Many electrolytes are also dissolved in plasma. They include sodium, potassium, calcium, magnesium, chloride, bicarbonate, phosphate, and sulfate. Molecules that contain nitrogen but are not proteins include amino acids, urea, and uric acid. Urea and uric acid are waste products produced by cells. Amino acids are the "building blocks" that combine to form proteins.

▶ Bleeding Control

LO 26.2

Hemostasis refers to the control of bleeding. The medical term *hemostasis* breaks down into *hemo,* meaning "blood," and *stasis,* meaning "stopping." Following an injury, four major events are involved in stopping the flow of blood at the injured site:

1. Blood vessel spasm
2. Platelet plug formation
3. Blood clotting
4. Fibrinolysis, or dissolving of the clot and return of the vessel to normal function

If the blood vessel is small and the injury is limited, a blood vessel spasm alone may stop the bleeding. At the time of injury, the involved blood vessel constricts (narrows in diameter), and this decreases the amount of blood flowing through the vessel, which stops or controls the bleeding. If bleeding continues in spite of the blood vessel spasms, platelets are called into action. The torn, inner lining of the blood vessels releases chemical signals, which stimulate platelets to gather at the injury site. These platelets clump together to form a platelet plug, which further decreases the flow of blood from the injured site. This process occurs within seconds after an injury and is known as primary hemostasis.

A blood clot eventually replaces the platelet plug. The formation of a blood clot is called blood **coagulation.** In this process, the plasma protein fibrinogen is converted to fibrin. Once fibrin forms, it sticks to the damaged area of the blood vessel, creating a mesh that entraps blood cells and platelets (Figure 26-4). The resulting mass—the blood clot—stops the bleeding entirely. The clot stimulates the growth of fibroblasts and smooth muscle cells within the vessel wall. This begins the repair process, which includes the final step in hemostasis, *fibrinolysis,* ultimately resulting in the dissolution of the clot. The vessel finally returns to normal. See Figure 26-5.

When a blood vessel is injured, it is normal for a blood clot to form. However, sometimes blood clots form on the side

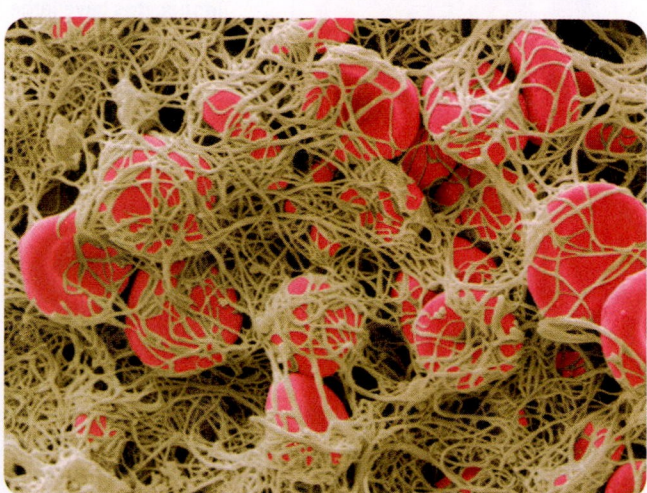

FIGURE 26-4 Scanning electron micrograph of a blood clot. Yellow fibrin threads are covering red blood cells.
© Science Photo Library/Alamy RF

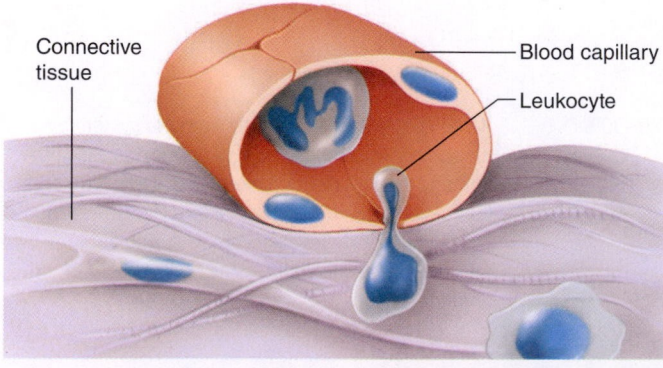

FIGURE 26-3 Diapedesis of white blood cells into surrounding tissue.

Connective tissue
Blood capillary
Leukocyte

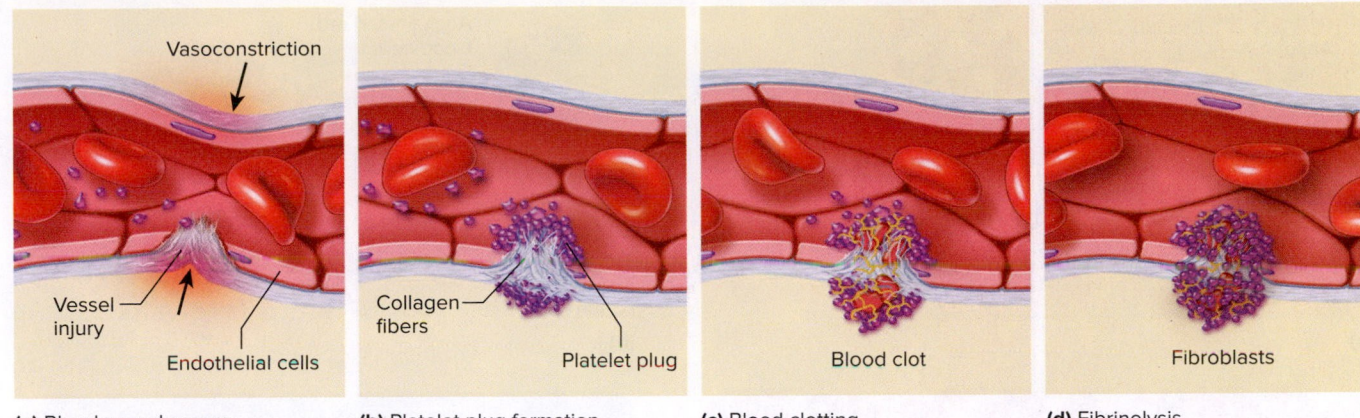

(a) Blood vessel spasm   (b) Platelet plug formation   (c) Blood clotting   (d) Fibrinolysis

FIGURE 26-5   Events in hemostasis.

of a blood vessel with no known injury; this abnormal blood clot is called a **thrombus.** A thrombus is dangerous because a portion of it can break off and start moving through the bloodstream. The moving portion of the thrombus is called an *embolus.* An embolus is dangerous because, as discussed in the chapter *The Cardiovascular System,* it can eventually block a small artery in the lungs, heart, or brain, causing pulmonary embolism, myocardial infarction, or CVA (stroke), respectively. All of these are serious and possibly fatal conditions if not treated, or if treatment cannot be initiated quickly enough to stop the condition from progressing.

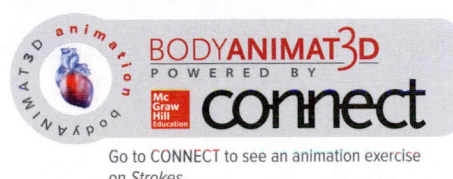

BODYANIMAT3D
POWERED BY
McGraw Hill Education
connect

Go to CONNECT to see an animation exercise on *Strokes.*

▶ ABO Blood Types   LO 26.3

When a patient needs a blood transfusion, the blood used in the transfusion must be compatible with the patient's blood type. If it is not, antigens on the patient's RBCs will bind to antibodies in the donor's plasma. This causes the RBCs to clump, resulting in severe anemia. This clumping process is called **agglutination** (see Figure 26-6).

The most widely used system to determine blood typing and compatibility is the ABO blood group system. This system places blood into one of four groups, or types, based on the antigens present on the red blood cells.

- Type A—blood that has antigen A on the surface of its RBCs and antibody B in its plasma
- Type B—blood that has antigen B on the surface of its RBCs and antibody A in its plasma
- Type AB—blood that has both antigen A and antigen B on the surface of its RBCs but has neither antibody A nor antibody B in its plasma
- Type O—blood that has neither antigen A nor antigen B on the surface of its RBCs but has both antibody A and antibody B in its plasma

	TABLE 26-2 ABO Blood Type Overview		
Blood Type	**Antigen Present**	**Antibody Present**	**Blood Type That Can Be Received**
A	A	B	A and O
B	B	A	B and O
AB	A and B	None	All blood types
O	None	A and B	O only

The reaction between these antigens and antibodies is very specific. Antibody A binds only to antigen A, and antibody B binds only to antigen B. If a person with type A blood is given type B blood, then the antibody B in the recipient's blood will bind with the RBCs of the donor blood because those cells have antigen B on their surfaces. As a result, agglutination occurs, and the donated RBCs are destroyed. This is why a person with type A blood should not be given type B blood (and vice versa).

People with type AB blood are called *universal recipients* because most of them can receive all ABO blood types. They can receive these blood types because they lack antibody A and antibody B in their plasma, so there is no reaction with antigens A and B of the donor blood.

People with type O blood are called *universal donors* because their blood can be given to most people, regardless of the recipient's blood type. Type O blood will not agglutinate when given to other people because it does not have the antigens to bind to antibody A or antibody B. Table 26-2 summarizes the ABO blood groups. Also see Figure 26-7 for a pictorial representation of each blood type.

▶ The Rh Factor   LO 26.4

The *Rh antigen* is a protein first discovered on RBCs of the rhesus monkey, hence the name Rh. People who are Rh-positive have RBCs that contain the Rh antigen. People who are Rh-negative have RBCs that do not contain the Rh antigen. If a person who is Rh-negative is given Rh-positive blood, then the Rh-negative person's blood will make antibodies that bind to the Rh antigens. If the Rh-negative person

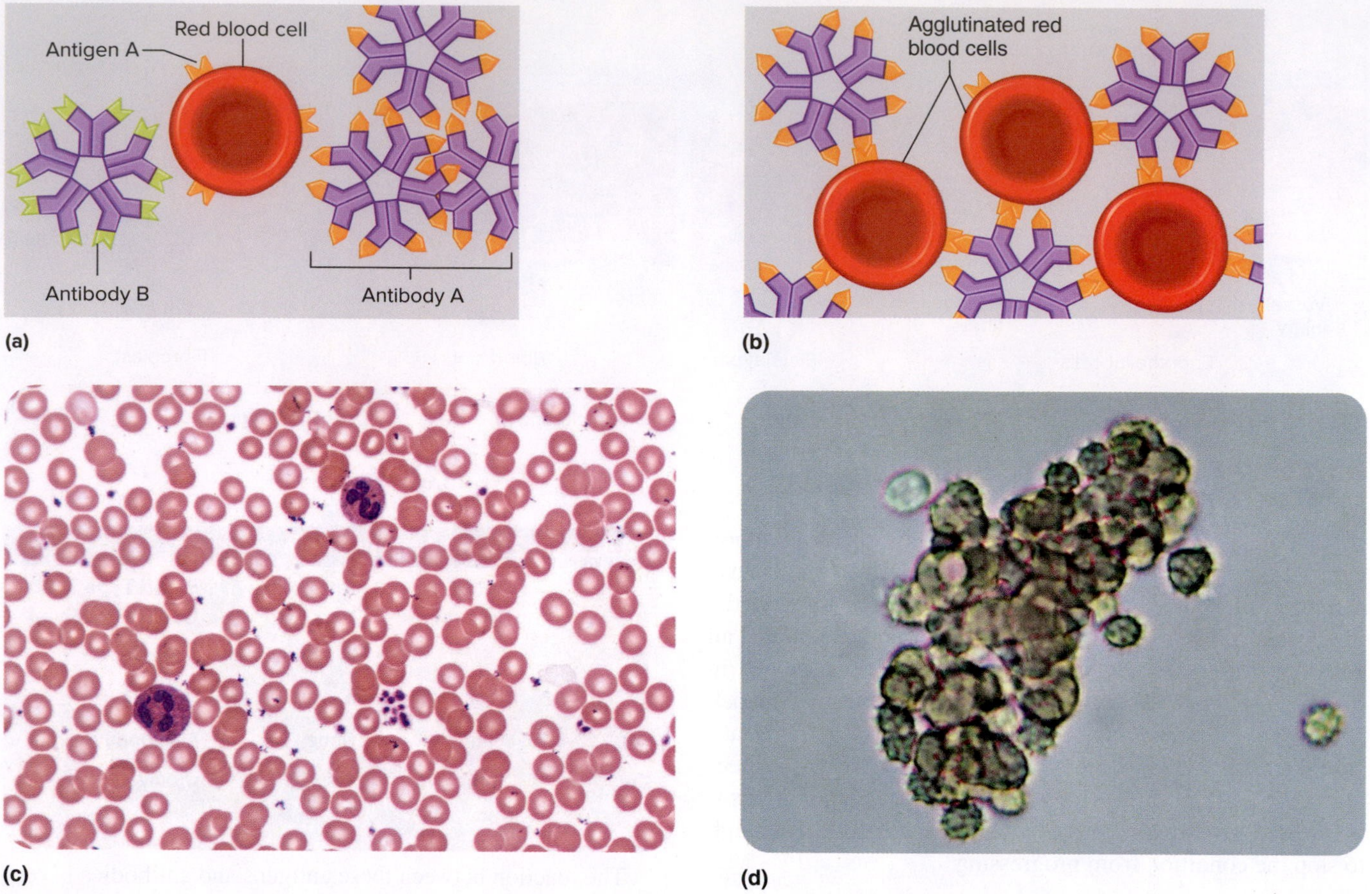

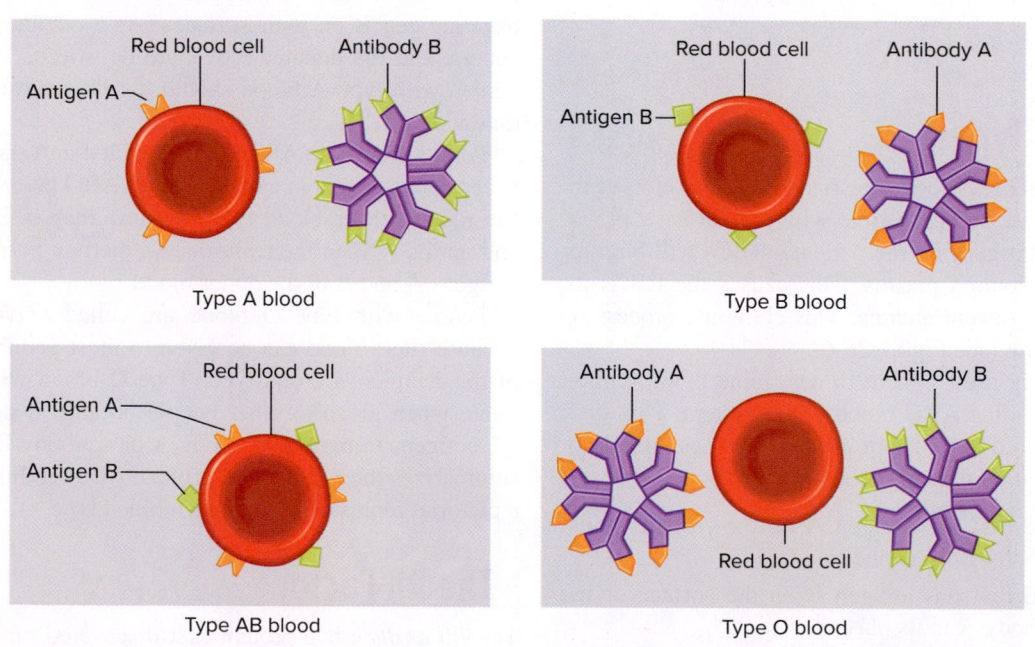

FIGURE 26-6 Agglutination: (a) red blood cells with antigen A are added to blood that contains antibody A; (b) antibody A reacts with antigen A, causing the agglutination of blood; (c) normal blood; and (d) agglutinated blood.

© McGraw-Hill Education/Al Telser, photographer; © Ed Reschke/Getty Images

FIGURE 26-7 Blood Types A, B, AB, and O.

is given Rh-positive blood a second time, the antibodies will bind to the donor cells and agglutination will occur.

Clinically, it is very important for a female to know her Rh type if she is pregnant or wishes to become pregnant. If an

Rh-negative female mates with an Rh-positive male, there is a 50% chance her fetus will be Rh-positive. When the blood of an Rh-positive fetus mixes with the blood of a mother who is Rh-negative, the mother develops antibodies against the

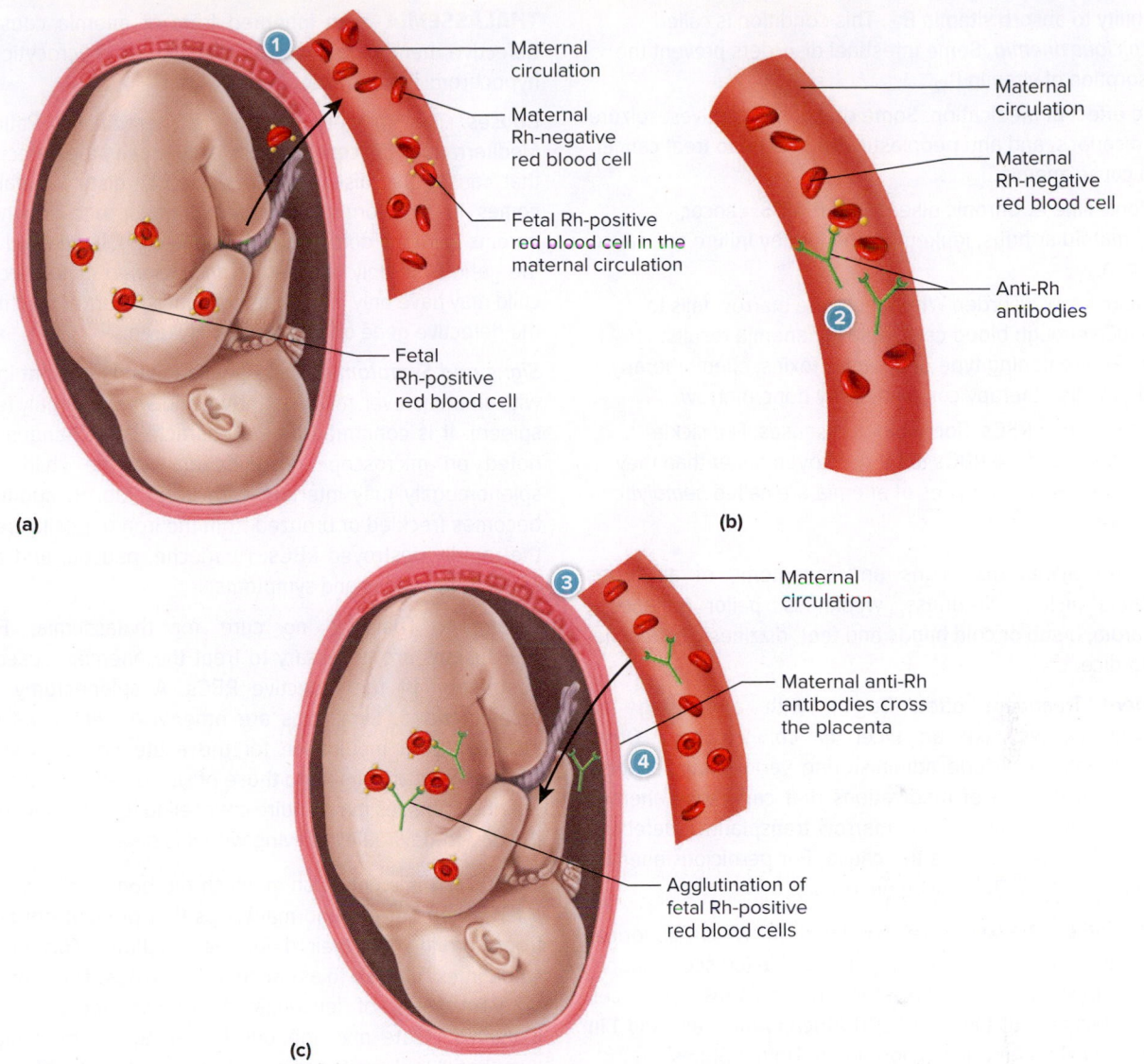

Maternal
circulation

Maternal
Rh-negative
red blood cell

Fetal Rh-positive
red blood cell in the
maternal circulation

Fetal
Rh-positive
red blood cell

(a)

Maternal
circulation

Maternal
Rh-negative
red blood cell

Anti-Rh
antibodies

(b)

Maternal
circulation

Maternal anti-Rh
antibodies cross
the placenta

Agglutination of
fetal Rh-positive
red blood cells

(c)

FIGURE 26-8   Development of antibodies in an Rh-negative woman in reaction to the blood of her Rh-positive fetus.

fetus's RBCs. Typically, the first Rh-positive fetus (infant) does not suffer any effects from these antibodies because it takes so long for the mother's body to generate them. However, if the mother conceives a second Rh-positive fetus, her antibodies will attack this fetus's blood right away. The second fetus then develops a condition called *erythroblastosis*

fetalis, and the baby is born severely anemic, often needing multiple blood transfusions at birth and often several times as a neonate (see Figure 26-8). Erythroblastosis fetalis is prevented by giving an Rh-negative woman the drug RhoGAM. RhoGAM prevents an Rh-negative mother from making antibodies against the Rh antigen.

PATHOPHYSIOLOGY

LO 26.5

Common Diseases and Disorders of the Blood System

ANEMIA is a condition in which a person does not have enough RBCs or hemoglobin in the blood to carry an adequate amount of oxygen to the body's cells. It is the most common blood disorder in the United States and can be a sign of a more serious disorder. It generally affects more women than men. Many types of anemia can be prevented through a healthy diet high in iron, vitamin B_{12}, and folic acid. Other types of anemia require medical attention for more serious, underlying conditions.

Causes. The many causes of this condition include the following:

- Iron deficiency. This is the most common cause of anemia. Iron is needed to make hemoglobin, which is the pigment that carries most oxygen in the blood. Pregnant women and women with heavy menstrual cycles are most susceptible to this type of anemia.
- Chronic blood loss. Slow blood loss can occur in conditions such as ulcers, colon polyps, or colon cancer.
- Vitamin deficiency. Vitamin B_{12} and folic acid are needed to make enough RBCs.

- Inability to absorb vitamin B$_{12}$. This condition is called *pernicious anemia*. Some intestinal disorders prevent the absorption of vitamin B$_{12}$.
- Side effect of medication. Some oral contraceptives, seizure medications, and anti-neoplastic drugs used to treat cancer can cause anemia.
- Chronic illness. Chronic diseases like AIDS, cancer, rheumatoid arthritis, leukemia, and kidney failure can cause anemia.
- Bone marrow disorder. When the bone marrow fails to produce enough blood cells, aplastic anemia results. This is a life-threatening type of anemia. Toxins, chemotherapy, and radiation therapy can all destroy bone marrow.
- Destruction of RBCs. Some blood diseases, like sickle cell disease, cause RBCs to be destroyed faster than they can be made. These types of anemia are called *hemolytic anemias*.

Signs and Symptoms. Signs and symptoms of all forms of anemia include tiredness, weakness, pallor (paleness), tachycardia, numb or cold hands and feet, dizziness, headache, and jaundice.

Treatment. Treatment often begins with addressing the underlying causes, like an ulcer or colon polyps. Other treatment options include administering various medications, discontinuing the use of medications that can cause anemia, and blood transfusions or bone marrow transplants if defective or diseased bone marrow is the cause. For pernicious anemia, injections of vitamin B$_{12}$ may be necessary.

SICKLE CELL ANEMIA is a condition in which abnormal hemoglobin causes RBCs to change to a sickle (crescent) shape. These sickle-shaped RBCs get stuck in capillaries. Sickle cell anemia affects about 1 in every 500 African Americans and 1 in every 1,400 Latino Americans born in the United States.

Causes. The primary cause is hereditary. As an autosomal recessive disorder, a person with this disease must inherit a sickle cell gene from both parents. If only one sickle cell gene is inherited, the person is said to have sickle cell trait and may have only mild symptoms of the disease. However, the person with sickle cell trait may pass on the trait or the disease to his or her children. This condition may be prevented through genetic screening of the parents.

Signs and Symptoms. The many signs and symptoms include anemia, periodic episodes of pain called *crises,* chest pain, numbness in the hands or legs, fainting, fatigue, swollen hands and feet, jaundice, frequent infections, sores on the skin, delayed growth, stroke, seizures, and breathing difficulties. Retinal damage, which causes visual problems, and spleen, liver, or kidney and lung damage also may be seen.

Treatment. There is no cure for sickle cell disease. The goal of treatment is to control the effects of the disease. Treatment includes antibiotics to treat infections, blood transfusions, pain medications, bone marrow transplants, supplemental oxygen, and medications to promote the development of normal hemoglobin.

THALASSEMIA is an inherited form of anemia caused by a defective hemoglobin chain, resulting in microcytic (small), hypochromic (pale), short-lived RBCs.

Causes. The primary cause is hereditary. Patients of Mediterranean descent are most likely to carry the defective gene that causes this disease. Like sickle cell disease, thalassemia comes in two forms. *Thalassemia major* occurs when both parents send the defective gene to the child. If the child receives the gene from only one parent, *thalassemia minor* occurs. The child may have only mild symptoms but is a carrier who may pass the defective gene on to his or her children.

Signs and Symptoms. Thalassemia major is evident in infancy with anemia, fever, failure to thrive, and splenomegaly (enlarged spleen). It is confirmed by the characteristic changes in RBCs noted on microscopic examination. As the child matures, splenomegaly may interfere with breathing. In addition, skin becomes freckled or bronzed from the iron deposits created by the rapidly destroyed RBCs. Headache, nausea, and anorexia are common signs and symptoms.

Treatment. There is no cure for thalassemia. Frequent transfusions are necessary to treat the anemia caused by the destruction of the defective RBCs. A splenectomy may be recommended. Symptoms are otherwise treated as needed, including pain medication for the acute episodes known as crises, which are similar to those of sickle cell patients. Patients and their families may require counseling to help them deal with the day-to-day reality of living with this disease.

LEUKEMIA is a condition in which the bone marrow produces a large number of abnormal WBCs that prevent normal WBCs from carrying out their defensive functions. This disorder is sometimes referred to as cancer of the WBCs. There are several different kinds of leukemia: acute lymphocytic (lymphatic) leukemia, acute myelogenous leukemia, chronic lymphocytic (lymphatic) leukemia, and chronic myelogenous leukemia.

Causes. Causes include mutations (changes) in WBCs, chemotherapy for the treatment of other cancers, genetic factors (for example, the inheritance of abnormal genes), and exposure to environmental and chemical agents that cause changes in the WBCs.

Signs and Symptoms. The many signs and symptoms include fatigue, dyspnea on exertion (DOE), an enlarged liver (hepatomegaly) or spleen (splenomegaly), swollen (nontender) lymph nodes, abnormal bruising, cuts that heal slowly, frequent infections, nosebleeds, bleeding gums, chronic fever, unexplained weight loss, and excessive sweating.

Treatment. Treatment options include chemotherapy, radiation therapy, medications to strengthen the immune system, antibodies to destroy mutated WBCs, bone marrow transplant, and stem cell transplant.

POLYCYTHEMIA VERA is a disease of the bone marrow that results in an abnormally high number of blood cells, especially red blood cells, causing the blood to thicken. It occurs more often in men than in women, and it usually occurs after the age of 40.

Causes. A genetic mutation causes polycythemia. However, the cause of the mutation is not known.

Signs and Symptoms. The signs and symptoms of polycythemia include difficulty breathing and shortness of breath, dizziness, excessive bleeding, enlarged spleen, and headache. Itching and a reddened skin color, especially in the face, may also be seen.

Treatment. Treatment involves reducing the thickness of the blood. Up to a pint of blood may be removed each week until the blood count becomes normal. Frequent blood counts are performed to monitor the blood, and further bloodletting, known as *therapeutic phlebotomy,* is performed when needed. Chemotherapy may also be used in some cases to reduce production of red blood cells, and aspirin may be prescribed to help prevent clots.

SUMMARY OF LEARNING OUTCOMES

LEARNING OUTCOMES	KEY POINTS
26.1 Describe the components of blood, giving the function of each component listed.	The formed elements in blood include red blood cells responsible for oxygen and carbon dioxide transport; white blood cells responsible for working with the immune system by fighting infection; and platelets, which assist in blood clotting. The liquid component of blood is called *plasma;* when all clotting factors and formed elements are spun out of plasma, the remaining liquid is called *serum.*
26.2 Explain how bleeding is controlled.	Hemostasis is the control of bleeding. Four basic processes occur during hemostasis: blood vessel spasm, platelet plug formation, blood coagulation, and fibrinolysis. Coagulation is the formation of a blood clot. It involves fibrinogen converting to fibrin, which sticks to the damaged area of the blood vessel, creating a mesh that traps blood cells and platelets.
26.3 Differentiate among blood types A, B, AB, and O related to their compatibility.	The four ABO blood types are A, B, AB, and O, based on the type of antigen present on the RBCs. Types A, B, and O have antibodies in the plasma that react to other antigens, so each of these types must receive only the same blood type during a transfusion. Type AB is considered the universal receiver because it has no antibodies in the plasma and is therefore compatible with all blood types. Type O has no antigens, so it is considered the universal donor. However, because it has antibodies to both antigen A and antigen B, people with type O blood can receive only type O blood.
26.4 Explain the difference between Rh-positive blood and Rh-negative blood.	The Rh factor (named for the rhesus monkey) is an antigen that may be attached to any blood type. Its importance arises during transfusions (Rh-negative blood cannot receive Rh-positive blood) and during pregnancy if the mother is Rh-negative but the fetus received the Rh-positive antigen from the father. The first fetus will not be much affected; unless treated, however, any subsequent Rh-positive fetus will suffer effects of erythroblastosis fetalis because the mother's blood developed antibodies against the Rh-positive factor during the initial pregnancy.
26.5 Describe the causes, signs and symptoms, and treatments of various diseases and disorders of the blood.	The blood can be affected by many common diseases and disorders with varied signs, symptoms, and treatments. Some of these include anemia, leukemia, sickle cell anemia, polycythemia vera, and thalassemia.

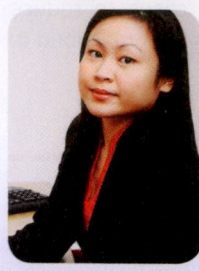

Recall Cindy Chen from the beginning of the chapter. Now that you have completed the chapter, answer the following questions regarding her case.

1. What information about Cindy's blood can be gained by the CBC and platelet count?

2. A helper T cell is a type of white blood cell (WBC). Why would information about Cindy's WBCs, particularly T cells, be of interest to her physician, considering her HIV status?

© Red Chopsticks/Getty Images RF

1. (LO 26.1) Which of the following is the hormone responsible for regulating the production of RBCs?
   a. Hemoglobin
   b. Erythropoietin
   c. Biliverdin
   d. Oxyhemoglobin
   e. Hematocrit

2. (LO 26.1) Which blood cell type does not contain a nucleus?
   a. RBCs
   b. Eosinophils
   c. Agranulocytes
   d. Basophils
   e. Neutrophils

3. (LO 26.2) Which term refers to control of bleeding?
   a. Hemoglobin
   b. Hematocrit
   c. Platelets
   d. Agglutination
   e. Hemostasis

4. (LO 26.2) The other term for blood coagulation is
   a. Plug
   b. Fibrin
   c. Clotting
   d. Granulation
   e. Agglutination

5. (LO 26.3) Which blood type is the universal donor?
   a. Blood type A
   b. Blood type B
   c. Blood type AB
   d. Blood type O
   e. Rh-negative

6. (LO 26.3) Which process could indicate a transfusion reaction because of a blood typing mismatch?
   a. Coagulation
   b. Clotting
   c. Hemorrhage
   d. Bleeding
   e. Agglutination

7. (LO 26.4) Which combination could be a problem for an unborn fetus?
   a. Rh-negative mom/Rh-positive dad/first pregnancy
   b. Rh-positive mom/Rh-negative dad/first pregnancy
   c. Rh-negative mom/Rh-positive dad/second pregnancy
   d. Rh-positive mom/Rh-negative dad/second pregnancy
   e. Rh-negative mom/Rh-negative dad/second pregnancy

8. (LO 26.4) RhoGAM is used to prevent
   a. Iron deficiency anemia
   b. Erythroblastosis fetalis
   c. Leukemia
   d. Transfusion reactions
   e. Hemophilia

9. (LO 26.5) Which of the following is *not* a cause of anemia?
   a. Vitamin B_{12} deficiency
   b. Blood loss
   c. RBC destruction
   d. Bone marrow destruction
   e. Low WBC count

10. (LO 26.5) Which blood disorder is hereditary?
    a. Sickle cell anemia
    b. Thalassemia
    c. Leukemia
    d. Sickle cell anemia and thalassemia
    e. Thalassemia and leukemia

Analyze the following medical terms, presented throughout the chapter. Using a medical dictionary (or Appendix I) place a / mark between each word part. Define each word part and then define the whole word.

EXAMPLE: **hemo / rrhage** = hemo means "blood" + rhagge means "excessive flow"
 HEMORRHAGE means "excessive flow of blood."

1. erythrocytes
2. leukocytes
3. granulocytes
4. agranulocytes

5. anemia
6. thrombocytes
7. hemostasis
8. erythroblastosis fetalis

9. leukemia
10. hemolytic
11. hematoma
12. venogram

The Lymphatic and Immune Systems

CASE STUDY

PATIENT INFORMATION			
Patient Name	**DOB**	**Allergies**	
Cindy Chen	7/15/19XX	NKA	
Attending	**MRN**	**Other Information**	
Alexis N. Whalen, MD	324-86-542	T-cell count 396 cells/mm³ Retest in 3 months	

Cindy Chen is a 28-year-old Asian female complaining of inability to sleep and nervousness. She tested positive for HIV in 2014 and is asymptomatic and on antiviral drugs. She currently lives with her aunt and is going to school

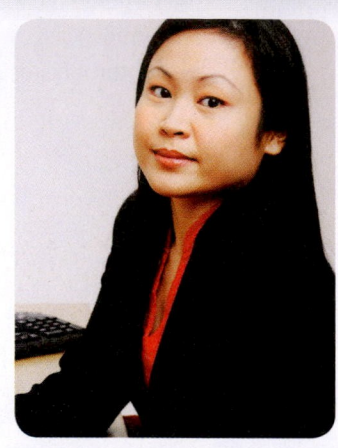

© Red Chopsticks/Getty Images RF

to become a phlebotomist. When looking at her chart, you notice she has lost 20 pounds since her last visit. Dr. Whalen has ordered a series of blood tests, including helper T-cell tests and CBC with platelet count.

Keep Cindy in mind as you study the chapter. There will be questions at the end of the chapter based on the case study. The information in the chapter will help you answer these questions.

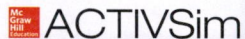

LEARNING OUTCOMES

After completing Chapter 27, you will be able to:

27.1 Describe the pathways and organs of the lymphatic system.

27.2 Compare the nonspecific and specific body defense mechanisms.

27.3 Explain how antibodies fight infection.

27.4 Describe the four different types of acquired immunities.

27.5 Describe the causes, signs and symptoms, and treatments of major immune disorders.

KEY TERMS

anaphylaxis
antibodies
antibody-mediated response
antigens
autoimmune disease
cell-mediated response
complements
cytokines
hapten
immunoglobulins
innate immunity
interstitial fluid

lymph
lymph node
lymphocytes
lymphokines
macrophages
major histocompatibility complex (MHC)
monokines
natural killer (NK) cells
phagocytosis
spleen
thymus
tonsils

MEDICAL ASSISTING COMPETENCIES

CAAHEP

I.C.4 List major organs in each body system

I.C.6 Compare structure and function of the human body across the life span

I.C.7 Describe the normal function of each body system

I.C.8 Identify common pathology related to each body system including
(a) signs
(b) symptoms
(c) etiology

I.C.9 Analyze pathology for each body system including:
(a) diagnostic measures
(b) treatment modalities

V.C.10 Define medical terms and abbreviations related to all body systems

ABHES

2. Anatomy & Physiology

a. List all body systems, their structure and functions

b. Describe common diseases, symptoms, and etiologies as they apply to each system

c. Identify diagnostic and treatment modalities as they relate to each body system

3. Medical Terminology

b. Build and dissect medical terms from roots/suffixes to understand the word element combinations that create medical terminology

c. Apply various medical terms for each specialty

d. Define and use medical abbreviations when appropriate and acceptable

▶ Introduction

Your immune system works as a personal coat of armor, responsible for protecting your body against bacteria, viruses, fungi, toxins, parasites, and cancer. This important system, present in every human being, works with the organs of the lymphatic system—the thymus, spleen, and lymph nodes—to clear the body of various disease-causing agents.

▶ The Lymphatic System   LO 27.1

The lymphatic system is a network of connecting vessels that collects the interstitial (or tissue) fluid found between cells. These lymphatic vessels then return this fluid, now called **lymph,** to the bloodstream. See Figure 27-1. The lymphatic system also picks up lipids and fat-soluble vitamins (A, D, E, and K) from the digestive tract and transports them to the bloodstream. The third function of the lymphatic system is to protect the body against disease-causing agents.

Interstitial (Tissue) Fluid and Lymph

Fluid constantly leaks out of blood capillaries into the spaces between cells. This fluid is high in nutrients, oxygen, and small proteins. Most of this fluid is picked up by body cells. However, some of the fluid persists between cells. Increased tissue hydrostatic pressure moves **interstitial** (tissue) **fluid** into the lymphatic vessels. This fluid is destined to become lymph.

Lymphatic Vessels and Lymph Circulation

The lymphatic vessels transport lymph and excess fluid away from the interstitial spaces toward the heart. Smaller lymphatic capillaries join to form larger lymphatic vessels.

Lymphatic Capillaries The lymphatic capillaries are similar in structure to blood capillaries except that lymphatic capillaries are larger in diameter and facilitate drainage of interstitial fluids—fluids between the cells—from the tissues. This is facilitated by the thin, very permeable lymphatic capillary walls, which are lined by a single layer of squamous epithelial cells called endothelium. The epithelial cells of the lymphatic capillary wall overlap, creating flap-like valves that allow fluid to enter the capillary but do not allow fluid to exit under normal conditions. However, under some conditions, lymph can leak out of the vessels, causing *edema,* or fluid buildup, in the interstitial spaces. Lymphatic capillaries converge to form lymphatic trunks, which in turn merge to form lymphatic ducts. This is similar to the structure of the venous system, but lymphatic vessels have thinner walls and more valves than do veins. The lymphatic pathway is illustrated in Figure 27-2.

Lymphatic Trunks and Ducts Lymphatic trunks are typically named after the region in which they are found. For example, the *jugular trunks* (left and right) drain the head and neck region. The *lumbar trunk* drains the lymph from the lower extremities, the *subclavian trunk* drains the upper limbs, and the *bronchomediastinal trunk* drains lymph from the thorax. The trunks eventually empty into the two lymphatic ducts. The *right lymphatic duct* receives lymph from the upper right side of the body. It empties its contents into the right internal jugular and right subclavian veins. These veins return the lymph to the right atrium by way of the superior vena cava. The other duct is the *thoracic duct,* which is the largest lymphatic vessel in the body. It drains lymph from all parts of the body that are not drained by the right lymphatic duct. The thoracic duct begins at the level of the second

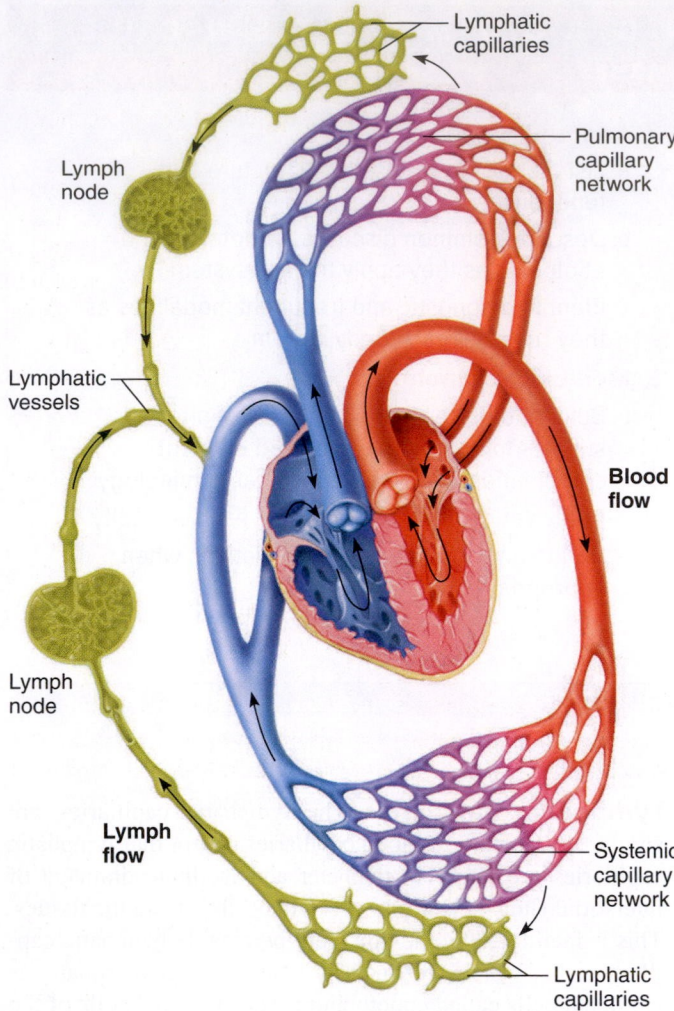

FIGURE 27-1 Schematic flow of lymph from the lymphatic capillaries to the bloodstream.

Labels in figure:
- Lymphatic capillaries
- Lymph node
- Pulmonary capillary network
- Lymphatic vessels
- Blood flow
- Lymph node
- Lymph flow
- Systemic capillary network
- Lymphatic capillaries

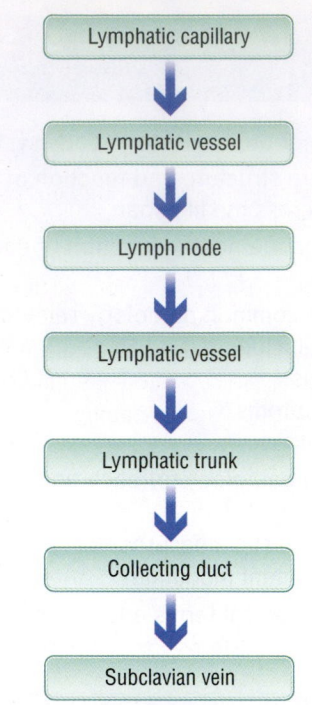

FIGURE 27-2 Lymphatic pathway.

Flow diagram:
Lymphatic capillary → Lymphatic vessel → Lymph node → Lymphatic vessel → Lymphatic trunk → Collecting duct → Subclavian vein

lumbar vertebra. The thoracic duct passes through the diaphragm beside the aorta. The thoracic duct empties into the junction of the left internal jugular and left subclavian veins (see Figure 27-3).

Lymph is moved along by two pumps and flows in only one direction—toward the heart. The *skeletal muscle pump* utilizes skeletal muscle contractions to move the lymph toward the heart. The other pump is the *respiratory pump*, which utilizes pressure changes in the thorax to assist circulation. Along its way to the venous blood, lymph will pass through more than 600 *lymph nodes* throughout the body.

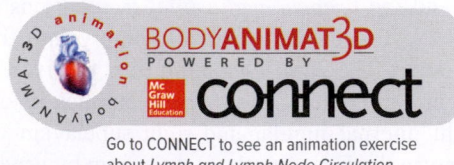

BODYANIMAT3D
POWERED BY
McGraw Hill Education
connect

Go to CONNECT to see an animation exercise about *Lymph and Lymph Node Circulation.*

Lymphoid Organs and Tissues

Lymphoid organs and tissues are widespread throughout the body and consist of lymph nodes, the thymus, and the spleen.

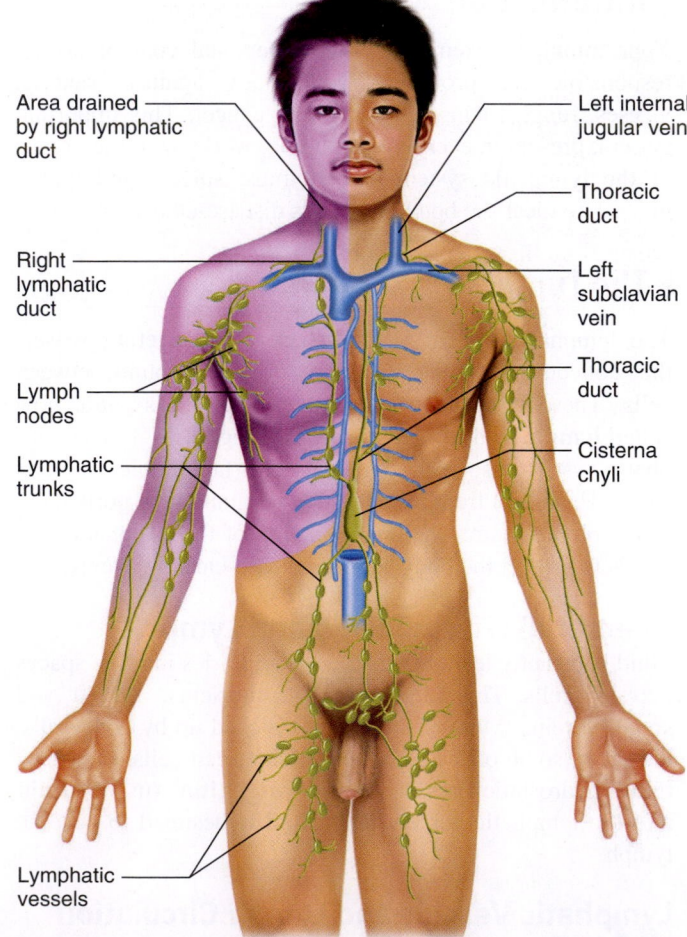

Labels in figure:
- Area drained by right lymphatic duct
- Left internal jugular vein
- Thoracic duct
- Right lymphatic duct
- Left subclavian vein
- Lymph nodes
- Thoracic duct
- Lymphatic trunks
- Cisterna chyli
- Lymphatic vessels

FIGURE 27-3 Areas drained by the right lymphatic duct (shaded) and thoracic duct (not shaded).

Lymph Nodes **Lymph nodes** are very small, glandular structures that usually cannot be felt, or palpated, very easily (Figure 27-4). They are located along the paths of larger lymphatic vessels and are spread throughout the body. A major exception is that no lymph nodes are found in the nervous system. There is a greater concentration of nodes in certain places in the body such as the cervical (neck), axillary (armpit), inguinal (groin), supratrochlear (medial side of the elbow), pelvic, thoracic, and aortic (thorax) nodes. The indented side of a lymph node is called the hilum. Nerves and blood vessels enter the node through the hilum. The lymphatic vessels that carry lymph to the node and are located opposite the hilum are called afferent (meaning "toward") lymphatic vessels. About four or five afferent vessels are associated with each node. The lymphatic vessels that carry lymph out of a node are called efferent (meaning "away from") vessels.

A lymph node usually has only one or two efferent vessels. Because more lymph enters the node than can exit at one time, lymph tends to concentrate in the node and pressure builds up that assists in the filtration process. Lymph nodes are also surrounded by a fibrous capsule of connective tissue. The lymph node is divided into an inner portion called the medulla and an outer portion called the cortex.

Two important cell types are found inside the nodes—macrophages and lymphocytes. Together these form the *lymph nodules,* the functional units of the lymph node. Lymph nodules are found in the cortex of the lymph node. **Macrophages** digest unwanted pathogens in the lymph and the **lymphocytes** are part of the immune response against the pathogen. Lymph nodes are also responsible for the generation of some lymphocytes.

When someone has a viral or bacterial infection, he or she may have *lymphadenitis,* an inflammation of the lymph nodes. Any disease of the lymph nodes is called *lymphadenopathy.* The terms *lymphadenitis* and *lymphadenopathy* are often used interchangeably by healthcare professionals, but it is important to remember that the suffix *-itis* refers to inflammation and the suffix *-pathy* refers to disease. Other causes of lymphadenopathy are autoimmune disease and malignancy.

Thymus The **thymus** is a soft, bilobed organ located behind the sternum, just below the thyroid gland and above the heart in the mediastinum (a space between the right and left lungs) (See Figure 27-5). The thymus is large in the infant and reaches its maximum size of 1 to 2 ounces when the child is about 2 years of age. After adolescence the thymus starts to atrophy (waste away) or *involute* (turn in on itself). In older adults, the thymus is tiny, almost nonexistent. Starvation or acute disease can sometimes accelerate this process. The outer portion of the thymus is called the cortex. This is where T lymphocytes (T cells) that have been produced in the bone marrow proliferate. They then move to a more central portion of the gland called the medulla, where they mature. The thymus also produces the hormone *thymosin,* which stimulates the production of mature lymphocytes.

Spleen The **spleen** is the largest lymphoid organ. It is located in the upper-left quadrant of the abdominal cavity, just below the diaphragm and behind the stomach. It is protected by the rib cage and normally is not palpable. The spleen is divided into lobules with two types of tissues: white pulp and red pulp. The white pulp is concentrated with lymphocytes similar to those seen in lymph nodes. Red pulp has an abundance of red blood cells, lymphocytes, and macrophages. The spleen filters blood in much the same way that lymph nodes filter lymph. The spleen also removes senescent (old), worn-out red blood cells from the bloodstream. If the spleen is injured or becomes enlarged due to disease, a condition known as *splenomegaly,* the spleen is often removed (a *splenectomy*) to prevent rupture of the spleen if trauma were to occur. When a splenectomy is performed, the patient's liver takes over most of its functions. Table 27-1 summarizes the characteristics of the major organs of the lymphatic system.

Lymph Nodules Lymph nodules are masses of lymphoid tissue not surrounded by a capsule. These are often referred to as *mucosa-associated lymphoid tissue (MALT)* because they are distributed in the connective tissue of mucosa. The **tonsils** are three sets of lymphoid tissue. These three sets include

- Pharyngeal tonsils, or adenoids, located at the junction of the mouth and oropharynx.
- Palatine tonsils, located at the junction of the nasal cavity and nasopharynx.
- Lingual tonsils, located at the base of the tongue.

The appendix, or *vermiform appendix,* is usually located in the lower-right quadrant at the junction of the large and small intestines. It was once thought that the appendix had no function. We now know it is part of the immune system. There are also lymph nodules in the small intestine.

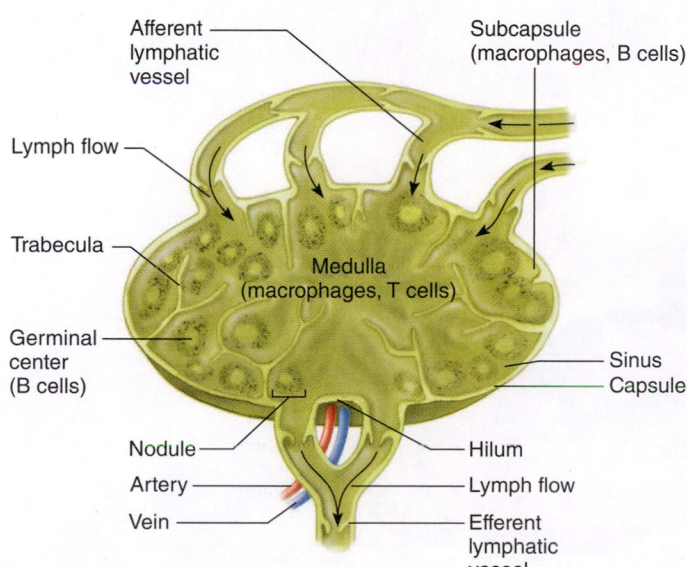

Afferent lymphatic vessel
Subcapsule (macrophages, B cells)
Lymph flow
Trabecula
Medulla (macrophages, T cells)
Germinal center (B cells)
Sinus
Capsule
Nodule
Hilum
Artery
Lymph flow
Vein
Efferent lymphatic vessel

FIGURE 27-4 Section of a lymph node.

TABLE 27-1   Major Organs of the Lymphatic System

Organ	Location	Functions
Thymus	In the mediastinum posterior to the upper portion of the body of the sternum	Houses lymphocytes; differentiates thymocytes into T lymphocytes
Spleen	In the upper-left portion of the abdominal cavity inferior to the diaphragm, posterior and lateral to the stomach	Blood reservoir; houses macrophages that remove foreign particles, damaged red blood cells, and cellular debris from the blood; contains lymphocytes
Lymph nodes	In groups or chains along the paths of the larger lymphatic vessels	Filter foreign particles and debris from lymph; produce and house lymphocytes that destroy foreign particles in lymph; house macrophages that engulf and destroy foreign particles and cellular debris carried in lymph

▶ Defenses Against Disease   LO 27.2

An infection is the presence of a pathogen—a disease-causing agent such as a bacterium, virus, toxin, fungus, or protozoan—in or on the body. The body has mechanisms called nonspecific defenses, or **innate immunity,** to protect itself from pathogens in general. The body also has mechanisms to protect itself against specific pathogens; these mechanisms, called immunities, are considered specific defenses.

Nonspecific Defenses

The nonspecific mechanisms that protect the body against pathogens include species resistance, mechanical and chemical barriers, and phagocytosis. Fever and inflammation are also effective in protecting the body from invading organisms. These defenses are described in this section and summarized in Table 27-2.

Species Resistance   Species resistance means that a species typically gets only diseases unique to that species. For example, humans do not get diseases that affect plants. Humans also do not get most diseases that affect animals.

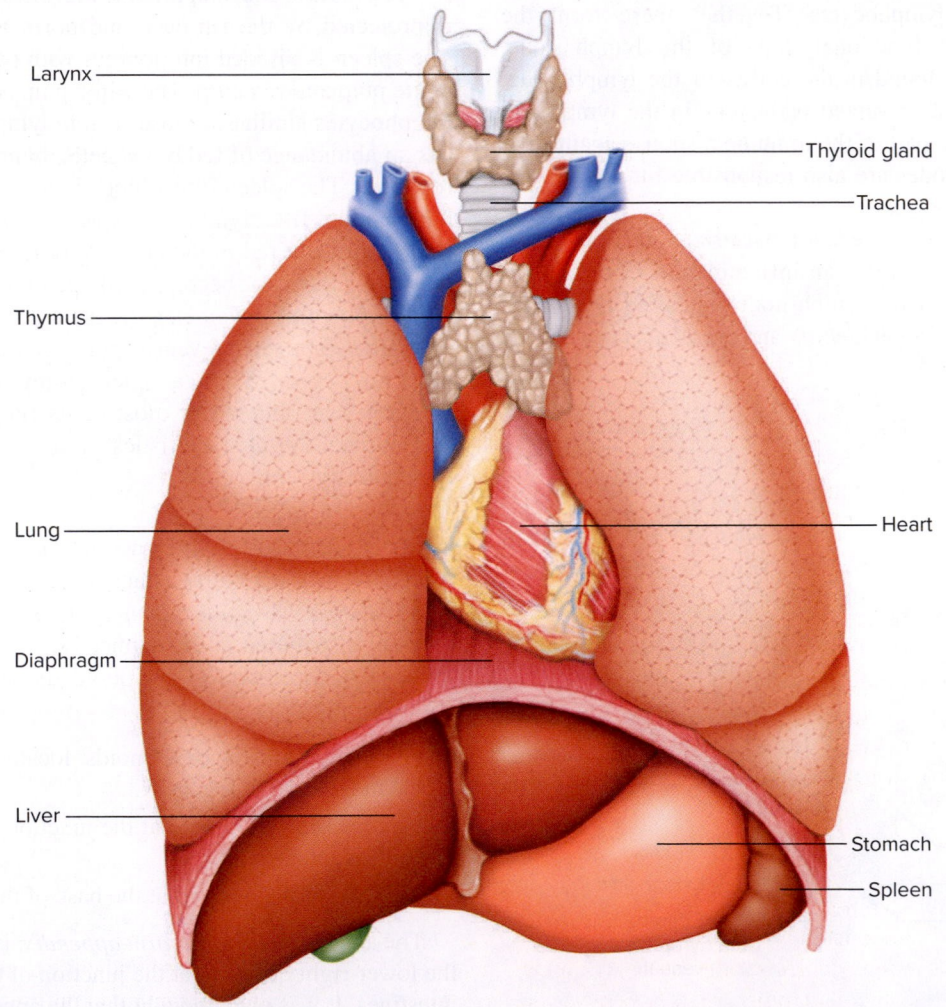

Larynx

Thymus

Lung

Diaphragm

Liver

Thyroid gland

Trachea

Heart

Stomach

Spleen

FIGURE 27-5   The bilobed thymus is located between the lungs and superior to the heart; the spleen is inferior to the diaphragm and posterior and lateral to the stomach.

TABLE 27-2 Nonspecific Defenses

Species resistance	A species is resistant to certain diseases to which other species are susceptible.
Mechanical barriers	Unbroken skin and mucous membranes prevent the entrance of some infectious agents; fluids wash away microorganisms before they can firmly attach to tissues.
Chemical barriers	Enzymes in various body fluids kill pathogens; pH extremes and high salt concentration also harm pathogens; interferons induce production of other proteins that block reproduction of viruses, stimulate phagocytosis, and enhance the activity of cells to resist infection and the growth of tumors; defensins damage bacterial cell walls and membranes; collectins attach to microbes; complement stimulates inflammation, attracts phagocytes, and enhances phagocytosis.
Phagocytosis	Neutrophils, monocytes, and macrophages engulf and destroy foreign particles and cells.
Fever	Elevated body temperature inhibits microbial growth and increases phagocytic activity.
Inflammation	Inflammation is a tissue response to injury that helps prevent the spread of infectious agents into nearby tissues.
Natural killer cells	Natural killer cells are a distinct type of lymphocyte that secretes perforins that lyse virus-infected cells and cancer cells.

Mechanical Barriers The covering of the body (skin) and the linings of the tubes of the body (mucous membranes) provide mechanical barriers against pathogens. Intact skin is impermeable or resistant to most pathogens. Intact mucous membranes, although generally impermeable, do permit the entry of a few pathogens.

Chemical Barriers Chemicals and enzymes in body fluids provide chemical barriers that destroy pathogens. For example, acids in the stomach destroy pathogens that are swallowed. Lysozymes in tears destroy pathogens on the surface of the eye. Salt in sweat kills bacteria, and interferon in blood blocks viruses from infecting cells.

Phagocytosis Phagocytes are cells that surround and destroy pathogens and unwanted debris in the body. Neutrophils and monocytes are the most active phagocytes in blood. They can also leave the bloodstream to attack pathogens in other tissues. When a monocyte leaves the bloodstream, it becomes a macrophage, which is simply a larger phagocytic cell. The process of destroying pathogens by this method is called **phagocytosis.**

Fever An elevated body temperature is a fever. It causes the liver and spleen to take iron out of the bloodstream. Many pathogens need iron to survive in a body, so when their iron sources are gone, they die. Fever also activates phagocytic cells in the body to attack pathogens.

Inflammation When an area of the body becomes injured or infected with a pathogen, inflammation can result. In inflammation, blood vessels in the injured area dilate and become leaky. Because blood vessels dilate, more blood enters the area, bringing phagocytic white blood cells (WBC) to the area to attack the pathogen. The blood also brings proteins to replace injured tissues and clotting factors to stop any bleeding. The clotting factors also "wall off" the area so that pathogens cannot spread. Because blood vessels become leaky, more fluid accumulates in the injured area, which leads to edema. The excess fluid often irritates pain receptors. The four cardinal signs of inflammation are redness, heat, swelling, and pain.

Natural Killer Cells Natural killer (NK) cells are another type of lymphocyte. They primarily target cancer cells but also protect the body against many types of pathogens. Like cytotoxic T cells, NK cells kill harmful cells on contact. They secrete chemicals that produce holes in the membranes of harmful cells, which cause the cells to burst. Unlike B cells and T cells, NK cells do not have to recognize a specific antigen to start destroying pathogens. B cells and T cells are discussed later in the chapter.

Specific Defenses

Specific defenses are called immunities. They protect the body against specific pathogens. For example, a person who has chickenpox develops a specific defense that prevents him or her from getting chickenpox again. However, this specific defense does not protect the person from any other disease. For example, a person who has measles will not get the measles again but if she is exposed to the mumps virus and has not been vaccinated, she can get the mumps.

Antigens are simply defined as foreign substances in the body. Pathogens have many antigens on their surfaces. The immune system is programmed to recognize antigens in the body. Foreign substances in the body that are too small to start an immune response by themselves are called **haptens.** Haptens often attach to proteins in the blood, where they are then able to trigger an immune response. Penicillin is an example of a hapten.

Antibodies and complements are the major proteins involved in specific defenses. **Antibodies** are proteins the body produces in response to specific antigens, and **complements** are proteins in serum that work with antibodies to eliminate or destroy antigens.

Lymphocytes and macrophages are the major WBCs involved in specific defenses. The cells of the lymphatic system produce proteins known as **cytokines,** which assist in immune response regulation. Cytokines are special messenger proteins that send signals to other parts of the immune system so that the immune response is coordinated. These messengers can act as on/off switches for certain immune cells or they can attract immune cells to a specific area of need, such as a wound, that needs immune cells to heal. Lymphocytes and macrophages produce cytokines known as **monokines.** Monokines assist in regulation of the immune response by increasing B-cell production and stimulating red bone marrow to produce more WBCs.

B Cells and T Cells   Two major types of lymphocytes are B cells and T cells. Although both B cells and T cells circulate in the blood, most of the lymphocytes in blood are T cells. B cells and T cells are also found in lymph nodes, the spleen, the thymus, the lining of digestive organs, and bone marrow.

Both T cells and B cells recognize antigens in the body; however, they respond to antigens in different ways. T cells bind to antigens on cells and attack them directly. This type of response is called a **cell-mediated response.** T cells also respond to antigens by secreting cytokines called **lymphokines,** which increase T-cell production and directly kill cells that have antigens.

B cells, on the other hand, do not attack antigens directly. They respond to antigens by becoming plasma cells. The plasma cells then make antibodies against the specific antigen. The antibodies attach to antigens in the humors (fluids) of the body; this response is called a humoral, or **antibody-mediated, response.** B cells become activated when a specific antigen binds to receptors on their surfaces. Each group of B cells recognizes only one type of antigen. Once activated, B cells divide to make plasma cells and memory B cells. Plasma cells make antibodies, which travel through the fluids of the body and bind to the antigens that activated the B cells. Memory B cells trigger a faster and stronger immune response the next time the person is exposed to the same antigen because they already know to respond to the antigen—just as you know what to expect the second time you play a computer game and can thus play faster and better. (See Figures 27-6 and 27-7.)

As seen in Figure 27-6, before a T cell can respond to an antigen, it must be activated. T-cell activation begins when a macrophage ingests and digests a pathogen that has antigens on it. The macrophage then takes some of the antigens from the pathogen and puts them on its cell membrane next to a large protein complex called a **major histocompatibility complex (MHC).** Every human being has a unique MHC (similar to an internal fingerprint), and it is present on every cell in the body. A T cell that has a receptor for the antigen recognizes and binds to the antigen and the MHC on the surface of the macrophage. The T cell is now activated and begins to divide to form other types of T cells and T memory cells. It is important to note that T cells cannot be activated without macrophages and MHC proteins. MHC is also involved in recognizing foreign cells versus host cells. This is important in keeping the immune system from attacking the body's own cells by mistake.

Some activated T cells form cytotoxic T cells that are important in protecting the body against viruses and cancer cells.

Other activated T cells become helper T cells that carry out many important roles in immunity. Helper T cells increase antibody formation, memory cell formation, B-cell formation, and phagocytosis. Some activated T cells become memory T cells that "remember" the pathogen that activated the original T cell. When a person is later exposed to the same pathogen, memory cells trigger an immune response that is more effective than the first immune response. The production of memory cells prevents a person from suffering from the same disease twice.

▶ Antibodies   LO 27.3

Antibodies are also called **immunoglobulins.** The following is a list of different types of immunoglobulins (Ig):

- IgA is an antibody found in secretions of the body like breast milk, sweat, tears, saliva, and mucus. It prevents pathogens from entering the body.
- IgD is an antibody found on the cell membranes of B cells. IgD has an important role in activating basophils, a type of white blood cell.
- IgE is an antibody found wherever IgA is located. It is involved in triggering allergic reactions.
- IgG is an antibody that primarily recognizes bacteria, viruses, and toxins. It can also activate complements.
- IgM is a large antibody that primarily binds to antigens on food, bacteria, or incompatible blood cells. It also activates complements.

When antibodies bind to antigens, they take one of the following actions:

- They allow phagocytes to recognize and destroy antigens.
- They make antigens clump together, causing them to be destroyed by macrophages. This is how incompatible blood cells are destroyed.
- They cover the toxic portions of antigens to make them harmless.
- They activate complements, which are proteins in serum that attack pathogens by forming holes in them. Complement proteins also attract macrophages to pathogens and can stimulate inflammation.

▶ Immune Responses and Acquired Immunities   LO 27.4

A primary immune response occurs the first time a person is exposed to an antigen. This response is slow and takes several weeks to occur. In this response, memory cells are made. A secondary immune response occurs the next time a person is exposed to the same antigen. This response is quick and usually prevents a person from developing a disease from the antigen. Memory cells carry out the secondary immune response.

A person is born with very few immunities but normally develops or acquires them as long as his immune system is healthy. The four types of immunities a person can acquire are (1) naturally acquired active immunity, (2) artificially acquired

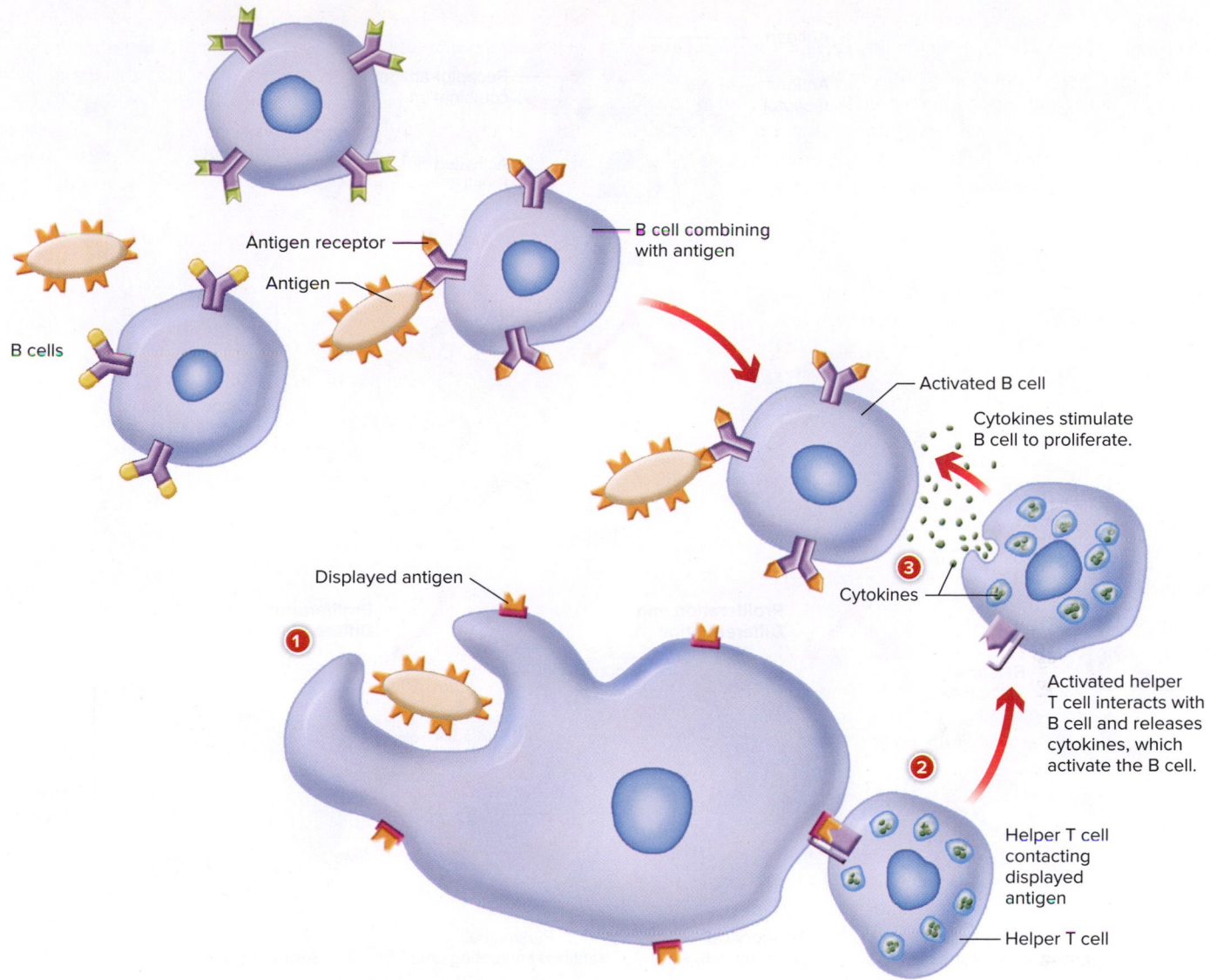

FIGURE 27-6   T-cell and B-cell activation. (1) A macrophage displays an antigen on its cell membrane. (2) A helper T cell binds to the antigen on the macrophage and becomes activated. (3) An activated helper T cell releases cytokines to help an activated B cell proliferate. Notice that the B cell must also bind to an antigen to become activated.

In the figure, the following labels appear: Antigen receptor, Antigen, B cells, B cell combining with antigen, Activated B cell, Cytokines stimulate B cell to proliferate., Cytokines, Displayed antigen, Activated helper T cell interacts with B cell and releases cytokines, which activate the B cell., Helper T cell contacting displayed antigen, Helper T cell

active immunity, (3) naturally acquired passive immunity, and (4) artificially acquired passive immunity.

Naturally Acquired Active Immunity

A person develops this immunity by being naturally exposed to an antigen and subsequently making antibodies and memory cells against the antigen. Having an infectious disease caused by pathogens, leads to the development of this type of immunity, which is usually long-lasting.

Artificially Acquired Active Immunity

A person develops this immunity by being injected with a pathogen and subsequently making antibodies and memory cells against the pathogen. Immunizations and vaccines cause this type of immunity, which is also usually long-lasting.

Naturally Acquired Passive Immunity

A person receives this immunity from his mother. When a mother breast-feeds, she passes antibodies to her baby through breast milk. A mother also passes antibodies to her baby across the placenta, which is a short-lived immunity.

Artificially Acquired Passive Immunity

A person receives this immunity when she is injected with antibodies made by another person or an animal. For example, if a person is exposed to hepatitis A at a restaurant, she can be given antibodies from a person who has previously had the disease. The treatment must be administered in the first 2 weeks after exposure. This type of immunity is short-lived.

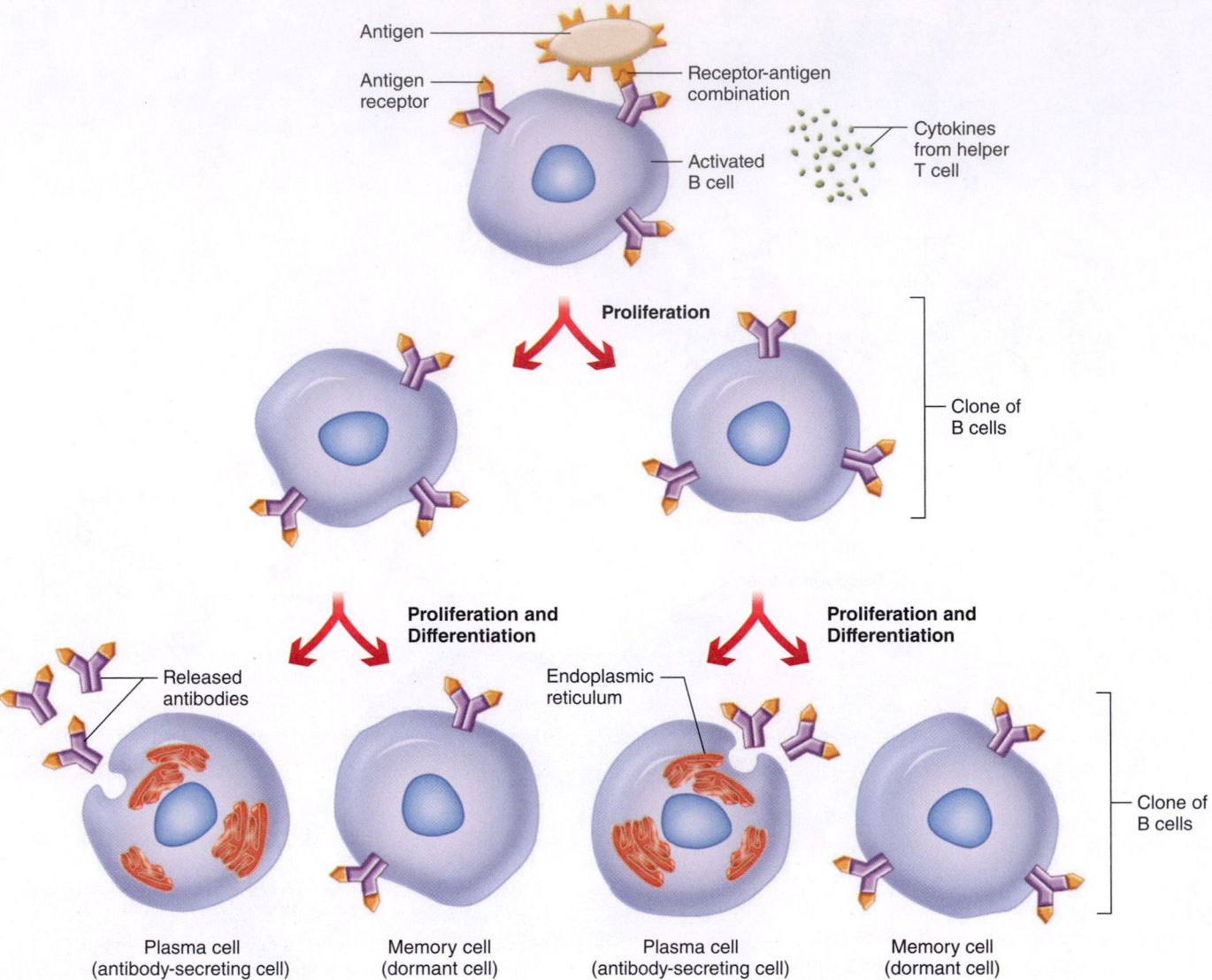

FIGURE 27-7 An activated B cell multiplies to become memory cells and plasma cells. Plasma cells secrete antibodies.

Labels in figure:
- Antigen
- Antigen receptor
- Receptor-antigen combination
- Activated B cell
- Cytokines from helper T cell
- Proliferation
- Clone of B cells
- Proliferation and Differentiation
- Released antibodies
- Endoplasmic reticulum
- Plasma cell (antibody-secreting cell)
- Memory cell (dormant cell)
- Plasma cell (antibody-secreting cell)
- Memory cell (dormant cell)
- Clone of B cells

PATHO PHYSIOLOGY

LO 27.5

Common Diseases and Disorders of the Immune System

As science and medicine develop a better understanding of the immune system and its relationship to causing disease, multiple diseases and disorders involving many body systems are now thought to have an autoimmune component.

An **autoimmune disease** is one in which the body begins to attack its own antigens. This happens when the immune system is no longer able to recognize itself and mounts an immune response against its own body cells. Examples of autoimmune diseases include scleroderma (integumentary system), rheumatoid arthritis (skeletal system), multiple sclerosis (nervous system), glomerulonephritis (urinary system), Crohn's disease (digestive system), and insulin-dependent (Type 1) diabetes mellitus (endocrine system). Although the reason is unknown, autoimmune disorders affect women almost 75% of the time, often during childbearing years.

A number of diseases and disorders can challenge the immune system. Among them, HIV infection, AIDS, cancer, and allergies are the most significant. HIV and AIDS are discussed in the *Microbiology and Disease* chapter. In this section, you will focus on specific immune system disorders. For other diseases with possible or probable autoimmune components, please refer to the appropriate body system in Appendix III.

CANCER is defined as the uncontrolled growth of abnormal cells. Healthy cells normally know when to stop reproducing, but cancer cells have lost this ability. Occasionally, normal cells create growths, but these are benign, which means they are not cancerous. Cancer cells, however, often form growths called malignant tumors, which may become fatal. In many cases, these cancerous cells or tumors damage normal cells of tissues and organs, causing organ systems to fail.

At least 200 different types of cancers are known. In the United States, the three most common cancer types in men are prostate, lung, and colon cancer. The three most common types in women are breast, lung, and colon cancer. Lung cancer kills more people in the United States than any other type of cancer.

Causes. The causes of cancer are mostly unknown, but certain risk factors have been identified, including a suppressed immune system, radiation, tobacco, and some viruses. Many other factors are suspected. One of the best ways to prevent cancer is to avoid smoking and other known risk factors. A factor known to cause the formation of cancer is called a carcinogen.

Diagnosis. Most cancers are diagnosed with a biopsy, which is a removal of tissues for examination. CT scans are also used to help diagnose most cancer types. Other diagnostic tests include blood counts, an analysis of blood chemistry, and X-rays.

Signs and Symptoms. The symptoms of different types of cancer vary, but the following symptoms are usually observed in most types: fever, chills, unintended weight loss, fatigue, and a general sense of not feeling well.

Treatment. The treatment of cancer differs depending on the type and stage of cancer. The stage of cancer refers to how large a tumor is and how far cancer cells have spread throughout the body. Table 27-3 provides a summary of cancer staging.

If tumors are localized and have not spread, the cancer can often be treated successfully by surgically removing the tumor. Other treatment options are chemotherapy, radiation therapy, newer immune therapies, and transplants, such as bone marrow transplant, which may be successful for curing certain types of cancer. Even if a cancer cannot be cured, its progression can sometimes be slowed, allowing the patient to live additional years.

ALLERGIES cause an allergic reaction, which is an immune response to a substance, like pollen, that is not normally harmful to the body. An allergy can also be an excessive immune response. Substances that trigger allergic responses are called *allergens.* Allergic reactions involve IgE antibodies and mast cells. IgE antibodies increase and respond when exposed to an allergen (trigger). The IgE antibodies bind to these allergens and cause mast cells to release histamine and heparin. These chemicals trigger allergic reactions such as sneezing or wheezing, or worse.

To help prevent this reaction, a patient receiving allergy shots is injected with tiny amounts of the allergen. This causes the body to produce IgG antibodies that will prevent IgE antibodies from binding to the allergen. IgG antibodies do not trigger immune responses because they do not activate mast cells.

Most allergies do not cause life-threatening conditions, but some do. One life-threatening condition that can result is **anaphylaxis,** when blood vessels dilate so quickly that blood pressure drops too fast for organs to adjust. Without treatment, patients may go into anaphylactic shock and die.

Signs and Symptoms. The signs and symptoms of allergies vary depending on what part of the body is exposed to allergens. Inhaled allergens often cause a runny nose, sneezing, coughing, or wheezing. Ingested allergens may cause nausea, diarrhea, or vomiting. Skin allergens cause rashes. Allergens in the blood, like penicillin, are often the most life-threatening for people who are allergic to them because the allergens can affect many organ systems.

Treatment. Many allergies are effectively treated with over-the-counter medications called antihistamines. Prescription-strength antihistamines are also available. Various types of nasal sprays and decongestants can also reduce allergy symptoms. When a person experiences anaphylaxis, an injection of epinephrine is usually an effective treatment. Epinephrine causes vasoconstriction, which increases blood pressure.

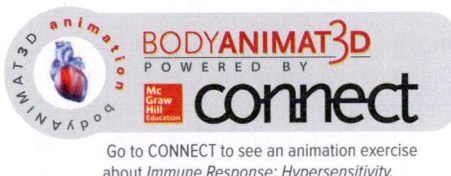

Go to CONNECT to see an animation exercise about *Immune Response: Hypersensitivity.*

ACQUIRED IMMUNODEFICIENCY SYNDROME (AIDS) is the development of severe signs and symptoms caused by the human immunodeficiency virus (HIV) as it destroys lymphocytes—particularly T lymphocytes—which leaves the immune system weakened and susceptible to many other diseases. Because a person may be infected with HIV for years before developing symptoms, it is important for all high-risk individuals to be tested.

Causes. AIDS is caused by the human immunodeficiency virus (HIV).

Signs and Symptoms. Symptoms of AIDS include T-cell counts below 200 (normal is more than 400); fever; diaphoresis; weakness; weight loss; frequent infections, including herpetic ulcers of the mouth, skin, and genitals; TB; yeast

TABLE 27-3	Cancer Staging
Stage	**Description**
Stage 0	Very early cancer. Cancer cells are localized in a few cell layers.
Stage I	Cancer cells have spread to deeper cell layers, or some may have spread to surrounding tissues.
Stage II	Cancer cells have spread to surrounding tissues but are considered contained in the primary cancer site.
Stage III	Cancer cells have spread beyond the primary cancer site to nearby areas.
Stage IV	Cancer cells have spread to other organs of the body.
Recurrent	Cancer cells have reappeared after treatment.

infections of the mouth, esophagus, and vagina; meningitis; and encephalitis. Cytomegalovirus (CMV), a specific type of herpetic virus, may also affect the eyes and other internal organs. Kaposi's sarcoma is a skin cancer commonly seen in AIDS patients.

Treatment. Although there is no cure for AIDS, treatments are available in the United States that significantly delay the progression of the disease for many patients. These treatments include the use of various antiviral drugs, but many of these drugs have serious side effects. Antibiotics are also used to treat infections.

CHRONIC FATIGUE SYNDROME (CFS) is a condition in which a person feels severe tiredness that cannot be relieved by rest and is not related to other illness.

Causes. The causes are primarily unknown, although a unique virus known as the Epstein-Barr virus (EBV) is suspected as a possible cause. This condition may also be caused by an autoimmune response against the nervous system.

Signs and Symptoms. The most common symptom is severe fatigue. Other signs and symptoms include mild fever, sore throat, tender lymph nodes in the neck or armpit, general body aches, joint pain, sleep disturbances, and depression.

Treatment. Treatment includes antiviral drugs, medications to treat the depression associated with this condition, and pain medications.

LYMPHEDEMA is the blockage of the lymphatic vessels that drain excess fluids from various areas of the body.

Causes. This condition may be caused by parasitic infections, trauma to the vessels, tumors, radiation therapy, cellulitis (a skin infection), and surgeries such as mastectomies and biopsies in which lymphoid tissues have been removed.

Signs and Symptoms. The common symptom is tissue swelling that lasts longer than a few days or increases over time.

Treatment. Treatment options include compression stockings for swelling in the legs or arms, elevation of the affected limb, and surgery to remove abnormal lymphoid tissue. Physical therapy and massage therapy are also helpful in the early stages of lymphedema to spread the fluid into surrounding tissues for reabsorption.

MONONUCLEOSIS is also known as mono. Because it frequently affects teenagers and is a highly contagious viral infection spread through the saliva of the infected person, it has earned the nickname "the kissing disease." Mono is also spread through coughing and sneezing.

Causes. Mononucleosis can be caused by either the Epstein-Barr virus or cytomegalovirus (CMV).

Signs and Symptoms. Unexplained fever, extreme fatigue, and sore throat are common. Other symptoms include weakness; headache; and swollen, tender lymph nodes (lymphadenopathy).

Treatment. Rest, proper nutrition, gargling with warm salt water, and taking acetaminophen for fever usually result in

recovery from acute symptoms in a week or two, although complete recovery may take a month or longer.

SYSTEMIC LUPUS ERYTHEMATOSUS (SLE), commonly referred to as lupus, is an autoimmune disorder that affects a few or, sometimes, many organ systems of the body. In this condition, people produce antibodies that target their own cells and tissues. As with many autoimmune disorders, lupus affects women much more often than men.

Causes. This disorder may be caused by some drugs or by bacterial infections. Except for its autoimmune component, its actual cause is unknown.

Signs and Symptoms. The list of signs and symptoms is extensive and may include any or all of the following:

- Fatigue
- General body aches
- Fever
- Weight loss (anorexia)
- Hair loss
- Arthritis
- Numbness of the fingers and toes
- "Butterfly" rash on the face
- Sensitivity to sunlight (photophobia)
- Vision problems
- Nausea
- Nosebleeds (epistaxis)
- Headaches
- Mental disorders
- Seizures
- Abnormal blood clots
- Chest pains
- Inflammation of heart tissues (carditis)
- Anemia
- Shortness of breath
- Fluid accumulation around the lungs
- Renal failure
- Blood in the urine (hematuria)

Treatment. Treatment options include anti-inflammatory medications, including steroids, and protective clothing and creams to prevent damage from sunlight. Dialysis, immunosuppressive medications, and kidney transplants may be necessary for more serious cases.

CELIAC DISEASE is an immune reaction to eating gluten, making it a diagnosable autoimmune disorder. Gluten is a protein substance found in wheat, barley, and rye.

Causes. When a person with celiac disease eats more than 10 milligrams of gluten (about 1/8 of a teaspoon of flour), this triggers an autoimmune reaction that causes the individual's body to attack the small intestinal mucosa. In the long term, if left untreated, a person with celiac disease will lose the ability to absorb nutrients and will increase his or her risk of developing another autoimmune disorder and/or cancer of the small intestine.

Signs and Symptoms. The intestinal damage from eating gluten can cause weight loss, bloating, and sometimes diarrhea. If left untreated, eventually the brain, nervous system, bones, liver, and other organs can be deprived of vital nutrients. In children, malabsorption in the small intestine can affect growth and development. The intestinal irritation can cause stomach pain, especially after eating.

Treatment. A strict, lifelong gluten-free diet is the only treatment. This means not only eating gluten-free foods but also being aware of gluten cross-contamination. For example, oats do not naturally contain gluten but can be contaminated during growth and manufacturing. The FDA regulations for labeling products as gluten free have tightened in the last 5 years. However, individuals with celiac disease should be aware that gluten can even be present in small quantities in more obscure additives, such as malt flavoring.

SUMMARY OF LEARNING OUTCOMES

LEARNING OUTCOMES	KEY POINTS
27.1 Describe the pathways and organs of the lymphatic system.	The lymphatic system is composed of pathways known as lymphatic vessels. In addition to the lymphatic vessels, the organs of the lymphatic system include lymph nodes, located throughout the body; the thymus, in the mediastinum; and the spleen, located in the upper-left quadrant of the abdominal cavity.
27.2 Compare the nonspecific and specific body defense mechanisms.	Nonspecific body defenses include species resistance, mechanical and chemical barriers, phagocytosis, fever, and inflammation. Specific defenses are immunities, or defenses, against specific antigens created by B cells, T cells, and natural killer (NK) cells.
27.3 Explain how antibodies fight infection.	Antibodies work in the following ways: phagocytosis, antigen clumping, covering (inactivating) toxic portions of antigens, and activating complements. Antibodies are also known as immunoglobulins. IgA prevents pathogens from entering the body; IgD controls B-cell activity; IgE works with IgA in triggering allergic reactions; IgG recognizes bacteria, viruses, and toxins and activates complements; and IgM binds to antigens on food, bacteria, or incompatible blood cells. IgM also activates complements.
27.4 Describe the four different types of acquired immunities.	The four types of immune response are naturally acquired active immunity, such as when a person becomes ill and develops immunity; artificially acquired active immunity, as when an injection is given against a pathogen, preventing illness; naturally acquired passive immunity, which occurs when an infant has its mother's immunity for a short while after birth and through breast milk; and artificially acquired passive immunity, which occurs after injection of antibodies such as an antivenom.
27.5 Describe the causes, signs and symptoms, and treatments of major immune disorders.	There are many common diseases and disorders of the immune system with varied signs, symptoms, and treatments. Some of these include cancer, allergies, AIDS and HIV infection, and other autoimmune diseases, in which the body attacks its own antigens.

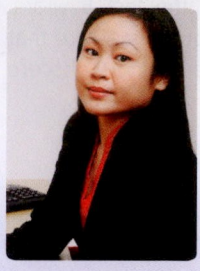

© Red Chopsticks/Getty Images RF

Recall Cindy Chen from the beginning of the chapter. Now that you have completed the chapter, answer the following questions regarding her case.

1. Explain the function of the helper T cell within her immune system.

2. Why might Cindy be more susceptible to other diseases than the general population?

3. If Cindy is HIV positive, does that mean she has visible symptoms? Why or why not?

4. Is Cindy's T-cell count normal? (Her T-cell count is reported in Other Information.) What T-cell count would be considered a symptom of AIDS?

EXAM PREPARATION QUESTIONS

1. (LO 27.1) The fluid found between cells is called
   a. Lymph
   b. Interstitial fluid
   c. Plasma
   d. CSF
   e. Cellular fluid

2. (LO 27.1) The thoracic duct collects lymph from which of the following areas of the body?
   a. Right side of the head and neck
   b. Right side of the chest
   c. Right leg
   d. Right arm
   e. Left side of the head and neck

3. (LO 27.2) Innate immunity is the other name for which type of body protection?
   a. Specific immunity
   b. Artificial immunity
   c. Humoral immunity
   d. Nonspecific immunity
   e. Temporal immunity

4. (LO 27.2) The types of white blood cells that are involved in specific defenses are lymphocytes and
   a. Macrophages
   b. Neutrophils
   c. Eosinophils
   d. Basophils
   e. Leukophils

5. (LO 27.3) Which of the following cells do not attack antigens directly
   a. Lymphokines
   b. B cells
   c. T cells
   d. NK cells
   e. Alpha cells

6. (LO 27.3) Which antibody is involved in triggering allergic reactions?
   a. IgA   d. IgM
   b. IgD   e. IgB
   c. IgE

7. (LO 27.4) A patient has been exposed to hepatitis A at a local restaurant and is treated with antibodies from a patient who previously had hepatitis A. What type of acquired immunity does this provide?
   a. Naturally acquired active immunity
   b. Artificially acquired active immunity
   c. Naturally acquired passive immunity
   d. Artificially acquired passive immunity
   e. Humorally acquired active immunity

8. (LO 27.5) Which of the following is a known carcinogen?
   a. Family history
   b. Weight gain
   c. Sedentary lifestyle
   d. Smoking
   e. Black vegetables

9. (LO 27.5) Which of the following is a life-threatening condition that can be caused by allergies?
   a. Anaphylaxis   d. Mononucleosis
   b. AIDS   e. HIV
   c. Lymphedema

10. (LO 27.5) An example of an autoimmune disease is
    a. Chickenpox
    b. Rheumatoid arthritis
    c. Influenza
    d. Atherosclerosis
    e. Strep throat

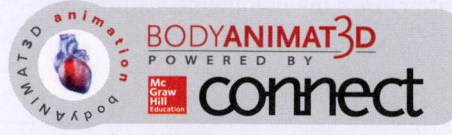

Go to CONNECT to see an animation exercise about *Inflammation*.

Analyze the following medical terms, presented throughout the chapter. Using a medical dictionary (or Appendix I) place a / mark between each word part. Define each word part and then define the whole word.

EXAMPLE: **patho** / **logy** = patho means "disease" + logy means "study of"
PATHOLOGY means "study of disease."

1. autoimmune
2. carcinogenic
3. cytotoxic
4. immunoglobulin

5. interstitial
6. leukocyte
7. lymphedema
8. lymphocyte

9. macrophage
10. mononucleosis
11. phagocytosis
12. thymectomy

CASE STUDY

Patient Name	DOB	Allergies
Mohammad Nassar	5/17/20XX	Animal dander?

Attending	MRN	Other Information
Elizabeth H. Williams, MD	423-90-687	Recently became sexually active

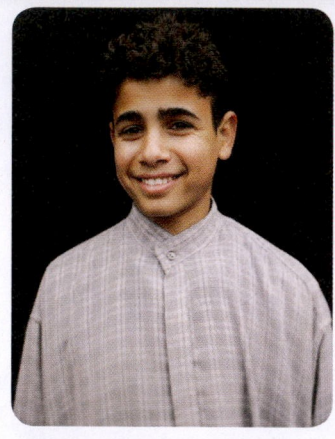

© David Sacks/Getty Images

Mohammad Nassar is a 16-year-old male complaining of increased difficulty breathing over the last 2 days. From his chart, you see that Mohammad has a history of asthma and is on a maintenance dose of albuterol 4 mg extended-release tablets twice a day. Mohammad states that he spent the weekend with his girlfriend's family at their summer home, with the family's two dogs and a cat. He is thinking that exposure to the pets may be connected to the worsening of his asthma. Dr. Williams has ordered a peak expiratory flow test and has referred Mohammad for allergy testing.

Keep Mohammad in mind as you study the chapter. There will be questions at the end of the chapter based on the case study. The information in the chapter will help you answer these questions.

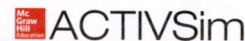

LEARNING OUTCOMES

After completing Chapter 28, you will be able to:

28.1 Describe the structure and function of each organ in the respiratory system.

28.2 Describe the events involved in the inspiration and expiration of air.

28.3 Explain how oxygen and carbon dioxide are transported in the blood.

28.4 Compare various respiratory volumes and tell how they are used to diagnose respiratory problems.

28.5 Describe the causes, signs and symptoms, and treatments of various diseases and disorders of the respiratory system.

KEY TERMS

alveoli
bronchi
bronchioles
dyspnea
epiglottis
expiration
glottis
inspiration
laryngopharynx
larynx
nares
nasal conchae

nasopharynx
oropharynx
paranasal sinuses
pharynx
pleura
respiratory capacity
respiratory volume
surfactant
thoracocentesis
thoracostomy
thorax
trachea

M E D I C A L   A S S I S T I N G   C O M P E T E N C I E S

CAAHEP

I.C.4   List major organs in each body system

I.C.5   Identify the anatomical location of major organs in each body system

I.C.6   Compare structure and function of the human body across the life span

I.C.7   Describe the normal function of each body system

I.C.8   Identify common pathology related to each body system including:
     (a) signs
     (b) symptoms
     (c) etiology

I.C.9   Analyze pathology for each body system including:
     (a) diagnostic measures
     (b) treatment modalities

V.C.9   Identify medical terms labeling the word parts

V.C.10   Define medical terms and abbreviations related to all body systems

ABHES

2. Anatomy & Physiology

a. List all body systems, their structures and functions

b. Describe common diseases, symptoms and etiologies as they apply to each body system

c. Identify diagnostic and treatment modalities as they relate to each body system

3. Medical Terminology

a. Define and use entire basic structure of medical words and be able to accurately identify in the correct context, i.e. root, prefix, suffix, combinations, spelling, and definitions

b. Build and dissect medical terms from roots/ suffixes to understand the word element combinations that create medical terminology

c. Apply various medical terms for each specialty

d. Define and use medical abbreviations when appropriate and acceptable

▶ Introduction

The function of the respiratory system is to move air in and out of the lungs. This process may be called ventilation, respiration, or breathing. The respiration process works with the cardiovascular system to deliver oxygen (O_2) to body cells via the bloodstream. It also removes a waste product—carbon dioxide (CO_2)—from the blood. This exchange of oxygen and carbon dioxide in the lungs is called *external respiration*. This same exchange, when it occurs within the hemoglobin of the red blood cells (RBCs), is known as *internal respiration*.

▶ Organs of the Respiratory System   LO 28.1

The organs of the respiratory system are the nose, pharynx, larynx, trachea, bronchial tree (including the bronchi and bronchioles), and lungs (see Figure 28-1). The nose is made of bones and cartilage and the skin covering them. The openings of the nose are the nostrils, which in medicine are referred to as the **nares.** The hairs within the nares prevent large particles from entering the nose.

The Nasal Cavity and Paranasal Sinuses

The nasal cavity is simply the hollow space behind the nose. The nasal cavity is divided into left and right portions by the cartilaginous nasal septum. Most of the nasal cavity is lined with a mucous membrane that warms and moistens air as it passes through the cavity. Three structures called **nasal conchae** extend from the lateral walls of the nasal cavity and support this mucous membrane by increasing the surface area of the nasal cavity. The three conchae are simply named by their position, as superior, middle, and inferior nasal conchae.

The nasal cavity is also lined with cells that possess *cilia,* which are microscopic, hair-like projections from the mucous membrane. As mucus traps dust and other particles in the nasal cavity, the cilia push the mucus toward the pharynx, where it is swallowed. The enzymes of the stomach then destroy these foreign particles and pathogens, thus helping to protect the respiratory system from disease.

The **paranasal sinuses** are air-filled spaces within the skull bones that open into the nasal cavity. The paranasal sinuses reduce the weight of the skull and equalize pressure between the inside of the skull and the outside environment. The sinuses also give your voice its tone. When your paranasal sinuses are "stopped up" with mucus, they cause the tone of your voice to change. The bones of the skull that contain the sinuses include the frontal, sphenoid, ethmoid, and maxillae bones. When sinus membranes become inflamed due to allergies or infection (sinusitis), they swell, which results in a sinus headache.

The Pharynx

The **pharynx** is a dual organ of the respiratory system as well as the digestive system. It consists of three separate sections:

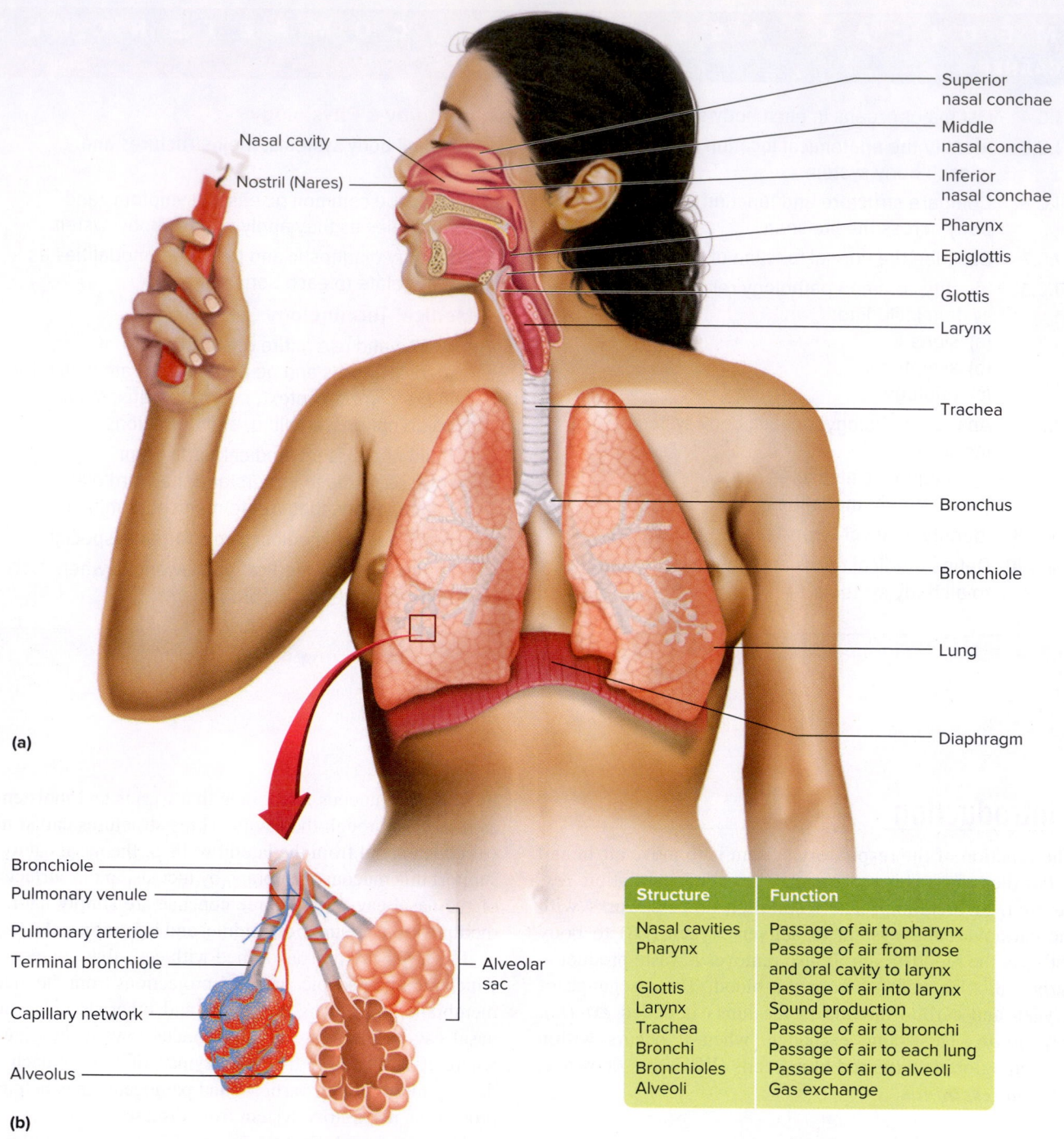

Structure	Function
Nasal cavities	Passage of air to pharynx
Pharynx	Passage of air from nose and oral cavity to larynx
Glottis	Passage of air into larynx
Larynx	Sound production
Trachea	Passage of air to bronchi
Bronchi	Passage of air to each lung
Bronchioles	Passage of air to alveoli
Alveoli	Gas exchange

FIGURE 28-1   (a) Organs of the respiratory system and (b) a bronchiole with alveolar sac, covered by capillary network, whole, and in cross section.

The **nasopharynx** is located at the junction of the nasal cavity and the pharynx; the **oropharynx** is the area at the junction of the oral cavity (mouth) and pharynx; and finally, the **laryngopharynx** is the area of the pharynx that contains the larynx, or "voice box." During inspiration, air flows from the nasal or oral cavity into the pharynx. From the pharynx, air flows into the larynx.

The Larynx and Vocal Cords

The **larynx** sits superior to and is continuous with the trachea, or windpipe. It moves air into and out of the trachea

and produces the sounds of a person's voice. The larynx consists mostly of cartilage and muscle tissue. There are three cartilages in the larynx (see Figure 28-2). The largest cartilage is called the *thyroid cartilage,* and it forms the anterior wall of the larynx. During the puberty of a male, testosterone causes the thyroid cartilage to enlarge to produce the "Adam's apple." A smaller cartilage called the *epiglottic cartilage* forms the framework of the **epiglottis,** the flaplike structure that closes off the larynx during swallowing so that food and liquids do not enter the respiratory system. The third cartilage of the larynx is called the *cricoid cartilage.*

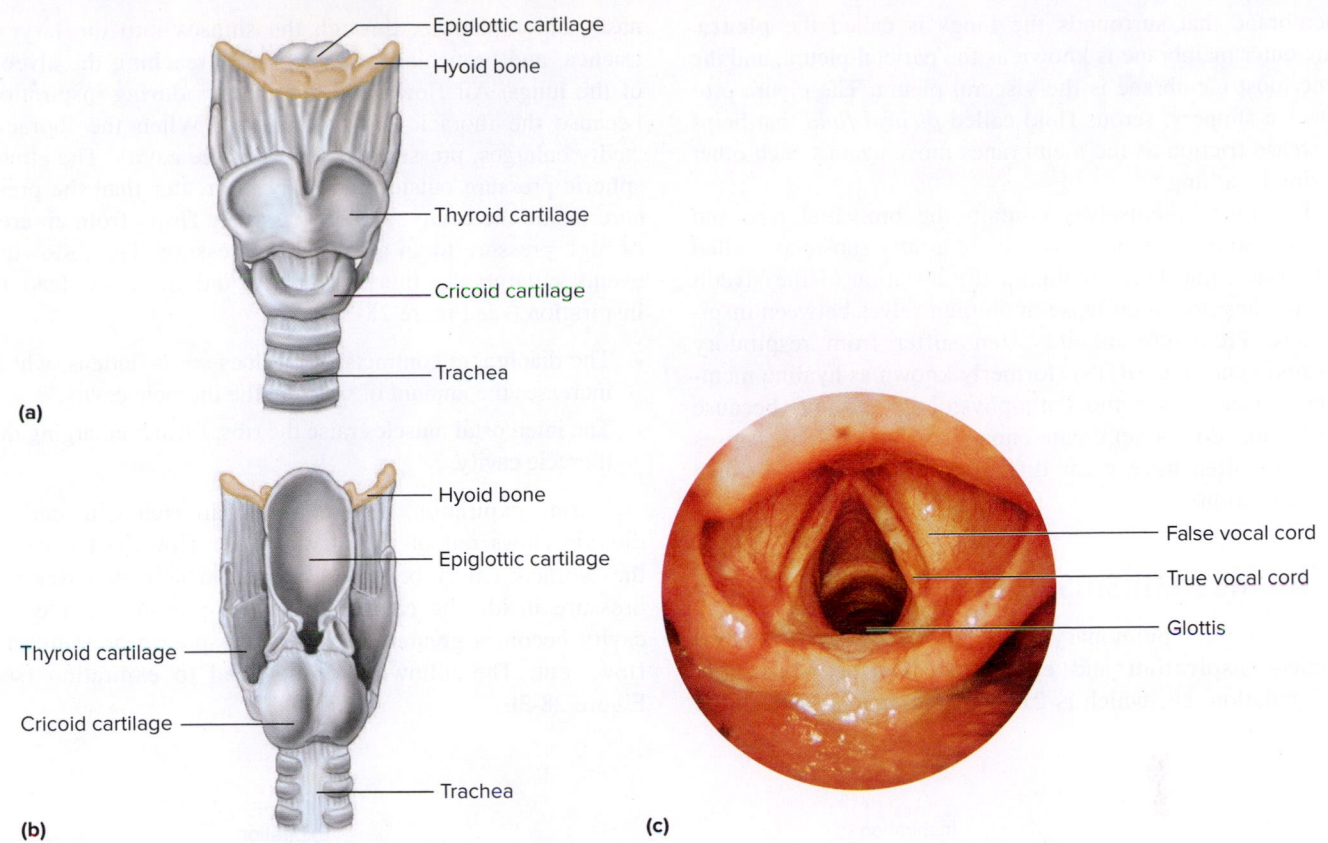

FIGURE 28-2 (a) Anterior view of larynx, (b) posterior view of larynx, and (c) photograph of the vocal cords and glottis.
© CNRI/Phototake

It forms most of the posterior wall of the larynx and a small part of the anterior wall.

The vocal cords stretch between the thyroid cartilage and the cricoid cartilage. The opening between the vocal cords is called the **glottis** (see Figure 28-2c). The upper vocal cords are referred to as *false vocal cords* because they do not produce sound. The lower vocal cords are called *true vocal cords* because muscles stretch and relax them to produce different types of sounds. When the true vocal cords are stretched, the voice becomes higher in pitch. When they are relaxed, the voice becomes lower in pitch. Males tend to have thicker vocal cords, which is why their voices are generally deeper than female voices.

The Trachea, Bronchi, and Bronchioles

The **trachea** (windpipe) is a tubular organ made of rings of cartilage and smooth muscle. It extends from the larynx to the bronchi. The trachea is lined with cells that possess cilia that constantly move mucus up to the pharynx and the esophagus, where it is swallowed. Mucus traps bacteria, viruses, and other harmful substances a person inhales. The digestive juices of the stomach then destroy the harmful substances.

Smoking destroys cilia, so the only way a smoker can get mucus out of his trachea is to cough. Smokers often feel the urge to cough more frequently than nonsmokers in an effort to move mucus to the pharynx.

The distal end of the trachea branches and starts a series of tubes called the *bronchial tree*. The first branches off the trachea are called primary, or main stem, **bronchi.** The branches of the primary bronchi are called secondary bronchi. The secondary bronchi branch into tertiary bronchi. Tertiary bronchi then branch into **bronchioles.** At the ends of the bronchioles are air sacs called alveoli (see Figure 28-1b).

Alveoli are thin sacs made of only one layer of simple squamous epithelial cells and are surrounded by capillaries. They are considered the "working tissue" of the lung because it is in the alveoli that the exchange of oxygen and carbon dioxide takes place. Many physicians refer to the alveoli as the *pulmonary parenchyma* (*parenchyma* means "working tissue"). Through the process of diffusion, red blood cells in the capillaries release carbon dioxide into the alveoli. Conversely, the alveoli release oxygen into the blood through the thin walls of the capillaries. This exchange is known as *internal* or *cellular respiration.*

The Lungs

The lungs are two cone-shaped organs that contain connective tissue, the bronchial tree, nerves, lymphatic vessels, and many blood vessels. The right lung is larger than the left because the heart is also located in the left **thorax,** or chest area. The right lung is divided into three lobes, known as the right upper, middle, and lower lobes. The left lung is divided into the left upper and lower lobes. The double-walled membrane that surrounds the lungs is called the **pleura.** The outer membrane is known as the parietal pleura, and the innermost membrane is the visceral pleura. The pleura produces a slippery, serous fluid called *pleural fluid* that helps decrease friction as the membranes move against each other during breathing.

The lungs themselves contain the bronchial tree and alveoli. Some alveolar cells secrete a fatty substance called **surfactant** that helps maintain the inflation of the alveoli so that they do not collapse in on themselves between inspirations. Premature infants often suffer from respiratory distress syndrome (RDS) (formerly known as hyaline membrane disease—see the Pathophysiology section) because their lungs do not yet create enough surfactant. This causes them to often have great difficulty maintaining adequate lung inflation.

▶ The Mechanisms of Breathing   LO 28.2

Breathing, or pulmonary ventilation, consists of two events—**inspiration** and **expiration.** During inspiration, or inhalation, air, which is 21% oxygen, enters through the naso- or oropharynx through the sinuses into the larynx, trachea, and bronchial tree, eventually reaching the alveoli of the lungs. Air flows into the airways during inspiration because the thoracic cavity enlarges. When the thoracic cavity enlarges, pressure decreases in the cavity. The atmospheric pressure outside the body is greater than the pressure inside the cavity, and air passively flows from an area of high pressure to an area of low pressure. The following events enlarge the thoracic cavity and therefore lead to inspiration (see Figure 28-3a):

- The diaphragm contracts. As it does so, it flattens, which increases the amount of space in the thoracic cavity.
- The intercostal muscles raise the ribs, further enlarging the thoracic cavity.

During expiration, or exhalation, air rich with carbon dioxide flows out of the airways. Air flows out because the thoracic cavity becomes smaller, which increases the pressure inside the cavity. When the pressure inside the cavity becomes greater than the atmospheric pressure, air flows out. The following events lead to expiration (see Figure 28-3b):

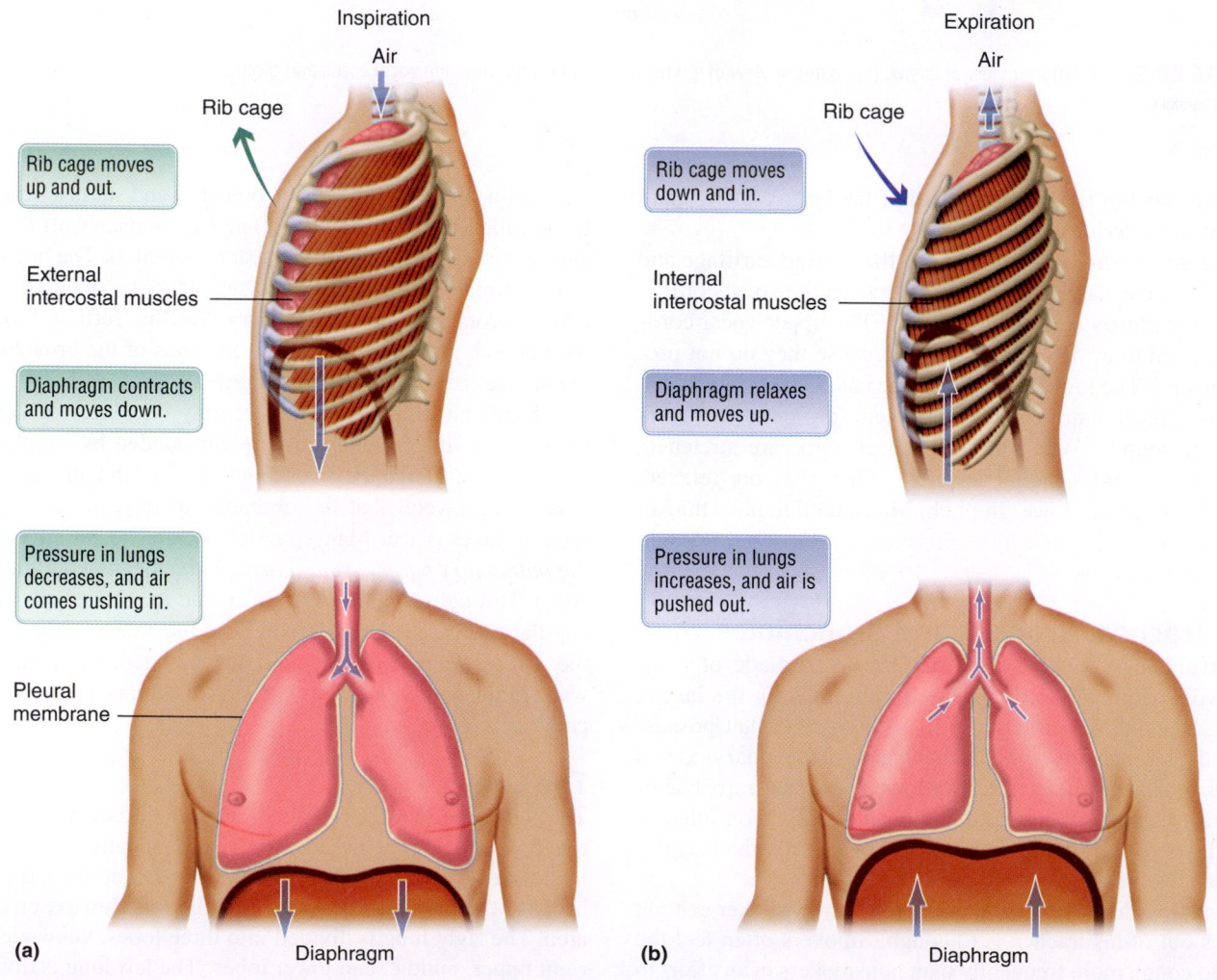

Inspiration
Air
Rib cage
Rib cage moves up and out.
External intercostal muscles
Diaphragm contracts and moves down.
Pressure in lungs decreases, and air comes rushing in.
Pleural membrane
(a)   Diaphragm

Expiration
Air
Rib cage
Rib cage moves down and in.
Internal intercostal muscles
Diaphragm relaxes and moves up.
Pressure in lungs increases, and air is pushed out.
(b)   Diaphragm

FIGURE 28-3   (a) Events of inspiration and (b) events of expiration.

- The diaphragm relaxes. As it does so, it domes up into the thoracic cavity, which decreases the space in the cavity.
- The intercostal muscles lower the ribs; this further decreases the size of the thoracic cavity.

Breathing is controlled by the respiratory center of the brain, which is located in the pons and medulla oblongata. The medulla oblongata controls both the rhythm and the depth of breathing. The pons controls the rate of breathing.

Other factors that affect breathing are the carbon dioxide levels in the blood and the pH of the blood. When carbon dioxide levels rise in the blood, the rate and depth of breathing increase. The rate and depth of breathing also increase when the blood pH drops. Fear and pain also increase the breathing rate. Breathing rapidly and deeply is called *hyperventilation,* which decreases the amount of carbon dioxide in the blood. However, it should be noted that in patients with chronic obstructive pulmonary disease (COPD), decreased oxygen levels stimulate respiratory rates. Therefore, giving a patient with COPD a high level of oxygen may actually decrease his or her breathing reflex.

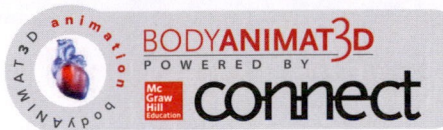

Go to CONNECT to see animation exercises about *Acid-Base Balance: Acidosis* and *Acid-Base Balance: Alkalosis.*

The inflation reflex also helps to regulate the depth of breathing. Stretch receptors in pleural membranes are activated when the lungs are stretched past a certain point. This triggers a decrease in the depth of breathing to prevent over-inflation of the lungs.

Normal, everyday situations also alter our breathing patterns. Consider these common occurrences:

- Coughing. A deep inspiration occurs and the glottis is closed. As the air forces the glottis open, a rush of air is forced up to clear the lower respiratory passages.
- Sneezing. The same process occurs as in coughing except that air is moved to the nasal passages by lowering the uvula. This causes a clearing of the upper respiratory passages.
- Laughing. A deep breath is expelled in short bursts, expressing happiness.
- Crying. The same respiratory process occurs as in laughing, but the expression is one of sadness.
- Hiccups. Also spelled hiccoughs, these are spasmodic contractions of the diaphragm against a closed glottis. Interestingly, the purpose for this is not known.
- Yawning. A deep inspiration that increases the amount of air brought to the alveoli aids in blood oxygenation.

- Speaking. Air is forced through the larynx, vibrating the vocal cords. Words are formed by the tongue, lips, and teeth, allowing for verbal communication.

Also, consider the common patient complaint of snoring. See the feature *Educating the Patient* for more information.

▶ The Transport of Oxygen and Carbon Dioxide in the Blood   LO 28.3

Once oxygen gets into the bloodstream, most of it binds to the heme portion of hemoglobin in red blood cells. Hemoglobin bound to oxygen is called *oxyhemoglobin* and is bright red in color. Some oxygen stays dissolved in plasma and does not bind to hemoglobin, but this is generally a lesser amount than that which attaches to the RBCs. Carbon dioxide also binds to hemoglobin, but at the globin or protein portion of the hemoglobin, forming *carboxyhemoglobin.* However, unlike oxygen, much of the carbon dioxide enters the plasma for transport through the body, after being converted into carbonic acid by the RBCs. Carbonic acid can quickly be converted into the buffer bicarbonate as needed by the blood to maintain its narrow, constant pH level of 7.35–7.45 (see *The Cardiovascular System* chapter).

Carbon monoxide is a colorless, odorless gas. Poisonous to humans, it is particularly dangerous because it binds to the same heme area of hemoglobin as does oxygen. In fact, it binds more tightly to this molecule than oxygen. When hemoglobin is exposed to carbon monoxide, the carbon monoxide "overrules" oxygen, leading to carbon monoxide poisoning.

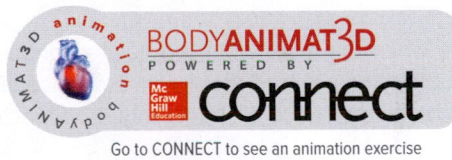

Go to CONNECT to see an animation exercise about *Oxygen Transport and Gas Exchange.*

▶ Respiratory Volumes   LO 28.4

The amount of air that moves into and out of the lungs when a person breathes is called **respiratory volume.** A person's respiratory volume varies depending on the depth and intensity of the breaths the person is taking. **Respiratory capacity,** or the amount of air the lungs can hold, is another common measure of respiratory health. It can be calculated by adding certain respiratory volumes together. In fact, several different measurements related to respiratory volume and capacity are commonly used to assess a person's lungs (see Table 28-1). You will learn more about these respiratory volumes and the process of measuring them in the *Electrocardiography and Pulmonary Function Testing* chapter.

TABLE 28-1 Respiratory Air Volumes and Capacities

Name	Volume*	Description
Tidal volume (TV)	500 mL	Volume moved into or out of the lungs during a respiratory cycle
Inspiratory reserve volume (IRV)	3,000 mL	Volume that can be inhaled during forced breathing in addition to resting tidal volume
Expiratory reserve volume (ERV)	1,100 mL	Volume that can be exhaled during forced breathing in addition to resting tidal volume
Residual volume (RV)	1,200 mL	Volume that remains in the lungs at all times
Inspiratory capacity (IC)	3,500 mL	Maximum volume of air that can be inhaled following exhalation of resting tidal volume: IC = TV + IRV
Functional residual capacity (FRC)	2,300 mL	Volume of air that remains in the lungs following exhalation of resting tidal volume: FRC = ERV + RV
Vital capacity (VC)	4,600 mL	Maximum volume of air that can be exhaled after taking the deepest breath possible: VC = TV + IRV + ERV
Total lung capacity (TLC)	5,800 mL	Total volume of air that the lungs can hold: TLC = VC + RV
Forced vital capacity (FVC)	Varies depending on gender, age, and height	Amount of air exhaled with force after inhaling as deeply as possible
Peak expiratory flow (PEF)	Varies depending on gender, age, and height	Greatest rate of flow during forced exhalation

*Values are typical for a tall, young adult.

EDUCATING THE PATIENT

Snoring

Snoring occurs when the muscles of the palate, tongue, and throat relax. Airflow then causes these soft tissues to vibrate. These vibrating tissues produce the harsh sounds characteristic of snoring.

Snoring causes daytime sleepiness and is sometimes associated with a condition known as obstructive sleep apnea (OSA). In OSA, the relaxed throat tissues cause airways to collapse, which prevents a person from breathing. Snoring affects approximately 50% of men and 25% of women older than age 40. The common causes of snoring include the following:

- Enlargement of the tonsils or adenoids
- Being overweight
- Alcohol consumption
- Nasal congestion
- A deviated (crooked) nasal septum

The severity of snoring varies among people. The Mayo Clinic's Sleep Disorders Center uses the following scale to determine the severity of snoring:

- Grade 1: Snoring can be heard from close proximity to the face of the snoring person.
- Grade 2: Snoring can be heard from anywhere in the bedroom.

- Grade 3: Snoring can be heard just outside the bedroom with the door open.
- Grade 4: Snoring can be heard outside the bedroom with the door closed.

You can educate patients about making lifestyle modifications and using aids to help reduce their snoring:

- Lose weight.
- Change the sleeping position from the back to the side.
- Avoid the use of alcohol and medications that cause sleepiness.
- Use nasal strips to widen the nasal passageways.
- Use dental devices to keep airways open.

In addition, patients may benefit from a continuous positive airway pressure (CPAP) machine if obstructive sleep apnea (OSA) is diagnosed as the underlying cause of the snoring. A CPAP machine, uses a mask attached to a pump that forces air into their passageways while they sleep. If these therapies are not effective, patients may need surgery such as a uvulotomy to trim excess tissues in the throat, or laser surgery to remove a portion of the soft palate.

PATHOPHYSIOLOGY

Common Diseases and Disorders of the Respiratory System

ALLERGIC RHINITIS is a hypersensitivity reaction to various airborne allergens.

Causes. There are many causes, which may be seasonal, such as hay fever, or continual, such as those caused by dust, molds, colognes, cigarette smoke, animal dander, and mites.

Signs and Symptoms. There are numerous signs and symptoms, which may include sneezing; itchy, watery eyes; red, swollen eyelids; congested nasal mucous membranes; and nasal discharge.

Treatment. Treatment commonly includes the use of over-the-counter (OTC) antihistamines and decongestants. Severe cases may be treated with prescription medication such as Allegra® and OTC medication such as Zyrtec®. Patients should also avoid known allergens. Air filters and air conditioners assist in keeping allergen counts down. Seeking the assistance of an allergist for desensitization injections may be an option for long-term management.

ASTHMA is a condition in which the tubes of the bronchial tree become obstructed as a result of inflammation.

Causes. The causes include allergens (pollen, pets, dust mites, etc.), cigarette smoke, pollutants, perfumes, cleaning agents, cold temperatures, and exercise (in susceptible individuals).

Signs and Symptoms. Symptoms include difficulty breathing, a tight feeling in the chest, wheezing, and coughing, all of which can cause a feeling of suffocation and increased anxiety.

Treatment. Treatment includes avoiding allergens, using steroidal and nonsteroidal inhalers such as Advair® and Flovent®, and taking oral medications such as Singulair® and other bronchodilators to reduce inflammation. See Figure 28-4. Patients should avoid smoky environments; those who smoke should stop. Strongly scented items such as perfumes, hair products, and cleaning agents should also be avoided.

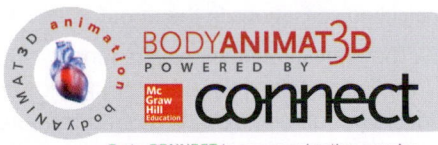

Go to CONNECT to see an animation exercise about *Asthma.*

ATELECTASIS is more commonly called collapsed lung. It may occur after abdominal or thoracic surgery or because of pleural effusion, which may consist of blood, fluid, air, or pus in the pleural cavity. The medical names for these conditions are hemothorax (blood in the pleural cavity), hydrothorax (fluid), pneumothorax (air), and pyothorax (pus).

Causes. These include underlying cystic fibrosis and COPD in which patients may have a chronic form of atelectasis. Cancer patients and those with inflammatory conditions such as

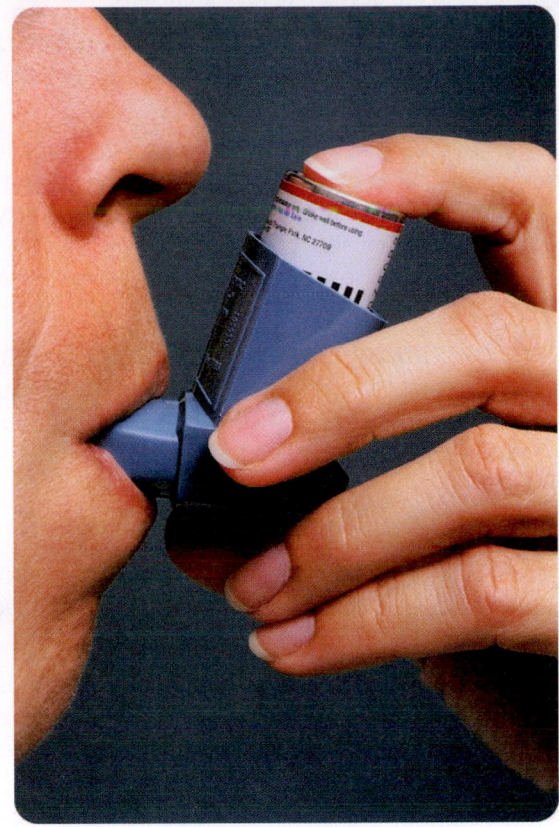

FIGURE 28-4 Individuals with asthma may use an inhaler with steroidal or nonsteroidal medication for treatment.
© Royalty-Free/Corbis

pleurisy (pleuritis) may also be subject to chronic atelectasis. Acute atelectasis may occur after any injury to the ribs or trauma to the thorax. Postsurgical patients are also susceptible.

Signs and Symptoms. These include **dyspnea** (difficulty breathing), cyanosis (a blue coloration of skin and mucous membranes), diaphoresis (excessive perspiration), anxiety, tachycardia, and intercostal muscle retraction. Depending on the cause of the atelectasis, there may also be chest pain.

Treatment. In acute cases, thoracocentesis may be needed to drain the pleural cavity. For chronic atelectasis, treatment may include chest percussion, postural drainage, coughing, deep breathing exercises, and intermittent positive-pressure breathing (IPPB).

BRONCHITIS is inflammation of the bronchi and often follows a cold. Bronchitis that occurs frequently often indicates more serious underlying conditions, such as asthma or emphysema. Smokers are much more likely to develop bronchitis than are nonsmokers. Repeated episodes of bronchitis increase a person's chance of eventually developing lung cancer.

Causes. This condition can be caused by viruses and gastroesophageal reflux disease (GERD), a condition in which acids move from the stomach into the esophagus. Exposure to cigarette smoke, pollutants, and household cleaner fumes can also contribute to the development of bronchitis.

Signs and Symptoms. The signs and symptoms include chills, fever, coughing up yellow-gray or green mucus, tightness in the chest, wheezing, and dyspnea.

Treatment. This condition can be treated with rest, fluids, nonprescription and prescription cough medicines, and the use of a humidifier. Antibiotics are usually prescribed only for smokers. Patients who also have asthma may need to use inhalers. They should also wear masks if they may be exposed to lung irritants.

CHRONIC OBSTRUCTIVE PULMONARY DISEASE (COPD)
is a group of lung disorders that limit airflow to the lungs and usually cause enlargement of the alveoli in the lungs. Emphysema and chronic bronchitis are the most common types of COPD.

Causes. The primary causes are smoking and air pollution.

Signs and Symptoms. Common signs and symptoms include dyspnea, hypoxia (inadequate oxygenation of the cells), fatigue, and frequent coughing.

Treatment. Treatment should first be focused on lifestyle changes, especially smoking cessation. Other treatment options include respiratory therapy and the use of inhalers. In more serious cases, a lung transplant may be necessary.

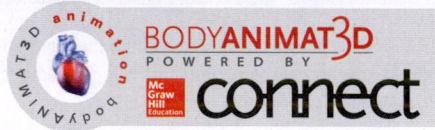

Go to CONNECT to see an animation exercise about *COPD*.

EMPHYSEMA is a chronic condition that damages the alveoli of the lungs. It is heavily associated with smoking, which causes stretching of the spaces between the alveoli and paralyzes the cilia of the respiratory system.

Causes. The most common causes are cigarette smoking and exposure to cigarette smoke; pollutants; and the dust from grains, cotton, wood, or coal.

Signs and Symptoms. Symptoms include shortness of breath that progresses over time, chronic cough, unintended weight loss, and fatigue. Pulmonary function tests and arterial blood gases become increasingly more abnormal as the disease progresses. In advanced cases, patients develop the characteristic barrel chest caused by the muscular changes in the chest as the patient struggles to breathe.

Treatment. Smoking cessation and prevention of exposure to cold environments and pollutants should be the first treatment measures. Vaccinations to prevent the flu and pneumonia as well as antibiotics to control the respiratory infections associated with emphysema may also be administered. In addition, patients can be treated with bronchodilators, supplemental oxygen, inhaled steroids, and respiratory therapy. The most serious cases may require either surgery to remove damaged lung tissue or a lung transplant, without which patients will develop respiratory and/or heart failure, resulting in death.

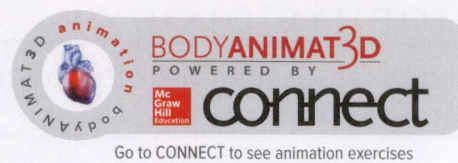

Go to CONNECT to see animation exercises about *Respiratory Tract Infections* and *Respiratory Failure.*

INFLUENZA is more commonly called the flu. Babies, the elderly, people with suppressed immune systems, and those with chronic respiratory illnesses, such as COPD, are at the highest risk of developing influenza. The flu normally lasts between 5 and 10 days.

Causes. This disease is caused by a number of different viruses that attack the respiratory system. It can be prevented or at the least the course shortened and symptoms lightened through a yearly flu vaccination. Note that each year there are multiple strains of influenza. Therefore, the vaccine available each year is for the known strains for that year. Explain this to patients so that they understand they need a flu shot each year for that year's specific strains of the virus.

Signs and Symptoms. Common symptoms include a runny nose (rhinorrhea), sore throat (pharyngitis), sneezing, fever or chills, dry cough, muscle pain, fatigue, anorexia (loss of appetite), and diarrhea.

Treatment. OTC analgesics and antipyretics can alleviate the aches and pains as well as the fever associated with the flu. Other treatment options include bed rest, fluids, and antiviral medications.

LARYNGITIS is an acute inflammation of the larynx. Chronic laryngitis is associated with lung cancer.

Causes. The causes of this condition are varied and include the following: viruses; bacteria; polyp formation in the larynx; excessive talking, shouting, or singing; allergies; smoking; frequent heartburn; the frequent use of alcohol; damage to nerves that supply the larynx; and a stroke (cerebrovascular accident, or CVA) that paralyzes vocal cord muscles.

Signs and Symptoms. Signs and symptoms include a hoarse voice (dysphonia), a sore throat (pharyngitis), a dry cough and throat, and tickling sensations in the throat.

Treatment. The most common treatment options are antibiotics, the management of heartburn, the avoidance of cigarettes and alcohol, and voice rest. The treatment of more serious cases includes the removal of laryngeal polyps and surgery to tighten the vocal cords.

LEGIONNAIRE'S DISEASE is an acute type of bacterial pneumonia. As with many respiratory diseases, smokers are much more susceptible to pneumonia than are nonsmokers.

Causes. This disease is caused by Legionnaire bacilli that usually grow in the standing water of air-conditioning systems.

Signs and Symptoms. The symptoms include fever, which may spike as high as 105.8°F, fatigue, anorexia, dyspnea, frequent coughing, chest pain, muscle aches, and headache. Complications may include hypotension, arrhythmia, respiratory and renal failure, and shock, which is often fatal.

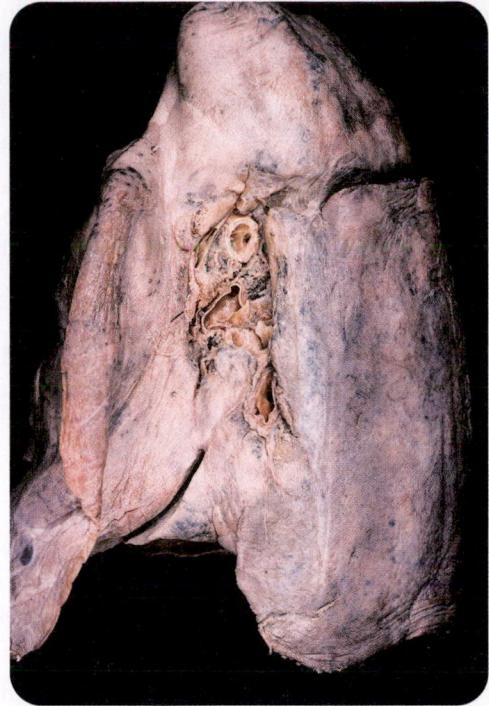

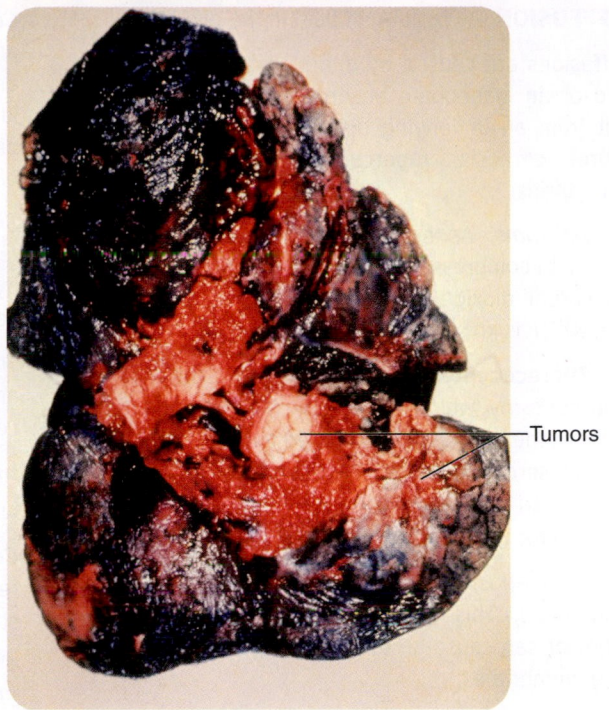

(a) Healthy lung, mediastinal surface

(b) Smoker's lung with carcinoma

Tumors

FIGURE 28-5 A healthy lung is pink, unlike a lung with cancer caused by smoking, as shown on the right.
© McGraw-Hill Education/Dennis Strete, photographer; © Biophoto Associates/Science Source

Treatment. Treatments include antibiotics, antipyretics, and respiratory therapy, including oxygen and ventilator support if needed. Supportive therapy, such as IV fluids, is also used.

LUNG CANCER kills more people in the United States than any other type of cancer. Although other causes of cancer exist, smoking and secondhand smoke account for approximately 85% of all lung cancer cases. See Figure 28-5.

Causes. The primary causes of lung cancer are smoking and exposure to radon, asbestos, and industrial carcinogens.

Signs and Symptoms. The respiratory symptoms include a cough that worsens over time, hemoptysis (coughing up blood), dyspnea, wheezing, shortness of breath, and recurrent bronchitis. Other symptoms are chest pain, dysphonia, unintended weight loss, and bone pain if the cancer has spread.

Classification. Lung cancer is classified as follows:

- *Small cell lung cancer.* This type occurs almost exclusively in smokers. It is the most aggressive type and spreads readily to other organs. Small cell lung cancer that spreads to other organs is termed *extensive*.
- *Squamous cell lung cancer.* This type of lung cancer arises from the epithelial cells that line the bronchi and bronchioles of the lungs. It occurs most commonly in men.
- *Adenocarcinoma.* This type arises from the mucus-producing cells of the lungs. It develops most commonly in women and nonsmokers.
- *Large cell carcinoma.* This type of lung cancer arises from the peripheral parts of the lungs.

Stages. Squamous cell lung cancer, adenocarcinoma, and large cell carcinoma are staged as follows:

- Stage 0: Cancer is found only in the lining of the bronchi and bronchioles of the lungs.
- Stage 1: Cancer has spread from the lining of the bronchi and bronchioles to lung tissues.
- Stage 2: Cancer has spread to the lymph nodes or the chest wall.
- Stage 3: Cancer has spread to the lymph nodes and to other organs within the chest.
- Stage 4: Cancer has spread to organs outside the chest.

Small cell lung carcinoma is staged as follows:

- Limited-stage small cell lung cancer: Cancer is found in one lung, the tissues between the lungs, and nearby lymph nodes only.
- Extensive-stage small cell lung cancer: Cancer has spread outside of the lung in which it began or to other parts of the body.

Treatment. Treatment varies, depending on the type of cancer and the stage. Stopping smoking and avoiding exposure to secondhand smoke should be the first treatment considerations. Common treatment options include chemotherapy and radiation therapy. More serious cases may require the surgical removal of tumors (if they are confined), a lobectomy (the removal of a lung lobe or lobes), or a pneumonectomy (the removal of an entire lung).

PLEURAL EFFUSION is a buildup of fluid in the pleural cavity.

Causes. Effusions are caused by either an overproduction of pleural fluid or an inadequate absorption of the fluid. These often result from an underlying disease, such as congestive heart failure, cirrhosis, tuberculosis, cancer, lupus, or rheumatoid arthritis.

Signs and Symptoms. As the fluid builds in the pleural space, the lungs begin to compress, reducing the gaseous exchange of oxygen and carbon dioxide. Infective processes may result in a pus buildup, which is known as empyema.

Treatment. **Thoracocentesis** is done to remove the fluid and/ or pus. **Thoracostomy,** which involves the insertion of a tube to continually drain the fluid, may be required to maintain drainage of the acute phase of the illness. Oxygen may be administered to increase oxygen concentration in the lung. Antibiotics may also be required for any infective process.

PLEURITIS, or *pleurisy,* is a condition in which the pleura becomes inflamed. This often causes the membranes to stick together or can cause an excess amount of fluid to form between the membranes.

Causes. Causes include viruses, pneumonia, autoimmune diseases such as lupus or rheumatoid arthritis, tuberculosis, a pulmonary embolism, inflammation of the pancreas, and trauma to the chest.

Signs and Symptoms. Symptoms include fever or chills; a dry cough; shortness of breath; and a sharp, stabbing chest pain during respiration.

Treatment. Analgesics may be prescribed to relieve chest pain. Anti-inflammatory drugs, antibiotics, and the removal of fluid around the lungs by thoracocentesis are the primary treatment options.

PNEUMOCONIOSIS is the name given to lung diseases that result from years of exposure to different environmental or occupational types of dust. There are three basic types: *anthracosis, asbestosis,* and *silicosis.*

Causes. Anthracosis (black lung disease) results from exposure to coal dusts. Asbestosis results from lung exposure to asbestos. Silicosis arises from exposure to silica sand from sand blasting and ceramic manufacture.

Signs and Symptoms. These include tachypnea, nonproductive cough, progressive dyspnea on exertion, pulmonary hypertension, recurrent respiratory infections, and eventual right ventricular hypertrophy. In all cases, fibrous tissue takes over healthy lung tissue, which destroys the alveoli and takes over the air passageways.

Treatment. Treatment for all types includes avoiding respiratory infections, using bronchodilators, and using supplemental oxygen as needed. Respiratory therapy can also be useful in helping patients rid themselves of respiratory secretions.

PNEUMONIA, also known as *pneumonitis,* is characterized by an inflammation of the lungs caused by a bacterial, viral, or fungal infection. There are at least 50 different types of pneumonia, and they range from mild to serious. *Double pneumonia* refers to inflammation of both lungs.

Causes. Pneumonia can be caused by bacteria, viruses, fungi, and parasites. It can also be caused by foreign matter that enters the lungs (for example, stomach contents that enter the lungs after vomiting), known as aspiration pneumonia. This disorder may be prevented by not smoking and, for some types of pneumonia, by pneumococcal vaccinations.

Signs and Symptoms. Common signs and symptoms include fever or chills, headache, chest or muscle pain, fatigue, dyspnea, and sputum consisting of rust-colored, green, or yellowish mucus.

Treatment. Rest, fluids, OTC pain medications, and antibiotics are the most common treatments. In severe cases, oxygen and ventilator support may be required.

PNEUMOTHORAX is a collection of air in the chest around the lungs, which may cause atelectasis.

Causes. Some causes of this disorder are unknown. Various respiratory diseases and trauma to the chest, such as a stabbing wound, can also contribute to the development of pneumothorax.

Signs and Symptoms. The primary symptoms include tightness in the chest or a sharp chest pain, shortness of breath, and a rapid heart rate.

Treatment. The insertion of a chest tube (thoracostomy) to remove air from the chest and surgery to repair chest wounds are the primary treatments.

PULMONARY EDEMA is a condition in which fluids fill spaces within the lungs. This disorder makes it very difficult for the lungs to oxygenate the blood. It most commonly occurs when the heart cannot pump all the blood it receives from the lungs. Left heart failure occurs when blood then backs up in the lungs, causing fluids to seep into lung spaces.

Causes. The many causes of this condition include the following: congestive heart failure, myocardial infarction (heart attack), cardiomyopathy, heart valve disorders, lung infections, allergic reactions, smoke inhalation, drowning, various drugs such as narcotics and heroin, chest injuries, and high altitudes. This disorder may be prevented by avoiding high altitudes and smoking. Preventing heart disease may also reduce the chance of developing this disorder.

Signs and Symptoms. The symptoms of pulmonary edema are shortness of breath; difficulty breathing, especially when lying down (a condition known as *orthopnea*); a feeling of suffocating; wheezing; a productive cough that produces pink mucus; rapid weight gain; pallor; and profuse sweating, which is known as diaphoresis.

Treatment. Treatment includes oxygen therapy, diuretics to eliminate excess fluids, and morphine to reduce anxiety and shortness of breath.

PULMONARY EMBOLISM is a blocked artery in the lungs. Usually the artery is blocked by a blood clot that has traveled from a vein in the legs. If an artery in the lungs is completely blocked, death can occur quickly from resultant respiratory failure.

Causes. People at the highest risk of developing this condition are those who have had previous heart attacks, cancer, a fractured hip, or chronic lung diseases. Women who use birth control pills and individuals who have a pacemaker may be at risk for developing a pulmonary embolism. In addition, long periods of inactivity, increased levels of clotting factors in the blood (usually caused by certain cancers), injury to veins, or a stroke that causes paralysis of the arms or legs may cause this condition. A sedentary lifestyle as well as auto or airplane travel—or any activity that requires prolonged sitting or standing—are also major risk factors for developing a pulmonary embolism. A half-dose aspirin (formerly known as a baby aspirin) taken daily, as well as plenty of fluids and frequent movement of the arms and legs, may help prevent the development of a pulmonary embolism.

Signs and Symptoms. Symptoms include fainting, a sudden shortness of breath, hemoptysis (coughing up blood), wheezing, tachycardia (a rapid heartbeat), diaphoresis (profuse sweating), and chest pain that may spread to a shoulder, an arm, or the face.

Treatment. Support stockings can be used to promote circulation. The patient should rest until the blood clot has dissolved and may be prescribed thrombolytic (clot-dissolving) medications, such as TPA. Anticoagulants, typically warfarin, may be used to prevent new blood clots from forming in the deep veins of the body. Finally, a filter may be surgically implanted in the vena cava to prevent blood clots from reaching the lungs.

RESPIRATORY DISTRESS SYNDROME (RDS), which was formerly known as hyaline membrane disease, kills apparently healthy infants. At highest risk are newborns to infants 8 months of age, especially "preemies."

Causes. The etiology is unknown. The underlying problem is known to be a lack of surfactant in the lungs. Surfactant helps prevent the alveoli from totally collapsing on expiration. Without it, the alveoli collapse, resulting in poor oxygenation due to difficulty with reinflation of the alveoli.

Signs and Symptoms. RDS is usually diagnosed soon after birth, when the infant's breathing becomes rapid and shallow. The infant's nares flare, and the accessory muscles are used to aid in respiration. The infant will also exhibit "grunting" noises in an attempt to breathe.

Treatment. Treatment must be immediate, preferably in a neonatal intensive care unit (NICU). Oxygen therapy, an endotracheal tube, ventilator support, and artificial surfactant are all used in an attempt to keep the alveoli inflated. Infants who survive RDS may be at higher risk for respiratory infections later, but this threat lessens as their lungs continue to mature.

SEVERE ACUTE RESPIRATORY SYNDROME (SARS) is a respiratory disease that is very contagious and sometimes fatal. It was first identified in 2003.

Causes. SARS is caused by viruses associated with the common cold as well as by unknown viruses. It can be prevented by thoroughly washing the hands, wearing a mask, and avoiding exposure to individuals with this disease.

Signs and Symptoms. Signs and symptoms include fever or chills, headache, a dry cough, and muscle aches.

Treatment. Rest and antiviral drugs are the primary treatments.

SINUSITIS is an inflammation of the membranes lining the sinuses of the skull.

Causes. Bacteria, excess mucus production in the sinuses (often from the "common cold"), the blockage of sinus openings, and the destruction of cilia that move mucus out of sinuses can cause this disorder.

Signs and Symptoms. Fever, cough, headache, pharyngitis, facial pain, and nasal congestion are the common signs and symptoms.

Treatment. Treatment options include the use of nasal decongestants, nasal steroid sprays, a humidifier, applications of heat to the face, and antibiotics. Surgery to clear the sinuses or unblock sinus openings may be required.

SUDDEN INFANT DEATH SYNDROME (SIDS) claims the life of more than 7,000 babies a year in the United States. There are no characteristic signs or symptoms. Usually a baby with this disorder simply goes to sleep and never wakes up.

Causes. The causes of SIDS are unknown, but certain risk factors have been identified:

- Male babies are more likely to die of SIDS.
- Babies are most susceptible between the ages of 2 weeks and 6 months.
- Premature or low birth weight babies are more likely to have SIDS.
- A baby with a sibling who died of SIDS is more likely to also die of this disorder.
- African American or Native American babies are more likely to die of SIDS.
- Babies who were prenatally exposed to alcohol, cocaine, heroin, or nicotine are at a higher risk of developing SIDS.
- Babies who sleep on their stomachs are approximately three times more likely to die of SIDS.

Treatment. Proper sleep positioning on the baby's back is best for all infants, especially those known to be at risk, those with previous apneic episodes, and those who have lost a sibling to SIDS. At-risk infants may also be sent home with an apnea monitor that will sound an alarm if breathing ceases. Research into this disease is ongoing. Support groups are available and are suggested for families who have experienced the tragedy of losing a child to SIDS.

TUBERCULOSIS (TB) kills more than 2 million people worldwide each year. Although it primarily affects the lungs, it can spread to other parts of the body.

Causes. This disease is caused by various strains of the bacterium *Mycobacterium tuberculosis.* Widespread tuberculosis may be complicated by the following factors:

- HIV infection. HIV infection makes a person more vulnerable to TB.
- Crowded living conditions. This factor allows TB to spread easily; TB, therefore, is found in some prisons and homeless shelters.
- Poverty. Poverty prevents some patients with TB from seeking or completing therapy.
- Drug-resistant bacterium. Drug-resistant strains of the bacterium that causes TB have increased.
- Long-term therapy. Current treatments require antibiotic therapy for many months, which some patients with TB do not complete.

Signs and Symptoms. The symptoms include a cough that lasts more than 3 weeks, unintended weight loss, fever or chills, fatigue, night sweats, pain when breathing or difficulty breathing, and pain in other affected areas.

Treatment. The first step should be TB testing to detect carriers of this disease, who should then be treated. Therapy for TB normally lasts 6 months to a year, but drug-resistant cases of TB may require years of drug therapy. Isolating the patient during the contagious phase of the disease (usually 2 to 4 weeks after treatment begins) is required. Also, during the initial stages of treatment, the patient should be encouraged to receive adequate bed rest and maintain an adequate, nutritious diet.

UPPER RESPIRATORY (TRACT) INFECTION (URI) is the term often used for *coryza,* or the common cold.

Causes. URIs are caused by a family of viruses known as *rhinovirus.* The viruses are airborne and transmitted by contact with contaminated surfaces and on the hands. Children are frequent sources of transmission.

Signs and Symptoms. This is a generally self-limiting condition of approximately 1 week's duration, which follows an initial incubation period of 2 to 5 days. Symptoms include pharyngitis, nasal congestion, rhinitis, headache, fever, and general malaise. There may be a nonproductive cough, especially at night.

Treatment. Care is usually symptomatic and includes antipyretics, analgesics, decongestants, and cough suppressants. Adequate rest and plenty of fluids to flush the system are also helpful. Antibiotics are ordinarily only prescribed for patients with an underlying illness or complication.

SUMMARY OF LEARNING OUTCOMES

LEARNING OUTCOMES	KEY POINTS
28.1 Describe the structure and function of each organ in the respiratory system.	The function of the respiratory system is to move air into and out of the lungs in a process known as ventilation, respiration, or breathing. The larynx contains the vocal cords, which stretch between the thyroid and cricoid cartilages. The lungs contain connective tissue, the bronchial tree, nerves, lymphatic vessels, and blood vessels. The bronchial tree consists of the primary, secondary, and tertiary branches of the bronchi, the bronchioles, and the alveoli.
28.2 Describe the events involved in the inspiration and expiration of air.	During inspiration, the diaphragm contracts and the intercostal muscles raise the ribs, increasing the space in the thoracic cavity. This decreases the pressure within the cavity so that the air outside the body passively flows into the thoracic cavity. During expiration, the diaphragm relaxes, pushing up into the thoracic cavity, and the intercostal muscles lower the ribs, forcing the air to flow out of the body. Breathing is controlled by the respiratory center of the brain, located in the pons and medulla oblongata.
28.3 Explain how oxygen and carbon dioxide are transported in the blood.	Most of the oxygen in the bloodstream binds to the hemoglobin within red blood cells, resulting in oxyhemoglobin, although a small amount does not bind to hemoglobin and remains dissolved in the plasma. Carbon dioxide binds to hemoglobin, resulting in carboxyhemoglobin. Most of the carbon dioxide that enters the blood reacts with water in plasma and cerebrospinal fluid to form carbonic acid. As carbonic acid ionizes, it releases hydrogen and bicarbonate ions, which attach to hemoglobin making its way back to the lungs to be exhaled.

LEARNING OUTCOMES	KEY POINTS
28.4 Compare various respiratory volumes and tell how they are used to diagnose respiratory problems.	Respiratory volumes are measured to check the health of the respiratory system. The volumes are tidal volume, inspiratory and expiratory reserve volumes, residual volume, inspiratory capacity, functional residual capacity, vital capacity, and total lung capacity. The normal capacities are found in the chapter.
28.5 Describe the causes, signs and symptoms, and treatments of various diseases and disorders of the respiratory system.	There are many common diseases and disorders of the respiratory system with varied signs, symptoms, and treatments. Some of these include allergic rhinitis, asthma, atelectasis, bronchitis, chronic obstructive pulmonary disease (COPD), emphysema, influenza, laryngitis, Legionnaire's disease, lung cancer, pleural effusion, pleuritis, pneumoconiosis, pneumonia, pneumothorax, pulmonary edema, pulmonary embolism, respiratory distress syndrome (RDS), severe acute respiratory syndrome (SARS), sinusitis, sudden infant death syndrome (SIDS), tuberculosis (TB), and upper respiratory (tract) infection (URI).

CASE STUDY CRITICAL THINKING

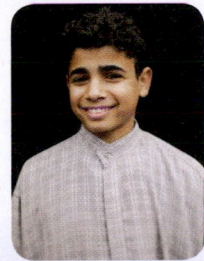

© David Sacks/Getty Images

Recall Mohammad from the beginning of the chapter. Now that you have completed the chapter, answer the following questions regarding his case.

1. Why is asthma considered a life-threatening condition?

2. Why did the doctor refer Mohammad for allergy testing?

3. In addition to the prescribed medication, what can Mohammad do to help reduce his symptoms?

EXAM PREPARATION QUESTIONS

1. (LO 28.1) Which of the following is/are known as the pulmonary parenchyma?
   a. Nares
   b. Bronchi
   c. Bronchioles
   d. Alveoli
   e. Larynx

2. (LO 28.2) What is responsible for raising and lowering the rib cage during respiration?
   a. Diaphragm
   b. Lungs
   c. Intercostal muscles
   d. Respiratory center
   e. Spinal cord

3. (LO 28.5) Lack of surfactant is responsible for which of the following in premature infants?
   a. SARS
   b. RDS
   c. COPD
   d. Pneumonia
   e. Asthma

4. (LO 28.1) Which structure covers the larynx during swallowing?
   a. Epiglottis
   b. Glottis
   c. Conchae
   d. Hyoid
   e. Uvula

5. (LO 28.5) Which condition is commonly known as a collapsed lung?
   a. Bronchitis
   b. Pleuritis
   c. Coryza
   d. Pneumonia
   e. Atelectasis

6. (LO 28.3) Most of the carbon dioxide in the blood remains in the plasma in which of the following forms?
   a. Carboxyhemoglobin
   b. Carbon monoxide
   c. Bicarbonate
   d. Carbonic acid
   e. Oxyhemoglobin

7. (LO 28.4) Which term refers to the total amount of air the lungs can hold?
   a. Total lung capacity
   b. Vital capacity
   c. Tidal volume
   d. Expiratory reserve volume
   e. Inspiratory reserve volume

8. (LO 28.2) Which of the following everyday occurrences alters our breathing patterns?
   a. Blinking
   b. Swallowing
   c. Yawning
   d. Watching TV
   e. Studying

9. (LO 28.5) The most common types of COPD are emphysema and which other disorder?
   a. Pleuritis
   b. Chronic bronchitis
   c. Asthma
   d. Pleural effusion
   e. Legionnaire's disease

10. (LO 28.2) Which of the following occurs during expiration?
    a. Air flows into the lungs
    b. The diaphragm contracts
    c. The diaphragm flattens
    d. The thoracic cavity enlarges
    e. The intercostal muscles lower the ribs

MEDICAL TERMINOLOGY PRACTICE

Analyze the following medical terms, presented throughout the chapter. Using a medical dictionary (or Appendix I) place a / mark between each word part. Define each word part and then define the whole word.

EXAMPLE: **pharyng / itis** = pharyng means "throat" + itis means "inflammation"
    PHARYNGITIS means "inflammation of the throat."

1. anthracosis
2. bronchitis
3. epiglottis
4. lobectomy

5. pneumothorax
6. pulmonary
7. pyothorax
8. rhinitis

9. thoracostomy
10. uvulotomy
11. costochrondritis
12. dyspnea

The Nervous System

CASE STUDY

Patient Name	DOB	Allergies
Nancy Evans	1/29/19XX	Amoxicillin

Attending	MRN	Other Information
Elizabeth H. Williams, MD	654-88-099	PET scan: Minor restrictions of blood flow in some areas MRI: WNL Lumbar puncture: WNL FH: Negative for Alzheimer's disease

In preparing for the patient interview, you check the chart and notice that at Nancy's previous visit, the physician ordered an MRI, a PET scan, and a lumbar puncture. She is here for a follow-up visit to find out the results of these tests. During the patient interview, you ask the patient her name and date of birth. She states, "I am Nancy Evans, I am Welsh, and I was born in January but I don't remember

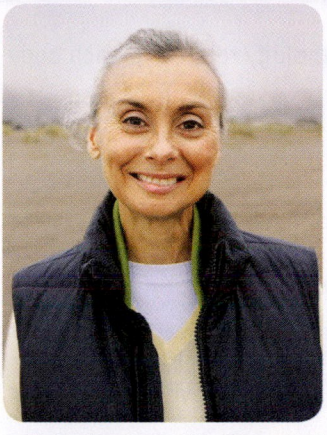

© John Lund/Sam Diephuis/Blend Images LLC RF

what year." You look at the chart and note that her name is Nancy Evans and she was born on January 29, 1945. Her husband is in the waiting room; after obtaining Nancy's permission, you ask him to come to the interview area. He confirms Nancy's complete name and date of birth and then states, "She seems to forget everything these days. I sure hope these tests last week will help you find out what is causing it."

Keep Nancy in mind as you study the chapter. There will be questions at the end of the chapter based on the case study. The information in the chapter will help you answer these questions.

LEARNING OUTCOMES

After completing Chapter 29, you will be able to:

29.1 Describe the general functions of the nervous system.

29.2 Summarize the structure of a neuron.

29.3 Explain the function of nerve impulses and the role of synapses in their transmission.

29.4 Describe the structures and functions of the central nervous system.

29.5 Compare the structures and functions of the somatic and autonomic nervous systems in the peripheral nervous system.

29.6 Recognize common tests that are performed to determine neurologic disorders.

29.7 Describe the causes, signs and symptoms, and treatments of various diseases and disorders of the nervous system.

KEY TERMS

afferent nerves

autonomic nervous system

axon

cell body

central nervous system (CNS)

cerebrospinal fluid (CSF)

dendrite

dermatome

efferent nerves

ganglia

interneurons

meninges

myelin sheath

neuroglia

neurotransmitter

parasympathetic branch

paresthesia

peripheral nervous system (PNS)

plexus

Schwann cells

somatic nervous system

sympathetic branch

synaptic knob

I.C.4 List major organs in each body system

I.C.5 Identify the anatomical location of major organs in each body system

I.C.6 Compare structure and function of the human body across the life span

I.C.7 Describe the normal function of each body system

I.C.8 Identify common pathology related to each body system including
    (a) signs
    (b) symptoms
    (c) etiology

I.C.9 Analyze pathology for each body system including:
    (a) diagnostic measures
    (b) treatment modalities

V.C.9 Identify medical terms labeling the word parts

V.C.10 Define medical terms and abbreviations related to all body systems

2. Anatomy & Physiology
  a. List all body systems, their structure and functions
  b. Describe common diseases, symptoms and etiologies as they apply to each system
  c. Identify diagnostic and treatment modalities as they relate to each system

3. Medical Terminology
  b. Build and dissect medical terms from roots/ suffixes to understand the word element combinations that create medical terminology
  c. Apply various medical terms for each specialty
  d. Define and use medical abbreviations when appropriate and acceptable

Introduction

The nervous system is highly complex. It controls all other organ systems and is important for maintaining balance within those systems. Disorders of the nervous system are often difficult to diagnose and treat because of this system's complexity.

General Functions of the Nervous System
LO 29.1

The nervous system is divided into two major parts—the **central nervous system (CNS)** and the **peripheral nervous system (PNS).** The CNS consists of the brain and the spinal cord; the peripheral nervous system consists of peripheral nerves, which are located throughout the rest of the body.

The peripheral nervous system is further divided into two separate sections: the **somatic nervous system,** which governs your body's skeletal (or voluntary) muscles, and the **autonomic nervous system,** which is in charge of your body's automatic functions, such as breathing and digesting food.

Three different types of nerve cells carry out the functions of the nervous system:

- **Afferent nerves**—sensory nerves responsible for detecting information from the environment or from inside the body and taking it to the CNS for interpretation

- **Efferent nerves**—motor nerves that take information or impulses from the CNS to the PNS to control the movement or action of a muscle or gland

- **Interneurons**—neurons in the brain and spinal cord that lie between the sensory and motor nerves and act as go-betweens, or interpreters, between the afferent and efferent nerves

An example of how the nervous system works would be noting a red light while driving. The afferent (sensory) neurons in your eyes note the color and send the information to the brain's cerebral cortex, where the interpretation takes place. The interneurons pick up the signal, interpret it, and send the information to the efferent (motor) neurons that you are supposed to stop your vehicle, which in turn sends the instructions to your right foot to step on the brake pedal of your vehicle. This entire transaction, of course, takes place in milliseconds, allowing you to stop in time.

The nervous system also includes a type of cell called *neuroglial cells,* or **neuroglia.** These cells do not transmit impulses. Instead, they function as support cells for neurons. (See Figure 29-1.) Neuroglial cells never lose their ability to divide. The three types of neuroglia are

- *Astrocytes*—star-shaped cells that anchor blood vessels to the nerve cells.

- *Microglia*—small cells that detect, engulf, and destroy invaders.

- *Oligodendrocytes*—cells that assist in the production of the myelin sheath, which will be discussed in further detail later.

Neuron Structure
LO 29.2

Neurons are the functional cells of the nervous system. They transmit electrochemical messages called *nerve impulses* to other neurons and *effectors* (muscles or glands). An important

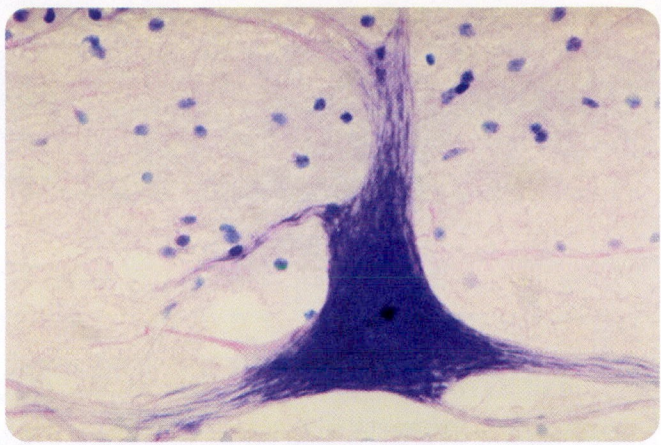

FIGURE 29-1 A typical neuron surrounded by neuroglial cells.
© Allen Bell/Corbis RF

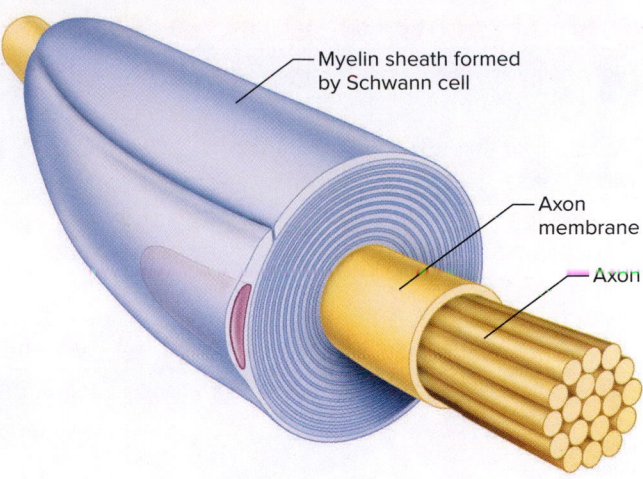

FIGURE 29-2 Schwann cells wrap around the axons of some neurons to create an insulating sheath that speeds up impulse transmission.

characteristic of neurons is that they lose their ability to divide. Therefore, when neurons are destroyed by disease, they cannot be replaced.

All neurons have a **cell body** and nerve fibers that extend from the cell body. The cell body is the portion of the neuron that contains the nucleus and the organelles typical of any cell. (Refer to the *Organization of the Body* chapter.) It is responsible for generating the large amount of protein and energy the neuron needs to carry out its functions.

Extending from the cell body are two types of nerve fibers: **axons** and **dendrites.** A neuron may have one or more dendrites but typically has only one axon. Dendrites are usually short and branch profusely near the cell body. Their function is to receive information for the neuron. Axons are typically long and branch profusely after they have extended far away from the cell body. Their function is to send information (nerve impulses) away from the cell body.

In the PNS, cells called **Schwann cells** wrap themselves around the axons of some of the neurons (see Figure 29-2). Schwann cells contain a large amount of myelin, a fatty substance that insulates the axons. This insulation, called a **myelin sheath,** allows nerve impulses to move more quickly through the axons.

▶ Nerve Impulse and Synapse LO 29.3

Neuron cell membranes have a *cell membrane potential.* This means the membrane is *polarized.* Just as a battery is polarized—one end is negative and the other end is positive—neuron cell membranes are polarized, because the inside is negatively charged and the outside is positively charged. This is true in most other types of body cells as well. The outside of cell membranes is positively charged because more positive ions are on the outside. The inside of cell membranes is negatively charged because more negative ions are on the inside. This membrane potential is very important for the function of neurons (see Figure 29-3).

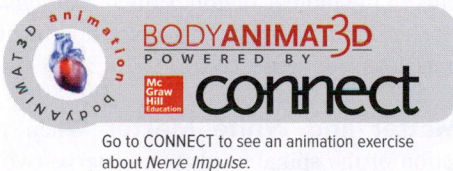

Go to CONNECT to see an animation exercise about *Nerve Impulse.*

Potassium and sodium ions are both positively charged and play important roles in generating nerve impulses. When a neuron is at rest or without stimulation, the outside of its membrane is relatively positive and the inside is relatively negative because the number of sodium and potassium ions is greater outside the membrane. As long as the neuron is at rest, it remains in this polarized state.

When a neuron detects a stimulus, such as heat or pressure, some of the sodium ions on the outside of the membrane move inside. This changes the polarization of the cell membrane, making the outside less positive and the inside more positive. There is now less difference between the inside and outside of the membrane, so it is said to be *depolarized.* The depolarization creates a nerve impulse, or electric current. The nerve impulse moves along the length of the axon as small areas along the axon become depolarized and then almost immediately repolarize, as shown in Figure 29-4. Repolarization begins when potassium moves outside the membrane, followed by sodium. Eventually, the potassium moves back inside the membrane and the cell is once again polarized (see Figure 29-3).

The speed of a nerve impulse depends on several factors. Myelinated axons conduct impulses faster than those that do not have a myelin sheath. The diameter of the axon also affects the speed of transmission. The larger the diameter, the faster the nerve impulse travels through the axon.

When traveling down an axon, a nerve impulse eventually reaches the **synaptic knob** at the end of the axon branches. Synaptic knobs contain small sacs called *vesicles* that produce chemicals called **neurotransmitters.** Neurotransmitters are released by the synaptic knob to transport the nerve impulse from the end of the axon to the dendrites of other neurons (see Figure 29-5). This allows the impulse to be conducted along a chain of neurons to reach its destination.

There are about 50 different neurotransmitters. In addition to helping transmit nerve impulses, many neurotransmitters perform other functions. These include causing muscles to contract or relax, causing glands to secrete products, activating

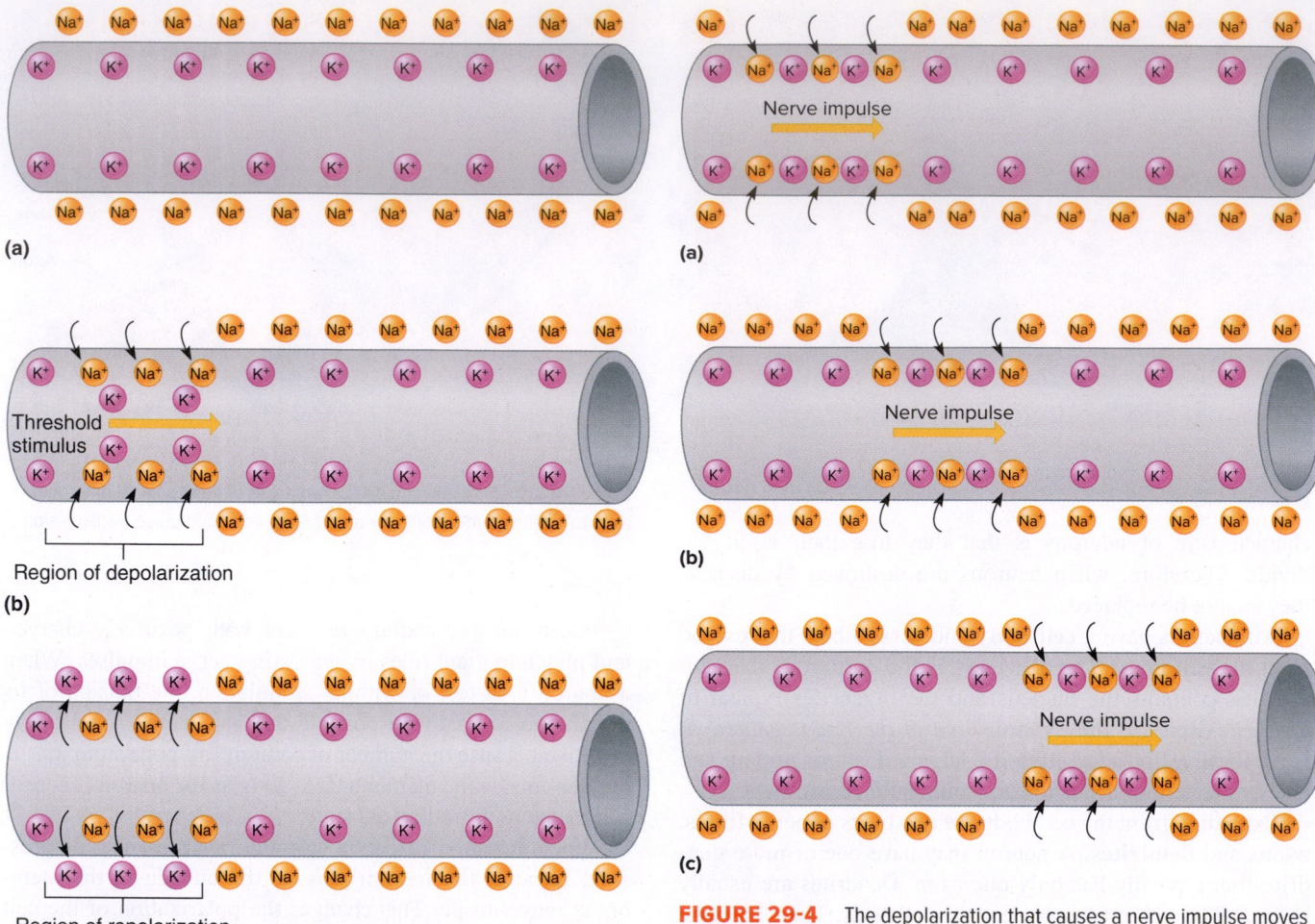

(a)

(b)

Region of depolarization

(c)

Region of repolarization

FIGURE 29-3 Nerve impulse: (a) At rest, or in its polarized state, more sodium (Na$^+$) is on the outside of the membrane, which makes the outside positive and the inside relatively negative (less positive). (b) When Na$^+$ moves into the cell, the membrane depolarizes, and the inside becomes more positive. (c) The membrane repolarizes when potassium (K$^+$) and later Na$^+$ move to the outside of the cell membrane.

neurons to send nerve impulses, and inhibiting neurons from sending nerve impulses.

Central Nervous System

LO 29.4

The CNS includes the spinal cord and brain (see Figure 29-6). The tissues of the CNS are so delicate that a *blood-brain barrier* and layers of membranes protect them. Tight capillaries form the blood-brain barrier, which prevents certain substances from entering the tissues of the CNS. For example, various waste products and drugs do not cross the blood-brain barrier well. Inflammation, however, can make this barrier more permeable.

Meninges are membranes that protect the brain and spinal cord. The three layers of meninges are dura mater, arachnoid mater, and pia mater. *Dura mater* is the toughest and outermost layer of the meninges. The space above the dura mater is called the *epidural space;* below the dura mater is the *subdural space.* The middle layer, named for its spider

(a)

Nerve impulse

(a)

Nerve impulse

(b)

Nerve impulse

(c)

FIGURE 29-4 The depolarization that causes a nerve impulse moves rapidly through the axon, with only a small portion of the axon depolarizing at a time. *Note:* For clarity, the repolarization process is not shown in this illustration.

web-like appearance, is the *arachnoid mater. Pia mater* is the innermost and most delicate layer. It sits directly on top of the brain and spinal cord and holds blood vessels onto the surface of these structures. Between the arachnoid mater and pia mater is an area called the *subarachnoid space.* It contains **cerebrospinal fluid (CSF),** sometimes referred to simply as *spinal fluid,* which cushions the CNS.

Spinal Cord

The spinal cord is a slender structure that is continuous with the brain. The spinal cord descends into the vertebral canal and ends around the level of the first or second lumbar vertebra. The spinal cord is divided into 31 spinal segments: 8 cervical segments, 12 thoracic segments, 5 lumbar segments, 5 sacral segments, and 1 coccygeal segment. The thickening of the spinal cord in the neck region is called the *cervical enlargement* and contains the motor neurons that control the arm muscles. Another thickening of the spinal cord occurs in the lumbar region. Called the *lumbar enlargement,* this thickening contains the motor neurons that control the leg muscles (see Figure 29-6).

Gray Matter and White Matter When you view a cross section of the spinal cord, you observe two differently

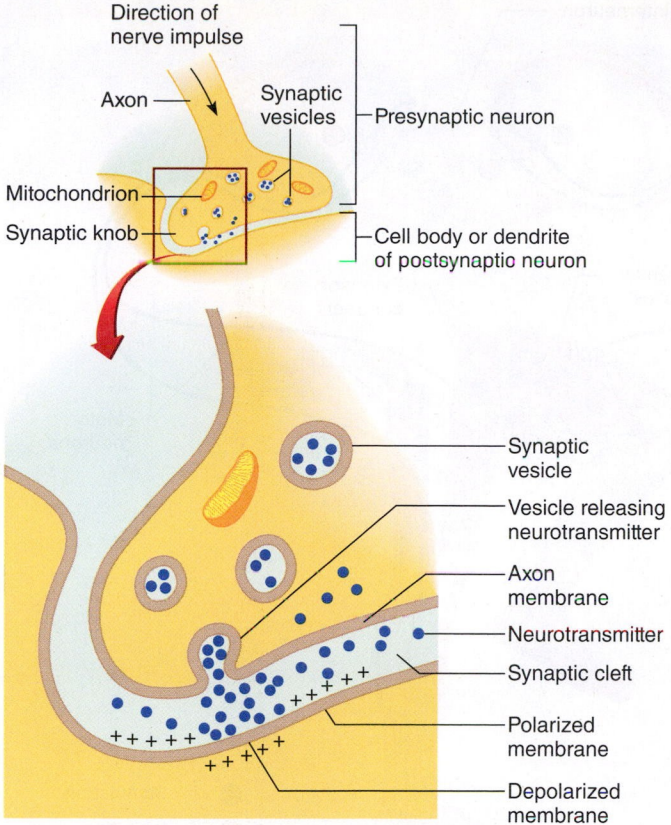

FIGURE 29-5 Synapse. When a nerve impulse reaches a synaptic knob, it releases a neurotransmitter that transports the impulse to the dendrites of the next neuron.

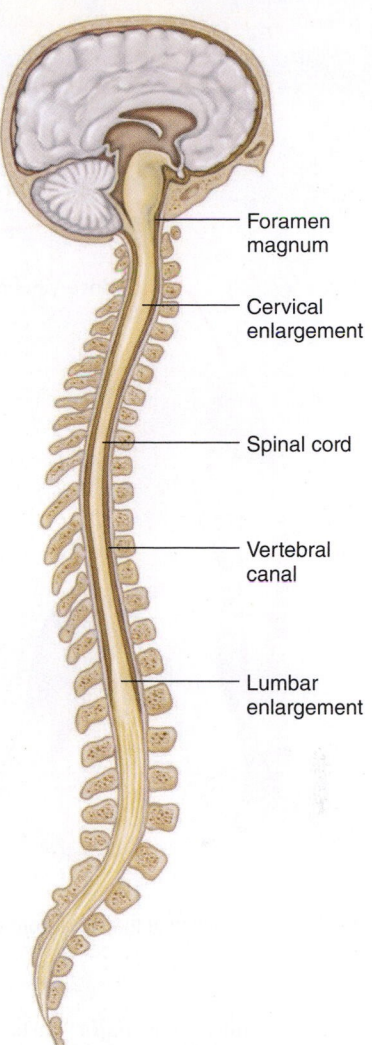

FIGURE 29-6 The central nervous system (CNS) consists of the brain and spinal cord. The spinal cord ends at the level of the third lumbar vertebra.

colored areas (see Figure 29-7). The inner tissue is termed *gray matter* because it is darker than the outer tissue, which is termed *white matter*. The white matter contains the myelinated axons of neurons. It is divided into columns that contain groups of axons called *nerve tracts*. The gray matter contains the neuron cell bodies and dendrites, as well as unmyelinated axons. A canal called the *central canal* contains CSF and runs through the center of the gray matter down the entire length of the spinal cord.

Ascending and Descending Tracts One function of the spinal cord is to carry sensory information up to the brain. The tracts that carry sensory information up to the brain are called *ascending tracts*. Another function of the spinal cord is to carry motor information down from the brain to muscles and glands in tracts called *descending tracts*.

Reflexes Another important function of the spinal cord is to provide reflexes. A *reflex* is a predictable, automatic response to a stimulus. For example, if you touch something hot, the predictable response is that you will pull your finger away from the hot surface in a withdrawal reflex. The information that flows through a typical reflex moves in the following order: from receptors to sensory neurons to interneurons to motor neurons to effectors. Figure 29-8 shows what happens in a typical reflex action. When a person steps on a tack, the receptors at the ends of the sensory neurons generate a nerve

impulse that travels through the sensory neurons directly to the interneurons in the spinal cord. The interneurons interpret the impulse and determine which muscles must be activated to remove the foot from the tack. They immediately trigger the motor neurons to act, inhibiting some muscle movements and stimulating others and coordinating the muscle movements to move the foot away from the painful stimulus.

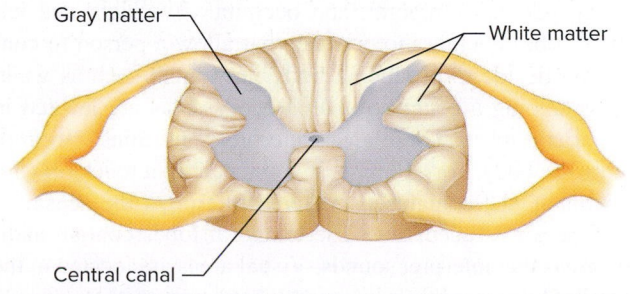

FIGURE 29-7 A cross section of the spinal cord shows the gray matter and the white matter that surrounds it. The central canal is located at the center of the spinal cord, in the gray matter.

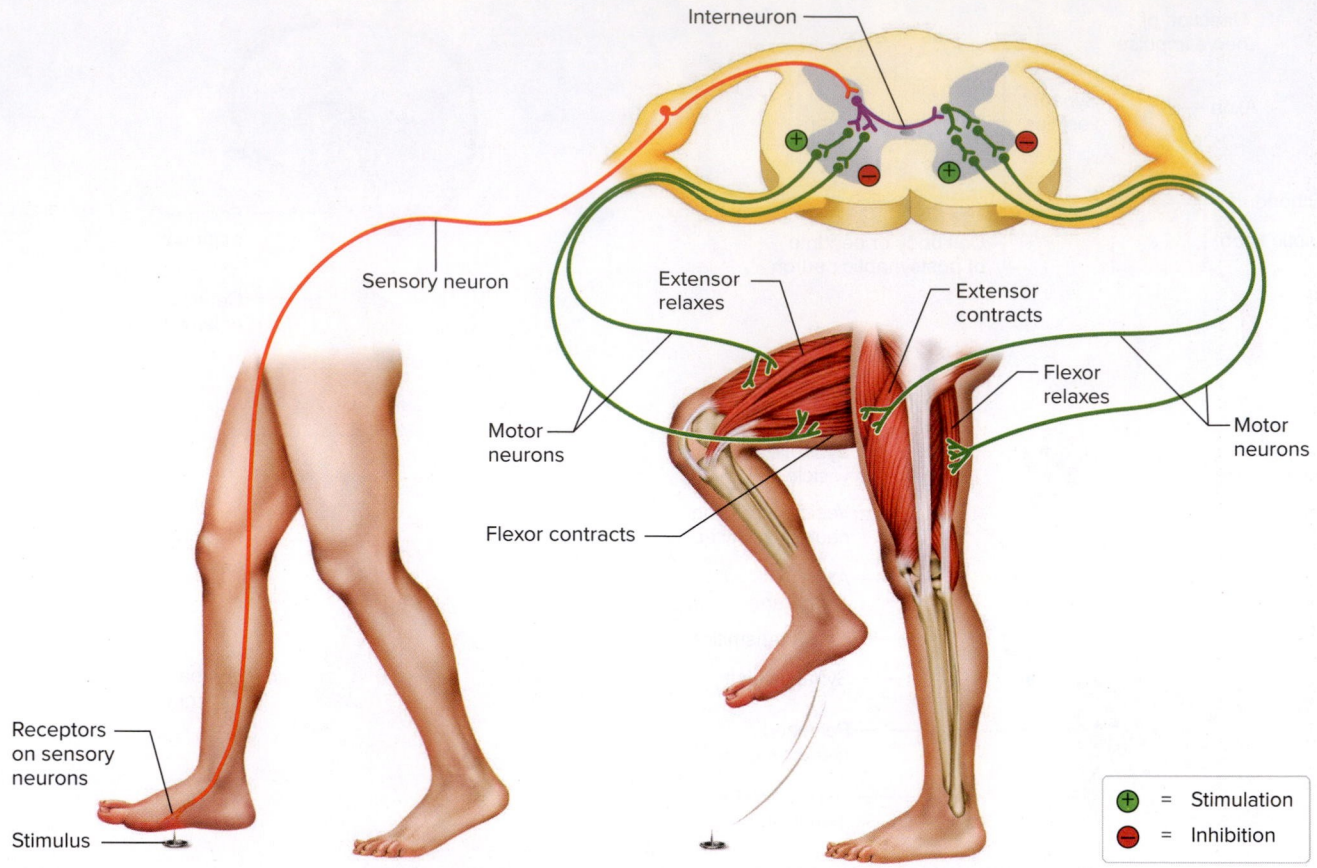

Interneuron

Sensory neuron

Extensor relaxes

Extensor contracts

Flexor relaxes

Motor neurons

Motor neurons

Flexor contracts

Receptors on sensory neurons

Stimulus

⊕ = Stimulation
⊖ = Inhibition

FIGURE 29-8   The cross section of the spinal cord and a spinal nerve illustrates a reflex arc.

Brain

The brain is divided into four major parts: the cerebrum, the diencephalon, the brainstem, and the cerebellum (see Figure 29-9).

Cerebrum The cerebrum is the largest part of the brain. It is divided into two halves called *cerebral hemispheres.* A thick bundle of nerve fibers called the *corpus callosum* connects the two hemispheres. The grooves on the surface of the cerebrum are called *sulci.* The "bumps" of brain matter between the sulci are called *gyri,* or convolutions. A deep groove called the *longitudinal* fissure runs between the two longitudinal hemispheres.

Lobes Each cerebral hemisphere is divided into *lobes*— frontal, parietal, temporal, and occipital. The right and left frontal lobes contain motor areas that allow a person to consciously decide to produce a body movement such as walking or tapping a pencil. Somatosensory areas are located in the parietal lobes. These areas interpret sensations felt on or within the body. For example, if you feel a light touch on your right hand, the somatosensory area interprets the sensation and where it is occurring. The temporal lobes contain auditory areas that interpret sounds. Visual areas are located in the occipital lobes, and they interpret what a person sees.

Cortex The outermost layer of the cerebrum is called the *cerebral cortex.* It is composed of gray matter and therefore contains neuron cell bodies and dendrites. This layer contains nearly 75% of all neurons in the entire nervous system. Beneath the cerebral cortex is white matter. Besides interpreting sensory information and initiating body movements, the cortex also stores memories and creates emotions.

Ventricles The *ventricles* are the cavities in the brain that produce cerebrospinal fluid (CSF). The two lateral ventricles are the largest and are located in the cerebrum (see Figure 29-10). The third ventricle is located in the diencephalon, and the fourth ventricle is located in the brainstem. All four ventricles are responsible for producing and circulating CSF to cushion and protect the brain and spinal cord. CSF also delivers nutrients to the brain and carries away wastes.

Diencephalon The *diencephalon* is located between the cerebral hemispheres and is superior to the brainstem. The diencephalon includes the thalamus and hypothalamus. The *thalamus* serves as a relay station for sensory information that heads to the cerebral cortex for interpretation. If sensory information does not pass through the thalamus before it reaches the cerebral cortex, it cannot be interpreted correctly. For example, say you are feeling pain in your left forearm. This information goes up the spinal cord and through the thalamus, and then to the cerebral cortex for interpretation. If the information did not go through the thalamus, the cerebral cortex might interpret that you are feeling cold instead of pain in your left forearm. The *hypothalamus* maintains homeostasis by

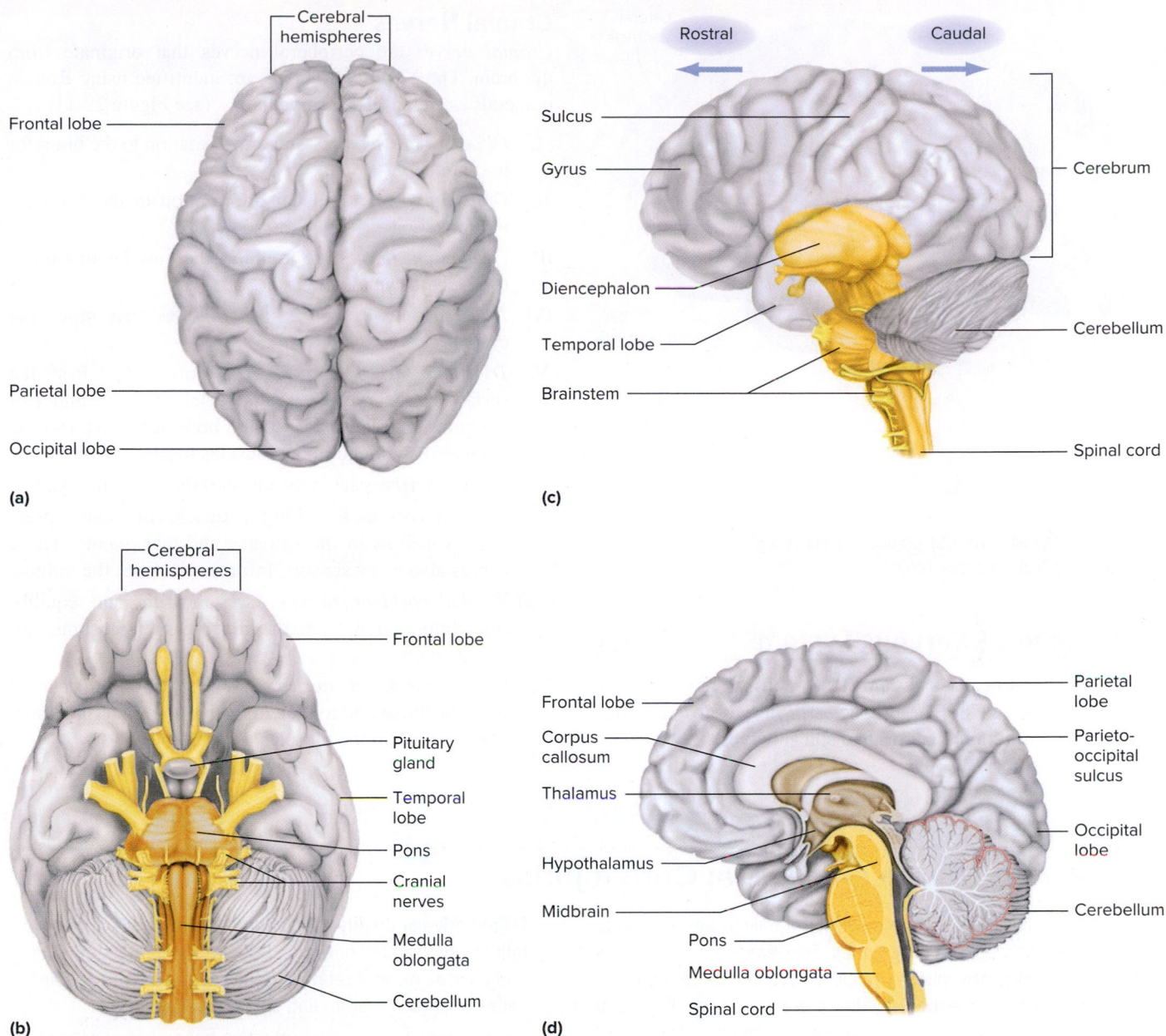

FIGURE 29-9 Four views of the brain: (a) superior, (b) inferior, (c) left lateral, and (d) sagittal section.

regulating hunger, thirst, and body temperature. It also provides a link between the nervous system and the endocrine system.

Brainstem The *brainstem* is a structure that connects the cerebrum to the spinal cord. The three parts of the brainstem are the midbrain, the pons, and the medulla oblongata. The *midbrain* lies just beneath the diencephalon. It controls both visual and auditory reflexes. Seeing something in your peripheral vision and automatically turning your head to view it more clearly is an example of a visual reflex.

The *pons* is a rounded bulge on the underside of the brainstem between the midbrain and the medulla oblongata. It contains nerve tracts to connect the cerebrum to the cerebellum. The pons also regulates respiration.

The *medulla oblongata* is the most inferior portion of the brainstem and is directly connected to the spinal cord. It controls many vital activities such as heart rate, blood pressure, and respiration. It also controls reflexes associated with coughing, sneezing, and vomiting.

Cerebellum The cerebellum is inferior to the occipital lobes of the cerebrum and posterior to the pons and medulla oblongata. It coordinates the complex skeletal muscle contractions needed for body movements. For example, when you walk, many muscles have to contract and relax at appropriate times. Your cerebellum coordinates these activities. The cerebellum also coordinates fine movements such as threading a needle, playing an instrument, and writing.

Maintaining the health of the central nervous system is vital. See the feature *Educating the Patient* for more information on preventing brain and spinal cord injuries.

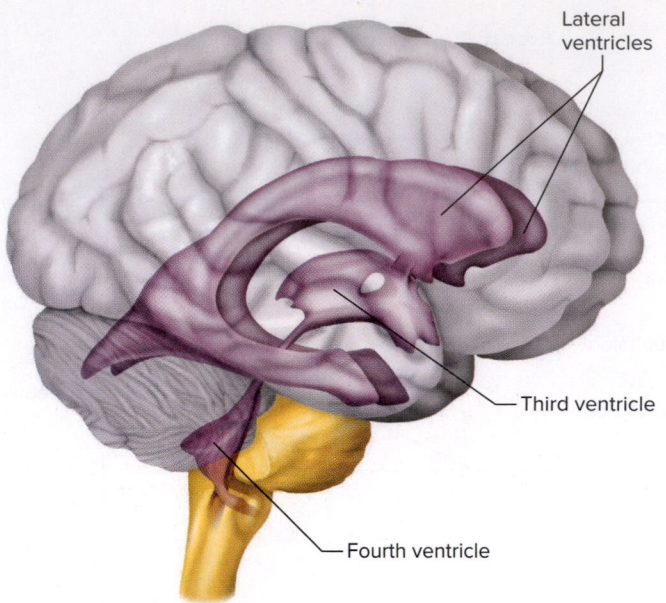

Lateral
ventricles

Third ventricle

Fourth ventricle

FIGURE 29-10   The CSF produced in the ventricles cushions and protects the brain and spinal cord.

▶ Peripheral Nervous System   LO 29.5

The peripheral nervous system (PNS) consists of nerves that branch off the CNS. These *peripheral nerves* are classified into two types: cranial nerves and spinal nerves.

Cranial Nerves

Cranial nerves are peripheral nerves that originate from the brain. The 12 cranial nerves are identified using Roman numerals as well as descriptive names (see Figure 29-11):

I.   *Olfactory nerves* carry smell information to the brain for interpretation.

II. *Optic nerves* carry visual information to the brain for interpretation.

III. *Oculomotor nerves* are found in the muscles that move the eyeball, eyelid, and iris.

IV. *Trochlear nerves* act in the muscles that move the eyeball.

V.   *Trigeminal nerves* carry sensory information from the surface of the eye, the scalp, facial skin, the lining of the gums, and the palate to the brain for interpretation. They also are found in the muscles needed for chewing.

VI. *Abducens nerves* act in the muscles that move the eyeball.

VII. *Facial nerves* are found in the muscles of facial expression as well as in the salivary and tear glands. These nerves also carry sensory information from the tongue.

VIII. *Vestibulocochlear nerves* carry hearing and equilibrium information from the inner ear to the brain for interpretation.

IX. *Glossopharyngeal nerves* carry sensory information from the throat and tongue to the brain for interpretation. They also act in the muscles of the throat.

EDUCATING THE PATIENT

Preventing Brain and Spinal Cord Injuries

In the United States alone, almost half a million people a year suffer brain and spinal cord injuries. The most common causes of these injuries are motor vehicle accidents, sports and recreational accidents—especially diving—and violence. People at the highest risk for spinal cord injuries are children and teens. However, most brain and spinal cord injuries can be prevented. Use the following tips to educate patients on preventing these types of injuries.

Prevention Tips

•   Buy and use approved head gear or a helmet when riding a bike or motorcycle, or doing any sporting activity in which you might fall such as horse riding or skateboarding. Your risk of brain injury is 85% greater during a biking accident if you are not wearing a helmet. Make sure your helmet fits properly. Replace your helmet if you have hit your head while wearing it; the helmet may be compromised from the fall and thus unsafe.

•   Know the depth of water into which you are diving. More than 90% of diving injuries occur in 5 feet of water or less.

•   Explore diving areas before diving. For example, know where rocks are located before you dive.

•   Do not drive or do any recreational activity while under the influence of alcohol or drugs. Both affect good judgment and control. Alcohol-related traffic crashes are the leading cause of disabling brain and spinal cord injuries.

•   Always wear appropriate protective gear while playing any sport.

•   Always wear your safety belt in the car.

•   Make sure children use car seats appropriate for their age and weight.

•   Be familiar with ways to get help quickly in emergencies.

•   Follow traffic rules and signs while walking, biking, or driving.

•   Follow safety rules posted on playgrounds, swimming pools, public beaches, and parks.

•   Store firearms and ammunition in separate and locked places.

•   Teach children the safety rules to follow if they find a gun.

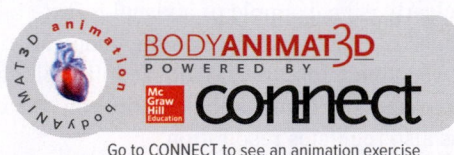

Go to CONNECT to see an animation exercise about *Spinal Cord Injury.*

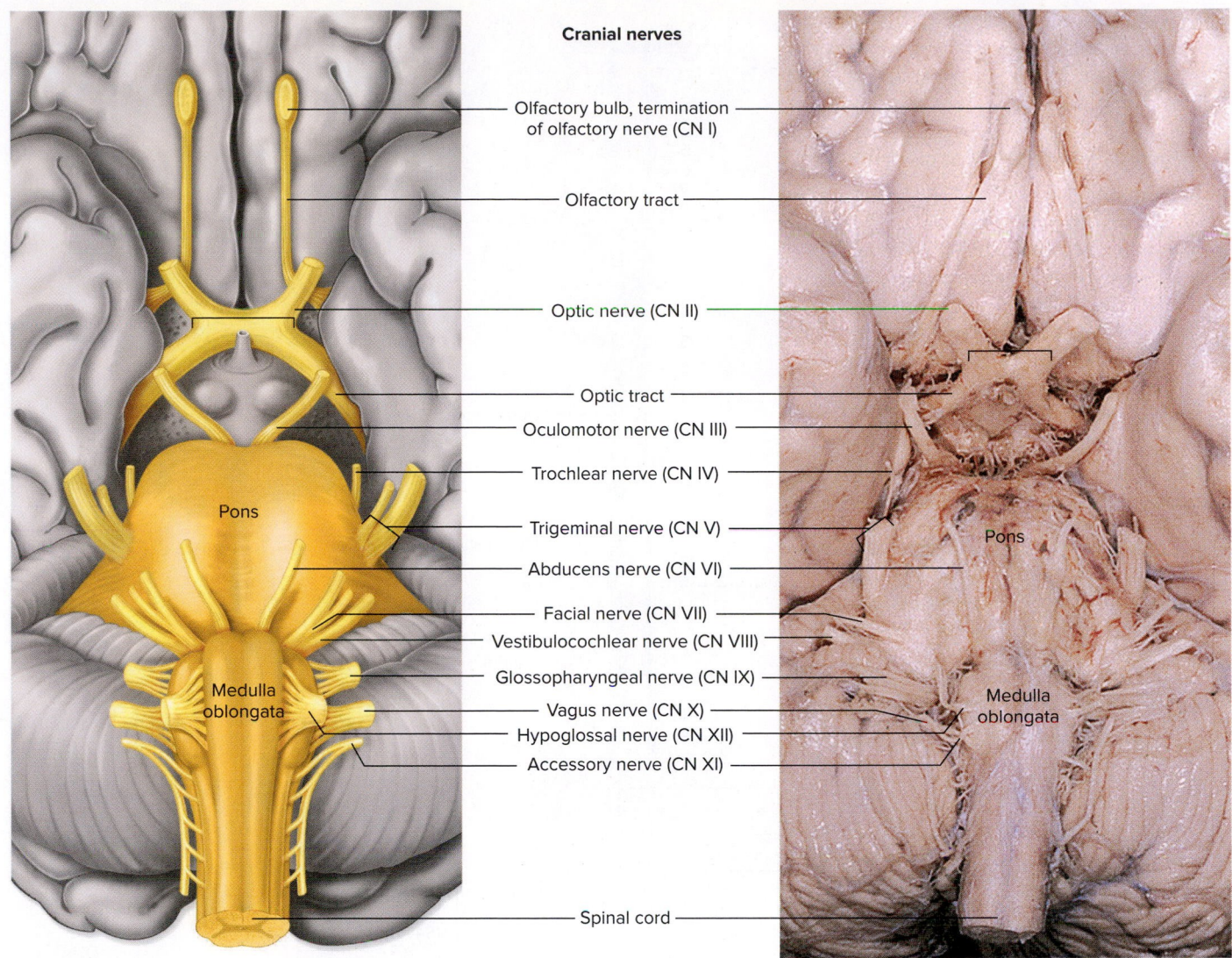

Cranial nerves

- Olfactory bulb, termination of olfactory nerve (CN I)
- Olfactory tract
- Optic nerve (CN II)
- Optic tract
- Oculomotor nerve (CN III)
- Trochlear nerve (CN IV)
- Trigeminal nerve (CN V)
- Abducens nerve (CN VI)
- Facial nerve (CN VII)
- Vestibulocochlear nerve (CN VIII)
- Glossopharyngeal nerve (CN IX)
- Vagus nerve (CN X)
- Hypoglossal nerve (CN XII)
- Accessory nerve (CN XI)
- Spinal cord

Pons

Medulla oblongata

FIGURE 29-11 A view of the inferior surface of the brain shows the 12 pairs of cranial nerves.
© McGraw-Hill Education/Rebecca Gray, photographer/Don Kincaid, dissections

X. *Vagus nerves* carry sensory information from the thoracic and abdominal organs to the brain for interpretation. These nerves are also found in the muscles in the throat, stomach, intestines, and heart.

XI. *Accessory nerves* are found in the muscles of the throat, neck, back, and larynx.

XII. *Hypoglossal nerves* are found in the muscles of the tongue.

Spinal Nerves

Spinal nerves are peripheral nerves that originate from the spinal cord (see Figure 29-12). There are 31 pairs of spinal nerves: 8 pairs of cervical nerves (numbered C1 through C8), 12 pairs of thoracic nerves (numbered T1 through T12), 5 pairs of lumbar nerves (numbered L1 through L5), 5 pairs of sacral nerves (numbered S1 through S5), and 1 pair of coccygeal nerves (Cx). Except for C1, each spinal nerve innervates a skin segment known as a **dermatome.** A map of the dermatomes with the spinal nerve responsible for the skin area is shown in Figure 29-13.

The spinal nerves are formed from two roots, or nerve fibers. The ventral, or anterior, root consists of efferent (motor) nerve fibers. The dorsal, or posterior, root consists of afferent (sensory) nerve fibers. Because these two roots combine to form the spinal nerves, these nerves can carry both sensory and motor information.

Except in the thoracic region, the main portions of spinal nerves fuse together to form complex networks called nerve **plexuses.** The major nerve plexuses are the cervical, brachial, and lumbosacral plexuses. Nerves coming off the cervical plexus supply the skin and the muscles of the neck. The phrenic nerve also originates from the cervical plexus. This nerve controls the diaphragm, which is a muscle needed for breathing.

The brachial plexus includes nerves that control muscles in the arms. The lumbosacral plexus supplies the lower abdominal wall, external genitalia, buttocks, thighs, legs, and feet. The largest nerve of the body, the sciatic nerve, originates from this plexus. This nerve controls the leg muscles. The coccygeal plexus is the source of the anococcygeal nerve, which controls the muscles in the anus and the back of the thighs.

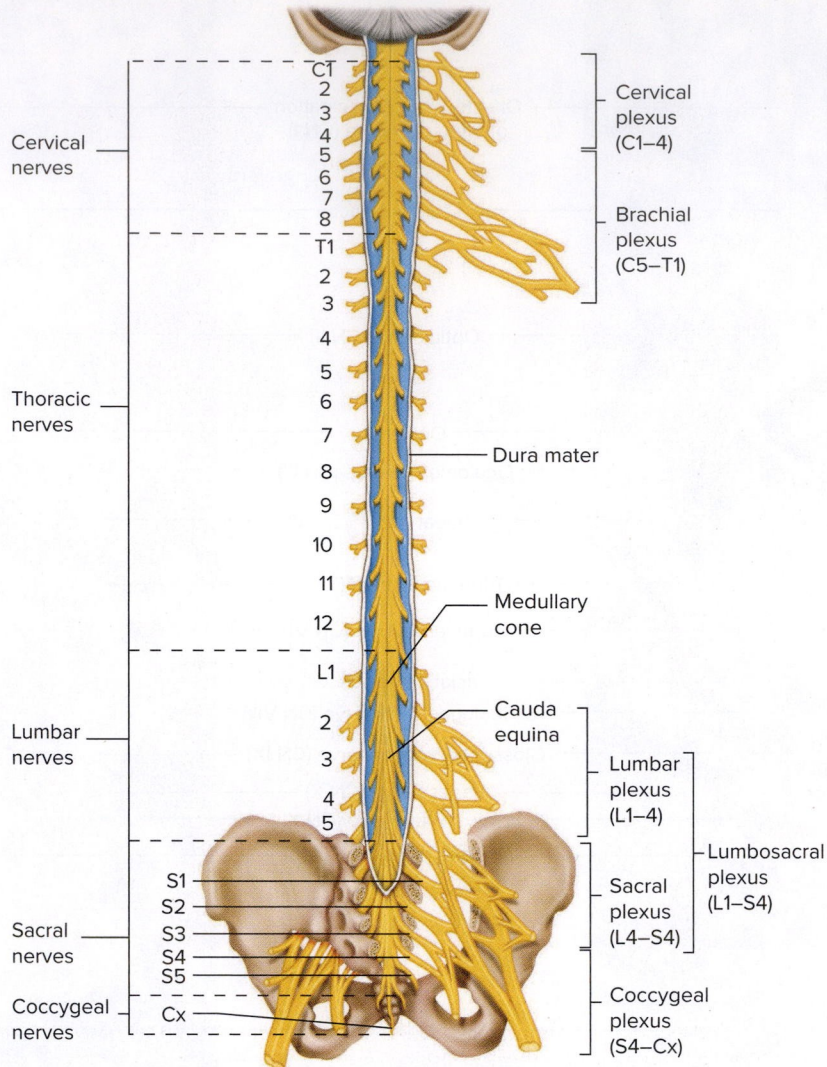

Cervical
nerves

Thoracic
nerves

Lumbar
nerves

Sacral
nerves

Coccygeal
nerves

C1
2
3
4
5
6
7
8
T1
2
3
4
5
6
7
8
9
10
11
12
L1
2
3
4
5
S1
S2
S3
S4
S5
Cx

Cervical
plexus
(C1–4)

Brachial
plexus
(C5–T1)

Dura mater

Medullary
cone

Cauda
equina

Lumbar
plexus
(L1–4)

Sacral
plexus
(L4–S4)

Coccygeal
plexus
(S4–Cx)

Lumbosacral
plexus
(L1–S4)

FIGURE 29-12   Spinal cord, spinal nerves, and plexuses.

Somatic and Autonomic Nervous Systems

The peripheral nervous system contains two subparts: the somatic nervous system (SNS) and the autonomic nervous system (ANS). The somatic nervous system consists of nerves that connect the central nervous system (CNS) to skin and skeletal muscle. Because it controls the skeletal muscles, which are under a person's direct (voluntary) control, this system is sometimes called the "voluntary" nervous system. The autonomic nervous system connects the central nervous system to body organs such as the heart, stomach, intestines, and bladder, as well as glands and blood vessels. Because these organs are not under a person's voluntary (direct) control, the autonomic nervous system is sometimes referred to as the "involuntary" nervous system.

In the autonomic nervous system, motor neurons from the brain and spinal cord communicate to other motor neurons located in ganglia. **Ganglia** are collections of neuron cell bodies outside the CNS. The motor neurons of ganglia then communicate to various organs and blood vessels.

The autonomic nervous system is further divided into the sympathetic and parasympathetic branches (see Figure 29-14). The **sympathetic branch** responds to stressful or emergency situations by increasing the heart rate. This is often called the "fight-or-flight" response because it increases blood flow throughout the body in preparation for immediate action. Most sympathetic neurons release the neurotransmitter norepinephrine into organs and glands. Norepinephrine increases heart and breathing rates; slows down the activity of the digestive glands, stomach muscles, and intestines; and dilates the pupils. It also constricts the blood vessels, increasing the blood pressure, which is a needed response during an emergency situation.

The **parasympathetic branch** of the autonomic nervous system does just the opposite. It keeps the heart rate relatively low, preparing the body for resting and digesting nutrients. Most of the body's organs are under parasympathetic control. All parasympathetic neurons release the neurotransmitter acetylcholine to organs and glands. Acetylcholine has

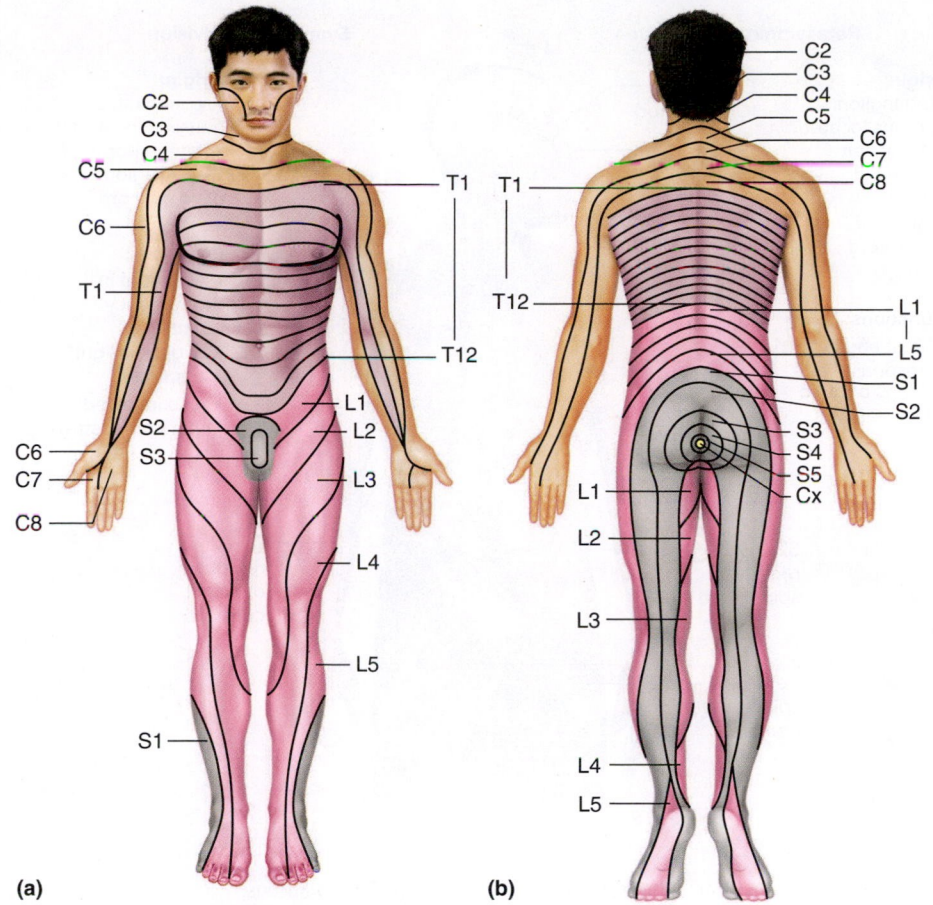

FIGURE 29-13 Dermatome maps. A dermatome is an area of skin supplied by a single spinal nerve. These diagrams only approximate the dermatomal distribution.

the opposite effect from norepinephrine. It slows the heart and breathing rates; activates the digestive glands, stomach muscles, and intestines; and constricts the pupils. It has little effect on the blood vessels, however, because most blood vessels do not receive input from the parasympathetic nerves.

▶ Neurologic Testing

LO 29.6

Patients with nervous system disorders may have a wide variety of signs and symptoms, but the most common are headache, muscle weakness, and **paresthesia** (loss of feeling). A typical neurologic examination can determine the following:

- State of consciousness. This state can vary from normal to a state of coma. A patient in a coma cannot respond to stimuli and cannot be awakened. Other terms used to describe states of consciousness include *stupor* (difficulty being awakened), *delirium* (loss of function of the cerebral cortex), *vegetative* (having no cortical function), and *asleep* (can be aroused with normal stimulation).
- Reflex activity. Reflex tests primarily determine the health of the peripheral nervous system.

- Speech patterns. Abnormal speech patterns include a loss of the ability to form words correctly or to form sentences that make sense.
- Motor patterns. Abnormal motor patterns include the loss of balance, abnormal posture, and inappropriate, involuntary movements of the body. For example, chorea is an exaggerated and sudden jerking of a body part.

Diagnostic Procedures

Common diagnostic procedures to determine neurologic disorders include the following tests:

- Lumbar puncture (spinal tap). When a physician needs to examine cerebrospinal fluid (CSF), a lumbar puncture is performed. A needle is used to remove CSF from the subarachnoid space, usually below the third lumbar vertebra of the spinal column. Analysis of this fluid provides a great deal of information about the patient's health. For example, cancer cells in CSF often indicate a brain tumor or spinal cord tumor. White blood cells in this fluid indicate infections such as meningitis. Red blood cells indicate abnormal bleeding.

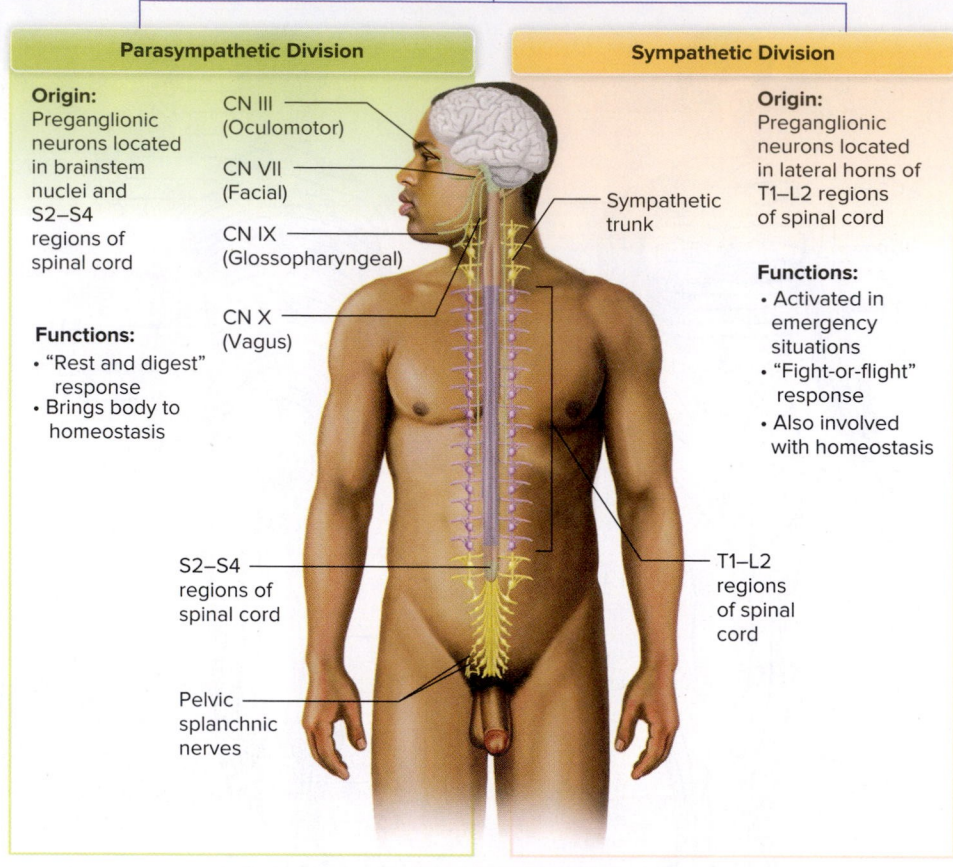

FIGURE 29-14 Comparison of the parasympathetic and sympathetic branches.

- Magnetic resonance imaging (MRI). This procedure allows the brain and spinal cord to be visualized from many angles. It uses powerful magnets to generate images and is useful in detecting tumors, bleeding, and other abnormalities.

- Positron emission tomography (PET) scan. This procedure uses radioactive chemicals that collect in specific areas of the brain. These chemicals allow images of those areas to be generated. This test is useful in detecting brain tumors, checking blood flow to different areas of the brain, and diagnosing diseases such as Parkinson's and Alzheimer's.

- Cerebral angiography. This procedure uses contrast material that can be visualized in the blood vessels of the brain. It is useful in detecting aneurysms (abnormal, blood-filled bulges in blood vessels).

- Computerized tomography (CT) scan. This procedure produces images that provide more information than a standard X-ray. It is useful in detecting tumors, abnormal structures, and bleeding.

- Electroencephalogram (EEG). This test detects electrical activity in the brain. It is useful in diagnosing various states of consciousness.

- X-ray. This procedure is useful in detecting skull or vertebral fractures.

Cranial Nerve Tests

Disorders of the cranial nerves can be determined using the following tests:

- The olfactory nerves (I) are tested by asking a patient to smell various substances.

- Cranial nerves III, IV, and VI are tested by asking a patient to track the movement of the physician's finger. If a patient cannot move her eyeballs properly, there may be damage to one of these nerves. Recall that these nerves control the muscles that move the eyeballs.

- Cranial nerve V controls the muscles needed for chewing. To assess this nerve, a patient is asked to clench his teeth. The physician then feels the jaw muscles. If the muscles feel limp or weak, this nerve may be damaged.

- If a person can no longer make facial expressions, then cranial nerve VII may be damaged. This nerve controls the muscles needed to make facial expressions.

- If a patient cannot extend his tongue and move it from side to side, cranial nerve XII may be damaged. This nerve controls tongue movement.

Reflex Testing

Testing a patient's reflexes allows a physician to evaluate the components of a reflex as well as the overall health of the individual's nervous system. The absence of a reflex is called *areflexia*. *Hyporeflexia* is a decreased reflex, and *hyperreflexia* is a stronger than normal reflex. The following are common reflex tests:

- Biceps reflex. The absence of this reflex may indicate spinal cord damage in the cervical region.
- Knee reflex. The absence of this reflex may indicate damage to lumbar or femoral nerves.
- Abdominal reflexes. These reflexes are tested to evaluate damage to thoracic spinal nerves.

PATHOPHYSIOLOGY

LO 29.7

Common Diseases and Disorders of the Nervous System

ALZHEIMER'S DISEASE is a progressive, degenerative disease that occurs in the brain.

Causes. Fiber tangles within neurons, degenerating nerve fibers, and a decreased production of neurotransmitters cause the symptoms of this disorder. Alzheimer's is associated with advanced age, family history, certain genes, and possibly some environmental factors. Many causes have not yet been determined.

Signs and Symptoms. Common symptoms include memory loss, confusion, personality changes, language deterioration, impaired judgment, and restlessness.

Treatment. There is no cure, but with medications such as Aricept®, Cognex®, Razadyne®, and Namenda®, as well as proper nutrition, physical exercise, social activity, and calm environments, the disease progress may be slowed and managed.

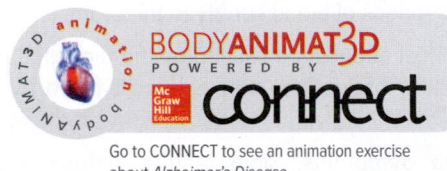

Go to CONNECT to see an animation exercise about *Alzheimer's Disease*.

AMYOTROPHIC LATERAL SCLEROSIS (ALS), commonly known as Lou Gehrig's disease, is a fatal disorder characterized by the degeneration of neurons in the spinal cord and brain.

Causes. Most causes are unknown, but researchers suspect that they involve hereditary and environmental factors.

Signs and Symptoms. Early symptoms include cramping of hand and feet muscles, persistent tripping and falling, chronic fatigue, and slurred speech. Signs and symptoms that appear in later stages include breathing difficulty and muscle paralysis.

Treatment. There is no cure for this disorder; however, physical, speech, and respiratory therapies help to manage the symptoms. Some medications relieve muscle cramping, but currently only the drug riluzole is approved by the US Food and Drug Administration (FDA) specifically for ALS.

BELL'S PALSY is a disorder in which facial muscles are very weak or totally paralyzed.

Causes. This condition can result from damage to cranial nerve VII (the facial nerve), but many times the cause is unknown. It is more common in people with diabetes, the flu, or a cold.

Signs and Symptoms. The most common signs and symptoms are a loss of feeling in the face, the inability to produce facial expressions, headache, and excessive tearing or drooling.

Treatment. Treatments include the use of eyedrops, anti-inflammatory medications, and pain relievers. Symptoms usually diminish or go away within 5 to 10 days.

BRAIN TUMORS AND CANCERS are abnormal growths in the brain. A brain tumor with cancer cells is termed malignant. Malignant tumors that start in any tissue of the brain are called primary brain cancers. Those that start in other body parts and spread to the brain are classified as secondary brain cancers. The most common primary brain tumors are *gliomas* that arise from neuroglial cells.

Causes. Like most cancers, the causes are gene mutations. Factors associated with gene mutations include exposure to toxins, an impaired immune system, and hereditary factors.

Signs and Symptoms. The signs and symptoms depend on the size and location of the tumor. Common symptoms include headache, seizures, nausea, weakness in the arms or legs, fatigue, changes in speech patterns, and a loss of memory.

Treatment. Treatment options include surgery, radiation therapy, chemotherapy, and gene therapy. The success of the treatment depends on the type of tumor, the location and extent of the tumor, the tumor's response to treatment, and the patient's overall health.

EPILEPSY AND SEIZURES occur when parts of the brain receive a burst of electrical signals that disrupt normal brain functioning. Seizures may be either petit mal (partial) or grand mal (generalized). Petit mal seizures may appear as loss of awareness of the present, whereas grand mal seizures result in the classic tonic-clonic seizure, in which the person becomes unconscious and muscles twitch sporadically. Epilepsy is the condition of having repeated seizures over a long period of time.

Causes. Causes vary but may include birth trauma, high fevers, alcohol and drug withdrawal, head trauma, infections, brain tumors, and certain medications. Many causes are unknown.

Signs and Symptoms. The signs and symptoms may include visual disturbances, nausea, generalized abnormal feelings, a loss of consciousness, and uncontrolled muscle contractions and tremors.

Treatment. The primary treatment is medication to prevent seizures. Surgery is sometimes an option in patients with partial seizures.

GUILLAIN-BARRÉ SYNDROME is a disorder in which the body's immune system attacks part of the peripheral nervous system. It usually has a sudden and unexpected onset.

Causes. The destruction of myelin by the body's immune system produces the signs and symptoms. Viral infections, immunizations, and pregnancy sometimes trigger the disease.

Signs and Symptoms. Symptoms may include weakness or tingling sensations in the legs or arms that can progress to paralysis. Difficulty breathing and an abnormal heart rate are more dangerous signs and symptoms. The disease normally runs its course, and with proper medical treatment, it is not fatal.

Treatment. Various supportive therapies, such as the use of respirators and heart machines, are necessary until the disease subsides. Physical therapy is used to keep muscles strong.

MENINGITIS is an inflammation of the meninges.

Causes. Causes include bacterial, viral, and fungal infections. Some types of meningitis can be prevented with vaccines.

Signs and Symptoms. Fever, headache, vomiting, stiffness in the neck, sensitivity to light, drowsiness, and joint pain usually accompany this disorder.

Treatment. The treatment varies depending on the type of meningitis. Intravenous antibiotics are used for bacterial meningitis, supportive therapy for viral meningitis, and antifungal drugs for fungal meningitis. Bacterial meningitis can be fatal.

MULTIPLE SCLEROSIS (MS) is a chronic disease of the central nervous system in which myelin is destroyed.

Causes. The causes are mostly unknown, but some known causes are viruses, genetic factors, and immune system abnormalities.

Signs and Symptoms. Depending on the type of MS, symptoms can range from mild to severe. In severe cases, a person loses the ability to walk or speak.

Treatment. There is no cure for MS, but supportive treatments may lessen the symptoms. Some medications, including interferon, Copaxone®, prednisone, and Solu-Medrol®, are available to treat and slow the progression of symptoms.

NEURALGIAS are a group of disorders commonly referred to as nerve pain. They most frequently occur in the nerves of the face.

Causes. There are many causes of neuralgia, including trauma, chemical irritation of the nerves, bacterial infections, and diabetes. Many times the causes are unknown.

Signs and Symptoms. Sudden and severe skin pain is the most common symptom. The pain occurs repeatedly in the same body area. Numbness of skin areas is also common.

Treatment. Many times the disorder goes away spontaneously, and treatment, other than pain medication, is not needed. Other treatments include injections of anesthetics or surgery to remove the affected nerves.

PARKINSON'S DISEASE is a motor system disorder. It is slowly progressive and degenerative.

Causes. Most causes are undetermined, although it is known that patients with this disease lack certain chemicals (neurotransmitters) in the brain. Brain tumors, certain drugs, carbon monoxide, or repeated head trauma may produce Parkinson's disease.

Signs and Symptoms. The most common signs and symptoms include tremor and stiffness of the arms and legs as well as a lack of coordination and balance. A mask face, where the patient shows little or no facial emotion, is also common, as is stooped posture with a shuffling gait.

Treatment. There is no cure, but medications such as dopamine, selegiline, and Symmetrel® alleviate some symptoms and slow the progression of this disease. Surgery is useful in some cases of Parkinson's.

SCIATICA occurs when the sciatic nerve is damaged.

Causes. The sciatic nerve is commonly damaged by excessive pressure on the nerve from prolonged sitting or lying down. It is also easily damaged from trauma to the pelvis, buttocks, or thighs.

Signs and Symptoms. The most usual symptoms include numbness, pain, or tingling sensations on the back of a leg or foot. Weakness of leg and foot muscles can also develop.

Treatment. This disorder is usually treated with pain and anti-inflammatory medication or steroids. Physical therapy is also needed following trauma to the nerve.

STROKE occurs when brain cells die because of an inadequate blood flow. The medical term is *cerebrovascular accident* (*CVA*). It is not uncommon for a stroke to be preceded by *transient ischemic attacks* (*TIAs*), or *"mini strokes,"* which are caused by brief interruptions of blood supply to the brain.

Causes. Most strokes are caused by the blockage of an artery in the neck or brain. They may also be caused by aneurysms that burst.

Signs and Symptoms. Signs and symptoms may include paralysis, speech problems, memory and reasoning deficits, coma, and possibly death. Symptoms vary depending on the location of the stroke within the brain.

Treatment. Because neurons in the brain cannot be replaced, the effects of a stroke can be permanent. However, physical, occupational, and speech therapy are often very useful in lessening the effects of a stroke.

HEADACHES

Headaches affect almost everyone at some point in life. A wide variety of factors produce headaches. Most headaches do not require medical attention, but a physician should evaluate repetitive and severe headaches. Headache types commonly include tension headaches, migraines, and cluster headaches.

EPISODIC TENSION *headaches* are the most common type of tension headache.

Causes. This type of headache is often the result of temporary stress or anger.

Signs and Symptoms. Symptoms include pain or soreness in the temples and the contraction of head and neck muscles.

Treatment. Most of these headaches can be managed by taking an over-the-counter (OTC) medicine, and relief usually occurs in 1 or 2 hours.

CHRONIC TENSION HEADACHES occur almost daily and persist for weeks or months.

Causes. This type of headache may be the result of stress or fatigue, but it may also be associated with physical problems, psychological issues, or depression.

Signs and Symptoms. As with episodic tension headaches, the symptoms include pain or soreness in the temples and the contraction of head and neck muscles.

Treatment. People who suffer from chronic headaches should seek medical treatment. Treatment may begin by identifying situations or actions that trigger the tension that causes the headaches and then developing healthy habits to remove the source of the tension. When this is not possible, or if the source of the headaches or tension is unknown, medications may be prescribed to prevent or relieve tension headaches.

MIGRAINES are the most severe type of headache. They are responsible for more "sick days" than any other headache type. Almost 30 million people in the United States suffer from migraines.

Causes. Hormones may influence migraines, which may explain why women experience migraines at least three times more often than men do. Migraines are considered vascular headaches because they are associated with the distension of the arteries of the brain.

Signs and Symptoms. Migraines often begin as dull pains that develop into throbbing pains accompanied by nausea and sensitivity to light and noise. There are many types of migraines, but the two most common classifications are migraine with aura and migraine without aura. Auras may include the appearance of jagged lines or flashing lights, tunnel vision, hallucinations, or the detection of strange odors. The auras may last up to an hour and usually go away as the headache begins. Most migraine headaches last about 4 hours, but some can last up to a week.

Treatment. When treating migraines, a physician may prescribe a drug to relieve the pain but also try to identify the factors that trigger it. Many medicines, both OTC and prescription, are available to prevent or treat migraines.

CLUSTER HEADACHES are so named because the attacks come in groups. More men than women experience these types of headaches.

Causes. Some research indicates that alcohol consumption can bring on attacks of cluster headaches.

Signs and Symptoms. Common symptoms include a runny nose, watery eyes, and swelling below the eyes. Cluster headaches normally last about 45 minutes to an hour, although they can last longer. It is common for a patient with this disorder to experience one to four headaches a day during a cluster time span. Cluster time spans can last weeks or months.

Treatment. One of the most effective treatments for cluster headaches is 100% oxygen administration. Several types of medications are available as well, including Imitrex® (which is also used for migraine headaches), as well as local anesthetics. Preventive treatments include verapamil and medications to reduce inflammation.

SUMMARY OF LEARNING OUTCOMES

LEARNING OUTCOMES	KEY POINTS
29.1 Describe the general functions of the nervous system.	The central nervous system (CNS) is composed of the brain and spinal cord. The peripheral nervous system (PNS) consists of the peripheral nerves located throughout the body. Three types of neurons carry out the functions of the nervous system: the afferent (sensory) nerves detect sensation or other stimuli from the body or environment and take it to the CNS for interpretation, the efferent (motor) nerves produce movement or other functions at the direction of the CNS, and the interneurons act as "interpreters" between the afferent and efferent nerves.
29.2 Summarize the structure of a neuron.	All neurons are composed of a cell body, the shorter and more numerous dendrites that receive information for the cell body, and the longer axons that take impulses from the cell body to the dendrite of the next neuron.

LEARNING OUTCOMES	KEY POINTS
29.3 Explain the function of nerve impulses and the role of synapses in their transmission.	Nerve impulses send information either from the central nervous system to the peripheral nervous system or vice versa. A synapse is the space between the axon of one neuron and the dendrite of the next. At the end of each axon is the synaptic knob, which contains vesicles that produce neurotransmitters. These are released by the synaptic knob to transmit the nerve impulse to the next neuron.
29.4 Describe the structures and functions of the central nervous system.	The brain consists of the cerebrum, diencephalon, brainstem, and cerebellum. The blood-brain barrier is a layer of tightly woven capillaries that protects the delicate brain tissues. The meninges are a triple-layered membrane protecting the brain and spinal cord. The spinal cord is continuous with the brain and consists of 31 spinal segments. The basic function of the spinal cord is to carry sensory information from the body to the brain and motor information from the brain to the muscles and glands of the body. Cerebrospinal fluid (CSF) is located within the subarachnoid space of the brain and within the central canal of the spinal cord. It cushions the brain and spinal cord.
29.5 Compare the structures and functions of the somatic and autonomic nervous systems in the peripheral nervous system.	The somatic nervous system connects the central nervous system to the skin and skeletal muscle (voluntary functions). The autonomic nervous system connects the CNS to the internal organs (involuntary functions). The autonomic nervous system is divided into the sympathetic branch, which prepares the body for "fight or flight" (stressful) situations, and the parasympathetic branch, which is the body's everyday "resting" system for normal situations.
29.6 Recognize common tests that are performed to determine neurologic disorders.	Tests commonly used to determine neurologic disorders include tests of the reflexes and cranial nerves, as well as diagnostic procedures such as lumbar puncture (spinal tap), MRI, PET, cerebral angiography, CT scan, EEG, and X-ray.
29.7 Describe the causes, signs and symptoms, and treatments of various diseases and disorders of the nervous system.	There are many common diseases and disorders of the nervous system with varied signs, symptoms, and treatments. Some of these include Alzheimer's disease, amyotrophic lateral sclerosis (ALS), Bell's palsy, brain tumors, cancer, epilepsy, seizures, Guillain-Barré syndrome, episodic and chronic tension headaches, migraines, cluster headaches, meningitis, multiple sclerosis (MS), neuralgias, Parkinson's disease, sciatica, and stroke (cerebrovascular accident, or CVA).

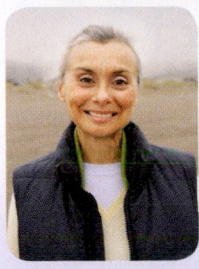

© John Lund/Sam Diephuis/
Blend Images LLC RF

Recall Nancy Evans from the beginning of the chapter. Now that you have completed the chapter, answer the following questions regarding her case.

1. Forgetfulness is a common sign of what types of neurologic disorders?

2. What are some of the possible causes of these disorders?

3. What information might the physician hope to gain from the ordered MRI, PET scan, and lumbar puncture?

4. What are the treatment options for these disorders?

E X A M   P R E P A R A T I O N   Q U E S T I O N S

1. (LO 29.6) Which of the following is *not* a common symptom of patients with neurologic disorders?
   a. Headache
   b. Paresthesia
   c. Fever
   d. Muscle weakness
   e. Numbness

2. (LO 29.6) Which of the following diagnostic procedures is done to detect blood flow within the brain for diagnosing brain tumors, Parkinson's disease, and Alzheimer's disease?
   a. MRI
   b. PET scan
   c. CT scan
   d. Cerebral angiography
   e. X-ray

3. (LO 29.4) The _____ are interconnecting cavities of the brain that produce and circulate CSF.
   a. Ventricles
   b. Lobes
   c. Convolutions
   d. Gyri
   e. Sulci

4. (LO 29.1) What kind of neurons connect the neurons that carry messages to the central nervous system with those that carry messages from the central nervous system to the muscles and glands?
   a. Efferent neurons
   b. Sensory neurons
   c. Afferent neurons
   d. Motor neurons
   e. Interneurons

5. (LO 29.2) Which type of neuroglial cells anchor blood vessels to the nerve cells?
   a. Microglia
   b. Oligodendrocytes
   c. Astrocytes
   d. Schwann cells
   e. Satellite cells

6. (LO 29.4) What is the name of the tough, outer layer of the meninges?
   a. Dura mater
   b. Epidural space
   c. Arachnoid mater
   d. Subdural space
   e. Pia mater

7. (LO 29.3) Which two ions are responsible for cell membrane depolarization and repolarization?
   a. Na^+ and Ca^{++}
   b. Na^+ and Cl^-
   c. Ca^{++} and Cl^-
   d. K^+ and Na^+
   e. K^+ and SO_4^-

8. (LO 29.5) Collections of neuron cell bodies outside the central nervous system that communicate with organs and blood vessels are called
   a. Ganglia
   b. Plexuses
   c. Dermatomes
   d. Ventral roots
   e. Dorsal roots

9. (LO 29.5) Which of the following cranial nerves are found in the muscles of the tongue?
   a. Olfactory nerves (I)
   b. Oculomotor nerves (III)
   c. Trigeminal nerves (V)
   d. Facial nerves (VII)
   e. Hypoglossal nerves (XII)

10. (LO 29.7) In which nervous system disorder are the facial muscles paralyzed?
   a. Amyotrophic lateral sclerosis
   b. Epilepsy
   c. Bell's palsy
   d. Guillain-Barré syndrome
   e. Meningitis

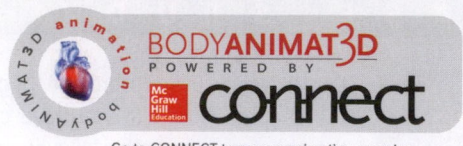

Go to CONNECT to see an animation exercise about *Strokes*.

M E D I C A L   T E R M I N O L O G Y   P R A C T I C E

Analyze the following medical terms, presented throughout the chapter. Using a medical dictionary (or Appendix I) place a / mark between each word part. Define each word part and then define the whole word.

EXAMPLE: **crani/ otomy** = crani means "skull" + otomy means "incision"
CRANIOTOMY means "incision into the skull."

1. angiography
2. areflexia
3. astrocyte
4. cerebral
5. electroencephalogram
6. hyperreflexia
7. hypothalamus
8. interneuron
9. neuralgia
10. neurotransmitter
11. meningitis
12. anesthesia

The Urinary System

CASE STUDY

PATIENT INFORMATION

Patient Name	DOB	Allergies
Peter Smith	3/28/19XX	NKA

Attending	MRN	Other Information
Paul F. Buckwalter, MD	428-69-544	Today's Vital Signs BP: 138/92 R: 18 P: 84 T: 101.2°

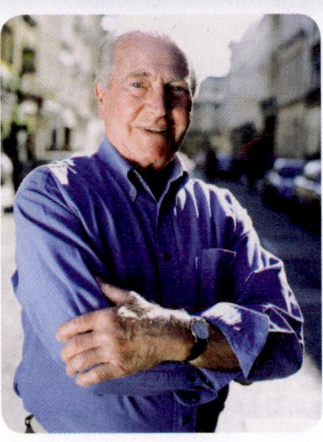
© Image Source/Getty Images RF

when he urinates. He has also been very tired lately. Based on the vital signs you measured and Peter's current complaints, the physician ordered a fasting blood glucose and a urinalysis.

Keep Peter in mind as you study the chapter. There will be questions at the end of the chapter based on the case study. The information in the chapter will help you answer these questions.

Peter Smith is a 73-year-old male with mild Type 2 diabetes. He states that he has needed to urinate more frequently during the last 2 weeks, and he feels a burning sensation

ACTIVSim

LEARNING OUTCOMES

After completing Chapter 30, you will be able to:

30.1 Describe the structure, location, and functions of the kidneys.

30.2 Explain how nephrons filter blood and form urine.

30.3 Compare the locations, structures, and functions of the ureters, bladder, and urethra.

30.4 Describe the causes, signs and symptoms, and treatments of various diseases and disorders of the urinary system.

KEY TERMS

Bowman's capsule	renal column
detrusor muscle	renal corpuscle
distal convoluted tubule	renal cortex
glomerulus	renal medulla
hilum	renal pelvis
lithotripsy	renal pyramids
loop of Henle	renal sinus
metabolic wastes	renal tubule
micturition	trigone
nephrons	ureters
proximal convoluted tubule	urethra

I.C.4 List major organs in each body system

I.C.5 Identify the anatomical location of major organs in each body system

I.C.6 Compare structure and function of the human body across the life span

I.C.7 Describe the normal function of each body system

I.C.8 Identify common pathology related to each body system including
   (a) signs
   (b) symptoms
   (c) etiology

I.C.9 Analyze pathology for each body system including:
   (a) diagnostic measures
   (b) treatment modalities

V.C.9 Identify medical terms labeling the word parts

V.C.10 Define medical terms and abbreviations related to all body systems

2. Anatomy & Physiology
   a. List all body systems, their structure and functions
   b. Describe common diseases, symptoms, and etiologies as they apply to each system
   c. Identify diagnostic and treatment modalities as they relate to each system

3. Medical Terminology
   b. Build and dissect medical terms from roots/suffixes to understand the word element combinations that create medical terminology
   c. Apply various medical terms for each specialty
   d. Define and use medical abbreviations when appropriate and acceptable

▶ Introduction

The organs of the urinary system are the kidneys, ureters, urinary bladder, and urethra (see Figure 30-1). This system removes waste products from the bloodstream. These waste products are excreted from the body in the form of urine. **Nephrons** are microscopic structures within the kidneys that filter blood, remove waste products, and form urine.

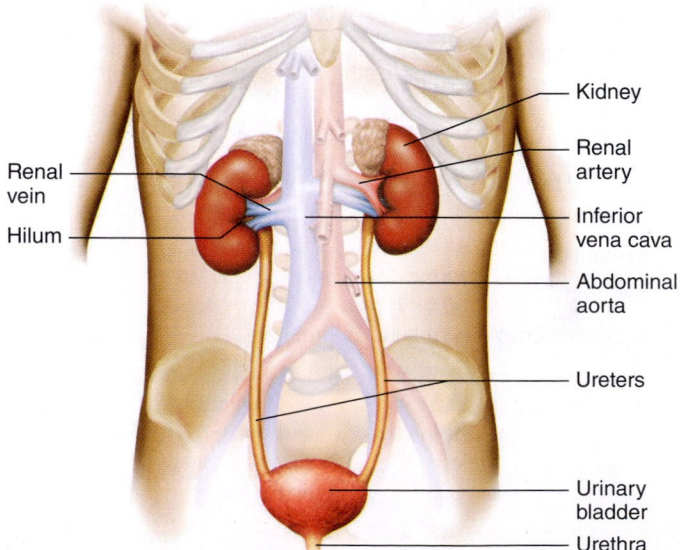

Renal vein

Hilum

Kidney

Renal artery

Inferior vena cava

Abdominal aorta

Ureters

Urinary bladder

Urethra

FIGURE 30-1 Organs of the urinary system.

▶ The Kidneys

LO 30.1

The kidneys remove metabolic waste products from the blood. **Metabolic wastes** are the waste products produced during normal operations such as converting food into a form that is usable by the body cells for energy. In the kidneys, metabolic wastes are combined with water and ions to form urine, which is excreted from the body. The kidneys also secrete the hormone *erythropoietin,* which stimulates the red bone marrow to produce red blood cells, and the hormone *renin,* which helps to regulate blood pressure. All three of these functions are important in maintaining the body's internal environment at homeostasis, which is a balanced, stable state within the body.

The kidneys are reddish-brown, bean-shaped organs. Tough, fibrous capsules cover them. The kidneys are *retroperitoneal* in position, which means they lie behind the peritoneal cavity. They lie on either side of the vertebral column at about the level of the lumbar vertebrae; the left kidney is slightly higher than the right, which is displaced by the liver.

The surface area of the concave depression of the kidney is called the **renal sinus.** The renal artery, renal vein, and ureter enter the kidney here in the area known as the **hilum.** The ureter is the tube that drains urine from the kidney, carrying it to the bladder. Inside the kidney, the same area is called the **renal pelvis,** formed by the expansion of the ureter inside the kidney. The renal pelvis itself further divides into small tubes known as *calyces* (*calyx* is the singular).

The outermost layer of the kidney is the **renal cortex,** and the middle portion is the **renal medulla** (see Figure 30-2). The renal medulla is divided into triangular-shaped areas called

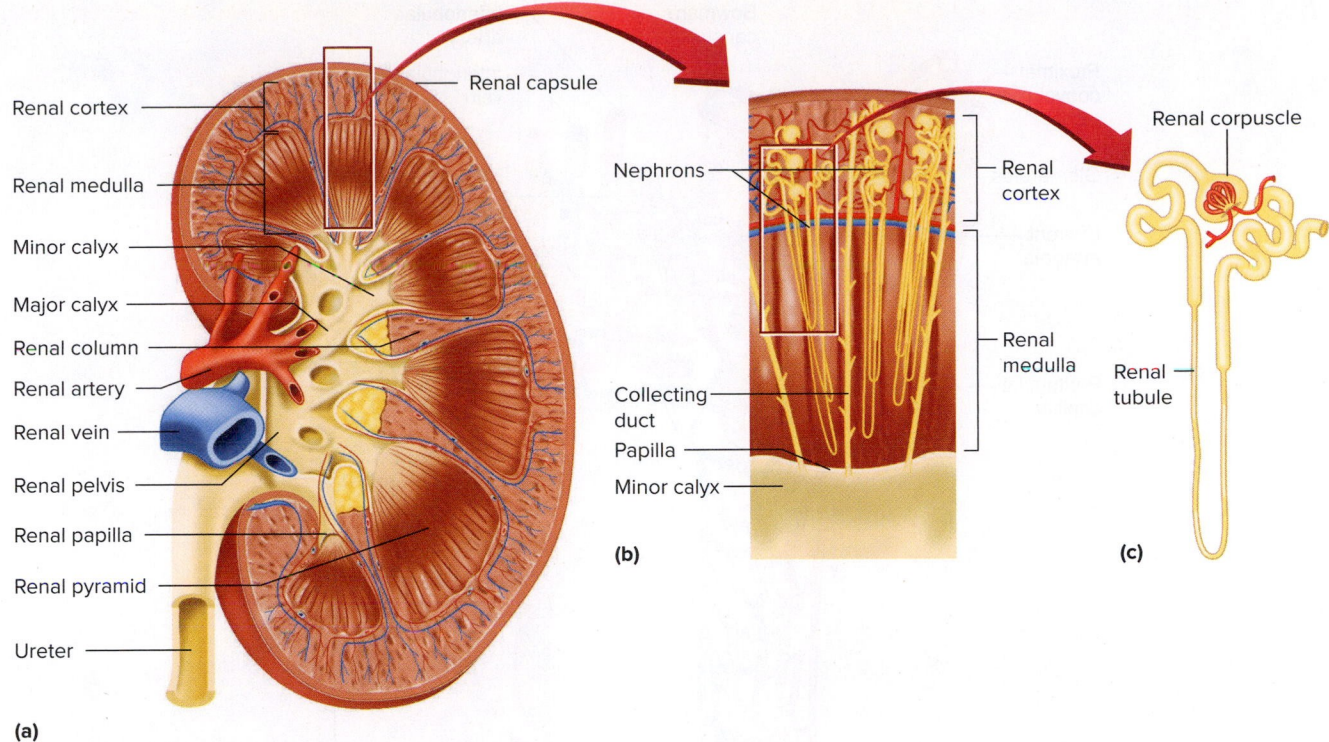

Renal cortex
Renal medulla
Minor calyx
Major calyx
Renal column
Renal artery
Renal vein
Renal pelvis
Renal papilla
Renal pyramid
Ureter

Renal capsule

(a)

Nephrons
Collecting duct
Papilla
Minor calyx

Renal cortex
Renal medulla

(b)

Renal corpuscle
Renal tubule

(c)

FIGURE 30-2   (a) Longitudinal section of a kidney, (b) the location of nephrons, and (c) a single nephron.

renal pyramids. The renal cortex covers the pyramids and dips down between them. The portions of the cortex located between pyramids are called **renal columns.**

Blood enters the kidney through the renal artery and goes through the filtration process explained in the next section. It then exits the kidney via the renal vein.

Nephrons

Nephrons remove waste products from the blood. Each kidney contains about 1 million nephrons, which are located in the renal medulla. Nephrons are made up of a **renal corpuscle** and a **renal tubule** (see Figure 30-2). A renal corpuscle is composed of a mass of capillaries called a **glomerulus;** the capsule that surrounds the glomerulus is called the **Bowman's capsule,** or *glomerular capsule.* Blood filtration occurs in the renal corpuscle.

Renal tubules extend from the Bowman's capsule of a nephron. The three parts of a renal tubule are the **proximal convoluted tubule,** the **loop of Henle** (*nephron loop*), and the **distal convoluted tubule** (see Figure 30-3). The proximal convoluted tubule is directly attached to the Bowman's capsule and eventually straightens out to become the loop of Henle. The loop of Henle curves back toward the renal corpuscle and starts to twist again, becoming the distal convoluted tubule. Distal convoluted tubules from several nephrons merge to form collecting ducts. These ducts collect urine and deliver it to the renal pelvis, which in turn empties urine into the ureters.

Afferent arterioles take blood to the tightly packed, increasingly narrow capillaries of the glomeruli. This narrowing causes the filtration of the blood. The blood is forced through the capillary walls, similar to what occurs when water drips through a coffee filter in a drip coffee-maker. Efferent arterioles deliver blood to *peritubular capillaries,* which are wrapped around the renal

tubules of the nephron. Blood leaves the peritubular capillaries through the veins of the kidneys. By the time the blood leaves the peritubular capillaries, it has been cleansed of waste products. Blood flows through a nephron in the following pathway:

afferent arteriole → glomerulus → efferent arteriole → peritubular capillaries → veins of the kidney

▶ Urine Formation   LO 30.2

The three processes of urine formation are glomerular filtration, tubular reabsorption, and tubular secretion.

Glomerular Filtration

Glomerular filtration takes place in the renal corpuscles of nephrons. In this process, the fluid part of blood is forced from the glomerulus (the capillaries) into Bowman's capsule (see Figure 30-4). The fluid in Bowman's capsule is called the *glomerular filtrate.*

Glomerular filtration depends on filtration pressure, which is the pressure that forces substances (filtrate) out of the glomerulus into Bowman's capsule. Filtration pressure is largely determined by blood pressure. If a person's blood pressure is too low, glomerular filtrate will not form. If the blood pressure increases, filtration pressure also increases, causing the rate of filtration and the amount of glomerular filtrate to increase as well.

The sympathetic branch of the autonomic nervous system largely controls the rate of filtration. If blood pressure or blood volume drops, the sympathetic nervous system causes the afferent arterioles in the kidneys to constrict. When this constriction occurs, glomerular filtration pressure decreases and less glomerular filtrate is formed. When less glomerular

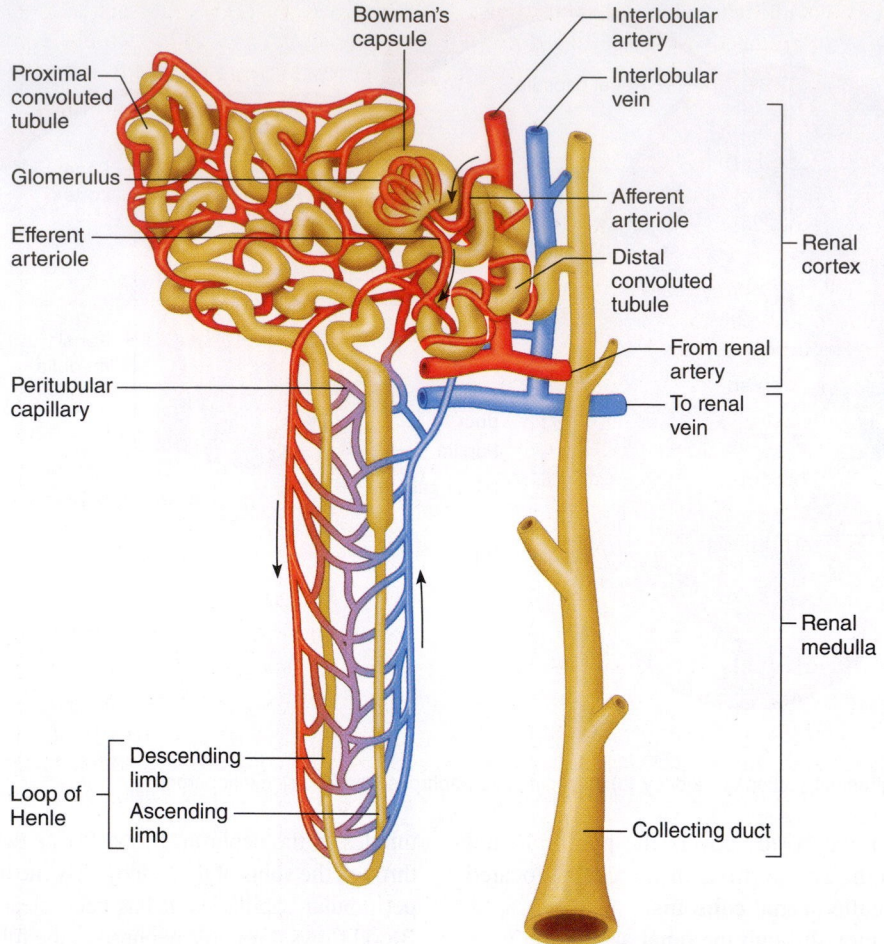

FIGURE 30-3   Structure of a nephron and its associated blood vessels.

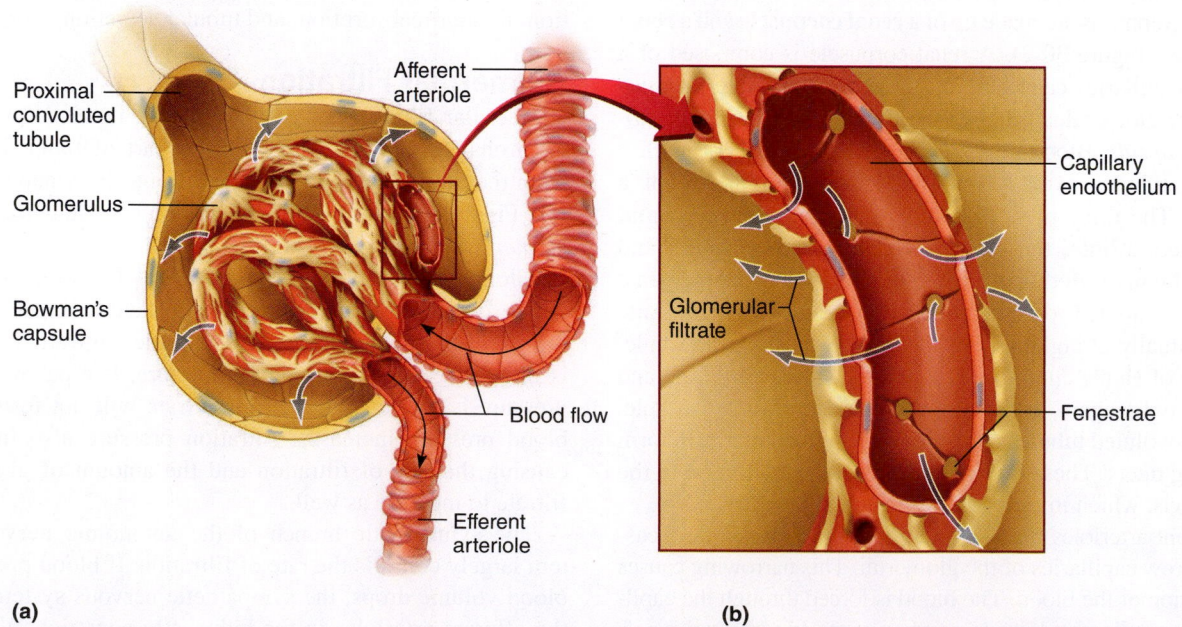

(a)   **(b)**

FIGURE 30-4   Glomerular filtration. (a) Substances move out of glomerular capillaries and into Bowman's capsule. (b) Glomerular capillaries have large holes called *fenestrae* that allow substances to move out of them and into Bowman's capsule.

filtrate is formed, less urine is ultimately formed. This allows the body to retain fluids that are needed to raise blood pressure and blood volume.

Tubular Reabsorption

Tubular reabsorption is the second process in urine formation. In this process, the glomerular filtrate flows into the proximal convoluted tubule (see Figure 30-5a). The body needs to keep many of the substances (nutrients, water, and ions) that are found in glomerular filtrate. In tubular reabsorption, all the substances to be kept pass through the wall of the renal tubule into the blood of the peritubular capillaries.

Water reabsorption varies depending on the presence of two hormones: antidiuretic hormone (ADH) and aldosterone. Both of these hormones increase water reabsorption, which decreases urine production. This fluid retention and the resultant increase in blood pressure is one of the reasons diuretics, which rid the body of excess fluid, are successful in treating some forms of hypertension.

Tubular Secretion

Tubular secretion is the third process of urine formation. In tubular secretion, substances move from the blood in the peritubular capillaries into the renal tubules (see Figure 30-5b). Substances that are secreted include drugs, hydrogen ions, and waste products, all of which will be excreted in the urine.

Urine Composition

The final solution that reaches the collecting ducts of the kidneys is urine. Urine is mostly made of water but also normally contains urea, uric acid, trace amounts of amino acids, and various ions. *Urea* and *uric acid* are waste products formed by the breakdown of proteins and nucleic acids. The secretion of these waste materials helps maintain the body's acid-base balance.

▶ The Ureters, Urinary Bladder, and Urethra   LO 30.3

The remaining organs in the urinary system transport and store urine after it is formed in the kidneys.

The Ureters

The **ureters** are long, muscular tubes that carry urine from the kidneys to the urinary bladder. They propel urine toward the bladder through rhythmic muscular contractions of the ureters called *peristalsis.*

The Urinary Bladder

The urinary bladder is a distensible (expandable) organ located in the pelvic cavity. Its function is to store urine (up to 600 mL on average) until it is eliminated from the body. The internal floor of the bladder contains three openings—one for the urethra and two for the ureters. These three openings form a triangle called the **trigone** of the bladder. The wall of the bladder contains smooth muscle, called the **detrusor muscle.** This muscle contracts to push urine from the bladder into the urethra (see Figure 30-6).

Micturition is the process of urination. The stretching of the bladder triggers this process—usually when the bladder

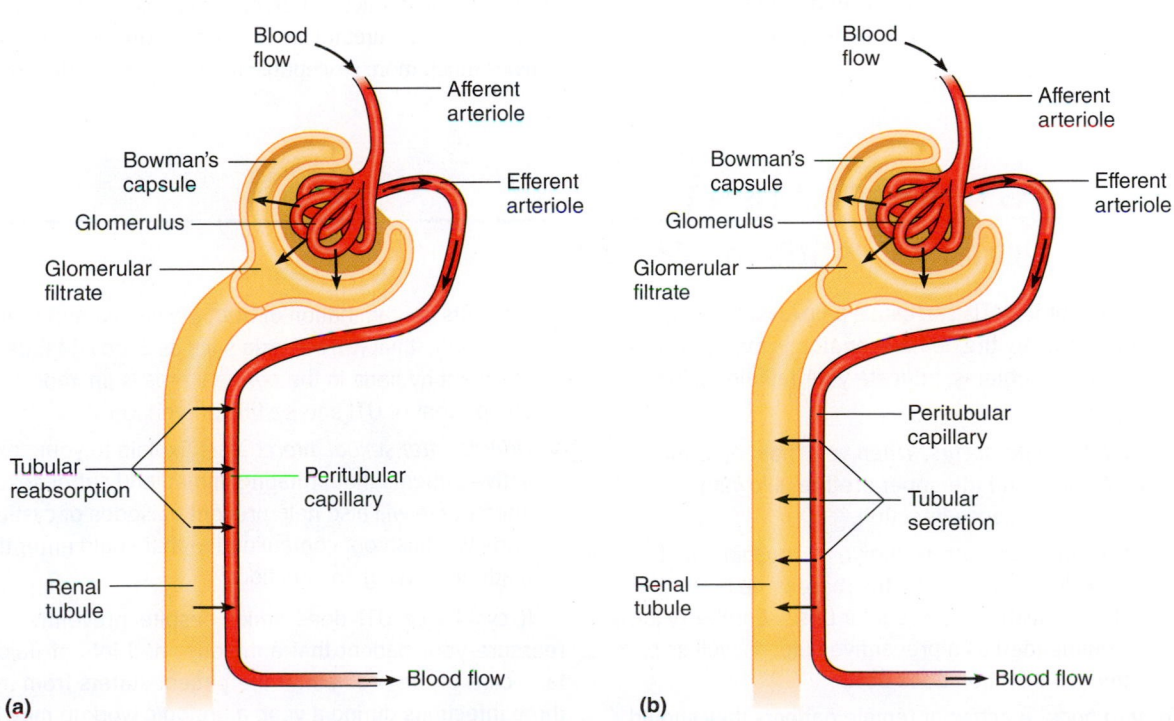

FIGURE 30-5 (a) Tubular reabsorption. Substances move from the glomerular filtrate into the blood of peritubular capillaries. (b) Tubular secretion. Substances move out of the blood of the peritubular capillaries into the renal tubule.

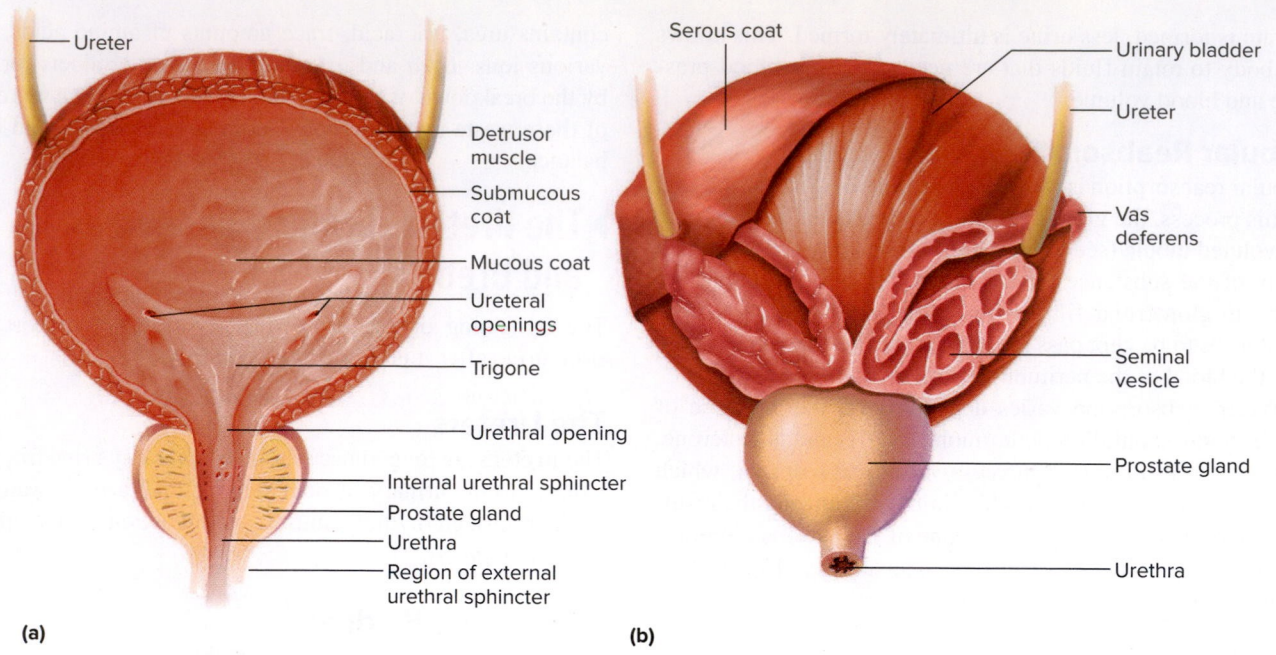

FIGURE 30-6   Male urinary bladder: (a) anterior view and (b) posterior view.

contains approximately 150 mL of urine. The major events of micturition are the following:

1. The urinary bladder distends as it fills with urine.
2. The distension stimulates stretch receptors in the bladder wall, which sends a nerve impulse to in the spinal cord.
3. Parasympathetic nerves stimulate the detrusor muscle, which begins rhythmic contractions that trigger the sense of the need to urinate.
4. The brainstem and cerebral cortex send impulses to voluntarily contract the external urethral sphincter and to inhibit the micturition impulse.

5. Upon the decision to urinate, the external urethral sphincter is relaxed and impulses from the pons and hypothalamus start the micturition reflex.
6. Contraction of the detrusor muscle occurs and urine is expelled through the urethra.

The Urethra

The **urethra** is a tube that moves urine from the bladder to the outside world. In females, the urethra is much shorter than in males. This anatomical difference, combined with the fact that the anus, vagina, and urethra are in close proximity in females, makes females much more susceptible to urinary tract infections (UTIs).

EDUCATING THE PATIENT

Preventing Urinary Cystitis in Women

Urinary cystitis and other UTIs can cause pain (dysuria), urgency, and frequency. Because the female anatomy makes women more prone to these problems, educate your female patients to take these steps:

1. *Urinate when the urge occurs.* When you "hold it," urine stays in the bladder and the upper urethra, allowing bacteria to grow and cause infection.
2. *Drink lots of clear fluids.* This is known as "pushing fluids." The more clear liquids you drink, the more urine is created and the system is flushed on a regular basis. Cranberry juice is highly recommended as a preventive fluid, as well as part of the treatment if infection does occur.
3. *Wipe front to back.* Teach your female patients they should wipe "front to back" after a bowel movement. Doing so

prevents contamination of both the vagina and urethra by gastrointestinal (GI) bacteria such as *E. coli*. Maintaining excellent hygiene in the perineal area is an important component of UTI and cystitis prevention.

4. *Urinate after sexual intercourse.* Explain to your sexually active patients that urinating immediately after sexual intercourse will also help prevent episodes of cystitis. The urine will flush out contamination that could enter the bladder, causing an infection.

If cystitis or UTI does strike despite preventive methods, reassure your patient that antibiotics and lots of fluids should take care of the problem. If the patient suffers from more than three infections during a year, a urologic workup may be advisable to look for underlying anatomical anomalies.

Common Diseases and Disorders of the Urinary System

ACUTE KIDNEY (RENAL) FAILURE is a sudden loss of kidney function.

Causes. There are many causes and risk factors of kidney failure, including burns, dehydration, low blood pressure, hemorrhaging, allergic reactions, obstruction of the renal artery, various poisons, alcohol abuse, trauma to the kidneys and skeletal muscles, blood disorders, blood transfusion reactions, kidney stones, urinary tract infections, enlarged prostate, childbirth, immune system disorders, and food poisoning involving the bacterium *E. coli.*

Signs and Symptoms. The signs and symptoms include decreased or no urine production, excessive urination, swelling of the extremities, bloating, mental confusion, coma, seizures, hand tremors, nosebleeds, easy bruising, pain in the back or abdomen, hypertension, abnormal heart or lung sounds, abnormal urinalysis, and an increase in potassium levels.

Treatment. The first treatment measure is modifying the diet to decrease the amount of protein consumed. Controlling fluid intake and potassium levels is also recommended. Antibiotics and dialysis may also be needed. If the underlying cause can be treated, acute renal failure may be reversed and kidney function returned to normal.

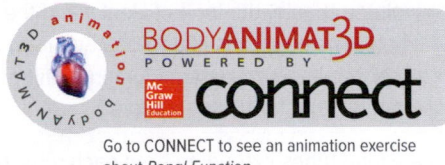

Go to CONNECT to see an animation exercise about *Renal Function.*

CHRONIC KIDNEY (RENAL) FAILURE is a condition in which the kidneys slowly lose their ability to function. The patient may be asymptomatic until the kidneys have lost about 90% of their function.

Causes. This disorder results from diabetes, hypertension, glomerulonephritis, polycystic kidney disease, kidney stones, obstruction of the ureters, and acute kidney failure.

Signs and Symptoms. The list of signs and symptoms is extensive and includes headache, mental confusion, coma, seizures, fatigue, frequent hiccups, itching, easy bruising, abnormal bleeding, anemia, excessive thirst, fluid retention, nausea, hypertension, abnormal heart or lung sounds, weight loss, white spots on the skin or increased pigmentation, high potassium levels, an increased or decreased urine output, urinary tract infections, and abnormal urinalysis results.

Treatment. This disorder can be treated with antibiotics; blood transfusions; medications to control anemia; restriction of fluids, electrolytes, and protein; control of high blood pressure; and dialysis. The most serious cases may require surgery to repair a ureteral obstruction or a kidney (renal) transplant.

CYSTITIS is a urinary bladder infection. Women are much more likely to develop this disorder than men because of the short length of their urethras. The urethral opening in women is also close to the anal opening, allowing bacteria from this area to be more easily

introduced into the urinary tract. For more information on preventing urinary cystitis in women, see the *Educating the Patient* feature.

Causes. This infection is caused by various types of bacteria (especially those found in the rectum), as well as by the placement of a catheter in the bladder. Good hygiene, urinating promptly when the urge occurs, and, for females, wiping from front to back can help to prevent this infection.

Signs and Symptoms. Common symptoms include fatigue, chills, fever, and a painful, frequent need to urinate, often with only small amounts of urine produced. Urine is often cloudy and blood may be present in the urine.

Treatment. This infection is treated with antibiotics and, when needed, pain medication. The patient should also be urged to drink lots of clear liquids.

GLOMERULONEPHRITIS is an inflammation of the glomeruli of the kidney. Chronic glomerulonephritis is one of the causes of chronic renal failure.

Causes. This disorder is caused by renal diseases, immune disorders, and bacterial infections.

Signs and Symptoms. The signs and symptoms are hiccups, drowsiness, coma, seizures, nausea, anemia, high blood pressure, increased skin pigmentation, abnormal heart sounds, abnormal urinalysis results, blood in the urine, and a decreased or increased urine output.

Treatment. Treatment begins with a low-sodium, low-protein diet. Medications to control high blood pressure, corticosteroids to reduce inflammation, and dialysis are other treatment options.

INCONTINENCE is a temporary or long-lasting condition in which a person (other than a child) cannot control urination. Women are more likely to develop incontinence than men are.

Causes. This condition can be caused by various medications, excessive coughing (for example, in smokers), UTIs, nervous system disorders, and bladder cancer. In men, prostate problems can lead to the development of this disorder. Weakness of the urinary sphincters from surgery, trauma, or pregnancy can also cause incontinence. It may be prevented by avoiding urinary bladder irritants such as coffee, cigarettes, diuretics, and various medications.

Signs and Symptoms. The primary symptom is the involuntary leakage of urine.

Treatment. Treatment includes various medications, incontinence pads, removal of the prostate, Kegel exercises to increase the control of urinary sphincters, and surgery to repair damaged bladders or urethral sphincters.

POLYCYSTIC KIDNEY DISEASE is a disorder in which the kidneys enlarge because they are filled with cysts. The disease develops relatively slowly, with symptoms worsening over time.

Causes. The causes are hereditary (via an inherited dominant gene from a parent).

Signs and Symptoms. Fatigue, hypertension, anemia, pain in the back or abdomen, joint pain, heart murmurs, the formation of kidney stones, kidney failure, blood in the urine, and liver disease are the symptoms of this disorder.

Treatment. Treatment includes medications to control anemia and high blood pressure, blood transfusions, draining of the cysts, dialysis, and surgery to remove one or both kidneys.

PYELONEPHRITIS is a complicated UTI. It begins as a bladder infection and spreads to one or both kidneys. This condition can develop suddenly, or it may be chronic.

Causes. This disorder is caused by bacteria, a bladder infection, kidney stones, or an obstruction of the urinary system ducts.

Signs and Symptoms. Signs and symptoms include fatigue, mental confusion, fever, nausea, pain in the back or abdomen, enlarged kidneys, painful urination, and cloudy or bloody urine.

Treatment. Treatment includes intravenous fluids, pain medication, and antibiotics.

RENAL CALCULI are commonly called *kidney stones*. They can become lodged in the ducts within the kidneys or ureters, causing more severe disorders such as pyelonephritis and chronic kidney failure.

Causes. This condition is caused by gouty arthritis, defects of the ureters, overly concentrated urine, and UTIs.

Signs and Symptoms. The signs and symptoms include fever, nausea, severe back or abdominal pain, a frequent urge to urinate, blood in the urine, and abnormal urinalysis results.

Treatment. Treatment includes pain medication, intravenous fluids, medications to decrease stone formation, surgery to remove kidney stones, and **lithotripsy** (a procedure that uses shock waves to break up stones).

SUMMARY OF LEARNING OUTCOMES

LEARNING OUTCOMES	KEY POINTS
30.1 Describe the structure, location, and functions of the kidneys.	The retroperitoneal kidneys are composed of the outer renal cortex and inner renal medulla. Their function is to remove metabolic wastes from the body.
30.2 Explain how nephrons filter blood and form urine.	A nephron is a single kidney cell. It is composed of a renal corpuscle, which consists of the glomerulus and the Bowman's capsule, and the renal tubule, which has three parts: the proximal convoluted tubule, the loop of Henle, and the distal convoluted tubule. The nephrons filter blood and form urine through three consecutive processes: glomerular filtration, tubular reabsorption, and tubular secretion.
30.3 Compare the locations, structures, and functions of the ureters, bladder, and urethra.	The ureters are long tubes extending from each renal pelvis that bring urine to the bladder for storage. The urethra is the muscular tube extending from the bladder that transports urine to be expelled from the body.
30.4 Describe the causes, signs and symptoms, and treatments of various diseases and disorders of the urinary system.	There are many common diseases and disorders of the urinary system with varied signs, symptoms, and treatments. Some of these include acute kidney (renal) failure, chronic kidney (renal) failure, cystitis, glomerulonephritis, incontinence, polycystic kidney disease, pyelonephritis, and renal calculi.

CASE STUDY CRITICAL THINKING

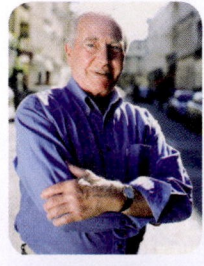

© Image Source/Getty Images RF

Recall Peter Smith from the beginning of the chapter. Now that you have completed the chapter, answer the following questions regarding his case.

1. What is the likely diagnosis for Mr. Smith?
2. Why did the physician order both a urinalysis and a blood glucose test?

3. Why might Mr. Smith's vital signs show that his temperature is slightly elevated?
4. Based on the laboratory test results, the physician prescribed an antibiotic for Mr. Smith. What can you advise Mr. Smith to do in addition to taking the antibiotic as prescribed?

1. (LO 30.4) _____ is a complicated UTI that begins as a bladder infection and spreads to one or both kidneys.
   a. Cystitis
   b. Glomerulonephritis
   c. Pyelonephritis
   d. Polycystic kidney disease
   e. Chronic renal failure

2. (LO 30.2) In which of the following processes do substances move into the renal tubules?
   a. Glomerular filtration
   b. Tubular secretion
   c. Tubular reabsorption
   d. Micturition
   e. Urination

3. (LO 30.2) Distal convoluted tubules from several nephrons merge together to form the
   a. Bowman's capsule
   b. Glomerulus
   c. Loop of Henle
   d. Collecting ducts
   e. Renal pyramids

4. (LO 30.2) Water reabsorption amounts vary depending on which two hormones?
   a. ADH and aldosterone
   b. ADH and erythropoietin
   c. Aldosterone and renin
   d. Angiotensin and ADH
   e. Erythropoietin and renin

5. (LO 30.1) _____ is the hormone from the kidneys that stimulates the bone marrow to produce RBCs.
   a. Renin
   b. ADH
   c. Aldosterone
   d. Hematopoietin
   e. Erythropoietin

6. (LO 30.1) The outermost layer of the kidney is the renal
   a. Cortex
   b. Pelvis
   c. Medulla
   d. Tubule
   e. Sinus

7. (LO 30.1) The _____ is the structure that surrounds the glomerulus.
   a. Loop of Henle
   b. Proximal convoluted tubule
   c. Distal convoluted tubule
   d. Bowman's capsule
   e. Renal pyramid

8. (LO 30.2) The rate of glomerular filtration is controlled mainly by the
   a. Blood pressure
   b. Sympathetic branch of the autonomic nervous system
   c. Somatic nervous system
   d. Parasympathetic branch of the autonomic nervous system
   e. Central nervous system

9. (LO 30.2) Which of the following is *not* a normal component of urine?
   a. Water
   b. Ions
   c. Glucose
   d. Uric acid
   e. Urea

10. (LO 30.3) The _____ is a triangular area formed by the urethral and ureteral openings into the bladder.
    a. Detrusor muscle
    b. Renal pyramid
    c. Trigone
    d. Hilum
    e. Calyx

M E D I C A L   T E R M I N O L O G Y   P R A C T I C E

Analyze the following medical terms, presented throughout the chapter. Using a medical dictionary (or Appendix I) place a / mark between each word part. Define each word part and then define the whole word.

EXAMPLE: **nephro/logy** = nephro means "kidney" + logy means "study of"
           NEPHROLOGY means "study of the kidney."

1. antidiuretic
2. cystitis
3. dysuria
4. erythropoietin

5. glomerulonephritis
6. lithotripsy
7. nephritis
8. peristalsis

9. peritubular
10. pyelonephritis
11. retroperitoneal
12. uric

The Reproductive Systems

CASE STUDY

PATIENT INFORMATION	Patient Name	DOB	Allergies
	Raja Lautu	8/3/19XX	Benzalkonium Chloride
	Attending	**MRN**	**Other Information**
	Elizabeth H. Williams, MD	224-86-564	BP slightly elevated: 132/88. Other vital signs within normal limits.

Raja Lautu, a 46-year-old woman, has come to the office complaining of vaginal itching and a greenish vaginal discharge with a "fishy" smell. She is sexually active and recently changed partners, but she says her partner has no symptoms. Dr. Williams obtains a vaginal fluid specimen and sends it to the lab for testing.

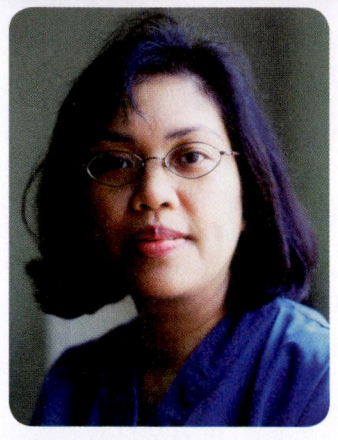

© ERproductions Ltd/Blend Images LLC RF

Keep Raja in mind as you study the chapter. There will be questions at the end of the chapter based on the case study. The information in the chapter will help you answer these questions.

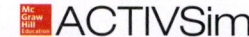

ACTIVSim

LEARNING OUTCOMES

After completing Chapter 31, you will be able to:

31.1 Summarize the organs of the male reproductive system, including the locations, structures, and functions of each.

31.2 Describe the causes, signs and symptoms, and treatment of various disorders of the male reproductive system.

31.3 Summarize the organs of the female reproductive system, including the locations, structures, and functions of each.

31.4 Describe the causes, signs and symptoms, and treatment of various disorders of the female reproductive system.

31.5 Explain the process of pregnancy, including fertilization, the prenatal period, and fetal circulation.

31.6 Describe the birth process, including the postnatal period.

31.7 Compare several birth control methods and their effectiveness.

31.8 Explain the causes of and treatments for infertility.

31.9 Describe the causes, signs and symptoms, and treatments of the most common sexually transmitted infections.

KEY TERMS

amnion
APGAR
Bartholin's glands
blastocyst
Cowper's glands
ductus arteriosus
ductus venosus
embryo
fetus
foramen ovale
infundibulum

menarche
menopause
oogenesis
ovulation
placenta
primary germ layer
seminiferous tubules
spermatogenesis
testes
zygote

M E D I C A L   A S S I S T I N G   C O M P E T E N C I E S

CAAHEP

I.C.4 List major organs in each body system

I.C.5 Identify the anatomical location of major organs in each body system

I.C.6 Compare structure and function of the human body across the life span

I.C.7 Describe the normal function of each body system

I.C.8 Identify common pathology related to each body system including
(a) signs
(b) symptoms
(c) etiology

I.C.9 Analyze pathology for each body system including:
(a) diagnostic measures
(b) treatment modalities

V.C.9 Identify medical terms labeling the word parts

V.C.10 Define medical terms and abbreviations related to all body systems

ABHES

2. Anatomy & Physiology
a. List all body systems, their structure and functions

b. Describe common diseases, symptoms, and etiologies as they apply to each system

c. Identify diagnostic and treatment modalities as they relate to each system

3. Medical Terminology
b. Build and dissect medical terms from roots/ suffixes to understand the word element combinations that create medical terminology

c. Apply various medical terms for each specialty

d. Define and use medical abbreviations when appropriate and acceptable

▶ Introduction

The male and female reproductive systems function together to produce offspring. The female reproductive system nurtures a developing offspring. If a female breast-feeds, her breasts, considered accessory organs of both her reproductive and integumentary systems, are also used to nurture the newborn baby. The male and female reproductive systems also produce a number of important hormones before and during the reproductive years.

▶ The Male Reproductive System   LO 31.1

The male reproductive system is responsible for developing sperm. Accessory organs also produce substances that provide an environment for the sperm that allows it to reach the female ova (eggs).

Testes

Testes are considered the primary organs of the male reproductive system because they produce the male sex cells (sperm) (see Figure 31-1). They also produce the male hormone *testosterone*. Most males have two testes that are held just below the pelvic cavity in the *scrotum*. During the fetal stage, the testes develop in the abdominopelvic cavity of the fetus. Shortly before or soon after birth, the testes descend into the scrotal sac. A fibrous capsule encloses each testis and invades the testis to divide it into lobules. Each lobule is filled with **seminiferous tubules,** which are filled with *spermatogenic cells*. These cells give rise to sperm

cells. Between the seminiferous tubules are the *interstitial cells,* which are the cells within the testes that produce testosterone.

Sperm Cell Formation Spermatogenic cells of the seminiferous tubules begin the process of making sperm cells, but the sperm cells do not mature until they travel to the *epididymis*. **Spermatogenesis** is the process of sperm cell formation. At the beginning of spermatogenesis, the cells are called *spermatogonia*. Spermatogonia contain 46 chromosomes. These cells undergo mitosis, as discussed and shown in the *Organization of the Body* chapter, and the resulting cells are called *primary spermatocytes*. Primary spermatocytes also contain 46 chromosomes. At about the time of puberty, primary spermatocytes undergo a process called *meiosis* (see Figures 31-2 and 31-3a). In meiosis, each primary spermatocyte divides to make two secondary spermatocytes. Each secondary spermatocyte divides to make two *spermatids*. Therefore, from one primary spermatocyte, four spermatids are formed. Spermatids develop flagella to become mature sperm cells. They contain only 23 chromosomes.

Structure of Sperm Cells A mature sperm (see Figure 31-3b) has the following three parts: the head, the midpiece, and the tail.

The Head The head is oval in structure and holds a nucleus with 23 chromosomes. The head is covered with an enzyme-filled sac called an *acrosome,* which helps the sperm penetrate an ovum at the time of fertilization.

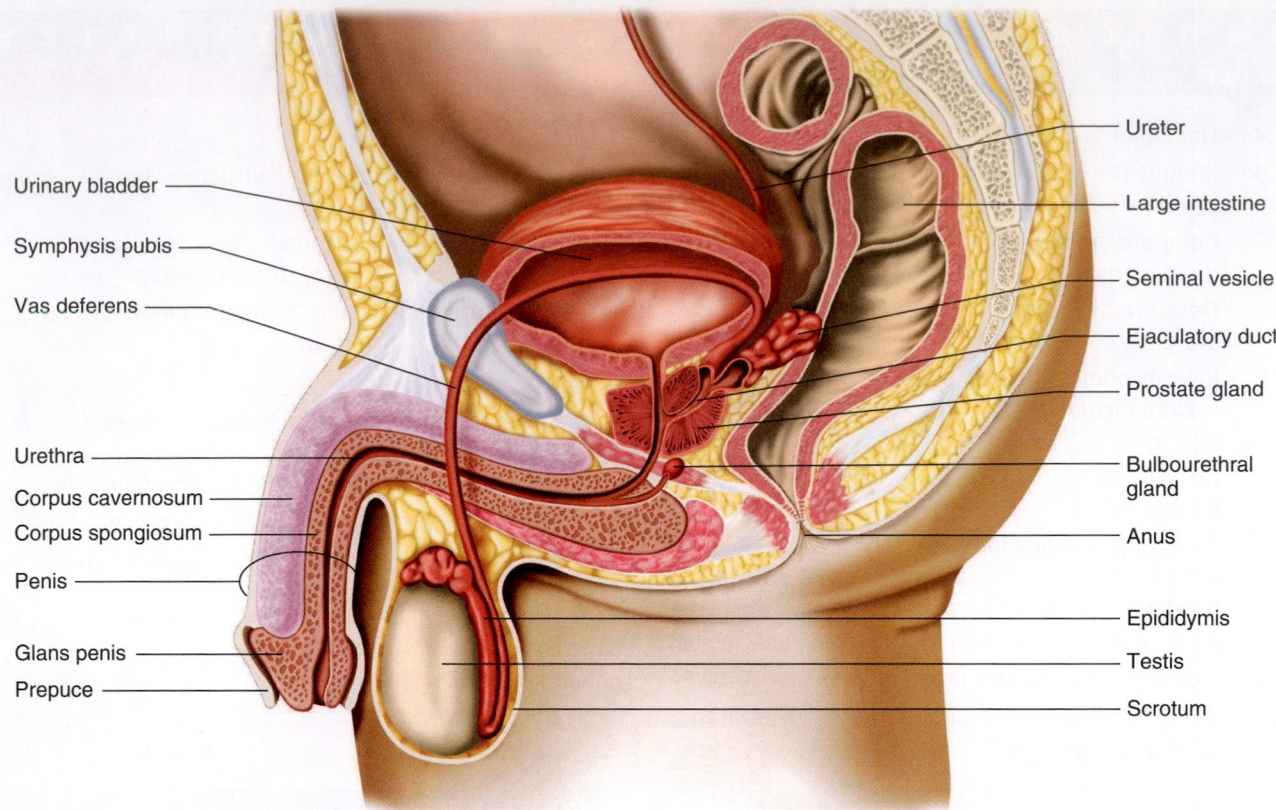

Urinary bladder

Symphysis pubis

Vas deferens

Urethra

Corpus cavernosum

Corpus spongiosum

Penis

Glans penis

Prepuce

Ureter

Large intestine

Seminal vesicle

Ejaculatory duct

Prostate gland

Bulbourethral gland

Anus

Epididymis

Testis

Scrotum

FIGURE 31-1   Sagittal view of male reproductive organs. The male reproductive system produces sperm and delivers them in a form that keeps them viable long enough to fertilize an ovum.

The Midpiece   This portion of the sperm is between the head and tail. It is filled with mitochondria that generate the energy the cell needs to move.

The Tail   The tail is a flagellum that propels the sperm forward in the female reproductive tract.

Internal Accessory Organs of the Male Reproductive System

The internal accessory organs of the male reproductive system are the epididymis, vas deferens, seminal vesicles, prostate gland, and bulbourethral, or Cowper's, glands.

Epididymis   An epididymis sits on top of each testis. It is a highly coiled tube that receives spermatids from seminiferous tubules as the spermatids are formed. Inside the epididymis, spermatids mature to become sperm cells.

Vas Deferens   A tube called a *vas deferens* is connected to each epididymis. These tubes carry sperm cells from the epididymis to the urethra in the male pelvic cavity. When a male has a vasectomy, these tubes are cut and tied to prevent sperm from reaching the ovum.

Seminal Vesicles   Seminal vesicles are sac-like organs that secrete an alkaline *seminal fluid* that is rich in sugars and *prostaglandins.* Sperm cells use the sugars to make

energy, and the prostaglandins stimulate muscular contractions in the female reproductive system. These muscular contractions, known as *peristalsis,* help to propel sperm forward in the female reproductive tract. Seminal vesicles release their product into the vas deferens just before ejaculation. Seminal fluid makes up approximately 60% of semen volume.

Prostate Gland   The muscular prostate gland surrounds the proximal portion of the urethra. It produces a milky, alkaline fluid and secretes this fluid into the urethra just before ejaculation. The alkaline nature of this fluid helps to protect the sperm when they enter the acidic environment of the female vagina. Prostatic fluid makes up approximately 40% of semen volume. During ejaculation, the muscular contractions of the prostate help expel semen.

Bulbourethral Glands   Bulbourethral glands, or **Cowper's glands,** are inferior to the prostate gland. They produce a mucus-like fluid that is secreted into the urethra before ejaculation. This fluid lubricates the end of the penis in preparation for sexual intercourse.

Semen   Semen is a mixture of sperm cells and fluids from the seminal vesicles, prostate gland, and bulbourethral glands. This alkaline mixture contains nutrients and prostaglandins. Total semen volume is between 1.5 and 5.0 mL per ejaculate,

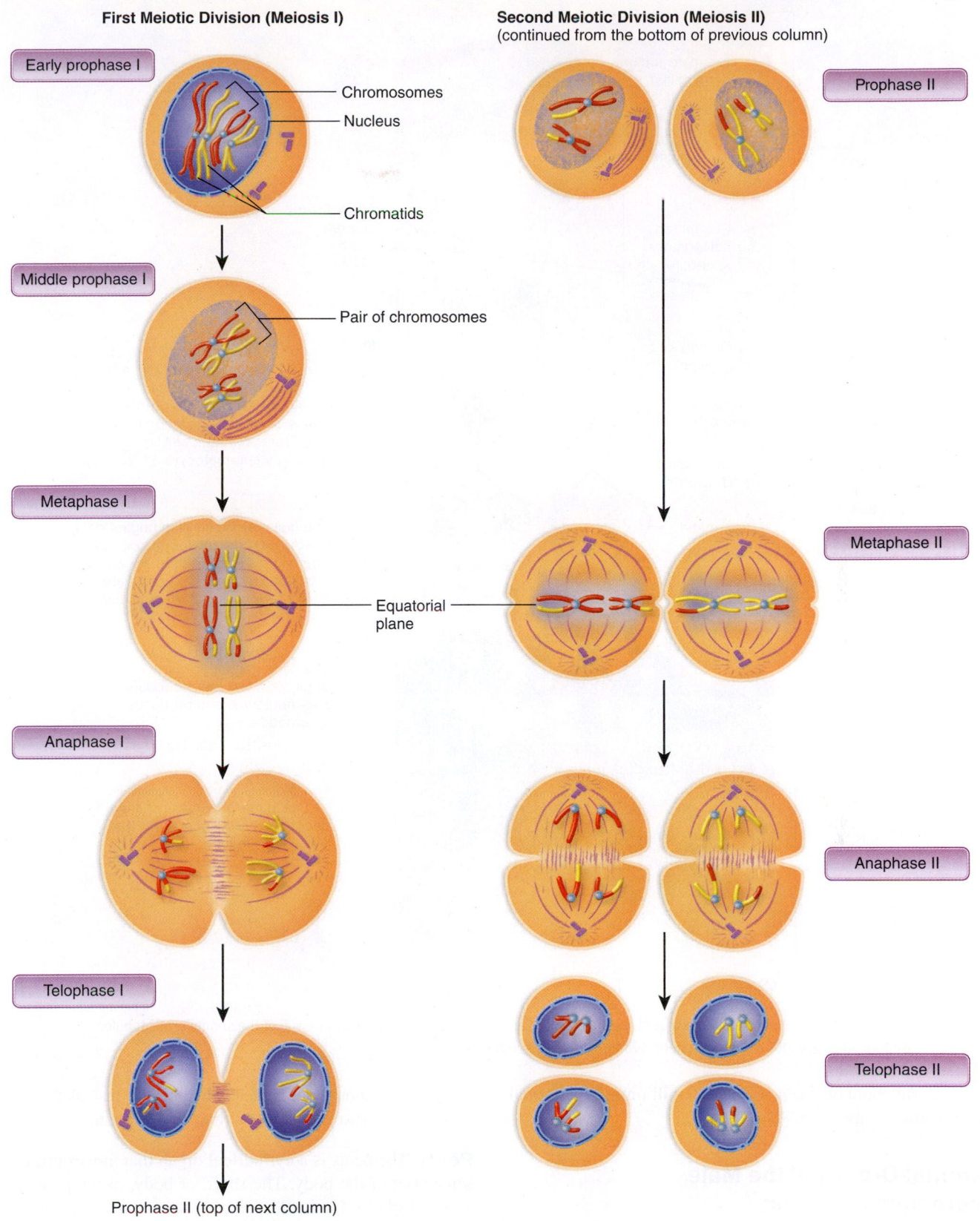

First Meiotic Division (Meiosis I)

Early prophase I

Chromosomes

Nucleus

Chromatids

Middle prophase I

Pair of chromosomes

Metaphase I

Equatorial plane

Anaphase I

Telophase I

Prophase II (top of next column)

Second Meiotic Division (Meiosis II)
(continued from the bottom of previous column)

Prophase II

Metaphase II

Anaphase II

Telophase II

FIGURE 31-2 The process of meiosis, including prophase, metaphase, anaphase, and telophase.

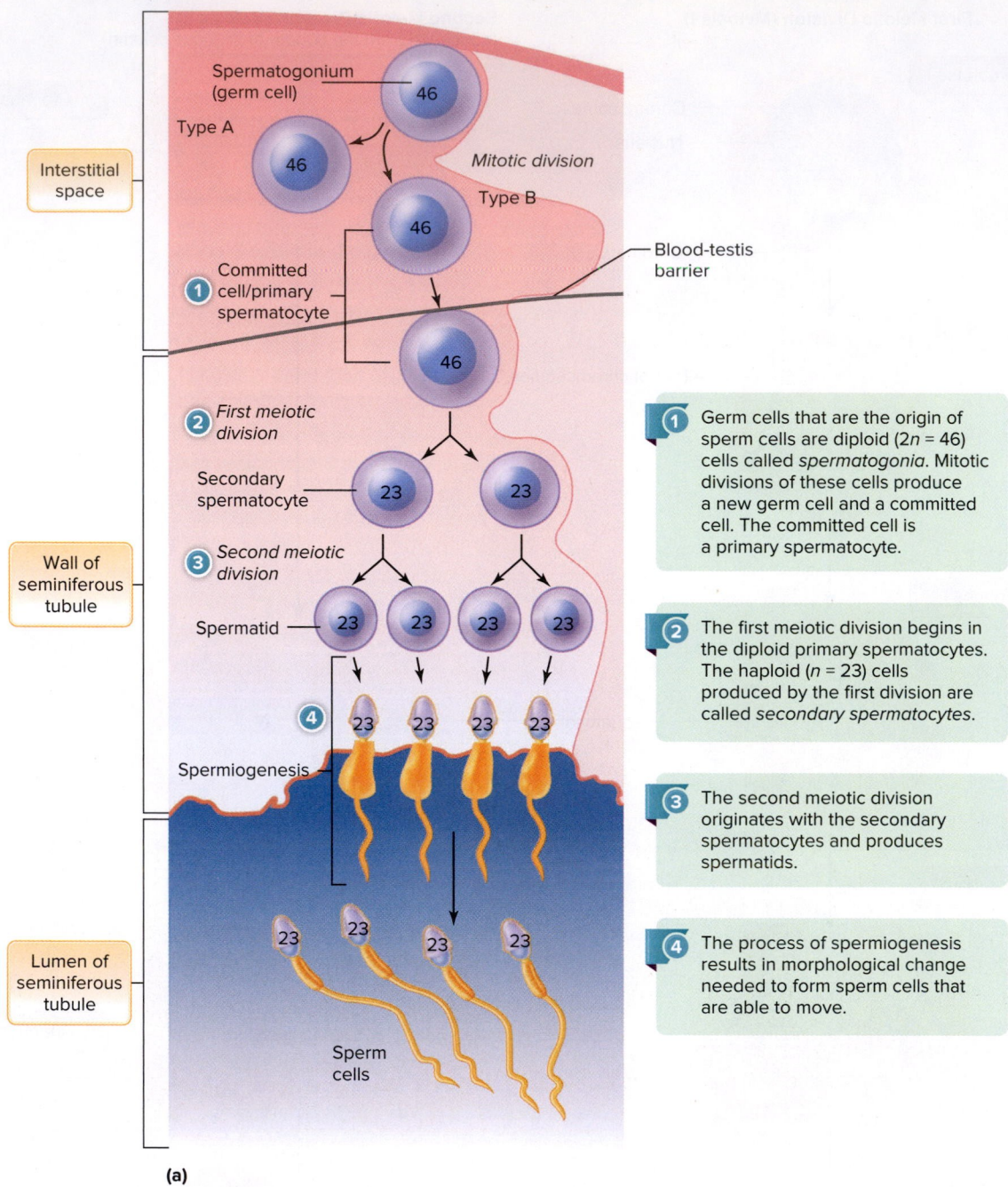

Interstitial space

Spermatogonium (germ cell)

Type A

Mitotic division

Type B

Blood-testis barrier

① Committed cell/primary spermatocyte

② *First meiotic division*

Secondary spermatocyte

③ *Second meiotic division*

Spermatid

④

Spermiogenesis

Wall of seminiferous tubule

Lumen of seminiferous tubule

Sperm cells

(a)

① Germ cells that are the origin of sperm cells are diploid ($2n = 46$) cells called *spermatogonia*. Mitotic divisions of these cells produce a new germ cell and a committed cell. The committed cell is a primary spermatocyte.

② The first meiotic division begins in the diploid primary spermatocytes. The haploid ($n = 23$) cells produced by the first division are called *secondary spermatocytes*.

③ The second meiotic division originates with the secondary spermatocytes and produces spermatids.

④ The process of spermiogenesis results in morphological change needed to form sperm cells that are able to move.

FIGURE 31-3 Spermatogenesis: (a) The process of spermatogenesis takes place in the wall of the seminiferous tubule. (b) Structural changes occur as a sperm cell forms from a spermatid.

with a sperm count between 40 and 250 million/mL. A normal sperm count is more than 80 million.

External Organs of the Male Reproductive System

The two male external reproductive organs are the scrotum and the penis (see Figure 31-1).

Scrotum The scrotum is a pouch of skin that holds the testes. It is lined with a serous membrane that secretes fluid to ensure that the testes move freely within it. The scrotum holds the testes away from the rest of the body, keeping their

temperature about 1 degree lower than the rest of the body, which is necessary for the viability of the sperm.

Penis The penis is a cylindrical organ that moves urine and semen out of the body. The shaft, or body, of the penis contains specialized *erectile tissue* that surrounds the urethra, which runs the length of the penis. The end of the penis is enlarged into a cone-shaped structure called the *glans penis*. If a male has not been circumcised, a piece of skin, called the *prepuce,* covers the glans penis. The function of the penis is to deliver sperm to the female reproductive tract. The penis also functions in urination because it contains the urethra, which drains urine from the bladder.

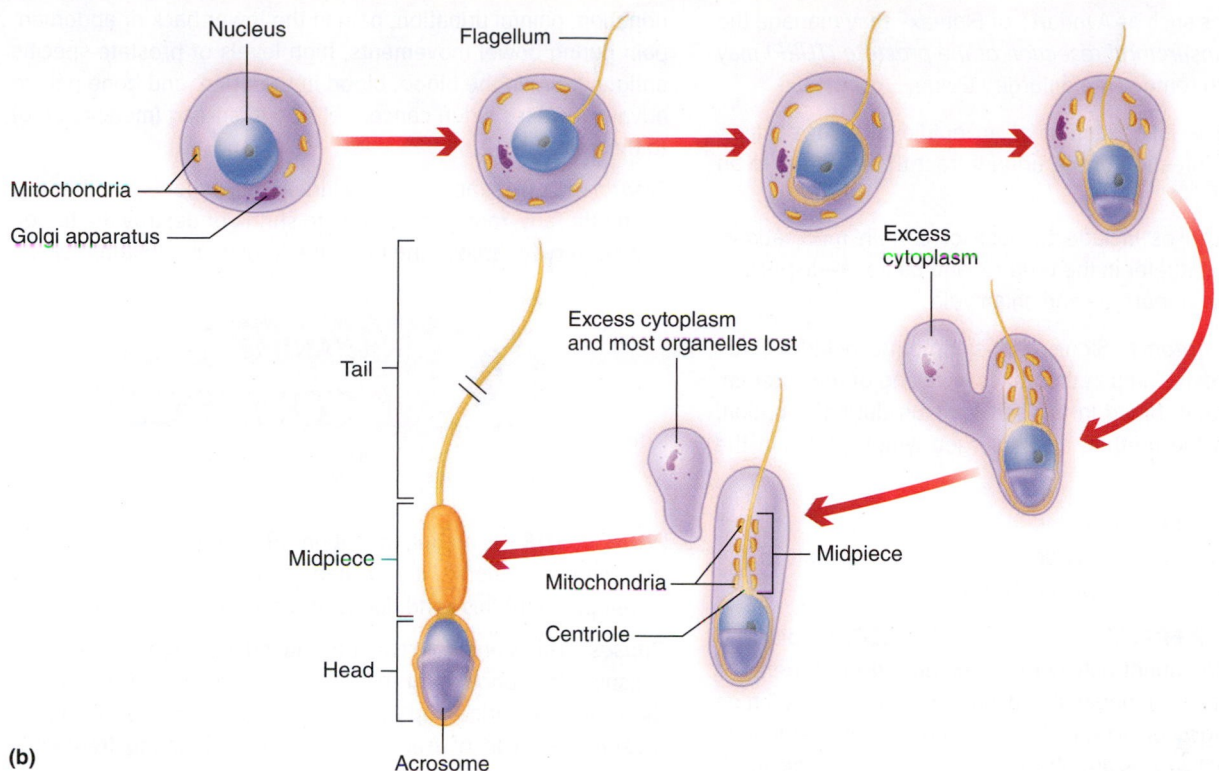

(b)

FIGURE 31-3 (concluded)

Erection, Orgasm, and Ejaculation

During sexual arousal, the parasympathetic nervous system causes erectile tissue of the penis to become engorged with blood, which produces erection of the penis. During orgasm, sperm cells are propelled out of the testes toward the urethra. The secretions of the prostate, seminal vesicles, and bulbourethral glands are also released into the urethra. The movement of the sperm and secretions into the urethra is called *emission*. The process of *ejaculation* occurs when semen is forced out of the urethra. After ejaculation, sympathetic nerve fibers cause the erectile tissue to release blood, and the penis gradually returns to a flaccid, or nonerect, state.

Male Reproductive Hormones

The hypothalamus, the anterior pituitary gland, and the testes secrete hormones that regulate male reproductive functions. At the onset of puberty and throughout life, the hypothalamus releases a hormone called *gonadotropin-releasing hormone (GnRH)*. GnRH stimulates the anterior pituitary gland to release *follicle-stimulating hormone (FSH)* and *luteinizing hormone (LH)*. FSH causes spermatogenesis to begin, and LH stimulates interstitial cells to produce *testosterone*.

Testosterone is responsible for the development of male secondary sex characteristics that are typically unique to males. Examples of these characteristics include chest hair, thick facial hair, a thickening and strengthening of muscles and bones, and the thickening of vocal cords that produces a deeper voice. Testosterone also stimulates the maturation of male reproductive organs.

Testosterone levels are regulated by negative feedback in the following cycle: Blood testosterone levels increase to above normal levels, which causes the hypothalamus to release GnRH. In response, the anterior pituitary ceases the secretion of LH and FSH, in turn causing the testosterone level to fall. When the testosterone level falls below normal, GnRH is again secreted by the hypothalamus, triggering the release of LH and FSH by the anterior pituitary, and the cycle begins again.

PATHOPHYSIOLOGY

LO 31.2

Common Diseases and Disorders of the Male Reproductive System

BENIGN PROSTATIC HYPERTROPHY, OR BPH, is the non-malignant enlargement of the prostate gland. This condition is common in older men.

Causes. BPH is related to the hormonal changes that occur as part of the aging process.

Signs and Symptoms. Men with BPH often complain of frequent urination, especially at night, as well as painful urination and difficulty starting or stopping the urinary stream, including "dribbling" at the end of urination.

Treatment. Diagnosis is often confirmed by digital rectal exam (DRE), in which the licensed practitioner inserts a gloved finger into the rectum and palpates the prostate. Blood tests (PSA) and a biopsy may be done to rule out cancer. Once cancer is ruled out, medications such as Avodart® or Flomax® may manage the problem, or *transurethral resection of the prostate (TURP)* may be performed to remove the enlarged tissue.

EPIDIDYMITIS is inflammation of an epididymis. Most cases start out as an infection of the urinary tract that spreads to an epididymis.

Causes. The causes include the use of certain medications, placement of a catheter in the urethra, and bacteria—especially those that cause gonorrhea and chlamydia.

Signs and Symptoms. Signs and symptoms include fever, pain in the testes, a lump in the testes, swelling of the scrotum, painful ejaculation, blood in the semen, pain during urination, discharge from the urethra, and enlarged lymph nodes in the pelvic area.

Treatment. Treatment includes pain medication, antibiotics for both the patient and his sexual partner, elevation of the scrotum, and ice packs applied to the scrotum.

IMPOTENCE, OR ERECTILE DYSFUNCTION (ED), is a disorder in which a male cannot achieve or maintain an erect penis to complete sexual intercourse. It is estimated that half of all men between the ages of 40 and 70 years have some degree of impotence. Most causes are physical and not psychological.

Causes. Psychological causes include anxiety, stress, and depression. Common physical causes include diabetes; high blood pressure; anemia; coronary artery disease (CAD); peripheral vascular disease (PVD); low testosterone production; various medications; smoking; excessive alcohol consumption; and drugs such as cocaine, marijuana, and heroin.

Signs and Symptoms. Signs and symptoms include an inability to achieve an erection and an inability to maintain an erection long enough to complete sexual intercourse.

Treatment. The first treatment step should be lifestyle changes to quit smoking and stop using alcohol and/or drugs. Counseling to reduce anxiety and depression may also be helpful. Other treatment options include oral medications such as Viagra® or Cialis®, penile injections of medications, and penile implants if oral medications do not work.

PROSTATE CANCER is one of the most common cancers in men older than age 40, and the risk of developing prostate cancer increases with age. Awareness about this malignancy is growing, and access to screenings such as digital rectal exam (DRE) is becoming widely available. Therefore, many cases in the United States are being diagnosed even before symptoms occur.

Causes. The causes are mostly unknown, although decreased testosterone production may contribute to the development of this disease, explaining why risk increases with age.

Signs and Symptoms. Common symptoms include anemia, weight loss, incontinence, difficulty starting or stopping

urination, painful urination, pain in the lower back or abdomen, pain during bowel movements, high levels of prostate-specific antigen (PSA) in the blood, blood in the urine, and bone pain in advanced cases when cancer cells have spread (metastasized) to the bone.

Treatment. Treatments include hormone therapy, chemotherapy, radiation therapy to shrink or destroy the tumor, and surgery to remove the prostate, known as *prostatectomy.*

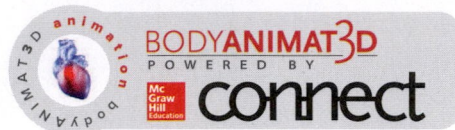

Go to CONNECT to see an animation exercise about *Prostate Cancer.*

PROSTATITIS is an inflammation of the prostate gland. If it develops suddenly, it is called *acute prostatitis.* The slow development of this condition is termed *chronic prostatitis.*

Causes. This condition can be caused by excessive alcohol consumption, bacterial infection, a catheterization, trauma to the urethra or urinary bladder, and scarring of the urethra or prostate because of frequent infections. Urinating frequently can help to prevent this infection.

Signs and Symptoms. Signs and symptoms include fever; pain in the scrotum, pelvic area, or abdomen; difficult, frequent, and/or painful urination; blood in the urine; painful ejaculation; blood in the semen; discharge from the urethra; a low sperm count; and white blood cells in urine or semen.

Treatment. This condition is treated with antibiotics. Surgery may also be required to repair any damage to the urethra.

TESTICULAR CANCER is a malignant growth of one or both testicles. Unlike prostate cancer, which tends to occur in older males, testicular cancer occurs in males ages 15 to 30 and is a much more aggressive malignancy.

Causes. Predisposing factors include cryptorchidism (undescended testicles during infancy). Family history may also be a factor.

Signs and Symptoms. A hard, painless lump in one testicle is a common early symptom. Patients may complain of groin or abdominal pain as the disease progresses.

Treatment. Orchiectomy, or removal of the involved testis, is usually performed, followed by radiation therapy and chemotherapy. Caught in the early stages, testicular cancer has up to a 95% success rate. It is therefore very important for males to perform testicular self-exams on a monthly basis. You will learn how to instruct patients in this important exam technique in the *Assisting in Reproductive and Urinary Specialties* chapter.

▶ The Female Reproductive System LO 31.3

Ovaries and Ovum Formation

The ovaries are considered the primary female sex organs because they produce the female sex cells, called *ova* (see Figures 31-4 and 31-5). They also produce *estrogen* and *progesterone,* the female hormones. Most females have two ovaries. They are oval in shape and are located in the pelvic cavity. Each ovary is divided into an inner area called the *medulla* and an outer area called the *cortex.* The medulla contains nerves, lymphatic vessels, and many blood vessels. The cortex contains small masses of cells called *ovarian follicles.* Epithelial tissue and dense connective tissue cover each ovary.

Before a female child is born, *primordial follicles* develop in her ovarian cortex. Each primordial follicle contains a large cell called a *primary oocyte* (immature ovum) and smaller cells called *follicular cells.* Unlike males, who make sperm cells throughout their entire life, a female is born with the maximum number of primary oocytes she will ever produce.

Oogenesis is the process of ovum formation. At the onset of puberty, some primary oocytes are stimulated to continue meiosis (see Figure 31-2). When a primary oocyte divides, it produces one *polar body* (a nonfunctional cell) and a *secondary oocyte.* The secondary oocyte is released from an ovary each month during a process called **ovulation.** When the secondary oocyte is fertilized, it divides to form a mature, fertilized ovum. Therefore, the process of meiosis begins before a female is born and is completed only if a secondary oocyte is fertilized. The mature ovum contains 23 chromosomes; when it combines with a sperm cell, the resulting cell contains 46 chromosomes.

Internal Accessory Organs of the Female Reproductive System

The female reproductive internal accessory organs are the fallopian tubes, uterus, and vagina.

Fallopian Tubes A fallopian tube, or *oviduct,* opens near each ovary, and the other end connects to the uterus. The fringed, expanded end of a fallopian tube near an ovary is called an **infundibulum.** The infundibulum ends in *fimbriae,* or finger-like projections. The infundibulum and its fimbriae "catch" an ovum as it leaves an ovary. Fallopian tubes are muscular tubes that are lined with mucous membrane and cilia. This construction allows the tube to propel the ovum toward the uterus using peristalsis and the sweeping motions of cilia.

Uterus The uterus is a hollow, muscular organ that receives a developing embryo and sustains its development. The upper, domed portion of the uterus is called the *fundus,* the main portion is called the *body,* and the narrow, lower portion that extends into the vagina is called the *cervix.* The opening of the cervix is called the *cervical orifice.*

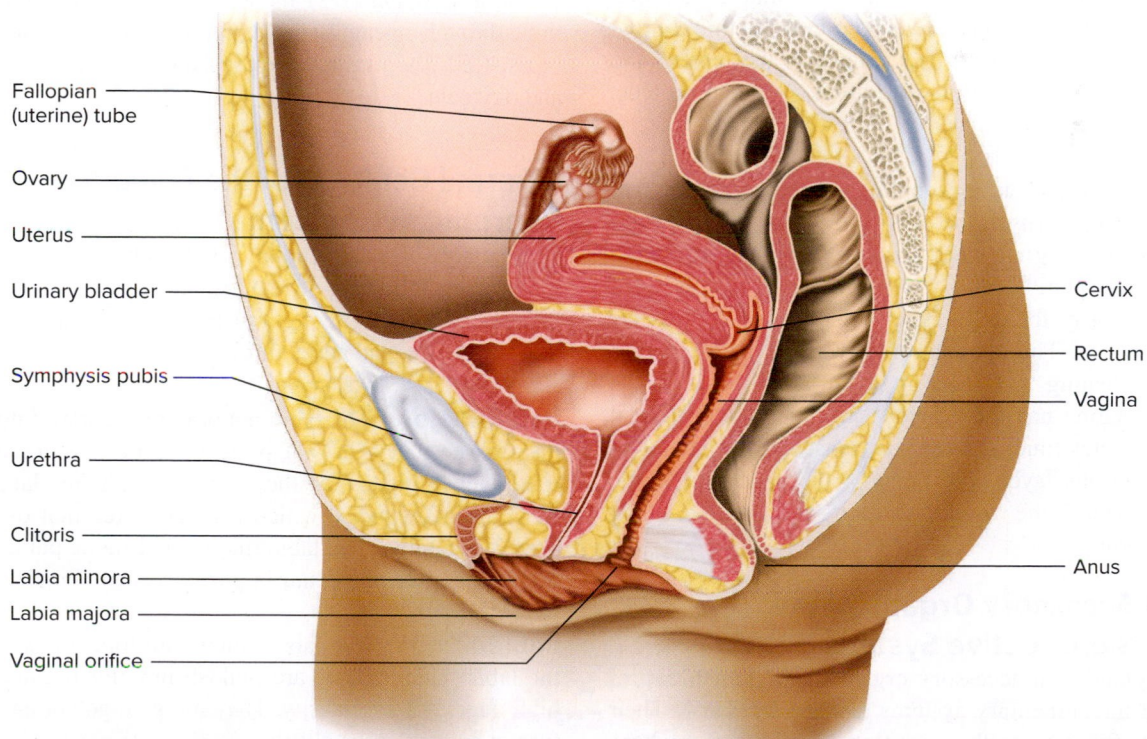

FIGURE 31-4 Sagittal view of female reproductive organs. The female reproductive system produces ova for fertilization and provides the place and means for a fertilized ovum to develop.

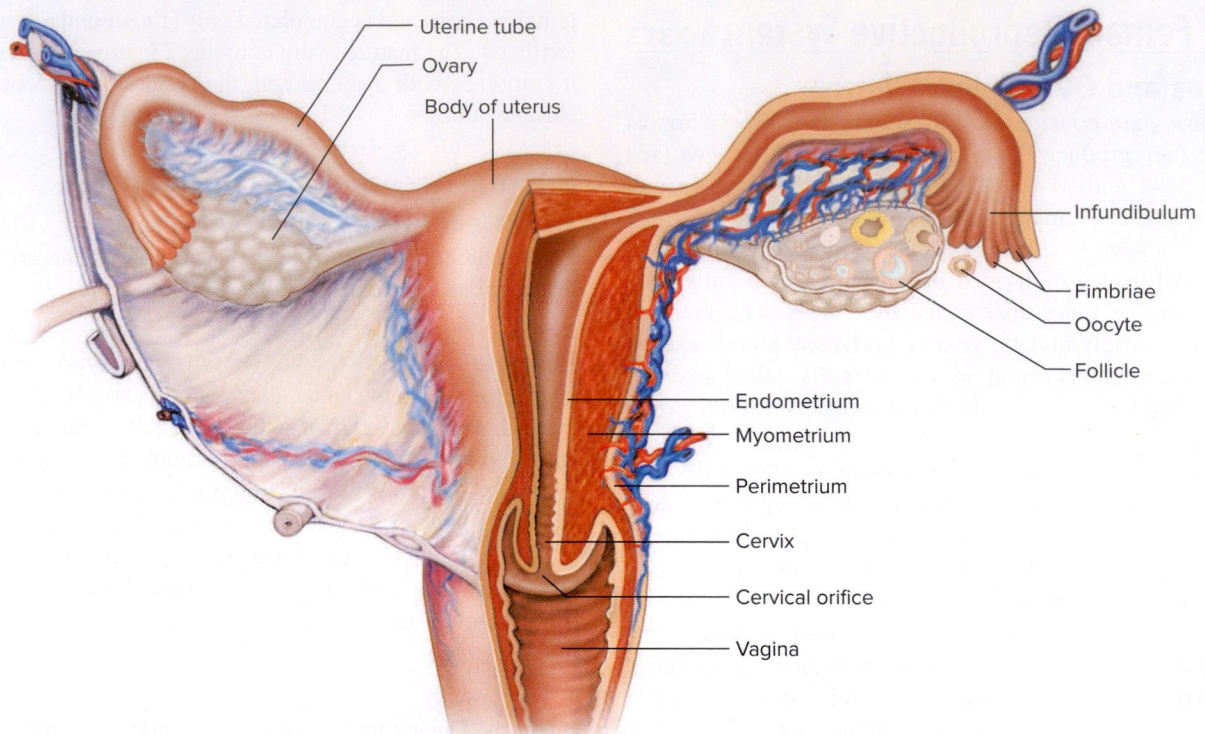

FIGURE 31-5 Anterior view of internal female reproductive organs, showing ovulation of an oocyte.

The wall of the uterus has three layers: the endometrium, myometrium, and perimetrium. The *endometrium* is the innermost lining of the uterus. It is vascular with a rich blood supply, and it contains numerous tubular glands that secrete mucus. The *myometrium* is the middle, thick, muscular layer. The *perimetrium* is a thin layer that covers the myometrium. It secretes serous fluid that coats and protects the uterus.

Vagina The vagina is a tubular, muscular organ that extends from the uterus to the outside of the body. The muscular folds of the vagina, called *rugae,* allow it to expand to receive an erect penis during sexual intercourse and to provide a passageway for delivery of offspring as well as for uterine secretions. The opening of the vagina is posterior to the urinary opening and anterior to the anal opening. The wall of the vagina has three layers: an innermost, mucosal layer that secretes mucus; a middle, muscular layer; and an outermost, fibrous layer. The opening of the vagina to the outside is known as the *vaginal os,* the *vaginal orifice,* or the *vaginal introitus.*

External Accessory Organs of the Female Reproductive System

Mammary glands are accessory organs of the female reproductive and integumentary systems (see Figure 31-6). Their reproductive function is the secretion of milk for newborn offspring.

Mammary glands are located beneath the skin in the breast area. A nipple is near the center of each breast. The pigmented area that surrounds the nipple is called the *areola.* Each gland is made of 15 to 20 lobes and contains *alveolar glands* that make milk under the influence of the hormone *prolactin.* The hormone *oxytocin (OT)* induces *lactiferous ducts* to deliver milk through openings in the nipples. If a woman wants to breast-feed, she must produce adequate amounts of prolactin and oxytocin.

External Genitalia of the Female Reproductive System

The female external genitalia, collectively known as the *vulva,* include the following structures: mons pubis, labia majora, labia minora, clitoris, urethral meatus, vaginal orifice, Bartholin's glands, and perineum.

Labia Majora The labia majora are rounded folds of adipose tissue and skin that protect the other external female reproductive organs. At their anterior ends, the labia majora form the *mons pubis,* which is a fatty area that overlies the symphysis pubis. The labia majora and mons pubis are typically covered in pubic hair in postpubescent females.

Labia Minora The labia minora are folds of skin between the labia majora. They are pinkish in color because of their high degree of vascularity. They merge together anteriorly to form a hood over the clitoris.

The space enclosed by the labia minora is called the *vestibule.* The **Bartholin's glands,** sometimes referred to as the *vestibular glands,* secrete mucus into this area during

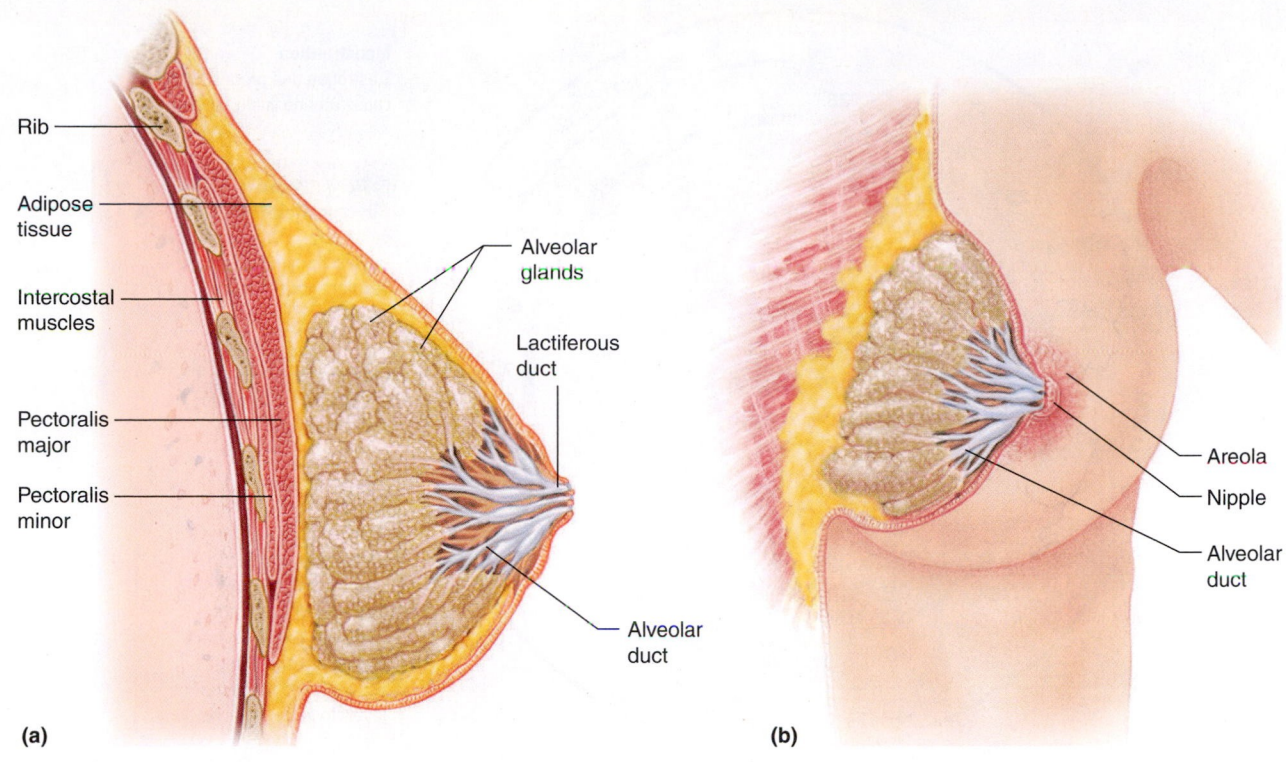

FIGURE 31-6 Mammary glands: (a) sagittal view and (b) anterior view.

In figure (a):
Rib
Adipose tissue
Intercostal muscles
Pectoralis major
Pectoralis minor
Alveolar glands
Lactiferous duct
Alveolar duct
(a)

In figure (b):
Areola
Nipple
Alveolar duct
(b)

sexual arousal. This mucus eases insertion of the penis into the vagina.

Clitoris The clitoris is anterior to the urethral meatus. It contains the female erectile tissue and is rich in sensory nerves.

Perineum The perineum is the area between the vagina and the anus. This is the area that is sometimes "clipped" during the birth process, in a procedure known as an *episiotomy*.

Erection, Lubrication, and Orgasm

During sexual arousal, nervous stimulation causes the clitoris to become erect and the Bartholin's glands to become active. At the same time, the vagina elongates. If the clitoris is sufficiently stimulated, an orgasm occurs. During orgasm, the walls of the uterus and fallopian tubes contract to help propel sperm toward the upper ends of the fallopian tubes.

Female Reproductive Hormones

Beginning at puberty, the hypothalamus secretes increasing amounts of GnRH. This causes the anterior pituitary gland to release FSH and LH, which stimulate the ovary to produce estrogen and progesterone, as well as to mature the ovarian follicles. The estrogen and progesterone are responsible for the female secondary sex characteristics: breast development, increased vascularization of the skin, and increased fat deposits in the breasts, thighs, and hips.

Female Reproductive Cycle

The female reproductive cycle is also called the *menstrual cycle*. See Figure 31-7. It consists of regular changes in the uterine lining that leads to a monthly "period," or shedding of the uterine lining, along with bleeding. The first menstrual period is known as **menarche. Menopause** is the termination of the menstrual cycle because of normal aging of the ovaries. The following steps are the major hormonal changes that occur during one reproductive cycle:

1. The anterior pituitary gland releases FSH, which stimulates an ovarian follicle to mature.

2. The maturing follicle secretes estrogen. Estrogen causes the uterine lining to thicken.

3. The anterior pituitary gland releases a sudden surge of LH, which triggers ovulation.

4. Following ovulation, follicular cells of the follicle become a *corpus luteum*.

5. The corpus luteum secretes progesterone, which causes the uterine lining to become more vascular and glandular.

6. If the released oocyte is not fertilized, the corpus luteum degenerates, causing estrogen and progesterone levels to fall.

7. The decline in estrogen and progesterone levels causes the uterine lining to break down, and menses (elimination of the uterine lining, with bleeding) starts.

8. When the anterior pituitary releases FSH, the reproductive cycle begins again.

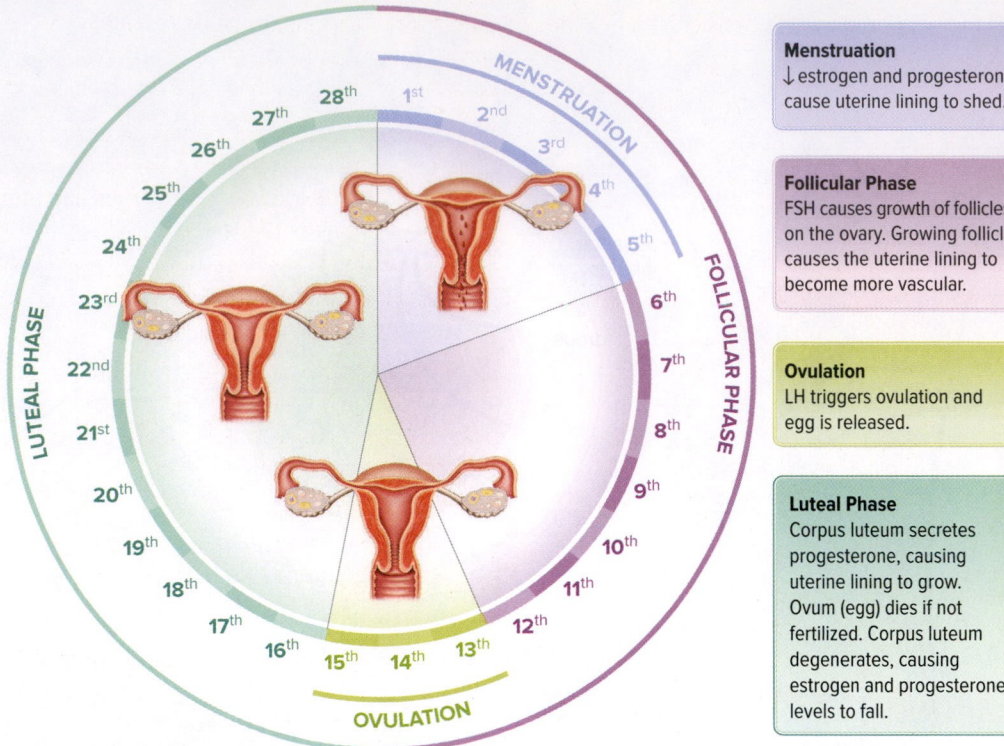

Menstruation
↓ estrogen and progesterone cause uterine lining to shed.

Follicular Phase
FSH causes growth of follicles on the ovary. Growing follicle causes the uterine lining to become more vascular.

Ovulation
LH triggers ovulation and egg is released.

Luteal Phase
Corpus luteum secretes progesterone, causing uterine lining to grow. Ovum (egg) dies if not fertilized. Corpus luteum degenerates, causing estrogen and progesterone levels to fall.

FIGURE 31-7 A typical 28-day menstrual cycle.

PATHOPHYSIOLOGY

LO 31.4

Common Diseases and Disorders of the Female Reproductive System

BREAST CANCER, according to the American Cancer Society, is the second leading cause of cancer deaths in women after lung cancer. Depending on tumor size and how far cancer cells have spread, breast cancer is classified in stages from 0 to 4, with stage 4 cancer being the most serious. Early diagnosis through regular mammograms and breast self-exams greatly increases the success of treatment. Teaching female patients about breast self-exam and its importance in the early detection of breast cancer is an important aspect of being a medical assistant. You will learn how to teach women this technique in the *Assisting in Reproductive and Urinary Specialties* chapter.

Causes. The causes are largely unknown, although breast cancer may be related to hormonal changes or the presence of certain genes.

Signs and Symptoms. Signs and symptoms include a lump in the breast that is usually painless and firm, a lump in the armpit, discharge from the nipples, dimpled skin on the breast or nipple, and breast pain. Swelling of the breast into the adjacent arm and bone pain may be present in advanced cases. Inflammatory breast cancer may present only as a painless rash of the affected breast with none of the other typical symptoms.

Treatment. Nonsurgical treatment methods include hormone therapy, radiation therapy, and chemotherapy. Surgical options include surgery to remove affected lymph nodes, lumpectomy

(surgery to remove a lump), and mastectomy (surgery to remove a breast).

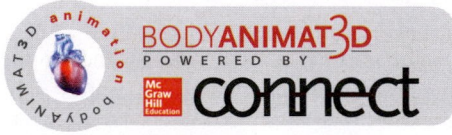

Go to CONNECT to see an animation exercise about *Breast Cancer.*

CERVICAL CANCER generally develops slowly, although adenocarcinoma of the cervix, which tends to be a more rapidly spreading cancer, is the exception to this rule. With early detection by a yearly Pap smear (a test looking for abnormal cervical cells), treatment is often successful. Note that the new recommendation for Pap smear screenings is now every other year if a woman's previous screenings have been negative for 5 years and if the woman is in a monogamous relationship and not on birth control pills.

Causes. A weak immune system may be a factor in the development of this cancer. Risk factors also include sexual intercourse early in life, multiple sexual partners, and infection with the human papillomavirus (HPV).

Signs and Symptoms. Primary symptoms include frequent vaginal discharge, sporadic vaginal bleeding, vaginal bleeding after sexual intercourse, and abnormal cells in the cervix. Patients who are in later stages of this disease may experience pain in the pelvic area or legs, or bone fractures.

Treatment. Radiation therapy, chemotherapy, the removal or destruction of diseased tissue with cryosurgery or laser surgery, and the removal of the uterus (hysterectomy) are the treatments for this disease.

CERVICITIS is an inflammation of the cervix, which is usually caused by an infection.

Causes. Causes include bacterial or viral infections and allergic reactions to spermicidal creams and latex condoms.

Signs and Symptoms. Frequent vaginal discharge, pain during intercourse, and vaginal bleeding after intercourse are common signs and symptoms.

Treatment. This condition is treated with antibiotics and by changing the contraception method.

DYSMENORRHEA is the condition of experiencing severe menstrual cramps that limit normal daily activities.

Causes. Causes include anxiety, endometriosis, pelvic inflammatory disease (PID), fibroid tumors in the uterus, ovarian cysts, abnormally high levels of prostaglandins, and multiple sexual partners.

Signs and Symptoms. Common symptoms are abdominal pain, including sharp or dull pain in the pelvic area just prior to and during the menstrual period.

Treatment. Nonsurgical treatments include pain medication, anti-inflammatory drugs, medications that inhibit prostaglandin formation, oral contraceptives, and antibiotics in the case of PID. Surgical treatments include hysterectomy and surgery to remove cysts or fibroids.

ENDOMETRIOSIS is a condition in which tissues that make up the lining of the uterus grow outside the uterus.

Causes. The cause of this disorder is unknown; it may be inherited.

Signs and Symptoms. Signs and symptoms include infertility, heavy bleeding from the uterus, pain in the abdomen or pelvis, painful periods, spotting between periods, and pain during sexual intercourse.

Treatment. Oral contraceptives, pain medications, and various hormone therapies may be prescribed. Surgical treatments include laser surgery to remove endometrial tissue outside the uterus and hysterectomy.

FIBROCYSTIC BREAST DISEASE is the presence of abnormal cystic tissues in the breasts. The cysts vary in size related to the menstrual cycle. It is a common disorder and occurs in more than 60% of women in the United States between age 30 and 50. It is rare in women who have gone through menopause because it is related to hormonal changes occurring during the menstrual cycle. It is important to note that fibrocystic breast disease is not considered to put a woman at higher risk of breast cancer.

Causes. This disorder is caused by hormonal changes associated with the menstrual cycle and ingestion of various dietary substances, including caffeine, nicotine, and sugar. Birth control pills may also aggravate this condition.

Signs and Symptoms. Common symptoms include breasts that feel "lumpy," breast tenderness or pain, itchy nipples, and dense tissues as seen in a mammogram.

Treatment. Treatments include changing one's diet and taking supplements such as vitamin E, B complex, and magnesium. Wearing support bras may help with pain control.

UTERINE FIBROIDS are benign (noncancerous) tumors that grow in the uterine wall. They are known to affect one out of four women in their thirties and forties and appear to be more common in women of African descent.

Causes. The causes are mostly unknown, although it has been found that the tumors enlarge as estrogen levels increase. Heredity appears to play a role.

Signs and Symptoms. The signs and symptoms are pressure in the abdomen, severe menstrual cramps, abdominal gas, heavy menstrual bleeding, and intermenstrual bleeding. Back and leg pain may also occur.

Treatment. Treatment includes pain medications, hormone treatments to shrink tumors, surgery to remove tumors, hysterectomy, and surgery to decrease the blood supply to the uterus.

OVARIAN CANCER is considered more deadly than other types of cancer because its signs and symptoms are usually mild or indistinct until the disease has spread to other organs, making early detection difficult. Current statistics suggest that about 1 woman in 67 will develop ovarian cancer. Women with a family history of ovarian cancer may be counseled to consider prophylactic *oophorosalpingectomy* (removal of the ovaries and fallopian tubes) prior to actually developing ovarian cancer.

Causes. The causes are unknown, although the presence of certain genes has been indicated as a risk factor. Some oral contraceptives may lower the risk of developing this disease.

Signs and Symptoms. Abdominal and pelvic discomfort, unusual menstrual cycles, indigestion, bloating, nausea, and excessive hair growth are signs and symptoms. Diagnosis is made after ultrasound, a CA-125 blood test, and an ovarian biopsy.

Treatment. Treatment options include radiation therapy, chemotherapy, and surgery to remove the ovaries and reproductive organs.

PREMENSTRUAL SYNDROME (PMS) is a collection of symptoms that occur just before a menstrual period.

Causes. The causes are mostly unknown, although hormone fluctuations during the menstrual cycle are implicated.

Signs and Symptoms. The signs and symptoms include anxiety, depression, irritability, acne, fatigue, food cravings, bloating, aches in the head or back, abdominal pain, breast tenderness, muscle spasms, diarrhea, weight gain, and loss of sex drive.

Treatment. PMS is commonly treated with pain medications, diuretics, medications to treat depression or anxiety, and oral contraceptives. Many women have also found changes in diet to be helpful, including limiting caffeine, sugar, and sodium. The addition of B complex vitamins may also be helpful.

UTERINE (ENDOMETRIAL) CANCER is most common in postmenopausal women. In the United States, it accounts for approximately 6% of cancer deaths in women.

Causes. The causes are mostly unknown, although it may be related to increased levels of estrogen.

Signs and Symptoms. Signs and symptoms include abdominal pain; abnormal bleeding from the uterus; pelvic pain; and a thin, white vaginal discharge in postmenopausal women.

Treatment. Treatment includes radiation therapy, chemotherapy, and surgery to remove the uterus, fallopian tubes, and ovaries.

VULVOVAGINITIS (inflammation of the vulva and vagina) and **VAGINITIS** (inflammation of the vagina) are usually associated with an abnormal vaginal discharge. Some vaginal discharge is normal for all women, and it varies throughout the menstrual cycle. Normal vaginal discharge is clear, whitish, or yellowish in color.

Causes. This condition can be caused by yeast infections, tampon use, poor hygiene, bacteria, antibiotics, and sexually transmitted infections (STIs). Vaginitis may be prevented through good hygiene and safe sex practices.

Signs and Symptoms. Common symptoms include fever, vulvar and vaginal itching and swelling, an abnormal increase or decrease in the amount of vaginal discharge, an abnormal color of vaginal discharge (brown, green, or pinkish), a change in the consistency of vaginal discharge (frothy or cheese-like), and vaginal discharge that has an abnormal odor.

Treatment. The patient may be given medications for fungal or bacterial infections, or the patient and her sexual partner may be treated for STIs.

▶ Pregnancy

LO 31.5

Pregnancy is defined as the condition of having a developing offspring in the uterus. Pregnancy results when a sperm cell unites with an ovum in a process called fertilization (see Figure 31-8).

Fertilization

Prior to fertilization, an ovum is released from an ovary and travels through a fallopian tube. During sexual intercourse, the male deposits semen into the vagina. Sperm cells must travel up through the uterus to the fallopian tubes to fertilize the ovum.

Prostaglandins in semen stimulate the flagella of sperm cells to undulate, causing the swimming action of sperm. Prostaglandins also stimulate muscles in the uterus and fallopian tubes to contract. These contractions (peristalsis) help the sperm reach the ovum. Normally about 10 to 14 days after ovulation, high estrogen levels stimulate the uterus and cervix to secrete a thin, watery fluid that also promotes the movement of sperm toward the ovum.

Although many sperm cells normally reach an ovum, only one sperm cell unites with the ovum, penetrating the follicular cells and a layer called the *zona pellucida,* which surrounds the cell membrane of the ovum. The acrosome of this sperm releases enzymes to help the sperm penetrate the membrane

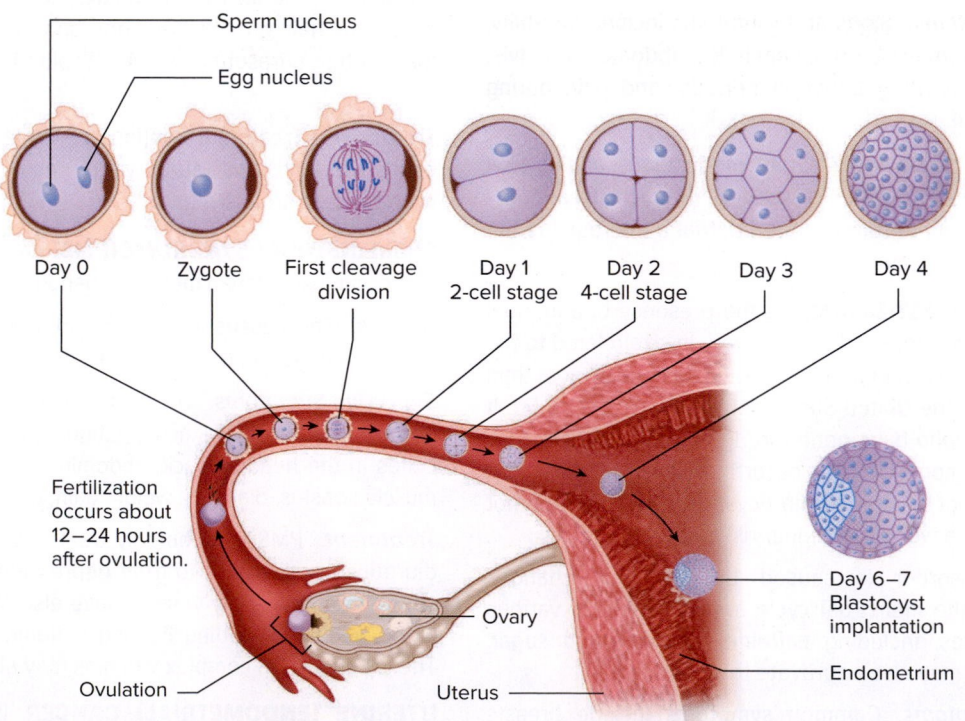

FIGURE 31-8 Stages of early embryo development.

of the ovum. Once a sperm unites with an ovum, the ovum releases enzymes to prevent other sperm from invading it. The enzymes cause the zona pellucida to become hard and therefore impenetrable to other sperm.

The nucleus of the ovum (with 23 chromosomes) and the nucleus of the sperm (with 23 chromosomes) fuse together to make one nucleus that contains 46 chromosomes. The cell that is formed by this union is called a **zygote.**

The Prenatal Period

The prenatal period is the time before the offspring is born. It is divided into an *embryonic period* (weeks 2 through 8 of pregnancy) and a *fetal period* (week 9 to the delivery of the offspring). It is further divided into three periods known as trimesters, which consist of 3 calendar months each. See *Points on Practice*: The Pregnant Patient.

About 1 day after the zygote forms, it begins to undergo mitosis at a relatively rapid rate. This rapid cell division is called *cleavage,* and the resulting ball of cells is called a *morula.* The morula travels down the fallopian tube to the uterus. Fluid then invades the morula, and this organism is called a **blastocyst.** The blastocyst implants in the endometrial wall of the uterus. The process of moving from zygote formation to implantation of the blastocyst takes about 1 week. Once the blastocyst implants, a group of cells in the blastocyst, called the *inner cell mass,* gives rise to an **embryo.** Other cells in the blastocyst, along with cells of the uterus, eventually form the **placenta.**

The Embryonic Period The embryonic period extends from the second week of pregnancy to the end of the eighth week of development. During this stage, the placenta, *amnion, umbilical cord,* and *yolk sac* form, along with most of the internal organs and external structures of the embryo (see Figure 31-9). The cells of the inner cell mass organize into

layers called **primary germ layers.** All organs are formed from the primary germ layers, which include the ectoderm, mesoderm, and endoderm.

- The *ectoderm* develops into nervous tissue and some epithelial tissue.
- The *mesoderm,* the middle layer, develops into connective tissues and some epithelial tissue.
- The *endoderm* develops into epithelial tissues only.

The placenta allows nutrients and oxygen from maternal blood to pass to embryonic blood. It also allows waste products from the fetal blood to pass into maternal blood. The **amnion** is a protective, fluid-filled sac that surrounds the embryo. The *umbilical cord* contains three blood vessels—one umbilical vein that carries oxygenated blood from the placenta to the embryo, and two umbilical arteries that carry deoxygenated blood from the embryo back to the placenta.

The yolk sac makes new blood cells for the fetus, as well as cells that eventually become the sex cells of the baby. By the end of the embryonic stage, the baby closely resembles a human because all external structures (arms, hands, legs, feet, etc.) have formed.

The Fetal Period The fetal period begins at the end of the eighth week of development and ends at birth. During this period, the growth of the offspring, which is now called a **fetus,** is rapid. By the twelfth week, bones have begun to harden and the external reproductive organs are distinguishable as male or female.

The growth rate of the fetus slows down in the fifth month but skeletal muscles become active. In the sixth month, the fetus starts to gain substantial weight. In the seventh month, the eyelids open. In the last 3 months of pregnancy, fetal brain cells divide rapidly and organs continue to grow. The testes of the male descend into the scrotum. The last organ systems to

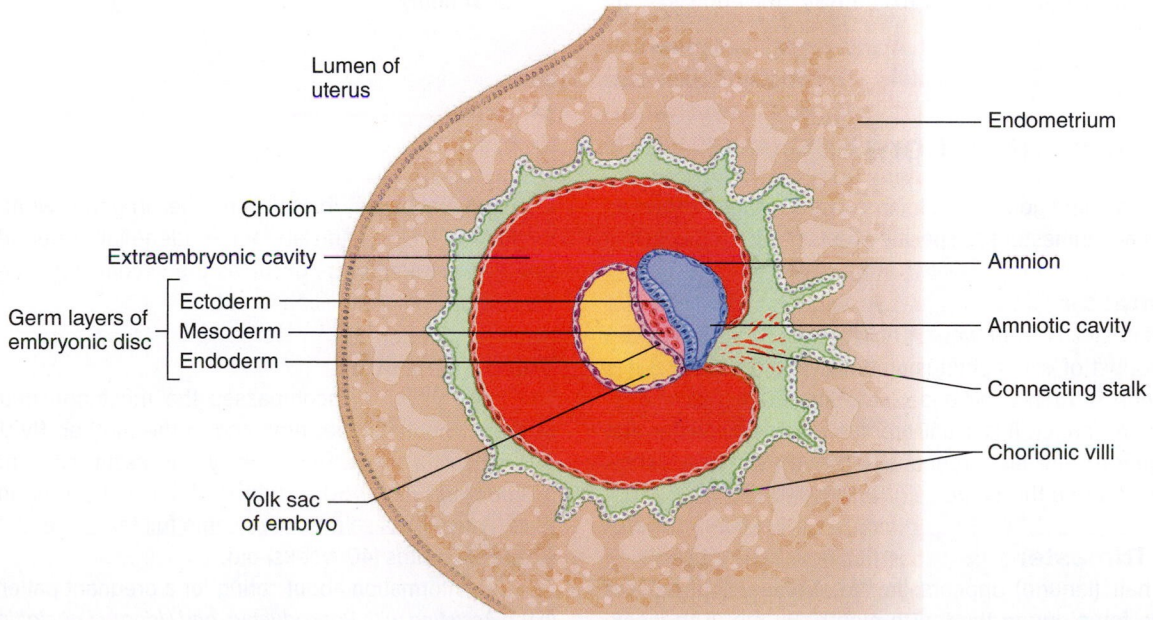

FIGURE 31-9 Primary germ layers and membranes associated with an embryo.

completely develop are the digestive and respiratory systems. By the end of the ninth month, the fetus is usually positioned upside down in the uterus in preparation for delivery.

Fetal Circulation

Throughout prenatal development, the placenta and umbilical blood vessels carry out the exchange of nutrients, oxygen, and waste products between maternal and fetal blood. Therefore, the fetus does not need to send blood to the lungs to pick up oxygen, nor does it need to send blood to the liver to process nutrients.

Fetal circulation has some important differences from normal circulation, which are illustrated in Figure 31-10. In the adult heart, blood flows from the right atrium into the right ventricle so that it can be pumped to the lungs. In the fetal heart, a hole called the **foramen ovale** is located between the right and left atria. This hole allows most of the fetal blood to flow from the right atrium into the left atrium. However, some fetal blood does flow from the right atrium into the right ventricle, and the right ventricle then delivers the blood to the pulmonary trunk.

In the fetus, there is also a connection between the pulmonary trunk and the aorta called the **ductus arteriosus.** This connection allows blood to flow from the pulmonary trunk into the aorta. In the adult, this connection closes and blood flows from the pulmonary trunk to the lungs. The fetus also contains a blood vessel called the **ductus venosus** that allows most of the blood to bypass the liver. After a baby is born, the foramen ovale, ductus arteriosus, and ductus venosus normally close.

Hemoglobin within the fetus has a much higher affinity for oxygen than does the normal hemoglobin that is found after birth and during growth. Therefore, the fetus's blood is adapted to carry more oxygen.

Hormonal Changes During Pregnancy

Many hormonal changes take place when a woman is pregnant. Following implantation of the embryo, the embryo cells begin to secrete *human chorionic gonadotropin (HCG).* HCG maintains the corpus luteum in the ovary so it will continue to secrete estrogen and progesterone. The placenta also secretes large amounts of progesterone and estrogen.

Progesterone and estrogen stimulate the uterine lining to thicken and inhibit the anterior pituitary gland from secreting FSH and LH to prevent ovulation during pregnancy. Estrogen and progesterone also stimulate the development of the mammary glands, inhibit uterine contractions, and stimulate the enlargement of female reproductive organs.

A hormone called *relaxin,* which comes from the corpus luteum, inhibits uterine contractions and relaxes the ligaments of the pelvis in preparation for childbirth. The placenta also secretes *lactogen,* a hormone that stimulates the enlargement of mammary glands. *Aldosterone,* which is secreted from the adrenal gland, increases sodium and water retention. The secretion of *parathyroid hormone (PTH)* increases, helping to maintain high calcium levels in the blood.

▶ The Birth Process   LO 31.6

The birth process ends pregnancy. This process begins when progesterone levels fall. When this happens, uterine contractions are no longer inhibited and the uterus secretes prostaglandins that stimulate uterine contractions, which cause the posterior pituitary gland to release oxytocin. Oxytocin stimulates stronger uterine contractions until the birth process ends. The birth process itself occurs in three stages after the fetus settles into position in the mother's pelvis (see Figure 31-11a).

1. *Dilation* (see Figure 31-11b). The cervix thins and softens, known as *effacement,* dilating to approximately 10 cm. Regular contractions occur at this stage and the amniotic sac ruptures. If rupture does not occur, the sac may be surgically punctured. This stage normally lasts 8 to 24 hours.

POINTS ON PRACTICE

The Pregnant Patient

The pregnant patient goes through three distinct stages known as *trimesters.* Each trimester has specific events associated with it.

First Trimester

The first trimester is from week 1 to week 12. During weeks 1 to 8 the product of conception is an embryo; after week 8 it is a fetus. Week 12 marks the end of the first trimester, or one-third of the pregnancy. It is usually during the first trimester that women confirm they are pregnant. "Morning sickness" commonly occurs during this stage.

Second Trimester

Fine, soft hair (lanugo) appears on the shoulders, back, and head of the fetus during the fourth month. By the 20th week, fetal movement may be felt, and the pregnant woman begins to show fullness in the abdomen. Identifiable periods of fetal sleep and wakefulness occur as the second trimester ends at the completion of the sixth month.

Third Trimester

The last trimester encompasses the most noticeable period of growth, both in the fetus and in the mother. By the end of 30 weeks, the fetus most likely has assumed a head-down position and has a 50% chance of survival if it is born at this time. The fetus is said to have come full term after it is approximately 9 months (40 weeks) old.

More information about caring for a pregnant patient is found in the *Assisting with Reproductive and Urinary Specialties* chapter.

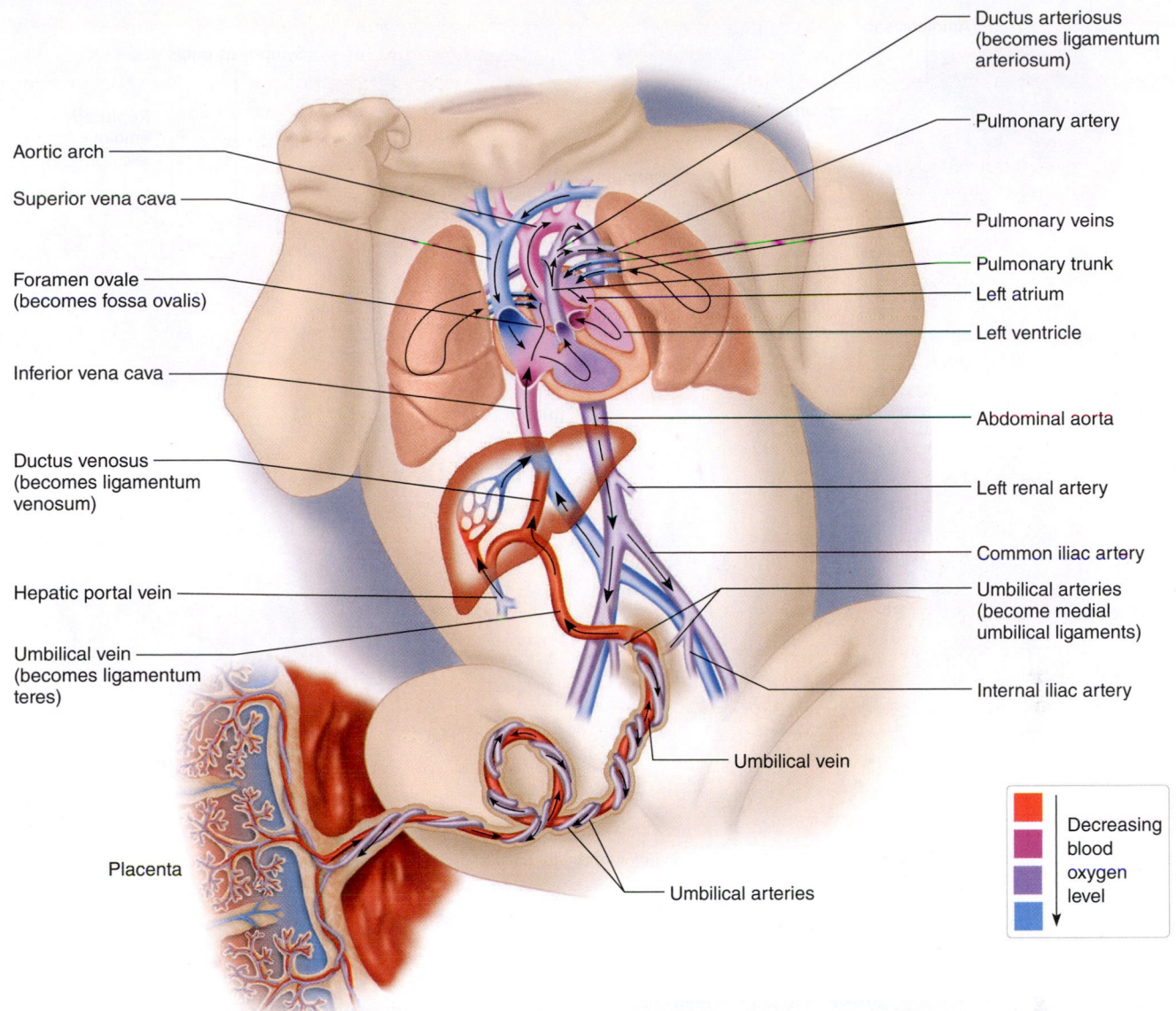

Aortic arch

Superior vena cava

Foramen ovale
(becomes fossa ovalis)

Inferior vena cava

Ductus venosus
(becomes ligamentum
venosum)

Hepatic portal vein

Umbilical vein
(becomes ligamentum
teres)

Placenta

Ductus arteriosus
(becomes ligamentum
arteriosum)

Pulmonary artery

Pulmonary veins

Pulmonary trunk

Left atrium

Left ventricle

Abdominal aorta

Left renal artery

Common iliac artery

Umbilical arteries
(become medial
umbilical ligaments)

Internal iliac artery

Umbilical vein

Umbilical arteries

Decreasing
blood
oxygen
level

FIGURE 31-10   Fetal circulation.

2. *Expulsion* (see Figure 31-11c). Also known as *parturition,* this is the actual childbirth stage. Forceful contractions and abdominal compressions force the fetus from the uterus into the vagina. This stage may take 30 minutes or only a few minutes.

3. *Placental stage* (see Figure 31-11d). This stage is also referred to as the *afterbirth.* Approximately 10 to 15 minutes after the birth, the placenta separates from the uterine wall and is expelled. Uterine contractions continue during this stage and the blood vessels constrict to prevent hemorrhage. Normal blood loss is less than 350 mL (12 oz).

If the fetus is not in the usual head-down position, the child is said to be *breech,* in which the buttocks or feet present first. If the fetus cannot be turned manually, forceps may be used to assist in the birth. Alternately, a *cesarean section* (C-section) may be performed to deliver the infant through the abdominal wall.

At 1 minute and 5 minutes after the baby is born, an **APGAR** test is performed to determine how well the baby is breathing and how well the heart is working. The test has five categories: respiratory effort, heart rate, skin color, reflexes, and muscle tone. In each category, the baby is given a score of 0, 1, or 2, with 2 being the best score. Table 31-1 shows how the scores are applied. The individual scores are added together to provide the APGAR score. A score of 7 to 9 is considered normal. Babies rarely score a 10 because their extremities are normally blue immediately after birth. An APGAR score below 7 indicates that the baby may need medical support, such as supplemental oxygen or physical stimulation.

The Postnatal Period

The *postnatal period* is the 6-week period following birth. The first 4 weeks of the postnatal period are called the *neonatal period* and the offspring is called a *neonate.* The neonatal

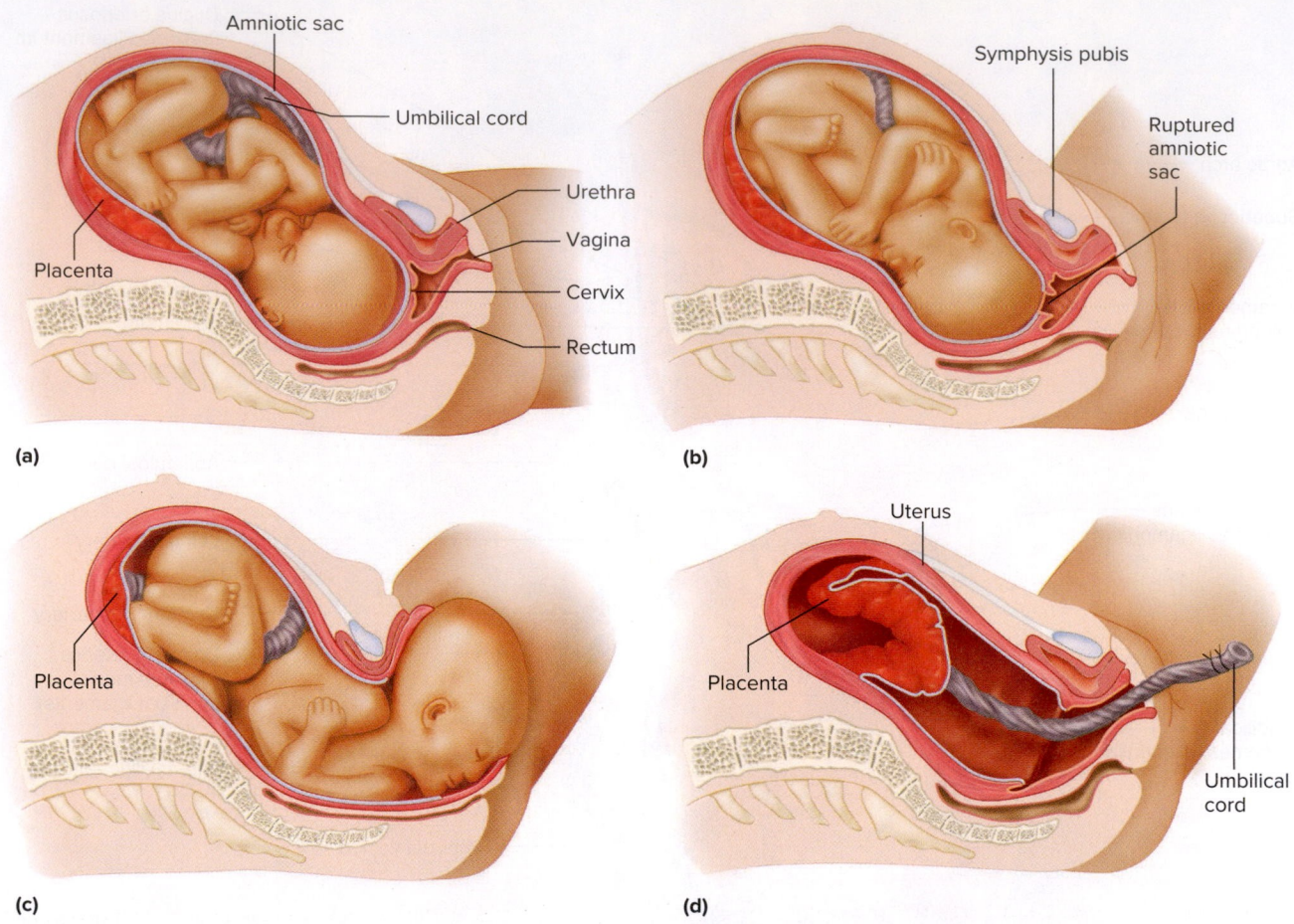

Amniotic sac
Umbilical cord
Urethra
Vagina
Cervix
Rectum
Placenta

(a)

Symphysis pubis
Ruptured amniotic sac
Placenta

(b)

Placenta

(c)

Uterus
Placenta
Umbilical cord

(d)

FIGURE 31-11 Stages of the birth process: (a) the fetal position before birth, (b) dilation of the cervix, (c) delivery of the fetus, and (d) delivery of the placenta.

TABLE 31-1	APGAR Scores		
	0	**1**	**2**
Respiratory Effort	Baby is not breathing.	Baby is breathing, but breaths are slow or irregular.	Baby is breathing well enough to cry successfully.
Heart Rate	Baby's heart is not beating.	Heart rate is less than 100 beats per minute.	Heart rate is 100 beats per minute or greater.
Skin Color	The skin is cyanotic (pale blue).	The skin is pink except in the extremities, which are cyanotic.	The skin is entirely pink.
Reflexes	Baby does not respond to stimulation such as a light pinch.	Baby grimaces in response to stimulation.	Baby grimaces and sneezes, coughs, or cries in response to stimulation.
Muscle Tone	Muscles are flabby or loose.	Muscles have some muscle tone.	The baby actively moves.

period is marked by adjustment to life outside the uterus. The lungs of the neonate must expand, which is why the baby's first breath is forceful. The newborn's liver is immature, so the baby must obtain most of its glucose from fat stores in the skin. The newborn urinates a lot because the kidneys are too immature to concentrate urine well. In addition, body temperature tends to be unstable. The newborn's umbilical vessels constrict, and the foramen ovale, ductus arteriosus, and ductus venosus close.

Milk Production and Secretion

After childbirth, prolactin causes the mammary glands to produce milk. The hormone oxytocin stimulates the ejection of milk from mammary gland ducts. As long as milk is removed from the mammary glands, milk production continues. Once a female stops breast-feeding, the hypothalamus inhibits the release of prolactin and oxytocin, and milk production stops.

▶ Contraception   LO 31.7

Birth control methods, also referred to as *contraception*, reduce the risk of pregnancy (see Figure 31-12). Although many birth control methods are available, some are more

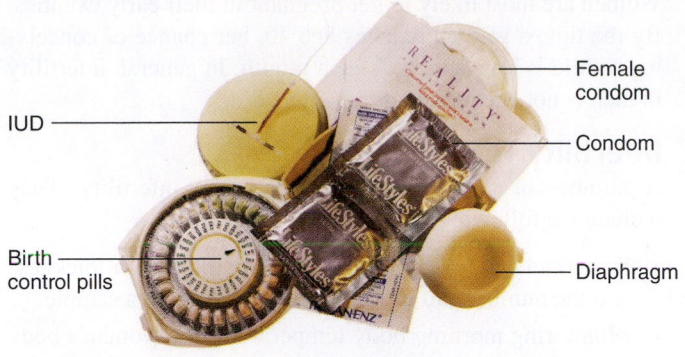

IUD

Birth control pills

REALITY

Female condom

Condom

Diaphragm

FIGURE 31-12 Couples use various forms of contraception. To provide adequate patient teaching, you should be knowledgeable of these methods.

© Peter Ardito/Getty Images

reliable than others. The following are the most commonly used birth control methods:

- Coitus interruptus (withdrawal). The male physically withdraws the penis from the vagina before ejaculation. This method is not reliable because small amounts of semen may enter the vagina before ejaculation.
- Rhythm method (periodic abstinence). This method requires abstinence from sexual intercourse around the time a female is ovulating. However, predicting ovulation can be difficult; therefore, this type of contraception can be unreliable.
- Mechanical barriers. Mechanical barriers prevent sperm from entering the female reproductive tract. They include condoms, diaphragms, and cervical caps. Spermicides are often used in conjunction with barrier methods, particularly condoms and diaphragms.
- Chemical barriers. Chemical barriers destroy sperm in the female reproductive tract. They primarily include spermicides.

- Oral contraceptives. Birth control pills are oral contraceptives. They normally include low doses of estrogen or progesterone that prevent the LH surge necessary for ovulation. These pills therefore prevent ovulation. Newer oral contraceptives have been developed in which the woman takes the pill daily for 3 months and then is off for 1 week, so that a period occurs only four times a year.
- Injectable contraceptives. Depo-Provera® is one brand of injectable contraceptive. It prevents ovulation and alters the lining of the uterus so that implantation of a blastocyst is not likely.
- Insertable contraceptives. NuvaRing® is one of the newest forms of contraception. The woman inserts the ring vaginally and leaves it in for 3 weeks. She removes the ring at the beginning of the fourth week to allow for menstruation on the same schedule she would experience using most oral contraceptives. However, this method has been associated with increased chances for blood clots, stroke, and heart attack, especially in women who smoke.
- Contraceptive implants. Contraceptive implants are small rods of progesterone that are implanted beneath the skin to prevent ovulation.
- Transdermal contraceptives. Commonly called "the patch," transdermal contraceptives are applied to the skin once a week and removed on the seventh day for a 3-week cycle. No patch is applied during the fourth week to allow for the menstrual period.
- Intrauterine devices. An intrauterine device (IUD) is a small, solid device that a licensed practitioner places in the uterus. It prevents the implantation of a blastocyst.
- Surgical methods. *Tubal ligation* is a surgical method used in females to prevent pregnancy. In this process, each fallopian tube is cut and tied to prevent sperm from reaching the oocyte. *Vasectomy* is a surgical method used in males to prevent pregnancy. In this process, each vas deferens is cut and tied to prevent sperm from being ejaculated. Figure 31-13 illustrates these birth control methods.

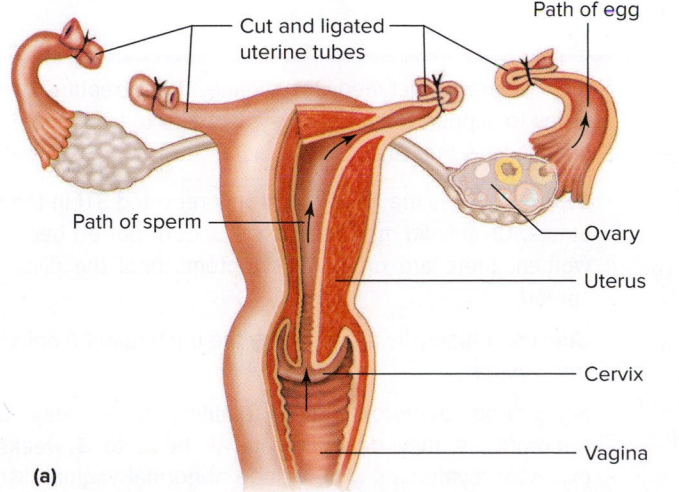

Cut and ligated uterine tubes

Path of egg

Path of sperm

Ovary

Uterus

Cervix

Vagina

(a)

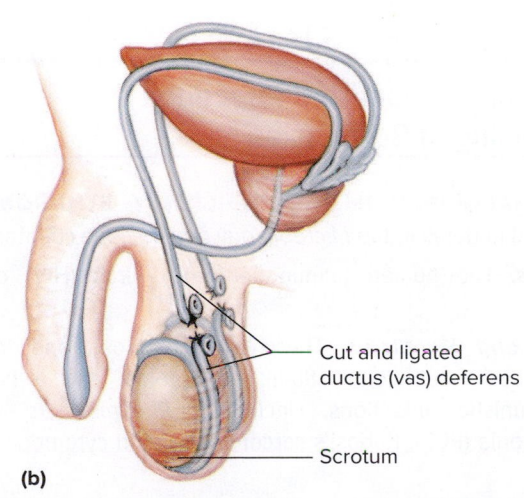

Cut and ligated ductus (vas) deferens

Scrotum

(b)

FIGURE 31-13 (a) Tubal ligation involves cutting and ligating each fallopian tube. (b) Vasectomy involves cutting and ligating the vas deferens.

▶ Infertility

LO 31.8

Infertility is the inability to conceive a child. A couple that has never been pregnant and has tried for 12 months to achieve pregnancy is said to have *primary infertility*. If a couple has had at least one pregnancy but has not been able to get pregnant again after 1 year, they are said to have *secondary infertility*.

In the United States, about 15% of infertility causes are unknown, about 35% are the result of problems in the male, and about 50% are because of problems in the female. Common causes of infertility as a result of male factors include the following:

- Impotence
- Retrograde ejaculation
- Low or absent sperm count
- Use of various medications or drugs
- Decreased testosterone production
- Scarring of the male reproductive tract from STIs
- Previous mumps infection that infected the testes
- Inflammation of the epididymis or testes

Infertility because of female factors includes these common causes:

- Scarring of fallopian tubes from sexually transmitted infections (STIs)
- Pelvic inflammatory disease (PID)
- Inadequate diet
- Lack of ovulation
- Lack of menstrual cycles
- Endometriosis
- Abnormal shape of the uterus or cervix
- Hormone imbalances
- Cysts in ovaries
- Being older than age 40

Women are most likely to get pregnant in their early twenties. By the time a woman reaches age 40, her chance of conceiving a child is less than 10% each month. In general, infertility in men is not age related.

Infertility Tests

A number of tests are used to diagnose infertility. They include the following:

- Semen analysis. This test determines the semen thickness and the number and motility of sperm cells in a sample.
- Monitoring morning body temperature. If a woman's body temperature does not rise slightly once a month, which is best determined by taking her temperature first thing in the morning, she may not be ovulating.
- Blood hormone measurements. In females, various hormone levels can be monitored to predict ovulation and the general health of the ovaries. In males, testosterone levels are measured.
- Endometrial biopsy. This test determines the health of the uterine lining.
- Urinary analysis for luteinizing hormone. The absence of this hormone in urine may indicate a lack of ovulation.
- Hysterosalpingogram. This type of X-ray uses contrast media to visualize the shape of the uterus and the fallopian tubes. If a woman has excess scar tissue in her fallopian tubes, the contrast cannot run through them.
- Laparoscopy. Laparoscopy is a procedure used to visualize pelvic organs.

Treatment of Infertility

Many treatments are available for infertility, but often there is no cure for this condition. Common treatments include surgery to repair abnormal or scarred fallopian tubes, fertility drugs to increase ovulation, and hormone therapies. When infertility cannot be cured, procedures such as artificial insemination, in vitro fertilization, or the use of a surrogate may help a couple to have a child.

PATHOPHYSIOLOGY

LO 31.9

Sexually Transmitted Infections Occurring in Both Sexes

AIDS (ACQUIRED IMMUNODEFICIENCY SYNDROME) is covered in detail in the *Microbiology and Disease* chapter.

Causes. The human immunodeficiency virus (HIV) causes AIDS.

Signs and Symptoms. These are numerous and include decreased T-cell count; flu-like symptoms; and a host of opportunistic infections, including *Pneumocystis carinii* pneumonia (PCP), Kaposi's sarcoma (KS), and cytomegalovirus (CMV).

Treatment. Antiviral medications have been successful in decreasing the viral load and maintaining T-cell counts in some patients, but there are many side effects to these drugs, and they require a strict medicine regime. Other treatments include drugs to support the immune system and to treat opportunistic infections as they arise.

CHLAMYDIA is the most commonly reported STI in the United States. Chlamydia may be grossly underreported because, for women, there are often no symptoms until the disease has spread.

Causes. Chlamydia is caused by the bacterium *Chlamydia trachomatis*.

Signs and Symptoms. For females, there may be no symptoms. If they do occur, it will be 2 to 3 weeks after exposure. Symptoms may include abnormal vaginal discharge and burning on urination. As the disease progresses to other reproductive organs, pelvic inflammatory disease (PID) occurs and can cause abdominal pain, pain during intercourse, and intermenstrual bleeding. Men may have a penile discharge and pain on urination. In women, PID is a common cause of infertility; men seldom have serious complications related to chlamydia.

Treatment. Both partners must be treated to avoid reinfection. Effective antibiotics against chlamydia include azithromycin and doxycycline. Patients must complete the medication cycle and avoid sexual contact until both partners are cured. Because of the high rate of reinfection, women should be retested 3 to 4 months after treatment.

GENITAL WARTS, also known as *Condyloma acuminata,* are one of the most common STIs in the world affecting both men and women. The virus that causes genital warts has been implicated in an increased risk of cervical cancer in women.

Causes. Human papillomavirus (HPV) is the cause of genital warts.

Signs and Symptoms. Not everyone infected with HPV has symptoms. Genital warts may appear weeks or months after infection in the vulva, vagina, and cervix in women. In men, warts appear on the scrotum and penis. They have also been known to appear around the anus and on the thighs and groin. It is important to note that HPV can be spread even if the patient has no outward signs of the disease.

Treatment. Imiquimod cream, 20% podophyllin anti-miotic solutions, and TCA (trichloroacetic acid) may be used to remove warts. Cryosurgery, cautery, and laser surgery may also be used; however, the virus remains in the patient's body. Currently, there is no treatment to rid the body of the virus. Vaccines to prevent infection with some strains of HPV have been approved by the FDA and are considered highly effective.

GONORRHEA is a bacterial STI that is common in the United States. The Centers for Disease Control and Prevention (CDC) estimates 700,000 new infections per year.

Causes. Gonorrhea is caused by *Neisseria gonorrhoea,* a bacterium that thrives in the warm, moist areas of the reproductive tract, urethral tract, mouth, throat, eyes, and anus.

Signs and Symptoms. Men often have no symptoms. If they do appear, it will be 2 to 3 days after exposure, when the patient will experience burning on urination and/or white, yellow, or greenish penile discharge. Women may also be asymptomatic, but common symptoms include dysuria, increased vaginal discharge, and intermenstrual bleeding. Gonorrheal infections, like chlamydia, may lead to PID in women. In men, it may lead to epididymitis.

Treatment. Antibiotics are effective against gonorrhea, and both partners must be treated. However, drug-resistant strains of gonorrhea are developing, making successful treatment more difficult. It is not unusual for a patient with gonorrhea to also be diagnosed with chlamydia or other STIs, which also need to be tested for and treated if found to be present. In addition, gonorrhea lives well and actively in the throat, even if there is not an active genitourinary infection, which can lead to additional co-infection.

HERPES SIMPLEX infections include those caused by both herpes simplex 1 and herpes simplex 2.

Causes. Herpes viruses cause both infections. In most cases, herpes simplex 1 causes oral blisters known as cold sores, and herpes simplex 2 causes what is commonly known as genital herpes, although herpes simplex 1 has also been known to cause the genital type of infection. The herpes infection may also be passed from an infected mother to her child during pregnancy and birth with potentially fatal outcomes.

Signs and Symptoms. Many infected persons, both male and female, have minimal or no symptoms. Typical symptoms of genital herpes include blisters on or around the genitals or rectum. These blisters break, leaving tender ulcers in their wake for 2 to 4 weeks. The number and severity of outbreaks tend to decrease over a period of years.

Treatment. There is no treatment to rid the patient of the herpes virus; however, antiviral medications such as acyclovir may shorten outbreaks when they occur. Daily suppressive therapies with medications like Valtrex® may reduce the risk of transmission. Pregnant women with active outbreaks should deliver the child via a C-section.

PUBIC LICE are known commonly as *crabs* and medically known as *Pediculosis pubis.*

Causes. Pubic lice are caused by a parasitic infestation in the genital area, most commonly spread through sexual contact.

Signs and Symptoms. Symptoms include itching in the genital area with visible evidence of eggs known as *nits,* as well as crawling lice. Lice only live while on a human body. If they fall off the body, they will die in 24 to 48 hours.

Treatment. Patients should use a lice-killing shampoo of 1% permethrin or pyrethrin. All laundry and clothing must be washed in hot water and dried using the hot dryer cycle for at least 30 minutes. Nits remaining in hair may be removed by hand. All partners should be treated and sexual contact should be avoided until treatment is completed.

SYPHILIS is the one bacterial STI whose incidence in women is decreasing, according to the CDC. However, it is increasing in males, especially in those who have sex with other males.

Causes. Syphilis is caused by the bacterium *Treponema pallidum.*

Signs and Symptoms. Primary-stage syphilis usually involves the appearance of a painless sore known as a *chancre,* which appears 10 to 90 days after exposure. It remains for 3 to 6 weeks, disappearing even without treatment. If untreated, the disease lies dormant, progressing to the second stage, which is characterized by a nonpruritic rash and lesions in the mucous membranes. The rash may be associated with flu-like symptoms. Again, all symptoms disappear without treatment. After a long latent period without symptoms, often years later, the third stage becomes apparent, with damage to the brain, eyes, heart, blood vessels, liver, and bones. This damage may lead to muscular incoordination, paralysis, numbness, blindness, dementia, and, finally, death.

Treatment. The cure for syphilis in its early stage is a single dose of intramuscular penicillin. Additional doses are needed for disease present longer than a year. Other antibiotics are also effective for patients allergic to penicillin. The patient must avoid sexual contact until treatment is completed to avoid further spread of the disease.

TRICHOMONIASIS (also known as *trichomonas* infection or the abbreviation *trich*) is a common, curable STI.

Causes. Trichomoniasis is caused by the protozoan parasite *Trichomonas vaginalis*.

Signs and Symptoms. The vagina is the most common site of infection for females; the urethra is the most common site for males. Male patients may have penile irritation, dysuria, or a mild penile discharge, but more often than not, men have no symptoms. Females often have a frothy, yellow-green vaginal discharge with a strong "fishy" odor to it. Itching and irritation of the vulva are also common.

Treatment. Oral metronidazole (Flagyl®) is the treatment of choice. Both partners, even those who are asymptomatic, must be treated to avoid reinfection. Sexual contact should be avoided until after treatment is completed.

SUMMARY OF LEARNING OUTCOMES

LEARNING OUTCOMES	KEY POINTS
31.1 Summarize the organs of the male reproductive system, including the locations, structures, and functions of each.	The organs of the male reproductive system include the testes, responsible for sperm and hormone production; accessory organs of vas deferens, seminal vesicles, prostate gland, and bulbourethral glands; scrotum; and penis.
31.2 Describe the causes, signs and symptoms, and treatment of various disorders of the male reproductive system.	The diseases of the male reproductive system vary widely from simple inflammation to cancers, with varied signs, symptoms, and treatments. Some of these include benign prostatic hypertrophy, epididymitis, impotence (also called erectile dysfunction, or ED), prostate cancer, prostatitis, and testicular cancer.
31.3 Summarize the organs of the female reproductive system, including the locations, structures, and functions of each.	The organs of the female reproductive system include the ovaries, fallopian tubes, uterus, and vagina. The accessory organs and structures include the mons pubis, labia majora and labia minora, clitoris, urethral meatus, vaginal orifice, Bartholin's glands, perineum, and mammary glands.
31.4 Describe the causes, signs and symptoms, and treatment of various disorders of the female reproductive system.	The diseases of the female reproductive system vary widely from simple inflammation to cancers, with varied signs, symptoms, and treatments. Some of these include breast cancer, cervical cancer, cervicitis, dysmenorrhea, endometriosis, fibrocystic breast disease, ovarian cancer, premenstrual syndrome (PMS), uterine (endometrial) cancer, vaginitis, and vulvovaginitis.
31.5 Explain the process of pregnancy, including fertilization, the prenatal period, and fetal circulation.	Fertilization occurs with the union of a sperm cell and an ovum, usually within the fallopian tubes, but it may occur anywhere in the female reproductive tract. The fertilized ovum, now a blastocyst, implants in the endometrial wall of the uterus. The embryonic period occurs from week 2 through week 8 of the pregnancy; the fetal period is from week 9 through delivery.
31.6 Describe the birth process, including the postnatal period.	The birth process ends pregnancy and occurs in three stages: dilation (effacement), in which the cervix thins and softens and dilates up to 10 cm; expulsion (parturition), in which the baby is expelled from the vagina; and placental stage (afterbirth), in which the placenta is expelled through the vagina. The postnatal period is the 6-week period following birth, when the baby's organs continue to mature and the baby adjusts to life outside the uterus.

LEARNING OUTCOMES	
31.7 Compare several birth control methods and their effectiveness.	Some of the contraceptive methods include coitus interruptus; the rhythm method; mechanical barriers; chemical barriers; oral contraceptives; injectable, implantable, and insertable contraceptives; transdermal contraceptives; and surgical methods.
31.8 Explain the causes of and treatments for infertility.	The causes of infertility are varied, with about 15% of infertility from unknown causes. There are a number of infertility tests and treatments; the treatment plan depends on the reason for the infertility.
31.9 Describe the causes, signs and symptoms, and treatments of the most common sexually transmitted infections.	There are many sexually transmitted infections occurring in both sexes, all passed between sexual partners (both heterosexual and same-sex partners), with varied signs, symptoms, and treatments. Some of these include AIDS (acquired immunodeficiency syndrome), chlamydia, genital warts, gonorrhea, pubic lice, syphilis, and trichomoniasis.

CASE STUDY CRITICAL THINKING

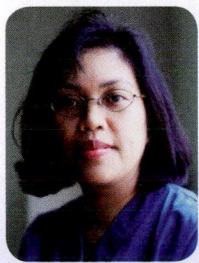

© ERproductions Ltd/Blend Images LLC RF

Recall Raja Lautu from the beginning of the chapter. Now that you have completed the chapter, answer the following questions regarding her case.

1. From Raja's symptoms, which STI might you suspect she is experiencing?

2. What causes this STI, and how is it treated?

3. Why is it important for her sexual partner to be treated?

EXAM PREPARATION QUESTIONS

1. (LO 31.1) Testosterone is produced in the _____ of the testes.
   a. Seminiferous tubules
   b. Epididymis
   c. Vas deferens
   d. Interstitial cells
   e. Bulbourethral gland

2. (LO 31.3) The innermost layer of the uterus is the
   a. Endometrium
   b. Myometrium
   c. Perimetrium
   d. Infundibulum
   e. Cervical orifice

3. (LO 31.4) In _____, the normal uterine lining is found outside of the uterus.
   a. PID
   b. Endometriosis
   c. PMS
   d. Dysmenorrhea
   e. Trichomoniasis

4. (LO 31.6) A newborn is described as a neonate until it reaches the age of
   a. 4 weeks
   c. 2 months
   b. 6 weeks
   d. 6 months
   e. 1 year

5. (LO 31.7) "The patch" is a _____ method of contraception.
   a. Barrier
   b. Mechanical
   c. Transdermal
   d. Chemical
   e. Surgical

6. (LO 31.2) An enlargement of the prostate gland due to normal hormonal changes as a man ages is known as
   a. Epididymitis
   b. Erectile dysfunction
   c. Prostatitis
   d. Testicular cancer
   e. Benign prostatic hypertrophy

7. (LO 31.3) The union of the nucleus of an ovum and a the nucleus of a sperm to create one nucleus containing 46 chromosomes results in a(n)
   a. Blastocyst
   b. Embryo
   c. Zygote
   d. Inner cell mass
   e. Morula

8. (LO 31.8) Which of the following is *not* a test performed to diagnose infertility?
   a. Semen analysis
   b. Endometrial biopsy
   c. Hysterosalpingogram
   d. Amniocentesis
   e. Blood hormone measurement

9. (LO 31.9) The most commonly reported STI in the United States is
   a. Gonorrhea
   b. Chlamydia
   c. Syphilis
   d. AIDS
   e. Trichomoniasis

10. (LO 31.5) The structure in a fetus that allows most of the blood to bypass the liver is the
   a. Ductus venosus
   b. Foramen ovale
   c. Ductus arteriosus
   d. Fossa ovalis
   e. Ligamentum arteriosum

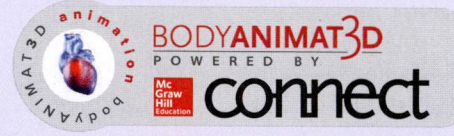

Go to CONNECT to see an animation exercise about *Meiosis vs. Mitosis.*

M E D I C A L   T E R M I N O L O G Y   P R A C T I C E

Analyze the following medical terms, presented throughout the chapter. Using a medical dictionary (or Appendix I) place a / mark between each word part. Define each word part and then define the whole word.

EXAMPLE: **spermato/cyte** = spermato means "sperm" + cyte means "cell"
   SPERMATOCYTE means "sperm cell."

1. blastocyst
2. ectoderm
3. endometrium
4. episiotomy

5. hysterectomy
6. lactiferous
7. neonate
8. oogenesis

9. oviduct
10. vasectomy
11. vaginosis
12. oophorectomy

The Digestive System

CASE STUDY

PATIENT INFORMATION

Patient Name	DOB	Allergies
Sylvia Gonzales	9/1/19XX	Penicillin

Attending	MRN	Other Information
Alexis N. Whalen, MD	341-73-792	NIDDM blood sugars erratic

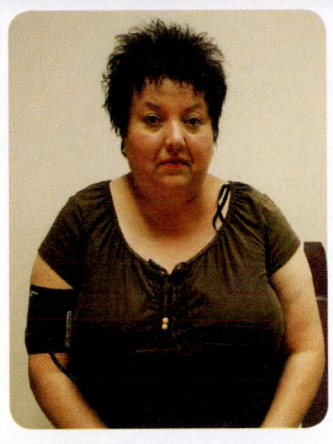

© McGraw-Hill Education

Yesterday afternoon, Sylvia Gonzales, a 51-year-old female, came to the gastroenterologist's office complaining of severe pain in her upper right abdomen. She was nauseated and stated that for several months—and especially following meals—she had been having periodic abdominal pain. After several tests, she was diagnosed as having gallstones and was scheduled for the surgical removal of her gallbladder.

Keep Sylvia in mind as you study this chapter. There will be questions at the end of the chapter based on the case study. The information in the chapter will help you answer these questions.

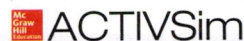
ACTIVSim

LEARNING OUTCOMES

After completing Chapter 32, you will be able to:

32.1 Describe the organs of the alimentary canal and their functions.

32.2 Explain the functions of the digestive system's accessory organs.

32.3 Identify the nutrients absorbed by the digestive system and where they are absorbed.

32.4 Describe the causes, signs and symptoms, and treatments of various common diseases and disorders of the digestive system.

KEY TERMS

alimentary canal	feces
bile	glycogen
bolus	lipid
cardiac sphincter	mechanical digestion
chemical digestion	nutrient
cholesterol	palate
chyme	peritoneum
diverticula	triglycerides
esophageal hiatus	uvula

CAAHEP

I.C.4 List major organs in each body system

I.C.5 Identify the anatomical location of major organs in each body system

I.C.8 Identify common pathology related to each body system including:
(a) signs
(b) symptoms
(c) etiology

I.C.9 Analyze pathology for each body system including:
(a) diagnostic measures
(b) treatment modalities

V.C.9 Identify medical terms labeling the word parts

V.C.10 Define medical terms and abbreviations related to all body systems

ABHES

2. Anatomy & Physiology
a. List all body systems, their structures and functions
b. Describe common diseases, symptoms and etiologies as they apply to each body system
c. Identify diagnostic and treatment modalities as they relate to each body system

3. Medical Terminology
a. Define and use entire basic structure of medical words and be able to accurately identify in the correct context, i.e. root, prefix, suffix, combinations, spelling, and definitions
b. Build and dissect medical terms from roots/suffixes to understand the word element combinations that create medical terminology
c. Apply various medical terms for each specialty
d. Define and use medical abbreviations when appropriate and acceptable

▶ Introduction

Digestion is the mechanical and chemical breakdown of foods into forms that your body cells can absorb. The digestive system's organs carry out the digestive process and can be divided into two categories: organs of the alimentary (digestive) canal and accessory organs. Organs of the **alimentary canal** form a tube or pathway that extends from the mouth to the anus. These organs include the mouth, pharynx, esophagus, stomach, small intestine, large intestine, and anal canal. The accessory organs include the teeth, tongue, salivary glands, liver, gallbladder, and pancreas (Figure 32-1). You may find it helpful to review the *Organization of the Body* chapter to revisit the abdominal regions and quadrants while studying the organs described in this chapter.

▶ Characteristics of the Alimentary Canal

LO 32.1

The wall of the alimentary canal consists of four layers:

- *Mucosa.* The mucosa is the innermost layer of the canal wall. It is made mostly of epithelial tissue that secretes enzymes and mucus into the lumen, or passageway, of the canal. This layer also is active in absorbing nutrients.
- *Submucosa.* The submucosa is the layer just outside the mucosa. It contains loose connective tissue, blood vessels, glands, and nerves. The blood vessels in this layer carry absorbed nutrients throughout the body.
- *Muscular layer.* This layer lies between the submucosa and the canal's outermost layer. It is made of layers of smooth muscle tissue and contracts to move materials through the canal.

- *Serosa.* The serosa is the double-walled, outermost layer of the canal and is also known as the **peritoneum.** The innermost wall of the serosa is known as the *visceral peritoneum.* It secretes serous fluid to keep the outside of the canal moist, preventing it from sticking to other organs or to its outer layer, the *parietal peritoneum,* also called the abdominal lining.

Smooth muscle in the canal's wall can contract to produce two basic types of movements: churning and peristalsis. Churning mixes substances in the canal. Peristalsis propels substances through the tract (Figure 32-2).

The Mouth

The mouth, also known as the *buccal cavity,* takes in food and reduces its size through chewing—a process known as **mechanical digestion.** The mouth also starts the process of **chemical digestion** of food because saliva (spit) contains the enzyme amylase, which breaks down carbohydrates.

The cheeks consist of skin, adipose tissue, skeletal muscles, and an inner lining of moist, stratified squamous epithelium. The cheeks hold food in the mouth. The lips contain sensory nerve fibers that can judge the temperature of food before it enters the mouth. The tongue is made mostly of skeletal muscles and is covered by a mucous membrane. The body of the tongue is held to the floor of the oral cavity by a flap of mucous membrane called the *lingual frenulum.* The tongue mixes food in the mouth and holds it between the teeth. It also contains taste buds. The back of the tongue contains two lumps of lymphoid tissue called *lingual tonsils,* which destroy bacteria and viruses on the back of the tongue.

The **palate** is the roof of the mouth. It separates the oral cavity from the nasal cavity. The front of the palate—the hard

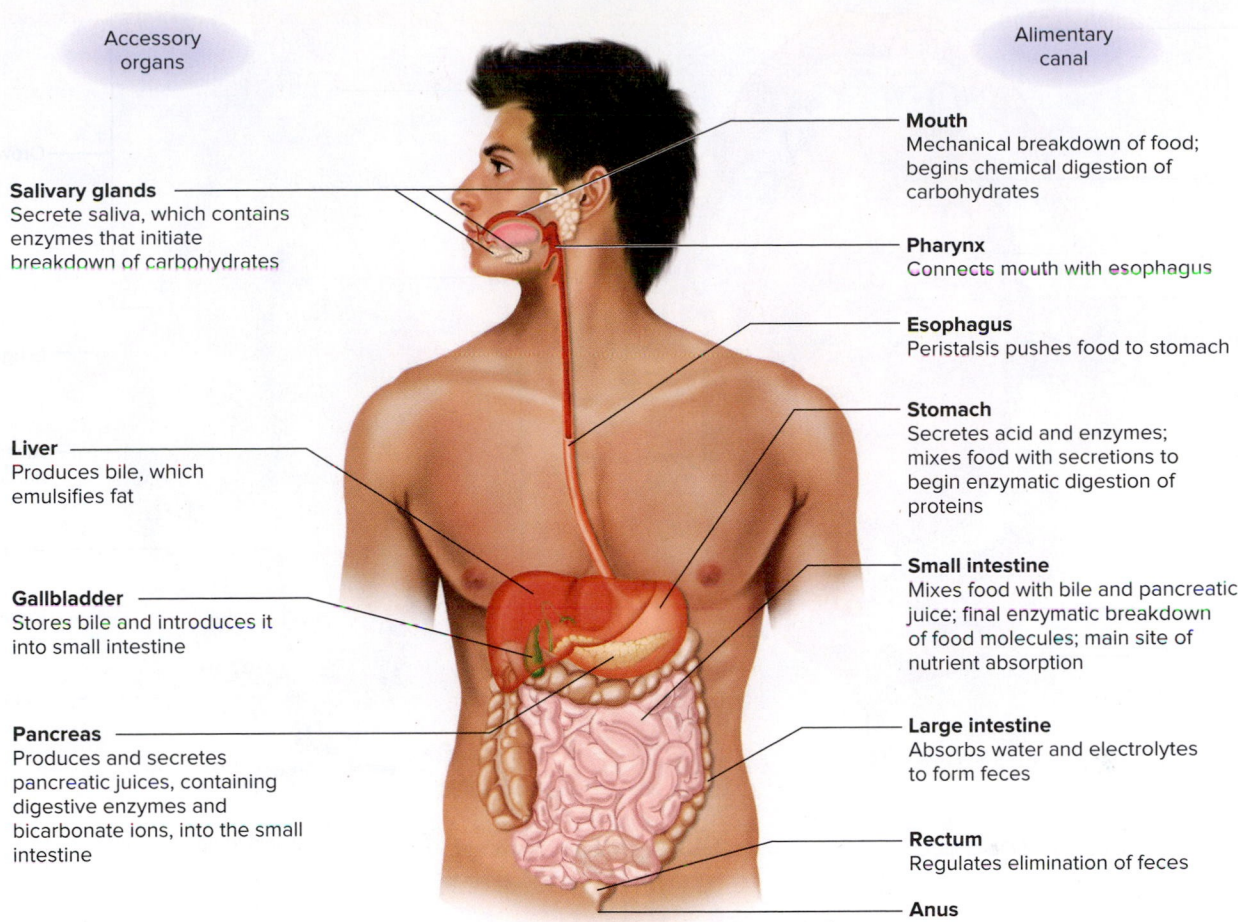

Mouth
Mechanical breakdown of food; begins chemical digestion of carbohydrates

Salivary glands
Secrete saliva, which contains enzymes that initiate breakdown of carbohydrates

Pharynx
Connects mouth with esophagus

Esophagus
Peristalsis pushes food to stomach

Stomach
Secretes acid and enzymes; mixes food with secretions to begin enzymatic digestion of proteins

Liver
Produces bile, which emulsifies fat

Small intestine
Mixes food with bile and pancreatic juice; final enzymatic breakdown of food molecules; main site of nutrient absorption

Gallbladder
Stores bile and introduces it into small intestine

Large intestine
Absorbs water and electrolytes to form feces

Pancreas
Produces and secretes pancreatic juices, containing digestive enzymes and bicarbonate ions, into the small intestine

Rectum
Regulates elimination of feces

Anus

FIGURE 32-1 Major organs of the digestive system.

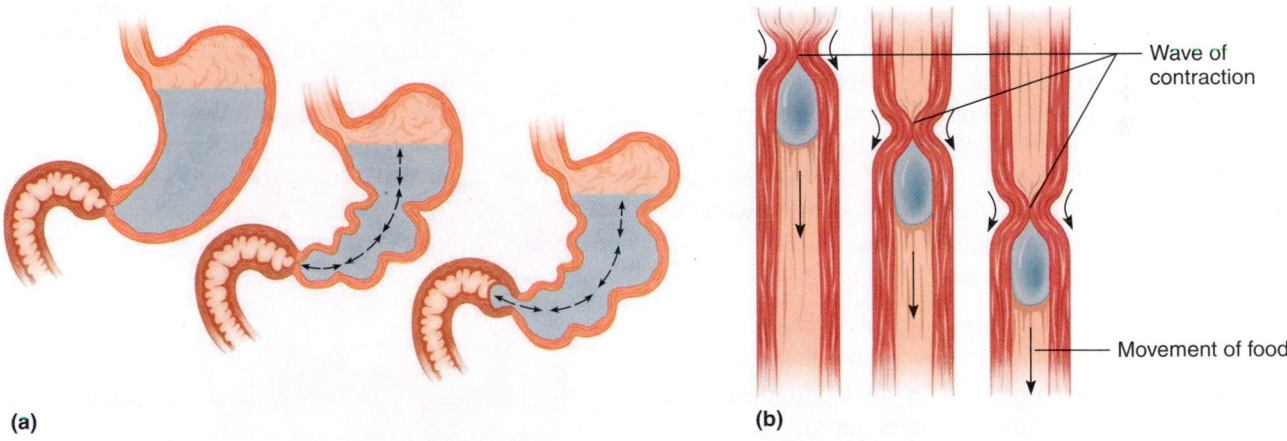

Wave of contraction

Movement of food

(a) **(b)**

FIGURE 32-2 Movements through the alimentary canal: (a) Churning movements move substances back and forth to mix them. (b) Peristalsis moves contents along the canal.

palate—is rigid because it has bony plates in it. The back of the palate, or soft palate, lacks bony material, so it is not rigid. The back of the soft palate hangs down into the throat. This portion of the soft palate is called the **uvula.** It prevents food and liquids from entering the nose during swallowing (Figure 32-3).

At the back of the mouth, where the oral cavity joins the pharynx in the area known as the *oropharynx,* are two masses of lymphoid tissue called *palatine tonsils.* Just above the

palatine tonsils, in the area known as the *nasopharynx* (the nasal cavity joins the pharynx here), are two more masses of lymphoid tissue called the *pharyngeal tonsils,* or *adenoids.* These masses of lymphoid tissue protect the area from bacteria and viruses.

Humans have 32 teeth—16 on the upper jaw and 16 on the lower jaw—which through mastication (chewing) work to decrease the size of food particles. Different types of teeth are adapted to handle food in different ways. The most

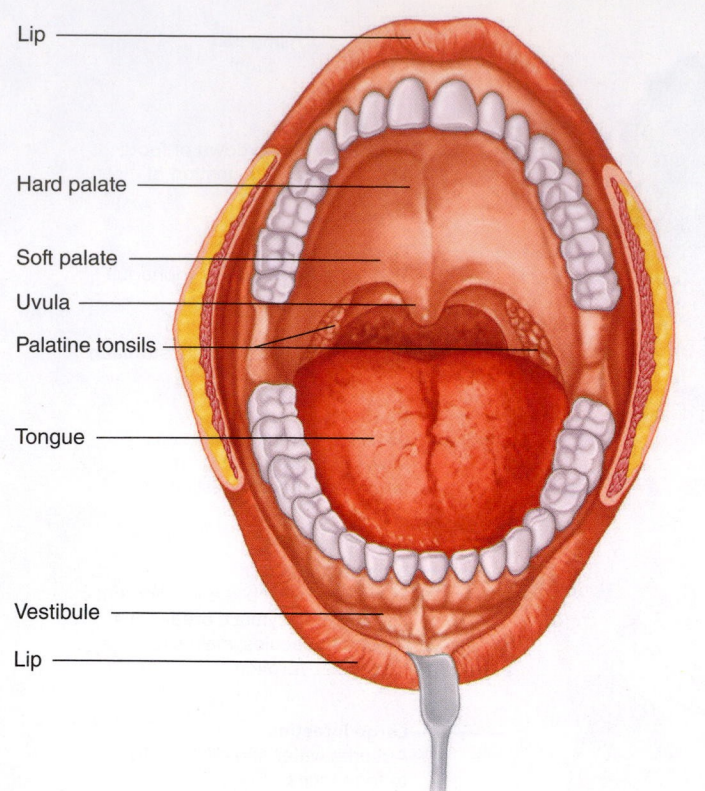

FIGURE 32-3 Structures of the mouth.

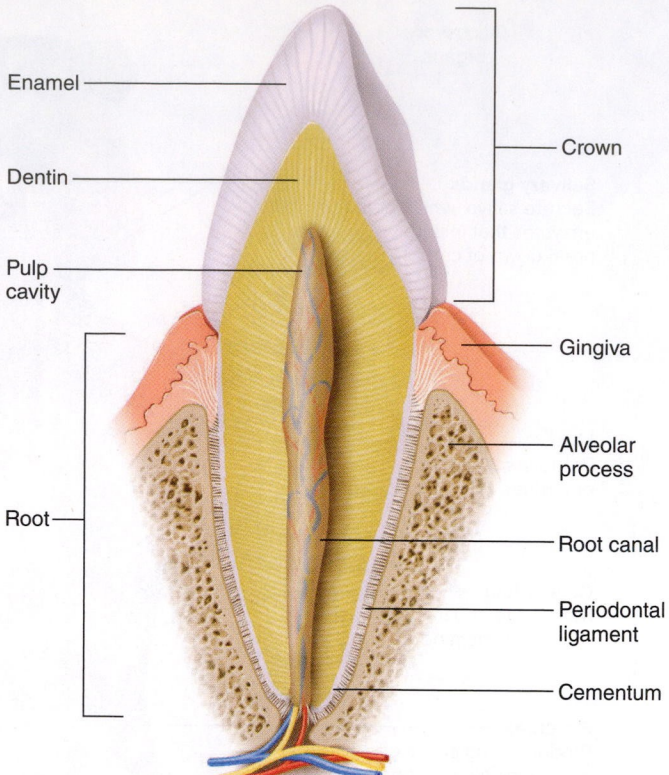

FIGURE 32-4 Structure of a cuspid tooth.

medial teeth, called *incisors,* act as chisels to bite off food pieces. Teeth called *cuspids,* also known as the canines, are the sharpest teeth and designed to tear tough food (Figure 32-4). The back teeth, called *bicuspids* and *molars,* are flat and designed to grind food (Figure 32-5).

Salivary glands secrete saliva—a mixture of water, enzymes, and mucus—and are made of two types of cells: serous cells and mucous cells. Serous cells secrete a fluid made mostly of water, and they secrete amylase. Mucous cells secrete mucus. The mass created by food mixed with the saliva and mucous mixture is called a **bolus.**

All major salivary glands are paired (Figure 32-6):

- *Parotid glands* are the largest of the salivary glands, located beneath the skin just in front of the ears.
- *Submandibular glands* are located in the floor of the mouth just inside the surface of the mandibles (jaws).
- *Sublingual glands* are the smallest of the salivary glands, located in the floor of the mouth beneath the tongue.

The Pharynx

The pharynx, commonly called the throat, is a long, muscular structure that extends from the area behind the nose to the esophagus. It connects the nasal cavity with the oral cavity for breathing through the nose. It also pushes food into the esophagus (Figure 32-7).

The divisions of the pharynx are the:

- *Nasopharynx:* the portion behind the nasal cavity.

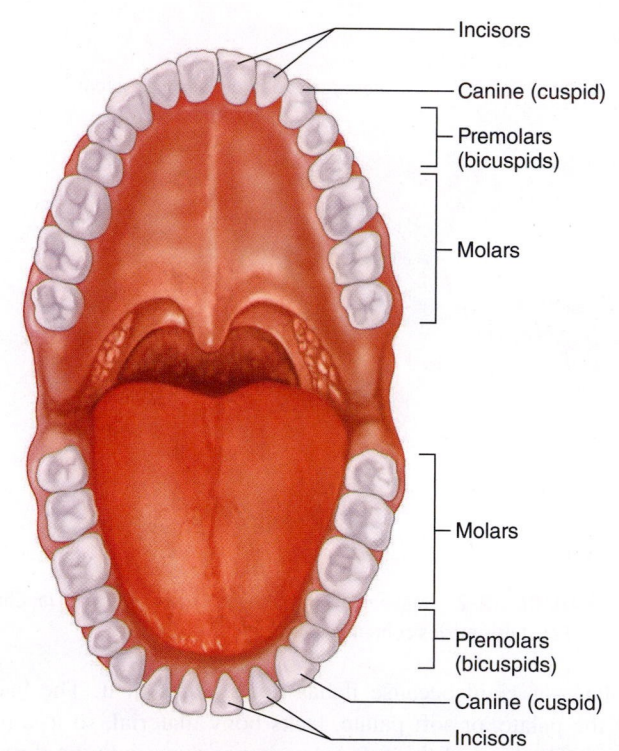

FIGURE 32-5 Types of teeth.

- *Oropharynx:* the portion behind the oral cavity.
- *Laryngopharynx:* the portion behind the larynx. The laryngopharynx continues as the esophagus.

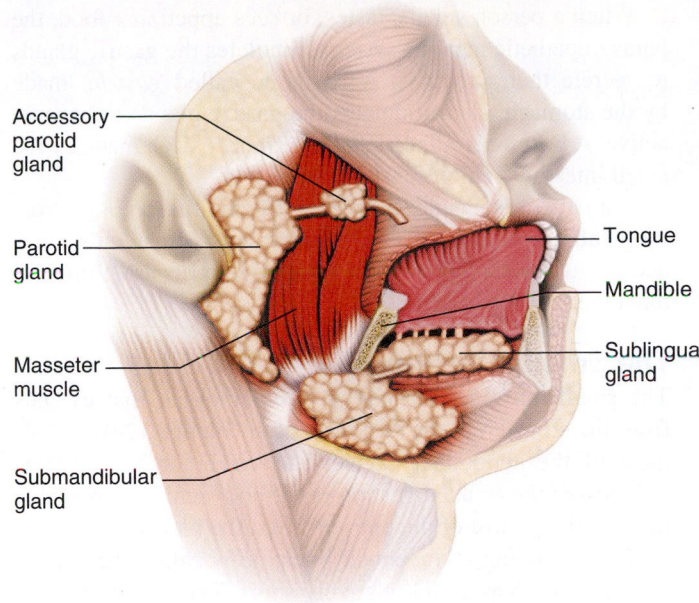

FIGURE 32-6   Major salivary glands.

Swallowing is largely a reflex. In other words, it is an automatic response that does not require much thought. The following events occur during swallowing:

1. The soft palate rises, causing the uvula to cover the opening between the nasal cavity and the oral cavity.
2. The epiglottis covers the opening of the larynx so that food does not enter it (see Figure 32-7).
3. The tongue presses against the roof of the mouth, forcing food into the oropharynx.
4. The muscles in the pharynx contract, forcing food toward the esophagus.
5. The esophagus opens.
6. The muscles of the pharynx push food into the cardiac sphincter.

The Esophagus

The esophagus is a muscular tube that connects the pharynx to the stomach (Figures 32-7 and 32-8). It descends through the thoracic cavity, through the diaphragm, and into the abdominal cavity, where it joins the stomach. The hole in the diaphragm that the esophagus goes through is called the **esophageal hiatus.** This hiatus is a place where hernias commonly occur.

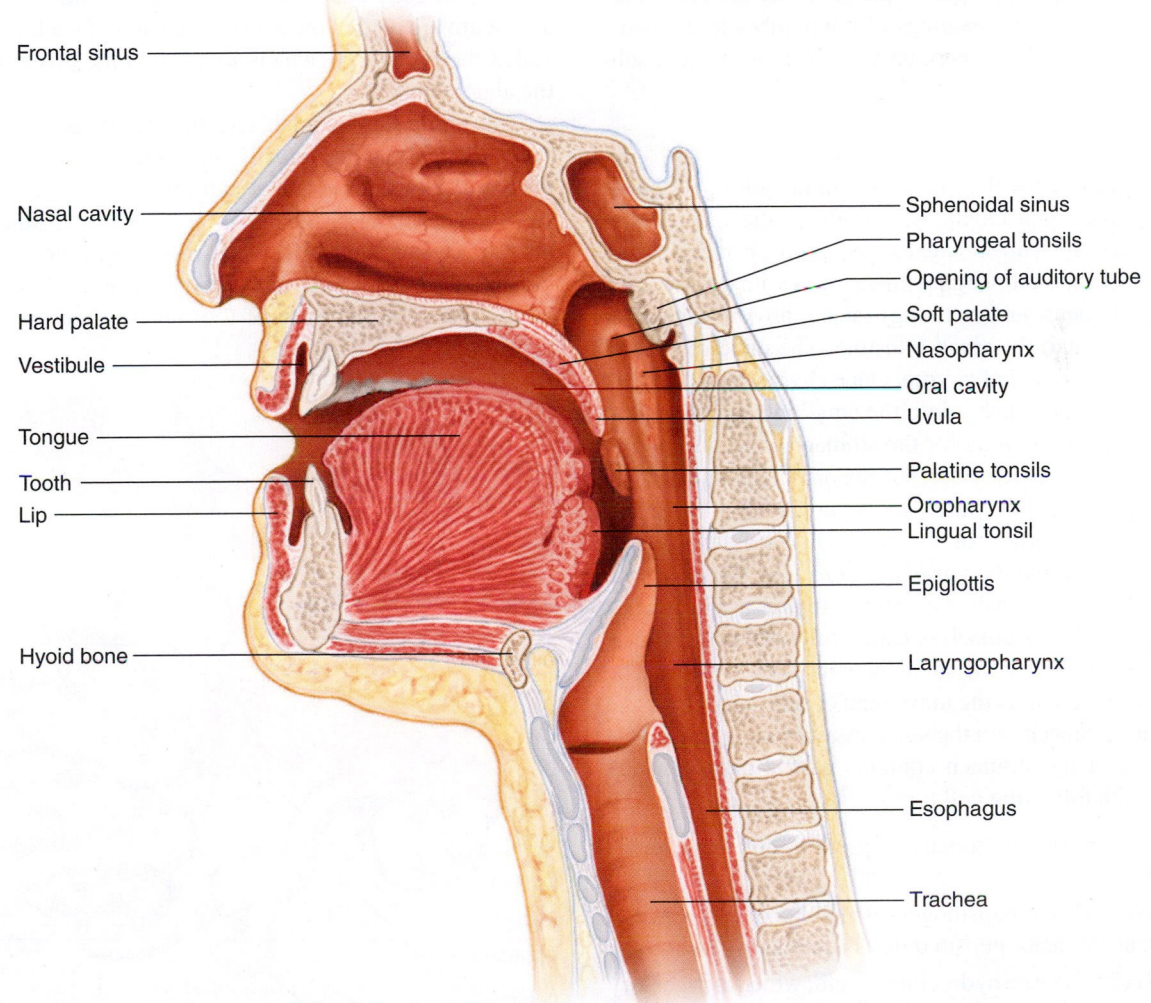

FIGURE 32-7   Sagittal section of the mouth, nasal cavity, and pharynx.

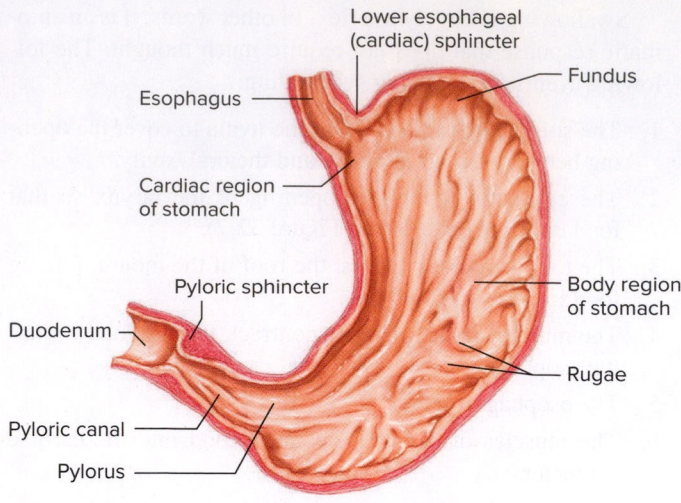

FIGURE 32-8 Regions of the stomach.

A hernia develops when an organ pushes through a wall that contains it. A hiatal hernia occurs when the stomach gets pushed up into the thoracic cavity through the esophageal hiatus.

The **cardiac sphincter,** also known as the *lower esophageal sphincter,* controls the movement of food into the stomach. As stated in earlier chapters, sphincters are circular bands of muscle located at the openings of many tubes in the body. They open and close to allow or prevent the movement of substances out of a tube.

The Stomach

The stomach lies below the diaphragm in the left upper quadrant of the abdominal cavity. The folds of the inner lining of the stomach are called *rugae.* The stomach receives the food bolus from the esophagus, mixes food with gastric juice (secretions of the stomach lining), starts protein digestion, and moves food into the small intestine. The mixture of food and gastric juices is called **chyme.** Once chyme is well mixed, stomach contractions push it into the small intestine a little at a time. It takes 4 to 8 hours for the stomach to empty following a meal. The stomach does not absorb many substances, but it can absorb alcohol, water, and some fat-soluble drugs.

The beginning portion of the stomach that is attached to the esophagus is called the *cardiac region.* The portion of the stomach that balloons over the cardiac region is the *fundus.* The main part of the stomach is called the *body,* and the narrow portion connected to the small intestine is the *pylorus.* The *pyloric sphincter* controls the movement of substances from the pylorus of the stomach into the small intestine (Figure 32-8).

The lining of the stomach contains gastric glands, which are made of the following cell types:

*   *Mucous cells:* secrete mucus to protect the lining of the stomach
*   *Chief cells:* secrete pepsinogen, which becomes *pepsin* in the presence of acid; pepsin digests proteins
*   *Parietal cells:* secrete hydrochloric acid, which is necessary to convert pepsinogen to pepsin; they also secrete *intrinsic factor,* which is necessary for vitamin B_{12} absorption

When a person smells, tastes, or sees appetizing food, the parasympathetic nervous system stimulates the gastric glands to secrete their products. A hormone called *gastrin,* made by the stomach, also stimulates the gastric glands to become active. A hormone called *cholecystokinin (CCK),* made by the small intestine, inhibits gastric glands.

If a patient is unable to swallow for any reason, a gastrostomy tube, or G tube, may be inserted into the patient's stomach so that he can be fed liquid meals, like Ensure®, through this tube.

The Small Intestine

The small intestine is a coiled, tubular organ that extends from the stomach to the large intestine (Figure 32-9). It fills most of the abdominal cavity. The small intestine carries out most of the actual digestion in the body and is responsible for absorbing most of the nutrients into the bloodstream.

The beginning of the small intestine is called the *duodenum.* It is C-shaped and relatively short. The middle portion of the small intestine is called the *jejunum.* It is coiled and forms the majority of the small intestine. If a patient's stomach is diseased or removed, a jejunostomy, or J, tube may be inserted into the jejunum to allow her to receive nutrition.

The last portion of the small intestine is called the *ileum,* and it is directly attached to the large intestine. The jejunum and ileum are held in the abdominal cavity by a fan-like tissue called the *mesentery,* which attaches to the posterior wall of the abdomen.

The lining of the small intestine contains cells that have *microvilli.* Microvilli greatly increase the surface area of the small intestine so that it can absorb nutrients more efficiently. The lining of the small intestine also contains glands that secrete various substances, including mucus and water. Water aids in digestion, but infections or exposure to some toxins cause the secretion of too much water, and this leads

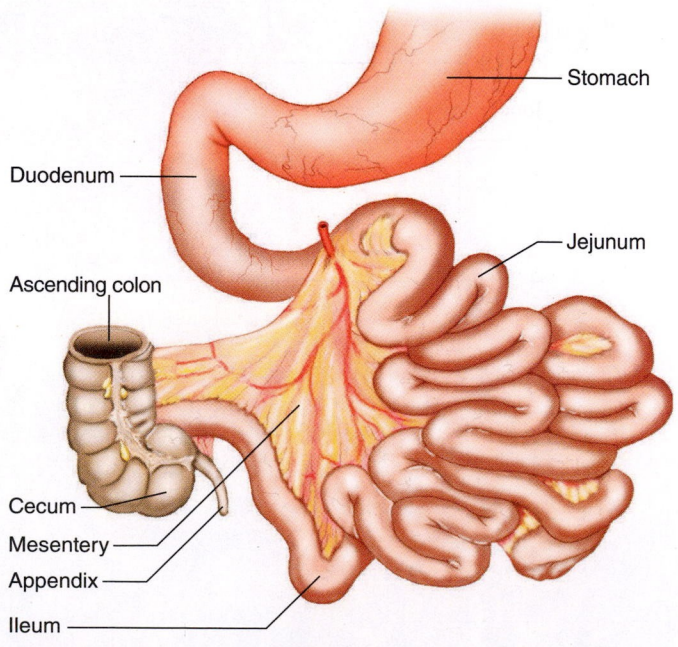

FIGURE 32-9 Parts of the small intestine.

to diarrhea—which in turn aids the body in eliminating the toxins. It also means, however, that needed nutrients are not absorbed in the small intestine as usual. The mucus secreted by the small intestine helps protect its lining. The parasympathetic nervous system and the stretching of the wall of the small intestine as it fills are the primary factors that trigger the small intestine to secrete its products. The following are the major enzymes the small intestine secretes:

- *Peptidases.* These enzymes digest proteins.
- *Sucrase, maltase, and lactase.* These enzymes digest sugars. A person who cannot produce lactase will not be able to digest lactose, which is the sugar in dairy products. This causes a condition called *lactose intolerance.*
- *Intestinal lipase.* This enzyme digests fats.

The small intestine absorbs almost all nutrients (water, glucose, amino acids, fatty acids, glycerol, and electrolytes) as the wall of the small intestine contracts to mix chyme and to propel it toward the large intestine. The *ileocecal sphincter* controls the movement of chyme from the ileum to the *cecum,* which is the beginning of the large intestine.

The Large Intestine

The large intestine begins at the ileum of the small intestine and ends where it opens to the outside of the body as the anus. The beginning of the large intestine is called the cecum. Projecting off the cecum is the *vermiform appendix,* which is made mostly of lymphoid tissue. It was once thought to have no function, but it is now thought to have a role in immunity. The cecum eventually gives rise to the ascending colon, which is the portion of the large intestine that runs up the right side of the abdominal cavity. If you remember that the appendix is in the right lower quadrant (RLQ), it will be easy to remember that the ascending colon also goes up the right side of the abdomen. The ascending colon becomes the transverse colon as it crosses the abdominal cavity; from there, it becomes the descending colon as it descends the left side of the abdominal cavity. In the pelvic cavity, the descending colon then forms the S-shaped tube called the *sigmoid colon.*

The Rectum and Anal Canal

Eventually, the sigmoid colon straightens out to become the *rectum.* The last few centimeters of the rectum are known as the *anal canal,* and the opening of the anal canal to the outside of the body is called the *anus* (Figure 32-10).

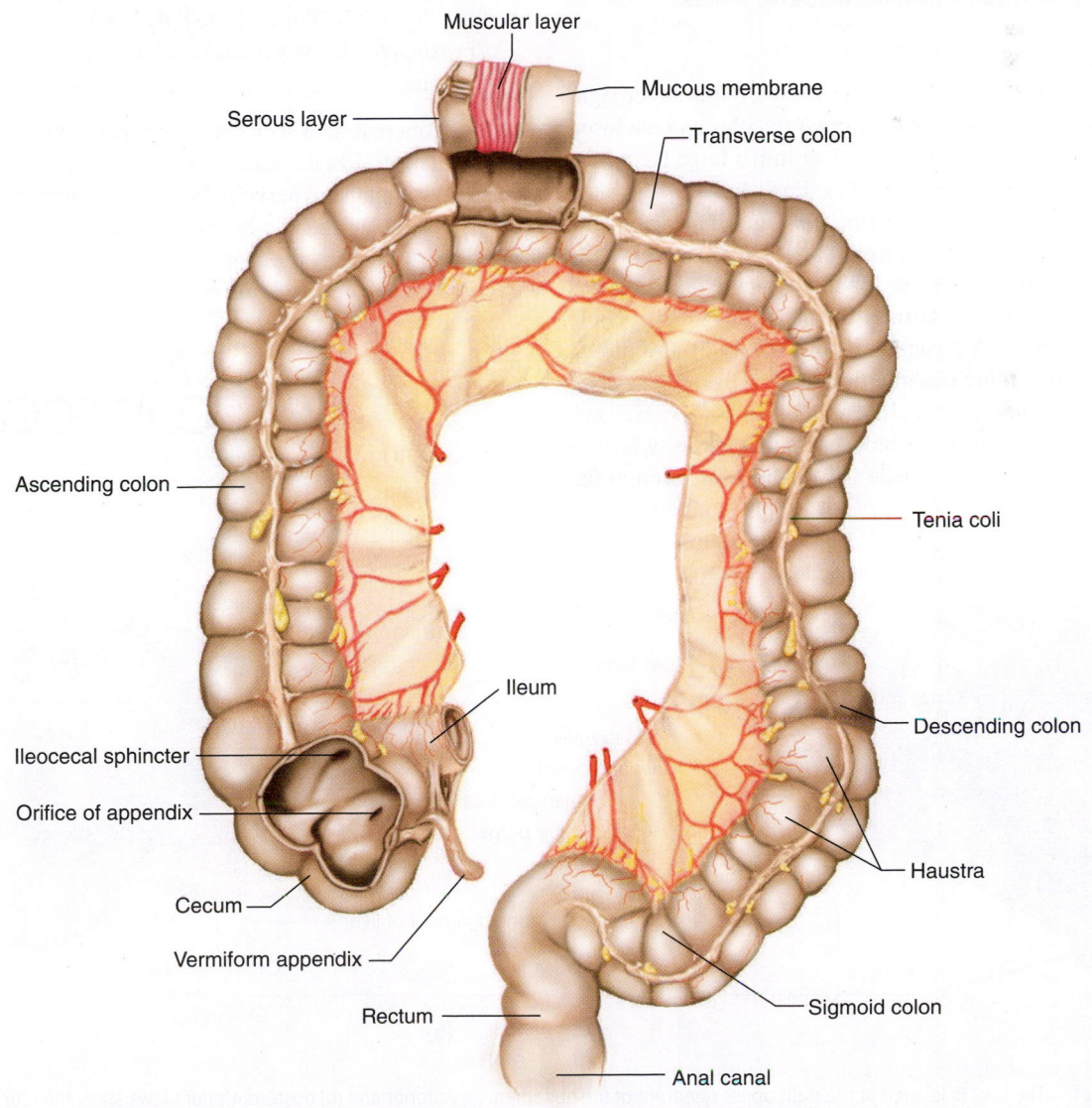

FIGURE 32-10   Parts of the large intestine.

The lining of the large intestine secretes mucus to aid in the movement of substances. As chyme leaves the small intestine and enters the large intestine, the proximal portion of the large intestine absorbs water and a few electrolytes from it. The leftover chyme is then called **feces,** which are made of undigested solid materials, a little water, ions, mucus, cells of the intestinal lining, and bacteria.

The contractions of the large intestine propel feces forward, but these contractions normally occur periodically and as mass movements. Mass movements trigger the *defecation reflex,* which allows the anal sphincters to relax and feces to move through the anus in the process of elimination. The squeezing actions of the abdominal wall muscles also aid in emptying the large intestine.

▶ Characteristics of the Digestive Accessory Organs   LO 32.2

Although they do not form part of the alimentary canal, the digestive system's accessory organs play important roles in digestion. They deliver enzymes and other substances to the alimentary canal to assist with the digestive process.

The Liver

The liver is a large organ that fills most of the upper-right abdominal quadrant. It is reddish-brown in color and enclosed by a tough capsule that divides the liver into a large right lobe and a small left lobe (Figure 32-11). Each lobe is separated into smaller divisions called *hepatic lobules.* Branches of the *hepatic portal vein* carry blood from the digestive organs to the hepatic lobules. These hepatic lobules contain macrophages that destroy bacteria and viruses in the blood. Most people associate the liver with cleansing and detoxifying the blood, but it also has other functions important to the digestive system. Each lobule contains many cells called *hepatocytes.* Hepatocytes process the nutrients in blood and make **bile,** which is used in the digestion of fats. Bile leaves the liver through the

hepatic duct. The *hepatic duct* merges with the *cystic duct* (the duct from the gallbladder) to form the *common bile duct.* This duct delivers bile to the duodenum. Another important function of the liver is to store vitamins and iron.

The Gallbladder

The gallbladder is a small, sac-like structure located beneath the liver (Figures 32-11 and 32-12). Its only function is to store bile, which leaves the gallbladder through the cystic duct. The hormone cholecystokinin causes the gallbladder to release bile. The salts in bile break large fat globules into smaller ones so that the digestive enzymes can more quickly digest them. Bile salts also increase the absorption of fatty acids, cholesterol, and fat-soluble vitamins into the bloodstream.

The Pancreas

The pancreas is located behind the stomach. Pancreatic *acinar cells* produce pancreatic juices, which ultimately flow through the pancreatic duct to the duodenum (Figure 32-12). Pancreatic juices contain the following enzymes:

- *Pancreatic amylase,* which digests carbohydrates
- *Pancreatic lipase,* which digests lipids
- *Nucleases,* which digest nucleic acids
- *Trypsin, chymotrypsin,* and *carboxypeptidase,* which digest proteins

The pancreas also secretes bicarbonate ions into the duodenum that neutralize the acidic chyme arriving from the stomach. The parasympathetic nervous system stimulates the pancreas to release its enzymes. The hormones secretin and cholecystokinin also stimulate the pancreas to release digestive enzymes. Secretin and cholecystokinin come from the small intestine.

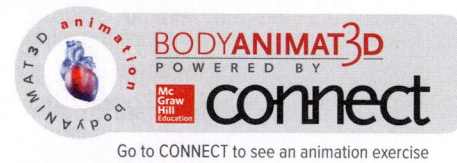

Go to CONNECT to see an animation exercise about *Food Absorption.*

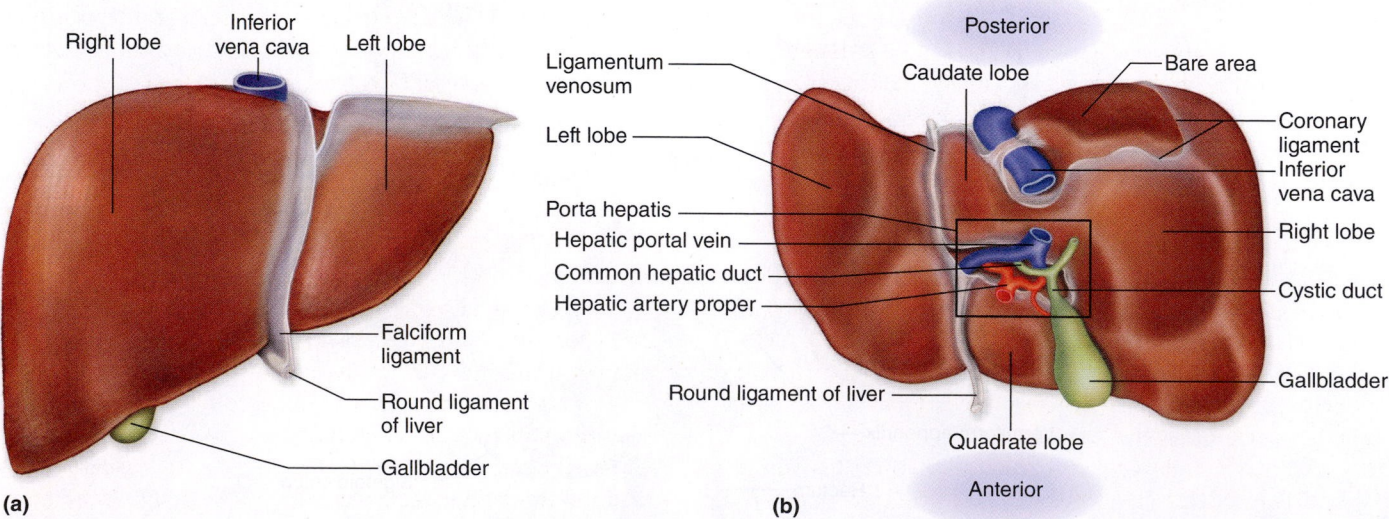

(a)

(b)

FIGURE 32-11   The liver is located in the right upper quadrant of the abdomen. (a) Anterior and (b) posteroinferior views show the four lobes of the liver, gallbladder, inferior vena cava, hepatic portal vein, and hepatic artery.

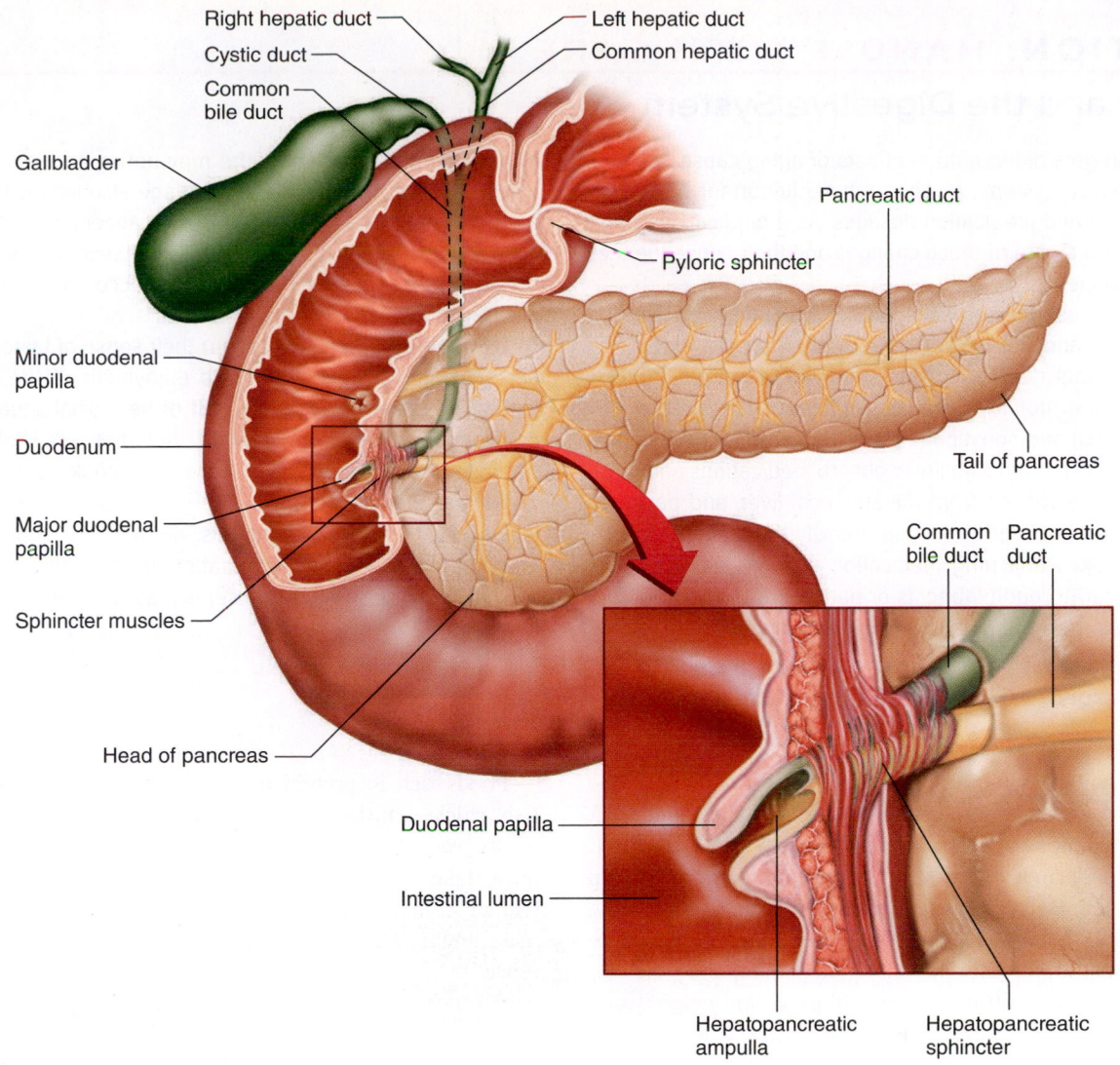

Right hepatic duct
Cystic duct
Common bile duct
Gallbladder
Minor duodenal papilla
Duodenum
Major duodenal papilla
Sphincter muscles
Head of pancreas

Left hepatic duct
Common hepatic duct
Pancreatic duct
Pyloric sphincter
Tail of pancreas
Common bile duct
Pancreatic duct
Duodenal papilla
Intestinal lumen
Hepatopancreatic ampulla
Hepatopancreatic sphincter

FIGURE 32-12   Pancreas and its connections to the gallbladder and duodenum.

▶ The Absorption of Nutrients   LO 32.3

Necessary food substances are known as **nutrients.** They include carbohydrates, proteins, lipids, vitamins, minerals, and water.

Three types of carbohydrates that humans ingest are starches (polysaccharides), simple sugars (monosaccharides and disaccharides), and cellulose. Starches come from foods such as pasta, potatoes, rice, and breads.

Monosaccharides and disaccharides are obtained from sweet foods and fruits. Most body cells use the monosaccharide glucose to make adenosine triphosphate (ATP). ATP provides a type of chemical energy needed by the body. When a person has an excess of glucose, it can be stored in the liver and skeletal muscle cells as **glycogen.**

Cellulose is a type of carbohydrate that humans cannot digest; it is found in many vegetables. It is necessary for digestion because it provides fiber or bulk for the large intestine, which helps the large intestine to empty more regularly. According to Harvard Medical International, a connection

has been made between higher-fiber diets and a decrease in colon diseases, including cancer. This may be because fiber increases water absorption and bulk, causing more rapid emptying of the colon and decreasing the production of benign growths, such as adenomas or polyps, which increase the risk of cancer. Fiber may also neutralize toxins produced by gastrointestinal (GI) tract bacteria.

Lipids (fats) are obtained through various foods. The most abundant dietary lipids are **triglycerides.** They are found in meats, eggs, milk, and butter. **Cholesterol** is another common dietary lipid and is found in eggs, whole milk, butter, and cheeses. Lipids are used by the body primarily to make energy when glucose levels are low. Excess triglycerides are stored in adipose tissue. Cholesterol is essential to cell growth and function; cells use it to make cell membranes and some hormones. People should have the essential fatty acid linoleic acid in their diet because the body cannot make it. This fatty acid is found in corn and sunflower oils. People also need a certain amount of fat to absorb fat-soluble vitamins.

The fat-soluble vitamins are vitamins A, D, E, and K; the water-soluble vitamins are all the B vitamins and vitamin C. The many functions of vitamins are summarized in Table 32-1.

Minerals—primarily found in bones and teeth—make up about 4% of total body weight. Cells use minerals to make enzymes, cell membranes, and various proteins like hemoglobin. The most important minerals to the human body are calcium, phosphorus, sulfur, sodium, chlorine, and magnesium. The body needs trace elements, including iron, manganese, copper, iodine, and zinc, in very small amounts.

Foods rich in protein include meats, eggs, milk, cheese, fish, chicken, turkey, nuts, seeds, and beans. Protein requirements vary from individual to individual, but all people must take in proteins that contain certain amino acids (called *essential amino acids*) because the body cannot make them. The body uses proteins for growth and tissue repair.

Keep in mind that an individual's ability to absorb nutrients changes over the course of his or her lifetime. See the feature *Caution: Handle with Care* for more information.

TABLE 32-1	Common Vitamins and Their Importance in the Body
Vitamin	**Function**
Vitamin A	Needed for the production of visual receptors, mucus, the normal growth of bones and teeth, and the repair of epithelial tissues
Vitamin B_1 (thiamine)	Needed for carbohydrate metabolism
Vitamin B_2 (riboflavin)	Needed for carbohydrate and fat metabolism and for the growth of cells
Vitamin B_6	Needed for protein, antibody, and nucleic acid synthesis
Vitamin B_{12} (cyanocobalamin)	Needed for myelin production and carbohydrate and nucleic acid metabolism
Biotin	Needed for protein, fat, and nucleic acid metabolism
Folic acid	Needed for the production of amino acids, DNA, and red blood cells
Pantothenic acid	Needed for carbohydrate and fat metabolism
Niacin	Needed for carbohydrate, protein, fat, and nucleic acid metabolism
Vitamin C (ascorbic acid)	Needed for the production of collagen, amino acids, and hormones and for iron absorption
Vitamin D	Needed for calcium absorption
Vitamin E	Antioxidant that prevents the breakdown of certain tissues
Vitamin K	Needed for blood clotting

Common Diseases and Disorders of the Digestive System

APPENDICITIS is an inflammation of the appendix. If not treated promptly, it can be life-threatening.

Causes. This disorder may be caused by an appendix blocked by feces or tumor, infection, or other *idiopathic* (unknown) cause.

Signs and Symptoms. The signs and symptoms include lack of appetite, pain in the RLQ that may radiate throughout the abdomen and even down the right leg, nausea, slight fever, and an increased white blood cell (WBC) count.

Treatment. The primary treatments are antibiotics to prevent infection and an *appendectomy* to remove the appendix.

CIRRHOSIS is a chronic liver disease in which normal liver tissue is replaced with nonfunctional scar tissue.

Causes. This disease is often an autoimmune disease. It may also be caused by some medications and alcohol consumption. Hepatitis B and C infections can also contribute to the development of cirrhosis.

Signs and Symptoms. This disease has many symptoms, including anemia, fatigue, mental confusion, fever, vomiting, blood in the vomit, an enlarged liver, jaundice, unintended weight loss, swelling of the legs or abdomen, abdominal pain, decreased urine output, and pale feces.

Treatment. Alcohol consumption should be discontinued. A patient with cirrhosis may be given various medications, including antibiotics and diuretics. A liver transplant may be needed for the most seriously ill patients.

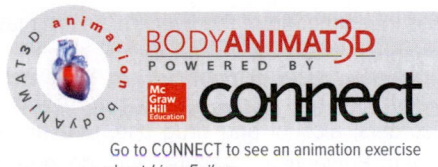

Go to CONNECT to see an animation exercise about *Liver Failure.*

CHOLELITHIASIS, or gallstones, are hard deposits that usually consist of either cholesterol or bilirubin. They are more common in women than in men.

Causes. Gallstones can be caused by a variety of factors, including diabetes, cirrhosis, and other medical conditions; rapid weight loss; failure of the gallbladder to empty completely, which may occur during pregnancy; and organ transplant.

Signs and Symptoms. Some people who have gallstones do not have symptoms. If symptoms do occur, they may include pain in the right upper quadrant (RUQ) of the abdomen, fever, jaundice, nausea and vomiting, and clay-colored feces.

Treatment. Surgery to remove the stones is the most common treatment for people who have symptoms associated with gallstones. The most commonly used procedure is *laparoscopic cholecystectomy.* Another procedure, *lithotripsy,* is also a treatment option. It uses electrohydraulic shock waves to dissolve or break up the stones without the need for surgery. Medications are also used in some cases, but they take a long time to work.

COLITIS is inflammation of the large intestine. This condition can be chronic or short lived, depending on the cause.

Causes. Colitis can be caused by a viral or bacterial infection or the use of antibiotics. Ulcers in the large intestine, Crohn's disease, various other diseases, and stress may also contribute to the development of this disorder.

Signs and Symptoms. The primary symptoms are abdominal pain, bloating, and diarrhea.

Treatment. The first goal of therapy is to treat the underlying causes. Changing antibiotics, treating existing ulcers, and drinking plenty of fluids are treatment options. In advanced cases, surgery to remove the affected area of the colon, known as a *colectomy,* may be recommended. If too much of the colon is affected, a *colostomy* may be performed. In this procedure, the majority of the colon is removed and the opening to the outside of the body is moved to the abdomen, where an appliance known as an ostomy, usually with a collecting device commonly called a bag, collects fecal material.

COLORECTAL CANCER usually comes from the lining of the rectum or colon. This type of cancer is curable if treated early.

Causes. The causes are mostly unknown, although research is putting some blame on high-fat/low-fiber diets. Polyps in the colon or rectum can become cancerous, leading to this disease. Colorectal cancer may be prevented through regular screenings for polyps, which is done with a procedure known as a colonoscopy.

Signs and Symptoms. Anemia, unintended weight loss, abdominal pain, blood in the feces, narrow feces, or changes in bowel habits are all common symptoms.

Treatment. Chemotherapy is the first line of treatment. Surgery to remove a cancerous tumor or the affected portions of the colon or rectum (colectomy or colostomy) may be needed in more advanced cases.

CONSTIPATION is the condition of difficult defecation, which is the elimination of feces.

Causes. The primary causes are lack of physical activity, lack of fiber and adequate water in the diet, the use of certain medications, and thyroid and colon disorders.

Signs and Symptoms. Common signs and symptoms include infrequent bowel movements (for example, no bowel movement for 3 days), bloating, abdominal pain and pain during bowel movements, hard feces, and blood on the surface of feces.

Treatment. Treatment includes an increase in dietary fiber; adequate fluid intake; regular exercise; and the use of stool softeners, laxatives, and enemas (for extreme cases only).

CROHN'S DISEASE is a common disorder called *inflammatory bowel disease.* It typically affects the end of the small intestine.

Causes. This is an autoimmune disorder.

Signs and Symptoms. The signs and symptoms of Crohn's disease include fever, tender gums, joint pain, GI ulcers, abdominal pain and gas, constipation or diarrhea, abnormal abdominal sounds, weight loss, intestinal bleeding, and blood in the feces.

Treatment. The first treatment is to change the patient's diet. Other treatments include medications to reduce inflammation, including steroids, as well as antibiotics and bowel "rest" in which IV (intravenous) feedings are given so that the patient's digestive system is not used. For the most serious cases, surgery to remove the affected part of the intestine may be needed. This procedure is known as an *enterectomy*.

DIARRHEA is the condition of watery and frequent feces. Many cases of diarrhea do not require treatment because they usually stop within a day or two.

Causes. The causes of diarrhea include bacterial, viral, or parasitic infections of the digestive system. It may also be caused by the ingestion of toxins; food allergies, including lactose intolerance; ulcers; Crohn's disease; laxative use; antibiotics; chemotherapy; and radiation therapy. Diarrhea related to infections may be prevented by washing hands thoroughly and cooking food properly.

Signs and Symptoms. The symptoms include abdominal cramps, watery feces, and the frequent passage of feces.

Treatment. Patients should drink fluids to prevent dehydration. The underlying causes, if known, should be treated. Medications and dietary changes are the primary treatment options. In severe cases, antidiarrheal medications such as Lomotil® may be prescribed.

DIVERTICULITIS is inflammation of diverticula in the intestine. **Diverticula** are abnormal dilations or pouches in the intestinal wall. When the diverticula are not inflamed, the condition is known as **DIVERTICULOSIS.**

Causes. The causes are mostly unknown. Lack of fiber in the diet and a bacterial infection of the diverticula can cause this disorder. Patients may find that certain foods, like peanuts and seeds, aggravate this disorder.

Signs and Symptoms. Signs and symptoms include fever, nausea, abdominal pain, constipation or diarrhea, blood in the feces, and a high WBC.

Treatment. Treatments include a high-fiber diet, antibiotics, and keeping a food diary to track foods that cause flare-ups. A *colectomy* (surgery to remove the affected portion of the intestine) may be necessary in severe cases.

GASTRITIS is an inflammation of the stomach lining. It is often referred to as an "upset stomach."

Causes. Gastritis can be caused by bacteria or viruses, some medications, alcohol use, spicy foods, excessive eating, poisons, and stress. Cooking food properly to kill harmful bacteria and viruses can help to prevent this condition.

Signs and Symptoms. Symptoms include nausea, lack of appetite, heartburn, vomiting, and abdominal cramps. An upper

endoscopy may be done to confirm the diagnosis and rule out more serious conditions, such as an ulcer or cancer.

Treatment. Lifestyle changes should be implemented to avoid foods or medications that irritate the stomach lining. Treatment with various medications to reduce the production of stomach acids, such as Pepcid® and Nexium®, can provide relief from the symptoms of this disorder.

GASTROESOPHAGEAL REFLUX DISEASE (GERD) is more commonly known as heartburn. It occurs when stomach acids are pushed into the esophagus.

Causes. Alcohol, some foods, a defective cardiac sphincter, pregnancy, obesity, a hiatal hernia, and repeated vomiting can contribute to the development of this disease.

Signs and Symptoms. Common symptoms include frequent burping, difficulty swallowing, a sore throat, a burning sensation in the chest following meals and nausea when lying down, and blood in the vomit.

Treatment. Treatment includes weight loss, making dietary changes, reducing alcohol consumption, taking medications such as Pepcid® and Nexium®, and elevating the head, neck, and chest when lying down.

HEMORRHOIDS are varicose veins of the rectum or anus.

Causes. Hemorrhoids are caused by constipation, excessive straining during bowel movements, liver disease, pregnancy, and obesity.

Signs and Symptoms. Signs and symptoms include itching in the anal area, painful bowel movements, bright red blood on feces, and veins that protrude from the anus.

Treatment. Constipation can be avoided or lessened by eating a high-fiber diet. Other treatments include stool softeners, medications to reduce hemorrhoid inflammation, and the surgical removal of hemorrhoids (*hemorrhoidectomy*).

HEPATITIS is inflammation of the liver. There are many different types of hepatitis.

Causes. Causes include bacteria, viruses, parasites, immune disorders, alcohol and drug use, and an overdose of acetaminophen. Preventive measures include getting hepatitis B (HBV) vaccinations, practicing safer sex, avoiding undercooked food (especially seafood), and using prescription or over-the-counter drugs (especially those containing acetaminophen) at their recommended dosages or as prescribed by a physician.

Signs and Symptoms. Symptoms include mild fever, bloating, lack of appetite, nausea, vomiting, abdominal pain, weakness, jaundice, itching in various body parts, an enlarged liver, dark urine, and breast development in males.

Treatment. Patients should avoid using alcohol and drugs as the inflamed liver cannot detoxify them. Various medications may be prescribed.

A **HIATAL HERNIA** occurs when a portion of the stomach protrudes into the chest cavity through an opening in the diaphragm.

Causes. The causes are mostly unknown, although obesity and smoking are considered risk factors. Eating small meals can be an effective preventive measure.

Signs and Symptoms. Signs and symptoms include excessive burping, difficulty swallowing, chest pain, and heartburn.

Treatment. Treatments are weight reduction, medications to reduce stomach acid production, and surgical repair of the hernia.

INGUINAL HERNIAS occur when a portion of the large intestine protrudes into the inguinal canal (groin), which is located where the thigh and the body trunk meet. In males, the hernia can also protrude into the scrotum.

Causes. The causes are mostly unknown, although these hernias may be caused by weak muscles in the abdominal walls.

Signs and Symptoms. A lump in the groin or scrotum and pain in the groin that gets worse when bending or straining are the common symptoms.

Treatment. Pain medications may be prescribed. Surgery to repair the hernia is needed, in which the large intestine is pushed back into the abdominal cavity.

ORAL CANCER usually involves the lips or tongue but can occur anywhere in the mouth. This type of cancer tends to spread rapidly to other organs.

Causes. The causes are mostly unknown, although the use of tobacco products and alcohol are known risk factors. Poor oral hygiene and ulcers in the mouth can also cause oral cancer.

Signs and Symptoms. Signs and symptoms include difficulty tasting; problems swallowing; and ulcers on the tongue, lip, or other mouth structures. Leukoplakia, or hardened white patches in the mucous membrane of the mouth, is considered a precancerous lesion. A healthcare professional should examine any abnormal patch and biopsy it if it looks suspicious.

Treatment. Radiation therapy, chemotherapy, and surgical removal of the malignant area are the treatment options.

PANCREATIC CANCER is the fourth leading cause of cancer deaths in the United States.

Causes. The causes are mostly unknown, although smoking and alcohol consumption are considered risk factors.

Signs and Symptoms. Common signs and symptoms include depression, fatigue, lack of appetite, nausea or vomiting, abdominal pain, constipation or diarrhea, jaundice, and unintended weight loss.

Treatment. Treatment includes radiation therapy, chemotherapy, and surgical removal of the tumor.

STOMACH CANCER most commonly occurs in the uppermost, or cardiac, portion of the stomach. It appears to occur more frequently in Japan, Chile, and Iceland than in the United States.

Causes. The causes are mostly unknown, although stomach ulcers may contribute to the development of stomach cancer.

Signs and Symptoms. Signs and symptoms include frequent bloating, lack of appetite, feeling full after eating small amounts, nausea, vomiting (with or without blood), abdominal cramps, excessive gas, and blood in the feces.

Treatment. Treatment includes radiation therapy, chemotherapy, and surgical removal of the tumor.

STOMACH ULCERS occur when the lining of the stomach breaks down.

Causes. Bacteria (particularly *Helicobacter pylori*), smoking, alcohol, excessive aspirin use, and hypersecretion of stomach acid can all cause stomach ulcers. They may be prevented by stopping smoking and avoiding aspirin, certain foods, and alcohol.

Signs and Symptoms. Symptoms include nausea, abdominal pain, vomiting (with or without blood), and weight loss. Diagnosis can be confirmed by an upper endoscopy.

Treatment. Treatment options include antibiotics, medications to reduce stomach acid production, *partial gastrectomy* (surgery to remove the affected portion of the stomach), and *vagotomy* (cutting the vagus nerve) to reduce the production of stomach acid.

SUMMARY OF LEARNING OUTCOMES

LEARNING OUTCOMES	KEY POINTS
32.1 Describe the organs of the alimentary canal and their functions.	The pathway of food through the alimentary canal starts with the mouth and continues through the pharynx, esophagus, stomach, small intestine, large intestine, and anal canal. The mouth takes in food and the teeth assist in reducing its size through chewing. The tongue mixes food and holds it between the teeth. The salivary glands produce saliva to moisten and break down food. The pharynx is a long, muscular tube connecting the oral and nasal cavities. It pushes food into the esophagus. The esophagus is a muscular tube that pushes food toward the stomach through muscular contractions. The stomach receives the food, mixes it with gastric juices to start protein digestion, and moves it into the small intestine. The small intestine carries out most of the nutrient absorption. The large intestine's primary job is to rid the body of solid waste by defecation.

LEARNING OUTCOMES	KEY POINTS
32.2 Explain the functions of the digestive system's accessory organs.	The accessory organs to the digestive system include the liver, gallbladder, and pancreas. As a digestive organ, the liver stores vitamins and iron and produces macrophages to fight infection. It also secretes bile for fat digestion. The gallbladder stores the bile produced by the liver. The pancreas produces pancreatic juices that assist in carbohydrate, lipid, and protein digestion.
32.3 Identify the nutrients absorbed by the digestive system and where they are absorbed.	Nutrients absorbed by the body include carbohydrates, proteins, lipids, vitamins, minerals, and water. Most of the absorption takes place in the small intestine.
32.4 Describe the causes, signs and symptoms, and treatments of various common diseases and disorders of the digestive system.	There are many common diseases and disorders of the digestive system with varied signs, symptoms, and treatments. Some of these include appendicitis, cirrhosis, cholelithiasis, colitis, colorectal cancer, constipation, Crohn's disease, diarrhea, diverticulitis, diverticulosis, gastritis, gastroesophageal reflux disease or GERD (commonly known as heartburn), hemorrhoids, hepatitis, hiatal hernia, inguinal hernia, oral cancer, pancreatic cancer, stomach cancer, and stomach ulcers.

CASE STUDY CRITICAL THINKING

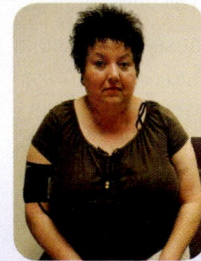

© McGraw-Hill Education

Recall Sylvia Gonzales from the beginning of this chapter. Now that you have completed the chapter, answer the following questions regarding her case.

1. What is the function of the gallbladder?

2. If Sylvia does not want to have surgery, what other treatment options are available?

3. Will Sylvia need to change her diet once her gallbladder is removed?

EXAM PREPARATION QUESTIONS

1. (LO 32.1) Which layer of the digestive tract is the most active in absorbing nutrients?
   a. Mucosa
   b. Submucosa
   c. Muscular
   d. Serosa
   e. Visceral

2. (LO 32.2) Which of the following is an accessory organ of the digestive process?
   a. Stomach
   b. Small intestine
   c. Liver
   d. Esophagus
   e. Pharynx

3. (LO 32.1) Although it hangs from the soft palate, the _____ is not one of the tonsils.
   a. Lingual
   b. Uvula
   c. Palatine
   d. Pharyngeal
   e. Adenoid

4. (LO 32.1) When an organ pushes through the wall that contains it, a(n) _____ develops.
   a. Sphincter
   b. Aneurysm
   c. Ulcer
   d. Hernia
   e. Bolus

5. (LO 32.4) Also known as inflammatory bowel disease, _____ often affects the end of the small intestine.
   a. Diverticulitis
   b. Crohn's disease
   c. GERD
   d. Colitis
   e. Cholelithiasis

6. (LO 32.2) Which of the following is made by the liver?
   a. Amylase
   b. Trypsin
   c. Secretin
   d. Bilirubin
   e. Bile

7. (LO 32.3) Which of the following is *not* a type of carbohydrate?
   a. Monosaccharides
   b. Polysaccharides
   c. Cellulose
   d. Disaccharides
   e. Triglycerides

8. (LO 32.3) Why do people need to include fiber in their diet?
   a. To help the large intestine empty more regularly
   b. To make energy when glucose levels are low
   c. To make cell membranes and hormones
   d. To help the body absorb fat-soluble vitamins
   e. To help synthesize antibodies and nucleic acids

9. (LO 32.4) Which of the following terms is used to describe difficult defecation?
   a. Cirrhosis
   b. Constipation
   c. Cholelithiasis
   d. Diarrhea
   e. Crohn's disease

10. (LO 32.4) Which disorder is commonly referred to as an "upset stomach"?
   a. GERD
   b. Diverticulitis
   c. Gastritis
   d. Hiatal hernia
   e. Crohn's disease

MEDICAL TERMINOLOGY PRACTICE

Analyze the following medical terms, presented throughout the chapter. Using a medical dictionary (or Appendix I) place a / mark between each word part. Define each word part and then define the whole word.

EXAMPLE: **gastr/oid** = gastr means "stomach" + oid means "resembling"
   GASTROID means "resembling the stomach."

1. bicuspid
2. carboxypeptidase
3. diverticulosis
4. hepatocyte

5. idiopathic
6. laryngopharynx
7. nuclease
8. polysaccharide

9. pyloric
10. sublingual
11. hematemesis
12. gastroenteritis

The Endocrine System

CASE STUDY

	Patient Name	DOB	Allergies
PATIENT INFORMATION	Ken Washington	12/1/19XX	Sulfa
	Attending	**MRN**	**Other Information**
	Paul F. Buckwalter, MD	891-12-743	Recent CVA w/ residual foot drop

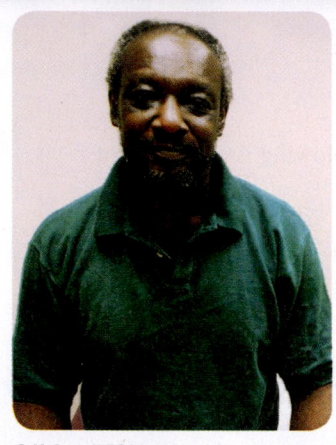

© McGraw-Hill Education

Ken Washington, a 61-year-old man, comes to the office today complaining of feeling "odd." His symptoms include weight loss for no apparent reason, "jitteriness" with a feeling like his heart is racing, and overall irritability. You notice that the patient's eyes appear more prominent than normal. Ken is particularly concerned about his new symptoms, as he was only recently discharged from the hospital after suffering a CVA. He has a residual foot drop, for which he wears a brace and is receiving physical therapy.

Keep Ken Washington in mind as you study this chapter. There will be questions at the end of the chapter based on the case study. The information in the chapter will help you answer these questions.

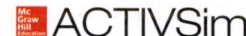

LEARNING OUTCOMES

After completing Chapter 33, you will be able to:

33.1 Describe the general functions of hormones and the endocrine system.

33.2 Identify the hormones released by the pituitary gland, thyroid gland, parathyroid glands, adrenal glands, pancreas, and other hormone-producing organs and give the functions of each.

33.3 Explain the effect of stressors on the body.

33.4 Describe the causes, signs and symptoms, and treatments of various endocrine disorders.

KEY TERMS

endocrine gland
exocrine gland
feedback loop
gonads
G-protein
hormone
islets of Langerhans
nonsteroidal hormone

parathyroid glands
pineal body
prostaglandins
steroidal hormone
stressor
thymus
thyroid gland

MEDICAL ASSISTING COMPETENCIES

CAAHEP

I.C.4 List major organs in each body system

I.C.5 Identify the anatomical location of major organs in each body system

I.C.7 Describe the normal function of each body system

I.C.8 Identify common pathology related to each body system including:
(a) signs
(b) symptoms
(c) etiology

I.C.9 Analyze pathology for each body system including:
(a) diagnostic measures
(b) treatment modalities

V.C.9 Identify medical terms labeling the word parts

V.C.10 Define medical terms and abbreviations related to all body systems

ABHES

2. Anatomy & Physiology
a. List all body systems, their structures and functions
b. Describe common diseases, symptoms and etiologies as they apply to each body system
c. Identify diagnostic and treatment modalities as they relate to each body system

3. Medical Terminology
a. Define and use entire basic structure of medical words and be able to accurately identify in the correct context, i.e. root, prefix, suffix, combinations, spelling, and definitions
b. Build and dissect medical terms from roots/ suffixes to understand the word element combinations that create medical terminology
c. Apply various medical terms for each specialty
d. Define and use medical abbreviations when appropriate and acceptable

▶ Introduction

The endocrine (*endo-,* meaning "within," and *-crine,* meaning "to secrete") system includes the organs of the body that secrete hormones directly into body fluids such as blood. Hormones help to regulate the chemical reactions within cells. They therefore control the functions of the organs, tissues, and other cells. In this chapter, you will learn about the processes and organs of the endocrine system. Figure 33-1 shows the organs of the endocrine system, as well as the heart and kidney, both of which secrete a hormone, although hormone secretion is not the primary function of either of them. As shown, the gastrointestinal (GI) tract also secretes hormones, but again hormone secretion is not its primary function.

▶ Hormones   LO 33.1

Endocrine glands are ductless glands. This means they release their hormones directly into the tissues they act upon, or into the bloodstream, which carries the hormone to the target cells. As you study each gland discussed in this chapter, refer to Figure 33-1 for its location.

Hormones are chemicals secreted by a cell that affect the functions of other cells. Once released, most hormones enter the bloodstream, which transports them to their target cells. A hormone's target cells are those that contain the receptors for the hormone. A hormone cannot affect a cell unless the cell has receptors for it, in much the same way that a locked door needs the key specifically cut to open its lock. Table 33-1 outlines the endocrine glands, the hormone(s) secreted by each, and the action resulting from each hormone.

Types of Hormones

Many hormones in the body are derived from steroids. Steroids are soluble in lipids (fats) and can therefore cross cell membranes easily. Once a **steroidal hormone** is inside a cell, it binds to its receptor, which is commonly in the cell's nucleus. The hormone-receptor complex turns a gene on or off. When new genes are turned on or off, the cell begins to carry out new functions, and this is ultimately how steroidal hormones affect their target cells. Examples of steroidal hormones are estrogen, progesterone, testosterone, and cortisol.

Nonsteroidal hormones are made of amino acids or proteins. Proteins cannot easily cross the cell membrane. Therefore, these hormones bind to receptors on the cell's surface. The hormone-receptor complex in the membrane usually activates a G-protein. The **G-protein** causes enzymes inside the cell to be turned on. Different chemical reactions then begin inside the cell, and the cell takes on new functions.

Prostaglandins (tissue hormones) are local hormones. They are derived from lipid molecules and typically do not need to travel in the bloodstream to find their target cells. Instead, their target cells are located in the same area of tissue where the prostaglandin hormone is created. Prostaglandins have the same effects as other hormones and are produced by many body organs, including the kidneys, stomach, uterus, heart, and brain.

Negative and Positive Feedback Loops

Hormone levels are controlled by a mechanism known as a **feedback loop,** which can be negative or positive (see Figure 33-2). In a negative feedback loop, a stimulus such as eating raises blood sugar levels. This increase is detected by the

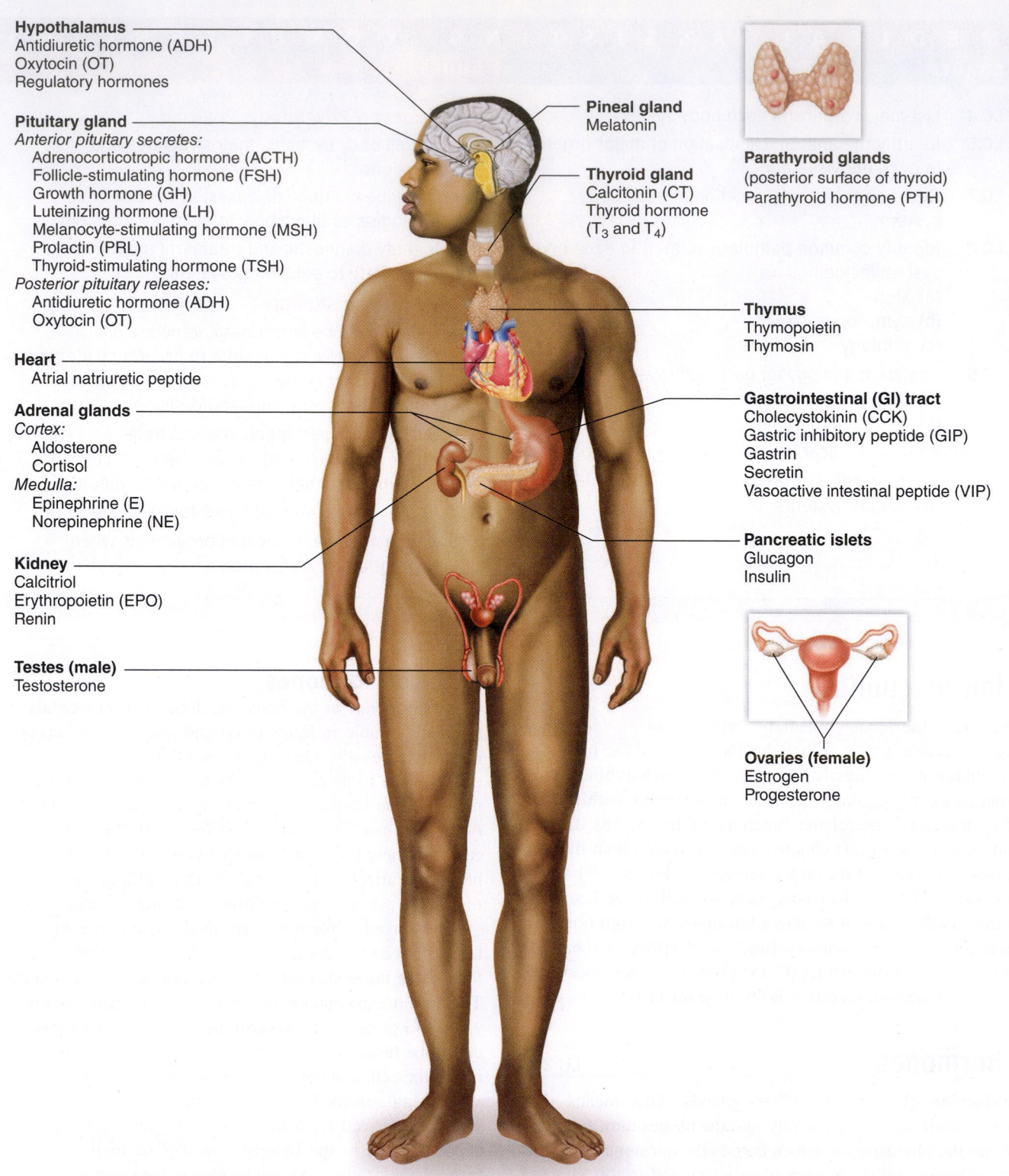

Hypothalamus
Antidiuretic hormone (ADH)
Oxytocin (OT)
Regulatory hormones

Pituitary gland
Anterior pituitary secretes:
  Adrenocorticotropic hormone (ACTH)
  Follicle-stimulating hormone (FSH)
  Growth hormone (GH)
  Luteinizing hormone (LH)
  Melanocyte-stimulating hormone (MSH)
  Prolactin (PRL)
  Thyroid-stimulating hormone (TSH)
Posterior pituitary releases:
  Antidiuretic hormone (ADH)
  Oxytocin (OT)

Heart
  Atrial natriuretic peptide

Adrenal glands
Cortex:
  Aldosterone
  Cortisol
Medulla:
  Epinephrine (E)
  Norepinephrine (NE)

Kidney
Calcitriol
Erythropoietin (EPO)
Renin

Testes (male)
Testosterone

Pineal gland
Melatonin

Thyroid gland
Calcitonin (CT)
Thyroid hormone
(T_3 and T_4)

Parathyroid glands
(posterior surface of thyroid)
Parathyroid hormone (PTH)

Thymus
Thymopoietin
Thymosin

Gastrointestinal (GI) tract
Cholecystokinin (CCK)
Gastric inhibitory peptide (GIP)
Gastrin
Secretin
Vasoactive intestinal peptide (VIP)

Pancreatic islets
Glucagon
Insulin

Ovaries (female)
Estrogen
Progesterone

FIGURE 33-1 Endocrine system—endocrine glands and other organs that secrete hormones are found throughout the body. They produce various types of hormones.

pancreas, which secretes the hormone insulin in response. As cells of the liver take up glucose to store it as glycogen and the body cells take up glucose for energy, the blood glucose levels decline and the insulin release stops as blood glucose levels normalize.

In a positive feedback loop, a stimulus also begins the process, as when a nursing infant suckles at the mother's breast. The suckling sends an impulse to the hypothalamus, which in turn signals the posterior pituitary to release oxytocin. The oxytocin stimulates milk production and ejection from the

TABLE 33-1 Endocrine Glands: Their Hormones and Actions

Gland	Hormone	Action Produced
Hypothalamus (produces)	Antidiuretic hormone (ADH)	Stored and released by posterior pituitary
	Oxytocin (OT)	Stored and released by posterior pituitary
Anterior pituitary	Growth hormone (GH)	Promotes growth and tissue maintenance
	Melanocyte-stimulating hormone (MSH)	Stimulates pigment regulation in epidermis
	Adrenocorticotropic hormone (ACTH)	Stimulates adrenal cortex to produce its hormones
	Thyroid-stimulating hormone (TSH)	Stimulates the thyroid to produce its hormones
	Follicle-stimulating hormone (FSH)	(F) Stimulates ovaries to produce ova and estrogen (M) Stimulates spermatogenesis
	Luteinizing hormone (LH)	(F) Stimulates ovaries for ovulation and estrogen production (M) Stimulates testes to produce testosterone
	Prolactin (PRL)	(F) Stimulates breasts to produce milk (M) Works with and complements LH
Posterior pituitary (releases)	Antidiuretic hormone (ADH)	Stimulates kidneys to retain water
	Oxytocin (OT)	Stimulates uterine contractions for labor and delivery
Pineal body	Melatonin	Regulates biological clock; linked to onset of puberty
Thyroid	T_3 and T_4	Protein synthesis and increased energy production for all cells
	Calcitonin	Increases bone calcium and decreases blood calcium
Parathyroid	Parathyroid hormone (PTH)	Agonist to calcitonin; decreases bone calcium and increases blood calcium
Thymus	Thymosin and thymopoietin	Both hormones stimulate the production of T lymphocytes
Adrenal cortex	Aldosterone	Stimulates body to retain sodium and water
	Cortisol	Decreases protein synthesis; decreases inflammation
Adrenal medulla	Epinephrine and norepinephrine	Prepare the body for stress; increase heart rate, respiration, and blood pressure
Pancreas (islets of Langerhans)	Alpha cells—glucagon	Increases blood sugar; decreases protein synthesis
	Beta cells—insulin	Decreases blood sugar; increases protein synthesis
Gonads: Ovaries (Female)	Estrogen and progesterone	Secondary sex characteristics; female reproductive hormones
Testes (Male)	Testosterone	Secondary sex characteristics; male reproductive hormone

mammary glands. Milk continues to be released as long as the infant continues to nurse.

▶ Hormone Production   LO 33.2

Hormones are produced in various organs and glands throughout the body. For example, the brain has several sites of hormone production, including the hypothalamus, pituitary gland, and pineal body. The pancreas, kidneys, stomach, and reproductive organs also produce important hormones.

The Hypothalamus

The hypothalamus is located in the diencephalon of the brain (see the chapter *The Nervous System*) and produces the hormones *oxytocin* and *antidiuretic hormone (ADH)*. These hormones are transported to the posterior pituitary, where they are stored and released as directed by the hypothalamus.

The Pituitary Gland

The pituitary gland, also known as the *hypophysis,* is located at the base of the brain and controlled by the hypothalamus. This gland is well protected by a bony structure called the sella turcica. The pituitary is divided into two lobes: the anterior lobe and the posterior lobe (see Figures 33-1 and 33-3).

Anterior Lobe of the Pituitary Gland The anterior lobe of the pituitary gland, also known as the *adenohypophysis,* secretes the following hormones:

- *Growth hormone (GH).* As its name suggests, this hormone stimulates an increase in the size of the body's muscles and bones. It is important in childhood for growth. It also stimulates tissue repair. Growth hormone is also known as *somatotropin.*
- *Melanocyte-stimulating hormone (MSH).* This hormone stimulates synthesis of melanin and its disbursement to the skin cells of the epidermis.

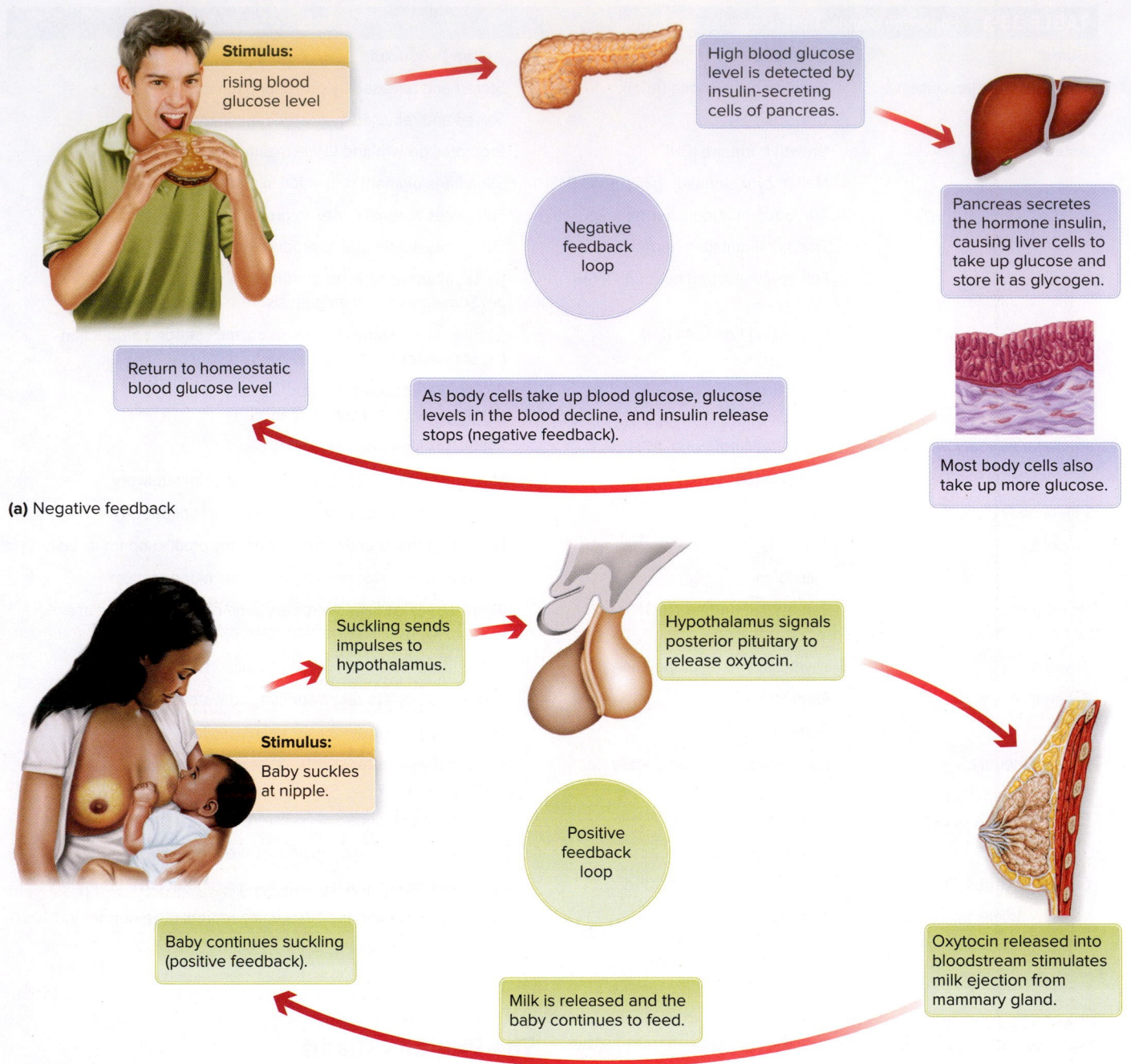

(a) Negative feedback

Stimulus: rising blood glucose level

High blood glucose level is detected by insulin-secreting cells of pancreas.

Pancreas secretes the hormone insulin, causing liver cells to take up glucose and store it as glycogen.

Negative feedback loop

Return to homeostatic blood glucose level

As body cells take up blood glucose, glucose levels in the blood decline, and insulin release stops (negative feedback).

Most body cells also take up more glucose.

(b) Positive feedback

Suckling sends impulses to hypothalamus.

Hypothalamus signals posterior pituitary to release oxytocin.

Stimulus: Baby suckles at nipple.

Positive feedback loop

Baby continues suckling (positive feedback).

Milk is released and the baby continues to feed.

Oxytocin released into bloodstream stimulates milk ejection from mammary gland.

FIGURE 33-2 Positive and negative feedback loops in the endocrine system—the initial step in any feedback pathway is the stimulus. (a) A negative feedback loop occurs when the end product of a pathway turns off or slows down the pathway, whereas (b) a positive feedback loop is involved when the end product of a pathway stimulates further pathway activity.

- *Adrenocorticotropic hormone (ACTH).* This hormone stimulates the adrenal cortex to release its hormones.
- *Thyroid-stimulating hormone (TSH).* This hormone stimulates the thyroid gland to release its hormones.
- *Follicle-stimulating hormone (FSH).* In females, this hormone stimulates the production of estrogen by the ovaries. More significantly, FSH stimulates maturation of the ova (eggs) before ovulation. In males, it stimulates sperm production (spermatogenesis).

- *Luteinizing hormone (LH).* In females, this hormone stimulates ovulation (the release of an egg from the ovaries) and the production of estrogen. In males, it stimulates the production of testosterone.
- *Prolactin (PRL).* In females, this hormone stimulates milk production by the mammary glands. Because of this function, it is sometimes called the lactogenic hormone. In males, prolactin is known to enhance the functioning of LH.

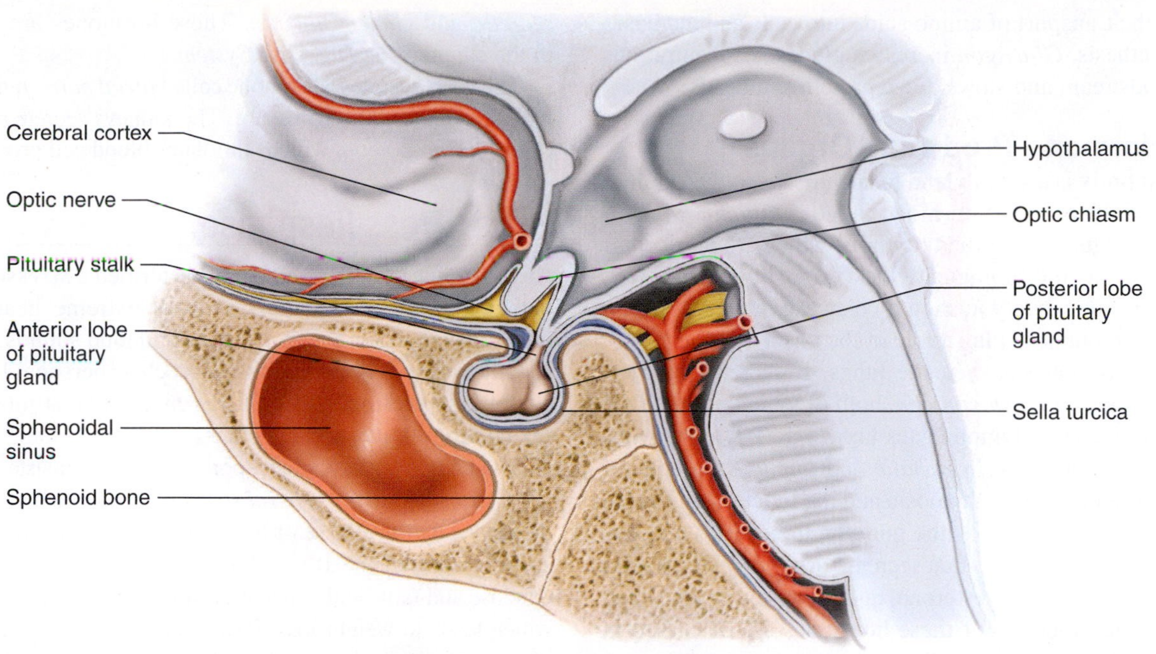
Cerebral cortex
Optic nerve
Pituitary stalk
Anterior lobe of pituitary gland
Sphenoidal sinus
Sphenoid bone
Hypothalamus
Optic chiasm
Posterior lobe of pituitary gland
Sella turcica

FIGURE 33-3 Location of the pituitary gland.

Posterior Lobe of the Pituitary Gland The posterior lobe of the pituitary gland, also known as the *neurohypophysis,* secretes the following two hormones:

- *Antidiuretic hormone (ADH).* This hormone stimulates the kidneys to conserve water. It therefore decreases urine output and helps to maintain blood pressure. You may find it easier to remember the purpose of this hormone by remembering your terminology word parts: *anti* = against, *dia* = complete, and *uresis* = urination.
- *Oxytocin (OT).* In females, this hormone causes contractions of the uterus during childbirth. It also causes the ejection of milk from mammary glands during breast-feeding. In males, oxytocin stimulates the contraction of the prostate and vas deferens during sexual arousal.

The Thyroid Gland and Parathyroid Glands

The **thyroid gland** sits below the larynx (voice box) and consists of two lobes. The lobes are divided into follicles, which store some of the hormones this gland produces. Two major types of hormones produced by the thyroid gland are *thyroid hormones* and *calcitonin.* There are two main thyroid hormones: *triiodothyronine* (T_3) and *thyroxine* (T_4). The *T* stands for *thyroid,* and the numeral refers to the number of iodine atoms that are needed for each of these hormones to work properly.

Thyroid hormones increase cells' energy production, stimulate protein synthesis, and speed up the repair of damaged tissues. In children, they are important for normal growth and the development of the nervous system. Calcitonin lowers blood calcium levels by pulling excess calcium from the blood to activate osteoblasts to build new bone tissue.

Most people have four **parathyroid glands.** They are small glands embedded into the posterior surface of the thyroid gland. The only hormone secreted by the parathyroid glands is called *parathormone,* or *parathyroid, hormone (PTH).* This hormone acts as an agonist to calcitonin by raising blood calcium levels through the activation of osteoclasts. Osteoclasts are bone-dissolving cells. When they dissolve bone, calcium levels in bone decrease as calcium is released into the bloodstream. This action raises blood calcium levels.

The Adrenal Glands

An adrenal gland sits on top of each kidney. It is divided into two portions: the adrenal medulla and the adrenal cortex. The adrenal medulla is the central portion of the gland and secretes *epinephrine* and *norepinephrine.* These hormones produce the same effects that the sympathetic nervous system produces. They increase heart rate, breathing rate, blood pressure, and all the other actions that prepare the body for stressful situations.

The adrenal cortex is the outermost portion of the adrenal gland. It secretes many hormones, but the two major ones are aldosterone and cortisol. *Aldosterone* stimulates the body to retain sodium, which helps it to retain water. This retention of fluid is important for maintaining blood pressure. *Cortisol* is released when a person is stressed. It decreases protein synthesis, and so it slows down the repair of tissues. Its advantage is that it also decreases inflammation, which decreases pain.

The Pancreas

The pancreas is located behind the stomach. It is an endocrine gland as well as an exocrine gland. It is considered an **exocrine gland** because it secretes digestive enzymes into a duct that leads to the small intestine. It is considered an endocrine gland because it contains structures known as **islets of Langerhans** that secrete hormones into the bloodstream. The islets of Langerhans consist of two types of cells: alpha cells, which secrete glucagon, and beta cells, which secrete insulin.

Insulin promotes the cells' uptake of glucose. It therefore reduces glucose concentrations in the bloodstream. It also promotes the transport of amino acids into cells and increases protein synthesis. *Glucagon* increases glucose concentrations in the bloodstream and slows down protein synthesis.

Other Hormone-Producing Organs

The **pineal body** is a small gland located between the cerebral hemispheres. It secretes a hormone called *melatonin*. Melatonin helps to regulate circadian rhythms, which are more commonly known as the biological clock. Your biological clock helps you decide when you should be awake or asleep. Melatonin is also thought to play a role in the onset of puberty.

The **thymus** lies between the lungs. It secretes the hormones *thymosin* and *thymopoietin*, both of which promote the production of certain lymphocytes known as T lymphocytes. Refer to the chapter *The Lymphatic and Immune Systems* for further information about thymosin and the function of T cells.

Sometimes referred to as the **gonads,** the ovaries and testes are reproductive organs that secrete hormones. The ovaries release estrogen and progesterone, and the testes produce testosterone. The functions of these hormones are discussed in the chapter *The Reproductive Systems.*

The stomach and small intestine also secrete hormones. The stomach produces gastrin, and the small intestine releases *secretin* and *cholecystokinin.* These hormones are discussed in the chapter *The Digestive System.*

The heart secretes a hormone called *atrial natriuretic peptide,* which regulates blood pressure. The kidneys secrete a hormone called *erythropoietin,* which stimulates blood cell production.

▶ The Stress Response
LO 33.3

Any stimulus that produces stress is termed a **stressor.** Stressors include physical factors such as extreme heat or cold, infections, injuries, heavy exercise, and loud sounds. Stressors also include psychological factors such as personal loss, grief, anxiety, depression, and guilt. Even positive stimuli such as sexual arousal, joy, and happiness can be stressors.

The body's physiologic response to stress consists of a group of reactions called the *general stress syndrome,* which is primarily caused by the release of hormones. This syndrome results in an increase in the heart rate, breathing rate, and blood pressure. Glucose and fatty acid concentrations also increase in the blood, which leads to weight loss. Prolonged stress causes the release of cortisol. Cortisol slows down body repair because it prevents protein synthesis and inhibits immune responses, which is why a person under stress becomes more susceptible to illness.

PATHOPHYSIOLOGY
LO 33.4

Common Diseases and Disorders of the Endocrine System

Refer to Table 33-2 for a quick reference to diseases and disorders of the endocrine system. The table lists hormones according to the hyposecretion or hypersecretion of individual hormones. They are listed in "head-to-toe" order according to the organ that makes the hormone.

ACROMEGALY is a disorder in which too much growth hormone is produced in adults (see Figure 33-4).

Causes. This disorder is caused by an increased production of growth hormone or by a tumor of the pituitary gland.

Signs and Symptoms. The primary signs and symptoms include enlargement of the bones in the entire skull as well as in the hands and feet, and thickening of the skin. Other symptoms

TABLE 33-2	Endocrine System Diseases/Conditions: Quick Reference Guide	
Hormone	**Hypo- or Hypersecretion**	**Disease or Condition**
GH (somatotropin)	Hyposecretion (children)	Dwarfism
	Hypersecretion (children)	Gigantism
	Hypersecretion (adults)	Acromegaly
ACTH	Hyposecretion (adrenal cortex—cortisol)	Addison's disease
	Hypersecretion (adrenal cortex—cortisol)	Cushing's syndrome
ADH	Hyposecretion	Diabetes insipidus (dehydration)
	Hypersecretion	Edema, hypertension
T₃/T₄	Hyposecretion (congenital/children)	Cretinism
	Hyposecretion (adults)—*severe cases*	Hypothyroidism and *myxedema*
	Hypersecretion (adults or children)	Graves' disease (hyperthyroidism)
Glucagon	Hyposecretion	Hypoglycemia
	Hypersecretion	Hyperglycemia
Insulin	Hyposecretion	Hyperglycemia (diabetes mellitus)
	Hypersecretion	Hypoglycemia (hyperinsulinism)

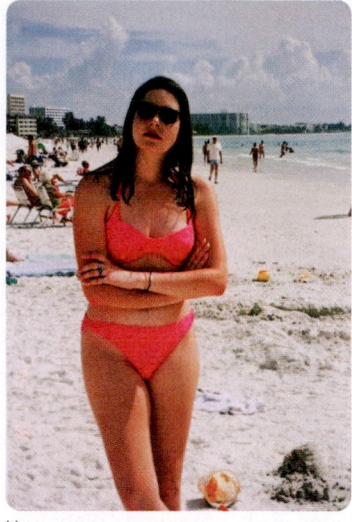

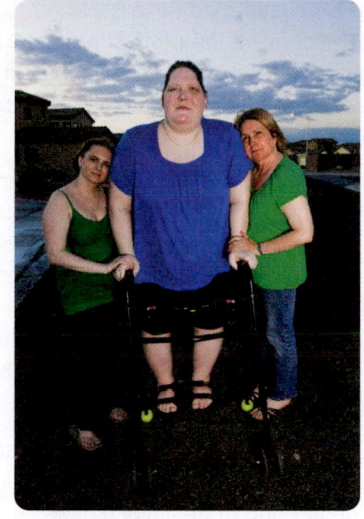

FIGURE 33-4 Acromegaly is caused by the secretion of excessive growth hormone (GH) in adulthood. The face and hands are most notably affected, as seen in this individual at ages 16 and 30.

© Incredible Features/Barcroft Media/Getty Images

include headache, fatigue, profuse sweating, pain (especially in the arms and legs), gaps between the teeth, weight gain, excessive hair production, cardiovascular diseases, arthritis, and vision problems.

Treatment. Treatment includes medications to lower the production of growth hormone, radiation therapy to reduce the size of a pituitary tumor, and surgery to remove a pituitary tumor.

ADDISON'S DISEASE is a condition in which the adrenal glands, specifically the adrenal cortex, fail to produce enough corticosteroids. It affects about 1 in every 25,000 people (see Figure 33-5).

Causes. The cause of this disease is most often unknown. It may be caused by an autoimmune dysfunction. It can be caused

by cancer and other serious diseases that damage the adrenal glands.

Signs and Symptoms. The signs and symptoms may begin long before a diagnosis is made. They include weakness, fatigue, and dizziness after rising from a sitting or reclining position. Other symptoms include weight loss, muscle pain, lack of appetite, nausea, vomiting, diarrhea, and dehydration.

Treatment. Because this disease can be life-threatening, the first treatment is to administer corticosteroids. Medications or other hormones may be prescribed to help balance the levels of sodium and potassium.

CUSHING'S SYNDROME is also known as *hypercortisolism*. In this condition, a person produces too much cortisol (see Figure 33-6).

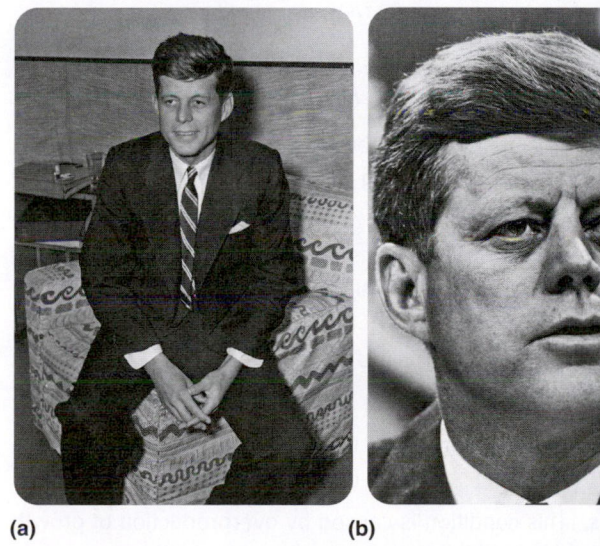

(a)   (b)

FIGURE 33-5 Addison's disease. (a) John F. Kennedy prior to being treated for Addison's disease. (b) In 1960, Kennedy's face shows the facial swelling that was one of the effects of cortisone treatment for Addison's disease.

© Evening Standard/Getty Images; © Hulton Archive/Getty Images

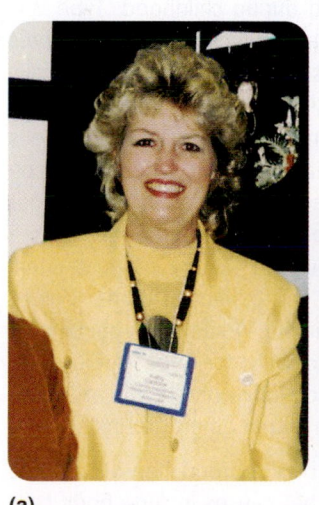

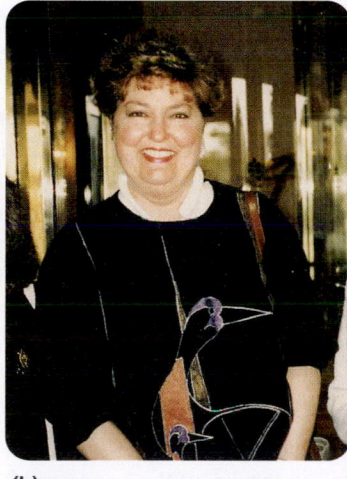

(a)   (b)

FIGURE 33-6 Cushing's syndrome. (a) Photo prior to the onset of Cushing's syndrome. (b) The same person after the onset of Cushing's syndrome. Notice the rounding, or fullness, of the face.

Courtesy of the Cushing's Support and Research Foundation, www.CSRF.new and Kathy Carbone

Causes. This syndrome is caused by an excessive production of ACTH (a hormone that increases the production of cortisol), a tumor of the adrenal gland (the source of cortisol), a tumor of the pituitary gland (the source of ACTH), or the long-term use of steroidal hormones.

Signs and Symptoms. Common symptoms include a round, or full, face ("moon face"), a hump of fat between the shoulders ("buffalo hump"), thin arms and legs with a large abdomen, fatigue, thin skin, acne, frequent thirst (polydipsia), frequent urination (polyuria), mental disabilities, a loss of menstrual cycle in females (amenorrhea), high blood pressure (hypertension), high blood glucose levels (hyperglycemia), and body aches in the muscles, back, or head.

Treatment. The first treatment includes lifestyle changes, especially stopping the use of steroidal hormones. Radiation therapy or surgery may be needed to treat any tumors.

DIABETES INSIPIDUS is a condition in which the kidneys fail to reabsorb water, causing excessive urination. Diabetes insipidus is not related to diabetes mellitus, the pancreatic disorder causing hyperglycemia.

Causes. The primary cause is the hyposecretion of ADH.

Signs and Symptoms. These include excessive thirst, even with a more-than-adequate fluid intake. Other signs and symptoms include excessive urination and, in severe cases, muscle cramps and cardiac arrhythmias related to electrolyte imbalances caused by the excessive fluid loss.

Treatment. The primary treatment is increased fluid intake. Other treatments include surgery for any tumor of the pituitary that may cause the inadequate secretion of ADH. Changes in diet and medication help increase water retention.

DIABETES MELLITUS is a chronic disease characterized by high glucose levels in the blood (hyperglycemia). There are at least three different types of diabetes mellitus. Type 1 is referred to as *early-onset diabetes* or *insulin-dependent diabetes mellitus* (IDDM), and it often is diagnosed during childhood. Type 2 is the most common type and is often called *late-onset diabetes* or *noninsulin-dependent diabetes mellitus* (NIDDM). Historically this type of diabetes was primarily diagnosed in older adults but there has been a surge in the number of adolescents and teens being diagnosed with Type 2 diabetes. This surge has been linked to excessive weight and lack of exercise in the younger population. Gestational diabetes occurs only in pregnant women and is usually temporary, although a history of gestational diabetes has been found to put the patient at higher risk of developing Type 2 diabetes later in life. Women with gestational diabetes should be monitored closely for Type 2 diabetes. African Americans, Hispanics, and Native Americans are more likely to develop diabetes than any other ethnic groups.

Causes. This disease is caused by the production of too little or no insulin by the pancreas. Other causes include body cells having too few insulin receptors, obesity, high blood pressure, pregnancy, and high cholesterol levels in the blood.

Signs and Symptoms. There are many signs and symptoms of this disease. They include high levels of glucose in the blood, excessive thirst (polydipsia), frequent urination (polyuria), fatigue, increased appetite, unexplained weight loss, blurry vision, impotence in men, nausea, skin wounds that heal slowly, high glucose and ketone levels in the urine, and lower extremity problems (due to poor circulation).

Treatment. Treatment includes daily injections of insulin, oral medications to increase insulin production, oral medications to increase the body's sensitivity to insulin, frequent monitoring of glucose levels in the blood, and frequent monitoring of ketone levels in the urine. Lifestyle changes are important and should include reducing weight (especially if obese), changing eating habits, and getting regular exercise. Lifestyle changes to prevent injury to legs and feet may also be needed. More information on diet and treatment for diabetic patients may be found in the *Nutrition and Health* chapter.

Complications. Left untreated, diabetes can result in long-term and life-threatening complications. Blood vessels become thickened, which can damage vital organs, including the kidneys, eyes, heart, and brain. Long-term damage can result in kidney disease, blindness, and atherosclerosis (the buildup of fatty deposits in blood vessels). Circulation worsens, which not only affects organs but also may result in slower overall healing and ulcers that develop in the lower extremities, particularly the feet. Because of the body's decreased ability to heal, these ulcers may require amputation of the affected foot and possibly part of the leg (below-knee amputation, or BKA). Further information on diabetic emergencies, including insulin shock and diabetic coma, may be found in the *Emergency Preparedness* chapter.

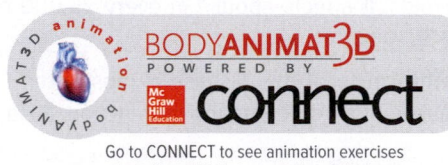

Go to CONNECT to see animation exercises about *Type 1 Diabetes* and *Type 2 Diabetes*.

DWARFISM is a condition in which too little growth hormone (somatotropin) is produced in childhood (see Figure 33-7).

Causes. This condition can be caused by an underproduction of the growth hormone during childhood, trauma to the pituitary gland, or a pituitary tumor.

Signs and Symptoms. Signs and symptoms include short height, abnormal facial features, cleft lip or palate, delayed puberty, headaches, frequent urination, and excessive thirst.

Treatment. Treatment is the administration of supplemental growth hormone.

GIGANTISM is a condition in which too much growth hormone is produced during childhood (see Figure 33-8).

Causes. This condition is caused by overproduction of growth hormone during childhood. It can also be caused by a tumor in the pituitary gland.

Signs and Symptoms. Very tall height, delayed sexual maturity, thick facial bones, thick skin, weakness, and vision problems are common symptoms.

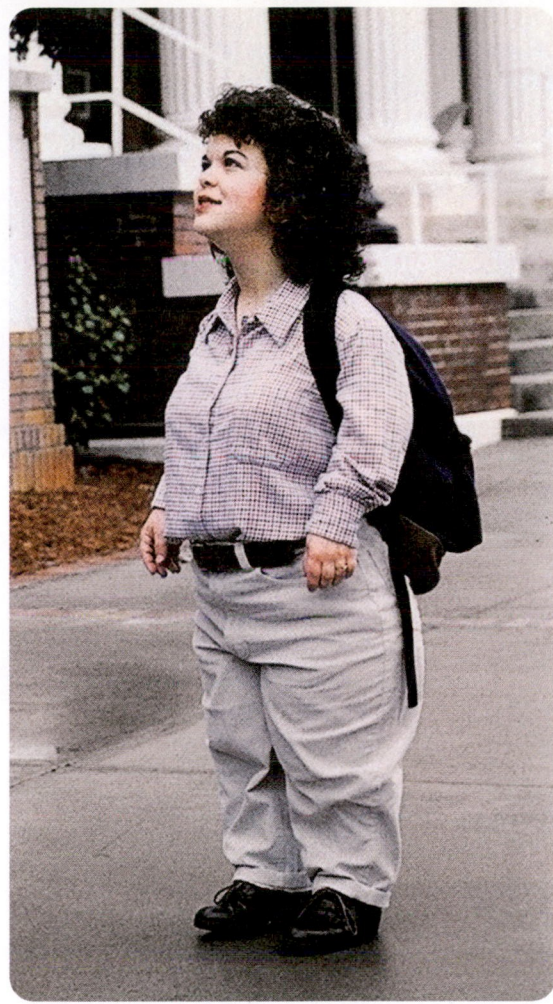

FIGURE 33-7 Pituitary dwarfism is caused by hyposecretion of growth hormone.
© McGraw-Hill Education/Joe DeGrandis, photographer

Treatment. Treatment includes medications to reduce growth hormone levels, radiation therapy, and surgery to remove the tumor.

GOITER is an enlargement of the thyroid gland, causing (sometimes disfiguring) swelling of the neck (see Figure 33-9).

Causes. Typically, a simple goiter is caused by a deficiency of iodine in the diet. Iodine is needed for the thyroid to produce thyroid hormones.

Signs and Symptoms. These include overgrowth of the follicles of the thyroid gland, which causes enlargement of the gland and of the neck, and abnormal thyroid function tests (TFTs).

Treatment. The most common treatment is iodine supplementation in the diet. In the United States, salt contains iodine, so goiters are seldom seen. Because a goiter may not shrink even after adequate iodine is introduced into the diet, surgery may be required to remove some or most of the enlarged gland.

GRAVES' DISEASE is a disorder in which a person develops antibodies that attack the thyroid gland (see Figure 33-10). This attack causes the thyroid to produce too many thyroid

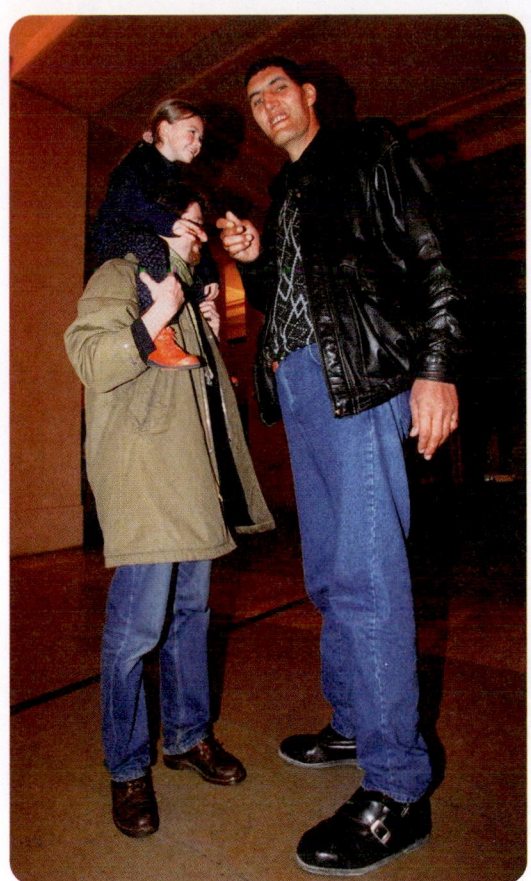

FIGURE 33-8 Gigantism results from hypersecretion of growth hormone.
© Eric Robert/Sygma/Corbis

hormones. Graves' disease is the most common type of hyperthyroidism in the United States.

Causes. This disease is caused by an overproduction of thyroid hormones. It is also considered an autoimmune disorder.

Signs and Symptoms. The most common signs and symptoms include exophthalmos (protrusion of the eyes) and goiter (thyroid

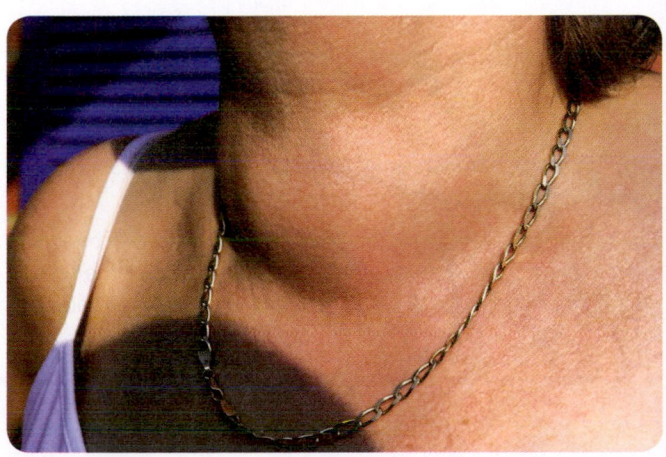

FIGURE 33-9 An iodine deficiency causes simple (endemic) goiter and results in high levels of TSH.
© Chris Pancewicz/Alamy RF

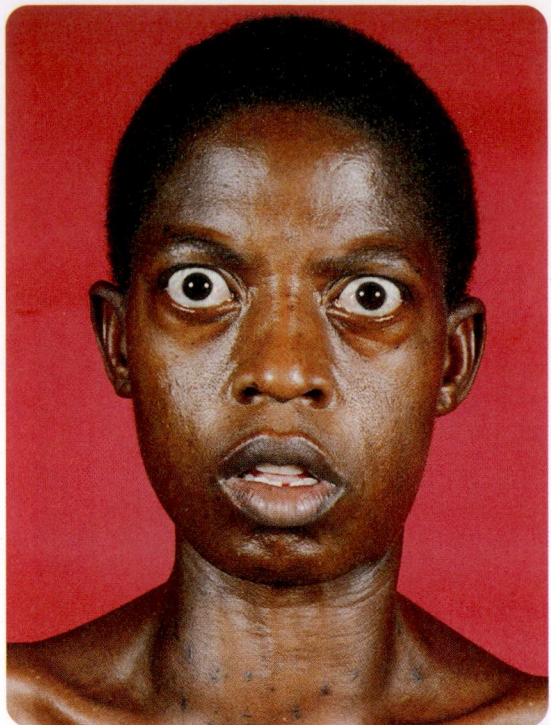

FIGURE 33-10 Signs of Graves' disease, a form of hyperthyroidism, include protruding eyes and goiter.

© Dr. M. A. Ansary/Science Source

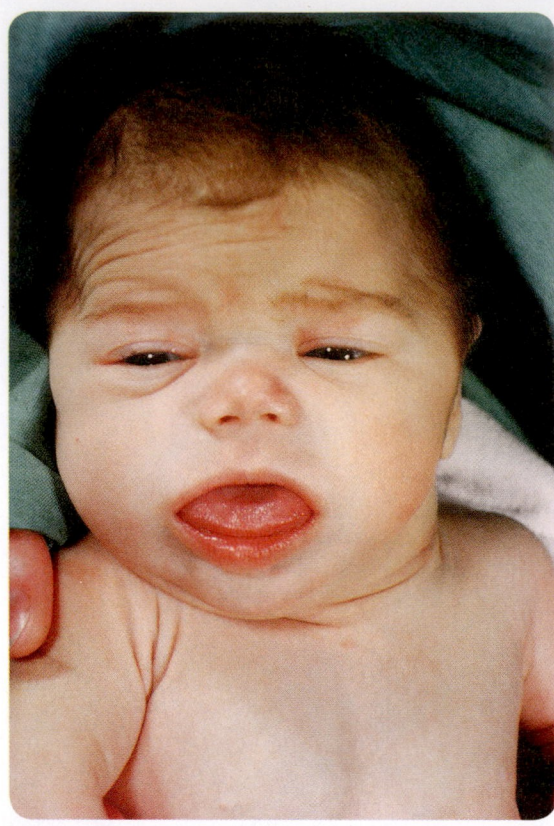

FIGURE 33-11 Cretinism is the result of an underactive thyroid gland during infancy and childhood.

© Mediscan/Alamy

enlargement). Other symptoms include insomnia, unexplained weight loss, anxiety, muscle weakness, increased appetite, excessive sweating, vision problems, and an increased heart rate.

Treatment. Treatment includes medications to reduce heart rate, sweating, and nervousness; radiation to destroy the thyroid gland; surgery to remove the thyroid gland (thyroidectomy); and supplemental thyroid hormones if the gland is destroyed or removed.

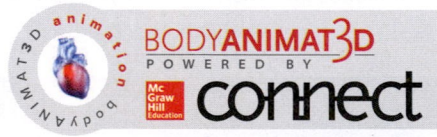

Go to CONNECT to see an animation exercise about *Hyperthyroidism.*

CRETINISM is an extreme form of hypothyroidism that is present prior to or soon after birth (see Figure 33-11).

Causes. The cause is hypothyroidism at birth (a congenital anomaly) related to the absence or malformation of the thyroid gland, abnormal formation of thyroid hormones, or pituitary failure that results in a lack of thyroid stimulation.

Signs and Symptoms. Stunted growth, abnormal bone formation, mental retardation, low body temperature, and overall sluggishness are the primary signs and symptoms.

Treatment. The treatment is thyroid hormone replacement.

MYXEDEMA is a disorder in which the thyroid gland does not produce adequate amounts of thyroid hormone. It is a severe type of hypothyroidism that is most common in females over age 50.

Causes. Causes include the removal of the thyroid, radiation treatments to the neck area, and obesity. This disorder may be congenital.

Signs and Symptoms. Signs and symptoms include weakness, fatigue, weight gain, depression, general body aches, dry skin and hair, hair loss, puffy hands or feet, a decreased ability to taste food, abnormal menstrual periods, pale or yellow skin, a slow heart rate, low blood pressure, anemia, an enlarged heart, high cholesterol levels, and coma.

Treatment. Treatment consists of giving supplemental thyroid hormones intravenously or orally and closely monitoring the levels of thyroid hormones.

LEARNING OUTCOMES	KEY POINTS
33.1 Describe the general functions of hormones and the endocrine system.	Endocrine glands are ductless glands, releasing hormones directly into the bloodstream and tissues. The organs of the endocrine system produce hormones that regulate the chemical reactions within cells, controlling the functions of organs, tissues, and other cells. Hormone levels are controlled by positive and negative feedback loops.
33.2 Identify the hormones released by the pituitary gland, thyroid gland, parathyroid glands, adrenal glands, pancreas, and other hormone-producing organs and give the functions of each.	The pituitary gland releases the following hormones: GH, MSH, ACTH, TSH, FSH, LH, PRL, ADH, and OT. The thyroid gland releases calcitonin, T_3, and T_4, which are important in growth and protein synthesis. The parathyroid gland releases PTH, which balances the action of calcitonin. The adrenal medulla secretes epinephrine and norepinephrine, which work with the sympathetic nervous system. The adrenal cortex produces many hormones, but the two major ones are aldosterone and cortisol. The two types of hormone-releasing cells in the pancreas are alpha cells, which release glucagon, and beta cells, which release insulin. The pineal body releases melatonin; the thymus releases thymosin and thymopoietin; ovaries release estrogen and progesterone (females); and the testes (males) release testosterone. The kidneys produce erythropoietin, and the heart produces atrial natriuretic peptide. Each hormone's specific function may be found in Table 33-1.
33.3 Explain the effect of stressors on the body.	Stressors are stimuli that produce a stress response, a physiologic response to the stimulus that changes the body's functioning in some way.
33.4 Describe the causes, signs and symptoms, and treatments of various endocrine disorders.	The diseases and disorders of the endocrine system are as varied as the organs and hormone dysfunctions that cause them. An overview of these conditions is found in Table 33-2.

CASE STUDY CRITICAL THINKING

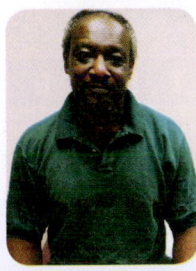

© McGraw-Hill Education

Recall Ken Washington from the beginning of the chapter. Now that you have completed this chapter, answer the following questions regarding his case:

1. What gland is likely to be causing Ken's problems?

2. Based on what you have learned in this chapter, what diagnosis do you think Dr. Buckwalter will have for Ken?

3. What treatment options are available?

4. What other condition is often caused by treating this condition, and how is it managed?

1. (LO 33.1) Which of following hormone types is also known as a tissue hormone?
   a. Steroidal hormones
   b. Nonsteroidal hormones
   c. G-proteins
   d. Prostaglandins
   e. Thyroid hormones

2. (LO 33.2) Which endocrine organ also has a digestive function?
   a. Adrenal medulla
   b. Adrenal cortex
   c. Pancreas
   d. Pineal body
   e. Thymus

3. (LO 33.2) Which hormone assists the kidneys in retaining fluid?
   a. ACTH
   b. ADH
   c. PTH
   d. FSH
   e. MSH

4. (LO 33.2) The numeral in "T_3" and "T_4" stands for the number of _____ atoms needed for the hormones to work properly.
   a. Chloride
   b. Potassium
   c. Calcium
   d. Iodine
   e. Sodium

5. (LO 33.4) From which endocrine disease did President John F. Kennedy suffer?
   a. Cushing's syndrome
   b. Addison's disease
   c. Acromegaly
   d. Hypothyroidism
   e. Graves' disease

6. (LO 33.3) Which hormone is released when a person is under prolonged stress?
   a. Glucagon
   b. Aldosterone
   c. Melatonin
   d. Oxytocin
   e. Cortisol

7. (LO 33.2) Which of the following hormones is not produced by the anterior pituitary?
   a. Growth hormone
   b. Follicle-stimulating hormone
   c. Oxytocin
   d. Luteinizing hormone
   e. Prolactin

8. (LO 33.1) Nonsteroidal hormones require which of the following to turn on enzymes inside target cells?
   a. Amino acids
   b. Prostaglandins
   c. Calcitonin
   d. G-protein
   e. Prolactin

9. (LO 33.4) A condition in which the body produces too much cortisol is
   a. Cushing's syndrome
   b. Graves' disease
   c. Myxedema
   d. Gigantism
   e. Diabetes insipidus

10. (LO 33.4) When too much growth hormone is produced in adults, the result is
    a. Dwarfism
    b. Gigantism
    c. Cretinism
    d. Myxedema
    e. Acromegaly

MEDICAL TERMINOLOGY PRACTICE

Analyze the following medical terms, presented throughout the chapter. Using a medical dictionary (or Appendix I) place a / mark between each word part. Define each word part and then define the whole word.

EXAMPLE: **aden/ oma** = aden means "gland" + oma means "tumor"
ADENOMA means "tumor of a gland."

1. acromegaly
2. adrenocorticotropic
3. antidiuretic
4. exocrine
5. hypothalamus
6. melanocyte
7. natriuretic
8. nonsteroidal
9. parathyroid
10. thymopoietin
11. hyperparathyroidism
12. endocrine

Special Senses

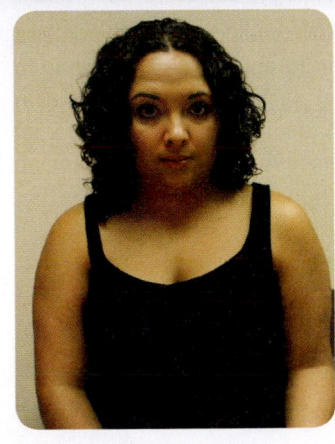
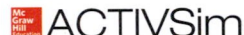
LEARNING OUTCOMES

After completing Chapter 34, you will be able to:

34.1 Describe the anatomy of the nose and the function of each part.

34.2 Describe the anatomy of the tongue and the function of each part.

34.3 Describe the anatomy of the eye and the function of each part, including the accessory structures and their functions.

34.4 Explain the visual pathway through the eye and to the brain for interpretation.

34.5 Describe the causes, signs and symptoms, and treatments of various disorders of the eyes.

34.6 Describe the anatomy of the ear and the function of each part, and explain the role of the ear in maintaining equilibrium.

34.7 Explain how sounds travel through the ear and are interpreted in the brain.

34.8 Describe the causes, signs and symptoms, and treatments of various disorders of the ears.

KEY TERMS

auricle
cerumen
choroid
cochlea
conjunctiva
cornea
eustachian tube
external auditory canal
gustatory cortex
labyrinth
lacrimal apparatus
organ of Corti
ossicles
oval window
papillae
refraction
retina
semicircular canals
sensory adaptation
tympanic membrane
vestibule

▶ Introduction

The special senses are smell, taste, vision, hearing, and equilibrium. They are called special senses because their sensory receptors are located within relatively large sensory organs in the head—the nose, tongue, eyes, and ears. Although the skin is also considered a sense organ (in fact, it is the largest sense organ), touch is not considered a special sense but rather a generalized one (refer to the chapter *The Integumentary System*). This chapter introduces the structure and function of the special sense organs.

As a medical assistant, you will likely be asked to assist with or perform examinations and treatments for common disorders of the eyes and ears. So you will need to understand how these important sense organs function.

▶ The Nose and the Sense of Smell   LO 34.1

Smell receptors, also called *olfactory receptors,* are located in the olfactory organ, found in the upper part of the nasal cavity. See Figure 34-1. Smell receptors are chemoreceptors, which mean that they respond to changes in chemical concentrations. Chemicals that activate smell receptors must be dissolved in the mucus of the nose. Once smell receptors are activated, they send their information to the olfactory nerves. Refer to the chapter *The Nervous System* for more information about these nerves and the various parts of the brain. The olfactory nerves send the information along olfactory bulbs and tracts to different areas of the cerebrum in the brain. The cerebrum interprets the information as a particular type of smell.

Consider the following information related to our sense of smell.

- When individuals have either a "dry nose" or excessive mucus related to an upper respiratory tract infection or allergies, they may have trouble smelling. This is due to the inability of the chemicals (odors) that cause our sense of smell to be dissolved in the mucus of the nose.

- Humans have a relatively poor sense of smell compared to certain animals for two reasons. The chemicals (odors) that activate smell must diffuse all the way up the nasal cavity. Also, the human nose has fewer smell receptors than most animal noses.

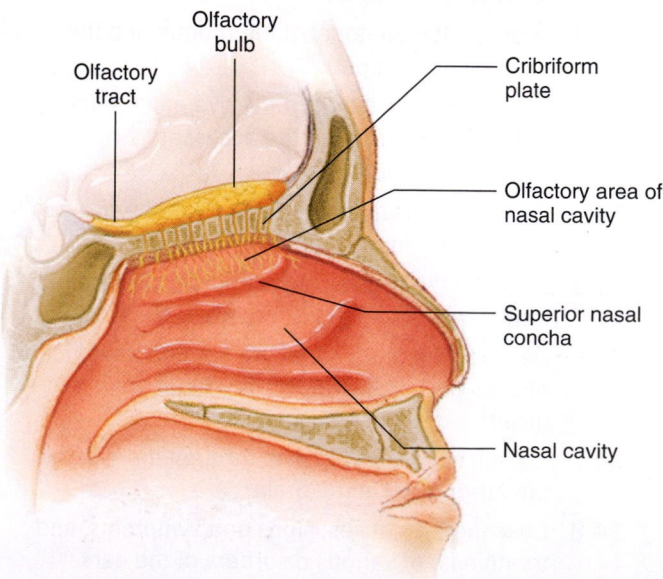

FIGURE 34-1 The olfactory area (organ) is located in the superior part of the nasal cavity.

- Our sense of smell undergoes **sensory adaptation,** which means that the same chemical can stimulate smell receptors for only a limited amount of time. In a relatively short period of time, the smell receptors fatigue and no longer respond to the same chemical (odor), and it can no longer be smelled. Sensory adaptation explains why you smell a strong odor, such as perfume, when you first encounter it, but after a few minutes, you cannot smell it or may be less aware of it.

▶ The Tongue and the Sense of Taste

LO 34.2

Taste, or gustatory, receptors are located on taste buds. Taste buds are microscopic structures found mostly on the **papillae** (bumps) of the tongue. They cannot be seen with the naked eye. Some taste buds are also scattered on the roof of the mouth and in the walls of the throat. Recent research has indicated that a few taste receptors are also found in the lungs.

Each taste bud is made of taste cells and supporting cells (see Figure 34-2). The taste cells function as taste receptors, and the supporting cells simply fill in the spaces between the taste cells. Like the olfactory cells of smell, taste cells are

types of chemoreceptors. They are activated by chemicals found in food and drink that must be dissolved in saliva as part of the digestive process.

There are five types of taste sensations. Each sensation is recognized by a different type of taste cell:

- Sweet: taste cells with receptors that respond to "sweet" chemicals
- Sour: taste cells with receptors that respond to "sour" chemicals
- Salty: taste cells with receptors that respond to "salty" chemicals
- Bitter: taste cells with receptors that respond to "bitter" chemicals
- Umami: taste cells with receptors that respond to a savory, meaty sensation

For many years, it was thought that each type of taste cell was concentrated in a different area on the tongue. However, research has shown that all five types of taste cells are typically located within each taste bud. The sensory nerve at each taste bud is responsible for transmitting all of the taste sensations to the cranial nerves in the brain. There, the information is processed by the **gustatory cortex,** an area of the brain

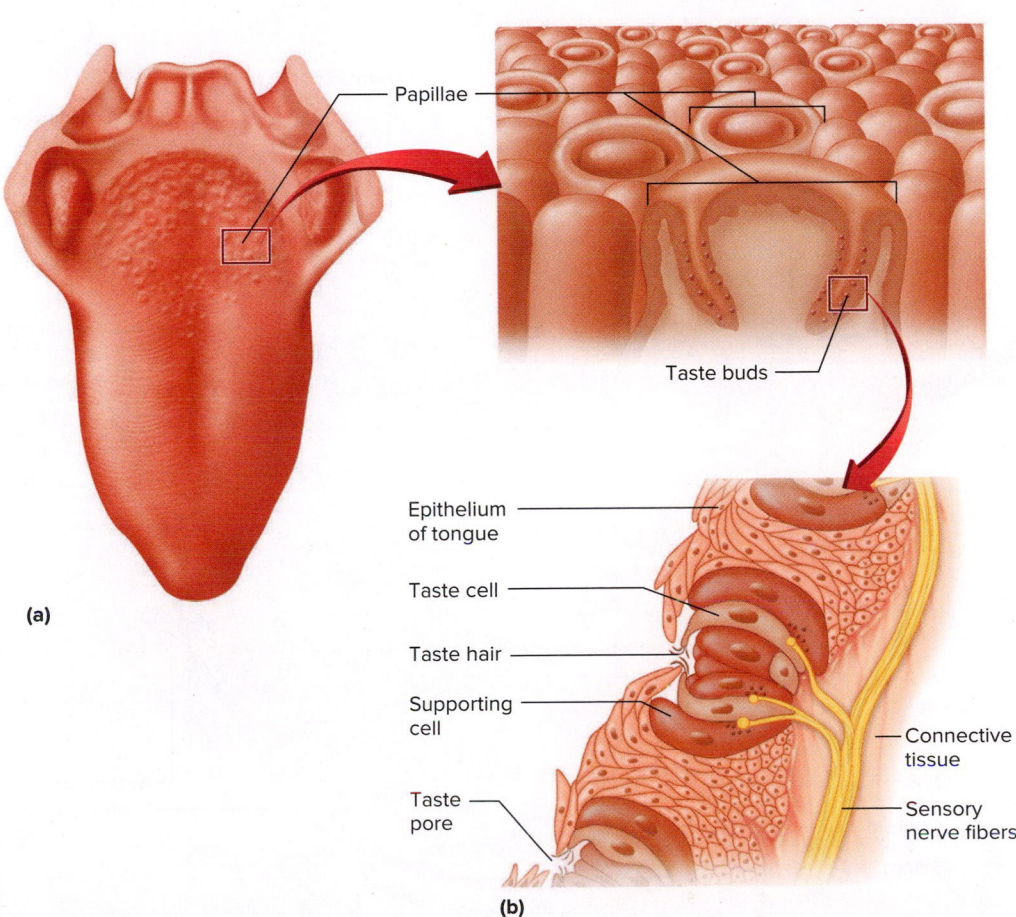

FIGURE 34-2   (a) Taste buds are located on and near the papillae on the tongue. (b) Each taste bud has several taste cells corresponding to the various taste sensations.

that is responsible for interpreting taste sensations. The gustatory cortex integrates information from the taste cells with other information to provide a more complete interpretation. For example, eating spicy foods may activate pain receptors on the tongue that are interpreted by the gustatory cortex as "spicy."

▶ The Eye and the Sense of Sight   LO 34.3

The sense of sight comes from the eyes and is supported by visual accessory organs.

Vision

Your visual system consists of the eyes; the optic nerve, which connects the eyes to the vision center of the brain; and several accessory structures. If these parts of the system are healthy and normal, you are able to see normally.

Structure of the Eye

The eye is a complex organ that processes light to produce images. It is made up of three main layers, two chambers, and a number of specialized parts, as shown in Figure 34-3.

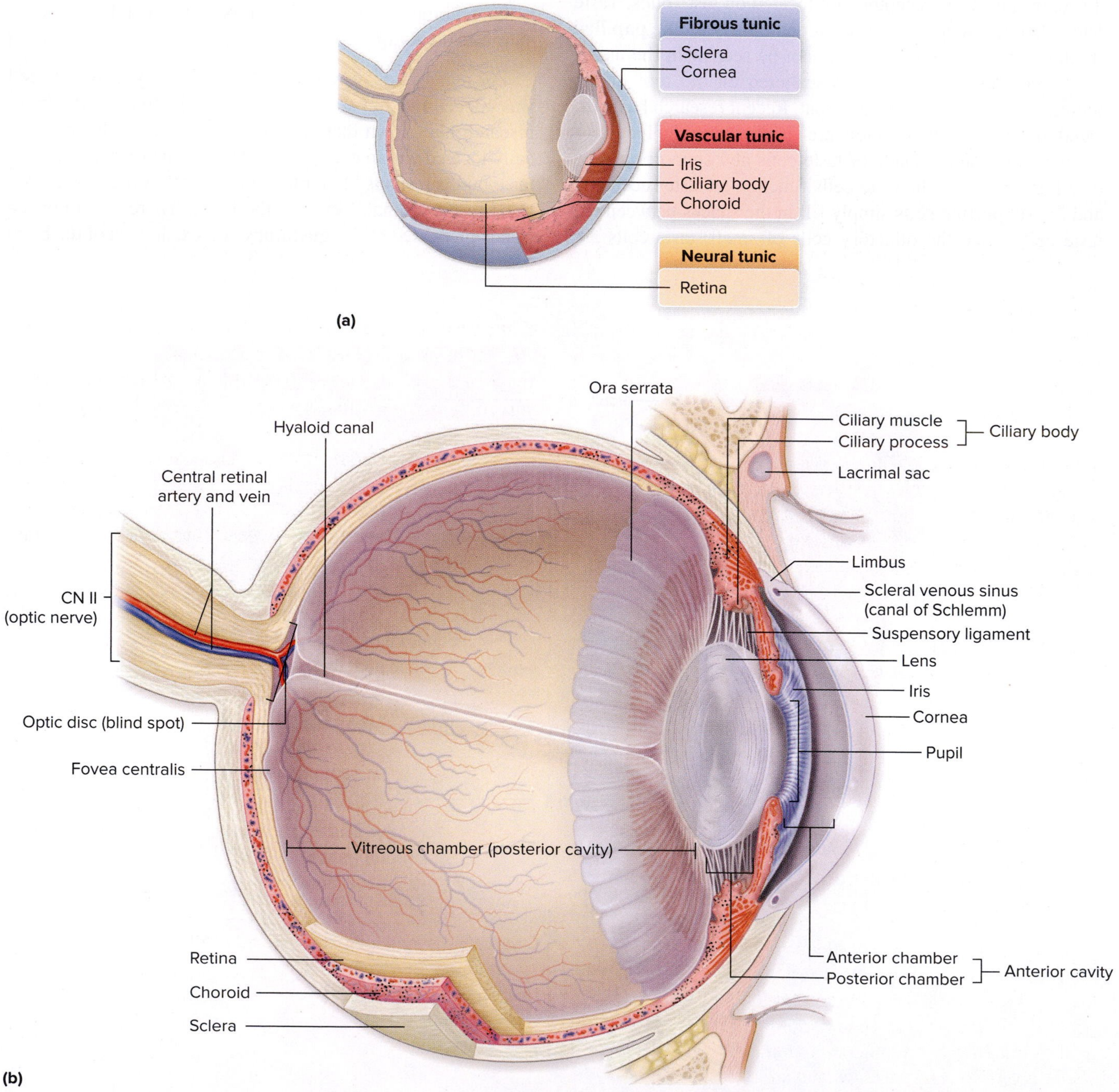

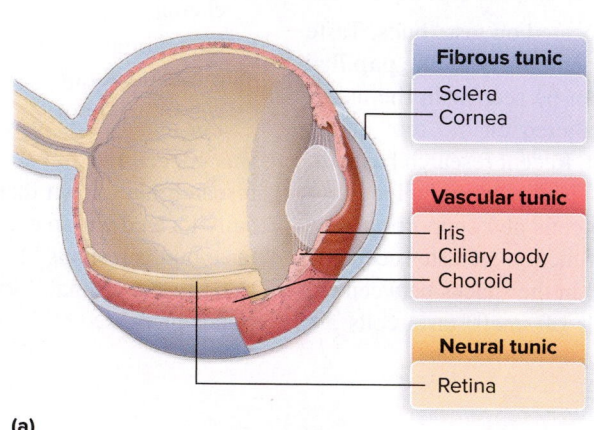

Fibrous tunic
Sclera
Cornea

Vascular tunic
Iris
Ciliary body
Choroid

Neural tunic
Retina

(a)

Ora serrata

Hyaloid canal

Central retinal artery and vein

CN II (optic nerve)

Optic disc (blind spot)

Fovea centralis

Ciliary muscle
Ciliary process — Ciliary body

Lacrimal sac

Limbus

Scleral venous sinus (canal of Schlemm)

Suspensory ligament

Lens

Iris

Cornea

Pupil

Vitreous chamber (posterior cavity)

Retina

Choroid

Sclera

Anterior chamber
Posterior chamber — Anterior cavity

(b)

FIGURE 34-3   Anatomy of the internal eye—sagittal views depict (a) the three layers of the eye and (b) internal eye structures.

The Outer Layer The white of the eye—the *sclera*—is the tough, outermost layer of the eye. This layer, through which light cannot pass, covers all except the front of the eye. Here, the sclera gives way to the cornea in an area known as the corneal-scleral junction, or *limbus*. The **cornea** is a transparent area on the front of the eye that acts as a window to let light into the eye. Although there are no blood vessels in the sclera, numerous sense receptors detect even the smallest particles on the eyeball's surface.

The Middle Layer The **choroid** is the middle layer of the eye, which contains most of the eye's blood vessels. In the anterior part of the choroid are the iris and the ciliary body. The iris is the colored part of the eye. It is made of muscular tissue. As this tissue contracts and relaxes, an opening at its center (the pupil) grows larger or smaller. The size of the pupil regulates the amount of light that enters the eye. In bright light, the pupil becomes constricted (smaller). In dim light, it becomes dilated (larger).

The ciliary body is a wedge-shaped thickening in the eyeball's middle layer. Muscles in the ciliary body control the shape of the lens—making the lens more or less curved for viewing either near or distant objects. The lens is a clear, circular disk located just posterior to the iris. Because the lens can change shape, it helps the eye focus images of near or faraway objects. This process is called *accommodation.* Clouding and hardening of the lens, which often occur with aging, lead to visual changes in a condition known as *cataracts.* This condition will be discussed in more detail later in the *Assisting with Eye and Ear Care* chapter.

The Inner Layer The eye's inner layer consists of the **retina.** Nerve cells at the posterior of the retina sense light. The area where the optic nerve enters the retina is known as the optic disc. This area contains no sensory nerves itself and is referred to as the *blind spot.* There are two types of nerve cells, each named for its shape. *Rods* are highly sensitive to light. They function in dim light but do not provide a sharp image or detect color, only black, white, and shades of gray. They give you your limited "night vision" as well as peripheral vision. *Cones* function best in bright light. They are sensitive to color and provide sharper images. They are responsible for the ability to differentiate tones and hues of color. Deficiencies in the number or types of cones are responsible for the various types of color blindness, which is generally an inherited condition.

The Chambers of the Eye Each eyeball is divided into two chambers: anterior and posterior.

The Anterior Chamber The anterior chamber is in front of the lens and is filled with a watery fluid called *aqueous humor.* Aqueous humor provides nutrients to and bathes the structures in the anterior chamber of the eyeball. When there is an accumulation of aqueous humor, a person develops a visual condition known as *glaucoma.* This disorder will be discussed in more detail in the *Assisting with Eye and Ear Care* chapter.

The Posterior Chamber The posterior chamber of the eyeball is behind the lens and is filled with a thick, jelly-like fluid called *vitreous humor.* Vitreous humor keeps the retina flat and helps to maintain the eye's shape.

Visual Accessory Organs

Visual accessory organs assist and protect the eyeball. They include the orbits, eyebrows, eyelids and eyelashes, conjunctiva, lacrimal apparatus, and extrinsic eye muscles.

Eye Orbits and Eyebrows The eye sockets, or *orbits,* form a protective shell around the eyes. Eyebrows protect the eyes by reducing the chances that sweat and direct sunlight will enter them.

Eyelids and Eyelashes Each eyelid is composed of skin, muscle, and dense connective tissue. The muscle in the eyelid is called the *orbicularis oculi* and is responsible for blinking and squinting. Blinking the eyelids prevents the mucous membrane surface of the eyeball from drying. A moist eyeball surface is much less likely to grow bacteria than a dry one is. Blinking also protects the eyes, keeping foreign material from entering them with the assistance of the eyelashes, which catch foreign substances, including perspiration and dust.

Conjunctiva The **conjunctiva** is the mucous membrane that lines the inner surfaces of the eyelids and covers the anterior surface of each eyeball. Mucous membranes produce mucus, which keeps the surface of the eyeballs moist.

The Lacrimal Apparatus The **lacrimal apparatus** consists of lacrimal glands and nasolacrimal ducts (see Figure 34-4). *Lacrimal glands,* located on the lateral edge of each eyeball, produce tears. Tears are mostly water, but they

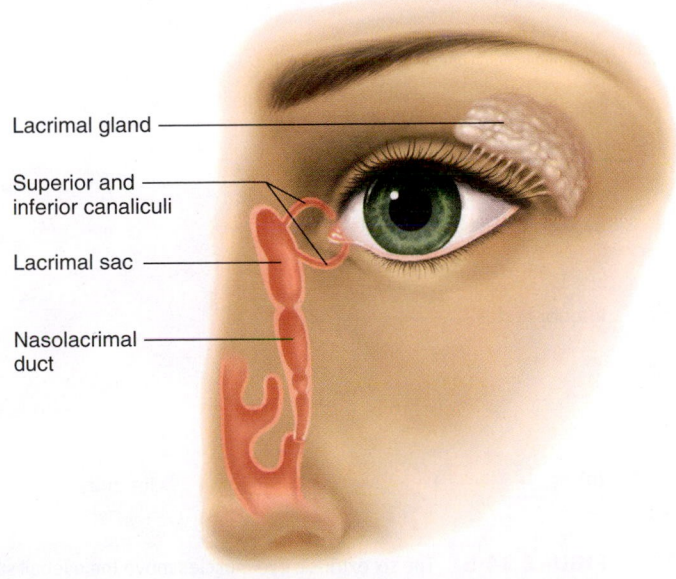

Lacrimal gland

Superior and inferior canaliculi

Lacrimal sac

Nasolacrimal duct

FIGURE 34-4 Lacrimal apparatus.

also contain enzymes that can destroy bacteria and viruses. Tears also have an outer, oily layer that prevents them from evaporating. *Nasolacrimal ducts,* located on the medial aspect of each eyeball, drain tears into the nose. When a person cries, the abundance of tears entering the nose produces the "runny nose" associated with crying.

Extrinsic Eye Muscles Extrinsic eye muscles are skeletal muscles that move the eyeball. Each eyeball has six extrinsic eye muscles attached to it that move the eyeball superiorly, inferiorly, laterally, or medially. (See Figure 34-5.)

▶ Visual Pathways   LO 34.4

The eye works much as a camera does. Light reflected from an object, or produced by one, enters the eye from the outside and passes through the cornea, pupil, lens, and fluids in the eye. The cornea, lens, and fluids help focus the light onto the retina by bending it in a process known as **refraction.** As in a camera, light patterns carry an image of an object. The image is projected upside-down—on film in a camera and on the retina in an eye (see Figure 34-6). The retina converts the light into nerve impulses. These impulses are transmitted along the optic nerve to the brain. This nerve, which consists of about a million fibers, serves as a flexible cable connecting the eyeball to the brain.

Parts of the optic nerve fuse together, then cross at a structure called the *optic chiasm*—an x-shaped structure located at the base of the brain. The visual area in the occipital lobes of the cerebrum is responsible for interpreting vision. Because visual information crosses in the optic chiasm, about half of the visual information detected in each eye is interpreted on

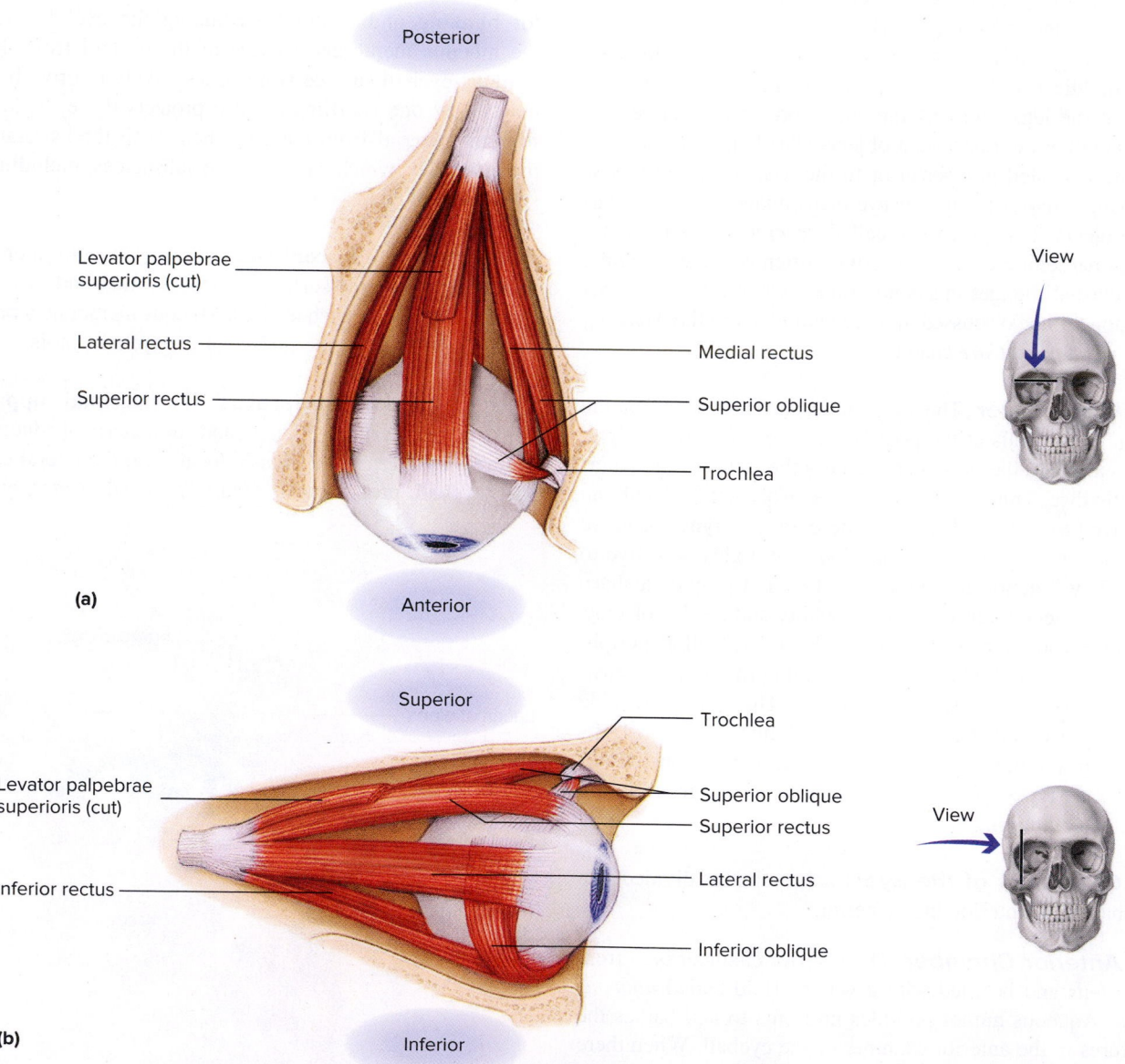

FIGURE 34-5   The six extrinsic eye muscles move the eyeball superiorly, inferiorly, laterally, or medially.

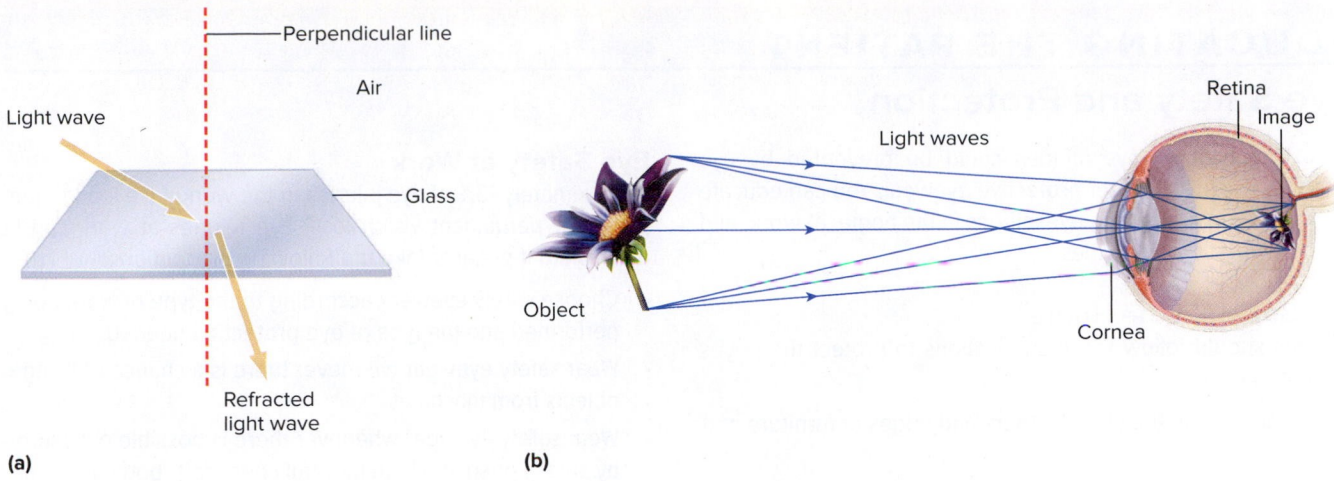

FIGURE 34-6 Visual pathways. (a) Refraction is the process of bending light. (b) The image forms upside-down on the retina.

the opposite side of the brain. So half of what a person sees in the right eye is interpreted in the left side of the brain and vice versa, where it is brought together as one image. The brain interprets these impulses, turns the image right-side up, and "develops" a picture of the object from which the light originally came. See Table 34-1 for a summary of the parts of the eye and their functions.

TABLE 34-1	The Functions of the Parts of the Eye
Structure	**Function**
Aqueous humor	Nourishes and bathes structures in the anterior eye cavity
Vitreous humor	Holds the retina in place; maintains the shape of the eyeball
Sclera	Protects the eye
Cornea	Allows light to enter the eye; bends light as it enters the eye (refraction)
Choroid	Supplies nutrients and provides a blood supply to the eye
Ciliary body	Holds the lens; controls the shape of the lens for focusing
Iris	Controls the amount of light entering the eye
Lens	Focuses light onto the retina (accommodation)
Retina	Contains visual receptors
Rods	Allow vision in dim light; detect black, white, and gray images; detect broad outlines of images
Cones	Allow vision in bright light; detect colors; detect details
Optic nerve	Carries visual information (stimuli) from rods and cones toward the brain

The Aging Eye

With age, a number of changes occur in the structure and function of the eye, including the following:

- The amount of fat tissue diminishes; this loss may cause the eyelids to droop.
- The quality and quantity of tears decrease.
- The conjunctiva becomes thinner and may be drier because of a decrease in tear production.
- The cornea begins to appear yellow, and a ring of fat deposits may appear around it.
- The sclera may develop brown spots.
- Changes in the iris cause the pupil to become smaller, limiting the amount of light entering the eye.
- The lens becomes denser and more rigid; this trend reduces the amount of light that reaches the retina and makes focusing more difficult.
- Yellowing of the lens causes problems in distinguishing colors.
- Changes in the retina may make vision fuzzy.
- The ability of the eye to adapt to changes in light intensities may be reduced; glare can become painful as this ability diminishes.
- Night vision may be impaired.
- Peripheral vision is reduced, limiting the area a person can see and reducing depth perception.
- The vitreous humor breaks down, producing tiny clumps of gel or cellular material that cause floaters—dark spots or lines—that appear in a person's field of vision.
- Rubbing of the vitreous humor on the retina produces flashes of light, or "sparks."

Because of changes that impair vision—such as reductions in the field of vision, in depth perception, and in visual clarity—elderly people may fall more often than younger people.

Eye Safety and Protection

Almost 90% of all eye injuries could be prevented by eye safety practices or proper protective eyewear. You can educate patients about preventing eye injuries in the home, at work, and during recreational activities.

Eye Safety in the Home
Patients should follow these suggestions to protect their eyes in the home:

- Pad or cushion the sharp corners and edges of furniture and home fixtures.
- Make sure adequate lighting and handrails are available on stairs.
- Keep personal use items (like cosmetics and toiletries), kitchen utensils, and desk supplies out of the reach of children.
- Keep toys with sharp edges out of the reach of children. Also, make sure toys intended for older children are kept away from younger children.
- Remove dangerous debris from the lawn before mowing it.
- Wear safely goggles when operating any type of power equipment.
- Keep dangerous solvents, paints, cleaners, fertilizers, and other chemicals out of the reach of children.
- Never mix cleaning agents.

Eye Safety at Work
Approximately 15% of eye injuries in the workplace lead to temporary or permanent vision loss. Eye injuries at work can be diminished if patients take the following precautions:

- Choose safety eyewear according to the type of work being performed and the type of eye protection needed.
- Wear safety eyewear whenever there is a chance of flying objects from machines.
- Wear safety eyewear whenever there is possible exposure—by splash or splatter—to harmful chemicals, body fluids, or radiation.

Eye Safety During Sports and Recreational Activities
Eye injuries that commonly occur while playing a sport include scratched corneas, inflamed irises and retinas, bleeding in the anterior chamber of the eye, traumatic cataracts, and fractures of the eye socket. Wearing sports eye guards or goggles can prevent most sports eye injuries. These guards are recommended for baseball, basketball, soccer, football, rugby, and hockey. Protective goggles are recommended for mountain biking, motocross, and snow skiing. Virtually any type of contact sport requires appropriate eye protection.

PATHOPHYSIOLOGY

LO 34.5

Common Diseases and Disorders of the Eyes

As with all the body's organs, the sense organs are also susceptible to various diseases and disorders. Many eye injuries, however, are preventable. See the *Educating the Patient* feature for general tips about eye safety and protection. The following common diseases and disorders are specific to the eyes. Additional information about diseases and disorders of the eyes is found in the chapter *Assisting with Eye and Ear Care*.

ASTIGMATISM occurs when the lens has an abnormal shape or the cornea is unevenly curved. This abnormality causes blurred images in near or distant vision. Astigmatism may cause vertical or horizontal lines to appear out of focus.

Causes. This condition is considered to be congenital.

Signs and Symptoms. There are no symptoms with this condition other than blurred vision. However, it can be diagnosed during an ophthalmic (eye) exam.

Treatment. Treatment includes corrective lenses or surgery, such as photorefractive keratectomy (PRK) or, more commonly now, laser-assisted in situ keratomileusis (LASIK) to reshape the cornea (see Figure 34-7). This procedure—done on an outpatient basis under local anesthesia—involves reshaping the cornea with a special laser. After LASIK surgery, 70% of patients have normal vision. A very small percentage of patients have postsurgical complications that cause their vision to worsen.

DRY EYE SYNDROME is one of the most common eye problems physicians treat. This syndrome results from a decreased production of the oil within tears, which normally occurs with age.

Causes. Dry eye can be caused by cigarette smoke; air conditioning; eye strain created by long hours at a computer monitor; some medications; contact lenses; hormonal changes associated with menopause; and hot, dry, or windy climates.

Signs and Symptoms. The common eye symptoms include burning, irritation, redness, itching, and excessive tearing.

Treatment. Artificial tears may provide relief to many patients, and drugs like Restasis® have helped patients with this condition make more of their own tears. People with this condition should drink 8 to 10 glasses of water a day and make a conscious effort to blink more frequently and avoid rubbing their eyes. In addition, punctal plugs can be inserted to trap tears on the eyes, which prevents the tears from entering the nasolacrimal duct and being drained.

ECTROPION is characterized by eversion (turning inside-out) of the lower eyelid.

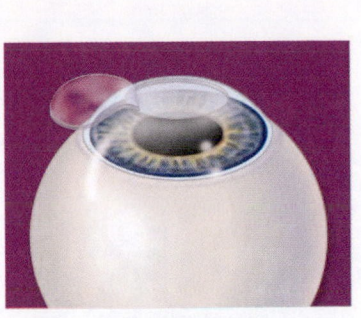
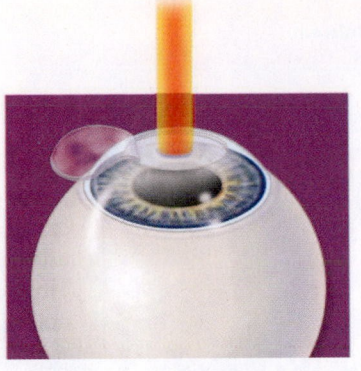
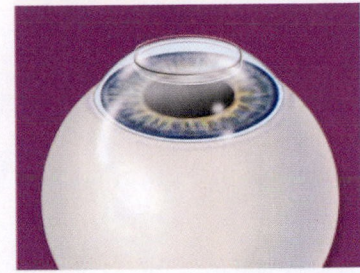

① Cornea is sliced with a sharp knife. Flap of cornea is reflected, and deeper corneal layers are exposed.

② A laser removes microscopic portions of the deeper corneal layers, thereby changing the shape of the cornea.

③ Corneal flap is put back in place, and the edges of the flap start to fuse within 72 hours.

FIGURE 34-7 LASIK laser vision correction procedure.

Causes. Aging and skin relaxation or scar tissue may cause this condition.

Signs and Symptoms. Common signs and symptoms include redness, irritation, and drying of the conjunctiva. Poor tear drainage through the nasolacrimal system may also be present.

Treatment. Surgery to repair the defect may be needed if the condition is bothersome to the patient.

ENTROPION is characterized by an inversion (turning outside-in) of the lower eyelid.

Causes. Aging and scar tissue may cause this condition.

Signs and Symptoms. Signs include irritation of the sclera as the lashes brush against it, which may lead to corneal ulceration or scarring.

Treatment. Surgery is the only treatment option to correct this problem.

NYSTAGMUS is rapid, involuntary eye movements.

Causes. Alcohol and some drug use may cause nystagmus. Inner ear disturbances may also result in involuntary eye movements. Brain lesions and injury (including those that may occur during birth) and cerebrovascular accidents (CVA), or strokes, may also cause nystagmus.

Signs and Symptoms. These include rapid, irregular eye movements that may be horizontal, vertical, or rotary, depending on the underlying cause of the nystagmus.

Treatment. Treatment focuses on the underlying cause of the disorder.

RETINAL DETACHMENT occurs when the layers of the retina separate. It is considered a medical emergency and, if not treated right away, leads to permanent vision loss.

Causes. Retinal detachment is rare; however, it is more common as people age. This disorder is sometimes caused by fluids that seep between layers of the retina; this occurs most commonly in nearsighted people. In diabetics, vitreous body or scar tissue pulls the retina loose. Another cause is eye trauma that causes fluid to collect underneath the layers of the retina.

Signs and Symptoms. Signs and symptoms include light flashes, wavy vision, a sudden loss of vision (particularly of peripheral vision), and a larger amount of floaters.

Treatment. When detected early, a hole in the retina can be "sealed" so that the retina does not completely detach. Sealing the hole is usually accomplished through the use of lasers or a procedure called cryopexy—surgical fixation with cold.

If the retina has already detached, some vision can often be restored with the following procedures.

- Pneumatic retinopexy, which involves injecting a gas bubble into the posterior segment of the eye; the pressure from the gas bubble flattens the retina, and the retina is later fixed in place with a laser
- Scleral buckle, which involves using a silicone band to hold the retina in place
- Replacing the vitreous body with silicone oil to reattach the retina

▶ The Ear and the Senses of Hearing and Equilibrium   LO 34.6

The organ of hearing is the ear. In addition to providing the sense of hearing, the ear aids the body in maintaining balance, or equilibrium. To assist with ear exams and procedures, you need to understand ear anatomy and the hearing process.

Structure of the Ear

The ear is divided into three parts: the external ear, middle ear, and inner ear (see Figure 34-8).

External Ear The external ear is composed of the **auricle,** or pinna, and the **external auditory canal.** The auricle is the flap of skin and cartilage that extends from the side of the head. It collects sound waves. The external auditory canal is

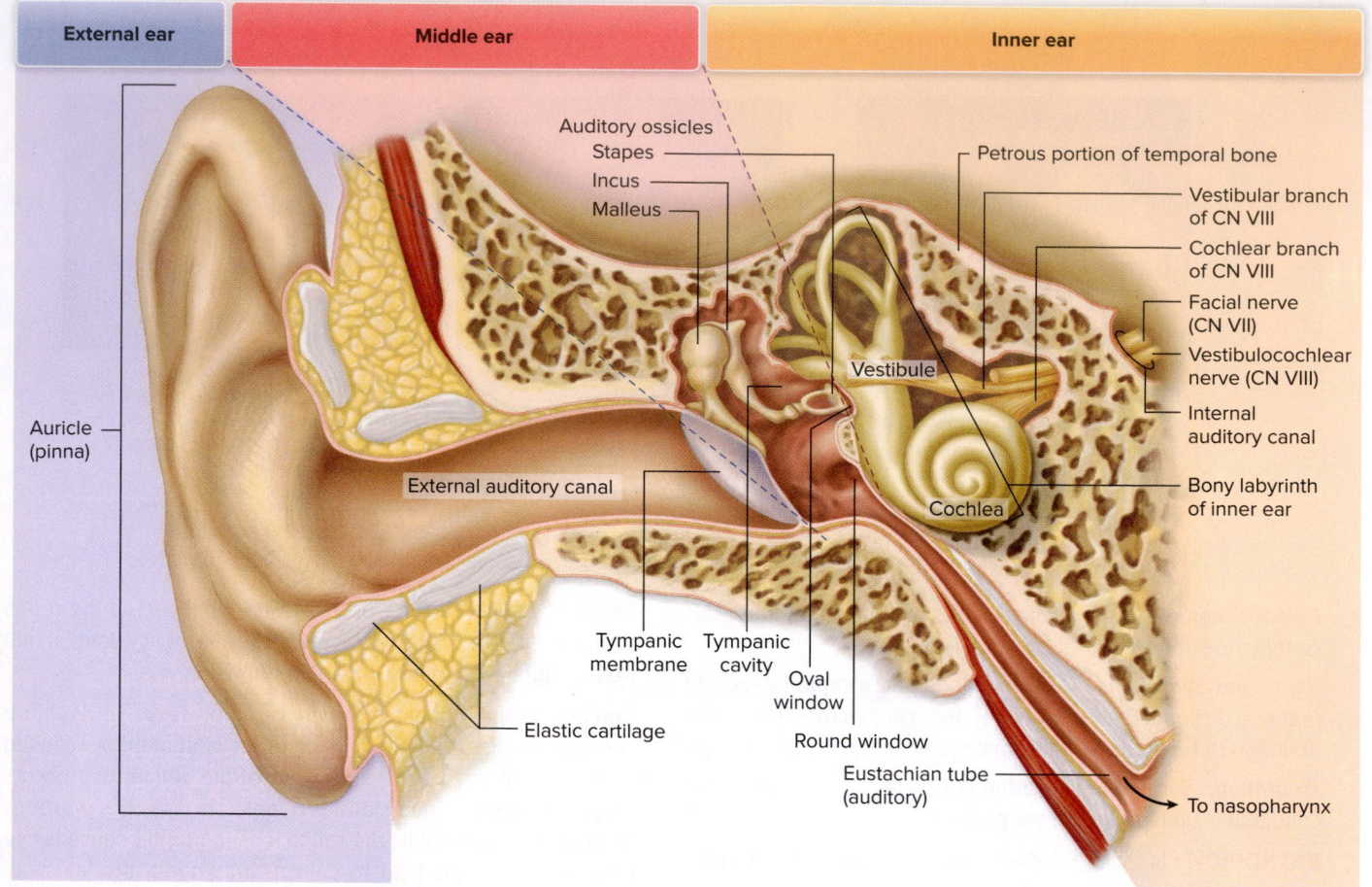

FIGURE 34-8 Anatomical regions of the right ear—the ear is divided into external, middle, and inner regions.

more commonly called the ear canal and is lined with skin that contains hairs and glands that produce **cerumen,** a wax-like substance commonly known as earwax. Cerumen lubricates the ear and protects it by trapping dirt, dust, and other microbes. This canal carries sound waves to the **tympanic membrane,** or eardrum. The tympanic membrane is a fibrous partition located at the inner end of the external auditory canal. It separates the external ear from the middle ear.

Middle Ear The middle ear includes the tympanic membrane, the ossicles, and the oval window. The tympanic membrane is thin and vibrates when sound waves hit it. On the other side of the tympanic membrane are three tiny bones called ear **ossicles**—the *malleus* (hammer), *incus* (anvil), and *stapes* (stirrup). When the tympanic membrane vibrates, it causes the ossicles to vibrate and hit a membrane called the **oval window.** The oval window ends the middle ear and marks the beginning of the inner ear.

The middle ear is connected to the throat by a tube called the **eustachian** (auditory) **tube.** This tube helps maintain equal pressure on both sides of the eardrum, which is important for normal hearing. Because the middle ear is connected to the throat by this tube, any throat infection can easily spread to the ear and vice versa.

Inner Ear The inner ear is a complex system of communicating chambers and tubes known as the **labyrinth.** It is divided into three portions: **semicircular canals,** a **vestibule,** and a **cochlea** (see Figure 34-9). Each ear has three semicircular canals that detect the body's balance. The cochlea is shaped like a snail's shell and contains hearing receptors, including the **organ of Corti,** which is known as the organ of hearing. The vestibule is the area between the semicircular canals and the cochlea. Like the semicircular canals, it functions in equilibrium. When the head moves, the *perilymph* and *endolymph* fluids in the semicircular canals and vestibule move. This activates both equilibrium and hearing receptors. The equilibrium receptors send the information along vestibular nerves to the cerebrum for interpretation. The cerebrum can then advise the body if it needs to make any adjustments to prevent a fall.

When sound waves of different volumes and frequencies activate the hearing receptors in the cochlea, they send their information to auditory nerves. Auditory nerves (vestibulocochlear nerves) deliver the information to the auditory cortex in the cerebrum's temporal lobe. The auditory cortex interprets the information as sounds.

▶ The Hearing Process   LO 34.7

A sound consists of waves of different frequencies that move through the air. The external ear initiates sound conduction when it collects these waves and channels them to the tympanic membrane. Here, the waves make the tympanic membrane vibrate. The vibrations, in turn, are amplified by the middle ear's ossicles. The amplified waves enter the inner ear and the cochlea. These waves cause tiny hairs that line the cochlea to bend. Movements of the hairs trigger nerve impulses. The auditory nerve transmits these impulses to the brain, where they are perceived as sound.

Sound waves are also conducted through the bones of the skull directly to the inner ear—a process called bone conduction. This alternative pathway for sound bypasses the external and middle ears. When you hear your own voice, the sound has reached your inner ear mainly through bone conduction. By comparing a person's ability to sense sounds by bone conduction and through the entire ear, doctors can often identify what part of the ear is causing a hearing problem. For example, if bone conduction is normal, a hearing problem likely involves the middle or external ear rather than the inner ear.

The Aging Ear

As a person grows older, a number of changes occur in the ear. The external ear appears larger because of continued cartilage growth and the loss of skin elasticity. The earlobe gets longer and may have a wrinkled appearance. The glands that produce cerumen become less efficient, producing earwax that is much drier and prone to impaction. The ear canal also becomes narrower.

In the middle ear, changes in the eardrum cause it to shrink and appear dull and gray. The joints between the bones of the middle ear degenerate, so they do not move as freely. In the inner ear, the semicircular canals become less sensitive to changes in position, and this reduced sensitivity affects balance.

Problems with equilibrium make the elderly prone to falls. Some ear disorders, like hearing loss and Ménière's disease, are also more common in older individuals. Additional information about diseases and disorders of the ear are found in the chapter *Assisting with Eye and Ear Care.*

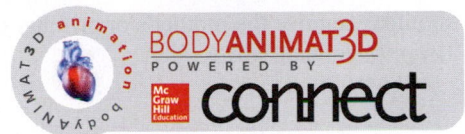

Go to CONNECT to see an animation exercise about *Hearing Loss: Sensorineural.*

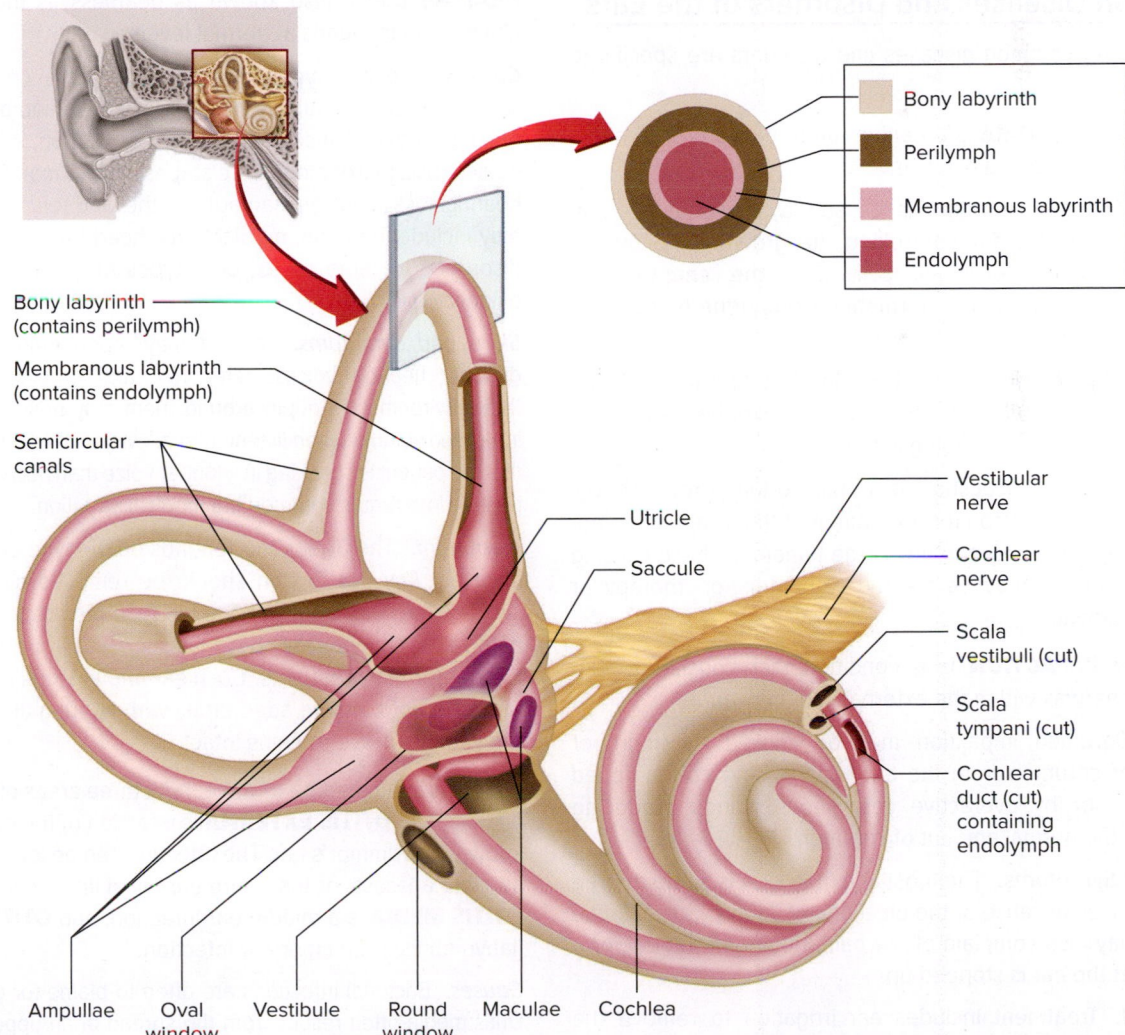

FIGURE 34-9 Right inner ear—the inner ear is composed of a bony labyrinth cavity that houses a fluid-filled, membranous labyrinth. Within the bony labyrinth are the vestibular organs for equilibrium and balance and the cochlea for hearing.

How to Recognize Hearing Problems in Infants

Hearing problems in infants are not easy to recognize. The following general guidelines can be used to teach parents how to identify normal hearing in infants. Any deviations from these guidelines may indicate a hearing loss.

Infants Up to 4 Months Old

- They should be startled by loud noises (barking dog, hand clap, and so on).
- When sleeping in a quiet room, they should wake up at the sound of voices.
- Around the fourth month of age, they should turn their head or move their eyes to follow a sound.
- They should recognize the mother's or primary caregiver's voice better than other voices.

Infants 4 to 8 Months of Age

- They should regularly turn their head or move their eyes to follow sounds.
- Their facial expressions should change at the sound of familiar voices or loud noises.
- They should begin to enjoy certain sounds such as rattles or ringing bells.
- They should begin to babble at people who talk to them.

Babies 8 to 12 Months of Age

- They should turn quickly to the sound of their name.
- They should begin to vary the pitch of the sounds they produce in their babbling.
- They should begin to respond to music.
- They should respond to the instruction "no."

PATHOPHYSIOLOGY

LO 34.8

Common Diseases and Disorders of the Ears

The following common diseases and disorders are specific to the ears.

ACOUSTIC NEUROMA is a benign tumor of the cranial nerve involved in hearing and balance.

Causes. Acoustic neuroma is caused by a malfunction in a gene responsible for controlling the growth of Schwann cells—a type of neuroglial cell. (See the chapter *The Nervous System* for more information.) This gene is found on chromosome 22.

Signs and Symptoms. Gradual hearing loss in one ear is the most common symptom. Patients may also experience balance problems and tinnitus—ringing in the ears.

Treatment. Since acoustic neuromas often grow slowly, the physician may monitor the tumor if the patient is not experiencing severe symptoms. Large tumors or those causing severe symptoms may be treated with radiation therapy or surgical removal.

CERUMEN IMPACTION is a condition that consists of the buildup of earwax within the external auditory canal.

Causes. Cerumen impaction may be caused by improper cleaning of cerumen from the ear canal—using cotton-tipped applicators—or by overactive ceruminous glands producing more than the normal amount of cerumen.

Signs and Symptoms. The most common sign is some degree of hearing loss because of the blockage of sound waves. Some patients may also complain of ear pain, ringing in the ear, or a feeling that the ear is stopped up.

Treatment. Treatment includes ear irrigation to remove the blockage. Severely hardened cerumen may require an earwax softener such as Debrox® to soften and loosen the cerumen before the impaction can be removed.

HEARING LOSS, also known as deafness, is the loss of the ability to hear sounds at normal levels.

Causes. The two types of hearing loss are conductive and sensorineural. Conductive hearing loss is caused by a blockage of sound waves caused by cerumen impaction, a foreign body, otosclerosis (hardening of the stapes), or a tumor. Sensorineural hearing loss involves damage to the auditory nerve. Causes may include infection, medications, head trauma, and vascular disorders. In some cases, both types of hearing loss may be evident.

Signs and Symptoms. Patients may report gradual or sudden difficulty hearing voices, television, and other sounds within their environment. People around them may notice the need for increased volume when listening to television or the radio, or notice that the patient is speaking in a louder voice than necessary. Sudden hearing loss requires immediate medical attention.

Treatment. The treatment depends on the type of hearing loss involved. Any obstruction should be removed by irrigation or surgery if necessary. If hearing loss is a medication side effect, medication changes may be necessary. Hearing aids may be the answer for many patients. Cochlear implants may be an option for those not assisted adequately with hearing aids, as long as the auditory nerve remains intact.

OTITIS is inflammation of the ear. All three areas of the ear may be inflamed. **OTITIS EXTERNA** is infection of the outer ear, also known as swimmer's ear. The infection can be localized, as with a boil or abscess, or the entire ear canal lining can be affected. **OTITIS MEDIA** is a middle ear infection, and **OTITIS INTERNA** (labyrinthitis) is an inner ear infection.

Causes. Bacterial infections are often to blame for otitis externa. Otitis media often results from the spread of an upper respiratory infection from the throat that enters the eustachian tube and infects the middle ear. Labyrinthitis, especially the purulent or infective type, results from a spread of otitis media to the inner ear.

Signs and Symptoms. Pain in the ear with associated hearing loss is the primary symptom. Patients with otitis externa may also report itching and pus in the ear. Purulent (pus-containing) drainage may also occur in some forms of otitis media. Labyrinthitis often causes vertigo and nausea.

Treatment. Antibiotics or antifungals are given to treat the causative agent. Anti-inflammatory or pain medication and fever reducers may also be given to make the patient more comfortable. Antihistamines and anti-nausea medications may also be used to treat otitis interna.

OTOSCLEROSIS is the immobilization of the stapes within the inner ear, which is a common cause of conductive hearing loss.

Causes. Genetics seems to play a role. This disease occurs more frequently in females than in males.

Signs and Symptoms. These include a slow and progressive hearing loss that may be accompanied by tinnitus.

Treatment. Surgical removal of the stapes (stapedectomy) with insertion of a prosthetic stapes may result in at least a partial hearing restoration.

PRESBYCUSIS is hearing loss because of the aging process.

Causes. Factors like prolonged exposure to loud noise, infection, injury, certain medications, and some diseases are thought to be causes of presbycusis. Also, as part of the natural aging process, the auditory system deteriorates, resulting in a loss of hair cells (sensory receptors) in the organ of Corti. Changes in the blood supply to the ear and reduced function of the tympanic membrane or ossicles are also contributing factors.

Signs and Symptoms. Signs and symptoms include gradual, progressive hearing loss, usually of high-frequency sounds first. Typically both ears are affected and the patient has difficulty hearing high-pitched tones as well as normal conversation. Tinnitus may accompany this loss and the patient may become depressed and frustrated at the developing inability to communicate well as a result of the hearing loss.

Treatment. In most cases, hearing aids are prescribed to alleviate some of the hearing loss, although the condition itself is irreversible.

SUMMARY OF LEARNING OUTCOMES

LEARNING OUTCOMES	KEY POINTS
34.1 Describe the anatomy of the nose and the function of each part.	Olfactory receptors—the sense receptors for the sense of smell—are found in the olfactory organ located in the upper part of the nasal cavity.
34.2 Describe the anatomy of the tongue and the function of each part.	Gustatory receptors are found on the taste buds, which are located on the papillae (bumps) of the tongue.
34.3 Describe the anatomy of the eye and the function of each part, including the accessory structures and their functions.	The eye is composed of three layers. The sclera is the outer, protective layer and includes the cornea. The middle, vascular layer is the choroid consisting of the iris, pupil, ciliary body, and lens and is the area of light regulation and focusing. The innermost layer is the retina containing the rods and cones, the optic nerve, and the optic disc. This is where the nerve impulse is picked up and taken to the brain for interpretation. The accessory organs are the orbits and eyebrows, eyelids and eyelashes, conjunctiva, lacrimal apparatus, and extrinsic eye muscles.
34.4 Explain the visual pathway through the eye and to the brain for interpretation.	The cornea, lens, and fluids focus light on the retina. The retina converts the image into nerve impulses, which the optic nerve transmits to the brain for interpretation.
34.5 Describe the causes, signs and symptoms, and treatments of various disorders of the eyes.	There are many common diseases and disorders of the eyes with varied signs, symptoms, and treatments. Some of these include astigmatism, dry eye syndrome, ectropion, entropion, nystagmus, and retinal detachment.

LEARNING OUTCOMES	KEY POINTS
34.6 Describe the anatomy of the ear and the function of each part, and explain the role of the ear in maintaining equilibrium.	There are three parts to the ear. The external ear includes the auricle, or pinna, and the external auditory canal to the tympanic membrane. The middle ear begins at the tympanic membrane and ends at the oval window and includes the ear ossicles. The inner ear is composed of the labyrinth and contains the organ of Corti as well as perilymph and endolymph—the fluids of hearing. The semicircular canals and vestibule in the inner ear function in the body's equilibrium and balance, sending impulses to the vestibular nerves, which take information to the cerebrum for interpretation.
34.7 Explain how sounds travel through the ear and are interpreted in the brain.	The outer ear collects sound waves and channels them to the tympanic membrane, which vibrates. The vibrations are amplified by the ear ossicles and enter the inner ear and cochlea. The movements of the hairs in the cochlea trigger nerve impulses, which the auditory nerve transmits to the brain.
34.8 Describe the causes, signs and symptoms, and treatments of various disorders of the ears.	There are many common diseases and disorders of the ears with varied signs, symptoms, and treatments. Some of these include acoustic neuroma, cerumen impaction, hearing loss, otitis, otitis externa, otitis media, otitis interna, otosclerosis, and presbycusis.

CASE STUDY CRITICAL THINKING

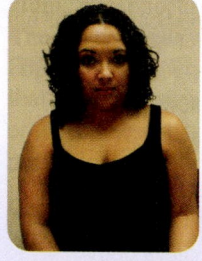

© McGraw-Hill Education

Recall Valarie Ramirez from the beginning of the chapter. Now that you have completed the chapter, answer the following questions regarding her case.

1. Describe the structures of the eye that might be affected by Valarie's motorcycle injury.

2. What can you tell Valarie about protecting her eyes when she rides her motorcycle again?

3. When you enter the examination room, you see Valarie and her boyfriend. You also notice a strong body odor smell and you are not sure where it is coming from. You consider reporting it to the licensed practitioner but after you have been in the room awhile the odor goes away. What, if anything, should you do about this odor? Why do you think the odor went away?

EXAM PREPARATION QUESTIONS

1. (LO 34.1 and LO 34.2) Which of the special senses utilize chemoreceptors?
   a. Smell and hearing
   b. Taste and vision
   c. Smell and taste
   d. Vision and hearing
   e. Smell and vision

2. (LO 34.3) Which of the following is the other name for the corneal-scleral junction?
   a. Optic chiasm
   b. Limbus
   c. Blind spot
   d. Orbicularis oculi
   e. Ciliary body

3. (LO 34.3) The changing of the lens shape is called
   a. Astigmatism
   b. Accommodation
   c. Refraction
   d. Focusing
   e. Ectropion

4. (LO 34.3) The fluid in the anterior eye chamber is
   a. Aqueous humor
   b. Lacrimal humor
   c. Vitreous humor
   d. Orbital humor
   e. Vestibular humor

5. (LO 34.2) Taste buds are found on the
   a. Supporting cells
   b. Papillae
   c. Chemoreceptors
   d. Esophagus
   e. Gingiva

6. (LO 34.3) The mucous membranes that line each eye are known as
   a. Lacrimal glands
   b. Cornea
   c. Conjunctivas
   d. Aqueous tissues
   e. Chonchae

7. (LO 34.6) Which of the following marks the beginning of the inner ear?
   a. Tympanic membrane
   b. Eustachian tube
   c. Stapes
   d. Auditory canal
   e. Oval window

8. (LO 34.6) Another name for the auricle of the ear is the
   a. Exteral auditory canal
   b. Pinna
   c. Malleus
   d. Eustachian tube
   e. Earlobe

9. (LO 34.7) The process by which sound waves bypass the external ear and middle ear is known as
   a. Bone conduction
   b. Tympanic conduction
   c. Sensorineural conduction
   d. Air conduction
   e. Ossicular pathway

10. (LO 34.6) Which of the following structures is involved with equilibrium?
    a. Limbus
    b. Ossicles
    c. Eustachian tube
    d. Organ of Corti
    e. Semicircular canals

M E D I C A L   T E R M I N O L O G Y   P R A C T I C E

Analyze the following medical terms, presented throughout the chapter. Using a medical dictionary (or Appendix I) place a / mark between each word part. Define each word part and then define the whole word.

EXAMPLE: **ophthalmo/scope** = ophthalmo means "eye" + scope means "instrument used to examine"
OPHTHALMOSCOPE means "instrument used to examine the eye."

1. amblyopia
2. auditory
3. conjunctivitis
4. ectropion
5. endolymph

6. entropion
7. glaucoma
8. ophthalmologist
9. optician
10. optometrist

11. otosclerosis
12. perilymph
13. semicircular
14. sensorineural
15. tympanic

Infection Control Practices

CASE STUDY

PATIENT INFORMATION

Patient Name	DOB	Allergies
Ken Washington	12/1/19XX	Sulfa

Attending	MRN	Other Information
Paul F. Buckwalter, MD	891-12-743	U/A with microscopic exam and culture ordered

Ken Washington, a 61-year-old male patient, arrived today for a follow-up visit from a recent hospitalization for a stroke. Up until his hospitalization, he had hypertension but no other major health issues. He now has weakness in his left arm and leg and his speech is difficult to understand. His wife tells you that she has noticed some blood in the toilet after he urinates. She also tells you that he has had some pain when he urinates and often only urinates a small amount. While he was in the hospital, Ken had a urinary catheter in place for 6 days.

Keep Ken in mind as you study this chapter. There will be questions at the end of the chapter based on the case study. The information in the chapter will help you answer these questions.

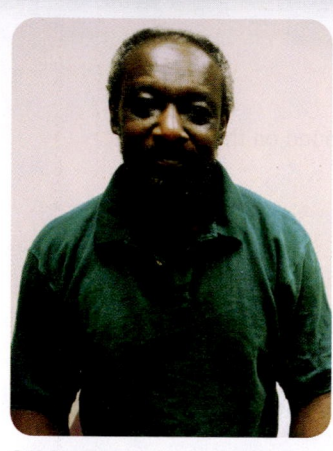

© McGraw-Hill Education

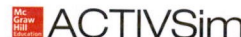
ACTIVSim

LEARNING OUTCOMES

After completing Chapter 35, you will be able to:

35.1 Identify various healthcare-associated infections specific to the ambulatory care setting.

35.2 Describe methods of infection control, including those for preventing healthcare-associated infections.

35.3 Describe various methods of injection safety, including safety-engineered devices and work practice controls.

35.4 Summarize proper respiratory hygiene/cough etiquette practices utilized in the medical office.

35.5 Describe infection control procedures related to medical equipment.

35.6 Describe surgical site infections (SSIs) and ways to prevent them.

35.7 Discuss the procedures used in a medical office to sterilize surgical instruments and equipment.

35.8 Describe Centers for Disease Control and Prevention (CDC) requirements for reporting cases of infectious disease.

KEY TERMS

- add-on safety feature
- autoclave
- biological indicator
- catheter-associated urinary tract infection (CAUTI)
- central line
- central line–associated bloodstream infections (CLABSI)
- invasive procedure
- medical asepsis
- personal protective equipment (PPE)
- re-sheathing scalpel
- respiratory hygiene/cough etiquette
- retractable needle
- self-blunting/blunt tip blood drawing needle
- self-sheathing needle
- sterilization indicator
- surgical asepsis
- surgical site infection (SSI)

CAAHEP

III.C.1 List major types of infectious agents

III.C.3 Define the following as practiced within an ambulatory care setting:
(a) medical asepsis
(b) surgical asepsis

III.C.4 Identify methods of controlling the growth of microorganisms

III.C.5 Define the principles of standard precautions

III.C.6 Define personal protective equipment (PPE) for:
(a) all body fluids, secretions, and excretions
(b) blood
(c) non-intact skin
(d) mucous membranes

III.C.7 Identify Centers for Disease Control (CDC) regulations that impact healthcare practices

III.P.1 Participate in bloodborne pathogen training

III.P.2 Select appropriate barrier/personal protective equipment (PPE)

III.P.4 Prepare items for autoclaving

III.P.5 Perform sterilization procedures

III.P.10 Demonstrate proper disposal of biohazardous material
(a) sharps

III.A.1 Recognize the implications for failure to comply with Centers for Disease Control (CDC) regulations in healthcare settings

ABHES

9. Clinical Procedures
a. Practice standard precautions and perform disinfection/sterilization techniques
e. Perform specialty procedures including but not limited to minor surgery, cardiac, respiratory, OB-GYN, neurological, gastroenterology

10. Medical Laboratory Procedures
c. Dispose of biohazardous materials

▶ Introduction

As a medical assistant, you have a responsibility to protect the patient from exposure to infectious agents found in the medical environment. Following certain guidelines set forth by the Centers for Disease Control and Prevention (CDC) will help you meet this responsibility. These guidelines were introduced in the *Infection Control Fundamentals* chapter. In this chapter you will learn about the most common healthcare-associated infections (HAI) found in outpatient settings. A healthcare-associated infection is one acquired by a patient in a healthcare setting, sometimes called a nosocomial infection. The CDC uses the more current term *healthcare-associated infection*.

It is essential that you apply CDC guidelines and OSHA regulations in order to protect the patient, your coworkers, and yourself from exposure to infectious microorganisms. This requires strict adherence to standard precautions (including hand hygiene, which is covered in detail in the *Infection Control Fundamentals* chapter), proper selection and use of PPE, injection safety, and respiratory hygiene/cough etiquette. Also covered in this chapter are infection control practices related to medical equipment, sterilization procedures for surgical equipment, and reporting guidelines for infectious disease.

▶ Healthcare-Associated Infections LO 35.1

Increasingly, people are having surgery and complex diagnostic and treatment procedures in outpatient facilities instead of hospitals. This puts them at risk for infection caused by numerous pathogens found in the healthcare environment. No matter the level of care, all facilities must make infection control their top priority. As a medical assistant, you should be familiar with the most common types of healthcare-associated infections that occur in the outpatient setting, the risk factors associated with them, and ways to prevent them.

Risk Factors for Healthcare-Associated Infections

Patients can acquire healthcare-associated infections at hospitals, ambulatory surgical centers, physicians' offices, dialysis centers, and long-term healthcare facilities. Several common risk factors are associated with increased incidence of HAI in both outpatient and inpatient facilities:

- Use of catheters and other indwelling (fixed within the body for a period of time) devices
- Surgical procedures

- Healthcare environment contamination
- Communicable disease transmission (for example, influenza) between patients and healthcare workers
- Improper antibiotic use
- Immunocompromised patients

Common Healthcare-Associated Infections in Outpatient Settings

As you learned in the *Infection Control Fundamentals* chapter, touching is the most common means of transmission of infectious agents. As a medical assistant, your duties will include activities that require you to touch patients. If standard precautions are not followed during procedures that require touching, such as obtaining vital signs, changing a dressing, and removing sutures, you and the patient are at risk for infection. HAI are also associated with the devices used during medical procedures and testing, surgical site infections, and improper use of needles, syringes, and blood collection devices. You should use the utmost care when performing any patient procedure or test, no matter how small the risk.

Methicillin-Resistant *Staphylococcus aureus*

Methicillin-resistant *Staphylococcus aureus* (MRSA) is an infection caused by a specific type of staph bacteria. These bacteria have become resistant to most of the antibiotics used to treat the infection. For this reason, MRSA infections are difficult to treat and can have devastating consequences. Skin infections, the most common type of infection caused by MRSA, can begin as small bumps or pimples and quickly develop into a large abscess (Figure 35-1). Additionally, MRSA infections can occur in the bloodstream, lungs, heart, bones, or joints. Anyone who has an **invasive procedure** (any procedure that requires entry into a body cavity or cutting into skin or mucous membranes) is at risk for MRSA infection.

The key to stopping the transmission of MRSA in the healthcare setting is proper hand hygiene and contact precautions (discussed in the *Infection Control Fundamentals* chapter). When assisting a patient with a known or suspected MRSA infection, put on gloves and a gown prior to entering the exam room. Once you are finished assisting with the patient care, remove your gloves and gown (in that order) before leaving the room. Perform proper hand hygiene immediately after removing your PPE.

***Clostridium difficile* Infection** *Clostridium difficile,* also known as C. diff, is a type of bacterium that causes diarrhea. It is of great concern in the elderly but can affect anyone taking antibiotics for prolonged periods of time and receiving medical care. It is transmitted by the fecal/oral route (touching a surface or patient contaminated with feces and then touching the mouth or mucous membranes). Symptoms of C. diff include watery diarrhea, fever, loss of appetite, nausea, and abdominal pain. Healthcare workers can transmit C. diff to patients by touching if proper hand hygiene is not followed. Since C. diff is found in feces, any surface or device contaminated with feces is a potential source of infection. This includes toilets, sinks, and rectal thermometers. For this reason, proper environmental cleaning in the healthcare facility is essential. Bathrooms and surfaces that may be contaminated with C. diff must be thoroughly decontaminated. You should wear gloves when assisting with a patient with known

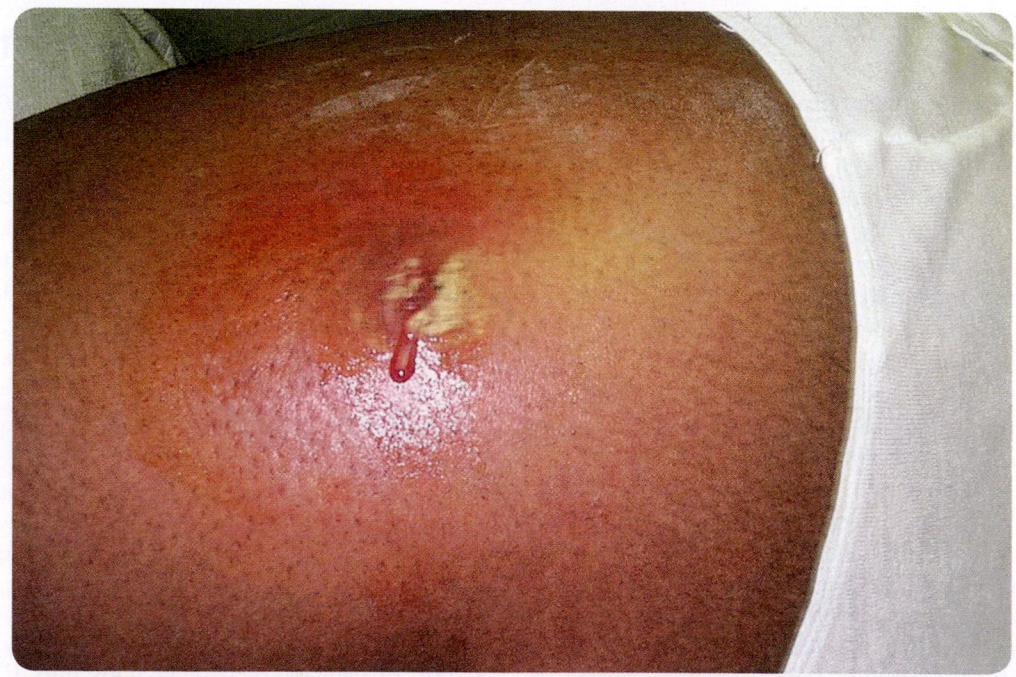

FIGURE 35-1 A wound infected with MRSA is difficult to treat and can lead to tissue loss and sepsis.
CDC

or suspected C. diff infection or when cleaning and disinfecting the exam room and equipment. Alcohol does not kill C. diff; therefore, the CDC recommends handwashing with soap and water after caring for a patient with C. diff. If C. diff is diagnosed or suspected, alcohol hand disinfectants are not recommended. Surfaces and equipment that are likely to be contaminated should be cleaned and disinfected. A solution of 1:10 bleach or an EPA-approved disinfectant with sporicidal (able to kill spores) properties is recommended. (See the *Examination and Treatment Areas* chapter for more information about mixing a 1:10 bleach solution.)

Central Line–Associated Bloodstream Infections

Central line–associated bloodstream infections (CLABSI) are caused by the entry of infectious microorganisms into the bloodstream by way of a **central line.** A central line is a catheter placed in a large vein, usually in the neck, chest, or groin, used to give fluids or medications. A central line differs from a normal intravenous (IV) catheter in several ways. IVs are usually placed for short amounts of time and are located in surface veins, whereas central lines are generally left in place for longer periods of time (weeks or months) and are placed in deep veins that are close to the heart. Though central lines are most often used in intensive care settings, they are also seen in patients receiving outpatient treatments such as chemotherapy.

Healthcare practitioners must follow strict infection control practices when inserting, checking, or changing a bandage of a central line:

- Following hand hygiene procedures
- Performing appropriate skin antisepsis at the site of insertion
- Allowing the skin prep agent to dry thoroughly before inserting the catheter
- Wearing gloves, gown, cap, and mask when inserting the catheter
- Using a large drape to cover the site during the procedure
- Washing hands before and after checking the central line

The CDC recommends removing the central line as soon as it is no longer needed.

As a medical assistant, you should instruct patients with central lines to contact the office immediately if

- The dressing covering the central line comes off or becomes wet or dirty.
- The site around the central line becomes red, hot, or sore.
- They have a fever or chills.

Additionally, you should instruct patients to

- Not touch the catheter insertion site.
- Avoid touching the tubing as much as possible.
- Not let visiting family and friends touch the tubing or site.
- Ask visiting family and friends to wash their hands when they arrive and before they leave.
- Tell the healthcare practitioner if they have concerns about the central line or the infection control practices of the healthcare personnel caring for them.

Catheter-Associated Urinary Tract Infections

Anyone who uses urinary catheters on a long-term basis is at risk for **catheter-associated urinary tract infections (CAUTI).** Bacteria can enter the urinary tract by way of the catheter. The longer a catheter is in place, the more chance a patient has of contracting a CAUTI. For this reason, the CDC recommends that catheters be used for the least possible amount of time and only when necessary and no alternative is available. Catheters must be placed only by trained individuals using aseptic techniques. As a medical assistant, you can help patients with indwelling catheters to avoid CAUTI by teaching them to take the following precautions:

- Wash hands thoroughly with soap and water before and after touching the catheter.
- Ensure that the urine collection bag is always below the level of the bladder.
- Do not pull on the tubing.
- Do not kink or twist the tubing.

▶ Infection Control Methods   LO 35.2

As you learned in the previous section, there are numerous healthcare-associated infections that patients can be exposed to. The best way to keep patients from being infected is to consistently apply infection control methods. As a medical assistant, you must have a thorough knowledge of the two types of asepsis:

- **Medical asepsis,** or clean technique, is based on maintaining cleanliness to prevent the spread of microorganisms and to ensure that there are as few microorganisms in the medical environment as possible. The goal of medical asepsis is to reduce/control microorganisms after they leave the body.
- **Surgical asepsis,** or sterile technique, depends on a completely sterile environment that eliminates all microorganisms. The goal of surgical asepsis is to keep organisms from entering the body. (More information about surgical asepsis can be found later in this chapter and in the *Assisting with Minor Surgery* chapter.)

Medical asepsis and surgical asepsis are required by law. Each individual who works in a medical setting must recognize the importance of asepsis and strictly adhere to aseptic procedures in daily routines.

Medical Asepsis

Because the medical office can be a host to many pathogens, strict, controlled asepsis is crucial. All employees in the medical office must observe and practice the principles of asepsis to ensure a safe environment for patients and staff.

You can promote asepsis through vigilant cleanliness. Every day before patients arrive, you must inspect the office for any surfaces or objects that may be dirty or contaminated. Keeping the office clean reduces the number of microorganisms on surfaces.

Transmission from Healthcare Workers

There may be times when a healthcare worker has a serious infection that could be transmitted to a patient. OSHA has special recommendations for workers who perform procedures that could result in a patient's exposure to disease. Although the risk of a healthcare worker's transmitting an infection to a patient is small if OSHA standards are followed, these additional precautions are advised for high-risk procedures. High-risk procedures include the following:

- Those that are thought to have caused the transmission of infection from a medical worker to a patient in the past
- Those that may carry a high risk of infection, such as oral, obstetric, and gynecologic procedures
- Those that involve needles, especially if a needle is in a body cavity or a body space that is difficult to see and the healthcare worker's fingers are nearby (if the worker's skin is cut, the patient could be exposed to the worker's blood)

Workers who perform high-risk procedures should know their HIV and HBV status. HBV vaccination is strongly recommended. Also, workers who have skin conditions characterized by sores that secrete fluid should forgo direct patient care and the handling of equipment used for exposure-prone procedures until their condition has healed.

HIV or HBV infection should not necessarily keep an individual from practicing as a healthcare worker, but some special measures may need to be taken. A member of the medical staff who is infected with HIV or HBV should not perform procedures that might result in exposure for the patient without the advice of an expert review panel. This panel could include the healthcare worker's own physician, someone with expert knowledge about the transmission of infectious disease, a medical professional with expert knowledge about the procedures in question, public health officials, and a member of the infection control committee of the institution, if applicable.

The panel advises the worker on whether procedures may be performed. The advice includes requiring the worker to inform potential patients of the infection before the procedure. Each medical facility has policies in place outlining if and how patients will be notified of a healthcare professional's HIV or HBV status. The notification may be in writing from the panel, or the healthcare worker may speak directly to the patient. It is the healthcare worker's ethical duty to protect a patient from known exposure to bloodborne pathogens. However, the panel also must protect the healthcare worker's confidentiality if possible.

Although great controversy has surrounded the subject of required testing of all healthcare workers for HIV or HBV, no recommendations are in place for such testing. The risk of infection transmission from worker to patient is not considered great enough to justify the extensive resources that mandatory testing would require.

Office Procedures

Other physical aspects of the medical office that contribute to asepsis include

- A reception room that has designated waiting areas for well and sick people. If there is not enough space, sick patients

should be led immediately to an examination room. You may need to explain this policy to well people who have been waiting so that no one thinks other patients are getting preferential treatment.
- An office that is cleaned daily.
- An office that is well lit and ventilated, has no drafts, and has a temperature of approximately 72°F.
- Furniture that is kept in good repair and is replaced when necessary.
- A strict "no eating or drinking" policy in the lab, clinical, and other patient areas.
- Trash that is emptied as necessary, at least once daily.
- An insect-free environment.
- A sign stating that any safety or health hazard should be reported to the receptionist.
- A sign asking that patients use tissues for coughs or sneezes, put all waste in the trash can, and tell the receptionist if they are nauseated or have to use the restroom. (Ideally, the reception area should be equipped with a restroom for emergencies.) See Figure 35-2.

Asepsis During Medical Assistant Procedures

Many of the procedures you perform require aseptic techniques to prevent cross-contamination from one place to another. For instance, when opening a sterile container, you should rest its lid face-up instead of facedown. Placing it facedown contaminates the inside of the lid by picking up materials on the surface of the counter such as dust, dirt, blood, or body fluids, making it unsuitable to be put back on the sterile container. When administering tablets or capsules, you should pour them into the bottle cap or a cup rather than into your hand to prevent the transfer of microorganisms from your hand onto the medication. To prevent cross-contamination, you also must follow guidelines about the types of protective gear to wear during a procedure. (Personal protective equipment is discussed later in this chapter.)

Other Aseptic Precautions

You need to make certain precautions part of your daily routine. For example, take these safeguards:

- Avoid leaning against sinks, supplies, or equipment.
- Avoid touching your face or mouth.
- Use tissues when you cough or sneeze, and always wash your hands afterward.
- Whenever possible, avoid working directly with patients when you have a cold.
- Wear gloves and a mask if you have a cold and must work with patients.
- Stay home if you have a fever, and remain there until you have maintained a normal temperature for 24 hours.

Personal Protective Equipment

Employers are required by law to supply **personal protective equipment (PPE)** at no charge to their employees. PPE is any type of protective gear worn to guard against physical

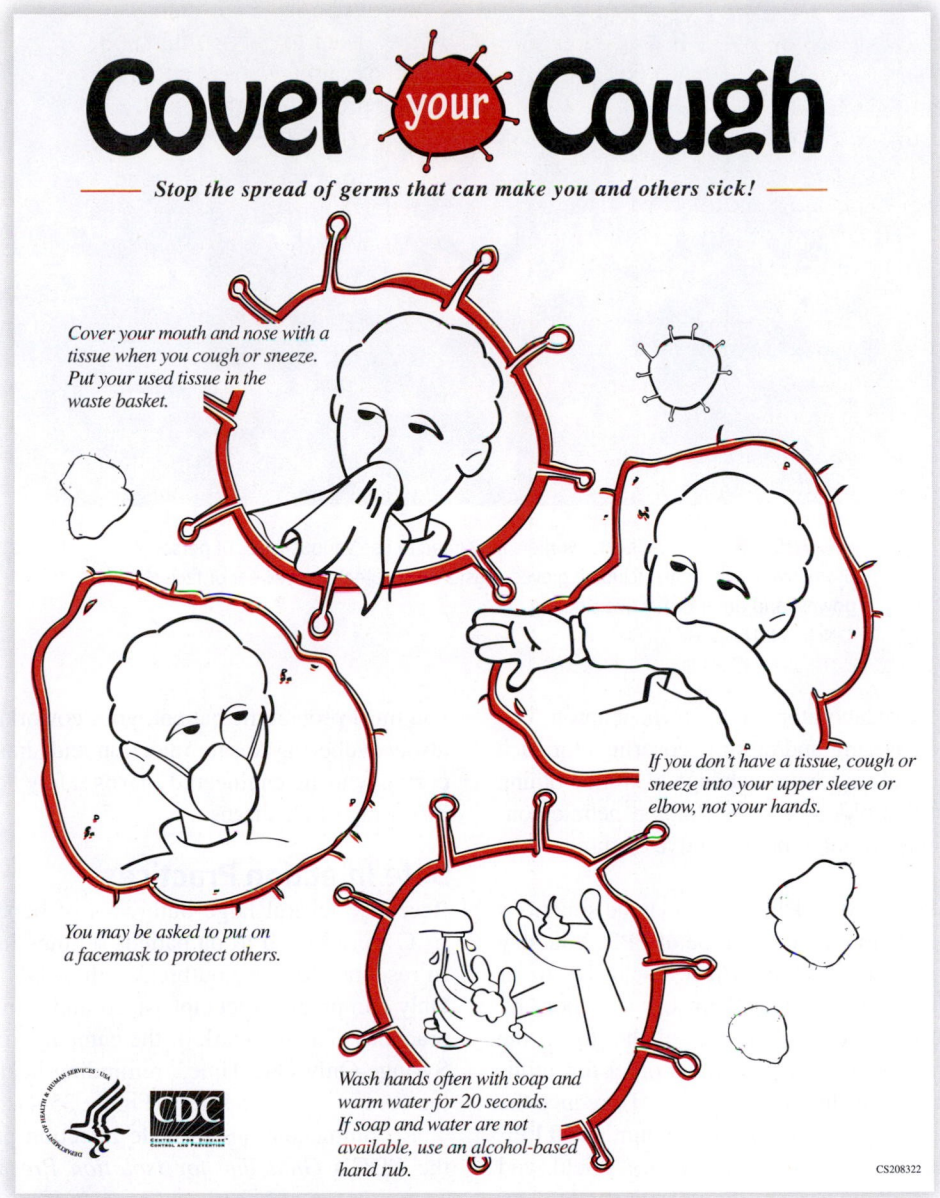

FIGURE 35-2 Posting notices like this CDC poster in patient reception areas reminds patients to use tissues and cover their coughs to reduce the spread of infectious agents.

hazards. Healthcare workers require many kinds of personal protective equipment to do their jobs, including gloves, masks and protective eyewear or face shields, and protective clothing (Figure 35-3). During each procedure, keep in mind that the greater your chances of exposure to blood or other body fluids, the more pieces of PPE you will need to wear.

Gloves You must wear gloves for all procedures that involve exposure to blood, other body fluids, or broken skin. Several kinds of gloves for different situations are

- Disposable gloves—worn once and discarded. They cannot be used if they are torn, punctured, or otherwise damaged. Both examination and sterile gloves are disposable.
- Examination gloves—worn during procedures that do not require a sterile environment.

- Sterile gloves—used for sterile procedures such as minor surgery or urinary catheterization.
- Utility gloves—used when cleaning up. They are stronger than disposable gloves and may be decontaminated and reused if they show no signs of deterioration (including discoloration) after use.

Masks and Protective Eyewear or Face Shields
You must wear appropriate masks and protective eyewear or face shields for procedures in which your eyes, nose, and mouth may be exposed. These procedures are ones that have a potential for spraying or splashing blood, such as surgery or dental procedures.

Protective Clothing If you are likely to have blood or body fluids sprayed or splashed on your clothing during a procedure,

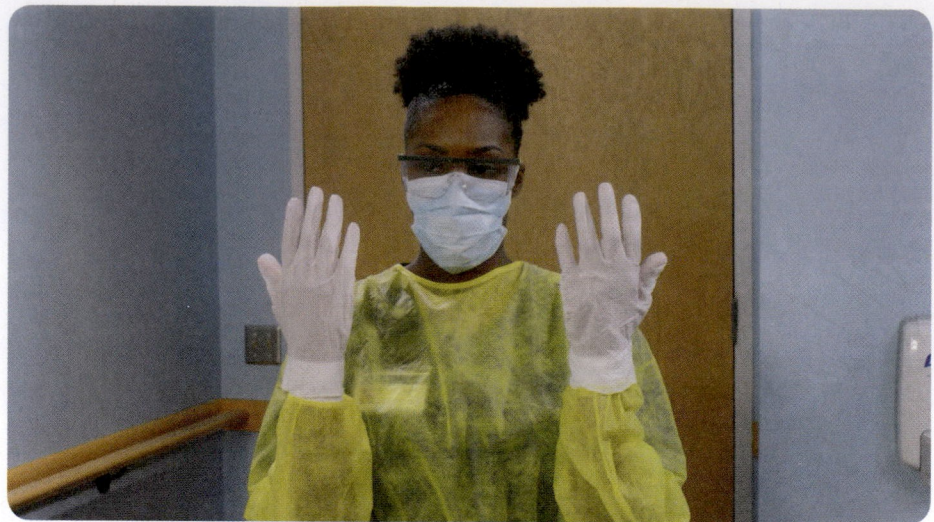

FIGURE 35-3 Healthcare workers may need to use various types of personal protective equipment, including gloves, masks and protective eyewear or face shields, gowns, and other protective clothing.
© McGraw-Hill Education

you must wear a protective laboratory coat, gown, or apron. You also may wear a hair covering and/or shoe coverings for such procedures. You should always have a change of work clothing available in the event that blood or body fluids penetrate your regular clothes around or through the protective clothing.

Use of Multiple Types of PPE There may be situations that require you to wear more than one type of PPE. You may have to wear gloves, a gown, and a mask/face shield. The order in which you put these on and take them off is important. Since the gloves must go over the sleeves of the gown, the gown must go on first. The proper placement order for multiple PPE is gown, mask/face shield, and gloves. To reduce the possibility of cross-contamination, remove contaminated PPE in the opposite order; that is, gloves, mask/face shield, and gown. Procedure 35-1 demonstrates the correct method for removing contaminated gloves, and Procedure 35-2 demonstrates the proper method for removing a contaminated gown.

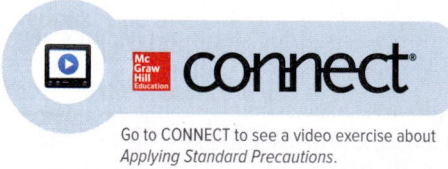

Go to CONNECT to see a video exercise about *Applying Standard Precautions.*

▶ Safe Injection Practices and Sharps Safety

LO 35.3

According to the World Health Organization (WHO), a safe injection does not cause injury to the patient, expose the provider to an avoidable risk, or create dangerous environmental/community waste. As a medical assistant, you may perform tasks, such as giving an injection, that require you to use needles or other sharp devices. During the course of these tasks,

you must protect the patient, your coworkers, and yourself by always adhering to safe injection and sharps safety practices, correctly using engineered sharps safety devices, and properly disposing of all sharps.

Safe Injection Practices

Recently, several large outbreaks of hepatitis B and hepatitis C were linked to outpatient settings in the United States. In response to these outbreaks, the CDC began the One and Only campaign to reemphasized and reinforce safe injection practices. The hallmark of the campaign is "One Needle One Syringe Only One Time," reminding healthcare providers of the core of injection safety (Figure 35-4).

Recommendations for safe injection practices are part of the CDC's *Guideline for Isolation Precautions: Preventing Transmission of Infectious Agents in Healthcare Settings 2007* and include the following:

- Use aseptic technique to avoid contamination of sterile injection equipment.
- Clean the top of medication vials with 70% isopropyl alcohol before withdrawing medications.
- Do not administer medications from a syringe to multiple patients.
- Use single-dose vials for parenteral medications whenever possible.
- Do not administer medications from single-dose vials or ampules to multiple patients or combine leftover contents for later use.
- If multi-dose vials must be used, both the needle or cannula and syringe used to access the multi-dose vial must be sterile.
- Do not keep multi-dose vials in the immediate patient treatment area and store in accordance with the manufacturer's recommendations; discard if sterility is compromised or questionable.

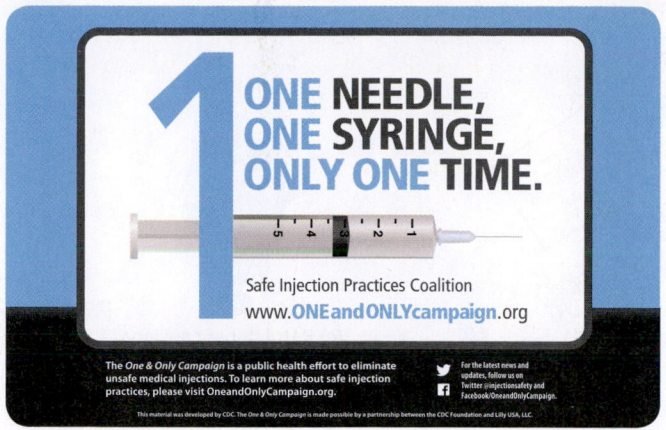

FIGURE 35-4 Posting notices like this CDC One and Only poster reminds healthcare providers to follow safe injection practices.

Protecting Against Needlestick Injuries

OSHA estimates that there are approximately 800,000 needlestick injuries each year and 2% of these are most likely contaminated with human immunodeficiency virus (HIV). Needlestick injuries are completely preventable if you follow OSHA and CDC guidelines. In order to protect yourself from exposure to bloodborne pathogens when handling contaminated sharps, there are certain work practice controls that you should always follow:

- Do not recap needles unless there is no alternative. If no alternative exists, use a one-handed "scoop" technique.
- Do not bend or break needles.
- Use engineered safety devices whenever possible.
- Engage safety devices on needles and scalpels immediately after use.
- Dispose of sharps promptly using approved sharps containers.
- Have sharps containers easily accessible and as close as is feasible for patient safety.
- Use only OSHA-approved sharps containers.
- Do not overfill sharps containers.
- Close sharps containers before removing for disposal so that the contents do not spill.
- Never try to open a sharps container.

If you treat any needle or sharp device as if it were contaminated with a bloodborne pathogen, you have a greater chance of staying safe in the medical office.

Safety-Engineered Devices As you learned in the *Infection Control Fundamentals* chapter, work practice and engineering controls are the key to any needlestick safety program. There are a variety of safety-engineered devices (devices specifically engineered to reduce the incidence of needlesticks) available, including self-sheathing, retractable and self-blunting needles, re-sheathing scalpels, needleless devices, and needles with hinged safety features. According to OSHA, healthcare employers are required to evaluate new safety-engineered devices on a yearly basis and implement the use of devices that reasonably reduce the risk of needlestick injuries. Employers must also solicit input from employees using the devices. As a medical assistant, you may be asked to evaluate and provide input about safety-engineered devices. It is important that you familiarize yourself with the various types and categories of safety-engineered devices.

Self-Sheathing Needles **Self-sheathing needles** have a sheath over the barrel of the syringe. After injecting the patient, the user slides the sheath forward over the needle and locks it into place. The sheath completely covers the needle and, once locked, cannot be slid back over the barrel (Figure 35-5a). The disadvantage of this type of safety device is that it requires two hands to activate.

Retractable Needles and Capillary Puncture Devices Syringes with **retractable needles** such as the BD Integra™ have a needle that retracts inside the barrel of the syringe after it is activated. Once the medication is injected, the plunger is pushed again and the needle withdraws inside the syringe (Figure 35-5b). Capillary puncture devices are single-use devices. The lancet retracts into the device after use, keeping it away from the user (Figure 35-5c).

Self-Blunting Needles **Self-blunting,** or **blunt tip, blood drawing needles** have a blunt tip that slides forward through the needle past the sharp point. This puts the sharp point of the needle below the blunt tip, removing the danger of a needlestick injury. Once the tube is filled with blood, the device can be activated while still in the patient's vein and then removed (Figure 35-5d). Blunt tip devices are available for blood collection systems and winged steel needles.

Re-sheathing Scalpels **Re-sheathing scalpels** are single-use, disposable devices. After use, the healthcare practitioner slides a sheath over the blade, locking it in place. This is done using one hand, keeping the hands clearly away from the blade. Once the sheath is activated, the blade is safely out of the way and the blade is discarded in a sharps container (Figure 35-5e).

Needles with Add-On Safety Devices Injection, phlebotomy, and winged steel needles are available with **add-on safety features.** The device is either a hinged or sliding sheath attached to the needle. Activating the device is done with one hand by either moving the hinged sheath into place or sliding the sheath up and over the needle tip. This keeps the user's hands behind the needle (Figure 35-5f).

▶ Respiratory Hygiene/Cough Etiquette Practices   LO 35.4

As you learned in the *Infection Control Fundamentals* chapter, many infectious diseases can be transmitted through respiratory droplets. Influenza, measles, whooping cough, and meningitis are all transmitted through respiratory droplets. A sneeze or a cough can send virus-filled droplets into the air and onto surfaces several feet away, putting anyone in

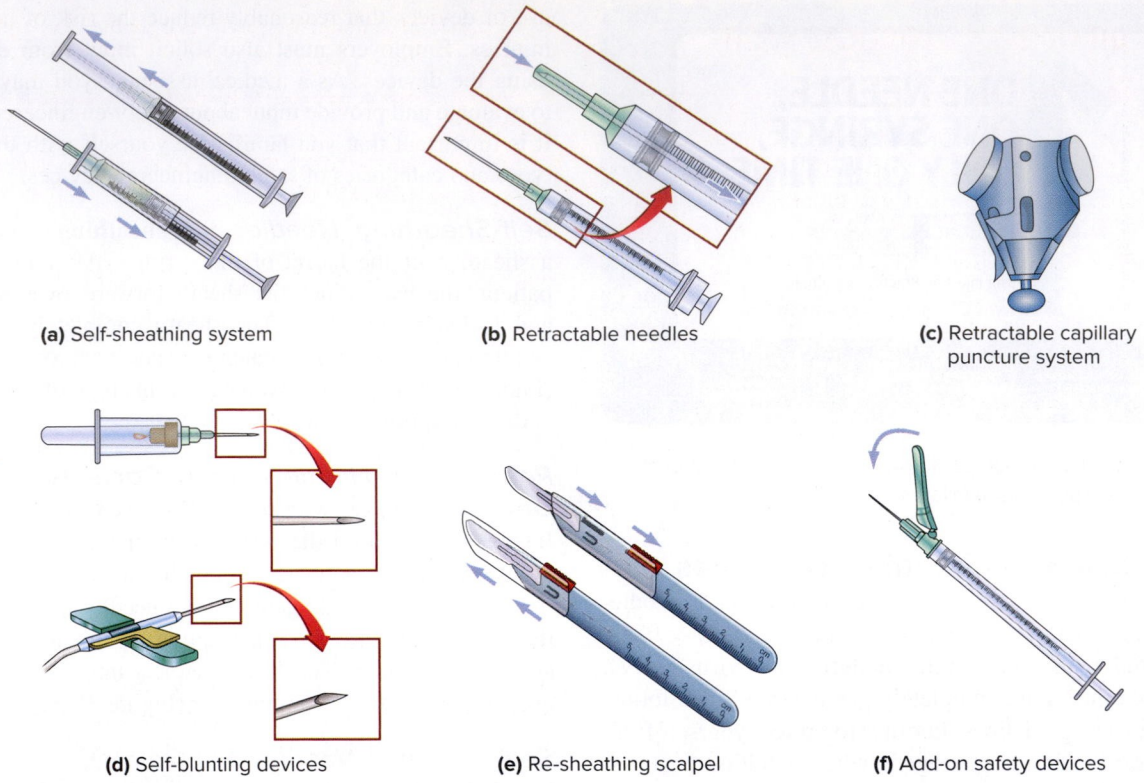

(a) Self-sheathing system

(b) Retractable needles

(c) Retractable capillary puncture system

(d) Self-blunting devices

(e) Re-sheathing scalpel

(f) Add-on safety devices

FIGURE 35-5 These are some of the safety-engineered devices available for use in healthcare settings.

the area at risk for exposure. Anyone who coughs or sneezes into her hand and then touches surfaces such as doorknobs, light switches, pens, papers, and exam tables is spreading viruses throughout the environment. As a medical assistant, you will need to take measures to protect patients, coworkers, and yourself from exposure to infectious agents transmitted by droplets. **Respiratory hygiene/cough etiquette** practices are simple and effective, commonsense approaches to defending yourself and others against infectious agents spread by respiratory droplets.

Using Reminders, Alerts, and Education to Stop the Spread of Respiratory Infection

Patients, their family members, and office staff all need to be reminded what they should do in case they are ill with a fever, cough, and sneezing. As mentioned earlier, posters should be displayed at the front door of the medical office reminding patients and their families to let the staff know if they suspect they have a respiratory illness. They may also be posted in exam rooms, bathrooms, and reception areas. The CDC has a variety of posters in several languages that may be obtained either free of charge or for a nominal fee. These posters should remind everyone to

- Cough and sneeze into a disposable tissue and immediately discard the tissue in an appropriate waste receptacle.
- Perform hand hygiene after coughing or sneezing to prevent the spread of germs.

Healthcare facilities should have tissues and alcohol-based hand rubs readily accessible in the reception area and

in exam rooms and laboratory areas. No-touch waste receptacles should be placed so that patients can easily access them. Additionally, give patients educational materials to take home, reminding them of ways to reduce the spread of respiratory infection to family and friends.

Masks, Isolation, and Decontamination

During local or regional outbreaks of respiratory illness, special precautions may be necessary. Ask patients who are coughing to wear a mask. Have masks readily available for patients, including in sizes that fit children. If possible, isolate patients who are coughing in a separate reception area. If this is not possible, ask patients who are coughing to sit at least 3 feet away from other patients. If a patient is coughing and has a high fever, ask him to put on a mask and move him to an exam room as quickly as possible.

When assisting with a patient who is coughing, put on a mask before entering the room. If a patient is coughing uncontrollably and there is considerable spray, you should wear gloves, a gown, and goggles. Perform hand hygiene before and after touching the patient or items or surfaces likely contaminated with respiratory droplets. Once the patient has left the room, you should wash your hands, put on gloves, and thoroughly clean and disinfect the exam room using an EPA-approved disinfectant of a 1:10 bleach solution. Include any surface the patient may have touched, including the doorknob, chair, desk, and exam table. If you are unsure if a patient touched a surface or an item, treat it as contaminated and clean and disinfect it. Medical equipment used to examine the patient should be disinfected according to office policy and procedure.

▶ Infection Control Practices with Medical Equipment
LO 35.5

There is a vast array of medical equipment used in patient care. Much of it is single use, meaning it is designed to be used for one patient during one test or procedure and then discarded in an approved container. Some equipment is reusable and must be appropriately disinfected or sterilized. This equipment is categorized based on the level of disinfection or sterilization necessary for reuse. Equipment is categorized as one of the following:

- Noncritical (such as blood pressure cuffs and reflex hammers)—these items only come in contact with intact skin and require low-level disinfection
- Semi-critical (such as endoscopes)—these items come in contact with mucous membranes and non-intact skin and require high-level disinfection at a minimum
- Critical (such as surgical instruments)—these items enter sterile tissue, body cavities, and veins and arteries and must be sterilized prior to use

CDC key recommendations for cleaning, disinfecting, and/or sterilizing medical equipment in ambulatory care settings include the following:

- Reusable medical equipment should be cleaned and reprocessed prior to use with each patient.
- Cleaning and reprocessing reusable equipment must be done according to the manufacturer's recommendations. If no recommendations exist, the device may not be considered appropriate for use on multiple patients.
- Equipment reprocessing should only be done by trained professionals.
- Copies of the manufacturer's reprocessing recommendations should be kept on file and posted in the reprocessing area.
- Equipment reprocessing should be routinely monitored.
- Personnel responsible for reprocessing equipment should wear appropriate PPE.
- Equipment must be cleaned to remove organic material (blood and tissue) prior to disinfection.
- Single-use equipment should never be used on more than one patient. It is not designed for reprocessing and reuse.

▶ Surgical Site Infections (SSIs)
LO 35.6

An infection that occurs after a surgical procedure at the site of surgery is considered a **surgical site infection (SSI).** Approximately 3% of patients will develop an infection at the surgical site. The most common microorganism associated with SSIs is the bacterium *Staphylococcus aureus;* however, other bacteria also can cause infections at surgical sites. Most SSIs are endogenous—caused by microorganisms found on the skin or in the body of the patient—but they also can be exogenous—brought into the surgical site by medical instruments or equipment. Classifications of SSIs are dependent on the location and extent of the surgical wound. The three classifications are

- Superficial incisional—involves only the skin and subcutaneous tissue.
- Deep incisional—involves deep tissues such as fascia and muscle.
- Organ/space—excludes skin, fascia, and muscle; includes organs or body cavities.

In the medical office, you will most often see superficial incisional SSIs. Symptoms of superficial infections include

- Purulent drainage from the surgical wound.
- Positive wound culture from the site.
- Redness, swelling, and heat at the wound site.

Adherence to CDC guidelines, careful sterile technique during office procedures, and comprehensive patient education are the keys to preventing SSIs in the medical office. For more information about sterile technique, see the *Assisting with Minor Surgery* chapter.

Educating the Patient Prior to Surgery
Because most SSIs are endogenous, it is important that the patient be involved in reducing the occurrence of infection. You can help patients avoid an infection after surgery by giving them clear instructions about what to do before and after the surgical procedure:

Before the Procedure

- Report any previous postsurgical infections to the healthcare practitioner.
- Stop smoking as soon as possible before the surgery.
- Tell your doctor if you have diabetes.
- Eat well and get plenty of rest.
- Shower with an antibacterial soap before the procedure.
- Do not shave near the surgical site before your surgery.
- Stay warm while on the way to the hospital by starting the car and getting it warm before leaving for your surgery, wearing warm clothes and covering with a blanket if needed.

The Day of Surgery

- Take any prescribed medications as instructed by your healthcare practitioner.
- Do not be afraid to speak up if you see healthcare workers fail to wash their hands.
- If a healthcare worker tells you she is going to shave the site with a razor, question her and ask to speak to the surgeon before allowing her to shave you. (The CDC recommends the use of clippers for hair removal, not razors.)

After the Surgery

- Do not allow family or friends to touch the wound.
- Care for the wound as directed by your healthcare practitioner.
- Wash your hands before and after caring for your wound.
- Call the office if you see any signs of infection.

You should give the patient all instructions in writing and verbally before the surgical procedure. Provide enough time for the patients to ask questions of you and the healthcare practitioner. Well-informed patients will be better prepared to care for themselves after surgery. Knowing how to care for their surgical wounds helps reduce the incidence of SSIs.

▶ Sterilization
LO 35.7

Sterilization is required for all instruments and supplies that will penetrate a patient's skin or come in contact with any other normally sterile areas of the body. Sterilization is also required for all instruments that will be used in a sterile field, even if they will not be used on a patient. An item is considered either sterile or unsterile. If you doubt the status of an item, consider it unsterile.

Before sterilizing an item, you must first sanitize it and, sometimes, disinfect it. Instruments and equipment that need to be sterilized include the following:

- Curettes (spoon-shaped instruments for removing material from a cavity wall or other surface)
- Instruments used during surgical procedures
- Suture removal instruments
- Vaginal specula (instruments used to enlarge the opening of the vagina and allow examination of the vagina and cervix)

Sterilize instruments and equipment by one of the following methods:

- Autoclaving
- Chemical (cold) processes

The Autoclave

The primary method for sterilizing instruments and equipment is the use of pressurized steam in an **autoclave** (Figure 35-6). This device forces the temperature of steam above the boiling point of water (212°F, or 100°C). Sterilization by autoclave is a widely accepted method of sterilization for two reasons:

1. Steam autoclaves can operate at a lower temperature than is required for dry heat sterilization. The moist heat from steam more quickly permeates the clean, porous wrappings in which all instruments are placed prior to loading them into the unit.

2. The moisture causes coagulation of proteins within microorganisms at a much lower temperature than is possible with dry heat. When cells containing coagulated protein cool, their cell walls burst; this kills the microorganisms.

General Autoclave Procedures   In general, the sterilization process using an autoclave involves the following steps:

1. Prepare sanitized and disinfected instruments and equipment for loading into the autoclave by wrapping them in muslin, special porous paper, plastic bags, or envelopes and labeling each pack. (Include sterilization indicators.)

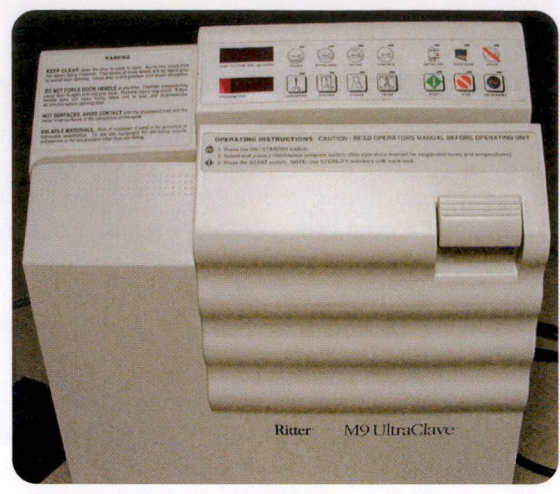

FIGURE 35-6   Steam autoclaving is the most common method of sterilizing instruments and equipment. Understanding the gauges and timer is essential to proper operation of an autoclave.
© *Total Care Programming, Inc.*

2. Check the water level in the autoclave; add distilled water if necessary.

3. Preheat the autoclave according to the manufacturer's guidelines. (Some models require putting instruments in before preheating.)

4. Perform any required quality control procedures (in addition to sterilization indicators in instrument packs).

5. Load the instruments and equipment into the autoclave. Allow adequate space around the items to ensure that steam reaches all areas.

6. Choose the correct setting based on the load type (unwrapped items, pouches, packs, liquids, and so on). If the autoclave is not automatic, set the autoclave for the correct time after the correct temperature and pressure have been reached.

7. Run the autoclave through the sterilization cycle, including drying time.

8. Remove the instruments and equipment from the autoclave.

9. Store the instruments and equipment properly for the next use. Rotate stored items so that packages with the oldest date are used first. Do not use packages past their expiration date.

10. Clean the autoclave and the surrounding work area.

During the autoclave process, assume the instruments and equipment are contaminated, and follow standard precautions:

- Wear gloves to avoid contamination by blood, body fluids, or tissues.
- Take measures to protect against needlesticks or cuts—for example, use forceps to handle sharps.
- Wash your hands thoroughly after all cleaning procedures.

Wrapping and Labeling All Items   Wrap items in porous fabric, paper, or plastic before placing them in the autoclave. This material helps surround the items with the correct levels of moisture and heat. Instruments and equipment to be used immediately after autoclaving can be placed on trays with material above and below the items. Items that must be stored in a sterile state for later use are wrapped and sealed before autoclaving. Refer to Procedure 35-3 at the end of this chapter, for wrapping and labeling instructions.

A number of products are available for wrapping items for sterilization. Muslin (140 count) may be used. However, because it is woven, it is more susceptible to contamination. All packs wrapped in muslin must be double wrapped. Other products include permeable paper, disposable nonwoven fabric, and clear plastic envelopes with one side made of permeable material. Figure 35-7 shows several common wrapping products and sterilization indicators.

Instruments that will be used together should be wrapped together to form a sterile pack. Wrap the pack loosely so that the steam can reach the instruments inside. After using a pack, consider all items (even those not used) unsterile and return them for sanitization, disinfection, and sterilization.

Clearly label each pack with a nontoxic marker to identify the item or items inside the wrapping and the person who completed the procedure. The label also must include the date to prevent use after expiring.

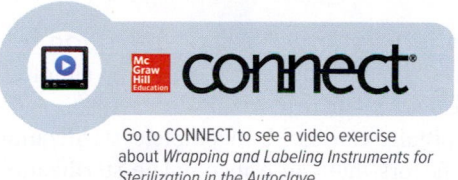

Go to CONNECT to see a video exercise about *Wrapping and Labeling Instruments for Sterilization in the Autoclave.*

Preheating the Autoclave
Check for solutions that may have boiled over and for deposits that may have formed on any of the inner surfaces. Make sure the water reservoir is filled to the proper level with distilled water. Also check the discharge lines and valves to make sure there are no obstructions. If lines or valves are blocked, air may remain trapped inside the chamber, rendering the load unsterile.

Following this inspection, preheat the unit according to the manufacturer's guidelines. Loading cold instruments into an overheated chamber can cause excess condensation, so be sure to understand and follow the preheating instructions.

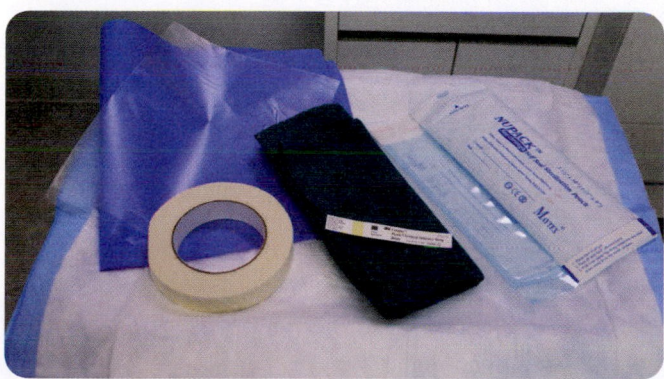

FIGURE 35-7 Common wrapping products and sterilization indicators.
© McGraw-Hill Education

Understanding Autoclave Settings
Modern autoclaves are designed to operate as automatically as possible; however, manual autoclaves are still used. Because you are responsible for the sterility of the items processed by the autoclave, you must be able to identify the various gauges and interpret their readings correctly.

Manual autoclaves have three gauges and a timer. The jacket pressure gauge shows the outer chamber's steam pressure. The chamber pressure gauge shows the inner chamber's steam pressure. The temperature gauge shows the temperature inside the inner, or sterilization, chamber. The timer allows you to control the number of minutes the load is exposed to the high-temperature, pressurized steam.

Exact temperature and pressure requirements vary with the model and type of autoclave, and with the instruments and packaging in the load. In general, the temperature must reach 250°F to 270°F (121°C to 132°C) and the chamber pressure gauge must show 15 to 30 pounds of pressure. Follow the manufacturer's instructions precisely for each autoclave load. Procedure 35-4, at the end of this chapter, describes the general steps to follow for running a load through the preheated autoclave.

Sterilization Indicators and Quality Control
It is important to monitor all sterilization procedures. This is accomplished through the use of various types of indicators and quality control measures.

Sterilization indicators include special packages, tags, inserts, tapes, tubes, and strips that confirm the items in the autoclave have been exposed to the correct volume of steam at the correct temperature for the correct length of time. Several types of indicators are available (Figure 35-8).

For example, you place tags or inserts within the load, whereas you affix tapes to the outside of wrapped instrument packs. Indicators have designated areas or words that change color when the correct temperature, pressure, and proper length of time have been reached. Although it is generally acceptable to rely on indicators as a guarantee of sterility, in reality, they are only indicators that the load has been exposed to conditions that usually result in sterile surfaces. They do not guarantee that the autoclave contents are actually sterile.

Biological indicators—containing bacterial spores—are used as a quality control method to confirm that sterilization has occurred. Bacterial spores come in various forms, including strips, disks, and ampules. They are used because they are more resistant to common sterilization processes than non-spore-forming organisms. The general procedure for using biological indicators is as follows:

- Place a biological indicator in a load to be sterilized.
- Place another biological indicator outside the autoclave as a positive control.
- Run the load as usual.
- Interpret the biological indicator and positive control as directed by the manufacturer or send to an outside lab for processing.
- Incubate as recommended by the manufacturer.

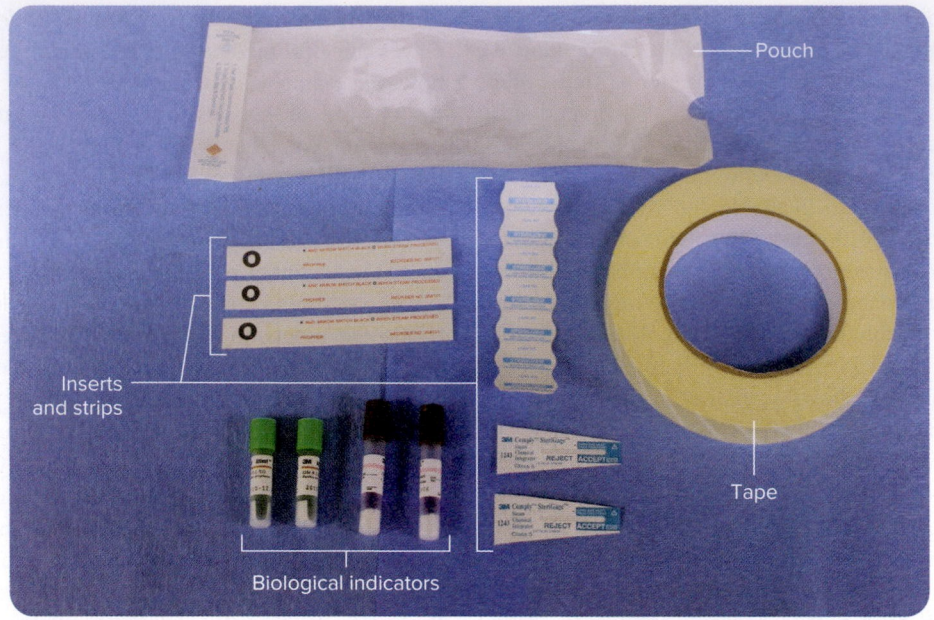

FIGURE 35-8 Sterilization indicators are manufactured in various types, sizes, and shapes.

© McGraw-Hill Education

In general, place indicators in a sufficient number of places in the load so that you can be reasonably confident of the sterility of all items in the chamber. The following locations are suitable for indicator positioning:

- Within instrument packs
- On the outside of wrapped instrument packs
- Inside containers, especially those that cannot be positioned to allow steam to surround the item
- Near the air exhaust valve
- In any other areas into which steam might not be able to flow freely

For information on interpreting the results of a biological indicator, see the *Caution: Handle with Care* feature.

Preventing Incomplete Sterilization Although the autoclave is generally considered the simplest and most effective method for sterilizing instruments and equipment, certain pitfalls can cause incomplete sterilization. The four leading factors that cause incomplete sterilization are incorrect timing, insufficient temperature, overcrowding of packs, and inadequate steam levels. Once again, the manufacturer's guidelines provided with the autoclave unit are the best source of accurate information on how to operate it correctly.

Timing Guidelines After loading the autoclave, make sure the heating cycle lasts long enough to allow the steam to permeate all wrappings to reach the instruments and equipment inside. Timing for items to be sterilized should not be started until the unit has reached the proper temperature. Automatic

CAUTION: HANDLE WITH CARE

Interpreting the Results of a Biological Indicator

In some cases, you may be asked to interpret the results of a biological indicator. If the indicator exposed to the sterilization cycle is positive for bacterial growth, then sterilization has not occurred. The load should be held, the chemical indicators checked, and the biological indicator test repeated. If the second test is positive, have the sterilizer serviced. Once the sterilizer has been serviced, retest with three consecutive tests in an empty chamber. If all three tests are negative, the sterilizer can be returned to service. If the indicator exposed to the cycle shows no bacterial growth, check the growth of the positive control. The positive control should show bacterial growth because it has not been exposed to the sterilization cycle. If there is no growth on the positive control, you should repeat the quality control procedure with biological indicators from another manufactured lot number. Record the results of each biological indicator monitoring procedure in the sterilization log. Biological indicators should be used at the following times:

- If a new type of packaging material is used
- If you have a new autoclave
- After autoclave maintenance or repair
- On a weekly basis as a general quality control measure

autoclaves have preset timing for each load type. You should keep up with the amount of time an automatic autoclave takes to complete a cycle, noting any differences between loads. Large differences in the amount of time it takes to complete a load cycle should alert you to a problem with the autoclave. Although following timing guidelines helps ensure sterilization, you also should use sterilization indicators.

If you have any doubt about the sterility of an instrument or a piece of equipment, do not use it. Instead, put it aside for another cycle of sanitization, disinfection, and sterilization. The risks to patients and to you are too great to take chances.

Temperature Guidelines The length of the sterilization cycle is only one factor that has an impact on the final quality of autoclave operations. If the autoclave is manual, the unit must operate at the correct temperature. Unit thermometers and sterilization indicators help confirm that correct temperatures have been reached.

Temperatures that are too high can cause problems as easily as those that are too low. If the temperature is too high inside the autoclave compartment, the steam does not have the correct level of moisture. The heat and moisture will not penetrate wrapped instrument packs, resulting in an unsterilized load.

If the temperature is too low, the steam contains too much moisture. Packs will be oversaturated and the drying cycle will be insufficient. Wet packs can easily pick up contaminants from surfaces they touch after you unload them from the autoclave. Common causes of low temperature are failing to preheat the autoclave chamber, loading cold instruments into an overheated chamber, opening the unit door too wide during drying, and overfilling the water reservoir. Always make sure you are familiar with the manufacturer's recommendations before running a load through an autoclave.

Overcrowding Packs or instruments placed in too close proximity in the autoclave chamber may not be sterilized because of the inability of the steam to penetrate or reach all surfaces.

Steam Level Guidelines Steam under pressure is necessary for sterilization. If the correct level of steam is not present during the autoclave cycle, items will not be sterile at the end of the cycle. It is vital that the unit force all air out of the chamber at the beginning of the sterilization cycle. It is also essential that you place items in the chamber in positions that will not cause the formation of air pockets.

To help ensure proper operation of the unit, check all release valves and discharge lines to make sure they are free from obstruction. Clogged valves and lines may prevent elimination of all air from the chamber.

To prevent the formation of air pockets, load items in the autoclave so that the steam can circulate freely around all sides of the items. Place containers on their sides to avoid trapping air. Besides allowing the free flow of steam, careful positioning helps ensure that all items dry thoroughly before you remove them from the autoclave.

Storing Sterilized Supplies Sterilized packs and instruments must be stored in a clean, dry location where they will not be disturbed or shuffled around. This keeps the wrapping material from being torn or otherwise compromised.

The method you use to wrap an item for sterilization determines the item's sterile shelf life. As a general rule, double-layer fabric- or paper-wrapped packages are considered sterile for 30 days. The manufacturers of other wrapping products provide their own guidelines for sterile shelf life.

Return items for sanitization, disinfection, and sterilization after the sterile shelf life period has elapsed. Do not reuse any wrapping or labeling products. Instead, open the packs or wrappings and process each item as if it had never been cleaned.

Cleaning the Autoclave and Work Area Clean the autoclave after each use to prevent accumulation of deposits that might affect the unit's operation. You may use a nontoxic all-purpose cleaner, although specific cleaning products are available for autoclave use.

You are responsible for ensuring that routine cleaning is done correctly and thoroughly. When you clean the unit, also check for signs of cracking or wear in gaskets, drain valves, and tubing. Check the level of distilled water in the reservoir. Service representatives who specialize in the maintenance of your unit should periodically clean and check all seals and gauges.

The work area around the autoclave unit should be divided into two clearly marked areas: one for nonsterile, not-yet-autoclaved items and one for sterile equipment as it is removed from the unit. Do not use supplies from one area in the other. Be sure to move any sterile packs or equipment to the correct storage areas when cleaning the counters and other work surfaces. If anything is spilled on a sterile pack or instrument, return the item for sanitization, disinfection, and sterilization.

Chemical Sterilization

Chemical, or cold, sterilization involves the use of liquids to eliminate microorganisms. It is used on instruments and equipment that are sensitive to heat and steam. For example, in a gastroenterologist's office, you may need to disinfect or sterilize an endoscope. Although each facility may perform this process differently, the process involves five steps after performing a leak test on the endoscope:

1. Clean: Mechanically clean internal and external surfaces, including brushing internal channels and flushing each internal channel with water and a detergent or enzymatic cleaners.

2. Disinfect: Immerse the endoscope in a high-level disinfectant or chemical sterilant and ensure contact of the germicide into all accessible channels, such as the suction/biopsy channel and air/water channel. Expose for the time recommended for specific products.

3. Rinse: Rinse the endoscope and all channels with sterile water, filtered water, or tap water (high-quality potable water that meets federal clean water standards at the point of use).

4. Dry: Rinse the insertion tube and inner channels with alcohol, and dry with forced air after disinfection and before storage. Drying the endoscope is essential to greatly reduce the chance of recontamination of the endoscope by microorganisms that may be present in the rinse water.

5. Store: Store the endoscope in a way that prevents recontamination and promotes drying, such as hanging it vertically.

▶ Reporting Guidelines for Infectious Diseases
LO 35.8

The CDC requires the reporting of certain diseases to the state or county department of health. This information, which is forwarded to the CDC, helps research epidemiologists control the spread of infection. Table 35-1 lists diseases that must be reported to the National Notifiable Disease Surveillance System of the CDC, through your state or county health department. When you report a communicable disease, you must fill out a report form. Your state health department may have a different form for each reportable disease. You must obtain the correct form and a disease identification number from the health department every time you report a communicable disease. To fill out such a form, you need access to the following information:

- Disease identification (usually a code number as well as the name of the disease)
- Patient identification (including name, address, date of birth, sex, ethnic origin, and occupational or educational status) if required
- Infection history (date of onset, vaccination history, laboratory results)
- Reporting-institution information (name of person completing report, title, contact information)

Each state and each medical facility has specific guidelines for filling out such a form. Procedure 35-5 describes, in general, how to notify state and county agencies about reportable diseases. This procedure uses a paper form; however, electronic reporting may be available in the facility where you are employed.

Reporting guidelines also must be followed if a worker comes in contact with a substance that may transmit infection. These guidelines, which are explained in OSHA's Bloodborne Pathogens Standard, include reporting exposure incidents to employers immediately.

TABLE 35-1 The National Notifiable Disease Surveillance System	
Anthrax	Giardiasis
Arboviral neuroinvasive and non-neuroinvasive diseases	Gonorrhea
Babesiosis	*Haemophilus influenzae,* invasive disease
Botulism, foodborne	Hansen disease (leprosy)
Botulism, infant	Hantavirus pulmonary syndrome
Botulism, other (wound and unspecified)	Hemolytic uremic syndrome, post-diarrhea
Brucellosis	Hepatitis A, acute
Chancroid	Hepatitis B, acute
Chlamydia trachomatis, genital infections	Hepatitis B, chronic
Cholera	Hepatitis B virus, perinatal infection
Coccidioidomycosis	Hepatitis C, acute
Cryptosporidiosis	Hepatitis C, past or present
Cyclosporiasis	HIV infection*
Dengue fever	• HIV infection, adult/ adolescent (age > = 13 years)
Dengue hemorrhagic fever	• HIV infection, child (age > = 18 months and < 13 years)
Dengue shock syndrome	• HIV infection, pediatric (age < 18 months)
Diphtheria	Influenza-associated pediatric mortality
Ehrlichiosis/anaplasmosis	Legionellosis
• *Ehrlichia chaffeensis*	Listeriosis
• *Ehrlichia ewingii*	Lyme disease
• *Anaplasma phagocytophilum*	Malaria
• Undetermined	Measles

(continued)

TABLE 35-1 The National Notifiable Disease Surveillance System

Meningococcal disease	Syphilis, congenital
Mumps	Syphilitic stillbirth
Novel influenza A virus infections	Tetanus
Pertussis	Toxic-shock syndrome (other than Streptococcal)
Plague	Trichinellosis (trichinosis)
Poliomyelitis, paralytic	Tuberculosis
Poliovirus infection, nonparalytic	Tularemia
Psittacosis	Typhoid fever
Q fever, acute and chronic	Vancomycin-intermediate *Staphylococcus aureus* (VISA)
Rabies, animal	Vancomycin-resistant *Staphylococcus aureus* (VRSA)
Rabies, human	Varicella (deaths only)
Rubella	Varicella (morbidity)
Rubella, congenital syndrome	Vibriosis
Salmonellosis	Viral hemorrhagic fevers, due to
Severe acute respiratory syndrome–associated coronavirus (SARS-CoV) disease	• Ebola virus
Shiga toxin–producing *Escherichia coli* (STEC)	• Marburg virus
Shigellosis	• Arenavirus
Smallpox	• Crimean-Congo hemorrhagic fever virus
Spotted fever rickettsiosis	• Lassa virus
Streptococcal toxic-shock syndrome	• Lujo virus
Streptococcus pneumoniae, invasive disease	• New world arena viruses
Syphilis, all stages	Yellow fever

*Acquired immunodeficiency syndrome (AIDS) (reclassified as HIV stage III).

Source: From Centers for Disease Control and Prevention Nationally Notifiable Infectious Conditions US 2011.

PROCEDURE 35-1 Removing Contaminated Gloves

Procedure Goal: To remove gloves contaminated with blood, body fluids, or other potentially hazardous substances while avoiding cross-contamination of your hands or other surfaces

OSHA Guidelines: This procedure does not involve exposure to blood, body fluids, or tissue if performed correctly.

Materials: Contaminated gloves, lined trash container or biohazardous waste container

Method:

1. Using your dominant hand, grasp the palm of the glove of your nondominant hand.
2. Gently pull the glove downward off the nondominant hand, turning it inside out and holding it in your dominant hand.
3. Encase the removed glove completely in the dominant hand.

RATIONALE: *To contain any contaminants in the glove so that they are not accidently transferred to your hands; encasing the glove also limits the possibility of splattering contaminants by flipping the glove*

4. Place the thumb or two fingers of the ungloved hand under the cuff of the remaining glove, being careful not to touch the outside of the glove with your bare hand.
   RATIONALE: *The inside of the glove is most likely not contaminated.*
5. Pull the glove over your hand, turning it inside out over the other glove, leaving no outside surface exposed.
6. Throw the gloves away in the appropriate waste container.
7. Wash your hands.

PROCEDURE 35-2 Removing a Contaminated Gown

Procedure Goal: To remove a gown contaminated on the front and sleeves with blood, body fluids, or other potentially hazardous substances while avoiding cross-contamination of your hands, body, or other surfaces

OSHA Guidelines: This procedure does not involve exposure to blood, body fluids, or tissue if performed correctly.

Materials: Contaminated gown, lined trash container or biohazardous waste container

Method:

1. Unfasten ties from the neck, then from behind your back.

2. Peel the gown down and away from neck and shoulders, touching inside of gown only.
   RATIONALE: *You should always move from clean to dirty to avoid cross-contamination.*

3. Continue pulling the gown down from the neck and shoulders and away from your body.

4. Turn gown inside out, making sure you do not touch the outer surface of the gown.
   RATIONALE: *To avoid contaminating your hands*

5. Slowly fold or roll into a bundle and discard.

6. Wash your hands if they become visibly contaminated; otherwise use an alcohol-based hand sanitizer.

PROCEDURE 35-3 Wrapping and Labeling Instruments for Sterilization in the Autoclave

Procedure Goal: To enclose instruments and equipment to be sterilized in appropriate wrapping materials to ensure sterilization and to protect supplies from contamination after sterilization

OSHA Guidelines:

Materials: Dry, sanitized, and disinfected instruments and equipment; wrapping material (paper, muslin, gauze, bags, envelopes); sterilization indicators; autoclave tape; labels (if wrapping does not include space for labeling); and a waterproof pen

Method:

For Wrapping Instruments or Equipment in Pieces of Paper or Fabric

1. Wash your hands and don gloves before beginning to wrap the items to be sterilized.

2. Place a square of paper or muslin on the table with one point toward you. With muslin, use a double thickness. The paper or fabric must be large enough to allow all four points to cover the instruments or equipment you will be wrapping. It also must be large enough to provide an overlap, which will be used as a handling flap.

3. Place each item to be included in the pack in the center area of the paper or fabric "diamond." Items that will be used together should be wrapped together. Make sure, however, that surfaces of the items do not touch each other inside the pack so that steam can penetrate every surface of all instruments in the pack. Inspect each item to ensure it is operating correctly. Place hinged instruments in the pack in the open position. Wrap a small piece of paper, muslin, or gauze around delicate edges or points to protect against damage to other instruments or to the pack wrapping.

4. Place a sterilization indicator inside the pack with the instruments. Position the indicator correctly, following the manufacturer's guidelines (Figure a).
   RATIONALE: *A sterilization indicator must always be placed inside the pack to ensure the contents have been sterilized properly.*

5. Fold the bottom point of the diamond up and over the instruments in to the center (Figure b). Fold back a small portion of the point (Figure c).
   RATIONALE: *This "handle" will be used later, when the sterile pack is opened.*

6. Fold the right point of the diamond in to the center. Again, fold back a small portion of the point to be used as a handle (Figure d).

7. Fold the left point of the diamond in to the center, folding back a small portion to form a handle. The pack should now resemble an open envelope (Figure e).

8. Grasp the covered instruments (the bottom of the envelope) and fold this portion up, toward the top point (Figure f). Fold the top point down over the pack, making sure the pack is snug but not too tight.

9. Secure the pack with autoclave tape (Figure g). A "quick-opening tab" can be created by folding a small portion of the tape back onto itself. The pack must be snug enough to prevent instruments from slipping out of the wrapping or damaging each other inside the pack but loose enough to allow adequate steam circulation through the pack.

10. Label the pack with your initials and the date. Then list the contents of the pack. If the pack contains syringes, be sure to identify the syringe size(s).

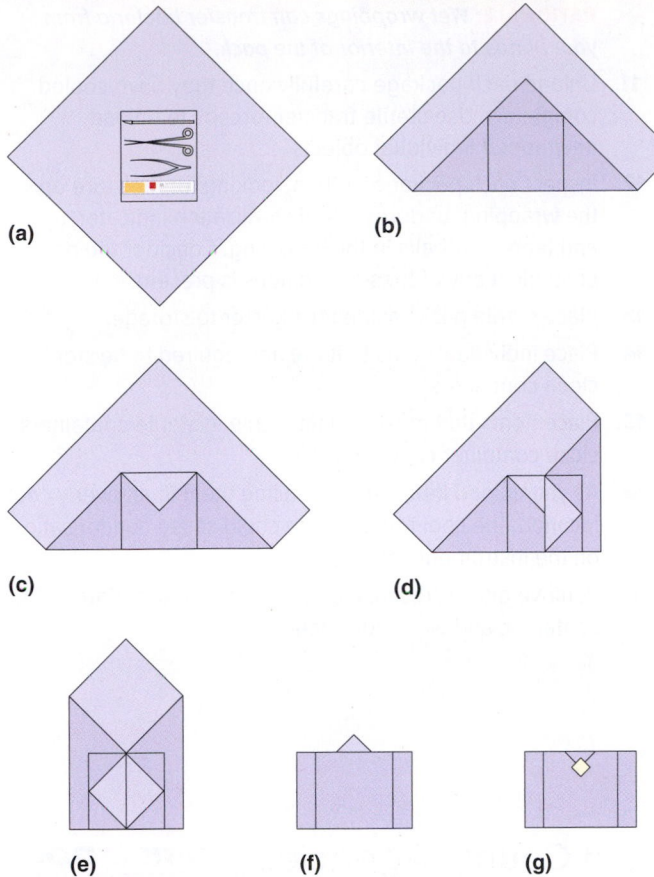

(a)

(b)

(c)

(d)

(e)

(f)

(g)

FIGURE Procedure 35-3 Steps 4 through 9 Follow the sequence in this figure when you wrap instruments in a paper or fabric pack for sterilization in an autoclave.

RATIONALE: *Dating helps you keep up with the date the pack expires. Items should be easily identified without opening the pack.*

11. Place the pack aside for loading into the autoclave.

12. Remove gloves, dispose of them in the appropriate waste container, and wash your hands.

For Wrapping Instruments and Equipment in Bags or Envelopes

1. Wash your hands and put on gloves before beginning to wrap the items to be sterilized.

2. Insert the items into the bag or envelope as indicated by the manufacturer's directions. Hinged instruments should be opened before insertion into the package.
   RATIONALE: *This allows steam to penetrate inside the hinge.*

3. Close and seal the pack. Make sure the sterilization indicator is not damaged or already exposed.
   RATIONALE: *If the sterilization indicator is damaged or already exposed, you have no way of knowing if the sterilization cycle was completed.*

4. Label the pack with your initials and the date. Then list the contents of the pack. The pens or pencils used to label the pack must be waterproof; otherwise, the contents of the pack and date of sterilization will be obliterated.
   RATIONALE: *Dating helps you keep up with the date the pack expires. Items should be easily identified without opening the pack.*

5. Place the pack aside for loading into the autoclave.

6. Remove gloves, dispose of them in the appropriate waste container, and wash your hands.

PROCEDURE 35-4   Running a Load Through the Autoclave

Procedure Goal: To run a load of instruments and equipment through an autoclave, ensuring sterilization of items by properly loading, drying, and unloading them

OSHA Guidelines:

Materials: Dry, sanitized, and disinfected instruments and equipment, both individual pieces and wrapped packs; oven mitts; sterile transfer forceps; and storage containers for individual items

Method:

1. Wash your hands and don gloves before beginning to load items into the autoclave.

2. Rest packs on their edges and place jars and containers on their sides.

3. Place lids for jars and containers with their sterile sides down.

4. If the load includes plastic items, make sure no other item leans against them.
   RATIONALE: *Pressure that results from the high temperatures can cause plastic items to bend or warp.*

5. If your load is mixed—containing both wrapped packs and individual instruments—place the tray containing the instruments below the tray containing the wrapped packs.
   RATIONALE: *This arrangement prevents any condensation that forms on the instruments from dripping onto the wrapped packs and saturating the wrapping.*

6. Close the door and start the unit. For automatic autoclaves, choose the cycle based on the type of load you are

running. Consult the manufacturer's recommendations before choosing the load type.

7. For manual autoclaves, start the timer when the indicators show the recommended temperature and pressure.

8. Right after the end of the steam cycle and just before the start of the drying cycle, open the door to the autoclave slightly (between ¼ and ½ inch).

   RATIONALE: *Opening the door more than ½ inch causes cold air to enter the autoclave, possibly creating excessive condensation in the chamber. This condensation would cause incomplete drying. Consult the manufacturer's recommendations regarding opening the door. Some automatic autoclaves do not require opening the door during the drying cycle.*

9. Dry according to the manufacturer's recommendations. Packs and large items may require up to 45 minutes for complete drying.

10. Unload the autoclave after the drying cycle is finished. Do not unload any packs or instruments with wet wrappings, or the objects inside will be considered unsterile and must be processed again.

RATIONALE: *Wet wrappings can transfer bacteria from your hands to the interior of the pack.*

11. Unload each package carefully once they have cooled completely. Use sterile transfer forceps to unload unwrapped individual objects.

12. Inspect each package or item, looking for moisture on the wrapping, underexposed sterilization indicators, and tears or breaks in the wrapping. Consider the pack unsterile if any of these conditions is present.

13. Place sterile packs aside for transfer to storage.

14. Place individual items that are not required to be sterile in clean containers.

15. Place items that must remain sterile in sterile containers; close container covers tightly.

16. As you unload items, avoid placing them in an overly cool location; the cool temperature could cause condensation on the instruments or packs.

17. Remove gloves, dispose of them in the appropriate waste container, and wash your hands.

PROCEDURE 35-5 Notifying State and County Agencies About Reportable Diseases WORK // DOC

Procedure Goal: To report cases of infection with reportable disease to the proper state or county health department

OSHA Guidelines: This procedure does not involve exposure to blood, body fluids, or tissues.

Materials: Communicable disease report form, pen, envelope, and stamp

Method:

1. Check to be sure you have the correct form. Some states have specific forms for each reportable infectious disease or type of disease. CDC forms also may be used for reporting specific diseases.

2. Fill in all blank areas unless they are shaded (generally for local health department use).

3. Follow office procedures for submitting the report to a supervisor or physician before sending it out.

4. Sign and date the form. Address the envelope, put a stamp on it, and place it in the mail.

MICHIGAN DEPARTMENT OF PUBLIC HEALTH
Division of Disease Surveillance

ENTERIC ILLNESS CASE INVESTIGATION
(Please check appropriate illness)

_____ Shigellosis	_____ Giardiasis
_____ Non-typhoid Salmonellosis	_____ Amebiasis
_____ Campylobacter enteritis	

CASE INFORMATION

Name: _____ Age or Birthdate: _____ Sex: _____ Race: _____

Address: _____ Phone: _____
        (Street)   (City)   (County)   (Zip)

Occupation: _____ *High Risk: Y N
               (What)   (Where)
(If infant or student list school, nursery or day care center)

Attending   Address or   Was the patient
Physician: _____ Phone: _____ hospitalized: Y N

Hospital: _____ Dates: _____
                                        (Admission)   (Discharge)

Onset: _____ Date recovered: _____ Symptom Summary: _____

_____

_____

Suspected Causative Agent: _____
(include species or serotype if known)

HOUSEHOLD CONTACTS INFORMATION

Name	Age	Family Relationship	Occupation	*High Risk Y N	Provide date of onset for all household members with concurrent similar illness
1)					
2)					
3)					
4)					
5)					
6)					
7)					
8)					
9)					
10)					

*"High Risk" = occupation as food handler, direct patient care worker, day care center worker or person attending day care or who is institutionalized. Stool specimens should be obtained on "high risk" cases and "high risk" household contacts as appropriate for the illness. Results may be recorded in Laboratory Information Section of this form (see over).

Name of the person who completed this form: _____ County: _____

Information obtained from: _____ Date: _____

Telephone Interview: _____ Home Visit: _____ Outbreak Investigation: _____

C-30 Rev. 10/83   AUTH: Act 368, P.A. 1978

FIGURE Procedure 35-5 Step 1 Some states have specific forms for use with particular communicable diseases or diseases of a certain type. (*Continued*)

NON-HOUSEHOLD CONTACTS WITH A CONCURRENT SIMILAR ILLNESS

Name	Approximate date of onset of symptoms	Address and/or Phone	Relationship to case (Nature of contact)
1)			
2)			
3)			
4)			
5)			

ADDITIONAL EXPOSURES OR COMMENTS

Home Sewage System: Municipal   Septic Tank   Other_____

Home drinking Water Type: Municipal   Private Well   Other_____

As appropriate for the illness, ask about meals eaten away from home, stores where groceries bought, brand of poultry, meat, dairy products consumed, overnight travel, recent foreign travel, group functions, exposure to raw milk, untreated water, animals, etc. within one incubation period before onset.

   (shigellosis to 7 days, salmonellosis - up to 3 days, Campylobacter enteritis - up to 10 days)

Be specific, provide place name(s) and date(s).

_____

FOLLOW-UP FECAL CULTURE RESULTS FOR "HIGH RISK" CASE AND/OR CONTACTS.

Name or Initials	Date(s) Obtained and Findings
1)	
2)	
3)	
4)	
5)	

FIGURE Procedure 35-5 Step 1   Some states have specific forms for use with particular communicable diseases or diseases of a certain type.

SUMMARY OF LEARNING OUTCOMES

LEARNING OUTCOMES	KEY POINTS
35.1 Identify various healthcare-associated infections (HAI) specific to the ambulatory care setting.	The most common HAI specific to the ambulatory care setting is MRSA. Other types of HAI that occur in outpatient settings include *Clostridium difficile* (C. diff), central line–associated bloodstream infections (CLABSI), catheter-associated urinary tract infections (CAUTI), and surgical site infections (SSIs).
35.2 Describe methods of infection control, including those for preventing healthcare-associated infections.	The two basic methods of infection control are medical asepsis (clean technique) and surgical asepsis (sterile technique). OSHA recommends that healthcare workers who work with high-risk patients know their HIV and HBV status, participate in an HBV vaccination program, and avoid direct patient contact if they have a skin condition characterized by sores that secrete fluid. Any healthcare worker who is HIV- or HBV-positive should not perform procedures that might expose a patient without first consulting an expert review panel.

LEARNING OUTCOMES	KEY POINTS
35.3 Describe various methods of injection safety, including engineered safety devices and work practice controls.	Injection safety procedures include always following strict aseptic procedures and standard precautions when administering injections. In addition, use safety-engineered devices whenever feasible.
35.4 Summarize proper respiratory hygiene/cough etiquette practices utilized in the medical office.	Post reminders for patients and staff to always cover their coughs and sneezes with a tissue and properly dispose of the tissue in an appropriate waste container. When assisting with a patient who has symptoms of a respiratory infection, ask patients to wear masks and use isolation precautions to stop the spread of infections.
35.5 Describe infection contol procedures related to medical equipment.	Multi-use medical equipment should be properly cleaned, disinfected, and sterilized according to the manufacturer's recommendations before use with every patient. Single-use medical equipment should be properly disposed of and never reused with a different patient.
35.6 Describe surgical site infections (SSIs) and ways to prevent them.	A surgical site infection (SSI) is an infection that occurs after a surgical procedure at the site of the surgery. The signs of an SSI include purulent drainage, heat and redness at the site, and fever. Giving patients clear instructions about what to do before and after surgery and always following surgical aseptic procedures reduces the incidence of SSI.
35.7 Discuss the procedures used in a medical office to sterilize surgical instruments and equipment.	Instruments and equipment that must be sterilized before use should be sanitized to remove blood and gross tissue and then sterilized either in an autoclave or by chemical means.
35.8 Describe Centers for Disease Control and Prevention (CDC) requirements for reporting cases of infectious disease.	The CDC requires the reporting of certain diseases to the state or county department of health, which then reports the information to the National Notifiable Disease Surveillance System of the CDC.

C A S E   S T U D Y   C R I T I C A L   T H I N K I N G

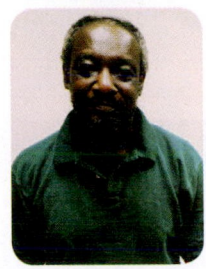

Recall Ken Washington from the beginning of the chapter. Now that you have completed the chapter, answer the following questions regarding his case.

1. Is it significant that Ken had a urinary catheter in place for 6 days while he was in the hospital?

2. Dr. Buckwalter plans to send Ken home with a urinary catheter in place. What information can you give him to help him prevent infection?

3. You note on the chart that Dr. Buckwalter wants to see Ken again in 2 days. You ask Ken to schedule an appointment for that time. Ken's wife states that they are going out of town for a week and will not be able to return until after that time. What should you tell Ken about making an appointment for more than a week?

1. (LO 35.2) When opening a sterile container, you should place the lid
   a. On the sterile field
   b. Facedown on the counter
   c. On a separate sterile field
   d. In your opposite hand
   e. Face-up on the counter

2. (LO 35.1) Which of the following best describes a CAUTI?
   a. An infection at the site of surgery
   b. An infection caused by microorganisms entering the bladder by way of a catheter
   c. A blood infection caused by a central line
   d. A procedure to stop bleeding
   e. A skin infection caused by antibiotic-resistant bacteria

3. (LO 35.4) All of the following are considered good respiratory hygiene *except*
   a. Isolating patients with respiratory infections in a separate reception area
   b. Placing a mask and goggles on anyone with symptoms of a respiratory infection
   c. Performing hand hygiene after coughing or sneezing
   d. Asking patients who are coughing to sit at least 3 feet away from other patients
   e. Immediately discarding used tissues into appropriate waste containers

4. (LO 35.6) A superficial incisional surgical site infection is one that involves
   a. Only the skin and subcutaneous tissue
   b. Organs and body cavities
   c. Muscles and fascia
   d. Bones and joints
   e. Intestinal tissue

5. (LO 35.8) All of the following are reportable diseases *except*
   a. Hantavirus
   b. Giardiasis
   c. Chickenpox
   d. Adenovirus
   e. Malaria

6. (LO 35.6) Which of the following is the term for surgical site infections caused by microorganisms found on the skin?
   a. Remote
   b. Exogenous
   c. Purulent
   d. Endogenous
   e. Extrinsic

7. (LO 35.1) A procedure that requires entry into a body cavity or cutting into skin or mucous membranes is known as
   a. Infectious
   b. Systemic
   c. Invasive
   d. Internal
   e. Vital

8. (LO 35.3) Self-blunting, or blunt tip, blood drawing needles have
   a. A device that slides through the lumen of the needle past the sharp point
   b. A sheath that slides over the needle and locks
   c. A needle that retracts into the syringe
   d. A needle that automatically breaks off after removing from the patient
   e. A needle with a hinged safety cover

9. (LO 35.7) The sterile shelf life of a paper-wrapped surgical pack is
   a. 1 month
   b. 1 year
   c. 6 months
   d. 2 months
   e. 14 days

10. (LO 35.2) Another name for medical asepsis is
    a. Sterile technique
    b. Aseptic principles
    c. Safe technique
    d. Clean technique
    e. Surgical cleaning

SOFT SKILLS SUCCESS

Recall Ken Washington from the case study at the beginning of the chapter. While you are giving Ken Washington care instructions for urinary catheterization, his wife states that she is not happy that Ken has to have another urinary catheter. She tells you that she thinks that the "man in the hospital" did not insert his urinary catheter properly and that is what has caused Ken's problem. She asks you if you think it is possible that Ken was "damaged" at the hospital when he had his urinary catheter inserted. What should you tell Ken's wife?

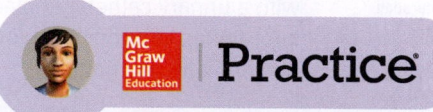

Go to PRACTICE MEDICAL OFFICE and complete the module Admin: Check Out - Privacy and Liability.

Patient Interview and History

CASE STUDY

PATIENT INFORMATION

Patient Name	DOB	Allergies
Peter Smith	3/28/19XX	NKA

Attending	MRN	Other Information
Paul F. Buckwalter, MD	428-69-544	Sleep study scheduled with Metro Sleep Specialists

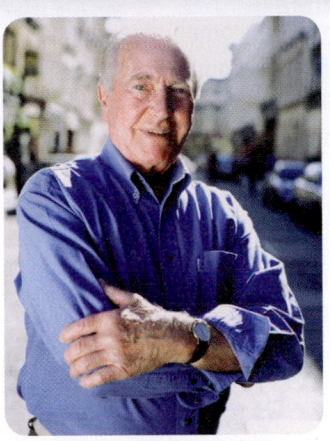

© Image Source/Getty Images RF

Peter Smith, a 73-year-old male with mild Type 2 diabetes, calls to schedule an appointment. He states that he is feeling very anxious and fatigued and is having difficulty eating and sleeping. He arrives at the clinic with his wife and needs to check in.

During the patient interview, he states that he wakes up in the middle of the night almost nightly. He also has many nights when he cannot even fall asleep. In addition, he has lost about 8 pounds in the last month. His symptoms started when his son died 6 months ago.

Keep Mr. Smith in mind as you study this chapter. There will be questions at the end of the chapter based on the case study. The information in the chapter will help you answer these questions.

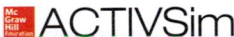

LEARNING OUTCOMES

After completing Chapter 36, you will be able to:

36.1 Identify the skills necessary to conduct a patient interview.

36.2 Recognize the signs of anxiety; depression; and physical, mental, or substance abuse.

36.3 Use the six Cs for writing an accurate patient history.

36.4 Carry out a patient history using critical thinking skills.

KEY TERMS

addiction

clarification

mirroring

objective data

reflection

restatement

subjective data

substance abuse

verbalizing

I.P.3	Perform patient screening using established protocols
I.A.1	Incorporate critical thinking skills when performing patient assessment
I.A.2	Incorporate critical thinking skills when performing patient care
V.C.2	Identify types of nonverbal communication
V.C.4	Identify techniques for overcoming communication barriers
V.C.15	Differentiate between adaptive and non-adaptive coping mechanisms
V.C.16	Differentiate between subjective and objective information
V.P.1	Use feedback techniques to obtain patient information including: (a) reflection (b) restatement (c) clarification
V.P.2	Respond to nonverbal communication
V.P.3	Use medical terminology correctly and pronounced accurately to communicate information to providers and patients
V.A.1	Demonstrate (b) active listening (c) nonverbal communication
X.P.2	Apply HIPAA rules in regard to: (a) privacy (b) release of information
X.P.3	Document patient care accurately in the medical record
X.P.4	Apply the Patient's Bill of Rights as it relates to: (a) choice of treatment (b) consent for treatment (c) refusal of treatment
X.A.1	Demonstrate sensitivity to patient rights

3. Medical Terminology

   d. Define and use medical abbreviations when appropriate and acceptable

4. Medical Law and Ethics

   a. Follow documentation guidelines

   b. Institute federal and state guidelines when releasing medical records or information

   f. Comply with federal, state, and local health laws and regulations as they relate to healthcare settings

   g. Display compliance with Code of Ethics of the profession

5. Psychology of Human Relations

   a. Respond appropriately to patients with abnormal behavior patterns

   c. Intervene on behalf of the patient regarding issues/concerns that may arise, i.e. insurance policy information, medical bills, physician/provider orders, etc.

9. Clinical Procedures

   b. Obtain vital signs, obtain patient history, and formulate chief complaint

11. Career Development

   b. Demonstrate professional behavior

▶ Introduction

As a medical assistant, it is your job to prepare the patient and the patient's chart before the physician enters the exam room to examine the patient. You are the first contact with the patient in the exam room. How you conduct yourself during those first few moments can make a major difference in the patient's attitude and perception of the medical office. The patient must cooperate fully to provide the information the physician needs for an accurate diagnosis and successful treatment. Conducting the patient interview and recording the necessary medical history are essential to the practitioner's exam process.

▶ The Patient Interview and History LO 36.1

The first step in the exam process is the patient interview. A well-conducted initial interview in the exam room helps establish a beneficial relationship between you and the new patient while providing a detailed exchange of pertinent information. Subsequent interviews with established patients may take less time; however, all patient interviews require good communication skills.

When you interview a patient, you will ask the patient (or an attending family member) for specific information about the reason for his or her visit. If the visit is for a medical problem, you will ask about his or her symptoms and determine the patient's chief complaint. The chief complaint is a subjective statement made by the patient describing the patient's most significant symptoms or signs of illness. Medicare and most insurers require this information. When a patient makes an office visit for a routine checkup, you will ask the patient about general health and lifestyle and about any changes in health status since the last visit.

A patient's medical and health history is the basis for all treatment rendered by the practitioner. The history also provides information for research, reportable diseases, and insurance claims. The information contained on the chart becomes a legal record of the treatment rendered to the patient. It must be complete and accurate to be a good defense in case of legal action. Document all information regarding the patient precisely and accurately.

Patient Rights, Responsibilities, and Privacy

It is important to remember that all the data you obtain are subject to legal and ethical considerations. Most states have adopted a version of the American Hospital Association's (AHA) Patient's Bill of Rights, written in 1973 and revised in 1992. Although AHA has replaced this bill of rights with "The Patient Care Partnership: Understanding Expectations, Rights, and Responsibilities," each state encourages healthcare workers to be aware of and provide for the patient's rights. Familiarize yourself with the information about patient rights contained in the following list. All patients have the right to

- Receive considerate and respectful care.
- Receive complete and current information concerning his or her diagnosis, treatment, and prognosis.
- Know the identity of physicians, nurses, and others involved with his or her care as well as know when those involved are students, residents, or trainees.
- Know the immediate and long-term costs of treatment choices.
- Receive information necessary to give informed consent prior to the start of any procedure or treatment.
- Have an advance directive concerning treatment or be able to choose a representative to make decisions.
- Refuse treatment to the extent permitted by law.
- Receive every consideration of his or her privacy.
- Be assured of confidentiality.
- Obtain reasonable responses to requests for services.
- Obtain information about his or her healthcare and be allowed to review his or her medical record and to have any information explained or interpreted.
- Know whether treatment is experimental and be able to consent or decline to participate in proposed research studies or human experimentation.
- Expect reasonable continuity of care.
- Ask about and be informed of the existence of business relationships between the hospital and others that may influence the patient's treatment and care.

- Know which hospital policies and practices relate to patient care, treatment, and responsibilities.
- Be informed of available resources for resolving disputes, grievances, and conflicts, such as ethics committees or patient representatives.
- Examine his or her bill and have it explained, and be informed of available payment methods.

Medical assistants also should know that patients have certain responsibilities when they seek medical care. Patients are responsible for

- Providing information about past illnesses, hospitalizations, medications, and other matters related to their health status. If an incorrect diagnosis is made because a patient fails to give the physician the proper information, the physician is not liable.
- Participating in decision making by asking for additional information about their health status or treatment when they do not fully understand information and instructions.
- Providing healthcare agencies with a copy of their written advance directive if they have one.
- Informing physicians and other caregivers if they anticipate problems in following a prescribed treatment.
- Following the physician's orders for treatment. If a patient willfully or negligently fails to follow the physician's instructions, that patient has little legal recourse.
- Providing healthcare agencies with necessary information for insurance claims and working with the healthcare facility to make arrangements to pay fees when necessary.

Additionally, in April 2003, enforcement of the Health Insurance Portability and Accountability Act (HIPAA) began. If this act is not followed, individual healthcare workers can be subject to fines up to $250,000 and 10 years in jail. The privacy standards of this act ensure the following:

- Healthcare facilities must provide patients with a written notice of their practices regarding the use and disclosure of all individually identifiable health information.
- Healthcare facilities may not use or disclose protected health information for any purpose that is not in the privacy notice.
- Patient consent is required when protected information is used or disclosed for purposes of treatment, payment, or health operations.
- Written authorization is required for other types of disclosures.
- Hospitals must make the privacy notice available either prior to or at the time of the delivery of care.
- A privacy notice must be posted in a clear and prominent location within the hospital facility.

Communicating with Professionalism

Remember, the first impression you make with patients in the exam room can be everlasting, as it can affect the way patients view the entire office's practice, including the physicians. As a medical assistant, communicating with professionalism is key. In addition to your awareness of patient rights, responsibilities, and privacy, your overall professionalism and poise can be a direct result of your verbal communication skills. If you use improper language skills, such as poor grammar or slang, or appear to have sloppy body language, you may give the patient the perception that you are not educated or intelligent. Your communication skills will have a direct impact on your career. Take care and pride in what you know and how you communicate. Think before you speak or react and you will learn to avoid communication pitfalls.

Interviewing Skills

To conduct a successful patient interview and obtain history and health information, you will need to apply a variety of skills, including the following:

- Using effective listening
- Being aware of nonverbal clues and body language
- Using a broad knowledge base
- Summarizing to form a general picture

Using Effective Listening Listening attentively is one of the most important skills you will need for a successful interview. When you listen to what the patient is saying, you not only listen for details but also try to get an overall view of the patient's situation. As you become more experienced in conducting patient interviews, these skills will improve. One way to be a good listener is to hear, think about, and respond to what the patient has said. This technique is called *active listening*. Passive listeners simply sit back and hear. When you are an active listener, you look at the patient, pay attention, and provide feedback. For example, you may use the technique of **restatement.** Simply repeat what the patient says, in your own words, back to the patient. This helps to ensure that you have understood the meaning of the patient's words.

Being Aware of Nonverbal Clues and Body Language Verbal communication is the asking and answering of questions. To conduct a successful interview, you also must be aware of nonverbal communication. The patient's tone of voice, facial expression, and body language are examples of nonverbal communication. These signs often communicate more than words could ever say. For example, a patient who has difficulty making eye contact may be embarrassed by some symptoms and may need your extra patience and encouragement to report symptoms fully. A child or adolescent may deny or exaggerate pain. Pay attention to the patient's facial expression and how much the patient guards the area in question.

Using a Broad Knowledge Base To conduct a successful interview, you must have a broad knowledge base so that you can ask questions that will elicit the most meaningful information about the patient. You must take every opportunity to expand your knowledge base by learning more about medical terminology, anatomy and physiology, symptoms, and diseases.

Summarizing to Form a General Picture You will gather a variety of subjective and objective data as you conduct a patient interview. You must consider the relative importance of each piece of information so that you can summarize the data to formulate a general picture of the patient. It is always

a good idea to repeat back a summary of information to the patient. This will ensure that all important data are recorded. Patients will sometimes forget to add something, and repeating the summary may jog their memory.

Interviewing Successfully

One of the main goals of the patient interview is to give the patient an opportunity to fully explain, in her own words, the reason for the current office visit. These eight steps will help you conduct a successful interview.

1. Do your research before the patient interview.
2. Plan the interview.
3. Approach the patient and request the interview.
4. Make the patient feel at ease.
5. Conduct the interview in private without interruptions.
6. Deal with sensitive topics with respect.
7. Do not diagnose or give a diagnostic opinion.
8. Formulate the general picture.

Doing Research Before the Patient Interview Before the interview, review the patient's medical record for history, medications, and chronic problems (for example, diabetes or high blood pressure). Note whether the patient has family problems that might have an impact on health issues. Make sure that all currently ordered diagnostic testing, laboratory work, and consultation results are in the chart. If you discover that you are missing a result, you have some time to retrieve it from the facility while the patient is in the office.

Planning the Interview Develop an interview plan by having a general idea of the questions you will ask. For example, if a patient is being treated for high blood pressure, you might ask about headaches or tinnitus (ringing in the ears), which are common signs of high blood pressure. Planning the interview helps you maintain your focus and ensures that you will obtain all the necessary information.

It is important to be organized before the interview takes place. Follow the office policies when gathering patient information. For example, you may record the patient's height, weight, and vital signs before you begin the interview. Make sure that you follow office policy on the types of information you will need to ask the patient during the interview. For example, some physicians prefer that you record the patient's medication list before the exam, whereas others prefer to record the medication list themselves. Planning for the types of information that you need to collect will save time for the visit itself.

Approaching the Patient and Requesting the Interview Ask the patient for permission before conducting the interview. You may need to explain that questions about the reason for the visit and the patient's current health situation are necessary to plan the most effective care. It is more courteous to seek permission to ask questions than to say that you "need to take a history." Asking permission helps the patient feel more comfortable and emphasizes the importance of the interview process. It also makes the patient feel more like a participant in the medical care being provided.

Making the Patient Feel at Ease Using certain words or phrases known as icebreakers can help set the stage for the interview. Icebreakers put the patient at ease and create a relaxed atmosphere. Examples of icebreakers include acknowledging the patient's reason for the visit, introducing yourself, and commenting about the weather. Icebreakers that also convey a sincere and sensitive interest in the patient are asking the patient how she prefers to be addressed and clarifying the pronunciation of a difficult name.

Another way to convey an image of a professional who is sensitive to the patient's needs is to sit with the patient and appear relaxed. By appearing relaxed, you help the patient relax and encourage a more open and comfortable interview. Eye contact is important when interviewing a patient. Sometimes patients will feel intimidated if they are forced to look up at you. If the patient sits in a chair, then it is best that you sit; if the patient sits on the examining table, then it is appropriate to stand while recording the visit. Remember, if you are entering data into an electronic record, there is a patient in the room with you. If you pay more attention to inputting information into the computer than looking at and speaking with your patient, she may feel as if she is just another patient and not an individual being cared for by you.

Conducting the Interview in Private Without Interruptions After setting the stage for the interview, ensure privacy by showing the patient to a private room or area or by closing the door if the patient is already in a private room. You can then begin to ask relevant questions. Some approaches are more effective than others, as shown in Table 36-1. Listening carefully to the patient's responses may lead you to ask questions other than those in your interview plan.

Developing a rapport with the patient is essential. Keep the atmosphere relaxed, do not rush, maintain eye contact, and

TABLE 36-1	Methods of Collecting Patient Data
Effective Methods	**Characteristics**
Asking open-ended questions	Requires more than a yes or no answer; allows the patient to more fully explain the situation, resulting in more relevant data. Instead of asking, "Do you have a cough?" ask, "Can you tell me about your symptoms?"
Asking hypothetical questions	Allows you to determine the patient's knowledge of the situation and whether it is accurate. For example, ask a patient who has been prescribed nitroglycerin for chest pain, "What would you do if you had chest pain?"
Mirroring patient's responses and verbalizing the implied	Allows nonthreatening ways for the patient to discuss the situation further and to provide underlying meaning. **Mirroring** means restating what the patient says almost exactly as the patient says it. **Verbalizing** means stating what you believe the patient is suggesting by his response. If the patient says, "I have been hurting for 3 days and it is just getting worse and worse. It hasn't quit all day," you might say, "So the pain started about 3 days ago and has been getting worse each day, and today it has not let up at all."
Focusing on patient	Shows the patient that you are really listening to what he is saying. You maintain eye contact (as culturally appropriate), assume a relaxed and open body posture, and use the proper responses.
Encouraging patient to take the lead	Motivates the patient to discuss or describe the situation in his own way. Ask a question such as "Where would you like to begin?"
Encouraging patient to provide additional information	Conveys sincere interest in the patient by continuing to explore topics in more detail when appropriate. You might ask the patient if he has experienced a symptom before or if he associates it with a change in routine. This provides for **clarification,** or increased understanding of the problem.
Encouraging patient to evaluate his situation	Provides an idea of the patient's point of view about the situation; allows you to determine the patient's knowledge of the situation and possible fears. Ask the patient, "What do you think is going on here?" This will allow you and the patient to use **reflection.** Reflection is when a thought, an idea, or an opinion is formed as a result of deeper thought, in this case stimulated by a question.
Ineffective Methods	**Characteristics**
Asking closed-ended questions	Provides little information because closed-ended questions offer the patient little freedom to explain his answers. Closed-ended questions require only yes or no answers.
Asking leading questions	Leading questions suggest a desired response instead of the patient's true response. The patient tends to agree with such statements instead of elaborating on them. An example of a leading question is "You seem to be making progress, don't you agree?" This type of question limits the patient's response.
Challenging patient	The patient may feel you are disagreeing with what he is saying if you ask an emotional or challenging question or use a certain tone of voice. The patient may become defensive, which might block further communication. An example of challenging the patient is "You are not having that much pain from this small wound, are you?"
Probing	Continuing to question a patient after he appears to have finished giving information can make him feel that you are invading his privacy. The patient may become defensive and withhold information.
Agreeing or disagreeing with patient	When you agree or disagree with a patient, it implies that the patient is either "right" or "wrong." This action can block further communication.

use the patient's name in conversation. Avoid interruptions, like taking phone calls and letting people walk in and out of the room. Make sure that you do not use "pet names" for your patients, such as "honey" or "sweetie." Doing so can offend some patients and can be misinterpreted as being insincere.

Dealing with Sensitive Topics with Respect Sometimes you will have to ask patients questions about sensitive topics. Such topics may be related to sexuality, lifestyle, or behaviors that put a person at risk for diseases. You must approach these topics gently so that the patient does not feel threatened by the questioning. You can show respect for the patient's rights and privacy by knowing when to stop. Both verbal and nonverbal clues can guide you in this area. It is also important to be conscious of your body language when dealing with sensitive subjects. You may find yourself exposed to situations that you do not have any experience with, and "shock" may register on your face.

Avoiding Making a Diagnosis or Giving a Diagnostic Opinion Only the physician can make a diagnosis, based on the patient's symptoms and complaints. If the patient asks for your opinion about a diagnosis, explain that the physician should be asked about diagnoses. If pressed, you may need to say you are not able to give opinions about a diagnosis and the physician will answer any questions he or she may have. Never go beyond your scope of practice or job description. Remember, your role as a medical assistant is to observe and report.

Formulating the General Picture Summarize the key points of the interview. Ask the patient whether he or she has questions or other information to add. You will be most successful with the interview process if you remain alert and organized but flexible. Procedure 36-1, at the end of the chapter, demonstrates the proper approach to an interview.

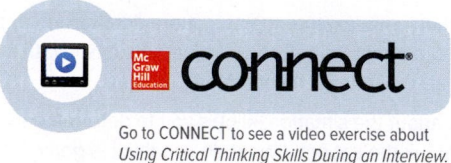

Go to CONNECT to see a video exercise about *Using Critical Thinking Skills During an Interview.*

▶ Your Role as an Observer   LO 36.2

During the pre-exam stage of the office visit, you will gather most of your information through verbal and nonverbal communication. The nonverbal communication that occurs during the interview and history taking, however, sometimes reveals more about a patient than the patient's words. Listening attentively and observing the patient closely may help you detect a problem that might otherwise go unnoted.

Anxiety

Anxiety is a common emotional response in patients. Some patients respond with anxiety to a specific fear, such as fear of pain. Others simply feel anxious when they are in an unfamiliar situation. For example, many patients have what is called "white coat syndrome," which is anxiety related to seeing a physician.

To recognize anxiety, you must understand that it varies from mild to severe. A patient with mild anxiety may have a heightened ability to observe and to make connections. A patient with severe anxiety has difficulty focusing on details, feels panicky, and is virtually helpless. Whether a patient has a heightened focus or a lack of focus, it can hinder your ability to get the information and cooperation you need. A patient may use an adaptive (helpful) or a non-adaptive (harmful) coping mechanism to relieve the anxiety. When you observe signs of anxiety in a patient, make every effort to help her use adaptive coping mechanisms such as deep breathing to help her relax and reduce the anxious feelings. You may be able to help by allowing the patient to describe her feelings. If a patient becomes agitated while discussing a physical complaint, you may need to postpone talking about the matter until the patient is calmer. In either situation, give support in nonverbal ways by trying to make the patient as comfortable as possible. Give the patient time to respond and then wait quietly, provide privacy, make eye contact, and communicate at the patient's level of understanding.

Depression

Depression can be difficult to recognize, as some of its symptoms are the same as those of many common illnesses. For example, fatigue and sleep disturbances are symptoms of both depression and hypothyroidism. To complicate matters, many patients with major depression develop great skill in hiding depression or are unaware they are suffering from it. Consequently, many patients—especially the elderly—have undiagnosed depression.

To recognize depression, you must be aware of common symptoms associated with the condition. Classic symptoms of depression are profound sadness and fatigue. In addition, a depressed person may have difficulty falling asleep at night or getting up in the morning. The depressed patient may suffer from loss of appetite, loss of energy, or both.

Depression seems to occur most frequently during late adolescence, in middle age, and after retirement. In late adolescence, depression can be difficult to distinguish from addiction and substance abuse. Depression in middle age is often triggered by life events like financial troubles or death of a family member. It is sometimes confused with midlife crises. And in the elderly, depression is common but often mistaken for senility. If you observe any signs of depression, indicate them in the patient's chart and alert the physician.

As mentioned in the previous paragraph, depression, addiction, and substance abuse in adolescents can be difficult to distinguish, as the signs of substance abuse or addiction can be mistaken for those of depression. The reverse is also true. And sometimes all three conditions exist simultaneously. If you have any clues that point to one of these conditions in an adolescent patient, notify the physician immediately. For symptoms that may be signs of these disorders, see the *Caution: Handle with Care* feature.

Physical and Psychological Abuse

Abuse can involve people from all walks of life and of all ages. Abuse can be physical, psychological, or both. As a medical assistant, you are in a unique position to detect abuse in the patients you see.

CAUTION: HANDLE WITH CARE

Signs of Depression, Substance Abuse, and Addiction in Adolescents

Signs of depression, substance abuse, and addiction are often hard to distinguish in adolescents. Part of the difficulty is that adolescents are particularly skilled at hiding signs of all three disorders.

Various signs may indicate depression in an adolescent. One teenager may lose interest in or be unable to enjoy everyday activities. Another may sleep for long periods and have difficulty getting up in the morning, whereas yet another may sleep very little. Chronic fatigue or aches and pains may signal depression, as may trouble with concentration or school absenteeism. These signs also may indicate substance abuse or addiction.

It is important to know the difference between substance abuse and addiction. **Substance abuse** refers to the use of a substance, even an over-the-counter drug, in a way that is not medically approved. Inappropriate use includes such practices as using diet pills to stay awake and consuming large quantities of cough syrup that contains codeine. It also includes taking larger-than-prescribed doses of a medication. Substance abusers are not necessarily addicts, however.

Addiction refers to a physical or psychological dependence on a substance. Addiction usually involves a pattern of behavior that includes an obsessive or compulsive preoccupation with a substance and the security of its supply, as well as a high rate of relapse after withdrawal.

As a medical assistant, you should not try to make a diagnosis. Quite likely, an adolescent with one or more of these disorders will be uncooperative and refuse to answer relevant questions. You must be aware, however, of physical signs or behaviors that may be associated with depression, substance abuse, or addiction in an adolescent patient. The following signs or behaviors are important clues that you should report immediately to the doctor.

- The patient complains of altered eating habits or disturbed sleep patterns (either too much or too little sleep).
- The patient's weight has changed drastically (either up or down) since the previous office visit.
- The patient appears lethargic or sullen, or exhibits radical mood changes.
- The patient has slurred speech.
- The patient appears to have illogical thought patterns.
- The patient appears to have needle tracks (anywhere on the body, especially on the arms or legs).
- The patient has pinpoint (highly constricted) pupils.

Although you must not make hasty judgments, you may suspect abuse when a patient speaks in a guarded way. An unlikely explanation for an injury also may be a sign of abuse. There may be no history of the injury, or the history may be suspicious. In either case, the following injuries may be signs of physical abuse:

- Head injuries and skull fractures
- Burns (especially those that appear to be deliberate, such as from a cigarette or an iron)
- Broken bones
- Bruises (especially multiple bruises, those that are clearly in the shape of an object, and those in various stages of healing)

Although a patient can recover physically from abuse, the emotional and psychological scars may last a lifetime. Other signs of physical abuse (including sexual abuse and neglect) and signs of psychological abuse include the following:

- A child's failure to thrive
- Severe dehydration or being underweight
- Delayed medical attention
- Hair loss
- Drug use
- Genital injuries

Women, children, and elderly patients are more likely to be abused. Pay extra attention to these patients when performing the interview. If you suspect abuse, report it to your supervisor or physician. Prepare a list of local abuse hotline numbers for potential abuse victims.

The Interview and Abuse

Again, because women, children, and the elderly are more likely to be victims of abuse, it is crucial to pay extra attention to them during the interview.

Women According to the Domestic Violence Resource Center, 85% of victims of domestic violence are women, and those ages 20 to 24 are at the greatest risk. Victims stay in abusive relationships for a variety of reasons, including fear of the abuser, threats of suicide by the abuser, financial dependence, lack of housing options, low self-esteem, and isolation. Women who are abused often feel shame. They may make excuses for their abuser or simply will not talk about it. It is important that you not be embarrassed to approach the subject of abuse with the patient. As with any other sensitive topic, you should not worry about embarrassing or insulting the patient by asking sensitive questions. Be kind, supportive, and nonjudgmental while interviewing a woman you suspect may be a victim of abuse. Careful listening and encouragement will build rapport with the patient, making the interview easier for the patient and more productive for you.

Children Children pose a unique situation during the patient interview. For infants and younger children, you will be asking the parent or other caregiver about the child's condition.

However, no matter what the age of the child, you should consider the child first. Communicate with the child, observe the child for nonverbal signs of pain or other problems, and ask questions whenever possible.

Remember, children are often the targets of violence, much of which occurs in the home. In addition to being physically, emotionally, or sexually abused, children can be abused by being neglected. In addition to watching for physical signs of abuse during the interview, watch for any problems in the relationship between the child and the caregiver. If you suspect a problem, report it to the physician.

The Elderly Physical and mental disabilities can make elderly people dependent on a caregiver. So elderly patients may or may not be able to communicate with you verbally during the patient interview. You may need to speak with their caregiver. However, always observe elderly patients for nonverbal signs of problems, such as grimacing, foul odors, or bruising, even if they cannot speak to you verbally. The caregiver may perceive the patient as a burden and abuse can occur. Disabilities may make the elderly person defenseless against abuse. If you suspect a problem, report it to the physician.

Drug and Alcohol Abuse

Substance abuse and addiction to drugs or alcohol are serious social problems. Individuals often use drugs or alcohol as a non-adaptive coping mechanism to relieve anxiety or emotional pain. Symptoms of substance abuse or addiction differ from drug to drug, as indicated in Table 36-2. Addiction, however, typically causes a gradual decline in the quality of someone's work or relationships. The patient may behave erratically, have frequent mood changes, suffer from loss of appetite, and be constantly tired.

Someone who is abusing alcohol may have no apparent signs or symptoms at first. As time goes on, however, that person may suffer from blackouts (failure to remember what happened while drinking) or may become secretive and guilty about drinking and deny that there is a problem. She may suffer from bruises she does not remember getting, trembling hands, or chronic stomach problems. Even though the patient may feel she does not have a substance abuse or addiction problem, healthcare team members may recognize a problem. When this occurs, their job is to try to persuade the patient to seek help.

▶ Documenting Patient Information LO 36.3

Whenever you interview a patient, keep in mind that the patient chart is a legal document. The chart can be used as evidence in a court of law, so you must meet certain guidelines when recording data.

TABLE 36-2	Symptoms Associated with Commonly Abused Drugs	
Drug Names/Type	**Trade or Other Name**	**Symptoms, Effects**
Amphetamines/stimulants	Benzedrine, Dexedrine®, methamphetamine, beans, black beauty, speed, uppers, uppies	Altered mental status, from confusion to paranoia; hyperactivity, then exhaustion; insomnia; loss of appetite
Anabolic steroids	Anadrol®, Depo®-testosterone, roids, juice	Irritability, aggression, nervousness, male-pattern baldness
Barbiturates/sedatives	Amobarbital, phenobarbital, Butisol®, secobarbital, yellow jackets, red birds	Slowed thinking, slowed reflexes, slowed respiration, loss of anxiety
Benzodiazepines/sedatives	Ativan®, diazepam, Librium®, Valium®, downers, candy	Poor coordination, drowsiness, increased self-confidence
Cocaine/stimulant	Coke, snow, crack	Alternating euphoria and apprehension, intense craving for more of the drug
Ecstasy/psychoactive	Adam, XTC, MDMA	Confusion, depression, anxiety, paranoia, increased heart rate and blood pressure
GHB/depressants	G, liquid ecstasy, Georgia homeboy	Slow pulse and breathing, lowered blood pressure, drowsiness, poor concentration
Heroin	Big H, black tar, dope, nanoo, nickel deck, smack	Track marks, slowed or slurred speech, vomiting
Inhalants	Solvents: paint thinner Gases: aerosol, butane, or propane	Stimulation, intoxication, hearing loss, arm or leg spasms
LSD (lysergic acid diethylamine)/hallucinogen	Acid, battery acid, microdot	Heightened sense of awareness, grandiose hallucinations, mystical experiences, flashbacks
Marijuana/cannabinoids/hashish	Pot, grass, joints, reefer, weed, chronic, Mary Jane, hash, boom	Altered thought processes, distorted sense of time and self, impaired short-term memory
Opium, morphine, codeine/opiate narcotics	Monkey, white stuff	Decreased level of consciousness, detachment, drowsiness, impaired judgment
PCP (phencyclidine)/hallucinogen	Angel dust, angel mist, hog, rocket fuel, DOA, peace pill	Decreased awareness of surroundings, hallucinations, poor perception of time and distance, possible overdose and death

The Six Cs of Charting

To help ensure that you record patient data accurately, you must follow the six Cs of charting. These guidelines are as follows:

1. *Client's words* must be recorded exactly. The doctor may uncover clues to use in diagnosing the patient's condition. Place quotation marks to indicate what the patient said.

2. *Clarity* is essential when you describe the patient's condition. You must use medical terminology and precise descriptions.

3. *Completeness* is required on all the forms used in the patient record.

4. *Conciseness* can save time and space when you are recording information.

5. *Chronological order* and dates on all entries in patient records are critical in the documentation of patient care. This information also can be used for legal questions regarding medical services. Most charts are arranged with the most recent information on top. This type of charting is known as *reverse chronological order*.

6. *Confidentiality* is essential to protect the patient's privacy. You cannot discuss a patient's records, forward them to another office, fax them, or show them to anyone except the doctor unless the patient gives you written permission to do so. The only exception is when the records must be sent to ensure continuity of care of the patient and the patient is unable to grant permission.

Contents of Patient Charts

In most medical offices, patient records are electronic. Whether they are electronic or paper, all records must contain the following standard information:

- The patient registration form contains general information, including the date of the patient's current visit, and generally lists the patient's age, address, medical insurance, occupation, education, racial or ethnic background, marital status, number of children, and nearest relative. There is a section that allows the patient to indicate his or her preference about telephone contact, such as leaving messages, or relaying information to designated family members or friends. Some medical offices also use e-mail to communicate with patients. Make sure the patient understands the privacy information section and chooses the appropriate action.

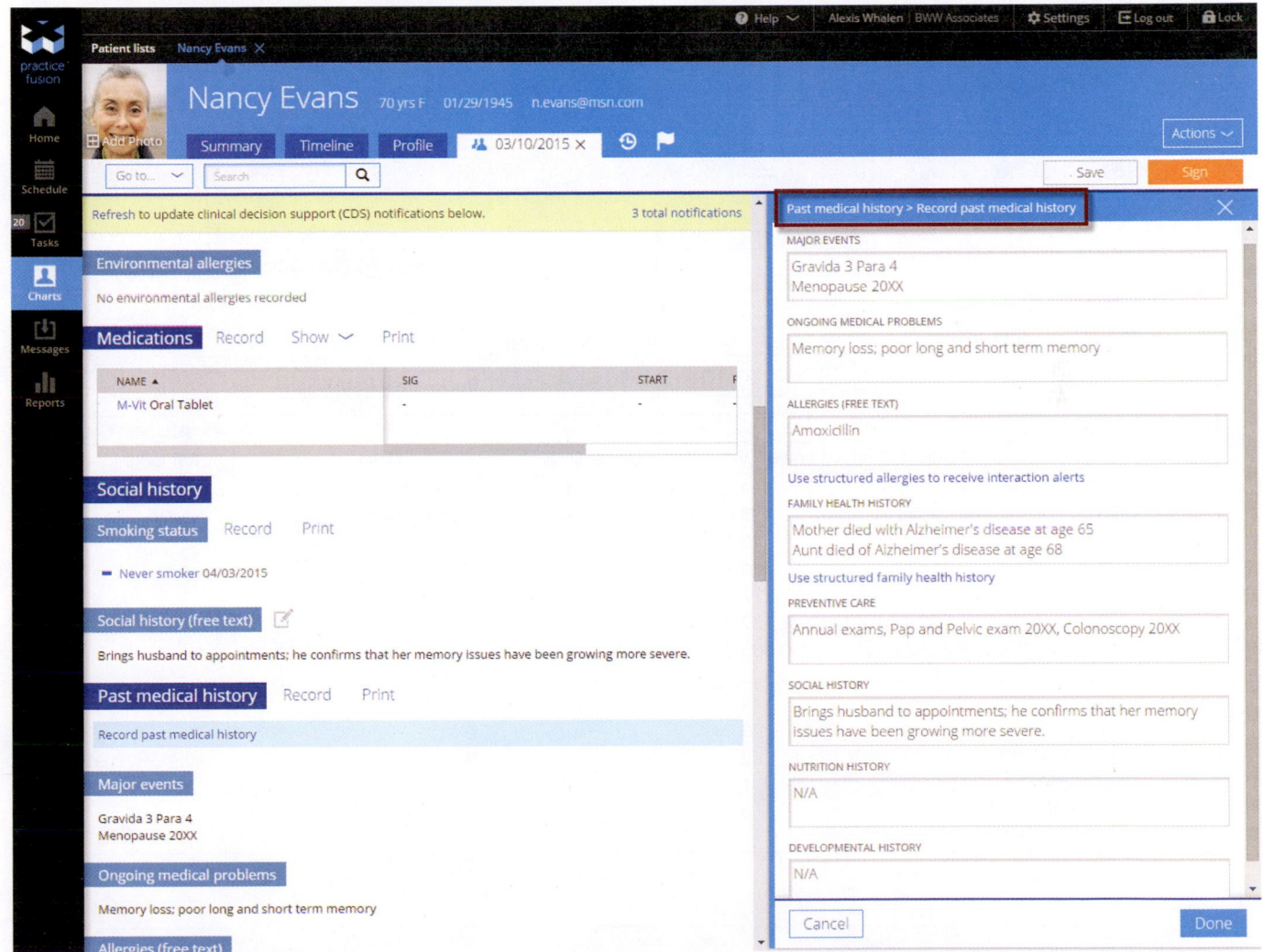

FIGURE 36-1 Medical history forms in an electronic health record, like this one from Practice Fusion®, allow you to select, enter, or delete items based upon your patient interview.

© Practice Fusion®

- Patient medical history usually includes the chief complaint, history of the present illness, past medical history (including medical treatment, surgeries, known allergies, and current medications), family history, and social and occupational history (including diet, exercise, smoking, and use of alcohol or drugs). This section also may be used to record the results of a general physical exam. See Figure 36-1 for one example.
- Test results include those performed in the office and those received from other physicians, hospitals, or independent laboratories. Physicians may have tests run on a patient's blood, urine, or tissue samples to aid in their diagnoses. Figure 36-2 shows examples of laboratory reports of a panel of chemical tests on blood performed by an outside laboratory.
- Records from other physicians or hospitals are accompanied by a copy of the patient's written authorization to release the records.
- The physician's diagnosis and treatment plan are specific and detailed.
- Operative reports include a record of all procedures, surgeries, follow-up care, and additional notes the physician makes

regarding the patient's case. Continuation forms can be used for additional information. Some medical offices also keep a separate log of telephone calls to and from the patient.
- Informed consent forms verify that the patient has understood the treatment offered and the possible outcomes or side effects of it. The patient signs the consent form but may withdraw consent if she decides to change or discontinue treatment.
- A discharge summary form is used when a patient is hospitalized. This form includes information that summarizes the reason the patient entered the hospital; tests, procedures, or operations performed in the hospital; medications administered; and the disposition, or outcome, of the case.
- Correspondence with or about the patient is marked or stamped with the date the physician's office received the document.

When recording information in the patient chart, be sure to date and initial every entry. This documentation makes it easy to tell which items you entered into the chart and which items others entered. The physician usually initials reports before they are filed to prove that she saw them.

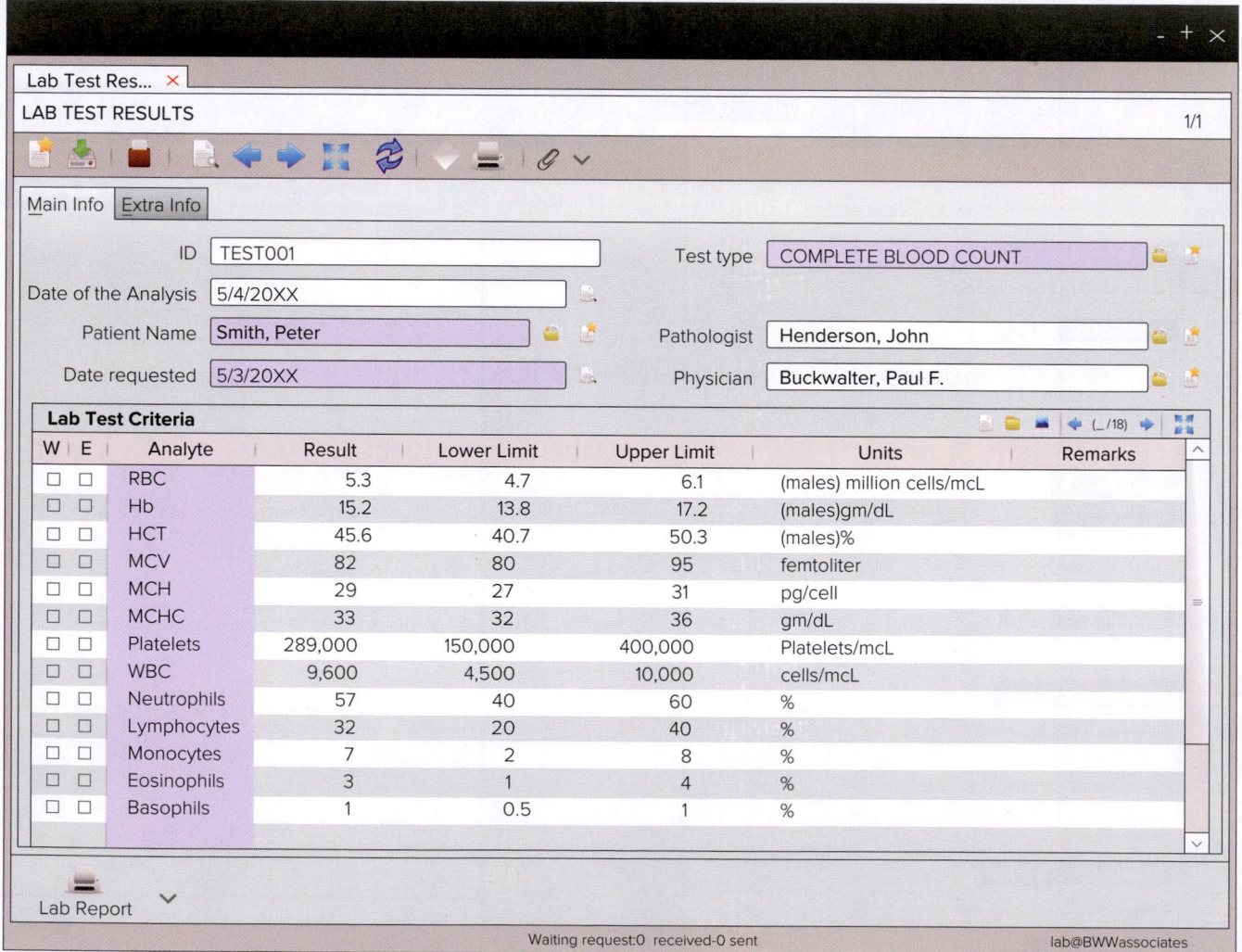

(a)

FIGURE 36-2   Laboratory reports (a) EHR laboratory reports includes normal ranges appropriate for the laboratory's testing procedures.

John Miller	09/12/XX	09/12/XX	09/13/XX
Patient Name	Date Drawn	Date Received	Date of Report
Sex **M** Age **65**	Alexis N. Whalen, MD BWW Medical Associates, PC 305 Main Street Port Snead, YZ 12345-9876	**23341** ID Number	**67294** Account Number
166241809 Patient ID, Soc. Sec. Number			**897211** Specimen Number

Test name	Result Abnormal	Result Normal	Units	Reference range
Chem-screen panel				
Glucose		76.0	MG/DL	65.0–115
Sodium		139.0	MMOL/L	134–143
Potassium		4.00	MMOL/L	3.60–5.10
Chloride		107.0	MMOL/L	96.0–107
BUN		17.0	MG/DL	6.00–19.0
BUN/creatinine ratio		14.2		
Uric acid		4.30	MG/DL	2.20–6.20
Phosphate		2.40	MG/DL	2.40–4.50
Calcium		9.50	MG/DL	6.60–10.0
Magnesium		1.75	MEG/L	1.40–2.00
Cholesterol	237.0		MG/DL	130–200
Chol. percentile	90.0		PERCENTILE	1.00–75.0
HDL cholesterol	41.0		MG/DL	48.0–89.0
Chol./HDL ratio		5.80		
LDL Chol., calculated	175.0		MG/DL	65.5–130
Triglycerides		104.0	MG/DL	00.0–200
Total protein		6.60	GM/DL	6.40–8.00
Albumin		4.10	GM/DL	3.70–4.80
Globulin		2.50	GM/DL	2.20–3.60
Alb/glob ratio		1.64		1.10–2.10
Total bilirubin		0.60	MG/DL	0.20–1.30
Direct bilirubin		0.15	MG/DL	0.00–0.20
Alk. phosphatase		44.0	UNITS/L	25.0–125
G-glutamyl transpep		8.00	UNITS/L	1.00–63.0
AST (SGOT)		21.0	IU/L	1.00–40.0
ALT (SGPT)		14.0	IU/L	1.00–50.0
LD		134.0	IU/L	90.0–250
Iron		130.0	MCG/DL	35.0–180

(b)

FIGURE 36-2 Laboratory reports (b) Laboratory results paper reports also include normal ranges. All laboratory reports provide valuable information about patients' health.

Methods of Charting

Various methods of charting are used on the medical record. Most methods are based on a series of steps to document the information. These steps are referred to as the SOAP method of documentation (Figure 36-3). Understanding the parts of SOAP will help you document information in a logical manner.

1. *Subjective data.* You obtain **subjective data** from conversation with the patient or an attending family member. Subjective data include thoughts, feelings, and perceptions, including the chief complaint. Such data are based on the patient's interpretation and opinion. They are not measurable by an outside observer; however, you should remember that they are real to the patient. An example of subjective

OUTLINE FORMAT PROGRESS NOTES

Patient Name Chen / Cindy / M.   Date of Birth 07 / 15 / XX Chart # H234
Last — First — Middle

Prob. No. or Letter	Date	Subjective	Objective	Assess	Plans
	6/16/XX	Patient complaining of pain in lower right quadrant. Has been running fever of between 100.5° F and 101.3° F since Sunday morning. Has queasy feeling in stomach and has been unable to eat since yesterday morning.			
			BP 125/75. Temperature 101.2° F. Abdominal exam revealed rebound tenderness and distension in lower right quadrant.		
				Appendicitis	
					1. Admit to hospital
					2. Surgically remove appendix.

Signature Paul F. Buckwalter, MD

Start each progress note (Subjective, Objective, Assessment, and Plans) at the appropriate shaded column to create an outline form. Write through the intervening columns to the right margin of the page.

© 1976 BIBBERO SYSTEMS, INC., PETALUMA, CA

TO REORDER CALL TOLL FREE: (800)BIBBERO (800 242-2376)
FORM # 26-7215-01

PROGRESS NOTES

FIGURE 36-3 When you use the SOAP approach to documenting patient information, start each progress note at the appropriate shaded column to create an outline form. Write through the intervening columns to the right margin of the page.
Reprinted with permission from Bibbero Systems, Inc., An InHealth Company, Petaluma, CA (800) 242–2376, www.bibbero.com.

information is the patient's statement about his or her chief complaint: "I have an itchy, red rash on my left hand that I noticed 3 days ago." The patient states that the rash is itchy; since itchiness cannot be observed or measured by the physician, it is considered subjective. The chief complaint should always be recorded in the patient's own words.

2. *Objective data.* **Objective data** are readily apparent and measurable, such as vital signs, test results, and the physician's exam. An example of objective data is the examination of the rash by the physician.

3. *Assessment.* Assessment is the physician's diagnosis or impression of the patient's problem.

4. *Plan of action.* Options for treatment, the type of treatment chosen, medications, tests, consultations, patient education, and follow-up are included in a plan of action. The plan of action may include an order for injection or other treatment that you as the medical assistant will need to perform.

The following are three common methods for maintaining notes on a patient chart:

1. Conventional or source-oriented medical records (SOMR). Information is arranged according to who supplied the data or the source. This could be the patient, the doctor, a specialist, or someone else. The medical form may have a space for patient remarks followed by a section for the doctor's comment.

2. Problem-oriented medical records (POMR). This method is used more extensively by large clinics or practices that may have more than one physician who may see the same patient. POMR includes a problem list that is dated, and numbers are assigned to each patient condition or problem. At the patient's initial visit, conditions or problems are identified by a number throughout the record until the problem is resolved. The POMR has four components:

- *Database.* This includes the patient's medical history, diagnostic and laboratory results, and physical exam reports. This is the foundation of the problem-oriented medical record.

- *Problem list.* Each patient condition or problem is listed individually, assigned a number, and dated.

- *Diagnostic and treatment plan.* Laboratory and other diagnostic tests are completed and the physician's treatment plan for the condition is documented.

- *Progress notes.* The physician enters notes on every condition or problem recorded on the problem list. Progress notes are entered chronologically and include

TABLE 36-3　Common Medical Abbreviations

Abortion	Ab	Headache	HA
Abnormal	Abnl	History of	H/O
Antibiotics	Abx	History and physical	H & P
Against medical advice	AMA	Hypertension	HTN
As much as possible	AMAP	Left	L
Awake and oriented	A&O	Right	R
Both	B	Low back pain	LBP
Biopsy	BX	Low birth weight	LBW
Childhood diseases	CHD	Last menstrual period	LMP
Complains of	C/O	No known allergies	NKA
Cause of death	COD	Packs per day	PPD
Chest X-ray	CXR	Rule out	R/O
Date of birth	DOB	Range of motion	ROM
Date of conception	DOC	Shortness of breath	SOB
Diagnosis	Dx	Sudden unexplained/ unexpected death	SUD
Digital rectal exam	DRE	Seizure	Sz
Estimated delivery date	EDD	Tonsillectomy and adenoidectomy	T & A
Follow-up	F/U	Years old	Y/O
Fracture	FX	Within normal limits	WNL
Growth and development	G & D		

the chief complaint, problems, conditions, treatments, and responses to treatment.

3. Computerized medical records. This method uses a combination of SOMR and POMR but provides accessibility by the physician or other healthcare workers at any time from a computer terminal. This accessibility enhances the patient's continuity of care between departments and specialty physicians in other practices because everyone is looking at the same record.

Common Chart Terminology and Abbreviations

Most of the information that you collect verbally from a patient will be documented in the patient's medical record. Table 36-3 lists some of the most common abbreviations used in the medical chart. Abbreviations used must be accepted by the facility where you are employed as well as The Joint Commission (TJC).

The Joint Commission (TJC) and the Institute for Safe Medication Practice (ISMP) are two healthcare organizations whose mission includes promotion of patient safety. These organizations have identified frequently misinterpreted abbreviations, acronyms, and symbols that have contributed to harmful medical errors. TJC, in 2005, published the *Official "Do Not Use" List*, a standardized list of abbreviations, acronyms, and symbols that are not to be used. See Table 36-4. The ISMP publishes the more comprehensive *ISMP's List of Error-Prone Abbreviations, Symbols, and Dose Designations,*

which is updated periodically. This list includes all of the abbreviations on TJC's "Do Not Use" list, denoting them with a double asterisk (**). It is found at http://www.ismp.org/tools/abbreviations/. Although you may see some of these on preprinted order sheets, *do not use* the error-prone abbreviations when charting.

▶ Recording the Patient's Medical History　LO 36.4

A patient's medical history includes pertinent information about the patient and the patient's family. Age, previous illnesses, surgical history, allergies, medication history, and family medical history are key items.

When recording a patient history, you must do more than just fill out the form (Figure 36-4). You must review the pieces of information, organize them, determine their importance, and document the facts. When you write your first histories, you may find it to be a lengthy process. When you become more experienced, however, you will be able to write histories more quickly. Whenever you write information on the chart, you must consider its completeness and accuracy. First determine the chief complaint, or the main reason for the patient visit. For example, the patient may have a rash or pain. Then ask more questions. A good interview technique is the "PQRST" interview technique. It will help you remember the types of questions that are appropriate for the condition. Each letter stands for a word that will remind you to ask more specific questions about the chief complaint or problem the patient is having:

P: Provoke or Palliative

Q: Quality or Quantity

R: Region or Radiation

S: Severity Scale

T: Timing

See Table 36-5 for questions and charting examples using the PQRST interview technique.

You will need to chart other information prior to the physician visit. Figure 36-5b shows a form used by the medical assistant and the licensed practitioner when seeing a patient. When keying information in an electronic record, it is just as important to correctly type the information into the record. Pay special attention to spelling when entering data into the chart or electronic record. If you do not know how to spell a word, look it up. Use only TJC-approved and office-recognized abbreviations (see Tables 36-3 and 36-4). Many facilities have a document identifying these abbreviations. Electronic health records often use drop-down menus with common medical information provided. Take care to click the correct box when using drop-down menus. Remember, the chart is a legal document, so special attention to detail is required when charting.

The Progress Note

Many offices use a variation of the progress note for established patients who are seen for routine visits or follow-ups like hypertension, arthritis, or flu (see Figures 36-3 and 36-5).

TABLE 36-4 TJC "Do Not Use" Abbreviations, Acronyms, and Symbols

Abbreviation	Potential Problem	Preferred Term
U (for unit)	Mistaken as zero, four, or cc.	Write "unit."
IU (for international unit)	Mistaken as IV (intravenous) or 10 (ten).	Write "international unit."
Q.D., QD, qd, q.d., Q.O.D., QOD, q.o.d, qod (Latin abbreviation for once daily and every other day)	Mistaken for each other. The period after the Q can be mistaken for an "I" and the "O" can be mistaken for "I."	Write "daily" and "every other day."
Trailing zero (X.0 mg), lack of leading zero (.X mg) except when trailing zero is used to indicate a level of precision when reporting a lab value	Decimal point is missed.	Never write a zero by itself after a decimal point (X mg), and always use a zero before a decimal point (0.X mg) when writing medication documentation.
MS MSO$_4$ MgSO$_4$	Confused for one another. Can mean morphine sulfate or magnesium sulfate.	Write "morphine sulfate" or "magnesium sulfate."
Other Abbreviations, Acronyms, and Symbols to Avoid		
μg (for microgram)	Mistaken for mg (milligrams), resulting in one-thousand-fold dosing overdose.	Write "mcg."
c.c. (for cubic centimeter)	Mistaken for U (units) when poorly written.	Write "mL" for milliliters.
> (greater than) < (less than)	Misinterpreted as the number "7" or the letter "L"; confused for one another.	Write "greater than" and "less than."
Abbreviations for drug names	Misinterpreted due to similar abbreviations for multiple drugs.	Write drug names in full.
Apothecary units	Unfamiliar to many practitioners. Confused with metric units.	Use metric units.
@	Mistaken for the number "2" (two).	Write "at."
H.S. (for half-strength or Latin abbreviation for bedtime)	Mistaken for either half-strength or hour of sleep (at bedtime). qH.S. mistaken for every hour. All can result in a dosing error.	Write out "half-strength" or "at bedtime."
T.I.W. (for three times a week)	Mistaken for three times a day or twice weekly, resulting in an overdose.	Write "3 times weekly" or "three times weekly."
S.C. or S.Q. (for subcutaneous)	Mistaken as SL for sublingual, or "5 every."	Write "Sub-Q," "subQ," or "subcutaneously."
D/C (for discharge)	Interpreted as discontinue whatever medications follow (typically discharge meds).	Write "discharge."
A.S., A.D., A.U. (Latin abbreviation for left, right, or both ears) O.S., O.D., O.U. (Latin abbreviation for left, right, or both eyes)	Mistaken for each other (such as AS for OS, AD for OD, AU for OU, etc.).	Write "left ear," "right ear," or "both ears"; "left eye," "right eye," or "both eyes."

The medical history form is primarily used for new patients the physician is seeing for the first time. The following are some important guidelines to consider when using a progress note:

- It must be arranged in reverse chronological order.
- Every entry must be initialed and signed by the person making the entry. Typically, the first initial, last name, and credentials are used—for example, K. Haddix, RMA (AMT).
- Entries most commonly made on progress notes include documentation for prescription refills, follow-up visits, telephone conversations with patients, appointment cancellations or no shows, and referrals and consultation efforts made by the office for the patient.

- The patient name must be recorded on every progress note along with any other identifying information such as birth date or chart number.
- All entries must be dated. All entries typically include the time and must always include the date.

Procedure 36-2, at the end of this chapter, will guide you in how to use a progress note.

Polypharmacy

Many patients will take a variety of medications to treat several conditions, such as hypertension, elevated cholesterol, and diabetes. Some patients take several medications for the same condition, with each one treating a different aspect of the condition. The chapters *Principles of Pharmacology* and

HEALTH HISTORY
(Confidential)

Name _____ Birthdate _____ Today's Date _____

Age _____ Date of last physical examination _____

What is your reason for visit? _____

SYMPTOMS Check (✓) symptoms you currently have or have had in the past year.

GENERAL
- Chills
- Depression
- Dizziness
- Fainting
- Fever
- Forgetfulness
- Headache
- Loss of sleep
- Loss of weight
- Nervousness
- Numbness
- Sweats

MUSCLE/JOINT/BONE
Pain, weakness, numbness in:
- Arms
- Back
- Feet
- Hands
- Hips
- Legs
- Neck
- Shoulders

GENITO-URINARY
- Blood in urine
- Frequent urination
- Lack of bladder control
- Painful urination

GASTROINTESTINAL
- Appetite poor
- Bloating
- Bowel changes
- Constipation
- Diarrhea
- Excessive hunger
- Excessive thirst
- Gas
- Hemorrhoids
- Indigestion
- Nausea
- Rectal bleeding
- Stomach pain
- Vomiting
- Vomiting blood

CARDIOVASCULAR
- Chest pain
- High blood pressure
- Irregular heart beat
- Low blood pressure
- Poor circulation
- Rapid heart beat
- Swelling of ankles
- Varicose veins

EYE, EAR, NOSE, THROAT
- Bleeding gums
- Blurred vision
- Crossed eyes
- Difficulty swallowing
- Double vision
- Earache
- Ear discharge
- Hay fever
- Hoarseness
- Loss of hearing
- Nosebleeds
- Persistent cough
- Ringing in ears
- Sinus problems
- Vision – Flashes
- Vision – Halos

SKIN
- Bruise easily
- Hives
- Itching
- Change in moles
- Rash
- Scars
- Sore that won't heal

MEN only
- Breast lump
- Erection difficulties
- Lump in testicles
- Penis discharge
- Sore on penis
- Other

WOMEN only
- Abnormal Pap smear
- Bleeding between periods
- Breast lump
- Extreme menstrual pain
- Hot flashes
- Nipple discharge
- Painful intercourse
- Vaginal discharge
- Other

Date of last menstrual period _____

Date of last Pap smear _____

Have you had a mammogram? _____

Are you pregnant? _____

Number of children _____

CONDITIONS Check (✓) conditions you have or have had in the past.

- AIDS
- Alcoholism
- Anemia
- Anorexia
- Appendicitis
- Arthritis
- Asthma
- Bleeding Disorders
- Breast Lump
- Bronchitis
- Bulimia
- Cancer
- Cataracts
- Chemical Dependency
- Chickenpox
- Diabetes
- Emphysema
- Epilepsy
- Glaucoma
- Goiter
- Gonorrhea
- Gout
- Heart Disease
- Hepatitis
- Hernia
- Herpes
- High Cholesterol
- HIV Positive
- Kidney Disease
- Liver Disease
- Measles
- Migraine Headaches
- Miscarriage
- Mononucleosis
- Multiple Sclerosis
- Mumps
- Pacemaker
- Pneumonia
- Polio
- Prostate Problem
- Psychiatric Care
- Rheumatic Fever
- Scarlet Fever
- Stroke
- Suicide Attempt
- Thyroid Problems
- Tonsillitis
- Tuberculosis
- Typhoid Fever
- Ulcers
- Vaginal Infections
- Venereal Disease

MEDICATIONS List medications you are currently taking

ALLERGIES To medications or substances

Pharmacy Name _____ Phone _____

(All information is strictly confidential)

FAMILY HISTORY Fill in health information about your family.

Relation	Age	State of Health	Age at Death	Cause of Death	Check (✓) if your blood relatives had any of the following: Disease	Relationship to You
Father					Arthritis, Gout	
Mother					Asthma, Hay Fever	
Brothers					Cancer	
					Chemical Dependency	
					Diabetes	
Sisters					Heart Disease, Strokes	
					High Blood Pressure	
					Kidney Disease	
					Tuberculosis	
					Other	

HOSPITALIZATIONS

Year	Hospital	Reason for Hospitalization and Outcome

PREGNANCY HISTORY

Year of Birth	Sex of Birth	Complications if any

Have you ever had a blood transfusion? ☐ Yes ☐ No
If yes, please give approximate dates. _____

SERIOUS ILLNESS/INJURIES

	DATE	OUTCOME

HEALTH HABITS Check (✓) which substances you use and describe how much you use.
- Caffeine
- Tobacco
- Drugs
- Other

OCCUPATIONAL CONCERNS Check (✓) if your work exposes you to the following:
- Stress
- Hazardous Substances
- Heavy Lifting
- Other

Your occupation: _____

I certify that the above information is correct to the best of my knowledge. I will not hold my doctor or any members of his/her staff responsible for any errors or omissions that I may have made in the completion of this form.

Signature _____ Date _____

Reviewed By _____ Date _____

FIGURE 36-4 The health history form must be complete and accurate. The patient should start the form and the medical assistant should check and complete it.

TABLE 36-5   Example Questions When Using the PQRST Interview Technique

PQRST Interview Technique	Chief Complaint: *Itching/Rash Under Arms*	Chief Complaint: *Pain in the Left Shoulder*	Chief Complaint: *Persistent Cough*
P: Provoke or Palliative	• What causes the itching to occur? • Does anything make the itching go away?	• When did you first notice the pain? • Is there anything you do that reduces the pain?	• When is the cough worse? Morning? Night? • Is there anything that relieves the cough? Aggravates it?
Q: Quality or Quantity	• How severe is the rash/itching? • How often does the itching occur?	• Can you describe the pain: dull, aching, burning, or sharp? • When does the pain occur?	• Is the cough productive or nonproductive? • Are you coughing anything up? If so, does it have any color? • Do you have pain when you cough?
R: Region or Radiation	• Where is the itching/rash?	• Where do you feel the pain? • Does the pain move from one location to another?	• Is the pain on one side or both? • Does the pain radiate?
S: Severity Scale	• Is the rash/itching interfering with your daily life?	• Is the area red or tender to the touch? • Is there any swelling? • Rate the pain on a scale of 1 to 10, with 10 being the worst. (See Figure 36-6.)	• Rate the pain on a scale of 1 to 10, with 10 being the worst. • Does the cough disturb your sleep?
T: Timing	• When did you first notice the rash/itching?	• How long have you had the pain? • Is the pain intermittent or continuous? • How long does the pain last?	• Does the cough come in bouts or fits or is it continuous? • How long have you had the cough?

Medication Administration provide detailed information regarding various medications. During the patient interview, it is important to document medications the patient is currently taking. The patient will often see several physicians or specialists, and it is important for your office to be up to date on the treatments a patient is receiving. This reduces the likelihood of polypharmacy or unnecessarily repeating medical tests.

Some offices may use a medication flowsheet for the physicians to record patient medication histories. In some cases, the medical assistant gathers the information for the current medication flowsheet (see Figure 36-7). A helpful hint for organizing this task is to develop a form or card for the patient to use (if the office does not already have a form) and gather the initial medication history. Then instruct the patient to use the list and to have it updated by the other physicians whom he or she sees. A drug reference guide or the Internet will assist you with the spelling of medications.

The Health History Form

The medical office usually has a standard medical history form that is used for all patients. The specific arrangement and wording of items on this form, however, may vary from office to office. The following sections contain brief descriptions of each of the parts of this form. Procedure 36-3, at the end of this chapter, will assist in your practice of obtaining medical histories.

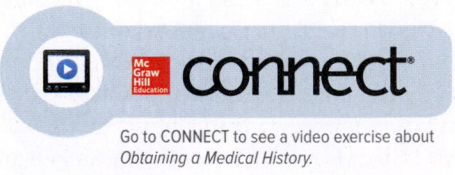

Go to CONNECT to see a video exercise about *Obtaining a Medical History.*

Personal Data This information is obtained from the administrative sheet and includes the patient's name, birth date, and other basic data.

Chief Complaint Abbreviated as CC, the chief complaint is the reason the patient came to visit the practitioner. It should be short and specific and should cover subjective and/or objective data stated by the patient.

History of Present Illness This history includes detailed information about the chief complaint, including when the problem started and what the patient has done to treat the problem (including any medications taken). For example, a chief complaint might be "sore throat" and the history of the present illness would include when the sore throat started (such as 3 days ago), how severe the pain is on a scale of 1 to 10 (such as pain scale rating of 6 out of 10), and what treatments have been used (such as throat lozenges and four to six aspirin daily).

Past Medical History The past medical history includes any and all health problems both present and past, including major illnesses and surgery. The past medical history also includes important information about medications and allergies. It should list any medications taken by the patient, including their dosages and the reasons for taking them. Over-the-counter and herbal medications should be listed as well. Known or suspected allergies to medications or other substances should be listed and clearly visible. Some facilities use a red sticker or other means on charts to identify allergies immediately. Most electronic health record programs

BWW

BWW Medical Associates, PC
305 Main Street, Port Snead YZ 12345-9876
Tel: 555-654-3210, Fax: 555-987-6543
Web: BWWAssociates.com

Paul F. Buckwalter, MD
Alexis N. Whalen, MD
Elizabeth H. Williams, MD

PROGRESS NOTES

Name _____Cindy Chen_____ Chart # ___01769___

DATE	
10/12/XX	Patient c/o headache and cough X 3 days. HA is dull ache, pain scale 7/10
	cough — nonproductive. ———————— Kaylyn Haddix RMA (AMT)

(a)

Name _____Cindy Chen_____ DOB __07/15/XX__ Date __08/28/XX__
ALLERGIES ___NKA___

Review of Systems

Systems	NL	Note	Systems	NL	Note
Constitutional			Musculoskeletal		
Eyes			Skin/breasts		
ENT/mouth			Neurologic		
Cardiovascular			Psychiatric		
Respiratory			Endocrine		
GI			Hem/lymph		
GU			Allergy/immun		

Current Medicines	Date	Current Diagnosis
ClaritinD PRN		
MVI †qd		
Ortho Novum 7/7/7		
†qd		

Note

H: _5'7"_ W: _140_ T: _97.8_ P: _88_ R: _20_
B/P Sitting _122/78_ or Standing _____Supine _____

Last Tetanus _06/12/XX_
L.M.P. _08/20/XX_

O2 Sat: _98%_
Pain Scale: _6/10_

Social Habits	Yes	No
Tobacco		✓
Alcohol	✓	
Rec. Drugs		✓

CC: (L) shoulder pain X 3 days due to fall.
"sharp pain that hurts when I move"

HPI:

(b)

FIGURE 36-5 These forms are completed by the medical assistant prior to the physician visit. All information must be complete and accurate. (a) Progress note. (b) Medical visit form.

automatically run drug allergy and drug-drug interaction checks. If you are entering medication data into an EHR program that does not have this feature, make sure you flag patient drug allergies according to office policy.

Family History This section includes information about the health of the patient's family members. Many times, the family history can help lead a practitioner to the cause of a current medical problem. Obtain specific information about family members' current ages and medical conditions or, if deceased, their age at death and the cause. Ask open-ended questions about the siblings, parents, and grandparents. Because the death of a parent or sibling or the limited knowledge of an adopted child can be difficult to discuss, use great care and sensitivity when asking these questions.

Social and Occupational History Information like marital status, sexual behaviors and orientation, occupations, hobbies, and the use of chemical substances helps determine a patient's risk for disease. Patients should be asked about their use of alcohol, tobacco, recreational drugs, or other chemical substances. Be aware that patients may feel uncomfortable

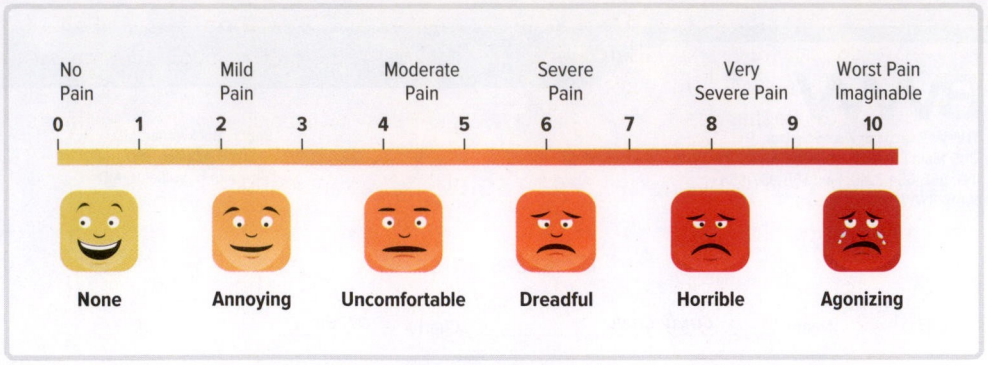

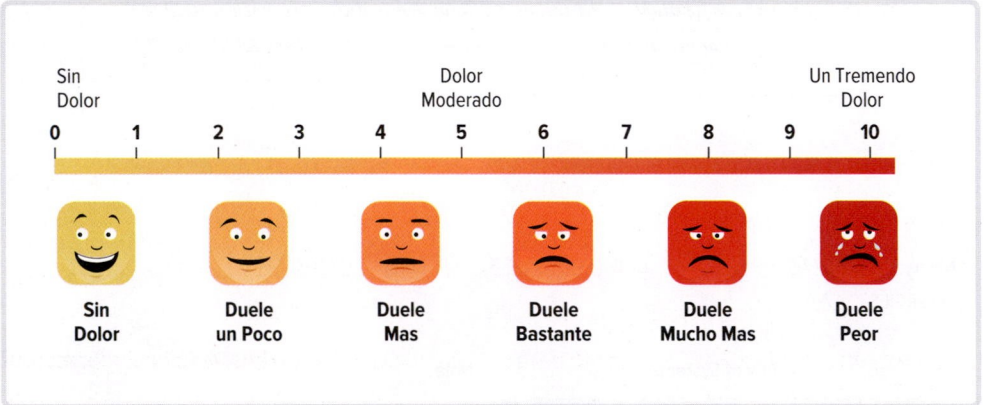

FIGURE 36-6 Assessing a patient's pain, considered the fifth vital sign, is part of the interview and history-taking process. A chart similar to this is used to make the process easier for the patient and the medical assistant.

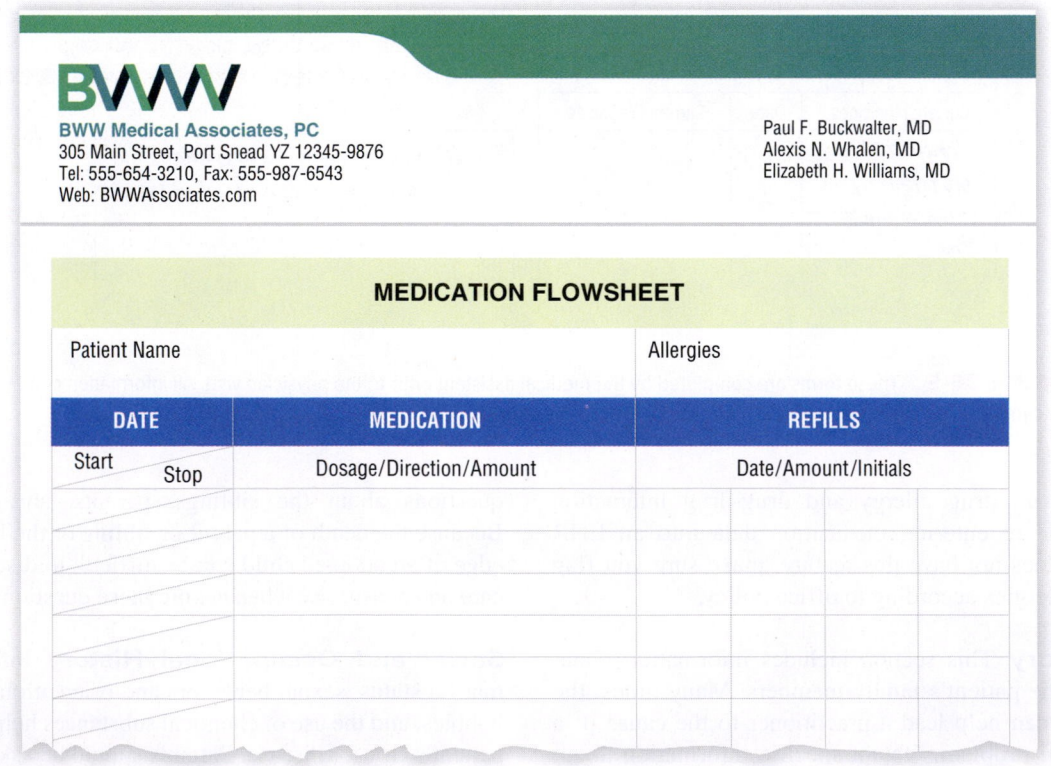

FIGURE 36-7 Medication flowsheet.

or may refuse to provide certain information. Depending on the circumstances, you may ask the question later in the interview. For example, an adolescent child may not want to answer questions about his sexual behaviors in front of his parents. Occupational information regarding the patient's level of stress, exposure to hazardous substances, and heavy lifting also may be included here.

Review of Systems Some of this information may be started by the patient but is completed by the practitioner. This systematic review of each of the body systems includes questions and an exam by the practitioner. The information is obtained in an orderly fashion but may vary depending on the physician or practitioner.

PROCEDURE 36-1 Using Critical Thinking Skills During an Interview   WORK // DOC

Procedure Goal: To be able to use verbal and nonverbal clues and critical thinking skills to optimize the process of obtaining data for the patient's chart

OSHA Guidelines: This procedure does not involve exposure to blood, body fluids, or tissues.

Materials: Progress note, patient chart or electronic health record, pen (if using a paper record)

Method:

Example 1: Getting at an Underlying Meaning

1. You are interviewing a female patient with Type 2 diabetes who has recently started insulin injections. She is in the office for a follow-up visit.
2. Use open-ended questions such as "How are you managing your diabetes?"
   RATIONALE: *Open-ended questioning allows the patient to explain the situation in her own words and often provides more information than closed-ended questioning.*
3. The patient states that she "just can't get used to the whole idea of injections."
4. To encourage her to verbalize her concerns more clearly, you can mirror her response or restate her comments in your own words. For example, you might say, "You seem to be having some difficulty giving yourself injections."

RATIONALE: *This response should encourage her to verbalize the specific area in which she is having problems such as loading the syringe, injecting herself, finding the time for the injections, and so on.*

5. Verbalize the implied, which means that you state what you think the patient is suggesting by her response.
   RATIONALE: *Restating her response ensures you have understood.*
6. After you determine the specific problem, you will be able to address it in the interview or note it in the patient's chart for the doctor's attention.

Example 2: Dealing with a Potentially Violent Patient

1. You are interviewing a 60-year-old male patient who is new to the office. He appears agitated. You ask his reason for seeing the doctor today.
2. The patient explains that he does not want to talk to "some assistant" about his problem. He just wants to see the doctor.
3. You say that you respect his wish not to discuss his symptoms but explain that you need to ask him a few questions so that the doctor can be prepared to provide the proper medical care. Ask questions that help the patient reflect on his or her situation.
   RATIONALE: *The patient has the right to refuse to answer a question, even if it is a reasonable one.*
4. The patient begins to yell at you, saying he wants to see the doctor and does not "want to answer stupid questions."

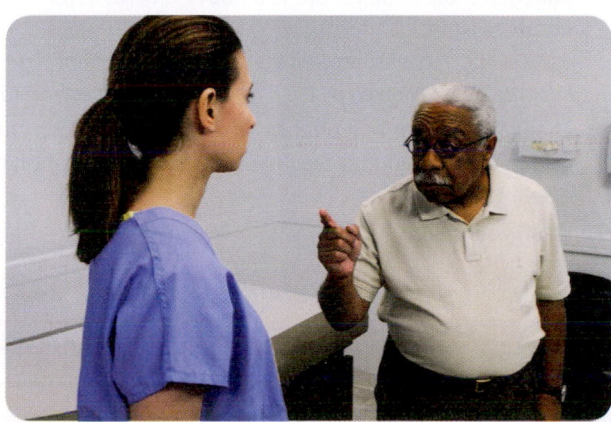

FIGURE Procedure 36-1 Example 2 Step 4   Do not try to handle by yourself a patient who may become violent. Ask for help from other staff members.
© McGraw-Hill Education

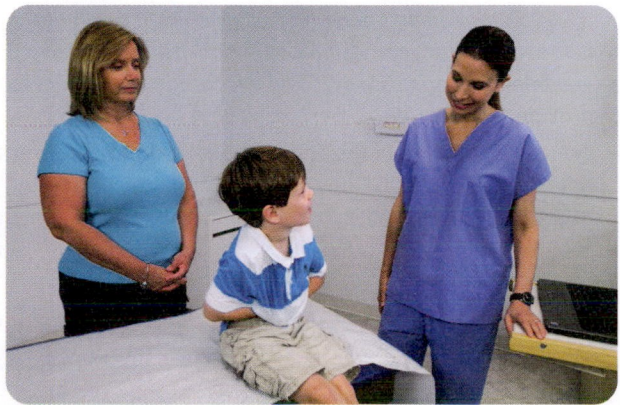

FIGURE Procedure 36-1 Example 3 Step 2   Gather any symptom information you can from the child. Then ask the parent or caregiver similar questions.
© McGraw-Hill Education

5. The fact that the patient appears agitated and begins to raise his voice in anger should be a warning to you that he may become violent. It would be best not to handle this patient by yourself.

6. If you are alone with the patient, leave the room and request assistance from another staff member.

Example 3: Gathering Symptom Information About a Child

1. A parent brings a 5-year-old boy to the office because the child is complaining about stomach pain.

2. To gather the pertinent symptom information, ask the child various types of questions.
   RATIONALE: *Talking to the child first allows him to feel that his view of the problem is important.*
   a. Can he tell you about the pain?

RATIONALE: *Open-ended questioning allows him to tell you about his problem in his own words.*
   b. Can he tell you exactly where it hurts?
   c. Is there anything else that hurts?

3. To clarify the child's answers, ask the parent to answer similar questions.

4. You should then ask the parent additional questions. Begin with an open-ended question, as above. Follow up with specific questions such as these:
   a. How long has he had the pain?
   b. Is the pain related to any specific event (like going to school)?

5. Ask the child to confirm the parent's answers. He may be able to provide additional information at this time.

PROCEDURE 36-2 Using a Progress Note

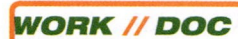

Procedure Goal: To accurately record a chief complaint on a progress note

OSHA Guidelines: This procedure does not involve exposure to blood, body fluids, or tissues.

Materials: Progress note, patient chart or electronic health record, pen (if using a paper record)

Method:

1. Wash your hands.

2. Review the patient's chart notes from the patient's previous office visit. Verify that all results for any previously ordered laboratory work or diagnostics are in the chart.
   RATIONALE: *Ensures that all reports have been reviewed by the physician*

3. Greet the patient and escort her to a private exam room.

4. Introduce yourself and ask the patient her name.

5. Using open-ended questions, find out why the patient is seeking medical care today.
   RATIONALE: *Asking open-ended questions like "What is the reason for your visit today?" and "How long have you been feeling this way?" will encourage the patient to provide more details.*

6. Accurately document the chief complaint on the progress note. Document vital signs. Initial or sign the chart entry according to office policy.

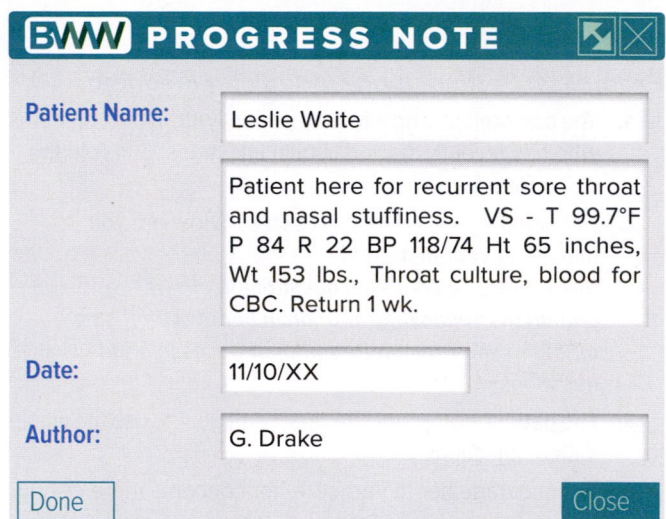

BWW PROGRESS NOTE

Patient Name: Leslie Waite

Patient here for recurrent sore throat and nasal stuffiness. VS - T 99.7°F P 84 R 22 BP 118/74 Ht 65 inches, Wt 153 lbs., Throat culture, blood for CBC. Return 1 wk.

Date: 11/10/XX

Author: G. Drake

Done   Close

7. File the progress note in chronological order within the patient's chart if the record is a paper record. Refer to Progress Note.
   RATIONALE: *This ensures that the most current patient information is reviewed by the physician and the medical staff.*

8. Thank the patient and offer to answer any questions she may have. Explain that the physician will come in soon to examine her.

9. Wash your hands.

PROCEDURE 36-3 Obtaining a Medical History

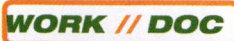

Procedure Goal: To obtain a complete medical history with accuracy and professionalism

OSHA Guidelines: This procedure does not involve exposure to blood, body fluids, or tissues.

Materials: Medical history form, physical examination form, patient chart, pen or electronic medical record

Method:

1. Wash your hands.

2. Assemble the necessary materials. Review the medical history form and plan your interview.
RATIONALE: *This saves time and improves the effectiveness of the visit; plus, it will assist in determining the appropriate questions to ask.*

3. Invite the patient to a private exam room and correctly identify the patient by introducing yourself and asking his or her name and date of birth.

4. Explain the medical history form while maintaining eye contact. Make the patient feel at ease.

5. Using language that the patient can understand, ask appropriate, open-ended questions related to the medical history form. Listen actively to the patient's response using reflection, restatement, and clarification.

6. Accurately document the patient's responses.

7. Thank the patient for his or her participation in the interview. Offer to answer any questions.

8. Sign or initial the medical history form and file it in the patient's chart.

9. Inform the physician that you are finished with the medical history according to the physician's office policy.

10. Wash your hands.

SUMMARY OF LEARNING OUTCOMES

LEARNING OUTCOMES	KEY POINTS
36.1 Identify the skills necessary to conduct a patient interview.	The skills necessary to conduct an interview include effective listening, awareness of nonverbal cues, use of a broad knowledge base, and the ability to summarize a general picture.
36.2 Recognize the signs of anxiety; depression; and physical, mental, or substance abuse.	Anxiety can range from a heightened ability to observe to a difficulty in being able to focus. Depression can be demonstrated through severe fatigue, sadness, difficulty sleeping, and loss of appetite. Abuse can be physical (such as an injury) or psychological (such as neglect).
36.3 Use the six Cs for writing an accurate patient history.	The six Cs for writing an accurate patient history are client's words, clarity, completeness, conciseness, chronological order, and confidentiality.
36.4 Carry out a patient history using critical thinking skills.	When obtaining a patient history, you can use open-ended questions, active listening, clarification, restatement, reflection, and the PQRST interview technique; review the information obtained; determine the importance; and then document the facts accurately.

CASE STUDY CRITICAL THINKING

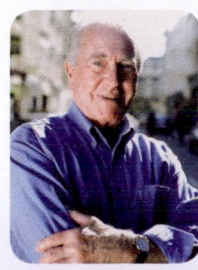

Recall Peter Smith from the beginning of the chapter. Now that you have completed the chapter, answer the following questions regarding his case.

1. What diagnosis will the licensed practitioner most likely give this patient?

2. What specific symptoms make you suspect this condition?

3. Mr. Smith complains of not being able to fall asleep. Is this information objective or subjective data?

4. Why do you think a sleep study was ordered?

1. (LO 36.3) Which of the following represents objective data?
   a. Headache
   b. Pain
   c. Itching
   d. Rash
   e. Nausea

2. (LO 36.1) Which of the following is an open-ended question?
   a. How long have you had the rash under your arm?
   b. So, have you had a headache for 3 days on the left side of your head?
   c. Can you tell me more about your symptoms?
   d. How long does your pain last?
   e. Does your left arm hurt?

3. (LO 36.1) Which of the following is the most effective question to use during a patient interview?
   a. Do you agree that you are getting better when you use the medicine?
   b. Have you had a headache every day this week?
   c. Do you agree you should not have taken so much medication?
   d. What do you think is going on here?
   e. You haven't been taking your medicine, have you?

4. (LO 36.2) Which type of patient is the *least* likely victim of abuse?
   a. A 2-year-old child
   b. A 48-year-old male
   c. A 78-year-old male
   d. A 35-year-old female
   e. An 85-year-old female

5. (LO 36.3) Which of the following is an accepted abbreviation?
   a. HA
   b. OU
   c. HS
   d. ASA
   e. AU

6. (LO 36.4) In the PQRST interview technique, the "P" stands for
   a. Prescription
   b. Problem
   c. Provoke
   d. Plan
   e. Prevent

7. (LO 36.2) The intentional use of a medication or other substance in a way that is not medically approved is known as
   a. Medication error
   b. Substance abuse
   c. Polypharmacy
   d. Addiction
   e. Palliation

8. (LO 36.3) Which of the following is considered subjective data?
   a. Rash
   b. Fever
   c. Increased pulse rate
   d. Headache
   e. Hypertension

9. (LO 36.1) "You seem to be having trouble taking your medication, don't you agree?" is an example of
   a. Asking a leading question
   b. Asking an open-ended question
   c. Asking a hypothetical question
   d. Focusing on the patient
   e. Mirroring the patient's response

10. (LO 36.4) Asking a patient if his pain moves from one location to another is an example of which part of the PQRST interview technique?
    a. P
    b. Q
    c. R
    d. S
    e. T

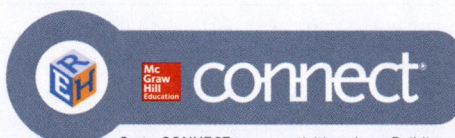

Go to CONNECT to see activities about *Building a Patient's Face Sheet*, *Printing a Patient's Face Sheet*, and *Documenting in a Patient's Progress Note*.

Mrs. Smithers, an 83-year-old established patient, is in today for follow-up after falling and breaking her arm 2 weeks ago. Her daughter is with her and insists on going back to the exam room. During the patient interview, you notice that each time you ask Mrs. Smithers a question her daughter answers before she is able to. How should you handle this situation?

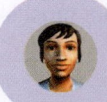

Go to PRACTICE MEDICAL OFFICE and complete the module Clinical - Interactions.

Vital Signs and Measurements

CASE STUDY

PATIENT INFORMATION

Patient Name	DOB	Allergies
Mohammad Nassar	5/17/20XX	Animal dander

Attending	MRN	Other Information
Elizabeth H. Williams, MD	423-90-687	Current medication: albuterol 4 mg bid

Mohammad Nassar, a 16-year-old male, comes to the office because he has had several episodes of what he describes as "my heart is beating too fast." Mohammad has a known history of asthma that is being managed using albuterol. You measure his vital signs and record that his blood pressure is 104/62, his pulse is currently 88 beats per minute, his oral temperature is 99.1°F, and his respirations are 18

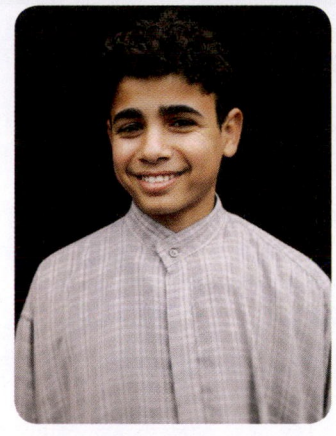
© David Sacks/Getty Images

breaths per minute. He is 5'10" tall and weighs 140 lb. When you ask about the episodes he has experienced, he says they often occur in the evening while he is studying for a big exam. He says he drinks coffee in order to stay awake later and is worried about keeping his grades up so that his parents will continue to allow him to play sports.

Keep Mohammad in mind as you study this chapter. There will be questions at the end of the chapter based on the case study. The information in the chapter will help you answer these questions.

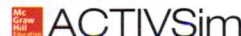

LEARNING OUTCOMES

After completing Chapter 37, you will be able to:

37.1 Describe the vital signs.
37.2 Identify various methods of taking a patient's temperature.
37.3 Describe the process of obtaining pulse and respirations.
37.4 Carry out blood pressure measurements.
37.5 Summarize orthostatic, or postural, vital signs.
37.6 Illustrate various body measurements.

KEY TERMS

afebrile	hypotension
apnea	orthostatic hypotension
auscultated blood pressure	palpatory method
body mass index (BMI)	positive tilt test
bradycardia	postural hypotension
calibrate	rales
dyspnea	rhonchi
febrile	sphygmomanometer
hyperpnea	stethoscope
hyperpyrexia	tachycardia
hypertension	tachypnea
hyperventilation	thermometer

I.P.1   Measure and record:
- (a) blood pressure
- (b) temperature
- (c) pulse
- (d) respiration
- (e) height
- (f) weight
- (i) pulse oximetry

I.P.6   Analyze healthcare results as reported in:
- (a) graphs
- (b) tables

II.P.4   Document on a growth chart

V.P.11   Report relevant information concisely and accurately

X.P.3   Document patient care accurately in the medical record

2. Anatomy and Physiology
- c. Identify diagnostic and treatment modalities as they relate to each body system

4. Medical Law and Ethics
- f. Comply with federal, state, and local health laws and regulations as they relate to healthcare settings

9. Clinical Procedures
- b. Obtain vital signs, obtain patient history, and formulate chief complaint
- j. Make adaptations with patients with special needs

▶ Introduction

Vital signs are one of the most important assessments you can make when preparing the patient to be examined by the practitioner. Temperature, pulse, respirations, and blood pressure give information about how a patient will adjust to changes within the body and in the environment. Changes in the vital signs can indicate an abnormality.

Measurements such as height, weight, and head circumference can indicate physical growth and development, especially in infants and children. These measurements also are used to evaluate health problems such as obesity, and other measurements are completed to evaluate a patient's condition. For example, you may need to measure the size of a wound or bruise or the diameter of an arm or a leg. In all cases, you must be accurate when performing and recording vital signs and body measurements. The practitioner uses your results when making a diagnosis.

▶ Vital Signs   LO 37.1

As a medical assistant, you will usually take the vital signs before the doctor examines the patient. Vital signs include temperature, pulse, respirations, and blood pressure. Pain assessment, which was discussed in the *Patient Interview and History* chapter, is considered by some practitioners to be the "fifth vital sign." Pain level is typically evaluated during the patient interview and recorded along with the vital signs. These measurements provide the doctor with information about the patient's overall condition.

In some offices, pre-exam procedures such as vital signs are performed in a general area outside the patient exam room. In other offices and in most pediatric offices, these measurements are taken in the exam room. In either case, you typically take the measurements before the patient disrobes. Follow the standard procedure used in your office and be sure to follow the HIPAA regulations and provide for the privacy of your results.

Vital signs are usually measured at every office visit. There is a standard range of values for each measurement, as shown in Table 37-1, and each patient has an individual baseline value that is normal for that patient. The difference between a patient's current values and normal values can help the licensed practitioner in making a diagnosis. You must follow closely the guidelines from the Department of Labor's Occupational Safety and Health Administration (OSHA) for taking measurements of vital signs (Table 37-2). These guidelines are intended to prevent transmission of disease to or from the patient. They help protect the patient and you, and they keep the workplace safe.

▶ Temperature   LO 37.2

When you take a patient's temperature, you will determine whether the patient is **febrile** (has a body temperature above the patient's normal range) or **afebrile** (has a body temperature within the patient's normal range). A fever is usually a sign of inflammation or infection. An exceptionally high fever is known as **hyperpyrexia**. Body temperature is the balance between heat produced by metabolic processes and heat lost from the body; it varies based on numerous factors. These factors include the time of day (usually higher at night due to exercise and food intake), age, gender, physical exercise, emotion, pregnancy, drugs, food, environmental changes, and

TABLE 37-1 Normal Ranges for Vital Signs*

Vital Sign	Age					
	0–1 Year	1–2 Years	2–5 Years	6–12 Years	Greater Than 12 Years	Adult
Temperature						
Oral (°F)	—	—	—	97.4–99.5	97.6–99.6	97.8–99.1
Rectal (°F)	99–100	97.9–100.4	97.9–100.4	97.9–100.4	98.6–100.6	98.8–100.1
Pulse (beats per minute)	100–160	90–150	80–140	70–120	60–100	60–100
Respirations (per minute)	30–60	24–40	22–34	18–30	12–16	12–18
Blood pressure (mmHg)***†						
Systolic	80–106	80–106	84–112	91–123	101–136	Less than 120
Diastolic	34–54	34–59	39–70	53–79	59–84	Less than 80

*Normal vital signs vary. Always compare your results with previous results obtained on the patient.

**Classifications for adult blood pressure are shown in Table 37-4.

†Pediatric blood pressure ranges vary greatly based on height percentiles and gender. Always consult the licensed practitioner regarding specific ranges for each patient.

TABLE 37-2 OSHA Guidelines for Taking Measurements of Vital Signs

Situation	OSHA Guidelines
Before and after all patient contact	• Examination area cleaned according to OSHA standards • Aseptic handwashing
Temperature by oral or rectal route Contact with patient with lesions Contact with patient suspected of having infectious disease	• Gloves always worn for rectal route • Gloves worn for oral route if contact precautions exist • Biohazard bags used for disposal of used thermometer sheaths, otoscope tips, alcohol swabs, dressings, and bandages
In presence of patient suspected of having an airborne infectious disease (particularly sneezing)	• Mask worn • Patient weighed, measured, and examined in room away from staff and other patients • Protective clothing (laboratory coat, gown, or apron) worn • Biohazard bags used as above

metabolism (a slow metabolism, as seen in hypothyroidism, would cause a lower temperature). The body location where the temperature is measured also can affect the result.

Temperature is measured with either an electronic or a disposable **thermometer.** You can take a temperature in one of five locations: mouth (oral), ear (tympanic), rectum (rectal), armpit or axilla (axillary), and temporal artery (temporal). Temperature can be measured in degrees Fahrenheit (°F) or degrees Celsius (°C). Table 37-3 gives equivalent values for these two temperature scales. Normal adult oral temperature is considered to be about 98.6°F or 37.0°C. See the *Points on Practice* box to review formulas and example conversions.

Electronic Digital Thermometers

Electronic digital thermometers are used frequently in medical offices. These thermometers provide a digital readout of the patient's temperature (Figure 37-1). They are accurate, fast, easy to read, and comfortable for the patient. Separate probes and tips are available for oral and rectal use. Most units beep or have another audible indicator to let you know when the temperature has registered and is displayed.

Another type of electronic thermometer is the tympanic thermometer, which is designed for use in the ear. See Figure 37-2. This thermometer measures infrared energy

TABLE 37-3 Fahrenheit and Celsius Equivalents for Temperature

°F	°C	°F	°C	°F	°C	°F	°C
95.0	35.0	98.4	36.9	101.8	38.8	105.2	40.7
95.2	35.1	98.6	37.0	102.0	38.9	105.4	40.8
95.4	35.2	98.8	37.1	102.2	39.0	105.6	40.9
95.6	35.3	99.0	37.2	102.4	39.1	105.8	41.0
95.8	35.4	99.2	37.3	102.6	39.2	106.0	41.1
96.0	35.6	99.4	37.4	102.8	39.3	106.2	41.2
96.2	35.7	99.6	37.6	103.0	39.4	106.4	41.3
96.4	35.8	99.8	37.7	103.2	39.6	106.6	41.4
96.6	35.9	100.0	37.8	103.4	39.7	106.8	41.6
96.8	36.0	100.2	37.9	103.6	39.8	107.0	41.7
97.0	36.1	100.4	38.0	103.8	39.9	107.2	41.8
97.2	36.2	100.6	38.1	104.0	40.0	107.4	41.9
97.4	36.3	100.8	38.2	104.2	40.1	107.6	42.0
97.6	36.4	101.0	38.3	104.4	40.2	107.8	42.1
97.8	36.6	101.2	38.4	104.6	40.3	108.0	42.2
98.0	36.7	101.4	38.6	104.8	40.4		
98.2	36.8	101.6	38.7	105.0	40.6		

Math for Measurements

When performing vital signs and measurements, certain basic math conversions may be required. You may need to convert a temperature from Fahrenheit (°F) to Celsius (°C), weight from pounds (lb) to kilograms (kg), or inches to feet and inches. Review the following formulas and examples in preparation for practice.

To convert °C to °F, use this formula:
°F = (°C × 9/5) + 32

Example: Convert 37.6°C to °F:

°F = (37.6 × 9/5) + 32

°F = (338.4/5) + 32

°F = 67.68 + 32

°F = 99.68, rounded to the nearest tenth equals 99.7

To convert °F to °C, use this formula:
°C = (°F − 32) × 5/9

Example: Convert 99.6°F to °C:

°C = (99.6 − 32) × 5/9

°C = 67.6 × 5/9

°C = 338/9

°C = 37.55, rounded to the nearest tenth equals 37.6

To convert kg to lb, use this formula:
lb = kg × 2.205

Example: Convert 52.4 kg to lb:

lb = 52.4 × 2.205

lb = 115.542, rounded to the nearest tenth equals 115.5

To convert lb to kg, use this formula:
kg = lb × 0.454

Example: Convert 134 lb to kg:

kg = 134 × 0.454

kg = 60.836, rounded to the nearest tenth equals 60.8

To convert inches to feet and inches:

Divide the number of inches by 12 and carry the remainder. The answer is the number of feet and the remainder indicates the number of inches. For example, 66/12 = 5 with a remainder of 6, so a person who is 66 inches tall is 5 feet, 6 inches tall.

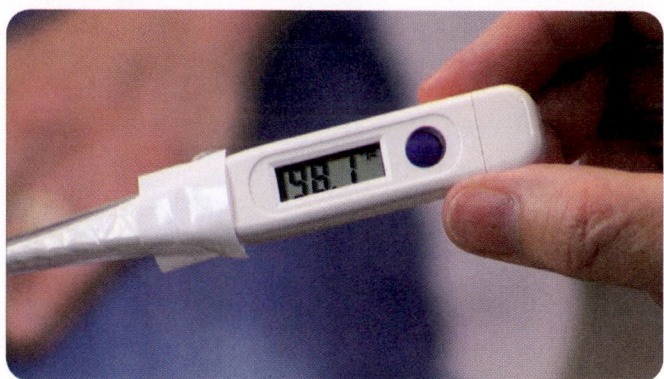

FIGURE 37-1 An electronic digital thermometer provides a digital readout of the patient's temperature.
© McGraw-Hill Education

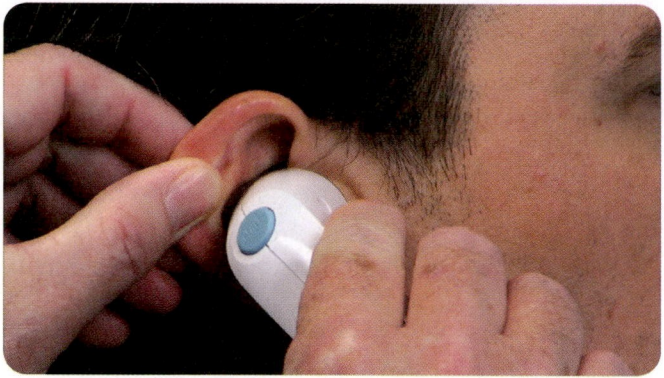

FIGURE 37-2 The tympanic thermometer measures infared energy emitted from the tympanic membrane. The result, converted to body temperature, is displayed within seconds of insertion of the shielded tip into the ear.
© McGraw-Hill Education

emitted from the tympanic membrane (eardrum). This energy is converted into a temperature reading. The tip is covered with a disposable sheath to prevent cross-contamination.

A third type of electronic thermometer is a temporal scanner (Figure 37-3). This thermometer measures the infrared heat of the temporal artery and the ambient temperature (the temperature around the area) at the site where the temperature is taken. These two readings are processed to calculate the body temperature, which is then displayed on the screen.

Disposable Thermometers

Disposable, single-use thermometers are usually made of thin strips of plastic with specially treated dot or strip indicators (Figure 37-4). The indicators change color according to the temperature. This type of thermometer is used for oral and

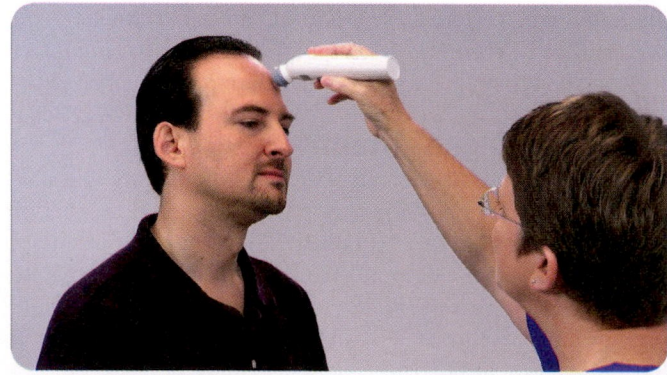

FIGURE 37-3 This temporal scanner is passed across the forehead to measure the temperature of the blood in the temporal artery.
© McGraw-Hill Education

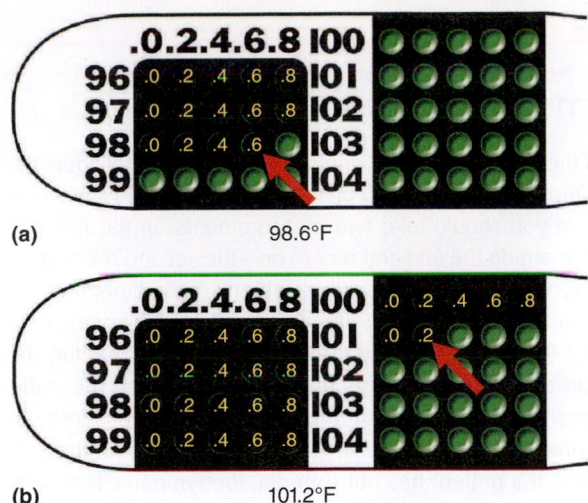

(a)   98.6°F

(b)   101.2°F

FIGURE 37-4   A disposable thermometer like this one is a convenient method for taking temperature. Thermometer reading after taking (a) a normal temperature and (b) an elevated temperature.

axillary or skin temperature measurements, particularly in children. Although not as accurate, disposable thermometers are useful for patients in their homes.

Taking Temperatures

Using the proper instrument and technique provides the most accurate temperature readings and prevents the spread of infection. All temperature measurements should be recorded to the nearest one-tenth of a degree. The procedure for taking temperatures is described in Procedure 37-1 at the end of this chapter.

Measuring Oral Temperatures   To take an oral temperature, make sure the patient is able to hold the thermometer in the mouth. The patient also must be able to breathe through the nose. Place the thermometer under the tongue in either pocket just off-center in the lower jaw (Figure 37-5). The patient should hold the thermometer with lips closed. Wait at least 15 minutes after a patient has been eating, drinking, or smoking before taking an oral temperature; otherwise, you may obtain an inaccurate result.

Measuring Tympanic Temperatures   Proper technique must be used when measuring a tympanic temperature. These thermometers are easy to use, but you must follow manufacturers' instructions precisely. First, remove the thermometer from its recharging cradle and then wait for the indicator light to show that the unit is ready. Attach a disposable sheath and place the thermometer in the opening of the ear so that the fit is snug. To make sure you have a tight fit and the thermometer is pointing at the eardrum, pull the ear up and back for adults; pull the ear down and back for children. Pull the ear correctly for each age group to ensure that the thermometer is aiming directly at the eardrum. Press the button and the result will be displayed within seconds. Be certain to press the correct button to read the temperature. Another button on the thermometer releases the sheath. You do not want to release the sheath into the patient's ear. See the *Caution: Handle with Care* box for problems that can occur with tympanic thermometers.

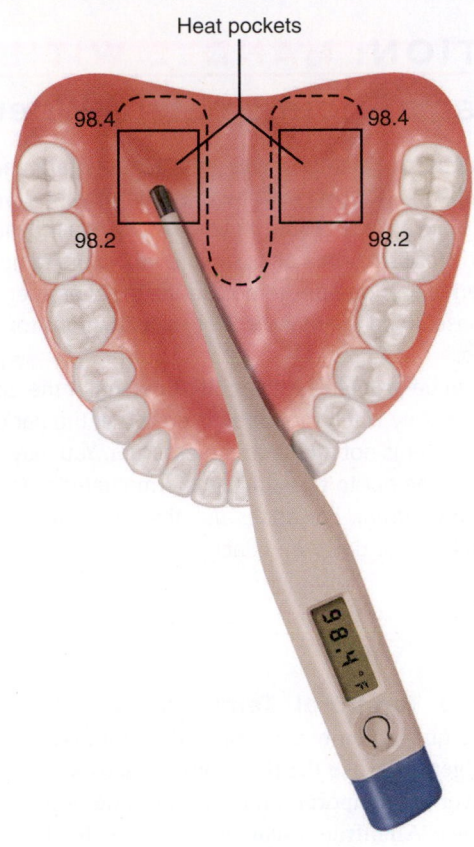

Heat pockets

98.4   98.4

98.2   98.2

FIGURE 37-5   When taking an oral temperature, place the thermometer under the tongue to the side of the mouth, as shown here.

Measuring Rectal Temperatures   Rectal temperatures are usually 1°F higher than oral temperatures and are considered the most accurate measurement of body temperature. Temperatures are sometimes measured rectally in infants and in adults in whom an oral temperature cannot be taken. Gloves are always worn and the patient is placed on his or her side. The left side is the preferred position because the rectum is angled in this direction. This position promotes comfort and prevents accidental puncture of the rectal wall. The tip of the thermometer should be inserted slowly and gently until it is covered or until you feel resistance, at approximately 1 inch for adults and ½ inch for infants and small children. For safety, always hold the thermometer in place while taking the temperature.

Measuring Axillary Temperatures   To take an axillary temperature, first have the patient sit or lie down. Place the tip of the thermometer in the middle of the axilla (armpit), with the shaft facing forward. The patient's upper arm should be pressed against his side and his lower arm should be crossed over the stomach to hold the thermometer in place. Make sure the tip of the thermometer touches skin on all sides of the probe. The axillary temperature is 0.5 to 1 degree lower than the oral temperature and 2 degrees lower than the rectal temperature. Therefore, if the patient's axillary temperature is 99 degrees or higher, verify the patient's temperature using another method, because the patient may have a fever. Be sure to note the location of temperature measurement on the patient's chart.

Measuring Temporal Temperatures The temporal scanner is a quick, noninvasive procedure for taking temperatures. You gently stroke the thermometer across the forehead, crossing over the temporal artery (on the side of the forehead at the temple). An infrared scanner measures the difference in the temperature of the forehead and that of the temporal artery and then electronically calculates the patient's body temperature. As with all electronic devices, check the manufacturer's instructions before using.

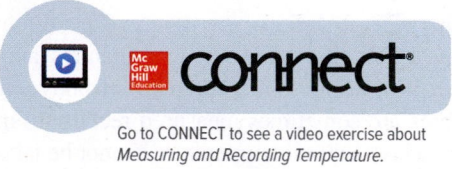

Go to CONNECT to see a video exercise about *Measuring and Recording Temperature.*

▶ Pulse and Respiration   LO 37.3

Pulse and respiration are related because the circulatory and respiratory systems work together. Pulse is measured as the number of times the heart beats in 1 minute. Respiration is the number of times a patient breathes in 1 minute. One breath, or respiration, equals one inhalation and one exhalation. Usually, if either the pulse or respiration rate is high or low, the other is also. The usual ratio of the pulse rate to the respiration rate is about 4:1 (for example, a pulse of 80 and a respiration of 20). In general, the younger the patient, the higher the normal pulse and respiration rate. Additionally, adult female rates tend to be faster than those for males. You should be familiar with these rates and how to perform the procedure. See Table 37-1 and Procedure 37-2, at the end of this chapter.

Pulse

A pulse rate gives information about the patient's cardiovascular system. It is an indirect measurement of the patient's cardiac output or the amount of blood the heart is able to

pump in one minute. If the pulse is weak or irregular, or if the patient has **tachycardia** (abnormally fast pulse) or **bradycardia** (abnormally slow pulse), the patient may have a medical problem.

Measure the pulse of adults at the radial artery, where it can be felt in the groove on the thumb side of the inner wrist. Press lightly on this pulse point with your fingers and not your thumb (a pulse is located in your thumb, and you may feel it instead of the patient's pulse). Count the number of beats you feel in a set period of time (up to 1 minute). Also note the rhythm and volume. The rhythm can be regular or irregular. The volume can be weak, strong, or bounding. A bounding pulse feels like it is leaping out and then quickly disappearing with each pulse beat and sometimes can be seen at the pulse site. You may be asked to document the pulse volume on a numerical scale from 0 to 4+. Following are the characteristics of this scale.

- 0 = no palpable pulse
- 1+ = weak
- 2+ = faint pulse
- 3+ = normal pulse
- 4+ = bounding pulse

Count the pulse for 30 seconds and, if the beat is regular, multiply the results by 2 to obtain the beats per minute. If the pulse is irregular, weak, or bounding, you must count for a full minute and document the irregularities. In some cases, you may be able to count the pulse for as little as 15 seconds and multiply by 4 to obtain the beats per minute. However, this should only be done when you are comfortable with the procedure and you are certain the pulse is normal (3+) and regular.

Pulse sites other than the radial pulse may be used for various reasons. For example, in young children, the radial artery may be hard to feel. You may instead take the pulse at the brachial artery, which is in the medial aspect of the antecubital fossa (the bend of the elbow) or on the medial (inner) side of the upper arm. If you cannot feel the brachial pulse, then take the pulse over the apex (the left lower corner) of the heart, where the strongest heart sounds can be heard. Count the apical pulse (the heartbeat at the apex of the heart) while you listen with a **stethoscope,** an instrument that amplifies body sounds. The apex is located in the fifth intercostal space between the ribs on the left side of the chest, directly below the center of the clavicle. Consult Figure 37-6 for placement of the stethoscope. Though the condition is rare, you may encounter a patient with *dextrocardia*—a congenital condition in which the heart is pointed toward the right side of the chest. In this case, you will find the apical pulse on the right side of the chest, directly below the clavicle in the fifth intercostal space. You also may use other locations to take a pulse. Figure 37-7 shows the location of common pulse points.

Electronic Pulse The pulse may be measured electronically using a device attached to the finger or sometimes the nose or earlobe. Figure 37-8 shows one type of device used as part of an electronic blood pressure machine. A pulse oximeter machine, which measures the oxygen level of the blood, also can be used (Figure 37-9).

When using these devices, be certain to attach the clip firmly to the finger, lobe, or nose. When using a nose bridge pulse oximeter, make sure there is good skin contact. The nose bridge pulse oximeter should only be used with patients who have good peripheral circulation. See Figure 37-10. The finger clip uses an infrared light to measure the pulse and

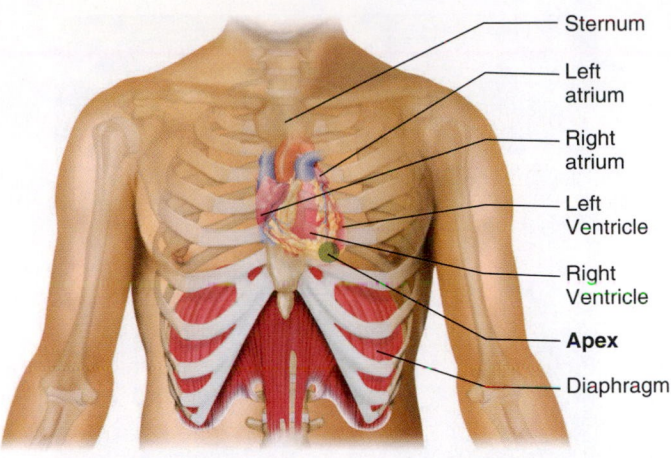

FIGURE 37-6   A stethoscope is used over the apex of the heart to listen for the heart sounds and measure the heart rate in patients in whom pulse is not otherwise detectable.

oxygen levels, so it works best when no nail polish is present on the patient's finger. The pulse reading and the oxygen saturation of the blood will display on the screen. If the pulse is outside the normal range (see Table 37-1), it should be taken again or performed manually. If the oxygen level is less than 92%, the patient should be asked to take deep breaths during the procedure to increase her oxygen level. An oxygen level below 92% that does not improve with deep breaths should be reported.

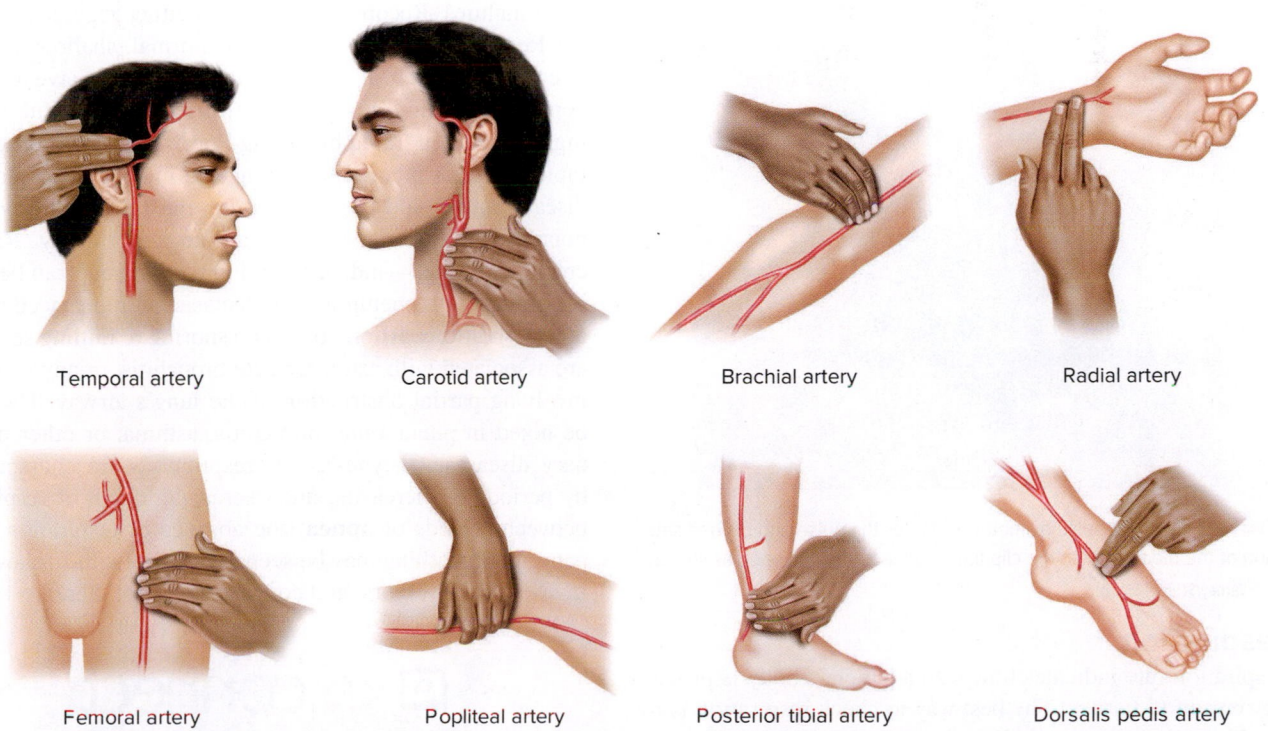

FIGURE 37-7   There are many locations on the body where major arteries are close enough to the surface to allow a pulse to be felt and counted.

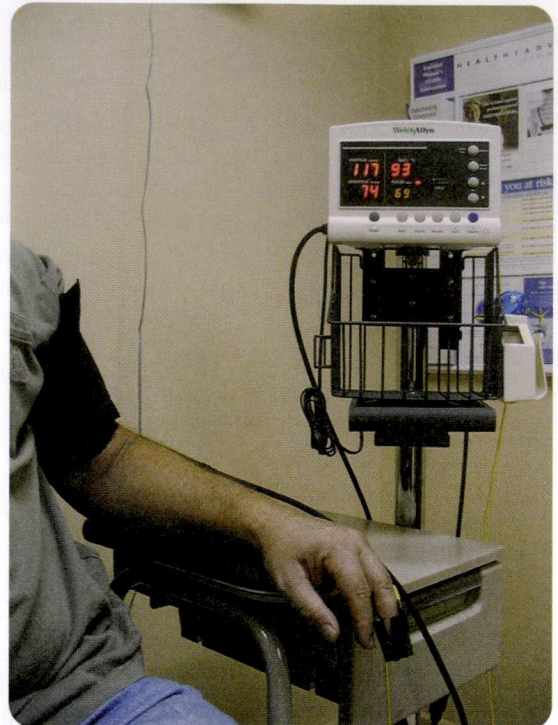

FIGURE 37-8 Pulse, blood pressure, and oxygen saturation can all be measured with this electronic blood pressure device.
© Total Care Programming, Inc.

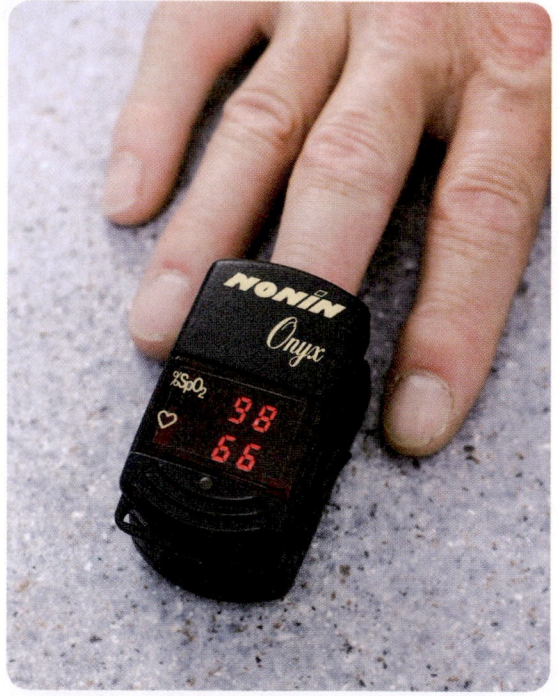

FIGURE 37-9 A pulse oximeter measures the pulse and oxygen saturation of the blood. Attach the clip firmly to the patient's finger, as shown.
© Jim Varney/Science Source

Respiration

Respiration rate indicates how well a patient's body is providing oxygen to tissues. The best way to check respiration is by watching, listening, or feeling the movement at the patient's chest, stomach, back, or shoulders. If you cannot see the chest

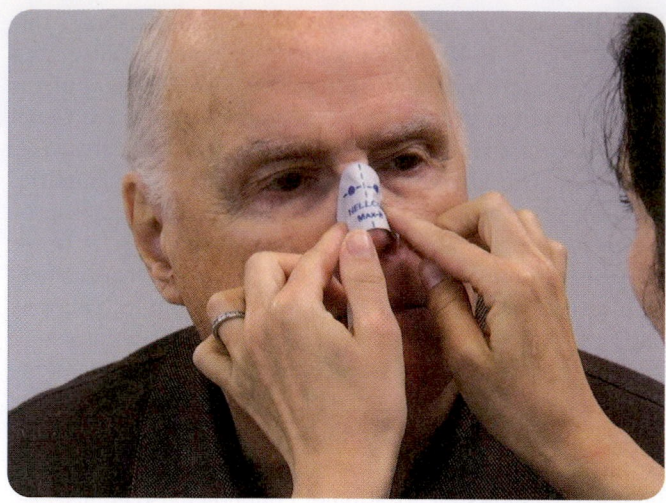

FIGURE 37-10 Make sure there is good skin contact when using a nose bridge pulse oximeter.
© McGraw-Hill Education

movement, then place your hand over the patient's chest, shoulder, or abdomen and listen and feel for the movement of air.

Respirations also may be counted with a stethoscope. Place the stethoscope on one side of the patient's spine in the middle of the back to count respirations. You need to count respirations subtly because once the patient is aware that respiration is being measured, he may unintentionally alter his breathing. If using a stethoscope, tell the patient that you want to listen to his lungs. When you are not using a stethoscope, count the respirations while you have your hand on the pulse site.

Respirations are counted for 1 full minute in order to determine the rate, rhythm, and effort (quality). Counting for less than a minute may cause you to miss certain breathing abnormalities. Record the rhythm as either regular or irregular. Record the quality of effort as normal, shallow, or deep. Irregularities such as **hyperventilation** (excessive rate and depth of breathing), **dyspnea** (difficult or painful breathing), **tachypnea** (rapid breathing), or **hyperpnea** (abnormally rapid, deep, or labored breathing) are indications of possible disease and should be noted. Rales and rhonchi are types of noisy breathing that can indicate an abnormality. **Rales**—crackling sounds—indicate fluid in the lung and can be heard in patients with pneumonia, atelectasis, pulmonary edema, or other conditions. **Rhonchi**—deep snoring or rattling sounds—are associated with asthma, acute bronchitis, or any condition involving partial obstruction of the lung's airway. They may be noted in pneumonia, bronchitis, asthma, or other pulmonary diseases. Cheyne-Stokes respirations are characterized by periods of increasing and decreasing depth of respiration between periods of **apnea** (the absence of respiration). This pattern of breathing may be seen in patients with strokes, head injuries, brain tumors, and congestive heart failure.

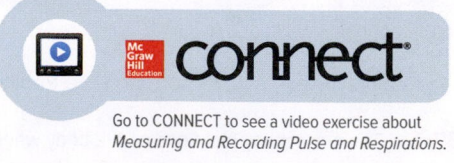

Go to CONNECT to see a video exercise about *Measuring and Recording Pulse and Respirations.*

▶ Blood Pressure
LO 37.4

Blood pressure (also known as arterial blood pressure) is the force at which blood is pumped against the walls of the arteries. The standard unit for measuring blood pressure is millimeters of mercury (mmHg). The pressure measured when the left ventricle of the heart contracts is known as the systolic pressure. The pressure measured when the heart relaxes is known as the diastolic pressure. The diastolic pressure indicates the minimum amount of pressure exerted against the vessel walls at all times.

According to the Joint National Committee of Prevention, Detection, Evaluation, and Treatment of High Blood Pressure, expected adult systolic readings are less than 120 mmHg and adult diastolic readings are less than 80 mmHg. These values may increase with advancing age. Table 37-4 outlines blood pressure classifications.

Factors Affecting Blood Pressure

High blood pressure, known as **hypertension**, is a common health problem. If the blood pressure reading is consistently elevated after two or more office visits, the patient may be diagnosed with hypertension. According to the American Heart Association, more than 76 million Americans over the age of 20 have high blood pressure. Hypertension may be categorized as essential or secondary. There is no identifiable cause for essential hypertension. According to the Joint National Committee, 95% of all hypertension is essential. Secondary hypertension occurs as a result of some other condition, such as kidney or heart disease.

Many factors affect the blood pressure. Internal factors such as cardiac output (amount of blood pumped by the heart), blood volume (amount of blood in the body), vasoconstriction (peripheral resistance), and blood viscosity (thickness) regulate the blood pressure within the body.

Malignant hypertension is high blood pressure that is high enough to cause renal or heart failure, *papilledema* (swelling of the optic nerve), or other vital organ damage. Patients with elevated blood pressure are frequently checked more than once during an office visit and may be monitoring their blood pressure at home.

Hypotension, or low blood pressure, is not generally a chronic health problem. Slightly low blood pressure may be normal for some patients and does not usually require treatment. Severe hypotension may be present with shock, heart failure, severe burns, and excessive bleeding.

Blood Pressure Measuring Equipment

Blood pressure is measured with an instrument called a **sphygmomanometer.** A sphygmomanometer consists of an inflatable cuff, a pressure bulb or automatic device for inflating the cuff, and a manometer to read the pressure. The three basic types of sphygmomanometers differ in how the pressure is displayed.

Aneroid Sphygmomanometers Aneroid sphygmomanometers have a circular gauge that registers pressure. The needle on the gauge rotates as pressure rises. This type of sphygmomanometer is very accurate as long as calibration is done on a regular basis. Each measurement line indicates 2 mmHg (Figure 37-11).

Electronic Sphygmomanometers Electronic sphygmomanometers provide a digital readout of blood pressure (Figure 37-12). Unlike aneroid sphygmomanometers, these devices do not require use of a stethoscope to determine blood pressure. They are easy to use but can be costly. Accuracy can sometimes be an issue, so maintain the equipment according to the manufacturer's instructions. If you question the results of an electronic blood pressure measurement, take it again with an aneroid cuff.

Mercury Sphygmomanometers Mercury sphygmomanometers contain a column of mercury that rises with an increase in pressure as the cuff is inflated. Mercury instruments are gradually being replaced because the government has restricted the use of mercury due to its effects on people and the environment. In 2007, the World Health Organization, in conjunction with Healthcare Without Harm, began an initiative to eliminate the use of mercury thermometers and sphygmomanometers by the year 2017. Consequently, no new mercury sphygmomanometers are being manufactured in the United States.

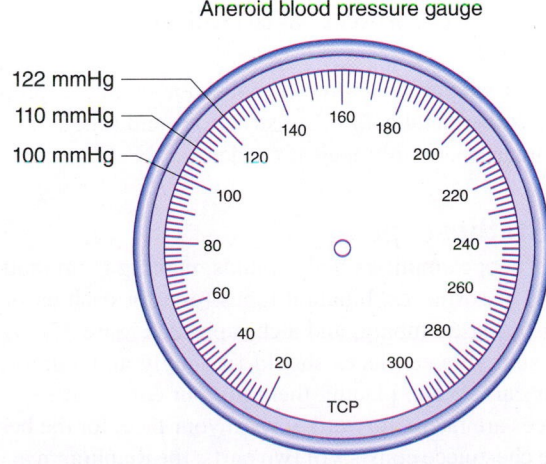

Aneroid blood pressure gauge

FIGURE 37-11 Each line on the aneroid gauge indicates 2 mmHg. To prevent inaccuracies, look directly at this gauge when performing a blood pressure test.

TABLE 37-4	Blood Pressure Classifications	
Classification	**Systolic (mmHg)**	**Diastolic (mmHg)**
Normal	Less than 120	AND less than 80
Prehypertension	120–139	OR 80–89
Stage 1 hypertension	140–159	OR 90–99
Stage 2 hypertension	Greater than 160	OR greater than 100
Hypertensive crisis (emergency care needed)	Greater than 180	OR greater than 110

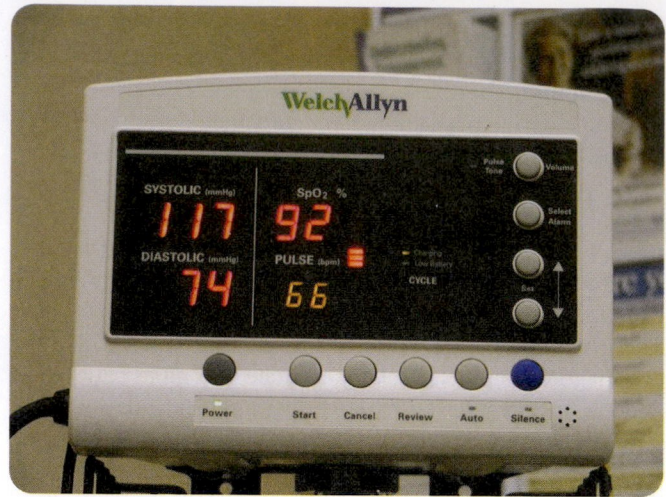

FIGURE 37-12 This electronic sphygmomanometer displays the patient's blood pressure, pulse, and oxygen saturation. If you question any of the results, repeat the test using a manual method.
© Total Care Programming, Inc.

Calibrating the Sphygmomanometer

To ensure that sphygmomanometers are working properly, you or a medical supply dealer must calibrate them regularly. To **calibrate** means to standardize a measuring instrument. Follow the manufacturer's instructions for an electronic sphygmomanometer.

Using an uncalibrated sphygmomanometer will result in inaccurate blood pressure readings, so do not use a sphygmomanometer unless you are certain it is calibrated. To calibrate an aneroid sphygmomanometer, follow these steps:

1. Check that the needle on the dial rests within the small square at the bottom of the dial when no pressure is applied to the cuff.

2. To calibrate the dial, use a Y connector to attach the dial to a pressure bulb and a calibrated manometer.

3. Use the pressure bulb to elevate both manometer readings to 250 mmHg. As you let the pressure fall, record both readings at four different points.

4. The difference between paired readings should not exceed 3 mmHg.

5. If the sphygmomanometer does not calibrate properly, check the manufacturer's instructions and send the sphygmomanometer for repair if needed.

The Stethoscope

A stethoscope amplifies body sounds, making them louder. It consists of earpieces, binaural tubes (one for each earpiece), rubber or plastic tubing, and a chestpiece (Figure 37-13). For best results, the earpieces should fit snugly and comfortably in your ears. When placing them in your ears, make sure the earpieces are facing forward, toward your face, for the best fit.

The chestpiece consists of two parts: the diaphragm and the bell. The diaphragm is the larger, flat side of the chestpiece, which is covered by a thin, plastic disk. The diaphragm—best at amplifying high-pitched sounds, such as bowel and lung

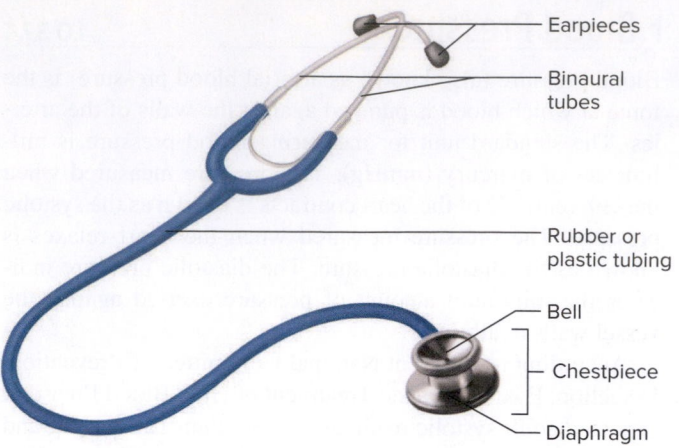

FIGURE 37-13 The stethoscope amplifies body sounds.

sounds—must be placed firmly against the skin for proper amplification of sound.

The bell is the cone-shaped side of the stethoscope chestpiece. It must be held lightly against the skin to amplify sound. The bell is best at amplifying low-pitched sounds, such as vascular and heart sounds. With practice, you may find you prefer to use one side rather than the other for various purposes.

Measuring Blood Pressure

To measure blood pressure, wrap the cuff of the sphygmomanometer around the patient's upper arm, just above the brachial artery's pulse point (Figure 37-14). This pulse point is located in the antecubital fossa (bend of the elbow). When measuring blood pressure, you should first determine the palpatory pressure that represents the target peak inflation. With the cuff placed just above the brachial artery pulse, palpate the radial pulse. This **palpatory method** provides an approximation of the systolic blood pressure to ensure an adequate level of inflation when the actual measurement is made. Inflate the cuff until you can no longer feel the radial pulse and note the pressure at that point. Allow the arm to rest for 30 to 60 seconds or remove the cuff and replace. Checking the chart or asking the patient his or her usual blood pressure may be helpful if you have difficulty obtaining a palpatory result. Then determine the **auscultated blood pressure,** a precise measurement of blood pressure

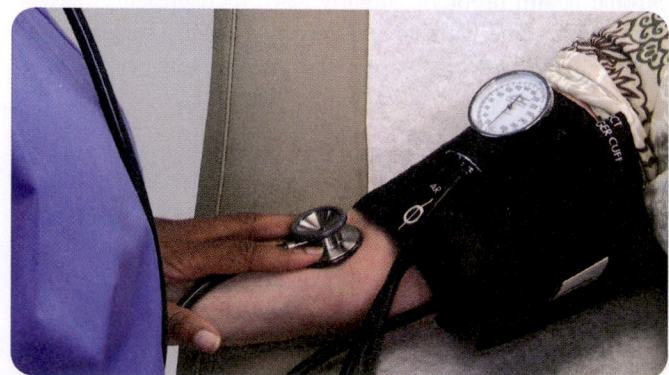

FIGURE 37-14 The blood pressure cuff should be 1 inch above the elbow with the center of the bladder directly above the brachial pulse.
© McGraw-Hill Education

obtained by using the sphygmomanometer with a stethoscope to amplify the heart sounds. Inflate the cuff to 30 mmHg above the palpatory result, or no more than 180 to 200 mmHg. Then, while you release the air in the cuff, listen with the stethoscope placed over the brachial pulse point. The sounds you hear are the result of blood flowing through the circulatory system. Refer to the chapter *The Cardiovascular System* for more information about heart sounds and their relationship to blood pressure readings. The heart sounds will change as the pressure in the blood pressure cuff decreases. These sounds are called Korotkoff sounds and they have five phases:

- Phase 1: The first tapping sound you hear represents the systolic pressure.
- Phase 2: A strong heartbeat changes to a softer, swishing sound.
- Phase 3: A crisp, tapping sound resumes.
- Phase 4: Sounds become muffled.
- Phase 5: The point at which the sound disappears; this represents the diastolic pressure.

Sometimes the sound will vanish temporarily between phase 1 and phase 2. This happens when the blood vessels beneath the cuff become congested and is often a sign of hypertension. When the congestion clears, the sound resumes. The period during which the sound either changes or vanishes is called the *auscultatory gap*.

Blood pressure is usually recorded with the systolic and diastolic sounds separated by a slash—for example, 116/76. If there is a pressure difference greater than 10 mmHg between the muffled sound and its disappearance, the blood pressure may be recorded with all three sounds, noted as 120/80/60. The process of taking blood pressure is described in Procedure 37-3, at the end of this chapter.

Special Considerations in Adults Blood pressure is elevated during and just after exercise. If a patient has engaged in strenuous activity before the exam, you should wait 15 minutes before taking blood pressure measurements. This waiting period also applies to patients with ambulatory disabilities, to those who are obese, and to those who have a known blood pressure problem. If you ensure that patients have relaxed for 15 minutes before you measure their blood pressure, you should get an accurate reading.

Blood pressure also may be elevated when a patient is anxious or under stress. The patient may be aware that a blood pressure reading is high or low and upset about the reading. If the patient seems stressed or upset, allow him to rest for about 5 minutes before measuring his blood pressure. To help the patient relax, try to engage the person in conversation rather than calling attention to the fact that you are waiting to take his blood pressure. If the patient still appears anxious or under stress, take his blood pressure anyway and make a notation for the licensed practitioner (who may want to repeat the measurement later in the visit).

However, there are certain instances when you should not take a blood pressure measurement on a particular arm. Blood pressure should not be taken on an arm that is on the same side as a mastectomy (breast removal) or on an arm that has an injury, a blocked artery, or a device under the skin (implant) at the site. In such cases, use the other arm or the upper leg, placing the stethoscope over the popliteal artery behind the knee. Note the measurements and their locations in the patient's chart.

Be sure you use the proper size cuff when taking blood pressure. The bladder inside the cuff should encircle 80% to 100% the distance around the arm or leg. Although the standard adult cuff can be used for most adults, some may require the larger size. Using an improper size may result in an inaccurate reading.

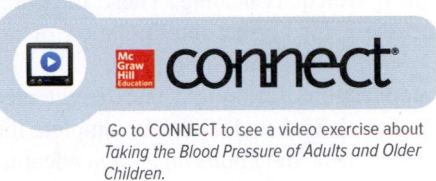

Go to CONNECT to see a video exercise about *Taking the Blood Pressure of Adults and Older Children.*

▶ Orthostatic, or Postural, Vital Signs   LO 37.5

Orthostatic vital signs are taken in different positions to assess for **orthostatic,** or **postural**, **hypotension.** This means that as the patient moves from a lying to sitting or standing position, the blood pressure becomes lower and, as a result, the pulse increases. This usually indicates some sort of fluid loss or malfunctioning of the cardiovascular system, which may be the result of vomiting, diarrhea, or prolonged bed rest.

Orthostatic vital signs are taken in three different positions. Blood pressure and pulse are taken with the patient lying down, then sitting up, and then standing. The recommended interval between checking the blood pressure in the various positions is 2 to 5 minutes. This allows the body's systems to adjust between readings. Do not allow the patient's arm to hang down while taking the blood pressure because this could cause a false blood pressure increase. Instead, rest the patient's arm on the bed or table. Watch the patient carefully, because the patient is at increased risk for passing out during these position changes. If there is an increase in the pulse rate of more than 10 bpm and the blood pressure drops more than 20 points, then the patient is considered to have orthostatic hypotension. This is sometimes documented as a **positive tilt test.** A positive tilt test may be due to dehydration, heart disease, diabetes, medications, or a nervous system disorder.

▶ Body Measurements   LO 37.6

Certain measurements are obtained before the patient is seen by the practitioner. These include height and weight for adults and older children, and weight, length, and head circumference for infants. Usually, these measurements are taken before or after the vital signs, depending on the office policy. Depending on the patient, you may choose to take the patient's vital signs first. For example, if a patient may become upset about her weight, you should take her vital signs first so that the patient's vital signs will not be affected by the weight results. Anxiety can cause a patient's pulse, respirations, and blood pressure to increase. Follow the policy at your facility.

Measurements taken at each visit provide baseline values for a patient's current condition. Any extreme or abnormal changes may indicate a disease or disorder and should be noted for the practitioner. For children and adolescents, these measurements should be taken at each office visit, which allows the licensed practitioner to follow growth and development.

Measurements are also important in determining the extent of an injury or illness and help define certain treatment regimens. For example, dosages of some medications are based on patient weight; a wound or bruise may be measured to determine how well it is healing. These measurements also may be necessary for correct interpretation of certain diagnostic tests, such as electrocardiography.

Metric conversions for weight and height measurements are given in Tables 37-5 and 37-6. To complete these conversions yourself, review the *Points on Practice* feature, Math for Measurements.

Measuring the Weight of Adults

Measure the weight of adults and older children at each office visit. Weight should be listed in the patient's chart to the nearest quarter of a pound. In some cases it will need to be converted to metric units. See Table 37-5. The steps for weighing an adult or child are described in Procedure 37-4.

Measuring the Height of Adults

The height of an adult should be measured at the patient's initial visit and whenever a complete physical exam is performed or at least yearly. Height for older children is typically measured at each visit. Height should be measured to the nearest quarter of an inch. In some cases it will need to be converted to metric units. See Table 37-6. Measure the patient's height

TABLE 37-6	Metric Conversions for Height				
in	**cm**	**in**	**cm**	**in**	**cm**
20	51	42	107	62	157
22	56	44	112	64	163
24	61	46	117	66	168
26	66	48	122	68	173
28	71	50	127	70	178
30	76	52	132	72	183
32	81	54	137	74	188
34	86	56	142	76	193
36	91	58	147	78	198
38	97	60	152	80	203
40	102				

Note: cm = in × 2.54; in = cm × 0.394. Conversions are rounded to the nearest whole number.

after weighing the patient. Most office scales have a height bar located in the center of the scale. This bar is calibrated in inches and quarter inches. The steps for measuring the height of an adult are described in Procedure 37-4.

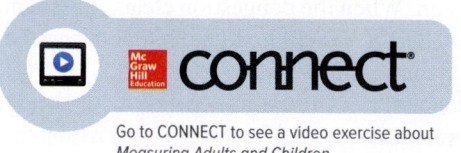

Go to CONNECT to see a video exercise about *Measuring Adults and Children.*

Body Mass Index

A reliable indicator of healthy weight is **body mass index (BMI),** which is calculated based on height and weight. If you are asked to calculate a patient's BMI, use the CDC's BMI chart (Figure 37-15). Hand-held BMI calculators are

TABLE 37-5	Metric Conversions for Weight				
lb	**kg**	**lb**	**kg**	**lb**	**kg**
10	4.5	95	43.1	180	81.7
15	6.8	100	45.4	185	84.0
20	9.1	105	47.7	190	86.3
25	11.4	110	49.9	195	88.5
30	13.6	115	52.2	200	90.8
35	15.9	120	54.5	205	93.1
40	18.2	125	56.8	210	95.3
45	20.4	130	59.0	215	97.6
50	22.7	135	61.3	220	99.9
55	25.0	140	63.6	225	102.2
60	27.2	145	65.8	230	104.4
65	29.5	150	68.1	235	106.7
70	31.8	155	70.4	240	109.0
75	34.1	160	72.6	245	111.2
80	36.3	165	74.9	250	113.5
85	38.6	170	77.2		
90	40.9	175	79.5		

Note: kg = lb × 0.454; lb = kg × 2.205. Conversions are rounded to nearest tenth.

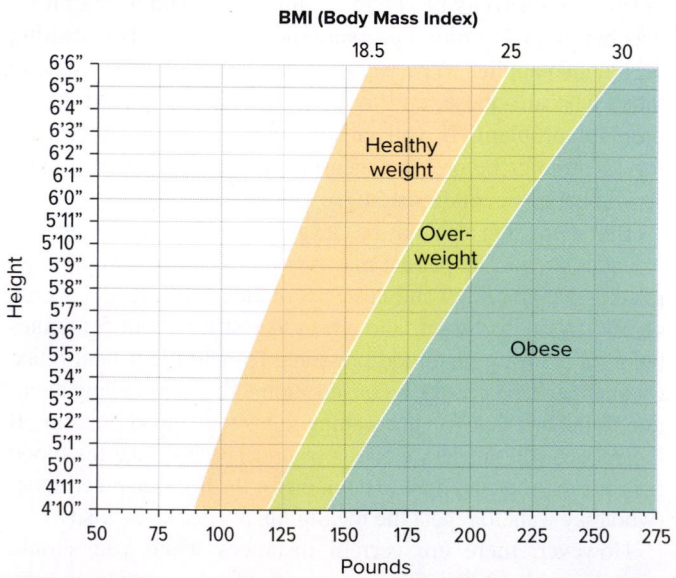

FIGURE 37-15 Use a BMI chart to calculate a patient's body mass index.

also available. See the chapter *Nutrition and Health* for more information on healthy weight management.

Other Body Measurements

In some facilities, you may be asked to obtain other body measurements. For example, if a patient has edema (swelling) of an arm or a leg, you might be asked to measure the diameter. You should measure both arms or legs to determine the difference in size. If a patient has a wound, bruise, or other injury, you may need to measure its length and width to evaluate the healing process. Additionally, sometimes an infant will need her chest circumference measured, or an adult may require a measurement around his abdomen, which is known as *abdominal girth*. Infant vital signs and measurements are described in more detail in the *Assisting in Pediatrics* chapter.

PROCEDURE 37-1 Measuring and Recording Temperature

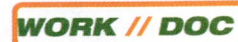

Procedure Goal: To accurately measure patient temperature while preventing the spread of infection

OSHA Guidelines:

 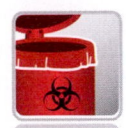

Materials: Thermometer, probe cover if required by thermometer, lubricant for rectal temperature, gloves, trash receptacle, patient's chart or progress note, and a black pen if recording in a paper record

Method:

1. Gather the equipment and make sure the thermometer is in working order.
2. Identify the patient and introduce yourself.
3. Wash your hands and explain the procedure to the patient.
4. Prepare the patient.
   a. *Oral.* If the patient has had anything to eat or drink, or has been smoking, wait at least 15 minutes before measuring the temperature orally.
   RATIONALE: *Inaccurate reading could result.*
   b. *Rectal.* Have the patient remove the appropriate clothing; assist as needed. Have the patient lie on his or her left side and drape for comfort.
   RATIONALE: *Proper positioning is necessary for the patient's safety and comfort.*
   c. *Axillary.* Assist the patient to expose the axilla. Provide for privacy and comfort. Pat dry the axilla.
   RATIONALE: *Perspiration or heavy deodorant prevents the thermometer from coming in direct contact with the skin.*
   d. *Temporal or tympanic.* If the patient is wearing a hat, ask the patient to remove it.
5. Prepare the equipment.
   a. Prepare an electronic thermometer by inserting the probe into the probe cover if necessary.

RATIONALE: *Probe covers are needed to prevent contamination of the probe.*
   b. Prepare a disposable thermometer by removing the wrapper to expose the handle end. Avoid touching the part of the thermometer that goes in the mouth or on the skin.
   RATIONALE: *Touching the thermometer could interfere with an accurate reading.*
   c. Prepare a temporal scanner by removing the protective cap and making sure the lens is clean.
   RATIONALE: *This will ensure an accurate reading.*
6. Measure the temperature.
   a. *Oral.* Place the thermometer under the tongue in the back of the mouth on one side. Have the patient hold it in place with his or her lips and tongue. Wait for the electronic thermometer to beep or indicate completion. For a disposable thermometer, wait the required time, usually 60 seconds.
   b. *Rectal.* Put on gloves. Lubricate the thermometer tip. Raise the buttock with one hand to expose the anus and insert the thermometer into the anal canal using your other hand, approximately 1 inch for adults and ½ inch for infants and children. Hold the thermometer securely in place until the indicator beeps or blinks.
   RATIONALE: *Injury could occur if the thermometer is inserted too far or if the patient moves during the procedure.*
   c. *Axillary.* Place the thermometer into the axilla, making sure the tip is in direct contact with the top of the axilla and is touching skin on all sides. Hold the arm firmly against the body until the indicator light blinks or beeps or the proper amount of time has passed.
   RATIONALE: *Ensures accuracy.*
   d. *Tympanic.* Hold the outer edge of the ear (pinna) with your free hand. Gently pull the pinna up for adults and down for children (see figure). Insert the probe into the ear canal directed toward the eardrum and sealing the ear canal. Press the scan button.

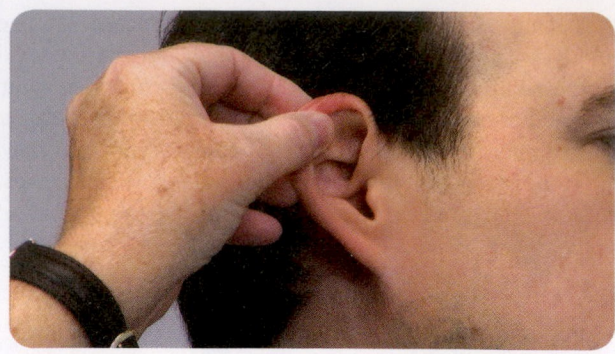

(a)

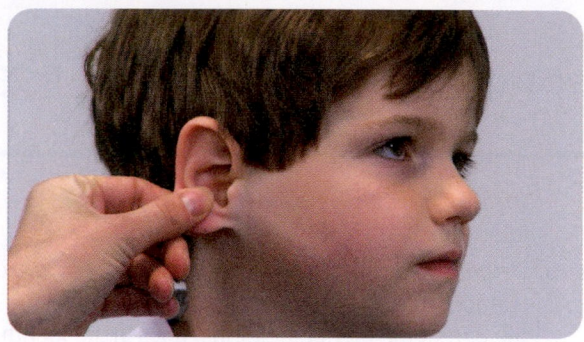

(b)

FIGURE Procedure 37-1 Step 6d When placing a tympanic thermometer, seal the ear canal by holding the pinna (outer ear) upward and outward for an adult (a) and downward and backward for a child (b).
© McGraw-Hill Education

RATIONALE: *Ensures accuracy.*

e. *Temporal.* Position the probe flat on the center of the exposed forehead. Press and hold the SCAN button and then slide the thermometer straight across the forehead until it beeps and the red light blinks.

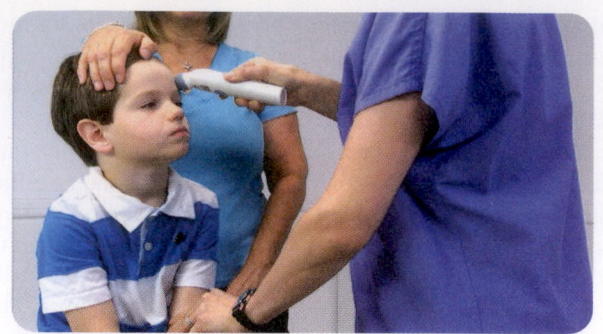

FIGURE Procedure 37-1 Step 6e A temporal scanner is a safe, fast, and noninvasive method for taking temperature.
© McGraw-Hill Education

7. Remove and read the measurement in the display or on the thermometer. Discard the disposable thermometer. Eject and discard the probe cover for an electronic thermometer. Replace the cap and/or place the thermometer into the charging base.
   RATIONALE: *Contaminated items should be removed and the thermometer should be protected and charged until the next use.*

8. Record the results. Chart by including the date and location where the temperature was taken.
   - Oral: 98.6
   - Rectal: 99.6 R
   - Axillary: 97.6 Ax
   - Temporal: 97.6 Temp or TA
   - Tympanic: 97.6 Tymp

   RATIONALE: *The temperature varies depending upon the location; this location should be charted to ensure an accurate diagnosis.*

9. Help the patient to replace clothing as necessary. Clear the area and provide for safety and comfort for the patient.

10. Wash your hands.

PROCEDURE 37-2 Measuring and Recording Pulse and Respirations

WORK // DOC

Procedure Goal: To accurately measure a patient's pulse and respirations while keeping the patient unaware the respirations are being counted

OSHA Guidelines:

 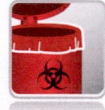

Materials: Watch with a second hand, patient's chart or progress note, and black pen if recording in a paper chart

Method:

1. Gather the equipment and wash your hands.
2. Introduce yourself and identify the patient.
3. Explain the procedure, saying, "I am going to take your vital signs. We'll start with your pulse first." Do not tell him you are counting the respirations.
   RATIONALE: *If the patient is aware you are counting respirations, he may unconsciously change his breathing rate.*
4. Ask the patient to sit or lie in a comfortable position. Have the patient rest his arm on a table. The palm should be facing downward.

5. Position yourself so you can observe and/or feel the chest wall movements. You may want to lay the patient's arm over the chest to feel the respiratory chest movements.

6. Place two or three fingers on the radial pulse site. Find the radial bone on the thumb side of the wrist; then slide your fingers into the groove on the inside of the wrist to locate the pulse.

7. Count the pulse for 30 seconds if regular. Note the rhythm and volume. If irregular, count for a full minute. Remember or note the number.
   RATIONALE: *An irregular pulse is counted for a full minute to ensure accuracy and to note abnormalities.*

8. Without letting go of the wrist, observe and feel the respirations, counting for 1 full minute. Observe for rhythm, volume, and effort.

9. Once you are certain of both numbers, release the wrist and record them. If the pulse was measured for less than 1 minute, obtain the number of beats per minute. Multiply the number of beats counted in 30 seconds by 2.

10. Document results with the date and time (example: 6/18/16 P 88 regular and strong R 16 regular).

11. Report any findings that are a significant change from a previous result or outside the normal values, as shown in Table 37-1.

PROCEDURE 37-3 Taking the Blood Pressure of Adults and Older Children

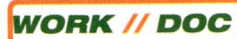

Procedure Goal: To accurately measure blood pressure in adults and older children

OSHA Guidelines:

 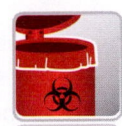

Materials: Sphygmomanometer, stethoscope, alcohol gauze squares, patient's chart or progress note, and black pen if recording in a paper chart

Method:

1. Gather the equipment and make sure the sphygmomanometer is in working order and correctly calibrated.
   RATIONALE: *Calibration helps ensure an accurate result.*

2. Identify the patient and introduce yourself.

3. Wash your hands and explain the procedure to the patient.

4. Have the patient sit in a quiet area. If she is wearing long-sleeved clothing, have her loosely roll up one sleeve. If she cannot, have her change into a gown.

5. Have the patient rest her bared arm on a flat surface so that the midpoint of the upper arm is at the same level as the heart.
   RATIONALE: *Doing so helps ensure an accurate reading.*

6. Select a cuff that is the appropriate size for the patient. The bladder inside the cuff should encircle 80% of the arm in adults and 100% of the arm in children younger than the age of 13. If you are not sure about the size, use a larger cuff.
   RATIONALE: *Using the proper cuff size helps ensure an accurate reading.*

7. Locate the brachial artery in the antecubital space.

8. Position the cuff so that the midline of the bladder is above the arterial pulsation. Then wrap and secure the cuff snugly around the patient's bare upper arm. The lower edge of the cuff should be 1 inch above the antecubital space, where the head of the stethoscope is to be placed.
   RATIONALE: *If the blood pressure cuff touches the stethoscope, it could interfere with your ability to hear.*

9. Place the manometer so that the center of the aneroid dial is at eye level and easily visible and so that the tubing from the cuff is unobstructed.

10. Close the valve of the pressure bulb until it is finger-tight.

11. Inflate the cuff rapidly to 70 mmHg with one hand and increase this pressure in 10 mmHg increments while palpating the radial pulse with your other hand. Note the level of pressure at which the pulse disappears and subsequently reappears during deflation. This procedure is the palpatory method.

12. Open the valve to release the pressure, deflate the cuff completely, and wait at least 30 seconds or remove and replace the cuff.
    RATIONALE: *If you do not deflate the cuff completely and wait, blood may pool in the artery and give a falsely high reading.*

13. Place the earpieces of the stethoscope in your ear canals and adjust them to fit snugly and comfortably. When placed in the ears, they should point toward the nose. Switch the stethoscope head to the diaphragm position. Confirm the setting by listening as you tap the stethoscope head gently.

14. Place the head of the stethoscope over the brachial artery pulsation, just above and medial to the antecubital space but below the lower edge of the cuff. Hold the stethoscope firmly in place using your index and middle fingers, making sure the head is in contact with the skin around its entire circumference.
    RATIONALE: *Do not hold the stethoscope with your thumb because the pulse of your thumb can interfere with the reading.*

15. Inflate the bladder rapidly and steadily to a pressure 30 mmHg above the level previously determined by the palpatory method. Then partially open (unscrew) the valve and deflate the bladder at approximately 2 mm per second while you listen for the Korotkoff sounds.

16. As the pressure in the bladder falls, note the level of pressure on the manometer at the first appearance of repetitive sounds. This reading is the systolic pressure.

17. Continue to deflate the cuff gradually, noting the point at which the sound changes from strong to muffled.

18. Continue to deflate the cuff, and note when the sound disappears. This reading is the diastolic pressure.

19. Continue to listen for an additional 10 mmHg, listening carefully for a return of the repetitive sounds.
    RATIONALE: *Continue listening to ensure that the lack of sound is not the result of an auscultatory gap.*

20. Deflate the cuff completely and remove it from the patient's arm.

21. Record the systolic and diastolic numbers, separated by a slash, in the patient's chart. Chart the date and time of the measurement, the arm on which the measurement was made, the subject's position, and the cuff size when a nonstandard size is used. The value recorded is an exact measurement of the auscultated blood pressure.

22. Fold the cuff and replace it in the holder.

23. Inform the patient that you have completed the procedure.

24. Disinfect the earpieces and diaphragm of the stethoscope with gauze squares moistened with alcohol.

25. Properly dispose of the used gauze squares and wash your hands.

PROCEDURE 37-4 Measuring Adults and Children

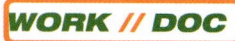

Procedure Goal: To accurately measure weight and height of adults and children

OSHA Guidelines:

Materials: For an adult or older child, adult scale with height bar, disposable towel; for toddler, adult scale with height bar or height chart, disposable towel, patient chart/progress note

Method:

Adult or Older Child: Weight

1. Identify the patient and introduce yourself.

2. Wash your hands and explain the procedure to the patient.

3. Check to see whether the scale is in balance by moving all the weights to the left side. The indicator should be level with the middle mark. If not, check the manufacturer's directions and adjust it to ensure a zero balance. If you are using a scale equipped to measure either kilograms or pounds, check to see that it is set on the desired units and that the upper and lower weights show the same units.
   RATIONALE: *Proper functioning of the scale helps ensure an accurate result.*

4. Ask the patient to remove her shoes, if that is the standard office policy.
   RATIONALE: *Follow the policy and use the same procedure for all visits for consistency of results.*

5. Place a disposable towel on the scale or have the patient leave her socks on.
   RATIONALE: *Prevents cross-contamination of the scale from various patients' feet*

6. Ask the patient to step on the center of the scale, facing forward. Assist as necessary.

7. Place the lower weight at the highest number that does not cause the balance indicator to drop to the bottom.
   RATIONALE: *To ensure accuracy*

8. Move the upper weight slowly to the right until the balance bar is centered at the middle mark, adjusting as necessary.
   RATIONALE: *To ensure accuracy*

9. Add the two weights together to get the patient's weight.

10. Record the patient's weight in the chart to the nearest quarter of a pound or tenth of a kilogram.

11. Return the weights to their starting positions on the left side.

Adult or Older Child: Height

12. With the patient off the scale, raise the height bar well above the patient's head and swing out the extension. (This can also be done before the patient steps on the scale for his weight measurement.)
    RATIONALE: *Doing so prevents hitting the patient with the extension bar.*

13. Ask the patient to step on the center of the scale and to stand up straight and look forward.
    RATIONALE: *Standing straight is necessary for accuracy.*

14. Gently lower the height bar until the extension rests on the patient's head.

15. Have the patient step off the scale while you hold the height bar before reading the measurement.
    RATIONALE: *To better visualize the height measurement*

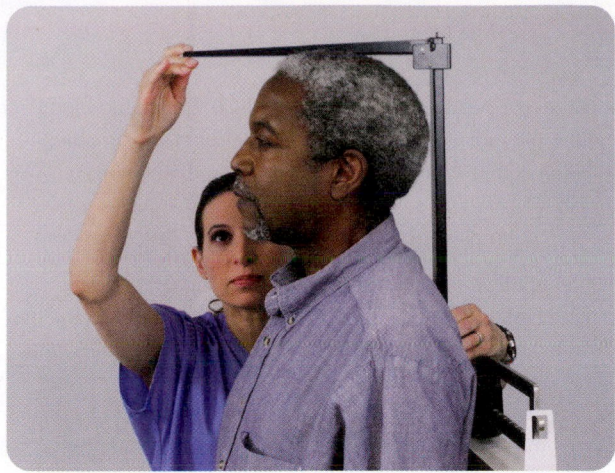

FIGURE Procedure 37-4 Step 14 The medical assistant adjusts the height bar to meet the top of the patient's head.
© McGraw-Hill Education

16. If the patient is fewer than 50 inches tall, read the height on the bottom part of the ruler; if the patient is more than 50 inches tall, read the height on the top, movable part of the ruler at the point at which it meets the bottom part of the ruler. Note that the numbers increase on the bottom part of the bar and decrease on the top, movable part of the bar. Read the height in the right direction.

17. Record the patient's height.

18. Have the patient put shoes back on, if necessary.

19. Properly dispose of the used towel and wash your hands.

Toddler: Weight

1. Identify the patient and obtain permission from the parent to weigh the toddler.

2. Wash your hands and explain the procedure to the parent.

3. Check to see whether the scale is in balance and place a disposable towel on the scale or have the patient wear shoes or socks, depending on the facility's policy.

4. Ask the parent to hold the patient and to step on the scale. Follow the procedure for obtaining the weight of an adult.

5. Have the parent put the child down or hand the child to another staff member.

6. Obtain the parent's weight.
   RATIONALE: *This is done to find the difference between the two weights.*

7. Subtract the parent's weight from the combined weight to determine the child's weight.

8. Record the patient's weight in the chart to the nearest quarter of a pound or tenth of a kilogram.

Toddler: Height

9. Measure the child's height in the same manner as you measure adult height, or have the child stand with her back against the height chart. Measure height at the crown of the head.

10. Record the height in the patient's chart.

11. Properly dispose of the towel (if used) and wash your hands.
    RATIONALE: *Doing so prevents infection.*

SUMMARY OF LEARNING OUTCOMES

LEARNING OUTCOMES	KEY POINTS
37.1 Describe the vital signs.	Vital signs include temperature, pulse, respirations, and blood pressure; some practitioners also consider pain assessment to be one of the vital signs.
37.2 Identify various methods of taking a patient's temperature.	Using either an electronic digital or disposable thermometer, a patient's temperature may be measured by the oral, tympanic, rectal, axillary, or temporal method.
37.3 Describe the process of obtaining pulse and respirations.	Pressing lightly at the radial artery using your fingers, count the number of beats you feel in 1 minute to get the pulse. While still keeping fingers on the patient's pulse site, observe and feel the patient's respirations, and count the respirations for 1 full minute. See Procedure 37-2.
37.4 Carry out blood pressure measurements.	To obtain a blood pressure, have the patient sit in a quiet area, rest his or her bared arm on a flat surface at heart level, locate the brachial artery, snugly secure the cuff above the brachial artery, use the palpatory method to determine the approximate systolic pressure, and use a stethoscope to auscultate the systolic and diastolic blood pressure.

LEARNING OUTCOMES	KEY POINTS
37.5 Summarize orthostatic, or postural, vital signs.	Orthostatic, or postural, vital signs consist of taking the blood pressure and pulse in different positions, from lying to sitting to standing, waiting 2 to 5 minutes between repositioning to allow the body's systems to adjust to the change.
37.6 Illustrate various body measurements.	For adults and older children, the measurements obtained are the height and weight; for infants, they are the weight, length, and head circumference. See Procedure 37-4. BMI, extremities, and wounds are also measured according to facility policy and patient condition.

C A S E   S T U D Y   C R I T I C A L   T H I N K I N G

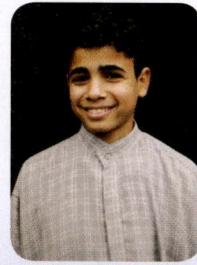

© David Sacks/Getty Images

Recall Mohammad from the beginning of the chapter. Now that you have completed the chapter, answer the following questions regarding his case.

1. Why is an accurate measurement and recording of Mohammad's vital signs critical in this case?

2. After examining Mohammad and ordering and reviewing the results of an ECG test, Dr. Williams indicates that Mohammad's heart appears to be normal. What factors might be contributing to Mohammad's episodes of tachycardia?

3. The physician is going to give Mohammad an injection and needs to know his weight in kilograms. You measured his weight as 140 pounds. Convert this weight to kilograms.

E X A M   P R E P A R A T I O N   Q U E S T I O N S

1. (LO 37.4) If a patient's blood pressure is 138/82, it is considered
   a. Normal
   b. Hypotension
   c. Prehypertension
   d. Stage 1 hypertension
   e. Stage 2 hypertension

2. (LO 37.1) When taking a patient's oral temperature, you should wear gloves if
   a. The patient is in for a routine physical exam
   b. There are contact precautions for the patient
   c. The patient is less than 5 years old
   d. You suspect the patient has a fever
   e. The patient cannot hold the thermometer in her mouth

3. (LO 37.2) Using the formula to convert degrees Fahrenheit to degrees Celsius, determine which of the following is equal to 99.8°F (round to the nearest tenth).
   a. 37.7°C
   b. 37.7°F
   c. 37.6°C
   d. 35.8°C
   e. 36.7°C

4. (LO 37.2) How would you abbreviate a rectal temperature of 99.7° Fahrenheit?
   a. T 97.9 R
   b. P 99.7 R
   c. T 99.7 Ax
   d. T 99.7 R
   e. T 99.7

5. (LO 37.3) The average ratio of the pulse rate to the respiration rate is
   a. 1:4
   b. 1:2
   c. 3:1
   d. 4:1
   e. 5:2

6. (LO 37.3) Abnormally rapid, deep, or labored breathing is known as
   a. Hyperpyrexia
   b. Hyperpnea
   c. Tachypnea
   d. Hypertension
   e. Bradypnea

7. (LO 37.3) Which of the following are crackling noises heard when the patient breathes?
   a. Rhonchi
   b. Apnea
   c. Cheyne-Stokes
   d. Asthma
   e. Rales

8. (LO 37.4) Low blood pressure is known as
   a. Papilledema
   b. Hypertension
   c. Tachycardia
   d. Hypotension
   e. Bradycardia

9. (LO 37.6) When measuring a patient's weight in pounds, it is important to round to the nearest
   a. ¼ pound
   b. Pound
   c. ½ pound
   d. Ounce
   e. ⅛ pound

10. (LO 37.5) Taking a patient's blood pressure in different positions is used to assess for
   a. Heart failure
   b. Hypertension
   c. Postural hypotension
   d. Vasoconstriction
   e. Kidney disease

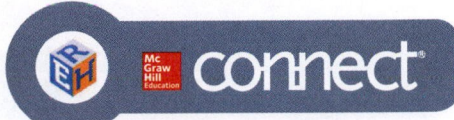

Go to CONNECT to see activities about *Documenting Vital Signs, Adding Vital Signs as Part of an Office Visit, Recording Vital Signs for Pediatric Patients, and Viewing Vital Signs in a Patient's Chart.*

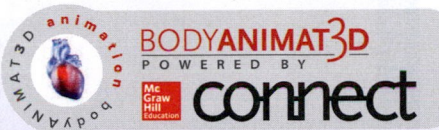

Go to CONNECT to see an animation exercise about *Hypertension.*

SOFT SKILLS SUCCESS

The electronic pulse oximeter is in use and, although you would rather not do it, you take the patient's pulse manually. While counting the pulse you notice it seems irregular and every so often it seems to feel stronger. You look at the patient who appears pale and has a slight grimace on his face. What should you do?

Go to PRACTICE MEDICAL OFFICE and complete the module Clinical - Office Operations.

Assisting with a General Physical Examination

38

CASE STUDY

Valarie Ramirez, a 33-year-old female, is at the office for a pre-employment general physical exam. Her vital signs are BP 122/80, T 98.6 P 84 R 20, height 62 inches, and weight 140 pounds. While you are interviewing her, she shows you a wart on her right hand and says it is very painful and would like it taken off.

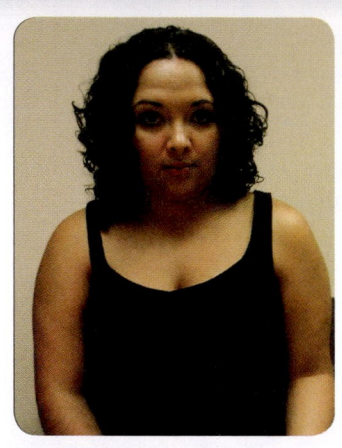

© McGraw-Hill Education

Keep Valarie Ramirez in mind as you study this chapter. There will be questions at the end of the chapter based on the case study. The information in the chapter will help you answer these questions.

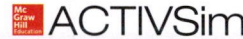
McGraw-Hill Education **ACTIVSim**

LEARNING OUTCOMES

After completing Chapter 38, you will be able to:

38.1 Identify the purpose of a general physical exam.

38.2 Describe the role of the medical assistant in a general physical exam.

38.3 Explain safety precautions used during a general physical exam.

38.4 Carry out the steps necessary to prepare the patient for an exam.

38.5 Carry out positioning and draping a patient in each of the nine common exam positions.

38.6 Apply techniques to assist patients from different cultures and patients with physical disabilities.

38.7 Identify the six examination methods used in a general physical exam.

38.8 List the components of a general physical exam.

38.9 Describe follow-up steps after a general physical exam.

KEY TERMS

auscultation
body mechanics
clinical diagnosis
culture
differential diagnosis
digital examination
fenestrated drape
hyperventilation
inspection
kyphosis
manipulation

mensuration
nasal mucosa
palpation
percussion
prognosis
quadrant
scoliosis
sign
symmetry
symptom

CAAHEP

I.P.8 Instruct and prepare a patient for a procedure or a treatment

I.P.9 Assist provider with a patient exam

III.P.2 Select appropriate barrier/personal protective equipment (PPE)

V.P.3 Use medical terminology correctly and pronounced accurately to communicate information to providers and patients

V.P.5 Coach patients appropriately considering:
(a) cultural diversity
(c) communication barriers

X.P.3 Document patient care accurately in the medical record

ABHES

2. Anatomy and Physiology
c. Identify diagnostic and treatment modalities as they relate to each body system

5. Psychology of Human Relations
c. Intervene on behalf of the patient regarding issues/concerns that may arise, i.e. insurance policy information, medical bills, physician/provider orders, etc.

8. Medical Office Business Procedures Management
f. Display professionalism through written and verbal communications

9. Medical Office Clinical Procedures
a. Practice standard precautions and perform disinfection/sterilization techniques
b. Obtain vital signs, obtain patient history, and formulate chief complaint
c. Assist provider with general/physical examination
h. Teach self-examination, disease management and health promotion
j. Make adaptations with patients with special needs

▶ Introduction

Whether a patient comes for a regular checkup or to have a problem diagnosed and treated, the physical exam is the first step in the process for the physician or other licensed practitioner. As the medical assistant, your role during the physical exam is to make the patient comfortable and assist the physician as necessary. A skilled medical assistant who is sensitive to patient needs and proficient in performing these skills can create an atmosphere that results in a positive outcome for the patient during the exam.

▶ The Purpose of a General Physical Exam
LO 38.1

Physicians perform general physical exams for two purposes. The first is to examine a healthy patient to confirm an overall state of health and to provide baseline values for vital signs and measurements. The second is to examine a patient to diagnose a medical problem.

To confirm a patient's health status, physicians usually perform exams on a routine basis, such as once a year. Some exams are done to fulfill a requirement before an individual starts school, begins a new job, or starts an exercise program.

When a physician performs an examination to diagnose medical problems, she usually focuses on a particular organ system. The organ system is indicated to the physician by the patient's condition and chief complaint. Because organ systems are so interdependent, however, physicians generally perform an overall physical exam even when a specific medical problem exists.

During a general physical exam, physicians check all the major organs and body systems. They can determine much about a patient's general condition of health from the exam. If appropriate, they also try to make an initial, or **clinical, diagnosis**—a diagnosis based on the signs and symptoms of a disease. A **sign** is objective information that can be detected by a person other than the affected person. Some examples of signs are blood in the stool and a bloody nose. A **symptom** is subjective information supplied by the patient. Anxiety, back pain, abdominal pain, and fatigue are examples of symptoms. Only the patient can perceive these sensations, which are typically part of the chief complaint.

After forming an initial diagnosis of a patient's problem, physicians may order laboratory or other diagnostic tests. These tests are done to confirm a clinical diagnosis or to rule out other possible disorders and are necessary when a patient has symptoms that may indicate more than one condition. Determining the correct diagnosis when two or more diagnoses are possible is called making a **differential diagnosis.**

Laboratory and diagnostic tests also may aid physicians in developing a **prognosis,** or a forecast of the probable course and outcome of the disorder and the prospects of recovery.

In addition, such tests help physicians formulate a treatment plan or appropriate drug therapy. Physicians may ask to have these tests repeated as part of the follow-up evaluation of a patient's progress.

▶ The Role of the Medical Assistant LO 38.2

Your job as a medical assistant is to assist both the licensed practitioner and the patient during the general physical exam. Your role starts before the actual exam. First, you interview the patient, document an accurate history, determine vital signs, and measure weight and height.

Generally, your responsibilities during the exam include ensuring all instruments and supplies are readily available to the licensed practitioner. You also ensure that patients are physically and emotionally comfortable during the exam by helping them into position and keeping them aware of what is going to happen. It is important to observe the patient for signs that indicate distress or the need for assistance. Providing comfort and safety to the patient and competent assistance to the physician are key during a general physical exam.

▶ Safety Precautions LO 38.3

As you prepare for and assist with a general physical exam, you will practice safety measures. Some of these are outlined by the Department of Labor's Occupational Safety and Health Administration (OSHA) and the Department of Health and Human Services' Centers for Disease Control and Prevention (CDC). Recall that OSHA standards and guidelines are designed to protect employees and make the workplace safe. The CDC establishes the guidelines intended to protect both patients and healthcare professionals in the medical office and the hospital setting. Taken together, these safety measures help protect you, the physician, and the patient from disease transmission.

Safety measures that you must take before, during, and after a general physical exam include the following:

- Perform a thorough aseptic handwashing before and after contact with each patient and before and after each procedure. Waterless, alcohol-based hand cleanser may be used between patients if no gross contamination or visible soilage is on your hands. Refer to the chapter *Infection Control Fundamentals* for a review of these procedures.

- Wear gloves whenever there is a possibility that you may come in contact with blood, body fluids, nonintact skin, or moist surfaces, both during the patient exam and when handling specimens.

- Instruct symptomatic patients to maintain respiratory hygiene/cough etiquette by covering their mouth and nose when coughing; using tissues and disposing of them in a no-touch receptacle; observing hand hygiene; and wearing a surgical mask or maintaining a distance of greater than 3 feet if possible. See the chapter *Infection Control Practices* for more information about respiratory hygiene/cough etiquette.

- Wear a mask in the presence of a patient suspected of having an infectious disease that is transmitted by airborne droplets, such as tuberculosis (TB) or meningitis.

- Patients with highly contagious infectious diseases, such as diphtheria or chickenpox, must be examined under isolation precautions, such as in a private room. Wear personal protective equipment (PPE) during contact. Table 38-1 provides a summary of necessary PPE based on specific diseases. Refer to the chapter *Infection Control Practices* for additional information.

- Discard in biohazardous waste containers all disposable equipment and supplies that come in contact with a patient's blood or body fluids.

- Clean and disinfect the exam room following each patient's exam.

- Sanitize, disinfect, and sterilize equipment, as appropriate, after each patient's exam.

▶ Preparing the Patient for an Exam LO 38.4

As a medical assistant, you will need to prepare the patient both emotionally and physically.

Emotional Preparation

To prepare patients, begin by explaining exactly what will occur during the exam. Use simple, direct language that patients can understand. Describe what patients can expect to feel and how their cooperation can contribute to the procedure's success. As discussed in the *Assisting in Pediatrics* chapter, emotional preparedness is particularly important when dealing with children, who deserve to have the same sort of information and reassurance as adults. Mature adults may require special attention to communication during emotional preparation, as discussed in the *Assisting in Geriatrics* chapter.

If you are a male medical assistant, a female physician may ask you to remain in the room when she examines a male patient. Likewise, if you are a female medical assistant, a male physician may ask you to remain in the room when he examines a woman. These measures are for the protection of both the patient and the physician. Such policies depend on the standard procedures in each medical practice or facility.

Physical Preparation

To ensure the patient is physically prepared before the physician enters the exam room, give the patient an opportunity to empty his bladder and/or bowels in order to be more comfortable during the exam. Collect a urine specimen at this time, if needed.

Ensure the room temperature is comfortable and when the patient is ready, ask him to disrobe and put on an exam gown or cover himself with a drape. The extent of disrobing depends on the type of exam and the physician's preference. If the physician requests a gown for the patient, show the patient how to put on the gown. Include specific instructions

TABLE 38-1	PPE for Infection and Precaution Type	
Infection	**Precaution Type**	**Appropriate PPE**
Abscess	Contact	Gloves and gown
AIDS	Standard	Use appropriate PPE when exposed to blood or body fluids.
Anthrax	Standard	Use appropriate PPE when exposed to blood or body fluids.
Chickenpox (varicella)	Airborne/contact	Respirator (or mask and goggles) and gloves
Diphtheria • Cutaneous • Pharyngeal	Contact droplet	Gloves and gown Mask and goggles when working within 3 feet of patient
Gastroenteritis	Standard/contact	Use appropriate PPE when exposed to blood or body fluids; avoid contact with fecal material by donning gloves and gown.
Hepatitis		
• A	Contact	Gloves and gown
• B	Standard	Use appropriate PPE when exposed to blood or body fluids.
• C	Standard	Use appropriate PPE when exposed to blood or body fluids.
• E	Standard	Use appropriate PPE when exposed to blood or body fluids.
Herpes zoster (shingles)	Contact	Gloves and gown; *note:* individuals who have not had chickenpox should avoid contact with patients with shingles.
Influenza	Droplet	Mask and goggles when working within 3 feet of patient
Measles	Airborne	Mask and goggles or respirator
Meningitis	Standard/droplet	Use appropriate PPE when exposed to blood or body fluids; use mask and goggles when working within 3 feet of patient.
Mumps	Droplet	Mask and goggles when working within 3 feet of patient
Pertussis	Droplet	Mask and goggles when working within 3 feet of patient
Poliomyelitis	Standard	Use appropriate PPE when exposed to blood or body fluids.
Rotavirus	Contact	Gloves and gown
Rubella	Droplet	Mask and goggles when working within 3 feet of patient
Scabies	Contact	Gloves and gown
Staphylococcal disease	Contact	Gloves and gown
Streptococcal disease	Contact/droplet	Gloves, gown, mask, and goggles
Tuberculosis	Airborne	Mask and goggles or respirator

on whether the gown should open in the back or front and whether it should be left open or tied. Leave the exam room while the patient disrobes to give him privacy, unless he needs and requests assistance.

Be aware of the patient's modesty and comfort at all times. Imagine what it feels like to visit a physician and, as you disrobe and put on the gown, you notice that it is too small and it's beginning to tear. In order to ensure patient comfort, make sure a variety of sizes are available for patient use. Use your critical thinking skills when selecting a patient gown. Your patient will remember this gesture and appreciate your consideration.

▶ Positioning and Draping   LO 38.5

During the exam, the patient may need to assume a variety of positions, which facilitate the physician's exam of certain areas of the body. The physician will indicate which positions

are needed for specific exams. You may need to help the patient assume these positions. Depending upon the patient's mobility (ability to move), you may need to help transfer, lift, and move the patient. To protect yourself from injury when helping to positioning a patient, always follow the basic rules of good **body mechanics.** Body mechanics is the application of physical principles to help prevent stress and injury to healthcare practitioners who are lifting, moving and positioning patients:

• Lifting with your strongest muscles, including your legs and arms, rather than your back
• Keeping your feet apart
• Bending from the hip and knees

Some positions are embarrassing or physically uncomfortable for patients. If you perceive embarrassment, explain the need for the position and help the patient assume the position when necessary. Consider cultural differences and be understanding to each individual's needs. Most important, help minimize the time a patient spends in any embarrassing or uncomfortable position.

If a patient is physically uncomfortable in a position, you may be able to ease the discomfort by using a small pillow to support part of the body. You may have to help the patient maintain a position during the exam. Always try to make the patient as comfortable as possible.

When you need to make changes in the patient's position, do so gradually. If your office is equipped with an examining table that can be adjusted automatically, learn to use the controls efficiently to maximize patient comfort. Always tell the patient what movement to expect.

When patients have assumed the correct position, cover them with an appropriate drape. Drapes vary in size. Make sure you choose one that will help keep the patient warm and maintain privacy. You will position drapes differently depending on the exam position and the parts of the patient's body that the physician examines.

Exam Positions

The following are the positions commonly used during a medical exam (see Figure 38-1):

- Sitting
- Supine (recumbent)
- Dorsal recumbent
- Lithotomy
- Fowler's
- Prone
- Sims'
- Knee-chest or knee-elbow
- Proctologic

Sitting In the sitting position, the patient sits at the edge of the examining table without back support (see Figure 38-1a). The physician examines the patient's head, neck, chest, heart, back, and arms. While the patient is in the sitting position, the physician evaluates the patient's ability to fully expand the

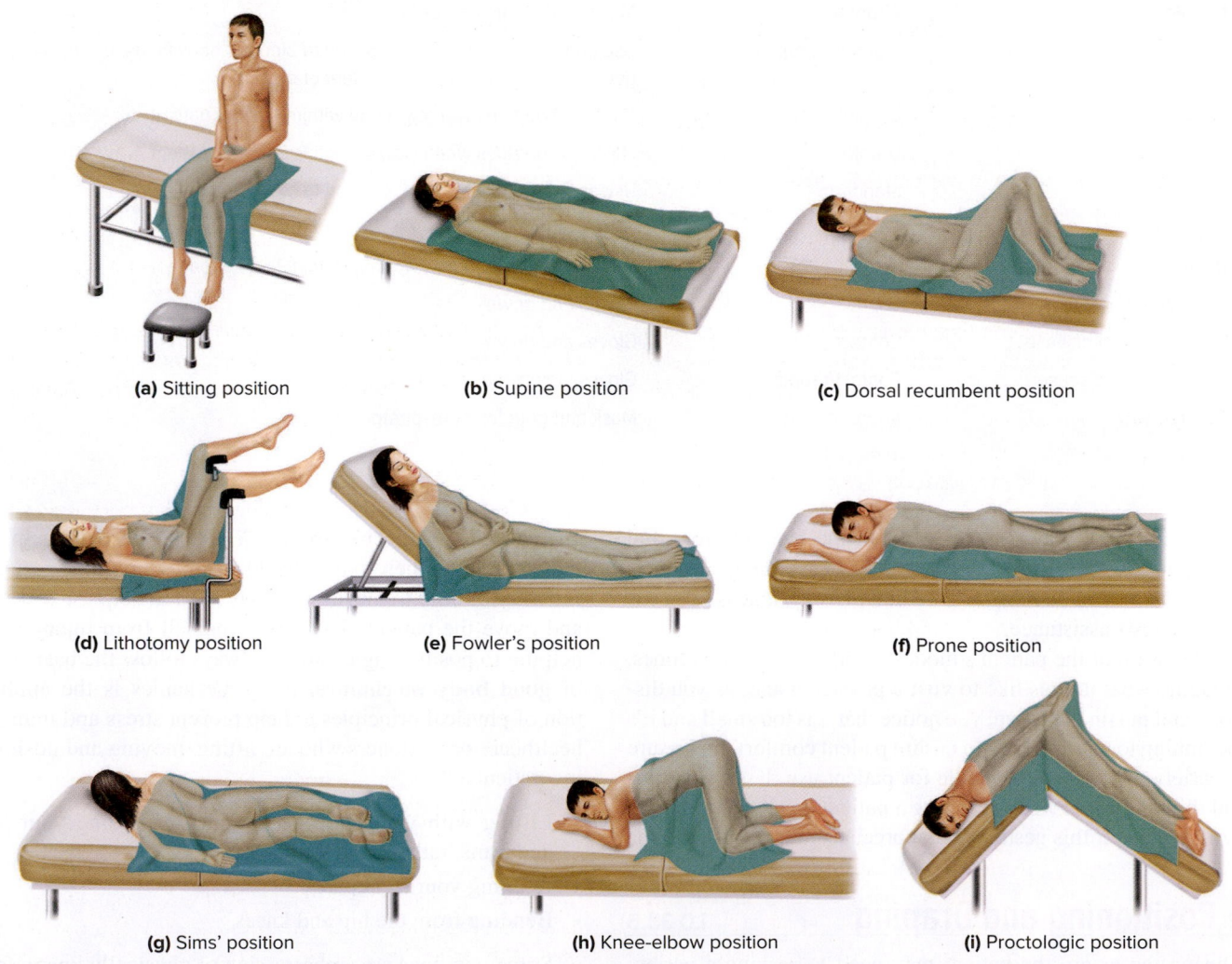

(a) Sitting position   (b) Supine position   (c) Dorsal recumbent position

(d) Lithotomy position   (e) Fowler's position   (f) Prone position

(g) Sims' position   (h) Knee-elbow position   (i) Proctologic position

FIGURE 38-1 These positions may be used during the general physical examination.

lungs. She then checks the upper body parts for **symmetry,** the degree to which one side is the same as the other. In the sitting position, the drape is placed across the patient's lap for men or across the patient's chest and lap for women.

If a patient is too weak to sit unsupported, another position is necessary, such as the supine position.

Supine (Recumbent)
In the supine, or recumbent, position, the patient lies flat on the back with the hands to the side (Figure 38-1b) or on the abdomen. (*Supine* means "lying down face-up"; *recumbent* means "lying down." Both terms are used to describe this position.) This is the most relaxed position for many patients. A physician can examine the head, neck, chest, heart, abdomen, arms, and legs when a patient is in this position. The patient is normally draped from the neck or underarms down to the feet.

The supine position may not be comfortable for patients who become short of breath easily or for a pregnant patient late in her pregnancy. Also, patients with a back injury or lower back pain may find it uncomfortable. You can make these patients more comfortable by placing pillows under their head and knees. Some patients, however, may need to be placed in the dorsal recumbent position.

Dorsal Recumbent
In the dorsal recumbent position, the patient lies face-up, with the back supporting all the weight. (The term *dorsal* refers to the back.) This position is the same as the supine position, except the patient's knees are drawn up and the feet are flat on the table, as shown in Figure 38-1c. Again, the hands can be at the patient's side or on the abdomen. The physician may examine the head, neck, chest, and heart while a patient is in this position. The patient is normally draped from the neck or underarms down to the feet.

Patients who have leg disabilities may find the dorsal recumbent position uncomfortable or even impossible. On the other hand, patients who are elderly or have painful disorders such as arthritis or back pain may find the dorsal recumbent position more comfortable than the supine position because the knees are bent. This position is sometimes used as an alternative to the lithotomy position when patients have severe arthritis or joint deformities.

Lithotomy
The lithotomy position is used during examination of the female genitalia. In this position, the patient lies on her back with her knees bent and her feet in stirrups attached to the end of the examining table. You may need to help the patient place her feet in the stirrups. She should then slide forward to position her buttocks near the edge of the table, as shown in Figure 38-1d.

Many women are embarrassed and physically uncomfortable in this position, so you should not ask a patient to remain in this position any longer than necessary. Use a large drape that covers the patient from the breasts to the ankles. Placing the drape with one point or corner between the legs will make the exam easier in this position.

A patient with severe arthritis or joint deformities in the hips or knees may have difficulty assuming the lithotomy position. She may be able to place only one leg in the stirrup, or she may need your assistance in separating her thighs. An alternative position for such a patient is the dorsal recumbent position. Other patients who may have difficulty with the lithotomy position are those who are obese or in the late stages of pregnancy.

Fowler's
In Fowler's position, the patient lies back on an examining table on which the head is elevated at a 45-degree angle, as shown in Figure 38-1e. The physician may examine the head, neck, and chest areas while the patient is in this position. The patient is usually draped from the neck or underarms down to the feet.

Fowler's position is one of the best positions for examining patients who are experiencing shortness of breath or and patients with a lower back injury.

Prone
In the prone position, the patient is lying flat on the table, facedown. The patient's head is turned to one side, and the arms are placed at the sides or bent at the elbows, as shown in Figure 38-1f. The patient is normally draped from the upper back to the feet.

With the patient in this position, the physician can examine the back, feet, or musculoskeletal system. The prone position is unsuitable for women in advanced stages of pregnancy, obese patients, patients with respiratory difficulties, and the elderly.

Sims'
In the Sims' position, the patient lies on the left side. The patient's left leg is slightly bent, and the left arm is placed behind the back so the patient's weight is resting primarily on the chest. The right knee is bent and raised toward the chest, and the right arm is bent toward the head for support, as shown in Figure 38-1g. The patient is draped from the upper back to the feet.

Sims' position is used during anal or rectal exams and may also be used for perineal and certain pelvic exams. Patients with joint deformities of the hips and knees may have difficulty assuming this position.

Knee-Chest or Knee-Elbow
In the knee-chest position, the patient is lying on the table facedown, supporting the body with the knees and chest. The patient's thighs should be at a 90-degree angle to the table and slightly separated. The head is turned to one side, and the arms are placed to the side or above the head. The patient may need your assistance to assume this position correctly and to maintain it during the exam.

The knee-chest position is used during exams of the anal and perineal areas and during certain proctologic procedures. Some patients—those who are pregnant, obese, or elderly—may have difficulty assuming this position. An alternative that puts less strain on the patient and is easier to maintain is the knee-elbow position, shown in Figure 38-1h. This position is the same as the knee-chest position except that the patient supports body weight with the knees and elbows rather than the knees and chest. In either of these two positions, the patient is commonly covered with a **fenestrated drape,** in which a special opening provides access to the area to be examined.

Proctologic The proctologic, or jackknife, position may be used as an alternative to the Sims' or knee-chest position. In the proctologic position, the patient is bent at the hips at a 90-degree angle. The patient can assume this position by standing next to the examining table and bending at the waist until the chest rests on the table. If an adjustable examining table is available, the patient can assume the position by lying prone on the table, which is then raised in the middle with both ends pointing down. This places the patient at the correct 90-degree angle, as shown in Figure 38-1i. In either variation of this position, the patient is draped with a fenestrated drape, as in the knee-chest position.

The steps for placing patients into these positions are described in Procedure 38-1 at the end of this chapter.

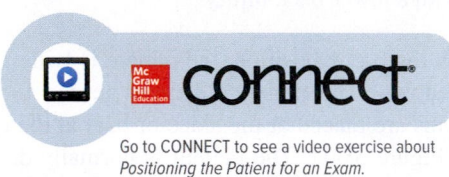

Go to CONNECT to see a video exercise about *Positioning the Patient for an Exam.*

▶ Special Patient Considerations   LO 38.6

Patients from other cultures and patients with disabilities may require special considerations during a general physical exam.

Patients from Different Cultures

You can expect to assist with a general physical exam for patients from other cultures. A **culture** is defined as a pattern of assumptions, beliefs, and practices that shapes the way people think and act. Avoid the temptation to stereotype an individual or group on the basis of a single patient's behavior. Stereotyping can lead to incorrect judgments, which may influence the care you provide to patients. Avoid making judgments about patients or cultural groups on the basis of your experience with other patients or with your own family and friends. Remember, if their culture is different from yours, then your culture also seems different to them.

Patients from different cultures may not be familiar with the medical exam and may not know what to expect. These patients may be more modest than other patients and may have a greater need for privacy. They may not want the physician to examine certain areas of their bodies. Procedure 38-2, at the end of this chapter, describes techniques you can use to help ensure effective communication with patients from other cultures while meeting their privacy needs.

Patients with Physical Disabilities

Patients with physical disabilities have different strengths and weaknesses and vary in their ability to ambulate (move from place to place). Many patients with physical disabilities require the use of wheelchairs, canes, walkers, or other equipment that permits or enhances mobility.

Depending on the extent of their disability, these patients may require extra assistance in preparing for a general physical exam. You may need to help them disrobe, move from a

mobility device to the examining table, and assume certain positions on or off the examining table. At all times, you should ask another staff member for assistance if you are not sure whether you can safely move or lift a patient on your own. Procedure 38-3, at the end of this chapter, outlines the steps you would take to transfer a patient from a wheelchair to the examining table.

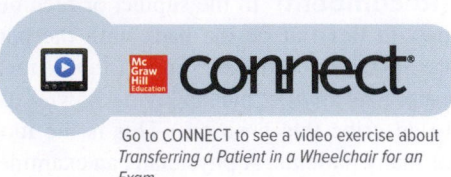

Go to CONNECT to see a video exercise about *Transferring a Patient in a Wheelchair for an Exam.*

▶ Exam Methods   LO 38.7

The six methods for examining a patient during a general physical exam enable the practitioner to gather important information about the patient's condition. Although practitioners may have their own preference, the methods are normally performed in the following sequence:

1. Inspection
2. Auscultation
3. Palpation
4. Percussion
5. Mensuration
6. Manipulation

Inspection

Inspection is the visual exam of the patient's entire body and overall appearance. During inspection, the physician assesses posture, mannerisms, and hygiene. The physician also inspects parts of the body for size, shape, color, position, symmetry, and the presence of abnormalities like rashes or growths. You can help the physician perform the inspection by making sure good lighting is available and that the patient's body parts are properly exposed.

Auscultation

Auscultation is the process of listening to body sounds. Physicians use auscultation to detect the flow of blood through an artery and perform auscultation extensively in the general exam to assess sounds from the heart, lungs, and abdominal organs. They use a stethoscope to hear most of these sounds (see Figure 38-2).

Palpation

The physician uses **palpation** (touch) extensively in the general physical exam to assess characteristics such as texture, temperature, shape, and the presence of vibrations or movements. The physician may palpate superficially (on the skin surface), or she may palpate with additional pressure. She uses extra pressure when assessing characteristics of underlying tissues and organs. Depending on the characteristic the physician is measuring, she may perform palpation using the fingertips, one hand, two hands (bimanual), or the palm of the hand.

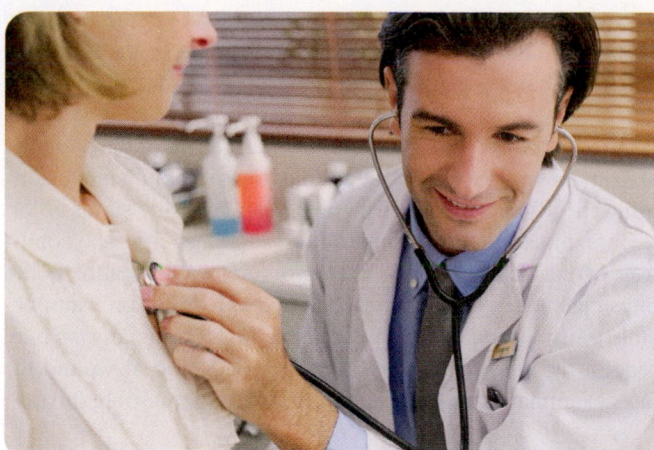

FIGURE 38-2 Auscultation, or listening to body sounds, can be done using a stethoscope.
© Chris Ryan/age fotostock

Percussion

Percussion involves tapping or striking the body to hear sounds or feel vibrations. Physicians use percussion to determine the location, size, or density of a body structure or organ under the skin. For example, physicians use percussion to determine whether the lungs contain air or fluid.

The physician may perform percussion by striking the body directly with one or two fingers. More commonly, however, he performs indirect percussion by placing one finger of one hand on the area and striking it with a finger from the other hand.

Mensuration

Mensuration is the process of measuring. In addition to the measurements you take before the exam—weight and height—you may need to take other measurements during the exam. For example, measurements may be done to monitor the growth of the uterus during pregnancy or to note the length and diameter of an extremity or a wound. You will usually use a tape measure or small ruler to take measurements.

Manipulation

Manipulation is the systematic moving of a patient's body parts. Physicians may palpate an area of the body while manipulating it to check for abnormalities that affect movement. Physicians often use manipulation to determine a joint's range of motion (ROM).

▸ Components of a General Physical Exam

LO 38.8

Each physician performs the general physical exam in a certain order. Most physicians begin by assessing the patient's overall appearance and the condition of the patient's skin, nails, and hair. They usually then proceed with the exam in the following order, using the exam methods described in the previous section:

1. Head
2. Neck
3. Eyes
4. Ears
5. Nose and sinuses
6. Mouth and throat
7. Chest and lungs
8. Heart
9. Breasts
10. Abdomen
11. Genitalia
12. Rectum
13. Musculoskeletal system
14. Neurologic system

Learn the standard order that licensed practitioners in your facility follow when performing the general exam. You also should be familiar with the components of the exam and the instruments and supplies needed for each component (see Table 38-2 and Figure 38-3).

The following are the basic items needed for a general physical exam:

- Penlight
- Otoscope/ophthalmoscope
- Vision chart
- Color vision chart

TABLE 38-2	Components and Materials for a General Physical Exam
Component	**Materials Required***
General appearance (skin, nails, hair)	No special materials needed
Head	No special materials needed
Neck	No special materials needed
Eyes and vision	Penlight, ophthalmoscope, and vision and color vision charts
Ears and hearing	Otoscope and audiometer
Nose and sinuses	Penlight and nasal speculum
Mouth and throat	Gloves and tongue depressor
Chest and lungs	Stethoscope
Heart	Stethoscope
Breasts	No special materials needed
Abdomen	Stethoscope
Genitalia (women)	Gloves, vaginal speculum, and lubricant
Genitalia (men)	Gloves
Rectum	Gloves and lubricant
Musculoskeletal system	Tape measure
Neurologic system	Reflex hammer and penlight

*Gloves should always be worn if your hands will come in contact with the patient's nonintact skin, blood, body fluids, or moist surfaces. Additional appropriate PPE should be worn when patients have a suspected or actual infectious disease.

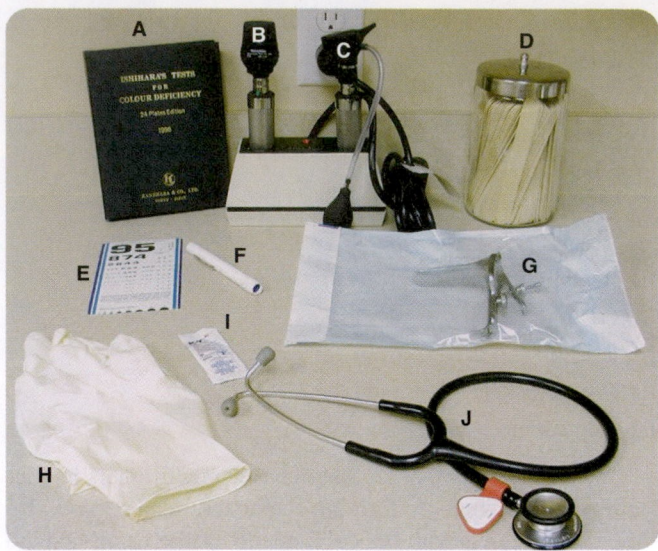

FIGURE 38-3 Some common instruments and supplies for the general physical examination are (A) color vision chart, (B) ophthalmoscope, (C) otoscope, (D) tongue blades (depressors), (E) near vision chart, (F) penlight, (G) vaginal speculum, (H) gloves, (I) lubricant, and (J) stethoscope.
© Total Care Programming, Inc.

- Audiometer
- Nasal speculum
- Gloves
- Tongue depressor
- Stethoscope
- Vaginal speculum (for female internal exam only)
- Lubricant (for rectal exam)
- Tape measure

Certain parts of the exam may be your responsibility and you should know how to perform them. You also should understand the physician's responsibilities. Part of the medical assistant's role in the general exam is to ensure the patient is as comfortable as possible. You can do this by helping to protect the patient's modesty as much as you can. For example, when the physician removes a drape or gown to expose an area for inspection, watch the patient for signs of embarrassment. If you notice any such signs, do your best to keep the patient covered without hindering the physician's exam. The steps for assisting the physician with a general physical exam are outlined in Procedure 38-4 at the end of this chapter.

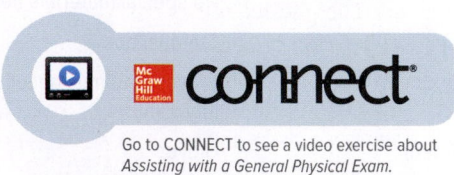

Go to CONNECT to see a video exercise about
Assisting with a General Physical Exam.

General Appearance

The physician usually begins the exam by reviewing the patient's general appearance and noting whether the patient appears to be in good health and of an acceptable weight. The physician also notes whether the patient appears to be

distressed or in pain and assesses the level of the patient's alertness. Then the physician examines the patient's skin, nails, and hair.

Skin The physician may prefer to examine all of the patient's skin at one time or to look at certain areas of skin while examining specific body parts. The physician notes the skin's color, texture, moisture level, temperature, and elasticity. The condition of the skin is a good indicator of overall health. If the physician notices any lesions, he wears gloves to prevent possible transmission of microorganisms. The physician also may request that a specimen be taken from a lesion or wound for later examination to determine the infecting microorganism.

Nails When the physician examines the patient's nails, he looks at both the nails and the nail beds. The condition of the nails may indicate poor nutrition, disease, infection, or injury. If needed, remind the patient to remove nail cosmetics prior to the appointment.

Hair The physician notes the patient's pattern of hair growth and the texture of the hair on the patient's scalp and on the rest of the body. Sudden hair loss or changes in hair growth may be indicators of an underlying disease.

Head

After reviewing the patient's general appearance, the physician examines the patient's head. He looks for any abnormal condition of the scalp or skin, puffiness around the eyes or lips or in other areas of the face, or any abnormal growths.

Neck

The physician checks the neck for symmetry and range of motion. He also palpates the neck to check the patient's lymph nodes, thyroid gland, and major blood vessels. Enlarged lymph nodes may be a sign of infection or blood cancer.

Eyes

The physician examines the patient's eyes—particularly the eyelids and conjunctiva—for the presence of disease or abnormalities. He checks eye muscles by observing the patient's ability to follow the movement of a finger. He checks the pupils for their response to light (the pupils should constrict—become smaller—when a penlight is directed toward them). Then he uses an ophthalmoscope to examine the patient's retinas and other internal structures of the eyes. You may be required to perform various vision tests either before or after the general physical exam.

Ears

The physician checks the patient's outer ears for size, symmetry, and the presence of lesions, redness, or swelling. Using an otoscope, he then examines the inner structures of the patient's ears. The physician may ask you to assist in keeping the patient's head still during the otoscopic exam, particularly if the patient is a young child. Although this procedure is usually painless, patients with an ear infection may find it uncomfortable or painful.

The physician checks the patient's ear canals for redness, drainage, lesions, foreign objects, or the presence of excessive cerumen (a waxy secretion from the ear, also known as earwax). During the most important part of the ear exam, the physician assesses the color, shape, and reflectiveness of the eardrums. If an eardrum bulges outward or reflects light abnormally, the middle ear could be infected. One of your responsibilities may be to perform various hearing tests either before or after the general physical exam.

Nose and Sinuses

When examining the nose, the physician checks for the presence of infection or allergy. She uses a penlight to view the color of the **nasal mucosa** (lining of the nose) and notes any discharge, lesions, obstructions, swelling, or inflammation. Mucosa that is red or swollen and is accompanied by a yellowish discharge usually indicates an infection. A pale, swollen mucosa accompanied by a clear discharge indicates an allergy. When examining adults, the physician uses the nasal speculum to view the structures of the nose.

The physician may use palpation to check for tenderness in a patient's sinuses. Tenderness is an indication of inflammation or swelling.

Mouth and Throat

The condition of the patient's mouth provides a general impression of overall health and hygiene. Using a tongue depressor to draw back the patient's cheeks, the physician examines the lining of the cheeks, the underside of the tongue, and the floor of the mouth. Changes in color or any lesions in these areas may indicate possible infection or oral cancer. The physician also assesses the condition of the teeth and gums. When examining children, he counts the number of teeth. Most physicians leave this part of the exam of infants and toddlers until last because children of this age tend to resist opening their mouths.

The physician also examines the patient's throat carefully, as it is a common site of infection. He uses a tongue depressor to press the patient's tongue down and out of the way while asking the patient to say "ah." This procedure allows the physician to view the throat and tonsils more clearly while checking them for redness or swelling, which can indicate the presence of infection.

Chest and Lungs

The physician usually assesses the patient's chest and lungs while the patient sits at the end of the examining table. The physician may remove the patient's gown or lower the drape from the waist up. Then he asks the patient to breathe normally or to take deep breaths. A patient who becomes dizzy during deep breathing may be hyperventilating. **Hyperventilation** is overly deep breathing that leads to a loss of carbon dioxide in the blood. You can help by having the patient breathe into a paper bag. If no bag is available, the patient can breathe into cupped hands.

The physician inspects the patient's chest from the back, side, and front. He checks its shape, symmetry, and postural position and looks for the presence of any type of deformity.

For example, **kyphosis,** better known as humpback, is commonly seen in the elderly.

The physician then uses a stethoscope to auscultate the chest from the back, side, and front. He listens to the lung sounds during both normal and deep breathing. The stethoscope allows him to hear abnormal breathing that may result from disorders such as bronchitis, asthma, or pneumonia. The physician also palpates the chest and performs percussion to check for the presence of fluid or a foreign mass in the lungs.

Heart

The physician usually examines the patient's heart and vascular system at the same time as, or immediately after, the lung exam. He may palpate the area first to locate the correct anatomical landmarks for placing the stethoscope. He may use percussion to check the heart's size. The patient should not speak while the physician auscultates the heart sounds with the stethoscope. The physician notes the heart's rate, rhythm, intensity, and pitch.

Breasts

During a general physical exam, every woman should have a complete breast exam to check for signs of cancer. The physician begins the exam with the patient in a sitting position. The physician asks the patient to hold her arms at her sides while he inspects the breasts for symmetry, contour, masses, and retracted areas. He then asks the patient to raise her arms above her head while he palpates the lymph nodes under her arms.

Next, the physician asks the patient to lie down and place her hand under her head on the first side to be examined. (The physician may ask you to place a small pillow or folded towel under the patient's shoulder blade on the same side.) This procedure allows the breast tissue to flatten evenly against the chest wall, permitting easier palpation. The physician then palpates the breast in a circular, systematic manner to check for lumps, examines the areola and nipple, and then repeats the procedure on the other side.

The breasts of men are also checked. When examining male patients, the physician palpates the patient's breasts and lymph nodes in the same manner that he does with his female patients. He also checks the breasts for lesions or swelling.

Abdomen

The physician examines the patient's abdomen while the patient is in a supine position with arms down at the sides. The abdominal muscles should be completely relaxed for this part of the exam. The physician may ask you to place a small pillow under the patient's head or knees (or both) to help keep the abdomen relaxed. If the patient is wearing a gown, it is raised to just under the breasts. If the patient is draped, the drape must be lowered to just above the genitalia to allow a complete view of the area. A separate drape should be placed to cover a female patient's breasts.

The order of exam methods for the abdomen should be followed correctly. The physician begins with inspection and auscultation, followed by percussion and palpation. Following this order allows the physician to listen to bowel sounds before palpating the abdominal organs. Palpation of the abdominal area can change bowel sounds in such a way that the physician could misdiagnose a patient's condition.

The physician begins with an inspection of the abdominal skin's color and surface and follows with an inspection of the abdomen's shape and symmetry. He then uses auscultation to check bowel and vascular sounds and uses percussion to note the size and position of the organs. Finally, he uses palpation to check muscle tone and to determine the presence of any tenderness or masses.

The physician describes observations based on a system of landmarks that map out the abdominal region. The abdomen is typically divided into four equal sections, or **quadrants.** Some physicians divide the abdomen into nine sections, similar to a tic-tac-toe board. For example, if a patient has had her appendix removed, the physician might note that the patient has an abdominal scar on the right lower quadrant.

Female Genitalia

Female patients may feel self-conscious or anxious in the lithotomy position—most commonly used during examination of the genitalia. The medical assistant may help the patient relax during this procedure to assist the patient in maintaining the position. This type of exam may be performed by a specialist or by a primary care physician. The procedure for a gynecologic exam is described in detail in the *Assisting in Reproductive and Urinary Specialties* chapter.

Male Genitalia

During the genitalia exam, men may be just as embarrassed or uncomfortable as women. If the physician performing the assessment is female, a male medical assistant, if available, should be in the room to protect both the patient and the physician from potential lawsuits.

The procedure begins with the patient in the supine position. The physician puts on gloves and visually inspects the patient's penis for signs of infection or structural abnormalities, palpating any lesions. The physician then examines the scrotum in the same manner, palpating the testicles for lumps. The patient is asked to stand while the physician checks for any bulges in the groin that may indicate a hernia. At the same time, the physician palpates the local lymph nodes to check for any abnormality.

Rectum

The physician usually examines the rectum after examining the genitalia. You may need to assist an adult patient into a dorsal recumbent or Sims' position. Female patients may already be in the lithotomy position for this exam. The physician normally examines a child when the child is in the prone position and inspects only the external areas of the rectum.

In adults, the physician may perform a **digital examination** to palpate the rectum for lesions or irregularities. Physicians recommend that patients older than age 40 have a yearly digital examination for early detection of colorectal cancer. For this exam, the physician puts on a clean pair of gloves. You may assist by applying lubricant to the physician's gloved index finger before the exam begins.

After performing the procedure, the physician may request that any stool found on the glove be tested for the presence of occult blood using a guaiac-based fecal occult blood test. The presence of occult blood in the stool is a possible indication of colorectal cancer or gastrointestinal bleeding. This test—often called by its brand name, Hemoccult® or Seracult® test—involves placing a sample of stool on a cardboard slide. You assist by presenting the slide to the physician. To produce an accurate test, three consecutive bowel movements are tested; this sample is usually the first. After the exam, you may be responsible for instructing the patient on how to collect the additional two samples. The procedure is outlined on the package of the occult blood-testing kit and in the *Collecting, Processing, and Testing Urine and Stool Specimens* chapter.

After the rectal exam, offer the patient the opportunity to clean the anal area before you adjust the drape. Dispose of gloves and soiled materials in a biohazardous waste container.

Musculoskeletal System

If the physician did not examine the patient's back during the chest exam, he does so during the musculoskeletal assessment. The physician checks for good posture from the back and side. He may ask the patient to walk so he can assess her gait. The physician always asks a child to bend at the waist so that he can check for the presence of **scoliosis,** a lateral curvature of the spine.

During the musculoskeletal assessment, the physician determines range of motion, the strength of various muscle groups, and body measurements. The physician also examines the arms, hands, legs, and feet for any lesions, deformities, or circulatory problems.

The physician checks a patient's range of motion to detect joint deformities and to learn whether the patient has any limitations in movement caused by an injury or other conditions, such as arthritis. Checking a patient's range of motion also allows the physician to follow a patient's progress during recovery from an injury or surgery.

Neurologic System

The physician's neurologic assessment includes an evaluation of the patient's reflexes, mental and emotional status (including intelligence, speech, and behavior), and sensory and motor functions. The physician often performs the neurologic assessment at the same time as the musculoskeletal assessment because both systems are involved in movement and coordination.

The physician may incorporate certain aspects of the neurologic assessment into other parts of the exam. For example, testing how a patient's pupils react to light is part of an eye exam, but because this test also examines the patient's light reflex, the test includes a neurologic assessment as well. To check reflexes, the physician uses a reflex hammer to tap tendons in different areas of the patient's body.

Most exams of children also include an intellectual assessment, in which the physician asks the child general questions appropriate to the child's age. Physicians may also test the mental status and memory of older adults to detect disorders such as senility and Alzheimer's disease in patients who show signs of confusion or complain of memory loss.

▶ After the Exam

After the physician completes the exam, you should assist in making the patient comfortable. Help her into a sitting position; then allow her to perform any necessary self-hygiene. Additionally, tests and procedures may be ordered. Depending upon what is ordered, you will complete them either before the patient dresses or after she is dressed. In addition, you may be responsible for patient education as well as follow-up care based on the physician's recommendations.

Additional Tests and Procedures

Post-exam procedures may include taking body fat measurements, obtaining blood samples, or preparing the patient for a diagnostic or therapeutic procedure, such as an X-ray or a physical therapy session. Other procedures medical assistants may perform before the patient dresses include administering cold or heat therapy, applying a bandage, collecting specimens, and administering certain medications.

If the physician has not ordered any additional procedures—or if wearing clothing does not interfere with the procedures ordered—the patient may dress. Help the patient get off the examining table and allow her to dress in privacy. Make sure she knows you are available to assist if she needs help dressing. Tests and procedures that can be done after the patient has dressed include urinalysis, pulmonary function tests, administration of oral medications, and eye or ear irrigation or medication administration.

Patient Education

The general physical exam provides you with the opportunity to assess the patient's educational needs. Based on the findings of the patient's interview, history, and exam, you may identify areas in which the patient will benefit from additional education.

Pay special attention to educating patients about risk factors for disease. For example, women are often instructed about the risk factors for breast cancer, and men are instructed about the risk factors for prostate cancer. The physician also may request that you teach patients how to administer certain medications or how to perform self-help or diagnostic techniques. These procedures may involve collecting samples for occult blood testing or urine testing, applying cold or hot packs, or instilling eye drops. It is important to teach the patient the correct way to perform a diagnostic test. If a specimen is incorrectly obtained, the test results will be inaccurate.

Regardless of the type of instruction, be sure to address patients at a language level they can understand without talking down to them. To ensure they understand fully, ask patients to repeat each instruction and to perform each demonstration. Give patients written instructions they can refer to at home.

Follow-Up

After the exam, you must help the patient follow up on all of the physician's recommendations. Follow-up may include these actions:

- Scheduling the patient for future visits at the office
- Making outside appointments for certain diagnostic tests, such as mammograms or other radiologic procedures, or for therapeutic procedures, such as physical therapy
- Helping the patient and the patient's family plan for home nursing care after an illness or a surgical procedure
- Helping the patient obtain assistance from community or social service organizations, such as adult day care, counseling, or meal programs

Follow-up appointments can vary depending on the outcome of the patient visit. Patient follow-up can be scheduled to review diagnostic testing or laboratory results and to discuss possible treatment methods for any abnormal test results. Another type of follow-up visit is to monitor previous treatments for diagnosed conditions, such as hypertension or diabetes.

During the follow-up exam, it is important to make sure patient preparation is appropriate for the type of exam scheduled. For example, it is not necessary for a patient to disrobe for a follow-up exam for hypertension. Use your critical thinking skills and follow office procedures to prepare patients correctly for the various types of patient visits.

PROCEDURE 38-1 Positioning a Patient for an Exam

Procedure Goal: To effectively assist a patient in assuming the various positions used in a general physical exam

OSHA Guidelines:

Materials: Adjustable examining table or gynecologic table, stepstool, exam gown, and drape

Method:

1. Identify the patient and introduce yourself.
2. Wash your hands.
3. Explain the procedure to the patient.
4. Provide a gown or drape, if the physician has requested one, and instruct the patient in the proper way to wear it after disrobing. Allow the patient privacy while disrobing and assist only if the patient requests help.

RATIONALE: *Taking an extra minute to explain to the patient how to wear the gown will make the visit more efficient and the patient more comfortable.*

5. Explain to the patient the necessary exam and the position required.

6. Ask the patient to step on the stool or the pullout step of the examining table. If necessary, assist the patient onto the examining table.

7. Assist the patient into the required position:

   a. *Sitting.* Do not use this position for patients who cannot sit unsupported.

   b. *Supine (recumbent).* Do not use this position for patients with back injuries, low back pain, or difficulty breathing. Place a pillow or other support under the head and knees for comfort, if needed.

   c. *Dorsal recumbent.* This position may be difficult for someone with leg disabilities. It may be used for patients when lithotomy is difficult.

   d. *Lithotomy.* This position is used to examine the female genitalia, with the patient's feet placed in stirrups. Assist as necessary. The patient's buttocks should be near the edge of the table. Drape the patient with a large drape to help prevent embarrassment.

   e. *Fowler's.* Adjust the head of the table to the desired angle. Help the patient move toward the head of the table until the patient's buttocks meet the point at which the head of the table begins to incline upward.

   f. *Prone.* In this position, the patient lies facedown. It is not used for later stages of pregnancy, obese patients, patients with respiratory difficulty, or certain elderly patients.

   g. *Sims'.* In this position, the patient lies on her left side with her left leg slightly bent and her left arm behind her back. Her right knee is bent and raised toward her chest and her right arm is bent toward her head. This position may be difficult for patients with joint deformities.

   h. *Knee-chest or knee-elbow.* This position is difficult for patients to assume. The patient is facedown, supporting his weight on his knees and chest, or in an alternative knee-elbow position. These positions are used for rectal and perineal exams. Keep the patient in this position for the shortest amount of time possible.

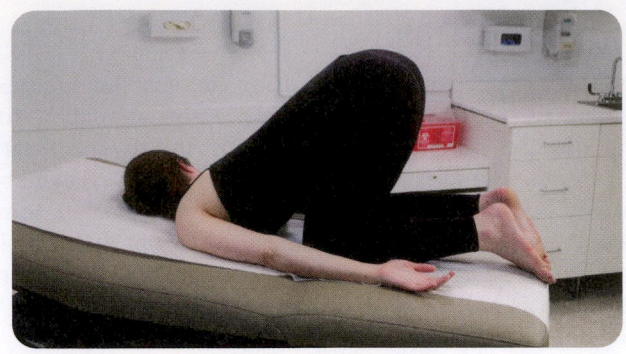

FIGURE Procedure 38-1 Step 7h   Patient in the knee-chest position on examining table.
© McGraw-Hill Education

   i. *Proctologic.* This position also is used for rectal and perineal exams. In this position, the patient bends over the examining table with his chest resting on the table.

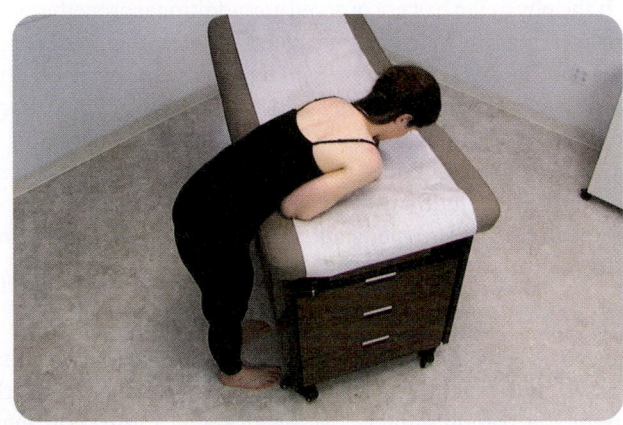

FIGURE Procedure 38-1 Step 7i   Patient in the proctologic position.
© McGraw-Hill Education

8. Drape the patient to prevent exposure and avoid embarrassment. Place pillows for comfort as needed.
   RATIONALE: *The patient's comfort and safety are mandatory.*

9. Adjust the drapes during the exam.

10. On completion of the exam, assist the patient out of the position as necessary and provide privacy as the patient dresses.

PROCEDURE 38-2 Communicating Effectively with Patients from Other Cultures and Meeting Their Needs for Privacy

Procedure Goal: To ensure effective communication with patients from other cultures while meeting their privacy needs

OSHA Guidelines: This procedure does not involve exposure to blood, body fluids, or tissue.

Materials: Exam gown and drapes

Method:

Effective Communication

1. When it is necessary to use a translator, direct conversation or instruction to the translator.
   RATIONALE: *Translators will reduce the risk of litigation and improve patient outcomes.*

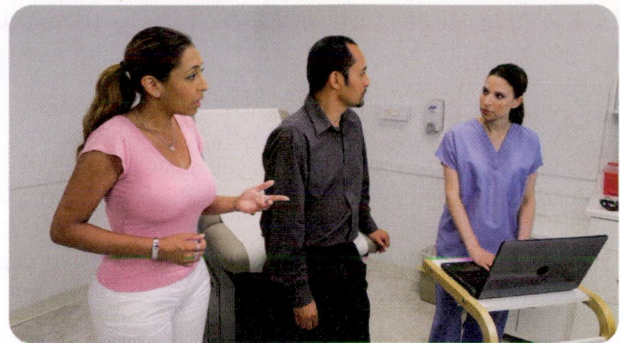

FIGURE Procedure 38-2 Step 1   Medical assistant using a translator for effective communication with the patient.
© McGraw-Hill Education

2. Direct conversation and demonstrations of what to do, such as putting on an exam gown, to the patient.

3. Confirm with the translator that the patient has understood the instruction or demonstration.

4. Allow the translator to be present during the exam if the patient prefers.

5. If the patient understands some English, speak slowly, use simple language, and demonstrate instructions whenever possible.

Meeting the Need for Privacy

6. Before the procedure, thoroughly explain to the patient or translator the reason for disrobing. Indicate that you will allow the patient privacy and ample time to undress.

7. If the patient is reluctant, reassure him that the physician respects the need for privacy and will look at only what is necessary for the exam.
   RATIONALE: *Some patients from certain cultures are embarrassed when exposed.*

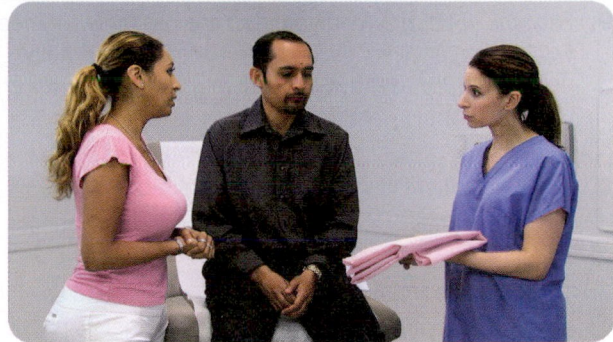

FIGURE Procedure 38-2 Step 7   Medical assistant providing a gown to the patient.
© McGraw-Hill Education

8. Provide extra drapes if you think doing so will make the patient feel more comfortable.

9. If the patient is still reluctant, discuss the problem with the physician; the physician may be able to negotiate a compromise with the patient.

10. During the procedure, ensure that the patient is undraped only as much as necessary.

11. Whenever possible, minimize the amount of time the patient remains undraped.

PROCEDURE 38-3   Transferring a Patient in a Wheelchair for an Exam

Procedure Goal: To assist a patient in transferring from a wheelchair to the examining table safely and efficiently

OSHA Guidelines:

Materials: Adjustable examining table or gynecologic table, stepstool (optional), exam gown, and drape

Method: *Caution:* Never risk injuring yourself; call for assistance when in doubt. As a rule, you should not attempt to lift more than 35% of your body weight.

Preparation for Transfer

1. Identify the patient and introduce yourself.

2. Wash your hands.

3. Explain the procedure in detail.

4. Position the wheelchair at a right angle to the end of the examining table. This position reduces the distance between the wheelchair and the end of the examining table across which the patient must move.

5. Lock the wheels of the wheelchair.
   RATIONALE: *To prevent the wheelchair from moving during the transfer.*

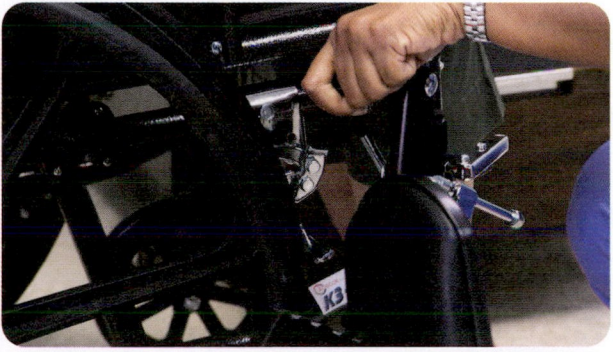

FIGURE Procedure 38-3 Step 5   Lock the wheels on the wheelchair before a transfer.
© McGraw-Hill Education

6. Lift the patient's feet and fold back the foot and leg supports of the wheelchair.

7. Place the patient's feet on the floor. The patient should have shoes or slippers with nonskid soles. Place your feet in front of the patient's feet.

RATIONALE: *These actions prevent the patient from slipping.*

8. If needed, place a stepstool in front of the table and place the patient's feet flat on the stool.

Transferring the Patient by Yourself

9. Face the patient, spread your feet apart, align your knees with the patient's knees, and bend your knees slightly.
RATIONALE: *If you lift while bending at the waist instead of bending your knees, you can cause serious injury to your back.*

10. Have the patient hold on to your shoulders.

11. Place your arms around the patient, under the patient's arms.

12. Tell the patient you will lift on the count of 3, and ask the patient to support as much of her own weight as possible (if she is able).

13. At the count of 3, lift the patient.

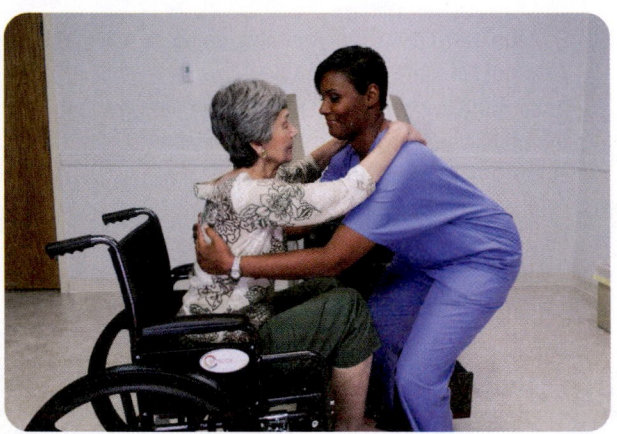

FIGURE Procedure 38-3 Step 13   Medical assistant transferring the patient by herself from wheelchair to exam table.
© McGraw-Hill Education

14. Pivot the patient to bring the back of the patient's knees against the table.

15. Gently lower the patient into a sitting position on the table. If the patient cannot sit unassisted, help her move into a supine position.

16. Move the wheelchair out of the way.

17. Assist the patient with disrobing as necessary, providing a gown and drape.

Transferring the Patient with Assistance

18. Working with your partner, both of you face the patient, spread your feet apart, position yourselves so that one of each of your knees is aligned with the patient's knees, and bend your knees slightly.
RATIONALE: *If you lift while bending at your waist instead of bending your knees, you can cause serious injury to your back.*

19. Have the patient place one hand on each of your shoulders and hold on.

20. Each of you places your outermost arm around the patient, one under each of the patient's arms. Then interlock your wrists.

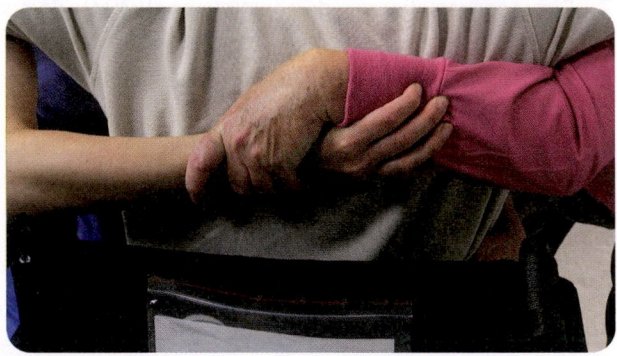

FIGURE Procedure 38-3 Step 20   Interlock your wrists to lift the patient when transferring the patient with assistance.
© McGraw-Hill Education

21. Tell the patient you will lift on the count of 3, and ask the patient to support as much of her own weight as possible (if she is able).

22. At the count of 3, you should lift the patient together.

23. The stronger of the two of you should pivot the patient to bring the back of the patient's knees against the table.

24. Working together, gently lower the patient into a sitting position on the table. If the patient cannot sit unassisted, help her move into a supine position.

25. Move the wheelchair out of the way.

26. Assist the patient with disrobing as necessary, providing a gown and drape.

PROCEDURE 38-4   Assisting with a General Physical Exam   WORK // DOC

Procedure Goal: To effectively assist the physician with a general physical exam

OSHA Guidelines:

  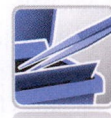 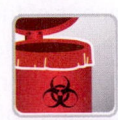

Materials: Supplies and equipment will vary depending on the type and purpose of the exam and the physician's practice preferences. Supplies may include the following: patient chart/progress note, gown, drape, adjustable examining table, gloves, laryngeal mirror, lubricant, nasal speculum, otoscope and ophthalmoscope, pillow, reflex hammer, tuning fork, sphygmomanometer, stethoscope, tape measure, tongue depressors, and a penlight.

Method:

1. Wash your hands and adhere to standard precautions throughout the procedure.
   RATIONALE: *Safe, aseptic technique greatly reduces the transmission of an infectious disease.*

2. Gather and assemble the equipment and supplies.

3. Arrange the instruments and equipment in a logical sequence for the physician's use.

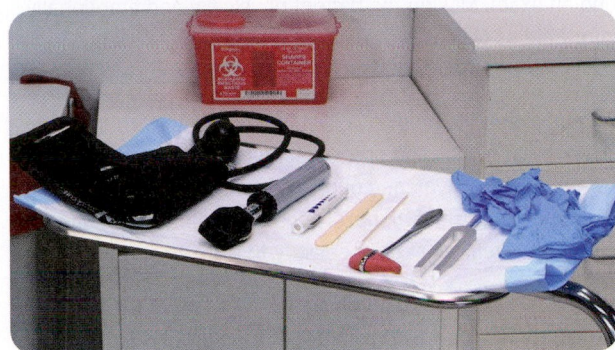

FIGURE Procedure 38-4 Step 3   Assemble and arrange equipment for a general physical exam.
© McGraw-Hill Education

4. Greet and properly identify the patient using at least two patient identifiers.
   RATIONALE: *To prevent treatment errors.*

5. Review the patient's medical history with the patient if office policy requires it.

6. Obtain vital statistics according to the physician's preference.

7. Obtain the patient's weight and height (with shoes removed).

8. Obtain a urine specimen before the patient undresses for the exam.

9. Explain the procedure and exam to the patient.
   RATIONALE: *This builds the patient's confidence with the office and prepares the patient physically and emotionally.*

10. Obtain blood specimens or other laboratory tests according to the chart or verbal order.

11. Provide the patient with an appropriate gown and drape, and explain where the opening for the gown is placed.

12. Obtain the ECG if ordered by the physician.

13. Assist the patient to a sitting position at the end of the table with the drape placed across her legs.

14. Inform the physician the patient is ready and remain in the room to assist the physician.

15. You may be asked to shut off the light in the exam room to allow the patient's pupils to dilate sufficiently for a retinal exam.

16. Hand the instruments to the physician as requested.

17. Assist the patient to a supine position and drape her for an exam of the front of the body.

18. If a gynecologic exam is needed, assist and drape the patient in the lithotomy position.

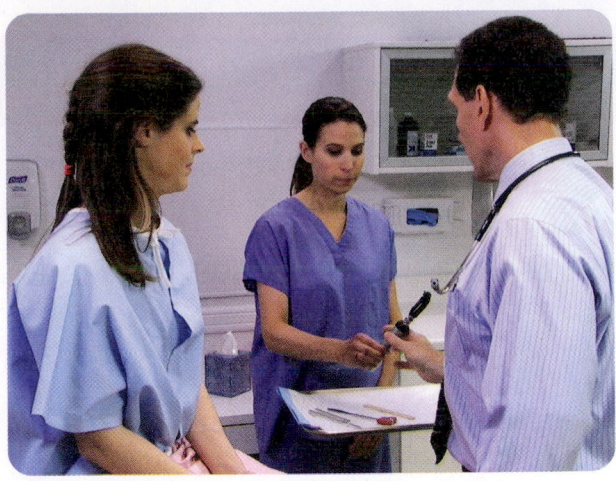

FIGURE Procedure 38-4 Step 16   Hand the instruments to the physician as needed.
© McGraw-Hill Education

19. If a rectal exam is needed, assist and drape the patient in the Sims' position.

20. Assist the patient to a prone position for a posterior body exam.

21. When the exam is complete, assist the patient to a sitting position and ask the patient to sit for a brief period of time.
    RATIONALE: *Some patients experience dizziness when they first sit up.*

22. Ask the patient if she needs assistance in dressing.

23. After the patient has left, dispose of contaminated materials in an appropriate container.

24. Remove the table paper and pillow covering and dispose of them in the proper container.

25. Disinfect and clean the counters and the examining table.

26. Sanitize and sterilize the instruments, if needed.

27. Prepare the room for the next patient by replacing the table paper, pillowcase, equipment, and supplies.

28. Document the procedure (refer to Progress Note).

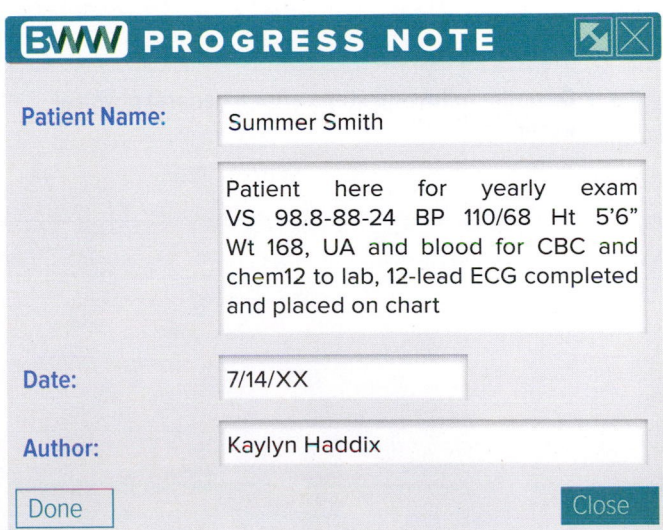

BWW PROGRESS NOTE

Patient Name:	Summer Smith
	Patient here for yearly exam VS 98.8-88-24 BP 110/68 Ht 5'6" Wt 168, UA and blood for CBC and chem12 to lab, 12-lead ECG completed and placed on chart
Date:	7/14/XX
Author:	Kaylyn Haddix

Done   Close

LEARNING OUTCOMES	KEY POINTS
38.1 **Identify the purpose of a general physical exam.**	A general physical exam is done either to confirm an overall state of health or to examine a patient to diagnose a medical problem.
38.2 **Describe the role of the medical assistant in a general physical exam.**	The medical assistant assists the patient and the physician during an exam. Making the patient physically and emotionally comfortable as well as providing materials and assistance to the physician are essential to a successful exam.
38.3 **Explain safety precautions used during a general physical exam.**	During an exam, the medical assistant should perform hand hygiene, wear gloves and other personal protective equipment, ensure respiratory hygiene/cough etiquette, use isolation precautions, dispose of biohazardous waste, and clean and disinfect the exam room as necessary to provide for safety.
38.4 **Carry out the steps necessary to prepare the patient for an exam.**	The medical assistant should prepare the patient for an exam emotionally, by using simple direct language, and physically, by providing for the patient's comfort and privacy when positioning him or her according to the type of exam or procedure and by modifying techniques to meet the needs of special patients.
38.5 **Carry out positioning and draping a patient in each of the nine common exam positions.**	The nine common exam positions include sitting, supine, dorsal recumbent, lithotomy, Fowler's, prone, Sims', knee-chest/knee-elbow, and proctologic.
38.6 **Apply techniques to assist patients from different cultures and patients with physical disabilities.**	When assisting with the physical exam, avoid judging and stereotyping patients from different cultures and obtain a translator for proper communication if necessary. Assist patients who have physical disabilities with transfers and other tasks they cannot accomplish themselves.
38.7 **Identify the six examination methods used in a general physical exam.**	The six examination methods used in a general physical exam include inspection, auscultation, palpation, percussion, mensuration, and manipulation.
38.8 **List the components of a general physical exam.**	A general physical exam typically includes an evaluation of the general appearance, head, neck, eyes, ears, nose and sinuses, mouth and throat, chest and lungs, heart, breasts, abdomen, genitalia, rectum, musculoskeletal system, and neurologic system.
38.9 **Describe follow-up steps after a general physical exam.**	In order to assist the patient with follow-up after the exam, you may schedule future visits, schedule visits outside of the office, help plan for home care, and, if within your scope of practice, provide education related to the patient's condition.

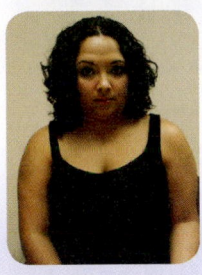

© McGraw-Hill Education

Recall Valarie Ramirez from the beginning of the chapter. Now that you have completed the chapter, answer the following questions regarding her case.

1. What would you chart as her chief complaint?

2. What things will you do during her exam to make her more comfortable?

3. What are the most likely position(s) she will be put in during her examination, and why would these positions be used?

4. If you were unable to communicate with Valarie successfully, what measures should you take to improve communication and meet her privacy needs?

EXAM PREPARATION QUESTIONS

1. (LO 38.7) When the physician uses a stethoscope to listen to body sounds, he is performing
   a. Auscultation
   b. Percussion
   c. Inspection
   d. Palpation
   e. Mensuration

2. (LO 38.3) Which safety measure should the medical assistant perform with every patient?
   a. Wear gloves
   b. Use isolation precautions
   c. Perform hand hygiene
   d. Transfer the patient to the exam table
   e. Place all waste in a biohazardous container

3. (LO 38.5) Which of the following positions would be used to examine the female genitalia?
   a. Prone
   b. Sims'
   c. Fowler's
   d. Proctologic
   e. Lithotomy

4. (LO 38.1) The patient is complaining of pain in her left foot. This would be considered a
   a. Sign
   b. Symptom
   c. Prognosis
   d. Clinical diagnosis
   e. Differential diagnosis

5. (LO 38.2) You are asked to do all of the following during a general physical exam. Which one is outside your scope of practice?
   a. Prepare the instruments and supplies
   b. Give the patient a pillow while the physician conducts the exam
   c. Determine the vital signs, height, and weight
   d. Provide the patient with emotional support
   e. Check the patient's abdomen when he complains of pain

6. (LO 38.4) What would be your best response to a nervous, young female patient who is going to have a general physical exam by a male physician when she asks, "Will this hurt?"
   a. An exam is not painful; you don't need to worry
   b. No, you just have to lie still; I will be here with you the whole time
   c. Yes, you can expect a lot of pain, but I will be here with you the whole time
   d. You won't have any discomfort; Dr. Buckwalter is very gentle
   e. The exam may be uncomfortable at times, but I will be here to help keep you comfortable

7. (LO 38.6) When assisting with a patient from another culture during an exam, which of the following would *least* likely be necessary?
   a. Extra drapes
   b. Translator
   c. Wheelchair
   d. Direct demonstrations
   e. Thorough explanations

8. (LO 38.8) What is the purpose of a digital examination?
   a. To check for blood in the urine
   b. To determine if a female patient has breast cancer
   c. To check for rectal lesions or irregularities
   d. To locate a landmark on the abdomen
   e. To listen to the patient's breathing

9. (LO 38.9) Which of the following would *not* be one of your duties after the physician has completed a general physical exam?
   a. Schedule a future visit to check the blood pressure
   b. Administer a medication
   c. Provide patient education
   d. Document a chief complaint
   e. Help the family plan for in-home care

10. (LO 38.3) A patient is suspected of having TB. What PPE should you wear?
  a. Mask only
  b. Mask and goggles when working within 3 feet of the patient
  c. Gown and gloves
  d. Gloves, gown, mask, and goggles
  e. Mask and goggles or respirator

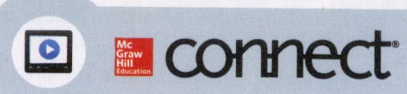

Go to CONNECT to see a video exercise about *Communicating Effectively with Patients from Other Cultures and Meeting Their Needs for Privacy.*

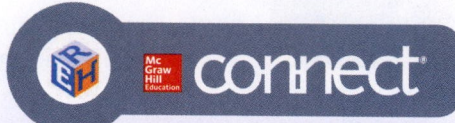

Go to CONNECT to see EHR activities about *Documenting a Physical Exam* and *Documenting a Procedure.*

SOFT SKILLS SUCCESS

A 59-year-old female patient who has generalized weakness in her extremities and is in a wheelchair has arrived at the office for her yearly physical. She is here for a pelvic exam, which will require her to be placed in lithotomy position.

1. What would you say to the patient when you enter the room to prepare her for the examination?

2. Once you transfer her to the examination table, she blushes and does not seem willing to be placed in the correct position. What should you do?

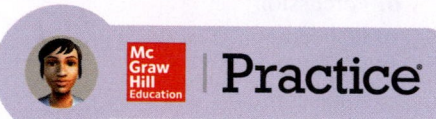

Go to PRACTICE MEDICAL OFFICE and complete the module Clinical - Interactions.

CASE STUDY

PATIENT INFORMATION		
Patient Name	**DOB**	**Allergies**
Raja Lautu	2/23/19XX	Benzalkonium chloride
Attending	**MRN**	**Other Information**
Elizabeth H. Williams, MD	224-86-564	Nonsmoker, occasional wine with meals

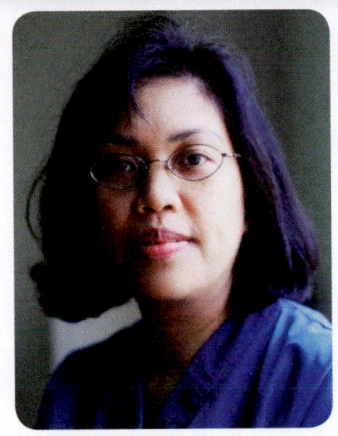

© ERproductions Ltd/Blend Images LLC RF

Raja Lautu, a 42-year-old woman, has arrived at the office for her annual gynecologic physical and the results of her annual digital mammogram. The digital mammogram results reveal a small, abnormal density close to the chest wall on the right breast. Dr. Williams speaks to Ms. Lautu and then schedules an ultrasound to determine if the density is fluid-filled or solid. The right breast ultrasound reveals a solid mass close to the chest wall. Since the mass is solid, the physician orders a right stereotactic fine-needle breast biopsy, which reveals a grade II infiltrating ductal carcinoma (IDC).

Keep Raja Lautu in mind as you study the chapter. There will be questions at the end of the chapter based on the case study. The information in the chapter will help you answer these questions.

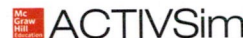

ACTIVSim

LEARNING OUTCOMES

After completing Chapter 39, you will be able to:

39.1 Carry out the role of the medical assistant in the medical specialty of gynecology.

39.2 Carry out the role of the medical assistant in the medical specialty of obstetrics.

39.3 Identify diagnostic and therapeutic procedures performed in obstetrics and gynecology.

39.4 Relate the role of medical assisting to the medical specialty of urology.

39.5 Identify diagnostic tests and procedures performed in urology.

39.6 Recognize diseases and disorders of the reproductive and urinary systems.

KEY TERMS

amenorrhea

dysmenorrhea

induction

infertility

last menstrual period (LMP)

loop electrosurgical excision procedure (LEEP)

menarche

menopause

menorrhagia

menstruation

metrorrhagia

postcoital

speculum

vasectomy

wet mount

CAAHEP

I.C.6	Compare structure and function of the human body across the life span
I.C.8	Identify common pathology related to each body system including: (a) signs (b) symptoms (c) etiology
I.C.9	Analyze pathology for each body system including: (a) diagnostic measures (b) treatment modalities
I.P.8	Instruct and prepare a patient for a procedure or a treatment
I.P.9	Assist provider with a patient exam
V.C.6	Define coaching a patient as it relates to: (e) adaptations relevant to individual patient needs
X.P.3	Document patient care accurately in the medical record

ABHES

2. **Anatomy and Physiology**
   a. List all body systems, their structure and functions
   b. Describe common diseases, symptoms and etiologies as they apply to each system
   c. Identify diagnostic and treatment modalities as they relate to each body system

3. **Medical Terminology**
   c. Apply various medical terms for each specialty

4. **Medical Law and Ethics**
   a. Follow documentation guidelines

9. **Clinical Procedures**
   d. Assist provider with specialty examination including cardiac, respiratory, OB-GYN, neurological, gastroenterology procedures
   e. Perform specialty procedures including but not limited to minor surgery, cardiac, respiratory, OB-GYN, neurological, gastroenterology
   g. Recognize and respond to medical office emergencies
   h. Teach self-examination, disease management and health promotion
   j. Make adaptations with patients with special needs

10. **Medical Laboratory Procedures**
    b. Perform selected CLIA-waived tests that assist with diagnosis and treatment
       (6) Kit testing
          (a) Pregnancy

▶ Introduction

Obstetrics (OB) involves the study of pregnancy, labor, delivery, and the period following labor, called postpartum. This field is often combined with gynecology (GYN), which is care of the female reproductive system. An OB/GYN practices both specialties. A urologist diagnoses and treats disorders and diseases of both the female and the male urinary systems, as well as the male reproductive system. For this reason, the specialty fields of OB/GYN and urology are discussed together in this chapter. Excellent knowledge of the reproductive and urinary systems (both male and female) is a must to work in these specialties. As a medical assistant, you will need to recall diseases and disorders, examinations, diagnostic tests, and treatments for each of these systems. Most importantly, you must be able to assist the physician, physician assistant, nurse practitioner, midwife, or other licensed practitioner during exams, treatments, and procedures and be able to provide patient education unique to these specialties.

▶ Assisting with the Gynecologic Patient

LO 39.1

Gynecologic patients are females, and as females mature, they experience many physical changes throughout their bodies. These changes, including menstruation and menopause and the hormones that cause them, are common reasons for women to visit their OB/GYN licensed practitioner.

Menstruation

Menstruation is a woman's normal cycle of preparation for conception (the union of egg and sperm that initiates pregnancy). The normal age range of **menarche**—the beginning of menstruation—is 10 to 15 years of age. Each month (averaging every 28 days), the endometrium, which lines the uterus, is shed in vaginal bleeding. If the woman becomes pregnant, this shedding does not occur and the woman misses her menstrual period.

A period lasts an average of 5 days, with durations of 3 to 7 days considered normal. Menstrual cycles are prompted by changes in hormonal (estrogen and progesterone) levels.

Menopause

Menopause, like menstruation, is a natural occurrence. It is the cessation (the end) of the menstrual cycle. Menopause usually occurs between ages 45 and 55. Several stages surround menopause. Premenopause is the time period before menopause, during which the menstrual periods may be irregular. The time just before and after menopause is called perimenopause. During perimenopause, a woman may experience irregular periods, hot flashes, and vaginal dryness, all caused by changing levels of estrogen. Because hormonal change is occurring, the woman may experience mood swings or other psychological changes. Menopause can also be brought on by the surgical removal of the uterus and ovaries, known as a hysterectomy and discussed later in this chapter. The symptoms and treatment for menopause are the same for both surgical and naturally occurring menopause.

The Gynecologic Exam

The gynecologic exam is intended to provide an overview of a woman's health and to offer the opportunity for important cancer-screening exams and tests. The American College of Obstetricians and Gynecologists (ACOG) has specific recommendations regarding when a woman should have a gynecologic exam and tests related to the female reproductive system. These recommendations are outlined in Table 39-1.

During the exam, a female medical assistant should be in the exam room to assist a male licensed practitioner. In this case, the medical assistant can act as a witness to provide legal protection. Your role during the exam is similar to that for the general physical exam. In this role, you will complete the following:

TABLE 39-1	ACOG Examination and Screening Recommendations	
Age	**Exam(s) Needed**	**Frequency**
<21	Cervical cytology	Three years after onset of sexual activity, then annually
	Pelvic exam	As medical history dictates
21–29	Pelvic exam and cervical cytology	Annually
<25	Chlamydia screening	When sexually active
Adolescents	Gonorrhea screening	When sexually active (can use urine-based screening)
19–64	HIV screening	When sexually active
30–64	Pelvic exam and cervical cytology	Annually; under certain conditions, decrease to every 2 to 3 years after 3 normal tests
>65	Pelvic exam	Annually
	Cervical cytology	Discontinue after 3 normal tests under certain conditions

- Ask the patient to empty her bladder; if a urine specimen is needed, it should be collected at this time.
- Provide the patient with a gown before the exam and give her privacy while she changes.
- During the interview, discuss her gynecologic and general health and inquire about any changes in appetite, weight, or emotional status.
- Observe for signs of problems such as substance abuse, sexually transmitted infections, or domestic violence. It is crucial that you bring to the licensed practitioner's attention any clues you notice during your interview. See the *Caution: Handle with Care* feature Detecting Domestic Violence.
- Determine the first day of her **last menstrual period (LMP).**
- Then have her sit on the examining table while you check her vital signs. For accurate results, keep the patient's arm elevated during the blood pressure measurement. For example, you may have her rest her arm on your shoulder.

The Licensed Practitioner's Interview

The gynecologic physical exam is more than an internal pelvic exam. It is an evaluation of the patient's total health and a review of factors that could be an indication of possible cancer or sexually transmitted infections (STIs). STIs, previously known as STDs (sexually transmitted diseases), are discussed later in this chapter. The licensed practitioner asks questions about the patient's menstrual cycle and about any abnormal discharge or discomfort during sexual intercourse. These questions help the licensed practitioner determine what tests need to be ordered. The licensed practitioner also examines the breasts and listens to the patient's heart and lungs before beginning the gynecologic exam.

Breast Exam

While reviewing the patient's chart, the licensed practitioner checks to see when the last mammogram was performed. He will also ask the patient about any other concerns or changes in her breasts. Since the breast self-exam is now an optional screening tool for breast cancer, the physician may or may not ask whether she knows how to perform a breast self-exam (BSE) and how often she is performing this exam. The licensed practitioner will then perform a clinical breast exam (CBE) by examining the patient's breasts and underarm areas to check for abnormal lumps that could be cancerous.

Patients must understand the need for regular breast exams including mammograms (discussed later in this chapter), clinical breast exams, optional breast self-exams, and additional tests if needed. When interviewing the patient and after the exam, you should take a moment to emphasize the following breast cancer detection guidelines of the American Cancer Society and National Cancer Institute:

- Yearly mammograms are recommended starting at age 40 and continuing for as long as a woman is in good health.
- A clinical breast exam is recommended about every 3 years for women in their 20s and 30s and every year for women 40 and over.

Detecting Domestic Violence

Licensed practitioners and medical assistants are in a position to detect signs of domestic violence. These signs can be seen in unusual bruising or injuries that the patient may try to hide or excuse. You may hear signs in a patient's tone of voice or choice of words during a conversation in the office or over the telephone. Many times patients who are abused blame themselves. When the patient's injuries do not match his or her story, this may indicate the likelihood of abuse. Observe the male or female who constantly answers questions for his or her partner. You play an important role in noticing these signs, and you must inform the licensed practitioner of any signs that you detect.

You must also create a supportive office environment where the patient can seek help. Encourage the licensed practitioner to join the American Medical Association's National Coalition of Physicians Against Family Violence if not already a member. This organization provides posters—which often help patients feel encouraged to discuss domestic violence—in addition to pamphlets and other information. Reporting suspected domestic violence is mandatory in some states. You should have a folder that contains lists of the phone numbers for domestic violence hotlines, women's shelters, and other helpful resources. You can offer the following general guidelines to women.

- Ignoring the problem never works—silence does not help anyone.
- Understand that abusive family members may not be able to help themselves.
- Call for help if a physical threat exists.

- Women should know how their breasts normally look and feel and report any breast change promptly to their healthcare provider. A breast self-exam is an option for women starting in their 20s.
- Women with a family history, a genetic tendency, or certain other factors should be screened with an MRI (discussed later in the chapter) in addition to mammograms. The number of women who fall into this category is less than 2% of all the women in the United States.

In some cases, you may be asked to instruct the patient in performing the BSE. Review the *Educating the Patient* feature How to Perform a Breast Self-Exam.

Pelvic Exam

During the pelvic exam, the licensed practitioner checks the external genitalia, cervix, vaginal wall, internal reproductive organs, and rectum. Exam methods include palpation and inspection. Inspection is done with a **speculum,** which is an instrument that expands the vaginal opening to permit viewing of the vagina and cervix (see Figure 39-1). The licensed practitioner wears gloves and may use a lubricant for patient comfort.

Your role is to assist the patient into position, with her feet in the stirrups of the examining table and her buttocks at the end of the table. Drape her so that only the area between the thighs is exposed. Assist the licensed practitioner by having gloves and instruments ready for use and by applying lubricant, if indicated, to the licensed practitioner's gloved fingers.

You also may warm the speculum for the patient's comfort. Be prepared to provide reassurance and explanation to a patient who appears to be uncomfortable or nervous. Encourage her to breathe deeply to help relax the pelvic muscles and reduce discomfort. After checking the vagina and cervix and while the speculum is still in place, the licensed practitioner

EDUCATING THE PATIENT

How to Perform a Breast Self-Exam

The breast self-exam, although now considered an optional screening method for breast cancer, is still an important part of breast cancer prevention. As a medical assistant, you may be responsible for coaching the patient about the monthly breast self-exam. Check the office policy to see which of several methods it recommends for teaching BSE.

Consider the following when teaching the BSE:

1. Explain the purpose of the BSE. Make sure the patient knows that she should perform the BSE around the same date of each month after her period ends, if she is still menstruating. (At this time, the breasts are most normal and least swollen and lumpy.) Have the patient mark her calendar as a monthly reminder.

2. Emphasize that the BSE is not a substitute for mammograms or regular breast exams by a licensed practitioner.

3. Demonstrate the breast self-exam according to the method used at your facility. For example, the National Cancer Institute has established one method and provides the instructions on its Internet site.

4. Observe the patient's self-exam technique. (If the patient is reluctant to examine herself in front of you, have her repeat the highlights of the procedure or use the synthetic model.)

5. Review and reinforce teaching as needed. Provide patient educational materials that explain how to perform the BSE.

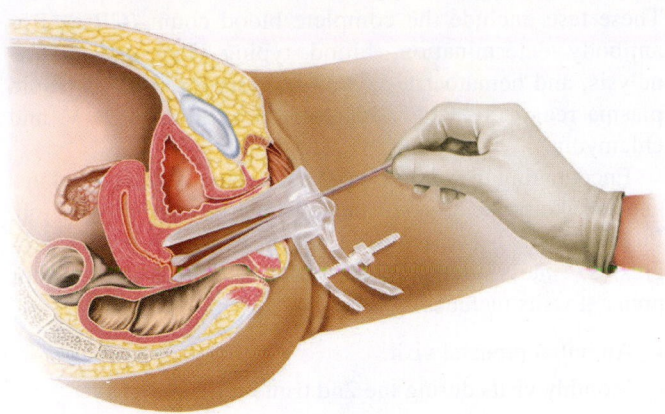

FIGURE 39-1 A speculum is used to expand the vaginal opening to help view the vagina and cervix and obtain specimens.

obtains a specimen. The most common type of specimen the licensed practitioner will obtain is a Papanicolaou (Pap) smear. This test is discussed later in the chapter.

Sometimes a sample is taken by the licensed practitioner to test for infections. These specimens are usually prepared by the medical assistant during the procedure and viewed by the licensed practitioner after the exam. To check for fungus, a sample may be mixed with potassium hydroxide (KOH) on a slide. The slide is viewed under a microscope. The KOH helps dissolve the cells and mucus in the sample so that the fungus can be better visualized. A **wet mount** is prepared by mixing a sample with a saline solution. The slide is viewed to check for bacteria, yeast, and trichomoniasis. Trichomoniasis, commonly called "trich," is a vaginal infection caused by a microscopic organism and is transferred during sexual intercourse.

The licensed practitioner then removes the speculum and begins the bimanual phase of the exam. *Bimanual* means using two hands rather than the speculum. The practitioner may ask for your assistance in removing the examining

gloves, putting on new gloves, and lubricating two fingers. Placing those fingers in the vagina and using the other hand to palpate the abdomen, the licensed practitioner assesses the position of the uterus. She may then place a lubricated finger in the rectum and palpate for abnormal growths with the other hand by pressing on the lower abdomen.

When the licensed practitioner completes the exam, she usually asks the patient if she has any questions or concerns. After the licensed practitioner leaves the exam room, be sure to ask the patient whether she has additional questions. You may need to provide written information in addition to answering the patient's questions orally. Materials are available from a variety of sources, including the AMA, government agencies, and pharmaceutical companies. The website of the National Women's Health Information Center is one excellent resource. See Procedure 39-1, at the end of this chapter, on how to assist with a gynecologic exam. The *Caution: Handle with Care* feature Guidelines for Cervical Specimen Collection and Submission provides information about how to ensure an adequate specimen for optimal screening.

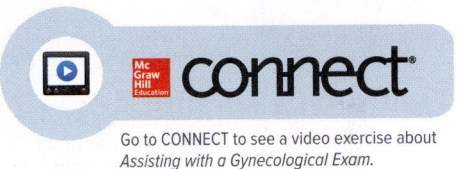

Go to CONNECT to see a video exercise about *Assisting with a Gynecological Exam.*

▶ Assisting with the Obstetric Patient   LO 39.2

When a woman discovers she is pregnant, one of the first things she wants to know is the baby's due date. One simple method to estimate the delivery date for a pregnant woman is called Nägele's rule. Begin with the first day of the patient's last menstrual period, subtract 3 months, and add 7 days plus

---

CAUTION: HANDLE WITH CARE

Guidelines for Cervical Specimen Collection and Submission

In order to ensure that the cervical specimen collected is adequate for optimal screening, the American Society of Cytopathology has clinical guidelines for collecting patient information. As a medical assistant, you will be responsible for helping the licensed practitioner implement these guidelines, which include

- Scheduling a patient appointment about 2 weeks after the patient's last menstrual period.
- Instructing patients not to douche; use tampons, foams, or jellies; or have sexual intercourse 48 hours prior to the test.
- Completing a lab requisition form, which includes the following information:
  - Patient name (note any recent name changes)
  - Date of birth

- Menstrual status (last menstrual period, hysterectomy, and so on)
- Any patient risk factors
- Specimen source
- Completing a specimen label, which includes the following materials and information:
  - Liquid samples
  - Complete all requested information on the label and affix it to the vial.
- Glass slide
  - Label the frosted end of the slide with the patient's first and last name.
  - Include an additional patient identifier, such as the patient record number.

1 year. For example, if the first day of the last menstrual period was June 30, 2014, subtracting 3 months would give you March 30, 2014. After the addition of 7 days plus 1 year, April 6, 2015, would be the estimated delivery date.

Prenatal Care

Pregnant women should be attentive to nutrition, exercise, medical monitoring, and childbirth classes. They should avoid using tobacco, alcohol, and drugs. Normal changes occur during pregnancy, such as morning sickness (usually in the first trimester), weight gain, urinary frequency, fatigue, depression, constipation, and swollen hands and feet. Review Figure 39-2 and Table 39-2 regarding the trimesters of pregnancy and what changes may be expected.

You may perform or assist with routine tests for pregnant women, or you may send them to an outside laboratory. These tests include the complete blood count (CBC), Rh-antibody determination, blood typing, Pap smear, urinalysis, and hematocrit, as well as tests for syphilis (rapid plasma reagin, or RPR), hepatitis B antibodies, HIV, and chlamydia.

Encouraging the obstetric patient to have regular checkups and to take proper care of herself may be part of your job. Prenatal visits become more frequent as the pregnancy progresses. Unless complications occur, a typical schedule for prenatal visits includes

- An initial prenatal visit.
- Monthly visits during the 2nd trimester.
- Visits every other week during the 3rd trimester up to 36 weeks' gestation.
- Once-a-week visits from 36 weeks until delivery.

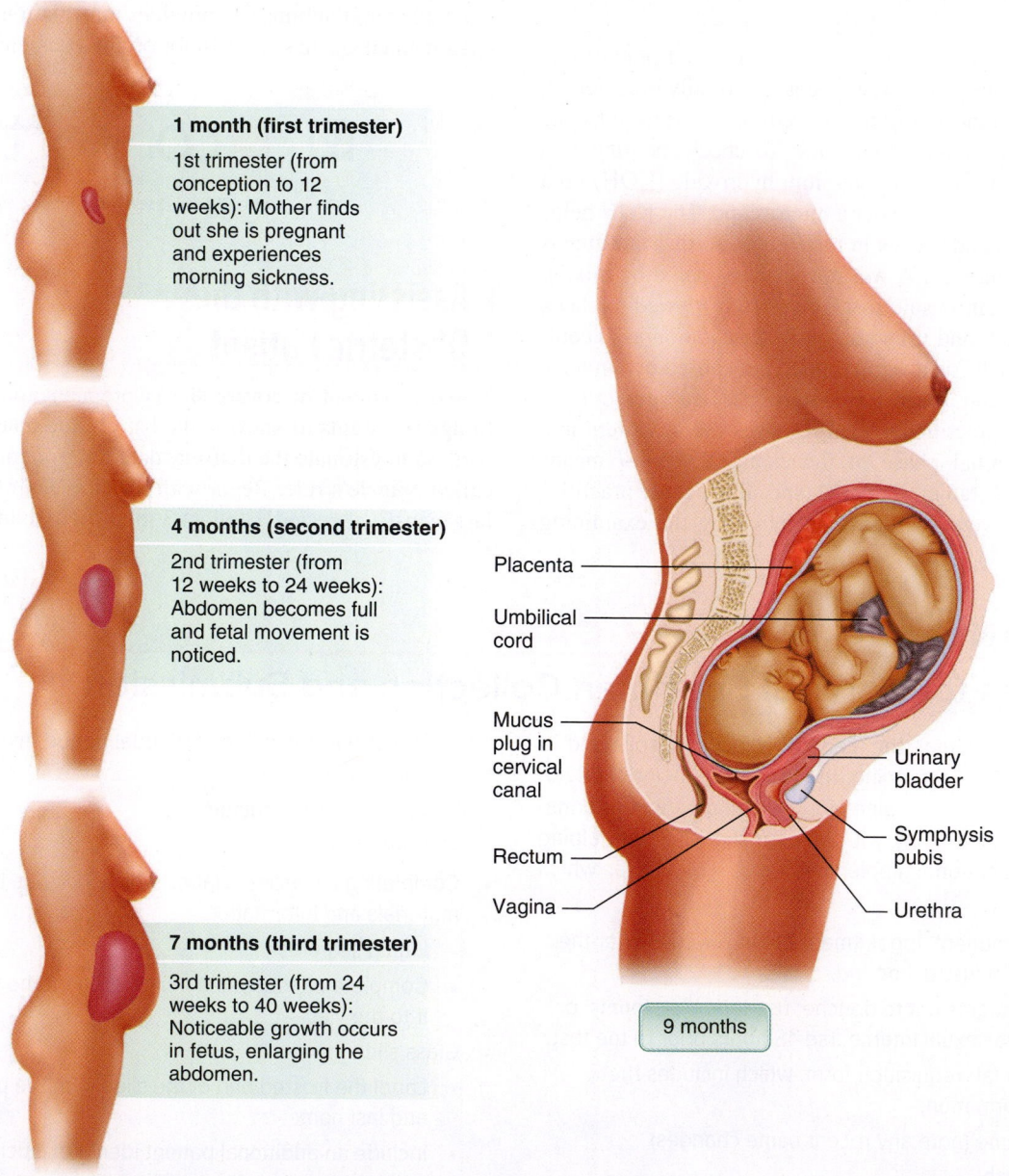

1 month (first trimester)

1st trimester (from conception to 12 weeks): Mother finds out she is pregnant and experiences morning sickness.

4 months (second trimester)

2nd trimester (from 12 weeks to 24 weeks): Abdomen becomes full and fetal movement is noticed.

7 months (third trimester)

3rd trimester (from 24 weeks to 40 weeks): Noticeable growth occurs in fetus, enlarging the abdomen.

Placenta
Umbilical cord
Mucus plug in cervical canal
Rectum
Vagina
Urinary bladder
Symphysis pubis
Urethra

9 months

FIGURE 39-2 The fetus develops over the course of three trimesters.

TABLE 39-2 Changes During Pregnancy

Stage of Pregnancy	Normal Changes	Example Complications
1st trimester (weeks 1 to 12)	Missed period, fatigue, morning sickness, frequent urination, moodiness, heartburn, constipation, swollen and tender breasts	Ectopic pregnancy—severe dizziness with vaginal bleeding and abdominal pain
2nd trimester (weeks 12 to 24)	Weight gain up to 4 pounds a month; fetal movement around 16 weeks; stretched, enlarging breasts; back, pelvis, and hip pain; mild contractions known as Braxton Hicks or "false labor"	Deep vein thrombosis—blood clot in a leg vein causing pain and swelling; Preterm labor—painful uterine contractions that have a regular pattern and don't go away with movement
3rd trimester (weeks 24 to 40)	Unable to sleep on back; leg cramps; frequent urination; strange dreams; nasal congestion; heartburn; constipation; hemorrhoids; varicose veins; puffiness, especially the feet	Pregnancy-induced hypertension—extreme swelling of the hands and face, headache, blurred vision

In addition to assisting with prenatal examinations, you may also help teach and support both parents throughout the pregnancy. You must document all information given to or taken from the patient. Providing information on the effects of using drugs or alcohol during pregnancy is particularly important. See the *Caution: Handle with Care* feature Alcohol and Drugs During Pregnancy.

The following are your responsibilities when assisting with routine prenatal patient visits:

- Ask the patient about any problems and record any symptoms she reports.
- Ask the patient to empty her bladder and obtain a urine specimen in the cup you provide.
- Weigh the patient and note her weight in the chart.
- Perform the reagent urine test (chemical analysis) and note the results in her chart.
- Give the patient a drape and ask her to undress from the waist down if the licensed practitioner will be performing an internal exam.
- Assist the patient to the examining table. Some positions (such as the prone—on the stomach—and lithotomy—on the back with the feet up—positions) are not recommended for a pregnant patient, especially during late stages of pregnancy. Other positions may be difficult or impossible for a pregnant woman to achieve.
- Take her vital signs. Record them in her chart.

- Assist the licensed practitioner as needed with the exam. Provide the flexible centimeter tape measure and Doppler, an instrument used to listen to the fetal heartbeat.
- Assist the patient from the examining table after the exam.

Procedure 39-2, at the end of this chapter, outlines steps to take that ensure that a pregnant woman's needs are addressed during an exam.

Prenatal Care by the Licensed Practitioner

The licensed practitioner carefully monitors the progress of a pregnancy. She monitors the patient's blood pressure, weight changes, and urinalysis results for possible signs of preeclampsia. Preeclampsia is a serious condition that can occur during pregnancy. Signs of this condition include increased blood pressure (hypertension), unusual weight gain because of edema, and protein in the urine. The licensed practitioner examines urine specimens for possible urinary tract infections (UTIs) and occasionally asks for other laboratory tests, such as a CBC. She may prescribe special vitamins and iron as dietary supplements.

During the prenatal period, the licensed practitioner will monitor for many conditions, including placenta previa, abruptio placenta, and gestational diabetes. Placenta previa is indicated by bright red vaginal bleeding that is painless. Abruptio placenta is a more serious condition that includes vaginal bleeding and back and abdominal pain. Gestational diabetes is indicated by an increase in glucose in the blood or urine.

CAUTION: HANDLE WITH CARE

Alcohol and Drugs During Pregnancy

Everything a pregnant woman eats, drinks, or smokes will affect her developing baby. Alcohol, for example, crosses the placental barrier and directly affects fetal development. Drinking alcohol during pregnancy can cause fetal alcohol syndrome (FAS). This syndrome may include fetal growth deficiencies, mental retardation or learning disabilities, heart defects, cleft palate, a small head, a small brain, and deformed limbs.

Preventing FAS by teaching all pregnant patients about the potential effects of alcohol on their unborn babies is crucial.

Drugs used during pregnancy can also pose problems for the unborn fetus. Whether the drugs are illegal, over-the-counter, or prescription, pregnant women should be aware of the potential effects. See the chapter *Principles of Pharmacology* for information about prescription drug pregnancy labeling.

Labor

When working in an OB/GYN office, you will need to know the signs of labor and when to tell the patient to go to the hospital. Most practices provide patient instructions regarding when to seek medical care and procedures to follow if they believe they are in labor. For example, most patients will be told to go to the hospital if they are having regular contractions—six or more per hour for at least 2 hours. Also, a sudden surge of fluid from the uterus indicates that the "water broke," which signals impending labor and requires the patient to go to the delivering healthcare facility.

Delivery

Delivery of an infant is typically through the vagina. After the labor process and delivery, the licensed practitioner clamps, ties, and cuts the umbilical cord and presents the baby to the mother. Women either go into labor spontaneously or may need to have their labor induced. **Induction** of labor means that the patient is admitted to the delivering healthcare facility, then given medication to start uterine contractions. If labor is spontaneous, most women go to the delivering facility as directed by their licensed practitioner. However, the medical assistant may need to schedule inductions at the delivering healthcare facility.

If the pregnant woman cannot deliver the baby vaginally, the licensed practitioner may deliver the baby by performing an operation known as a cesarean section, or C-section. Several conditions may require a cesarean section, such as a large baby or a breech position. Again, the medical assistant may need to schedule C-sections with the delivering healthcare facility.

Deliveries can be an emergency. Although not a common occurrence or a typical job responsibility for a medical assistant, if you are working in a busy obstetric practice, knowing the steps of emergency childbirth may be appropriate. You could be called upon to assist a physician during an in-office emergency delivery.

Breastfeeding

Human milk is the preferred form of nutrition for an infant. Colostrum, the first milk the mother produces after delivery, is rich in antibodies that provide passive natural immunity to the baby. Breastfeeding is economical and convenient. There is no need to buy or make formula or wash bottles and nipples. Breast milk is always available to the baby at the correct temperature.

A woman's success at breastfeeding depends largely on her desire to breastfeed, her satisfaction with it, and her available support systems. You can support patients who choose to breastfeed by providing them with pamphlets and other written materials. Emphasize how essential the mother's nutritional intake is and explain that she needs to follow a high-protein, high-calorie diet. Patients who need help can be referred to lactation consultants or support groups such as the La Leche League.

Bottle Feeding

Bottle feeding is an acceptable alternative for women who choose not to breastfeed or for one reason or another are unable to breastfeed. There are several acceptable formulas available,

including milk-based, soy-based, and special formulas for low-birth-weight infants. The type of formula is recommended by the licensed practitioner. If an infant is to be bottle-fed, parents must be given instruction about the type of formula and how to prepare it correctly. Regular, full-fat cow's milk should not be given to a child until after his or her first birthday.

Postpartum

Postpartum is a period after the delivery of an infant. During this time women experience many changes and challenges as their body is trying to get back to normal. These include

- Shrinking of the uterus back to its prepregnancy size, which typically takes about 6 weeks.
- Sharp abdominal pains, known as afterpains, that occur while the uterus is shrinking. These usually subside about the third day.
- Sore muscles of the arms, neck, or jaw for women who have labored and/or delivered vaginally.
- Difficulty with urination and bowel movements.
- Postpartum bleeding (lochia), which may last up to 4 weeks and can come and go up to 2 months.
- Recovery from a vaginal tear, episiotomy (surgical incision for a vaginal delivery), or abdominal incision for C-section.
- Pain that may occur from pelvic bone separation during vaginal delivery.
- Emotional stress related to coping with the physical changes and the needs of the new family.

The postpartum patient returns to the licensed practitioner at least once after the delivery of her baby to be evaluated. As a medical assistant you will need to ask questions regarding her recovery and document any complaints or concerns. You also may need to assist with a physical exam or provide information about birth control if asked to do so by the physician. Recall methods of birth control from the chapter *The Reproductive Systems.*

▶ OB/GYN Diagnostic and Therapeutic Tests and Procedures   LO 39.3

Many OB/GYN offices have their own small laboratories for immediate results, especially for pregnancy-related tests. Other diagnostic tests and procedures are sent to outside laboratories or performed at outpatient surgery centers or hospitals.

Pregnancy Test

Pregnancy tests are done on a specimen of blood or urine (the patient's first urine of the morning). These tests detect whether or not the hormone human chorionic gonadotropin (HCG)—produced during pregnancy—is present. A variety of testing kits are available, including over-the-counter urine self-test kits that the patient can use at home. These tests are not foolproof; false positives and false negatives do occur. For example, an abnormal pregnancy can result in a lower level of HCG that is not detectable by the tests. Urine specimens that contain blood, protein, or drugs also can give a false-positive result. False negatives may result from testing too early after getting pregnant or from a urine specimen that is too dilute. Dilute urine occurs when the woman has consumed too much fluid and the urine does not have enough HCG to cause the test to react as a positive. The tests are also subject to human error. The licensed practitioner confirms pregnancy after taking the patient's history, performing an exam, and ordering a pregnancy test. You can review and practice this procedure, presented in the *Collecting, Processing, and Testing Urine and Stool Specimens* chapter.

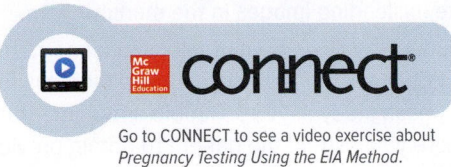

Go to CONNECT to see a video exercise about *Pregnancy Testing Using the EIA Method.*

Tests for Sexually Transmitted Infections

The licensed practitioner diagnoses and treats sexually transmitted infections (STIs) by taking bacterial and tissue cultures, examining lesions, ordering blood tests, and discussing the patient's history, as appropriate for the specific disease. Some facilities do not permit the release of these results, even to the parents of a minor, without the patient's written consent. Be sure you are familiar with your state's regulations regarding the reporting of STIs to the state epidemiology department.

Radiologic Tests

Several radiologic tests are used in obstetrics and gynecology. The gynecologist uses X-ray, ultrasonography, CT scan, and MRI. X-rays are avoided when a patient is pregnant. If it is crucial for a pregnant woman to have an X-ray, a lead apron must cover her abdomen, and she must be made aware that the X-ray could cause an abnormality in the fetus. As a medical assistant, you will usually schedule the appointment for radiologic tests. Tell the patient when and where to go for the test and answer her questions about the procedure. Medical assistants need further training to assist with X-ray procedures.

Hysterosalpingography Hysterosalpingography is an X-ray exam of the fallopian or uterine tubes and the uterus that uses a contrast medium, such as dye or air. Because the procedure is quite uncomfortable, the licensed practitioner may prescribe a sedative.

Mammogram A mammogram is a picture of the breast on film or digital media. Digital mammograms are more easily stored and transported and require less radiation. Mammography can detect cancer about 2 years before it can be palpated with a BSE. A baseline or first mammogram is done so that later mammograms can be compared. The mammogram procedure involves compressing the breast to obtain a clear X-ray (Figure 39-3). Recall our patient Raja Lautu, whose routine mammogram revealed an abnormality that was later found to be cancerous. Detailed information may need to be discussed with the patient before she has a mammogram. Review the *Educating the Patient* feature Checking for Breast Cancer to help you prepare the patient for a mammogram.

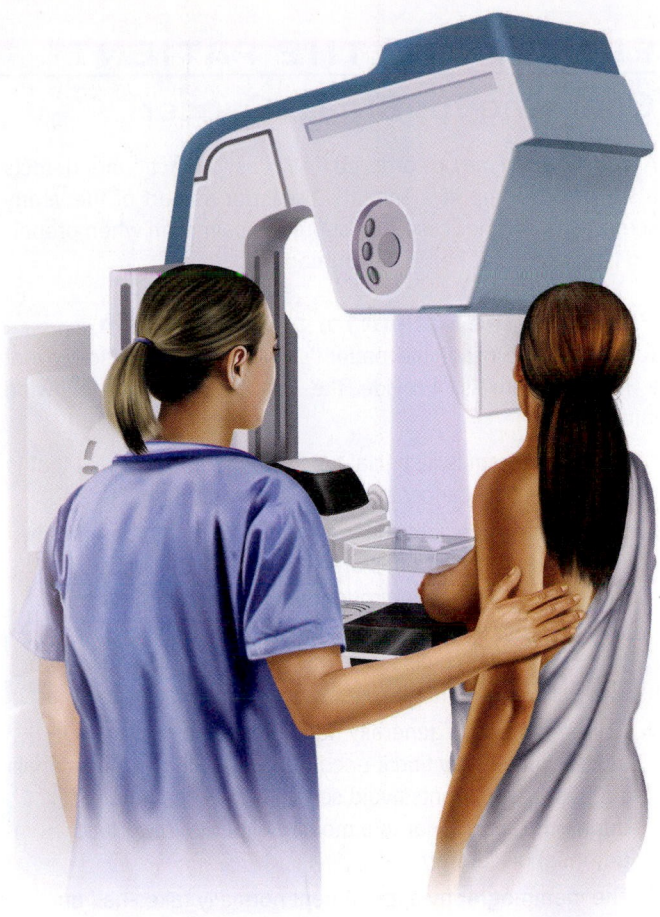

FIGURE 39-3 Mammography consists of two views of each breast and is achieved by compressing the breast between the radiography plates.

Fetal Screening

Fetal screening tests can indicate the presence of several types of birth defects, including Down syndrome and spina bifida. The licensed practitioner will consider the patient's age and medical history and the age of the unborn baby when ordering fetal screening tests. Tests for determining the health of an unborn child are performed on many women. Some, like an ultrasound, may be performed routinely. Other tests are used only for women whose unborn babies are at high risk of having birth defects. This includes women over 35, couples with a family history of genetic defects, and couples who have had a previous child with a birth defect.

Alpha Fetoprotein Alpha fetoprotein (AFP) is a protein produced by the unborn child that normally passes into the mother's blood. A blood test determines whether the AFP level in the blood is normal. Too little or too much AFP in the blood can indicate a fetal abnormality known as a neural tube defect. A neural tube defect is a developmental abnormality of the brain or spinal cord. AFP is also measured in amniotic fluid collected by amniocentesis. The licensed practitioner may order a blood test known as a triple screen or triple test. In addition to AFP, maternal levels of human chorionic gonadotropin and estriol are tested. These substances, like AFP, are only present during pregnancy. The triple test is used to detect neural tube defects and is a better indicator of Down syndrome than AFP alone. This test is generally done between the 15th and 22nd weeks of pregnancy.

Ultrasound Ultrasound translates the echoes of sound waves into a picture of an internal part of the body. The picture, or image, is called a sonogram, and it can help identify and diagnose cysts and tumors in the abdominal cavity or obstructions of the urinary tract. Ultrasound is painless and safe to use on pregnant women to determine fetal size and position. It is also used to guide a licensed practitioner in performing amniocentesis as well as chorionic villus sampling (CVS) for chromosomal abnormalities and other inherited disorders. A patient who is going to have an ultrasound exam during early pregnancy should be instructed not to urinate before the test because a full bladder allows a better view of the uterus. The patient is asked to lie on an examining table and a gel or lotion is applied to the surface of her skin on the abdomen. This gel or lotion helps enhance sound wave conduction and reduce friction of the transducer on the skin (Figure 39-4).

Invasive Procedures

Many surgical OB/GYN procedures require the use of needles or other instruments to obtain tissue or amniotic fluid samples. Some procedures are used for obstetric reasons only; others may be used gynecologically and obstetrically.

Pap Smear A Pap smear is used to determine the presence of abnormal or precancerous cells. As discussed earlier, during a pelvic exam, cells from the cervix, endocervix, and vagina are smeared on a special, properly labeled slide. They are then sprayed with a fixative and sent to a laboratory for microscopic analysis. Obtaining accurate Pap smear results is an important tool in the successful treatment of cervical cancer. See the *Points on Practice* feature Pap Smear Technologies. The Pap test results are classified according to level of abnormality. The Bethesda system is used for interpreting the results. Review Table 39-3 to better understand Pap smear results.

Amniocentesis Amniocentesis is a procedure performed when a genetic or metabolic defect is suspected in a fetus. The test involves removing from the uterus a small amount of amniotic fluid, which surrounds the fetus. The licensed practitioner inserts a needle, which is guided with ultrasonography,

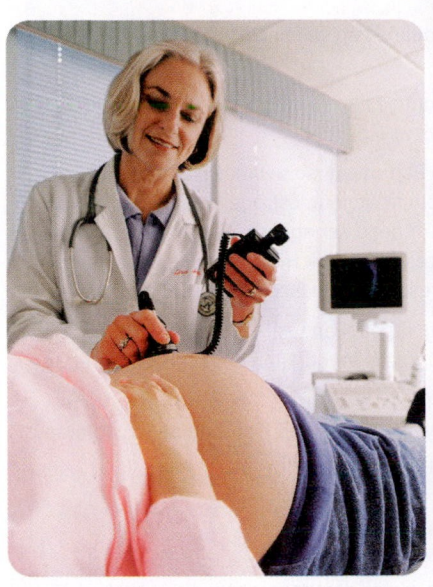

(a)

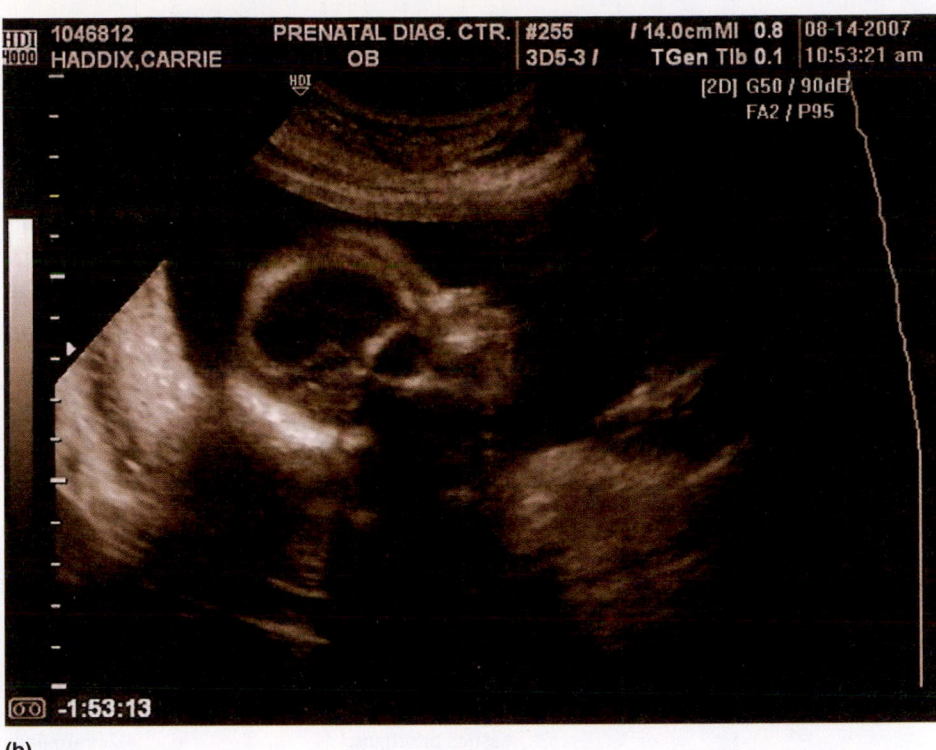

(b)

FIGURE 39-4 (a) An ultrasound technician lightly rubs the transducer over a pregnant woman's abdomen to reveal the anatomy of her fetus. (b) Routine ultrasounds are usually two-dimensional, as shown here; however, three-dimensional ultrasounds can be done.

© Andersen Ross/Getty Images RF; © Total Care Programming, Inc.

POINTS ON PRACTICE

Pap Smear Technologies

During a Pap smear, a false-negative test occurs when abnormal cells are not detected. This can occur as a result of the following:

- Too many cells left on the sampling device (brush, broom, or spatula)
- Too many cells piled on top of one another on the slide
- Epithelial cells hidden by extraneous material (blood, mucus, and so on)

A false-negative result could cause a delay in treatment of a year or more, depending on the timing of the next Pap smear. Different types of tests have been developed to help reduce false negatives. The thin-layer preparation of cells is a liquid-based sampling technique. The licensed practitioner collects cervical cells in much the same way as for traditional Pap smears, using a brush- or broom-like device. Once collected, the cells are suspended in a liquid preserving medium rather than being smeared directly onto a glass slide. The cells are then sent to an outside laboratory, where they are filtered or centrifuged and placed on a slide in a thin layer. This method

has been shown to produce samples that are more accurately interpreted by cytotechnologists. A cytotechnologist is a healthcare professional who uses a microscope to examine cells for changes that might indicate the presence of cancer. The advantages of thin-layer preparation over conventional specimen preparation include the following:

- Artifacts caused by air-drying are reduced because cells are placed in a fixative solution immediately.
- The possibility of hidden cells is reduced because cells are placed on the slide in a single layer.
- Blood and cellular debris are removed from the field of view because they are washed away or filtered out.
- The fluid left over after the thin-layer slide preparation may be used for additional testing (for instance, DNA testing for human papillomavirus).

If your office uses a thin-layer cell preparation system, make sure you read and follow all instructions for handling specimens. These instructions can be found in the package inserts for the individual tests.

TABLE 39-3 Understanding Pap Smear Results[*]

Classification	What It Means	Tests and Treatments That May Be Indicated
Unsatisfactory	Inadequate sampling or other interfering substance	The test must be repeated.
Negative	Cells appear normal and no identifiable infection is evident.	Continue routine Pap smears.
Benign	Noncancerous cells, but smear shows infection, irritation, or normal cell repair.	Continue routine Pap smears.
Atypical cells of uncertain significance: either ASC-US or ASC-H	Abnormal cells are present but it is uncertain what these cells may indicate.	Repeat the Pap smear; sometimes changes can go away without treatment. Estrogen cream for women who are at or near menopause. Follow-up test of cells for presence of high-risk HPV (human papillomavirus). If HPV is present, a colposcopy is performed.
Low-grade changes (mild dysplasia)	Cells have changes that are not cancer but have the potential to be cancer. Cell changes may be caused by HPV infection.	HPV testing; repeat Pap test; colposcopy, and if abnormal tissue is found, then endocervical curettage or biopsy
High-grade changes (moderate to severe dysplasia or carcinoma in situ, depending upon amount and location of cells)	Cells have more evident changes and look very different than normal cells.	Colposcopy and biopsy; LEEP procedure, cryotherapy, laser therapy, or conization
Squamous cell carcinoma	Cells invade deep into the cervix and other tissues or organs.	Immediate treatment including surgical removal; rare finding in well-screened populations such as the United States

*Based on the Bethesda System for Classification of Papanicolaou Smear.

through the anesthetized lower abdominal wall. Fetal skin cells obtained from the fluid are then grown in a culture and examined for chromosomal abnormalities. The level of AFP also may be measured in amniotic fluid.

Chorionic Villus Sampling Chorionic villus sampling (CVS) is a test done on patients over 35 or those with a history of genetic disorders to determine problems with the fetus. A sample of the chorionic villi (finger-shaped projections) of the placenta is collected either through amniocentesis or directly through the vagina. Collection through the vagina and cervix is done by using a small flexible tube with a long thin needle. As in amniocentesis, an ultrasound is used as a guide to locate the correct spot for sampling. Unlike amniocentesis, which is usually done between 15 and 20 weeks, a sampling can be taken through the vagina as early as 10 to 12 weeks. This provides parents the results earlier in the pregnancy so a decision can be made whether to continue or end the pregnancy.

Biopsy Biopsy is the surgical removal of tissue for later microscopic exam. It is the most accurate and, in some cases, the only way to diagnose breast and other cancers. Biopsy of the endometrium, which is the mucous membrane lining the uterus, may help the licensed practitioner diagnose uterine cancer and show whether ovulation is occurring. It also may indicate whether infection, polyps, or abnormal cells are present. If a patient's Pap smear indicates abnormal cells, a cervical or endocervical biopsy may be performed to rule out or diagnose cervical cancer. Procedure 39-3, at the end of this chapter, explains how to assist with a cervical biopsy.

To assist with these biopsies, you must have knowledge of the female anatomy, the order of the procedure, and the instruments used. You also will need to instruct patients about having an escort, appropriate clothing, and any special dietary restrictions. A careful medical history must be obtained to screen for problems like possible allergic reactions. The day before the biopsy, you might call the patient to confirm the appointment and address any concerns. A biopsy is considered minor surgery and consequently requires observance of standard precautions and sterile technique. Depending on the extent and site of the biopsy, the patient may receive sedation or local anesthesia. During the procedure, you may be responsible for clipping excess material from sutures (stitches) and any other special assistance the licensed practitioner requests. You must place the biopsy specimen in a sterile, solution-filled container provided by the laboratory. You also may assist with or perform the cleaning and bandaging of the site after the procedure. Because of the nature of the procedure, emotional support should be provided as needed during any biopsy.

Colposcopy Colposcopy is the exam of the vagina and cervix with an instrument called a colposcope. See Figure 39-5. The licensed practitioner first cleanses the cervix with saline solution. She then cleanses the cervix with acetic acid, which makes abnormal tissue appear white. The licensed practitioner inserts the colposcope into the vagina and uses the attached magnifying lens to identify abnormal cells, such as cancerous or precancerous cells. The abnormal cells may not be cancerous but may be caused by infection or medication.

This procedure is often performed prior to a biopsy or LEEP procedure after results of a Pap smear show the

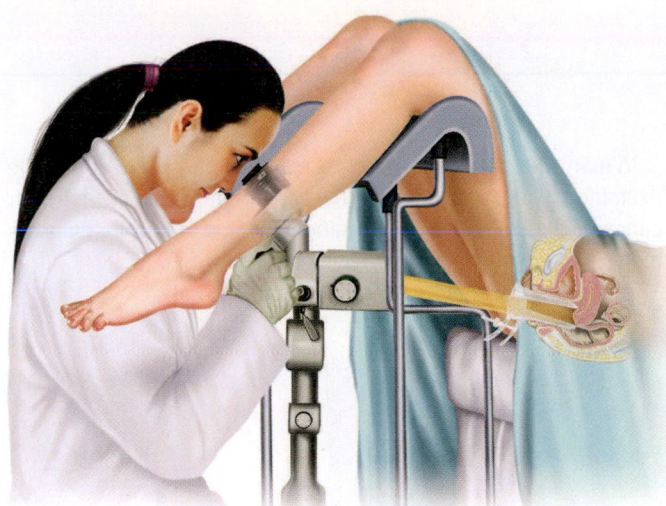

FIGURE 39-5 A colposcope is used to examine the vagina and cervix for abnormal cells.

presence of abnormal cells. LEEP procedures are described later in this chapter.

Dilation and Curettage (D&C) A D&C consists of widening the opening of the cervix (dilation) and scraping the uterine lining (curettage). Reasons for the D&C procedure include assessing the size and shape of the uterus, removing polyps and fibroids from the endometrium, obtaining endometrial specimens for biopsy, performing an abortion, and completing an incomplete miscarriage. Other diagnoses for which a D&C may be performed include abnormal uterine bleeding, abnormal menstrual bleeding, **postcoital** bleeding, spotting between periods, postmenopausal bleeding, and an imbedded intrauterine device (IUD).

The procedure is usually performed in a hospital or outpatient surgical facility. You must inform the patient that she will need to have someone take her to and from the facility and that she will have anesthesia before the licensed practitioner performs a routine pelvic exam. For the D&C procedure, the licensed practitioner swabs the vagina with an antiseptic and inserts a speculum. After dilating the cervix, the licensed practitioner uses a curette to remove a portion of the endometrium to assess the texture. Both cervical and endometrial tissue may be sent to a laboratory for examination. Exploration of the uterine cavity and removal of any abnormal growths complete the procedure. Instruct the patient not to have intercourse, take tub baths, or use tampons for 1 week after the procedure. She should also avoid strenuous activity.

Stereotactic Core Biopsy/Fine-Needle Aspiration In a fine-needle aspiration, the licensed practitioner uses a fine needle to remove by vacuum a sample of tissue from a cyst, lump, or tumor of the breast. The term *stereotactic* means that the licensed practitioner finds the target to aspirate using three-dimensional coordinates from a radiographic mammogram, computed tomography, or MRI. This procedure may be used instead of mammography to diagnose breast

disorders in pregnant patients, thus avoiding the use of radiation. Patients with fibrocystic breast disease (involving multiple cystic lumps within the breast tissue) may have needle aspiration of a cyst followed by replacement of the cystic fluid with a steroid to prevent recurrence.

Hysterectomy A hysterectomy is the surgical removal of the uterus. If surgery includes removal of one or both fallopian tubes, it is called a hysterosalpingectomy. Surgical removal of the uterus, the fallopian tubes, and the ovaries is called a hysterosalpingo-oophorectomy. A hysterectomy or a related surgery may be performed for the following reasons: cervical or endometrial cancer; severe endometriosis; unusual bleeding; a leiomyoma, or fibroid; defects of pelvic supports; pregnancy-related problems; and pelvic adhesions or other causes of uterine pain not controllable by other methods.

Inform the patient that an abdominal hysterectomy is major surgery that requires hospitalization. It also requires preadmission urine and blood tests, cleansing enemas, and shaving of the pelvic area. Normal activities, including sexual intercourse, can usually be resumed within a few weeks. Premenopausal women who have hysterectomies or hysterosalpingectomies may begin menopause sooner than they otherwise would have. Premenopausal women who have hysterosalpingo-oophorectomies will experience menopause immediately after the surgery.

Laparoscopy A laparoscope is a long, tubular instrument. It contains fiber-optic threads that illuminate the organs and a lens that resembles a small telescope. A licensed practitioner can use the laparoscope to view the internal female organs. Laparoscopy is used to help determine the cause of **infertility** (the inability to conceive), to obtain tissue samples, to remove abnormal growths, and to surgically sterilize a patient. It is also used in the treatment of ectopic pregnancies, endometriosis, and laparoscopy-assisted hysterectomy.

During laparoscopy the patient is anesthetized and the laparoscope tube is inserted through a small incision in or around the navel. Carbon dioxide or another gas is pumped into the abdomen to spread the organs apart, making them easier to see. The patient's body is then tilted with her head lower than her hips to allow the intestines to move away from the lower abdomen. This positioning permits a clearer view of the ovaries, uterus, and fallopian tubes.

Loop Electrosurgical Excision Procedure (LEEP) A **loop electrosurgical excision procedure (LEEP)** is when a thin wire loop electrode attached to the speculum is inserted in the vagina and used to cut away abnormal cervical tissue that was discovered during a Pap smear. The tissue is then sent to a lab for further testing. This procedure may last about 20 to 30 minutes and may be done as part of a colposcopy. A small amount of smoke may be seen during this procedure.

Cryosurgery Cryosurgery is using extremely cold temperatures to freeze and destroy abnormal tissues such as venereal warts, to treat precancerous tumors, and to control bleeding. The procedure is done through the vagina using a vaginal

Testicular Self-Exam

Although testicular cancer is rare, it is currently the most common cancer in American males between the ages of 15 and 34. The American Cancer Society recommends that all men perform a monthly testicular self-exam from age 15 on to increase the chances of early detection. Although testicular cancer is one of the most curable cancers, early detection is vital to its treatment.

A TSE should be performed in the following manner after a warm shower or bath, when scrotal skin is relaxed. A medical assistant may be responsible for coaching the patient through the steps of this technique.

1. The man first observes the testes for changes in appearance, such as swelling. He then manually examines each testicle, gently rolling it between the fingers and thumbs of both hands to feel for hard lumps (see Figure 39-6).

2. After examining each testicle, the man should locate the area of the epididymis and spermatic cord and know these are normal structures. This area can be felt as a cord-like structure originating at the top back of each testicle.

A man who perceives an abnormality during a TSE should be examined by a physician right away. Warning signs of testicular cancer include a heavy or dragging feeling in the groin, enlargement of one testicle, and a dull ache in the groin.

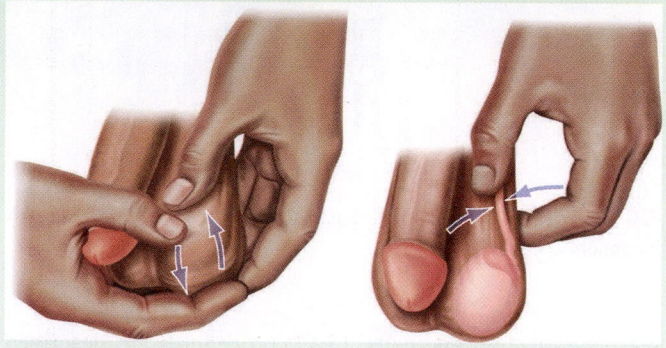

FIGURE 39-6   Males from age 15 on should perform a monthly testicular self-exam.

---

speculum and a probe. Compressed gases flow through the probe, making it as low as −50°C. The extreme cold freezes and kills the tissues. A second treatment might be done after 3 minutes. Patients may experience slight cramping during the procedure. After the procedure, sexual intercourse and douching are avoided for up to two weeks, and discharge may be seen.

Assisting in Urology   LO 39.4

The urologist focuses on the male and female urinary systems as well as the male reproductive system. Urologists perform surgical procedures such as hernia repairs and vasectomies. In a urologist's office, you would assist with general exams; collect and process urine, blood, and other specimens; obtain cultures; and participate in patient education about conditions and about presurgical and postsurgical care. So you need to understand the urinary system and the diseases and disorders you are likely to encounter.

You must be thorough when you take a patient's history for a urologist. Much information about urinary problems is obtained by questioning the patient about changes in frequency or urgency of urination, difficulty or pain with urination (dysuria), and incontinence. The physical exam usually includes palpation of the kidneys and bladder and visual inspection of the external genitalia. Women are usually examined in the lithotomy position. Men are typically seated when the exam begins. During the examination of the male reproductive system, the urologist inspects and palpates the patient's penis and scrotum. The genitalia are usually examined with the patient standing and the chest and abdomen

draped. The physician usually examines the inguinal region for a hernia and, in men over 40, checks the prostate gland. This gland is examined by digital insertion into the rectum. The physician instructs the patient as needed in performing a regular testicular self-exam (TSE). This instruction, discussed in the *Educating the Patient* feature Testicular Self-Exam, may also be your responsibility.

Urologic Diagnostic Tests and Procedures   LO 39.5

Urologists sometimes use imaging techniques such as CT scans and MRIs. Pyelography is an X-ray of the kidney area with an iodine-based contrast agent. It is used to diagnose renal (kidney-related) disorders. Urologists also use several other diagnostic techniques.

Urine and Blood Tests

Urinalysis (analysis of the urine) is the most commonly ordered test in a urology practice. Urine can be tested for the presence of bacteria, blood, and other substances. Blood testing is also done for a variety of reasons, including monitoring for dysfunctions of the prostate gland and for certain sexually transmitted infections (STIs). For example, a PSA (prostate-specific antigen) blood test is done to screen for prostate cancer.

Semen Analysis and Smears

Semen samples may be obtained to determine fertility. This test is done if a couple finds themselves unable to conceive or if the patient has had a vasectomy. A **vasectomy** is surgical sterilization by cutting the vas deferens. This is the tube that allows semen to pass outside the body. The patient usually collects these samples at home, but you may be required to provide the patient with a container, written instructions, and laboratory paperwork. Smears are used in diagnosing infections.

Cystometry

Cystometry is used to measure urinary bladder capacity and pressure. A catheter is passed through the urethra into the bladder. Then the physician fills the bladder with carbon dioxide gas. The test results are examined to diagnose bladder function disorders.

Cystoscopy

In cystoscopy, the physician examines the walls of the bladder and urethra by visualization and inspection. A viewing instrument called a cystoscope is used for this procedure. The cystoscope is inserted into the bladder through the urethra.

Testicular Biopsy

Testicular biopsy, an invasive procedure, involves obtaining a tissue sample of a mass for laboratory examination. The patient will need your emotional support because he will most likely be very anxious about the nature of the lump.

▶ Diseases and Disorders of the Reproductive and Urinary Systems   LO 39.6

Many of the diseases and disorders encountered in OB/GYN and urology practices have been mentioned in the context of the procedures in this chapter. Tables 39-4 and 39-5 outline common obstetric, gynecologic, and urologic diseases and disorders.

TABLE 39-4	Common Obstetric and Gynecologic Diseases and Disorders	
Condition	**Description**	**Treatment**
Cancer	Common occurrence in cervix, endometrium (uterus), and ovaries; cells divide uncontrollably, eventually forming a tumor or other growth of abnormal tissue; most often seen in women between the ages of 50 and 60; symptoms differ for each type of cancer	Surgery (hysterectomy), radiation, chemotherapy, hormones; for ovarian cancer, surgical removal of all reproductive organs, affected lymph nodes, appendix, and some muscle tissue, followed by chemotherapy (to extend survival time)
Ectopic pregnancy	Fertilized egg unable to move out of fallopian tube into uterus for implantation; patient experiences pain within a few weeks of conception; can be fatal	Surgery to remove the embryo from the fallopian tube before the tube ruptures
Endometriosis	Endometrial tissue present outside uterus, usually in pelvic area; not life-threatening but may cause sterility; symptoms include abnormal menstruation and pain (sometimes severe) in lower abdominal area and back	Hormone therapy, hysterectomy for severe cases, endometrial ablation (1-day surgery, alternative to hysterectomy), leuprolide acetate injection
Fibrocystic breast disease	Benign, fluid-filled cysts or nodules in breast; sometimes confused with malignant growths in breast until complete diagnostic tests are performed; symptoms include pain and tenderness	Depending on severity, vitamin E supplements, hormones, compresses, analgesics, aspiration, biopsy, restricted caffeine intake
Fibroids, or leiomyomas	Common, benign, smooth tumors of muscle cells (not fibrous tissue) grouped in uterus; symptoms include excessive menstruation and bloating; diagnosis by bimanual examination and ultrasound	Surgery for severe cases
Menstrual disturbances	May be (1) **amenorrhea** (absence of menstruation), (2) **dysmenorrhea** (painful menstruation), (3) **menorrhagia** (excessive amount of menstrual flow or prolonged period of menstruation), or (4) **metrorrhagia** (bleeding between menstrual periods)	Treatment according to symptoms; analgesics; possibly D&C or cryosurgery; for severe cases, hysterectomy
Ovarian cysts	Sacs of fluid or semisolid material, usually benign and without symptoms; occur anytime between puberty and menopause; extensive ovarian cysts may cause pelvic discomfort, lower back pain, and abnormal bleeding	Analgesics and bed rest if severe pain; hormone therapy; surgery is usually reserved for cysts that rupture or are large enough to put pressure on surrounding organs
Pelvic inflammatory disease (PID)	Acute, chronic infection of reproductive tract; causes include untreated STIs, such as gonorrhea and chlamydia, and organisms such as staphylococci and streptococci; symptoms include vaginal discharge, fever, and general discomfort	Antibiotics

(Continued)

TABLE 39-4 Common Obstetric and Gynecologic Diseases and Disorders

Condition	Description	Treatment
Pelvic support problems (uterine prolapse, rectocele, cystocele)	Abnormal weakening of vaginal tissue, unusual increase in abdominal pressure, congenital weakening (weakness since birth); symptoms include urine leakage, pelvic heaviness ("bottom falling out"), pain or discomfort in pelvic area, pulling or aching feeling in lower back, abdomen, or groin	Kegel or perineal exercises to strengthen muscles, insertion of pessary (device to hold pelvic organs in place), surgery to repair muscles, physical therapy
Polyps	Red, soft, and fragile growths, with slender stem attachment, sometimes found on mucous membranes of cervix or endometrium; may cause pain	Depending on size and shape, may be removed in office or hospital
Premenstrual dysphoric disorder (PMDD)	A severe form of premenstrual syndrome that affects 5% of women; symptoms have a very disrupting effect on the patient's life; screening tests and physician evaluation are necessary for diagnosis	Medications, including antidepressants, anti-anxiety drugs, analgesics, hormones, and diuretics; exercise, relaxation, diet modification, vitamins, minerals, and herbal preparations are also useful
Premenstrual syndrome (PMS)	Symptoms include swelling, bloating, weight gain, breast tenderness, headaches, and mood shifts 1 week to 10 days before menstruation	Vitamins, diuretics, hormones, oral contraceptives, tranquilizers, other medications; stress-reduction methods as needed; restricted intake of dietary sodium, alcohol, and caffeine
Sexual function disorders	Interruption or lack of sexual response cycle (excitement, plateau, orgasm, and resolution); unhealthy view of one's feelings about oneself as a woman and feelings toward sex; sometimes caused by painful intercourse, abusive partner, unrealistic demands on oneself, or menopause	Counseling (for both woman and partner) to teach relaxation, effective communication, and identification of cycle stages and natural responses
Vaginitis	Inflammation of vagina caused by bacteria, viruses, yeasts, or chemicals in sprays, douches, or tampons; symptoms include itching, redness, pain, swelling	Treatment prescribed according to cause; avoiding douches, tampons, tight pants, wiping from back to front, sometimes avoiding sex during treatment

TABLE 39-5 Common Urologic Diseases and Disorders

Condition	Description	Treatment
Epididymitis	Bacterial infection of the epididymis; causes pain, swelling, and sometimes fever	Rest and antibiotic medications
Hydrocele	Excess fluid in the scrotum; usually caused by infection of the epididymis or testes; can also result from a congenital defect or after injury	Aspiration of fluid to relieve discomfort
Impotence	Inability either to achieve or to maintain an erection; the cause may be physical, as when it results from cardiovascular or endocrine disease, or it may be a side effect of a medication such as certain diuretics and chemotherapy agents; the cause may also be psychological or emotional	Depends on the cause or causes and may include medication, counseling, or surgical procedures
Incontinence	Loss of bladder control, which results in anything from mild urine leaking to uncontrollable wetting; most bladder-control problems happen when muscles are too weak or too active; stress incontinence occurs when the muscles that keep the bladder closed are too weak and urine leaks during a sneeze, when laughing, or when lifting a heavy object	Depends on the cause and severity of the problem; may include simple exercises, medicines, special devices or procedures prescribed by a licensed practitioner, or surgery
Kidney stones	Chemical substances in the urine form crystals in the kidney, ureter, or bladder; if kidney stones cannot pass through the ureter, they can cause excruciating pain	Some stones pass; however, large stones often must be removed surgically or broken up by means of sound waves (lithotripsy) or laser techniques
Prostate cancer	The most common type of cancer among men; often no symptoms are evident, but sometimes a nodule may be felt on palpation of the prostate; if the growth is large enough, problems with urination may occur; a blood test known as a prostate-specific antigen (PSA) is used for screening in men over 50 years of age; an abnormal elevation of the PSA could indicate prostate cancer	Radiation therapy, removal of the prostate, hormone therapy, chemotherapy, biologic therapy
Prostatic hypertrophy (hyperplasia)	Enlargement of the prostate gland; occurs most commonly in men over 50; may constrict the urethra, causing difficulty in urinating and repeated urinary infections	Medications to reduce the enlarged prostate, surgery

(Continued)

TABLE 39-5	Common Urologic Diseases and Disorders	
Condition	**Description**	**Treatment**
Prostatitis	Inflammation of the prostate, usually bacterial; symptoms are pain on urination and, often, fever; patients are instructed to avoid sitting for long periods	Antibiotic medications and sitz baths
Sexually transmitted infections (STIs)	Numerous diseases acquired through sexual contact; affect both reproductive and urinary systems	Prevention through education, specific treatments depending on the disease
Urethritis	Inflammation of the urethra; like cystitis, usually caused by bacterial infection	Antibiotics

Sexually Transmitted Infections (Diseases)

Sexually transmitted diseases (STDs)—diseases acquired through sexual contact with an infected person—are now frequently called sexually transmitted infections. You may have asked yourself why the term *sexually transmitted infection* is preferred instead of the term *sexually transmitted disease*. The term *infection* more accurately describes conditions in which sexual partners may not have symptoms and may not be aware that they have an infection. Many of these infections are actually curable. Also, the term *infection* carries less of a social stigma than the term *disease*. STI is now used by many leading sexual health organizations. Urologists and gynecologists are both involved in the diagnosis and treatment of STIs.

Your role as an educator is vital in dealing with patients who have STIs. Some patients may be hesitant to ask for information. Providing educational materials in the exam room will help answer their questions and put them at ease. These materials deal with sensitive or embarrassing topics, and the patient's privacy must be maintained. Patient education about prevention and treatment of STIs is needed. See the *Educating the Patient* feature Teaching Patients About Sexually Transmitted Infections for more information on this topic.

EDUCATING THE PATIENT

Teaching Patients About Sexually Transmitted Infections

You must provide complete and detailed information with a non-judgmental and supportive attitude when you teach patients about STIs. Begin with the principle that all STIs are preventable. The key to prevention is avoiding sexual activities in which blood, semen, or vaginal secretions pass from one person to another. Although there are various levels of protection in connection with STIs, the only absolute methods of "safe sex" are abstinence (no sex) and masturbation (self-stimulation). The next level is mutual monogamy, in which partners have sex only with each other. Emphasize that monogamy provides protection from STIs only if neither partner has an STI when the relationship begins. A final level of prevention applies to people who do not practice abstinence or mutual monogamy but wish to protect themselves and others from STIs. The following measures provide some protection:

- Use a latex condom and spermicide for every act of intercourse. (Use a latex condom during vaginal, oral, or anal sex.)
- Use only water-based lubricants with latex condoms. (Oil and petroleum-based lubricants can break down latex, causing the condom to tear or break.)
- Know all your sexual partners, and discuss STI prevention with them.
- Have a physician regularly screen you for STIs because many people, especially men, have no signs when they are infected.

- Consult a physician if any signs of STIs develop, such as a blister, a sore, discharge, a rash, or abdominal pain.

Encourage patients to ask questions and discuss any concerns they have. Explain the need to make follow-up appointments with a physician if appropriate. Teaching a patient who has been diagnosed with an STI how to treat or manage the disease is especially important. Make sure the patient understands all directions and the necessity for treatment. Bacterial infections such as chlamydia, gonorrhea, and syphilis can be cured with antibiotics as long as the patient takes all the medication in the prescribed manner. Viral infections such as AIDS, genital herpes, and genital warts cannot be cured, although they can be treated and managed to differing degrees.

Emphasize to patients with an STI that they should avoid all sexual contact until the infection has been treated completely. Many STIs can be spread through any type of genital contact, including vaginal intercourse, anal sex, and oral sex. Herpes can be spread through kissing if there are herpes sores in the mouth. Encourage patients to inform each person with whom they had sexual contact that they have contracted an STI. Explain that unless all sexual partners are treated successfully, the disease will pass back and forth indefinitely.

You can reinforce your education efforts by providing patients with materials on the prevention and treatment of STIs. Keep a variety of pamphlets, books, and other resources in your office to help patients cope with and manage STIs.

When assisting the licensed practitioner in treating a patient who has an STI, you will emphasize to the patient the importance of completing the course of therapy and avoiding sexual contact while the infection is still active. Sexual partners also must be treated to avoid reinfection. Several types of STIs are fairly common. Other types are very serious. Review the chapters *The Reproductive Systems* and *Microbiology and Disease* to become familiar with these infections.

PROCEDURE 39-1 Assisting with a Gynecologic Exam WORK // DOC

Procedure Goal: To assist the licensed practitioner and maintain the client's comfort and privacy during a gynecologic exam

OSHA Guidelines:

Materials: Patient chart/progress note, gown and drape; vaginal speculum; specimen collection equipment, including cervical brush, cervical broom, and/or scraper; cotton-tipped applicator; potassium hydroxide solution (KOH); exam gloves; tissues; laboratory requisition; water-soluble lubricant; examining table with stirrups; exam light; microscopic slide(s); thin-layer collection vial (or slides if used); tissues; spray fixative; pen; and pencil

Method:

1. Gather equipment and make sure all items are in working order.

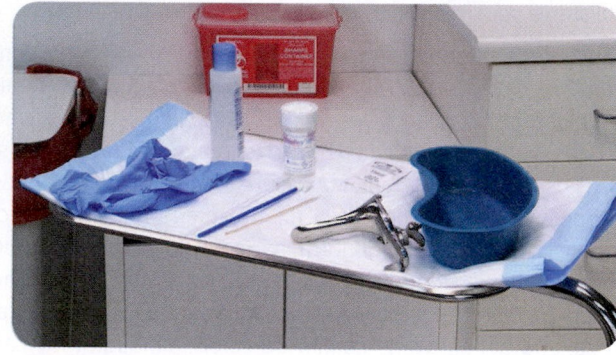

FIGURE Procedure 39-1 Step 1   Gather the necessary equipment.
© McGraw-Hill Education

2. Identify the patient and explain the procedure. The patient should remove all clothing, including underwear, and put the gown on with the opening in the front.

3. Ask the patient to sit on the edge of the examining table with the drape until the licensed practitioner arrives.

4. When the licensed practitioner is ready, have the patient place her feet into the stirrups and move her buttocks to the edge of the table. This is the lithotomy position.
   RATIONALE: *Putting the patient in the lithotomy position too early can cause the patient to experience back and leg cramps.*

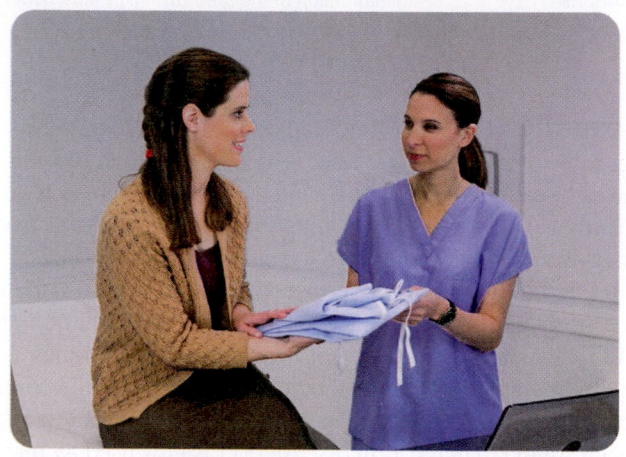

FIGURE Procedure 39-1 Step 2   Have the patient remove all clothing and put on the gown with the opening in the front.
© McGraw-Hill Education

5. Provide the licensed practitioner with gloves and an exam lamp as she examines the genitalia by inspection and palpation. Put on gloves per standard precautions guidelines.

6. Pass the speculum to the licensed practitioner. To increase patient comfort, you may place the speculum in warm water before handing it to the licensed practitioner. Lubricant is not typically recommended prior to the Pap smear because it may interfere with the test results.

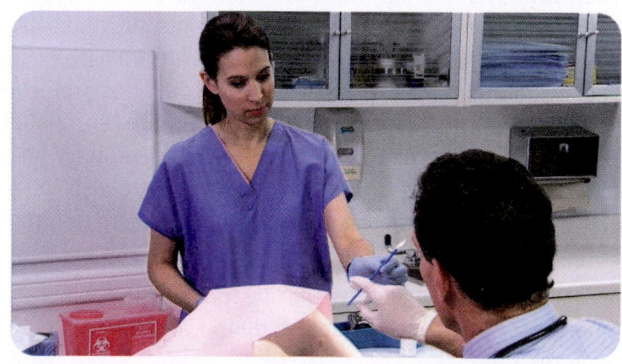

(a)

FIGURE Procedure 39-1 Step 6   Hand the speculum to the practitioner when needed.
© McGraw-Hill Education

7. For the Pap (Papanicolaou) smear, be prepared to pass a cotton-tipped applicator and cervical brush, broom, or scraper for the collection of the specimens. Have the slide or vial available for the licensed practitioner to place the specimen on the slide. Depending on

the licensed practitioner, the specimen collected, the method of collection, and the method of preparation, two or more slides or collection vials may be necessary. They may be labeled based on where the specimen was collected: endocervical (E), vaginal (V), and cervical (C).

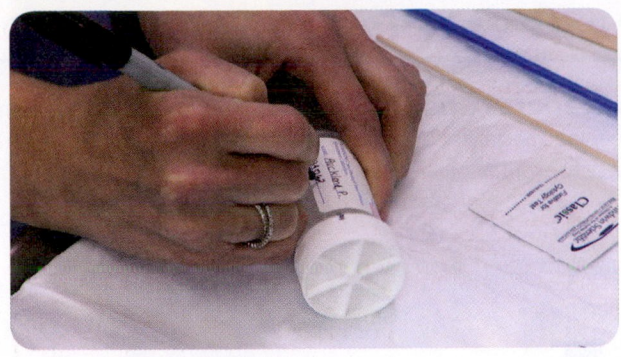

FIGURE Procedure 39-1 Step 9   Specimens should be labeled immediately after processing.
© McGraw-Hill Education

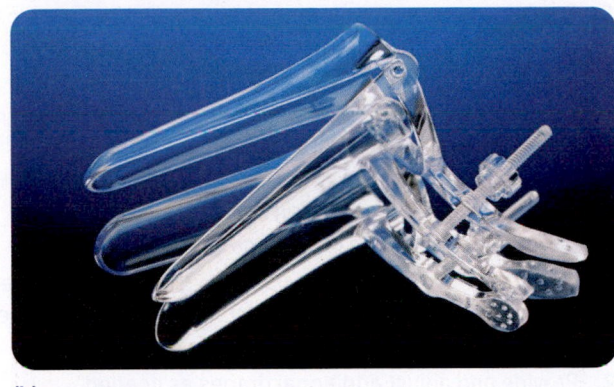

(b)

FIGURE Procedure 39-1 Step 6   A speculum is used to view the internal structures during a gynecologic exam.
© Doc-Stock/Corbis RF

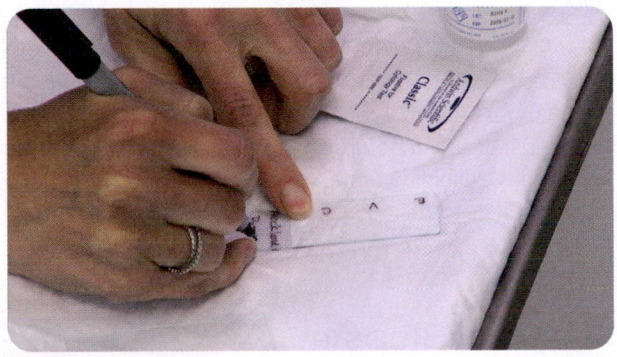

FIGURE Procedure 39-1 Step 7   Label the slide for the specimen using the office protocol.
© McGraw-Hill Education

10. After the licensed practitioner removes the speculum, a digital exam is performed to check the position of the internal organs. Provide the licensed practitioner with additional lubricant as needed.

11. Upon completion of the exam, help the patient switch from the lithotomy position to a supine or sitting position.

12. Provide tissues or moist wipes for the patient to remove the lubricant and ask the patient to get dressed. Assist as necessary or provide for privacy. Explain the procedure for communicating the laboratory results.

13. After the patient has left, don gloves and clean the exam room and equipment. Dispose of the disposable speculum, specimen collection devices, and other contaminated waste in a biohazardous waste container.

14. Store the supplies, straighten the room, and discard the used exam paper on the table.

15. Prepare the requisition slip and place the specimen and requisition slip in the proper place for transport to an outside laboratory.

16. Remove your gloves and wash your hands.

17. Document the specimen and complete the laboratory log if needed (refer to Progress Note).

8. Once the specimen is on the slide, a cytology fixative must be applied immediately. A spray fixative is common and should be held 6 inches from the slide and sprayed lightly with a back-and-forth motion. Allow the slide to dry completely.
   RATIONALE: *The fixative holds the cells in place until a microscopic exam is performed.*
   Cells collected for thin-layer preparation should be washed into the collection vial and transported to an outside lab for processing and analysis.

9. Label the slides/vials immediately after processing the specimen unless office protocol requires pre-labeling the container.
   RATIONALE: *Slides or vials should be immediately and properly labeled to avoid confusing one patient's specimen with another's.*

BWW PROGRESS NOTE

Patient Name:	Rita Huggins
	PAP smear specimen collected and labeled at 12:15pm. Sent to MedLAB lab with early afternoon shipment.
Date:	3/7/XX
Author:	K. Haddix

Done   Close

PROCEDURE 39-2 Assisting During the Exam of a Pregnant Patient

Procedure Goal: To assist the licensed practitioner and meet the special needs of the pregnant woman during the general physical exam

OSHA Guidelines:

Materials: Patient education materials, examining table, exam gown, drape

Method:

Providing Patient Information

1. Identify the patient and introduce yourself.

2. Assess the patient's need for education by asking appropriate questions and having the patient describe what she already knows about the information you are providing.

3. Provide any appropriate instructions or materials.

4. Ask the patient whether she has any special concerns or questions about her pregnancy that she might want to discuss with the licensed practitioner.

5. Communicate the patient's concerns or questions to the licensed practitioner; include all pertinent background information on the patient.
   RATIONALE: *Maintains your scope of practice and ensures that the patient receives correct information*

Ensuring Comfort During the Exam

6. Identify the patient and introduce yourself.

7. Wash your hands.

8. Explain the procedure to the patient.

9. Provide a gown or drape and instruct the patient in the proper way to wear it after disrobing. (Allow the patient privacy while disrobing and assist only if she requests help.)

10. Assist the patient onto the examining table. Ask the patient to step on either the stool or the pullout step of the examining table.
    RATIONALE: *Pregnant women may need assistance during the later stages of pregnancy.*

11. Help the patient into the position requested by the licensed practitioner, observing the patient for any difficulties she may have in achieving the requested position.

12. Provide and adjust additional drapes as needed.

13. Minimize the time the patient must spend in uncomfortable positions by making sure that the licensed practitioner has all supplies and equipment for the exam before it begins.

14. If the patient appears to be uncomfortable during the procedure, ask whether she would like to reposition herself or take a break; assist as necessary.

15. To prevent pelvic pooling of blood and subsequent dizziness or hyperventilation, allow the patient time to adjust to sitting before standing after she has been lying on the examining table. Assist the patient off the exam table if needed.

PROCEDURE 39-3 Assisting with a Cervical Biopsy

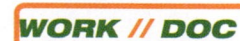

Procedure Goal: To assist the physician in obtaining a sample of cervical tissue for analysis

OSHA Guidelines:

  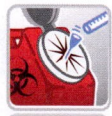 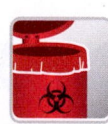 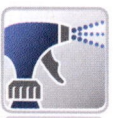

Materials: Patient chart/progress note, laboratory requisition form, gown and drape, tray or Mayo stand, disposable cervical biopsy kit (disposable forceps, curette, and spatula in a sterile pack), transfer forceps, vaginal speculum, biopsy specimen container, clean basin, sterile cotton balls, sterile gauze squares, sanitary napkin

Method:

1. Identify the patient and introduce yourself.

2. Look at the patient's chart and ask the patient to confirm information or explain any changes. Specific patient information you need to ask about and note in the chart includes the following:

   - Date of birth and Social Security number (verify that you have the correct chart for the correct patient)
   - Date of last menstrual period
   - Method of contraception, if any
   - Previous gynecologic surgery
   - Use of hormone replacement therapy or other steroids

3. If within your scope of practice, describe the biopsy procedure to the patient, noting that a piece of tissue will be removed to diagnose the cause of her problem. Explain that it may be painful but only for the brief moment during which tissue is taken.

4. Give the patient a gown, if needed, and a drape. Direct her to undress from the waist down and to wrap the drape around herself. Tell her to sit at the end of the examining table.

5. Wash your hands and put on exam gloves.

6. Using sterile method, open the sterile pack to create a sterile field on the tray or Mayo stand and arrange the instruments with transfer forceps. Add the vaginal speculum and sterile supplies to the sterile field.
RATIONALE: *The instruments and supplies must stay sterile because this is an invasive procedure.*

7. When the physician arrives in the exam room, ask the patient to lie back, place her heels in the stirrups of the table, and move her buttocks to the edge of the table.
RATIONALE: *Placing the patient in the lithotomy position too early can cause the patient's back and legs to cramp.*

8. Assist the physician by arranging the drape so that only the genitalia are exposed, and place the light so that the genitalia are illuminated.

9. Use transfer forceps to hand instruments and supplies to the physician as he requests them. You may don sterile gloves and hand the physician supplies and instruments directly.

10. When the licensed practitioner is ready to obtain the biopsy, tell the patient that it may hurt. If she seems particularly fearful, instruct her to take a deep breath and let it out slowly.

11. When the physician hands you the instrument with the tissue specimen, place the specimen in the specimen container and discard the instrument in the appropriate container.

12. Label the specimen container with the patient's name, the date and time, cervical or endocervical (as indicated by the physician), the physician's name, and your initials.

13. Place the container and the cytology laboratory requisition form in the envelope or bag provided by the laboratory.

14. When the physician has completed the procedure and removed the speculum, properly clean instruments as needed and dispose of used supplies and disposable instruments. Metal speculums, if used, should be placed in a clean basin for later sanitization, disinfection, and sterilization.

15. Remove the gloves and wash your hands.

16. Tell the patient that she may get dressed. Inform her that she may have some vaginal bleeding for a couple of days, and provide her with a sanitary napkin. Instruct her not to take tub baths or have intercourse and not to use tampons for 2 days. Encourage her to call the office if she experiences problems or has questions.

17. Document the procedure as appropriate (refer to Progress Note).

BWW PROGRESS NOTE

Patient Name:	Harriet Gibbers
	Cervical specimen labeled and sent to MedLAB lab.
Date:	4/9/XX
Author:	K. Haddix

Done · Close

SUMMARY OF LEARNING OUTCOMES

LEARNING OUTCOMES	KEY POINTS
39.1 Carry out the role of the medical assistant in the medical specialty of gynecology.	Medical assistants assist with gynecologic exams, provide patient teaching for OB/GYN and breast health issues, and must handle cervical and other specimens correctly.
39.2 Carry out the role of the medical assistant in the medical specialty of obstetrics.	Medical assistants assist with examinations for pregnant females, providing for their needs, and provide education for the pregnant patient and new mother.
39.3 Identify diagnostic and therapeutic procedures performed in obstetrics and gynecology.	Diagnostic and therapeutic procedures performed in OB/GYN include pregnancy tests, tests for STIs, radiologic tests such as mammograms, fetal screening, Pap smears, D&C, and fine-needle aspiration.
39.4 Relate the role of medical assisting to the medical specialty of urology.	Medical assistants assist with urologic exams and diagnostic tests. Patient education for urologic patients regarding TSE and other information is also the duty of a medical assistant working in urology.

LEARNING OUTCOMES	KEY POINTS
39.5 Identify diagnostic tests and procedures performed in urology.	Various urologic diagnostic tests and procedures are performed, including semen analysis, cystometry, cystoscopy, and testicular biopsy.
39.6 Recognize diseases and disorders of the reproductive and urinary systems.	Diseases and disorders of the reproductive and urinary systems are listed for review in Table 39-4, Common Obstetric and Gynecologic Diseases and Disorders, and Table 39-5, Common Urologic Diseases and Disorders.

CASE STUDY CRITICAL THINKING

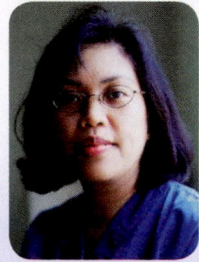

© ERproductions Ltd/Blend Images LLC RF

Recall Raja from the beginning of the chapter. Now that you have read the chapter, answer the following questions regarding her case.

1. How often should Raja have a pelvic exam, cervical cytology, HIV screen, and mammogram?

2. What should have been discussed with Raja before she had the mammogram?

3. How is stereotactic fine-needle biopsy performed?

EXAM PREPARATION QUESTIONS

1. (LO 39.2) A pregnant patient, Molly Holiday, has started feeling the movement of her baby. What is her current stage of pregnancy?
   a. 1st trimester
   b. Menarche
   c. 3rd trimester
   d. 2nd trimester
   e. 4th trimester

2. (LO 39.4) A TSE is
   a. Surgery that involves bypassing a blockage in the heart
   b. An imaging procedure that uses magnets and radio waves
   c. An examination of the testicles by the patient
   d. Scanning of the blood flow and metabolic activity in the brain
   e. An examination of the testicles by the physician

3. (LO 39.2) A pregnant patient is monitoring her blood glucose level with a glucometer. She most likely has
   a. Type 2 diabetes
   b. Type 1 diabetes
   c. Gestational diabetes
   d. Hyperthyroidism
   e. Diabetes mellitus

4. (LO 39.1) Which of the following indicates the LMP?
   a. The last day of the last menstrual period
   b. The first day of the last menstrual period
   c. A late menstrual period
   d. A likely menopausal pregnancy
   e. The heaviest flow day of the last menstrual period

5. (LO 39.1) A speculum is used to
   a. Evaluate for a DVT
   b. Evaluate the LMP
   c. Perform a basic physical exam
   d. Perform a vaginal exam
   e. Examine the breasts

6. (LO 39.3) Which of the following patients would *most* likely have an alpha fetoprotein test?
   a. 28-year-old male patient with urinary frequency and urgency
   b. 36-year-old female in her 3rd trimester of pregnancy
   c. 27-year-old female with vaginal discharge
   d. 54-year-old female with urinary incontinence
   e. 35-year-old female in her 2nd trimester of pregnancy

7. (LO 39.5) Which of the following diagnostic tests would *least* likely be performed on a male urologic patient?
   a. Colposcopy
   b. Testicular biopsy
   c. Semen analysis
   d. Urinalysis
   e. Cystoscopy

8. (LO 39.1) At what age should most women start having yearly mammograms, according to the American Cancer Society and National Cancer Institute?
   a. 20
   b. 30
   c. 40
   d. 50
   e. 65

9. (LO 39.6) Your 27-year-old female patient has a menstrual disturbance. Which of the following does she *least* likely have?
   a. Amenorrhea
   b. Menorrhea
   c. Dysmenorrhea
   d. Metrorrhagia
   e. Menorrhagia

10. (LO 39.6) Your male patient has an infection that is not an STI. Which of the following is most likely the problem?
   a. Hydrocele
   b. Vaginitis
   c. Epididymitis
   d. Gonorrhea
   e. Prostatic hypertrophy

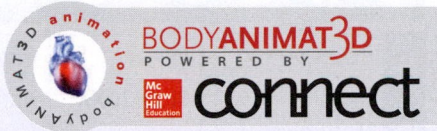

Go to CONNECT to see animation exercises about *Breast Cancer* and *Prostate Cancer*.

SOFT SKILLS SUCCESS

A young adult female patient begins asking you questions regarding birth control choices. She states she feels uncomfortable asking her physician, Dr. Buckwalter. Can you act as an "intermediary" for her with Dr. Buckwalter? Do you have any ideas to help her regarding her fears surrounding the need for this discussion?

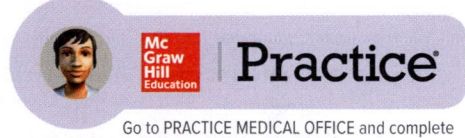

Go to PRACTICE MEDICAL OFFICE and complete the module Clinical - Interactions.

Assisting in Pediatrics

CASE STUDY

PATIENT INFORMATION

Patient Name	DOB	Allergies
Chris Matthews	11/19/20XX	NKA

Attending	MRN	Other Information
Alexis N. Whalen, MD	324-95-786	Home-schooled; parents refused immunizations

Chris Matthews is a 7-year-old male patient whose mother states he has had diarrhea for 3 days. He kept her up all night last night going to the bathroom at least three times. He says his stomach hurts but has not vomited, although he is eating very little. While you are preparing to weigh the patient, he initially does not want to get on the scale and begins to cry.

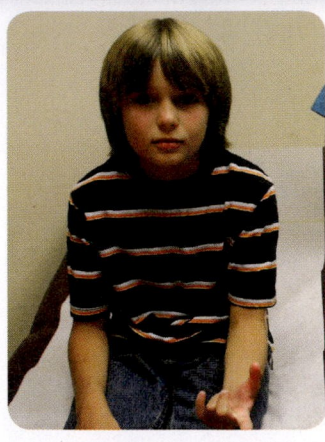

© McGraw-Hill Education

After his mother has persuaded him to get on the scale and you have obtained all the measurements and vital signs, you check his immunization record. While doing so, you see a note on Chris's chart indicating he is home-schooled and his parents are against immunizations.

Keep Chris in mind as you study this chapter. There will be questions at the end of the chapter based on the case study. The information in the chapter will help you answer these questions.

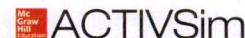

LEARNING OUTCOMES

After completing Chapter 40, you will be able to:

40.1 Relate growth and development to pediatric patient care.

40.2 Identify the role of the medical assistant during pediatric examinations.

40.3 Discuss pediatric immunizations and the role of the medical assistant.

40.4 Explain variations of pediatric screening procedures and diagnostic tests.

40.5 Describe common pediatric diseases and disorders and their treatment.

40.6 Recognize special health concerns of pediatric patients.

KEY TERMS

addiction

bilirubin

contraindication

enuresis

fontanels

growth chart

immunizations

jaundice

menarche

moro reflex

phenylketonuria (PKU)

puberty

substance abuse

I.C.6 Compare structure and function of the human body across the life span

I.C.8 Identify common pathology related to each body system including
(a) signs
(b) symptoms
(c) etiology

I.C.9 Analyze pathology for each body system including:
(a) diagnostic measures
(b) treatment modalities

I.P.1 Measure and record:
(a) blood pressure
(b) temperature
(f) weight
(g) length (infant)
(h) head circumference (infant)

I.P.3 Perform patient screening using established protocols

I.P.7 Administer parenteral (excluding IV) medications

I.P.8 Instruct and prepare a patient for a procedure or a treatment

I.P.9 Assist provider with a patient exam

I.A.1 Incorporate critical thinking skills when performing patient assessment

I.A.2 Incorporate critical thinking skills when performing patient care

I.A.3 Show awareness of a patient's concerns related to the procedure being performed

II.C.6 Analyze healthcare results as reported in:
(a) graphs

II.P.4 Document on a growth chart

X.C.12 Describe compliance with public health statutes
(b) abuse, neglect, and exploitation
(c) wounds of violence

X.P.3 Document patient care accurately in the medical record

2. Anatomy and Physiology
a. List all body systems, their structure and functions
b. Describe common diseases, symptoms and etiologies as they apply to each system
c. Identify diagnostic and treatment modalities as they relate to each body system

3. Medical Terminology
c. Apply various medical terms for each specialty

4. Medical Law and Ethics
a. Follow documentation guidelines

5. Psychology of Human Relations
a. Respond appropriately to patients with abnormal behavior patterns
c. Intervene on behalf of the patient regarding issues/concerns that may arise, i.e. insurance policy information, medical bills, physician/provider orders, etc.
d. Discuss developmental stages of life
e. Analyze the effect of hereditary, cultural, and environmental influences on behavior

9. Clinical Procedures
b. Obtain vital signs, obtain patient history, and formulate chief complaint
c. Assist provider with general/physical examination
d. Assist provider with specialty examination including cardiac, respiratory, OB-GYN, neurological, gastroenterology procedures
e. Perform specialty procedures including but not limited to minor surgery, cardiac, respiratory, OB-GYN, neurological, gastroenterology
f. Prepare and administer oral and parenteral medications and monitor intravenous (IV) infusions
j. Make adaptations with patients with special needs

▶ Introduction

Pediatrics is a specialty area of medicine that involves the care of children up to the age of 18, and in some cases 21. To be a good pediatric medical assistant, you must first like children of all ages. If you do, you will be better able to relate to them and to communicate with them effectively. The pediatrician specializes in the healthcare of children, monitoring their development and diagnosing and treating their illnesses. Just as with other specialty fields, there are subspecialties of pediatrics, such as surgery and oncology.

As a medical assistant working in pediatrics, your primary areas of responsibility include parent or caregiver education, adherence to immunization schedules, and recognition of special health concerns. You also will assist with the pediatric patient's physical exam and treatment. Relating to the child, as well as being a liaison between the parent or caregiver and the physician, is essential to your job.

▶ Developmental Stages and Care   LO 40.1

Different periods of childhood present different changes and challenges. As discussed in the *Interpersonal Communication* chapter, understanding lifespan development will, among other things, enhance your communication skills. This chapter focuses on the life stages from birth through the teenage years.

Understanding the child's stages of growth and development will improve your skills as a medical assistant. During each stage of growth, the following developmental milestones occur:

- Physical development is the actual bodily changes that occur.
- *Intellectual-cognitive development* refers to the thinking skills the child is developing.
- *Psycho-emotional development* refers to the changes in feelings experienced during a particular period.
- Social development is the way a person relates to others.

The stages of growth and development for pediatric patients include neonate, infant, toddler, preschooler, elementary school child, middle school child, and adolescent. As you explore each stage, you will also review the related aspects of care to help you provide the necessary care and patient education.

Neonate

An infant is called a *neonate* from birth to 1 month of age. Many changes take place in this short time.

Physical Development The full-term infant usually weighs between 7 and 9 pounds and is 18 to 22 inches in length. The newborn infant's head seems large in comparison to the rest of her body. No wonder—the head is usually one-fourth of the infant's entire length! An adult head is usually only about one-ninth of the body length. An infant's head has two soft spots, or **fontanels,** which are tough, fibrous cartilage (Figure 40-1). The anterior, or front, fontanel is diamond-shaped. The baby's pulse can sometimes be seen here. The infant can move her head from side to side. However, because the neck muscles are not strong enough to hold the head up, the person holding the infant must provide support.

The newborn baby's skin is usually loose, wrinkled, and somewhat red in appearance. During the first week of life, this skin may start to peel. This is not harmful, and nothing needs to be done about it. The part of the umbilical cord still attached to the baby's body is a "stump" about 1 to 1½ inches in length. At birth it has a white, waxy appearance, then turns darker and usually falls off around the tenth day of life (Figure 40-2).

Sometimes infants develop neonatal **jaundice**—a yellowish color of the skin—in the first few days of life. This is caused by an accumulation of **bilirubin,** the waste product from the normal breakdown of the red blood cells. Babies have large numbers of red blood cells at birth. Their immature liver is unable to handle the breakdown of these cells. The waste product accumulates, giving the skin a yellowish tint. The whites of the eyes also may appear yellow, and the urine and feces may have a dark yellow color.

Certain reflexes can be observed in the newborn. Some are protective. For example, blinking is a reflex that protects the eyes. Everyone, including newborns, has this reflex. Other reflexes are due to the infant's immature nervous system. For example, the **moro reflex** is one in which the infant feels as if she is falling. The arms spread out and then back in and crying often occurs. The physician will check reflexes as part of an examination.

Infants can see objects within 8 inches of their eyes. They probably detect brightness rather than color. Their eyes tend to turn outward or may even cross. Infants seem to prefer high-pitched tones.

Intellectual-Cognitive Development Newborns will become calm when picked up and held firmly. They tune out disturbing stimulation by sleeping.

Social Development Early on, infants respond to stimulation and establish an individual activity pattern. Generally, an infant responds to a soft, gentle voice and tries to focus

FIGURE 40-1 Be aware of the newborn's fontanels, or "soft spots." These areas are open at birth so that the brain can grow. They close as the infant ages.

Labels on figure:
- Frontal suture (metopic suture)
- Frontal bone
- Anterior fontanel
- Sagittal suture
- Posterior fontanel

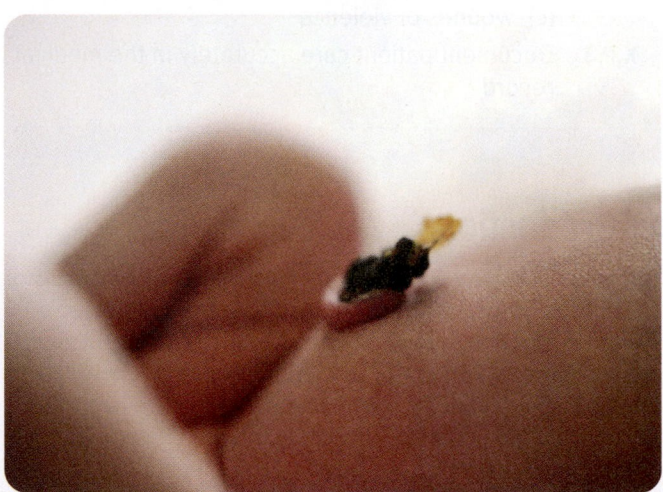

FIGURE 40-2 The umbilical cord usually falls off when the baby is about 10 days old.
© Ian Boddy/Science Source

on the voice and face. Newborns can show excitement and distress.

Aspects of Care: Neonate Consider the following when caring for neonates or providing parent or caregiver education.

- Sponge baths with tepid water and limited amounts of mild infant cleansing soap are given until the cord has fallen off. The infant's face should be washed with tepid water. No oil should be rubbed on the baby. Lotions and powders also should be avoided.

- If an infant is to be breast-fed, parents are given instruction about frequency of feedings, duration of feedings, and care of the mother and her breasts while breast-feeding. If an infant is to be bottle-fed, parents must be given instruction about the type of formula and how to prepare it correctly. Parents also should be taught about bowel movements and spitting up.

- The treatment for jaundice in the newborn is keeping the infant well hydrated with breast milk or formula. If necessary, the infant is placed under ultraviolet light. These bright lights can damage the infant's eyes, so eye protection is necessary during this treatment. Some neonates may need to use a bili-blanket, which is a type of phototherapy device that helps the infant eliminate the bilirubin, thus improving the jaundice (Figure 40-3). Blood tests will be performed fairly often to ensure that the bilirubin level does not become dangerously high. Other newborn blood tests are performed, including a screening test for phenylketonuria (PKU). See the *Points on Practice* box Testing for Phenylketonuria (PKU) for more information about this important test.

The Infant: 1 Month to 1 Year

Many changes occur in an infant during the first year. Parents cherish the wonder of their growing, developing child during this period.

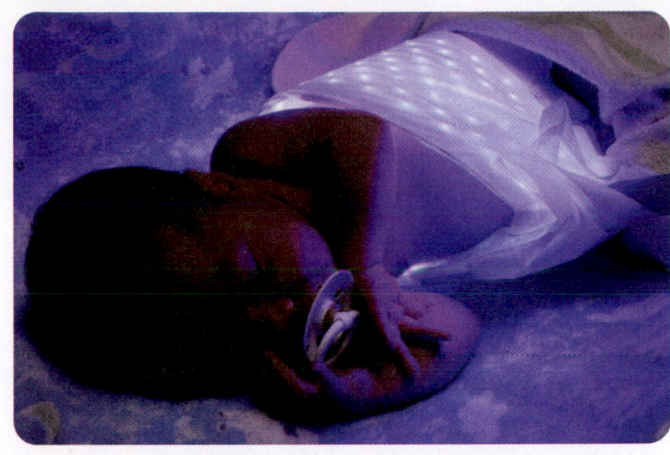

FIGURE 40-3 A newborn with excessive bilirubin may be sent home with an ultraviolet light bili-blanket to help reduce the jaundice.
© Aaron Haupt / Science Source

Physical Development Growth is rapid during the first year of life. Infants triple their birth weight by their first birthday. They develop in a cephalocaudal fashion, with the earliest development starting at the head and moving down. Infants first gain control of the head, neck, and shoulders, and then the arms, torso, and legs. This is why an infant finds and uses his hands before he finds and uses his feet. Larger groups of muscles develop before the smaller groups of muscles develop. The nervous system develops rapidly. Changes are seen in reflexes and in the development of coordinated movement and eye-hand coordination. The following is a brief look at some specific types of physical development in infants.

- By about 3 weeks of age, infants can focus on objects.

- By about 4 weeks, infants can follow an object with their eyes and make eye-to-eye contact. The infant can lift his head when lying on his abdomen.

- At 2 months, infants can follow objects with their eyes from one side to the other, listen to sounds, bat at objects, and respond to sounds. At this age, the infant may string together vowel sounds.

POINTS ON PRACTICE
Testing for Phenylketonuria (PKU)

Phenylketonuria (PKU) is a rare metabolic disorder. It is caused by a mutation in a gene that is responsible for creating an enzyme that breaks down phenylalanine, an amino acid found in protein-rich foods. If this amino acid is not broken down, it accumulates in the body and causes brain damage. Screening newborns for PKU is required in all states.

The screening test is a qualitative test for the presence of phenylalanine and related substances and is usually done 24–48 hours after birth. The newborn must ingest proteins prior to the test to ensure accuracy. Though this test is usually done in the hospital prior to discharge, there may be occasions when it is done in the physician's office.

To perform the test, a capillary puncture is done on the infant's heel. Three or four drops of blood are collected on a card or paper. Before the test is performed, the card must be filled out completely, including the following information:

- Mother's name and address
- Ordering physician's name and contact information
- Baby's name, date of birth, and weight
- Gestational age
- Date and time of the collection

- By 3 months, an infant may raise the head and shoulders while on the abdomen and may hold up the head (Figure 40-4). When the infant is pulled to a sitting position, the head remains in line with the backbone.
- By 4 months, the infant may roll from stomach to back and may begin to play with a rattle placed in the hand. Teething may begin at this time.
- By 5 months, the infant may transfer a rattle from one hand to the other.
- At 6 months, the infant rolls from back to stomach, may be able to sit up briefly, and can reach to retrieve a dropped object. The two bottom front teeth have probably erupted, or emerged, from the gums.
- At 9 months, the infant is able to sit and to creep on hands and knees. The infant is beginning to use the pincer grasp. The infant can put consonants with vowels and make repetitive sounds such as "mama" and "dada."
- At 12 months, the child can hold on to a piece of furniture and move around it, perhaps taking a step or two. With tooth development and the pincer grasp, the infant can pick up and eat small pieces of food.

Intellectual-Cognitive Development At 1 month of age, an infant can make contact. This progresses to recognition of familiar faces and then to "making faces" at 4 to 5 months. At around 6 months of age, the child is making babbling sounds and by 9 months is able to play games like peek-a-boo. The infant begins to understand cause and effect. If the infant drops a toy and someone retrieves it, the infant will drop it again. This becomes a game. At 12 months, an infant can follow simple directions.

Psycho-Emotional Development By the time a child is 1 month old, he or she can smile at another smiling face. By 3 months, the infant smiles spontaneously and displays pleasure in making sounds. At 4 months, the infant can vocalize a mood. At 6 months, there may be abrupt mood changes. At 9 months, the infant displays pleasure in playing simple

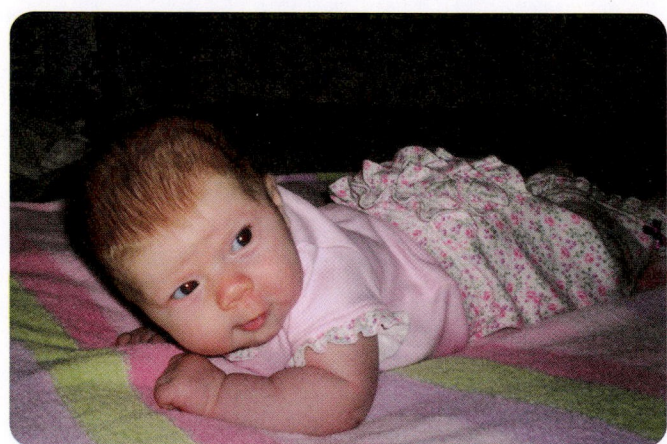

FIGURE 40-4 A 3-month-old infant should be able to hold up her head when lying on her stomach.
© Total Care Programming, Inc.

games and by 1 year has learned to express many emotions. For infants to develop physically and emotionally, it is important that their physical needs be addressed quickly and calmly.

Social Development Infants become social beings very quickly. By 1 month of age, infants are able to smile. At 3 months, the infant responds to voices. This can be seen when the infant pays attention and coos along with a person speaking in a quiet and gentle manner. At 6 months, the baby "babbles" and is interested in his or her own voice. Imitative play becomes an important part of the infant's interaction with others. At 9 months, the first development of words can be observed. This leads to increased interaction with family and others.

Aspects of Care: 1 Month to 1 Year Consider the following when caring for infants or providing parent or caregiver education.

- Regular health checkups and immunizations should be followed. Immunizations will be discussed later in this chapter.
- Infants need tactile stimulation for growth and development. Physical contact and cuddling, as well as prompt attention to their needs, help infants develop a sense of security and trust, which is necessary for them to thrive.
- In the first 4 to 6 months, the mother's breast milk or infant formula meets the growing infant's needs. The physician will provide guidance about the introduction of solid foods to the diet. You may be asked to assist the physician in guiding the parent or caregiver regarding the diet of a pediatric patient. Table 40-1 provides basic pediatric guidelines; however, always follow the policy of the facility where you are employed. In addition, be aware that dietary guidelines change with research.
- Ensure infant safety. See the *Educating the Patient* feature Keeping Infants and Toddlers Safe.

The Toddler: 1 to 3 Years
Children from the age of 1 to 3 years need constant attention from parents and others. Although they grow less rapidly during this period, their growth is still fast, and their communication skills begin to take shape in their use of language.

Physical Development Weight gain slows between 1 and 2 years. The arms and legs grow more than the trunk and head, and now seem to be in proportion to the child's overall size. Girls usually reach half of their adult height between 1½ and 2 years of age; boys reach half of their expected adult height between 2 and 2½ years.

Growth charts, as shown in Figure 40-5, are used to determine a child's growth in relation to average rates. The growth charts consist of percentile curves. Percentiles rank the position of an individual by indicating what percentage of the referenced population the individual would equal or exceed. For example, on the weight-for-age growth charts, an 18-month boy whose weight is at the 90th percentile weighs the same or more than 90 percent of the reference population

TABLE 40-1 Pediatric Dietary Guidelines*

AGE GROUP	RECOMMENDATIONS	SPECIFIC CONCERNS
Birth to 4 months	• Breast milk every 2 to 4 hours or formula six to eight times a day with 2 to 3 ounces per feeding.	• Never give infants honey; it may contain botulism spores. • Infants may need to be woken up at night if they are not eating enough during the day.
4 to 6 months	• Introduce 1 to 2 tablespoons of cereal mixed with formula or breast milk two times a day. Gradually increase to 3 to 4 tablespoons.	• Do not give cereal in a bottle unless directed by the physician. • Never put the infant to bed with a bottle in the mouth. This promotes tooth decay.
6 to 8 months	• Introduce strained vegetables and fruits. Give 2 to 3 tablespoons and offer about four servings per day. • Teething foods such as toast strips, unsalted crackers, and teething biscuits may also be introduced.	• Introduce finger foods if recommended by the physician, but avoid things such as apple chunks or slices, grapes, hot dogs, sausages, peanut butter, popcorn, nuts, seeds, round candies, and hard chunks of uncooked vegetables.
8 to 12 months	• Introduce strained or finely chopped meats. • Increase vegetables and fruits to 3 to 4 tablespoons, four times a day. • Include egg yolks 3 to 4 times per week.	• Start breast-fed babies on meat at 8 months to improve iron intake. • Start weaning off the bottle. • Do not give whole milk to infants under the age of 1.
1 to 2 years	• Whole milk can replace breast milk or formula. • Include fruits, vegetables, meats, breads, and grains.	• If a child does not like a food on the first attempt, try again later. • Offer one new food at a time.
2 years and older	• Balance dietary calories with physical activity to maintain normal growth. • Eat vegetables and fruits daily; limit juice intake. • Use vegetable oils and soft margarines low in saturated fat and trans fatty acids instead of butter or most other animal fats in the diet. • Eat whole-grain breads and cereals rather than refined-grain products. • Reduce the intake of sugar-sweetened beverages and foods. • Use nonfat (skim) or low-fat milk and dairy products daily. • Eat more fish, especially oily fish, broiled or baked. • Reduce salt intake, including salt from processed foods.	• Control when food is available and when it can be eaten. Regular meals and healthy snacks should be provided. • Have regular family meals that include social interaction with the family. • Teach about food and nutrition at the grocery store and when cooking meals. • Counteract inaccurate information from the media and other influences. • Teach other care providers (such as day care, babysitters) about what you want your children to eat. • Serve as role models and lead by example; "do as I do" rather than "do as I say." • Promote and participate in regular daily physical activity.

*Infants and children vary in growth and development; information intended as guidelines only. Adapted from Medline Plus http://www.nlm.hin.gov/medlineplus and American Academy of Pediatrics http://pediatrics.aappublications.org/.

of 18-month boys and weighs less than 10 percent of the 18-month boys in the reference population. Pediatric growth charts are used as a clinical tool for health professionals to determine if a child's growth is adequate. Procedure 40-2, at the end of this chapter, provides more information about how to record height, weight, and head circumference on a growth chart.

Most toddlers will walk independently by 15 months of age. At 18 months, a toddler can squat to reach for a toy, kneel and remain upright, and precisely perform the pincer grasp. The toddler may use a spoon for self-feeding. By 2 years of age, the child can run, throw a ball, and scribble with a pencil. The child may want to feed herself. At 3 years, the child is very active. Children of this age can dress themselves, ride a tricycle, draw simple shapes, and use a pair of child's scissors. Many children are toilet-trained between 2 and 3 years of age.

Intellectual-Cognitive Development During the toddler years, the child begins to learn about the world through play. Children enjoy imitating sweeping, raking, and making things they have seen adults make. A major task for the toddler is to develop independence. Toddlers are curious about their world, and their play may involve experimenting.

The toddler progresses with speech in the following ways:

• Speaks a few single words at 12 to 15 months

• Makes sentences containing 6 to 20 words at 2 years

• Repeats nursery rhymes at 3 years

At 15 months, the child enjoys looking at books. Between 2 and 3 years of age, the toddler seems to be constantly asking "Why?" By 3 years of age, the child may participate in the retelling of familiar stories and can draw and recognize simple shapes. During the toddler years, the child also enjoys playing with blocks.

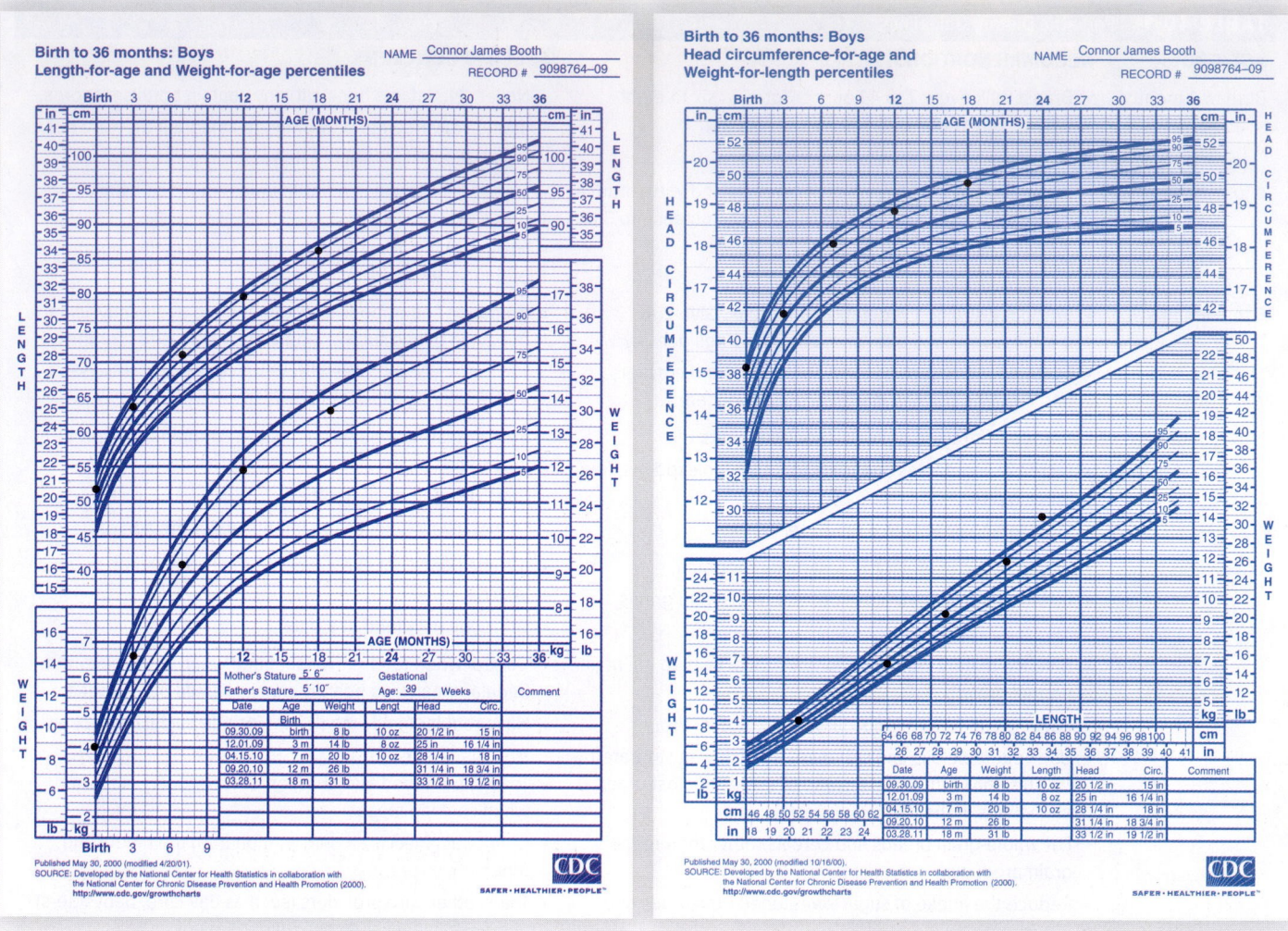

FIGURE 40-5 The curved lines on these growth charts are used to chart the growth for boys from birth to age 36 months. The child's length, height, and head circumference are measured and recorded, then plotted on this graph to show progress.

Psycho-Emotional Development At 1 year of age, children are able to express many emotions. As children move from 1 year to 3 years, they gain some control over ways of expressing their feelings. Temper tantrums may become a problem between 18 months and 2 to 2½ years of age. A child of 15 months may respond to "No," but by the time the toddler approaches 18 to 21 months, he or she is resisting authority and is the one who is saying "No!" Children of this age need consistent limits. If the child learns that a certain behavior will gain nothing, the behavior will stop fairly soon. As toddlers approach 3 years of age, they become sensitive to the feelings of others and may be characterized as affectionate.

Social Development Between 1 and 2 years, the toddler is unlikely to be able to truly play with another child. Play may involve taking toys from another child rather than sharing. Between 2 and 3 years, children become able to share and play with others. Adult guidance is necessary for the toddler to develop an awareness of what is appropriate when playing with other children. See the *Educating the Patient* feature Keeping Infants and Toddlers Safe.

Aspects of Care: 1 to 3 Years Consider the following when caring for toddlers or providing parent or caregiver education. Safety is of utmost importance. See the *Educating the Patient* feature Keeping Infants and Toddlers Safe. During the toddler years, it is also very important to allow a child to increase independence in a safe environment.

- Toddlers need opportunities to work on their fine-motor skills, such as those used in writing with crayons.
- Toddlers are developing their language skills, so simple explanations provide a positive environment for development.
- Setting limits helps the child to develop boundaries in relationships and behavior. At the same time, the environment should not be one in which the child is constantly told "No."

The Preschooler: 3 to 5 Years

The child of 3 to 5 years is preparing to go out into the world.

Physical Development Individual differences, such as heredity, account for differences in height and weight among

Keeping Infants and Toddlers Safe

Teaching the parents or caregivers of infants and children about safety may be the responsibility of the medical assistant. Use the following points when teaching parents or caregivers:

- Keep emergency phone numbers close to the phone for the family and sitters.
- Make sure the crib meets federal safety standards.
- Never hold the infant or toddler on your lap in a car. Use an approved car seat placed in the back of the vehicle. Use the current recommendations from the American Academy of Pediatrics (http://www.aap.org) for forward-facing or rear-facing infant car seats. (See Figure 40-6.)
- Never leave the child unattended in the car.
- Do not put pillows, comforters, or plush toys in the infant's crib.
- Prevent falls. Place the baby on a low surface and use correctly installed gates across stairs.
- Prevent choking. Check toys for small objects that might come loose. Be sure that clothing does not have cords around the neck.
- Do not leave hanging toys over the crib once the child begins to reach, pull, and roll over.
- Keep all cords on window blinds, lamps, and electrical equipment out of reach.
- Never leave a child unattended around, near, or in any kind of water, including the water in toilets, mop buckets, or pools.

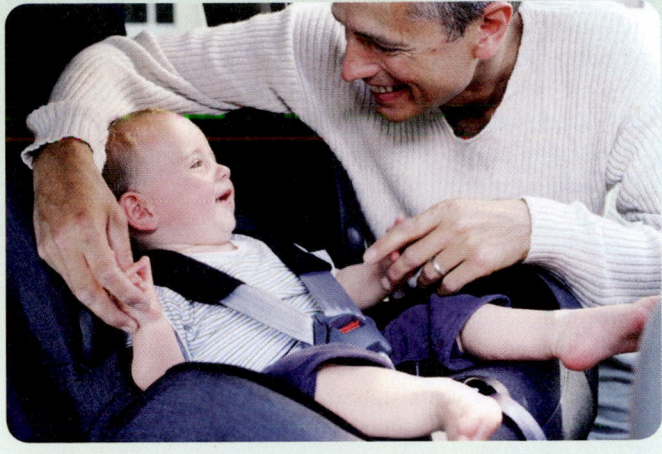

FIGURE 40-6 Infants and toddlers should be in approved car seats. Check the Internet site of the American Academy of Pediatrics for proper type and size.
© Lawrence Lawry/Getty Images RF

- Set the water temperature of the household hot water tank at 120°F. Turn pot handles inward, away from the edge of the stove, while cooking. Cover electrical outlets.
- Keep medicines and chemicals, including household cleaners, out of reach or in locked cabinets. Post the local poison control center's phone number in an accessible location.

---

children between the ages of 3 and 5 years. During this time, it is best not to compare the preschooler's size to that of another preschooler. Each child's growth should be monitored and compared to the size documented on his or her ongoing growth chart. Girls progress more rapidly toward their adult height and weight than do boys. The respiratory rate and heart rate begin to slow down, coming closer to the adult range. Bones begin to ossify, or harden, between the ages of 2 and 7. During these years, it is important for children to be active in their play. They also need adequate calcium intake for the development of strong bones. Most children will have achieved nighttime bowel and bladder control by the time they are 3 or 4 years of age. If lack of bowel and/or bladder control persists beyond 4 or 5 years, this should be brought to the physician's attention.

During the 3- to 5-year period, many skills are achieved, including going up and down stairs using an alternating step approach, riding a tricycle, skipping, hopping on one foot, and throwing a ball with accuracy. Girls are usually about a year ahead of boys in small muscle coordination and fine-motor skills. A child of 3 can draw simple shapes and use a pencil to imitate the way an adult writes. At 4, the child can draw a simple human figure and can cut with blunt scissors, though not well at this age. A child of 5 can reproduce some shapes, letters, and numbers. By the age of 5, some children also may have learned how to tie their shoes.

Intellectual-Cognitive Development Language grows by leaps and bounds during these years. The imaginative child of 3 years has a vocabulary of about 900 words, forms simple sentences, and can tell simple stories that may be very "I"-oriented. At 4 years of age, the child's vocabulary is about 1,600 words, sentences are complete, and the favorite question is "Why?" Parents need to give very simple answers such as "Because it will keep you safe right now." The child's vocabulary at age 5 exceeds 2,000 words, and the stories the child tells involve more detail. At this age, the child has learned the difference between telling stories and lying.

Psycho-Emotional Development The 3-year-old child is very easy and pleasant. Children of this age usually enjoy music. A child at this age has an increasing sense of self, but imagination may lead the child to have unfounded worries and fears, especially at night. At 4 years of age, negativity may increase. Parents hear more of the "Nos" that they heard when the child was 2 years old. The 4-year-old child is testing limits and needs guided opportunities for freedom. Once a child reaches 5 years, life settles down a little. The child is more self-assured, well adjusted, and home-centered. At this age, the child likes to follow the rules, may want to "play by the rules," and is capable of accepting some responsibility.

Social Development Three-year-old children know what gender they are. The child knows how to take turns and may enjoy brief activities in a group with other children. A 3-year-old child likes to "help." Four-year-old children are very social and enjoy playing simple group games, like tag and hide-and-seek. At 5 years, the child continues to be very social, enjoys playing with other children, and likes games in which the "rules" are observed.

Aspects of Care: 3 to 5 Years Consider the following when caring for children from 3 to 5 years or providing parent or caregiver education.

- The child of 5 years should receive a complete preschool developmental assessment and physical that includes an evaluation of hearing and vision.
- Immunizations, discussed later, must be up to date when the child enters kindergarten.
- Children of about 3 years may have night terrors. Parents should discuss these with the pediatrician if they are severe or persistent.
- Children may use delaying tactics at bedtime and may need to be shown repeatedly that there is nothing in the closet or under the bed. A nightlight is useful.
- Nighttime routines are important in helping a child feel secure.

The Elementary School Child: 6 to 10 Years
The following describes the stages of development of the 6- to 10-year-old child.

Physical Development During childhood, girls may be taller and heavier than boys. Bones continue to ossify. Permanent teeth replace "baby teeth." Muscles continue to develop. Regular exercise is needed to encourage strength and coordination. At 9 and 10 years of age, the reproductive system also will be developing.

Intellectual-Cognitive Development Knowledge explosion happens once a child enters school. On entering school, the 6-year-old child has a brief attention span. By 10 years old, she is able to focus for longer periods of time. Most children of this age like to talk. As children move from 5 or 6 years of age toward 9 and 10 years, they are better able to separate fantasy from reality. They develop a sense of what is right and wrong, of honesty and fairness.

Psycho-Emotional Development When children approach 10 years of age, they may be more influenced by their peers than by their parents. During these years, children are beginning to develop a sense of self and learn gender-related roles. Children of 6 to 8 years of age may have trouble thinking about disasters that they hear about. As children

approach 10 years of age, they are better able to grasp concepts of time and distance. A 9- to 10-year-old child may want to do something to help others. School-age children may be very sensitive to criticism and to what they see as failure.

Social Development School is central to the life of a child between 6 and 10 years of age. Although team sports and activities become important, parents need to avoid allowing the child to become overwhelmed with too many organized activities at this time. Children also need time to be quiet and alone. Outdoor activities help to use up some of the child's energy. Appropriate social behaviors are learned during this stage.

Aspects of Care: 6 to 10 Years Consider the following when caring for 6- to 10-year-olds or providing parent or caregiver education.

- Structure and a schedule help to maintain order and discipline.
- Monitor physical activities to prevent injury. The American Academy of Pediatrics advises against elementary-school-age children participating in contact sports.
- Consistency in daily activities and in discipline helps the child to develop intellectually, emotionally, and socially.
- Regular health and dental care and maintenance of immunizations are required.
- Communicable diseases are common.

The Middle School Child: 11 to 13 Years
The following sections will give you some insight into the stages of development of the 11- to 13-year-old child.

Physical Development In the United States and most other Western cultures, the onset of puberty occurs in females at around 12 or 13 years of age, but some may experience changes as early as 9. **Puberty** refers to the physiological changes that make a person capable of sexual reproduction. By the time a girl reaches middle school, a significant occurrence may be the onset of menstruation. It is important for everyone to remember that even though her body may be maturing, she is still only between 9 and 12 years old. Males tend to go through the changes of puberty later than females (Figure 40-7). The average age for males to experience these changes is around 14 years. Hormonal changes may contribute to development of skin problems and acne.

Intellectual-Cognitive Development Grades may slip during this time. So much physical growth is taking place and so many physiological changes are occurring that less energy is available to concentrate on academics. Preadolescents may tend to exaggerate and "bend the truth."

Psycho-Emotional Development Although preadolescents crave independence, they are also very unsure of themselves. They are experiencing a wide range of physical changes and, at the same time, are learning the roles of

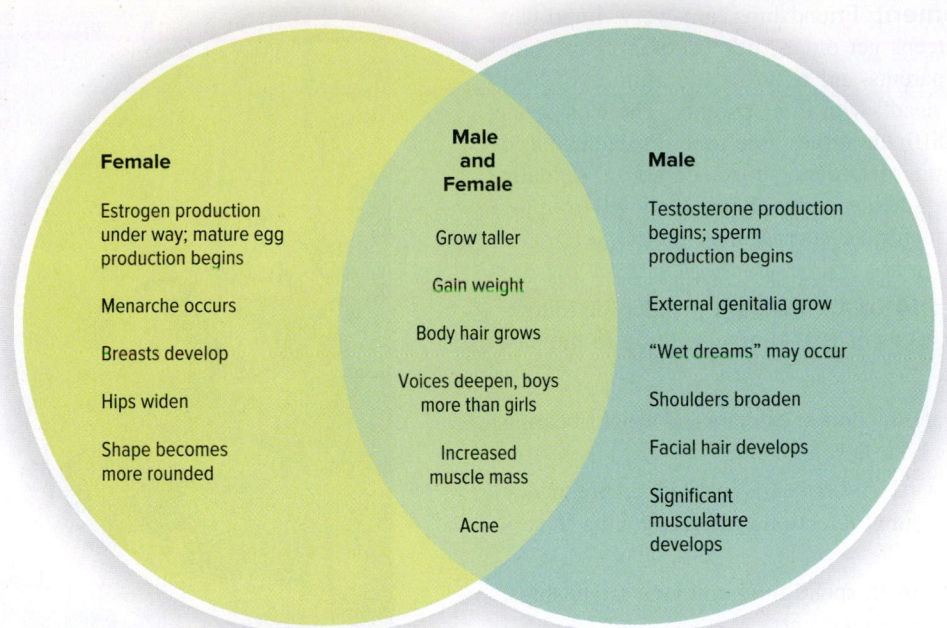

Female

Estrogen production under way; mature egg production begins

Menarche occurs

Breasts develop

Hips widen

Shape becomes more rounded

Male and Female

Grow taller

Gain weight

Body hair grows

Voices deepen, boys more than girls

Increased muscle mass

Acne

Male

Testosterone production begins; sperm production begins

External genitalia grow

"Wet dreams" may occur

Shoulders broaden

Facial hair develops

Significant musculature develops

FIGURE 40-7   Some changes during puberty are the same for males and females. Others are unique to one sex.

sexuality. It is very important for preadolescents to receive accurate information about their changing bodies and feelings from appropriate and reliable sources. Middle-school-age students may not be comfortable asking parents questions about sexuality. Conflict may arise at this time. Parents may find that the preadolescent is easily annoyed and may be temperamental. Frequently, the preadolescent child will take on the behaviors of his or her peer group.

Social Development   During the middle school years, children are learning about their own sexual identity and may not be comfortable in heterosexual relationships. Girls express an earlier interest in male-female relationships than do boys. Children of this age need to be able to turn to an adult with whom they are comfortable, so they can ask personal and intimate questions.

Aspects of Care: 11 to 13 Years   Consider the following when caring for preadolescents or providing parent or caregiver education.

- A preadolescent needs to be assured that he or she is valued and loved.
- Consistency in discipline is very important.
- Parents should not be hypercritical or make too many demands.
- Friendships and associations should be monitored.
- Overscheduling of the child's time should be avoided.

The Adolescent: 14 to 19 Years

The teen years can be full of excitement for teenagers and their family and friends. They also can be difficult years.

Tremendous physiological changes during this time may cause internal conflicts that can turn into external clashes. Parents may feel anxious about their child's quest for independence and about the child's upcoming departure from the home. The process of developing independence, a personal identity, and future plans is important during this stage.

Physical Development   During the later teen years, females attain their adult height and weight. Males may continue to grow in height until 25 years of age. Physical growth and development in the teenage years are centered on normal sexual change. Girls usually have reached **menarche,** the onset of menstruation. Boys may have nocturnal emissions of seminal fluid (also called wet dreams). Weight control can be a concern. Some health problems of adulthood can be traced back to lifelong habits of poor dietary choices and lack of exercise begun in adolescence.

Intellectual-Cognitive Development   During the early adolescent years, the child may have taken the word of an adult or a peer without question. Now, the teen asks questions and needs to work out answers that fit into his or her values. Adolescents often do not see the connection between behavior and consequences. This may lead to experimentation with drugs, alcohol, or sex.

Psycho-Emotional Development   An adolescent knows the socially acceptable and appropriate ways to express feelings, but the pressures felt by adolescents may result in angry outbursts. Anger that is directed inward can be harmful. Anxiety and sometimes depression are part of adolescence.

Social Development Friendships are very important to adolescents. As teens get older, they become more comfortable with their parents and outgrow the attitude of "not wanting to be seen dead" with their parents. The teen years are wonderful and difficult at the same time. Problems faced by teens include eating disorders, substance abuse, sexually transmitted infection, suicide, and violence. You will examine these special concerns further later in this chapter.

Aspects of Care: 14 to 19 Years Consider the following when caring for teens or providing education to the parents or caregiver.

- Teens need adequate amounts of calcium and weight-bearing exercise for strong bone development.
- Teens should know the risks of early, unplanned pregnancy and sexually transmitted infections when engaging in sexual activity.
- The adolescent needs to spend time enjoying friendships, sporting events, and social events.
- People who are caring for teens should
  - Listen.
  - Give them the facts.
  - Trust them.
  - Provide them with firm and friendly discipline.
  - Be consistent.
  - Educate them with their independence in mind.
  - Set limits and stick to them.
  - Set examples of good behavior and good taste.
  - Remember how it feels to be an adolescent.

▶ Pediatric Examinations

LO 40.2

Many of the exam procedures for a pediatric patient are the same as those for an adult. While you prepare the child or adolescent for the exam, you may discuss with the parent, caregiver, or child topics such as eating habits, sleep patterns, daily activities, immunization schedules, and toilet training. Discussions should be appropriate for the child's developmental stage. This discussion will provide important clues to possible abnormal physical, cognitive-intellectual, psycho-emotional, and social development. Additional discussion topics such as sexually transmitted infections, drugs, and alcohol may be appropriate for an adolescent. Point out potential problems to the licensed practitioner.

Some children are afraid of going to the doctor's office. You can help relieve a child's fear by calmly explaining procedures before they occur, giving the reason for each procedure and being cheerful and mindful of a child's feelings. Allowing a child to examine some of the blunt instruments may also lessen fear (Figure 40-8). If a patient is physically resistant to the exam, you may need to call for assistance from the licensed practitioner or caregiver, or the child may need to be restrained.

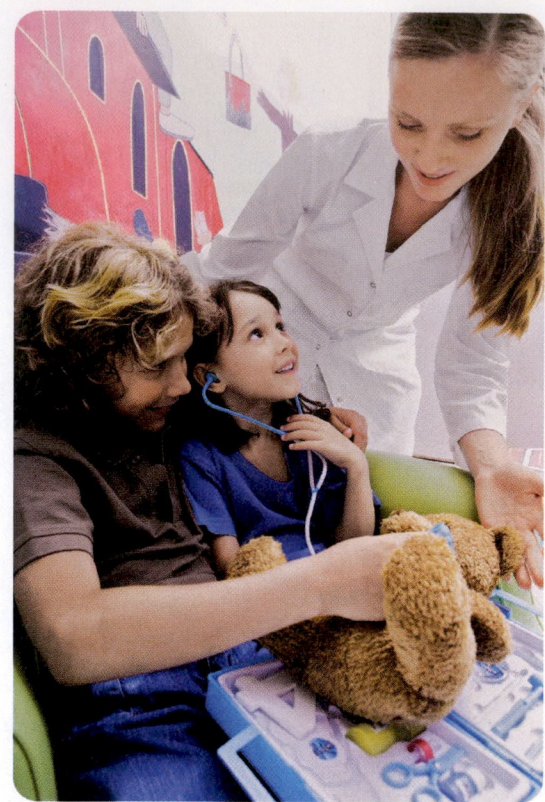

FIGURE 40-8 Providing a pediatric patient with a diversion may help lessen the child's fear.
© PhotoAlto/Laurence Mouton/Getty Images

Try to speak in terms aimed at the child's age level and kneel if necessary to make eye contact with the child. Treat the child with respect and provide positive reinforcement when a child is cooperative. Avoid making light of crying or pain. Make a game out of some aspect of a procedure and provide a small token reward at the end of a visit. For infants, a gentle approach, such as talking quietly and holding them comfortingly, is helpful.

Be mindful of adolescents' sensitivity toward rapid growth and physical, sexual, and social development when you prepare them for examination. Adolescents and preadolescents often feel awkward and self-conscious about being examined. They also may prefer to dress alone and to be alone with the licensed practitioner.

Well-Child Examination

Parents should bring their infants and children to the pediatrician for regular checkups and growth monitoring. The American Academy of Pediatrics (AAP) recommends the following frequency:

- Infants need seven well-baby exams during their first year, at these intervals: 3 to 5 days, 1 month, 2 months, 4 months, 6 months, 9 months, and 1 year.
- Children in the second and third years of life should have checkups at 15, 18, 24, and 30 months.
- From the age of 3, children should have checkups every year.

The AAP has developed recommendations for these examinations. See Table 40-2 for a summary of the components of the well-child examination based on the age of the child.

Follow standard precautions and prepare for the physical exam the same way you would for an adult, except for draping and positioning. Ask the parent of an infant or toddler to remove all the child's clothing except the diaper. Then keep the child covered until the physician enters the exam room. An infant or toddler may be crying during the exam. To assist the physician in hearing chest sounds with a stethoscope, ask the parent to allow the infant to suck on a pacifier, if used, to quiet the crying. Feeding the child during the exam is not encouraged because stomach sounds interfere with clear auscultation (listening to body sounds with a stethoscope). Distracting infants and toddlers with mobiles, shiny surfaces, or toys may help the exam go more smoothly. Review the *Points on Practice* feature Assisting with an Exam for an Infant or Child for additional information about the pediatric exam.

TABLE 40-2	Recommendations for Preventive Pediatric Healthcare*
Developmental Stage	**Components of the Examination**
Infancy (birth to 12 months)	History and physical Length/height and weight Head circumference Weight for length Immunizations Newborn metabolic/hemoglobin screening Developmental/behavioral assessments
Early childhood (12 months to 4 years)	History and physical Length/height and weight Head circumference up to 24 months Body mass index starting at 24 months Weight for length up to 18 months Blood pressure and vision screening starting at 3 years Hearing starting at 4 years Immunizations Developmental/behavioral assessments
Middle childhood (5 years to 10 years)	History and physical Length/height and weight Body mass index Blood pressure Vision and hearing screening Oral health at 6 years Immunizations
Adolescence (12 years to 21 years)	History and physical Length/height and weight Body mass index Blood pressure Vision and hearing screening Ages 18–21 dyslipidemia screening

*Adapted from the American Academy of Pediatrics, *Recommendations for Preventive Pediatric Health Care,* copyright 2008.

Assisting with an Exam for an Infant or Child

When assisting with an exam for an infant or child, you will need to take some special considerations. The techniques you use to prepare an infant or child emotionally and physically should be modified based on the patient's age and ability.

Emotional

Infants and toddlers are likely to be afraid of you because you are a stranger. Approach these children slowly, smile, and use a gentle voice. Children of preschool age are sometimes uncooperative and challenging. Remain calm, perform the procedures quickly, and restrain the child (with assistance from the parent) when appropriate. To prevent children from getting injured, watch them at all times.

Physical

Base your choice of an exam position for children on each child's age and ability to cooperate. Although young infants are usually examined on an examining table, older infants and toddlers may need to be examined while held on a parent's lap. Some toddlers may cooperate while standing on the examining table with a parent nearby. Some children may need to be restrained during parts of the examination or during an immunization. See Figure 40-9. Preschool children can usually be placed on the examining table if a parent is nearby. Regardless of their position, watch children at all times to prevent injury. When examining young children, licensed practitioners typically perform percussion (tapping on the surface to hear the underlying structures) and auscultation (listening) first, because children are more likely to be calm and quiet at the outset. Practitioners always examine painful areas last. Practitioners may examine older children's genitalia last because, after a certain age, children tend to find such an exam embarrassing.

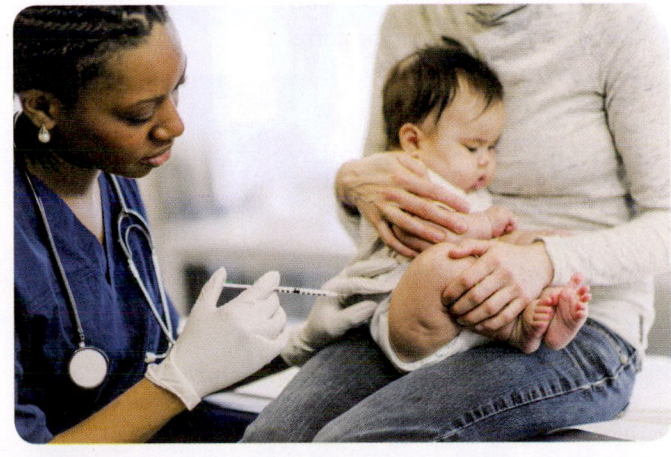

FIGURE 40-9   By fully immobilizing the child, you decrease the risk that his or her movement will result in injury.
© Christopher Futcher/Getty Images RF

▶ Pediatric Immunizations LO 40.3

As discussed in the *Infection Control Fundamentals* chapter, you should know that one of the necessary elements in the cycle of infection is the transmission of the pathogen to a susceptible host. To reduce the susceptibility of the host to infection, **immunizations** are given. An immunization is the administration of a vaccine to protect susceptible individuals from infectious diseases. When a healthy patient is vaccinated with a weakened strain of a virus, the patient's lymphocytes manufacture antibodies against that virus. These antibodies remain in the body, making it immune to that virus in the future. In general, there are two types of vaccines: live-attenuated and inactivated. Live-attenuated vaccines are a weakened form of the virus itself. Inactivated vaccines are either whole viruses, whole bacteria, or fractions of either. Inactivated vaccines usually require multiple doses for immunity to occur.

Immunizations are usually given during regular checkups (Figure 40-10). Immunizing children against diseases such as hepatitis B, diphtheria, tetanus, pertussis (whooping cough), poliomyelitis, measles, mumps, rubella (German measles), chickenpox, human papillomavirus (HPV), rotavirus, meningococcal disease, and *Haemophilus influenzae* type B (Hib) is recommended. Many vaccines have largely eliminated the threat of these once-prevalent, life-threatening diseases.

The first vaccine, for hepatitis B, is given to a newborn the day after birth. Some vaccines require a series of doses to give immunity. Booster doses may be required for a particular vaccine at a later age. The Centers for Disease Control and Prevention (CDC) recommends that physicians take every reasonable opportunity to vaccinate a child, to ensure that the child receives the protection he needs. If a child gets behind on his immunizations, a catch-up schedule is available.

As a medical assistant, you will play a vital role in the immunization process. Your duties may include

- Scheduling appointments and follow-up visits at the appropriate time based on the immunization schedule.
- Educating parents about the benefits and risks of vaccines and obtaining informed consent.
- Administering the vaccine correctly.

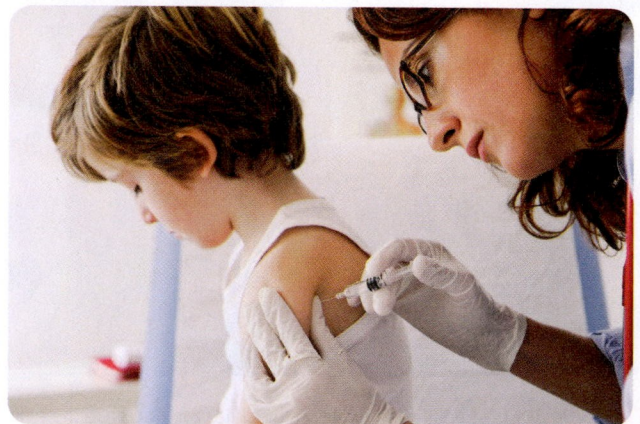

FIGURE 40-10 Immunizations are part of routine well-child visits in a pediatric practice.
© BSIP SA/Alamy Stock Photo

- Keeping careful immunization records, including the vaccine type, the date of vaccination, and the vaccine lot number.
- Ensuring proper vaccine storage and handling, including checking the temperature of the refrigerator and freezer daily.

Immunization Recommendations

The Advisory Committee on Immunization Practices, the American Academy of Pediatrics, and the American Academy of Family Physicians jointly publish immunization schedules for children. When working in a pediatrician's office, you should be familiar with the current vaccination schedule guidelines because they change occasionally. New guidelines, methods, and vaccines are constantly being developed. See Figure 40-11 for the birth to age 6 and the ages 7–18 immunization schedules. If you are responsible for administering immunizations, you should stay current with the most recent information found online at http://www.cdc.gov/vaccines/schedules/hcp/imz/child-adolescent.html.

Informed Consent

The licensed practitioner may ask you to explain the benefits and risks of an immunization to the parents. You will need to explain that the side effects of immunizations are usually mild, such as a slight fever or soreness, and of short duration. Review with the parent the vaccine information statement for the specific immunization you will be administering (Figure 40-12). Advise parents that the benefits of immunity greatly outweigh the risks. Then obtain informed consent for the child's immunization. Provide a copy of the vaccine information statement and then have the parent sign so the immunization can be given. Remember that religious or other personal beliefs may prevent parents from consenting to immunizations for their child. Some parents may want to delay or slow down the number of immunizations given at one time. Give immunizations as ordered and record all appropriate information in the patient's chart.

Administering Immunizations

In many states, medical assistants may administer immunizations. Most immunizations are given as injections. You might be required to give more than two vaccinations in a single visit. Careful site selection is important when giving multiple injections. Refer to the *Medication Administration* chapter for information about administering various types of injections and selecting an appropriate injection site. Some vaccines, such as live polio, are given orally. Most vaccinations may be administered even if the child has a mild illness. The physician will make the decision to vaccinate a child who is ill based on the disease and the severity of the symptoms. For the most part, if a child has a fever, the physician may postpone the immunization until the fever has subsided. However, do not postpone the visit if the child has an upper respiratory infection without a fever. Remember that the child does not need to restart a series of immunizations. He can simply receive the next scheduled immunization as soon as possible.

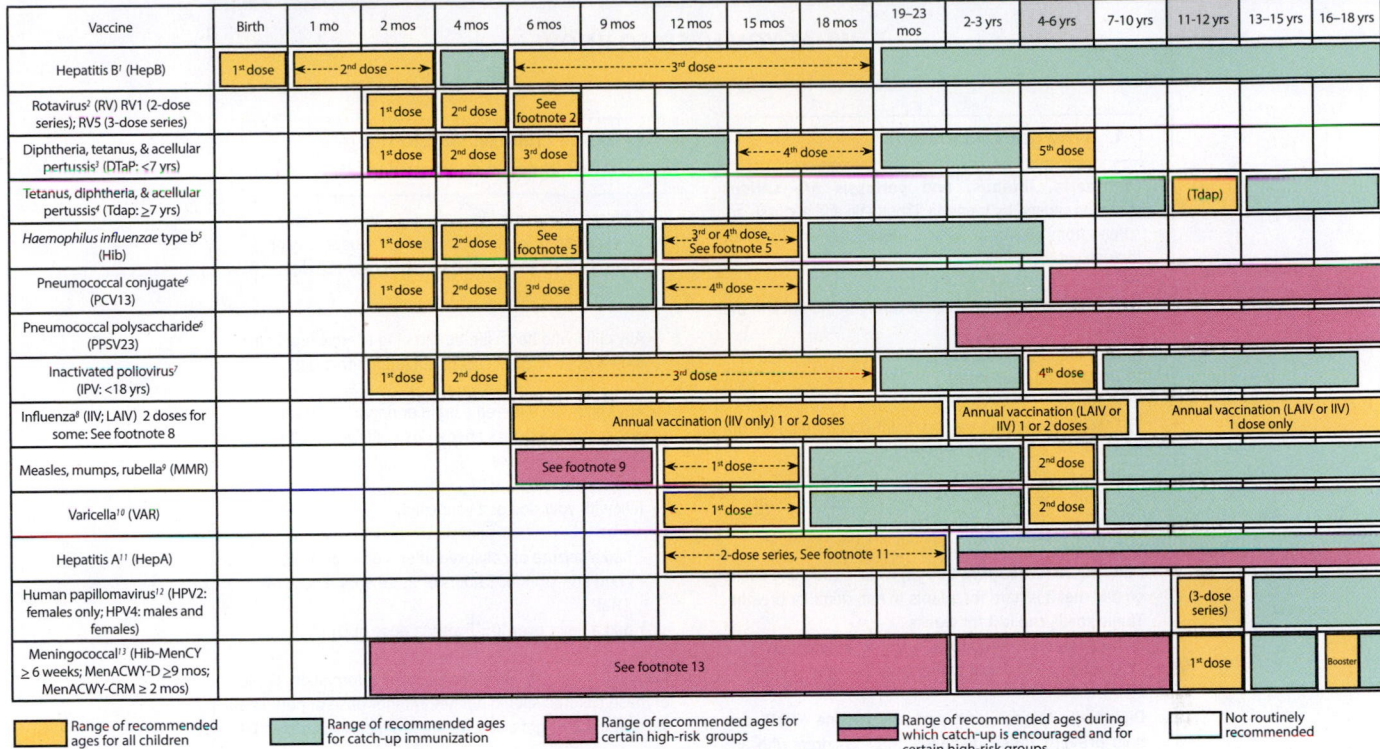

Figure 1. Recommended immunization schedule for persons aged 0 through 18 years – United States, 2015.

These recommendations must be read with the footnotes that follow. For those who fall behind or start late, provide catch-up vaccination at the earliest opportunity as indicated by the green bars in Figure 1. To determine minimum intervals between doses, see the catch-up schedule. School entry and adolescent vaccine age groups are shaded.

| Range of recommended ages for all children | Range of recommended ages for catch-up immunization | Range of recommended ages for certain high-risk groups | Range of recommended ages during which catch-up is encouraged and for certain high-risk groups | Not routinely recommended |

This schedule includes recommendations in effect as of January 1, 2015. Any dose not administered at the recommended age should be administered at a subsequent visit, when indicated and feasible. The use of a combination vaccine generally is preferred over separate injections of its equivalent component vaccines. Vaccination providers should consult the relevant Advisory Committee on Immunization Practices (ACIP) statement for detailed recommendations, available online at http://www.cdc.gov/vaccines/hcp/acip-recs/index.html. Clinically significant adverse events that follow vaccination should be reported to the Vaccine Adverse Event Reporting System (VAERS) online (http://www.vaers.hhs.gov) or by telephone (800-822-7967). Suspected cases of vaccine-preventable diseases should be reported to the state or local health department. Additional information, including precautions and contraindications for vaccination, is available from CDC online (http://www.cdc.gov/vaccines/recs/vac-admin/contraindications.htm) or by telephone (800-CDC-INFO [800-232-4636]).

This schedule is approved by the Advisory Committee on Immunization Practices (http://www.cdc.gov/vaccines/acip), the American Academy of Pediatrics (http://www.aap.org), the American Academy of Family Physicians (http://www.aafp.org), and the American College of Obstetricians and Gynecologists (http://www.acog.org).

FIGURE 40-11 Recommended immunization schedules for birth to 18 years. For more detail and the most current information, check the Centers for Disease Control and Prevention website.

Before administering a childhood immunization, check for any contraindications to its use. A **contraindication** is a known risk or reason not to give the immunization. For example, pertussis vaccine must not be given to a child with a progressive neurologic disorder. It also must not be administered to a child who developed seizures, persistent crying, or a high fever after receiving a previous pertussis vaccine. In such a situation, the doctor would direct you to administer diphtheria and tetanus toxoids instead of the diphtheria and tetanus toxoid and pertussis vaccine (DTaP).

Immunization Records

Under the National Childhood Vaccine Injury Act of 1988, you must record certain information about immunizations in a child's permanent medical record. Required information includes

- The vaccine's type, manufacturer, and lot number.
- The date on the vaccine information statement and the day and time the statement was given to the parent.
- The date of administration.

- The name, address, and title of the healthcare professional who administered the vaccine.

You also must document the vaccine type using standard abbreviations. For combination vaccines, such as Pediatrix™, you record the vaccine under all three components: DTaP, IPV, and hepatitis B. In addition, you must document

- The administration site, route, and dosage.
- The vaccine's expiration date.

Parents should maintain an accurate, up-to-date immunization record for each child. They should be encouraged to bring this record with them to each healthcare visit. Each state and/or the CDC issues an immunization record form, which may be available in languages other than English. Complete a form after each child's first immunization. Instruct the parents to keep the form and bring it with the child for each subsequent immunization so that you can update the record. The immunization record for Chris Matthews, our case study patient, is shown in Figure 40-13. Advise parents that this record is important to keep because it acts as proof of immunization,

DIPHTHERIA TETANUS & PERTUSSIS **VACCINES**

WHAT YOU NEED TO KNOW

Many Vaccine Information Statements are available in Spanish and other languages. See http://www.immunize.org/vis.

1. Why get vaccinated?

Diphtheria, tetanus, and pertussis are serious diseases caused by bacteria. Diphtheria and pertussis are spread from person to person. Tetanus enters the body through cuts or wounds.

DIPHTHERIA causes a thick covering in the back of the throat.
- It can lead to breathing problems, paralysis, heart failure, and even death.

TETANUS (Lockjaw) causes painful tightening of the muscles, usually all over the body.
- It can lead to "locking" of the jaw so the victim cannot open his mouth or swallow. Tetanus leads to death in up to 2 out of 10 cases.

PERTUSSIS (Whooping Cough) causes coughing spells so bad that it is hard for infants to eat, drink, or breathe. These spells can last for weeks.
- It can lead to pneumonia, seizures (jerking and staring spells), brain damage, and death.

Diphtheria, tetanus, and pertussis vaccine (DTaP) can help prevent these diseases. Most children who are vaccinated with DTaP will be protected throughout childhood. Many more children would get these diseases if we stopped vaccinating.

DTaP is a safer version of an older vaccine called DTP. DTP is no longer used in the United States.

2. Who should get DTaP vaccine and when?

Children should get <u>5 doses</u> of DTaP vaccine, 1 dose at each of the following ages:

- 2 months
- 4 months
- 6 months
- 15–18 months
- 4–6 years

DTaP may be given at the same time as other vaccines.

3. Some children should not get DTaP vaccine or should wait.

- Children with minor illnesses, such as a cold, may be vaccinated. But children who are moderately or severely ill should usually wait until they recover before getting DTaP vaccine.

- Any child who had a life-threatening allergic reaction after a dose of DTaP should not get another dose.

- Any child who suffered a brain or nervous system disease within 7 days after a dose of DTaP should not get another dose.

- Talk with your doctor if your child:
  - had a seizure or collapsed after a dose of DTaP,
  - cried non-stop for 3 hours or more after a dose of DTaP,
  - had a fever over 105°F after a dose of DTaP.

Ask your healthcare provider for more information. Some of these children should not get another dose of pertussis vaccine but may get a vaccine without pertussis, called **DT**.

4. Older children and adults

DTaP is not licensed for adolescents, adults, or children 7 years of age and older.

But older people still need protection. A vaccine called **Tdap** is similar to DTaP. A single dose of Tdap is recommended for people 11 through 64 years of age. Another vaccine, called **Td**, protects against tetanus and diphtheria, but not pertussis. It is recommended every 10 years. There are separate Vaccine Information Statements for these vaccines.

| Diphtheria/Tetanus/Pertussis | 5/17/2007 |

FIGURE 40-12 Review the vaccine information sheet with the parent and obtain a signature before administering a vaccine.

which may be required by day care centers, schools, the military, and other organizations. This record also may be helpful when parents consult another doctor, in case of emergency, or when moving to a new location.

Vaccine Storage and Handling

Vaccines must be stored properly. As a medical assistant, in order to ensure vaccine safety and effectiveness, you are responsible for proper storage and handling from the time a vaccine arrives at your facility until it is administered to the patient. Follow these general guidelines.

- Store vaccines at the recommended temperatures immediately upon arrival at your facility. Check and record temperatures of refrigerators and freezers daily. If the correct temperature is not maintained, the vaccine will lose its effectiveness. Live-attenuated virus vaccines are especially sensitive to heat.

- Store refrigerated vaccines between 35°F and 46°F (2°C and 8°C).

- Store frozen vaccines between −58°F and +5°F (−50°C and −15°C).

- Rotate your supply of vaccines so those with the shortest expiration date are used first. Place the vaccine with the longest expiration date behind the vaccine that will expire the soonest. Remove expired vaccines from usable stock immediately.

Vaccine (circle specific type given)	Date Given	Doctor or Clinic
1 Hep B	2/25/XX	BWW Assoc.
2 Hep B	3/21/XX	BWW Assoc.
3 Hep B	8/12/XX	BWW Assoc.
1 Hep A	5/12/XX	BWW Assoc.
2 Hep A		
Other		
Other		
Other		
Other		

Please fold on dotted line

Vaccine	Date Given	Doctor or Clinic
1 *Flu (TIV/LAIV)		
2 *Flu (TIV/LAIV)		
Yearly *Flu (TIV/LAIV)		
Yearly *Flu (TIV/LAIV)		
Other		
Other		
Other		

All children ages 6 months through 8 years who receive seasonal influenza vaccine for the first time should be given 2 doses. Children who receive only one dose in the first year of vaccination should receive two doses in their second year of vaccination.
*Seasonal   Please fold on dotted line

Immunization Record

Name ___Matthews, Chris___
                              (Last, First, MI)
Date of Birth ___11/19/XX___

Physician or Clinic___BWW Associates___
            ___Alexis M. Whalen MD___

Notice to Parents: Please take this card with you when you visit your doctor or clinic and have them fill in the information.

Vaccine (circle specific type given)	Date Given	Doctor or Clinic
1 DtaP/DT/Td	4/08/XX	BWW Assoc.
2 DtaP/DT/Td	6/10/XX	BWW Assoc.
3 DtaP/DT/Td	8/12/XX	BWW Assoc.
4 DtaP/DT/Td		
5 DtaP/DT/Td		
1 Tdap/Td		
1 Hib	4/08/XX	BWW Assoc.
2 Hib	6/10/XX	BWW Assoc.
3 Hib	8/12/XX	BWW Assoc.
4 Hib		
1 IPV	4/08/XX	BWW Assoc.
2 IPV	6/10/XX	BWW Assoc.
3 IPV	5/12/XX	BWW Assoc.
4 IPV		
5 IPV		
1 MMR/MMRV	5/12/XX	BWW Assoc.
2 MMR/MMRV		
1 Varicella	5/12/XX	BWW Assoc.
2 Varicella		
1 Rotavirus	4/08/XX	BWW Assoc.
2 Rotavirus	6/10/XX	BWW Assoc.
3 Rotavirus	8/12/XX	BWW Assoc.
1 PCV	4/08/XX	BWW Assoc.
2 PCV	6/10/XX	BWW Assoc.
3 PCV	8/12/XX	BWW Assoc.
4 PCV	5/12/XX	BWW Assoc.
1 MCV		
1 HPV		
2 HPV		
3 HPV		
other		

DH 686, 8/09 Stock Number 5740-000-0686-5

(a)   (b)

FIGURE 40-13 Example immunization record of Chris Matthews. (a) Front. (b) Back.

- Prepare vaccines just prior to administration to the patient.
- Follow infection control guidelines when preparing and administering vaccines.

Pediatric Screening and Diagnostic Tests   LO 40.4

Pediatricians look for any sign of growth abnormality during routine well-child visits. Physicians compare a child's physical, cognitive-intellectual, psycho-emotional, and social signs to charts showing national averages. In general, physicians look for signs that the child is in the appropriate stage of growth for her age. The medical assistant's role in pediatric exams is similar to the role in adult patient exams.

During the pediatric exam, the medical assistant may assist with or perform many tasks, including taking vital signs and body measurements, performing vision and hearing tests, collecting specimens, and administering medications and immunizations.

Vital Signs

Some variations in technique and results should be considered when performing vital signs on pediatric patients. In addition to the normal vital signs range variations (review Table 37-1 from the *Vital Signs and Measurements* chapter), some other things should be taken into account. Taking a child's or an infant's temperature can be a challenge. If the infant or child is likely to cry or become agitated, take the temperature last. Measure pulse, respiration, and blood pressure (if ordered) before you take the temperature to avoid having these measurements elevated because of the child's agitation. Oral thermometers are not appropriate for children younger than 5 years of age because these children are too young to safely hold the thermometer in their mouths. Instead, take axillary, rectal, tympanic, or temporal temperatures. If you use a rectal thermometer, hold it in place until the temperature registers to prevent the thermometer from being expelled or injuring the patient. Tympanic and temporal thermometers are especially useful in pediatric offices because of their speed and safety.

Blood pressure in children or infants is not routinely measured at each visit. Instead, the measurement is taken per the doctor's orders. The procedure is the same as that for taking blood pressure in adults, except for these modifications:

1. Ideally, take the patient's blood pressure before performing other tests or procedures that may cause anxiety. In this way, you can avoid a falsely high result.

2. Be sure to use the correct cuff size for the child or infant. The bladder width should not exceed two-thirds the length of the upper or lower arm. The bladder should cover three-fourths of the extremity's circumference.

3. Do not attempt to estimate an infant's blood pressure using the palpatory method (discussed in the *Vital Signs and Measurements* chapter). It is typically not used.

4. Inflate the pressure cuff to 20 mmHg above the point at which the radial pulse disappears.

5. Deflate the cuff at a rate of 2 mmHg per second.

6. You may continue to hear a heartbeat on a child or infant until the pressure reaches zero, so note when the strong heartbeat becomes muffled.

Body Measurements

Children and infants are weighed and measured at each office visit. Children who can stand may be weighed on an adult scale. If toddlers cannot remain still on an adult scale, weight may be determined by weighing an adult holding the toddler, then subtracting the adult's weight. Infants are weighed on infant scales, which typically measure pounds and ounces. Infant scales are sometimes built into a pediatric examining table.

The height of children and the length of infants are measured at each office visit. Measure children in the same manner as you measure an adult. Some offices are equipped with height bars or wall charts that are separate from a scale. Use these devices in the same way as those attached to a scale. Measure infants while they are lying down; in this instance, you are measuring length instead of height. Some pediatric examining tables have a built-in bar for measuring length. You also can use a tape measure or yardstick.

The circumference of an infant's head is an important measure of growth and development and is used to evaluate diseases such as hydrocephalus or excessive cerebrospinal fluid in the cranial cavity, which causes enlargement of the head. You may be asked to perform or assist with this measurement

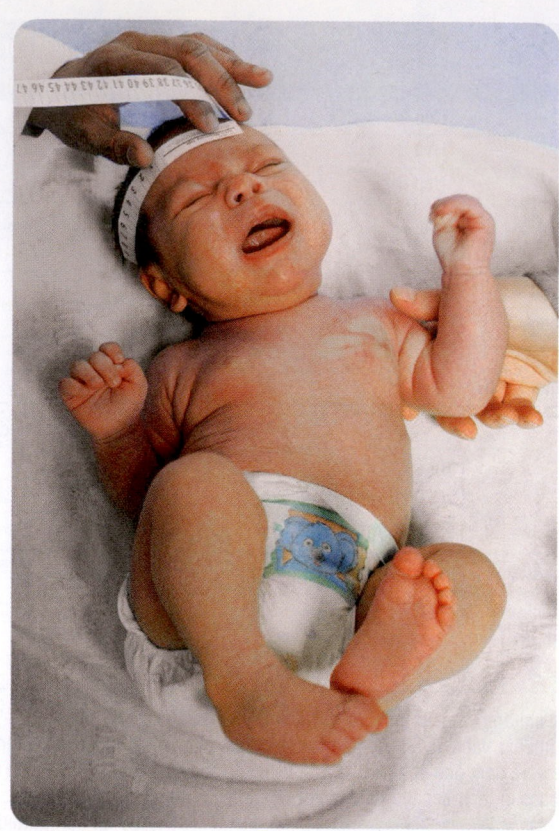

FIGURE 40-14   The medical assistant uses a flexible tape to measure the circumference of an infant's head.
© CMSP/Getty Images RF

when you measure the infant's length. Measurement of head circumference may be performed at the same time as weight and length, or it may be part of the general physical exam (Figure 40-14). The steps for measuring infants are described in Procedure 40-1, at the end of this chapter. Review the *Vital Signs and Measurements* chapter and the procedures for weighing and measuring children.

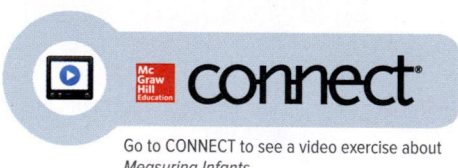

Go to CONNECT to see a video exercise about *Measuring Infants*.

General Eye and Vision Exam

As part of the general exam, the pediatrician examines the interior of the child's eyes with an instrument called an *ophthalmoscope*. You will probably perform the visual acuity test (Figure 40-15). Make a game of covering the child's eye if the child resists this part of the procedure. Use a pediatric vision chart as shown in Figure 40-16 for patients who cannot read. If the caregiver brought the child in specifically for a vision test, record in the child's chart whatever symptoms the caregiver mentions. Follow the procedure in the *Assisting with Eye and Ear Care* chapter and use these modifications when performing vision screening on a pediatric patient:

• Watch for signs of visual difficulty during the test, such as tilting the head in a certain direction, blinking, squinting,

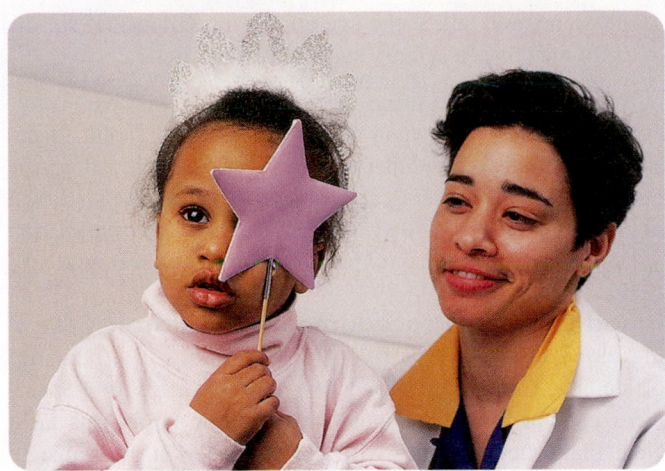

FIGURE 40-15 Making a game out of the visual acuity test helps put a child at ease.
© Ken Lax

or frowning. Observe the child for eyes that are misaligned or don't focus together. Keep in mind that some vision problems may have no warning signs. For example, amblyopia, or lazy eye, is a fairly common eye problem (affecting about 2 out of 100 children) that develops when a child has one eye that doesn't see well or is injured and he begins to use the other eye almost exclusively. The problem must be detected by the age of 3 in order to treat and restore normal vision in the affected eye by age 6. If this situation persists for too long (past 7 to 9 years of age), vision may be lost permanently in the unused eye.

- Use a pointer to select one symbol at a time in random order to prevent patients from memorizing the order.
- It is common to start with children at the 40- or 30-foot line or larger if low vision is suspected and then proceed to the 20-foot line.
- Note the smallest line on which the child can identify three out of four or four out of six symbols correctly.

General Ear and Hearing Exam

A pediatric ear exam is important because so many children have ear infections or upper respiratory infections involving the ear. Because children's eustachian tubes are more horizontal than those of adults, fluid collects more easily in the tubes and can promote bacterial growth. The tubes are also short and connected to the throat, making it easy for any upper respiratory infections to travel to the ear.

You may be asked to perform a hearing test on a pediatric patient. Use the procedure found in the *Assisting with Eye and Ear Care* chapter. When performing a hearing test on an infant or toddler, follow these general guidelines:

1. Have the patient sit, lie down, or be held by the parent in a quiet location.
2. Instruct the parent to be silent during the procedure.
3. Position yourself so that your hands are behind the child's right ear and out of sight.

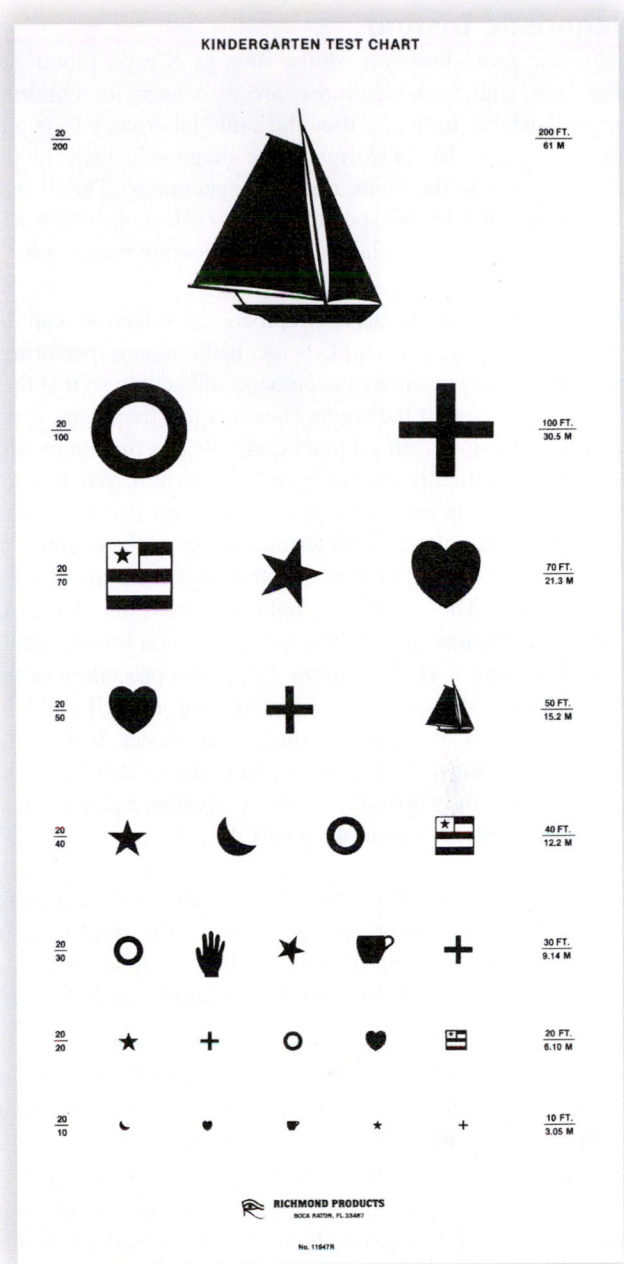

FIGURE 40-16 A kindergarten test chart is used to check the vision of a child who cannot read.
Reprinted with permission of Richmond Products, Inc.

4. Clap your hands loudly. You also may use a device such as a rattle or clicker to generate sounds of varying loudness. Observe the child's response. (Never clap or create noise directly in front of the ear because this can damage the eardrum.)
5. Record the child's response as positive or negative for loud noise.
6. Position one hand behind the child's right ear, as before.
7. Snap your fingers or make a softer noise using a device. Observe the child's response.
8. Record the response as positive or negative for moderate noise.
9. Repeat the steps for the left ear and record all results.

Diagnostic Testing

Diagnostic procedures on adults, such as X-rays, blood and urine tests, and throat cultures, are also used for children. The pediatrician basically uses the same laboratory tests and radiologic tests. He performs some diagnostic tests in the office and needs the same types of specimens. Throat cultures, urine, and blood specimens are collected with a few extra considerations, explained in the following paragraphs.

Throat Culture Because streptococcal infection can be especially serious in a child, some pediatricians perform a rapid test for the presence of streptococcal bacteria so that they can immediately start the appropriate medical treatment. If the test is positive, the licensed practitioner begins treatment with antibiotics specifically for this type of bacterium. Whether the test is positive or negative, the practitioner may also do a throat culture. A throat culture can determine which of the streptococcal bacteria are present or whether other organisms are causing the symptoms. The results can indicate a possible change in medication. Review the method for obtaining a throat culture in the Obtaining a Throat Culture Specimen procedure in the chapter *Microbiology and Disease*. Having a small child lie down rather than sit may make the process easier. If the child refuses to open the mouth, gently squeeze the nostrils shut. The child will eventually open the mouth to breathe. Enlist the parent's help to restrain the child's hands if necessary.

Pediatric Urine Specimen When you collect a urine specimen from a pediatric patient, involve the child (if age-appropriate) and the parents or guardians. Explain the procedure thoroughly and ask specific questions, including the following:

- If the child is in diapers, ask whether there is a problem of persistent diaper rash. (Rash may indicate a change in urine composition because of renal dysfunction.)
- Is the child excessively thirsty? (In this case, the patient may not be taking in enough fluids for the amount of urine being excreted. Excessive thirst, combined with increased urinary frequency and volume, is symptomatic of diabetes.)
- Has the child experienced any difficulty urinating or a urine stream change? (These signs may suggest an obstruction in the urinary tract.)
- Does the child cry when urinating? (If so, the child may have pain or burning on urination, which can indicate a urinary tract infection.)
- If the child is in diapers, ask how many diapers are wet each day. Has the number changed recently? (Responses to these questions can rule out or confirm a urine volume change. For example, a child with a fever and increased perspiration might experience decreased urine volume.)
- Has the child experienced deterioration in bladder control, such as bed-wetting (**enuresis**)? (The child may be under stress or may have a small bladder capacity or a urinary tract infection.)
- If the child is having problems with toilet training and is older than 4 years old, ask whether the child learned to sit, stand, and talk at the age-appropriate times. (If so, the child may have a urinary system dysfunction.)

When you collect a urine specimen from a child who is toilet-trained, follow the same procedures as for an adult. If the child is an infant or not toilet-trained, however, follow the steps outlined in Procedure 40-3, at the end of this chapter, and shown in Figure 40-17. The *Collecting, Processing, and Testing Urine and Stool Specimens* chapter provides additional information.

Blood-Drawing Procedures and Children Collecting blood may be part of your responsibility in a pediatric office. The *Collecting, Processing, and Testing Blood Specimens* chapter provides detailed information about this task. Note that when working with children, it is a challenge to explain blood-drawing procedures to them, and that many children become visibly upset by the situation. If possible, it is best to talk with the parents or caregivers before working with the child. The adults can provide the best insight into how their child handles stressful situations.

Your primary concern when working with infants is to complete tests accurately. Because an infant's veins are often too small for adequate blood collection, the best site for drawing blood is usually the heel, using a dermal puncture.

When working with children, address them directly. Speak clearly in a calm, soothing voice and explain the procedure briefly in terms they can understand. If they ask whether the process will hurt, be honest. A parent, guardian, or coworker should hold a very young child during a venipuncture or dermal puncture to prevent the child from moving. If a child is extremely distressed, it may be best to go on to another patient while the child calms down.

After you have begun the procedure, give the child status reports, such as "We're almost finished!" and make comments like "You've been very brave." This also helps to calm nervous parents or caregivers. When the procedure is complete, offer a compliment on some aspect of the child's behavior. Gather your supplies and samples as quickly as possible to avoid alarming the child with the sight of blood-collection tubes. If parents or caregivers have questions, encourage them to discuss the tests with the child's physician.

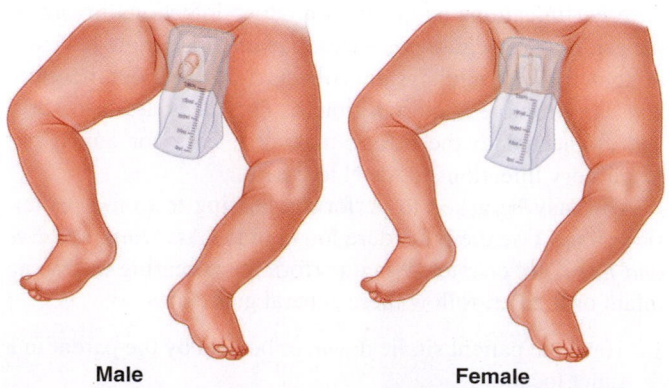

Male   Female

FIGURE 40-17 When you apply a pediatric urine bag, make sure there are no leaks. Follow the steps in Procedure 40-3, at the end of this chapter.

▶ Pediatric Diseases and Disorders LO 40.5

Many common disorders found in children are not specific diseases. Upper respiratory infections, including colds and viral influenza, occur frequently among children. Do not make assumptions regarding diagnosis or treatment. When reported symptoms include fever, sore throat, runny nose, and earache, any number of conditions could be the cause. Encourage the parent to bring the child to the office. You should, however, tell the doctor as soon as possible when a child has an extremely high fever. The doctor may want the child to go to an emergency room. Do not recommend aspirin for fever in children, as aspirin use in children has been associated with Reye syndrome, a potentially fatal disease of the central nervous system (CNS) and liver. Acetaminophen (Tylenol®) or ibuprofen (Motrin®) is preferred for treating fever in children. However, you should check with the doctor before recommending any fever-reducing medication such as Tylenol® or Motrin®.

Common Diseases and Disorders

When you work in a pediatric office, you should know the signs and symptoms of childhood diseases. These include infectious diseases such as chickenpox, influenza, croup, measles, mumps, pertussis, rubella, scarlet fever, and tetanus, which are discussed in the *Microbiology and Disease* chapter. In addition to infectious diseases, there are several other common diseases of childhood, which are outlined in Table 40-3.

Less Common Diseases and Disorders

Some less common diseases and disorders also can be found in children. You need to be aware of the basic symptoms and the treatments for these disorders.

AIDS Most childhood cases of human immunodeficiency virus (HIV) infection are transmitted from a mother to her infant. The transmission of HIV from an HIV-positive mother to her child during pregnancy, labor, delivery, or breast-feeding is called mother-to-child (*vertical*) transmission. In the absence of any interventions, transmission rates range from 15% to 45%. This rate can be reduced to levels below 5% with effective interventions. All babies born to HIV-positive mothers have HIV antibodies that are detectable through testing at birth. The antibodies persist for a period of 15 to 18 months, but not all of these babies remain permanently infected. AIDS has no cure, but treating the pregnant woman and newborn child with antiviral agents has been shown to lower the rate of HIV infection in the child.

Juvenile Rheumatoid Arthritis Juvenile rheumatoid arthritis (JRA) is an autoimmune disease of the joints that occurs in children aged 16 or younger. The symptoms of JRA include swelling, pain, and stiffness of the joints. The most common type of JRA affects four or fewer joints, typically the large joints such as the knees. A less common form of JRA affects five or more joints, most commonly the small joints of the hands and feet. The severity of the disease ranges from mild to severe and may affect the eyes and internal organs. A child with JRA will have periods of remission (a lessening of symptoms)

and flare-up (a worsening of symptoms). JRA is diagnosed based on the severity of symptoms, specific laboratory tests, and X-rays. Treatment of this disease includes nonsteroidal anti-inflammatory drugs (NSAIDs), disease-modifying anti-rheumatic drugs (DMARDs), corticosteroids, biologic agents, and physical therapy.

As a medical assistant, your role in caring for children with JRA includes emphasizing the value of exercise and physical therapy, stressing the importance of taking medications as directed, and offering assistance by providing patient education brochures and information about local support groups and organizations.

Attention Deficit Hyperactivity Disorder and Learning Disabilities Attention deficit hyperactivity disorder (ADHD) and learning disabilities (LD) are found in children, adolescents, and adults. These disorders can cause gross motor disability, inability to read or write, hyperactivity, distractibility, impulsiveness, and generally disruptive behavior. ADHD encompasses all conditions formerly identified as hyperactivity, or hyperkinesis, and attention deficit. LD encompasses a wide range of conditions that interfere with learning, including dyslexia (reading problems), dysgraphia (writing problems), and dyscalculia (math problems).

ADHD is misunderstood, misdiagnosed, and overdiagnosed in children. Some physicians fail to recognize ADHD as a cause of academic, social, and emotional problems. Others are quick to attribute too many such problems to ADHD. When ADHD is the correct diagnosis, methylphenidate hydrochloride (Ritalin®) and other drugs may alleviate the symptoms, but not without risk of adverse effects, such as insomnia, increased heart rate and blood pressure, and interference with growth rate. Successful treatment usually requires a combination of drug and behavioral therapies and educational, psychological, and emotional support tailored to the child.

Cerebral Palsy Cerebral palsy, a birth-related disorder of the nerves and muscles, is the most frequent crippling disease in children. It is caused by brain damage that occurs before, during, or shortly after birth or in early childhood. Signs of spastic cerebral palsy (the most common form) include hyperactive tendon reflexes, rapid alteration between muscular contraction and relaxation, permanent muscle shortening, and underdevelopment of extremities. Among people who have this disease, 40% are mentally retarded, 25% have seizures, and 80% have impaired speech. There is no known cure, but the effects of the disorder can be alleviated with physical therapy, speech therapy, orthopedic surgery, splints, skeletal muscle relaxants, and anticonvulsant medication.

Congenital Heart Disease Congenital heart disease is caused by a cardiovascular malformation in the fetus before birth. If the fetus survives, the newborn is usually small. The defect may be so small, however, that it may not be recognized until days, months, or even years later. Some patients have such a mild case of the disease that no treatment is necessary. Others require only low-risk surgery. In still others,

TABLE 40-3 Common Pediatric Diseases and Disorders

Condition	Description	Treatment
Asthma	Inflammation of the airways caused by triggers such as animals (hair or dander), dust, mold, pollen, tobacco smoke, exercise, strong emotions, and viral infection. Symptoms include tightness in the chest, chest retractions, shortness of breath, rapid breathing, and tiredness.	Avoidance of known triggers; measuring of peak flow to determine breathing function; inhaled medications for long-term treatment, including corticosteroids and leukotriene; for quick relief of symptoms, albuterol or Atrovent; allergy shots and oral medications
Head lice	Small insects easily spread among children by head-to-head contact and by sharing objects such as combs and hairbrushes. Lice live on the scalp and lay eggs strongly attached to hair shafts; symptoms include itchy scalp. Identify this condition by locating crawling lice or nits (eggs) attached to hair; examine parted hair carefully at the scalp and bottom of hair strands.	Anti-lice shampoo or 1% permethrin cream rinse; removal of eggs with fine-tooth comb; disinfection of clothing, bedding, and washable toys by machine washing and drying in hot cycles or by dry cleaning; tight bagging for 30 days of items that cannot be washed; disinfection of combs and brushes (used for hair) by washing in anti-lice shampoo
Herpes simplex virus (HSV)	The virus causes cold sore blisters on or near the mouth; diagnosis is made by inspecting lesions. The first stage (2–12 days before appearance of blister) involves tingling and itching sensations; later, the blister ruptures and forms a yellow crust. An outbreak takes about 3 weeks to heal completely.	Application of ice cube to blister, which may promote faster healing; ointments to alleviate cracking and discomfort; avoidance of sun exposure because it may trigger an outbreak
Impetigo	Highly contagious dermatologic disease caused by staphylococcal, or sometimes streptococcal, bacteria; transmitted by direct contact. Causes inflammation and pustules, which are small, lymph-filled bumps that rupture and become encrusted before healing; frequently seen around the mouth and nostrils.	Avoidance of scratching lesions and sharing utensils, towels, bed linens, or bath or pool water that could cause further transmission; careful washing of affected areas two or three times per day to keep lesions clean and dry; topical antibacterial cream
Infectious conjunctivitis ("pink eye")	Highly contagious streptococcal or staphylococcal bacterial infection of the conjunctiva of the eye; transmitted by direct contact. Causes redness, pain, swelling, and discharge; usually begins in one eye and spreads to other.	Avoidance of scratching eyes and sharing utensils, towels, or bed linens that could cause further transmission; warm compresses to relieve discomfort; antibiotic drops or ointment
Pinworms	Parasites transmitted by swallowing worm eggs, by touching something that the infected person has touched, or by putting infested sand or dirt into mouth. When the eggs hatch in the body, worms attach to intestinal lining; mature females travel to areas just outside the rectum to lay eggs, which causes itching.	Medication given to the whole family to treat and prevent further infestation
Ringworm	Contagious fungal infection of the scalp, groin, feet, or other areas of body, causing flat, dry, and scaly or moist and crusty lesions; lesions develop into a clear center with an outer ring. When the scalp is affected, may cause bald patches.	Oral and topical antifungal medication; isolation to prevent spreading; frequent changing of towels and bedding, with no sharing with others in family; caution that the child should not use others' combs or brushes
Scarlet fever ("scarlatina")	Red rash that starts as patches then turns to fine bumps. Occurs either before symptoms or up to 7 days after. Symptoms includes fever, sore throat, chills, vomiting, and abdominal pain.	Antibiotics to clear up the symptoms and to prevent long-term health problems such as rheumatic fever or kidney disease
Streptococcal sore throat ("strep throat")	Contagious disease spread by droplet. Symptoms include headache, high fever, vomiting, and extremely painful, swollen, and red or white sore throat; causes difficulty swallowing. Complications include progression to rheumatic fever (with arthritis, nephritis, and inflammation of the inner lining of heart).	Streptococci-specific antibiotics given as soon as possible; therapy based on the practitioner's experience is sometimes given without confirmed diagnosis; antibiotics are adjusted with confirmation of infecting organism; possible hospitalization in acute cases

major high-risk surgery is necessary. Many patients diagnosed with the problem are treated with antibiotics to avoid secondary infections.

A cardiovascular defect can be caused by genetic mutations (changes in the genes), maternal infections (such as rubella or cytomegalovirus), maternal alcoholism, or maternal insulin-dependent diabetes. Blue lips and fingernails—signs of cyanosis in a newborn—are obvious indications of a cardiac defect.

Down Syndrome Down syndrome is a congenital disorder resulting from one extra chromosome in each of the millions of cells formed during development of the fetus. It is the most common chromosomal abnormality in humans, and it

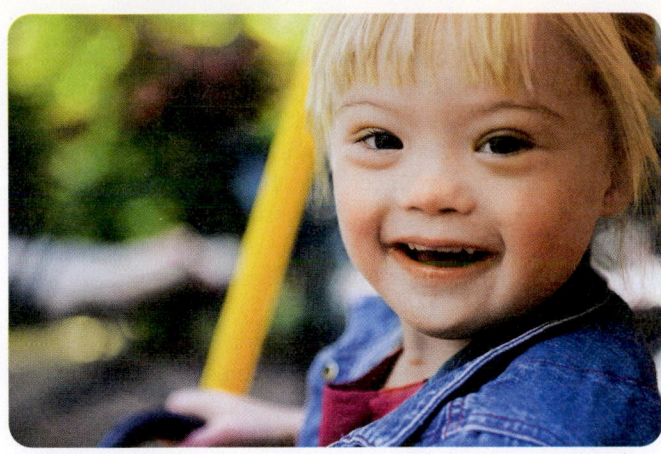

FIGURE 40-18 A child with Down syndrome usually has distinct facial features.
© Rhea Anna/Getty Images

is not caused by any parental behavior, such as diet or activity. The estimated risk for a Down syndrome birth increases, however, as maternal age increases. Down syndrome is characterized by low muscle tone, which can be alleviated with physical therapy. Characteristic facial features are also evident (Figure 40-18). These include broad face, flattened nasal bridge, narrow nasal passages (increasing the risk of congestion), slanting eyes (vision problems are common), and small teeth and ears. Mild to severe impaired intellectual disability is also a characteristic of Down syndrome.

Hepatitis B Infection with the hepatitis B virus (HBV) can lead to a serious and chronic liver infection. A child can carry the virus for years and only later develop liver failure or liver cancer. The virus can be transmitted across the placenta or during birth if the mother is infected. The disease also may be transmitted sexually, by blood transfusion, or by direct contact. It is frequently seen among drug abusers who share needles. Immunization is available, and children should be immunized starting the day after birth. Children who have not been immunized should begin to receive the series of immunizations for protection from infection.

Respiratory Syncytial Virus The respiratory syncytial virus (RSV) is a major cause of lower respiratory disease in infants and young children. RSV is most often seen in the winter and spring as outbreaks of pneumonia, bronchiolitis, and tracheobronchitis. It is highly contagious, and reinfection is common. Treatment is difficult because the infection is viral rather than bacterial. Antibiotics are thus effective for treating only the possible secondary infections that develop during or after contracting RSV. You may be asked to obtain nasal smears to assist in the diagnosis of RSV. More information about collecting specimens is found in the *Microbiology and Disease* chapter.

Sudden Infant Death Syndrome Sudden infant death syndrome (SIDS) is the sudden death of an infant, which occurs during sleep, that remains unexplained after all possible causes have been carefully ruled out. Most SIDS cases occur between

2 and 4 months of age. Victims appear to be healthy and are more likely to be male than female. When necessary, recommend and refer families to support groups that are helpful to the parents of a SIDS infant. The American SIDS Institute provides this advice as well as family support for victims of SIDS. Counseling and information are also available through local health organizations. Placing the infant on his back to sleep is highly recommended to help prevent SIDS. Other things that can be done to reduce the risk of SIDS include

- Obtain good prenatal care.
- Do not smoke, drink, or take drugs when pregnant.
- Avoid pregnancy during the teenage years.
- Wait at least 1 year between pregnancies.
- Use a firm mattress and avoid covers, toys, pillows, and bumper pads.
- Keep the baby's crib in the parent's room until the baby is 6 months old, or use a monitor.
- Do not let babies sleep in adult beds.
- Do not overheat the infant with covers or clothing while sleeping.
- Avoid exposing the baby to smoke.
- Breast-feed whenever possible.
- Avoid exposure to people with respiratory infections; wash hands and clean anything that comes in contact with the baby.
- Offer the baby a pacifier.

Spina Bifida Spina bifida is a defect of spinal development that occurs during the first trimester of pregnancy. The tissues and bones around the spinal cord do not form correctly or close properly. Neurologic symptoms are common because the spinal cord is not fully protected by the spine's bony and connective tissues. These symptoms may vary with the defect's severity, ranging from foot weakness and bladder or bowel problems to paralysis of the lower extremities and mental retardation. In less severe cases the skin over the spinal cord often has a depression, tuft of hair, or port wine stain. In more severe cases, the newborn has a sac sticking out of the mid to lower back (Figure 40-19).

The treatment and outcome of spina bifida are based on the extent of damage. Surgical closure or implants are sometimes required. Unfortunately, the neurologic conditions cannot be reversed. However, some research has indicated that taking folic acid while trying to get pregnant and during the first trimester of pregnancy may reduce the risk of spina bifida.

Viral Gastroenteritis Gastroenteritis is an inflammation of the stomach and intestines that is caused by a virus. Gastroenteritis caused by a virus may be called the flu, traveler's diarrhea, or food poisoning. Viral gastroenteritis usually subsides within 1 to 2 days. It can be serious in young children, however, because it can cause extreme fluid loss that results in dehydration and electrolyte imbalances.

Symptoms include fever, nausea, abdominal cramping, diarrhea, and vomiting. Gastroenteritis is treated with bed

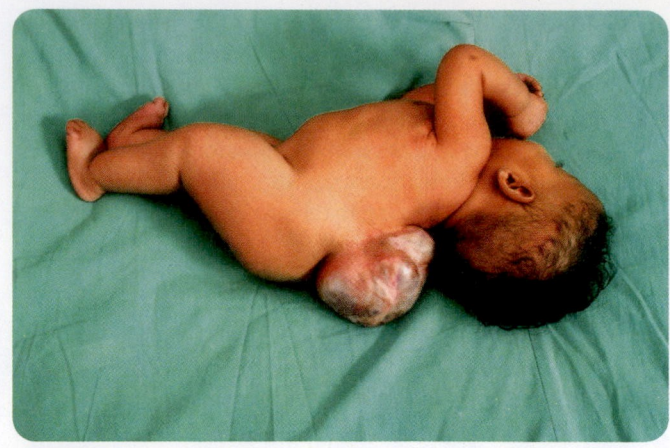

FIGURE 40-19 Spina bifida occurs when the tissue around the spinal cord does not develop completely. It can be mild, with no symptoms, or severe, causing neurologic symptoms such as paralysis of the lower extremities.
© Phototake

rest, increased fluid intake, dietary modifications (usually only clear liquids), and medication for vomiting and diarrhea if necessary. Antibiotics may be prescribed if evidence of bacterial involvement is present.

▶ Pediatric Patient Special Concerns   LO 40.6

In addition to well-child exams, immunizations, and the diseases discussed in the previous sections, there are some special concerns for pediatric patients. Medical assistants should be aware of problems such as child abuse or neglect; eating disorders; depression, substance abuse, and addiction; violence; suicide; sexually transmitted infections; and unwanted pregnancies.

Detecting Child Abuse or Neglect
Child abuse is an all-too-common and potentially fatal problem. It frequently goes unnoticed. Whenever a child comes to the office, you should watch for any signs of serious problems in the relationship between the parent or caregiver and the child. Also notice any signs of physical injury, such as unexplained bruises or burns. Any suspicious lesion on a child's genitalia also should prompt an investigation of sexual abuse. Possible signs of neglect include a dirty or neglected appearance, hunger, extreme sadness or fear, and an inability to communicate. Note any suspicions in the chart and report them to the licensed practitioner before he sees the patient. The practitioner will respond to your information by examining the child for clues to indicate the following:

- Internal injuries: tenderness when palpated or auscultated
- Malnutrition: tooth discoloration, unhealthy gums or skin color
- Lack of cognitive ability: dulled neurologic responses

Studies show that certain risk factors are usually present in parents who abuse their children. Risk factors for child abuse or neglect include stress, single parenthood, inadequate knowledge of normal developmental expectations, lack of family support, family hostility, financial problems, and mental health problems. Other risk factors include prolonged separation of parent and child, ambivalent feelings toward the child, and a mother younger than 16 years. Additional risk factors include an unhealthy or unsafe home environment, inappropriate supervision, substance abuse, a parental crime record, a negative attitude toward pregnancy, and a history of parents having been abused.

Intervention, such as home visits by healthcare professionals, can significantly lower the rate of child abuse. These professionals provide information on normal child growth and development and routine health needs, serve as informational support persons, and refer families to appropriate services when they require assistance. Keep in mind that according to the law, suspected child abuse and neglect must be reported. If you suspect that a child is being abused or neglected while you are working as a medical assistant, you must inform your supervising licensed practitioner. The practitioner may determine that a child protection agency should be contacted. Keep the child protection agency telephone number posted in your office.

Eating Disorders
Adolescents feel pressured to look good. Whether this pressure comes from modern media—magazines, television, movies, or the Internet—or from an adolescent's peer group, it's often focused on being slim and beautiful, which may include watching the scale and dieting, wearing stylish clothing, and having a certain hairstyle. This pressure may lead adolescents to develop abnormal eating behaviors such as anorexia nervosa. Although not limited to adolescents, patients with anorexia basically starve themselves by not eating. Males and females may suffer from anorexia, but it is more common in females.

Another eating disorder is bulimia nervosa—a pattern of binge eating and purging. Purging is done by vomiting, taking excessive doses of laxatives, abusing diuretics such as Diurex® water pills, or exercising excessively. However, a teen suffering from bulimia may still be of normal weight. Additional information about eating disorders is found in the *Nutrition and Health* chapter.

Depression, Substance Abuse, and Addiction
Signs of depression, addiction, and substance abuse in adolescents can be difficult to distinguish. Signs of substance abuse or addiction can be mistaken for depression. The reverse is also true. Sometimes all three conditions exist simultaneously. The use of alcohol, tobacco, club drugs, marijuana, cocaine, and heroin is an important concern with adolescents. Club drugs include GHB, a central nervous system (CNS) depressant; ecstasy, a mental stimulant that increases physical energy; and flunitrazepam, a sedative-hypnotic similar to Xanax®. The abuse of controlled prescription drugs, such as Ritalin® or Oxycontin®, is equally dangerous. Family members should be aware of and willing to discuss signs of adolescent depression, substance abuse, and addiction with the

Signs of Depression, Substance Abuse, and Addiction in Adolescents

Signs of depression, substance abuse, and addiction are often hard to distinguish in adolescents, partly because adolescents are particularly skilled at hiding the signs of all three disorders. However, various signs may indicate depression in an adolescent. One teenager may lose interest in or be unable to enjoy everyday activities. Another may sleep for long periods and have difficulty getting up in the morning, whereas another may sleep very little. Chronic fatigue or aches and pains may signal depression, as may trouble with concentration or school absenteeism. These signs also may indicate substance abuse or addiction.

It is important to know the difference between substance abuse and addiction. **Substance abuse** refers to the use of a substance, even an over-the counter drug, in a way that is not medically approved. Inappropriate use includes practices such as using diet pills to stay awake or consuming large quantities of cough syrup that contains codeine. It also includes taking larger-than-prescribed doses of a medication. Substance abusers are not necessarily addicts, however.

Addiction refers to a physical or psychological dependence on a substance. Addiction usually involves a pattern of behavior that includes an obsessive or compulsive preoccupation with a substance and the security of its supply, as well as a high rate of relapse after withdrawal.

As a medical assistant, you should not try to make a diagnosis. Quite probably, an adolescent with one or more of these disorders will be uncooperative and refuse to answer relevant questions. You must be aware, however, of physical signs and behaviors that may be associated with depression, substance abuse, or addiction in an adolescent patient. The following signs and behaviors are important clues that you should report immediately to the licensed practitioner:

- The patient complains of altered eating habits or disturbed sleep patterns (either too much or too little sleep).
- The patient's weight has changed drastically (either up or down) since the previous office visit.
- The patient appears lethargic or sullen or exhibits radical mood changes.
- The patient has slurred speech.
- The patient appears to have illogical thought patterns.
- The patient appears to have needle tracks (anywhere on the body, especially on the arms or legs).
- The patient has pinpoint (highly constricted) pupils.

---

licensed practitioner. Although these signs are difficult to evaluate in a short office visit, as the medical assistant, you should also be alert to them. If the practitioner determines that a teen has a substance abuse problem, medical and health counseling services should be provided. Review the *Caution: Handle with Care* feature Signs of Depression, Substance Abuse, and Addiction in Adolescents for more information about this pediatric special concern.

Violence

Violence takes many forms. Teens of many cultures are exposed to violence in movies, television, video games, and music. Excessive exposure leads to insensitivity toward violence. Teens also may be victims of physical, emotional, psychological, or sexual violence at home. Bullying, browbeating, or abusing is recognized as a cause of violence at school. Many youths who have carried out homicidal acts of violence were deeply disturbed by repeated bullying experiences such as being teased, taunted, and rejected by peers. Most students are able to tolerate moderate amounts of teasing, but students who are depressed and harbor resentment and anger for a long time may explode in a violent way. In other cases, the teen may turn inward and commit suicide, which is discussed later. The medical assistant should be aware of the following warning signs of potential violence:

- Frequent physical fighting
- Increased or serious use of drugs or alcohol
- Increase in risk-taking behavior
- Gang membership or strong desire to be in a gang
- Trouble controlling feelings such as anger
- Withdrawal from friends and usual activities
- Feeling rejected or alone
- Having been a victim of bullying
- Feeling constantly disrespected
- Failing to acknowledge the feelings or rights of others

Suicide

According to the Centers for Disease Control and Prevention, suicide is the third leading cause of death for people aged 15 to 24. Unintentional or accidental injury and homicide are the first and second causes, respectively. The suicide rate among young people is greater for males than for females. Females are more likely to attempt suicide than males, but males are more likely to be successful in their first attempt at suicide. Be alert for warning signs:

- Depression
- Anger that is directed inward, toward the self
- Alcohol and/or other substance abuse
- Changes in habit—carelessness, sloppiness, and a lack of interest in personal appearance
- Giving away personal possessions
- Giving verbal hints about committing suicide

If you notice these signs or if you hear someone talking about committing suicide, you should listen and take the person seriously. Never assume that it's "just talk." Discuss your concerns with the licensed practitioner immediately.

Sexually Transmitted Infections and Pregnancy Prevention

Sexually transmitted infections (STIs) threaten long-term health and well-being. They are spread by bloodborne pathogens and require public education for teens as well as adults. Since teens may engage in sex, they should be aware of STIs and their effects. Teens also should know about pregnancy prevention. Information and education are available through schools, local and state departments of health, television ad campaigns, the Internet, and the Centers for Disease Control and Prevention. Further information about STIs is found in the chapter *The Reproductive Systems*. Additional information about birth control is found in the chapter *Assisting in Reproductive and Urinary Specialties*.

PROCEDURE 40-1 Measuring Infants

Procedure Goal: To accurately measure weight and length of infants and infant head circumference

OSHA Guidelines:

Materials: Patient chart/progress note, growth chart, pediatric examining table or infant scale, cardboard, pencil, yardstick, tape measure, disposable towel

Method:

Weight

1. Identify the patient and obtain permission from the parent to weigh the infant.

2. Wash your hands and explain the procedure to the parent.

3. Ask the parent to undress the infant.
   RATIONALE: *The infant's clothing and diaper can affect the results.*

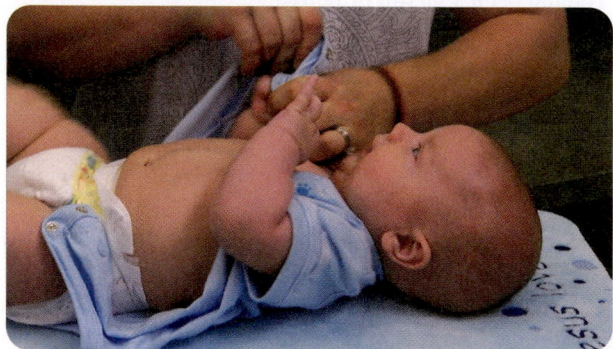

FIGURE Procedure 40-1 Step 3　Mother undressing her infant.
© McGraw-Hill Education

4. Place the disposable towel on the infant scale; then check to see whether it is in balance.
   RATIONALE: *Balancing the scale ensures accuracy.*

5. Have the parent place the child face-up on the scale (or on the examining table if the scale is built into it). Keep one hand over the infant at all times, and hold a diaper over a male patient's penis to catch any urine the infant might void.

RATIONALE: *Keeping one hand over the infant can prevent a fall, and holding a diaper over a male patient's penis prevents contamination of yourself and the weighing area with urine.*

6. Place the lower weight at the highest number that does not cause the balance indicator to drop to the bottom.
   RATIONALE: *Doing so ensures accuracy.*

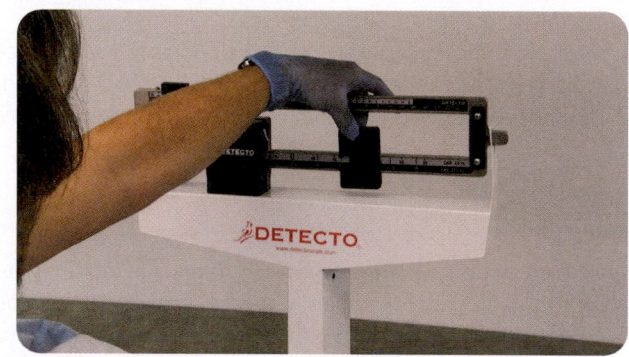

FIGURE Procedure 40-1 Step 6　Move the lower weight first.
© McGraw-Hill Education

7. Move the upper weight slowly to the right until the balance bar is centered at the middle mark, adjusting as necessary.
   RATIONALE: *Doing so ensures accuracy.*

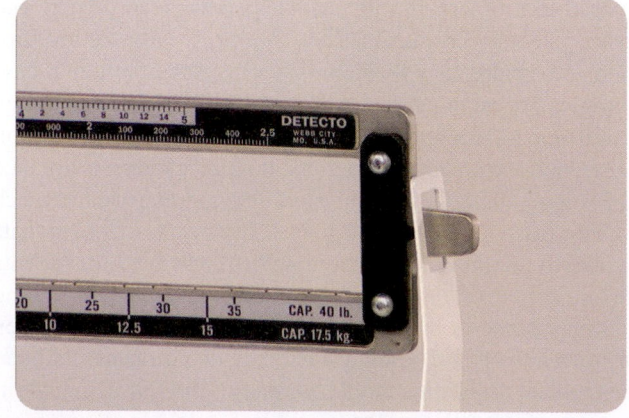

FIGURE Procedure 40-1 Step 7　Center the balance bar at the middle mark.
© McGraw-Hill Education

8. Add the two weights together to get the infant's weight.

9. Record the infant's weight in the chart or on the growth chart in pounds and ounces or to the nearest tenth of a kilogram.

10. Return the weights to their starting positions on the left side.

Length: Scale with Length (Height) Bar

11. If the scale has a height bar, move the infant toward the head of the scale or examining table until her head touches the bar.

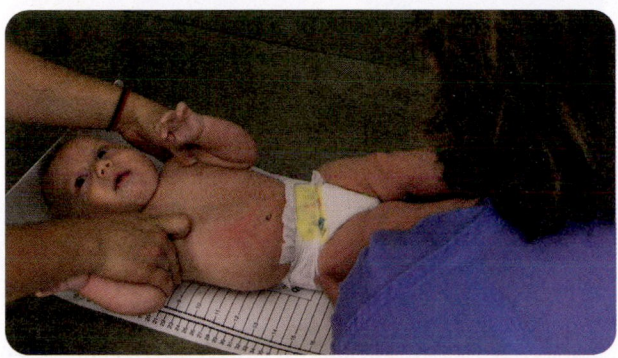

FIGURE Procedure 40-1 Step 11   Moving the infant toward the head of the scale to measure height.
© McGraw-Hill Education

12. Have the parent hold the infant by the shoulders in this position.

13. Holding the infant's ankles, gently extend the legs and slide the bottom bar to touch the soles of the feet.
    RATIONALE: *The legs are held to ensure that the correct length will be measured.*

14. Note the length and release the infant's ankles.

15. Record the length in the patient's chart or on the growth chart.

Length: Scale or Examining Table Without Length (Height) Bar

16. If neither the scale nor the examining table has a height bar, have the parent position the infant close to the head of the examining table and hold the infant by the shoulders in this position.

17. Place a stiff piece of cardboard against the crown of the infant's head and mark a line on the paper.

18. Holding the infant's ankles, gently extend the legs and draw a line on the paper to mark the heel, or note the measure on the yardstick.

RATIONALE: *The legs are held to ensure that the correct length will be measured.*

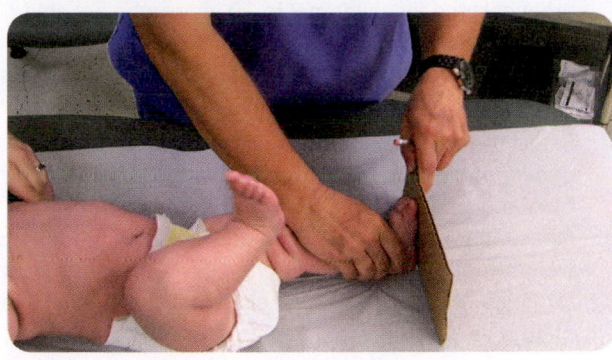

FIGURE Procedure 40-1 Step 18   Holding the infant's ankle to extend the leg and measure for correct length at the heel.
© McGraw-Hill Education

19. Release the infant's ankles and measure the distance between the two markings on the towel or paper using the yardstick or a tape measure.

20. Record the length in the patient's chart or on the growth chart.

Head Circumference

21. With the infant in a sitting or the supine position, place the tape measure around the infant's head at the forehead.

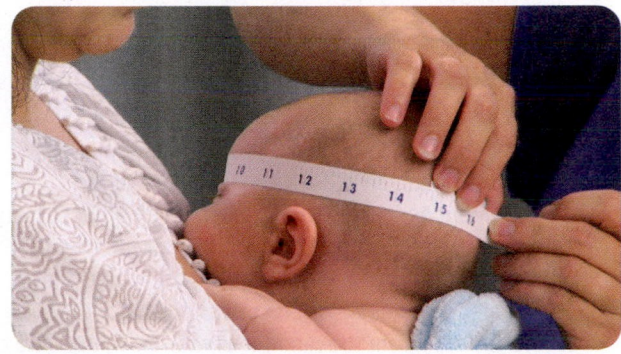

FIGURE Procedure 40-1 Step 21   Wrapping the tape measure around the infant's head at the forehead.
© McGraw-Hill Education

22. Adjust the tape so that it surrounds the infant's head at its largest circumference.

23. Overlap the ends of the tape and read the measure at the point of overlap.

24. Remove the tape and record the circumference in the patient's chart or on the growth chart.

25. Properly dispose of the used towel and wash your hands.

PROCEDURE 40-2 Maintaining Growth Charts

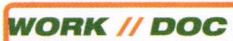

Procedure Goal: To accurately document the height, weight, and head circumference of a pediatric patient on a growth chart

OSHA Guidelines: This procedure does not involve exposure to blood, body fluids, or tissues.

Materials: Appropriate growth chart, calculator or BMI calculator, pencil, and pen

Method:

1. Obtain accurate measurements: Weight and stature (height) are measured for children 2 to 20 years who are able to stand. Weight, length, and head circumference are measured for children fewer than 36 months, or 3 years, who are measured while lying down.

2. Select the growth chart to use based on the age and gender of the child being weighed and measured. For boys and girls less than 36 months whom you will be measuring while they are lying down, use length-for-age, weight-for-age, head circumference-for-age, and weight-for-length. When measuring height in a standing position of boys and girls age 2 to 20 years, use weight-for-age, stature-for-age, and BMI-for-age. Charts are available in the workbook that accompanies this textbook or on the website of the Centers for Disease Control and Prevention.

   RATIONALE: *The correct growth chart must be used because growth charts are used as a comparison to other patients in the same age category.*

3. Record the patient's name and record number at the top of the form.

4. Record the mother's and father's stature (height) and the gestational age (pregnancy week) at which the infant was born.

5. Record the date of birth, birth weight, length, and head circumference, and add notable comments—for example, breast-feeding. *Note:* This data are not included for growth charts for children age 2 to 20 years.

6. Determine the age based upon the date of birth. For infants, determine the age to the nearest month by subtracting the birth date from the date of the measurement as follows: To subtract, it will be necessary to convert months to days and years to months if either the month or day in the birth data is larger than in the date of measurements. When converting 1 month to days, subtract 1 from the number of months in the date of measurement; then add 28, 30, or 31, as appropriate, to the number of days.

   a. Example A: Patient was born on March 26, 2013, and today is January 13, 2015.

	Year	Month	Day
Date of measurement	2015	1	13
Convert 1 month to days	2015	(−1)	(+31)
		0	44
Convert 1 year to months	(−1)	(+12)	44
	2014	12	
Birthday	2013	3	26
Child's age	1	9	18

   Round day to months: 0–15 days = 0 months and 16 to 31 days = 1 month.

   When charting for example A patient, you would use 1 year 10 months.

   b. Example B: Child was born on November 27, 2008, and today is May 15, 2015.

	Year	Month	Day
Date of measurement	2015	5	15
Convert 1 month to days	2015	(−1)	(+31)
		4	46
Convert 1 year to months	(−1)	(+12)	46
	2014	16	
Date of birth	2008	11	27
Child's age	6	5	19

   Round 5 months and 19 days to 6 months, making the patient 6 years and 6 months. Since the age is over 2 years, round months to nearest ¼ year:

   0–1 month = 0 year
   2–4 months = ¼ year
   5–7 months = ½ year
   8–10 months = ¾ year
   11–12 months = 1 year

   When charting for example B patient, you would use 6½ years.

7. Record the date, age, weight, height (stature), and head circumference. Add comments as appropriate, such as "patient uncooperative."

8. Calculate the body mass index (BMI) if using the BMI-for-age chart. First, convert weight and stature measurements to the correct decimal value using the following table.

Fraction	Ounces	Decimal
⅛	2	0.125
¼	4	0.25
⅜	6	0.375
½	8	0.5
⅝	10	0.625
¾	12	0.75
⅞	14	0.875

   Use a calculator and one of the following formulas to determine the BMI:

   - BMI = Weight (kg) ÷ Stature (cm) ÷ Stature (cm) × 10,000
     Example A: Weight = 3.6 kg; Stature = 98 cm
     BMI = 3.6 ÷ 98 ÷ 98 × 10,000
     BMI = 3.7
   - BMI = Weight (lb) ÷ Stature (in) ÷ Stature (in) × 703
     Example B: Weight = 36 lb; Stature = 44½ in
     BMI = 36 ÷ 44.5 ÷ 44.5 × 703
     BMI = 12.8 (rounded from 12.78)

Note: You can also calculate the BMI using an online calculator such as the one found on the National Lung and Blood Institute's website.

9. Plot the measurement on the graph using the data you entered on the chart from the current visit.

   - Find the child's age on the horizontal axis. When plotting weight-for-length, find the length on the horizontal axis. Use a straightedge or right-angle ruler to draw a vertical line up from that point.

   - Find the appropriate measurement (weight, length, stature, head circumference, or BMI) on the vertical axis. Use a straightedge or right-angle ruler to draw a horizontal line across from that point until it intersects the vertical line.

   - Make a small dot where the two lines intersect.

   To ensure accuracy, you may want to use a pencil first to mark the small dot, then mark over with pen or a fine tip marker to make the document part of the legal healthcare record.

PROCEDURE 40-3 Collecting a Urine Specimen from a Pediatric Patient

WORK // DOC

Procedure Goal: To collect a urine specimen from an infant or a child who is not toilet-trained

OSHA Guidelines:

  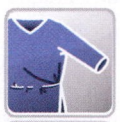

Materials: Patient chart/progress note, laboratory request form, urine specimen bottle or container, label, sterile cotton balls, soapy water, sterile water, plastic disposable urine collection bag

Method:

1. Confirm the patient's identity and be sure all forms are correctly completed.

2. Explain the procedure to the child (if age-appropriate) and to the parents or guardians.

3. Wash your hands and put on exam gloves.

4. Have the parent(s) pull the child's pants down and take off the diaper.

5. Position the child with the genitalia exposed.

6. Clean the genitalia. For a male patient, wipe the tip of the penis with a soapy cotton ball and then rinse it with a cotton ball saturated with sterile water. Allow to air-dry. For a female patient, use soapy cotton balls to clean the labia majora from front to back, using one cotton ball for each wipe. Again, use cotton balls saturated in sterile water to rinse the area and allow it to air-dry.
   RATIONALE: *The area must be thoroughly cleaned so that microorganisms from the head of the penis or vulva do not contaminate the specimen.*

7. Remove the paper backing from the plastic urine collection bag and apply the sticky, adhesive surface over the penis and scrotum (in a male patient) or vulva (in a female patient). Seal tightly to avoid leaks. Do not include the child's rectum within the collection bag or cover it with the adhesive surface.

8. Diaper the child.

9. Remove the gloves and wash your hands.

10. Check the collection bag every half-hour for urine. You must open the diaper to check; do not just feel the diaper.
    RATIONALE: *The diaper should not be wet, and feeling the diaper without looking could dislodge the bag.*

11. If the child has voided, wash your hands and put on exam gloves.

12. Remove the diaper, take off the urine collection bag very carefully so that you do not irritate the child's skin, wash off the adhesive residue, rinse, and pat dry.

13. Diaper the child.

14. Place the specimen in the specimen container and cover it.

15. Label the urine specimen container with the patient's name, ID number, and date of birth; the physician's name; the date and time of collection; and your initials.

16. Remove the gloves and wash your hands.

17. Complete the laboratory request form.

18. Record the collection in the patient's chart (refer to Progress Note).

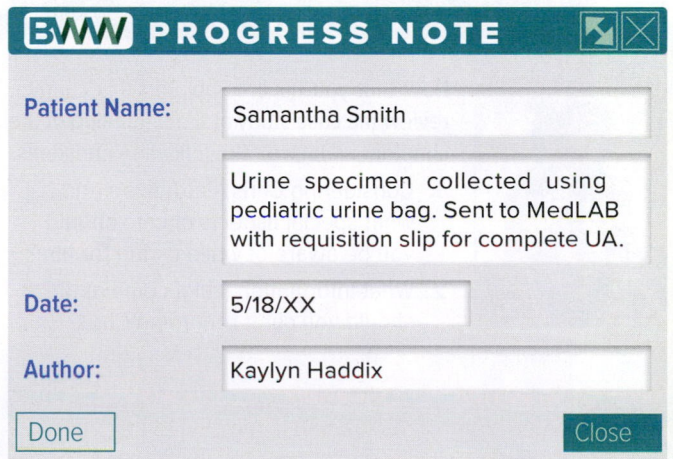

BWW PROGRESS NOTE

Patient Name: Samantha Smith

Urine specimen collected using pediatric urine bag. Sent to MedLAB with requisition slip for complete UA.

Date: 5/18/XX

Author: Kaylyn Haddix

Done | Close

LEARNING OUTCOMES	KEY POINTS
40.1 Relate growth and development to pediatric patient care.	Growth and development occur in stages throughout life, including neonate, infant, toddler, preschooler, elementary school child, middle school child, and adolescent. Each stage of development occurs through physical, cognitive-intellectual, psycho-emotional, and social milestones.
40.2 Identify the role of the medical assistant during pediatric examinations.	The medical assistant must be able to communicate with pediatric patients of all stages, gather and provide educational information to the parent or caregiver, assist with diagnostic and screening procedures, and serve as a liaison between the patient and the physician.
40.3 Discuss pediatric immunizations and the role of the medical assistant.	Immunizations provide patients with protection from infectious diseases. Throughout life, especially during childhood, immunizations are recommended. The medical assistant may schedule appointments, provide education, obtain informed consent, administer the medication, maintain the immunization record, and properly handle and store the immunizations.
40.4 Explain variations of pediatric screening procedures and diagnostic tests.	Screening procedures and diagnostic tests for pediatric patients vary depending upon the age and size of the child. When performing vital signs, body measurements, vision and hearing tests, specimen collection, or administration of immunizations and medications, follow the specific guidelines for the procedure and child.
40.5 Describe common pediatric diseases and disorders and their treatment.	There are many common childhood diseases including diseases include chickenpox, influenza, measles, mumps, rubella, and tetanus. Other diseases are outlined in Table 40-3.
40.6 Recognize special health concerns of pediatric patients.	The medical assistant should be alert to signs of special health concerns of pediatric patients, including child abuse and neglect; eating disorders; depression, substance abuse, and addiction; violence; suicide; sexually transmitted infections; and unwanted pregnancies.

CASE STUDY CRITICAL THINKING

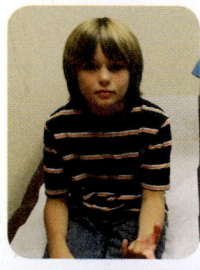

© McGraw-Hill Education

Now that you have completed this chapter, review the case study at the beginning of the chapter and answer the following questions.

1. Considering Chris Matthews's age, what special aspects of care should you be aware of while caring for him?

2. What information (chief complaint) should you chart regarding Chris?

3. According to his immunization record (see Figure 40-13), what immunizations are missing?

4. What screening and diagnostic tests would you perform or assist the licensed practitioner in performing?

1. (LO 40.1) When Chris was a neonate, he had a high level of bilirubin in his blood. As a medical assistant, you know that he had _____ and needed _____.
   a. Jaundice; hospitalization
   b. Jaundice; medication
   c. Hypobilirubinemia; a bili-blanket
   d. Jaundice; a bili-blanket
   e. Hyperbilirubinemia; hospitalization

2. (LO 40.1) Which of the following statements indicates that the parents of a 12-month-old, named Ian, understand the importance of safety for their child?
   a. "Ian loves to sit on my lap when we drive to the grocery store. It keeps him quiet and happy."
   b. "Ian got some new toys from his cousin. It says they are for 3-year-olds or older but he plays with them all the time."
   c. "Ian learned how to turn on the water in the bathtub, so I had my husband set the water temperature on the hot water tank to 140 degrees."
   d. "We put locks on all the cabinets to keep Ian from opening them."
   e. "Ian never puts anything in his mouth. He is such a good boy, we let him play with whatever he wants."

3. (LO 40.2) Which of the following would be the most important information to point out to a physician about a pediatric patient?
   a. A 3-year-old boy is not toilet-trained yet
   b. An 18-month-old girl just started having temper tantrums
   c. An adolescent patient does not want his parents to be in the room during his examination
   d. A 5-year-old girl doesn't want to go to bed at night
   e. A 7-year-old does not have any friends at school

4. (LO 40.2) If an infant is crying while you are counting respirations, which of the following would be the best course of action?
   a. Wait until the infant stops crying to continue
   b. Provide the infant with a pacifier if he uses one
   c. Have the parent leave the room
   d. Blow in the infant's face
   e. Hold the infant more tightly in your arms

5. (LO 40.3) Immunizations are
   a. Vaccines that protect susceptible individuals from infectious diseases
   b. Never given to a child who has minor cold symptoms
   c. Kept at room temperature
   d. Administered even if contraindications are present
   e. Recorded in the patient's chart only

6. (LO 40.4) Which method of temperature should *not* be used on a 2-year-old patient?
   a. Temporal
   b. Axillary
   c. Oral
   d. Rectal
   e. Tympanic

7. (LO 40.4) Which of the following vital signs would be taken last for an infant?
   a. Temperature
   b. Blood pressure
   c. Pulse
   d. Respiration
   e. Pain assessment

8. (LO 40.4) You are to collect a urine specimen on an infant in diapers. Which of the following questions would you *least* likely ask the infant's parent(s)?
   a. Has your baby experienced enuresis?
   b. How many diapers are wet each day?
   c. Does the baby have a persistent diaper rash?
   d. Does your baby cry when she wets her diaper?
   e. Has your baby had a fever?

9. (LO 40.5) A parent calls in, stating that her 5-year-old son has a fever of 102 degrees and will not eat. What should you do?
   a. Suggest that the parent take the child to the emergency room
   b. Tell the parent to give the child either Tylenol® or Motrin® right away
   c. Schedule the child for the first available appointment that day
   d. Tell the parent to give the child a cool bath to lower the child's temperature
   e. Have the parent call back if the child's fever goes over 102 degrees

10. (LO 40.6) Which of the following is an incorrect or untrue statement regarding child abuse and/or neglect?
    a. Report only cases of child abuse and/or neglect that you are sure occurred
    b. Unexplained bruises may be a sign
    c. Risk factors include young parent, single parent, financial problems, and family stress
    d. Intervention can lower the rate of child abuse
    e. Signs of abuse and neglect are not just physical

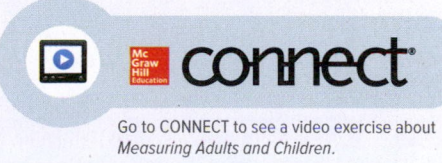

Go to CONNECT to see a video exercise about *Measuring Adults and Children.*

A 4-year-old child arrives at the clinic with his mother. She tells you that she recently moved in with her new boyfriend and that her son has been very quiet lately and has not been sleeping well. She also notes that the child has been holding his arm rather strangely since yesterday. What should you do or say?

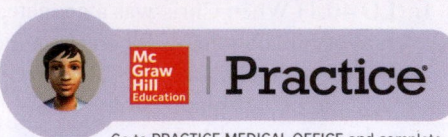

Go to PRACTICE MEDICAL OFFICE and complete the module Clinical - Interactions.

Assisting in Geriatrics

CASE STUDY

Patient Name	DOB	Allergies
Peter Smith	3/28/19XX	NKA

Attending	MRN	Other Information
Paul F. Buckwalter, MD	428-69-544	Vital signs at this visit: BP 136/88, P 76 and slightly irregular, R 16, T 97.8

Peter Smith, a 73-year-old male with mild Type 2 diabetes, calls to schedule an appointment. He states that he is feeling very anxious and fatigued and is having difficulty eating and sleeping since his wife passed away a few months ago. You notice in his medical record that his sleep issues are ongoing and were present before his wife's death. A sleep study was ordered several months ago, revealing mild nocturnal apnea. At that time, Mr. Smith was given a brochure and was educated on behavior modifications to help prevent apnea. When you ask if these seemed to help, Mr. Smith states that he lost the brochure and does not remember what it said.

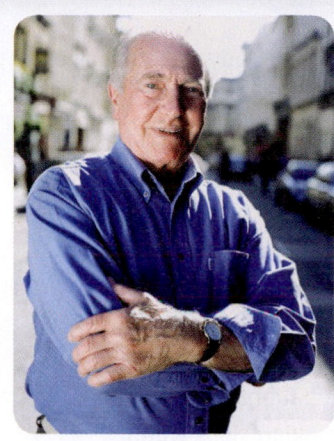
© Image Source/Getty Images RF

Keep Peter Smith in mind as you study this chapter. There will be questions at the end of the chapter based on the case study. The information in the chapter will help you answer these questions.

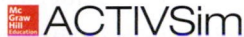
ACTIVSim

LEARNING OUTCOMES

After completing Chapter 41, you will be able to:

41.1 Relate developmental changes in geriatric patients to medical assisting practice.

41.2 Describe common geriatric diseases and disorders and their treatment.

41.3 Identify variations of care for geriatric patients during examinations, screening procedures, diagnostic tests, and treatments.

41.4 Explain special health concerns of geriatric patients.

KEY TERMS

elderly
geriatrician
incontinence
kyphosis
lentigos
nocturia
osteoarthritis

osteoporosis
patient compliance
polypharmacy
preventive medicine
prolapse
sleep apnea

I.C.6 Compare structure and function of the human body across the life span

I.C.8 Identify common pathology related to each body system including:
(a) signs
(b) symptoms
(c) etiology

I.C.9 Analyze pathology for each body system including:
(a) diagnostic measures
(b) treatment modalities

I.C.11 Identify the classifications of medications including:
(a) indications for use
(b) desired effects
(d) adverse reactions

I.P.8 Instruct and prepare a patient for a procedure or a treatment

I.P.9 Assist provider with a patient exam

I.A.1 Incorporate critical thinking skills when performing patient assessment

I.A.2 Incorporate critical thinking skills when performing patient care

V.P.4 Coach patients regarding:
(b) health maintenance

V.P.5 Coach patients appropriately considering:
(b) developmental life stage
(c) communication barriers

V.A.3 Demonstrate respect for individual diversity including:
(d) age

X.C.12 Describe compliance with public health statutes
(c) wounds of violence

X.P.3 Document patient care accurately in the medical record

2. Anatomy and Physiology
a. List all body systems, their structure and functions
b. Describe common diseases, symptoms and etiologies as they apply to each system
c. Identify diagnostic and treatment modalities as they relate to each body system

3. Medical Terminology
c. Apply various medical terms for each specialty

4. Medical Law and Ethics
a. Follow documentation guidelines

5. Psychology of Human Relations
a. Respond appropriately to patients with abnormal behavior patterns
c. Intervene on behalf of the patient regarding issues/concerns that may arise, i.e. insurance policy information, medical bills, physician/provider orders, etc.
d. Discuss developmental stages of life

9. Clinical Procedures
c. Assist provider with general/physical examination
d. Assist provider with specialty examination including cardiac, respiratory, OB-GYN, neurological, gastroenterology procedures
e. Perform specialty procedures including but not limited to minor surgery, cardiac, respiratory, OB-GYN, neurological, gastroenterology
h. Teach self-examination, disease management and health promotion
j. Make adaptations with patients with special needs

▶ Introduction

Geriatrics is the field of medicine concerned with the conditions related to aging. It is a subspecialty of internal medicine and family medicine. This field is growing because of increases in the average lifespan. Growing numbers of people are living longer, healthier lives. In fact, it is not uncommon now for people to live well into and beyond their 90s. Although there is no specific age at which a patient is prescribed geriatric treatment, in general, **elderly** patients (those over 65) will be cared for by a specialist in geriatrics. These specialists are called **geriatricians.**

According to the US Census Bureau, by the year 2030, more than 20% of the population will be 65 years of age or older. Given that older people typically have more health concerns, you may find that as a medical assistant, at least 50% of your time will be spent caring for older patients. Keep in mind that the elderly are not simply older versions of young adults. Geriatric patients have unique needs and concerns, which will be discussed in this chapter. Knowledge of the geriatric patient's needs will prepare you to work as a medical assistant in a geriatric practice, as well as in a general medical practice.

▶ The Geriatric Patient   LO 41.1

As individuals age, they experience changes unique to aging. As a medical assistant, you should be aware of the physical changes that make the geriatric patient more prone to certain diseases and disorders. In addition, geriatric patients experience cognitive-intellectual, psycho-emotional, and social changes. Some aspects of geriatric patient care are age specific.

Physical Changes of Aging

As the body ages, all body systems begin to show signs of aging. It is important to note that not all people experience all changes and that these changes occur at different rates. Let's explore the characteristic signs of aging for the body systems, outlined in the following paragraphs. The systems of the body include the integumentary, nervous, special senses, musculo-skeletal, cardiovascular, respiratory, immune, digestive, geni-tourinary, and endocrine.

Integumentary System Changes in the integumentary system that occur with aging include

- Thinning and wrinkling skin due to decreased amounts of collagen and elastin in the dermis.
- Atrophy, or degeneration, of the subcutaneous layer of skin due to a decrease in adipose tissue.
- Decreased number of cells that produce pigment, or melanocytes, which protect against ultraviolet light. Melanocytes that are still present gather in common locations, causing the brown spots known as **lentigos** or "liver spots" (Figure 41-1).
- Graying, thinning hair.
- Brittle nails.
- Decreasing inflammatory response, resulting in slower healing.

Nervous System Changes in the nervous system that occur with aging include

- Slower reaction time and thought processing.
- Decreased blood flow to the brain due to arteriosclerosis, a group of disorders that cause thickening of the artery walls.

- Shortened attention span and difficulty handling several tasks at one time, caused by decreased frontal lobe size.
- Shrinkage of temporal lobes, leading to weaker signals to the brain for processing.
- Impairment of fine motor activities such as writing, caused by shrinkage of the substantia nigra, a layer of gray matter in the brain.
- Memory loss caused by changes in the part of the brain called the *hippocampus* and a lack of acetylcholine—a chemical that transmits messages between nerve cells or between nerve cells and muscle cells.

Special Senses Changes in the special senses that occur with aging include

- Impaired vision and hearing.
- Altered or decreased taste sensations, which contribute to undereating and possible malnutrition.

Musculoskeletal System Changes in the musculoskel-etal system that occur with aging include

- **Osteoporosis,** or decreased bone density, leading to increased incidence of fracture, particularly fractures of the hip.
- **Osteoarthritis** (OA), or degenerative joint disease (DJD) (Figure 41-2).
- Decreased numbers of musculoskeletal fibers.

Cardiovascular System Changes in the cardiovascular system that occur with aging include

- Decreased cardiac output, especially during exercise.
- Arteriosclerosis.
- Postural hypotension, or loss of blood pressure when standing or sitting up abruptly.
- Increased risk of heart disease.

FIGURE 41-1 Fair-skinned individuals are more likely to have lenti-gos, also called liver spots because they are the color of the liver.
© Dr. P. Marazzi/Science Source

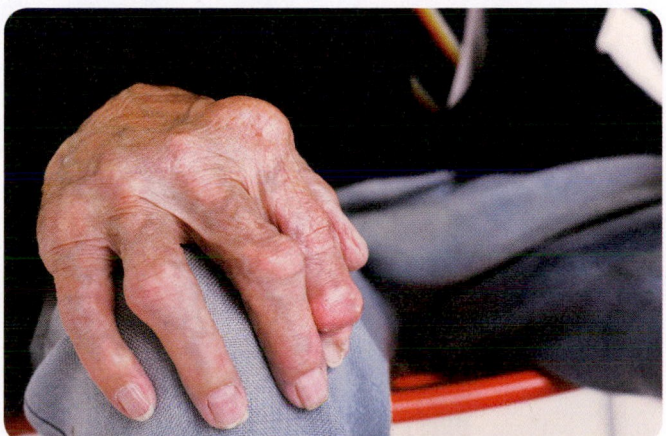

FIGURE 41-2 Also known as degenerative arthritis or degenerative joint disease, osteoarthritis occurs mostly in individuals over the age of 45 years and causes pain, stiffness, and swelling.
© Image Source/Getty Images RF

Respiratory System Changes in the respiratory system that occur with aging include

- Some loss of elasticity of the lungs.
- Calcification of the intercostal cartilage (located between the ribs) and the development of **kyphosis** (curvature of the spine), making it difficult for the lungs to expand properly (Figure 41-3).
- Increased shortness of breath, caused by the physical changes listed above.

Immune System Changes in the immune system that occur with aging include

- Susceptibility to infectious diseases.
- Susceptibility to autoimmune diseases such as cancer and rheumatoid arthritis.

Digestive System Changes in the digestive system that occur with aging include

- Constipation, caused by lack of exercise and poor diet.
- Fecal incontinence, caused by lack of muscle tone.

Genitourinary System Changes in the genitourinary system that occur with aging include

- Decreased number of nephrons, which are the functional units of the kidneys.

- The kidneys filter blood more slowly, causing reduced tolerance to stress, medications, and illness.
- Loss of voluntary control of urination.

Endocrine System Changes in the endocrine system that occur with aging include

- Decreased thyroid function.
- Loss of estrogen production in postmenopausal females.
- Decreasing levels of aldosterone, a hormone that has a role in regulating blood pressure.
- Increase in the time it takes for levels of the hormone cortisol to return to normal after stressful events.
- Deficiencies in response to insulin by various organs.

Cognitive-Intellectual Development

Age-related physical changes in geriatric patients may in turn cause changes in cognitive and intellectual development—how well the patients understand new concepts and learn new skills. Because of changes in the brain, geriatric individuals may take longer to process information. However, they can and do continue to learn. Long-term memory seems to remain intact. Short-term memory may be less acute. If they do not have a disease such as Alzheimer's, they can continue to perform the same functions as they always have. Their accumulated wealth of information and life experiences makes mature adults great teachers.

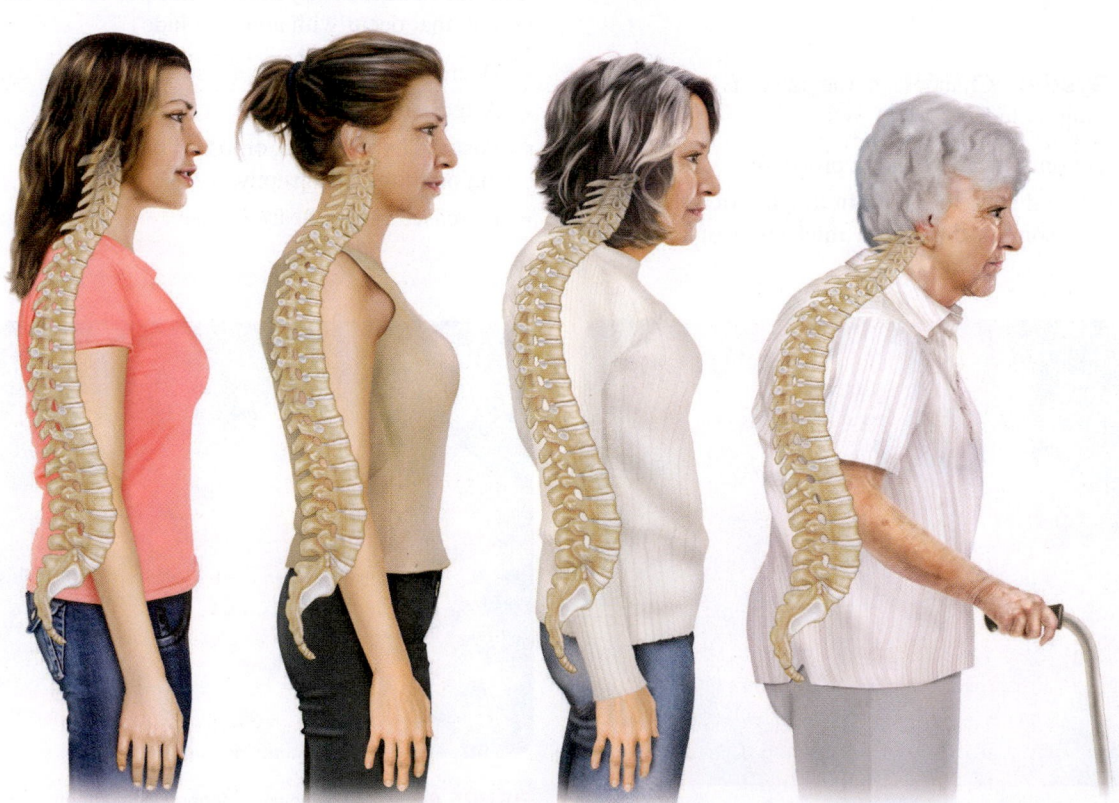

FIGURE 41-3 Kyphosis, a type of curvature of the spine also known as "humpback," occurs with age due to degeneration of the spine from a decrease in bone density.

Psycho-Emotional Development

Many changes may occur in the life of the mature adult. In Western cultures, people retire when they are about 65 to 70 years of age. Retirement is a major change that may have benefits or cause difficulties. For example, people who no longer have a career may feel an unexpected sense of loss and grief. Those who have developed interests outside of their careers may make a smoother transition to retirement. Today, however, many older adults keep working because of financial need.

The deaths of a spouse and of friends are more common life events as a person ages. These deaths may have a major effect on a person's emotional and psychological status. Dealing with the deaths of loved ones may also prompt mature adults to face the reality of their own eventual death. Sometimes, physical ailments and the inability to physically and mentally do what they used to do can lead to increasing dependence on other family members—frequently, middle-aged children. This may result in depression in the mature adult who does not want to "be a burden" to the family.

Social Development

Mature adults may experience an increased spirituality. Individuals who are financially and physically able may prefer to remain in their own home and familiar neighborhood. Others choose to move to their "dream" retirement home or community. Most mature adults in the United States live independently, contributing numerous volunteer hours to their communities. Frequently, relationships with grandchildren are a source of great pleasure.

Aspects of Care

Although all patient needs vary, as a medical assistant working with mature adults, you should consider the following points when caring for and providing patient education to geriatric patients:

- Encourage regular weight-bearing and aerobic exercises to reduce and prevent bone loss.
- Provide patient education regarding a balanced nutritional plan. Specifics of a nutritional plan may need to be discussed with a nutritionist or other licensed healthcare practitioner, particularly if there are complicating medical conditions, such as cardiovascular disease or diabetes.
- Question mature adults about their sleeping patterns. As adults reach the age of maturity, their periods of extended sleep may decrease, but short periods of rest during the day may help to offset that loss. Adequate rest helps an individual to be alert and better able to perform the tasks of the day. Disturbances in sleep or excessive fatigue should be reported to a healthcare practitioner.
- Encourage socialization. Social contact persists throughout adult life and should be encouraged. As an adult matures, retires from the world of work, and maybe even loses a spouse, opportunities for socialization may decrease. It is essential that an individual join with other community members to maintain social contact. Frequently, this can be accomplished through volunteer activities.

- Encourage the patient to continue to get regular healthcare checkups, dental care checkups, and breast and prostate exams.
- Remember that the old adage "Use it or lose it!" applies. Keeping the brain active is necessary and can sometimes even prevent loss of function. Studies have shown that individuals who maintain active interests in the world around them maintain mental function better than those individuals who do not.

▶ Diseases and Disorders of Geriatric Patients   LO 41.2

Aging-associated diseases, or diseases that increase in frequency as individuals age, include cardiovascular disease, hypertension, cancer, arthritis, cataracts, diabetes mellitus, and Alzheimer's disease. Other disorders, such as constipation, diarrhea, and osteoporosis—while not serious for young and middle-aged adults—can be major problems for the elderly. A complete discussion of diseases and disorders that commonly affect mature adults appears in Table 41-1.

▶ Assisting with Geriatric Care   LO 41.3

Usually, examination, screening, diagnostic procedures, and treatments for geriatric patients are similar to those for younger adults. However, as a medical assistant, you should be aware of variations in the care and treatment of elderly patients. Notice the vast differences in the capabilities of people of this age group, and do not stereotype all elderly patients as frail or confused (most are not). Each patient deserves to be treated according to her own individual abilities. Always treat geriatric patients with respect. Regardless of their physical or mental state, elderly patients are adults. Do not talk down to them. Good communication is necessary. For more information about communication with geriatric patients, see *Points on Practice:* Talking with the Geriatric Patient.

Patient Education

Patient education for elderly patients is especially valuable because it can help them prevent or manage health problems and remain independent. You may need to educate some older patients about the importance of taking measures to protect their health. You may work with elderly patients who have hearing or vision problems or physical limitations that restrict their ability to perform certain tasks. Practice good communication in addition to keeping the following suggestions in mind when educating elderly patients.

- Speak in clear, low-pitched tones. High-pitched voices are more difficult for people with hearing impairments to understand. When asking questions, give the patient time to answer and confirm the response to prevent misunderstandings. Avoid both overly simple "yes" or "no" questions that the patient might answer without thinking and overly complex questions that might confuse the patient.

TABLE 41-1   Diseases of the Elderly

Disease	Description	Treatment
Alzheimer's disease	Severely debilitating brain disorder, with warning signs that include changes in personality, mood, or behavior; recent memory loss and increased forgetfulness; decreased ability to perform familiar tasks; difficulty with use of language and abstract thinking; decreased powers of judgment; and disorientation to time or place	Because there is no cure, the primary role of caregivers is to provide comfort and safety to the patient. Medications such as Aricept® and Namenda® are available that can slow the symptoms of the disease.
Arthritis/osteoarthritis	Chronic inflammatory disease of joint tissues; symptoms include pain, swelling, and stiffness in joints (see Figure 41-2).	Anti-inflammatory medication for inflammation and pain; surgery, including joint replacement in severe cases
Cancer	Abnormal growth of cells that are able to invade other tissues	Surgery, chemotherapy, or radiation therapy; under-diagnosis and treatment as well as side effects of treatment are concerns for geriatric patients
Cardiovascular diseases	Dysrhythmias: abnormal heart rates	Medication or surgery to control the heart rate
	Coronary artery disease: blockages of the arteries surrounding the heart	Stop smoking, improve cholesterol with medication or diet and exercise, angioplasty and/or placement of stents, or coronary artery bypass surgery
	Valvular diseases: abnormalities of the heart valves	Most frequently, surgical repair of the affected valve
	Congestive heart failure	Medication to reduce excessive fluid and edema (diuretics) and to improve the beating of the heart (digoxin, beta blockers)
Cataracts	Lens of the eye becomes cloudy and opaque, causing decreased vision.	Sunglasses, improved lighting, and changing of glasses; cataract surgery to replace the lens
Constipation-diarrhea cycle	The cycle of constipation followed by diarrhea occurs when people's diets lack the fiber and liquids to maintain healthy bowel function and they use harsh laxatives to treat their constipation. The patient then complains of diarrhea and asks for antidiarrheal medication, which in turn causes constipation again.	Encourage elderly patients to eat more high-fiber foods, such as cereals, fruits, and vegetables, and to increase their fluid intake, as well as increase their activity level if possible.
Diabetes mellitus Type 2	High levels of sugar (glucose) in the blood; symptoms include fatigue, hunger, increased thirst, increased urination, and even blurred vision	Diet, exercise, and weight control; monitoring of blood sugar; oral medications such as metformin and, in rare cases, insulin
Hypertension	Elevation of blood pressure over 140 systolic and 90 diastolic; often, there are no symptoms or symptoms are mild	Medications to reduce blood pressure; dietary restrictions to reduce fat and sodium and lose weight; increased exercise to lose weight and strengthen the heart
Hyperlipidemia	A condition in which lipid (fat) levels are above normal. These include cholesterol and triglycerides. Although not just a disease of the elderly, it tends to be more common and serious with age. High cholesterol levels can lead to atherosclerosis, the accumulation of fatty deposits along the inner walls of arteries (Figure 41-4). These deposits, along with other substances in the blood, can form an atherosclerotic plaque. This plaque can narrow the opening in an artery to the point of obstructing blood flow. Atherosclerosis is a primary cause of cardiovascular disease and stroke.	Teach patients about eating foods with lower amounts of cholesterol and increasing exercise. Provide patients with printed materials about hyperlipidemia and cholesterol. The doctor may prescribe medication (statins) to lower cholesterol in patients when diet modification and exercise are not effective.
Osteomalacia	Softening of the bones due to vitamin D and calcium deficiency, especially in postmenopausal women	Teach patients about the need for proper nutrition; encourage postmenopausal women to take vitamin and mineral supplements as needed.
Osteoporosis	An endocrine and metabolic disorder of the musculoskeletal system. Thinning of bone tissue and loss of bone density occur over time, leading to fractures. More common in women than men, this disorder may be caused by inadequate calcium consumption, estrogen deficiency, or alcoholism.	Prevention methods include regular weight-bearing and strength exercises and a diet high in calcium (perhaps including supplemental calcium). Prescription medications, such as Fosamax® or Actonel®, and hormone replacement therapy also are used.

(Continued)

TABLE 41-1 Diseases of the Elderly

Disease	Description	Treatment
Sleep apnea	Sleep disorder in which the person stops breathing for several seconds at a time while sleeping; if not treated, can predispose the patient to other, more serious complications such as cardiovascular disease, depression, and even memory loss.	In mild cases, teach patients behavioral changes such as losing weight, avoiding alcohol, stopping smoking, avoiding sleeping pills, and avoiding sleeping on the back. In more severe cases, the licensed practitioner may recommend a continuous positive airway pressure (CPAP) machine, which provides the patient with a continuous flow of air into the nose to keep the airway open. Some practitioners also recommend dental devices to help keep the airway open. In very severe cases, surgery may be needed. See the *Educating the Patient* feature Sleep Disorders for more information about behavioral modification.

POINTS ON PRACTICE
Talking with the Geriatric Patient

Communication is key to successful practice as a medical assistant. The following tips will help you and the patient communicate with each other more effectively.

- Make sure you select a private setting for the patient interview.
- Many older patients are hard of hearing but not deaf. Speak slightly more slowly than you normally would. Speak clearly and loudly (but do not shout—shouting will insult and anger an older patient who does hear well). Enunciate well and use a lower tone of voice (elderly people lose the ability to hear high-frequency sounds first). If the patient asks you to repeat a question, rephrase it instead of repeating it verbatim.
- Look at the patient directly so that she knows you care about what she has to say and so that you can make sure she understands what you tell or ask her.
- You can show respect for the patient's age by addressing the patient with *Mr., Mrs., Ms.,* or *Miss,* unless the patient asks to be called by his or her first name.
- Be patient. Some older patients live alone or in relative isolation and may be out of practice with the two-way communication skills that make a conversation or interview go smoothly. The simple act of being interviewed, even for what may seem to you a straightforward medical history, may unsettle the older patient. For example, he may need to stop and think of a word here and there. Do not supply the word. Wait and let the patient think of it on his own. Also, do not rush through your questions. Rushing will only make the patient feel anxious and incompetent if he feels he cannot keep up with you.
- Practice active listening skills. Pay attention to the patient's verbal and nonverbal cues. Do not interrupt the patient.

After the patient finishes giving each answer, repeat it to give her a chance to correct you if you misheard or misunderstood.

- If you are interviewing the patient to obtain a medical history, before you begin, explain the type of questions you will ask and how the information will be used.
- If you need to use medical terminology, try also to express the same information in lay terms. For example, you might ask, "Do you use a diuretic, or pill to help you eliminate fluids?"
- Be cheerful and friendly but not sugary-sweet. Do not talk down to older patients; they are not stupid.
- Avoid sounding surprised or excited by any answer to a question or to any information the patient gives.
- Under no circumstances use endearments such as *dear, honey,* or *sweetie.*
- Look for ways to make a connection so that the patient feels relaxed and comfortable. For example, in the course of taking a patient's history, you might find out that he enjoys swimming. Ask him to tell you about it.
- Show an interest in the patient as a person. Ask about something she is interested in. For example, a patient might be wearing a piece of handmade jewelry. Ask where it came from. She might have a wonderful story to tell.

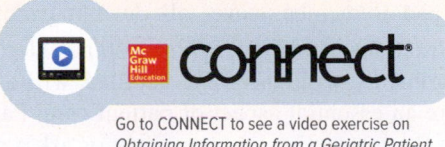

Go to CONNECT to see a video exercise on *Obtaining Information from a Geriatric Patient.*

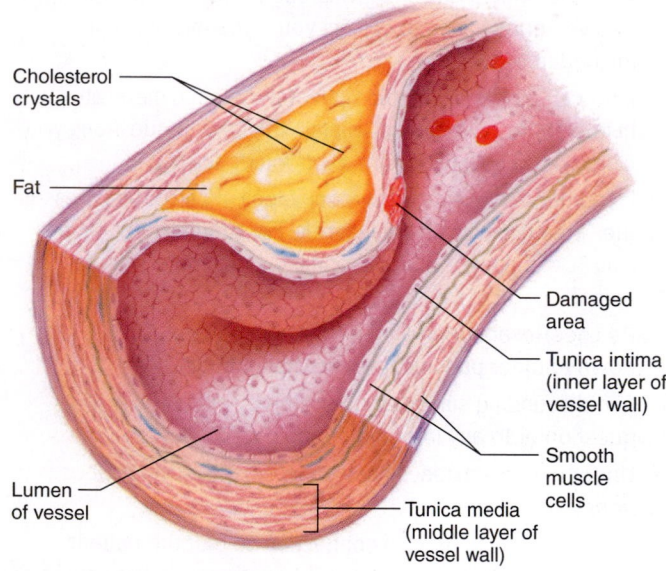

FIGURE 41-4 High cholesterol can lead to atherosclerosis. Help patients reduce their cholesterol through proper diet and exercise, along with medication, if prescribed.

Cholesterol crystals

Fat

Lumen of vessel

Damaged area

Tunica intima (inner layer of vessel wall)

Smooth muscle cells

Tunica media (middle layer of vessel wall)

- Some older people have trouble understanding directions. Try to communicate with them at the highest level they can understand. Remember, never talk down to patients.

- Put instructions in writing. Because some elderly patients have problems with memory, detailed written instructions are an essential aspect of patient care. Patients can refer to the instructions as necessary or ask a relative to do so.

- Adjust procedures as needed. When demonstrating a procedure to elderly patients, keep in mind any physical limitations they have and adjust the procedure accordingly. Make sure patients understand the instructions by asking them to perform the procedure for you.

Denial or Confusion

Sometimes elderly patients, just like many other adult patients, deny that they are ill. A patient's perception of how he feels may be quite different from his actual state of health. The reverse situation also can occur. Elderly patients may overreact to a problem and consider themselves sicker than they really are. They may become dependent, passive, or anxious.

Elderly patients also may over- or underestimate their ability to perform certain tasks or to deal with certain limitations. Elderly patients may be confused if they have some impairment in memory, judgment, or other mental abilities. Signs of confusion can occur with Alzheimer's disease and other types of dementia, depression, head injury, or misuse of medications or alcohol. Elderly patients may or may not be aware of their condition. They may have difficulty understanding instructions.

The Importance of Touch

Therapeutic touch is based on an ancient therapy called the laying on of hands. It was reconceived in the early 1970s by a registered nurse. Essentially, the hands are used to direct human energies to help or heal someone who is ill. Although little scientific evidence exists about the effectiveness of this therapy, it is known that touch can improve health and well-being.

Because they often live alone, many elderly patients experience a lack of physical touch. Using touch—offering to hold a patient's hand or placing an arm around his shoulder—communicates that you care about the patient, and it may improve his health and well-being (Figure 41-5).

Incontinence

Elderly patients may suffer from urinary **incontinence,** or involuntary leakage of urine. Many people are too embarrassed to ask for help or are unaware of possible solutions. In general, if a patient has urinary incontinence that interferes with day-to-day life, the licensed practitioner should be notified of the problem. Incontinence will sometimes cause a patient to drink less, making her prone to urinary tract infections and other problems.

Preventive Medicine

Many elderly patients may not be aware of or do not practice the concept of **preventive medicine** (measures taken to prevent illness). They are from environments in which people went to a doctor only when they were very ill. So they do not realize the importance of preventive measures such as regular checkups, digital rectal exams, immunizations, and colonoscopy. Also, older women often do not recognize the need for regular mammograms and Pap smears to detect cancers of the breast and cervix.

As a medical assistant, you should use any educational tools available to you to make elderly patients more aware of the importance of preventive measures. If you reinforce the doctor's recommendations with education, you increase the chance that patients will heed the advice they are given.

Lack of Compliance When Taking Medications

Often, geriatric patients need several medications, and many of them find it difficult to keep track and take the right medication at the right time. Sometimes patients have difficulty swallowing or simply decide not to take a medication because they feel they do not need it. In your role as a medical assistant, you can help by telling geriatric patients about available medication reminder boxes, timers,

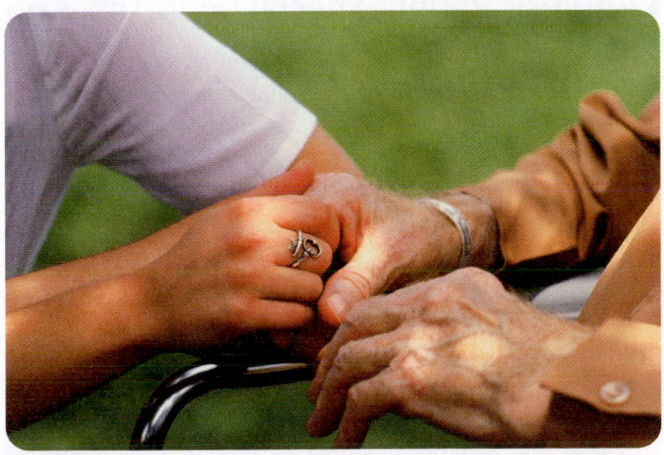

FIGURE 41-5 The importance of touch: Elderly patients may appreciate your touch as a sign of caring. Consider offering to hold their hand or placing an arm around their shoulder.
© Royalty-Free/Corbis

and medication organizers. These devices can help ensure **patient compliance** (obedience in following the orders of the licensed practitioner). Patient compliance helps patients remain healthier and get well faster.

Collecting Urine Specimens

Consider the following when you are collecting urine from a geriatric patient: Bladder muscles weaken with age, often leading to incomplete bladder emptying and chronic urine retention, which can cause urinary tract infection, **nocturia** (excessive nighttime urination), and incontinence.

Weakening of the supports of the uterus may cause it to **prolapse** (work its way down the vaginal canal). The uterus pulls with it the vaginal walls, bladder, and rectum. This weakening—often the result of several childbirths—may not occur until a woman is postmenopausal. Symptoms include pressure, incontinence, and urinary retention. Normal activities, such as walking up stairs, can aggravate the problem.

Find out whether the patient ever loses bladder control. If so, ask whether it occurs suddenly or whether a feeling of intense pressure precedes it. These symptoms can be a sign of weakening of the bladder muscles.

Keep in mind that some elderly patients need assistance in providing a urine specimen. For example, you may have to accompany the patient to the bathroom and hold the specimen container. (Wash your hands before and after doing so, and wear gloves while providing this help.)

Conditions of the urinary system, especially the bladder, in the elderly can interfere with collecting urine specimens. This is especially true for 24-hour urine specimens. Careful and repeated explanations or reminders about the procedure or the specimens needed may be necessary to ensure accuracy.

Blood-Drawing Procedures

The challenges presented by elderly patients may test your technical skills as well as your interpersonal skills. Physically, some older adults are frail and may not withstand blood-drawing procedures as easily as younger patients. Changes in skin condition often make elderly patients more prone to bruising and other injuries. Decreased circulation may make it difficult to collect enough blood for an adequate sampling. Be aware of these issues and take extra precautions when drawing blood on an elderly patient.

Hot and Cold Therapy

Elderly patients are usually more sensitive than others to cold and heat. As you may have noticed with elderly friends and relatives, there is a reduced ability to tolerate temperature changes. Sudoriferous (sweat-producing) glands of the skin decrease in number and, with less perspiration, high temperatures are more difficult to adjust to. At the same time, the loss of adipose tissue and decreased circulation result in a lessened ability to retain heat, which increases sensitivity to cold.

Along with possible poor circulation, geriatric patients also may have arthritis; impaired sensation; kidney, heart, or lung disease; or atherosclerosis. They also may have impaired skin integrity—thinning of the skin, resulting in increased risk of skin tearing, bruising, and burning. When administering cryotherapy (cold therapy) or thermotherapy (heat therapy), stay with an elderly patient during its application to check the patient's skin frequently for excessive paleness or redness.

Nutritional Guidelines

Universal nutritional guidelines for aging patients have not been developed. It is known, however, that energy and metabolic requirements usually decline with age, which calls for some dietary modification. The Food and Nutrition Board of the National Academy of Sciences recommends a 10% decrease in caloric intake for people over age 50 compared with that of young adults. Men and women older than age 75 should decrease their intake another 10% to 15%. The exact adjustment, however, depends on the individual patient's condition and needs.

Because protein requirements do not change, elderly patients should select foods that provide ample protein in a smaller quantity of food. To achieve daily nutritional goals, patients may require supplements for iron, calcium, and other minerals, such as phosphorus and magnesium.

Aging is often accompanied by decreased gastrointestinal muscle tone, so elderly patients should increase their intake of high-fiber foods and drink plenty of water. Of course, all people need to have an adequate amount of daily water. However, elderly patients sometimes restrict their fluid intake because they may need to urinate frequently, do not remember, or do not understand the importance of keeping the body well hydrated by consuming enough fluid. See Procedure 41-1 at the end of this chapter. Poor fluid intake also can quickly lead to urinary tract infections in mature adults.

Although all people need a certain amount of fat in their diet to help the body absorb vitamins, too much may lead to atherosclerosis. Elderly individuals should keep fat intake to 20% of their total calories.

Certain factors can impair or impede eating in this age group and may even lead to malnutrition. If you recognize any of these factors, discuss them with the patient's doctor:

- Physical factors, such as chewing difficulty caused by tooth loss or poorly fitting dentures, swallowing difficulty, and lack of appetite caused by altered taste, smell, or sight
- Medications, which may adversely affect food intake or nutrient use
- Social factors, including apathy toward food caused by depression, grief, or loneliness
- Economic factors, including homelessness or lack of money for food or transportation

Many types of adaptations can be used to help ensure that the nutritional needs of mature adults are met. To overcome physical factors, seeing to the patient's dental needs can help. Assistive devices such as plates with high edges that help keep food from falling onto the table can help the patient scoop food onto serving utensils. Using nonskid placemats may help keep the dishes from sliding around.

To counteract social factors such as loneliness and depression, it may help to suggest eating frequently with friends or neighbors. Patients who live alone may also benefit from using tablecloths, cloth napkins, and attractive centerpieces to make dining a more pleasant experience. Other healthcare team members, such as social workers, may need to be consulted if economic factors are interfering with a patient's nutritional status.

Immunizations

Influenza and influenza-related pneumonia represent a serious health risk for patients older than age 65. Although elderly patients can be immunized against influenza each year and against influenza-related pneumonia one time, they may have misconceptions about vaccinations. Another recommended vaccine for individuals over 60 is the shingles vaccine. No matter the vaccine, geriatric patients may worry about the expense, the possibility of getting the disease from the vaccine, or the need for a vaccination when they do not feel ill.

Explain to patients who are concerned about the cost of vaccinations that if they are not enrolled in one of the many insurance plans that cover immunization, Medicare Part B covers the cost. For those worried about the potential side effects of immunization, describe the mild symptoms they may encounter and emphasize that the symptoms are short-lived. You also might mention that compared to the potential dangers of contracting a serious infection, the symptoms are quite mild.

Because older patients are much more likely than younger patients to develop side effects as a result of immunizations, instruct older patients so that they recognize and immediately report any adverse reactions. That way, the licensed practitioner can treat elderly patients before their illness becomes severe.

▶ Geriatric Patient Special Concerns LO 41.4

As you can see, geriatric patients require a lot of special consideration. Four additional special concerns when working with the elderly are falls, depression, elder abuse, and polypharmacy.

Preventing Falls in the Elderly

Falls can occur at any age, but in the elderly, they can have especially serious consequences. Bones may become brittle with age due to osteoporosis, and falls can cause breaks in major bones, such as those in the hip and wrist. Complications from falls and bone fractures can lead to death in individuals in this age group.

The elderly are prone to falling because of vision problems, slowing reflexes, quick position changes that can lower the blood pressure, and changes in the ear that cause equilibrium problems. In addition, medications can increase the risk of falls because they may make the patient less alert or cause dizziness.

As a medical assistant, you should discuss a safety checklist with elderly patients and their families. Point out that by taking precautions, elderly patients can reduce the risk of falling. Make sure patients and their families understand the following instructions:

- Remove reading glasses before getting up and walking around.
- Make sure that potentially hazardous areas, such as stairs and doorway entrances, are well lit.
- Use night-lights in the bedroom and bathroom to help prevent night falls.
- When getting up from a reclining or recumbent position, sit at the edge of the bed for a few minutes before trying to stand to allow blood flow and blood pressure to adjust.
- Wear well-fitting shoes with low heels and slippers with nonslip soles.
- Use a cane or walker if you are unsteady on your feet.
- Secure rugs and floor coverings to the floor to prevent slippage.
- Attach all electrical cords to the walls or floor moldings.
- Place sturdy banisters along all stairs inside and outside the home.
- Install secure handrails near the bathtub and toilet.
- Apply nonslip appliques to the bathtub and shower floor.
- Minimize clutter in the home.
- Store frequently used items within easy reach.

Depression

Depression is common in the elderly, but many of the symptoms of depression mimic those of other conditions. As a medical assistant, you can help elderly patients—and their families—recognize the signs of depression. Recall Mr. Peter Smith from our case study at the beginning of the chapter. What symptoms does he have? Do you think he has depression? Knowing what to look for may help patients seek help sooner than they otherwise would and receive prompt diagnosis and treatment. See the *Caution: Handle with Care* feature Helping Elderly Patients with Depression for a discussion of the symptoms and treatment of depression in the elderly.

Elder Abuse

Even though you may need to communicate verbally with an elderly patient's caregiver, always observe the elderly patient for nonverbal signs of problems such as grimacing, foul odors, or bruising even if the patient cannot speak to you verbally. Disabilities may make the elderly person defenseless against abuse, and a medical assistant should be alert to signs of abuse.

It is difficult to detect elder abuse. There is no uniform and comprehensive definition of this type of abuse, and bruises from falls and other accidents can be mistaken for abuse. Also, the signs of neglect can be similar to the signs of some chronic medical conditions. There are three basic categories of elder abuse: domestic elder abuse, institutional elder abuse, and self-neglect, or self-abuse. Elders can be abused physically, sexually, or psychologically. Elders may also be neglected, abandoned, or exploited materially or financially. Elders may even choose to neglect or abuse themselves. More than one type of abuse can occur simultaneously. Elder abuse occurs in all racial, socioeconomic, and religious groups. However, most victims are older women with chronic illness or disabilities. Risk factors and situations that increase the possibility of elder abuse include

- History of alcoholism, drug abuse, or violence in the family.
- History of mental illness in the abuser or victim.
- Isolation of the victim from family members and friends other than the abuser.
- Recent stressful events affecting the abuser or victim.

Signs of neglect include

- Foul odor from the patient's body.
- Poor skin color.
- Inappropriate clothing for the season.
- Soiled clothing.
- Extreme concern about money.

You can assist the doctor by taking a careful history. Ask the patient about living arrangements, social contact, and emotional stress. Note the interaction between the caregiver and the patient. Be aware that a patient with dementia may be abused but is not able to report it and the caregiver may be able to cover it well. If you suspect abuse, inform the doctor. He will then be able to direct the physical exam toward possible internal injuries, malnutrition, or lack of cognitive ability. Most states require doctors who suspect elder abuse or neglect to report their concerns to a designated office. Early intervention usually results in better living arrangements for both the patient and the caregiver.

Polypharmacy

Age-related changes in the body can affect drug absorption, metabolism, distribution, and excretion. These normal changes can be exaggerated by various diseases or disorders. So as people age, they have an increased risk of drug toxicity, adverse reactions, or lack of therapeutic effects. Because of this risk, be especially alert when assessing an elderly patient who is on drug therapy.

Many elderly patients have complex, chronic diseases with unusual symptoms. This situation can make it difficult to tell whether a problem is caused by a drug. Listen closely to elderly patients and their family members; they are more likely to notice subtle changes than you are.

Patient and family education are important with elderly patients, particularly if they engage in **polypharmacy** (take several medications concurrently). Polypharmacy is common in elderly patients, and drug-drug interactions can be severe. See the *Caution: Handle with Care* feature Preventing Unsafe Polypharmacy.

CAUTION: HANDLE WITH CARE

Helping Elderly Patients with Depression

The National Institutes of Health (NIH) considers depression in people age 65 and older to be a major public health concern. In fact, suicide is more common among the elderly than any other age group. The NIH also indicates that only about 10% of elderly people who need treatment for depression ever receive it.

One reason for the low rate of treatment is that many older people—and their families—believe that depression is a normal consequence of growing old. After all, older people may experience many difficult life changes, including enduring the deaths of a spouse and siblings, adjusting to retirement, being alone, dealing with a relocation, suffering economic hardship, and managing a variety of physical ailments. Because of these circumstances, doctors and family may miss the signs of depression.

Recognizing the Symptoms

There is, unfortunately, no specific diagnostic test for depression, so a diagnosis must be made on the basis of symptoms. The symptoms of depression in the elderly are similar to those in other age groups and include the following:

- Decreased ability to enjoy life or to show an interest in activities or people
- Slow thinking, indecisiveness, or difficulty in concentrating
- Increased or decreased appetite
- Increased or decreased time spent sleeping
- Recurrent feelings of worthlessness
- Loss of energy and motivation
- Exaggerated feelings of sadness, hopelessness, or anxiety
- Recurrent thoughts of death or suicide

The failure to realize that symptoms like these indicate an illness prevents many older people from seeking help. However, there is evidence that treatment for depression in the elderly can be highly effective.

Treatment for Depression

Depression has been linked to poor diet, lack of exercise, and reduced social contacts. Modification to these things may improve symptoms of mild depression. However, treatment for clinical depression generally combines a course of antidepressant drugs with psychotherapy. Older patients generally respond to antidepressants more slowly than younger patients, so older patients may not experience relief until more than 6 weeks after starting treatment. For this and other reasons, compliance in taking medications for depression is a problem with the elderly. Many elderly patients do not understand depression and the importance of taking medications as prescribed. They also may be frightened by the idea of taking medication for a mental problem. Psychotherapy aims to help older patients talk through their anxieties, develop coping skills, and improve the quality of their lives. Again, compliance is a problem. Many older adults are unwilling to admit that they have a mental health problem and refuse to follow up on referrals to mental health professionals.

Benefits of Treatment

Elderly patients who follow a course of treatment for depression benefit in several of ways. They gain

- Relief from many of the symptoms associated with depression.
- Relief from some of the pain and suffering associated with physical ailments.
- Improved physical, mental, and social well-being.

Healthcare providers, including you as the medical assistant, can play a significant role in recognizing symptoms of depression in elderly patients and in encouraging them to get the treatment they need.

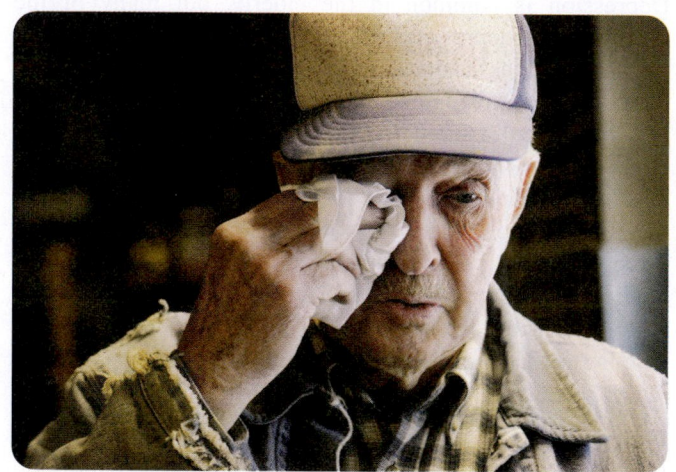

© Design Pics/Kristy-Anne Glubish RF

If an elderly patient is forgetful or confused, talk to the licensed practitioner about simplifying the medication schedule to reduce the risk of drug administration errors or omissions. If the patient has vision problems, provide drug instruction sheets in large type. To do this, type instructions on a word processor in a large type size, enlarge the instructions on a photocopier, or clearly handwrite the instructions in large block letters. You also might contact a local association for the blind or visually impaired for devices and tips.

CAUTION: HANDLE WITH CARE

Preventing Unsafe Polypharmacy

Before administering any drug by any route, you must know every drug, both prescription and nonprescription, that the patient is taking. Many patients, especially elderly ones, visit several doctors. It is possible that each doctor prescribes one or more drugs without being aware of other drugs the patient is taking. This practice can result in polypharmacy, which means taking several drugs at once. Polypharmacy can be safe, but if the doctor is unaware of the total drug profile, serious drug interactions can result.

When asking patients to identify *all* other drugs they are taking, including OTC drugs, keep in mind that patients may forget to mention all their medicines, OTC drugs, supplements, or herbal remedies to the doctor. Patients often forget to mention antacids (such as Tums® or Rolaids®), supplements that are part of a food or drink (such as flavored drinks with glucosamine-chondroitin), medicines that are used only as needed such as medicine for migraine headaches, vitamins, and herbal remedies such as ginkgo biloba or omega-3.

To help prompt patients about drugs they may have forgotten, ask patients who have seen an orthopedist or a cardiologist whether pain medication has been prescribed. Ask women who have seen a gynecologist if they are using a patch or other form of hormone replacement therapy. Ask all patients if they take any other dietary supplement, OTC medication, and/or herbal

remedy. If a patient has been referred to any other doctor for any reason, ask whether that doctor has prescribed medication. After determining the total drug profile, you should

- Update the patient's record (this should be done with every visit to your facility).
- Consider possible drug interactions, consulting online drug interaction checkers or other drug references, such as the *PDR*, if needed.
- Inform the licensed practitioner of your findings.

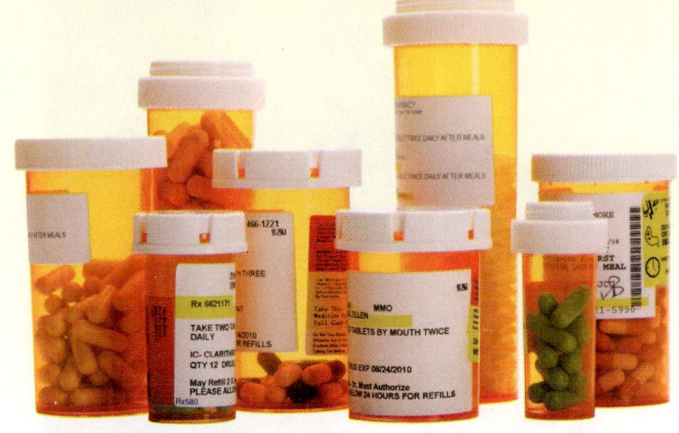
© Jeffrey Coolidge/Getty Images

PROCEDURE 41-1 Educating Adult Patients About Daily Water Requirements

WORK // DOC

Procedure Goal: To teach patients how much water their bodies need to maintain health

OSHA Guidelines: This procedure does not involve exposure to blood, body fluids, or tissues.

Materials: Patient education literature, patient's chart/progress note, and device to document education

Method:

1. Explain the importance of water to the body. Point out the water content of the body and the many functions of water in the body, including maintaining the body's fluid balance, lubricating the body's moving parts, and transporting nutrients and secretions.

2. Add any comments applicable to an individual patient's health status, such as issues related to medication use, physical activity, fluid limitation, or increased fluid needs. For example, geriatric patients have decreased gastrointestinal motility and require water to avoid constipation.

RATIONALE: *Some elderly patients purposely limit their fluid intake because of incontinence or physical limitations that make getting to a bathroom difficult, so it is necessary to provide specific comments about their exact fluid needs.*

3. Explain that people obtain water by drinking water and other fluids and by eating foods that contain water. On average, an adult should drink six to eight glasses of water a day to maintain a healthy water balance in which intake equals excretion. People's daily need for water varies with size and age, the temperatures to which they are exposed, the degree of physical exertion, and the water content of foods eaten. Make sure you reinforce the physician's or dietitian's recommendations for a particular patient's water needs.

4. Caution patients that soft drinks, coffee, and tea are not good substitutes for water and that it would be wise to filter out any harmful chemicals contained in the local tap water or to drink bottled water, if possible. A good rule

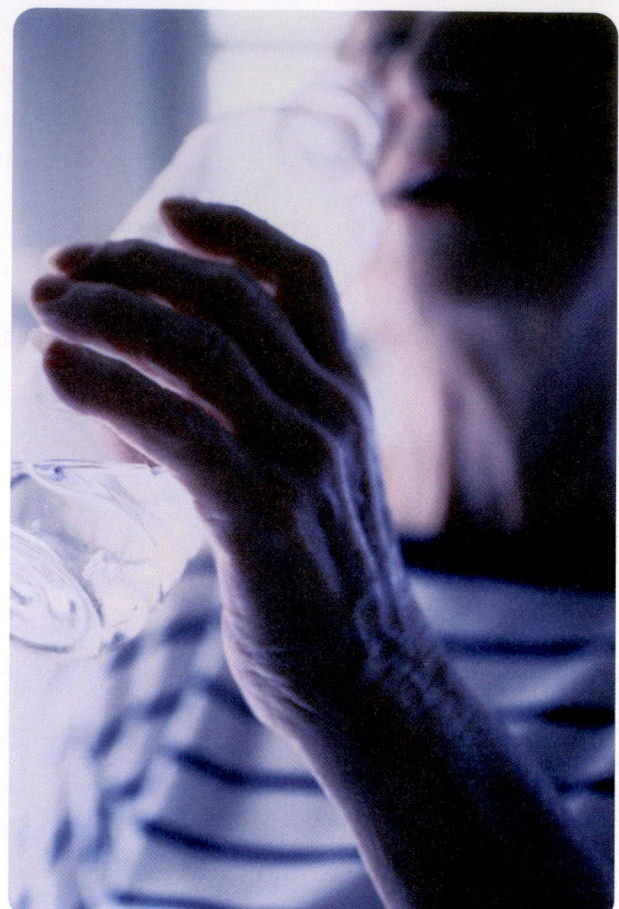

FIGURE Procedure 41-1 Step 5 Using a water bottle can help patients remember to drink a certain amount of water each day.
© Steven Puetzer/Getty Images RF

of thumb is that for every soft drink, coffee, or tea, the patient should drink the same amount of water to ensure hydration.

5. Provide patients with tips about reminders to drink the requisite amount of water. Some patients may benefit from using a water bottle of a particular size, so that they know they have to drink, say, three full bottles of

water each day. Another helpful tip is to make a habit of drinking a glass of water at certain points in the daily routine, such as first thing in the morning and after lunch or right before bedtime if it does not interrupt your sleep.

6. Provide patients with printed materials documenting the amount of water to drink and methods to ensure that their fluid intake is adequate.

7. Remind patients that you and the licensed practitioner are available to discuss any problems or questions.

8. Document any formal patient education sessions or significant exchanges with a patient in the patient's chart or on a progress note, noting whether the patient understood the information presented (refer to Progress Note).

   RATIONALE: *Many insurance companies require evidence of preventive health counseling, and documentation is an important aspect of patient insurance coverage.*

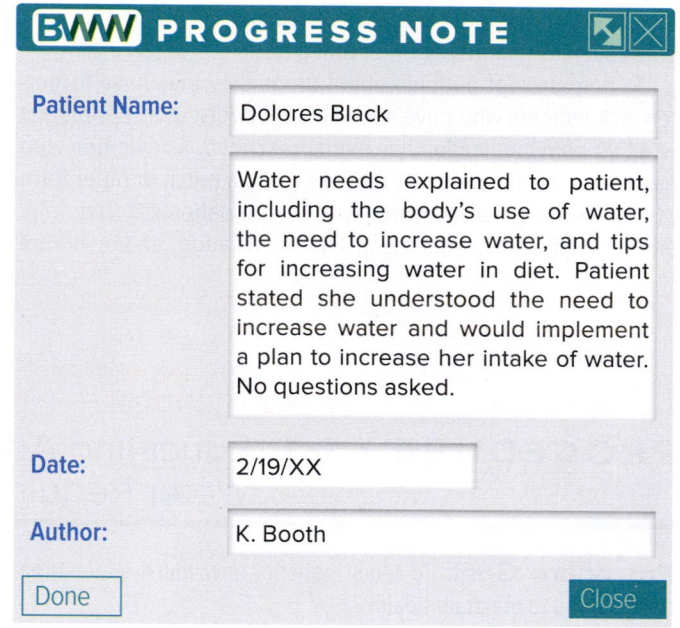

BWW PROGRESS NOTE

Patient Name:	Dolores Black
	Water needs explained to patient, including the body's use of water, the need to increase water, and tips for increasing water in diet. Patient stated she understood the need to increase water and would implement a plan to increase her intake of water. No questions asked.
Date:	2/19/XX
Author:	K. Booth

Done   Close

SUMMARY OF LEARNING OUTCOMES

LEARNING OUTCOMES	KEY POINTS
41.1 Relate developmental changes in geriatric patients to medical assisting practice.	Geriatrics is a subspecialty of internal medicine or family practice. Geriatricians typically care for patients over the age of 65. These patients have multiple physical changes as well as variations in psycho-emotional, cognitive-intellectual, and social development to consider when working as a medical assistant.
41.2 Describe common geriatric diseases and disorders and their treatment.	Common aging-associated diseases and disorders include cardiovascular disease, hypertension, cancer, arthritis, cataracts, diabetes mellitus, Alzheimer's disease, constipation, diarrhea, osteoporosis, osteomalacia, and sleep apnea. Understanding these will help you prepare to care for geriatric patients.

LEARNING OUTCOMES	KEY POINTS
41.3 Identify variations of care for geriatric patients during examinations, screening procedures, diagnostic tests, and treatments.	When working with geriatric patients, you must treat them with respect and dignity. Be aware of their physical and mental changes so that you can adapt your care to meet their needs.
41.4 Explain special health concerns of geriatric patients.	Each of the following special concerns should be handled appropriately when caring for the elderly: falls, elder abuse, depression, and polypharmacy.

CASE STUDY CRITICAL THINKING

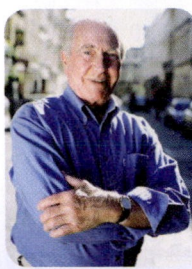

© Image Source/Getty Images RF

Recall Peter Smith from the beginning of the chapter. Now that you have completed this chapter, answer the following questions regarding his case.

1. Considering Mr. Smith's age, what special aspects of care should you be aware of while caring for him?

2. Why would Mr. Smith be prone to falls, and what can you do to help prevent them?

3. You need to collect a urine specimen from Mr. Smith. What special considerations should you take?

4. What symptoms does Mr. Smith have, and why is it important for you to recognize them?

EXAM PREPARATION QUESTIONS

1. (LO 41.1) Which of the following is the *least* likely to occur with a geriatric patient?
   a. Incontinence
   b. Kyphosis
   c. Hyperbilirubinemia
   c. Polypharmacy
   e. Lentigos

2. (LO 41.1) Your 68-year-old patient suffers from pain and swelling of his left knee. He also has poor vision and hearing. He needs education about how to care for his knee. Which of the following would be the best technique?
   a. Looking at your patient education sheet, give him simple directions at his level
   b. Perform patient education in an open area of the clinic to prevent him from being uncomfortable
   c. Have him go to a small class to teach him about his care
   d. Speak in clear, high-pitched tones so that he can hear you
   e. Look directly at the patient, speaking slightly slower in low-pitched tones

3. (LO 41.2) Which of the following patients is *most* likely to suffer from urinary incontinence?
   a. A 78-year-old female patient with a prolapsed uterus
   b. A 65-year-old male patient with nocturia due to an enlarged prostate
   c. A 76-year-old female patient taking 12 different prescription medications and 2 over-the-counter supplements
   d. A 68-year-old male patient with a history of alcoholism
   e. An 82-year-old patient who uses a walker for ambulation

4. (LO 41.2) Your 68-year-old patient suffers from disorientation to time and place. Which of the following is the *most* likely problem?
   a. Cataracts
   b. Valvular disease
   c. Depression
   d. Alzheimer's disease
   e. Osteoporosis

5. (LO 41.3) When speaking to Peter Smith, which of the following is the best way to address him?

    a. Hi, Pete, how are you doing today?

    b. Mr. Smith, how are you feeling today?

    c. Sir, I would like to take your vital signs.

    d. What is your chief complaint today, mister?

    e. Hi there, honey, will you sit down right here so we can start the interview?

6. (LO 41.3) Your elderly patient refuses an immunization. Which of the following is the *least* likely reason?

    a. He is worried about the expense

    b. He had a severe reaction to a previous immunization

    c. He does not feel bad and does not want to feel bad

    d. He does not have time to wait for the injection

    e. He is afraid he will get the disease from the vaccine

7. (LO 41.3) When providing nutritional education for an elderly patient, which of the following statements is *most* accurate?

    a. You will need to decrease the amount of protein in your diet

    b. As you age, you will require more calories in your diet

    c. High-fiber food and plenty of water should be included in your diet

    d. Your daily intake of fat should be at least 30% or more

    e. The medications you take will not affect your dietary intake

8. (LO 41.2) Which medication would *most* likely be given to an elderly patient with congestive heart failure?

    a. Statin

    b. Glucophage®

    c. Actonel®

    d. Aricept®

    e. Digoxin

9. (LO 41.4) Which of following is *not* a practice of preventive medicine?

    a. Biopsy

    b. Colonoscopy

    c. Mammogram

    d. Immunization

    e. Pap smear

10. (LO 41.4) Which of the following patients is engaging in polypharmacy?

    a. A 78-year-old female patient with a prolapsed uterus

    b. A 65-year-old male patient with nocturia due to an enlarged prostate

    c. A 76-year-old female patient taking 12 different prescription medications and 2 over-the-counter supplements

    d. A 68-year-old male patient with a history of alcoholism

    e. An 82-year-old patient who uses a walker for ambulation

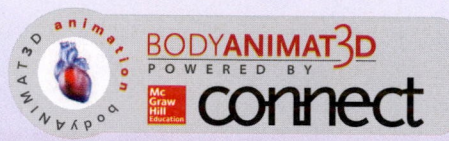

Go to CONNECT to see an animation exercise about *Alzheimer's Disease.*

SOFT SKILLS SUCCESS

You are assisting with an examination of an 80-year-old female patient who is at the clinic with her daughter. When the daughter steps out of the room to speak to the licensed practitioner, the patient states, "You know, she pinches me all the time." You note that she has some bruises on her left forearm. What should you do or say?

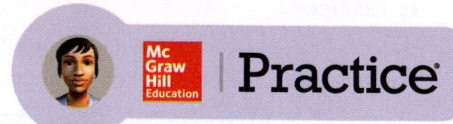

Go to PRACTICE MEDICAL OFFICE and complete the module Clinical - Interactions.

Assisting in Other Medical Specialties

CASE STUDY

Patient Name	DOB	Allergies
Valarie Ramirez	8/4/19XX	PCN

Attending	MRN	Other Information
Paul F. Buckwalter, MD	829-78-462	According to her chart, Valarie has lost 5 pounds in the last month but states that she has not been trying to diet.

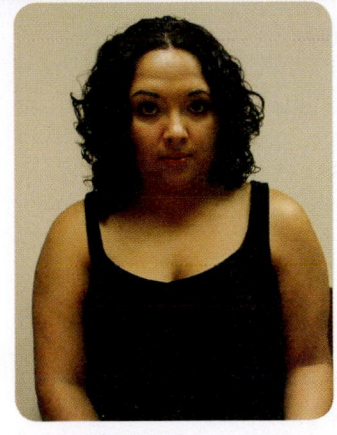

© McGraw-Hill Education

Valarie Ramirez, a 33-year-old female, arrives at the clinic for a follow-up check for the removal of a painful wart on her right hand. During the patient interview, she states she is not having trouble with her hand; however, she has noticed in the mirror that she has a lump on the front of her neck at the bottom. She is a little hoarse but denies any other symptoms. She thought she should tell the doctor. Her vital signs are BP 122/78 T 98.8 P 88 R 20 Ht. 5′ 2″ Wt. 135 lb. Dr. Buckwalter orders an ultrasound of the lump with needle biopsy if indicated. He also orders blood work, including TSH and CEA tests.

Keep Valarie in mind as you study this chapter. There will be questions at the end of the chapter based on the case study. The information in the chapter will help you answer these questions.

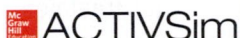

LEARNING OUTCOMES

After completing Chapter 42, you will be able to:

42.1 Describe the medical specialties of allergy, cardiology, dermatology, endocrinology, gastroenterology, neurology, oncology, and orthopedics.

42.2 Identify common diseases and disorders related to cardiology, dermatology, endocrinology, gastroenterology, neurology, oncology, and orthopedics.

42.3 Relate the role of the medical assistant in examinations and procedures performed in the medical specialties of allergy, cardiology, dermatology, endocrinology, gastroenterology, neurology, oncology, and orthopedics.

KEY TERMS

- angiography
- arthroscopy
- balloon angioplasty
- benign
- cardiac catheterization
- colonoscopy
- computed tomography
- coronary artery bypass graft (CABG)
- echocardiography
- endoscopy
- electroencephalography (EEG)
- electromyography
- intradermal test
- magnetic resonance imaging (MRI)
- malignant
- patch test
- positron emission tomography (PET)
- scratch test
- sigmoidoscopy
- stent
- Wood's light examination

I.C.8 Identify common pathology related to each body system including:
(a) signs
(b) symptoms
(c) etiology

I.C.9 Analyze pathology for each body system including:
(a) diagnostic measures
(b) treatment modalities

I.C.11 Identify the classifications of medications including:
(a) indications for use
(b) desired effects
(c) side effects
(d) adverse reactions

I.P.8 Instruct and prepare a patient for a procedure or a treatment

I.P.9 Assist provider with a patient exam

I.A.3 Show awareness of a patient's concerns related to the procedure being performed

V.P.4 Coach patients regarding:
(a) office policies
(b) health maintenance
(c) disease prevention
(d) treatment plan

V. A.3 Demonstrate respect for individual diversity including:
(a) gender
(b) race
(c) religion
(d) age
(e) economic status
(f) appearance

X.P.3 Document patient care accurately in the medical record

2. Anatomy and Physiology
a. List all body systems, their structure and functions
b. Describe common diseases, symptoms and etiologies as they apply to each system
c. Identify diagnostic and treatment modalities as they relate to each body system

3. Medical Terminology
c. Apply various medical terminology for each specialty

4. Medical Law and Ethics
a. Follow documentation guidelines

9. Medical Office Clinical Procedures
a. Practice standard precautions and perform disinfection/sterilization techniques
d. Assist provider with specialty examination including cardiac, respiratory, OB-GYN, neurological, gastroenterology procedures
e. Perform specialty procedures including but not limited to minor surgery, cardiac, respiratory, OB-GYN, neurological, gastroenterology
j. Make adaptations with patients with special needs

▶ Introduction

As a medical assistant, you may choose employment in a medical specialty. This chapter introduces you to many of the specialties, their diseases and disorders, the types of exams involved, and how the medical assistant can assist with diagnostic testing. Certain specialized tests and the correct methods to administer them also are included in this chapter. As with any other practice, when working in a medical specialty, keep in mind that you also perform basic administrative and clinical skills and will have the responsibility of communicating with and educating patients. Certain concerns and questions are common to patients within a specialty area. Being prepared to address these concerns and questions will allow you to help patients effectively and fulfill a vital role on the healthcare team.

▶ Working in Other Medical Specialties

LO 42.1

Licensed practitioners working in medical specialties focus on one body system (such as the skin) or a single type of disease (such as cancer). The medical specialties discussed here include allergy, cardiology, dermatology, endocrinology, gastroenterology, neurology, oncology, and orthopedics.

Using an Epinephrine Autoinjector

When working in a medical office that treats people with allergies, you must be familiar with epinephrine so that you can teach patients how to self-administer it. Epinephrine is a drug used to treat allergies so severe that exposure to the allergen may be life threatening. The following reactions indicate the possibility of anaphylaxis, or anaphylactic shock:

- Flushing
- Sharp drop in blood pressure
- Hives
- Difficulty breathing
- Difficulty swallowing
- Convulsions
- Vomiting
- Diarrhea and abdominal cramps

If a patient with a severe allergy experiences any or all of these symptoms, the reaction can be fatal unless emergency treatment is given immediately. So patients who cannot always control their exposure to an allergen—for example, bee or wasp venom—must have access to an epinephrine autoinjector for emergency intramuscular use. These prepackaged injectors (Figure 42-1) deliver either 0.3 mg of epinephrine—a single dose for an adult—or 0.15 mg of epinephrine—a single dose for a child. A patient who is exposed to the allergen should use the injector if the allergy is confirmed or if the allergy is suspected and signs of anaphylaxis appear. Teach the patient to follow these steps when using an autoinjector:

1. Remove the autoinjector from the packaging (box and/or plastic tube).
2. Pull back the gray cap.
3. Place the black tip of the injector on the outside of the upper thigh. (If needed, the injector can go through clothing.)
4. Press firmly into the thigh and hold for 10 seconds.
5. Remove the autoinjector and massage the injection site for a few minutes.
6. Call or have someone call 911 and go immediately to the nearest healthcare facility for follow-up care.

An autoinjector is for emergency supportive therapy only. It is not a replacement for immediate medical care. Make sure the patient is thoroughly familiar with the parts of the autoinjector, how to activate it, how to use it, and what to do next. Many injectors come packaged with a training injector for this task. If the patient is very young or otherwise unable to use the autoinjector reliably, teach a family member or companion how to use it. Additionally, "talking" autoinjectors are available and recommended for these patients.

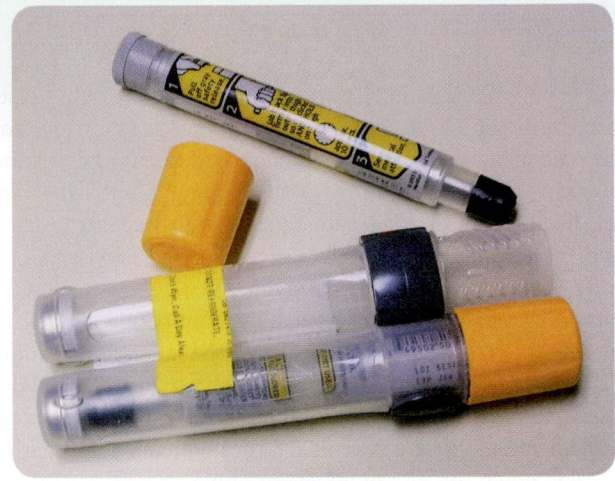

FIGURE 42-1 Epinephrine autoinjectors come prepackaged, containing the correct amount of the drug for an adult or a child.
© Leesa Whicker

Allergy

An allergist specializes in diagnosing and treating allergies. Allergies involve inappropriate immune system responses, or allergic reactions, to normally harmless substances called *allergens*. During an allergic reaction, inflammation and tissue damage occur. Common allergens include certain foods (such as eggs and nuts), pollens, medications, insect venom, and animal saliva or dander.

Allergic reactions may show themselves locally—with a skin rash or nasal congestion—or may manifest themselves throughout the body. The most severe kind of allergic reaction is anaphylaxis, or anaphylactic shock, which is life threatening. When anaphylaxis occurs, immediate medical intervention is needed to save the patient's life. You should know emergency medical intervention for anaphylaxis when preparing to work in an allergist's office. You may need to teach patients who have severe allergies how to use an epinephrine autoinjector. See the *Educating the Patient* feature.

Cardiology

A cardiologist is a physician who specializes in heart diseases and disorders. To assist a cardiologist, you must be familiar with the structure of the cardiovascular system and the typical exams and measurements associated with it. You also need to know about common heart diseases and their treatments. Many diagnostic tests are performed in this specialty, including electrocardiography and stress testing. Imaging techniques, such as X-rays and **echocardiography** (see Figure 42-2), also may be employed. You will assist with or perform some of these tests. Because managing a heart condition often involves many lifestyle changes, educating the patient about topics such as diet and exercise will be especially important in this specialty. You also will provide emotional support to patients with serious illnesses.

Dermatology

Dermatologists diagnose and treat skin diseases and disorders such as acne, eczema, and skin cancer. Some skin conditions

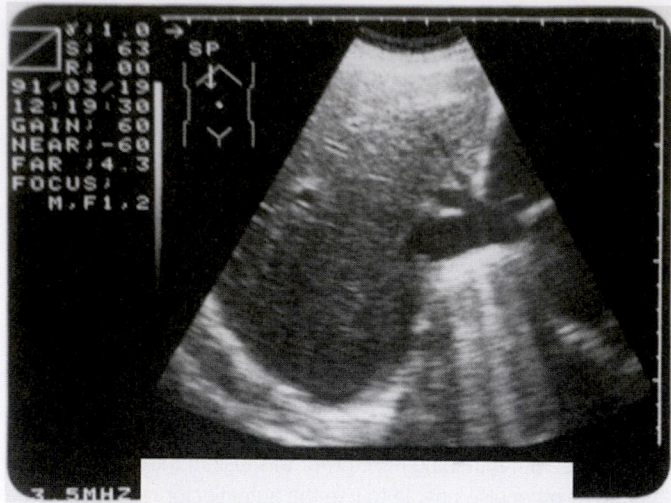

FIGURE 42-2 An echocardiograph shows the structures and function of the heart.

© Steve Allen/Getty Images RF

involve only the skin itself; others are a sign of disease else-where in the body. To assist in a dermatologist's office, you must understand the basic elements of dermatologic exams and procedures. In addition to developing familiarity with skin disorders and their treatments, you also need to under-stand the terminology used to describe skin lesions, as out-lined in the chapter *The Integumentary System.* Assisting with positioning and draping during a skin examination and taking skin scrapings or wound cultures might be among your duties in a dermatologist's office. You might perform procedures such as administering sunlamp treatments and applying topi-cal medications. You also will instruct patients about caring for a skin condition or wound site at home.

Endocrinology

Endocrinologists treat diseases and disorders of the endocrine system, which includes glands that regulate and coordinate the body's systems. Hormonal imbalances can affect the basic processes of growth, metabolism, and reproduction. Patients with thyroid imbalances, diabetes, or menopause frequently go to endocrinologists. In the endocrinologist's office, you will assist with exams and collect specimens for analysis.

Gastroenterology

Gastroenterologists diagnose and treat disorders of the entire gastrointestinal (GI) tract, from the mouth to the anus, as well as the liver and pancreas. Proctologists are another type of GI specialists. Unlike gastroenterologists, proctologists treat disorders of the rectum and anus only. A patient who sees a GI specialist has usually been referred by a family doctor, internist, or pediatrician who suspects a GI problem requiring additional expertise. You will need to understand the basic elements of GI exams and procedures to assist in a gastroenterologist's office. You also must be familiar with common GI disorders, their treatments, and the terminology used to describe them. In a gastroenterologist's office, you will tell patients how to prepare for a **colonoscopy** and other

exams and procedures performed in the office, a radiology facility, or a hospital. Colonoscopy is discussed later in this chapter.

Neurology

Neurologists diagnose and treat diseases and disorders of the central nervous system (CNS) and associated systems. Ner-vous system injuries or diseases can result in loss of sensa-tion, loss or impairment of voluntary movement, seizures, or mental confusion. Your duties in a neurologist's office include assisting with exams by readying equipment for use, positioning the patient, and handing the physician tools and other items. You may be asked to perform parts of these exams. You also may assist with certain diagnostic tests, such as **electroencephalography (EEG)** (see Figure 42-3). Your responsibilities may include instructing and educating patients and their families about procedures, disorders, and treatments.

Oncology

An oncologist specializes in the detection and treatment of tumors and cancerous growths. The term *cancer* refers to a number of oncologic diseases that affect different body sys-tems. All cancers are characterized by the uncontrolled growth and spread of abnormal cells. A tumor is a lump of abnormal cells. Tumors are classified as **benign** or **malignant.** Benign tumors contain abnormal cells, but the cells do not invade and actively destroy surrounding tissue. Malignant tumors contain cells that grow uncontrollably, invading and actively destroy-ing the tissue around them. Malignant, or cancerous, growths are capable of *metastasis*—the spreading of abnormal cells to body sites far removed from the original tumor. When cells become malignant, the process is called *carcinogenesis.* You will encounter patients with a variety of medical conditions in an oncologist's office, so you must be aware of the common types of cancer, what their symptoms are, and how they are treated (Table 42-1). Part of your job may involve preparing patients for the side effects of cancer treatment and helping patients deal with them. Patient and family education and sup-port are essential.

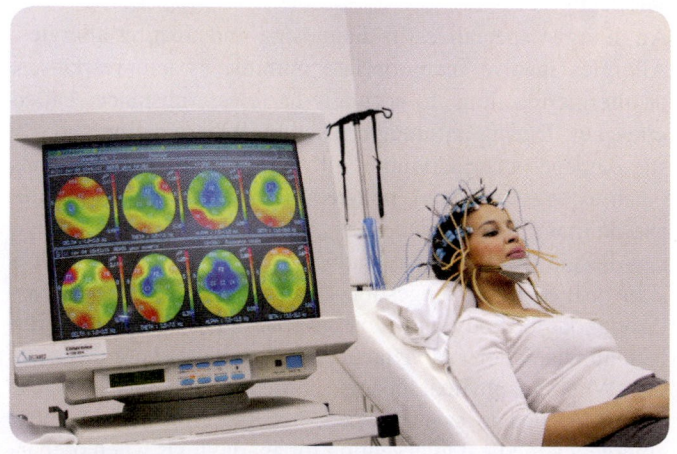

FIGURE 42-3 Electroencephalography (EEG) is performed by placing electrodes on the patient's forehead and scalp.

© AJ Photo/HOP Americain/SPL/Science Source

TABLE 42-1   Common Cancers by System

System	Cancer Type	Symptoms	Treatment
Reproductive (female)	Breast	Lump or thickening in breast, changed appearance, discharge	Surgery (lumpectomy or mastectomy), radiation, chemotherapy
	Endometrial	Postmenopausal bleeding	Surgery, radiation, chemotherapy
	Cervical	Usually none; possible painless vaginal bleeding and an abnormal Pap smear (Papanicolaou smear)	Surgery, radiation, chemotherapy
	Ovarian	Usually none; possible abdominal pain and bloating	Surgery, radiation, chemotherapy
Reproductive (male)	Prostate	Often none; possible difficult, frequent, or painful urination	Surgery, radiation, chemotherapy
	Testicular	Lump in testicle	Surgery, radiation, chemotherapy
Respiratory	Lung (including bronchus)	Often no early symptoms; later, new cough or cold that lingers; chest, shoulder, and/or back pain; wheezing and shortness of breath; hoarseness; coughing up blood; swelling in the face and neck; difficulty in swallowing; weight loss and anorexia; increased fatigue; recurrent respiratory infections	Surgery, radiation, chemotherapy
Digestive	Colorectal	Changes in bowel habits, blood in stools, rectal or abdominal pain	Surgery combined with radiation or chemotherapy
	Liver	Abdominal pain, fatigue, jaundice	Surgery, liver transplant
	Esophageal	Often no early symptoms; later, difficulty swallowing and/or regurgitation of food	Surgery, radiation, chemotherapy
	Oral (mouth and throat)	May begin with painless sore or mass; later, difficulty chewing or swallowing	Surgery, radiation, chemotherapy
	Stomach	Indigestion, weight loss, nausea	Surgery, chemotherapy
Circulatory	Leukemia (all types)	Fatigue, paleness, repeated infections	Chemotherapy, bone marrow transplants
	Non-Hodgkin's lymphoma	Enlarged lymph nodes, itching, fever, weight loss	Chemotherapy, radiation
Urinary	Kidney (renal cell)	Blood in urine, pain in side that does not go away; lump or mass in side or abdomen; weight loss for no known reason; fever; feeling very tired	Surgery, targeted therapy, radiation therapy
	Bladder	Blood in urine; urgent need to empty bladder; urinary frequency; feeling the need to empty the bladder without results; feeling pain when emptying the bladder	Surgery, chemotherapy, biological therapy, radiation therapy
Endocrine	Thyroid	A lump in the front of the neck; hoarseness or voice changes; swollen lymph nodes in the neck; trouble swallowing or breathing; pain in the throat or neck that does not go away	Surgery, thyroid hormone therapy, radioactive iodine therapy, external radiation therapy, chemotherapy
	Pancreatic	Dark urine, pale stools, and yellow skin and eyes from jaundice; pain in the upper part of the abdomen; pain in the middle part of the back that does not go away when shifting position; nausea and vomiting; stools that float in the toilet	Surgery, chemotherapy, targeted therapy, radiation therapy
Nervous	Malignant tumors of brain and brainstem	Headaches, nausea, and vomiting; changes in speech, vision, or hearing; problems balancing or walking; changes in mood, personality, or ability to concentrate; problems with memory; muscle jerking or twitching; numbness or tingling in the arms or legs	Surgery, radiation, chemotherapy
Skeletal	Osteosarcoma (most often in knee and upper arm)	Persistent, unusual pain or swelling in or near a bone	Surgery, chemotherapy, radiation therapy, immunotherapy, cryosurgery, vaccine therapy
	Chondrosarcomas: malignant tumors of cartilage (most often in hip, femur, humerus)	Usually no early symptoms; later, patients may feel a bony bump with pain, swelling, and limited movement of the affected bone	Surgery

Source: Adapted from American Cancer Society (http://www.cancer.org) and National Cancer Institute (http://www.cancer.gov).

Orthopedics

Orthopedics is the medical specialty focusing on disorders, injuries, and diseases of the muscular and skeletal systems. The two systems are so interdependent they are sometimes referred to as the musculoskeletal system, especially by orthopedists. In an orthopedist's office, you will be asked to assist with general exams. Other responsibilities may include assisting with X-rays, helping with casting, applying hot or cold treatments, and educating patients about therapy regimens.

▶ Diseases and Disorders of Medical Specialties   LO 42.2

The medical assistant working in medical specialties should have a basic knowledge of the diseases and disorders related to these specialties. Understanding the conditions that commonly occur in certain medical specialties will improve your ability to assist the licensed practitioner and patients.

Cardiology Diseases and Disorders

Cardiology is a common specialty practice because of the prevalence of cardiovascular diseases and disorders. Every year since 1918, the number one cause of death in the United States has been cardiovascular disease, or a disease of the heart and blood vessels. Approximately 2,500 Americans die every day from coronary artery disease (CAD)—narrowing of the blood vessels surrounding the heart that causes a reduction of blood flow to the heart. Cardiovascular disease claims more lives than the next four leading causes of death combined. Unbelievably, one of every three American adults has some form of CAD. You may know someone who has hypertension (high blood pressure) or other heart conditions. Maybe someone you know has had a myocardial infarction (MI), or heart attack. Several factors put patients at risk for heart disease, including inactivity, obesity, high blood pressure, cigarette smoking, high cholesterol, and diabetes. As a medical assistant working in a cardiology office, you should be able to teach patients about ways to reduce or prevent heart disease, stroke, and heart attack (see Table 42-2). Many of the diseases or disorders seen in a cardiology office are outlined in Table 42-3. Treatment for cardiovascular disease frequently includes medications, discussed in the *Principles of Pharmacology* chapter.

Dermatologic Conditions and Disorders

The condition of the skin plays a large part in a person's appearance. Patients with skin disorders, therefore, may worry about their attractiveness to and acceptance by others. Allow patients to express their anxieties; in return, provide encouragement about the course and outcome of their treatment. Table 42-4 discusses some of the most common dermatologic conditions and disorders. These and other diseases and disorders of the skin and accessory organs are discussed in the chapter *The Integumentary System*.

Endocrine Diseases and Disorders

The most common diseases and disorders seen in an endocrinologist's office are those related to the pancreas, thyroid, and

TABLE 42-2	Ways to Reduce or Prevent Heart Disease, Stroke, and Heart Attack

The American Heart Association now recommends that you watch your ABCs:

A. Avoid tobacco.
1. Stop smoking. A smoker's risk is twice that of a nonsmoker. Even exposure to environmental tobacco smoke (secondhand smoke, passive smoking) may increase heart disease risk.
2. Decrease stress.
3. Maintain healthy blood pressure. Find ways to lower blood pressure and to keep the numbers down. The goal is a blood pressure of less than 120/80 mmHg.
4. Maintain healthy blood cholesterol. Cholesterol will cause fat to lodge in your arteries, sooner or later causing a heart attack or stroke. Keep the total cholesterol less than 200 mg/dL.

B. Be more active.
1. Increase physical activity. The goal is to increase physical activity to 30 to 60 minutes on most days of the week. Increasing activity will decrease the following:
   a. Stress
   b. High blood pressure
   c. High blood cholesterol
   d. Obesity

C. Choose good nutrition. Maintain a well-balanced diet, which helps to decrease the following:
1. Alcohol consumption
2. Stress
3. High blood cholesterol
4. Diabetes
5. Obesity

Source: Adapted from The American Heart Association's guidelines.

reproductive organs. However, an endocrinologist would treat any disorder related to the endocrine system. Diabetes occurs when the pancreas does not secrete enough insulin or the body is resistant to insulin. A deficiency of insulin or a resistance to it interferes with the metabolism of carbohydrates, proteins, and fats, raising the glucose level in the blood. This condition is known as *hyperglycemia*. The symptoms of diabetes are often subtle and include frequent urination, excessive thirst, extreme hunger, unexplained weight loss, fatigue, and blurry vision. Common types of diabetes are Type 1, Type 2, and gestational diabetes, discussed in the chapter *The Endocrine System*. No matter the type of diabetes, the goal is basically the same: Keep blood sugar levels within a normal range, eat a healthy diet, exercise regularly, and see a healthcare provider routinely (see Figure 42-4).

Disorders related to the thyroid gland include hypothyroidism and hyperthyroidism. Hypothyroidism is characterized by decreased activity of the thyroid gland and underproduction of the hormone thyroxine. This shortage can cause cretinism in children, with resulting mental and physical disabilities. Underproduction of thyroxine in adults results in myxedema. Patients with this condition have fatigue, low blood pressure, dry skin and hair, facial puffiness, and goiter or an enlarged thyroid gland. Treatment for hypothyroidism consists of thyroid hormone supplements.

TABLE 42-3 Cardiovascular Diseases

Category of Disease/Disorder	Common Conditions*	Treatment
Arterial/vascular disorders	Aneurysm	Medication, surgery
	Arteriosclerosis	Medication, lifestyle and diet management, surgery
	Atherosclerosis	Medication, lifestyle and diet management, surgery
	Hypertension	Medication, lifestyle and diet management, stress management
	Varicose veins	Elastic stockings, weight loss, elevation of legs, surgery
Coronary artery disease	Angina pectoris	Medication, rest, lifestyle management
	Myocardial infarction	Medication, oxygen administration, rest, lifestyle management
Dysrhythmias	Atrial fibrillation	Medication, cardioversion (electric shock to the heart)
	Conduction delays or blocks (problems with electrical transmission within the heart)	Medication, pacemaker
	Tachycardia	Medication, diet management
Heart failure	Congestive heart failure	Medication, diet management, rest
	Cardiomyopathy (weakening of the heart muscle)	Medication, heart transplant
Inflammation of the heart tissue	Endocarditis (inflammation of heart lining and valves)	Medication, valve surgery
	Myocarditis	Specific treatment for underlying cause, medication, rest
	Pericarditis	Medication, rest
Valvular diseases	Aortic stenosis	Surgical replacement of valve
	Mitral stenosis	Medication, rest, valve surgery
	Mitral valve prolapse	Medication (usually antibiotic prophylaxis to prevent subacute bacterial endocarditis)

*Cardiovascular diseases and disorders are described in more detail in the chapter *The Cardiovascular System*.

Hyperthyroidism, also called Graves' disease, is characterized by increased thyroid gland activity. The patient has anxiety, irritability, elevated heart rate and blood pressure, tremors, and weight loss despite an increased appetite. Treatment includes the administration of radioactive iodine, antithyroid drugs, or surgery to remove part or all of the thyroid gland. Many patients require supplemental thyroid hormones following treatment for a hyperactive thyroid.

Gastrointestinal Diseases and Disorders

The level of discomfort from GI disorders can be misleading in relation to severity. There may be severe pain with intestinal gas, which is not serious, whereas there is virtually no pain in the initial stage of appendicitis, which is potentially life threatening. Be sure your notes are accurate and complete when a patient reports GI symptoms. Note the level of the patient's pain, whether over-the-counter (OTC) drugs have been administered, and if so, whether the OTC drugs provided any relief. Common diseases and disorders treated by a GI specialist are outlined in Table 42-5 and discussed in the chapter *The Digestive System*.

Neurologic Diseases and Disorders

Common diseases of the neurologic system are described in Table 42-6. Trauma can also cause damage to the nervous system; such injuries can result in loss of sensation and voluntary motion. You should know the terms related to the various types of sensation loss:

- Hemiplegia: paralysis on one side of the body commonly caused by a stroke, brain or spinal cord injury, or tumor
- Paraplegia: paralysis in the lower extremities
- Quadriplegia: paralysis of the arms, legs, and all muscles below a cervical (neck) spinal injury

Encephalopathy is a term for a disease of the brain that alters brain function or structure. Encephalopathy may be caused by an infectious agent, a metabolic dysfunction, a brain tumor, increased pressure in the skull, prolonged exposure to toxic elements, chronic progressive trauma, poor nutrition, or lack of oxygen or blood flow to the brain. The most prevalent sign of encephalopathy is an altered mental state. Common neurologic symptoms of encephalopathy are progressive loss of memory and cognitive ability, slight personality changes, inability to concentrate, lethargy, and progressive loss of consciousness.

Orthopedic Diseases and Disorders

Table 42-7 lists many of the diseases and disorders you will encounter in an orthopedic specialty. For example, back

TABLE 42-4   Common Dermatologic Conditions and Disorders

Condition	Description/Symptoms	Treatment/Prevention
Acne vulgaris (acne) © Dr. Harout Tanielian/Science Source	Inflammation of the follicles of the skin's sebaceous (oil) glands, causing skin eruptions. Pimples, blackheads, and cysts are seen on the face, back, and other areas.	Antibiotics, contraceptives, and retinoid are used to manage the outbreaks. Retinoid can damage a fetus, so it is not taken if a woman is pregnant or could get pregnant.
Contact dermatitis © John Kaprielian/Science Source	Caused by irritants such as rough fabrics, cosmetics, pollen, or plants such as poison ivy or poison oak. Symptoms include redness, itching, edema, and lesions.	Treatment depends on the cause and type of lesions. Anti-inflammatory medications or antihistamines; oral corticosteroids are prescribed for severe inflammation.
Eczema © Michel Jolyot/Science Source	Skin inflammation that may be an allergic response to allergens, such as chemicals or foods.	Combination of therapy and lifestyle changes to control flare-ups; oral or topical (applied to the skin) medication and phototherapy (light therapy).
Mole © Lea Paterson/Science Source	Raised or unraised brown, black, or tan spot less than 6 mm in diameter. Has even coloring and a round or oval shape and clear borders. Monitor for bleeding, itching, or changes in color, size, shape, or texture.	May be surgically removed.
Psoriasis © Biophoto Associates/Science Source	Patches of red, thickened skin with silver scales mostly found on the knees, elbows, scalp, face, palms, and soles of the feet. More common in adults than in children. Diagnosed through microscopic exam of skin scrapings.	Topical creams and ointments, light therapy, and systemic and combination therapies.
Ringworm © Dr. Lucille K. George/CDC	Most often affects the feet (athlete's foot, or tinea pedis), groin (jock itch, or tinea cruris), and scalp (tinea capitis). Flat lesions are dry and scaly or moist and crusty, and develop a clear center with an outer ring. Creates scaly bald patches on scalp.	Topical antifungal medications; oral medications if severe. Contagious, so patient should not share bedding, combs, towels, or other personal items.
Warts (verrucae) © Biophoto Associates/Science Source	Benign skin tumors that result from a viral skin infection. If a wart is scratched open, the virus may spread by contact to another part of the body or to another person. Several kinds: • Common warts are raised, rounded, flesh-colored lesions that usually occur on the hands and fingers. • Plantar warts appear on the soles of the feet. • Venereal warts appear on the genitalia and anus and are transmitted through sexual contact.	Treatment depends on the type of wart. Some warts go away without treatment. Removed by burning or freezing the wart tissue. Instruct the patient to keep the wart removal site clean and dry until a scab forms or the wart falls off.

(continued)

TABLE 42-4	Common Dermatologic Conditions and Disorders	
Condition	**Description/Symptoms**	**Treatment/Prevention**
Skin Cancer		
Basal cell carcinoma © Dr. P. Marazzi / Science Source	Risk factors: overexposure to the sun, X-rays, irritants, various chemical carcinogens, presence of premalignant lesions. Most common are malignant basal cell carcinomas on areas exposed to the sun, such as the face and neck. Higher-than-average risk of developing skin cancer: those who have had severe, blistering sunburns in their teens or 20s; those who have fair skin and hair and light-colored eyes; and those who work outdoors.	Treatments for skin cancer vary with the type of cancer and its extent. Treatments include surgery, electrosurgery, cryosurgery, radiation therapy, and chemotherapy.
Squamous cell carcinoma © Biophoto Associates/Science Source	Appears on sun-exposed areas and looks ulcerated or has a crust. Invades deeper into the skin and has a greater tendency to spread to other body areas.	Treatments for skin cancer vary with the type of cancer and its extent. Treatments include surgery, electrosurgery, cryosurgery, radiation therapy, and chemotherapy.
Malignant melanoma © Tom Myers/Science Source	Originates in cells that produce the pigment melanin; this is the most dangerous type of skin cancer. Malignant cells may spread through the bloodstream or lymphatic system to the liver, lungs, and other parts of the body. A sudden or continuous change in the appearance of a mole may signal melanoma.	Treatments for skin cancer vary with the type of cancer and its extent. Treatments include surgery, electrosurgery, cryosurgery, radiation therapy, and chemotherapy.

pain—especially lower back pain—is a common disorder. It can have many causes, including muscle strain, osteoarthritis, and the presence of a tumor. Treatments include the application of heat, the administration of analgesics or muscle relaxants, exercise therapy, special braces, traction, and surgery.

Another condition commonly encountered in the orthopedist's office is a fracture, or break in a bone. Fractures and their treatment are discussed in detail in the *Emergency Preparedness* chapter.

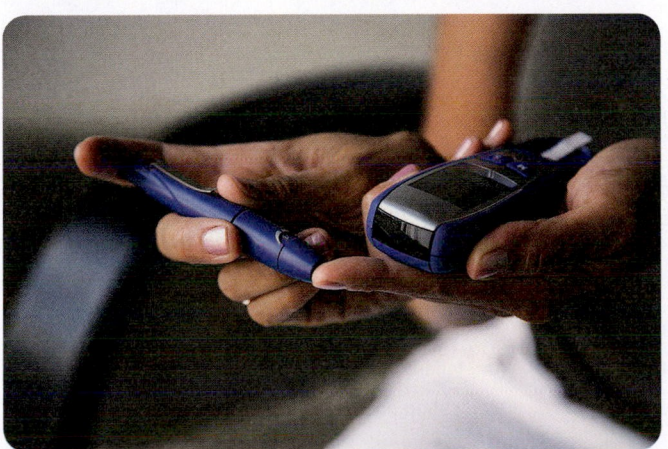

FIGURE 42-4 Patients with diabetes can use a glucometer to monitor their own blood glucose levels.
© Purestock/Getty Images RF

▶ Exams and Procedures in Medical Specialties
LO 42.3

As a medical assistant, understanding the anatomy and physiology of various body systems and the specific exam and procedural steps for each specialty area is key. Most specialists' offices have a procedure manual for you to use as a reference when learning new procedures. You will assist with exams and procedures and perform certain procedures on your own. This section will introduce you to basic exams and procedures performed in medical specialties.

Allergy Exams and Testing

An allergy exam involves a medical history and, usually, several diagnostic tests. You may assist with these tests or perform them yourself under a licensed practitioner's supervision. Skin tests, for example, involve introducing solutions containing suspected allergens onto or just below the skin. Any reaction is observed and assessed.

Allergy treatments include allergen avoidance, medications, and desensitization to a substance by means of injections. Part of your job will be to encourage patients to make necessary lifestyle changes to avoid allergens. See *Educating the Patient:* Creating a Dust-Free Environment. You also will help patients adhere to regimens of injections or medication.

TABLE 42-5 Common Gastrointestinal Diseases and Disorders

Condition*	Description	Treatment
Anal fissure	Ulcer in anal wall; may develop into fistula (an abnormal duct to the rectum)	Depends on extent; may require surgery to repair
Cholecystitis	Inflammation of the gallbladder caused by gallstones, tumor, or bile duct blockage; symptoms are pain, nausea, diarrhea	Avoidance of fatty foods if intolerant; lithotripsy to break up stones; antibiotic for bacterial infection
Cholelithiasis	Gallstones	Lithotripsy, antibiotics to prevent secondary infection or a cholecystectomy (removal of the gallbladder)
Colitis	Inflammation of the colon caused by bacteria, food intolerance, anxiety, or emotional disorder	Diet modification (clear liquid for acute phase), medication, psychotherapy, fluid replacement, colostomy for severe cases
Constipation	Having fewer than three bowel movements a week along with hard feces that are difficult and painful to pass.	Diet modification, stool-softener medication, enema, surgery if necessary for impaction
Diarrhea	Abnormally frequent, watery bowel movements	Diet modification, antibiotics for bacterial infection, fluids and medication to prevent dehydration
Diverticulitis	Inflammation of diverticulum	Diet modification, surgery for severe cases
Gastritis	Inflammation of stomach lining	Diet modification, drug therapy
Gastroesophageal reflux (GERD)	Gastric acid rising from stomach into esophagus	Diet modification, small meals, antacids, upright eating, remaining upright for several hours after eating, surgery (rarely)
Hemorrhoids	Enlargement of rectal or anal veins	Diet modification, surgery
Hernia	Organ pushes through a muscle or wall containing it; common abdominal hernias include hiatal hernia and inguinal hernia	Surgery to repair muscle
Stomatitis (canker sores)	Sore gums or other oral areas caused by herpes virus or acidic body chemistry; exacerbated by emotional distress, acidic foods; symptoms are ulcerations (canker sores) with burning, sometimes swelling	Bland diet, avoidance of stress, medicated mouth rinses, topical anesthetic

* Gastrointestinal diseases and disorders are described in more detail in the chapter *The Digestive System*.

TABLE 42-6 Common Diseases of the Neurologic System

Condition*	Description	Treatment
Alzheimer's disease	Disabling disease that involves dementia and deterioration of physical function	Frequent stimulation to possibly help slow deterioration, and medications that may slow progression of some symptoms
Bell's palsy	Disease that causes sudden weakness or paralysis on one side of the face because of damage to the facial nerve	Usually resolves without treatment in 1 to 8 weeks
Encephalitis	Inflammation of brain tissue usually caused by viral infection; symptoms: fever, headache, vomiting, stiff neck, drowsiness	Medication, rest
Epilepsy	Disease caused by misfiring of nerve groups in the brain, resulting in seizures	Medication
Herpes zoster	Disease caused by the virus that causes chickenpox; symptoms: painful blisters that form along path of one or more nerves	Medication to relieve pain
Meningitis	Inflammation of the meninges	Antibiotics and drugs to reduce swelling
Migraine headaches	Severe headaches caused by vascular disturbance	Medication
Multiple sclerosis	Degenerative disease of the central nervous system	Anti-inflammatory medications
Neuritis	Inflammation of one or more nerves; symptoms: severe pain and discomfort or paralysis of the affected area	Medication and rest
Parkinson's disease	Progressive neurological disease	Medication to relieve symptoms
Sciatica	Inflammation of the sciatic nerve	Medication to relieve pain, rest, heat applications

*Neurologic diseases and disorders are described in more detail in the chapter *The Nervous System*.

TABLE 42-7 Common Diseases and Disorders of the Musculoskeletal System

Condition*	Description	Treatment
Arthritis	Inflammation of joints	Anti-inflammatory medications, heat, rest, exercise, occupational and physical therapy, surgery (arthroplasty)
Bursitis	Inflammation of one or more bursae (sacs surrounding joints)	Anti-inflammatory medications
Carpal tunnel syndrome	Compression of the median nerve, causing wrist pain and numbness	Rest and occupational adjustments, splinting of wrists, injection of corticosteroids, surgical decompression of nerve
Dislocation	Displacement of bones at joint so that parts that are supposed to make contact no longer come together; occurs most often to fingers, shoulder, knee, and hip	Relocation, or shifting bones back into place; anti-inflammatory medications
Herniated intervertebral disk (HID)	Protruding contents of disk compress nerve roots, causing severe pain	Rest, traction, physical therapy, muscle relaxants, surgery
Osteomyelitis	Infection of bone; principal symptom is pain	Antibiotics and analgesics, surgery
Osteoporosis	Decreased bone mass, resulting in brittle, easily fractured bones	Exercise, dietary supplements, hormone therapy, drug therapy
Paget's disease	Chronic condition that causes bone deformities	Exercise, dietary supplements, hormone therapy, drug therapy
Scoliosis	Abnormal curving of spine	Back brace, surgery
Sprain	Injury to ligament caused by joint overextension	Rest, support, application of cold, anti-inflammatory medications
Tendonitis	Inflammation of tendon	Rest, support, anti-inflammatory medications

*Musculoskeletal diseases and disorders are described in more detail in the chapters *The Skeletal System* and *The Muscular System*.

Three tests are commonly performed in the allergist's office: the **scratch test,** the **intradermal test,** and the **patch test.** The *radioallergosorbent (RAST)* test is performed in a laboratory. Prior to a scratch, patch, or intradermal test, patients are asked to stop taking antihistamines and steroids. These medications could interfere with the test results. The RAST test has the advantage of allowing patients to continue to take antihistamines to control their allergies while being tested.

Scratch Test A scratch test tests the patient for specific allergies. Extracts of suspected allergens are applied to the patient's skin, usually on the arms or back. One site is always a negative control—a solution like the one used to carry the allergens but containing no allergen is applied. Then the skin is scratched to allow the extracts to penetrate. A scratch test may be performed using sterile needles or lancets. Some allergists prefer to use applicators that allow the tester to apply allergens to and puncture the skin in several places at once, as shown in Figure 42-5. Be sure to let the patient know the procedure may cause some discomfort and that itching afterward can be relieved with cold packs. See Procedure 42-1 at the end of this chapter. The licensed practitioner interprets the test results. Because a delayed reaction is possible, the practitioner may wish to recheck the scratch sites in 24 hours. When the results of the scratch test are inconclusive, another test, such as an intradermal test, may be ordered.

Intradermal Test This test introduces dilute solutions of allergens into the skin of the inner forearm or upper back with a fine-gauge needle. The intradermal test is more sensitive than the scratch test. A small blister, also known as a wheal, which is filled with the introduced fluid, appears on the skin over the injection site. The allergic reaction time is about 15

EDUCATING THE PATIENT

Creating a Dust-Free Environment

Patients with household dust allergies will need to reduce their dust exposure as much as possible. One way they can do this is to keep their environment, especially their bedroom, as clean as possible. Share these guidelines from The National Institute of Allergy and Infectious Diseases with your patients.

- Prepare the room by removing all contents, cleaning and scrubbing all woodwork, removing carpeting and drapery (if possible), and closing doors and windows. Maintain the room by cleaning it thoroughly once a week. This includes floors, the tops of doors, and windowsills and frames. Use a special vacuum filter and wash any curtains often.

- Keep the bed and bedding as dust free as possible by encasing box springs and mattress in a dustproof cover and washing all pajamas in 130°F water.

- Keep furniture in the room to a minimum, use furnace air filters (high-efficiency particulate absorption [HEPA] filters are best), avoid stuffed animals, and keep pets out of the bedroom.

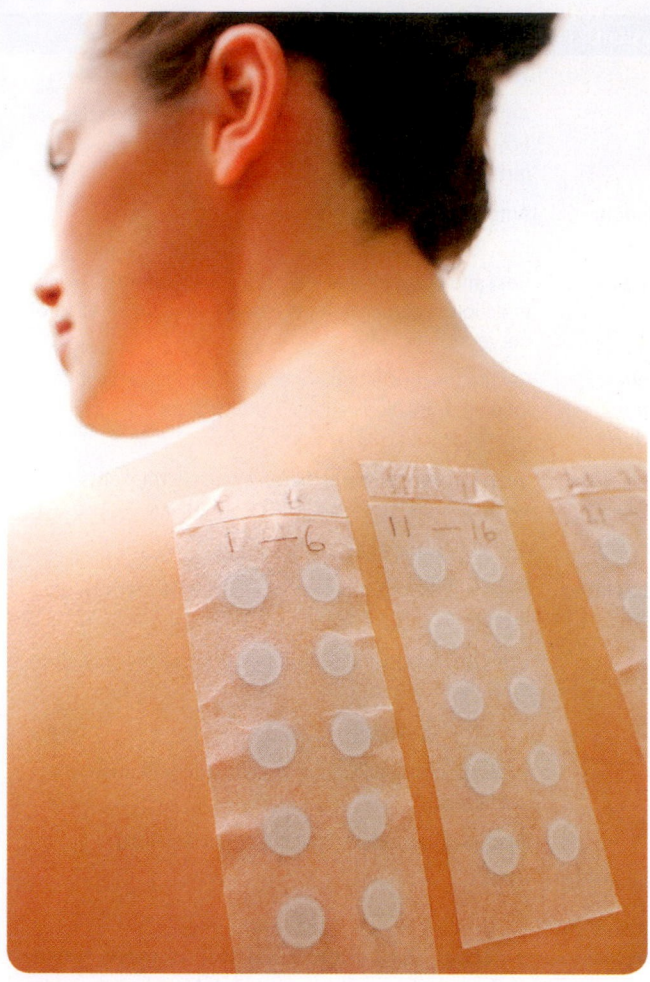

FIGURE 42-5 A multiple applicator allows the medical assistant to apply several allergens at one time.
© Science Photo Library/agefotostock RF

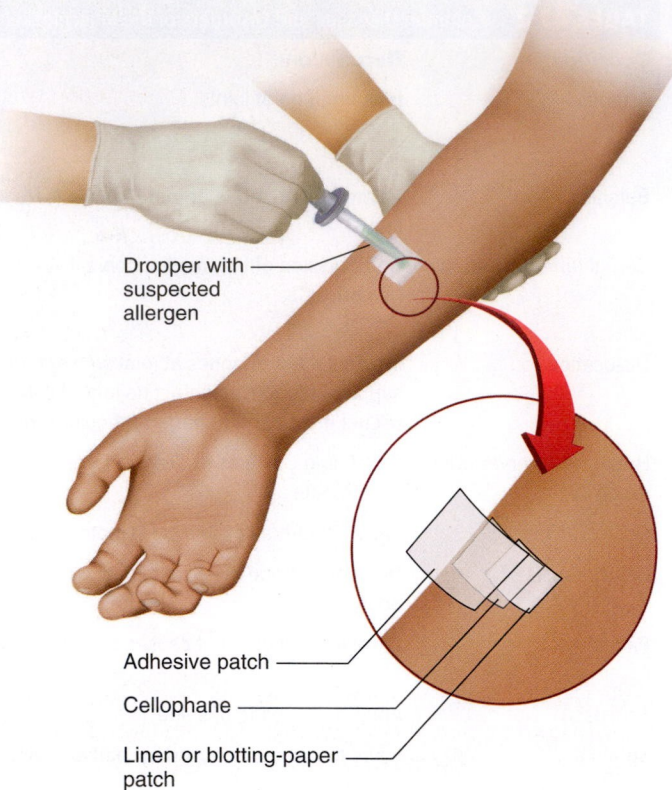

Dropper with suspected allergen

Adhesive patch

Cellophane

Linen or blotting-paper patch

FIGURE 42-6 A patch test is usually done on the arm and is read in 48 hours.

to 30 minutes, although some substances may cause delayed reactions. If no reaction appears, the test can be repeated with a more concentrated solution to confirm the result. If a severe reaction occurs, the licensed practitioner will order epinephrine to be administered.

The tuberculin test, or purified protein derivative (PPD) test, is a type of intradermal skin test. An extract from the tubercle bacillus is injected into the skin. The results are read in 48 to 72 hours. Raising and hardening of the skin around the area (induration), rather than redness alone, indicate a positive reaction. The procedure for administering an intradermal injection is found in the *Medication Administration* chapter.

Patch Test You perform a patch test by placing a linen or paper patch on uninvolved skin and then using a dropper to soak the patch with the suspected allergen (Figure 42-6). Cellophane or another occlusive material, usually covered with an adhesive patch, is then applied over the linen or paper patch. Among other things, this test is used to discover the cause of contact dermatitis.

Radioallergosorbent Test (RAST) The RAST measures blood levels of antibodies to specific allergens. You

obtain a blood sample from the patient and send it to a laboratory. There, the blood serum is exposed to suspected allergens and the levels of antibodies are measured. This test usually provides more information than skin testing but is more expensive.

Cardiology Exams

A general cardiovascular exam usually begins with a blood pressure reading and an evaluation of overall cardiac health. The cardiologist also palpates the chest wall and the vessels in the extremities to detect abnormal vibrations, pulses, swelling, or temperature. In addition, an electrocardiogram may be obtained.

Electrocardiogram An electrocardiogram (ECG or EKG) provides a measurement of the heart's electrical activity. Electrocardiography—a routine part of a cardiovascular exam—is a painless and safe diagnostic test. Electrodes are placed on the skin in particular areas of the chest and limbs. The heart's electrical activity is shown as a tracing on a strip of graph paper. Review the full procedure for performing an ECG in the *Cardiovascular and Respiratory Testing* chapter.

Stress Test An exercise stress test involves recording an ECG while the patient is exercising on a stationary bicycle, treadmill, or stair-stepping ergometer (see Figure 42-7). This test measures the patient's response to a constant or increasing workload. Part of your job may involve keeping the equipment properly maintained and calibrated. You also may be responsible for administering the test itself, but a licensed practitioner should always be present because of the risk of cardiac

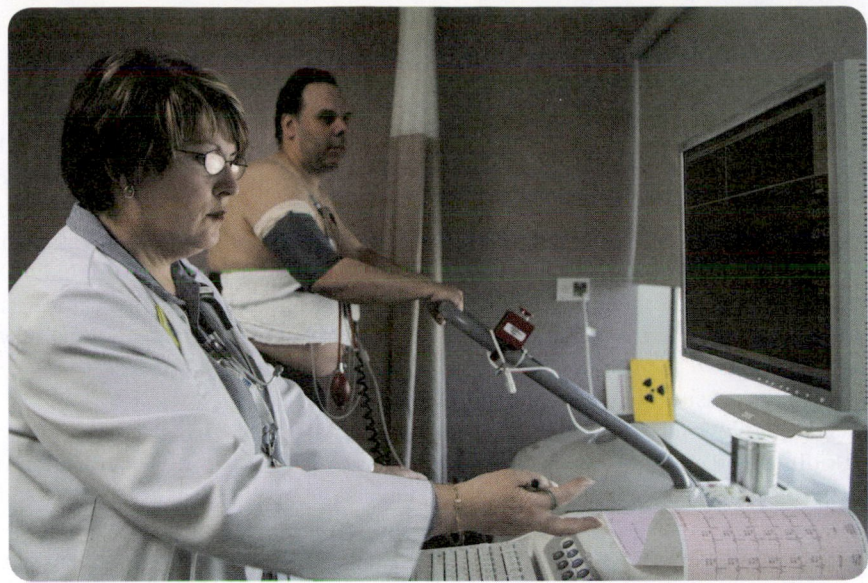

FIGURE 42-7 A stress test measures the electrical activity of the heart under a constant or increasing amount of exertion.
© BSIP/Newscom

crisis. Before the test, the patient has a screening appointment with the licensed practitioner, during which you take a careful medical history and explain pretest requirements. On the day of the test, be sure the patient has followed pretest directions, such as abstaining from smoking or consuming alcohol, and has signed the proper consent form. The patient is prepared as for an ECG by having electrodes attached to the skin. Show the patient how to use the exercise device. Review additional information regarding exercise electrocardiography (stress testing) in the *Cardiovascular and Respiratory Testing* chapter.

Variations on the basic stress test are the chemical stress test and the nuclear stress test. Chemical stress tests are performed when a patient is unable to perform the physical exercise required by a basic stress test. A chemical that mimics the effect of exercise on the heart is injected through an IV line. A nuclear stress test is similar to a chemical stress test, except that radioactive tracers (radionuclides) are injected so that the licensed practitioner can trace the path of blood through the heart.

Holter Monitor This is an ECG device that includes a digital recorder, allowing readings to be taken over a specific period of time. Electrodes are attached to the patient's chest in the licensed practitioner's office. Lead wires are attached to the electrodes and to the portable recording device, which the patient wears on a belt or sling (Figure 42-8). The patient returns home, and the device monitors heart activity for 24 or more hours. Review additional information regarding ambulatory electrocardiography (Holter monitoring) in the *Cardiovascular and Respiratory Testing* chapter.

Radiography and Imaging Techniques

Various radiographic techniques are used in cardiology. Chest X-rays can reveal conditions such as cardiac enlargement. In radionuclide studies, the patient ingests or is injected with a radioactive contrast medium, often referred to as a dye. X-rays are then taken. For example, fluoroscopy studies are X-ray exams

in which a contrast medium is injected and pictures of the heart in motion are projected onto a closed-circuit television screen. A venogram allows evaluation of the deep veins of the legs. **Angiography** is an X-ray examination of a blood vessel after the injection of a contrast medium. The test, performed in a hospital, evaluates the function and structure of one or more arteries.

Ultrasound, a noninvasive diagnostic method, is also used in cardiology. Doppler ultrasonography tests the body's main blood vessels for conditions such as weaknesses in vessel walls or blocked arteries. With the use of a handheld probe, sound waves are transmitted through the skin and are reflected by the blood cells moving through the blood vessels.

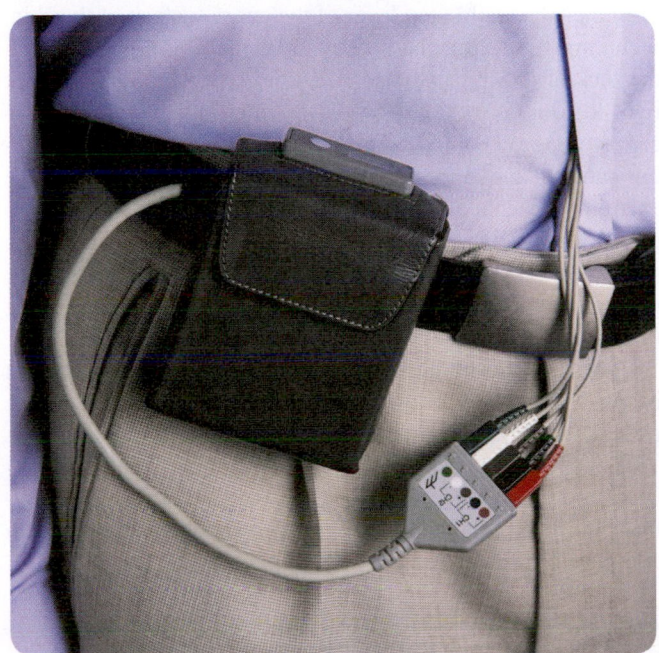

FIGURE 42-8 A Holter monitor allows the licensed practitioner to assess heart function during periods of normal activity.
© Sheila Terry/Science Source

Echocardiography tests the structure and function of the heart through the use of reflected sound waves, or echoes. Sound waves of an extremely high frequency are projected through the chest wall into the heart and are reflected back through a mechanical device. The echoes, recorded on paper or video, can indicate conditions such as structural defects and fluid accumulation.

Heart magnetic resonance imaging (MRI) is a diagnostic procedure that uses strong magnets and radio waves to produce images of the heart. This procedure is noninvasive and does not use ionizing radiation, so it is safer than other imaging techniques. Detailed pictures of the heart and heart vessels can be obtained using heart MRI.

Cardiac catheterization is an invasive diagnostic method in which a catheter (a slender, hollow tube) is inserted into a vein or an artery in the right or left arm or leg and passed through the blood vessels into the heart. The cardiologist can use this method to take blood samples for analysis, measure the pressure in the heart's chambers, and view the heart's motions with the aid of fluoroscopy. During cardiac catheterization, the cardiologist may choose to perform a **balloon angioplasty** to open partially blocked coronary arteries. This procedure involves passing a slender, hollow tube through the artery at the blockage site. The balloon at the end of the tube is then inflated, compressing the blockage and widening the artery. A metal mesh tube known as a **stent** may be placed in the artery in order to keep it open. These stents are usually coated with medications that prevent the reclosure of the blood vessel.

If the blockage is extensive, the patient may need surgery known as **coronary artery bypass graft (CABG),** which involves bypassing the blockage with a vessel taken from another area. All of these procedures are performed in the hospital.

Dermatology Exams

During a whole-body skin examination, the dermatologist examines the visible top layer of the entire surface of the skin, including the scalp, the genital area, and the areas between the toes. The physician uses a magnifying lens and a bright light to look for lesions, especially suspicious moles or precancerous growths. Your role in this exam includes preparing patients and helping them into the proper position before examining each skin area. During the exam, drape patients to protect their privacy as much as possible while exposing the area to be examined. The physician also may ask you to take photographs or make sketches of lesions to aid in detecting future changes.

Another type of dermatologic exam is the **Wood's light examination,** in which the licensed practitioner inspects the patient's skin under an ultraviolet lamp in a darkened room. This examination highlights certain abnormal skin characteristics and aids in diagnosis. The dermatologist also may perform more limited, focused exams to evaluate specific skin conditions or disorders.

Endocrine Exams and Tests

Before an exam, you will take a thorough medical history. The licensed practitioner will assess the patient's skin condition, weight, and cardiac functioning for clues about illness. An endocrinologist will perform a complete physical exam, including palpation of glands. Most of the endocrine glands are located deep within the body; only the thyroid, the testes, and, to some extent, the ovaries can be examined with palpation or auscultation. Therefore, you may need to collect specimens for essential diagnostic urine and blood tests.

Other diagnostic tools used in endocrinology include radiologic tests such as X-rays and iodine scans. In a thyroid scan, the patient receives an oral or intravenous (IV) dose of radioactive iodine, and the thyroid is X-rayed as the material is absorbed. Ultrasound also can be employed to view glands or detect tumors. Urine and blood may be tested for the presence of glucose or hormones.

Gastrointestinal Exams

The gastroenterologist's examination of the patient's GI tract covers the mouth (lips, oral cavity, and tongue), the abdomen and lower thorax, the lower sigmoid colon, the rectum, and the anus. Depending on the patient's symptoms, the physician may perform an invasive exam procedure during the patient's first visit. Formerly, such procedures were performed only in hospitals or special medical facilities. Now, many GI specialists' offices are equipped for these procedures and the management of possible resulting emergencies.

You must prepare the patient, provide reassurance during exams, and help patients be as comfortable as possible. Your duties during the procedures will vary according to your state's scope of practice and the physician for whom you work. Instruct patients in advance to arrange for someone to drive them to and from the exam. After a procedure in which patients have had a local anesthetic at the back of the throat, caution them to avoid eating until the drug has been eliminated from the body. Otherwise, they could choke or aspirate food particles into the trachea.

Endoscopy **Endoscopy** generally refers to any procedure in which a scope is used to visually inspect a canal or cavity within the body. Most endoscopic exams are performed with a flexible fiber-optic tube that has a lighted instrument on the end. These exams provide direct visualization of a body cavity and a means for collecting tissue biopsies and removing polyps, as in the colon. Endoscopy helps diagnose tumors, ulcers, structural abnormalities, and other problems. It is particularly useful in performing procedures that formerly would have required an incision, such as removing stones from the bile duct.

Peroral Endoscopy Peroral endoscopy involves inserting the scope by way of the mouth (Figure 42-9). The patient is sedated and the gag reflex is inhibited with a local anesthetic. The peroral endoscopic procedures include esophagoscopy (esophagus only), gastroscopy (stomach only), duodenoscopy (duodenum only), and panendoscopy (esophagus, stomach, and duodenum), also referred to as an EGD (esophagogastroduodenoscopy).

Colonoscopy Colonoscopy—performed by inserting a colonoscope through the anus—can provide direct visualization of the large intestine. The gastroenterologist uses this procedure to determine the cause of diarrhea, constipation,

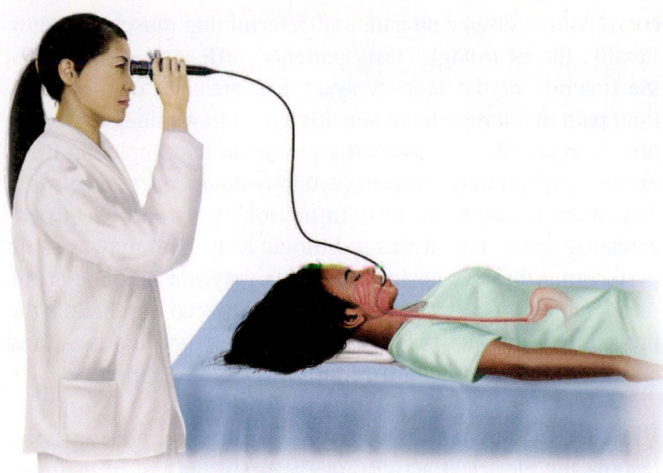

FIGURE 42-9 To perform a peroral endoscopy, the physician inserts a scope through the patient's mouth.

bleeding, or lower abdominal pain. A colonoscopy also is performed on patients over 50 to screen for abnormal growths called polyps that can lead to colon cancer.

Patient preparation is designed to clear the colon of fecal material so that the colon can be seen clearly. The type of preparation varies depending on the practice where you are working. For example, one regimen requires the patient to follow a liquid diet for 24 to 48 hours before the procedure, then take a cathartic on the two evenings prior to the colonoscopy. Patients may also need to use one or more prepackaged enema preparations the night before and the day of the procedure. Teach the patient the colon cleansing regimen and then tell him to expect diarrhea and possibly mild cramps.

Immediately before the procedure, instruct patients to empty the bladder. Patients should be given a sedative or an analgesic before undergoing the procedure. Patients lie in the Sims' position as the scope is guided through the large intestine. The licensed practitioner may manipulate the abdomen to facilitate passage of the scope.

Proctoscopy Proctoscopy is an examination of the lower rectum and anal canal. After an initial digital exam, the proctoscopy is performed with a 3-inch instrument called a proctoscope. This exam can detect hemorrhoids, polyps, fissures, fistulas, and abscesses.

Sigmoidoscopy Sigmoidoscopy is similar to colonoscopy, except that only the sigmoid area of the large intestine (the S-shaped segment between the descending colon and the rectum) is examined. Sigmoidoscopy also aids in diagnosing colon cancer, ulcerations, polyps, tumors, bleeding, and other lower intestinal problems. Patient preparation involves using one or two prepackaged enemas either the night before or the morning of the procedure, depending on the physician's instructions. The method for assisting the physician during a sigmoidoscopy is described in Procedure 42-2 at the end of this chapter.

Diagnostic and Laboratory Testing A GI specialist may order laboratory tests to determine the presence of

bacteria or bleeding in the stomach. GI specialists may also test the feces for occult, or hidden, bleeding from the intestinal tract. This is discussed in the *Collecting, Processing, and Testing Urine and Stool Specimens* chapter.

Gastroenterologists sometimes use imaging techniques, such as X-rays, ultrasound, radionuclide imaging, computed tomography (CT), and magnetic resonance imaging. Most GI radiologic exams are not performed in an office, but you should know enough about them to answer patients' questions. Generally, these exams are performed in a hospital X-ray laboratory or an outpatient facility. You may be responsible for scheduling tests at such facilities for patients. You also may help prepare the patient for these exams. However, in some cases, the patient should discuss specific preparation with personnel from the other facility.

Gallbladder Function Test Cholecystography is an older gallbladder function test performed by X-ray with a contrast agent. The patient swallows tablets of the contrast agent the night before the test. X-rays taken 12 to 14 hours later should show the contrast agent in the gallbladder. The patient then swallows a substance high in fat, which should make the gallbladder contract and empty the contrast agent into the duodenum.

Cholescintigraphy, also known as a HIDA scan test, uses a radioactive chemical injected into a vein. The test chemical then disperses everywhere that the bile goes–into the bile ducts, the gallbladder, and the intestine. A special camera is used to visualize where the chemical is dispersed to determine the functioning of these organs. See the *Diagnostic Imaging* chapter for more information.

Ultrasound Ultrasound is used commonly for diagnosing problems in the gallbladder, pancreas, spleen, and liver. The patient should have nothing to eat or drink after midnight of the night before and on the morning of the exam. Some gastroenterologists perform ultrasound exams in the office.

Barium Swallow The barium swallow (also called an upper GI series) is used to detect abnormalities in the esophagus, stomach, and small intestine. The patient swallows a liquid containing barium—an insoluble contrast agent. This material is viewed using fluoroscopy (moving X-ray images) as the liquid is swallowed and passes into the stomach. X-ray films are taken at frequent intervals to record the diagnostic images. The patient is asked to move into various positions while the barium is tracked through the small intestine. To prepare for this test, the patient should have nothing to eat or drink after midnight the night before and on the morning of the procedure. Refer to the *Diagnostic Imaging* chapter for more information.

Barium Enema A barium enema (also called a lower GI series) is used to detect abnormalities in the large intestine. Barium is given as an enema in this test. A balloon-like tube is inflated in the rectum during the X-ray and the patient is asked to move into various positions to ensure that the barium is distributed completely (Figure 42-10). Patients must eat no meats or vegetables for 1 to 3 days before the test to avoid

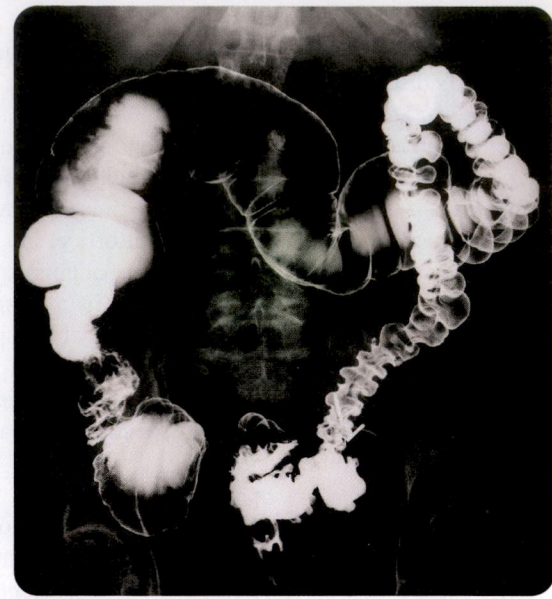

FIGURE 42-10 During a barium enema, the barium is tracked on X-rays.

© Jim Wehtje/Getty Images RF

incorrect indications on the X-ray. For 24 hours before the test, they must also follow a liquid diet, which includes drinking special liquid laxative preparations and more than a quart of water. Specific steps vary depending on the facility, but the intent is to cleanse the colon completely. See the *Diagnostic Imaging* chapter for more information.

Radionuclide Imaging Radiology subspecialists trained in nuclear medicine perform nuclear medicine studies with radionuclide imaging. The patient is first injected with a radioactive substance, then waits a prescribed length of time for the radioactive substance to be taken up by the body part being imaged. The patient is scanned or photographed with a gamma camera, which can read the radioactive areas to determine abnormalities in their composition. This technique is commonly used for liver, spleen, thyroid, and bone scans.

Neurologic Exams and Diagnostic Testing

The neurologist evaluates five categories of neurologic function in a complete exam:

- Cognitive function (mental status)
- Cranial nerves
- Motor system
- Reflexes
- Sensory system

Cognitive function can be assessed by observing general appearance and grooming as well as by asking patients specific questions. The neurologist also determines the status of the cranial nerves, which affect smell and taste, eye movements, hearing, voice quality, facial expression, and facial mobility. The physician may, for example, ask patients to close their eyes and then identify familiar smells. The neurologist observes patients' faces for symmetry of movement and tests visual and auditory acuity. The physician assesses motor ability by testing

coordination, observing gait, and determining muscle strength. Finally, the neurologist tests patients' reflexes and examines the function of the sensory system in areas of tactile sensation, pain and temperature sensitivity, and awareness of vibration. You are likely to assist the physician in completing these exams, and you may perform certain components yourself.

Common diagnostic tests in neurology include electroencephalography and various radiologic tests. You may assist in performing these tests. Invasive tests may not be done at the physician's office. In such cases, you will need to schedule the procedures, instruct patients about pretest preparations, and educate them about the procedure and what to expect.

Electroencephalography Electroencephalography records the electrical activity of the brain on a strip of graph paper. The tracing is an electroencephalogram (EEG). Electrodes are attached to the patient's scalp and readings are taken while the patient is at rest and engaged in specific activities. An EEG can be used to detect or examine conditions such as tumors, seizure disorders, or brain injury. You may assist with electrode placement or, after training, obtain the EEG on your own.

Imaging Procedures Several imaging techniques are used as neurologic diagnostic tools. Types of procedures include angiograms, brain scans, CT, MRI, myelography, and skull X-rays.

Cerebral Angiography Cerebral angiography (or angiogram) is a radiologic study of the cerebral blood vessels. After a contrast medium is injected into an artery, X-rays are taken to visualize the cerebral blood vessels.

Brain Scan A brain scan is performed by injecting the patient with radioisotopes and, after a period of time, using a scanner to detect the material. The radioisotopes tend to gather in areas of abnormality, such as tumors or abscesses.

Computed Tomography **Computed tomography,** often called a CT scan, is a radiographic exam that produces a three-dimensional, cross-sectional view of the brain. Often one scan is done without a contrast medium. Then a contrast medium is injected for greater clarity. CT scans can help diagnose a wide range of conditions, including tumors, blood clots, and brain swelling.

Magnetic Resonance Imaging **Magnetic resonance imaging (MRI)** is a viewing technique that enables licensed practitioners to see areas inside the body without exposing the patient to X-rays or surgery. The procedure, which takes 30 to 60 minutes, requires the patient to lie still on a padded table that is moved into a tunnel-like structure. A powerful magnetic field produces an image of internal body structures. Patients who are unable to tolerate being inside a tunnel-like structure can be examined with an MRI scanner that has a more open structure (Figure 24-11).

Positron Emission Tomography **Positron emission tomography,** often called a **PET** scan, studies the blood flow and metabolic activity in the brain to help licensed

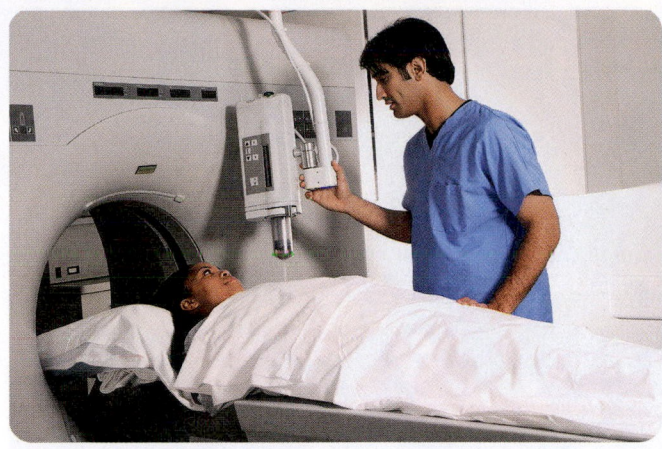

FIGURE 42-11 Magnetic resonance imaging is used to diagnose disorders in many specialties.
© Plush Studios/Getty Images RF

practitioners identify certain neurologic and CNS disorders. These disorders include Parkinson's disease, multiple sclerosis, Alzheimer's disease, transient ischemic attack (TIA), amyotrophic lateral sclerosis (ALS), Huntington's disease, epilepsy, stroke, cancer, and schizophrenia.

Myelography *Myelography* is an X-ray visualization of the spinal cord after the injection of a radioactive contrast medium or air into the spinal subarachnoid space (the space between the second and innermost of three membranes covering the spinal cord). Although an MRI is used more frequently, myelography can reveal tumors, cysts, spinal stenosis, and herniated disks.

Skull X-Ray Skull X-rays may be used to detect fractures in the skull and to locate tumors.

Other Tests Other diagnostic tests—including lumbar puncture and electromyography—do not involve imaging techniques. A lumbar puncture, or spinal tap, involves collecting a sample of cerebrospinal fluid (CSF) to diagnose infection, measure CSF pressure, and check for blood cells and proteins in the fluid. A needle is inserted between two lumbar vertebrae and into the subarachnoid space. The collected fluid is sent to a laboratory for analysis. **Electromyography** is used to detect neuromuscular disorders or nerve damage. Needle electrodes are inserted into some of the patient's skeletal muscles. When the muscles contract, a monitor records the nerve impulses and measures conduction time.

Oncology Exams and Diagnostic Testing

An exam in an oncologist's office focuses on the area of the body where a problem is suspected. The oncologist's goal is to detect, diagnose, and treat cancer, which is done through a variety of procedures. You will schedule some of these tests and provide pretest instructions and explanations to patients.

A biopsy is a common procedure an oncologist may perform, and you may assist with the procedure. There are several types of biopsies. A physician performs an incisional, or open, biopsy by making an incision and removing a piece of

tissue. A needle biopsy is performed by removing tissue with a needle inserted through the skin into the growth or area. Needle aspiration is performed by removing fluid from a lump or cyst with a needle. Procedure 42-3, at the end of this chapter, describes the steps in assisting with a needle biopsy. During a biopsy, standard precautions and sterile technique must be maintained. Always place the specimen in a prepared, labeled container provided by the laboratory. Transport it according to laboratory instructions, attaching the proper accompanying forms. After the biopsy, you might assist with or perform the cleaning and bandaging of the site.

In addition to a biopsy, you may obtain blood specimens for some tests and assist in other diagnostic procedures, such as the following:

- X-rays
- CT scans
- MRIs
- Blood tests, especially those to detect tumor markers, such as carcinoembryonic antigen (CEA) (increased levels of CEA indicate a variety of cancers), CA125, and CA15-3
- Ultrasonography

Cancer Treatment

Cancer treatments fall into three general categories: surgery, radiation therapy, and chemotherapy. Often, a combination of these treatment methods is used. All methods damage healthy as well as cancerous cells. The success of treatment depends on many factors, and recovery varies greatly from patient to patient.

Surgery Surgical removal of the tumor and some surrounding tissue is one method of cancer treatment. It is most effective when the tumor appears to be contained within a particular organ or is localized in an area of the skin. Surgery is often followed, however, by either radiation therapy or chemotherapy.

Radiation Therapy Radiation therapy uses radiation to kill and stop the growth of tumor cells. It is often used in conjunction with surgery or chemotherapy. Radiation therapy is effective because, although radiation affects all living cells, it has the most damaging effect on cells that are undergoing rapid division, including cancer cells.

Chemotherapy Chemotherapy is also used in conjunction with other therapies. Chemotherapy is the use of strong anticancer drugs to kill malignant cells. As with radiation therapy, rapidly dividing cells, such as like cancer cells, are most strongly affected by these medications. A variety of chemotherapy drugs are available, each with slightly different mechanisms of action. Table 42-8 lists common classes of chemotherapy drugs and outlines their major categories, their mechanism of action, and some examples in each category. These drugs may be used alone or in combination, depending on the type of cancer being treated. Although it is unlikely you will prepare or administer anticancer drugs, you need to

TABLE 42-8 Chemotherapy Drugs

Category	Mechanism of Action	Examples
Alkylating agents	Hinder cell division	Chlorambucil, cyclophosphamide
Antimetabolites	Interfere with folic acid and nucleic acid synthesis	Methotrexate, fluorouracil
Antibiotics	Break DNA strands	Actinomycin, bleomycin
Antimitotic agents	Affect cell division	Vinblastine, paclitaxel

be aware that they are highly toxic. General protective guidelines, including using PPE, must be followed whenever there is risk of contact with the drugs or patients' body fluids.

Orthopedic Exams and Procedures

An orthopedist uses inspection, palpation, and diagnostic tests to assess the structure and function of the musculoskeletal system. The patient is asked to stand, walk, and perform several range-of-motion exercises. The physician notes the degree of mobility the patient has, in some cases using a device called a *goniometer*. A complete exam takes some time, and you may need to help drape, position, or physically support the patient, especially if the patient is elderly or incapacitated. You also may be responsible for instructing the patient about care for a musculoskeletal condition, including how to perform therapeutic exercises.

Orthopedists use a variety of diagnostic tests. Bone and muscle biopsies may be performed to detect disorders such as bone infection and muscle atrophy. Electromyography is another diagnostic tool used in this specialty. An orthopedist also may order urine and blood tests to detect levels of substances such as calcium or phosphorus.

As in most other specialties, X-rays play a vital role in diagnosis and may be performed in the orthopedist's office. X-rays are especially useful in determining the nature and extent of a bone injury. Other common radiographic exams in the orthopedic specialty include the following:

- CT scan
- MRI
- Angiography (for affected vascular structures)

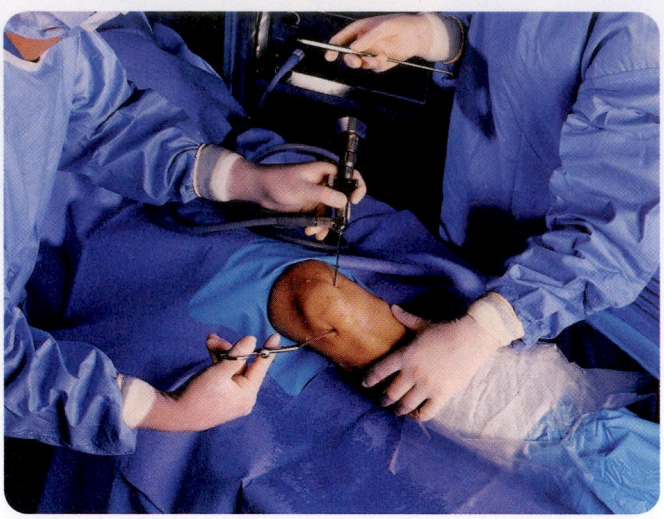

FIGURE 42-12 Arthroscopy can be used for diagnosis as well as biopsy and surgical repair.
© Royalty-Free/Corbis

- Myelography (for spinal disorders)
- Diskography (for intervertebral disk disorders)
- Arthrography (for joint disorders)
- Bone scans

These procedures are discussed in more detail in the *Diagnostic Imaging* chapter.

Arthroscopy enables the orthopedist to see inside a joint—usually the knee, shoulder, or hip—with an arthroscope. This tubular instrument includes an optical system; when the tube is inserted into the joint, it can be visualized (Figure 42-12). Arthroscopy is used to give the physician a closer look at conditions such as injuries and degenerative joint diseases and to guide surgical procedures.

Joint replacement surgery is often used to treat knee and hip joints severely damaged by arthritis, disease, or injury. Hip replacement may be indicated in cases of severe arthritis pain, femoral neck fractures, or hip joint tumors. Knee pain that does not respond to medications or physical therapy or a knee damaged by severe arthritis may indicate the need for knee replacement. Both surgeries require that the damaged joint be removed and an artificial joint inserted in its place. Physical therapy is usually started soon after surgery, and most patients fully recover in 3 to 12 months.

PROCEDURE 42-1 Assisting with a Scratch Test Examination

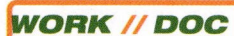

Procedure Goal: To assist a licensed practitioner in determining substances to which a patient has an allergic reaction

OSHA Guidelines:

  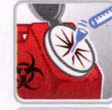 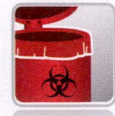 

Materials: Patient chart/progress note, disposable sterile needles or lancets, allergen extracts, control solution, cotton balls, alcohol, timer, adhesive tape, ruler, cold packs or an ice bag

Method:

1. Wash your hands and assemble the necessary materials.
2. Identify the patient and introduce yourself.

3. Show the patient into the treatment area. Explain the procedure and discuss any concerns. Confirm whether the patient followed pretesting procedures such as discontinuing medications.
   RATIONALE: *Antihistamines and steroids may interfere with the test.*

4. Assist the patient into a comfortable position and don exam gloves.

5. Swab the test site, usually the upper arm or back, with an alcohol prep pad.

6. Identify the sites with tape labels.
   RATIONALE: *The sites must be easily identified so that you can record reactions to individual antigens.*

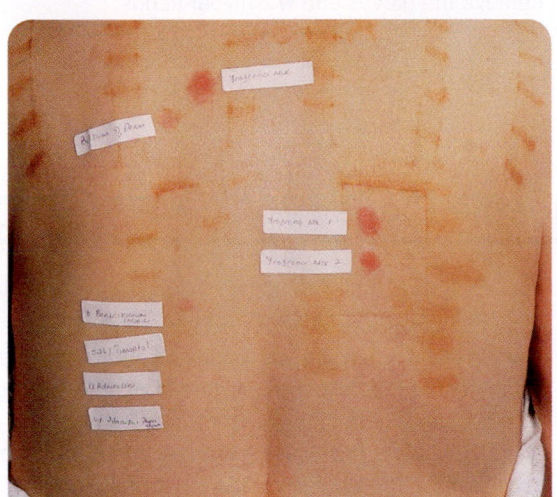

FIGURE Procedure 42-1 Step 6   Label each site with the name of the allergen or an accepted abbreviation.
© John Radcliffe/SPL/Science Source

7. Apply small drops of the allergen extracts and control solution onto the test site at evenly spaced intervals, about 1½ to 2 inches apart.

8. Open the package containing the first needle or lancet, making sure you do not contaminate the instrument.

9. Assist the licensed practitioner with the scratch procedure or perform the procedure if it is within your scope of practice. Using a new sterile needle or lancet for each site, scratch the skin beneath each drop of allergen, no more than ⅛-inch deep.

10. Start the timer for the 20-minute reaction period.

11. After the reaction time has passed, cleanse each site with an alcohol prep pad. (Do not remove identifying labels until the practitioner has checked the patient.)

12. Assist the practitioner or examine and measure the sites.

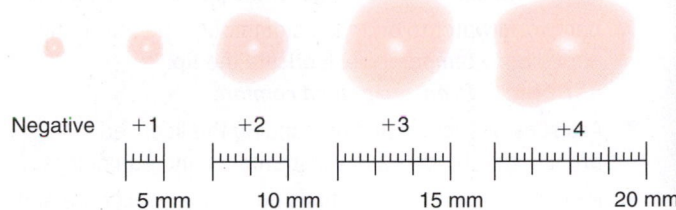

Negative   +1   +2   +3   +4
            5 mm   10 mm   15 mm   20 mm

FIGURE Procedure 42-1 Step 12   Physicians classify skin reactions as either negative (no greater than the reaction to the control) or positive. Positive reactions are rated on a scale of +1 to +4, depending on the size of the wheal.

13. Apply cold packs or an ice bag to sites as needed to relieve itching.

14. Properly dispose of used materials and instruments.

15. Clean and disinfect the area according to OSHA guidelines.

16. Remove the gloves and wash your hands.

17. Document the test results in the patient's chart, if required, and initial your entries (Refer to Progress Note).

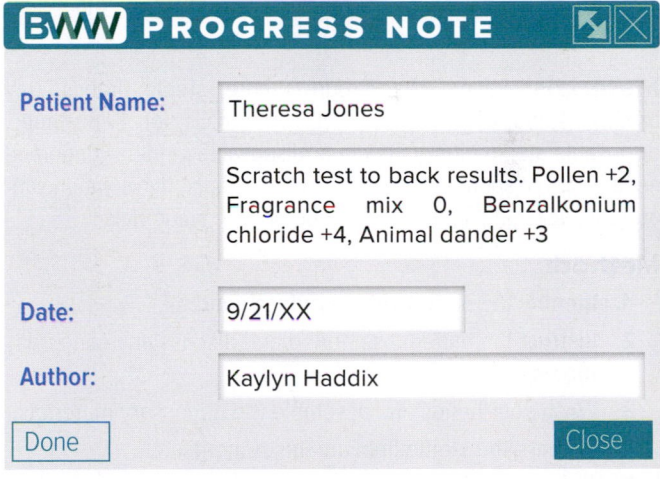

BWW **PROGRESS NOTE**

Patient Name: Theresa Jones

Scratch test to back results. Pollen +2, Fragrance mix 0, Benzalkonium chloride +4, Animal dander +3

Date: 9/21/XX

Author: Kaylyn Haddix

Done   Close

PROCEDURE 42-2   Assisting with a Sigmoidoscopy

Procedure Goal: To assist the licensed practitioner during the examination of the rectum, anus, and sigmoid colon using a sigmoidoscope

OSHA Guidelines:

 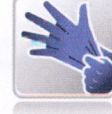 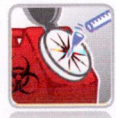  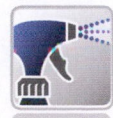

Materials: Sigmoidoscope, suction pump, lubricating jelly, drape, patient gown, and tissues

Method:

1. Wash your hands and assemble and position materials and equipment according to the licensed practitioner's preference.

2. Test the suction pump.

3. Identify the patient and introduce yourself.

4. Show the patient into the treatment room. Explain the procedure and discuss any concerns the patient may have.

5. Instruct the patient to empty the bladder, take off all clothing from the waist down, and put on the gown with the opening in the back.

6. Don exam gloves and assist the patient into the knee-chest or Sims' position. Immediately cover the patient with a drape.

7. Use warm water to bring the sigmoidoscope to slightly above body temperature; lubricate the tip.
   RATIONALE: *To ensure patient comfort.*

8. Assist as needed, including handing the licensed practitioner the necessary instruments and equipment.

9. Monitor the patient's reactions during the procedure and relay any signs of pain to the practitioner.

10. Clean the anal area with tissues after the exam.

11. Properly dispose of used materials and disposable instruments.

12. Remove the gloves and wash your hands.

13. Help the patient gradually assume a comfortable position.
    RATIONALE: *The patient should sit up slowly so that he does not become faint.*

14. Instruct the patient to dress.

15. Don clean gloves.

16. Sanitize reusable instruments and prepare them for disinfection and/or sterilization, as necessary.

17. Clean and disinfect the equipment and the room according to OSHA guidelines.

18. Remove the gloves and wash your hands.

PROCEDURE 42-3 Assisting with a Needle Biopsy

WORK // DOC

Procedure Goal: To assist the licensed practitioner with removing tissue from a patient's body so that it can be examined in a laboratory

OSHA Guidelines:

   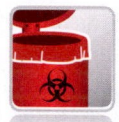 

Materials: Patient chart/progress note, sterile drapes, tray or Mayo stand, antiseptic solution, cotton balls, local anesthetic, disposable sterile biopsy needle or disposable sterile syringe and needle, sterile sponges, specimen bottle with fixative solution, laboratory packaging, and sterile wound-dressing materials

Method:

1. Identify the patient and introduce yourself.

2. Instruct the patient as needed and discuss any concerns the patient may have.

3. Wash your hands and assemble the necessary materials.

4. Prepare the sterile field and instruments.

5. Don exam gloves.

6. Position and drape the patient.

7. Cleanse the biopsy site. Prepare the patient's skin.
   RATIONALE: *To reduce the possibility of infection.*

8. Remove the gloves, wash your hands, and don clean exam gloves.

9. Assist the licensed practitioner as needed when she injects anesthetic.

10. Perform a surgical scrub and don sterile gloves if you will be handing the practitioner's sterile instruments.

11. Place the sample in the specimen container and label, complete the laboratory requisition form, and package the specimen for immediate laboratory transport.
    RATIONALE: *The specimen must be properly labeled and accompanied by a completed laboratory requisition form to ensure that the specimen is not lost and the appropriate tests are completed in the lab.*

12. Apply a dressing to the patient's wound site.

13. Properly dispose of used supplies and instruments.

14. Clean and disinfect the room according to OSHA guidelines.

15. Remove the gloves and wash your hands.

16. Document as needed (Refer to Progress Note).

BWW PROGRESS NOTE

Patient Name:	Mark Waters
	Needle biopsy performed by Dr. Buckwalter. Specimen labeled and sent to MEDLab.
Date:	12/10/XX
Author:	Kaylyn Haddix

Done   Close

LEARNING OUTCOMES	KEY POINTS
42.1 Describe the medical specialties of allergy, cardiology, dermatology, endocrinology, gastroenterology, neurology, oncology, and orthopedics.	The medical specialties discussed in this chapter include allergy, which is diagnosing and treating allergies (inappropriate immune system responses); cardiology, which is the study and treatment of heart diseases and disorders; dermatology, or the diagnosis and treatment of skin diseases and disorders such as acne, eczema, and skin cancer; endocrinology, or the treatment of diseases and disorders of the endocrine system, which includes glands that regulate and coordinate the body systems; gastroenterology, or the diagnosis and treatment of disorders of the entire gastrointestinal (GI) tract from the mouth to the anus, as well as the liver and pancreas; neurology, or the diagnosis and treatment of diseases and disorders of the central nervous system (CNS) and associated systems; oncology, which is concerned with the detection and treatment of cancerous growths; and orthopedics, which focuses on disorders, injuries, and diseases of the muscular and skeletal systems.
42.2 Identify common diseases and disorders related to cardiology, dermatology, endocrinology, gastroenterology, neurology, oncology, and orthopedics.	Many common diseases and disorders are identified in the specialty practices. You should have an understanding of the implications of these diseases on the patient and the necessary treatments.
42.3 Relate the role of the medical assistant in examinations and procedures performed in the medical specialties of allergy, cardiology, dermatology, endocrinology, gastroenterology, neurology, oncology, and orthopedics.	Exams and diagnostic tests performed in allergy, cardiology, dermatology, endocrinology, gastroenterology, neurology, oncology, and orthopedics specialties are numerous. During most of these exams and tests, your role may include ensuring patient safety and comfort, educating the patient about the necessary preparation and the procedure, and assisting the licensed practitioner.

CASE STUDY CRITICAL THINKING

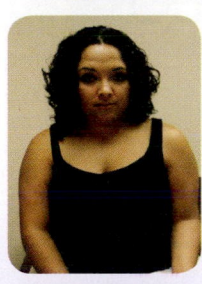

© McGraw-Hill Education

Recall Valarie Ramirez from the beginning of the chapter. Now that you have completed the chapter, answer the following questions regarding her case.

1. How would you chart Valarie's chief complaint?

2. The physician thinks Valarie has a thyroid nodule that may be cancerous. Which two types of specialists might she need to visit?

3. Based on the results of the ultrasound, the physician wants to evaluate the thyroid nodule by performing a needle biopsy. What will be your responsibilities during this procedure?

1. (LO 42.1) In which medical specialty practice would you *most* likely be working if you were assisting with a scratch test?
   a. Dermatology
   b. Cardiology
   c. Oncology
   d. Allergy
   e. Endocrinology

2. (LO 42.3) You just finished patient education for a patient who is to have a colonoscopy next week. At which of the following specialty practices do you *most* likely work?
   a. Cardiology
   b. Gastroenterology
   c. Surgery
   d. Urology
   e. Oncology

3. (LO 42.3) A patient has a growth on his arm and the licensed practitioner removes some of the tissue of the growth. He *most* likely had a
   a. Needle aspiration
   b. Wood's light examination
   c. Needle biopsy
   d. CABG
   e. RAST test

4. (LO 42.1) Which specialist would do a whole-body skin examination?
   a. Dermatologist
   b. Cardiologist
   c. Oncologist
   d. Allergist
   e. Endocrinologist

5. (LO 42.1) If a patient is suffering from Type 1 diabetes, what specialist would she *most* likely visit?
   a. Dermatologist
   b. Cardiologist
   c. Oncologist
   d. Allergist
   e. Endocrinologist

6. (LO 42.2) A patient has been diagnosed with the most dangerous type of skin cancer. What type of cancer does he have?
   a. Basal cell
   b. Melanoma
   c. Squamous cell
   d. Diabetic
   e. Arthritic

7. (LO 42.2) A patient has been diagnosed with Alzheimer's disease and will *most* likely see a specialist in
   a. Neurology
   b. Cardiology
   c. Endocrinology
   d. Oncology
   e. Dermatology

8. (LO 42.2) The type of medication used to treat cancer is
   a. Electroencephalogram
   b. Radiation
   c. Retinoid
   d. Contraceptives
   e. Chemotherapy

9. (LO 42.3) A patient has been instructed to sit up slowly after a sigmoidoscopy. What is the *most* likely reason?
   a. To prevent bleeding
   b. To maintain asepsis
   c. To prevent the patient from getting faint
   d. To check for a reaction
   e. To ensure that the test is done accurately

10. (LO 42.3) After a scratch test, you charted +4 pollen. What does this mean?
    a. The test was negative
    b. The test was mildly positive
    c. The test was +4 on a scale of 1 to 10
    d. The test was positive with a wheal of 10 mm
    e. The test was positive with a wheal of 20 mm

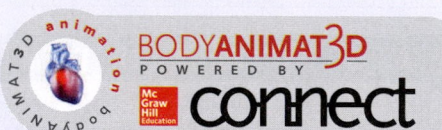

Go to CONNECT to see an animation exercise about *Coronary Artery Disease*.

SOFT SKILLS SUCCESS

You are working in a cardiologist's office with a patient who had an episode of angina and a stent placed for a 90% blockage of the anterior interventricular branch of the left coronary artery, also known as a widowmaker. The patient did not have heart damage but needs to follow a more heart-smart lifestyle to prevent any cardiovascular problems. The licensed practitioner has asked that you spend time doing patient education with this patient before he leaves the office. When you enter the exam room to begin your patient education, the patient makes the following comment: "I know why you are here, and I don't think you can do anything to help me." What should be your response?

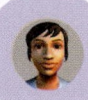

Go to PRACTICE MEDICAL OFFICE and complete the module Clinical - Interactions.

Assisting with Eye and Ear Care

43

CASE STUDY

PATIENT INFORMATION

Patient Name	DOB	Allergies
Valarie Ramirez	8/4/19XX	Penicillin

Attending	MRN	Other Information
Paul F. Buckwalter, MD	829-78-462	Vital Signs: 128/84 98.7-92 -18 Ht. 5' 2" Wt. 135 lb.

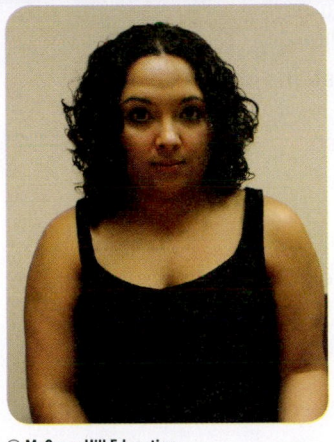

© McGraw-Hill Education

Valarie Ramirez, a 33-year-old female, has been examined by the physician after complaining that something flew into her eye while she was riding her motorcycle yesterday. The physician has examined the eye and determined that there is a small amount of debris in the eye. The physician has asked you to assist with eye irrigation.

Keep Valarie in mind as you study this chapter. There will be questions at the end of the chapter based on the case study. The information in the chapter will help you answer these questions.

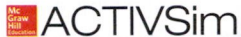
ACTIVSim

LEARNING OUTCOMES

After completing Chapter 43, you will be able to:

43.1 Describe the medical assistant's role in eye exams and procedures performed in a medical office.

43.2 Discuss various eye disorders encountered in a medical office.

43.3 Identify ophthalmic exams performed in the licensed practitioner's office.

43.4 Summarize ophthalmologic procedures and treatments.

43.5 Describe the medical assistant's role in otology.

43.6 Describe disorders of the ear encountered in the medical office.

43.7 Recall various hearing and other diagnostic ear tests.

43.8 Summarize ear procedures and treatments.

KEY TERMS

accommodation
astigmatism
audiologist
audiometer
cataract
cochlear implant
conductive hearing loss
conjunctivitis
decibels
frequency
glaucoma

hyperopia
Ménière's disease
myopia
ophthalmoscope
otologist
presbyopia
refraction examination
sensorineural hearing loss
slit lamp
tinnitus
tonometer

CAAHEP	ABHES

I.C.8 Identify common pathology related to each body system including:
(a) signs
(b) symptoms
(c) etiology

I.C.9 Analyze pathology for each body system including:
(a) diagnostic measures
(b) treatment modalities

I.C.11 Identify the classifications of medications including:
(a) indications for use
(b) desired effects
(c) side effects
(d) adverse reactions

I.P.4 Verify the rules of medication administration:
(a) right patient
(b) right medication
(c) right dose
(d) right route
(e) right time
(f) right documentation

I.P.8 Instruct and prepare a patient for a procedure or a treatment

I.P.9 Assist provider with a patient exam

I.A.2 Incorporate critical thinking skills when performing patient care

I.A.3 Show awareness of a patient's concerns related to the procedure being performed

V.P.4 Coach patients regarding:
(a) office policies
(b) health maintenance
(c) disease prevention
(d) treatment plan

V.A.3 Demonstrate respect for individual diversity including:
(a) gender
(b) race
(c) religion
(d) age
(e) economic status
(f) appearance

X.P.3 Document patient care accurately in the medical record

2. Anatomy and Physiology
a. List all body systems, their structure and functions
b. Describe common diseases, symptoms and etiologies as they apply to each system
c. Identify diagnostic and treatment modalities as they relate to each body system

3. Medical Terminology
c. Apply various medical terminology for each specialty

4. Medical Law and Ethics
a. Follow documentation guidelines

9. Medical Office Clinical Procedures
d. Assist provider with specialty examination including cardiac, respiratory, OB-GYN, neurological, gastroenterology procedures
j. Make adaptations with patients with special needs

▶ Introduction

Think about how often you use your eyes and ears. You use your eyes to *read* the words on this page and to watch the rise and fall of a patient's chest while counting respirations. Both your eyes and ears are needed when watching the dial on a sphygmomanometer while listening for the first Korotkoff sound while taking a blood pressure. These are daily activities for a medical assistant. Good eye and ear care is critical for you and for your patients. In this chapter, you will explore the role of ophthalmology and otology in patient care, various eye and ear disorders, and exams and procedures related to the eye and ear, including vision and hearing tests.

▶ Ophthalmology

LO 43.1

Ophthalmology is a branch of medicine specializing in the anatomy, function, and diseases of the eye. An ophthalmologist specializes in medical and surgical eye problems, treating the eyes and related tissues. The most common eye disorders that an ophthalmologist treats are visual defects, which are often correctable with eyeglasses or contact lenses. Ophthalmologists also treat eye injuries and remove foreign bodies from the eye. More serious disorders, such as cataracts and glaucoma, require medication or surgery. In an ophthalmologist's office, you may assist or perform some of the procedures that involve measuring various aspects and functions of the eye, such as visual acuity, color vision, and intraocular pressure. You also may perform some of these exams in a general practice office or an optometrist's office. Optometrists diagnose and treat visual defects only with glasses or contacts. Review eye anatomy and pathophysiology in the *Special Senses* chapter.

▶ Eye Diseases and Disorders

LO 43.2

You may encounter a wide range of eye diseases and disorders in an ophthalmologist's or general practitioner's office. Some, such as a sty or conjunctivitis, do not greatly affect vision and may be treated by a general practitioner. Others affect the eye's internal workings and require a specialist's attention.

Disorders of External Eye Structures

Some disorders affect external eye structures, such as the eyelid and the eyelashes.

Blepharitis Blepharitis is a chronic inflammation of the eyelid's edges, more common in older individuals than in younger people. It can be caused by infection or by the same skin condition that causes dandruff. Symptoms include red, swollen eyelids with scaling or crusting of skin at the edges. The patient's eyes may be irritated and itchy. Proper eye care and hygiene often clear up the condition successfully. Antibiotic creams may be necessary in severe cases.

Ptosis Ptosis is a drooping of the upper eyelid in which the lid partially or completely covers the eye. It is caused by weakness of or damage to the muscle that raises the eyelid or by problems with the nerve that controls the muscle. Often no treatment is required, although surgery may be performed if the condition interferes with vision or if the patient is concerned about appearance.

Sty A sty (external hordeolum) is the result of an eyelash follicle infection. The microorganism most often responsible for the infection is *Staphylococcus aureus*. A red, painful swelling appears on the eye's edge and typically forms a white head of pus. The head bursts and drains before it heals

in about a week. Applying warm, moist compresses to the sty may help it drain sooner.

Disorders of Structures at the Front of the Eye

Another group of disorders affects structures at the front of the eye, which include the conjunctiva and the cornea.

Conjunctivitis Conjunctivitis, or pinkeye, is an inflammation of the conjunctiva caused by an allergy, irritant, or infection. It is a common disorder that is annoying but normally not serious.

Allergic conjunctivitis occurs when a person has an allergic reaction to pollen, makeup, or other substance. The symptoms are itchy, red eyes. The licensed practitioner may prescribe medication to relieve troublesome symptoms and suggest avoidance of the trigger whenever possible. Irritants such as dust, smoke, wind, pollutants, and excessive glare also may cause conjunctivitis.

Infectious conjunctivitis can be caused by either a bacterial or a viral infection. Both forms are easily spread and have symptoms including redness and a gritty feeling in the eye. Bacterial infections typically produce pus, which may form a crust on the eye during sleep. Viral infections usually produce a watery discharge. Although eye irrigation or saline drops may be used to soothe eyes affected by either type of infection, only bacterial infections are treated with antibiotic drops or ointment.

Because you may not know the cause of a patient's conjunctivitis (allergies, irritants, bacteria, viruses), take precautions to avoid spreading infection. As with any potentially infectious disease, use standard precautions in medical settings. Wear appropriate personal protective equipment when dealing with any patient who has conjunctivitis.

Corneal Ulcers and Abrasions Ulcers (lesions) on the cornea may be the result of injury, infection, or both. An injury such as an abrasion (scratch) on the cornea can become infected with bacteria, viruses, or fungi. The symptoms of a corneal ulcer include pain or discomfort and unclear vision. Treatment consists of antibiotic eyedrops or ointments and drops that temporarily paralyze the eye's ciliary muscles—those that control the shape of the lens—to help control pain. Patching the eye is no longer recommended because doing so creates a warm, moist environment that supports further growth of microorganisms.

Disorders Involving Internal Eye Structures

Another group of disorders affects structures inside the eye. Cataracts, for example, affect the lens, while glaucoma can damage several internal eye structures.

Cataracts Cataracts are cloudy or opaque areas in the normally clear lens of the eye. Cataracts develop gradually, blocking the passage of light through the eye. The result is a progressive loss of vision in one or both eyes. In severe cases, you can see the cloudy lens through the eye's pupil (Figure 43-1).

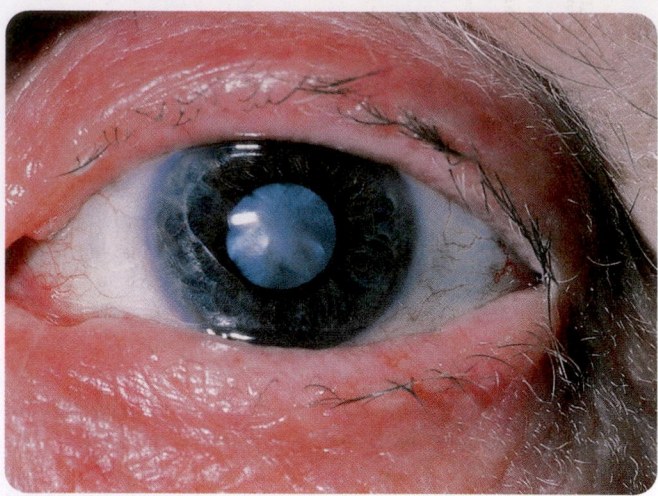

FIGURE 43-1   The lens of an eye with a cataract has a clouded appearance.
© Biophoto Associates/Science Source

Cataracts are more common in the elderly than in younger people, because the lens deteriorates with aging. Cataracts also can be caused by iritis, injury, ultraviolet radiation, or diabetes. Some cataracts are congenital. Treatment includes surgically removing the lens and using an artificial lens in its place. The artificial lens may be in the form of special eyeglasses, contact lenses, or an intraocular lens inserted at the time of cataract surgery.

Glaucoma **Glaucoma** is a condition in which fluid pressure builds up inside the eye. This pressure damages the eye's internal structures and gradually destroys vision. Glaucoma is the second leading cause of blindness in the United States and the first cause among African Americans. According to Prevent Blindness America, 2.3 million Americans over age 40 have glaucoma.

Capillaries in the ciliary body produce aqueous humor—a sticky, watery fluid that circulates between the lens and the cornea. In a patient with healthy eyes, this fluid drains out of this area through the angle formed by the iris and the cornea. The aqueous humor then diffuses into a vascular channel (Schlemm's canal) that encircles the cornea where it meets the sclera—the white of the eye (see the *Special Senses* chapter). The aqueous humor then returns to the systemic circulation (the circulation of the blood to body tissues). However, in a patient with glaucoma, the fluid drains out of the eye too slowly or fails to drain at all. The result is a buildup of intraocular pressure. Retinal nerve fibers are damaged and blood vessels are destroyed, leading to loss of vision and possible blindness.

Glaucoma is treated with medication that reduces pressure in the eye. Drops, pills, or both may be prescribed to reduce the production of aqueous humor. Sometimes, an iridotomy—a type of laser surgery procedure in which a small hole is created in the iris to allow excess fluid to drain—is performed. If the surgery is not effective, an iridectomy (partial removal of the iris) is done to create a larger opening in the iris.

Uveitis Uveitis is inflammation of the uveal track, which includes the iris, ciliary body, and choroid (refer to the *Special Senses* chapter). The most common type of uveitis is known as anterior uveitis. The term *iritis* is used sometimes to describe anterior uveitis, even though anterior uveitis involves other parts of the eye. The cause is often unknown but may be associated with eye trauma, infection, and some autoimmune diseases. White blood cells from the inflamed area and protein that leaks from small blood vessels float in the aqueous humor. The symptoms of iritis are pain or discomfort in one or both eyes; pain may be worse in bright light. The eye is red and loss of vision may occur. Left untreated, uveitis can lead to other complications, such as glaucoma and cataracts. Anti-inflammatory drops or ointment are used to treat this condition.

Disorders of the Retina

Several serious disorders affect the retina—the internal layer of the back of the eye. These disorders include retinal detachment, diabetic retinopathy, and macular degeneration.

Retinal Detachment Retinal detachment occurs when the retina separates from the underlying choroid layer—the middle, vascular layer of the eye. When this separation occurs, vision is damaged.

Early symptoms of detachment include flashes of light or floating black shapes, both of which can occur as the hole in the retina forms. Patients occasionally describe their field of vision as being like a window shade that has been pulled down. Peripheral vision is lost as the retina detaches. Vision becomes progressively blurred as detachment continues.

A hole in the retina can be fixed with cryopexy—surgical fixation with cold. During the procedure, the physician places a freezing probe on the outside of the eye over the area of the retinal tear, freezing the area and creating a thin scar that seals the hole. If the retina has already detached, some vision can often be restored with surgical and laser treatments.

Diabetic Retinopathy Diabetic retinopathy is a complication of diabetes. People who have had diabetes for a long time or who do not keep their condition under control experience damage to small blood vessels that supply the retina. The vessels initially leak fluid, which distorts vision. As the disease progresses, fragile new blood vessels grow on the retina and bleed into the vitreous humor—the thick, jelly-like fluid that fills the posterior eye chamber. Scar tissue also may form on the retina. The result is loss of vision. The damage usually cannot be repaired, but the disorder can be controlled to prevent further loss of vision.

Macular Degeneration The macula is the area of the retina responsible for the central area of a person's visual field. For unknown reasons, the macula begins to deteriorate as some individuals age. Macular degeneration causes loss of vision in the center of an image; peripheral vision remains intact. Macular degeneration is the leading cause of blindness among the elderly in the United States. According to the National Eye Institute, 1.75 million Americans have age-related macular degeneration.

When an individual develops macular degeneration, the loss of sharp vision occurs very gradually and without pain.

One of the first signs is difficulty in reading. The loss of vision often appears as a dark spot in the center of the field of vision. If macular degeneration is detected early, laser surgery may restore some vision or prevent further loss.

Disorders Involving Eye Movement

Normally, both eyes move together when people look at objects. However, a deviation of one eye is called strabismus. In young children, misaligned or unbalanced eye muscles cause strabismus. This misalignment makes it appear as though the child is looking in two different directions. A condition called amblyopia may occur as the misaligned eye becomes "lazy." The brain tends to ignore what the lazy eye sees; if the condition is not treated, vision will be affected in this eye. Treatment involves putting a patch over the fully working eye to force the child to use the other eye. Eyeglasses may be used along with the patch. In some cases, surgery on the eye muscle is required.

Strabismus in adults usually results from problems with the nerves connecting the brain and the eye muscles or with the muscles themselves. Conditions that can cause such problems include diabetes, high blood pressure, brain injury, muscular dystrophy, and inflammation of certain cerebral arteries. Treatment depends on the cause of the condition.

Refractive Disorders

Refraction refers to the way light from objects is focused through the eye to form an image on the retina. The normal eye focuses light exactly at the retina, producing a clear image (Figure 43-2). In some people, the eye focuses light either in front of or behind the retina, so the image is not clear. The problem may be the result of an abnormal shape of the eye or abnormal focusing of the light by the cornea and lens. The most common refractive disorders are nearsightedness, farsightedness, presbyopia, and astigmatism.

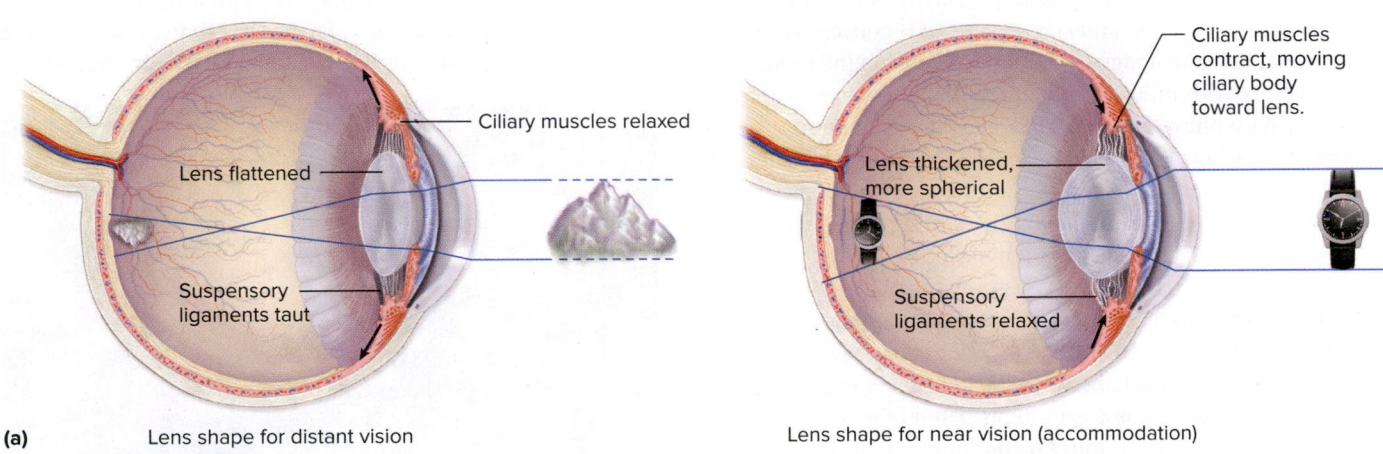

Ciliary muscles relaxed
Lens flattened
Suspensory ligaments taut

(a) Lens shape for distant vision

Ciliary muscles contract, moving ciliary body toward lens.
Lens thickened, more spherical
Suspensory ligaments relaxed

Lens shape for near vision (accommodation)

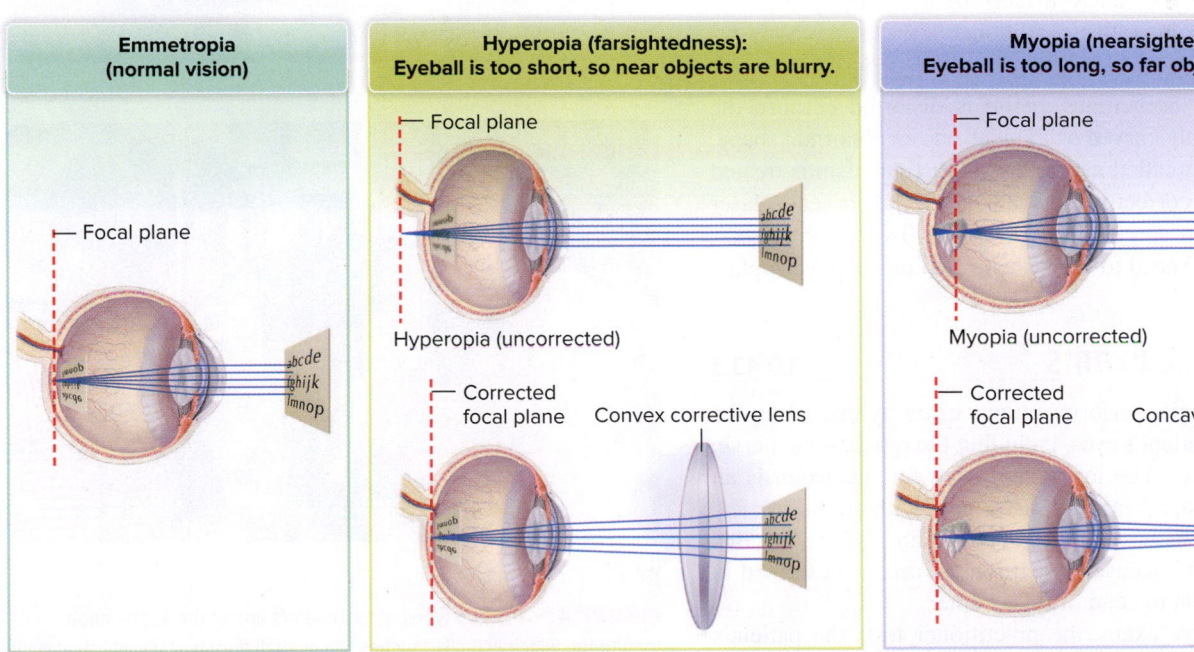

| Emmetropia (normal vision) | Hyperopia (farsightedness): Eyeball is too short, so near objects are blurry. | Myopia (nearsightedness): Eyeball is too long, so far objects are blurry. |

Focal plane

Focal plane
Hyperopia (uncorrected)
Corrected focal plane — Convex corrective lens

Focal plane
Myopia (uncorrected)
Corrected focal plane — Concave corrective lens

(b) Vision correction using (*center*) convex and (*right*) concave lenses

FIGURE 43-2 (a) Lens shape for distant vision and lens shape for near vision (accommodation). (b) Emmetropia, hyperopia, and myopia.

Myopia (Nearsightedness) Myopia is the condition in which images of distant objects come into focus in front of the retina and are blurred (Figure 43-2). This condition occurs if the eye is too long or if the cornea and lens bend light rays more than normally. Nearby objects are usually seen clearly, but objects far away are unclear.

Nearsightedness is corrected with eyeglasses or contact lenses that have inwardly curving (concave) lenses. The lenses correct the bending of light rays so that they focus on the retina. Surgical and laser techniques are also used to correct myopia by changing the shape of the cornea.

Hyperopia (Farsightedness) and Presbyopia

Hyperopia, or hypermetropia, causes images to come into focus behind the retina (Figure 43-2). The eyeball may be too short, or the cornea and lens may bend light rays less than normally. Faraway objects are usually seen clearly, but nearby objects are unclear. If the hyperopia is mild, young eyes can compensate for the problem by a process known as accommodation. The ciliary muscles contract during **accommodation,** thickening the lens and increasing its convexity. These changes allow the image to come into focus on the retina.

Patients with mild farsightedness may have no symptoms or may have blurred vision. They may have symptoms of eyestrain (an aching in the eye) because the ciliary muscles are overworked. Farsightedness is corrected with eyeglasses or contact lenses that have outwardly turning (convex) lenses. Aging usually causes the ciliary muscles to weaken, so a person may need stronger eyeglasses over time.

Presbyopia is a condition that most commonly affects people starting in their mid-40s. Older eyes tend to lose the ability to accommodate because the lens becomes more rigid. As a result, images come into focus behind the retina, as they do with farsightedness. Individuals find they must hold reading materials farther away to see them clearly. Corrective lenses are used to treat this condition.

Astigmatism Sometimes vision is distorted because the cornea is unevenly curved or the lens has an abnormal shape. This condition is called **astigmatism.** Astigmatism is treated with lenses that correct the unevenness of the cornea or laser vision correction surgery known as LASIK. After surgery, patients may still need to wear glasses to correct presbyopia.

▶ Ophthalmic Exams   LO 43.3

An ophthalmologist performs an eye exam by inspecting the interior of the patient's eyes, including the retina, optic nerve, and blood vessels. The instrument used for this exam is an **ophthalmoscope,** a handheld instrument with a light to view the inner eye structures. You will maintain and prepare this instrument for the licensed practitioner's use, as described in Procedure 43-1, at the end of this chapter.

During the eye exam, the practitioner tests the patient's visual fields. The visual field is the entire area visible to the eye when the patient looks at an object straight ahead. Visual fields are assessed by the confrontation method. The practitioner stands or sits about 2 feet in front of the patient. The patient covers one eye, and the practitioner closes her own opposite eye. (This makes the visual fields of the two individuals roughly the same.) Then the practitioner moves a pencil or other object into the patient's horizontal or vertical visual field, asking the patient to say "Now" when the object comes into view. Defects in the field of vision are noted. The practitioner then tests the convergence of the eyes (or how the eyes come together) by bringing the handheld object to the patient's nose as the eyes focus on it.

The ophthalmologist also routinely tests for glaucoma with the aid of a **tonometer** (Figure 43-3). The tonometer measures intraocular pressure, shown by the eyeball's resistance to indentation by either direct pressure or pneumatic pressure. Your role is to explain the procedure to the patient, instill anesthetizing eyedrops into the patient's eyes when required, assist the patient into position, and hand the instruments to the licensed practitioner.

Another instrument the ophthalmologist may use during the exam is the **slit lamp** (Figure 43-4). This instrument consists of a magnifying lens combined with a light source. It is used to examine the eye's anterior structures, including the eyelids, iris, lens, and cornea. Patients rest their chin on the

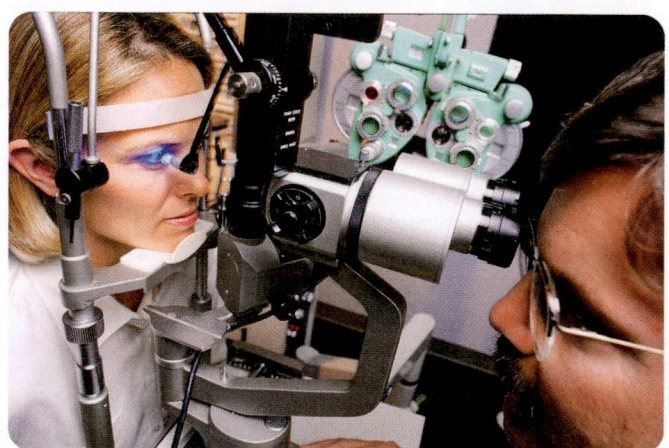

(a)

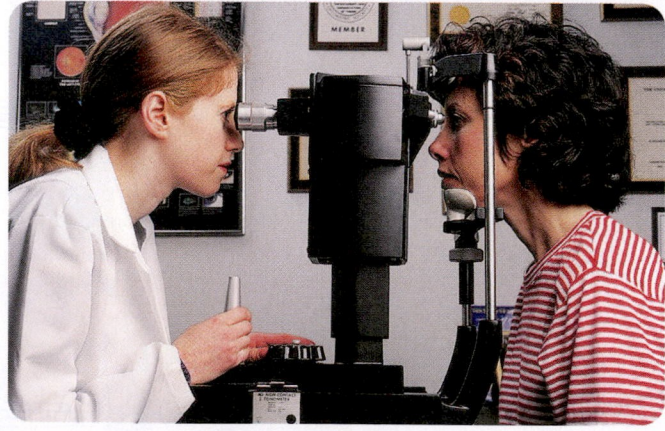

(b)

FIGURE 43-3 Two types of tonometers are (a) the applanation tonometer, which actually touches the eyeball during assessment, and (b) the noncontact, or airpuff, tonometer, which directs a puff of air at the cornea.

© Arthur Tilley/Getty Images; © Ken Lax

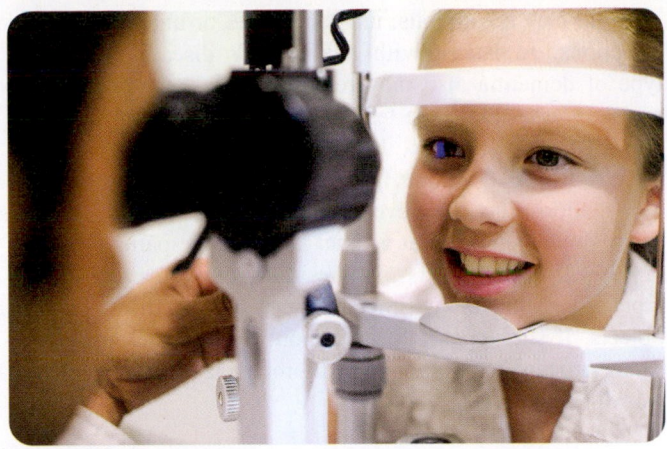

FIGURE 43-4 A slit lamp is used to examine the anterior structures of the eye.
© Ian Hooton/SPL/Getty Images

device's chin rest and stare straight ahead while the practitioner shines a narrow beam (slit) of light into the eye and looks at the eye through the instrument's lens. A special dye—fluorescein—may be used to help visualize foreign bodies or problems with the cornea.

The eye exam also may include a **refraction examination** to verify the need for corrective lenses. Normally, the lens and other parts of the eye work together to focus images on the retina. When errors of refraction exist, images are focused incorrectly, causing conditions such as farsightedness and nearsightedness.

A refraction examination is performed with a retinoscope or a phoropter, a device that contains many different lenses. The practitioner has the patient look through a succession of lens combinations to find out which one creates the clearest image (Figure 43-5).

Types of Vision Screening Tests

Screening tests are used to detect a number of common visual problems, including hyperopia, presbyopia, and myopia. Others test the ability to distinguish shades of gray or colors.

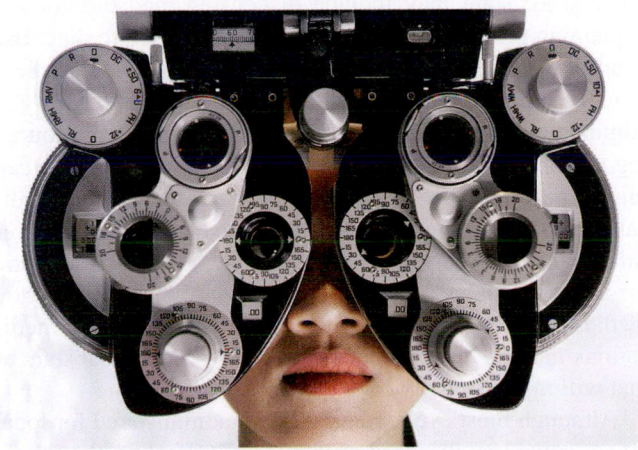

FIGURE 43-5 A phoropter helps the ophthalmologist assess errors of refraction.
© ERproductions Ltd/Getty Images RF

When you record the results of vision tests, be sure to document for which eye you are recording the results and note if the test was done with corrective lenses (glasses or contacts). If vision is tested with glasses or contacts, you will note this with the abbreviation (with correction). Details on how to perform various vision tests can be found in Procedure 43-2 at the end of this chapter.

Visual acuity screenings are procedures commonly performed by medical assistants either before or after the licensed practitioner's exam. These tests screen for distance vision, near vision, and color vision.

Distance Vision The Snellen chart is the most common screening tool for distance vision. You may be familiar with the Snellen letter chart used by many eye professionals. Snellen number charts and "tumbling E" charts are also available. (See Figure Procedure 43-2 Step 2 a and b.) These charts and similar charts that use symbols instead of numbers or letters are often used to test the visual acuity of children.

Near Vision To test for near vision, a Jaeger chart or similar chart is used (Figure Procedure 43-2 Step 21 b and c). These handheld cards contain letters, numbers, or paragraphs in various print sizes. They may be held and read at a normal reading distance (Figure Procedure 43-2 Step 21 a) or mounted in a frame and read through optical lenses. As you may recall, presbyopia is an age-related loss of lens elasticity that affects a person's near vision. The combination of myopia and presbyopia is the reason many people require bifocal lenses as they age.

Color Vision Color vision is commonly tested using a system of colored dots. The two most frequently used testing systems are the Ishihara Color Test (Figure 43-6) and the Richmond pseudoisochromatic color test. Both contain letters, numbers, or symbols made up of colored dots that appear among dots of other colors. The patient is asked to identify what he sees. A patient who is color-blind will not be able to see the items. Color blindness may be inherited; it occurs more commonly in males. Changes in one's ability to see colors, however, may indicate a disease of the retina or optic nerve.

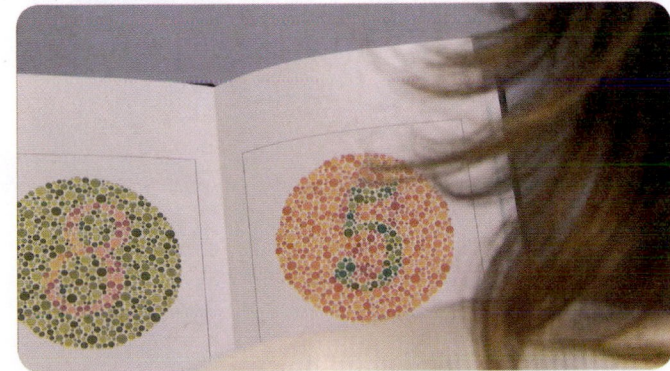

FIGURE 43-6 The Ishihara Color Test, one of the most common color vision tests, uses a system of colored dots to test for color blindness.
© McGraw-Hill Education

Contrast Sensitivity To test for the ability to distinguish shades of gray (contrast sensitivity), Evans Letter Contrast Test (ELCT) and the CSV-1000E contrast sensitivity test are widely used. Some systems provide contrast variations in a projected image (Figure 43-7). These tests can detect cataracts or problems in the retina even before the sharpness of the patient's vision is impaired.

Patients with Special Needs Certain patients may need special attention when having vision tests. For example, children may be anxious, uncooperative, or unable to follow directions. A patient with Alzheimer's disease or another type of dementia also may require special attention during a vision test. Before the test, encourage a family member to stay with the patient so that she is more comfortable. During the test, use simple language to explain the procedure and demonstrate whenever possible. Proceed through the exam slowly, one step at a time. Because the patient's memory and language skills may be impaired, you may need to repeat directions many times and help her to name particular objects. If she appears to have trouble with one part of the exam, proceed to another part and return later to the part that was difficult for her.

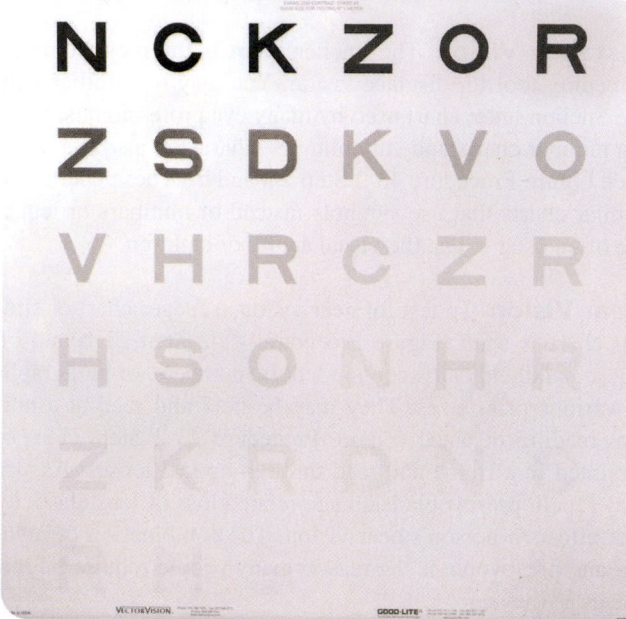

(a) Evans Letter Contrast Test (ELCT)

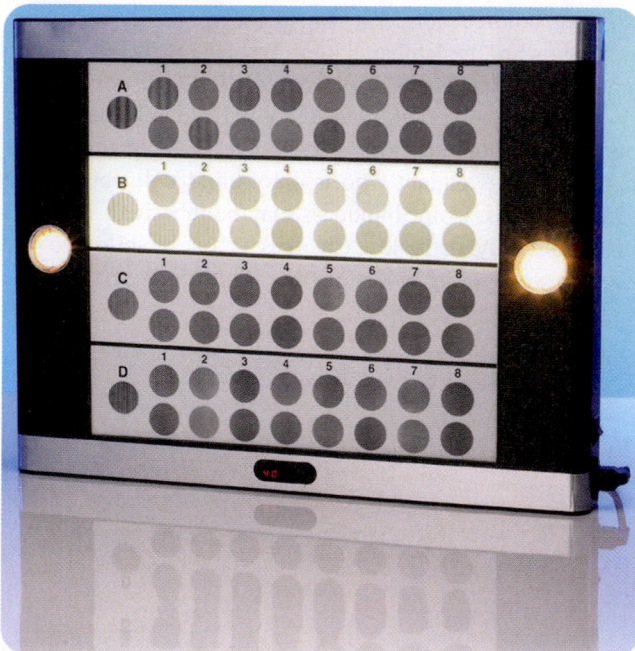

(b) CSV-1000E contract sensitivity test

FIGURE 43-7 Contrast sensitivity, or the ability to distinguish between shades of gray, is most commonly tested with the (a) ELCT and (b) the CSV-1000E.

Courtesy Vector Vision

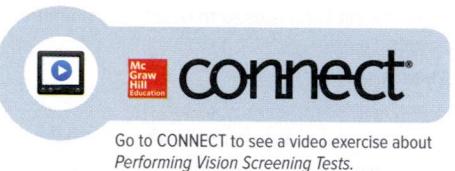

Go to CONNECT to see a video exercise about *Performing Vision Screening Tests.*

▶ Ophthalmologic Procedures and Treatments

LO 43.4

The eye is an extremely delicate organ. Even what seems to be a minor injury or infection can have lasting consequences. You must use the greatest caution as well as proper technique—including sterile technique—when treating a patient's eyes. You also should provide patients with information on how to routinely care for their eyes. See the *Educating the Patient* feature for specific guidelines to follow when presenting eye care information.

Administering Medications to the Eye

Licensed practitioners commonly administer eye medications or perform eye irrigations to assist patients in eye tests, reduce pressure in the eyes, relieve eye pain, and treat eye infections and inflammation. Your responsibility as a medical assistant may include dispensing medications and explaining their use. Some medications are used to diagnose conditions; others are used to treat conditions. Only medications for ophthalmic use should be used in the eye. If you administer eye medications as part of your job, avoid touching a dropper or ointment tube tip to the eye. Doing so can injure the eye, cause infection, and contaminate the medication. Teach patients how to check medication labels carefully before administering them at home. For example, optic medications for eye use could easily be confused for otic medications for the ear. Medications other than optic medications may be too concentrated or may contain substances that will injure sensitive eye tissue.

Although most eye medications are administered for local effect, some are absorbed systemically (affecting the whole body). To prevent systemic absorption, the practitioner may request that you apply pressure with one finger just below the inner corner of each eye after instilling medications.

Preventive Eye Care Tips

You can help patients take care of their eyes and protect their vision by providing them with the following guidelines. Go over each item slowly and carefully. Ask whether the patient has questions before moving on to the next item. Answer all questions and make sure the patient understands the answers.

1. Get regular health checkups. Patients may not appreciate the connection between their general health and their eyes. Point out that high blood pressure and diabetes can cause eye problems.

2. Get regular eye examinations. Most people need eye examinations every 1 to 2 years. Patients with diabetes should see their eye care specialists more frequently.

3. Be alert for eye disease warning signs. Tell patients to call their eye care specialist immediately if they experience any of these signs:
   - Eye pain
   - Loss of vision
   - Double or blurred vision
   - Headache with blurred vision
   - Redness of the eye or eyelid
   - A gritty or sticky feeling around the eye
   - Excessive tearing
   - Difficulty seeing in the dark
   - Flashes of light
   - Halos around lights
   - Sensitivity to light
   - Loss of color perception

4. Wear sunglasses with ultraviolet protection to shield the eyes from bright sunlight, even in the winter. Recommend that patients ask to have ultraviolet protection added when purchasing new distance prescription glasses. Explain to patients that the cornea can get sunburned, which can be painful and damaging. Also tell patients that excessive exposure to the sun is a contributing factor in the development of cataracts and malignant melanoma of the eye—a dangerous type of skin cancer that may spread through the bloodstream or lymphatic system.

5. Wear protective eye equipment to prevent eye injury. Indicate to patients that they should wear protective eyewear every time they participate in sports, work with chemicals, or encounter a situation in which they may be exposed to flying debris.

6. Use nonprescription eye medications properly. Show patients how to use eyedrops, emphasizing that the tip of the dropper should never touch the eye. Explain that medications should be used only as indicated on the label and discarded after the condition has cleared up.

7. Never share eye makeup, because bacterial infections can be passed via the applicators. To minimize contamination of the applicators, patients should take care of the applicators by storing them in a clean container and changing the applicator often. Patients should never place applicators on a dirty countertop.

Continue applying pressure for 2 to 3 minutes, as directed. Procedure 43-3, at the end of this chapter, provides information on administering eye medications.

Eye Irrigation

When foreign materials such as dust, sand, or chemicals enter the eye, they must be flushed out. Flushing—irrigation—should be done, whenever possible, with a sterile solution especially formulated for this purpose. Someone's eye also may need to be irrigated to relieve discomfort from irritating substances such as smog, pollen, chemicals, or chlorinated water. Procedure 43-4, at the end of this chapter, provides details about irrigating an eye. See the *Infection Control Fundamentals* chapter for more information on using an eyewash station.

▶ Otology   LO 43.5

An **otologist** treats diseases and disorders of the ears. Procedures common to this specialty are sometimes performed by other physicians as well, especially general practitioners, internists, and allergists. In your role as a medical assistant, you also may assist with or perform auditory screening, administer ear medications, perform ear irrigations, and help with diagnostic tests such as tympanometry. Otology specialists whose practices include problems affecting the nose and throat are called otorhinolaryngologists.

▶ Ear Diseases and Disorders   LO 43.6

When assisting licensed practitioners in administering various tests, treatments, and procedures, you may encounter a wide range of ear disease and disorder. Some—such as cerumen impaction and otitis externa—do not have lasting effects on hearing and may be treated by a general practitioner. Others affect the ear's middle or inner parts and may require a specialist's attention. Figure 43-8 shows the major parts of the ear. For more detailed information, refer to the *Special Senses* chapter.

Common Disorders of the Outer Ear

Several disorders affect the ear's external parts. These include cerumen impaction, otitis externa, and pruritus.

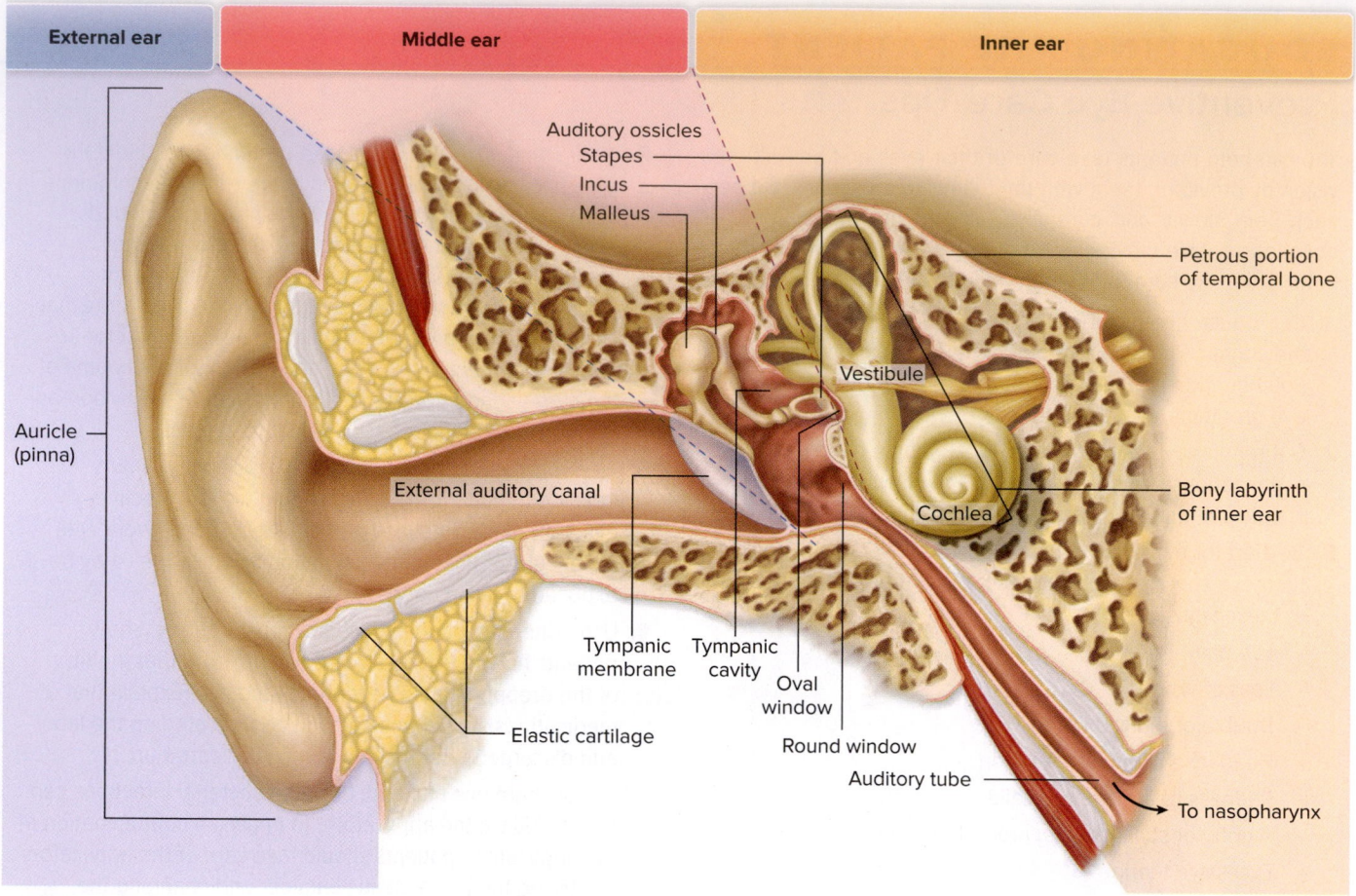

| External ear | Middle ear | Inner ear |

Auditory ossicles
Stapes
Incus
Malleus

Petrous portion
of temporal bone

Vestibule

Auricle
(pinna)

External auditory canal

Bony labyrinth
of inner ear

Cochlea

Tympanic
membrane

Tympanic
cavity

Oval
window

Elastic cartilage

Round window

Auditory tube

To nasopharynx

FIGURE 43-8 The major parts of the ear.

Cerumen Impaction A condition called cerumen impaction occurs when the ear canal becomes blocked by a buildup of cerumen (earwax). The wax can be softened with eardrops, and irrigation can be performed to remove the wax. Refer to Procedure 43-7, at the end of this chapter, for more information about ear irrigation.

Otitis Externa Otitis externa is an infection of the outer ear, usually caused by bacteria or fungi. Also known as swimmer's ear, fungal infections are common in swimmers due to persistent moisture in the ear canal. This infection is treated with a combination of antibiotic or antifungal eardrops and an anti-inflammatory medication.

Pruritus A common problem in the elderly is pruritus—or itching—of the ear canal. Because the sebaceous glands produce less wax with aging, the ear becomes dry and itchy. Dryness can be overcome by a regular routine of lubricating the ear canal with a few drops of mineral oil.

Common Disorders of the Middle Ear

Middle ear disorders involve the eardrum and the chamber behind it. They include otitis media, mastoiditis, otosclerosis, and ruptured eardrum.

Otitis Media Otitis media is an inflammation of the middle ear characterized by fluid buildup, most commonly referred to as an ear infection. For detailed information on otitis media, see the *Points on Practice* feature Otitis Media: The Common Ear Infection.

Mastoiditis The mastoid bone is located just behind the ear. It is connected to the middle ear by air cells, or sinuses, in the bone. Sometimes, if left untreated, an infection in the middle ear can spread to the mastoid bone through these air cells. Although mastoiditis is fairly rare, it may be serious because the mastoid air cells are close to the organs of hearing, important nerves, the covering of the brain, and the jugular vein. Severe cases of mastoiditis may require removal of the affected bone.

Otosclerosis Otosclerosis occurs when bone tissue grows abnormally around the stapes, or stirrup (the innermost of the three tiny bones that connect the eardrum and the inner ear). This overgrowth of tissue prevents the stapes from transmitting sound vibrations to the inner ear. The result is hearing loss in one or both ears. The condition is often hereditary.

Symptoms of otosclerosis include gradual loss of hearing and **tinnitus**—ringing in the ears. Surgery to replace

Otitis Media: The Common Ear Infection

Otitis media, commonly referred to as an ear infection, affects almost all children by age 6. This inflammation of the middle ear accounts for 22 million doctor visits each year—second only to routine well-child health exams.

Ear infections typically start when fluid becomes trapped in the middle ear. The lining of the middle ear and eustachian tube contains fluid similar to the mucus within the nasal passages. The normal flow of this fluid from the ear into the back of the nose where it joins the pharynx helps keep the middle ear and eustachian tube free of bacteria. When a child gets a cold or flu, the lining of the eustachian tube and middle ear can become inflamed and can trap the fluid, which becomes infected.

There are four distinct types of otitis media. One or both ears may be affected.

1. Acute otitis media typically is a bacterial infection of the middle ear that comes on suddenly. This type is common in children and typically follows an upper respiratory tract infection. The symptoms include pain, a feeling of fullness in the ear, some loss of hearing, and possibly fever. In severe cases, the eardrum may rupture because of the fluid pressure. Acute infections are not usually treated with oral antibiotics at first. Most infections will resolve on their own without treatment, so physicians usually wait 48–72 hours before prescribing antibiotic treatment for a patient with acute otitis media.

2. Recurrent otitis media is diagnosed when a child contracts acute otitis media repeatedly, perhaps once or twice every month.

3. Otitis media with effusion, also known as OME, involves an accumulation of fluid in the middle ear. Children with OME do not exhibit any symptoms, and they may not experience any discomfort.

4. Chronic otitis media is diagnosed when fluid is present in the ear and fails to clear up after 3 months or more. Infection may or may not be present. Without treatment, the undrained fluid thickens, possibly resulting in changes in the shape of the eardrum, erosion of the ossicles (tiny bones of hearing), and mastoiditis. Chronic otitis media left untreated for a sufficient amount of time can result in facial paralysis, brain infections, and balance problems. These changes may cause temporary or permanent hearing loss if not treated. Antibiotics and reconstructive surgery may be used to treat this condition.

If a child suffers from recurrent or chronic otitis media, myringotomy—surgical incision of the eardrum with insertion of tubes—may be recommended to keep the fluid draining continuously. This procedure usually removes enough fluid to clear up the infection. Depending on the type of tube, it falls out on its own within 3 to 18 months of insertion. See Figure 43-9.

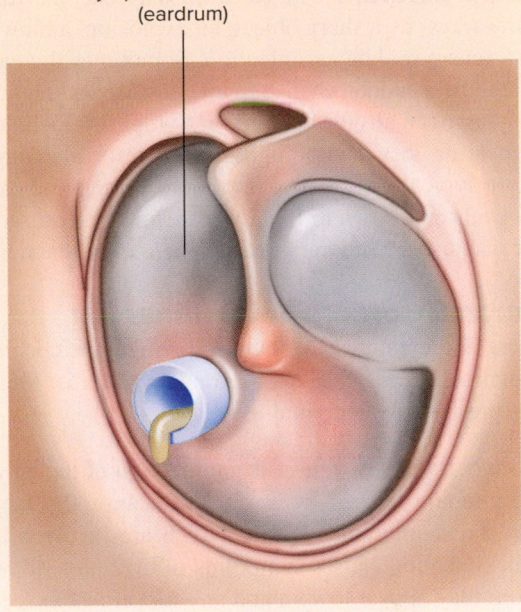

Tympanic membrane (eardrum)

FIGURE 43-9 A pressure-equalizing tube is inserted in the eardrum to help keep fluid from building up behind the eardrum.

Ear infections may be difficult to identify, especially in a young child who cannot talk. The following symptoms are indications of a possible ear infection, particularly if more than one is present:

- Tugging or rubbing of the ear
- Fever ranging from 100°F to 104°F
- Difficulty balancing
- Excessive crankiness
- Difficulty hearing or speaking
- An unwillingness to lie down (the pain may become more severe in a reclining position because of increased pressure against the eardrum)

Preventing ear infections is the best course of action. Several measures can be taken to reduce the likelihood of ear infections, including

- Preventing colds by teaching children to wash their hands often and not share cups and other eating utensils.
- Limiting a child's exposure to secondhand smoke.
- Breastfeeding for at least 6 months.
- Bottle feeding in an upright position—*never* put a baby to bed with a bottle.
- Keeping immunizations such as flu shots and pneumococcal vaccines up to date.

the stapes—ossicular replacement prosthesis surgery—can restore or improve hearing in almost 90% of patients with otosclerosis. Alternatively, a hearing aid may improve hearing for some patients.

Ruptured Eardrum The eardrum may become ruptured in several ways: by a sharp object, an explosion, a blow to the ear, or a severe middle ear infection. Sometimes the eardrum is ruptured by a sudden change in air pressure, as might occur when flying in an airplane or diving. Symptoms include pain, partial hearing loss, and a slight discharge or bleeding. The symptoms typically last only a few hours. A ruptured eardrum usually heals on its own in 1 to 2 weeks, but the licensed practitioner may use a temporary patch to help close the defect.

Common Disorders of the Inner Ear

Disorders of the inner ear, or labyrinth, affect the cochlea and the semicircular canals. They include labyrinthitis, Ménière's disease, presbycusis, and tinnitus.

Labyrinthitis Labyrinthitis is an infection of the labyrinth, most commonly caused by a virus. Because the labyrinth includes the semicircular canals, which are involved in balance, this infection causes symptoms of dizziness or vertigo. The room may appear to spin and any movement exacerbates (worsens) the sensation, sometimes to the point of nausea and vomiting. Although disturbing, labyrinthitis disappears on its own within 1 to 3 weeks. The patient may need to rest in bed for a few days, and medication can be given for symptoms.

Ménière's Disease Ménière's disease is caused by increased fluid in the labyrinth. The pressure of the fluid disturbs the sense of balance and may even rupture the labyrinth wall or damage the cochlea with its hearing receptors. One or both ears may be affected. Symptoms of this disorder include vertigo, nausea, vomiting, distorted hearing, and tinnitus. Some people may suffer hearing loss ranging from mild to severe. Medications may be used to combat vertigo, nausea, and vomiting. Other treatments that help some people include using diuretics and following a low-sodium diet.

Presbycusis Presbycusis is a type of sensorineural hearing loss. It is the most common form of hearing loss in older adults, affecting about 25% of people by the age of 60 or 70. Men are affected more often than women. Hearing loss can be treated effectively, however, with a hearing aid.

Tinnitus Tinnitus is more commonly called a ringing in the ears. This "ringing" can take several forms, including a buzzing, whistling, or hissing sound. The most common causes of tinnitus are damage to the hearing receptors from noise or toxins, age-related changes in the ear's organs, and long-term use of nonsteroidal anti-inflammatory drugs (NSAIDs) such as aspirin and ibuprofen. Tinnitus can affect people at any age but is more common as people get older. If tinnitus becomes chronic, the patient may find relief by listening to quiet, soothing music or other distracting sounds or by using a device similar to a hearing aid that masks the noise with more pleasant sounds.

Hearing Loss

Hearing loss is actually a symptom of a disease, not a disease in itself. Contrary to what most people believe, hearing loss is not a normal part of the aging process and should always be evaluated for proper treatment. There are two types of hearing loss: conductive and sensorineural. The two types differ in the point at which the hearing process is interrupted.

A **conductive hearing loss** is caused by an interruption in the transmission of sound waves to the inner ear. Conditions that can cause conductive hearing loss include obstruction of the ear canal (as with cerumen impaction or a tumor), infection of the middle ear, and otosclerosis or reduced movement of the ossicles.

A **sensorineural hearing loss** occurs when there is damage to the inner ear, to the nerve that leads from the ear to the brain, or to the brain itself. In this kind of loss, sound waves reach the inner ear, but the brain does not perceive them as sound. This type of hearing loss can be hereditary, can be caused by repeated exposure to loud noises or viral infections, or can occur as a side effect of medications such as NSAIDs and some antibiotics. Tinnitus suggests damage to the auditory nerve.

Sensorineural hearing loss can be differentiated from conductive hearing loss by hearing tests. It is also possible for both types of hearing loss to occur together.

Noise Pollution Prolonged exposure to loud noises is a common cause of hearing loss because of damage to the sensitive cells in the cochlea. People who work around noisy equipment—such as construction workers, aircraft personnel, and machine operators—are likely to suffer from this type of hearing loss unless they protect their ears (Figure 43-10). Repeatedly listening to loud music from a personal stereo or car radio set at too high a volume also can damage the ears.

Working with Patients with a Hearing Impairment

You may come in contact with patients of all ages who have hearing impairments. Many patients wear hearing aids to amplify normal speech. Some patients, however, may not

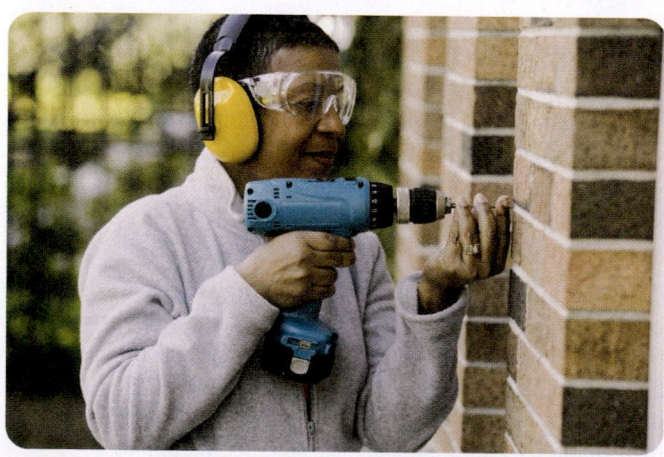

FIGURE 43-10 Loud noises, such as those produced by power tools, can damage hearing unless appropriate ear protectors are worn.
© Wave Royalty Free/age fotostock RF

admit they have a problem—out of fear, vanity, or misinformation. It is estimated that one-third of patients between the ages of 65 and 74 and one-half of those between the ages of 75 and 79 suffer from some loss of hearing.

To improve communication with a patient whose hearing is impaired, you can do the following:

- Speak at a reasonable volume. Do not shout. Shouting can actually make your words harder to understand. A hearing aid filters out loud sounds, so the patient may not hear everything you say if you shout.

- Speak in clear, low-pitched tones. Elderly patients may lose the ability to hear high-pitched sounds.

- Avoid speaking directly into the patient's ear. Stand 3 to 6 feet away and face the patient so that she can see your lip movements and facial expressions. Avoid covering your mouth with your hands. Speak at a normal rate.

- Avoid overemphasizing your lip movements, which makes lip reading difficult.

- Avoid hand gestures unless they are appropriate.

- If the patient does not understand what you say, restate the message in short, simple sentences. Have the patient repeat the message to verify that your words were understood.

- Treat patients who have a hearing impairment with patience and respect.

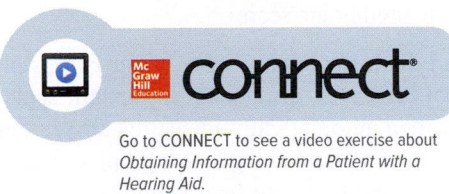

Go to CONNECT to see a video exercise about *Obtaining Information from a Patient with a Hearing Aid.*

▶ Hearing and Other Diagnostic Ear Tests   LO 43.7

Various tests are performed to find out whether a person hears normally. If the tests reveal a problem, follow-up tests are conducted to determine the cause of the problem. You may assist with the testing or educate the patient about caring for her ears.

Hearing Tests

As part of a general examination, licensed practitioners may perform simple hearing tests to determine whether a patient's stated hearing loss is conductive or sensorineural. The most common of these are the Weber test and the Rinne test. Both involve the use of tuning forks (see Figure 43-11).

In the Weber test, the licensed practitioner strikes a tuning fork against a hard surface to produce a sound and then places the tuning fork in the middle of the patient's head (Figure 43-12a). She then asks the patient whether the sound is coming from the right or the left, or both. In conductive hearing loss, the sound will be heard best through the ear with hearing loss. In sensorineural hearing loss, the sound travels toward the ear without hearing loss.

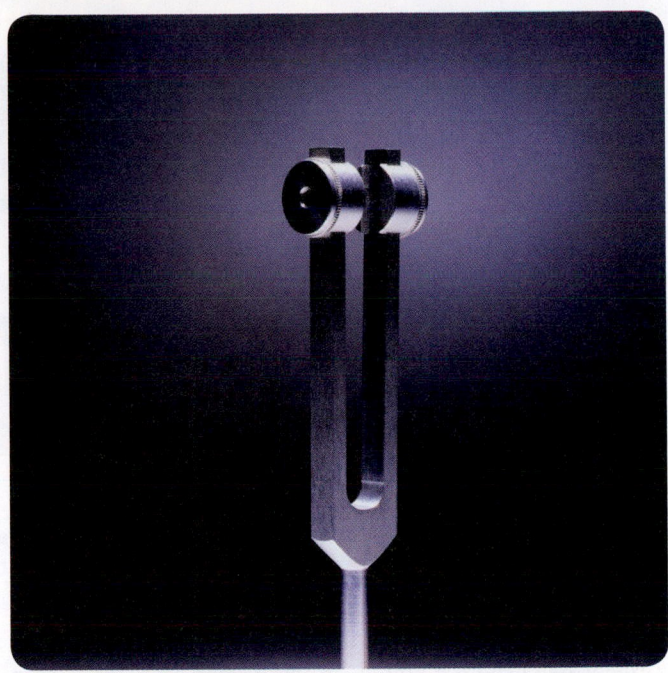

FIGURE 43-11 A tuning fork is used to perform simple hearing tests.
© Spike Mafford/Getty Images RF

To perform the Rinne test, the practitioner measures the amount of time the patient can hear the sound from a tuning fork placed near the mastoid bone (see Figure 43-12b). This measures sound conducted through the bone. She then measures the amount of time the patient can hear the sound when the tuning fork is placed near the ear canal to measure sound conducted through the air (see Figure 43-12c). The two times are then compared. A normal ear will hear the air-conducted sound twice as long as the bone-conducted sound. In a patient with conductive hearing loss, the bone-conducted sound will be at least as long as the air-conducted sound. In a patient with sensorineural hearing loss, the air-conducted sound will last slightly longer than the bone-conducted sound, but not twice as long.

If you have the necessary training, you may help perform a test that uses an audiometer. An **audiometer** is an electronic device that measures hearing acuity by producing sounds in specific frequencies and intensities. A **frequency** is the number of complete fluctuations—waves—of energy that pass a specific point in 1 second (Figure 43-13). Frequency is best described as the pitch of sound. High frequency is high-pitched and low frequency is low-pitched. The audiometer allows a licensed practitioner to test a person's hearing and to determine the nature and extent of hearing loss.

Many types of audiometers are available. Some machines automatically generate the various tones at different **decibels** (units for measuring the relative intensity—loudness—of sounds on a scale from 0 to 130) and print out the patient's responses. Others must be manually adjusted and the results charted by hand. During the test, the patient wears a headset to hear the sounds produced by the audiometer. Depending on the unit, the patient indicates hearing a sound by raising

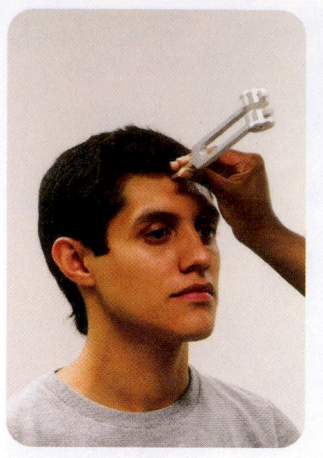
(a)

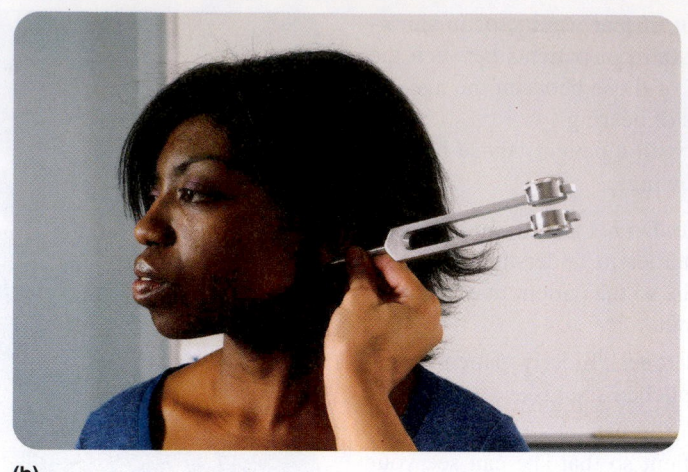
(b)

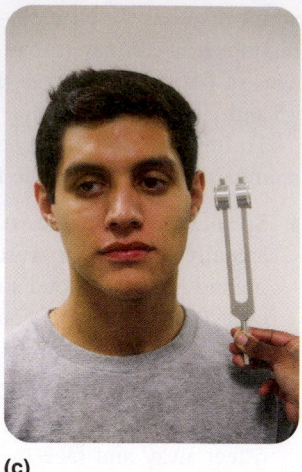
(c)

FIGURE 43-12   (a) During the Weber hearing test, the tuning fork is placed on the patient's forehead. (b) Place the tuning fork on the mastoid bone during the Rinne hearing test. (c) Place the tuning fork near the ear during the Rinne hearing test. Compare how long the patient can hear the sound during each step.

© McGraw-Hill Education. Jill Braaten, photographer

a finger or pushing a button. In the former case, the person administering the test records the response. In the latter case, the response may be recorded automatically or by the test giver. Procedure 43-5, at the end of this chapter, provides additional information about measuring auditory acuity.

Adults and children who can understand directions and respond appropriately can be screened in this manner. If you work in a pediatrician's office, you also may help to check an infant's response to sounds. These tests require special techniques, as infants cannot understand directions. The general steps involved in performing hearing tests on infants are outlined in the *Assisting in Pediatrics* chapter.

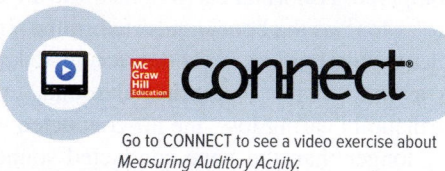

Go to CONNECT to see a video exercise about *Measuring Auditory Acuity.*

Tympanometry

A diagnostic test called tympanometry measures the eardrum's ability to move. This is an indication of the amount of pressure in the middle ear. Tympanometry is used to detect the following diseases and abnormalities of the middle ear or ear canal.

- Cerumen impaction
- Middle ear fluid
- Middle ear tumor
- Ossicular detachment
- Tympanic membrane perforation
- Tympanic membrane scars

To perform the test, a small, soft-rubber cuff is placed over the external ear canal, producing an airtight seal. The tympanometer then automatically measures air pressure against the tympanic membrane and prints a graph of the results. Let patients know that they will hear sounds during the test that may seem loud, but they need to remain as still as possible.

▶ Ear Treatments and Procedures   LO 43.8

Licensed practitioners use various approaches, devices, and techniques with each type of ear problem to improve patients' hearing and maintain or improve their ear health. As a medical assistant, you can provide patients with information on preventive ear care techniques, as described in the *Educating the Patient* feature Preventive Ear Care Tips.

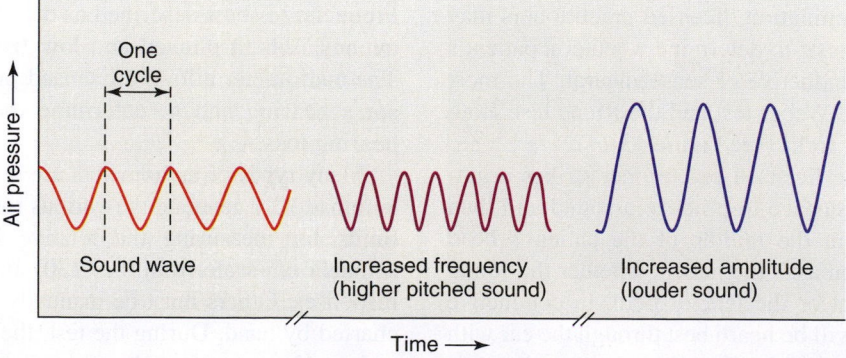

FIGURE 43-13   Sound frequency is determined by the number of waves per second that pass a specified point.

You also may administer ear medications, perform ear irrigations, and assist the physician in earwax removal.

Administering Medications to the Ear

Licensed practitioners often administer eardrops or perform ear irrigations to treat patients' ear infections or inflammation, relieve ear pain, or loosen earwax. Like eye medications, eardrops are used primarily for their local effects. They are not usually absorbed systemically, nor do they cause systemic effects. It is important that you warm the eardrops slightly before administration to avoid making the patient dizzy. Holding them in your hand for a minute or two will usually warm them enough. Procedure 43-6, at the end of this chapter, provides instructions for this procedure.

Earwax and Foreign Body Removal

Cerumen, or earwax, may build up in the ear canal, causing a full feeling in the ear, ear pain, partial hearing loss, and tinnitus. Cerumen normally protects the ear, but if a person produces too much, it can harden and block the ear canal. Also, cleaning your ear with cotton-tipped swabs can push the cerumen down into the ear canal. There are several treatments for removing earwax. In some cases, if the wax is close enough to reach, the licensed practitioner may be able to remove the wax with an ear curette, a small instrument with a scoop or loop on one end. Home remedies include over-the-counter wax softening drops, mineral oil, and glycerin. These may work if the impaction is not too severe. But if the wax is extremely hard or is stuck to the ear canal, irrigation may be the best treatment.

Ear Irrigation Irrigating the ear may relieve inflammation or irritation of the ear canal and help loosen and remove impacted earwax or a foreign body. This procedure is performed in the licensed practitioner's office. Irrigation is contraindicated in (inadvisable for) patients who

- Currently have or have had a ruptured eardrum.
- Have pressure equalizing tubes in their eardrum.
- Have an ear infection.
- Have had ear surgery, including mastoidectomy.

Always ask the patient about ear surgeries and other conditions before beginning the irrigation and make sure the irrigation solution is at body temperature before starting. This helps reduce the possibility of the patient becoming dizzy during the procedure. Procedure 43-7, at the end of this chapter, provides instructions for ear irrigation.

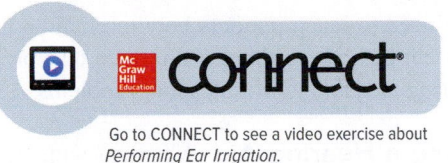

Go to CONNECT to see a video exercise about *Performing Ear Irrigation*.

EDUCATING THE PATIENT

Preventive Ear Care Tips

You can help patients protect their ears and their hearing by providing them with the following guidelines. As with any patient education, go over items slowly, ask patients whether they have questions before moving on, and answer all questions completely.

1. Get routine hearing exams. Screening for hearing problems is often part of a comprehensive physical exam. Encourage patients who have not had their hearing screened or who suspect they have hearing problems to arrange for testing by their licensed practitioner. Older patients, who may not admit they have a problem, may need special encouragement.

2. Avoid injury when cleaning the ears. Instruct patients in proper ear care. Point out that they should not put objects in the ear that might injure the eardrum or ear canal, which includes vigorous probing with cotton-tipped swabs.

3. Avoid injury from nonprescription ear care products. Tell patients to check with a licensed practitioner before using nonprescription products for softening earwax.

4. Use proper ear protection. Urge patients to wear ear protectors around loud work equipment and to avoid listening to loud music. It is especially important to keep the volume at a reasonable level when listening through earphones and through earbuds that fit directly into the external auditory canal.

5. Use all medications properly. Show patients how to use eardrops; emphasize that they must follow instructions precisely. Explain to patients that following instructions applies to all medications because many, including NSAIDs and some antibiotics, can cause hearing loss if used improperly.

6. Be alert for warning signs. Tell patients to call their licensed practitioner immediately if they experience any of these signs of ear problems:
   - Ear pain
   - Stuffiness
   - Discharge from the ear
   - Vertigo (dizziness)

   Also have patients notify the licensed practitioner if they have any of these signs of hearing problems:
   - Tinnitus (ringing)
   - Hearing others' speech as mumbled sounds
   - Speaking in a very loud voice without being aware of it

Microscopic Earwax and Foreign Body Removal

Occasionally, irrigation does not work to remove a cerumen impaction. With the help of a microscope, an otologist can use suction or an instrument to remove the wax. Foreign bodies in the ear also are removed with the aid of a microscope. During the procedure, the licensed practitioner looks through the microscope into the patient's ear canal. This gives her a better view of the ear, allowing her to get deeper into the ear canal without damaging the delicate structures within the ear. The patient must remain extremely still during this procedure. Your role as a medical assistant is to help keep the patient at ease and comfortable and to make sure the practitioner has the necessary instruments.

Hearing Aids

Hearing aids may be worn inside or outside the ear. If worn outside, they may be located behind the ear, mounted on eyeglasses, or worn on the body (Figure 43-14). Hearing aids consist of the following parts:

- A tiny microphone to pick up sounds
- An amplifier to increase the volume of sounds
- A tiny speaker to transmit sounds to the ear

You may need to teach patients how to obtain a hearing aid. You also can pass along tips to help them take proper care of their hearing aids and to troubleshoot problems.

Obtaining a Hearing Aid A patient with signs of hearing loss should be referred to an otologist, a medical doctor specializing in the health of the ear, or an **audiologist,** a specialist who focuses on evaluating and correcting hearing problems. Audiologists are not medical doctors and do not treat diseases of the ear. Instead, they evaluate the patient's hearing, fit hearing aids, give instruction in the use of hearing aids, and provide service for hearing aids if necessary. It is important for hearing aids to fit properly. If they do not, sounds may not be transmitted well into the ear.

Care and Use of Hearing Aids Hearing aids run on batteries that typically last about 2 weeks. So the patient must keep a fresh supply of batteries on hand. The hearing aid itself must be routinely cleaned or the microphone, switches, or dials may not work properly. Moisture can damage the aid, so it must not get wet. Hair sprays can clog hearing aid openings or interfere with the operation of moving parts. For these reasons, spray should be applied before a hearing aid is inserted. Cerumen often builds up behind hearing aids that are worn in the ear, reducing sound transmission. If buildup does occur, the cerumen plug should be removed by ear irrigation.

Other Devices and Strategies

People whose hearing cannot be substantially improved by hearing aids may need to use other devices or strategies to

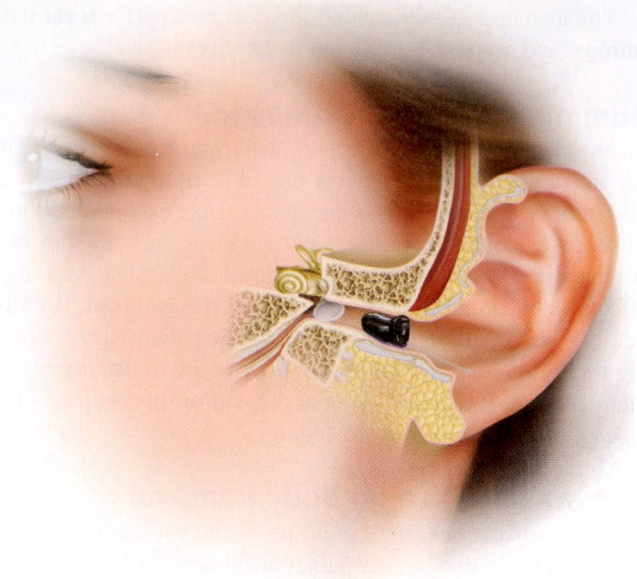

FIGURE 43-14 A hearing aid can be so small that it is inserted inside the ear canal.

overcome the problem. These devices include appliances that light up as well as ring—such as telephones, doorbells, smoke detectors, alarm clocks, and burglar alarms. Patients can purchase amplifiers for the telephone, television, and radio. Many closed-captioned television programs are also available. To benefit from closed captioning, the patient must have a television with a decoder that translates the captioning and displays the captions on the screen.

Cochlear Implants

A person who is profoundly deaf and cannot benefit from using a hearing aid may be a candidate for a **cochlear implant,** an electronic device that stimulates the auditory nerve. A cochlear implant has an external and an internal component. The external portion sits just behind the ear and the internal portion has an array of electrodes implanted directly into the cochlea. Cochlear implants do not amplify sound like a hearing aid but send signals through the auditory nerve to the brain. This gives patients the ability to detect warning signals such as smoke alarms and recognize speech patterns so that they can be better understood. Hearing with a cochlear implant is not the same as normal hearing; patients have to learn to recognize sounds. Adults with cochlear implants can often learn to understand speech without using visual cues such as lip reading. Children can learn to speak with extensive speech therapy. More than 42,000 adults and 28,000 children in the United States have cochlear implants.

PROCEDURE 43-1 Preparing the Ophthalmoscope for Use

Procedure Goal: To ensure that the ophthalmoscope is ready for use during an eye exam

OSHA Guidelines: This procedure does not involve exposure to blood, body fluids, or tissues.

Materials: Ophthalmoscope, lens, spare bulb, spare battery

Method:

1. Wash your hands.
2. Take the ophthalmoscope out of its battery charger. In a darkened room, turn on the ophthalmoscope light.
3. Shine the large beam of white light on the back of your hand to check that the instrument's tiny lightbulb is providing strong enough light.
4. Replace the bulb or battery if necessary. (The battery is located in the ophthalmoscope's handle.)
5. Make sure the instrument's lens is screwed into the handle. If it is not, attach the lens.

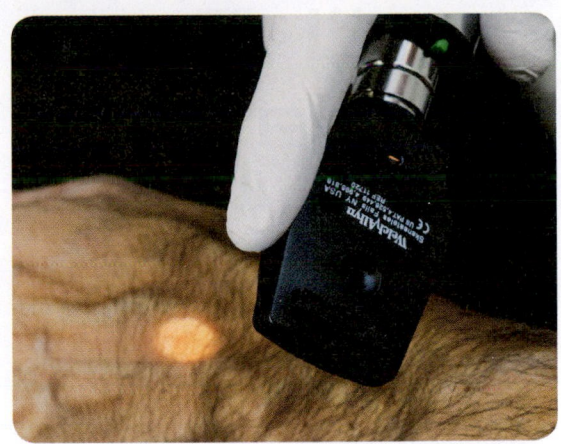

FIGURE Procedure 43-1 Step 3   Shine the ophthalmoscope light on your hand to check the strength of the beam.
© McGraw-Hill Education. Aaron Roeth, photographer

PROCEDURE 43-2 Performing Vision Screening Tests   WORK // DOC

Procedure Goal: To screen a patient's ability to see distant or close objects, to determine contrast sensitivity, or to detect color blindness

OSHA Guidelines:

 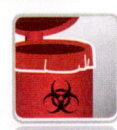

Materials: Eye occluder or card to block vision in one eye; alcohol; gauze squares; appropriate vision charts to test for distance vision, near vision, and color blindness; patient chart/progress note

Method:

Distance Vision

1. Wash your hands, clean the occluder with a gauze square dampened in alcohol, identify the patient, introduce yourself, and explain the procedure.
2. Mount one of the following eye charts at eye level: Snellen letter or similar chart (for patients who can read); Snellen tumbling E, Landolt C, pictorial, or similar chart (for patients who cannot read).

   If using the Snellen letter chart, verify that the patient knows the letters of the alphabet. With children or nonreading adults, use demonstration cards to verify that they can identify the pictures or direction of the letters.

   RATIONALE: *If the patient does not understand the instructions, the results will not be accurate.*

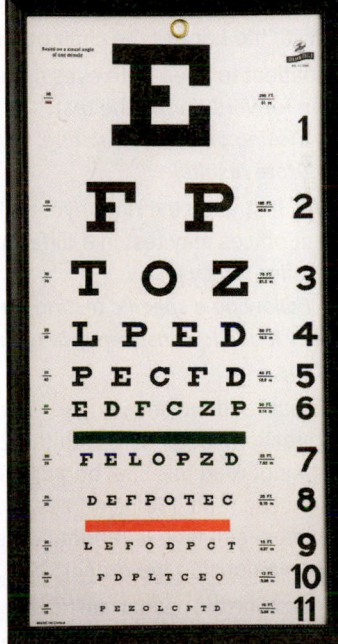

(a)

FIGURE Procedure 43-2 Step 2   (a) The Snellen letter chart is used to test the vision of people who can read.
© McGraw-Hill Education/Rick Brady, photographer

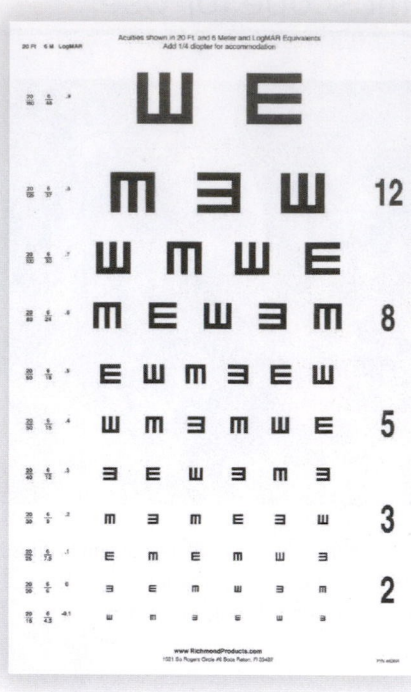

(b)

FIGURE Procedure 43-2 Step 2 (b) The Snellen "tumbling E" chart is used to test the vision of children and nonreading adults.

Reprinted with permission of Richmond Products, Inc.

3. Make a mark on the floor 20 feet away from the chart.

4. Have the patient stand with his or her heels at the 20-foot mark, or sit with the back of the chair at the mark.

5. Instruct the patient to keep both eyes open and not to squint or lean forward during the test.
   RATIONALE: *Closing one eye, squinting, or leaning will lead to inaccurate results.*

6. Test both eyes first, then the right eye, and then the left eye. (Different offices may test in a different order. Follow your office policy.)
   RATIONALE: *Following a specific testing order based on office policy leads to consistency in the results of all medical records.*

7. Have the patient read the lines on the chart (or identify the picture/direction), beginning with the 20-foot line. If the patient cannot read this line, begin with the smallest line the patient can read. (Some offices use a pointer to select one symbol at a time in random order to prevent patients from memorizing the order.)

8. Note the smallest line the patient can read or identify with no more than two errors. (Some offices only allow one error per line. Follow office policy when performing this test.)

9. Record the results as a fraction (for example, Both Eyes 20/40−1 if the patient misses one letter on a line or Both Eyes 20/40 −2 if the patient misses two letters on a line).

10. Show the patient how to cover the left eye with the occluder or card. Again, instruct the patient to keep both eyes open and not to squint or lean forward during the test.

11. Have the patient read the lines on the chart.

12. Record the results of the right eye (for example, Right Eye 20/30).

13. Have the patient cover the right eye and read the lines on the chart.

14. Record the results of the left eye (for example, Left Eye 20/20).

15. If the patient wears corrective lenses, record the results using c̄c̄ (if your office uses this abbreviation for "with correction") in front of the abbreviation (for example, c̄c̄ Both Eyes 20/20).
    RATIONALE: *For charting accuracy, vision correction must be noted using your office format.*

16. Note and record any observations of squinting, head tilting, excessive blinking, or tearing.

17. Ask the patient to keep both eyes open and to identify the color of the two colored bars on the Snellen chart, and record the results in the patient's chart.
    RATIONALE: *This step is sometimes done as a basic color vision screening.*

18. Clean the occluder with a gauze square dampened with alcohol.

19. Properly dispose of the gauze square and wash your hands.
    RATIONALE: *Maintain principles of aseptic technique at all times.*

Near Vision

20. Wash your hands, identify the patient, introduce yourself, and explain the procedure.

21. Have the patient hold one of the following at normal reading distance (approximately 14 to 16 inches): Jaeger, Richmond pocket, or similar chart or card.

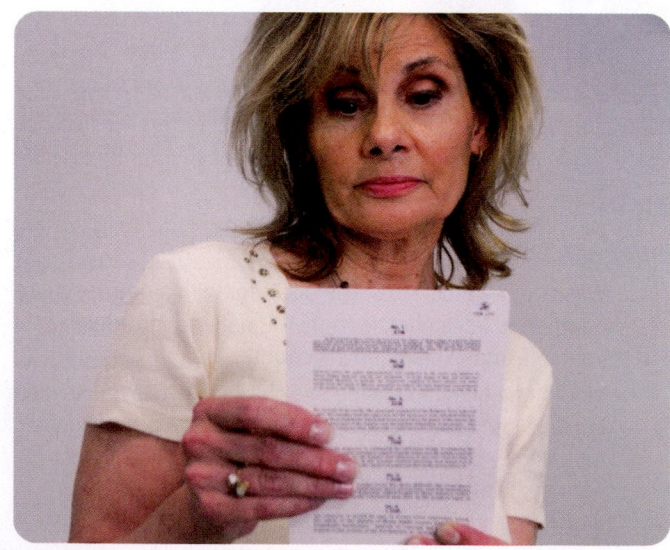

(a)

FIGURE Procedure 43-2 Step 21 (a) Have the patient hold the card at a comfortable reading distance.

© McGraw-Hill Education

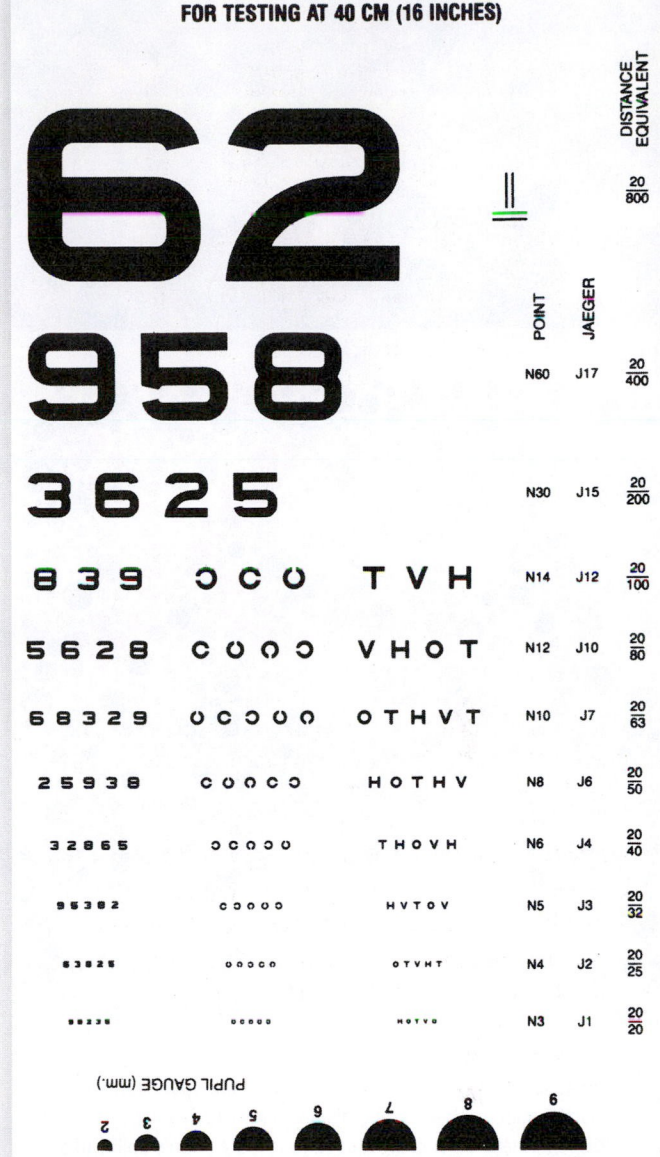

(b)

Text panel (b), near vision chart:

V = .50 D.

The fourteenth of August was the day fixed upon for the sailing of the brig Pilgrim, on her voyage from Boston round Cape Horn, to the western coast of North America. As she was to get under way early in the afternoon, I made my appearance on board at twelve o'clock in full sea-rig, and with my chest, containing an outfit for a two or three years voyage,

which I had undertaken from a determination to cure, if possible, by an entire change of life, and by a long absence from books and study, a weakness of the eyes which had obliged me to give up my pursuits, and which no medical aid seemed likely to cure. The change from the tight dress coat, silk cap and kid gloves of an undergraduate at Cambridge, to the

V = .75 D.

loose duck trousers, checked shirt and tarpaulin hat of a sailor, though somewhat of a transformation, was soon made, and I supposed that I should pass very well for a Jack tar. But it is impossible to deceive the practiced eye in these matters; and while I supposed myself to be looking as salt as Neptune himself, I was, no doubt, known for a landsman by every one on board, as soon as I hove in sight. A sailor has a peculiar cut to his clothes, and a way of wear-

V = 1. D.

ing them which a green hand can never get. The trousers, tight around the hips, and thence hanging long and loose around the feet, a superabundance of checked shirt, a low-crowned, well-varnished black hat, worn on the back of the head, with half a fathom of black ribbon hanging over the left eye, and a peculiar tie to the black silk neckerchief, with sundry other *details*, are signs the want of which betray the beginner at once.

V = 1.25 D.

Beside the points in my dress which were out of the way, doubtless my complexion and hands would distinguish me from the regular *salt*, who, with a sun-browned cheek, wide step and rolling gait, swings his bronzed and toughened hands athwartships half open, as though just to ready to grasp a rope. "With all my imperfections

V = 1.50 D.

on my head," I joined the crew, and we hauled out into the stream and came to anchor for the night. The next day we were employed in preparation for sea, reeving and studding-sail gear, crossing royal yards, putting on chafing gear, and taking on board our powder. On the

V = 1.75 D.

following night I stood my first watch. I remained awake nearly all the first part of the night, from fear that I might not hear when I was called; and when I went on deck, so great were my ideas of the importance of my trust, that I

V = 2. D.

walked regularly fore and aft the whole length of the vessel, looking out over the bows and taffrail at each turn, and was not a little surprised at the unconcerned manner in which the billows turned up their

Your glasses are of value to you only as they accurately interpret your prescription and this only as they are fitted and serviced in accordance with these needs. They are a therapeutic device.

RICHMOND PRODUCTS
BOCA RATON. FL 33487
No. 11974 R

(c)

FIGURE Procedure 43-2 Step 21   (b) This near vision chart is used to test the ability to see objects at a normal reading distance.
Reprinted with permission of Richmond Products, Inc.

FIGURE Procedure 43-2 Step 21   (c) The Richmond pocket vision screener is also used to test near vision.
Reprinted with permission of Richmond Products, Inc.

22. Ask the patient to keep both eyes open and to read or identify the letters, symbols, or paragraphs.
    RATIONALE: *If both eyes are not open, results may not be accurate.*

23. Record the smallest line read without error.

24. If the card is laminated, clean it with a gauze square dampened with alcohol.

25. Properly dispose of the gauze square and wash your hands.
    RATIONALE: *Maintain principles of aseptic technique at all times.*

Color Vision

26. Wash your hands, identify the patient, introduce yourself, and explain the procedure.

27. Hold one of the following color charts or books at the patient's normal reading distance (approximately 14 to 16 inches): Ishihara, Richmond pseudoisochromatic, or similar color-testing system.

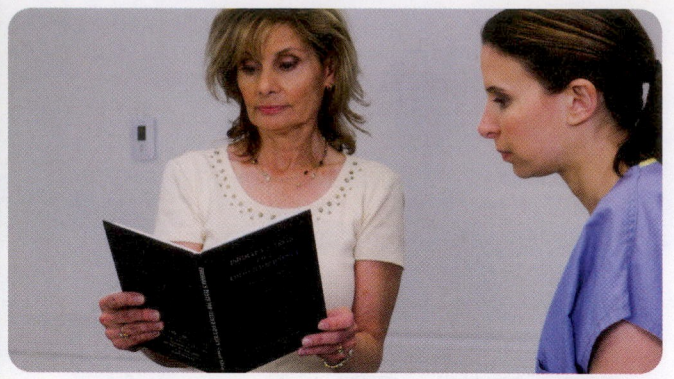

(a)

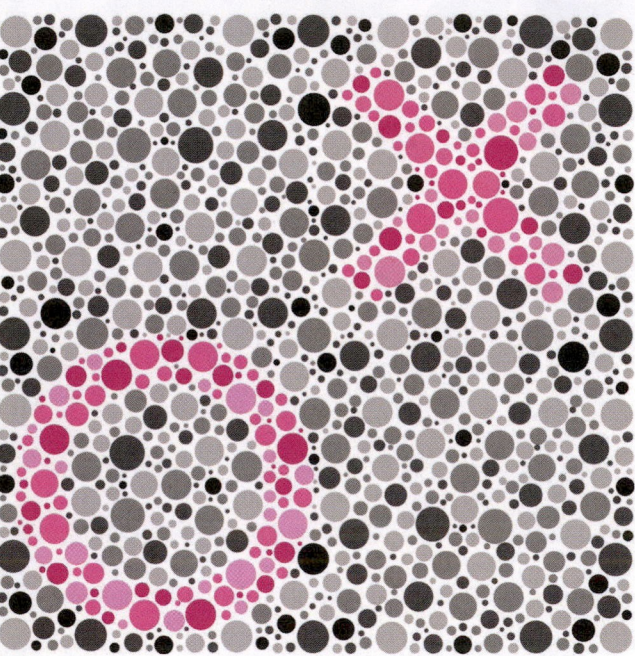

(b)

FIGURE Procedure 43-2 Step 27   (a) Have the patient hold the chart at a comfortable reading distance. (b) The Richmond pseudoisochromatic color chart is used to test a person's ability to see colors.

© **McGraw-Hill Education;** Reprinted with permission of Richmond Products, Inc.

28. Ask the patient to tell you the number or symbol within the colored dots on each chart or page.

29. Proceed through all the charts or pages, usually totaling 24.

30. Record the number correctly identified and failed with a slash between them (for example, 23 passed/1 failed).

31. If the charts are laminated, clean them with a gauze square dampened with alcohol.

32. Properly dispose of the gauze square and wash your hands.
    RATIONALE: *Maintain principles of aseptic technique at all times.*

33. Document the results after you have completed the procedure (Refer to Progress Note).

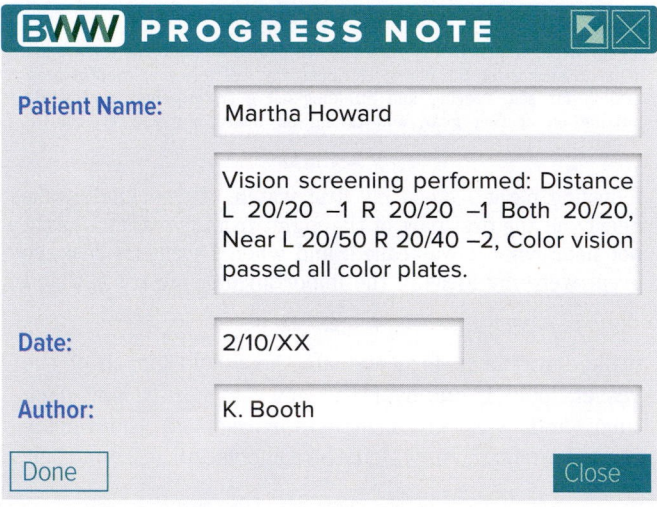

BWW **PROGRESS NOTE**

Patient Name: Martha Howard

Vision screening performed: Distance L 20/20 −1 R 20/20 −1 Both 20/20, Near L 20/50 R 20/40 −2, Color vision passed all color plates.

Date: 2/10/XX

Author: K. Booth

Done   Close

PROCEDURE 43-3 Administering Eye Medications   WORK // DOC

Procedure Goal: To instill (introduce) medication into the eye for treatment of certain eye disorders

OSHA Guidelines:

  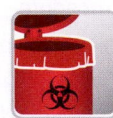

Materials: Medication (drops, cream, or ointment), tissues, eye patch (if applicable), progress note/patient chart

Method:

1. Identify the patient, introduce yourself, and explain the procedure.

2. Review the licensed practitioner's medication order. This should include the patient's name, drug name, concentration, number of drops (if a liquid), into which eye(s) the medication is to be administered, and the frequency of administration.
   RATIONALE: *The licensed practitioner's order must be followed exactly.*

3. Compare the drug with the medication order three times and complete a check of the rights of medication administration, including the right patient, medication, doses, route, time, and documentation.
   RATIONALE: *To ensure necessary accuracy.*

4. Ask whether the patient has any known allergies to substances contained in the medication.

5. Wash your hands and put on gloves.

6. Assemble the supplies.

7. Ask the patient to lie down or to sit back in a chair with the head tilted back.

8. Give the patient a tissue to blot excess medication as needed.

9. Remove an eye patch, if present.

10. Instruct the patient to look at the ceiling and to keep both eyes open during the procedure.

11. With a tissue, gently pull the lower eyelid down by pressing downward on the patient's cheekbone just below the eyelid with your nondominant hand. This pressure will open a pocket of space between the eyelid and the eye.

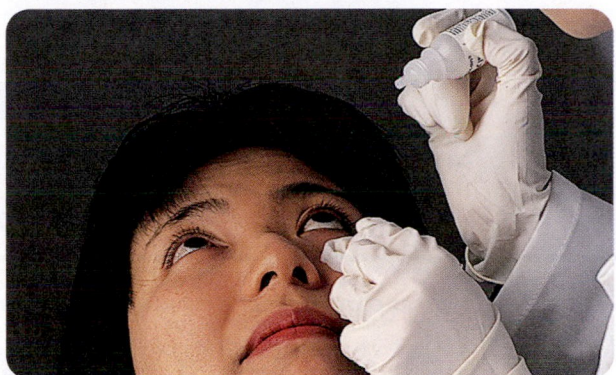

FIGURE Procedure 43-3 Step 11   Use a tissue to press down on the patient's cheekbone just below the eyelid, opening up a pocket of space between the eyelid and the eye.
© Ken Lax

Eyedrops

12. Resting your dominant hand on the patient's forehead, hold the filled eyedropper or bottle approximately ½ inch from the conjunctiva.
    RATIONALE: *Touching the patient's skin with the dropper or bottle tip will cause contamination.*

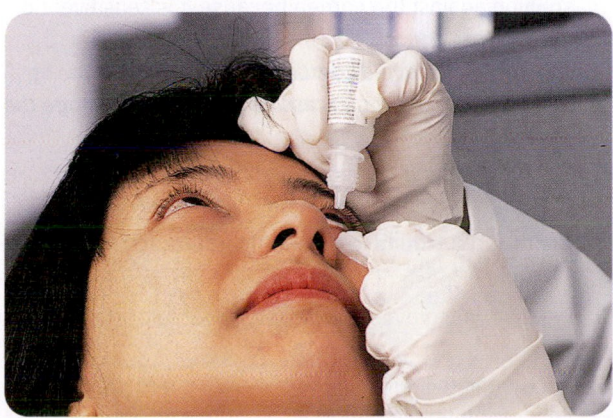

FIGURE Procedure 43-3 Step 12   The medication container should be approximately ½ inch from the conjunctiva as you prepare to instill drops into the patient's eye.
© Ken Lax

13. Drop the prescribed number of drops into the pocket. If any drops land outside the eye, repeat instilling the drops that missed the eye.

Creams or Ointments

14. Rest your dominant hand on the patient's forehead and hold the tube or applicator above the conjunctiva.

15. Without touching the eyelid or conjunctiva with the applicator, evenly apply a thin ribbon of cream or ointment along the inside edge of the lower eyelid on the conjunctiva, working from the medial (inner) to the lateral (outer) side.
    RATIONALE: *Touching the patient's skin with the applicator will cause contamination.*

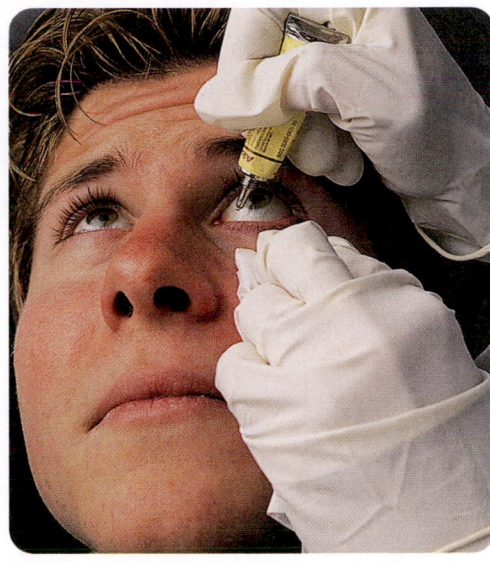

FIGURE Procedure 43-3 Step 15   Apply a thin ribbon of cream or ointment along the inside of the lower eyelid on the conjunctiva.
© Ken Lax

All Medications

16. Release the lower lid and instruct the patient to gently close the eyes.

17. Repeat the procedure for the other eye as necessary.

18. Remove any excess medication by wiping each eyelid gently with a fresh tissue from the medial to the lateral side.

19. Apply a clean eye patch to cover the entire eye, if ordered.

20. Ask whether the patient felt any discomfort and observe for any adverse reactions. Notify the licensed practitioner as necessary.

21. Instruct the patient on self-administration of medication and patch application, if ordered.

22. Ask the patient to repeat the instructions.

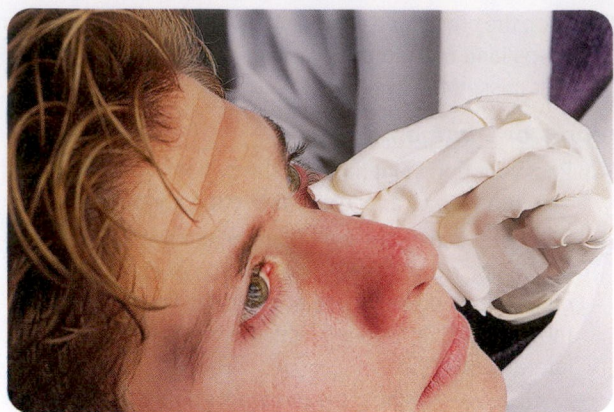

FIGURE Procedure 43-3 Step 18   Use a tissue to remove excess medication from the eyelid.
© Ken Lax

23. Provide written instructions.
24. Properly dispose of used disposable materials.
25. Remove gloves and wash your hands.

26. Document administration in the patient's chart. Include the drug, the concentration, the number of drops or amount, the time of administration, and the eye(s) that received the medication (Refer to Progress Note).

BWW PROGRESS NOTE ⤢ ✕

Patient Name:	Ken Carter
	Instilled Latanoprost 0.005% ophthalmic solution 1 drop both eyes at 4:30 pm.
Date:	10/01/XX
Author:	K. White

Done   Close

PROCEDURE 43-4   Performing Eye Irrigation   **WORK // DOC**

Procedure Goal: To flush the eye to remove foreign particles or relieve eye irritation

OSHA Guidelines:

  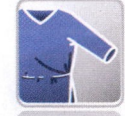 

Materials: Patient chart/progress note, sterile irrigating solution, sterile basin, sterile irrigating syringe and kidney-shaped basin, tissues

Method:

1. Identify the patient, introduce yourself, and explain the procedure.
2. Review the licensed practitioner's order. This should include the patient's name, the irrigating solution, the volume of solution, and for which eye(s) the irrigation is to be performed.
3. Compare the solution with the instructions three times, checking the rights of medication administration.
   RATIONALE: *To ensure necessary accuracy.*
4. Wash your hands and put on gloves, a gown, and a face shield.
   RATIONALE: *Splashing is possible when a syringe is used.*
5. Assemble supplies.
6. Ask the patient to lie down or to sit with the head tilted back and to the side that is being irrigated. The solution should not spill over into the other eye.

RATIONALE: *Cross-contamination between the eyes must be avoided.*

7. Place a towel or a disposable waterproof underpad over the patient's shoulder. Have the patient hold the kidney-shaped basin at the side of the head next to the eye to be irrigated.
8. Pour the solution into the sterile basin.
9. Fill the irrigating syringe with solution (approximately 50 mL).
10. Hold a tissue on the patient's cheekbone below the lower eyelid with your nondominant hand and press downward to expose the eye socket.
11. Holding the tip of the syringe ½ inch away from the eye, direct the solution onto the lower conjunctiva from the inner to the outer aspect of the eye. (Avoid directing the solution against the cornea because it is sensitive; do not use excessive force.)
    RATIONALE: *To avoid contamination, do not let the tip touch the eye or skin. Excessive force could damage the cornea.*
12. Refill the syringe and continue irrigation until the prescribed volume of solution is used.
13. Dry the area around the eye with tissues or gauze squares.
14. Properly dispose of used disposable materials.
15. Remove your gloves, gown, and face shield, and wash your hands.
16. Record the following in the patient's chart: procedure, type of solution, amount of solution used, time of administration, and eye(s) irrigated.
17. Put on gloves and clean the equipment and room according to OSHA guidelines.

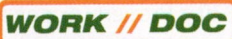

Procedure Goal: To determine how well a patient hears

OSHA Guidelines:

 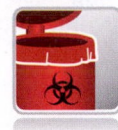

Materials: Patient chart/progress note, audiometer, headset, graph pad (if applicable), alcohol, gauze squares

Method:

Infants and Toddlers

1. Identify the patient and introduce yourself.
2. Wash your hands.
3. Pick a quiet location.
4. The patient can be sitting, lying down, or held by the parent.
5. Instruct the parent to be silent during the procedure.
6. Position yourself so that your hands are behind the child's right ear and out of sight.
   RATIONALE: *You want the child to respond to sound, not to sight.*
7. Clap your hands loudly. Observe the child's response. (Never clap directly in front of the ear because this can damage the eardrum. As an alternative to clapping, use devices such as rattles or clickers (which may be available in the office) to generate sounds of varying loudness.)
8. Record the child's response as positive or negative for loud noise.
9. Position one hand behind the child's right ear, as before.
10. Snap your fingers. Observe the child's response.
11. Record the response as positive or negative for moderate noise.
12. Repeat steps 6 through 11 for the left ear.
13. Document the information (Refer to Progress Note).

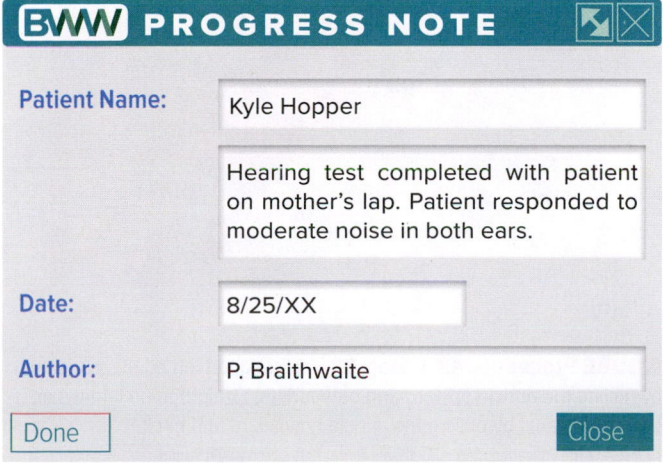

Adults and Children

1. Wash your hands, identify the patient, introduce yourself, and explain the procedure.
2. Clean the earpieces of the headset with a sanitizing wipe according to the manufacturer's instructions.
   RATIONALE: *Maintain aseptic technique at all times.*
3. Have the patient sit with his back to you.
   RATIONALE: *To prevent the patient from using visual clues to pass the hearing test*
4. Assist the patient in putting on the headset and adjust it until it is comfortable.
5. Tell the patient he will hear tones in the right ear.
6. Tell the patient to raise his finger or press the indicator button when he hears a tone.
7. Set the audiometer for the right ear.
8. Set the audiometer for the lowest range of frequencies and the first degree of loudness (usually 15 decibels). (When using automated audiometers, follow the instructions printed in the user's manual.)
9. Press the tone button or switch and observe the patient.
10. If the patient does not hear the first degree of loudness, raise it two or three times to greater degrees, up to 50 or 60 decibels.
11. If the patient indicates that he has heard the tone, record the setting on the graph.
12. Change the setting to the next frequency. Repeat steps 9, 10, and 11.
13. Proceed to the midrange frequencies. Repeat steps 9, 10, and 11.
14. Proceed to the high-range frequencies. Repeat steps 9, 10, and 11.
15. Set the audiometer for the left ear.
16. Tell the patient that he will hear tones in the left ear and ask him to raise his finger or press the indicator button when he hears a tone.
17. Repeat steps 8 through 14.
18. Have the patient remove the headset.
19. Clean the earpieces with a sanitizing wipe.

20. Properly dispose of the used sanitizing wipe and wash your hands.

RATIONALE: *Maintain aseptic technique at all times.*

21. Document the following information after you have completed the procedure (Refer to Progress Note).

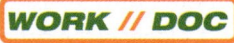

BWW PROGRESS NOTE

Patient Name:	Howard Tyler
	Audiometer hearing test completed, results charted on graph.
Date:	2/10/XX
Author:	M. Shaw

Done   Close

PROCEDURE 43-6 Administering Eardrops

WORK // DOC

Procedure Goal:
To instill medication into the ear to treat certain ear disorders

OSHA Guidelines:

  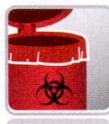

Materials:
Patient chart/progress note, liquid medication, cotton balls

Method:

1. Identify the patient, introduce yourself, and explain the procedure.

2. Check the licensed practitioner's medication order. It should include the patient's name, drug name, concentration, number of drops, into which ear(s) the medication is to be administered, and frequency of administration.

3. Compare the drug with the instructions three times, checking the rights of medication administration.

   RATIONALE: *To ensure necessary accuracy.*

4. Ask whether the patient has any allergies to ear medications.

5. Wash your hands and put on gloves.

6. Assemble supplies.

7. Warm the medication with your hands or by placing the bottle in a pan of warm water.

   RATIONALE: *Internal ear structures are very sensitive to extreme heat or cold. Administering cold medications can result in severe vertigo (dizziness) or nausea.*

8. Have the patient lie on his or her side with the ear to be treated facing up.

9. Straighten the ear canal by pulling the auricle upward and outward for adults, down and back for infants and children.

   RATIONALE: *Straightening the ear canal ensures that the medication reaches its destination.*

10. Hold the dropper ½ inch above the ear canal.

    RATIONALE: *The dropper must not be contaminated by touching the patient's skin or any other surface.*

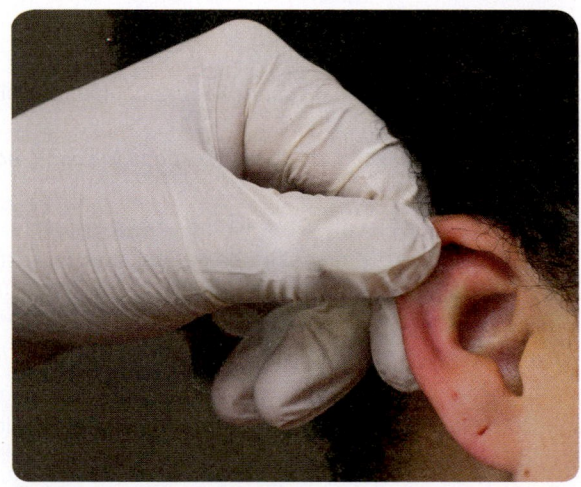

(a)

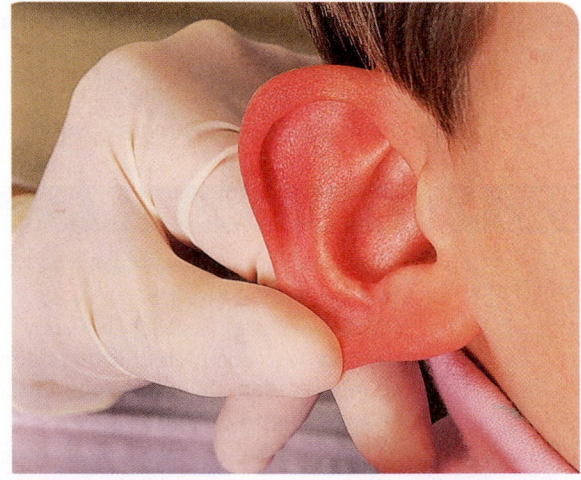

(b)

FIGURE Procedure 43-6 Step 9   (a) Straighten an adult's ear canal by pulling the auricle upward and outward. (b) Straighten an infant's or child's ear canal by pulling the auricle downward and back.

© McGraw-Hill Education. Aaron Roeth, photographer; © Terry Wild Studio

11. Gently squeeze the bottle or dropper bulb to administer the correct number of drops.

12. Have the patient remain in this position for 10 minutes.

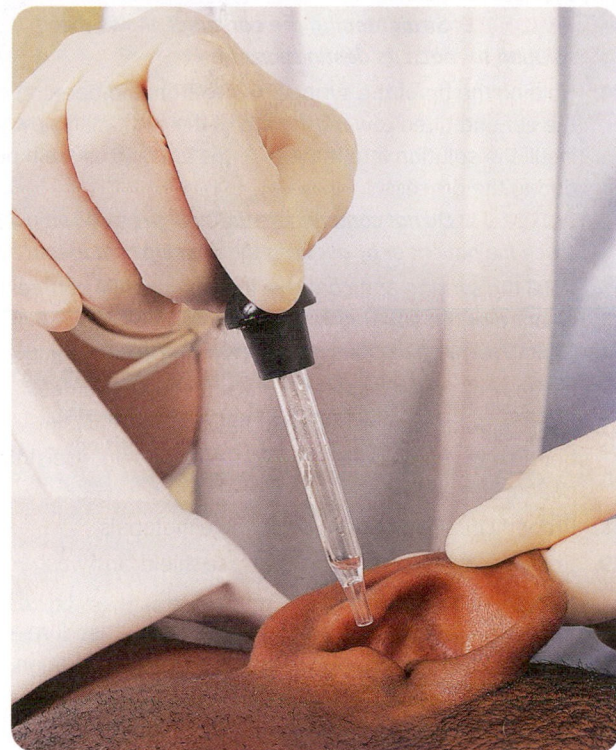

FIGURE Procedure 43-6 Step 11   Apply slow, gentle pressure to the dropper bulb so that you can count the drops and administer the prescribed number.
© Terry Wild Studio

13. If ordered, loosely place a small wad of cotton in the outermost part of the ear canal.

14. Note any adverse reaction, notifying the licensed practitioner as necessary.

15. Repeat the procedure for the other ear, if ordered.

16. Instruct the patient on how to administer the drops at home.

17. Ask the patient to repeat the instructions.
RATIONALE: *For maximum effectiveness, it is important that the patient understands how to correctly continue treatment at home.*

18. Provide written instructions.

19. Remove the cotton after 15 minutes.

20. Properly dispose of used disposable materials.

21. Remove gloves and wash your hands.

22. Record in the patient's chart the medication, the concentration, the number of drops, the time of administration, and which ear(s) received the medication (Refer to Progress Note).

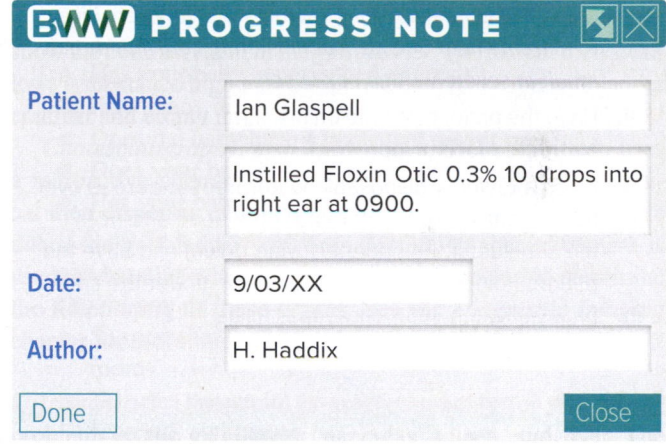

BWW PROGRESS NOTE

Patient Name: Ian Glaspell

Instilled Floxin Otic 0.3% 10 drops into right ear at 0900.

Date: 9/03/XX

Author: H. Haddix

Done   Close

PROCEDURE 43-7   Performing Ear Irrigation

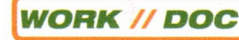
WORK // DOC

Procedure Goal:
To wash out the ear canal to remove impacted cerumen, relieve inflammation, or remove a foreign body

OSHA Guidelines:

 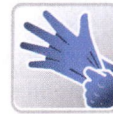 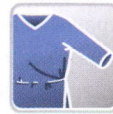 

 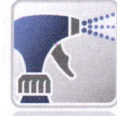

Materials:
Patient chart/progress note, fresh irrigating solution, clean basin, clean irrigating syringe, towel or absorbent pad, kidney-shaped basin, cotton balls

Method:

1. Identify the patient, introduce yourself, and explain the procedure.

2. Check the licensed practitioner's order. It should include the patient's name, the irrigating solution, the volume of solution, and for which ear(s) the irrigation is to be performed. If the practitioner has not specified the volume of solution, use the amount needed to remove the wax.

3. Compare the solution with the instructions three times, checking the rights of medication administration.
RATIONALE: *To ensure necessary accuracy.*

4. Wash your hands and put on gloves, a gown, and a face shield.
RATIONALE: *Splashing is possible when a syringe is used.*

5. Look into the patient's ear to identify cerumen or a foreign body needing to be removed. You will know when you have completed the irrigation when the cerumen or foreign body is removed.
RATIONALE: *Identifying the cerumen or foreign body visually will help you assess when you have successfully completed the irrigation.*

6. Assemble the supplies.

7. If the solution is cold, warm it to body temperature by placing the bottle in a pan of warm water.

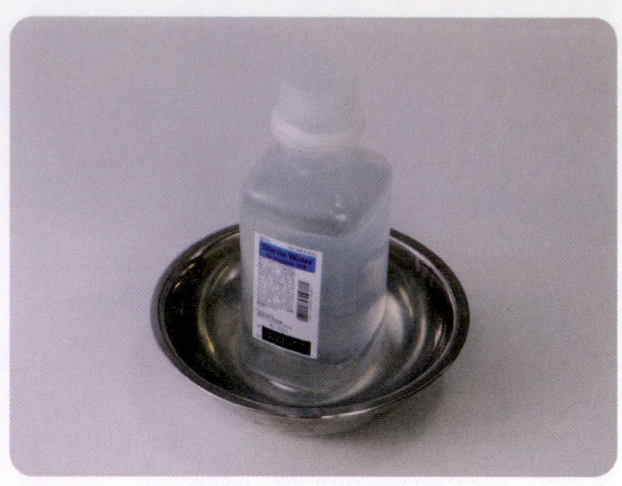

FIGURE Procedure 43-7 Step 7 — Warm the irrigation solution in a pan of warm water.
© McGraw-Hill Education

RATIONALE: *Internal ear structures are very sensitive to extreme heat or cold. Administering cold liquids can result in severe vertigo or nausea.*

8. Have the patient sit or lie on his or her back with the ear to be treated facing you.

9. Place a towel or disposable waterproof underpad over the patient's shoulder (or under the head and over the shoulder if the patient is lying down) and have the patient hold the kidney-shaped basin under the ear.

10. Pour the solution into the other basin.

11. If necessary, gently clean the external ear with cotton moistened with the solution.

12. Fill the irrigating syringe with solution (approximately 50 mL).

13. Straighten the ear canal by pulling the auricle upward and outward for adults.
    RATIONALE: *Straightening the ear canal allows the solution to reach its destination.*

14. Holding the tip of the syringe ½ inch from the opening of the ear and tilted toward the top of the ear canal, slowly instill the solution into the ear. Allow the fluid to drain out during the process.
    RATIONALE: *Do not contaminate the syringe by allowing it to touch the patient or by allowing the draining fluid to touch it.*

15. Refill the syringe and continue irrigation until the canal is cleaned or the solution is used up.

16. Dry the external ear with a cotton ball and, if ordered, leave a clean cotton ball loosely in place for 5–10 minutes.

17. If the patient becomes dizzy or nauseated, allow him or her time to regain balance before standing up. Assist the patient as needed.

18. Properly dispose of used disposable materials.

19. Remove your gloves, gown, and face shield, and wash your hands.

20. Record the following in the patient's chart: procedure and result, amount of solution used, time of administration, and ear(s) irrigated.

21. Put on gloves and clean the equipment and room according to OSHA guidelines.

SUMMARY OF LEARNING OUTCOMES

LEARNING OUTCOMES	KEY POINTS
43.1 Describe the medical assistant's role in eye exams and procedures performed in a medical office.	The medical assistant may assist or perform some of the procedures that involve measuring various aspects and functions of the eye, such as visual acuity, color vision, and intraocular pressure.
43.2 Discuss various eye disorders encountered in a medical office.	Disorders of the eye include those of the external eye structures, such as blepharitis, ptosis, and sty; disorders of the anterior eye structures, such as conjunctivitis and corneal abrasions; disorders involving internal eye structures, such as cataracts, glaucoma, iritis, and retinal disorders; and refractive disorders, such as myopia, hyperopia, astigmatism, and presbyopia.
43.3 Identify ophthalmic exams performed in the licensed practitioner's office.	Ophthalmic exams performed in the licensed practitioner's office include inspecting internal eye structures; testing visual fields; glaucoma testing; inspecting external eye structures; and refraction exams.
43.4 Summarize ophthalmologic procedures and treatments.	Ophthalmologic procedures and treatments include administering eye medications such as eyedrops and ointments and performing eye irrigation.
43.5 Describe the medical assistant's role in otology.	Medical assistants in an otology office may assist with or perform auditory screening, administer ear medications, perform ear irrigations, and help with diagnostic tests such as tympanometry.

LEARNING OUTCOMES	KEY POINTS
43.6 Describe disorders of the ear encountered in the medical office.	Ear diseases and disorders include those of the outer ear, such as cerumen impaction, otitis externa, and pruritus; middle ear disorders, such as otitis media, mastoiditis, otosclerosis, and ruptured eardrum; and those of the inner ear, such as labyrinthitis, Ménière's disease, presbycusis, tinnitus, and hearing loss.
43.7 Recall various hearing and other diagnostic ear tests.	Hearing and other diagnostic ear tests include audiometry and tympanometry.
43.8 Summarize ear procedures and treatments.	Ear treatments and procedures include administration of ear medications, ear irrigation, microscope-aided earwax or foreign body removal, hearing aid fitting, and cochlear implants.

CASE STUDY CRITICAL THINKING

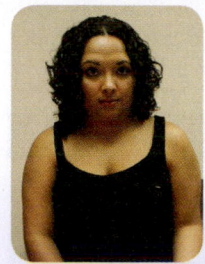

Recall Valarie from the beginning of the chapter. Now that you have completed the chapter, answer the following questions regarding her case.

1. What is the medical assistant's role during the eye irrigation?
2. What are some of the reasons a licensed practitioner might order an eye irrigation procedure?

EXAM PREPARATION QUESTIONS

1. (LO 43.2) Which of the following is the common name for an inflammation of the conjunctiva?
   a. Pruritus
   b. Pink eye
   c. Blepharitis
   d. Iritis
   e. Hordeolum

2. (LO 43.2) Drooping of the upper eyelid is known as
   a. Astigmatism
   b. Sty
   c. Ptosis
   d. Amblyopia
   e. Conjunctivitis

3. (LO 43.5) An otologist treats which of the following disorders?
   a. Glaucoma
   b. Refractive disorders
   c. Mastoiditis
   d. Cataracts
   e. Strabismus

4. (LO 43.6) Ringing in the ears is known as
   a. Presbycusis
   b. Tinnitus
   c. Ménière's disease
   d. Labyrinthitis
   e. Otitis media

5. (LO 43.2) The buildup of which fluid causes glaucoma?
   a. Aqueous humor
   b. Lacrimal fluid
   c. Vitreous humor
   d. Cerumen
   e. Perilymph

6. (LO 43.2) Which of the following is *not* a visual disturbance?
   a. Presbyopia
   b. Astigmatism
   c. Refractive error
   d. Presbycusis
   e. Hyperopia

7. (LO 43.3) Which of the following would be determined by a refraction exam?
   a. Astigmatism
   b. Blepharitis
   c. Corneal ulcers
   d. Diabetic retinopathy
   e. Strabismus

8. (LO 43.6) Which of the following would improve communication with a hearing-impaired patient?
   a. Speak very loudly
   b. Speak in clear, low-pitched tones
   c. Speak directly into the patient's ear
   d. Overemphasize your lip movements so that the patient can read your lips
   e. Write everything down for the patient to read

9. (LO 43.7) The units for measuring the relative intensity of sounds on a scale from 0 to 130 are
   a. Frequencies
   b. Waves
   c. Audiometers
   d. Periods
   e. Decibels

10. (LO 43.6) Sensorineural hearing loss is caused by
    a. Damage to the inner ear
    b. Impacted cerumen
    c. Otitis media
    d. Tinnitus
    e. Otosclerosis

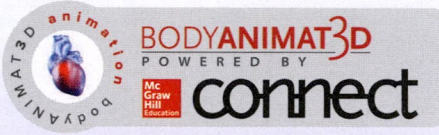

Go to CONNECT to see an animation exercise about *Hearing Loss: Sensorineural.*

SOFT SKILLS SUCCESS

You are assigned to assist with an audiogram on a patient. You have not yet used the new machine that the office just purchased for the audiogram. When you enter the room to introduce yourself to the patient, he looks at you blankly and does not appear to understand.

1. How should you proceed with the new equipment?
2. How should you interact with the patient?

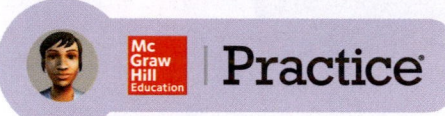

Go to PRACTICE MEDICAL OFFICE and complete the modules Clinical - Work Task Proficiencies and Clinical - Interactions.

Assisting with Minor Surgery

CASE STUDY

PATIENT INFORMATION	Patient Name	DOB	Allergies
	Peter Smith	3/28/19XX	NKA
	Attending	**MRN**	**Other Information**
	Paul F. Buckwalter, MD	428-69-544	Started swimming last week

Peter Smith is a 73-year-old male with a history of mild depression. He arrives at the clinic holding a bloody towel over his left forearm. He is taken immediately back to the treatment area. He states that he cut himself with a large knife while cutting a pineapple. You take his vital signs while waiting for the physician. You notice the blood is leaking through the towel. You need to control the bleeding.

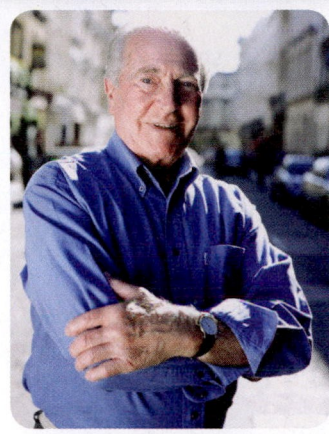

© Image Source/Getty Images RF

You put on PPE, most importantly gloves, and apply a large dressing over the area, holding firm pressure. The physician arrives, examines the patient, and determines that the patient will need sutures. While you are preparing Mr. Smith for his wound repair procedure, he tells you that he recently started swimming for exercise and is going to the Bahamas for a snorkeling trip in 2 weeks. He wants to know if this will ruin his trip.

Keep Mr. Smith in mind as you study this chapter. There will be questions at the end of the chapter based on the case study. The information in the chapter will help you answer these questions.

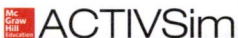
ACTIVSim

LEARNING OUTCOMES

After completing Chapter 44, you will be able to:

44.1 Define the medical assistant's role in minor surgical procedures.

44.2 Describe surgical procedures performed in an office setting.

44.3 Identify the instruments used in minor surgery and describe their functions.

44.4 Describe the procedures for medical and sterile asepsis in minor surgery.

44.5 Summarize the medical assistant's duties in preoperative procedures.

44.6 Describe the medical assistant's duties during an operative procedure.

44.7 Implement the medical assistant's duties in the postoperative period.

KEY TERMS

abscess	laceration
anesthesia	ligature
anesthetic	maturation phase
approximate	needle biopsy
cryosurgery	postoperative
debridement	preoperative
electrocauterization	proliferation phase
formalin	puncture wound
incision	sterile field
inflammatory phase	suture
intraoperative	swaged needle

I.P.8 Instruct and prepare a patient for a procedure or a treatment

I.P.9 Assist provider with a patient exam

III.C.3 Define the following as practiced within an ambulatory care setting:
(a) medical asepsis
(b) surgical asepsis

III.P.2 Select appropriate barrier/personal protective equipment (PPE)

III.P.3 Perform handwashing

III.P.6 Prepare a sterile field

III.P.7 Perform within a sterile field

III.P.8 Perform wound care

III.P.9 Perform dressing change

III.P.10 Demonstrate proper disposal of biohazardous material
(a) sharps
(b) regulated wastes

V.P.4 Coach patients regarding:
(b) health maintenance
(c) disease prevention
(d) treatment plan

X.P.3 Document patient care accurately in the medical record

2. Anatomy and Physiology
c. Identify diagnostic and treatment modalities as they relate to each body system

9. Clinical Procedures
a. Practice standard precautions and perform disinfection/sterilization techniques
e. Perform specialty procedures including but not limited to minor surgery, cardiac, respiratory, OB-GYN, neurological, gastroenterology

10. Medical Laboratory Procedures
c. Dispose of biohazardous materials

▶ Introduction

Minor surgical procedures are frequently performed in ambulatory care settings and office practices. Assisting with minor surgery requires a variety of duties and skills. As a medical assistant, you must be knowledgeable of the types of procedures performed where you are employed. You need to know how to prepare the patient for surgery, assist the practitioner during surgery, and care for the patient after surgery. Because all types of surgery require surgical asepsis, a working knowledge of this technique is mandatory.

▶ The Medical Assistant's Role in Minor Surgery   LO 44.1

Medical assistants play an important role in all aspects of minor surgical procedures. You will perform administrative tasks prior to the patient's surgery, including completing forms for insurance and obtaining signed informed consent from the patient. You will explain basic aspects of the surgical procedure and answer the patient's questions. Informing the doctor of all current prescription and over-the-counter (OTC) medications that the patient is currently taking is also an administrative task. Finally, you will make sure the patient knows how to follow the appropriate presurgical instructions.

In addition to presurgical administrative tasks, you also will perform many tasks directly related to the surgical procedure. You will make sure the surgical room is clean, neat, and properly lit. You will see that all the equipment, instruments, and supplies the doctor will use are clean, disinfected or sterilized, and properly arranged. You also may function as an unsterile assistant, ensuring the safety and comfort of the patient during the procedure and performing other duties. At other times, you may directly assist with the surgical procedure in a sterile capacity.

Following the surgical procedure, you will help dress the wound and perform other postoperative patient care, making sure the patient is not experiencing ill effects from the surgery or local anesthetic. You will educate the patient about wound care and proper procedures to follow after surgery and make sure the patient has safe transportation home. You also will clean the room and prepare it for the next patient.

Surgery in the Physician's Office LO 44.2

Minor surgical procedures are those that can be safely performed in the physician's office or clinic without general anesthesia. **Anesthesia** is a loss of sensation, particularly the feeling of pain. An **anesthetic** is a medication that causes anesthesia. A general anesthetic affects the entire body, whereas a local anesthetic affects only a particular area. Minor surgical procedures typically involve the use of a local anesthetic in the form of an injection or a cream applied to the skin.

Minor surgery is performed for many reasons, whether it be to diagnose an illness or repair an injury. Other procedures may be elective, or optional. Removal of a wart, skin tag (a small outgrowth of skin, occurring frequently on the neck as people get older), or other small growth for cosmetic reasons is an elective procedure. Some of the common minor surgical procedures you may assist the doctor with include the following:

- Repair of a laceration
- Irrigation and cleaning of a puncture wound
- Wound debridement
- Removal of foreign bodies
- Removal of small growths
- Removal of a nail or part of a nail
- Drainage of an abscess
- Collection of a biopsy specimen
- Cryosurgery
- Laser surgery
- Electrocauterization

Common Surgical Procedures

Many surgical procedures are routinely performed in a doctor's office. You may perform some of these procedures on your own. For example, you may change dressings for surgical wounds, and under a doctor's orders, you may remove sutures (commonly called stitches) or staples after wounds have healed. Any procedure that requires an **incision** (a surgical wound made by cutting into body tissue) must be performed by a doctor.

Draining an Abscess An **abscess** is a collection of pus (white blood cells [WBCs], bacteria, and dead skin cells) that forms as a result of infection. A protective lining can form around an abscess and prevent it from healing. In such a case, the physician may make an incision in the lining of the abscess. This procedure is known as an incision and drainage (I&D). The physician may allow the abscess to drain on its own or insert a drainage tube.

Obtaining a Biopsy Specimen A biopsy specimen is a small amount of tissue removed from the body for examination under a microscope. Most biopsies involve cutting the tissue. For a **needle biopsy,** the doctor uses a needle and syringe to aspirate (withdraw by suction) fluid or tissue cells. (The procedure in the *Assisting in Other Medical Specialties*

chapter describes how to assist with a needle biopsy.) All specimens must be placed in a preservative, most commonly a 10% **formalin** solution (a dilute solution of formaldehyde), to prevent changes in the tissue.

Mole Removal A mole, also called a *nevus,* is a small, discolored area of the skin. It may be raised or flat. Any mole that changes shape, size, or color should be evaluated for possible removal. Moles are typically removed by excision or by slicing flush with the skin. If the mole is excised, sutures are usually necessary. Moles that are removed by slicing flush with the skin do not require sutures but may need to be cauterized.

Caring for Wounds A wound is any break in the skin. The break may be accidental or intentional, as from a surgical procedure. There are several types of accidental wounds. A **laceration** is a jagged, open wound in the skin that can extend down into the underlying tissue. The jagged edges may have to be cut away before the wound is closed. A **puncture wound** is a deep wound caused by a sharp object. (See the *Emergency Preparedness* chapter for further information on types and care of accidental wounds.) Both surgical and accidental wounds require special care to prevent infection. Proper wound care that promotes healing without infection is discussed in the *Caution: Handle with Care* feature.

Cleaning a Wound The first step in preventing a nonsurgical wound from becoming infected is careful cleansing. First, clean around the wound with soap and water. Then, it must be irrigated with sterile saline solution or sterile water, applied with a syringe and needle.

Debridement is the removal of debris or dead tissue from a wound. This special type of cleaning may be required for a wound that has dead or sloughing tissue. This procedure helps to expose healthy tissue and promote healing. The doctor may use one of a number of wound debridement methods:

- Surgical—cutting away tissue with scalpel and scissors
- Chemical—using special compounds to dissolve tissue
- Mechanical—applying a dressing that sticks to the wound, removing dead tissue when the dressing is removed, or irrigating the wound with sterile saline
- Autolytic—applying a dressing that helps the body's natural fluids dissolve dead tissue

Wound Healing It is important to know how a wound heals so that you can care for it properly. A wound heals in three phases: inflammatory phase, proliferation phase, and maturation phase. The time it takes for a wound to heal depends on several factors, including the patient's age, nutritional status, and overall health. During the initial phase, or **inflammatory phase,** bleeding is reduced as blood vessels in the affected area constrict. Platelets, clotting factors, and WBCs play an important role in this phase. They seal the wound, clot the blood that has seeped into the area, and remove bacteria and debris from the wound. The wound contracts under the clot or scab that forms.

Conditions That Interfere with Fast, Effective Wound Healing

The goals for treating both surgical and nonsurgical wounds are similar: to heal the wound without infection and to preserve normal skin function and appearance. Nonsurgical wounds often involve conditions that do not promote fast, effective healing. In these cases, the wounds require special attention to ensure good results.

Many types of nonsurgical wounds contain foreign material that can lead to infection. For example, a child may have a deep laceration from landing on a dirty, broken bottle when falling off a bicycle. These types of wounds always need vigorous cleaning. Some may need debridement.

Wounds heal better when the edges are brought closely together, or approximated. Jagged edges in a laceration make approximation harder. It is also difficult to approximate crushed tissue, as you would see with fingers closed in a car door. Crushing disrupts a tissue's blood supply by rupturing blood vessels throughout the affected area. A physician might debride this type of wound with a scalpel to remove severely damaged tissue and achieve a clean wound edge before suturing.

After a surgical or nonsurgical wound is closed and sutured, it is essential to keep the wound clean and dry to help prevent infection. Infection delays the healing process and can have other serious consequences.

A sutured wound heals more quickly and smoothly when no scab forms because the migrating skin cells encounter no barrier to their movement. Proper postoperative care, including daily cleaning with soap and water or a mild antiseptic, keeps a wound scab-free. Although skin cells migrate across the space of a wound more easily in a somewhat moist environment, a wet wound offers the ideal conditions for bacteria to grow and cause infection. Covering a wound with a clean, dry dressing helps prevent infection.

Wound healing may be delayed in a number of instances not directly related to the surgery or injury. The presence of any of the following conditions can put a patient at risk for wound healing problems. Wounds in such patients may require extra attention and care.

- **Poor circulation.** This condition results in inadequate supplies of nutrients, blood cells, and oxygen to the wound, all of which delay the healing process.
- **Aging.** Physiologic changes that occur with age can decrease a person's resistance to infection.
- **Diabetes.** Patients with diabetes experience changes in their artery walls that result in poor circulation to peripheral tissues. These patients also may have a decreased resistance to infection.
- **Poor nutrition.** Patients who are undernourished, particularly those who are deficient in protein or vitamin C, do not have the physiologic resources for vigorous healing.
- **High levels of stress.** An increase in stress-related hormones can decrease resistance to infection.
- **Weakened immune system.** Patients who are on certain medications or who have certain chronic diseases may have weakened immune systems, putting them at increased risk of infection.
- **Obesity.** When someone is obese, the circulation directly under the skin is often poor, leading to slow healing.
- **Smoking.** Nicotine constricts the blood vessels in the skin, reducing circulation to the wound area and slowing healing.

During the second phase, or **proliferation phase,** new tissue forms. Skin cells at the edges of the wound begin to move together to close off the wound. The scab that often forms over a wound actually slows down this movement of skin cells. The edges of the wound eventually come together and form a continuous layer, closing off the wound.

The proliferation phase speeds up if the edges of an incision or a nonsurgical wound are **approximated,** or brought together so that the tissue surfaces are close. This intervention protects the area from further contamination and minimizes scab and scar formation. Small wounds can be held together with butterfly closures, sterile strips, or adhesive. Skin adhesive is a special type of glue used for closing small wounds. Larger wounds or those subject to strain may require suturing or stapling.

The **maturation phase** (the third phase) involves the formation of scar tissue. Scar tissue is important for closing large, gaping, or jagged wounds. The continuous layer of skin cells formed during the second phase becomes thicker and pushes off the scab, leaving a scar. Scar tissue contains no nerves or blood vessels and lacks the resilience of skin.

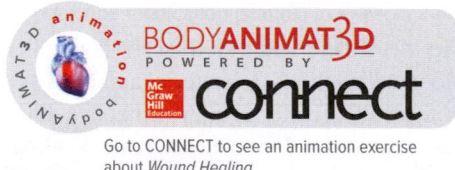

Go to CONNECT to see an animation exercise about *Wound Healing.*

Closing a Wound Sutures are surgical stitches a physician uses to close a wound. Suture materials, or **ligature,** can be either absorbable or nonabsorbable. The type and location of the wound will determine the type of suture material the healthcare practitioner chooses. The body breaks down absorbable sutures, so they do not require removal after the wound has healed. If a wound is particularly deep, the healthcare practitioner may need to suture in layers, from inside to outside. In this case, absorbable sutures are used for the inner suturing. Removable (nonabsorbable) sutures are generally used for the outside layer. Nonabsorbable ligature must be removed after wound healing is well under way. Sutures are discussed in greater detail later in the chapter.

Staples may be used to bring the edges of a wound together if there is considerable stress on the incision. For example, a long and deep surgical wound or a wound across the leg would have a strong tendency to gape open if not firmly secured. Surgical staples look somewhat like ordinary staples. They are inserted into the skin with a disposable staple unit.

Special Minor Surgical Procedures

Some types of minor surgical procedures require special surgical instruments. These procedures include laser surgery, cryosurgery, and electrocauterization. They all remove excess or abnormal tissue, as in the case of warts or skin lesions, and usually require surgical aseptic technique because they break the integrity of the skin.

Laser Surgery A laser emits an intense beam of light that is used to cut away tissue. Laser surgery is sometimes preferred over conventional surgery because it causes less damage to surrounding healthy tissue than does conventional surgery. Laser surgery also promotes quick healing and helps prevent infection.

When a laser is used in an office setting, close blinds and shades to keep out stray light. Remove any items—like the paper from wrapped sterile instruments or syringes—that could catch fire if they came in contact with the laser beam. Cover any shiny or reflective surfaces or use nonshiny instruments. Make sure that everyone in the room, including the patient, wears special safety goggles to protect the eyes. You should have a fire extinguisher in the room where it is out of the way but easily accessible. Post a standard laser warning placard in the room's entryway, per Occupational Safety and Health Administration (OSHA) regulations.

Position, drape, and prepare the patient as you would for conventional surgery. Place gauze around the surgical site and assist the physician with administration of a local anesthetic if requested. The physician uses the laser to vaporize the unwanted tissue; vaporized tissue is cleared away by the vacuum hose portion of the unit (see Figure 44-1). You may be asked to apply pressure to control any bleeding. Clean the wound with an antiseptic and apply a sterile dressing. Give the patient the normal instructions on wound care, including the recommendation to protect the site from sun exposure.

Cryosurgery The use of extreme cold to destroy unwanted tissue is called **cryosurgery.** Cryosurgery is often used to remove skin lesions and lesions on the cervix. Before cryosurgery, inform the patient that an initial sensation of cold will be followed by a burning sensation. Instruct the patient to remain as still as possible to prevent damage to nearby tissue.

The doctor may freeze the tissue by touching it with a cotton-tipped applicator dipped in liquid nitrogen or by spraying it with liquid nitrogen from a pressurized can. Sometimes,

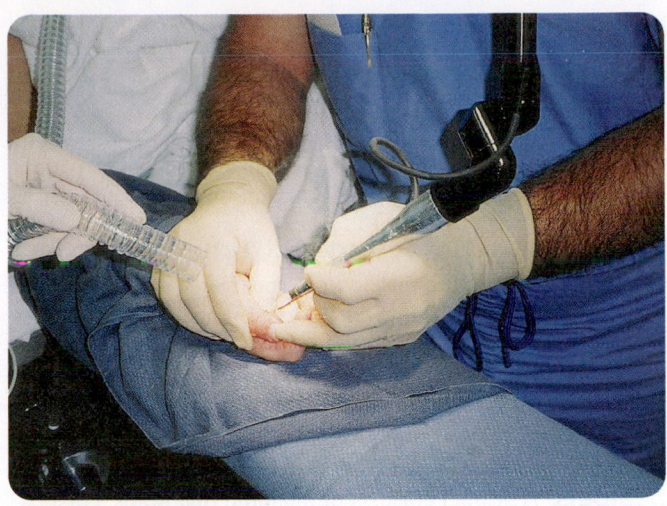

FIGURE 44-1 Suction eliminates vaporized tissue as a physician uses a laser to remove a wart from a patient's hand.
© Barry Slaven Photography

a special cryosurgical instrument is used, most often during surgery on the cervix.

Make the patient aware that more than one freezing cycle may be necessary. A local anesthetic is usually not required because the cold itself reduces sensation in the area. After the procedure, the area is cleaned with an antiseptic and a sterile dressing may be applied. An ice pack may be applied to reduce swelling and pain relievers given for pain.

Reassure the patient that some pain, swelling, or redness is normal after a cryosurgical procedure. Encourage the patient to use ice and pain relievers as necessary. Let the patient know that a large, painful, bloody blister may form. Left undisturbed, the blister usually ruptures in about 2 weeks. It should be left intact to promote healing and prevent infection. The patient should call the doctor if a blister becomes too painful. Be sure to provide the patient with complete wound care instructions.

Electrocauterization This is a technique whereby a needle, probe, or loop heated by electric current destroys the target tissue. A physician may use **electrocauterization** to remove growths such as warts, to stop bleeding, and to control nosebleeds that either will not subside or continually recur.

Several types of electrocautery units are in use. Some are small, handheld units powered by battery or by ordinary household electric current. Other, larger units are designed for countertop placement or wall mounting. Some units use disposable probes and others employ reusable ones.

With certain units, a grounding pad or plate is placed on or under the patient's body during the procedure. This grounding completes the circuit and prevents electric shock to the patient, the physician, and staff members. Reassure the patient that grounding causes no discomfort.

A local anesthetic may be administered before the procedure. After electrocauterization, a scab or crust generally forms over the area. Healing may take 2 to 3 weeks. General wound care instructions are appropriate for this procedure, except that a dressing may be omitted to keep the area drier.

▶ Instruments Used in Minor Surgery

LO 44.3

The type of minor surgical procedure determines which surgical instruments are used. Surgical instruments have specific purposes and may be classified by function.

Cutting and Dissecting Instruments

Cutting and dissecting instruments have sharp edges and are used to cut (incise) skin and tissue. Figure 44-2 illustrates some of the basic cutting and dissecting instruments you will encounter. You must be careful when cleaning, sterilizing, and storing these instruments to avoid injuring yourself and to protect the instruments' sharp edges.

Scalpels A scalpel consists of a handle that holds a disposable blade. Scalpel handles are either reusable or disposable and vary in width and length. A scalpel's specific use determines the shape and size of its blade. General-purpose scalpels have wide blades and a straight cutting surface (Figure 44-3). A no. 15 blade is the most common one for performing minor procedures.

Take special care when handling a scalpel. If the physician requests a reusable scalpel handle, it is essential that you load and unload the blade correctly on the handle. Carefully follow these steps when loading and unloading a scalpel blade:

Steps for Loading a Scalpel Handle

1. Carefully grasp the blade with a needle holder, staying away from the sharp edge.
2. Ensure that the blade edge is pointed away from you and you are gripping the blade just above the blade slot.
3. Firmly hold the scalpel handle in your nondominant hand. Hold the handle in the center, not close to the blade lock.
4. Carefully slide the blade over the grooves of the blade lock until it snaps into place.
5. The blade should slide smoothly down the groove. If it jams, carefully slide it back up the blade lock while grasping the blade with the needle holder, realign the blade slot, and slide the blade back down the blade lock.
6. Never use your fingers to load a blade on a scalpel handle. The blade is very sharp and may slip, causing serious injury.

Steps for Unloading a Scalpel Handle

1. Using your nondominant hand, hold the scalpel handle in the center.
2. With the blade lock facing up, point the blade and handle downward over a sharps container (make sure the sharps container is well below the blade and the blade is not pointed toward anyone in the room).
3. Using the needle holder, grasp the angled edge of the blade near the blade lock.

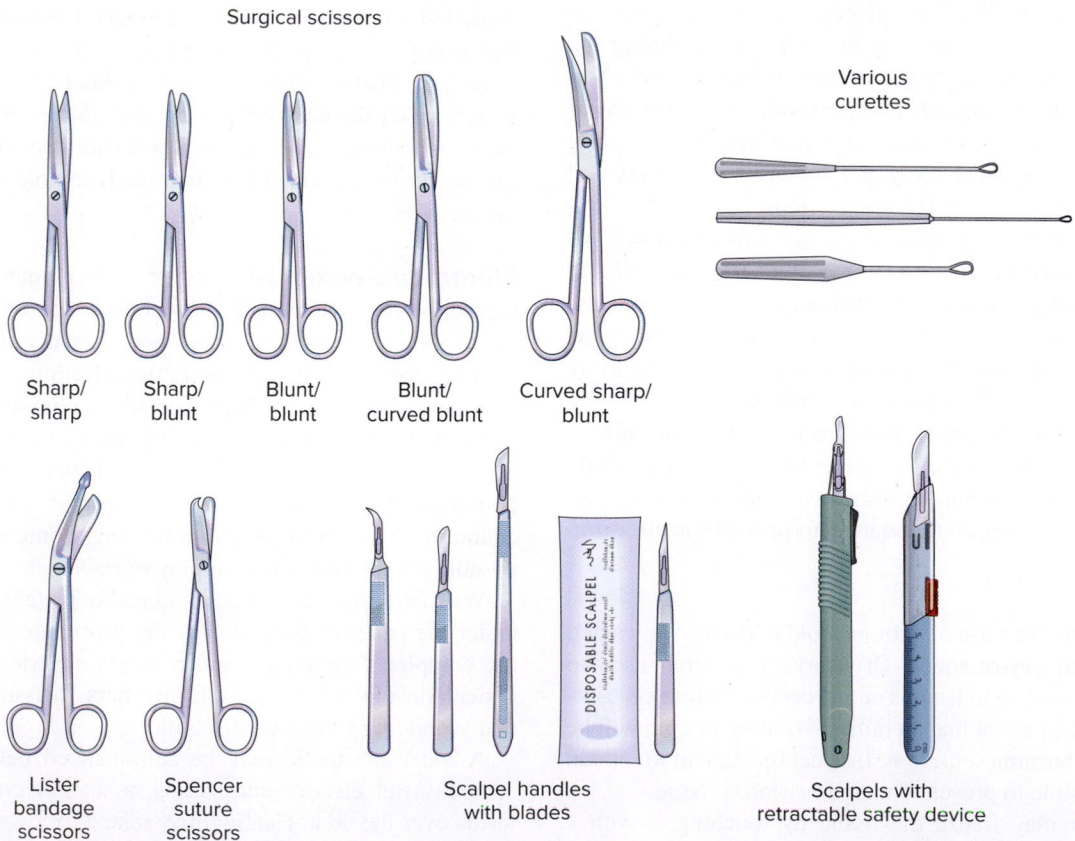

Surgical scissors

Sharp/ sharp Sharp/ blunt Blunt/ blunt Blunt/ curved blunt Curved sharp/ blunt

Various curettes

Lister bandage scissors Spencer suture scissors Scalpel handles with blades Scalpels with retractable safety device

FIGURE 44-2 These are typical cutting and dissecting instruments used in minor surgical procedures.

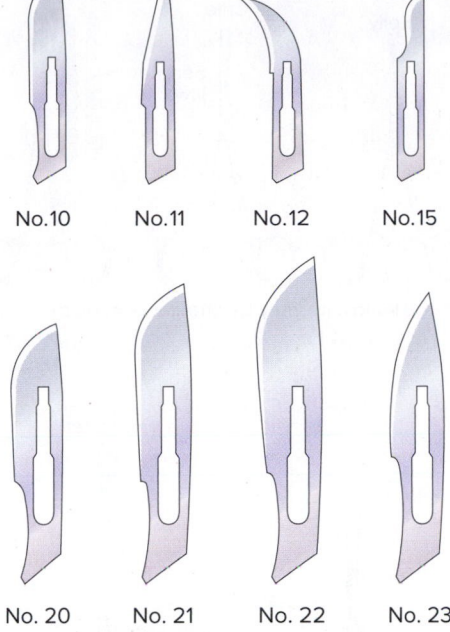

FIGURE 44-3 Scalpel blades come in various sizes and shapes, some of which are represented here.

4. Lift the blade slightly over the blade lock and slide it up to disengage the blade from the blade lock.

5. Immediately drop the blade into the sharps container.

6. Do not touch the blade with your fingers.

7. The blade handle is now ready for sanitization and sterilization.

A number of special blade removal devices are also available. These devices contain the blade in a case or box before removal. Follow the manufacturer's instructions for safe scalpel blade removal.

Scissors Surgical scissors come in various sizes. They may be straight or curved and have either blunt or pointed tips. Tissue scissors must be sharp enough to cut without damaging or ripping surrounding tissue. Suture scissors have blunt points and a curved lower blade. The lower blade is inserted under the suture material to cut it. Bandage scissors are used to remove dressings. They have a blunt lower blade to prevent injuring the skin next to the dressing. Clippers are scissor-like instruments used for cutting nails or thick materials.

Curettes The doctor uses a curette for scraping tissue. Curettes come in a variety of shapes and sizes and consist of a circular blade—actually a loop—attached to a rod-shaped handle. The blade is blunt on the outside and sharp on the inside. The inner part of the blade may also be serrated. Serrated blades may be used to take Pap (Papanicolaou) smears. Blunt curettes, known as Buck ear curettes, are used to remove wax from the ear canal when a large amount of cerumen has accumulated.

Grasping and Clamping Instruments

Special instruments are used for grasping and clamping tissue. Grasping instruments are used to hold surgical materials or to remove foreign objects, such as splinters, from the body. Clamping instruments are used to apply pressure and close off blood vessels. They also are used to hold tissue and other materials in position. Figure 44-4 shows some common grasping and clamping instruments.

Forceps Forceps are instruments that are commonly used to grasp or hold objects. Grasping types are usually shaped like tweezers and include thumb forceps and tissue forceps. Thumb forceps, also called smooth forceps, vary in shape and size. The blades of thumb forceps are tapered to a point and have small grooves at the tip. Tissue forceps (serrated forceps) have one or more fine teeth at the tips of the blades. When closed, these forceps hold tissue firmly. Holding forceps have handles with ratchets that lock the teeth in a closed position. Dressing, or sponge, forceps have ridges to hold a sponge or gauze when it is used to absorb body fluids.

Hemostats The most commonly used surgical instruments are hemostats. These surgical clamps vary in size and shape and are typically used to close off blood vessels. The serrated jaws of hemostats taper to a point. Like holding forceps, hemostats have handles that lock on ratchets, holding the jaws securely closed.

Towel Clamps Towel clamps are used to keep towels used for draping the surgical site in place during a surgical procedure. This stability is important in maintaining a sterile field.

Retracting, Dilating, and Probing Instruments

Retracting instruments are used to hold back the sides of a wound or an incision. Dilating and probing instruments may be used to enlarge, examine, or clear body openings, body cavities, or wounds. The shapes of these instruments vary with their functions. Some typical retracting, dilating, and probing instruments are shown in Figure 44-5.

Retractors The use of retractors allows greater access to and a better view of a surgical site. Some retractors must be held open by hand, while others have ratchets or locks to keep them open.

Dilators Dilators are slender, pointed instruments used to enlarge a body opening, such as a tear duct.

Probes A surgical probe is a slender rod with a blunt, bulb-shaped tip. Probes are used to explore wounds or body cavities and to locate or clear blockages.

Suture Material and Suturing Instruments

Suturing instruments are used to introduce suture materials into and retrieve them from a wound. Some carry the suture material, whereas others manipulate the suture carriers. Examples of suturing instruments are shown in Figure 44-6.

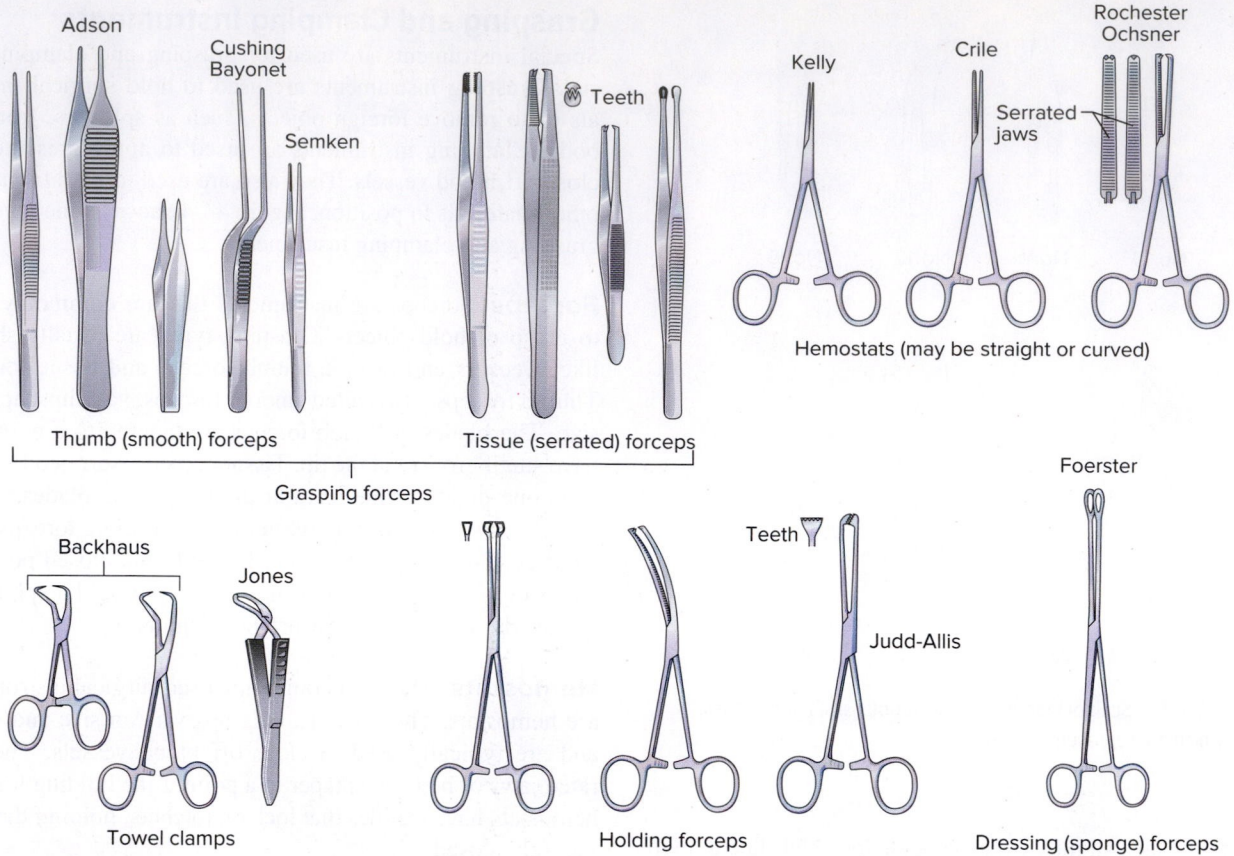

FIGURE 44-4 These are typical grasping and clamping instruments used in minor surgical procedures.

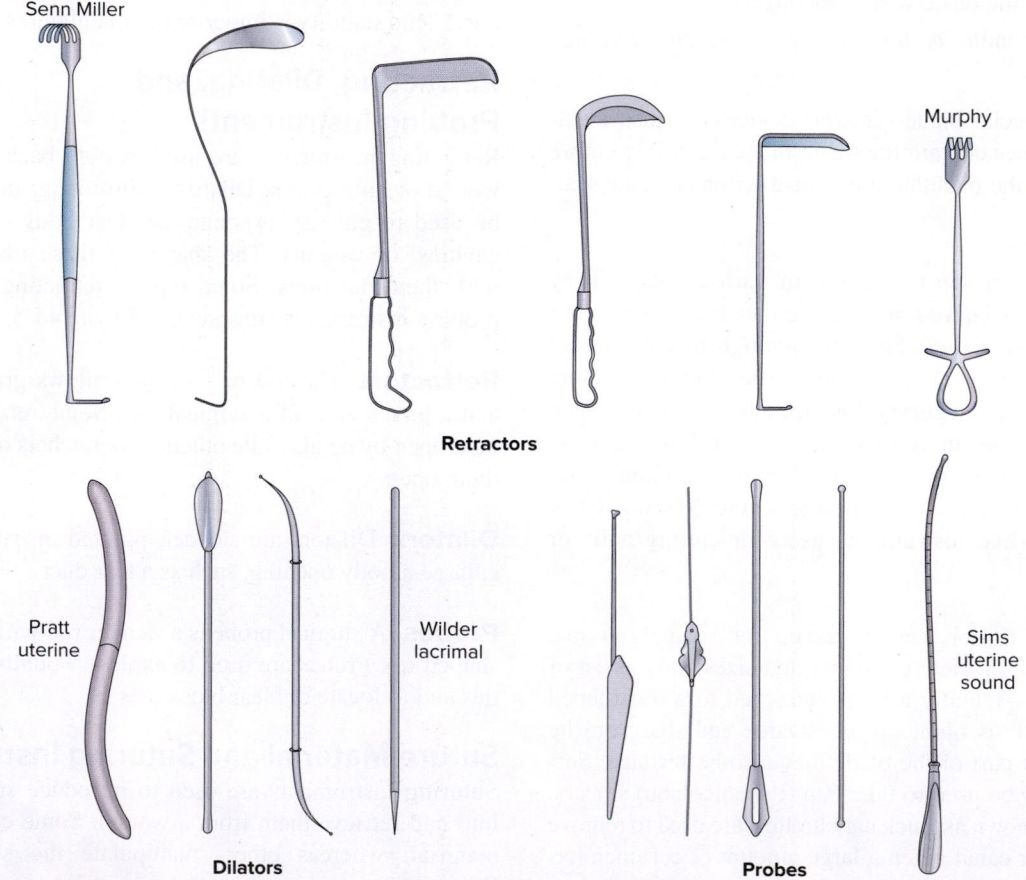

FIGURE 44-5 These are typical retracting, dilating, and probing instruments used in minor surgical procedures.

Suture Materials As a medical assistant, you need to be familiar with the various types of sutures. The health-care practitioner will ask for a specific suture type based on several considerations, including the type and location of the wound. Sutures may be natural or synthetic, absorbable or nonabsorbable. The healthcare practitioner will choose a needle that causes the least possible trauma to the tissues. The needle may be curved or straight, cutting, blunt, or tapered. A **swaged needle** has the suture material permanently attached to the needle. The needle may also have an eye where the suture material is manually threaded. It is important that you be able to quickly find information about the type of suture material in a package. Figure 44-7 illustrates the most common information found on a suture package.

General Features of Suture Materials Regardless of the type, suture materials have some general qualities in common:

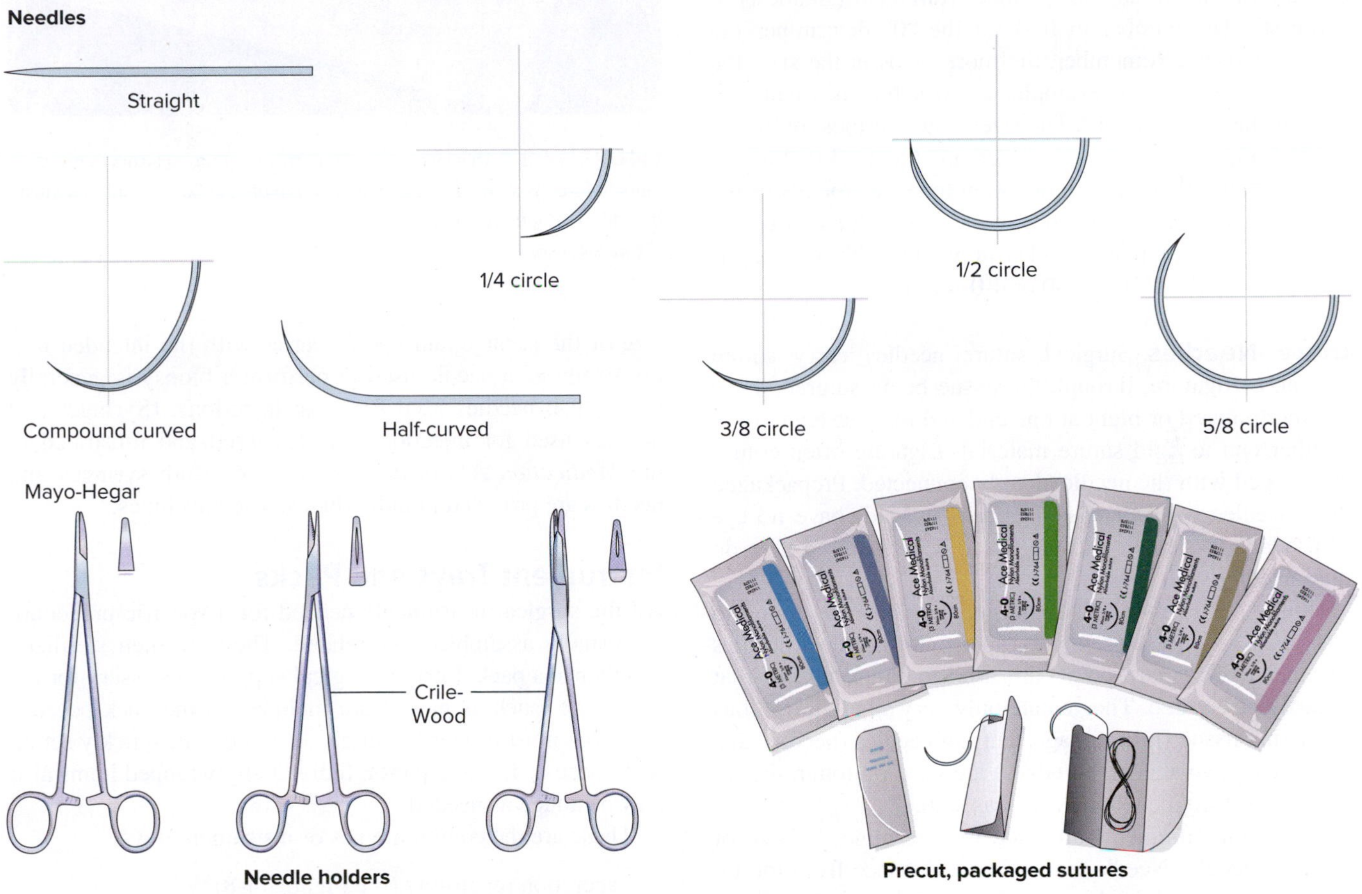

Needles

Straight

1/4 circle

1/2 circle

Compound curved

Half-curved

3/8 circle

5/8 circle

Mayo-Hegar

Crile-Wood

Needle holders

Precut, packaged sutures

FIGURE 44-6   These are typical suturing instruments.

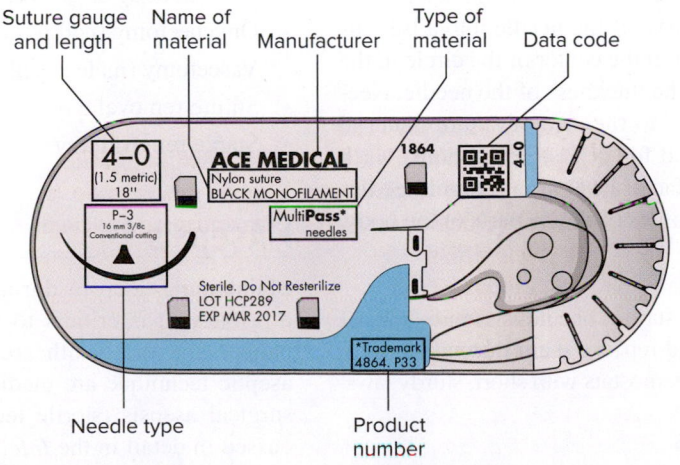

Suture gauge and length

Name of material

Manufacturer

Type of material

Data code

4–0
(1.5 metric)
18"

ACE MEDICAL
Nylon suture
BLACK MONOFILAMENT

1864

4-0

P–3
16 mm 3/8c
Conventional cutting

MultiPass*
needles

Sterile. Do Not Resterilize
LOT HCP289
EXP MAR 2017

*Trademark
4864, P33

Needle type

Product number

FIGURE 44-7   Information about the suture material can be found on the package.

- Sterility
- Uniform diameter
- Tensile strength (resistance to breaking under tension or pull)
- Flexibility
- Ability to retain or hold a knot
- Low incidence of tissue reactivity

Suture Size Suture size is determined by the diameter or thickness of the strand. Sizes range from 11-0 (smallest) to 7 (largest). The number in front of the "0" determines the number of zeros. Remember, the more zeros in the size, the smaller the suture. For example, a 6-0 suture is smaller in diameter than a 3-0 suture. The sizes you will most often see used for minor surgical procedures are 6-0 to 3-0. Sutures sized 6-0 and 5-0 are used most often to close wounds of the face, lips, and eyebrow. Wounds of the sole of the foot generally require a suture that is thicker in diameter. These wounds are usually repaired with a 3-0 or 4-0 suture.

Suture Needles Surgical suture needles carry suture material, or ligature, through the tissue being sutured. They are either pointed or blunt at one end and may have an eye at the other end to hold suture material. Ligature often comes prepackaged with the needle already connected. Prepackaged suture needles with attached ligature (swaged) have no eye and produce less trauma to the tissue being sutured than do suture needles with eyes.

Suture needles may be straight, or they may be curved to allow deeper suture placement. Taper point needles (needles that taper into a sharp point) are used to suture tissues that are easily penetrated. They create only very small holes, thus minimizing tissue fluid leakage. Cutting needles (needles that have at least two sharpened edges) are used on tough tissues that are not easily penetrated, such as skin.

Several measurements are used to determine the size of a surgical needle. Needle length is the distance from the tip to the end, measuring along the body of the needle. Chord length is the straight-line distance from the tip to the end of the needle. (Chord length is not the same as needle length in curved needles.) The radius of a curved needle is determined by mentally continuing the curve of the needle into a full circle and finding the distance from the center of the circle to the needle body. The diameter is the thickness of the needle. Needle size generally corresponds to the size of suture material used. Smaller needles are used for delicate procedures, such as eye surgery or repair of a facial laceration. Larger needles are used for suturing wounds of less delicate parts of the body, such as the hands or legs.

Needle Holders Curved suture needles require special instruments to hold, insert, and retrieve them during suturing. Most needle holders look like hemostats with short, sturdy jaws.

Syringes and Needles

Sterile syringes and needles are used to inject anesthetic solutions, withdraw fluids, and obtain biopsy specimens. The

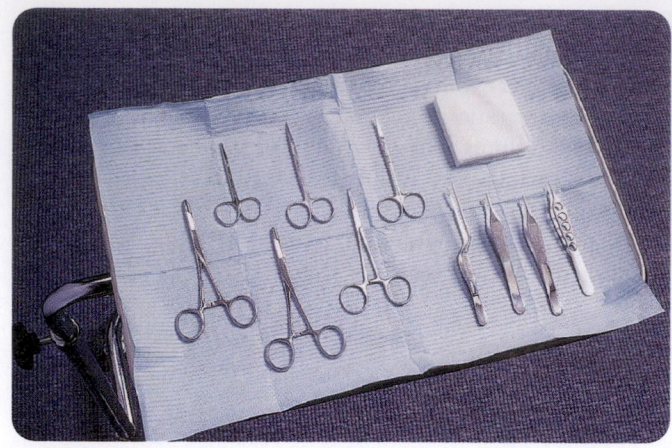

FIGURE 44-8 This laceration repair tray contains scissors, several pairs of forceps, a needle holder, and sterile gauze. Suture material must be added for the procedure.
© David Kelly Crow

size of the syringe and needle varies with the intended use. For example, a needle used to perform a biopsy is generally larger than needles used for most injections. (Syringes and needles used for injections are discussed and illustrated in the *Medication Administration* chapter.) Both syringes and needles are provided in individual sterile envelopes.

Instrument Trays and Packs

All the surgical instruments needed for a specific procedure are usually assembled beforehand. They are then sterilized together in a pack. Certain surgical supplies necessary for the procedure (such as gauze) are included in the pack because they, too, must be sterile. Surgical trays can be quickly set up with these instrument packs. Individually wrapped items also may be added as needed.

These are the common types of instrument trays:

- Laceration repair tray (see Figure 44-8)
- Laceration repair with debridement tray
- Incision and drainage tray
- Foreign body or growth removal tray
- Onychectomy (nail removal) tray
- Vasectomy (male sterilization procedure) tray
- Suture removal tray
- Staple removal tray

▶ Asepsis   LO 44.4

Maintaining asepsis during surgical procedures is always a priority. It is critical to the health and safety of both the patient and the healthcare professional. The two levels of aseptic technique are medical asepsis (clean technique) and surgical asepsis (sterile technique). Medical asepsis is discussed in detail in the *Infection Control Fundamentals* chapter. You will use both levels of asepsis when assisting with minor surgery.

Personal Protective Equipment

Personal protective equipment, or PPE, includes all items used as a barrier between the wearer and potentially infectious or hazardous medical materials. PPE includes gloves, gowns, and masks and protective eyewear or face shields. OSHA regulations regarding PPE are discussed in detail in the *Infection Control Fundaments* and *Infection Control Practices* chapters.

Gloves are of particular importance during surgical procedures. You should wear properly sized latex, nitrile, or vinyl gloves during any procedure that might expose you to potentially infectious or hazardous materials. (Gloves that are too big can catch on instruments or equipment and cause accidents.) When you wear gloves, you also protect the patient from any infectious organisms on your hands.

Vinyl, nitrile, and latex gloves can all prevent contamination of the hands with bacteria. Although latex gloves were the preference of healthcare professionals for many years, the incidence of latex allergy among healthcare professionals has grown. Allergic reactions to latex can range from a skin rash to shock and even death. Many healthcare institutions are switching to less allergenic low-powder or powderless non-latex gloves. The powder in latex gloves, which makes them easier to put on, is one of the primary sources of latex allergy. The latex protein that causes the allergy mixes with the powder. When the gloves are removed, the powder containing the latex protein becomes airborne and is inhaled.

If you work in a facility that uses latex gloves, take these steps to prevent latex allergy:

- If possible, use powder-free gloves only.
- Thoroughly dry hands after washing.
- Frequently apply non-oil-based lotion to the hands.
- Clean areas and equipment contaminated with latex-containing dust frequently.

If you notice latex allergy symptoms, consider consulting an allergist. You also should discuss your symptoms with your supervisor, who will recommend that you switch to hypoallergenic or vinyl gloves. If you have an allergy, the healthcare facility is required to provide nonlatex gloves for your use.

Sharps and Biohazardous Waste Handling and Disposal

Sharp medical and surgical instruments have great potential for transmitting infection through cuts and puncture wounds. Used scalpels, needles, syringes, and other sharp objects should be disposed of in a puncture-resistant sharps container.

All items other than sharps that have come in contact with tissue, blood, or body fluids must be disposed of in a leakproof plastic bag or container. The container must be either red or labeled with the orange-red biohazard symbol. The proper procedure for handling and disposing of sharps and biohazardous waste is discussed in detail in the *Infection Control Practices* chapter.

Surgical Asepsis

Surgical asepsis completely eliminates microorganisms. The goal of surgical asepsis is to control microorganisms before they enter the body. To accomplish this goal, the items used in healthcare must be sterile (completely free of microorganisms). Surgical instruments are sterilized before use, and sterile technique procedures must be followed.

You will be expected to perform the following common procedures involving sterile technique:

- Creating a sterile field
- Adding sterile items to the sterile field
- Performing a surgical scrub
- Putting on sterile gloves
- Sanitizing, disinfecting, and sterilizing equipment

Creating a Sterile Field A **sterile field** is an area free of microorganisms that is used as a work area during a surgical procedure. Always be aware that the sterile field is understood to become contaminated and must be redone in the following circumstances:

- An unsterile item touches the field.
- Someone reaches across the field.
- The field becomes wet.
- The field is left unattended and uncovered.
- You turn your back on the field.

For more rules of sterile technique, see the *Caution: Handle with Care* feature.

The sterile field is often set up on a Mayo stand—a movable, stainless steel instrument tray on a stand. Adjust the stand so that the tray is slightly above waist level. Remember, items placed below waist level are considered contaminated. Before beginning, disinfect the Mayo stand with 70% isopropyl alcohol and allow it to dry.

To create the sterile field, cover the stand with two layers of sterile material. This material can be sterile disposable drapes, separately sterilized muslin towels, or the muslin towels that the surgical instruments are wrapped in before autoclaving to produce office-sterilized sterile instrument packs. Commercially prepared sterile instrument packs, usually with disposable paper wrappings, are also used to create a sterile field. Procedure 44-1, at the end of this chapter, describes how to prepare a sterile field and how to open sterile packages.

When assembling the necessary supplies, place all unsterile items that may be used during the procedure outside the sterile field. Unsterile items include items that are sterile on the inside but not on the outside, such as a sterile gauze pack or a sterile liquid such as alcohol, saline, or peroxide inside an unsterile bottle. Unsterile supplies should be arranged on a counter away from the sterile field. A typical arrangement of unsterile items used in surgery is shown in Figure 44-9. If you place an unsterile item within the sterile field, the field is no longer sterile and you must repeat the entire process.

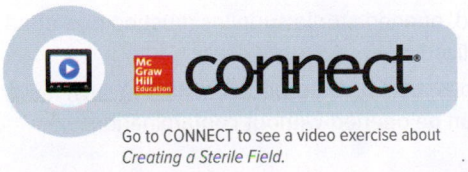

Go to CONNECT to see a video exercise about *Creating a Sterile Field.*

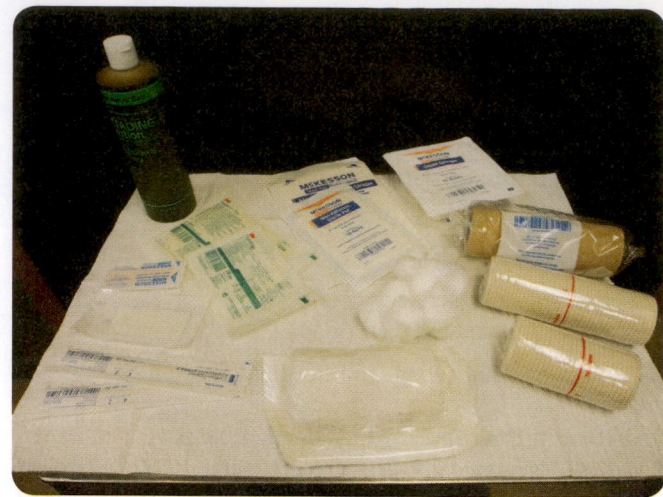

FIGURE 44-9   For each surgical procedure, unsterile surgical supplies must be gathered and arranged in an area separate from the sterile field.

© McGraw-Hill Education. David Moyer, photographer

Adding Sterile Items to the Sterile Field   The outer 1 inch of the sterile field is considered contaminated. So before you add sterile items to the sterile field, carefully plan where you will place the instruments so that they are within the sterile field.

Instruments and Supplies   If you have used sterile disposable drapes or separately sterilized muslin towels to create the sterile field, you will need to add the necessary instruments. Stand away from the sterile field and open the sterile instrument pack in the manner described in Procedure 44-1. Place the pack on a counter or hold it open in your hand. Transfer and arrange the instruments on the sterile field with sterile transfer forceps. Never reach across the sterile field.

Some instruments are sterilized individually in autoclave bags, and many sterile supplies are prepackaged. Stand away from the sterile field as you open an individual bag or package.

You can pull the flaps of the packaging partway apart, then snap (remove from position by a sudden movement) the item onto the sterile field from a distance of 8 to 12 inches. Alternatively, you can use sterile forceps to grasp and place the items in the sterile field.

Pouring Sterile Solutions   Sterile solutions are often required during the surgical procedure to rinse or wash the wound. These can be added to the sterile field after the sterile instruments. Several sterile solutions are commonly used during minor surgical procedures, including sterile water and normal saline (0.9% sodium chloride).

Bottles of these sterile solutions come in a variety of sizes. Choose the smallest size that will supply the amount of solution needed during the procedure to help minimize cost, because unused solutions are typically discarded.

When pouring a solution, cover the label on the bottle with the palm of your hand to keep the label dry. Pour a small amount of the liquid into a liquid waste receptacle to clean the lip of the bottle. As you pour the solution into a sterile bowl on the field, hold the bottle at an angle to avoid reaching over the sterile area. Hold the bottle fairly close to the bowl without touching it. Pour the contents slowly to avoid splashing the drape, which would contaminate the field (see Figure 44-10).

When a sterile solution bottle is opened and may be used again during the procedure, do not let any unsterile object touch the inside of its cap. To accomplish this, place the cap on a clean location with the sterile inside of the cap facing up.

Performing a Surgical Scrub and Donning Sterile Gloves   If you assist in a surgical procedure, you must perform a surgical scrub and wear sterile surgical gloves. Surgical scrub procedures are similar to those for aseptic handwashing, but there are several distinctions:

- A sterile scrub brush is used instead of a disposable nailbrush.
- Both the hands and the forearms are washed.

CAUTION: HANDLE WITH CARE

Rules for Sterile Technique

A sterile field is a microorganism-free area used during a surgical procedure. To maintain sterility throughout the procedure, follow surgical technique and adhere to these rules:

1. Do not touch a nonsterile article to a sterile article or area. This will cause the sterile area or article to be considered nonsterile.

2. If you are unsure about the sterility of an article or area, consider it nonsterile.

3. Unused, opened sterile supplies must be discarded or resterilized.

4. Packages must be wrapped or sealed in such a way that they can be opened without contamination.

5. The edges of wrappers (1-inch margin) covering sterile supplies and the outer lips of bottles and flasks containing sterile solutions are not considered sterile.

6. If a sterile surface or package becomes wet, it is considered contaminated and should not be used.

7. Do not reach over a sterile field when you are not wearing sterile clothing. This action contaminates the sterile field.

8. Keep your hands between your shoulders and your waist when wearing sterile gloves to maintain sterility.

9. Do not turn your back on a sterile field even if you are in a sterile gown. Your back is always considered contaminated.

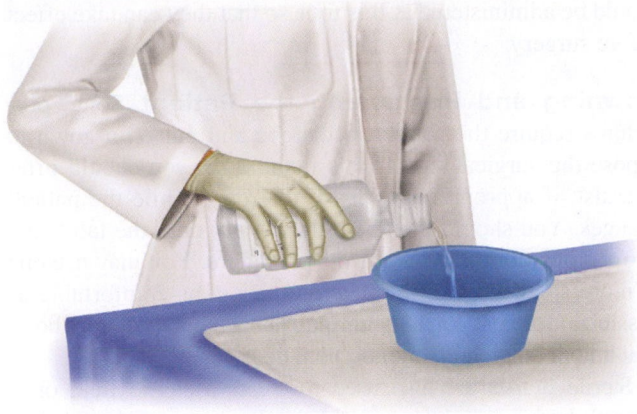

FIGURE 44-10 When pouring a sterile solution for use on a sterile field, be careful not to splash the solution.

- The hands are kept above the elbows to prevent water from running from the arms onto washed areas.
- Sterile towels are used instead of paper towels.
- Sterile gloves are put on immediately after the hands are dried.

You may wonder why a surgical scrub is necessary if you are planning to wear sterile gloves. The answer is that there is always the possibility that a glove may be punctured. If the skin is as clean as possible, the risk of contamination from a punctured glove is minimized. Nevertheless, if a glove is damaged during a sterile procedure, you must consider anything touched by that glove after it is damaged to be contaminated. Contaminated items must be resterilized or replaced before you continue.

A surgical scrub removes microorganisms more effectively than does routine handwashing. Routine handwashing removes bacteria present on the skin's surface, whereas the surgical scrub removes bacteria in deeper layers of the skin—where the hair follicles and oil-producing glands exist. Procedure 44-2, at the end of this chapter, describes the process for performing a sterile scrub.

Sterile gloves are required for many procedures. You don sterile gloves after you perform the surgical scrub. The process for donning sterile gloves is described in Procedure 44-3 at the end of this chapter.

Remember, once you are wearing sterile gloves, you may touch only the items in the sterile field. So you must remove any drape covering the sterile instrument tray before you glove. Sterile gloves provide a small margin of safety in preventing contamination; your movements must be controlled and precise to work within this margin to protect the sterile area.

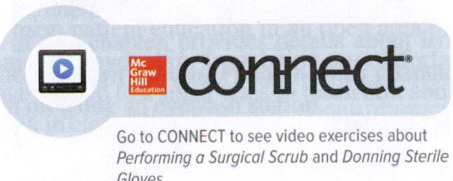

Go to CONNECT to see video exercises about *Performing a Surgical Scrub* and *Donning Sterile Gloves.*

Sanitizing, Disinfecting, and Sterilizing Equipment

Many supplies used in a doctor's office are disposable. Many surgical instruments, however, are made of steel and are reusable. Preparing surgical instruments for reuse involves cleaning them with germicidal soap and water (a process called *sanitization*), then disinfecting and/or sterilizing them, depending on how the equipment will be used. These procedures are described more fully in the *Examination and Treatment Areas* and *Infection Control Practices* chapters.

▶ Preoperative Procedures   LO 44.5

You must complete a number of steps before a surgical procedure, including performing various preliminary duties, preparing the surgical room, and physically preparing the patient for surgery.

Preliminary Duties

The first tasks you will perform before the surgery include providing **preoperative** (prior to surgery, or "pre-op") instructions to the patient, completing various administrative tasks, and easing the patient's fears.

Preoperative Instructions When a patient is scheduled for a minor surgical procedure in the doctor's office, you must explain the preoperative instructions. Be prepared to answer the patient's questions about the procedure and possible risks. The patient may ask you, rather than the doctor, such questions or may need clarification of information provided by the doctor.

A patient may need to follow certain dietary and fluid restrictions before a minor surgical procedure. Not eating or drinking for a specific period of time is a common restriction. The patient's medications may also be restricted because of anesthetic administration during the procedure. Non-English-speaking patients may need an interpreter who can help them understand the forms they must sign and their instructions.

Instruct the patient to wear either comfortable, loose-fitting clothes that will not interfere with the procedure or clothing that can be removed easily. In most cases, patients also need to arrange for someone to drive them home and stay with them for 24 hours after the procedure.

Administrative and Legal Tasks You must ensure that all the necessary paperwork is completed before surgery. Routine administrative tasks include completing the required insurance forms and obtaining prior authorization from the patient's insurance company.

Make absolutely certain the patient reads, understands, and signs the surgical consent form. The patient needs a clear understanding of what to expect during and after the surgery to give informed consent as required by law. Sometimes surgery is performed on a child or a patient with limited understanding of legal documents. In such cases, the consent form must be signed by the patient's parent or legal guardian.

Failure to obtain the necessary paperwork prior to a surgical procedure can cause serious legal problems. The doctor and other staff members could be held legally liable if problems were to develop during or after the procedure.

It is common practice to call the patient the day before the surgery to confirm the appointment. This call also provides a chance to ensure that the patient follows the preoperative instructions. You may be responsible for making this call.

Easing the Patient's Fears Knowing what to expect during and after a surgical procedure will ease the patient's fears. This information allows him or her to plan daily activities and, if necessary, to arrange for help at home during the recovery period.

Some offices have educational materials such as brochures, fact sheets, or videos about the procedure the patient will undergo. You may assist in preparing or acquiring these materials if your office's policy includes such participation for medical assistants. This type of information may increase patient compliance with pre- and postoperative instructions.

Much of a patient's fear about a surgical procedure can be overcome if you spend sufficient time before the procedure explaining what to expect. Be prepared to answer the patient's questions honestly, calmly, and confidently. Your calm and knowledgeable manner will reassure the patient. If the answer to a question requires experience or knowledge beyond your own, pass the question on to the healthcare practitioner.

Preparing the Surgical Room

Prior to surgery, the doctor should inform you of specific instructions concerning patient preparation. He also will tell you what special equipment or supplies are necessary for the procedure.

Because patients are likely to feel anxious before a procedure, it is best to have everything ready in the surgical room before you escort the patient into the room. Make sure the room is clean, neat, and free of waste from previous procedures. The examining table should have been cleaned and disinfected, and surface barriers (table paper and pillow covers) should have been changed.

Check to see that there is adequate lighting. Make sure that all equipment and supplies necessary for the procedure are available. Check the date and sterilization indicator on sterilized packs and supplies.

You will then wash your hands and prepare the sterile field as outlined in Procedure 44-1 at the end of this chapter. The sterile field and the instruments should be draped with a sterile towel.

Preparing the Patient

Just before the surgery, various concerns must be addressed and procedures completed in sequence. The initial tasks are followed by gowning and positioning the patient and preparing the patient's skin for surgery.

Initial Tasks Before leading the patient into the surgical room, give the patient an opportunity to use the bathroom. You must also find out whether she has followed the presurgical instructions. Restrictions on food and fluid intake are of particular concern. Also, ask what medications the patient is taking and whether she has taken that day's dosage.

Measure the patient's vital signs. Ask if there are any symptoms or problems the doctor should know about before the surgery. If any unusual signs or symptoms are present, notify the doctor. The doctor will want to examine the patient before proceeding.

Check the chart for medication orders, such as pain medication or a tranquilizer to calm the patient. Medications should be administered at this time so that they can take effect before surgery.

Gowning and Positioning the Patient Some procedures require the patient to disrobe and put on a gown to expose the surgical site. If this is the case, you should offer to assist, if appropriate, or leave the room while the patient changes. You should then help the patient onto the table and into the position required for the procedure. You may use one or more small pillows to make the patient as comfortable as possible. Then adequately drape the patient to retain body heat and preserve personal dignity.

Sterile drapes are also used to create a sterile field on a patient's body around the surgical site. Drapes come in a variety of sizes and styles. A fenestrated drape has a round or slit-like opening cut out in the center to provide access to the surgical site.

Surgical Skin Preparation Prior to surgery, the patient's skin must be prepared to reduce the number of microorganisms and the risk of surgical site infection. Preparation includes cleaning the area, removing the hair, and applying antiseptic. The area prepared should be 2 inches larger than the intended surgical field. The surgical field is the area exposed in the center of the fenestrated drape. The extra prepared skin area allows for draping without contaminating the surgical field.

Cleaning the Area Before proceeding with the surgical skin preparation, wash your hands and don exam gloves. Place a plastic-backed drape under the surgical site to absorb any liquids. Clean the site first with an iodine-based solution, using forceps and gauze sponges dipped in the solution. Begin at the center of the surgical site and work outward in a firm, circular motion (Figure 44-11). Discard the gauze sponge after each complete pass. Clean in concentric circles until you cover the full preparation area. Continue the process, repeating as

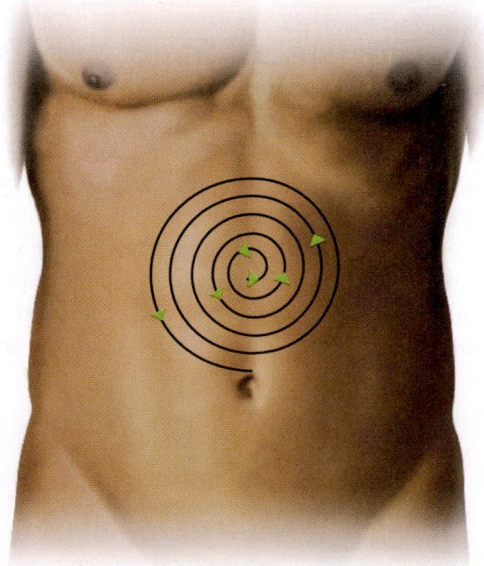

FIGURE 44-11 Clean the surgical site with an iodine-based solution. Begin at the center of the surgical site and work outward in a firm, circular motion. Clean in a circular, outward pattern 2 inches larger than the surgical field.

necessary, for at least 2 minutes or the amount of time specified in the office's procedure manual. Cleaning takes more time if a wound is dirty or contains foreign materials. When procedures are performed on a hand or foot, clean the entire hand or foot. The skin and body openings, particularly the nose, mouth, and perineum, cannot be considered sterile. Nevertheless, the principles of aseptic technique require that you try to keep the area as contamination-free as possible.

Removing Hair from the Area Depending on office policy, you may be required to remove hair from the surgical site. Shaving often causes many small wounds on the skin, which increases the risk of infection, and is not recommended. Some experts feel that hair should not be removed unless it is thick enough to interfere with surgery. If this is the case, hair may be trimmed with scissors or electric trimmers or smoothed out of the way. This should be done with care—to avoid damaging the skin—immediately before surgery.

Applying the Antiseptic Antiseptics are agents applied to the skin to limit the growth of microorganisms and to help prevent infection. Povidone iodine (Betadine®) is most commonly used, but chlorhexidine gluconate (Hibiclens®) or benzalkonium chloride (Zephiran®) may also be used, particularly if the patient is allergic to iodine. After cleaning or removing the hair when needed, swab an area 2 inches larger than the surgical field with the antiseptic solution in a circular, outward motion, starting at the surgical site. This is the same motion used for cleaning the surgical site. For surgery on a hand or foot, swab the entire hand or foot. Allow the antiseptic to air-dry; do not pat it dry—that would remove some of the solution's antiseptic properties.

When the area is dry, treat it as a sterile field. Instruct the patient not to touch the area. Cover the area with a sterile fenestrated drape, from front to back. Avoid reaching over the field. At this point, notify the physician that the patient is ready. Then prepare yourself to assist with the surgery.

▶ Intraoperative Procedures   LO 44.6

Intraoperative procedures are procedures that take place during surgery. You may be asked to perform a wide variety of unsterile and sterile tasks during surgery, such as preparing a local anesthetic, monitoring the patient, processing specimens, and handing instruments to the doctor. The doctor also may ask you to explain to the patient step by step what will be done next during the procedure.

Administering a Local Anesthetic

Before beginning the surgical procedure, the physician will administer a local anesthetic. Some local anesthetics are injected. An injected anesthetic is packaged in a sterile vial (a small glass bottle with a self-sealing rubber stopper). Other local anesthetics come in a cream, gel, or spray form. These anesthetics are topical (applied directly to the skin) and affect only the area to which they are applied. The choice of administration method depends on how invasive or painful the procedure is likely to be.

Lidocaine (Xylocaine®) is the most commonly used anesthetic, used as an injectable or a topical gel anesthetic.

Tetracaine hydrochloride (Pontocaine®), a long-acting anesthetic, is injected or topical.

Topical Application A topical anesthetic is useful when the pain will be mild or when only the skin's upper layers are affected. It is common to use such agents to anesthetize the area of a small laceration prior to suturing. Sometimes an anesthetic cream is applied before a local anesthetic is injected to reduce or eliminate the pain caused by the injection. A topical anesthetic must usually remain on the skin for 10 to 15 minutes for the area to become sufficiently anesthetized.

Injections If a local anesthetic is to be injected, it is typically administered after the skin is prepared but before the patient is draped. In some cases, however, the anesthetic is injected prior to skin preparation to allow time for it to take effect. In either case, it is important to note the time of anesthetic administration in the patient's chart.

If the doctor is already wearing sterile gloves, you may be asked to assist in administering the anesthetic. Because administering an anesthetic is an unsterile task (the outside of the vial is unsterile), when performing it, follow proper procedure to protect the sterility of the doctor's gloves and the anesthetic solution.

First, check the label of the anesthetic vial two times to confirm that it is the correct solution. Then, clean the vial's rubber stopper with a 70% isopropyl alcohol solution and leave the alcohol pad on top of the stopper. Present the requested needle and syringe to the doctor by peeling half the outer wrapper away and allowing the doctor to remove them from the wrapper.

Remove the pad from the rubber stopper and hold the vial so that the doctor can verify it is the proper medication. Turn the vial upside down and hold it securely around the base, without touching the sterile stopper. Be sure to hold the vial in front of you at shoulder height. Because significant force will be necessary to push the needle through the rubber stopper, brace the wrist of the hand holding the vial with your free hand. Hold the vial firmly so that the doctor can withdraw the anesthetic from it (Figure 44-12). Check the vial a third time to confirm that it is the correct solution.

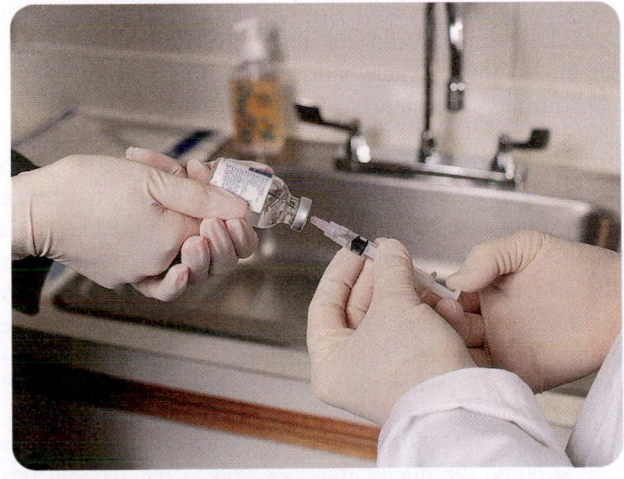

FIGURE 44-12 You must hold the anesthetic vial firmly to allow the physician to puncture the rubber stopper with the needle.
© Cliff Moore

Potential Side Effects of the Anesthetic Patients sometimes have reactions to anesthetic medications and should be informed of this prior to the procedure. Although rare, reactions may include dizziness, loss of consciousness, seizures, or cardiac arrest. Adverse reactions can occur if the anesthetic dose is too high or if it is absorbed too quickly. Reactions can also occur if the patient is taking other medications that should not be mixed with the anesthetic. All medications (including over-the-counter medications) that a patient is taking at the time of surgery must be documented to avoid possible reactions.

Use of Epinephrine Epinephrine is a sterile solution that is sometimes injected along with an anesthetic. It constricts the blood vessels, making them narrower, which reduces bleeding and prolongs the action of the local anesthetic. Epinephrine is used if the surgery site is an area with many small blood vessels that are expected to bleed profusely (such as the head). Reducing bleeding makes it easier to see and to repair the wound.

Epinephrine should be used with caution, however, in patients with heart disease or respiratory disease. Epinephrine also prolongs the anesthesia because epinephrine slows the rate at which the anesthetic spreads into the tissue. This effect may or may not be desirable. There is some concern that epinephrine may increase wound infection rates. If the wound is highly contaminated, the physician may choose to use anesthetic without epinephrine.

Assisting the Physician During Surgery

Your role in surgical assisting depends on the type of surgery and the physician's preference. You may assist the physician in one of two capacities with different duties: as a floater—an unsterile assistant who is free to move about the room and attend to unsterile needs—or as a sterile scrub assistant—who assists in handling sterile equipment during the procedure.

The Floater If you are assisting as a floater (sometimes called a circulator), you will perform a routine handwash and don exam gloves. Remember, you cannot touch sterile items in the sterile field because you have not performed a surgical scrub and are not wearing sterile gloves. Procedure 44-4, at the end of this chapter, outlines the tasks performed by a floater (unsterile assistant).

Monitoring and Recording One of a floater's most important duties is to monitor the patient during the procedure. You must measure vital signs regularly and observe the patient for reactions to the anesthetic. Record all observations in the patient's chart. Also, write down any information or notes the doctor requests. You must keep a record of time, including when the anesthetic is administered, when the procedure begins, and when the procedure is completed.

Processing Specimens When you serve as a floater during surgery, the doctor may ask you to receive and process specimens for laboratory examination. Most tissues are placed in a 10% formalin solution to preserve them before they are sent to the laboratory. If the container is not prefilled,

half-fill the specimen container with the formalin solution ahead of time. Remove the lid of the specimen container without touching the rim. Hold the container out toward the doctor so that she can place the tissue directly into it without contaminating the sample (Figure 44-13).

The container should be labeled with the following information:

- The patient's name and the doctor's name
- The date and time of collection
- The body site from which the specimen was obtained
- Your initials

If more than one specimen is obtained from a patient, place each specimen in a separate container. Label each container with the necessary information, along with a number to indicate the order in which the specimens are obtained (no. 1, no. 2, and so on). The physician will usually tell you the exact location of each specimen taken. You will also fill out a laboratory requisition slip to send along with the specimen(s). Specimen containers should be placed in a special transport bag labeled with the biohazard symbol. Most transport bags have an outside pouch for the lab requisition form. The form should accompany the sample but not be placed in contact with the specimen container. This protects lab personnel when they handle the requisition form.

Other Duties As a floater, you also may be asked to perform a number of other duties, including:

- Assisting with the injection of additional anesthetic
- Adding additional sterile items to the sterile tray
- Pouring sterile solutions
- Keeping the surgical area clean and neat during the procedure
- Repositioning the patient as necessary
- Adjusting lighting

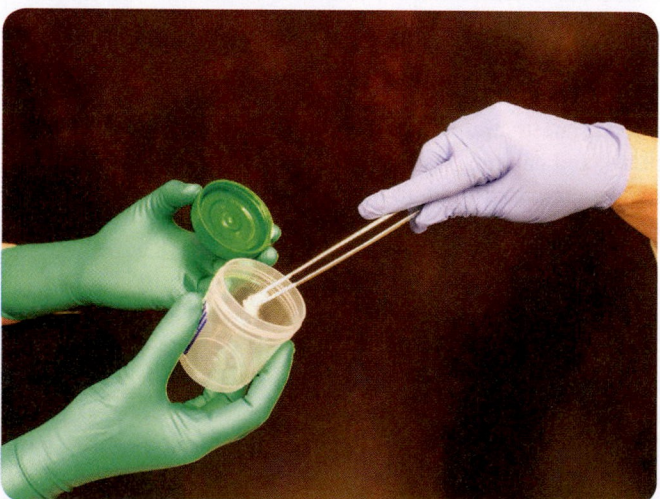

FIGURE 44-13 Be sure to hold the specimen container so that the doctor can place the tissue in it without touching the rim or outside of the container with the tissue.
© McGraw-Hill Education/David Moyer/photographer

The Sterile Scrub Assistant When serving as a sterile scrub assistant, you must perform a surgical scrub and wear sterile gloves. You may be asked to perform a variety of tasks under sterile conditions. Follow the rules of sterile technique listed earlier in this chapter, and remember not to touch unsterile items after putting on sterile gloves. Procedure 44-5, at the end of this chapter, and the sections that follow outline the tasks performed by a sterile scrub assistant.

Handling Instruments Your first duty as a sterile scrub assistant is, typically, to close the instruments on the sterile tray because they are left in the open position during sterilization. Your next duty is to rearrange the instruments on the tray in the order in which they will be used or according to the doctor's preference. Instruments are generally used in the following sequence:

- Cutting instruments
- Grasping instruments
- Retractors
- Probes
- Suture materials
- Needle holders and scissors

Prepare for swabbing by placing several sterile gauze squares in the dressing forceps, to be ready when needed. As the sterile scrub assistant, you will be asked to pass instruments to the doctor during the procedure. You must hold instruments so that the doctor can grasp them safely and securely, without needing to reposition them in her hands. At the same time, the instruments must be handled properly to maintain their sterility.

When passing scissors and clamps, hold them by the hinge (Figure 44-14). You will have a clear view of the instrument's tip and the doctor will have full use of the handles. Firmly slap the instrument handles into the doctor's extended palm. The doctor's hand will close around the handles as a reflex action to the slapping. This technique reduces the risk of dropping an instrument. If the scissors or clamp is curved, the curve should follow the same curve as the doctor's hand.

When passing a scalpel, hold it above and just behind the cutting edge of the blade with the blade facing away from your palm so that the doctor can grasp the entire handle (Figure 44-15). You should wait until the doctor has fully grasped the handle before taking your hand away. The doctor will wait until your hand is fully out of the way before moving the scalpel. This requires good communication between you and the doctor and helps avoid any injury while passing the scalpel. Pass a needle holder with suture material so that the needle is pointing up, and hold the end of the suture material with your other hand to prevent the material from becoming tangled in the handles. You may also use a sterile tray called a passing tray when passing sharp instruments to the doctor. Using a passing tray reduces the likelihood of having an exposure incident while passing instruments (Figure 44-16).

Other Duties As a sterile scrub assistant, you also may be asked to swab fluids from a wound or to retract the edges of a wound to help the doctor view the area. While the doctor is closing the wound, you may be required to cut the suture material after each stitch. The doctor may not verbalize every request to you. With practice and after experience with a particular doctor, you will learn how to respond to the doctor's actions.

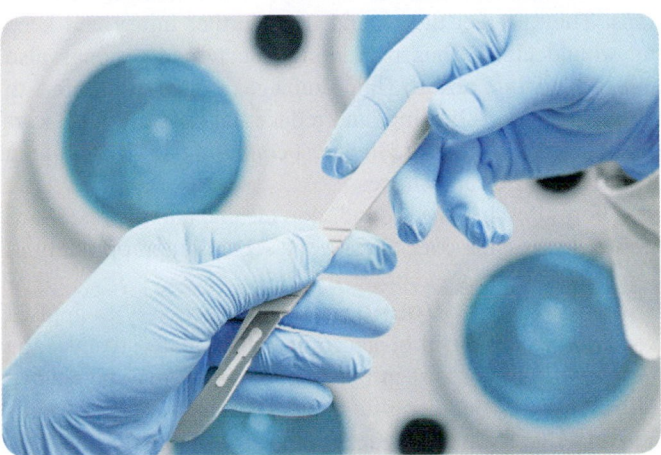

FIGURE 44-15 Hold a scalpel above and just behind the cutting edge as you pass the handle into the palm of the doctor's hand.
© Alexey Poprotskiy/Shutterstock

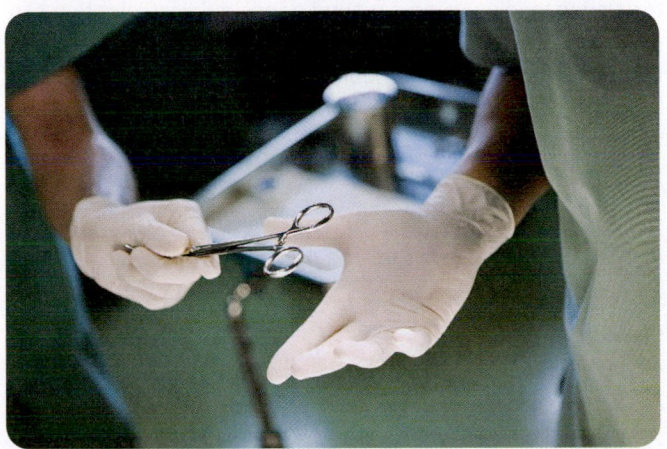

FIGURE 44-14 Holding the scissors by the hinge, slap the handles into the doctor's hand.
© MIXA/Getty Images RF

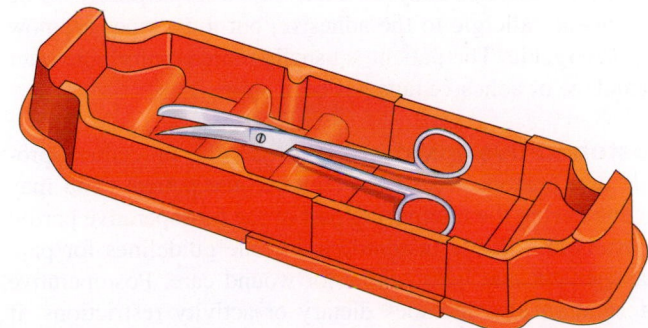

FIGURE 44-16 A passing tray may be used to safely pass sharp instruments during a surgical procedure.

When cutting suture materials, leave ⅛ inch of the material above the knot. This length prevents the suture from coming untied but is short enough that it does not bother the patient.

▶ Postoperative Procedures   LO 44.7

You will be responsible for the patient's **postoperative** ("post-op") follow-up after the surgical procedure. Your duties may include immediate care of the patient, proper cleaning of the surgical room, and follow-up care of the patient. Procedure 44-6, at the end of this chapter, outlines the tasks performed after a minor surgical procedure.

Immediate Patient Care

Patient care is your top priority as a medical assistant. Except for intravenous medications, you will administer postoperative medications the physician requests for the patient. You also will ensure that the patient remains lying down on the examining table for the prescribed length of time after the procedure. During this period, continue to monitor the patient's vital signs and watch for adverse reactions. Document your observations in the patient's chart.

Dressing the Wound You also may dress the wound during the monitoring period. Dressings are sterile materials used to cover an incision. They serve a number of functions. They protect the wound from further injury and keep the wound clean, thus preventing infection. Dressings also reduce bleeding, absorb fluid drainage, reduce discomfort to the patient, speed healing, and reduce the possibility of scarring. Gauze dressings are the most common type and come in a variety of sizes and shapes.

Before dressing the wound, don clean exam gloves. Place the sterile dressing over the site and secure it appropriately.

Bandaging the Wound It may be necessary to apply a bandage (a clean strip of gauze or elastic material) over the dressing to help hold it in place. Tube gauze may be needed for bandaging wounds on fingers or other extremities. Application of this type of gauze requires an applicator. The applicator is a wire cage on which the gauze is loaded. Bandages also may be used to improve circulation, to provide support or reduce tension on a wound or suture and prevent it from reopening, or to prevent movement of that area of the body. Adhesive tape also may be used for these purposes. Some patients are allergic to the adhesive, but most tapes are now hypoallergenic. The patient is usually more comfortable after a bandage or adhesive tape has been applied.

Postoperative Instructions After the procedure, provide oral postoperative instructions to the patient. You may do this during the monitoring part of the postoperative period or afterward. These instructions include guidelines for pain management and instructions for wound care. Postoperative information also includes dietary or activity restrictions, if any, and when to come in for a follow-up appointment. It is a good idea to ask patients to repeat what you have said so that you know they understand the information.

Instructions should be provided in writing as part of a complete postoperative information packet. You may be asked to help prepare or update packet materials, especially if you routinely assist patients as they recover from minor surgery. A postoperative information packet might include the following information:

- Proper wound care instructions
- Suggestions for pain relief and reduction of swelling, such as medications and hot or cold packs
- Dietary restrictions
- Activity restrictions
- Timing for a follow-up appointment or an appointment card

Wound care instructions include details on changing the dressing, keeping the wound clean, recognizing signs of infection, and protecting the wound. The instructions may vary depending on the depth and size of the wound. In general, the bandage should be removed after the first 24 hours or if it becomes soaked with blood, wet, or dirty. A wet dressing allows bacteria and other contaminants to enter the wound. In most cases, the wound may be cleaned with soap and water after 24 to 48 hours. Once cleaned, gently dry the incision with a sterile gauze and cover with a clean, dry bandage.

You should teach the patient about the signs of infection. For more information, see *Educating the Patient:* When to Call the Doctor About a Wound. Encourage the patient to protect the incision from sun exposure for the first 6 months; doing so helps prevent the incision line from becoming darker than the surrounding skin.

The length of time it takes for a wound to heal varies with the site, the patient's age and health status, and the severity

EDUCATING THE PATIENT

When to Call the Doctor About a Wound

Whether a wound is postsurgical or from an accident, it is important for patients to know when they should call the doctor. Understanding when a wound needs medical attention can reduce the instances of scarring and infection. You can help by teaching them what to look for when they have a wound. Patients with any wounds should call the office if they have any of the following:

- Jagged or gaping edges
- A face wound
- Limited movement in the area of the wound
- Tenderness or inflammation at the wound site
- Purulent drainage
- A fever greater than 100°F
- Red streaks near the wound
- A puncture wound
- Bleeding that does not stop after 10 minutes of pressure
- Sutures coming out on their own or too early

of the wound. So each patient needs specific instructions on how long to continue with the dressings and when to return for suture or staple removal. He or she also may need specific information about limiting activities.

Patient Release Notify the doctor when the patient is stabilized and ready to leave. The doctor may want to further observe and instruct the patient. Be sure to offer assistance if the patient needs help getting dressed.

Then help the patient check out. Schedule the next appointment for the patient. Make sure the patient has the correct discharge packet. Confirm arrangements to transport the patient home. Finally, assist the patient to the car or other transport if this is part of office procedure.

If a patient insists on driving himself home, enter this information on the chart. Indicate the time and have the patient initial the entry. This documentation is important for legal reasons. It would clarify liability, should an accident occur as a result of a reaction to the surgery or the anesthetic.

Surgical Room Cleanup

If there is time during the monitoring period, begin to clean up the surgical area. If time is not available then, perform the cleanup routine after the patient has been released. Refer to the *Examination and Treatment Areas* chapter for sanitization and disinfection guidelines.

Follow-Up Care

During a follow-up appointment, the physician examines the patient's surgical wound. The healthcare practitioner may ask you to change the dressing or remove the wound closures. Typically, suture or staple removal takes place 5 to 10 days after minor surgery. The sutures or staples are ready for removal when a clean, unbroken suture line is observed. There should be no scabs, no seepage from the wound, and no visible opening. Any of these signs may indicate unhealed areas. Suture removal is described in Procedure 44-7, at the end of this chapter. Staple removal is similar, except that staple removal forceps, rather than thumb forceps and scissors, are used to remove the staples.

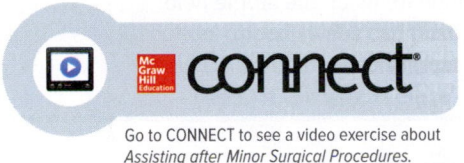

Go to CONNECT to see a video exercise about *Assisting after Minor Surgical Procedures.*

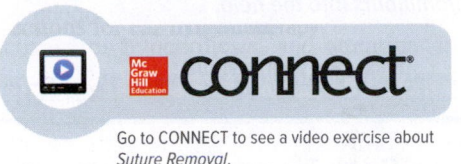

Go to CONNECT to see a video exercise about *Suture Removal.*

PROCEDURE 44-1 Creating a Sterile Field

Procedure Goal: To create a sterile field for a minor surgical procedure

OSHA Guidelines: This procedure does not involve exposure to blood, body fluids, or tissues.

Materials: Tray or Mayo stand, sterile instrument pack, sterile transfer forceps, cleaning solution, sterile drape, and additional packaged sterile items as required

Method:

1. Clean and disinfect the tray or Mayo stand.
2. Wash your hands and assemble the necessary materials.
3. Check the label on the instrument pack to make sure it is the correct pack for the procedure.
4. Check the date and sterilization indicator on the instrument pack to make sure the pack is still sterile.
   RATIONALE: *Using an out-of-date pack puts the patient at risk for surgical site infection.*
5. Place the sterile pack on the tray or stand and unfold the outermost fold away from yourself.
6. Unfold the sides of the pack outward, touching only the areas that will become the underside of the sterile field.
   RATIONALE: *Touching the inside of the pack will contaminate the sterile field.*
7. Open the final flap toward yourself, stepping back and away from the sterile field.

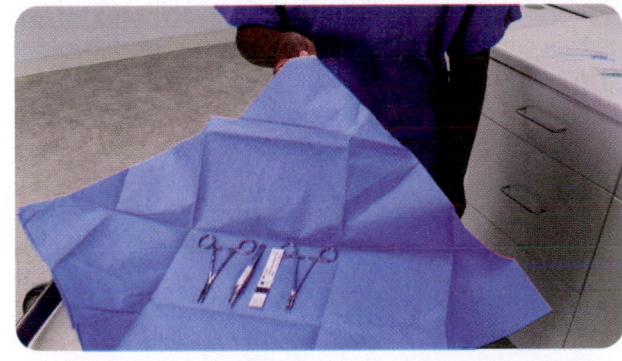

FIGURE Procedure 44-1 Step 7 Open the flap toward yourself last to avoid reaching over the sterile field.
© McGraw-Hill Education

8. Place additional packaged sterile items on the sterile field.
   - Ensure that you have the correct item or instrument and that the package is still sterile.
   - Stand away from the sterile field.
   - Grasp the package flaps and pull apart about halfway.
   - Bring the corners of the wrapping beneath the package, paying attention not to contaminate the inner package or item.
   - Hold the package over the sterile field with the opening down; with a quick movement, pull the flap completely open and snap the sterile item onto the field.

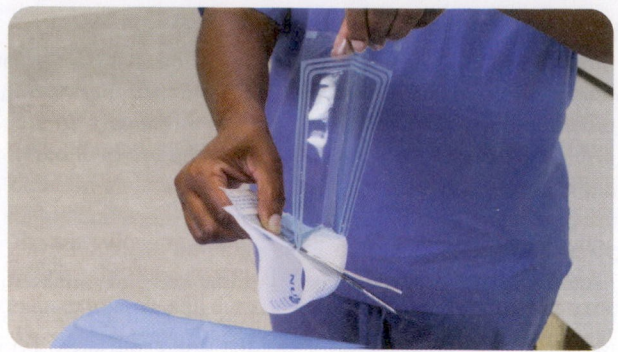

FIGURE Procedure 44-1 Step 8   Hold the package over the sterile field with the opening down. Pulling the flap open, snap the instrument onto the field.
© McGraw-Hill Education

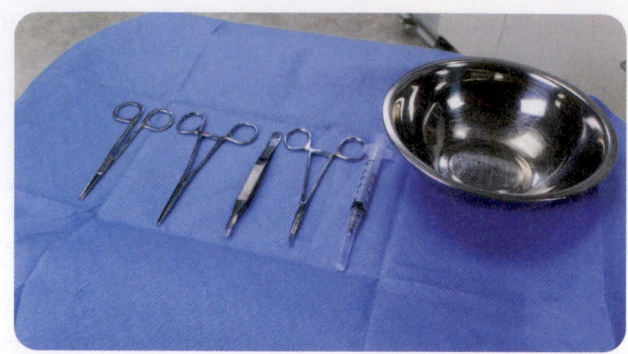

FIGURE Procedure 44-1 Step 9   Placing the bowl at the edge of the sterile field keeps you from reaching over the sterile field when you pour liquids into the bowl.
© McGraw-Hill Education

9. Place basins and bowls near the edge of the sterile field so that you can pour liquids without reaching over the field.
   RATIONALE: *Reaching over the field may drop contaminants into the field.*

10. Use sterile transfer forceps if necessary to add additional items to the sterile field.

11. If necessary, don sterile gloves after a sterile scrub to arrange items on the sterile field.

PROCEDURE 44-2   Performing a Surgical Scrub

Procedure Goal: To remove dirt and microorganisms from under the fingernails and from the surface of the skin, hair follicles, and oil glands of the hands and forearms

OSHA Guidelines: This procedure does not involve exposure to blood, body fluids, or tissues.

Materials: Dispenser with surgical soap, sterile surgical scrub brush or sponge, and sterile towels

Method:

1. Remove all jewelry and roll up your sleeves to above the elbow.

2. Assemble the necessary materials.

3. Turn on the faucet using the foot or knee pedal.

4. Wet your hands from fingertips to elbows, keeping your hands higher than your elbows.
   RATIONALE: *This prevents water from running down your arms and contaminating the washed area.*

5. Under running water, use a sterile brush to clean under your fingernails.

6. Apply surgical soap and scrub your hands, fingers, areas between the fingers, wrists, and forearms with the scrub sponge, using a firm, circular motion. Follow the manufacturer's recommendations to determine appropriate length of time (usually 2 to 6 minutes).
   RATIONALE: *Scrubbing all surfaces dislodges microorganisms so that they can be rinsed away.*

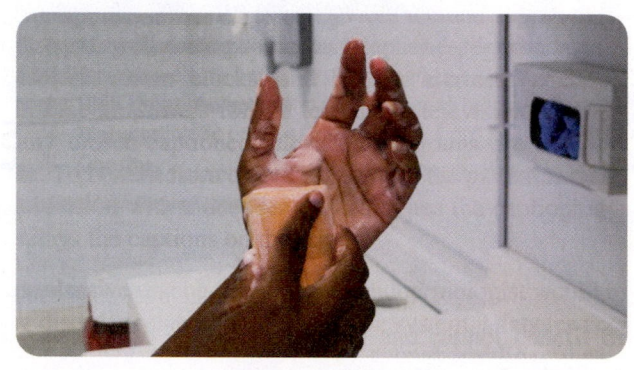

FIGURE Procedure 44-2 Step 6   With a sterile scrub brush, use a circular motion to scrub every surface of your hands and forearms.
© McGraw-Hill Education

7. Rinse from fingers to elbows, always keeping your hands higher than your elbows.

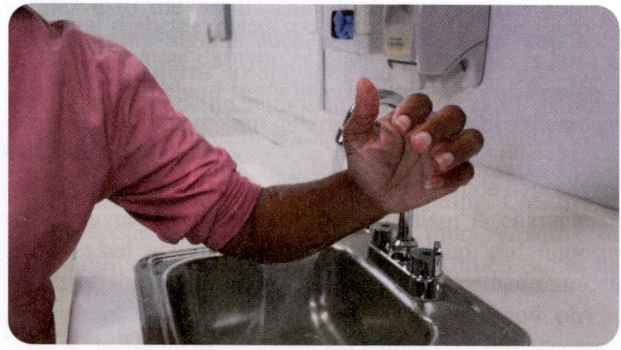

FIGURE Procedure 44-2 Step 7   Keep your hands higher than your elbows when rinsing after a surgical scrub so that water runs away from the fingertips.
© McGraw-Hill Education

8. Thoroughly dry your hands and forearms with sterile towels, working from the hands to the elbows.
   RATIONALE: *Using sterile towels prevents recontaminating your hands.*

9. Turn off the faucet with the foot or knee pedal. Use a sterile paper towel if a foot or knee pedal is not available.

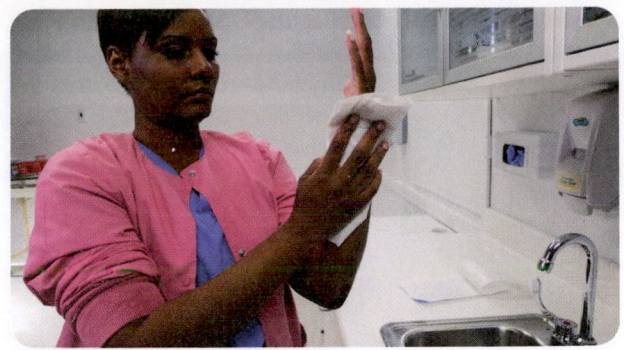

FIGURE Procedure 44-2 Step 8   Dry your hands with sterile towels, working from the hands to the elbows.
© McGraw-Hill Education

PROCEDURE 44-3 Donning Sterile Gloves

Procedure Goal: To don sterile gloves without compromising the sterility of the gloves' outer surface

OSHA Guidelines: This procedure does not involve exposure to blood, body fluids, or tissues.

Materials: Correctly sized, prepackaged, double-wrapped sterile gloves

Method:

1. Obtain the correct size gloves.

2. Check the package for tears and ensure that the expiration date has not passed.
   RATIONALE: *A torn package should be considered unsterile.*

3. Perform a surgical scrub.

4. Peel the outer wrap from the gloves and place the inner wrapper on a clean surface above waist level.

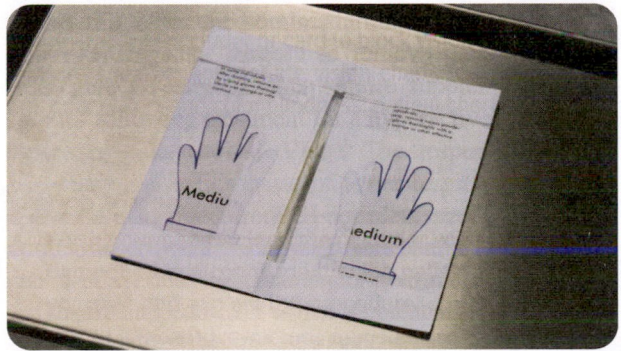

FIGURE Procedure 44-3 Step 4   Place the inner wrap on a clean surface, above waist level, with the cuff end closest to your body.
© McGraw-Hill Education

5. Position gloves so that the cuff end is closest to your body.

6. Touch only the flaps as you open the package.
   RATIONALE: *Touching the inside of the package could contaminate the gloves.*

7. Use instructions provided on the inner package, if available.

8. Do not reach over the sterile inside of the inner package.

9. Follow these steps if there are no instructions:
   a. Open the package so that the first flap is opened away from you.
   b. Pinch the corner and pull to one side.
   c. Put your fingertips under the side flaps and gently pull until the package is completely open.

10. Use your nondominant hand to grasp the inside cuff of the opposite glove (the folded edge). Do not touch the outside of the glove. If you are right-handed, use your left hand to put on the right glove first, and vice versa.
    RATIONALE: *Grabbing the inside of the glove allows you to put it on without contaminating its outside.*

11. Holding the glove at arm's length and waist level, insert the dominant hand into the glove, palm facing up. Do not let the outside of the glove touch any other surface.

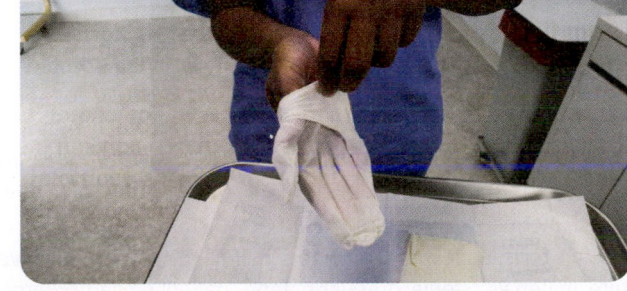

FIGURE Procedure 44-3 Step 11   When donning the glove, do not let the outside of the glove touch any other surface.
© McGraw-Hill Education

12. With your sterile gloved hand, slip the gloved fingers into the cuff of the other glove.

13. Pick up the other glove, touching only the outside. Do not touch any other surfaces.

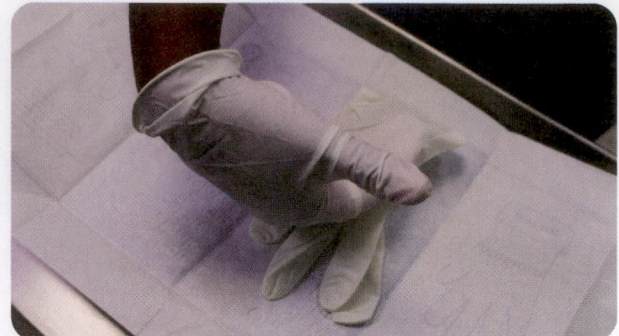

FIGURE Procedure 44-3 Step 13 Slip the fingers of your gloved hand into the other glove's cuff, touching only the outside.
© McGraw-Hill Education

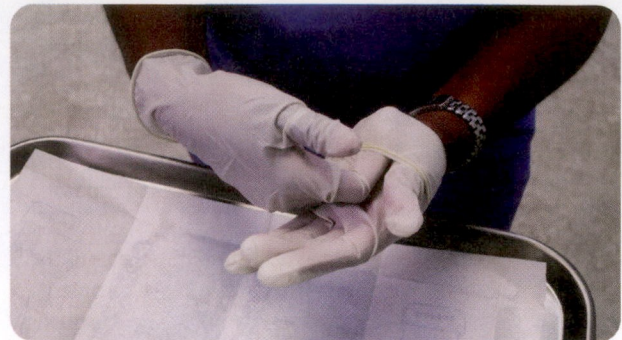

FIGURE Procedure 44-3 Step 14 Pull the glove up and onto your hand without touching the sterile gloved hand to your skin.
© McGraw-Hill Education

14. Pull the glove up and onto your hand, ensuring that the sterile gloved hand does not touch your skin.

15. Adjust your fingers as necessary, touching only glove to glove.

16. Do not adjust the cuffs because your forearms may contaminate the gloves.

17. Keep your hands in front of you, between your shoulders and waist. If you move your hands out of this area, they are considered contaminated.

18. If contamination or the possibility of contamination occurs, change gloves.

19. Remove these gloves the same way you remove clean gloves, by touching only the inside.
    RATIONALE: *Touching only the inside of the gloves reduces exposure to the patient's blood and body fluids.*

PROCEDURE 44-4 Assisting as a Floater (Unsterile Assistant) During Minor Surgical Procedures

WORK // DOC

Procedure Goal: To provide assistance to the doctor during minor surgery while maintaining clean or sterile technique as appropriate

OSHA Guidelines:

 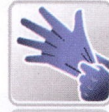  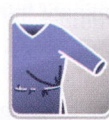

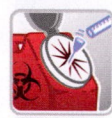  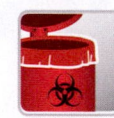 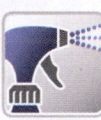

Materials: Sterile towel, tray or Mayo stand, appropriate instrument pack(s), needles and syringes, anesthetic, antiseptic, sterile water or normal saline, small sterile bowl, sterile gauze squares or cotton balls, specimen containers half-filled with preservative, suture materials, sterile dressings, tape, patient's chart/progress note, laboratory requisition form

Method:

1. Perform routine handwashing and don exam gloves.

2. Monitor the patient during the procedure; record the results in the patient's chart.

3. During the surgery, assist as needed.

4. Add sterile items to the tray as necessary.

5. Pour sterile solution into a sterile bowl as needed.

6. Assist in administering additional anesthetic.
   a. Check the medication vial two times.
   b. Clean the rubber stopper with an alcohol pad (write the date opened when using a new bottle); leave the pad on top.
   c. Present the needle and syringe to the doctor.
   d. Remove the alcohol pad from the vial and show the label to the doctor.
   e. Hold the vial upside down and grasp the lower edge firmly; brace your wrist with your free hand.
   RATIONALE: *This firmly supports the vial to sustain the force of the needle being inserted into the rubber stopper.*
   f. Allow the doctor to fill the syringe.
   g. Check the medication vial a final time.

7. Receive specimens for laboratory examination.
   a. Uncap the specimen container; present it to the doctor for the specimen's introduction.
   b. Replace the cap and label the container.
   c. Treat all specimens as infectious.
   d. Place the specimen container in a transport bag or other container.
   e. Complete the requisition form to send the specimen to the laboratory.

PROCEDURE 44-5 Assisting as a Sterile Scrub Assistant During Minor Surgical Procedures

Procedure Goal:

To provide assistance to the doctor during minor surgery while maintaining clean or sterile technique as appropriate

OSHA Guidelines:

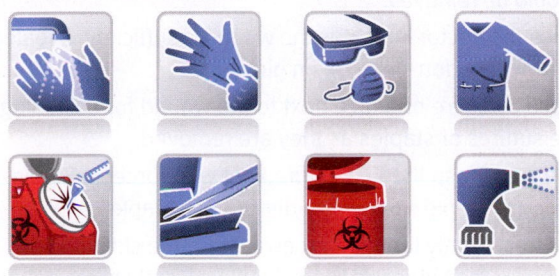

Materials:

Sterile towel, tray or Mayo stand, appropriate instrument pack(s), needles and syringes, anesthetic, antiseptic, sterile water or normal saline, small sterile bowl, sterile gauze squares or cotton balls, specimen containers half-filled with preservative, suture materials, sterile dressings, and tape

Method:

1. Perform a surgical scrub and don sterile gloves. (Remember, remove the sterile towel covering the sterile field and instruments before gloving.)
   RATIONALE: *You will be handling sterile instruments.*
2. Close and arrange the surgical instruments on the tray.
   RATIONALE: *They should be quickly and easily located.*
3. Prepare for swabbing by inserting gauze squares into the sterile dressing forceps.
4. Pass the instruments as necessary.
5. Swab the wound as requested.
6. Retract the wound as requested.
7. Cut the sutures as requested.

PROCEDURE 44-6 Assisting After Minor Surgical Procedures

Procedure Goal: To provide assistance to the doctor during and the patient after minor surgery while maintaining clean or sterile technique as appropriate

OSHA Guidelines:

  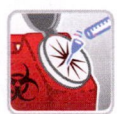 
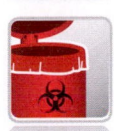 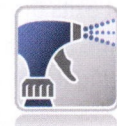

Materials: Examination gloves, antiseptic, tray or Mayo stand, sterile dressings, and tape

Method:

1. Monitor the patient.
2. Don clean exam gloves and clean the wound with antiseptic.
3. Dress the wound.
   RATIONALE: *To protect the wound.*
4. Remove the gloves and wash your hands.
5. Give the patient oral postoperative instructions in addition to the release packet.
   RATIONALE: *The patient will need to understand wound care, medication use, and dietary instructions for proper healing.*
6. Discharge the patient.
7. Put on clean exam gloves.
8. Properly dispose of used materials and disposable instruments.
9. Sanitize reusable instruments and prepare them for disinfection and/or sterilization as needed.
10. Clean equipment and the exam room according to OSHA guidelines.
11. Remove the gloves and wash your hands.

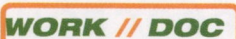
Procedure Goal: To remove sutures from a healing wound while maintaining sterile technique and protecting the integrity of the closed wound

OSHA Guidelines:

  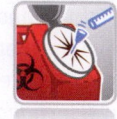 

Materials:

Tray or Mayo stand, patient chart/progress note, suture removal pack (suture scissors and thumb forceps or skin staple remover), sterile towel, antiseptic solution, hydrogen peroxide (3%), two small sterile bowls, sterile gauze squares, sterile strips or butterfly closures, sterile dressings, and tape

Method:

1. Clean and disinfect the tray or Mayo stand.
2. Wash your hands and assemble the necessary materials.
3. Check the date and sterilization indicator on the suture removal pack.
   RATIONALE: *You must ensure that the pack has been subjected to a sterilization procedure and has not expired.*
4. Unwrap the suture removal pack; place it on the tray or stand to create a sterile field.
   RATIONALE: *You need to maintain a sterile field to avoid contaminating the wound.*
5. Unwrap the sterile bowls; add them to the sterile field.
   RATIONALE: *You need to maintain a sterile field to avoid contaminating the wound.*
6. Pour a small amount of antiseptic solution into one bowl and a small amount of hydrogen peroxide into the other bowl.
7. Cover the tray with a sterile towel to protect the sterile field while you are out of the room.
8. Escort the patient to the exam room and explain the procedure.
9. Perform a routine handwash, remove the towel from the tray, and don exam gloves.
10. Remove the old dressing.
    a. Lift the tape toward the middle of the dressing to avoid pulling on the wound.
    b. If the dressing adheres to the wound, cover the dressing with gauze squares soaked in hydrogen peroxide. Leave the wet gauze in place for several seconds to loosen the dressing.
    c. Save the old dressing for the doctor to inspect.
11. Inspect the wound for signs of infection.

12. Clean the wound with gauze pads soaked in antiseptic; pat it dry with clean gauze pads.
13. Remove the gloves and wash your hands.
14. Notify the doctor that the wound is ready for examination.
    RATIONALE: *The doctor should determine if the sutures should be removed.*
15. Once the doctor indicates the wound is sufficiently healed to proceed, don clean exam gloves.
16. Place a square of gauze next to the wound for collecting the sutures or staples as they are removed.
17. Sutures: Grasp the first suture knot with forceps. Staples: Slide the staple remover under the first staple.
18. Sutures: Gently lift the knot away from the skin to allow room for the suture scissors. Staples: Gently press down on the staple remover handle.

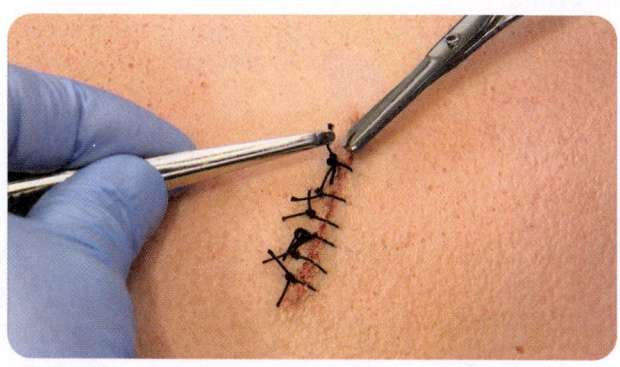

FIGURE Procedure 44-7 Step 18 Gently pulling each suture up and away from the skin creates room for the suture scissors.
© McGraw-Hill Education

19. Sutures: Slide the suture scissors under the suture material and cut the suture where it enters the skin.
    RATIONALE: *This minimizes the amount of exposed suture that travels beneath the skin during removal.*
    Staples: Continue pressing down on the staple remover to straighten the staple so that it exits the skin.
20. Sutures: Gently lift the knot up and toward the wound to remove the suture without opening the wound.

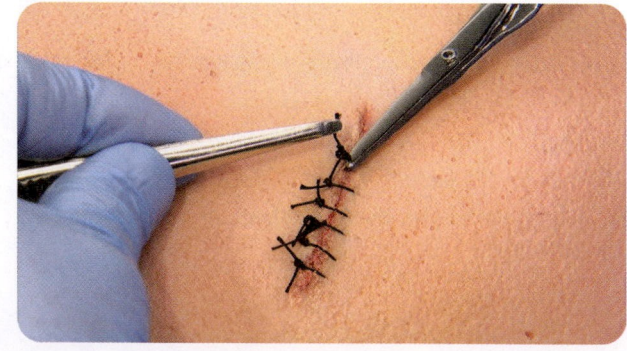

FIGURE Procedure 44-7 Step 20 Lift the knot up and toward the wound to prevent opening the wound.
© McGraw-Hill Education

Staples: Observe the staple on each side to ensure that it is completely out of the skin.

21. Place the suture or staple on the gauze pad; inspect to ensure that the entire suture or staple is present.
    RATIONALE: *Sutures inadvertently left in place may cause an infection.*

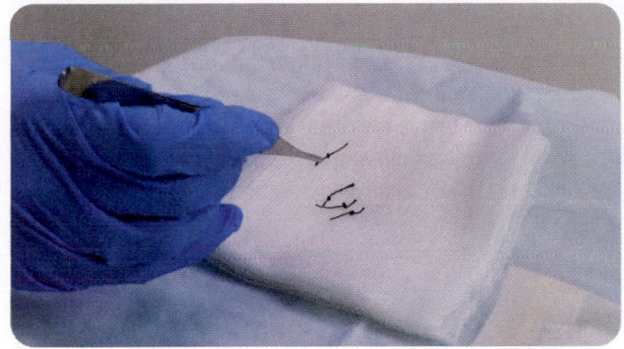

FIGURE Procedure 44-7 Step 21   Place sutures on a gauze square so that you can count and inspect them.
© McGraw-Hill Education

22. Repeat the removal process until all sutures or staples have been removed.

23. Count the sutures or staples and compare the number with that indicated in the patient's record.

24. Clean the wound with antiseptic; allow it to air-dry.

25. Dress the wound as ordered, or notify the doctor if sterile strips or butterfly closures are to be applied.

26. Observe the patient for signs of distress, such as wincing or grimacing.

27. Properly dispose of used materials and disposable instruments.

28. Remove the gloves and wash your hands.

29. Instruct the patient on wound care.

30. In the patient's chart, record pertinent information, such as the condition of the wound and the type of closures used, if any.

31. Escort the patient to the checkout area.

32. Don clean gloves.

33. Sanitize reusable instruments; prepare them for disinfection and/or sterilization as needed.

34. Clean the equipment and exam room according to OSHA guidelines.

35. Remove the gloves and wash your hands.

SUMMARY OF LEARNING OUTCOMES

LEARNING OUTCOMES	KEY POINTS
44.1 Define the medical assistant's role in minor surgical procedures.	The medical assistant's role in minor surgery includes both administrative and clinical tasks. These include but are not limited to completing insurance forms, obtaining signed patient consent, preparing the surgical room, and assisting during a procedure.
44.2 Describe surgical procedures performed in an office setting.	Several surgical procedures are performed in an office setting, including laser surgery, cryosurgery, and electrocauterization.
44.3 Identify the instruments used in minor surgery and describe their functions.	Various categories of instruments are used in minor surgery, including instruments for cutting and dissecting, grasping and clamping, retracting, dilating and probing, suturing, injecting, withdrawing fluids, and obtaining specimens.
44.4 Describe the procedures for medical and sterile asepsis in minor surgery.	Medical asepsis involves reducing the number of microorganisms to prevent the spread of disease. The goal of surgical asepsis is to eliminate all microorganisms.
44.5 Summarize the medical assistant's duties in preoperative procedures.	A medical assistant's preoperative duties include providing preoperative instructions to the patient, ensuring that all necessary paperwork is completed, easing the patient's fears, and preparing the surgical room.
44.6 Describe the medical assistant's duties during an operative procedure.	A medical assistant may serve in one of two capacities during a surgical procedure: either as an unsterile assistant known as a floater or as a sterile scrub assistant.
44.7 Implement the medical assistant's duties in the postoperative period.	A medical assistant's postoperative duties include giving immediate patient care, dressing and bandaging the wound, giving postoperative instructions, assisting with patient release, and cleaning the surgical room.

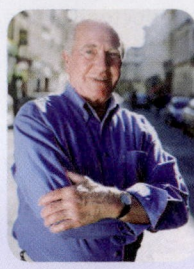

© Image Source/Getty
Images RF

Recall Peter Smith from the beginning of the chapter. Now that you have completed the chapter, answer the following questions regarding his case.

1. What is the medical assistant's role during this minor surgical procedure?

2. Why is it important to document the number of sutures Dr. Buckwalter uses to close Mr. Smith's wound?

3. How should you answer Mr. Smith's question about his trip to the Bahamas?

4. Knowing that Mr. Smith started swimming last week, what should you tell him about protecting his sutures?

E X A M   P R E P A R A T I O N   Q U E S T I O N S

1. (LO 44.2) The removal of dead tissue from a wound is known as
   a. Incision
   b. Debridement
   c. Ligature
   d. Cauterization
   e. Approximation

2. (LO 44.3) An instrument used to clear a blockage is a
   a. Probe
   b. Scalpel
   c. Retractor
   d. Syringe
   e. Forceps

3. (LO 44.4) Why is it important to keep your hands higher than your elbows when performing a surgical scrub?
   a. To avoid touching the sink
   b. So that the soap reaches the elbows
   c. To prevent water from contaminating the washed area
   d. It is not important to keep the hands higher than the elbows
   e. Your hands should be lower than your elbows

4. (LO 44.2) Another name for a mole is a
   a. Wart
   b. Hemangioma
   c. Ligature
   d. Birthmark
   e. Nevus

5. (LO 44.3) Which of the following is the suture with the smallest diameter?
   a. 2
   b. 2-0
   c. 3
   d. 3-0
   e. 4-0

6. (LO 44.2) A jagged, open wound of the skin is a(n)
   a. Incision
   b. Avulsion
   c. Laceration
   d. Puncture
   e. Abrasion

7. (LO 44.4) When adding solutions to a sterile field, you should cover the label with your palm to keep it
   a. Sterile
   b. Dry
   c. From pouring too quickly
   d. From dripping
   e. Visible

8. (LO 44.5) A medical assistant is working in the preoperative area. Which of the following duties would he most likely perform?
   a. Prepare the surgical room
   b. Perform a surgical scrub
   c. Clean the surgical room
   d. Work as a floater
   e. Work as a surgical scrub assistant

9. (LO 44.7) Sterile materials used to cover an incision are
   a. Bandages
   b. Sterile strips
   c. Sutures
   d. Drapes
   e. Dressings

10. (LO 44.3) What type of instrument is a curette?
    a. Probing and dilating
    b. Cutting and dissecting
    c. Grasping
    d. Retracting
    e. Clamping

You are assisting Dr. Sanford with a mole removal. You have already set up the surgical tray and are handing Dr. Sanford her sterile gloves. She tells you that she prefers a no. 11 scalpel blade for this procedure. You know you set up the tray with a no. 10 scalpel blade. How should you respond to Dr. Sanford, and what action should you take?

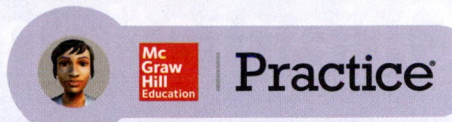

Go to PRACTICE MEDICAL OFFICE and complete the module Clinical - Work Task Proficiencies.

Orientation to the Lab

CASE STUDY

PATIENT INFORMATION

Patient Name	DOB	Allergies
Sylvia Gonzales	9/1/19XX	PCN

Attending	MRN	Other Information
Alexis N. Whalen, MD	341-73-792	Last Hemoglobin A1C 6.3%

Sylvia Gonzales, a 51-year-old female, is at the office for a 3-month return check for her newly diagnosed Type 2 diabetes. She states that she has taken the medication she received for her "sugar" and she knows the doctor wants to a do a special "sugar test" this time. Her medication list includes Januvia® 100 mg daily.

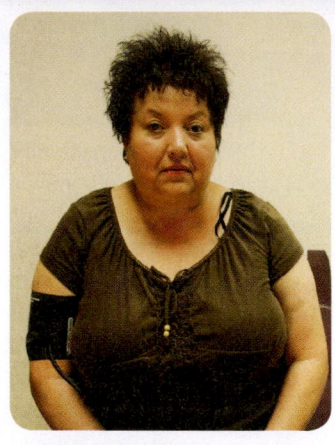

© McGraw-Hill Education

The physician has ordered a fasting blood sugar (FBS) and a hemoglobin A1C blood test. You will need to perform both of these waived tests in your office lab.

Keep Sylvia in mind as you study this chapter. There will be questions at the end of the chapter based on the case study. The information in the chapter will help you answer these questions.

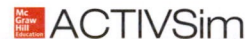

LEARNING OUTCOMES

After completing Chapter 45, you will be able to:

45.1 Describe the purpose of the physician's office laboratory.

45.2 Identify the medical assistant's duties in the physician's office laboratory.

45.3 Identify important pieces of laboratory equipment.

45.4 Illustrate measures to prevent accidents.

45.5 Explain the goal of a quality assurance program in a physician's office laboratory.

45.6 Carry out communication with patients regarding test preparation and follow-up.

45.7 Carry out accurate documentation, including all logs related to quality control.

KEY TERMS

10× lens
artifact
centrifuge
Certificate of Waiver tests
compound microscope
control sample
objectives
ocular
oil-immersion objective
optical microscope
photometer

physician's office laboratory (POL)
proficiency testing program
qualitative test response
quality assurance program
quality control program
quantitative test result
reagent
reference laboratory
standard

MEDICAL ASSISTING COMPETENCIES

CAAHEP

I.C.10 Identify CLIA waived tests associated with common diseases

I.C.12 Identify quality assurance practices in healthcare

I.P.10 Perform a quality control measure

III.C.5 Define the principles of standard precautions

IV.A.3 Use appropriate body language and other nonverbal skills in communicating with patients, family and staff

X.P.7 Complete an incident report related to an error in patient care

ABHES

3. **Medical Terminology**
   c. Apply various medical terms for each specialty
   d. Define and use medical abbreviations when appropriate and acceptable

4. **Medical Law and Ethics**
   a. Follow documentation guidelines

9. **Clinical Procedures**
   a. Practice standard precautions and perform disinfection/sterilization techniques

10. **Medical Laboratory Procedures**
    a. Practice quality control
    b. Perform selected CLIA-waived tests that assist with diagnosis and treatment
       (6) Kit testing
          c. Dip sticks
    c. Dispose of biohazardous materials

▶ Introduction

Laboratory testing of patients' specimens is an integral component of patient care. Medical assistants often perform a role in the clinical laboratory setting in the physician's office. This chapter will introduce you to the various types and uses of common laboratory equipment. You will learn about safety in the laboratory and steps to aid in preventing accidents. A discussion of the Clinical Laboratory Improvement Amendments of 1988 (CLIA '88) and this law's impact on the laboratory setting is included in this chapter to help you understand quality assurance, quality control procedures, and required recordkeeping.

▶ The Role of Laboratory Testing in Patient Care   LO 45.1

Laboratory analysis of blood, urine, or other body fluids and substances provides three kinds of information about a patient. First, regular monitoring through laboratory tests, like those that are part of an annual exam, can help a physician identify possible diseases or other problems. Second, specific tests can help confirm or contradict a physician's initial diagnosis. Third, laboratory testing can help a physician determine and monitor the proper dosage of a patient's medication.

Kinds of Laboratories

Some physicians prefer to have all laboratory tests performed by a **reference laboratory,** a laboratory owned and operated by an organization outside the practice. Other physicians choose to have some tests completed by the reference laboratory and some completed in the office in the **physician's office laboratory (POL).**

Each method of managing laboratory analyses has advantages and disadvantages. Reference laboratories often have more technological resources than those available in the POL. A reference laboratory offers a complete range of tests in all specialties, and subspecialties, including:

- Cytology—microscopic examination of cells to make a diagnosis; Pap smears (tests for detecting cervical cancer) are evaluated in the cytology department.

- Toxicology—testing to identify poisons or other chemicals in the body; workplace drug testing is a type of toxicology test.

- Immunology—testing to identify disorder and disease of the immune system; tests for autoimmune diseases are performed in the immunology department.

- Blood banking—the laboratory department responsible for processing and storing blood and blood products for transfusion and blood disorder treatments; this department would provide blood to someone with severe anemia who needs a transfusion.

- Urinalysis—testing urine for kidney diseases and disorders and certain metabolic disorders; testing for glucose in the urine (a test done on people with diabetes) is part of a urinalysis.

- Histology—microscopic evaluation of tissues to make a diagnosis; a biopsy of a skin lesion is sent to the histology department to examine the tissue for signs of cancer.

- Serology—testing the liquid part of the blood for antibodies against specific microorganisms; testing for malaria and viral hepatitis are serologic tests.

- Chemistry—testing for certain substances in the blood, urine, or other body fluids; substances tested for include cholesterol, electrolytes, glucose, calcium, and potassium; a lipid panel for cholesterol and triglycerides is a blood chemistry test.
- Microbiology—testing for the presence of pathogenic microorganisms such as bacteria, viruses, fungi, protozoans, and parasites in blood, urine, sputum, reproductive fluids, and fluids from wounds; a nasal culture for MRSA is a microbiology test.
- Hematology—testing of blood to identify problems with count, size, or number of blood cells to diagnose diseases and disorders; testing for anemia and leukemia are hematology tests.

Using a reference laboratory frees a physician's staff from testing duties and allows more time for patient care. It also reduces or eliminates the cost of running an in-house lab. Furthermore, some managed care companies have contracts with laboratory companies that require their subscribers to use a specific reference laboratory. An advantage of a POL is that processing tests produces a quicker turnaround and eliminates the need for the patient to travel to other test locations.

The Purpose of the Physician's Office Laboratory

Office policy determines which tests, if any, will be performed at your location and which tests will be performed by a reference laboratory. A POL, like the one shown in Figure 45-1, is responsible for accurate and timely processing of routine tests and for reporting test results to the physician. Tests most often performed in the POL include chemical analyses, hematologic tests, microbiologic tests, and urinalysis (discussed earlier in the chapter).

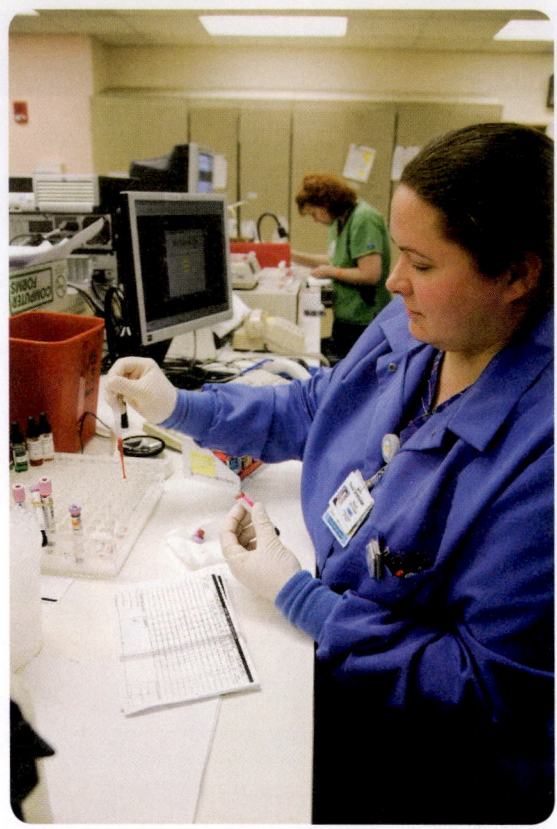

FIGURE 45-1 A physician's office laboratory (POL) may be simple or elaborate, depending on the tests the office performs.
© Jim West/Alamy

- Use of reference materials in the POL
- Screening and follow-up of test results

▶ The Medical Assistant's Role   LO 45.2

As a medical assistant, you may be responsible for processing tests done in the POL, including preparing the patient for the test, collecting the sample, completing the test, reporting the results to the physician, and communicating information about the test from the physician to the patient. Your role in the POL requires you to integrate a great deal of information to serve both the physician and the patient effectively. You will need to master the following subjects:

- Use of laboratory equipment
- Regulations governing laboratory practices and procedures
- Precautions for accident prevention
- Waste disposal requirements
- Housekeeping and maintenance routines
- Quality assurance and control procedures
- Technical aspects of specimen collection and test processing, including expected results
- Communication with patients
- Reporting of test results to the physician
- Recordkeeping of test specimens, procedures, and results
- Inventory and ordering of equipment and supplies

▶ Use of Laboratory Equipment   LO 45.3

As a medical assistant, you must be familiar with the operation of common laboratory equipment. Learning to use a specific piece of equipment may take the form of on-the-job training or attending training programs conducted by manufacturers' representatives. You may routinely use the following equipment:

- Autoclave
- Centrifuge
- Microscope
- Electronic equipment and software
- Equipment used for measurement

Autoclave

A steam autoclave is used to sterilize, or eradicate, all organisms on the surfaces of instruments and equipment before they are used on a patient or in testing procedures. Use of the autoclave is discussed in the *Infection Control Practices* chapter.

Centrifuge

A **centrifuge** is a device for spinning a specimen at high speed until it separates into its component parts. The centrifuge in a

POL is generally used to separate whole blood samples into blood components or to prepare urine samples for examination. Use of a centrifuge is described in greater detail in the *Collecting, Processing, and Testing Urine and Stool Specimens* chapter.

Microscope

An instrument often used in a POL is the microscope, commonly used for the examination of blood smears and identification of microorganisms in body fluid samples. Although on-site blood smear evaluation is convenient and fast for both patient and physician, it is important to know which procedures are routinely covered. Only CLIA-approved microscopy procedures are eligible for payment by Medicare and Medicaid. Table 45-1 lists CLIA-approved provider-performed microscopy procedures.

The **optical microscope,** also called the light microscope, is the type most often found in the POL (Figure 45-2). With this type of microscope, light is concentrated (condensed) through a condenser and then focused through the object being examined. This produces an image of the object. **Compound microscopes** use two lenses to magnify the image. The effect of the two lenses is compounded—added together—giving greater magnification than one lens can provide. Compound microscopes are the most common type of optical microscope used in the medical office.

You must be able to operate an optical microscope correctly. First, you need to become familiar with the component parts, described in the following paragraphs.

Oculars The **oculars** are the eyepieces through which you view the image. A microscope is either monocular, with a single eyepiece, or binocular, with two eyepieces. You can adjust the oculars on a binocular microscope to compensate for differences in visual acuity between your right and left eyes. You also can adjust the distance between oculars to match the distance between your eyes. The ocular contains a magnifying lens—called a **10× lens**—that usually magnifies an image 10 times.

Objectives Just below the ocular or oculars, the **objectives** are mounted on a swivel or rotating base called the *nosepiece.* These are known as objectives because they are closest to the

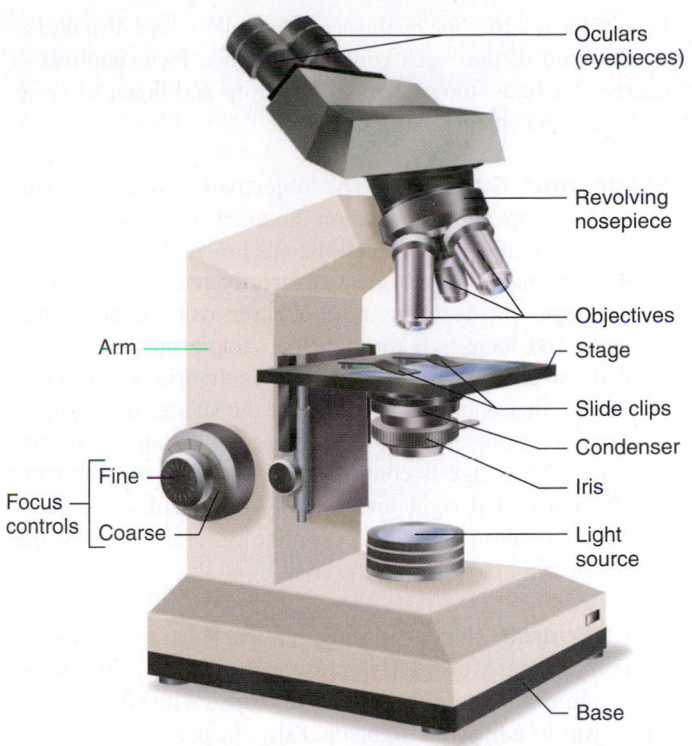

FIGURE 45-2 The microscope is an often used piece of equipment in a POL.

object being magnified. An objective contains another magnifying lens. Generally, microscopes used in the POL have a three-piece objective system with three different magnifications. An objective is moved into position directly under the ocular by rotating the nosepiece.

Two of the objectives are dry objectives; this means there is air space between the specimen under examination and the objective. Condensed (concentrated) light passes through the specimen and the air space above the specimen and then travels toward the objective lens. These dry objectives are low- and high-power lenses, usually 10× and 40×, respectively. When the low-power objective lens is combined with the ocular lenses, the total magnification factor is 100× (10× times 10×). The high-power lens and ocular lenses yield a magnification factor of 400× (10× times 40×).

The third objective is an **oil-immersion objective,** which is used for specimens that need extreme magnification, such as blood smears and bacteriologic slides. It is designed to be lowered into a drop of immersion oil placed directly on the slide above the prepared specimen under examination. This design eliminates the air space between the microscope slide and the objective, where some of the light scatters beyond the objective. Placing the end of the objective in oil reduces the loss of light by creating a column of oil that tightly focuses the light, keeping it from scattering. This results in a much sharper, brighter image, allowing for greater magnification. An oil-immersion objective has a magnification factor of 100×. Combined with the ocular lenses, the total magnification factor is 1,000×.

Arm and Focus Controls The ocular(s) and objectives, collectively referred to as the body tube, are attached to the

TABLE 45-1	CLIA-Approved Provider-Performed Microscopy Procedures
Wet mounts—vaginal, cervical, or skin specimens	
Potassium hydroxide preparations	
Pinworm examinations	
Fern test (for the presence of amniotic fluid in vaginal secretions)	
Urinalysis by dipstick with microscopy	
Urinalysis; two or three glass test (for the presence of blood 1—at the beginning of the urine stream, 2—midstream, and/or 3—at the termination of urination)	
Fecal leukocyte examination	
Semen analysis (for presence or motility of sperm)	
Nasal smears for eosinophils	

base of the microscope by the arm. The microscope arm is also the location of the focus controls. The two focus controls—coarse and fine—move the body tube up and down to bring into focus the object being examined.

Stage and Substage The objectives and oculars are focused on a specimen placed on the microscope's stage. The stage is the platform on which the specimen slide rests, held in place by metal clips. Located directly under the stage is the substage. This is where the condenser, which concentrates the light and focuses it through the sample on the slide, is located. Also located on the substage is the iris. The iris is a diaphragm that opens and closes like the shutter of a camera to increase or decrease the amount of light illuminating the specimen. The stage is controlled by the stage mechanisms, which control left-right and forward-backward movements of the stage, allowing you to examine different areas of the specimen without reseating the slide.

Light Source Under the stage and substage assemblies is the light source. Most POL microscopes use a built-in electric light source, and most of these are equipped with controls that allow you to adjust the light intensity. In place of a built-in light source, older microscopes use a mirror, which gathers and focuses light from a microscope lamp onto the specimen.

Specimen Slides and Coverslip Although the specimen slide is not technically part of the microscope assembly, it is necessary for using the microscope. All specimens must be placed on slides. Many specimens also require a coverslip, or cover glass. The slide and coverslip support and position the specimen. They also prevent contamination of the microscope by the specimen. Specimens that are to be stained or immersed in oil, such as blood smears, do not require coverslips.

Using an Optical Microscope To use an optical microscope, you must be able to focus it using each of the three objectives. Procedure 45-1, at the end of this chapter, describes how to operate an optical microscope correctly.

You also will be responsible for the proper care and maintenance of the optical microscope in your office. Related concerns and techniques are described in the *Caution: Handle with Care* feature.

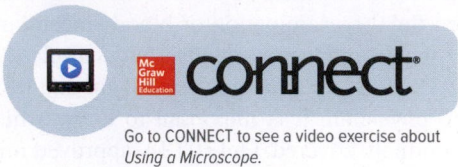

Go to CONNECT to see a video exercise about *Using a Microscope.*

Electronic Equipment and Software

Electronic equipment is used in the POL because it is safer, more accurate, and more efficient than manual methods; generally requires little maintenance; and does not require extensive training prior to its use. A wide variety of tasks, such as cell counting and complex chemical analyses, are performed with electronic equipment. A range of clinical laboratory software systems are available, which are used to create and maintain clinical data, making remote access and tracking between facilities easier. Manufacturers' instructions for operation and maintenance of these systems must be followed to ensure safety, efficiency, and reliable results.

A **photometer,** which measures light intensity, is a basic electronic component of many pieces of analytic laboratory equipment. A handheld glucometer (Figure 45-3), for example, contains a photometer that measures reflected light. Patients with diabetes and clinical personnel use a glucometer to monitor blood glucose levels.

Equipment Used for Measurement

Precise measurement is critical in the POL because it produces accurate test results. Much of this measurement is built into the electronic equipment or premeasured kits you will use. However, you will still need to perform various

---

CAUTION: HANDLE WITH CARE

Care and Maintenance of the Microscope

The microscope is the workhorse of the POL. For it to provide trouble-free service, however, it must be well cared for. Dust, oil, and other contaminants cause major problems with microscopes. Careless cleaning and haphazard storage will also eventually cause problems. These problems may include mechanical difficulties with the microscope or contamination of the specimen being examined. Foreign objects visible through a microscope, but unrelated to the specimen, are called **artifacts** and may be misinterpreted when the specimen is examined.

Clean the microscope after each use. Inspect the body tube, arm, and stage to make sure they are dust- and contaminant-free. Clean the ocular and objective lenses with lens paper, not tissue or other products. Tissue fibers are a common artifact. The eyepiece is an area in which skin oil, dust, and eye makeup may collect, posing a risk of disease transmission and making images difficult to see. Use lens-cleaning products according to the manufacturer's guidelines. Excess amounts of these products may dissolve the cement holding the lenses in place, rendering the microscope useless.

When not in use, the microscope should be stored under its plastic cover. If there is a power cord, wrap it loosely around the base and secure it with a twist-tie or elastic band. Lower the low-power objective close to the stage and center the stage.

If the microscope must be moved, hold it by the arm and support it under the base. Never carry a microscope with one hand or by just the arm. Carry the cord so that it does not dangle and pose a tripping hazard. Place the microscope on a sturdy table or bench, away from the edge.

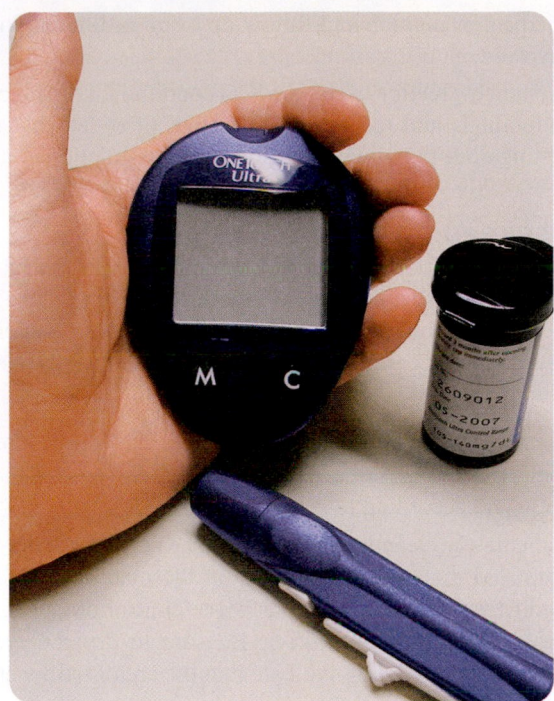

FIGURE 45-3 A handheld glucometer translates the amount of reflected light into the level of glucose in a blood sample.
© Leesa Whicker

measurements manually when blood, semen, urine, and other body fluids are analyzed using manual tests. Some reagents also require measuring.

Metric system units are commonly used in the POL. For information on metric system weight, height, and temperature measurements, see the *Vital Signs and Measurements* chapter. To learn how to convert between measurement systems, see the *Math and Dosage Calculation* chapter.

A variety of equipment is used to provide accurate measurements. You must take these measurements carefully for them to be of value in the final test results. Other types of measuring equipment include

- Pipettes (mechanical or manual)—used to measure small amounts of liquids.
- Volumetric or graduated flasks or beakers—used to measure the relatively large amounts (volumes) of liquids necessary for reagents and solutions.
- A hemocytometer—a specialized slide calibrated to the exact measurements needed to count blood cells and sperm under a microscope.
- Thermometers (generally in degrees centigrade)—used to provide legal documentation that refrigerators, bacterial incubators, and other appliances maintain the precise temperature range required for accurate laboratory work.

▶ Safety in the Laboratory   LO 45.4

Safety is a primary concern in any laboratory environment, and it is especially important in a physician's office laboratory because patients and laboratory workers may be at risk. For your own protection, as well as that of patients and coworkers, you must always be aware of and observe laboratory safety guidelines.

Use standard precautions when handling all body fluids, excretions, and secretions. If you have any doubt about whether you need to take precautions, take them. Even though some substances do not present a risk of transmitting bloodborne pathogens, they may present a high risk of transmitting other bacteria, viruses, or parasites. Follow these guidelines:

- Wear gloves when handling all body fluids, secretions, and excretions.
- Change gloves every time you move from patient to patient as you collect specimens for testing.
- Wash your hands immediately after removing used gloves.
- Wear other protective gear such as eye protection and face masks during procedures in which there is a risk that droplets or spray may come in contact with your eyes, nose, or mouth.
- Take special care to avoid injury from sharp or pointed instruments or equipment. Although gloves protect you from surface exposure to potentially infected substances, they offer little protection against exposure from needlesticks or cuts. Never use needles or other sharp instruments unnecessarily.
- Use only recommended instruments and equipment. A once-common laboratory technique that has been discontinued is the use of a mouth pipette (a type of calibrated glass or plastic straw) to transfer specimens. Under no circumstances should you use a mouth pipette to transfer blood from one collection device to another; doing so puts you at risk for getting blood or other hazardous fluids in your mouth.
- Take care to prevent spills and splashes when transporting specimens to the laboratory and when moving specimens in the laboratory.
- If a work surface becomes contaminated because of spilling or splashing, disinfect the area completely, using an approved solution such as 10% bleach, before beginning any other procedure.
- Dispose of waste products carefully and correctly.
- Be sure to remove protective gear before leaving the laboratory.

Biologic Safety

You will work with test specimens that may be contaminated with bloodborne or other pathogens. Treat every specimen as if it were contaminated. Additional information regarding OSHA's Bloodborne Pathogens Standard may be found in the *Infection Control Fundamentals* chapter. Follow standard precautions.

- If you have any cuts, lesions, or sores, do not expose yourself to potentially contaminated material. Consult your supervisor if you have any doubt about whether you can safely perform test procedures.
- Wash your hands before and after every procedure and whenever you come in contact with a potentially contaminated substance.

- Wear gloves at all times. Use other protective gear as appropriate to prevent exposing your eyes, nose, and mouth to potentially contaminated material.

- Mouth pipetting is prohibited at all times. Use specially made rubber suction bulbs to draw specimens mechanically.

- Work in a biologic safety cabinet (similar to a fume hood) when completing procedures that are likely to generate droplet sprays or splashes of potentially contaminated material.

- When transferring a blood specimen from a collection tube to another container, wear appropriate PPE (including a mask and goggles or a face shield) and cover the tube stopper with an absorbent pad or a commercial stopper remover to prevent spray or splatter from the tube. Do not rock the stopper back and forth because this could cause the tube to break. Always remove the stopper by opening it away from your face so that the vapor pressure flows away from you. Place the stopper on a sterile gauze pad while you work with the collection tube. Do not allow the stopper to come in contact with other work surfaces. Keep the collection tube stoppered unless you are actively using it.

- Establish clean and dirty areas in the laboratory. Place all used instruments and equipment in the dirty area for sanitization, disinfection, and sterilization.

- Disinfect your work area at least once a day with a 10% bleach solution or a germ-killing solution approved by the Environmental Protection Agency (EPA). If a spill occurs, immediately disinfect the work area.

- Dispose of waste products immediately.

- Dispose of needles in the appropriate sharps container.

- If an instrument or piece of equipment must be serviced, be sure it has been decontaminated first.

- If you use a bleach solution for disinfection, change it daily.

Accident Reporting

Despite all precautions, laboratory accidents still occur. Armed with an understanding of the materials with which you are working and basic first-aid procedures, you should be able to deal with most emergencies. Your office also should have written procedures to follow in the event of an accident. Familiarize yourself with the procedures beforehand so that you will know what to do if an accident occurs.

If the accident involves exposure to blood or blood products, OSHA regulations require that several steps be followed:

1. Immediate cleaning of the area, including disinfection of contaminated surfaces and sterilization of contaminated instruments and equipment

2. Notification of a designated emergency contact, as identified in your office's safety manual

3. Documentation of the incident on a form similar to that shown in Figure 45-4, including the names of all parties involved, the names of witnesses, a description of the incident, and a record of medical treatments given to those involved

4. Medical evaluation and follow-up exam of the employees involved

5. Written evaluation of the medical condition of the involved individuals and testing for infection, provided that such testing does not violate confidentiality regulations

Housekeeping

There is a high risk of serious contamination in the laboratory, and housekeeping duties are designed to reduce this risk. Great care must be taken by following these guidelines to ensure good operating procedures and to reduce the risk of infection:

- Refer to your office's written policies and procedures to ensure that you are performing housekeeping duties correctly and according to schedule.

- Immediately clean up spills or splashes of potentially contaminated material. Depending on the material, you may need to use special hazardous waste control products, like those shown in Figure 45-5. Be sure to dry the area if appropriate, or clearly indicate that the area is still wet.

- Clean laboratory equipment immediately after use. Contaminants often become hard to remove if they are left on for a long time.

- Dispose of waste products carefully and correctly.

- Use extreme caution when handling and disposing of sharps.

▶ Quality Assurance Programs   LO 45.5

The operation of a POL can have a significant impact on the health of the patients who depend on the medical practice for care. Accurate patient specimen testing is a primary concern. A **quality assurance program** is designed to monitor the quality of the patient care a medical laboratory provides. It also helps to ensure laboratory worker safety. An effective quality assurance program should be a written plan that includes both internal and external reviews of procedures. It assesses the quality of the tests performed in a clinical laboratory based on a set of written standards and procedures.

Clinical Laboratory Improvement Amendments

In response to public concern over the accuracy of laboratory tests, Congress enacted the Clinical Laboratory Improvement Amendments of 1988 (CLIA '88). This law placed all laboratory facilities that conduct tests for diagnosing, preventing, or treating human disease or for assessing human health under federal regulations administered by the Centers for Medicare and Medicaid Services (CMS) and the CDC. State governments may implement their own standards, which must be at least as stringent as federal standards. If your state has its own standards, your office will operate under those standards. The state health department provides information about which standards to follow in a given locale.

MILLSTONE
INDUSTRIES

Central State Division
Incident Report

Name of Injured Employee _____

Department _____ Job Title _____

Supervisor _____

Date of Accident _____ Time _____

Nature of Injury _____

Was injured acting in a regular line of duty? _____

Was first aid given? _____ By whom? _____

Was designated emergency contact notified? _____

Did injured receive medical treatment? _____

Was injured tested for infection? _____ If no, why not? _____

Did injured go to ER? _____ Other? _____

Did injured leave work? _____ Date _____ Hour _____ A.M.
P.M.

Did injured return to work? _____ Date _____ Hour _____ A.M.
P.M.

Other Parties Involved _____

Names of Witnesses _____

Describe where and how accident occurred. _____

_____

What, in your opinion, caused the accident? _____

Has anything been done to prevent a similar accident? _____

Has the hazard causing the injury been reported by telephone or in writing? _____

Date	Employee's Signature
Date	Supervisor's Signature

IF TREATMENT IS NEEDED, TAKE THE ORIGINAL AND DUPLICATE OF THIS FORM TO THE EMERGENCY ROOM.

This part for Employee Health Office use only

Was incident investigated? _____

Has injured had follow-up medical care? _____

Comments _____

Original copy to Employee Health Office   Duplicate copy to supervisor

FIGURE 45-4 In the event of an accident or exposure incident in the POL, OSHA regulations require completion of an incident report form.

CLIA '88 has had a major impact on office laboratories. Because of the complexity of the regulations and the expense required to meet them, many doctors have closed their laboratories or sharply reduced the number of tests they perform. Several attempts have been made to change the federal legislation, including an effort to exempt POLs from the regulations. As the healthcare debate continues, you may see changes in laboratory operations as a result of changes in CLIA '88 regulations.

CLIA '88 standards apply to four areas of laboratory operation:

• Standards—requirements for maintaining a laboratory; specific standards are determined by the complexity of the test

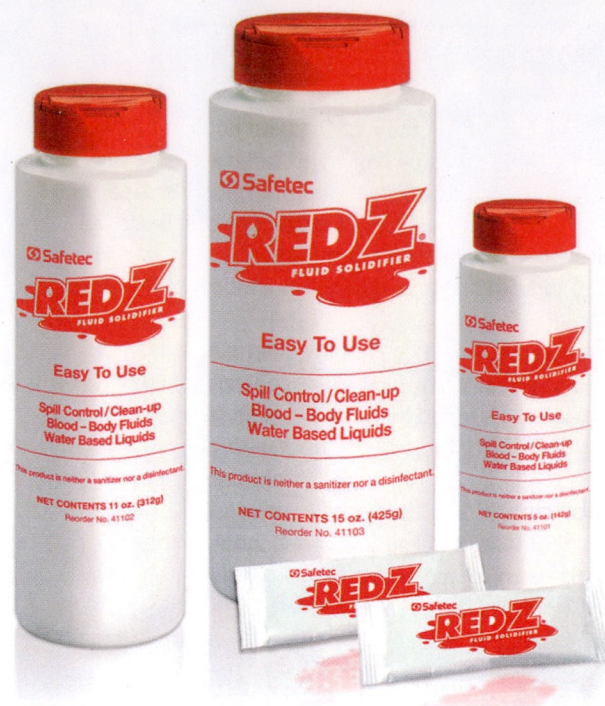

FIGURE 45-5 Certain substances require cleanup with specially formulated products such as these.
Courtesy Safetec of America

- Fees—charges for maintaining a laboratory
- Enforcement—penalties imposed for violating CLIA standards
- Proficiency testing programs—for laboratories that perform moderate- to high-complexity testing; labs in this category must go through a special inspection and assessment to perform tests that are moderately or highly complex

Most of the regulations relate to laboratory standards. Tests have been divided into these three categories, based on complexity: Certificate of Waiver tests, tests of moderate complexity, and tests of high complexity.

Certificate of Waiver Tests

The **Certificate of Waiver tests,** as listed in Table 45-2, are simple laboratory examinations and procedures that have an insignificant risk of an erroneous result. These tests are often performed in a POL. In order for a test to be classified as a waived test, it must

- Pose an insignificant risk to the patient if it is performed or interpreted incorrectly.
- Involve procedures that are simple and accurate so that the risk of obtaining incorrect results is minimal.
- Be approved by the Food and Drug Administration (FDA) for use by patients at home.

If laboratory management decides to perform these tests only, the office may apply for a Certificate of Waiver. When the certificate is granted, the laboratory is exempt from meeting various CLIA '88 standards that apply to the other two test categories. Such laboratories, however, are subject to the following: (1) random inspections to ensure that laboratories operating under a Certificate of Waiver are performing only those tests that qualify for the waiver and (2) investigation of the laboratory if there is any reason to believe the laboratory is not operating safely or if there have been complaints against the laboratory. See the *Caution: Handle with Care* feature Operating a Reliable Certificate of Waiver Laboratory for more information about good lab practice.

Tests of Moderate Complexity Tests of moderate complexity make up approximately 75% of all tests performed in the laboratory. Among these tests are blood cell counts and cholesterol screening. Test procedures falling into this category include studies involving bacteriology, mycobacteriology, mycology, parasitology, virology, immunology, chemistry, hematology, and immunohematology.

A laboratory that performs moderate-complexity testing must be run by a pathologist who has an MD or PhD degree. Technicians performing the tests must have training beyond the high school level as defined by CLIA '88 regulations. All personnel must participate in a quality assurance program for laboratory procedures, and the laboratory is subject to periodic unannounced inspections and proficiency testing.

Tests of High Complexity Tests of high complexity include more complicated tests in the specialties and subspecialties, including tests in clinical cytogenics, histopathology, histocompatibility, cytology, and any test not yet categorized by the CMS. Manufacturers' guidelines for testing products are often the best source for discovering a test's CMS determination. The CMS publishes a directory of all moderate- and high-complexity tests.

Like a laboratory that conducts moderate-complexity tests, a laboratory that conducts high-complexity tests is subject to inspection, proficiency testing, and participation in a quality assurance program, and it must be headed by a medical doctor or a scientist who has a PhD degree. Testing procedures can be performed only by qualified laboratory personnel whose training exceeds that provided by high schools and meets the requirements of CLIA '88 regulations. Medical assistants will need additional training and education to perform moderate- and high-complexity tests.

Components of Quality Assurance

Every quality assurance program must include the following components, in a measurable and structured system, to satisfy CLIA '88 requirements:

- Quality control
- Instrument and equipment maintenance
- Proficiency testing
- Training and continuing education
- Standard operating procedures documentation

Quality Control and Maintenance

A **quality control program** is one component of a quality assurance program. The focus of the quality control program is to ensure accuracy in test results through careful monitoring of test procedures. To be in compliance with quality control standards, a laboratory must follow certain procedures.

TABLE 45-2	**Certificate of Waiver Tests**
Urine Tests	Urinalysis by dipstick (reagent strip) or tablet reagent (nonautomated) for bilirubin, glucose, hemoglobin, ketone, leukocytes, nitrite, pH, protein, specific gravity, and urobilinogen
	Ovulation (visual color comparison tests)
	Pregnancy (visual color comparison tests)
	Home-screening tests for drugs (opioids, cocaine, methamphetamines, cannabinoids, phencyclidine, methadone, benzodiazepines, barbiturates, oxycodone)
	Nicotine detection tests
	Urine chemistry analyzer for microalbumin and creatinine (semi-quantitative)
	Tumor-associated antigen for bladder cancer (using devices approved by the FDA for home use)
	Catalase
	Ascorbic acid
Blood Tests	Erythrocyte sedimentation rate (ESR), nonautomated
	Hemoglobin by copper sulfate, nonautomated
	Spun microhematocrit
	Blood glucose (using devices approved by the FDA for home use)
	Hemoglobin by single analyte instruments, automated
	Prothrombin time
	Platelet aggregation
	Ketones in whole blood, over-the-counter test only
	Total cholesterol, high-density lipoprotein (HDL), low-density lipoprotein (LDL), and triglycerides
	Hemoglobin A1C
	Liver panel (alanine aminotransferase, alkaline phosphatase, amylase, gamma glutamyl transferase, aspartate aminotransferase, total bilirubin)
	Lactate in whole blood
	Chloride
	Carbon dioxide
	Calcium
	Sodium
	Potassium
	Urea
	Uric acid
	Creatinine
	Lead in whole blood
	Thyroid-stimulating hormone, rapid test
	Mononucleosis rapid test
	Helicobacter pylori rapid antibody test
	Lyme disease antibodies
	HIV antibody test
Fecal Tests	Fecal occult blood
Saliva Tests	Alcohol in saliva
Nasal Smear Tests	Adenovirus
	Influenza A and B antigens
	Respiratory syncytial virus
Vaginal Smear Tests	*Trichomonas vaginalis* antigens
	Vaginal pH
Throat Swab Tests	Strep A antigens
	Influenza A and B
Semen	Sperm concentration, home screening

Calibration Medical equipment used for testing patient specimens must be calibrated regularly, in accordance with manufacturers' guidelines. Calibration ensures that the equipment is operating correctly and is producing accurate results. In order to calibrate a medical instrument, you must have a set of known standards. A **standard** is a specimen, like the patient specimens you would normally process with the equipment, except that the value for each standard is already known. When you calibrate medical equipment, you run the standard with the known value. If the results do not match the known value, then the equipment is not in calibration. If the equipment does not yield the expected results during the calibration procedure, it must be adjusted until the expected results are obtained. Each calibration must be recorded in a quality control log like the one shown in Figure 45-6. Calibration routines are run on the standards alone, never with patient samples. They are used exclusively to ensure that the equipment is performing according to manufacturers' specifications. Check the manufacturer's instructions to determine how often the equipment should be calibrated. Calibration of some equipment must be performed by trained service personnel.

Control Samples **Control samples** are similar to standards in that they are specimens like those taken from a patient and have known values. Unlike standards, however, control samples are used before each patient sample is processed.

QUALITY CONTROL DAILY LOG

Name of Unit	Glucose Control Solution	Strip Lot No./ Exp. Date	Low Control Value 35–65 mg/dL	High Control Value 75–235 mg/dL	Analyzed By	Date	Remedial Action Taken If Control Values Abnormal	Retest After Remedial Action Taken
XYZ Glucometer	Check-strip control solution	Lot 851 10/15/XX	39 mg/dL	230 mg/dL	MSM	1/17/XX		
Mitchell Drugs Glucometer	Check-strip control solution	Lot 851 10/15/XX	50 mg/dL	267 mg/dL	MSM	1/17/XX	Machine cleaned	220 mg/dL high value
XYZ Glucometer	Check-strip control solution	Lot 851 10/15/XX	Unable to read	Unable to read	LMC	1/18/XX	Battery changed	38 mg/dL low 198 mg/dL high
Mitchell Drugs Glucometer	Check-strip control solution	Lot 851 10/15/XX	45 mg/dL	226 mg/dL	LMC	1/18/XX		

FIGURE 45-6 The quality control log shows the completion of every quality control check conducted on a piece of equipment.

Using a control sample serves as a check on the accuracy of the test. If the control tests do not fall within the manufacturer's prescribed ranges, patient samples should not be analyzed until the equipment is calibrated. This helps prevent erroneous patient test results.

The control samples for certain laboratory procedures show both normal (negative) and abnormal (positive) results. Generally, positive and negative control samples are used with tests that yield that **qualitative test response.** A qualitative test is testing to see if the substance is present in the specimen. It is not testing for the amount of a substance in the specimen, only if it is there or not.

Tests that yield **quantitative test results** require different control samples. Quantitative tests give the concentration or amount of a substance in a tested specimen. Control samples are formulated to show when results fall within a normal range. At least two control samples containing different concentrations—usually a high and a low value—of the test substance should be run for quantitative tests.

Reagent Control Control samples or standards are also run every time you open a new supply of testing products, such as staining materials, culture media, and reagents. **Reagents** are chemicals or chemically treated substances used in test procedures. A reagent is formulated to react in specific ways when exposed under specific conditions. One example of a reagent is the chemically coated strip used in blood glucose monitoring. A visual change on the reagent strip (also called a dipstick) occurs in the presence of glucose in a blood sample.

To ensure the quality of reagents, you should keep a reagent control log. If a defective reagent test is identified, it can be tracked to its source. A sample reagent control log is shown in Figure 45-7. Running controls on a routine basis

gives you information about the equipment and the reagents used during the test. If a control consistently yields unexpected results (for example, a positive control yields a negative result), you should check the reagents first and then the equipment calibration.

Maintenance Testing instruments and equipment must be properly maintained, and all maintenance procedures must be documented. Follow manufacturers' guidelines for performing instrument and equipment maintenance. A maintenance log provides a complete record of all work performed on an instrument or a piece of equipment (Figure 45-8).

Troubleshooting You may need to investigate the cause of a problem with a piece of equipment or a test. To do this, you should take a systematic approach to rule out the cause of the problem. For more information regarding investigating equipment and test malfunctions, see the *Caution: Handle with Care* feature Troubleshooting Problems in a Physician's Office Laboratory.

Documentation A quality control program depends first on careful adherence to procedures designed to identify problems with equipment calibration, errors in testing procedures, and defective testing supplies. The second component of a quality control program is the careful documentation of all procedures. Besides maintaining the quality control log, the reagent control log, and the equipment maintenance log, you also will complete the following records as part of a quality control program:

- Reference laboratory log, which lists specimens sent to another laboratory for testing
- Daily workload log, which shows all procedures completed during the workday

URINE REAGENT STRIP CONTROL LOG   Control Solution _____ Exp. Date _____ Lot # _____

Reagent Strip / Lot # & Exp. Date	Test	Specific Gravity	pH	Protein	Glucose	Ketone	Bilirubin	Blood	Nitrite	Urobi-linogen	Control Test Date	Remedial Action Taken If Reading Is Abnormal	Retest Date	Technician Initials
	Reagent Strip Expected Range													
	Test Results													
	Reagent Strip Expected Range													
	Test Results													

FIGURE 45-7 The reagent control log shows the quality testing performed on every batch or lot of reagent products.

Proficiency Testing

All laboratories that perform moderate- and high-complexity tests as identified by CLIA '88 must participate in a proficiency testing program. **Proficiency testing programs** measure test result accuracy and adherence to standard operating procedures. Generally, proficiency tests include two parts: (1) an unknown (testing) sample supplied by the proficiency testing organization contracted by your laboratory and (2) forms that must be completed to record the steps in the testing procedure. The unknown sample is processed normally, under the same conditions as any patient sample. The results, the forms, and sometimes the unknown samples are returned to the proficiency testing organization, which then informs your office whether it has passed or failed the test. A passing mark means that your laboratory can continue to perform that particular test. A failing mark can mean that your laboratory must discontinue that test and possibly other tests, too.

ACME MEDICAL SUPPLIES
Equipment Maintenance Record   Date 6/1/20XX

Practice	BWW Medical Associates
Name of Equipment	Acme Microscope Model ABC-123
Location	Lab Purchased 12/1/20XX

Date	Cleaning	Maintenance/Repair	Technician Initials
6/5	Microscope	Cleaned	CJC
6/11	Microscope high objective	Cleaned	DWM
6/14	Microscope	Changed bulb	CJC
6/16	Microscope eyepiece	Lens cover replaced	CJC
6/17	Microscope high objective	Cleaned	CJC

FIGURE 45-8 A maintenance log must be kept for every piece of laboratory equipment. All work done on the equipment must be recorded in the log.

CAUTION: HANDLE WITH CARE

Troubleshooting Problems in a Physician's Office Laboratory

Working in a physician's office laboratory can be exciting and challenging. Part of your job as a medical assistant is to make sure the tests you perform are accurate. Occasionally, you will encounter a piece of equipment that is not working or test results and controls that are consistently too high or too low. You will need to troubleshoot these problems to determine their cause. Troubleshooting is a thorough and logical investigation for the cause of a problem. You must eliminate possible causes of the problem one at a time. The general steps to troubleshooting a piece of equipment or test kit are

- Follow a written procedure for troubleshooting tests and equipment.
- Recognize the problem (controls give clues to possible problems).
- Think about possible causes.
- Start by investigating the simplest cause first.
- Document your findings.
- Call your service company after you have checked everything you know to check.

  When troubleshooting equipment, follow these steps:

- Check the power source at the machine, the wall outlet, the breaker box, or the battery.
- Check the equipment manual for troubleshooting information.
- Reboot the equipment by turning it off, waiting a few minutes, and then turning it back on.
- Check the service log for the date of the last maintenance.
- If you are able to repair the problem, run controls to verify that the problem is fixed before testing patient samples.

  When troubleshooting a test kit, follow these steps:

- Read the package insert to verify that you have performed the test correctly.
- Check to make sure you have used the correct reagents or test strips.
- Check the dates on the reagents or test strips to make sure they are not outdated.
- Make sure you are using the proper sample for the test.
- Repeat the test using control samples.
- If the controls are correct, repeat the test with the patient sample.

Training, Continuing Education, and Documentation

One of your employer's responsibilities is to provide opportunities for employee training and continuing education. Another is to provide written reference materials and documentation for all procedures conducted in the POL. Your responsibility is to consult reference materials and take part in available training to keep your skills sharpened and up to date.

It may seem unnecessary to refer to written instructions for procedures you perform many times a day. Changes can be made in a procedure for many reasons, however, and you must be aware of these changes. Here are some reference materials with which you should be familiar:

- Safety Data Sheets
- Standard operating procedures
- Safety manuals
- Equipment manufacturers' user or reference guides
- Clinical Laboratory Technical Procedure Manuals
- Regulatory documentation (OSHA standards, CLIA '88 requirements)
- Maintenance and housekeeping schedules

▶ Communicating with the Patient LO 45.6

In your job as a medical assistant, you will be involved with patients before they submit samples for laboratory testing, during the specimen collection procedure, and after the physician has interpreted the test results. It is your responsibility to ensure that patients understand what is expected of them every step of the way.

Before the Test

Certain tests require patients to prepare by fasting or restricting fluid intake. It is your duty to explain test preparations. Use simple, nontechnical language and check with patients to be sure they understand the information. In some cases, providing a written instruction sheet may be helpful.

Explaining the reason for the preparation can help ensure compliance or unearth potential problems. For example, if you explain to a patient that he is to refrain from drinking anything for a particular period, he might ask whether that includes the water he uses to take a certain medication. You can then make sure the patient receives the answers he will need for carrying out the physician's orders.

If you are the person who collects specimens, you need to determine whether patients have correctly completed the required test preparations. Test results are invalid in some cases if patients fail to follow test preparation guidelines. When preparations have not been completed correctly, discuss the situation with the physician or other appropriate staff member as required by your office to determine whether the specimen should still be collected. If the specimen is not collected, document the reason the test was not carried out as requested. Review the guidelines for specimen collection with the patient, and schedule another appointment if appropriate.

During Specimen Collection

Before collecting a specimen, you must first be sure you have the right patient. Proper patient identification is an essential part of good laboratory practice. You do not want to collect a blood sample from someone who only needs a urinalysis. Patients do not always understand the tests they are having. It is up to you to make sure you have the right patient and are performing the test as it is ordered.

The instructions you deliver to patients during specimen collection vary with the nature of the specimen. Always deliver instructions clearly and in language patients can understand. Do not assume that patients do not need to hear the instructions, even if they have had the test before. Explain what you must do and what patients must do before moving to each new step in the process.

Patients are understandably nervous during many collection procedures. In addition to communicating technical information, you should provide any helpful advice that may make the test easier. Also provide reassurance as appropriate. For example, if a patient asks whether the blood-drawing procedure is painful, explain that a sharp stick or stinging sensation may be experienced when the needle is inserted but that no pain should be felt after that. Let the patient be your guide in determining how much information to provide. Some people want to know every detail, whereas others prefer to know as little as possible.

One important aspect of communicating with patients about testing procedures is your nonverbal communication skills. Even if you deliver accurate technical information and answer every question patients have, there can still be a breakdown in communication if your nonverbal signals do not support your verbal message. Follow these guidelines to ensure that your nonverbal actions are helping, not hindering, the communication process:

- Strike a balance between a strict, business-like attitude and overly familiar friendliness. Your actions must impress on the patient that you are well informed about the procedure and that you care about the patient's understanding of it.
- Treat the patient with respect. Address the patient by name, using the appropriate courtesy title unless you have been invited to use the patient's first name or the patient is a child. Provide privacy during specimen collection. Privacy needs may be met by using a separate room or contained area for drawing blood, for example; a private bathroom is best for collecting urine specimens.
- Recognize that the patient may be under stress because of the test procedure or the pending results. Some patients may be familiar with the test procedures, but others may not know what to expect. You may need to repeat instructions or explain what you are doing more than one time. Remain calm and patient. Never be abrupt or condescending.
- Direct your attention to the patient, particularly during a procedure that might be uncomfortable, like drawing blood. Unless an emergency develops, pay attention to nothing else at that time.

After Specimen Collection

If the patient must follow particular guidelines after you collect the specimen, explain them. Commonly, post-test instructions deal with the care of venipuncture sites, signs and symptoms of infection, additional or continuing dietary restrictions, and the schedule for further testing if it is necessary.

When the Test Results Return

When you receive the test results, communicate them not to the patient but to the doctor. Only the doctor is qualified to interpret test results for the patient. Your role in reporting results comes after the doctor examines the test information and prepares a report. Sometimes, the doctor discusses the results with the patient. Other times, you will be asked to convey the test results to the patient along with instructions from the doctor. Answer only those patient questions that are within the range of your knowledge and experience. If the patient needs more information than you can provide, refer the patient to the doctor.

▶ Recordkeeping   LO 45.7

The importance of accurate and complete recordkeeping can be summed up in one statement: If it is not written down, it was not done. This motto applies to all your duties as a medical assistant. Besides recording information about quality control and equipment maintenance, you must keep track of every specimen that passes through your hands, or you may be called on to handle inventory control and record test results in patient records. You may need to use standard abbreviations for measures when recording test results. Table 45-3 provides a list of common abbreviations used in the laboratory.

Filling Out a Laboratory Requisition Form

As a medical assistant, it is your responsibility to ensure that the laboratory requisition form is properly completed. Missing information can lead to improper testing or lost results. The completed form should be included with the specimen collected or sent with the patient to the laboratory. Be sure to include the following information on all requisitions:

- Patient's full name, sex, date of birth, and address
- Patient's insurance information
- Physician's name, address, and phone number
- Source of the specimen
- Date and time of the specimen collection
- Test(s) requested
- Preliminary diagnosis
- Any current treatment that might affect the results

See Figure 45-9 for a sample laboratory requisition form.

Specimen Identification

All specimens must immediately be clearly identified with the patient's name, the patient's identification code (if your office uses one), the date and time the specimen was collected,

Laboratory Requisition

BWW
BWW Medical Associates, PC
305 Main Street, Port Snead YZ 12345-9876
Tel: 555-654-3210, Fax: 555-987-6543
Web: BWWAssociates.com

Laboratory Name and Address

_____
_____
_____

Requesting Provider
Paul F. Buckwalter, MD
Alexis N. Whalen, MD
Elizabeth H. Williams, MD

Please Indicate Bill Type Below
Attach Copy of Insurance Card

Patient Data (Please Print)

Last Name	First Name	Maiden Name

Address		Apt No.

City	State	Zip

SS#	Phone #

Date of Birth (Month, Day, Year) ☐ Male ☐ Female | Date Collected | Time Collected : ☐ a.m. ☐ p.m.

Physician 1	Physician 2

Billing Information (Please Print Clearly)

Please Bill to: ☐ Dr. Account (Client) ☐ Patient Self Pay ☐ Insurance Co

Responsible Party (Last, First) | Relationship to Subscriber ☐ Self ☐ Child ☐ Spouse ☐ Other

Primary Insurance Co. Name ☐ HMO ☐ PPO

Insurance Policy #	Insurance Group #

Primary Insurance Co: Address (Street, City, State, Zip)

Insured Date of Birth	Insured SS#

PLEASE PROVIDE MANDATORY ICD 10 CODE BELOW

1	2	3	4	5

CALL TEST RESULTS TO:

Test: _____
To: _____
Phone: (___) _____

FAX RESULTS TO:

To: _____
Fax: (___) _____

☐ Veni   Tech Code _____   Tubes Received _____

Please (X) desired Panel(s)/Profile(s)/Tests. See back of requisition for profile components.

PANELS/PROFILES

Hepatitis Panel, Acute	**2S**
Basic Metabolic Panel	MT
Comp Metabolic Panel	MT
Electrolyte Panel (Lytes)	MT
Hepatic Function Panel	MT
General Health Panel	MTL
Lipid Panel	**MT**
Obstetric Panel AMH	P2SL
Renal Panel	MT

MICROBIOLOGY

Source of Specimen:	
Culture, Anaerobe	
Chlamydia/GC Amp Probe	
Culture, Ear	
Culture, Eye	
Leukocytes Stool	
Culture, Fungal	
Culture, Genital	
Culture, Herpes	
Occult Blood Screen	
Ova & Parasites	
Rapid Strep Throat	
Culture, Stool	
Culture, GROUP A BetaStrep Screen	
Culture GROUP B Screen	
Culture, Throat	
Culture, Urine	
Culture, Wound / Abscess	
Culture, Viral	
C. Difficile Toxin A&B AMH	

INDIVIDUAL TESTS

ABO Group/RH	P
Acid Phosphatase, Prostatic	**S**
Albumin	MT
Alkaline Phosphatase	MT
Amylase	MT
Antinuclear Antibodies (ANA Send)	S
HCG, Beta Quant	**MT**
Bilirubin T / D Neonate	A
Bilirubin T / D Adult	MT
BNP Screen	**L**
BUN	MT
CA-125	**S**
CA-125 to Dianon	**S**
CRP	MT
CRP Cardio	MT
Calcium	**MT**
Carbamazepine/Tegretol	R
CBC & PLT w/o Diff	**L**
CBC & PLT w Diff	**L**
Carcino Embryonic Antigen (CEA)	**S**
Cholesterol Total	**MT**
Cortisol Level	MT
Creatine Kinase, Total (CK)	MT
CPK total w CKMB	MT
Creatinine Clearance	U
Creatinine	MT
D Dimer Quant	B
DNA AB Double Strand	S
Digoxin Level	**R**

INDIVIDUAL TESTS (cont.)

Drug Screen Urine	**U**	SGPT (ALT)	MT
Drug Screen Urine c Confirm	**U**	Testosterone	S
Estradiol Level	MT	Testosterone Free & Total	S
Ferritin Level	**MT**	TSH	MT
Fetal Fibronectin (FFN)	SWAB	**Total T3**	**MT**
Folic Acid (PROTECT)	MT	T3 Uptake	S
Follicle Stimulating Hormone	MT	**Free T3**	**MT**
GGT (Gamma Glut Trans)	**MT**	Free Thyroxine (FT4)	MT
Glucose	MT	Total T4	S
Glucose Fasting	**MT**	**Free Thyroxine index (FTI)**	**S**
Glucose Challenge 1° Preg	MT	Thyroid Antibodies	S
Glycosylated Hemoglobin (HA1C)	L	**Troponin/Quant**	**MT**
Hepatitis B Surface AG	**S**	Triglycerides	MT
Hepatitis B Surface AB	**S**	Uric Acid	MT
Hepatitis C Antibody	S	Urinalysis	U
Herpes Simplex 1 & 2 IgG AB	S	Valproic Acid / Depakote	R
Herpes Simplex 1 & 2 IgM AB	S	Vitamin B12 (PROTECT)	MT
HIV I & II Abs	**S**	Vitamin D 25 Hydroxy	S
Homocysteine	L		
Iron/TIBC	**MT**	**ADDITIONAL ORDERS**	
Lactate Dehydrogenase (LDH)	MT		
Lipase	MT		
Lithium	R		
Luteinizing Hormone	MT		
Microalbumin Random/24 Hr.	U		
Magnesium	**MT**		
MONO test heterophile	S		
Phenobarbital	R		
Phenytoin/Dilantin	R		
Phosphorous	**MT**		
Potassium	MT		
Progesterone	S		
Prolactin	MT		
PSA Free and Total	**S**		
PSA Screen (Medicare)	**S**		
PSA Diagnostic	**S**		
Prothrombin Time	**B**		
aPTT	**B**		
PTH Intact	**S**		
Reticulocyte Count	L		
Rheumatoid Factor (RF)	MT		
RPR QUAL	**S**		
Rubella, IgG	S		
ESR (Sed Rate)	**L**		
SGOT (AST)	MT		

FIGURE 45-9 The laboratory requisition form must be accurately completed.

TABLE 45-3	Abbreviations for Common Laboratory Measures
cm	centimeter
cm³	cubic centimeter
dL	deciliter
fl oz	fluid ounce
g	gram
L	liter
lb	pound
m	meter
mcg	microgram
mg	milligram
mL	milliliter
mm	millimeter
mmHg	millimeters of mercury
oz	ounce
pt	pint
QNS	quantity not sufficient
QS	quantity sufficient
qt	quart
wt	weight

the initials of the person who collected the specimen, the physician's name, and other information as required by the test procedure or your office. If you encounter an unidentified or incorrectly identified specimen, you must make an effort to track it to its source. The specimen will probably be discarded or destroyed, however, because there is no guarantee that it was identified correctly. Even if you do manage to identify it, it may have been compromised in some way.

Inventory Control
You will be responsible for taking inventory of equipment and supplies to ensure that the POL never runs out of them. To do so, you will keep a list of items that are used routinely and reordered systematically. Establish a regular schedule—perhaps weekly—for counting items in the POL. Then estimate when you will probably need to reorder an item—based on how quickly you use the item or material—and put the date on your calendar.

Patient Records
When recording test results, it may be your responsibility to identify unusual findings. Many offices require out-of-range test results to be circled or underlined in red. Follow the procedure established by your office. The physician usually initials or otherwise marks the records after examining them. Electronic health records automatically identify out-of-range tests when the results are entered.

PROCEDURE 45-1 Using a Microscope

Procedure Goal:
To correctly focus the microscope using each of the three objectives for examination of a prepared specimen slide

OSHA Guidelines:

  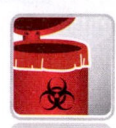 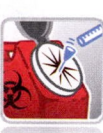

Materials:
Microscope, lens paper, lens cleaner, prepared specimen slide, immersion oil, and tissues

Method:
1. Wash your hands and don exam gloves.
2. Remove the protective cover from the microscope. Examine the microscope to make sure it is clean and that all parts are intact.
3. Plug in the microscope and make sure the light is working. If you need to replace the bulb, refer to the manufacturer's guidelines. (Be sure to note bulb replacements in the maintenance log for the microscope.) Turn the light off before cleaning the lenses.
4. Clean the lenses and oculars with lens paper. Avoid touching the lenses with anything except lens paper. Pay careful

attention to the oculars, as they are easily dirtied by dust and eye makeup. If a lens is particularly dirty, use a small amount of lens cleaner. Oil-immersion lenses are prone to oil buildup if not cleaned properly. Too much lens cleaner, however, can loosen the cement that holds the lens in place.
   RATIONALE: *The lenses must be clean to reduce artifacts.*
5. Place the specimen slide on the stage. Slide the edges of the slide under the slide clips to secure the slide to the stage.

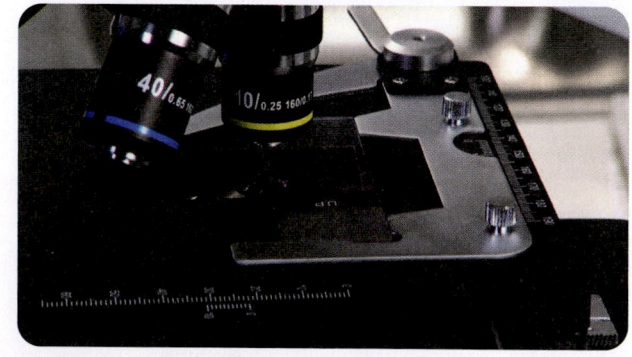

FIGURE Procedure 45-1 Step 5 Carefully secure the specimen slide on the stage of the microscope.
© McGraw-Hill Education

6. Adjust the distance between the oculars to a position of comfort.

7. Adjust the objectives so the low-power (10×) objective points directly at the specimen slide, as shown. Before swiveling the objective assembly, be sure you have sufficient space for the objective. Recheck the distance between the oculars, making sure the field you see through the eyepieces is a merged field, not separate left and right fields. Raise the body tube by using the coarse adjustment control and lower the stage as needed.
   RATIONALE: *If the objective assembly is too close to the stage, you may hit the specimen slide and crack it. The specimen is then contaminated and cannot be used. The objective also may be damaged.*

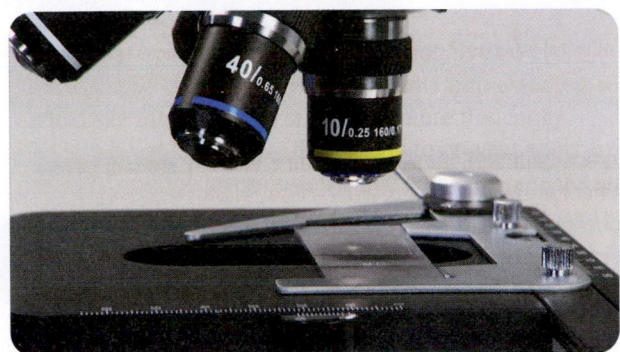

FIGURE Procedure 45-1 Step 7   Move the low-power objective into position above the specimen slide.
© McGraw-Hill Education

8. Turn on the light and, using the iris controls, adjust the amount of light illuminating the specimen so that the light fills the field but does not wash out the image. (At this point, you are not examining the specimen image for focus but adjusting the overall light level.)

9. Observe the microscope from one side and slowly lower the body tube to move the objective closer to the stage and specimen slide. This adjustment is shown below. If you used the stage controls to lower the stage away from the objectives, you also may need to adjust those controls. Again, take care not to strike the stage with the objective. The objective should almost meet the specimen slide but not touch it.

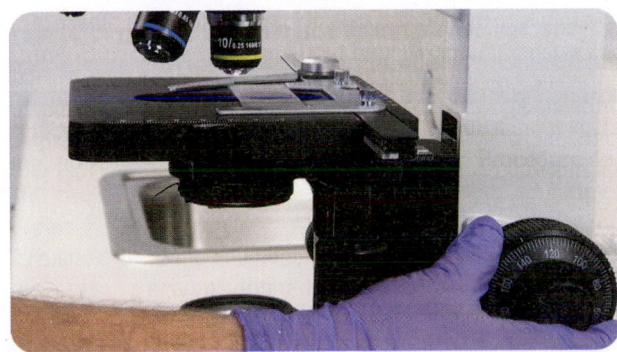

FIGURE Procedure 45-1 Step 9   When lowering the objective toward the stage and specimen slide, observe the microscope from the side to be sure you do not hit the stage with the objective and crack the slide.
© McGraw-Hill Education

10. Look through the oculars and use the coarse focus control to slowly adjust the image. If necessary, adjust the amount of light coming through the iris.

11. Continue using the fine focus control to adjust the image. When the image is correctly focused, the specimen will be clearly visible and the field illumination will be bright enough to show details but not so bright that it is uncomfortable to view or washed out.

12. Switch to the high-power (40×) objective. Use the fine focus controls to view the specimen clearly.
    RATIONALE: *Using the coarse adjustment could cause lens damage if the lens touches the slide.*

13. Rotate the objective assembly so that no objective points directly at the stage and specimen slide. You will now have enough room to apply a drop of immersion oil to the slide. (Only dry slides, without coverslips, are used with the oil-immersion objective.)

14. Apply a small drop of immersion oil to the specimen slide, as shown below.

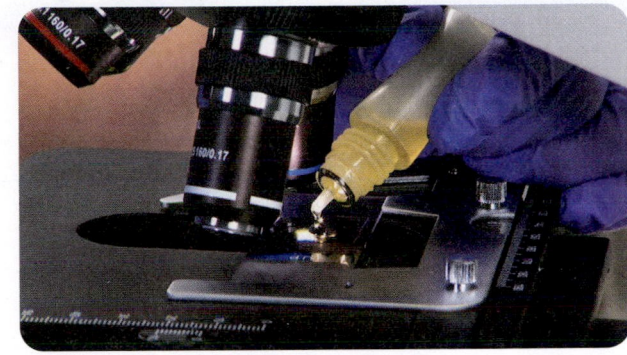

FIGURE Procedure 45-1 Step 14   Place a small drop of immersion oil directly on the dry specimen.
© McGraw-Hill Education

15. Gently swing the oil-immersion (100×) objective over the stage and specimen slide so that it is surrounded by the immersion oil.

16. Examine the image and adjust the amount of light and focus as needed. Only use the fine focus adjustment with this objective. To eliminate air bubbles in the immersion oil, gently move the stage left and right.

17. After you have examined the specimen as required by the testing procedure, lower the stage and raise the objectives.

18. Remove the slide. Dispose of it or store it as required by the testing procedure. If you must dispose of the slide, be sure to use the appropriate biohazardous waste container. If you must store the slide, remove the immersion oil with a tissue.

19. Turn off the light. Unplug the microscope if that is your laboratory's standard operating procedure.

20. Clean the microscope stage, ocular lenses, and objectives. Be careful to remove all traces of immersion oil from the stage and oil-immersion objective. Clean the oil-immersion lens last.

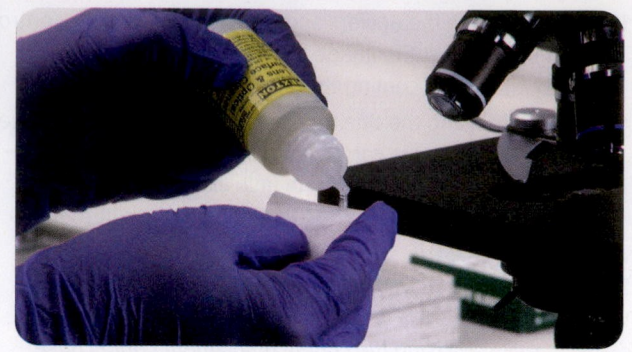

RATIONALE: *So that you do not get oil from the oil-immersion lens on the other lenses*

21. Rotate the objective assembly so that the low-power objective points toward the stage. Lower the objective so that it comes close to but does not rest on the stage.

22. Cover the microscope with its protective cover. Check the work area to be sure you have cleaned everything correctly and disposed of all waste material.

23. Remove the gloves and wash your hands.

FIGURE Procedure 45-1 Step 20 Clean the oil-immersion lens last using a small amount of lens cleaner.
© McGraw-Hill Education

SUMMARY OF LEARNING OUTCOMES

LEARNING OUTCOMES	KEY POINTS
45.1 Describe the purpose of the physician's office laboratory.	The physician's office laboratory (POL) is responsible for accurate and timely processing of routine tests, usually involving blood or urine, and for reporting test results to the physician.
45.2 Identify the medical assistant's duties in the physician's office laboratory.	The medical assistant's duties in a physician's office laboratory include preparing the patient for the test, collecting the sample, completing the test, reporting the results to the physician, and communicating information about the test from the physician to the patient.
45.3 Identify important pieces of laboratory equipment.	Common laboratory equipment includes autoclaves, centrifuges, microscopes, electronic equipment and software, and equipment used for measurement.
45.4 Illustrate measures to prevent accidents.	Preventing accidents in the physician's office laboratory begins by observing all safety guidelines, including standard precautions, reporting all laboratory accidents in a timely manner, and maintaining appropriate housekeeping in the lab setting.
45.5 Explain the goal of a quality assurance program in a physician's office laboratory.	The goal of a quality assurance program in a physician's office laboratory is to monitor the quality of the patient care that a medical laboratory provides.
45.6 Carry out communication with patients regarding test preparation and follow-up.	It is the medical assistant's responsibility to ensure that patients understand what is expected of them before a test. Providing clear pretest instructions in both oral and written form is an essential part of the test procedure.
45.7 Carry out accurate documentation, including all logs related to quality control.	Accurate quality control documentation in a physician's office laboratory includes a reference laboratory log and a daily workload log.

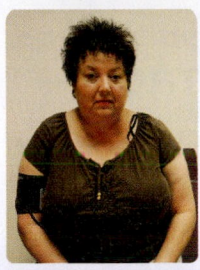

© McGraw-Hill Education

Recall Sylvia Gonzales from the beginning of the chapter. Now that you have completed the chapter, answer the following questions regarding her case.

1. Identify equipment used by a medical assistant in an office laboratory.

2. You will be measuring Sylvia's fasting blood glucose using a glucometer. You know this is classified as a waived test. What does the classification of waived test mean?

3. The glucometer contains an instrument called a photometer. How is blood glucose measured using a photometer?

4. Measuring blood glucose is a quantitative test. What does this mean?

5. What type of controls do you expect to use when measuring Sylvia's blood glucose?

6. When should you run the controls?

EXAM PREPARATION QUESTIONS

1. (LO 45.1) A laboratory owned by a company other than the physician's practice is a
   a. Physician's office laboratory
   b. Reference laboratory
   c. Pathology department
   d. Waived testing center
   e. High-complexity testing center

2. (LO 45.3) The eyepieces on a microscope are also called
   a. Objectives
   b. Condensers
   c. Oculars
   d. Irises
   e. Stages

3. (LO 45.3) An object visible through a microscope but unrelated to the specimen is a(n)
   a. Iris
   b. Aperture
   c. Artifact
   d. Speck
   e. Inclusion

4. (LO 45.5) A simple laboratory examination or procedure that has an insignificant risk of an erroneous result is a
   a. Waived test
   b. Moderate-complexity test
   c. High-complexity test
   d. Quality assurance test
   e. Reference test

5. (LO 45.5) Which of the following is a test to determine the amount of a substance in a specimen?
   a. Qualitative
   b. Waived
   c. Complex
   d. Quantitative
   e. Assurance

6. (LO 45.3) A device for spinning a specimen at high speed until it separates into its component parts is a
   a. Refractometer
   b. Photometer
   c. Concentrator
   d. Condenser
   e. Centrifuge

7. (LO 45.4) The most common disinfectant used in a physician's office laboratory is
   a. Germicidal soap
   b. 10% bleach
   c. Hydrogen peroxide
   d. Betadine®
   e. 70% alcohol

8. (LO 45.5) A laboratory that performs moderate-complexity testing must be run by a
   a. Pathologist
   b. Medical technologist
   c. Medical assistant
   d. Medical lab specialist
   e. CLIA-trained employee

9. (LO 45.5) Chemicals or chemically treated substances used in test procedures are known as
   a. Controls
   b. Standards
   c. Reagents
   d. Strips
   e. Negatives

10. (LO 45.3) An instrument used in a medical laboratory to measure light intensity is called a(n)
    a. Photometer
    b. Microscope
    c. Condenser
    d. Analyte
    e. Reflector

You are working in the lab today for Heather, who is out sick. Taylor brings you two tubes of blood and asks you to perform a blood glucose test for Mrs. Gonzales. After Taylor leaves the lab, you notice that one of the tubes is not labeled and the other tube has only the letter *S* written on it. What action should you take?

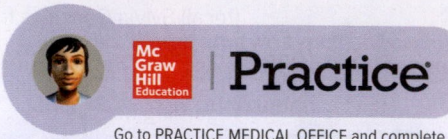

Go to PRACTICE MEDICAL OFFICE and complete the module Clinical - Privacy and Liability.

Microbiology and Disease

CASE STUDY

	Patient Name	DOB	Allergies
PATIENT INFORMATION	Cindy Chen	07/15/19XX	NKA
	Attending	**MRN**	**Other Information**
	Alexis N. Whalen, MD	324-86-542	Last CD4 count 250 cells/mm^3

Cindy Chen, a 28-year-old Asian female complaining of the inability to sleep and nervousness, arrives at the office. She tested positive for HIV in 2005. Currently, she lives with her aunt and is going to school to become a phlebotomist. She has lost 20 pounds since her last visit to the clinic. She

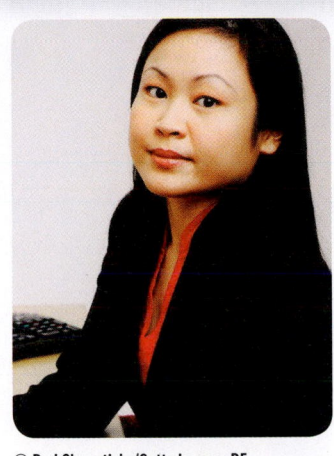

© Red Chopsticks/Getty Images RF

also has had a persistent cough and sore throat for the last 3 months. The physician orders a series of blood tests, including the helper T-cell test and a throat culture. Dr. Whalen asks you to send the throat culture to the reference lab for culture instead of doing a rapid strep test in the office.

Keep Cindy in mind as you study the chapter. There will be questions at the end of the chapter based on the case study. The information in the chapter will help you answer these questions.

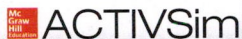

LEARNING OUTCOMES

After completing Chapter 46, you will be able to:

46.1 Explain the medical assistant's role in microbiology.

46.2 Summarize how microorganisms cause disease.

46.3 Describe how microorganisms are classified and named.

46.4 Discuss the role of viruses in human disease.

46.5 Discuss the role of bacteria in human disease.

46.6 Discuss the role of protozoans in human disease.

46.7 Discuss the role of fungi in human disease.

46.8 Discuss the role of multicellular parasites in human disease.

46.9 Describe the process involved in diagnosing an infection.

46.10 Identify general guidelines for obtaining specimens.

46.11 Carry out the procedure for transporting specimens to outside laboratories.

46.12 Compare two techniques used in the direct examination of culture specimens.

46.13 Carry out the procedure for preparing and examining stained specimens.

46.14 Carry out the procedure for culturing specimens in the medical office.

KEY TERMS

acid-fast stain	facultative
aerobe	Gram-negative
agar	Gram-positive
anaerobe	Gram stain
bacillus	KOH mount
coccus	mordant
colony	spirillum
culture	stain
culture and sensitivity (C&S)	vibrio
etiologic agent	

I.C.9	Analyze pathology for each body system including: (a) diagnostic measures
I.P.11	Obtain specimens and perform: (e) CLIA waived microbiology test
III.C.1	List major types of infectious agents
XII.P.1	Comply with: (a) safety signs (b) symbols (c) labels

3. Medical Terminology

   c. Apply various medical terms for each specialty

4. Medical Law and Ethics

   a. Follow documentation guidelines

9. Clinical Procedures

   a. Practice standard precautions and perform disinfection/sterilization techniques

10. Medical Laboratory Procedures

   a. Practice quality control

   b. Perform selected CLIA-waived tests that assist with diagnosis and treatment
     (4) Immunology testing
     (5) Microbiology testing
     (6) Kit testing
        b. Quick strep

   c. Dispose of biohazardous materials

   d. Collect, label, and process specimens
     (3) Perform wound collection procedures
     (4) Obtain throat specimens for microbiologic testing

▶ Introduction

Humans are surrounded by tiny, living organisms invisible to the naked eye. For the most part, these microorganisms cause no problems; however, when they are pathogenic in nature or are displaced from their natural environment, they can cause infections and disease. This chapter addresses the different life forms of microorganisms and how they may be identified; it also teaches you the proper collection techniques for common types of specimens. You will learn about the processes involved in identifying microorganisms, the types of culture media used for these processes, how antimicrobial testing is done, and how quality control fits into ensuring reliable patient results.

▶ Microbiology and the Role of the Medical Assistant
LO 46.1

Microbiology is the study of *microorganisms*—simple forms of microscopic (visible only through a microscope) life found everywhere. Most microorganisms are made up of a single cell. Some microorganisms, called resident normal flora, which are normally found on the skin and within the human body, perform a number of important functions and typically do not cause disease. For example, microorganisms in the intestines produce vitamins, help digest food, and help protect the body from infection.

Microorganisms capable of causing disease are known as pathogens. The infections caused by microorganisms can be mild, like the common cold, or they can lead to serious conditions. Their proper diagnosis and treatment are essential to restoring good health.

You may assist the physician in performing a number of microbiologic procedures in the medical office that aid in diagnosing and treating infectious diseases, including obtaining specimens or assisting the physician in doing so, preparing specimens for direct examination by the physician, and preparing specimens for transportation to a microbiology laboratory for identification.

▶ How Microorganisms Cause Disease
LO 46.2

Microorganisms live all around us—in and on our bodies, in the air we breathe, in the water we drink, and on almost every surface we touch. The variety of pathogenic microorganisms is extensive. Successful pathogens have developed ways to evade the host defenses. Each classification of microorganism contains pathogens. Some examples of these appear in Table 46-1.

Although everyone is surrounded by microorganisms, people are able to avoid infection most of the time for the following three reasons:

1. The majority of microorganisms are either beneficial or harmless. Pathogens comprise only a small portion of the total number of microorganisms that exist in a given environment.

TABLE 46-1 Microbial Pathogens and Their Characteristics

Classification	Characteristics	Example	Disease
Prions*	• Infectious particle made of protein • Very small • No nucleic acid • Reproduction unknown	PrP^{sc}	• Creutzfeldt-Jakob disease (CJD) • Bovine spongiform encephalopathy (BSE), or mad cow disease
Viruses	• DNA or RNA surrounded by a protein coat • Reproduced in living cells only • Very small • Acellular	Varicella-zoster virus	Chickenpox
Bacteria	• Single-celled • Reproduce quickly • Mostly asexual reproduction	*Vibrio cholerae*	Cholera
Protozoans	• Single-celled • Mostly asexual reproduction	*Entamoeba histolytica*	Amebic dysentery
Fungi	• Multicellular • Sexual and asexual reproduction	*Candida albicans*	Candidiasis
Helminths	• Multicellular • Parasitic • Contain specialized organs • Sexual reproduction	*Enterobius vermicularis*	Pinworms

*Although evidence exists that prions are directly responsible for several diseases that cause progressive brain degeneration, such as spongiform encephalopathies, some scientists believe prions merely aid another, unknown infectious agent in causing disease. Prion research is ongoing.

2. The human body has a variety of defenses that allow it to resist infection.

3. Conditions must be favorable for a pathogen to grow and to be transmitted to a person who is susceptible (sensitive) to infection.

Microorganisms and Disease Mechanisms

Microorganisms can cause disease in a variety of ways. They may use up nutrients or other materials needed by the cells and tissues they invade, they may damage body cells directly by reproducing themselves within cells, or their very presence may make body cells the targets of the body's own defenses. Some microorganisms produce cell- and tissue-damaging toxins or poisons. Infecting microorganisms, or the toxins they produce, may remain localized or travel throughout the body, damaging or killing cells and tissues. The resulting symptoms include local swelling, pain, warmth, and redness, along with generalized symptoms of fever, tiredness, aches, and weakness. Infection by certain organisms also may cause skin reactions, gastrointestinal upset, or other symptoms. Recall from the *Infection Control Fundamentals* chapter the chain of infection and how pathogenic organisms are transmitted from one person to another.

▶ Classification and Naming of Microorganisms
LO 46.3

Scientists classify microorganisms on the basis of their structure. Common classifications include the following:

- Subcellular microorganisms, which consist of hereditary material, either deoxyribonucleic acid (DNA) or ribonucleic acid (RNA), surrounded by a protein coat
- Prokaryotic microorganisms, which have a simple cell structure with no nucleus and no organelles in the cytoplasm
- Eukaryotic microorganisms, which have a complex cell structure containing a nucleus and specialized organelles in the cytoplasm

Table 46-2 lists the characteristics that distinguish these classifications and the types of microorganisms found in each classification. Types of microorganisms include:

- Viruses
- Bacteria
- Protozoans
- Fungi
- Multicellular parasites

These types may be further divided into groups that share certain characteristics. For example, within the bacteria classification are the mycobacteria and rickettsiae groups.

Specific microorganisms are named in a standard way, using two words. The first word refers to the *genus* (a category of biologic classification between the *family* and the *species*) to which the microorganism belongs. The second word refers to the particular species of the organism. Each species represents a distinct kind of microorganism. For example, within the bacteria classification is the *Staphylococcus* genus. Then within that genus are various species such as *Staphylococcus aureus* and *Staphylococcus epidermidis*. Although

TABLE 46-2	Classifications of Microorganisms	
Classification	**Characteristics**	**Examples**
Subcellular	• Noncellular • Nucleic acid surrounded by protein coat	Viruses
Prokaryotic	• Simple structure • Single chromosome, no nucleus • No organelles	Bacteria
Eukaryotic	• Highly structured • Nucleus and cytoplasm • Organelles	Protozoans, fungi, parasites

the two bacteria belong to the same genus, they differ greatly in their ability to cause disease. The first letter of the genus is always capitalized and the species name is always written in all lowercase letters.

▶ Viruses   LO 46.4

Viruses, which are among the smallest known infectious agents and cannot be seen with a regular microscope, are the cause of many common illnesses and conditions seen frequently in the medical office. Table 46-3 lists common viral pathogens. Because viruses are a simpler life form than the cell (see Figure 46-1), they can live and grow only within the living cells of other organisms.

Significant Viral Bloodborne Pathogens

In the medical office, you will likely encounter patients who are living with HIV and hepatitis. As you learned in the *Infection Control Fundamentals* chapter, proper technique is essential when handling blood and body fluids. You also must understand how HIV and hepatitis cause infection, and how to recognize the symptoms of each disease.

AIDS/HIV Infection HIV is a virus that infects and gradually destroys components of the immune system. AIDS is the condition that results from the advanced stages of this viral infection.

Over a period of time and in most cases, HIV infection develops into AIDS, which results in death. The pathogen gradually destroys helper T cells. *Helper T cells* are white blood cells that are a key component of the body's immune system, working in coordination with other white blood cells (B cells, macrophages, and so on) to combat infection.

The virus also attacks neurons, causing demyelination (destruction of the myelin sheath of a nerve), which results in neurologic problems, including dementia. Unlike a person with a properly functioning immune system, most AIDS patients are prone to various opportunistic infections—infections caused by microorganisms that do not ordinarily cause disease in people with properly functioning immune systems. Virtually everyone is at risk for contracting HIV. Although its initial outbreak in the United States appeared in the male homosexual population, and currently homosexual and bisexual men make up a large percentage of AIDS cases, the disease knows no limits.

Symptoms HIV infection can cause a variety of problems as it progresses to AIDS. Patients with AIDS may complain of any of the following symptoms:

- Systemic complaints, such as weight loss, fatigue, fever, chills, and night sweats
- Respiratory complaints, such as sinus fullness, dry cough, shortness of breath, difficulty swallowing, and sinus drainage
- Oral complaints, such as gingivitis, oral lesions, and hairy leukoplakia, which is a white lesion on the tongue
- Gastrointestinal complaints, such as diarrhea and bloody stool
- Central nervous system (CNS) complaints, such as depression, personality changes, concentration difficulties, and confusion or memory loss
- Peripheral nervous system complaints, such as tingling, numbness, pain, and weakness in the extremities
- Skin-related complaints, such as rashes, dry skin, and changes in the nail bed
- Kaposi's sarcoma, an unusual malignancy occurring in the skin and sometimes in the lymph nodes and organs and manifested by reddish purple to dark blue patches or spots on the skin

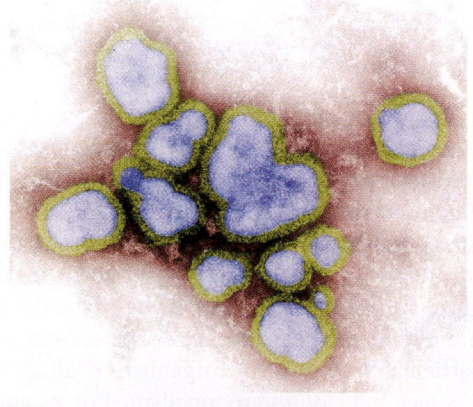

(a)

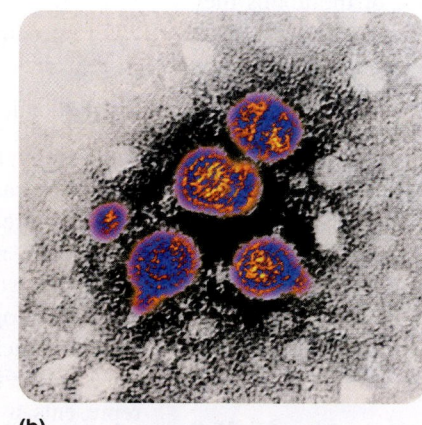

(b)

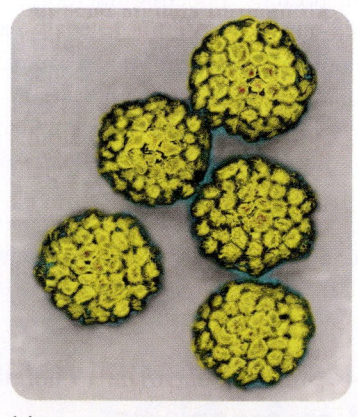

(c)

FIGURE 46-1 The three types of viral diseases often seen in medical offices are (a) influenza, (b) hepatitis, and (c) warts.

(a) CDC/F. A. Murphy; (b) © Kallista Images/Getty Images; (c) © BSIP/Corbis

TABLE 46-3 Viral Pathogens

Disease	Causative Organism	Route of Transmission	Signs and Symptoms
Viral pharyngitis	Adenovirus	Direct person-to-person contact and respiratory droplet contact	Colds, pharyngitis, bronchitis, pneumonia, diarrhea, pink eye, fever, cystitis, gastroenteritis, and/or neurologic disease
Infectious mononucleosis	Epstein-Barr virus	Direct contact with saliva from an infected person	Fever, sore throat, and swollen lymph glands
Hepatitis	Hepatitis A virus	Fecal-oral	Fever, fatigue, loss of appetite, nausea, vomiting, abdominal pain, dark urine, clay-colored bowel movements, joint pain, and jaundice
	Hepatitis B virus	Bloodborne, sexually transmitted infection (STI)	
	Hepatitis C virus	Bloodborne	
Cold sores	Herpes simplex virus, type 1	Direct contact with someone infected with *Herpes simplex,* type 1 (sharing eating utensils or drinking glasses, kissing)	Pain; tingling; small, painful, fluid-filled blisters on a raised, red area of the skin, typically around the mouth
Genital herpes	Herpes simplex virus, type 2	STI	Pain, itching, small red bumps, blisters, and ulcers
CMV	Cytomegalovirus	Direct contact, maternal-fetal transmission	Healthy adults: usually asymptomatic but may have mild hepatitis and prolonged fever Congenital: premature birth, liver problems, lung problems, spleen problems, small size at birth, small head size, seizures, hearing loss, vision loss, lack of coordination, and/or mental disability
AIDS	HIV	Bloodborne, STI	Initial: flu-like symptoms Untreated or advanced: heart, kidney, and liver disease; cancer; and opportunistic infections
Influenza	Influenza virus	Airborne, respiratory droplets	Fever, cough, sore throat, runny or stuffy nose, muscle or body aches, headaches, and fatigue
Measles	Measles virus	Airborne, respiratory droplets	Blotchy rash, fever, cough, runny nose, conjunctivitis, malaise, and tiny white spots with bluish-white centers inside the mouth
Mumps	Mumps virus	Airborne, respiratory droplets	Fever, headache, muscle aches, fatigue, loss of appetite, and swollen and tender salivary (parotid) glands
HPV infection	Human papillomavirus	STI	The majority of cases are asymptomatic; some strains cause genital warts; others are associated with cervical cancer
Upper respiratory infections, viral	Parainfluenza virus	Direct contact with respiratory secretions (droplets)	HPV1: croup HPV3: bronchiolitis and pneumonia
Polio	Poliovirus	Direct person-to-person contact	Fever, fatigue, nausea, headache, flu-like symptoms, back and neck stiffness, limb pain, and/or paralysis
Rabies	Rabies virus	Direct contact with saliva of rabid animal, usually through the bite of an infected animal	Initially: weakness, fever, and headache If untreated: cerebral dysfunction, anxiety, confusion, agitation, delirium, abnormal behavior, hallucinations, insomnia, and death
Norovirus infection, acute gastroenteritis	Norovirus	Fecal-oral; foodborne (most common cause of foodborne illness in the United States)	Diarrhea, nausea, stomach pain, vomiting, fever, headache, and body aches
Rotavirus infection	Rotavirus	Fecal-oral	Fever, diarrhea, abdominal pain, and vomiting
Fifth disease	Parvovirus B19	Direct contact with respiratory secretions (droplets); can be spread through blood or blood products	Fever, runny nose, headache, rash on face (slapped cheek appearance) and body, and arthralgia

(Continued)

TABLE 46-3 Viral Pathogens

Disease	Causative Organism	Route of Transmission	Signs and Symptoms
RSV	Respiratory syncytial virus	Airborne, respiratory secretions (droplets)	Cough, sneezing, runny nose, fever, loss of appetite, wheezing, and dyspnea
German measles (3-day measles)	Rubella virus	Airborne, respiratory secretions (droplets)	Fever and rash; if acquired during pregnancy, fetal symptoms may include deafness, cataracts, heart defects, mental retardation, and liver and spleen damage
Chickenpox	Varicella-zoster virus	Direct contact with respiratory secretions (droplets); airborne, respiratory secretions (droplets)	High fever, fatigue, loss of appetite, headache, and itchy rash that becomes blistered, then scabs over

Because many other diseases can cause these symptoms, the occurrence of any one symptom is not necessarily indicative of AIDS. Be aware, however, that patients exhibiting a combination of symptoms should be tested. The two symptoms most indicative of AIDS are hairy leukoplakia and Kaposi's sarcoma.

Chronic Disorders of the AIDS Patient The impaired immune system of the AIDS patient permits opportunistic infections, which further reduce the body's ability to fight off infection. These infections attack many different parts of the body.

One of the cornerstones of the care of patients who have AIDS is to prevent opportunistic infections and identify such infections as quickly as possible when they occur. Identifying malignancies, if they occur, is also of utmost importance. If you are familiar with the common disorders an AIDS patient faces, you will be better able to identify early signs of infection or malignancy and point them out to the doctor, in turn initiating early treatment, which is usually most effective. You can help patients who have been diagnosed with HIV to understand the risks they face and the measures best suited to preventing particular infections. Opportunistic infections and chronic disorders include:

- *Pneumocystis carinii* pneumonia
- Kaposi's sarcoma
- Non-Hodgkin's lymphoma
- Tuberculosis
- *Mycobacterium avium* complex (MAC) infection
- Meningitis
- Oral candidiasis
- Vaginal candidiasis
- Herpes simplex
- Herpes zoster

Hepatitis Hepatitis is a viral infection of the liver that can lead to cirrhosis and death. Hepatitis virus variants differ in their means of transmission and in their presenting symptoms of infection. Those variations commonly transmitted through the bloodborne route include the following:

- Hepatitis B is the most common bloodborne hazard healthcare workers face. It is spread through contact with contaminated blood or body fluids and through sexual contact.

Most patients recover fully from hepatitis B virus (HBV) infection, but some patients develop chronic infection or remain carriers of the pathogen for the rest of their lives. Adults and children with hepatitis B who develop lifelong infections may experience serious health problems, including cirrhosis (scarring of the liver), liver cancer, liver failure, and death. Preventing the spread of the infection is the most effective means of combating the disease. Following standard precautions and receiving HBV vaccinations are the most effective ways to control the spread of the infection.

- Hepatitis C is also spread through contact with contaminated blood or body fluids and through sexual contact. There is no cure for this variant, which has resulted in more deaths than hepatitis A and hepatitis B combined. Many people become carriers of hepatitis C without knowing it because they do not experience any symptoms. If the infection causes immediate symptoms, they often resemble the flu. Although treatment exists to suppress the virus, nothing can prevent or stop the virus from replicating. Over time, it is likely to damage the liver, causing cirrhosis, liver failure, and cancer. As with hepatitis B, preventing the spread of the infection is the best way to combat the disease.

- Hepatitis D (delta agent hepatitis) occurs only in people infected with HBV. Delta agent infection may make hepatitis B symptoms more severe, and it is associated with liver cancer. The HBV vaccine also prevents delta agent infection.

Symptoms People infected with hepatitis may show no symptoms, may experience such mild or subtle symptoms that they do not realize they are seriously ill, or may experience severe symptoms. When you treat patients with hepatitis, any of these signs and symptoms may be present:

- Jaundice (Figure 46-2)
- Diminished appetite
- Fatigue
- Nausea
- Vomiting
- Joint pain or tenderness
- Stomach pain
- General malaise

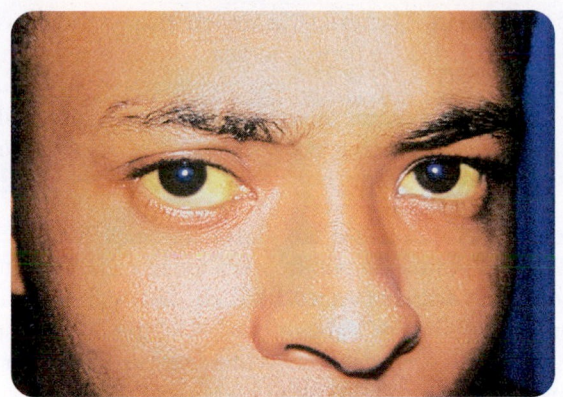

FIGURE 46-2   Jaundice is caused by excess bilirubin, which is produced in the liver and deposited throughout the body, resulting in the yellow appearance of the patient's eyes and skin.
CDC

▶ Bacteria

LO 46.5

Bacteria are single-celled prokaryotic (without a nucleus) organisms that reproduce very quickly and are one of the major causes of disease. Under the right conditions—the right temperature, the right nutrients, and moisture—bacterial cells can double in number in 15 to 30 minutes. This rapid reproduction is one reason that untreated infections can be dangerous.

Classification and Identification

Bacteria can be classified according to their shape, their ability to retain certain dyes, their ability to grow with or without air, and certain biochemical reactions.

Shape   The most common way to classify bacteria is according to their shape. The four common shape classifications are the coccus, bacillus, spirillum, and vibrio (see Figure 46-3).

A **coccus** (plural, *cocci*) is spherical, round, or ovoid. Cocci can be further divided into three types:

- *Staphylococci* are grape-like clusters of cocci commonly found on the skin (*staphylo* means "cluster of grapes"). One species of this microorganism causes a variety of infections, including boils, acne, abscesses, food poisoning, and a type of pneumonia. When viewed under a microscope, stained staphylococci look like clusters of purple grapes.

- *Diplococci* are pairs of cocci (*diplo-* means "double"). The causative agents for gonorrhea and some forms of meningitis are diplococci. When viewed under a microscope, stained diplococci are said to look like little boxing gloves.

- *Streptococci* are cocci that grow in chains (*strepto-* means "twisted chain"). These microorganisms are responsible for infections such as strep throat, certain types of pneumonia, and rheumatic fever. When viewed under the microscope, stained streptococci look like long chains of round beads.

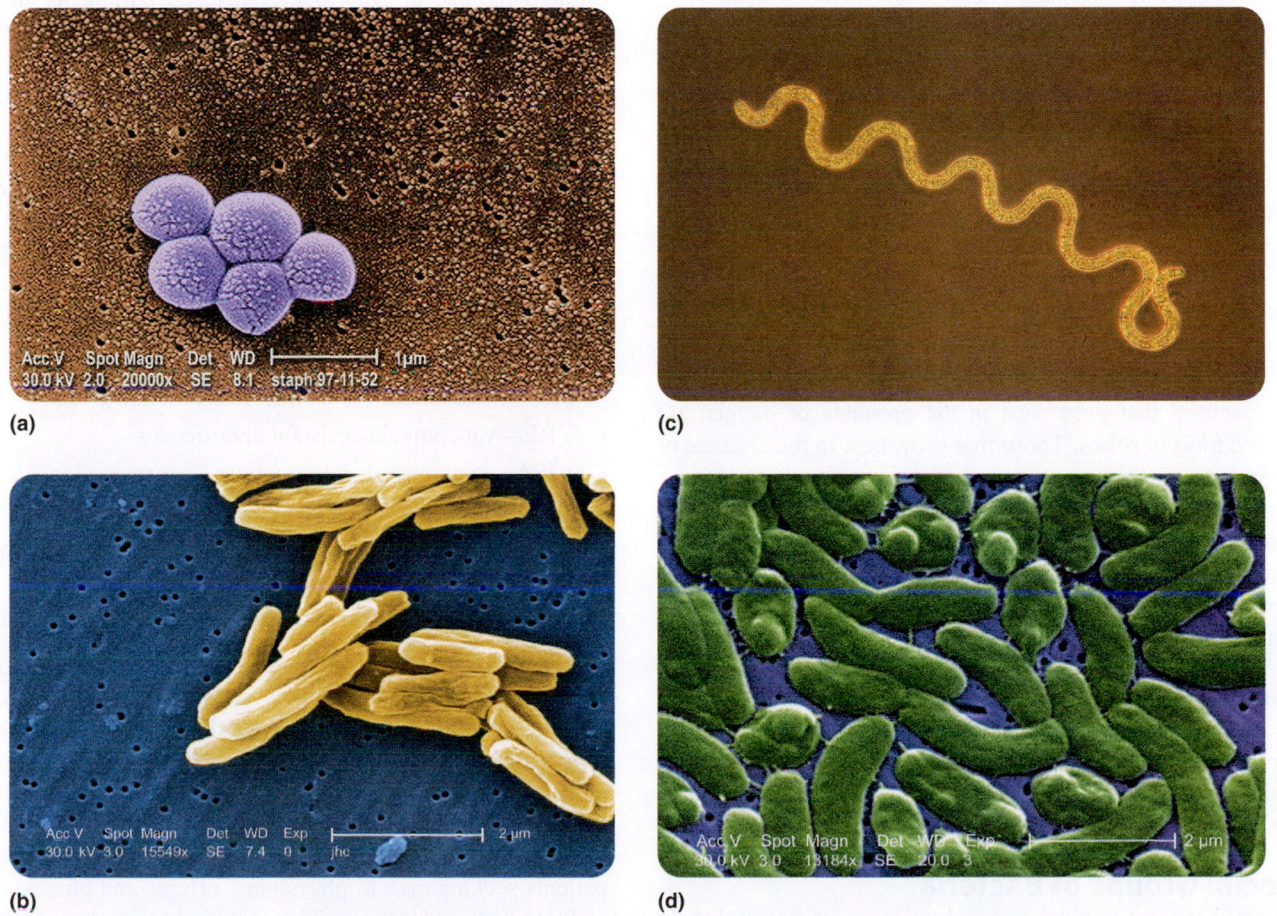

(a)

(c)

(b)

(d)

FIGURE 46-3   The four bacterial classifications by shape are (a) coccus, (b) bacillus, (c) spirillum, and (d) vibrio.
(a) © CDC/Janice Carr; (b) CDC/Janice Carr; (c) © Melba Photo Agency/Punchstock RF; (d) © Janice Carr/CDC

A **bacillus** (plural, *bacilli*) is rod-shaped (*bacillo-* is derived from the Latin word meaning "stick"). Bacilli are responsible for a wide variety of infections, including gastroenteritis, tuberculosis, pneumonia, whooping cough, urinary tract infections (UTIs), botulism, and tetanus. When viewed under the microscope, stained bacilli look like little rods or rounded sticks.

A **spirillum** (plural, *spirilla*) is spiral-shaped (*spira-* means "coil"). Spirilla are responsible for infections such as syphilis and Lyme disease. When viewed under a microscope, stained spirilla look like stretched-out springs or coils.

A **vibrio** (plural, *vibrios*) is comma-shaped (*vibrio* means "vibrate"). Most vibrio bacteria are found in water and are motile, meaning that they move. Vibrios are responsible for diseases such as cholera and some cases of food poisoning. When viewed under a microscope, stained vibrios look like commas or hooked structures.

Ability to Retain Certain Dyes In addition to their shape, bacteria are commonly classified by how they react to certain stains. A **stain** is a specific dye or group of dyes that imparts a color to microorganisms. The most common staining procedure in use today is the **Gram stain.** This method of staining uses a group of dyes and decolorizers to differentiate bacteria according to the chemical composition of their cell walls. Gram staining techniques separate bacteria into two groups, **Gram-positive** and **Gram-negative.** Gram-positive bacteria retain the crystal violet stain during the staining process causing them to appear blue when viewed under the microscope. Gram-negative bacteria do not retain the crystal violet stain during the staining process however, they do take up the red counter stain. This causes them to appear red when viewed under the microscope. The **acid-fast stain** is a staining procedure for identifying bacteria with a waxy cell wall. The bacteria that cause tuberculosis have waxy cell walls and can be stained with this procedure.

Ability to Grow in the Presence or Absence of Air Bacteria that grow best in the presence of oxygen are referred to as **aerobes.** Those that grow best in the absence of oxygen are referred to as **anaerobes.** Organisms that can grow in either environment are referred to as **facultative.** Although most common bacteria are aerobes, many of the bacteria that make up the body's resident normal flora are anaerobes. Not surprisingly, anaerobes are often responsible for infections within the body.

Biochemical Reactions Many closely related bacteria can be differentiated from one another only by certain biochemical reactions that occur within the bacterial cell. For example, one way to identify a particular bacterial strain is to look at what types of sugars the bacteria can grow on.

Special Groups of Bacteria

Several groups of bacteria have certain characteristics that set them apart from most other bacteria. These include the mycobacteria, rickettsiae, chlamydiae, and mycoplasmas.

Mycobacteria Mycobacteria are rod-shaped bacilli with a waxy cell wall, making them acid-fast. Certain types of mycobacteria cause disease in humans. For example, *Mycobacterium tuberculosis* causes the respiratory disease tuberculosis and *Mycobacterium leprae* causes leprosy, also known as Hansen's disease.

Rickettsiae Rickettsiae are unusually small bacteria that can live and grow only within other living cells. Rickettsiae are commonly found in insects like ticks and mites but may be transmitted to humans through bites. Rickettsiae are responsible for diseases such as Rocky Mountain spotted fever and typhus.

Chlamydiae Chlamydiae differ from other bacteria in the structure of their cell walls. Like rickettsiae, they can live and grow only within other living cells. In humans, chlamydiae can cause sexually transmitted infections (STIs), eye disease, certain types of pneumonia, and certain types of heart disease.

Mycoplasmas Mycoplasmas are unusually small bacteria that completely lack the rigid cell wall of other bacteria. These bacteria cause a variety of human diseases, including STIs and a form of pneumonia.

Bacterial Pathogens

In spite of our efforts to eradicate disease-causing bacteria through the use of antibiotics, bacterial pathogens are still with us. Table 46-4 lists some of these pathogens and the diseases they cause.

Drug-Resistant Microogranisms

Drug-resistant pathogens are the cause of many infections. Drug resistance has been linked to overuse of antibiotics. It is the responsibility of physicians, medical staff, and patients to use antibiotics wisely, as resistance to antimicrobial agents is a severe problem. Bacteria and other microorganisms that have developed resistance to antimicrobial drugs include the following:

- MRSA—methicillin/oxacillin-resistant *S. aureus*
- VRE—vancomycin-resistant enterococci
- VISA—vancomycin-intermediate *S. aureus*
- VRSA—vancomycin-resistant *S. aureus*
- ESBLs—extended-spectrum beta-lactamases, which are resistant to cephalosporins and monobactams
- PRSP—penicillin-resistant *Streptococcus pneumoniae*

MRSA and VRE are the most common multidrug-resistant organisms in patients who reside in nonhospital healthcare facilities (for example, nursing homes and other long-term care facilities). People outside of healthcare facilities are increasingly at risk for MRSA, as community-associated MRSA, an infection found in otherwise healthy individuals, is on the rise in the United States. PRSP is more common in patients seeking care in physicians' offices and clinics, especially in pediatric settings. This is thought to be because penicillin is the most commonly prescribed antibiotic in outpatient settings.

TABLE 46-4   Bacterial Pathogens

Disease	Causative Organism	Characteristics	Route of Transmission	Signs and Symptoms
Anthrax	*Bacillus anthracis*	Aerobic, Gram-positive, spore-forming bacillus	Contact with animals infected with or inhalation of *B. anthracis* spores, or consumption of raw or undercooked meat from infected animals	Cutaneous: raised, blistered skin lesion with development of black eschar (dead tissue) Inhalation: high fever, dyspnea, stridor, cyanosis, and shock
Whooping cough	*Bordetella pertussis*	Gram-negative bacterium	Airborne	Stage 1: runny nose, low-grade fever, and mild cough Stage 2: bursts of rapid, uncontrollable coughs with characteristic "whoops" at the end of the cough; cyanosis; and exhaustion Stage 3: recovery and less persistent cough
Lyme disease	*Borrelia burgdorferi*	Spirochete that does not have typical Gram stain characteristics	Tick-borne (Ixodes tick)	Red, expanding, "bull's-eye" rash; fatigue; fever; chills; headache; muscle and joint aches; and swollen lymph nodes
Campylobacteriosis	*Campylobacter jejuni*	Gram-negative, microaerophilic, spiral-shaped	Fecal-oral, foodborne	Diarrhea, sometimes bloody; abdominal cramps; and fever
Chlamydia	*Chlamydia trachomatis*	Coccus; does not have typical Gram stain characteristics but is considered Gram-negative; obligate, intracellular bacteria (must live within an animal cell)	STI	Women: often "silent"; possible vaginal discharge and dysuria Men: penile discharge and dysuria
Botulism	*Clostridium botulinum*	Anaerobic, Gram-positive, spore-forming bacillus	Foodborne	Double vision, blurred vision, drooping eyelids, slurred speech, difficulty swallowing, dry mouth, and muscle weakness
Pseudomembranous colitis	*Clostridium difficile*	Anaerobic, Gram-positive, spore-forming bacillus	Fecal-oral (healthcare-associated infection)	Watery diarrhea, fever, loss of appetite, nausea, and abdominal pain/tenderness
Tetanus	*Clostridium tetani*	Anaerobic, Gram-positive bacillus (sometimes forms spores)	Direct contact through a deep cut	Early: lockjaw, neck and abdomen stiffness, and difficulty swallowing Late: severe muscle spasms and generalized tonic-seizure-like activity
Diphtheria	*Corynebacterium diphtheria*	Gram-positive bacillus	Direct person-to-person contact with respiratory droplets or cutaneous lesions	Sore throat; low-grade fever; and presence of a pseudomembrane over the tonsils, throat, and nose
E. coli diarrhea	*Escherichia coli*	Gram-negative bacillus	Foodborne (some strains do not cause disease)	Diarrhea, severe abdominal cramps, and vomiting
Haemophilus influenzae Serotype b (Hib) disease (epiglottitis, pneumonia)	*Haemophilus influenzae*	Gram-negative coccobacillus	Direct contact with respiratory droplets	Epiglottitis: sore throat and difficulty breathing Pneumonia: difficulty breathing and fever
Peptic ulcer	*Helicobacter pylori*	Microaerophilic, Gram-negative bacillus	Not well understood; may be fecal-oral or oral-oral	Gnawing or burning stomach pain, nausea, bloating, and burping
Legionnaire's disease	*Legionella pneumophila*	Gram-negative bacillus	Water aerosol	High fever, chills, cough, chest pain, and pneumonia

(Continued)

TABLE 46-4   Bacterial Pathogens

Disease	Causative Organism	Characteristics	Route of Transmission	Signs and Symptoms
Leprosy	*Mycobacterium leprae*	Acid-fast bacillus	Airborne, respiratory droplets	Skin lesions, nodules, plaques, and thickened dermis
Tuberculosis	*Mycobacterium tuberculosis*	Acid-fast bacillus	Airborne, respiratory droplets	Bad cough lasting 3 weeks or longer, pain in the chest, coughing up blood or sputum, weakness or fatigue, weight loss, no appetite, chills, fever, and night sweats
Mycoplasma pneumonia	*Mycoplasma pneumoniae*	Wall-less bacteria, usually coccoid in shape with polar extensions	Direct contact with respiratory droplets	Fever, nonproductive cough, malaise, and headache
Gonorrhea	*Neisseria gonorrhoeae*	Gram-negative diplococcus	STI	Women: most have no symptoms; some have dysuria and vaginal discharge Men: dysuria and green, yellow, or white penile discharge Left untreated can cause complications in both women and men
Meningitis	*Neisseria meningitidis*	Gram-negative diplococcus	Direct contact with respiratory droplets	Stiff neck, fever, confusion, light sensitivity, nausea, and vomiting
	Haemophilus influenzae	Gram-negative coccobacillus		
	Group B Streptococcus (*Streptococcus agalactiae*)	Gram-positive coccus		
	Listeria monocytogenes	Gram-positive, flagellated bacillus		
Pseudomonas infection (hot tub rash)	*Pseudomonas aeruginosa*	Gram-negative bacillus	Direct contact with water contaminated with *P. aeruginosa*	Itchy, red rash and pustules around hair follicles
Rocky Mountain spotted fever	*Rickettsia rickettsi*	Gram-negative coccobacillus	Tick-borne (wood or dog tick)	Fever, rash (occurs 2–5 days after fever), headache, nausea, vomiting, abdominal pain, muscle pain, lack of appetite, and conjunctival inflammation
Shigellosis	*Shigella sonnei*	Gram-negative bacillus	Fecal-oral	Diarrhea, fever, and stomach cramps
Methicillin-resistant *Staphylococcus aureus* (MRSA) infection	*Staphylococcus aureus*	Gram-positive coccus	Direct contact	Red, swollen, painful pustules
Bacterial pneumonia	*Streptococcus pneumonia*	Gram-positive diplococcus	Direct person-to-person contact	Cough, chest pain, shortness of breath, malaise, and poor appetite
Strep throat	*Streptococcus pyogenes*	Gram-positive coccus	Direct contact with respiratory droplets	Sore throat and fever
Syphilis	*Treponema pallidum*	Gram-negative spirochete	STI	Primary stage: single sore (chancre) at site of the organism's entry into the body Secondary stage: skin rash and mucous membrane lesions Late stage: uncoordinated muscle movements, paralysis, numbness, gradual blindness, and dementia
Cholera	*Vibrio cholerae*	Gram-negative curved rod	Fecal-oral from contaminated water	Profuse watery diarrhea ("rice-water stools"), vomiting, rapid heart rate, loss of skin elasticity, dry mucous membranes, low blood pressure, thirst, muscle cramps, and restlessness or irritability

Risk Factors

There are a number of risk factors for both the development of and infection with drug-resistant organisms. These risk factors include:

- Advanced age
- Invasive procedures, which include dialysis, the presence of invasive devices, and urinary catheterization
- Previous use of antimicrobial agents
- Repeated contact with the healthcare system
- Severity of the illness
- Underlying diseases or conditions, especially chronic renal disease, insulin-dependent diabetes mellitus, peripheral vascular disease, and dermatitis or skin lesions

Preventing Antibiotic Resistance in Healthcare Settings

In response to a growing concern over the emergence of antibiotic-resistant infections, the CDC began the Campaign to Prevent Antimicrobial Resistance in Healthcare Settings. This campaign has four strategies to reduce the incidence of antibiotic-resistant microorganisms:

- Prevent infection
- Diagnose and treat infection appropriately
- Use antibiotics carefully
- Prevent transmission of infections

▶ Protozoans
LO 46.6

Protozoans are single-celled eukaryotic (with a nucleus) organisms that are generally much larger than bacteria. Found in soil and water, most do not cause disease in people. Certain protozoans are pathogenic, however, and cause diseases such as malaria, amebic dysentery (a type of diarrhea), and trichomoniasis vaginitis (a type of STI; see Figure 46-4). Protozoal diseases are a leading cause of death in developing countries because the lack of proper sanitation in some areas promotes their spread. These diseases are also common in patients with depressed immune systems. Table 46-5 lists some of the parasitic protozoans and multicellular parasites that affect humans.

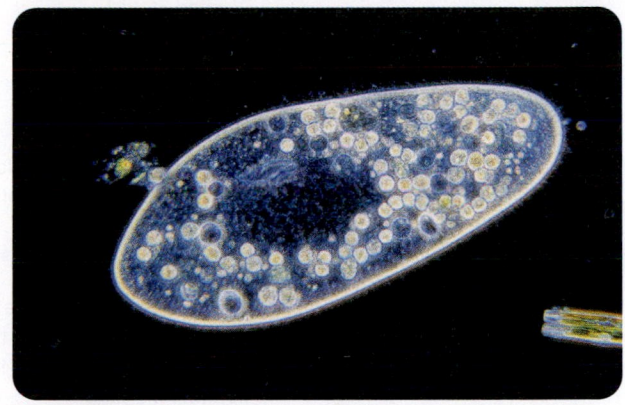

FIGURE 46-4 The protozoan *Trichomonas vaginalis* causes a common STI in humans.
© Melba Photo Agency/Punchstock RF

TABLE 46-5	Human Protozoal and Multicellular Parasites			
Disease	**Causative Organism**	**Notable Features**	**Route of Transmission**	**Signs and Symptoms**
Intestinal				
Amebiasis	*Entamoeba histolytica*	Can become invasive and cause liver abscess	Fecal-oral	Loose stool, abdominal pain, abdominal cramping, bloody diarrhea, and fever
Intestinal hookworm	*Necator americanus* and *Ancylostoma duodenale*	Larvae migrate to the intestinal tract.	Larvae in soil contaminated with feces from an infected person penetrate bare feet and cause infection.	Itching at the site of entry, abdominal pain, diarrhea, anorexia, and anemia due to loss of blood at the site of attachment in the intestine
Round worm	*Ascaris lumbricoides*	Most common helminthic (worm) infection in the world	Contact with contaminated soil	Can be asymptomatic; symptoms include abdominal discomfort and intestinal blockage
Cryptosporidiosis	*Cryptosporidium parvum* and *C. hominis*	Can be found in recreational water such as swimming pools and hot tubs contaminated with *Cryptosporidium*	Waterborne	Abdominal cramps and pain, dehydration, nausea, vomiting, fever, and weight loss
Cyclosporiasis	*Cyclospora cayetanensis*	Outbreaks in the United States have been linked to imported fresh produce.	Fecal-oral	Frequent, explosive, watery diarrhea; abdominal cramps; loss of appetite; weight loss; bloating; excessive gas; and fatigue
Fish or broad tapeworm	*Diphyllobothrium latum*	Longest human tapeworm, reaching up to 30 feet in length	Foodborne from eating raw or undercooked fish infected with *D. latum*	Abdominal discomfort, diarrhea, vomiting, weight loss, and vitamin B_{12} deficiency
Pinworm	*Enterobius vermicularis*	While the infected person is sleeping, female pinworms leave the intestine and lay their eggs on the skin surrounding the anus.	Fecal-oral	Anal itching, and nighttime restlessness due to anal itching

(Continued)

Disease	Causative Organism	Notable Features	Route of Transmission	Signs and Symptoms
TABLE 46-5 Human Protozoal and Multicellular Parasites				
Giardiasis	*Giardia intestinalis* (formerly *G. lamblia*)	Once outside the body, can live in soil or water for weeks or months	Fecal-oral	Greasy, floating stool; gas; diarrhea; abdominal pain and cramping; nausea; and dehydration
Lung fluke (Paragonimiasis)	*Paragonimus kellicotti*	Linked to eating raw or undercooked crab or crayfish infected with *P. kellicotti;* ingested larvae migrate to the lungs	Foodborne	Initially diarrhea and abdominal pain, followed by fever, chest pain, fatigue, and cough
Bloodborne/Vector-borne				
Chagas disease	*Trypanosome cruzi*	Found only in the Americas (mostly Latin America but also the United States)	Vector-borne (triatomine bug)	Acute phase: fever, fatigue, body aches, headache, and diarrhea Chronic phase: cardiomyopathy, heart failure, heart arrhythmia, enlarged esophagus, enlarged colon, and difficulty eating or passing stool
Malaria	*Plasmodium falciparum, P. vivax, P. ovale, P. malariae*	Fifth most common cause of death worldwide from infectious disease	Vector-borne (mosquito)	Fever, chills, sweats, headache, nausea, body aches, and general malaise
Skin				
Swimmer's itch (cercarial dermatitis)	*Austrobilharzia variglandis*	Ducks and geese are the most common host; however, the larvae will burrow into a human swimmer's skin.	Contact with larvae in water	Tingling, burning, or itching of the skin; small, reddish pimples; and small blisters
Head lice (pediculosis)	*Pediculus humanus capitis*	Can be transmitted by contact with clothing, combs, or brushes used by an infested individual	Direct contact with the hair of infested individual	Feeling that something is moving in your hair, itching, difficulty sleeping because of louse activity, and scalp sores
Pubic lice (pthiriasis)	*Phthirus pubis*	Infestation has been linked to casual contact with personal items—like combs or hairbrushes—used by infested individuals.	Direct contact with an infested individual (usually sexual contact)	Genital itching, visible nits (eggs), or crawling adult lice
Scabies	*Sarcoptes scabiei*	Symptoms worse at night	Prolonged, direct contact with an infested individual	Intense itching and papular rash
Bed bugs	*Cimex lectularius* and *C. hemipterus*	Not known to carry any disease and not considered a public health threat	Exposure to bedding or furniture infested with *C. lectularius* or *C. hemipterus*	Bite marks on the head, neck, face, hands, or other body parts occurring at night while sleeping
Muscle				
Trichinellosis	*Trichinella spiralis*	Currently uncommon in commercial pork; more cases in the United States are now associated with wild game.	Foodborne from eating raw or undercooked pork or wild animals	Nausea, diarrhea, vomiting, fatigue, fever, abdominal pain, headache, chills, coughing, eye swelling, and joint pain
Toxoplasmosis	*Toxoplasma gondii*	Forms cysts that may be found in skeletal muscle, myocardium, brain, and eyes	Foodborne, animal-to-human, mother-to-child (congenital)	Some have no or very mild symptoms; swollen lymph glands and muscle aches
Vagina, Vulva, Urethra				
Trichomoniasis	*Trichomonas vaginalis*	Considered the most common and most curable STI	Sexual contact	Women: itching, burning, redness or soreness of the genitals, dysuria, and watery discharge with an unusual smell Men: itching or irritation inside the penis, burning after urination or ejaculation, and some penile discharge

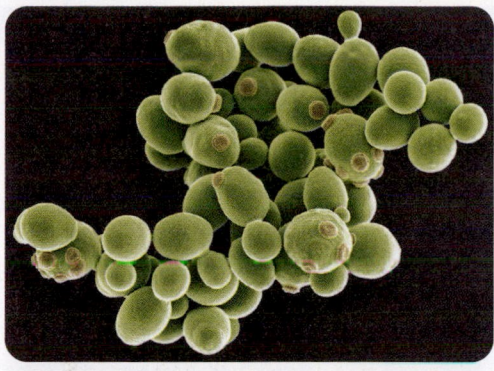

(a)

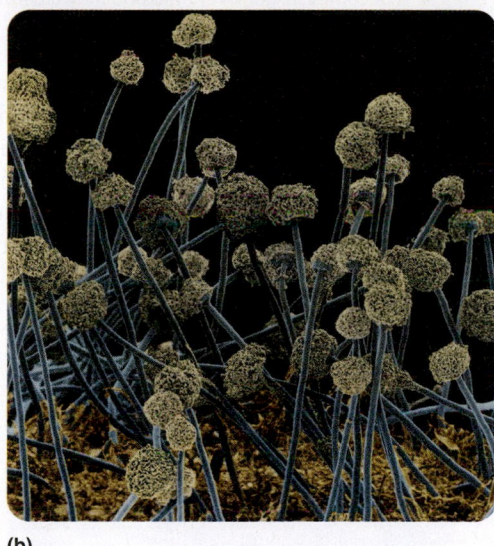

(b)

FIGURE 46-5 Because fungi lack the ability to make their own food, they depend on other life forms. (a) Single-celled fungi are called yeasts. (b) Multicelled fungi are called molds.

(a) © Science Photo Library RF/Getty Images; (b) © David Scharf/Science Source

▶ Fungi

LO 46.7

A *fungus* (plural, *fungi*) is a eukaryotic organism that has a rigid cell wall at some stage in the life cycle. Fungi that grow mainly as single-celled organisms and reproduce by budding are referred to as *yeasts,* whereas fungi that grow into large, fuzzy, multicelled organisms that produce spores are called *molds.* Figure 46-5 shows the differences between these two types of fungi.

Most fungi do not cause disease in humans. Of those that do, the majority produce superficial infections such as athlete's foot (tinea pedis), ringworm, thrush, and vaginal yeast infections. Fungi can produce serious, life-threatening illness, however, when they infect the internal tissues. This kind of infection can occur when patients have a depressed immune system, as in patients who are undergoing cancer treatment and patients with AIDS. Table 46-6 lists some of the most common fungal diseases and the organisms that cause them.

▶ Multicellular Parasites

LO 46.8

A *parasite* is an organism that lives on or in another organism and uses that other organism for food, or for some other advantage, to the detriment of the host organism. For example, a leech is a type of parasite that lives off of the host's blood. Viruses, rickettsiae, chlamydiae, and some protozoans are parasitic. Multicellular organisms also can be parasitic, and some of these organisms are microscopic during all or part of their lives. An infection caused by a parasite is called an *infestation.* Multicellular parasites that cause human disease include certain worms and insects, as illustrated in Figure 46-6 and listed in Table 46-5.

TABLE 46-6	Pathogenic Fungi		
Disease	**Causative Organism**	**Route of Transmission**	**Signs and Symptoms**
Aspergillosis	*Aspergillus fumigatus* and *A. flavus*	Airborne (inhalation of spores)	Wheezing, coughing, fever, chest pain, shortness of breath, and aspergilloma (fungus ball)
Blastomycosis	*Blastomyces dermatitidis*	Airborne (inhalation of spores)	Fever, chills, cough, muscle aches, joint pain, and chest pain
Candidiasis • Oropharyngeal (thrush) • Vaginal • Invasive	*Candida albicans*	*C. albicans* is part of the body's resident normal flora; conditions that cause an imbalance in the resident normal flora cause an overgrowth of the fungus.	• Oropharyngeal—white patches on the tongue and other oral mucous membranes, redness or soreness in the affected areas, difficulty swallowing, and cracking at the corners of the mouth • Vaginal—genital itching; burning; and thick, white vaginal discharge • Invasive—fever and chills
Coccidioidomycosis (valley fever)	*Coccidioides*	Airborne (inhalation of spores)	Fever, cough, headache, rash on upper trunk or extremities, muscle aches, joint pain in the knees or ankles, skin lesions, chronic pneumonia, meningitis, and bone or joint infection
Ringworm	Dermatophytes (*Trichophyton rubrum* and *T. tonsurans*)	Direct contact with an infected person	Redness, scaling, cracking of the skin, or a ring-shaped rash; loss of hair at the site of infection

(Continued)

TABLE 46-6	Pathogenic Fungi		
Disease	**Causative Organism**	**Route of Transmission**	**Signs and Symptoms**
Cryptococcosis	*Cryptococcus neoformans* and *C. gattii*	Airborne; *C. neoformans* is usually associated with large amounts of bird droppings.	Shortness of breath, cough, fatigue, fever, headache, and meningitis
Histoplasmosis	*Histoplasma capsulatum*	Airborne, usually associated with large amounts of bird or bat droppings	Fever, chest pains, and nonproductive cough
Pneumocystis pneumonia (PCP)	*Pneumocystis jirovecii*	Airborne, inhalation of spores; most common opportunistic infection in people with HIV/AIDS	Fever, dry cough, shortness of breath, and fatigue
Sporotrichosis	*Sporothrix schenckii*	Direct contact with spores	Small, painless nodule at contact site; lesion becomes larger over time and may ulcerate

Parasitic Worms

People can be infested with a parasitic worm by ingesting its eggs or an immature form of the worm or by having the parasite penetrate the skin. As with the protozoans, infestation by these parasites is more common in developing nations with poor sanitation.

Worms that infect people include roundworms, flatworms, and tapeworms. Roundworms can occur in the intestines, as in the case of pinworms, a common infection in children. Other roundworms, such as *Trichinella*, are found in muscle tissue. *Trichinella spiralis*, which causes the infection trichinosis, enters the human body in infected meat eaten raw or

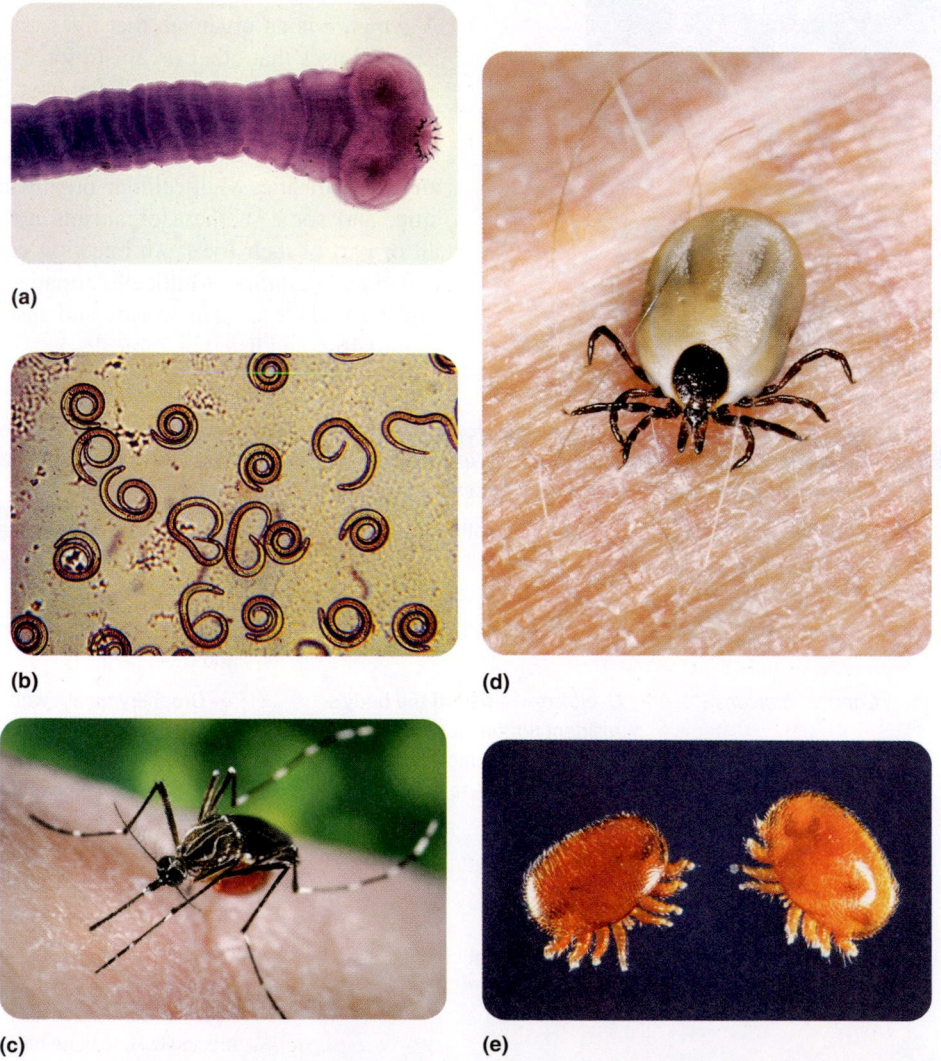

(a)

(b)

(c)

(d)

(e)

FIGURE 46-6 Parasitic worms, such as (a) tapeworms (Cestoda) and (b) *Trichinella*, cause disease in humans when they are ingested. Parasitic insects, such as (c) mosquitoes, (d) deer ticks, and (e) mites, cause disease by biting or burrowing into the skin.

(a) CDC; (b) © Dickson Despommier/Science Source; (c) CDC/James Gathany; (d) © The Image Bank/Getty Images; (e) © Photo by Scott Bauer/USDA

insufficiently cooked. People also may get flatworms and tapeworms by eating undercooked meats. A trained medical professional must inspect a patient's stool for the presence of the parasite or its eggs to diagnose an intestinal infection with a parasitic worm.

Parasitic Insects

Insects that can bite or burrow under the skin include mosquitoes, ticks, lice, and mites. These insects spread many viral, bacterial (including rickettsial), and protozoal diseases. The causative organisms can live in the insects' bodies and enter people's bodies when they are bitten by the insects. Such diseases include Lyme disease, malaria, Rocky Mountain spotted fever, and encephalitis. Lice are small insects that live on hair and skin and feed on blood. Scabies infestations are caused by mites that burrow under the skin.

▶ How Infections Are Diagnosed   LO 46.9

To assist with the diagnosis and treatment of an infection, a medical assistant must work closely with other medical team members. The basic steps in diagnosis and treatment are summarized in Figure 46-7.

Step 1. Examine the Patient

When a patient comes in to the office with signs or symptoms that suggest an infection, begin by taking the patient's vital signs and noting the patient's complaints. On the basis of these findings and the patient examination, the doctor can make a presumptive, or tentative, clinical diagnosis.

In many cases, signs and symptoms of a particular infection are so characteristic of the disease that the doctor need not perform additional tests to reach a diagnosis. An example is a case of chickenpox or mumps. At other times, however, the doctor needs to gather additional information to confirm a diagnosis and determine the cause.

Step 2. Obtain One or More Specimens

To determine the cause of an infection, you may need to obtain specimens from one or more areas of the patient's body. Label each specimen properly and include with it the physician's presumptive diagnosis. If the sample is to be transported to an outside laboratory, ensure that it is transported in such a way that any pathogenic organisms remain alive (and safely contained) during transit.

Step 3. Examine the Specimen Directly

You must sometimes obtain more than one specimen from each site. The doctor or specially trained laboratory or microbiology personnel will then directly examine one specimen under the microscope. The specimen may be viewed in one of two ways:

- As a wet mount, a preparation of a specimen in a liquid that allows the organisms to remain alive and mobile while they are being identified
- As a smear, in which a specimen is spread thinly and evenly across a slide

If you make a smear, allow it to dry and then treat or stain it as ordered before it is examined microscopically. In some cases, direct examination allows the doctor to make a presumptive diagnosis of the microorganism.

Step 4. Culture the Specimen

If the physician still needs a more definitive identification of the microorganism, you may perform a **culture,** in which a sample of the specimen is placed in or on a substance that allows microorganisms to grow. A *culture medium* is a substance that contains all the nutrients a particular type of microorganism needs. Most media come in the form of a semisolid gel. After inoculating (placing a sample of the specimen in or on) the medium, it is placed in an incubator (a chamber that can be set to a specific temperature and humidity) to allow the microorganism to grow This is often done by a laboratory technologist.

The culture is examined visually and microscopically after a specified time, and a preliminary identification is made. The physician sets up additional tests to confirm the identification of the microorganism that has been isolated from the specimen. Most microbiology laboratories and some physicians' office laboratories are equipped to grow routine bacterial cultures and some fungal cultures. Physicians' office laboratories, in particular, may have to send other types of cultures, such as virus cultures, to a specialized laboratory for identification.

Step 5. Determine the Culture's Antibiotic Sensitivity

In many cases of bacterial infection, a **culture and sensitivity (C&S)** is performed. This procedure involves culturing a specimen and then testing the isolated bacterium's susceptibility (sensitivity) to certain antibiotics. The results help the doctor determine which antibiotics might be most effective in treating the infection.

Step 6. Treat the Patient as Ordered by the Physician

On the basis of identification of the microorganism and antibiotic sensitivity, if determined, the physician can prescribe an *antimicrobial.* This agent, which kills microorganisms or suppresses their growth, should help clear up the patient's infection.

▶ Specimen Collection   LO 46.10

Perhaps the most important step in isolating and identifying a microorganism as the cause of an infection is collecting the specimen. If this is done incorrectly, the organism may not grow in culture in a way that it can be identified, resulting in an untreated infection. Furthermore, if the specimen becomes contaminated during collection and the contaminant is mistakenly identified as the cause of the infection, the patient may receive incorrect or even harmful therapy.

In addition to vaginal specimens (discussed in detail in the *Assisting in Reproductive and Urinary Specialties* chapter), the most common types of culture specimens involve the following:

- Throat
- Urine

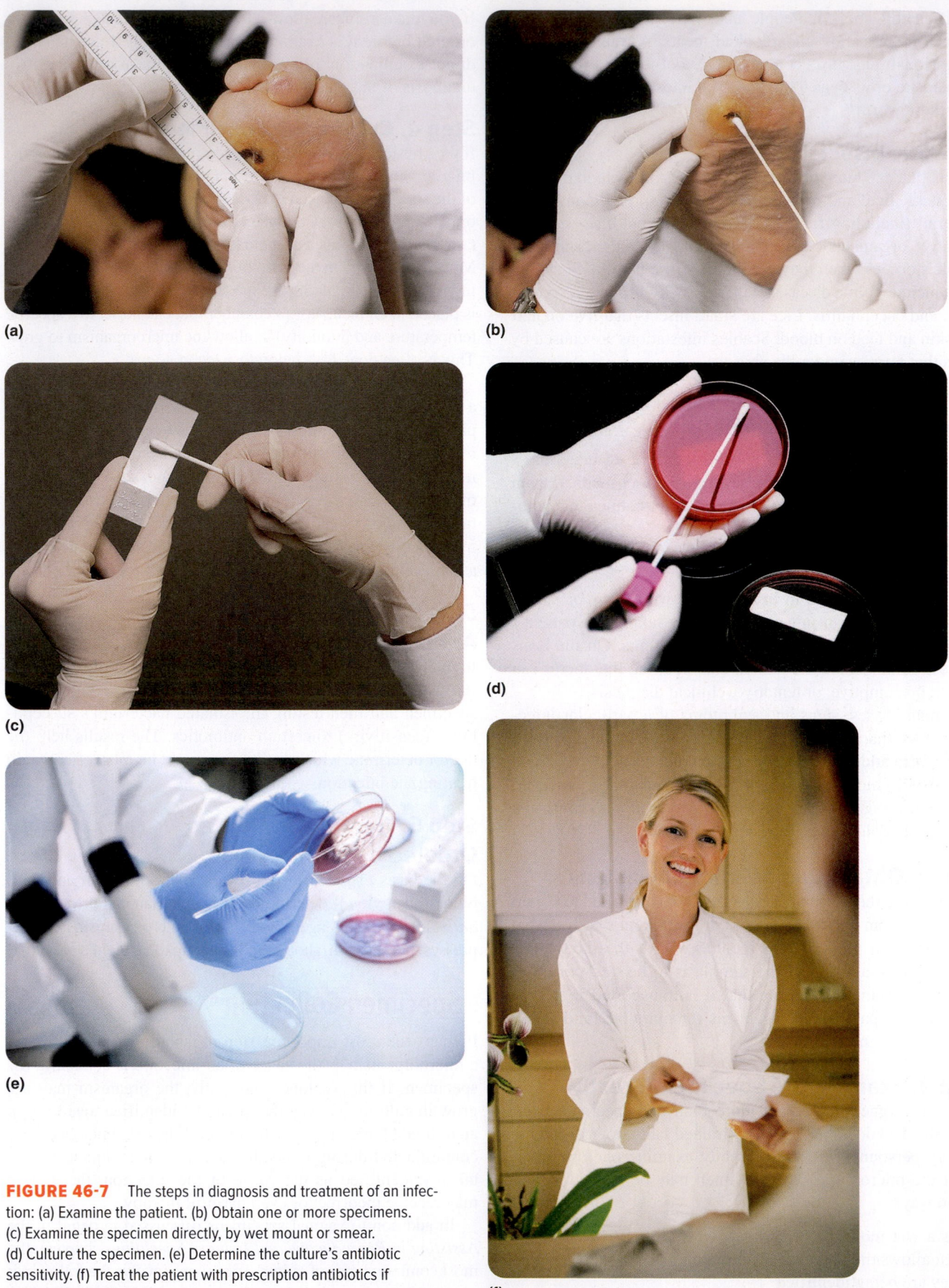

FIGURE 46-7 The steps in diagnosis and treatment of an infection: (a) Examine the patient. (b) Obtain one or more specimens. (c) Examine the specimen directly, by wet mount or smear. (d) Culture the specimen. (e) Determine the culture's antibiotic sensitivity. (f) Treat the patient with prescription antibiotics if ordered by the physician.

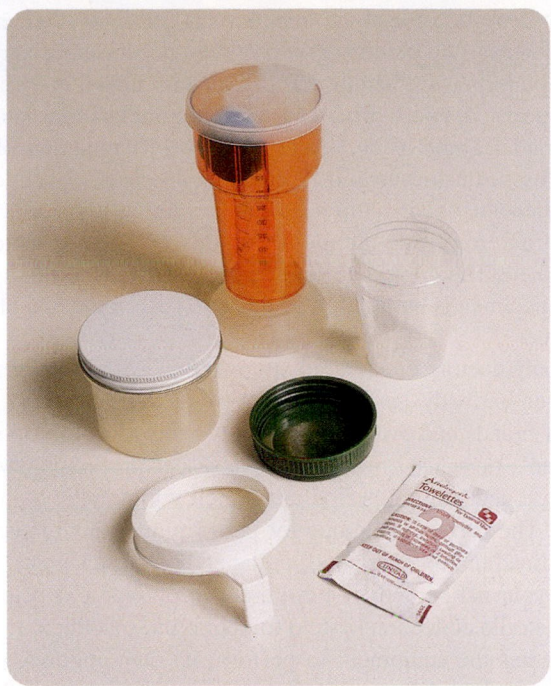

FIGURE 46-8 You may use specially designed collection containers to collect sputum, urine, and stool specimens.
© Cliff Moore

- Sputum
- Wound
- Stool

Specimen-Collection Devices

To help ensure optimal recovery of microorganisms, you must use the appropriate collection device and specimen container. Specimen-collection devices are available for the collection of sputum, urine, and stool specimens, as shown in Figure 46-8. These containers are designed with large openings to allow specimen collection with minimal chance of contamination. They also have tight-fitting caps to prevent leakage and contamination.

Sterile Swabs The most common device for obtaining cultures is the sterile swab. Sterile swabs vary in the absorbent material at the tip and in the composition of the shaft (Figure 46-9).

Although cotton is absorbent, it is no longer used for culture swabs because natural chemicals in cotton inhibit the growth of certain microorganisms. Polyester, rayon, or calcium alginate fibers are preferred. Most swabs used to collect routine specimens have a wooden or plastic shaft for rigidity. Swabs with a small tip and a flexible wire shaft are made especially for culturing hard-to-reach areas and obtaining pediatric specimens. Some collection containers contain two swabs—one for a culture and one for a smear.

Collection and Transport Systems

Sterile, self-contained systems for obtaining and transporting specimens are commercially available from many suppliers. The CULTURETTE Collection and Transport System, manufactured by Becton Dickinson Microbiology Systems of

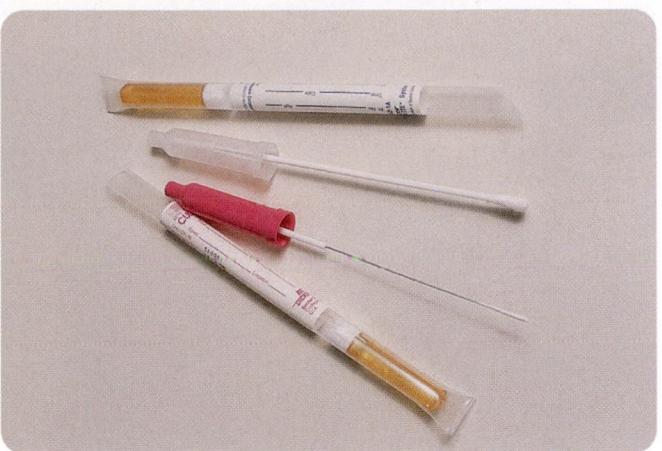

FIGURE 46-9 Sterile swabs vary in size and material.
© Cliff Moore

Sparks, Maryland, is a well-known example. The unit, shown in Figure 46-10, contains a polyester swab and a small, thin-walled vial of transport medium in a plastic sleeve. If a specimen will not be tested within 30 minutes after it is obtained, the swab is replaced in the sleeve and the vial is crushed between the thumb and the index finger. The moisture and nutrients provided by the transport medium help keep the bacteria alive during transport to the laboratory.

Several collection systems are also available for culturing anaerobic organisms. These systems provide a means of generating an oxygen-free environment so the anaerobic organisms remain viable (alive and able to reproduce) during transport.

Specimen-Collection Guidelines

To collect specimens properly, you should follow a number of general guidelines.

- Obtain the specimen with great care to avoid causing the patient harm, discomfort, or undue embarrassment. If patients are to collect specimens on their own, give them clear, detailed instructions along with the proper container.
- Collect the material from a site where the organism is most likely to be found and where contamination is least likely to occur. For example, the best location to obtain a specimen for diagnosing strep throat is at the back of the throat in the area of the tonsils. A properly collected sputum specimen should contain mucus coughed up from the respiratory tract but should not contain saliva, which is a contaminant.
- Obtain the specimen at a time that allows optimal chance of recovery of the microorganism. Knowledge of the infectious disease process allows the doctor to determine the best time to collect a specimen. For example, certain viruses are more readily isolated during the early, symptomatic stage of an illness.
- Use appropriate collection devices, specimen containers, transport systems, and culture media to ensure optimal microorganism recovery. The purpose of such equipment and materials is to preserve the viability of any microorganisms so that they will grow in culture. Special collection devices are available for certain body areas or suspected pathogens.

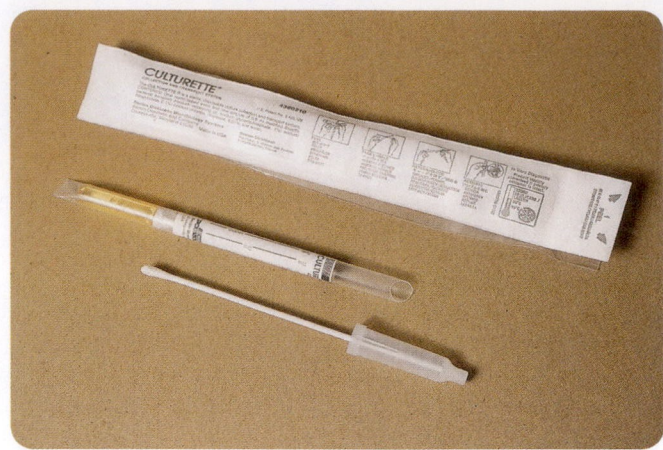

FIGURE 46-10 The CULTURETTE is used to obtain and transport microbiologic specimens to outside laboratories.
Source: Courtesy of Becton Dickinson Microbiology Systems.
© Cliff Moore

- Obtain a sufficient quantity of the specimen for performing the requested procedures. If, for example, both a culture and a direct examination of a swabbed specimen will be done, you must collect two specimens. Each procedure requires its own sample.
- Obtain the specimen before antimicrobial therapy begins. If the patient is already taking an antibiotic, note this fact on the laboratory request form or ask the doctor whether you should obtain the specimen.

After correctly collecting the specimen, you must label the container and include the appropriate requisition form. The label should contain the following information:

- Patient's name and identification number (if appropriate)
- Source (collection site) of the specimen
- Date and time of collection
- Doctor's name
- Your initials (if you obtained the specimen)

The requisition form should include the following information:

- Patient's name, address, and identification number
- Patient's age and gender
- Patient's insurance billing information
- Type and source of the microbiologic specimen (for example, discharge from wound, big toe)
- Date and time of microbiologic specimen collection
- Test requested
- Medications the patient is currently receiving
- Doctor's presumptive diagnosis
- Doctor's name, address, and phone number
- Special instructions or orders

Throat Culture Specimens

The doctor may request a throat culture on patients with signs or symptoms of an upper respiratory, throat, or sinus infection. In most cases, the doctor wants to determine whether the patient has strep throat, an infection caused by the bacterium *Streptococcus pyogenes,* a group A streptococcus. It is particularly important to diagnose and treat this infection because, left untreated, strep throat can lead to complications such as rheumatic fever. Rheumatic fever is an inflammation of the heart tissue that occurs most frequently in school-age children.

When you obtain a throat culture specimen, avoid touching any structures inside the mouth, as this will contaminate the specimen. The correct technique for obtaining a throat culture specimen is outlined in Procedure 46-1 at the end of this chapter.

Many doctors order rapid strep tests if strep is suspected. Antigen-antibody test kits for strep are available in a variety of brands and provide immediate indications of the strep antigen's presence on a throat swab, sparing the patient the expense and waiting period associated with having a culture done. The correct technique for performing a rapid strep test is outlined in Procedure 46-2 at the end of this chapter.

If your office does not culture microbiologic specimens, use a sterile collection system to obtain the specimen. If your office has the equipment to perform its own cultures, use a sterile swab and inoculate a culture plate directly with the swab. Specimens to be evaluated in the office should be cultured immediately after collection.

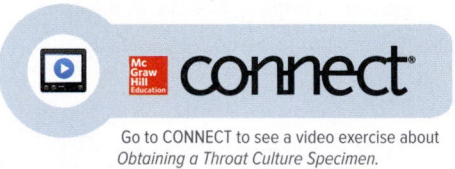

Go to CONNECT to see a video exercise about *Obtaining a Throat Culture Specimen.*

Urine Specimens

To minimize contaminants in urine specimens, it is important to obtain a clean-catch mid-stream specimen. You must process urine specimens within an hour of collection or refrigerate them to prevent continued bacterial growth. (Collection of urine specimens for culturing is discussed in detail in the *Collecting, Processing, and Testing Urine and Stool Specimens* chapter.)

Sputum Specimens

To obtain sputum specimens, have the patient expectorate (cough up) mucus from the lungs into a wide-mouthed specimen container. Beforehand, instruct the patient to avoid contaminating the specimen with saliva. If sputum specimens are not cultured right away, they should be refrigerated.

Observe standard precautions whenever you handle sputum samples and wear a face shield or mask and goggles when collecting such specimens, especially if the patient is coughing. Even when tuberculosis is not suspected, the potential for its transmission always exists.

Wound Specimens

You usually obtain specimens from infected wounds and lesions by swabbing. The procedure is similar to that of a throat culture. Be sure you obtain representative material from a deep area and a surface area of the wound without contaminating the swab by touching areas outside the site.

Transporting Specimens to an Outside Laboratory LO 46.11

Many physicians' offices do not perform microbiologic testing on-site, choosing instead to send their culture specimens to an outside laboratory. This is particularly true for many specialized microbiologic procedures like virus cultures and bacteria cultures (including chlamydia) that require special techniques and equipment rarely found in a physician's office laboratory.

Your Main Objectives

When you collect and transport a microbiologic specimen to an outside laboratory, you have three main objectives:

1. Making sure proper collection procedures are followed, including using the proper collection device. Improperly handled specimens will not be processed at the lab.

2. Maintaining the samples in a state as close to their original as possible. You must take specific steps to prevent them from deteriorating.

3. Protecting anyone who handles a specimen container from exposure to potentially infectious material. To do so, ensure that the specimen container has a tight-fitting lid. As extra protection against leakage, place the specimen container in a secondary container or zipper-type plastic bag (usually provided by the laboratory).

Methods of Transportation

Specimens to be tested by an outside laboratory may be transported in one of three ways:

- During regularly scheduled daily pickups by the laboratory
- During an as-needed pickup by the laboratory
- Through the mail

Pickup by the laboratory is the most reliable and timely method of transporting microbiologic specimens. Although each laboratory has its own procedure, the general steps for preparing specimens for transport to a laboratory are outlined in Procedure 46-3 at the end of this chapter.

Sending Specimens by Mail

There may be times when you must send a specimen through the mail to a special reference laboratory for a test not normally done by a local laboratory. The US Postal Service accepts a package containing microbiologic specimens as long as the total volume of specimen material is less than 50 milliliters and it is packaged under strict regulations specified by the US Public Health Service.

When sending specimens through the mail, pack them securely with adequate cushioning material to prevent breakage and leakage. Leakage can contaminate the specimen, putting mail handlers at risk of contamination with infectious materials. The proper technique for packaging and labeling microbiologic specimens is outlined by the Centers for Disease Control and Prevention (CDC) and is shown in Figure 46-11.

Securely close the primary culture container and surround it with enough absorbent packing material to absorb the entire fluid contents if the container were to leak. Place these items together in a secondary container, commonly a metal container with a screw-top or snap-on lid. Then place the secondary container in an outer shipping carton made of cardboard or Styrofoam®.

In addition to the address label, microbiologic specimens sent through the mail must have an etiologic agent label affixed to the package, as shown in Figure 46-11. This label uses the biohazard symbol to alert the mail carrier as to the nature of the contents. The term **etiologic agent** refers to a living microorganism or its toxin that may cause human disease.

Direct Examination of Specimens LO 46.12

At times, the physician may directly examine the specimen under a microscope to detect the presence of microorganisms or to identify them. Two types of procedures that allow direct

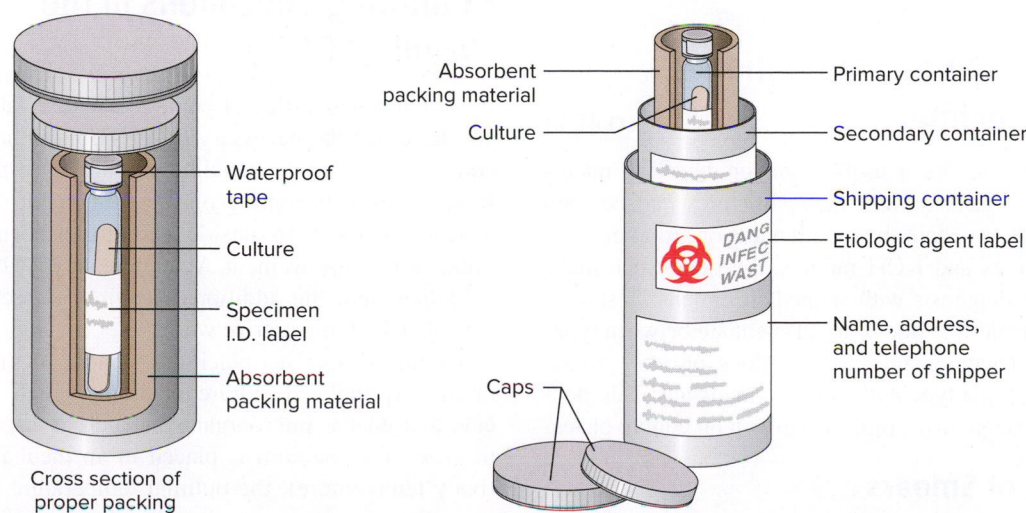

Waterproof tape
Culture
Specimen I.D. label
Absorbent packing material

Cross section of proper packing

Absorbent packing material
Culture
Primary container
Secondary container
Shipping container
Etiologic agent label
Name, address, and telephone number of shipper
Caps

DANGER INFECTIOUS WASTE

FIGURE 46-11 When packaging and labeling a specimen for mail delivery, you must follow the procedures set by the CDC, based on US Public Health Service regulations.

examination of microbiologic specimens are preparing wet mounts and preparing potassium hydroxide (KOH) mounts. You may be required to perform these procedures as part of your duties.

Wet Mounts

A wet mount permits quick identification of many microorganisms and is easy to prepare.

1. Wearing examination gloves, mix a small amount of the specimen with a drop of normal saline (0.9% sodium chloride [NaCl] solution) on a glass slide.
2. Apply a coverslip over the mixture.
3. Give the slide to the doctor for direct examination under the microscope.

If you obtain a specimen from a body site that is normally sterile, detection of microorganisms on a wet mount immediately tells the doctor whether there is infection. Wet mounts are also useful in determining whether a microorganism is motile, which helps in identifying the microorganisms.

Potassium Hydroxide (KOH) Mounts

A **KOH mount** is a type of wet mount used when a physician suspects that a patient has a fungal infection of the skin, nails, hair, or vagina. It is difficult to visualize a fungus directly in these types of specimens because the body produces a tough, hard protein called keratin, which often masks any fungus present. The chemical potassium hydroxide (KOH) is added to the specimen to dissolve the keratin and allow visualization of any fungus.

To prepare a KOH mount, follow these steps:

1. Wearing examination gloves, suspend the specimen in a drop of 10% KOH on a glass slide.
2. Apply a coverslip.
3. Allow the specimen to sit at room temperature for 30 minutes to dissolve the keratin.
4. Provide the physician with the slide to examine for microscopic evidence of fungal structures.

▶ Preparation and Examination of Stained Specimens   LO 46.13

Although wet mounts are a useful tool for detecting microorganisms, microorganisms and their structures can be seen more clearly when you stain them with a dye or group of dyes. As with wet mounts and KOH mounts, the doctor can make a quick, tentative diagnosis with stained specimens. A stained specimen also enables the doctor to differentiate between types of infections, like bacterial and yeast infections, or between bacterial infections of one type and another. Stains also help doctors identify microorganisms that have grown on culture plates.

Preparation of Smears

The first step in staining a microbiologic specimen is to prepare a smear. To do so, simply apply a small amount of the specimen in a thin layer on a glass slide. Allow the sample to dry and

then briefly heat the slide to "fix" the sample to the slide so that it does not wash off during the staining process. The steps are described in detail in Procedure 46-4 at the end of this chapter.

Gram Stain

The Gram stain is the most frequently used stain for microscopic examination of bacteriologic specimens. This stain is a moderate-complexity test that you may assist with in the medical office if you have additional training. The steps for performing a Gram stain are outlined in Procedure 46-5 at the end of this chapter.

A Gram stain involves performing a series of staining and washing steps on the heat-fixed smear. First, apply a purple stain called crystal violet (also known as gentian violet) to the smear. After washing the slide in water, apply iodine. The iodine acts as a **mordant,** a substance that fixes a stain, keeping it from being washed away. Iodine helps bind the dye to the bacterial cell wall.

After washing the slide again in water, apply a decolorizing solution (alcohol or acetone-alcohol). As you learned earlier in the chapter, certain bacterial species retain the purple dye even after the decolorizer is added. These bacteria appear blue or violet and are Gram-positive. (positive because they retained the purple dye).

Other bacteria lose their purple color when the decolorizer is added. To allow the physician to visualize these bacteria, apply a red counterstain (safranin) to the smear. Bacteria that lose the purple color and pick up the red color of the safranin are Gram-negative. Figure 46-12 illustrates Gram-positive and Gram-negative bacteria. It is important that you follow each step in the Gram stain process carefully to reduce the likelihood of misidentifying the microorganisms.

On the basis of a bacterium's staining characteristics and the shape and arrangement of cells, the physician can make a presumptive identification of an organism. For example, clusters of cocci that appear Gram-positive typically suggest an infection with staphylococci.

▶ Culturing Specimens in the Medical Office   LO 46.14

If your medical office is equipped with a laboratory and if you have had the necessary on-the-job training or additional courses, you may be required to culture certain specimens. It is, however, becoming more common for doctors' offices to send specimens to outside laboratories because of Clinical Laboratory Improvement Amendments of 1988 (CLIA '88) guidelines and the additional requirements concerning personnel and administrative work.

Culturing involves placing a sample of the specimen on or in a specialized culture medium, which contains nutrients that enable microorganisms such as bacteria and fungi to grow. The medium is placed in an incubator set at 37°C (body temperature), the optimal temperature for growth. As the microorganism multiplies, a **colony**—a distinct group of the organisms—can be seen on the culture medium's surface. The microorganism is identified according to the colony

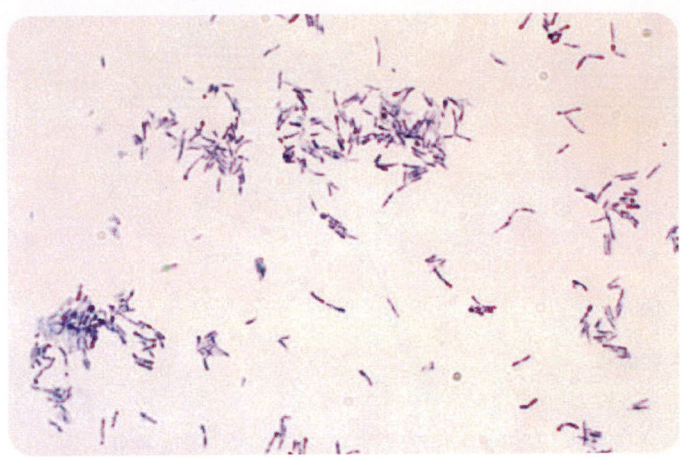

(a)

(b)

FIGURE 46-12 (a) Gram-positive organisms appear blue or violet after staining. (b) Gram-negative organisms appear red.
(a) CDC/P.B. Smith; (b) CDC

appearance, its staining characteristics, and certain biochemical reactions. A microorganism's biochemical reactions are determined by their growth on specific types of culture media.

Culture Media

Culture media come in liquid, semisolid, and solid forms. In the medical office, you will most likely work with a semisolid. The medium contains **agar,** a gelatin-like substance derived from seaweed, which gives the medium its consistency. This form of medium comes commercially prepared in culture plates—round, covered, glass or plastic dishes called *petri dishes.*

Handle petri dishes on the outside only, so that they do not become contaminated. You can avoid introducing contaminants by storing the petri dishes with the agar side up. Use the palm of your hand to pick up the agar-containing part of the dish when you are ready to inoculate it with a specimen.

Types of Media Many different types of semisolid media are commercially available. The type of medium used for culturing depends on the type of suspected organism and the site from which the specimen is obtained. Some types—called selective media—allow (select for) the growth of certain kinds of bacteria while inhibiting the growth of others. Selective

media are commonly used for specimens that normally contain bacteria, such as stool or vaginal samples. This is so that you can select for pathogenic organisms and not grow those that you expect to find.

Other types of media support the growth of most organisms and are referred to as nonselective media. The most common type of culture medium used in the laboratory is blood agar, a nonselective medium. Blood agar gets its red color from sheep's blood. Comparing the growth of a specimen on selective and nonselective media often provides important information about the microorganisms present.

You will typically use a blood agar plate when you culture a throat swab specimen. The organism that causes strep throat (*Streptococcus pyogenes*) can be identified when it grows on blood agar because it destroys the blood cells (hemolysis) in the agar, leaving a clear zone surrounding each colony.

Special Culture Units Small physicians' office laboratories often use commercial culture units with specific culturing purposes. Units for performing rapid urine culture, such as Uricult® (manufactured by Orion Diagnostica, Somerset, New Jersey), are typical. Uricult® consists of a small vial with a double-sided paddle attached to a screw-on top (Figure 46-13). Each side of the paddle contains a different type of medium on its surface. To culture a urine specimen, simply dip the media paddle into the clean-catch mid-stream urine specimen or catheterized specimen, coating both sides of the paddle. Then remove the paddle from the specimen, screw it into the vial, and place it upright in the incubator for 18 to 24 hours. If bacteria are present, they will grow on the surfaces of the media. Other units for culturing urine, throat specimens, vaginal specimens, and blood are also simple to use. These units usually enable you to obtain an estimate of the number of bacteria in the sample in addition to identifying the bacteria.

Inoculating a Culture Plate

Inoculating a culture plate involves transferring some or all of the specimen onto the plate. Before inoculating a plate, label it

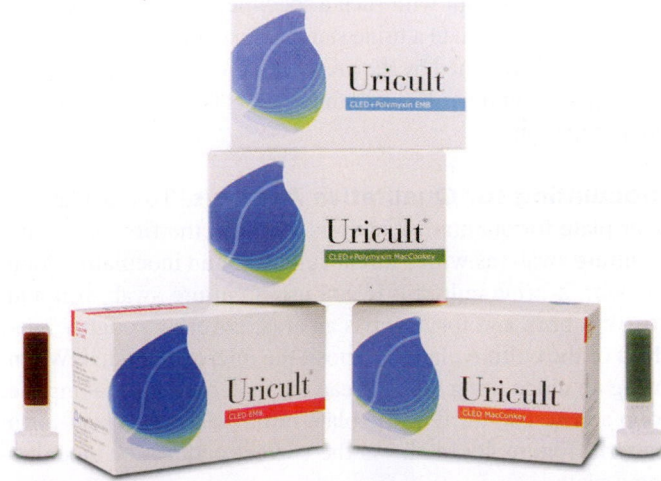

FIGURE 46-13 The Uricult® is one type of urine culture device consists of a lid and attached, double-sided paddle that screws into a vial.
Courtesy Orion Diagnostica

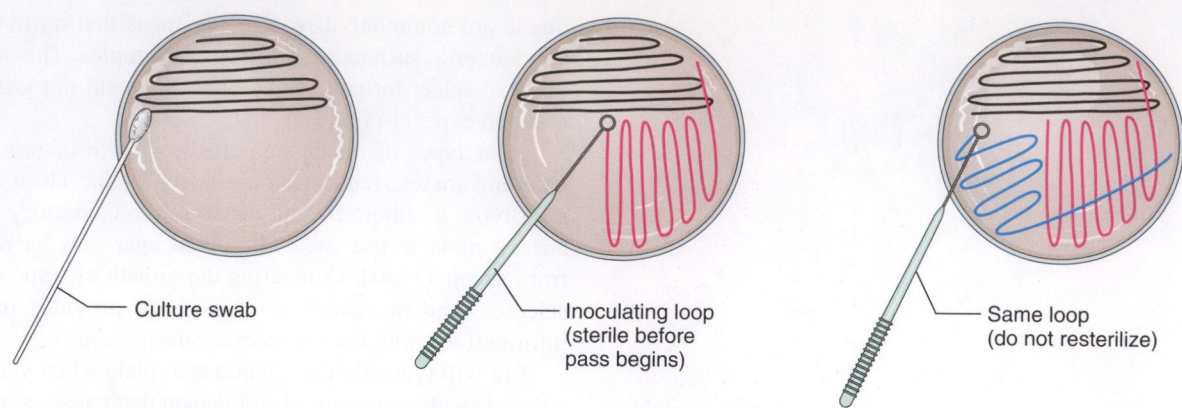

FIGURE 46-14 When inoculating a plate for qualitative analysis, roll and streak the culture swab or streak the inoculating loop of specimen material across one-third of the surface of the culture plate. Begin the next pass with a sterile loop.

on the bottom (agar side) rather than the lid because the lid can be lost or switched. Write close to the edge to avoid obscuring colony identification. Label the plate with the patient's name, doctor's name, source of the sample, date and time of inoculation, and your initials. You can apply a label or write the information with a grease pencil or permanent marker.

In the case of a specimen swab, inoculate the plate by streaking the swab across the plate. Bacterial colonies can be identified by their appearance. This determination of the type of pathogen is referred to as a qualitative analysis of the specimen.

To perform a qualitative analysis of a specimen such as urine, introduce only a small portion of the specimen onto the plate. A calibrated inoculating loop is used for this purpose. A loop is a small circle of wire or plastic attached to a long handle. When this loop is dipped into the specimen, a small, specific amount of liquid can be transferred to the plate. Different sizes of calibrated loops deliver different volumes of fluid. For example, calibrated loops may allow you to pick up either 0.01 or 0.001 milliliter of liquid.

In addition, you may need to perform a separate determination—called a quantitative analysis—of the number of bacteria present in specimens such as urine. A quantitative analysis is important with such a specimen because a few bacteria may contaminate a urine sample during collection. A true infection is confirmed by the presence of a specified number of bacteria; any number beneath this level is typically considered contamination.

Inoculating for Qualitative Analysis

To inoculate an agar plate for qualitative analysis, perform the first pass with a culture swab (as with a throat culture) or an inoculating loop (as with a urine culture). If you use a culture swab, roll and streak it back and forth across an area, covering roughly one-third of the culture plate to deposit the microorganisms. When using an inoculating loop, spread the material by streaking the loop across one-third of the plate in the same back-and-forth pattern. Figure 46-14 shows the correct pattern for inoculating a plate.

Because there may be several microorganisms in the specimen, you need to streak the inoculated (firstpass) area with a sterile loop to separate out individual colonies that can be

identified on the remaining areas of the culture plate. Unless you use a sterile disposable loop, first sterilize the loop by heating it in a bacterial loop incinerator until it glows red. Allow the loop to cool and then pass it once across the inoculated area of the plate to pick up a small number of microorganisms. Then streak it in a back-and-forth pattern over the second one-third of the plate. Next, sterilize the loop again, pass it once across the second inoculated area of the plate, and then streak it back and forth over the last one-third of the plate. Each successive pass reduces the microorganism concentration. This procedure allows isolated colonies, or colony-forming units, to be observed in the area of the last pass of the loop, as Figure 46-15 shows.

For throat cultures, the physician may simply want you to screen the sample for the presence of streptococcal organisms. You may not need to use a loop to spread the microorganisms; the swab will be sufficient, as described in Procedure 46-1, at the end of this chapter, when preparing the specimen for screening.

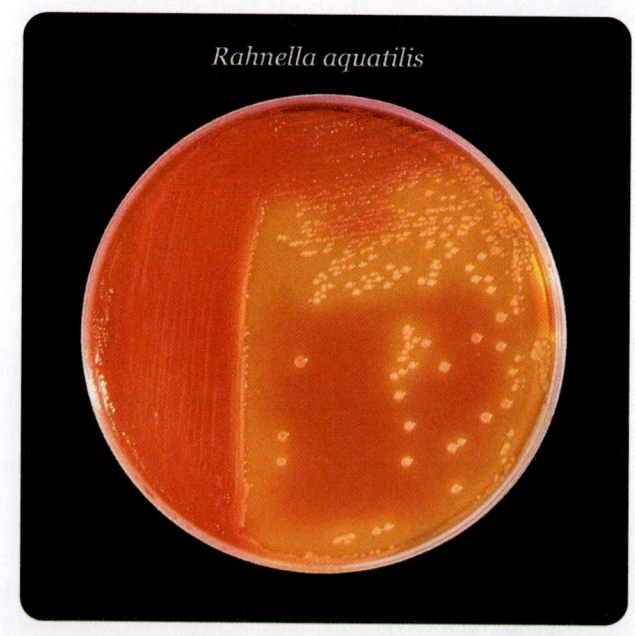

Rahnella aquatilis

FIGURE 46-15 You can see individual colony-forming units in the last third of an inoculated culture plate.
CDC

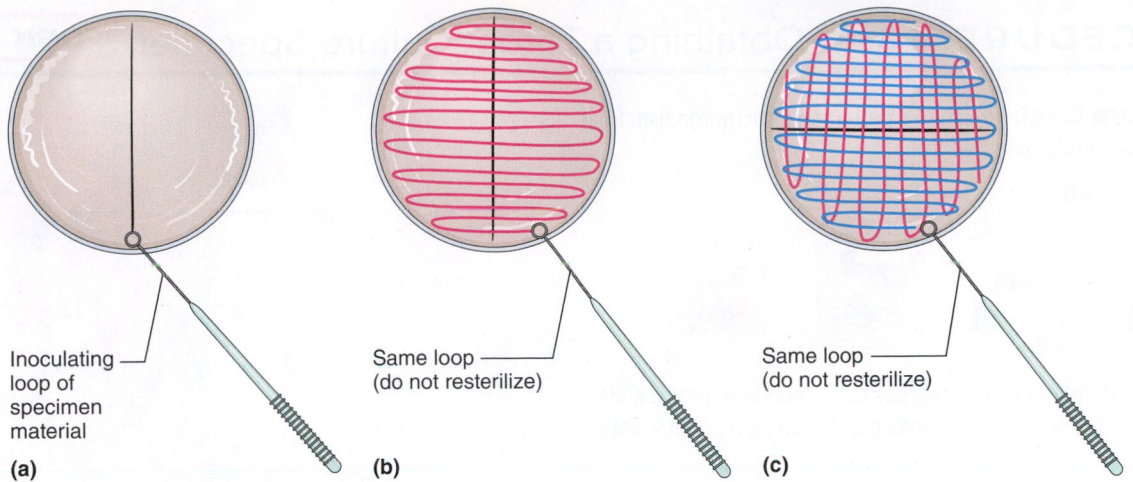

(a) Inoculating loop of specimen material

(b) Same loop (do not resterilize)

(c) Same loop (do not resterilize)

FIGURE 46-16 When inoculating a plate for quantitative analysis, (a) streak the loop down the center of the plate. Next, (b) streak the loop at right angles to the first inoculation. Then, (c) turn the plate 90° and streak the entire surface once more.

Inoculating for Quantitative Analysis To perform a quantitative analysis of a urine specimen, use a calibrated loop to withdraw a portion of urine from the sample. Be sure the urine specimen is well mixed before taking the sample, as the microorganisms may settle to the bottom of the specimen cup. Sterilize, cool, and dip the calibrated loop into the sample. Transfer the entire volume to the surface of an agar plate by making a single streak down the center of the plate. Next, spread the specimen evenly across the plate at a right angle to the initial streak, using the same loop (without sterilizing it). Turn the plate and spread the material again, at a right angle to the last streak, over the entire surface. Figure 46-16 illustrates this technique.

After the microorganisms are allowed to grow for 24 hours, estimate the number of microorganisms by counting the number of colonies that appear on the surface of the plate. For example, if you use a 0.001 milliliter calibrated loop to streak the plate and 50 colonies grow, multiply the 50 colonies by 1,000 to obtain the number of colonies per milliliter. In this case, you would estimate there are 50,000 colony-forming units per milliliter of urine. You must be especially careful that your counts and calculations are correct so that the doctor has accurate information on which to base a diagnosis.

Incubating Culture Plates

After inoculating a plate, place it in an incubator set at 35°C (95°F) to 37°C (98.6°F) (human body temperature) to allow the bacteria to grow. Plates are always incubated with the agar side up, so that any moisture that collects in the plate will fall on the inside of the lid and not on the microbes growing on the surface of the agar. How long plates are allowed to incubate varies with the type of culture. Most bacteria grow sufficiently within 24 hours, but some require 48 hours. Fungi typically take longer to grow than bacteria and may grow at a slightly lower temperature (95°F to 96.8°F).

Interpreting Cultures

After incubation, cultures are assessed for growth and are interpreted. This process requires considerable skill and practice because pathogens must often be differentiated from resident normal flora. This step may be performed by the physician, a microbiologist, or a technician who has been properly trained to do so through on-the-job training or additional coursework.

The process of interpreting a culture typically involves several determinations. The characteristics of the colonies growing on the agar are noted, along with their relative numbers. In addition, any changes in the media surrounding the colonies are noted because changes may reflect certain characteristics of the microorganism.

The physician decides at this point whether additional procedures are required. In the case of a throat culture, the presence of colonies of a characteristic shape, size, and color, surrounded by areas of hemolysis, suggests strep throat, as shown in Figure 46-17. A Gram stain and determination of bacterial shape may be all that is necessary for a confirmed diagnosis. Many cultures, however, require additional biochemical and, in some cases, serologic tests for definitive pathogen identification. Since this is an advanced skill, either the physician or an outside microbiology laboratory will make the final interpretation of the cultured microorganism.

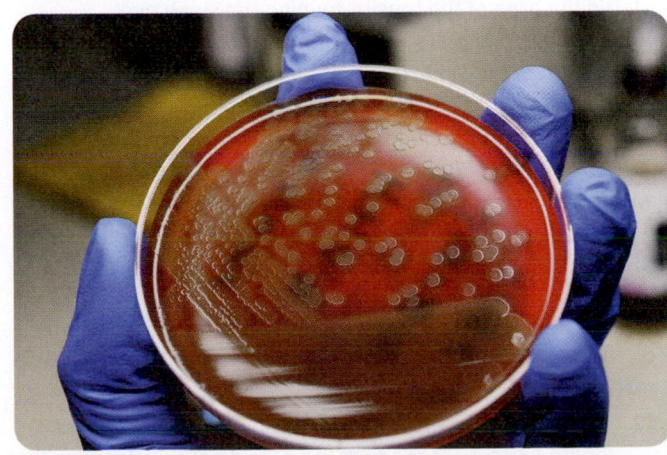

FIGURE 46-17 A positive strep throat culture contains distinctive colonies surrounded by areas of hemolysis.
© R Parulan Jr./Getty Images RF

PROCEDURE 46-1 Obtaining a Throat Culture Specimen WORK // DOC

Procedure Goal: To isolate a pathogenic microorganism from the throat or to rule out strep throat

OSHA Guidelines:

Materials: Patient chart/progress note, tongue depressor, sterile collection system or sterile swab plus blood agar culture plate

Method:

1. Identify the patient, introduce yourself, and explain the procedure.

2. Assemble the necessary supplies; label the culture plate if used.

3. Wash your hands and don examination gloves, goggles, and a mask or face shield.
   RATIONALE: *The patient may cough while you swab the throat.*

4. Have the patient assume a sitting position. (Having a small child lie down rather than sit may make the process easier. If the child refuses to open the mouth, gently squeeze the nostrils shut. The child will eventually open the mouth to breathe. Enlist the help of the parent to restrain the child's hands if necessary.)

5. Open the collection system or sterile swab package by peeling the wrapper halfway down; remove the swab with your dominant hand.

6. Ask the patient to tilt back her head and open her mouth as wide as possible.

7. With your other hand, depress the patient's tongue with the tongue depressor.

8. Ask the patient to say "Ah."

9. Insert the swab and quickly swab the back of the throat in the area of the tonsils, twirling the swab over representative areas on both sides of the throat. Avoid touching the uvula (the soft tissue hanging from the roof of the mouth), the cheeks, or the tongue.
   RATIONALE: *Touching these areas will contaminate the specimen.*

10. Remove the swab and then the tongue depressor from the patient's mouth.

11. Discard the tongue depressor in a biohazardous waste container.

To Transport the Specimen to a Reference Laboratory

12. Immediately insert the swab back into the plastic sleeve, being careful not to touch the outside of the sleeve with the swab.

13. Crush the vial of transport medium to moisten the tip of the swab.

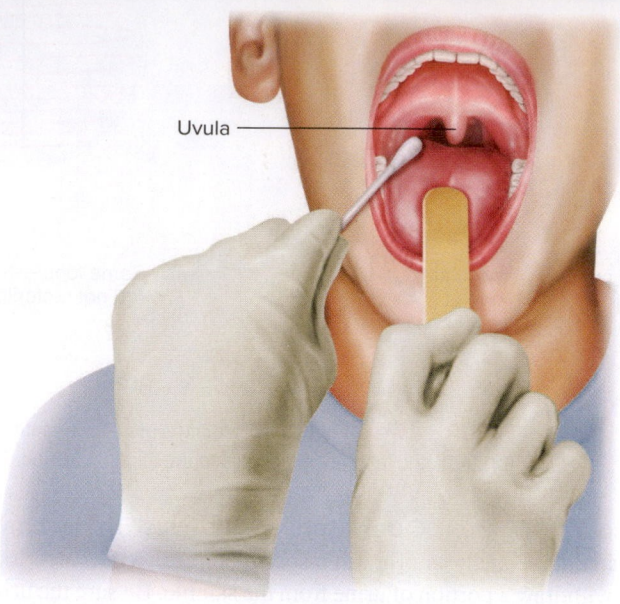

Uvula

FIGURE Procedure 46-1 Step 9   When obtaining a throat culture specimen, swab the back of the throat in the area of the tonsils on each side, taking care to avoid touching the uvula.

RATIONALE: *To keep the microorganisms alive during transport.*

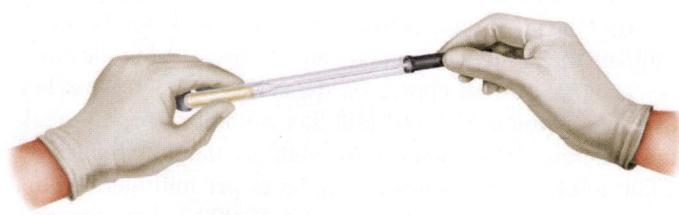

FIGURE Procedure 46-1 Step 13   The transport medium released from the crushed capsule keeps microorganisms alive while in transit to the laboratory for culturing.

14. Label the collection system and arrange for transport to the laboratory.

To Prepare the Specimen for Evaluation in the Physician's Office Laboratory

12. Immediately inoculate the culture plate with the swab, using a back-and-forth motion.

13. Discard the swab in a biohazardous waste container.

14. Place the culture plate in the incubator.

When Finished with All Specimens

15. Remove the gloves and wash your hands.

16. Document the procedure in the patient's chart.

PROCEDURE 46-2 Performing a Quick Strep A Test on a Throat Specimen

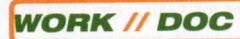

Procedure Goal: To determine the presence of strep A antigen in a throat specimen

OSHA Guidelines:

Materials: Patient chart/progress note, strep A testing kit, throat swab specimen, and a timer or watch

Method:

1. Review the laboratory requisition form and gather the supplies.
2. Confirm the patient's identity, introduce yourself, and explain the procedure.
3. Wash your hands and don gloves, goggles, and a mask or face shield.
4. Open the strep A testing kit and check the expiration date on the kit.
5. Obtain a throat specimen with a sterile swab, being careful not to touch the tongue, teeth, or cheeks.
   RATIONALE: *Swabbing only the throat reduces the likelihood of getting a false positive test result.*
6. Complete the quality control tests provided with the testing kit.
   RATIONALE: *To ensure the test is working correctly*
7. Put the required amount of the first reagent in the test tube or testing device provided in the kit.
8. Place the swab into the test tube or testing device. Following the manufacturer's instructions, swirl the swab and press it against the sides of the tube or device.
9. Add the second reagent as directed.
10. Read the results at the required time.
11. Dispose of testing supplies in the appropriate waste container according to OSHA requirements.
12. Remove your gloves and wash your hands.
13. Document the results in the patient's chart.

PROCEDURE 46-3 Preparing Microbiologic Specimens for Transport to an Outside Laboratory

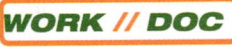

Procedure Goal: To properly prepare a microbiologic specimen for transport to an outside laboratory

OSHA Guidelines:

   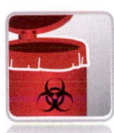

Materials:
Specimen-collection device, requisition form, secondary container or a zipper-type plastic bag

Method:

1. Wash your hands and don examination gloves (and goggles and a mask or face shield if you are collecting a microbiologic throat culture specimen).
2. Obtain the microbiologic culture specimen.
   a. Use the collection system specified by the outside laboratory for the test requested.
   b. Label the microbiologic specimen-collection device at the time of collection.
   c. Collect the microbiologic specimen according to the guidelines provided by the laboratory and office procedure.
   RATIONALE: *To ensure the specimen is correctly collected and handled.*
3. Remove the gloves and wash your hands.
4. Complete the test requisition form.
5. Place the microbiologic specimen container in a secondary container or zipper-type plastic bag.
   RATIONALE: *To prevent contaminating anyone who handles the specimen during transport.*
6. Attach the test requisition form to the outside of the secondary container or bag, per laboratory policy.
7. Log the microbiologic specimen in the list of outgoing specimens.
   RATIONALE: *So that you can follow up on lab tests sent to outside laboratories.*
8. Store the microbiologic specimen according to guidelines provided by the laboratory for that type of specimen (for example, refrigerated, frozen, or 37°C).
9. Call the laboratory for pickup of the microbiologic specimen, or hold it until the next scheduled pickup.
10. At the time of pickup, ensure that the carrier takes all microbiologic specimens that are logged and scheduled to be picked up.
11. If you are ever unsure about collection or transportation details, call the laboratory.

PROCEDURE 46-4 Preparing a Microbiologic Specimen Smear

Procedure Goal: To prepare a smear of a microbiologic specimen for staining

OSHA Guidelines:

   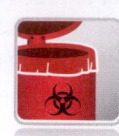

Materials: Glass slide with frosted end, pencil, specimen swab, Bunsen burner, and forceps

Method:

1. Wash your hands and don exam gloves.

2. Assemble all the necessary items.

3. Use a pencil to label the frosted end of the slide with the patient's name.

4. Roll the specimen swab evenly over the smooth part of the slide, making sure all areas of the swab touch the slide.
   RATIONALE: *To make sure a representative specimen is transferred to the slide.*

5. Discard the swab in a biohazardous waste container. (Retain the microbiologic specimen for culture as necessary or according to office policy.)

6. Allow the smear to air-dry. Do not wave the slide to dry it.
   RATIONALE: *Waving the slide may spread pathogens or contaminate the slide.*

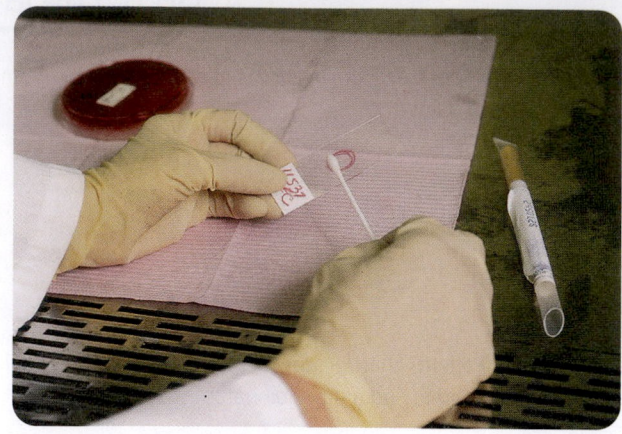

FIGURE Procedure 46-4 Step 4   Rolling the swab ensures that representative microorganisms collected on it are deposited on the slide. © Cliff Moore

7. Heat-fix the slide by holding the frosted end with forceps and passing the clear part of the slide, with the smear side up, through the flame of a Bunsen burner three or four times. (Your office may use an alternate procedure for fixing the slide, such as flooding the smear with alcohol, allowing it to sit for a few minutes, and either pouring off the remaining liquid or allowing the smear to air-dry. Chlamydia slides come with their own fixative.)
   RATIONALE: *The specimen must be fixed to the slide to prevent washing the microorganism off during staining or handling.*

8. Allow the slide to cool before the smear is stained.

9. Return the materials to their proper location.

10. Remove the gloves and wash your hands.

PROCEDURE 46-5 Performing a Gram Stain

Procedure Goal: To make bacteria present in a specimen smear visible for microscopic identification

OSHA Guidelines:

Materials: Heat-fixed smear, slide staining rack and tray, crystal violet dye, iodine solution, alcohol or acetone-alcohol decolorizer, safranin dye, wash bottle filled with water, forceps, and blotting paper or paper towels (optional)

Method:

1. Assemble all the necessary supplies.

2. Wash your hands and don examination gloves.

3. Place the heat-fixed smear on a level staining rack and tray, smear side up.

4. Completely cover the specimen area of the slide with the crystal violet stain.

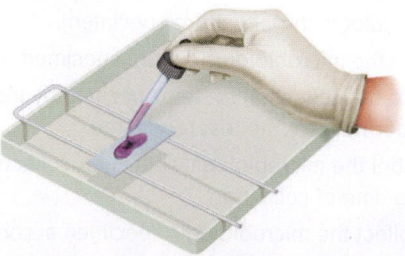

FIGURE Procedure 46-5 Step 4   Apply crystal violet. Wait 1 minute.

(Many commercially available Gram stain solutions have flip-up bottle caps that allow you to dispense stain by the drop. If the stain bottle you are using does not have an attached dropper cap, use an eyedropper.)

5. Allow the stain to sit for 1 minute; rinse the slide thoroughly with water from the wash bottle.

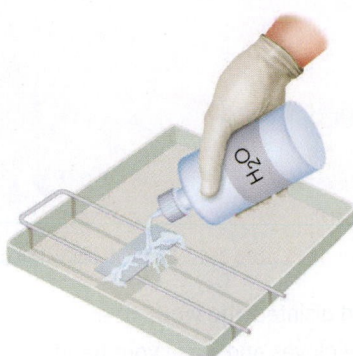

FIGURE Procedure 46-5 Step 5   Wash the slide with water.

RATIONALE: *Rinsing the slide after 1 minute stops the staining process and prevents overstaining.*

6. Use the forceps to hold the slide at the frosted end, tilting the slide to remove excess water.

7. Place the slide flat on the rack again and completely cover the specimen area with iodine solution.

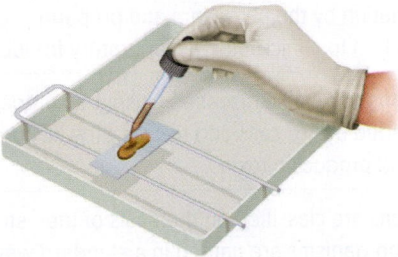

FIGURE Procedure 46-5 Step 7   Apply iodine solution. Wait 1 minute.

8. Allow the iodine to remain for 1 minute; rinse the slide thoroughly with water.
   RATIONALE: *The iodine helps increase cell staining.*

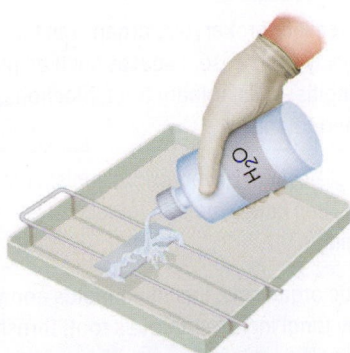

FIGURE Procedure 46-5 Step 8   Rinse the slide with water.

9. Use the forceps or a gloved hand to hold and tilt the slide to remove excess water.

10. While still tilting the slide, apply the alcohol or decolorizer drop by drop until no more purple color washes off. (This step usually takes 10 seconds to 30 seconds.)
    RATIONALE: *The decolorizing step is essential for differentiation between Gram-positive and Gram-negative bacteria.*

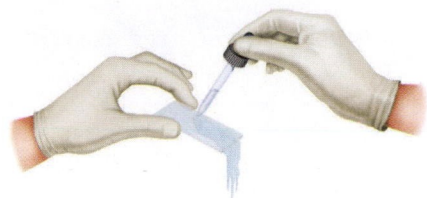

FIGURE Procedure 46-5 Step 10   Apply decolorizing solution.

11. Rinse the slide thoroughly with water; use the forceps to hold and tip the slide to remove excess water.

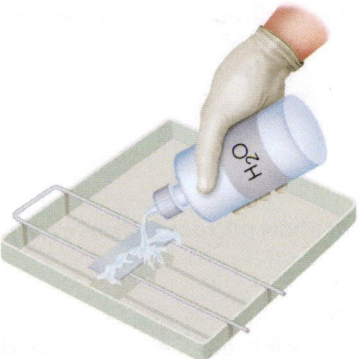

FIGURE Procedure 46-5 Step 11   Wash the slide with water.

12. Completely cover the specimen with safranin dye.

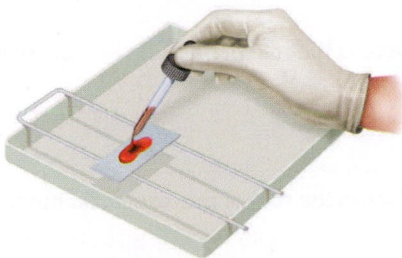

FIGURE Procedure 46-5 Step 12   Apply safranin dye to the slide. Wait 1 minute.

13. Allow the safranin to remain for 1 minute; rinse the slide thoroughly with water.
RATIONALE: *To counterstain the specimen so that Gram-negative organisms can be visualized.*

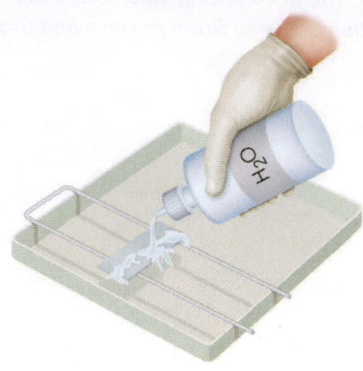

FIGURE Procedure 46-5 Step 13   Rinse the slide with water.

14. Use the forceps to hold the stained smear by the frosted end and carefully wipe the back of the slide to remove excess stain.

15. Place the smear in a vertical position and allow it to air-dry or blot it lightly between blotting paper to hasten drying. Take care not to rub the slide, or the specimen may be damaged.

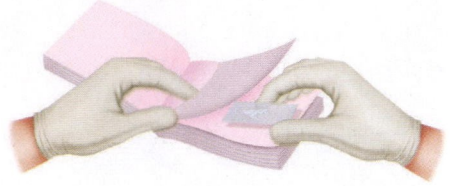

FIGURE Procedure 46-5 Step 15   Blot and allow the slide to air-dry.

16. Sanitize and disinfect the work area.

17. Remove the gloves and wash your hands.

SUMMARY OF LEARNING OUTCOMES

LEARNING OUTCOMES	KEY POINTS
46.1 Explain the medical assistant's role in microbiology.	As an office medical assistant, you may assist the physician with several microbiologic procedures that aid in diagnosing and treating infectious diseases, including obtaining specimens or assisting the physician in doing so; preparing specimens for direct examination by the physician; and preparing specimens for transportation to a microbiology laboratory for identification.
46.2 Summarize how microorganisms cause disease.	Microorganisms can cause disease by using up nutrients or other materials needed by the cells and tissues they invade, damaging body cells, and producing toxins.
46.3 Describe how microorganisms are classified and named.	Microorganisms are classified on the basis of their structure. Specific microorganisms are named in a standard way, using the genus (a category of biologic classification between the family and the species) to which the microorganism belongs and the particular species of the organism.
46.4 Discuss the role of viruses in human disease.	Viruses are among the smallest known infectious agents causing common diseases, including the common cold, influenza, chickenpox, croup, hepatitis, and warts.
46.5 Discuss the role of bacteria in human disease.	Bacteria are single-celled, prokaryotic organisms that reproduce very quickly and cause diseases such as pneumonia, tuberculosis, meningitis, boils, urinary tract infections, Lyme disease, cholera, and tetanus.
46.6 Discuss the role of protozoans in human disease.	Protozoans are single-celled, eukaryotic organisms found in soil and water. They can cause malaria, amebic dysentery, and trichomoniasis vaginitis.
46.7 Discuss the role of fungi in human disease.	Fungi are eukaryotic organisms, including molds and yeasts. Diseases caused by fungi include athlete's foot, thrush, ringworm, and vaginal yeast infections.

LEARNING OUTCOMES	KEY POINTS
46.8 **Discuss the role of multicellular parasites in human disease.**	Multicellular parasites include roundworms, tapeworms, flatworms, ticks, lice, and mites.
46.9 **Describe the process involved in diagnosing an infection.**	The steps involved in diagnosing an infection are to examine the patient, obtain one or more specimens, examine the specimen directly by either wet mount or smear, culture the specimen, and determine the culture's antibiotic sensitivity.
46.10 **Identify general guidelines for obtaining specimens.**	The general guidelines for obtaining specimens are to obtain the specimen with great care to avoid causing the patient harm, discomfort, or undue embarrassment; collect the material from a site; obtain the specimen at the proper time; use appropriate collection devices; obtain a sufficient quantity of the specimen; and obtain the specimen before antimicrobial therapy begins.
46.11 **Carry out the procedure for transporting specimens to outside laboratories.**	When transporting specimens to outside laboratories, the medical assistant should follow proper collection techniques using specific containers provided by the laboratory, maintain the samples in a state as close to their original as possible, and protect anyone who handles a specimen container from exposure to potentially infectious material.
46.12 **Compare two techniques used in the direct examination of culture specimens.**	Direct examination of culture specimens is accomplished in two ways: wet mounts and KOH mounts.
46.13 **Carry out the procedure for preparing and examining stained specimens.**	To prepare a stained specimen, the medical assistant must first prepare a smear, fix the sample to the slide so that it does not wash off during the staining process, and follow a specific staining procedure. The sample is then observed under a microscope for certain characteristics.
46.14 **Carry out the procedure for culturing specimens in the medical office.**	To culture a specimen, the medical assistant should place a sample of the specimen on or in a specialized culture medium and allow it to grow in an incubator for 24 to 48 hours.

CASE STUDY CRITICAL THINKING

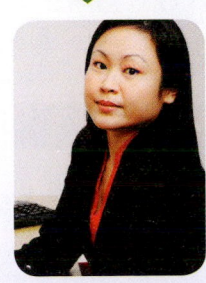

© Red Chopsticks/Getty Images RF

Recall Cindy Chen from the beginning of the chapter. Now that you have completed the chapter, answer the following questions regarding her case.

1. Why are Cindy's helper T cells being tested?
2. As Cindy's HIV infection progresses, what symptoms might she exhibit?
3. What special precautions should you take when drawing Cindy's blood?
4. Why do you think Dr. Whalen asked you to send the throat culture to the reference lab instead of doing a rapid strep test in the POL?

1. (LO 46.1) Microorganisms normally found on the skin and other body tissues are known as
   a. Tissue pathogens
   b. Viruses
   c. Resident normal flora
   d. Colonies
   e. Infections

2. (LO 46.3) Which of the following is an example of a subcellular microorganism?
   a. Bacterium
   b. Virus
   c. Fungus
   d. Helminth
   e. Multicellular organism

3. (LO 46.9) A specimen that is spread thinly and evenly across a slide is a
   a. Smear   d. Medium
   b. Wet prep   e. Streak
   c. Culture

4. (LO 46.12) A KOH mount is used to detect which of the following?
   a. Gonococci   d. Pinworms
   b. Fungi   e. HIV
   c. Viruses

5. (LO 46.10) Which of the following is an appropriate guideline for collecting specimens?
   a. The specimen label includes the patient's name and number, source of specimen, date and time, doctor's name, and your initials
   b. The best location to obtain a throat culture to diagnose strep throat is from the sides of the throat
   c. When a patient is collecting a specimen on her own, you should trust that she knows how to do it without an explanation
   d. When a patient is taking an antibiotic, you should never obtain a specimen
   e. Allow the patient to use a container from home to collect a sputum specimen

6. (LO 46.2) Organisms capable of causing disease are known as
   a. Commensals
   b. Flora
   c. Pathogens
   d. Facultative
   e. Aerobes

7. (LO 46.4) Infectious mononucleosis is caused by which of the following?
   a. Adenovirus
   b. Parvovirus
   c. Norovirus
   d. Epstein-Barr virus
   e. Rotavirus

8. (LO 46.7) Athlete's foot, thrush, and ringworm are all caused by types of
   a. Prions
   b. Parasites
   c. Bacteria
   d. Viruses
   e. Fungi

9. (LO 46.13) A substance that fixes a stain, keeping it from being washed away, is a
   a. Mordant
   b. Substrate
   c. Wash
   d. Dye
   e. Counterstain

10. (LO 46.8) An organism that lives on or in another organism and uses that other organism for its own nourishment is a(n)
    a. Obligate
    b. Eukaryote
    c. Resident
    d. Parasite
    e. Prokaryote

S O F T   S K I L L S   S U C C E S S

Recall Cindy Chen from the case study at the beginning of the chapter. After drawing Cindy's blood, you leave her lab requisition on the counter at the front of the lab while you escort her to the front office. When you return, Charlie Goodpasture is waiting to have his blood drawn for routine lab work. You notice he is glancing at the lab requisition you left on the counter. He asks you if that was Cindy Chen he saw. He also tells you that he knew Cindy from phlebotomy school and she has lost a lot of weight. Charlie asks if Cindy is sick. How should you handle this situation? What should you have done differently?

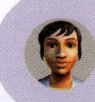

Go to PRACTICE MEDICAL OFFICE and complete the module Admin: Check Out - Privacy and Liability.

Collecting, Processing, and Testing Urine and Stool Specimens

47

CASE STUDY

PATIENT INFORMATION

Patient Name	DOB	Allergies
Ken Washington	12/1/19XX	Sulfa

Attending	MRN	Other Information
Paul F. Buckwalter, MD	891-12-743	Vital Signs: BP 142/88, T 99.2, P 76, R 16

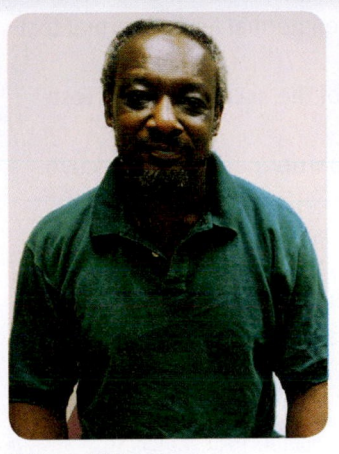

© McGraw-Hill Education

Ken Washington, a 61-year-old male patient, arrived today for a follow-up visit from a recent hospitalization for a stroke. Up until this hospitalization, he has had no major health issues. He now has weakness in his left arm and his speech is difficult to understand. His wife tells you that she has noticed some blood in the toilet after he urinates. She also tells you that he has had some pain when he urinates and often only urinates a small amount. Dr. Buckwalter would like for you to obtain a urine sample for a reagent test and have Ken collect a 24-hour urine sample for analysis.

Keep Ken in mind as you study this chapter. There will be questions at the end of the chapter based on the case study. The information in the chapter will help you answer these questions.

McGraw Hill Education ACTIVSim

LEARNING OUTCOMES

After completing Chapter 47, you will be able to:

47.1 Discuss the role of the medical assistant in collecting, processing, and testing urine and stool samples.

47.2 Carry out procedures for collecting urine specimens according to guidelines.

47.3 Describe the process of urinalysis and its purpose.

47.4 Carry out the proper procedure for collecting and processing a stool sample for fecal occult blood testing.

KEY TERMS

- anuria
- cast
- catheterization
- clean-catch mid-stream urine specimen
- crystal
- fecal occult blood test (FOBT)
- first morning urine specimen
- glycosuria
- hematuria
- O&P specimen
- oliguria
- proteinuria
- refractometer
- supernatant
- 24-hour urine specimen
- urinalysis
- urinary pH
- urine culture
- urine specific gravity
- urobilinogen

I.P.8 Instruct and prepare a patient for a procedure or a treatment

I.P.11 Obtain specimens and perform:
(c) CLIA waived urinalysis

I.A.3 Show awareness of a patient's concerns related to the procedure being performed

II.P.2 Differentiate between normal and abnormal test results

II.A.1 Reassure a patient of the accuracy of the test results

III.P.2 Select appropriate barrier/personal protective equipment (PPE)

III.A.1 Recognize the implications for failure to comply with Centers for Disease Control (CDC) regulations in healthcare settings

X.P.3 Document patient care accurately in the medical record

3. **Medical Terminology**
   d. Define and use medical abbreviations when appropriate and acceptable

4. **Medical Law and Ethics**
   f. Comply with federal, state, and local health laws and regulations as they relate to healthcare settings

9. **Clinical Procedures**
   a. Practice standard precautions and perform disinfection/sterilization techniques
   e. Perform specialty procedures including but not limited to minor surgery, cardiac, respiratory, OB-GYN, neurological, gastroenterology
   j. Make adaptations with patients with special needs

10. **Medical Laboratory Procedures**
    a. Practice quality control
    b. Perform selected CLIA-waived tests that assist with diagnosis and treatment
       (1) Urinalysis
       (6) Kit testing
          a. Pregnancy
          c. Dip sticks
    c. Dispose of biohazardous materials
    e. Instruct patients in the collection of a clean-catch mid-stream urine specimen
       (1) Clean-catch mid-stream urine specimen (CCMS, 24-hour, etc.)
       (2) Collection of fecal specimen

▶ Introduction

Proper collection and testing of urine and stool (fecal) samples is a crucial step in the diagnostic process. The routine analysis of a urine specimen is a simple, noninvasive diagnostic test that provides a healthcare provider with a window to a patient's health. Many significant conditions may be noted as a result of the physical, chemical, and microscopic examinations of a patient's specimen. In this chapter, you will learn about various types of urine specimens and how to properly instruct or assist patients with their collection. Additionally, you will learn how to correctly process a specimen, including a random specimen and a chain-of-custody drug screen. You will learn to identify normal and abnormal constituents of urine samples and what may cause these abnormal elements to be present in a specimen. You also will learn about stool samples, which are collected for a variety of reasons, including detecting bacterial infections, detecting parasites, and screening for cancer. Teaching patients proper techniques for collecting stool samples is key to getting accurate test results.

▶ The Role of the Medical Assistant LO 47.1

In your role as a medical assistant, you will help collect, process, and test urine and stool specimens. To perform your duties, you need to know about the anatomy and physiology of the kidneys, how urine is formed, and what its normal contents are. You also will need to understand the anatomy and physiology of the digestive system. This information will help you collect various specimen types, process them, and perform tests on them. Be sure to review the anatomy and physiology of the urinary system and the digestive system in chapters *The Urinary System* and *The Digestive System*. Also, see Table 47-1 for a list of abbreviations commonly used in urine analysis and stool testing. Dealing with a variety of patient groups who require special care, including elderly patients and pediatric patients, also will be an important part of your job.

When obtaining and processing urine and stool specimens, you will deal with potentially infectious body waste. For this reason, you must take precautions to protect yourself, the

TABLE 47-1   Abbreviations Common to Urine Analysis and Stool Testing

BIL; bili; BR	bilirubin	RBCs	red blood cells
Ca	calcium	SPG; sp gr; sp.gr.	specific gravity
CC	clean-catch (urine)	U/A	urinalysis
CCMS	clean-catch, mid-stream (urine)	UBG	urobilinogen
CL VOID	clean voided specimen (urine)	U/C	urine culture
CrCl	creatinine clearance	UC	urinary catheter
CSU	catheter specimen (urine)	UC&S	urine culture and sensitivity
Cys	cysteine	UcaV	urinary calcium volume
CYS	cystoscopy	UCRE	urine creatinine
EMU	early morning urine(s)	UFC	urinary free cortisol
FOBT	Fecal occult blood test	UK	urine potassium
HCG; hcg; hCG	human chorionic gonadotropin	UNa	urinary sodium
IVP	intravenous pyelogram	Uosm	urine osmolarity
K	potassium	UTI	urinary tract infection
Na	sodium	UUN	urinary urea nitrogen
O&P	Ova and parasites	UV	urinary volume
pH	hydrogen ion concentration	Vol	volume
PKD	polycystic kidney disease	WBCs	white blood cells
PKU	phenylketonuria		

patient, and others in the environment from transmitting disease-causing microorganisms. Most medical offices use standard precautions when dealing with urine. (See the *Infection Control Fundamentals* chapter for detailed information on these precautions.) During all procedures, you must be sure to wear adequate personal protective equipment (PPE); handle and dispose of specimens properly; dispose of used supplies and equipment properly; and sanitize, disinfect, and/or sterilize all reusable equipment according to facility policy.

▶ Obtaining Urine Specimens   LO 47.2

It is essential to collect, store, and preserve urine specimens in ways that do not alter their physical, chemical, or microscopic properties. You must follow guidelines each time you obtain specimens and instruct patients in the proper guidelines to follow.

General Collection Guidelines

When you collect urine specimens from patients, follow these guidelines:

- Follow the procedure specified for the urine test that will be performed.
- Use the type of specimen container indicated by the laboratory. If a patient must bring in a specimen, be sure the container is provided by the licensed practitioner's office or that it's appropriate for the testing protocol. If you provide the patient with a container that contains a preservative, make sure the appropriate warning labels are attached. You also should warn patients that the additive may contain acid and they should take care not to spill the acid on themselves.

- Label the specimen container before giving it to the patient or on receipt of a container the patient provides. Include the patient's name, the licensed practitioner's name, the date and time of collection, and your initials. Label the side of the specimen container, not the lid, because lids may be lost or switched.
- If the patient is having an invasive test, such as catheterization, always explain the procedure to the patient completely, using simple, clear language.
- If you are assisting in the collection process, wash your hands before and after the procedure and wear gloves during the procedure.
- If the urine specimen needs to be transferred to another container or if it is to be sent to a reference lab for testing, use a urine transfer straw or provide the patient with a container that has a transfer straw integrated into the collection cup. Label the container.
- Complete all necessary paperwork, recording the collection in the patient's chart and making sure you use the correct laboratory request slip for the ordered test.

In many instances, patients need to collect a urine specimen at home. It is your responsibility to give patients instructions for obtaining the specific type of specimen. In addition, provide them with the following general instructions:

- Urinate into the container indicated by the laboratory. In most instances, urinate into a wide-mouthed, throw-away, spouted specimen container as instructed. Do not add anything to the container except the urine.
- If the collection container contains liquid or powdered preservative, do not pour it out.

- If any of the preservative spills on you, wash the area immediately and contact the licensed practitioner's office.

- Always refrigerate the labeled collection container or keep it in a cooler or pail filled with ice.

- Be sure to keep the lid on the container.

Specimen Types

Many different tests are performed on urine. You may need to obtain different types of specimens for different tests, such as quantitative analysis or qualitative analysis. A quantitative analysis is a test that measures the amount of a specific substance in the urine. A qualitative analysis simply indicates the presence (or absence) of a substance in urine. Specimens vary in two ways: in the method used to collect them and in the time frame in which they are collected.

Quality assurance is essential in the licensed practitioner's office laboratory. As discussed in the *Orientation to the Lab* chapter, control samples must be used every time you test patient specimens. These are the types of urine specimens:

- Random
- First morning
- Clean-catch mid-stream
- Timed
- 24-hour

Random Urine Specimen The random urine specimen is the most common type of sample. It is a single urine specimen taken at any time of the day and collected in a clean, dry container.

If a random urine specimen collection is to be done at the licensed practitioner's office, supply the patient with a urine specimen container. Show the patient to the bathroom and ask the patient to void a few ounces of urine into the specimen cup and to leave the cup on the sink. Retrieve the specimen when the patient leaves the bathroom, and attach a properly completed label and requisition slip. Transport the specimen to the laboratory immediately. Urine specimens should be processed within 1 hour of collection. If this is not possible, refrigerate the specimen. Before processing refrigerated specimens, however, allow them to come to room temperature before processing them. If specimens will be shipped to an outside laboratory, chemical preservatives are added, or the specimens are transferred to a suitable container containing preservatives.

If patients are to collect a random urine specimen at home, have them use the container indicated by the laboratory. Either provide patients with a urine specimen container or instruct them to use a clean, wide-mouthed glass jar with a tight-fitting lid. Explain that a household dishwasher provides hot enough water to disinfect a jar adequately. Tell patients to refrigerate specimens until they bring them to the licensed practitioner's office and to keep them cool during transport.

First Morning Urine Specimen The **first morning urine specimen** is collected after a night's sleep. This type of specimen contains greater concentrations of substances that collect over time than do specimens taken during the day.

A urine specimen container or clean, dry jar is used to collect the urine as per the laboratory's request.

Clean-Catch Mid-Stream Urine Specimen The **clean-catch mid-stream urine specimen,** sometimes referred to as mid-void, may be collected and submitted for culturing to identify the number and types of pathogens present. A clean-catch mid-stream urine specimen may be collected at random or first thing in the morning. The presence of clinical symptoms or unexplained bacteria in a urinalysis specimen is an indication for urine culture.

The clean-catch mid-stream specimen method is not like other urine tests in which urine is simply voided into a specimen container. Instead, the clean-catch mid-stream method requires special cleansing of the external genitalia to avoid contamination by organisms residing near the urethral meatus (the external opening of the urethra). Voiding a small amount of urine into the toilet prior to collecting the mid-stream specimen flushes the normal flora out of the distal urethra to prevent possible contamination of the specimen. Procedure 47-1, at the end of this chapter, describes how to collect a clean-catch mid-stream urine specimen and how to instruct patients to perform this technique.

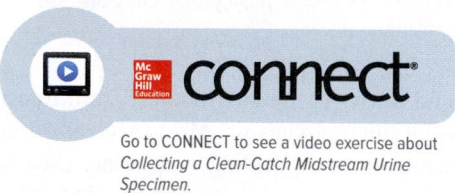

Go to CONNECT to see a video exercise about *Collecting a Clean-Catch Midstream Urine Specimen.*

Timed Urine Specimen A licensed practitioner may order a timed urine specimen to measure a patient's urinary output or to analyze substances. First, determine whether the required time period means that the patient must collect the specimen at home. If so, provide the patient with the proper collection container; written instructions on the process, including specimen preservation; and the following oral instructions:

- Discard the first specimen.
- Then collect *all* urine for the specified time (2 to 24 hours).
- Be sure the urine does not mix with stool or toilet paper.
- Keep the sample refrigerated until returning it to the licensed practitioner's office or laboratory.

24-Hour Urine Specimen A **24-hour urine specimen** is collected over a 24-hour period and is used to complete a quantitative and qualitative analysis of one or more substances, such as sodium, chloride, and calcium. You need to instruct the patient in the proper collection process. If an outside laboratory will be testing the specimen, you will receive protocols for collection, preservation, and transport. Procedure 47-2, at the end of this chapter, outlines the steps in collecting a 24-hour urine specimen.

Catheterization

A urinary catheter is a sterile plastic tube inserted into the kidney, ureter, or bladder to provide urinary drainage. **Catheterization** is the procedure during which the catheter is inserted, and it is performed for various reasons, including to

- Relieve urinary retention.
- Obtain a sterile urine specimen from a patient.
- Measure the amount of residual urine in the bladder to determine how much urine remains after normal voiding (patient voids and is then catheterized; more than 50 milliliters is considered abnormal).
- Obtain a urine specimen if the patient cannot void naturally.
- Instill chemotherapy as a treatment for bladder cancer.
- Empty the bladder before and during surgery and before some diagnostic exams.

The two primary types of urinary catheters are

- Drainage catheters, which are used to withdraw fluids. Drainage catheters include an indwelling urethral (Foley) catheter placed in the bladder; a retention catheter in the renal pelvis; a ureteral catheter; a catheter for drainage through a wound that leads to the bladder (cystostomy tube); and a straight catheter to collect specimens or instill medications.
- Splinting catheters, which are inserted after plastic repair of the ureter and must remain in place for at least a week after surgery.

Catheterization is not routinely recommended because it can introduce infection. Some states do not permit medical assistants to perform catheterization, and in most healthcare institutions, only a physician or nurse can insert or withdraw a catheter. Check the protocol in your state. If you are not permitted to perform the procedure, you may be asked to assemble the necessary supplies and to assist the licensed practitioner during the procedure.

Catheterization performed in a licensed practitioner's office is usually done for diagnostic purposes using a specially prepared catheterization kit. This kit contains all necessary instruments and supplies, including a sterile instrument pack that is used to create a sterile field for the procedure.

If a patient is incontinent, the licensed practitioner may use a bladder-drainage catheter to help drain the bladder and keep the patient dry. Another type of drainage catheter, the ureteral, is inserted into the ureter to help drain urine.

The indwelling urethral (Foley) catheter is designed to stay in place within the bladder (Figure 47-1). It consists of two tubes, one inside the other. The outside tube is connected to a balloon, which is filled with water or air to keep the catheter from slipping out of the bladder. Urine travels through the bladder and drains from the inside tube into a soft plastic container. The licensed practitioner may order a leg bag to attach to the patient's thigh. The bag is anchored to the leg by two bands placed around the thigh. Make sure the bag is positioned so that there is no tension on the catheter tube. To prevent back-flow into the patient's bladder, the container must always be lower than the bladder.

Special Considerations

When you obtain a urine specimen from a patient or take a history of a patient who may have a urinary problem, you need to consider the patient's sex, condition, and age. Some patients require special care during collection procedures.

Special Considerations in Male and Female Patients Depending on the test, you may need to alter guidelines for collecting urine specimens from a male or female patient. Procedure 47-1, at the end of this chapter, describes how to assist in collecting a clean-catch urine specimen from a female patient and from a male patient. In addition, when you take a medical history on a male or female patient, you will need to ask gender-specific questions as part of your assessment. For example, if a female patient leaks urine when laughing or coughing, she may have bladder dysfunction, which would affect the collection of a 24-hour urine specimen.

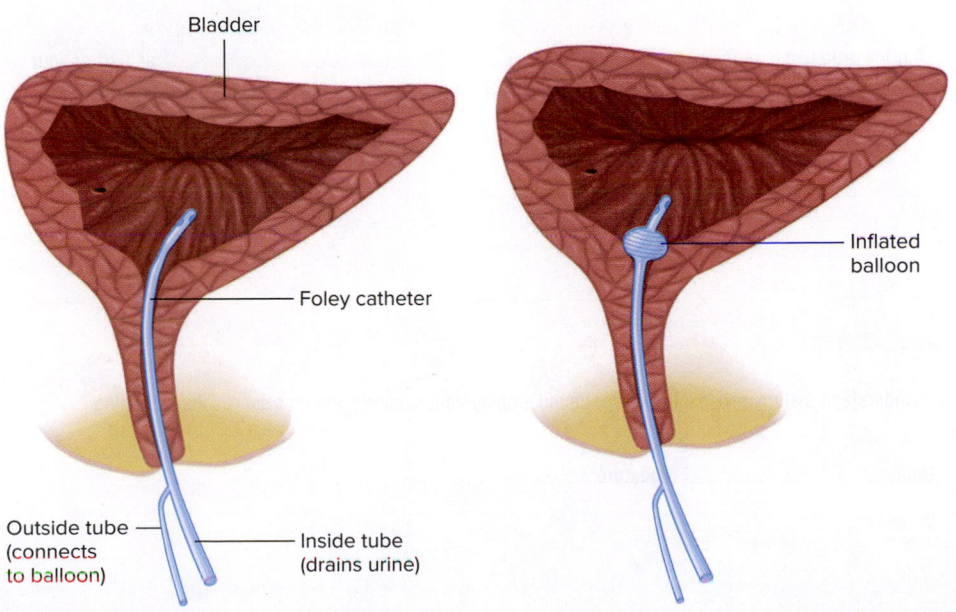

FIGURE 47-1 A Foley catheter stays in place within the bladder and has a collection container, which is emptied periodically.

Special Considerations in Pregnant Patients

Pregnant women normally have increased urinary frequency. They also may be prone to urinary tract infections. When a woman is pregnant, urine testing is done to screen for pregnancy-related issues. A pregnant woman's urine is checked for glucose. If this test shows elevated glucose (sugar) in the urine, it may indicate the possibility of gestational diabetes. When the urine tests positive for glucose, additional testing is performed. The woman's urine is also checked for abnormal levels of protein. Excess protein in her urine may indicate renal problems or preeclampsia, a condition brought on by pregnancy in which the blood pressure rises and other organs, such as the kidneys, may be damaged.

Ask a pregnant patient whether she has any pain during urination or in the kidney area. A positive response may indicate a urinary tract infection or kidney stones. Also ask about urine leakage and whether she has previously been pregnant. Leakage may occur in a woman who has had multiple births because the pressure of the fetus on the bladder or the delivery of the baby may have weakened the patient's bladder control. Additionally, ask whether any of the babies were delivered by forceps, which can injure urinary and genital structures.

Establishing Chain of Custody

Occasionally, you may need to obtain urine specimens for drug and alcohol analysis. These are considered legal specimens because they may be used in a court of law and they must be handled carefully. The specimen must be placed in a specimen transfer bag that permanently seals the specimen bag until it is cut open for analysis. The seal ensures that there has been no tampering with the bag's contents prior to reaching the lab for testing. A chain of custody must be established to document the handling of this specimen.

The specific steps to establish a chain of custody are described in Procedure 47-3 at the end of this chapter. Because medico-legal issues are involved when handling a legal specimen, it is important to follow the procedure exactly to avoid breaking the chain. Also, because supplying a specimen for drug or alcohol testing could be incriminating to the patient, it is important to thoroughly explain the procedure to the donor and have him or her sign a consent form (Figure 47-2). The consent form may be a part of the chain-of-custody form (CCF) (Figure 47-3), or it may be a separate form. The consent form states the purpose of the test and gives you permission to collect the specimen, prepare it for transport to the laboratory for analysis, and release the results to the agency requesting the test. Distribute copies of the CCF to the medical review officer, laboratory, patient, collector, and employer or other requesting party.

Inform the patient that medication (both prescription and nonprescription), drugs, and alcohol will show up in the test results. Encourage the patient to list on the consent form or CCF all substances consumed in the last 30 days, including what was taken and how much.

The CCF form indicates the source of the specimen. It verifies through signatures that the patient whose name is on the CCF and consent forms is the same person who provided the sealed specimen sent to the laboratory. Follow Procedure 47-3, at the end of this chapter, when collecting a urine sample for drug or alcohol testing.

BWW

BWW Medical Associates, PC
305 Main Street, Port Snead YZ 12345-9876
Tel: 555-654-3210, Fax: 555-987-6543
Web: BWWAssociates.com

DRUG SCREEN CONSENT FORM

A urine drug test is required by _____ as part of your pre-employment screening. Please provide us with a list of all medications that you are presently taking.

_____

_____

_____

_____

I understand that my prospective or continued employment is contingent on a successful screening.

Date: _____ Signature: _____

Witness: _____

FIGURE 47-2 A consent form is a legal requirement when urine is collected for drug testing.

Morris A. Turner, MD

C.L.I.A #21.1862

266 Line Road
Montelair, Delaware 00956
800-555-1567

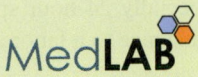

CHAIN-OF-CUSTODY FORM
SPECIMEN I.D.NO:

STEP 1—TO BE COMPLETED BY COLLECTOR OR EMPLOYER REPRESENTATIVE.

Employer Name, Address, and I.D. No.:   OR   Medical Review Officer Name and Address:

_____   _____

_____   _____

_____   _____

Donor Social Security No. or Employee I.D. No.: _____

Donor I.D. verified: ☐ Photo I.D.   ☐ Employer Representative _____

Signature

Reason for test: (check one)   ☐ Preemployment ☐ Random ☐ Postaccident

  ☐ Periodic ☐ Reasonable suspicion/cause

  ☐ Return to duty ☐ Other (specify)

Test(s) to be performed: _____ Total tests ordered: ☐

Type of specimen obtained: ☐ Urine ☐ Blood ☐ Semen ☐ Other (specify)

Submit only one specimen with each requisition.

STEP 2—TO BE COMPLETED BY COLLECTOR.

For urine specimens, read temperature within 4 minutes of collection.
Check here if specimen temperature is within range. ☐ Yes, 90°–100°F/32°–38°C
Or record actual temperature here: _____

STEP 3—TO BE COMPLETED BY COLLECTOR.

Collection site _____ Address _____
City _____ State _____ Zip _____ Phone _____
Collection date: _____ Time: _____ ☐ a.m. ☐ p.m.

I certify that the specimen identified on this form is the specimen presented to me by the donor identified in step 1 above, and that it was collected, labeled, and sealed in the donor's presence.

Collector's name: _____ Signature of collector: _____

STEP 4—TO BE INITIATED BY DONOR AND COMPLETED AS NECESSARY THEREAFTER.

Purpose of change	Released by Signature	Received by Signature	Date
A. Provide specimen for testing			
B. Shipment to Laboratory			
C.			

Comments:

STEP 5—TO BE COMPLETED BY THE LABORATORY.

Specimen package seal(s) intact when received in lab?   ☐ Yes ☐ No If no, explain.

Laboratory receiver's initials _____

Copy 1 - Original - Must accompany specimen to laboratory.

FIGURE 47-3 The chain-of-custody form provides documentation that specific specimen collection safeguards have been followed.

Preservation and Storage

Proper specimen preservation and storage are essential. Changes that can affect the physical, chemical, and microscopic properties of urine, and invalidate certain test results, occur in urine kept at room temperature for more than 1 hour.

Refrigeration is the most common method for storing and preserving urine. It prevents bacterial growth in a specimen for at least 24 hours. Refrigeration can cause other changes in the urine, however, that may affect the physical characteristics of sediment and specific gravity. Bringing the specimen back to room temperature before testing will correct these problems. You can also use chemical preservatives to preserve specimens, especially 24-hour specimens or those that must be sent a long distance to a laboratory.

- Physical
- Chemical
- Microscopic

▶ Urinalysis

LO 47.3

Urinalysis is the evaluation of urine by various types of testing methods to obtain information about body health and disease. Urinalysis consists of three types of testing:

There are normal values for all tests done on urine. The normal value for a specific substance may be negative or none, "normal," or a range in concentration. Urine test results within normal ranges indicate health and normality. Table 47-2 identifies normal values for a variety of urine tests.

TABLE 47-2	Standard Urine Values		
Physical Characteristics		**Microscopic Examination**	
Test	**Normal Values**	**Test**	**Normal Values**
Color	Pale yellow to yellow	*Epithelial cells*	
Clarity	Clear to slightly turbid	Renal	Negative
Reagent Strip Test		Squamous, adult females	Moderate
Bilirubin	Negative	Squamous, adult males	Few
Blood	Negative	Transitional	Rare
Glucose	Negative	Mucus	Rare–few
Ketone bodies (acetone)	Negative	Protozoa	Negative
Leukocytes	Negative	Red blood cells	0–3/high-powered field
Nitrites	Negative	White blood cells	0–8/high-powered field
pH	4.5–8.0	Yeast	Few
Protein	Negative to trace	*24-Hour*	
Specific gravity	1.002–1.028*	5-HIAA	2–8 mg
Urobilinogen	0.3–1.0 E.U.	Albumin (quantitative)	10–140 mg/L
Microscopic Examination		Ammonia	140–1,500 mg
Bacteria	Negative	Calcium (quantitative)	100–300 mg
Casts		Catecholamines, total	<100 mcg
Epithelial cell	Negative	Chloride	110–120 mEq
Granular	Negative	Cortisol	10–100 mcg
Hyaline	Few	Creatine, nonpregnant women/men	<100 mg
Red blood cell	Negative	Creatine, pregnant women	≤ 12% of creatinine
Waxy	Negative	Creatinine, men	1.0–1.9 g
White blood cell	Negative	Creatinine, women	0.8–1.7 g
Crystals		Cystine and cysteine	<38.1 mg
Amorphous phosphates	Normal	Glucose, quantitative	50–500 mg
Calcium carbonate	Normal	Phosphorus	0.4–1.3 g
Calcium oxalate	Normal	Potassium	25–120 mEq/L
Cholesterol	Negative	Protein (Bence Jones)	Negative
Cystine	Negative	Sodium	80–180 mEq
Leucine	Negative	Urea nitrogen	6–17 g
Sulfonamide	Negative	Uric acid	0.25–0.75 g
Triple phosphate	Normal	Urobilinogen, quantitative	1.0–4.0 mg
Tyrosine	Negative	Volume, adult females	600–1,600 mL
Uric acid	Normal	Volume, adult males	800–1,800 mL
		Volume, children	3–4 times adult rate/kg

Note: Individual laboratories may have slightly different reference values. Consult the reference values provided by the lab performing the test.

* Specific gravity is a physical property of urine.

Urinalysis is done as part of a general physical exam to screen for certain substances or to diagnose various medical conditions (Table 47-3). For example, daily urine output provides a picture of renal function. With adequate fluid intake, the average adult daily urine output is 1,250 milliliters, or approximately 5 cups per 24 hours. When total intake and output measurements are not approximately equal, urinary tract dysfunction may be the cause.

The urinary system works with other body systems to help the body function normally. So a disorder in another body system can affect urinary function. For example, the kidneys interact with the nervous system to help regulate blood

TABLE 47-3 Common Urine Tests According to Clinical Condition	
Clinical Condition or Suspected Disease	**Types of Urine Testing**
Acidosis	Reagent strip* for pH
	Specific gravity
Alkalosis (metabolic, respiratory)	Reagent strip* for pH
	Specific gravity
Diabetes mellitus	Odor (fruity)
	Microscopic examination for fatty, waxy casts
	Reagent strip* for ketonuria and glycosuria
	Specific gravity
Drug abuse	Gas chromatography
	Mass spectrometry**
Genitourinary infections (prostatitis, urethritis, vaginitis)	Cultures for bacteria, yeasts, and parasites
	Microscopic examination for bacteria and RBCs
Human immunodeficiency virus (HIV)	Culture for virus (antibiotic added to kill bacteria)
	Other tests as indicated by specific symptoms
Hypercalcemia	Microscopic examination for calcium oxalate crystals
	Specific gravity
Hypertension	Microscopic examination for casts (hyaline, RBC)
	Specific gravity
Infectious diseases (bacteria) or other inflammatory diseases	Color and odor
	Cultures for bacteria, yeasts, and viruses
	Microscopic examination for bacteria and WBCs
	RBC casts (in severe cases)
	Reagent strip* for bacteria
	Turbidity
Metabolic disorders (except diabetes mellitus)	Color
	Microscopic examination for cystine crystals
	Reagent strip* for ketonuria, fructosuria, galactosuria, pentosuria, and pH
Nephron disorders (nephrotic syndrome, glomerulonephritis, nephrosis, nephrolithiasis, pyelonephritis)	Color
	Microscopic examination for casts (epithelial, fatty, waxy, RBC) and RBCs
	Reagent strip* for proteinuria
	Specific gravity
	Turbidity
Phenylketonuria	Color
	Reagent strip* for pH

(Continued)

TABLE 47-3 Common Urine Tests According to Clinical Condition

Clinical Condition or Suspected Disease	Types of Urine Testing
Poisoning (arsenic, cadmium, lead, mercury)	Color
	Mass spectrometry**
Polycystic kidney disease	Proteinuria
	Urinary volume
Pregnancy	Reagent strip* for human chorionic gonadotropin (HCG)
Renal infections (acute glomerulonephritis, nephrotic syndrome, pyelonephritis, pyogenic infection)	Color
	Microscopic examination for epithelial cells (especially with tubular degeneration), numerous casts (granular, hyaline, WBC), RBCs, and WBCs
	Radioimmunoassay (RIA)**
	Reagent strip* for bacteria, albumin
	Specific gravity
	Turbidity
	Urinary volume
Renal disease, renal failure, severe renal damage, acute renal failure, renal tubular degeneration	Microscopic examination for epithelial cells (especially with tubular degeneration) and numerous casts (hyaline, fatty, waxy, RBC)
	Reagent strip* for proteinuria (albumin), pH
	Specific gravity
	Turbidity
	Urinary volume
Sickle cell anemia	RBC casts
Starvation, dietary imbalance, extreme change in diet, dehydration	Color
	Odor (fruity)
	Reagent strip* for ketonuria
	Specific gravity
Urinary tract infection or mild inflammation (cystitis, pyelonephritis)	Color and odor
	Cultures for bacteria, yeasts, and viruses
	Microscopic examination for bacteria, WBC casts, RBCs, and WBCs
	Reagent strip* for bacteria, albumin, and pH
	Specific gravity
	Turbidity
Urinary obstruction (tumor, trauma, inflammation)	Color
	Microscopic examination for RBCs
	Specific gravity
	Urinary volume

*Federal listings of waived tests refer to these as *dipstick tests*.

**Drug screening and some other common urine tests must be performed by a forensic laboratory or other laboratory capable of performing gas chromatography, mass spectrometry, and radioimmunoassay.

pressure and control urination. Thus, a nervous system disorder can affect the circulatory and urinary systems. The cardiovascular system delivers blood to the kidneys for filtration, and the kidneys regulate fluid balance, which helps maintain circulation of blood and myocardial function. A cardiovascular system disorder can allow blood to be delivered to the kidneys at a pressure inadequate for filtration, which would affect urinary system function.

Physical Examination and Testing of Urine Specimens

After confirming that the specimen is properly labeled, the first step in urinalysis is the visual examination of physical characteristics. As part of quality assurance, examine it to make sure there is no visible contamination and that no more than 1 hour has passed since collection (or since a refrigerated

TABLE 47-4 Urine Color and Turbidity: Possible Causes

Color and Turbidity	Pathologic Causes	Other Causes
Colorless or pale straw color (dilute)	Diabetes, anxiety, chronic renal disease	Diuretic therapy, excessive fluid intake (water, beer, and/or coffee)
Cloudy	Infection, inflammation, glomerular nephritis	Vegetarian diet
Milky white	Fats, pus	Amorphous phosphates, spermatozoa
Dark yellow, dark amber (concentrated)	Acute febrile disease, vomiting or diarrhea (fluid loss or dehydration)	Low fluid intake, excessive sweating
Yellow-brown	Excessive RBC destruction, bile duct obstruction, diminished liver cell function, bilirubin	Drugs (primaquine)
Orange-yellow, orange-red, orange-brown	Excessive RBC destruction, diminished liver cell function, bile, hepatitis, urobilinuria, obstructive jaundice, hematuria	Drugs (such as pyridium, rifampin), dyes
Salmon pink	No pathologic cause	Amorphous urates
Cloudy red	RBCs, excessive destruction of skeletal or cardiac muscle	None
Bright yellow or red	RBCs (hemorrhage, myoglobin, hemoglobin), excessive destruction of skeletal or cardiac muscle, porphyria	Beets, drugs (such as phenazopyridine hydrochloride), dyes (such as food coloring and contrast media)
Dark red, red-brown	Porphyria, RBCs (menstrual contamination, hemorrhage, hemoglobin), blood from previous hemorrhage	Menstrual contamination
Green, blue-green	Biliverdin, *Pseudomonas* organisms, oxidation of bilirubin	Vitamin B, methylene blue, asparagus (for green)
Green-brown	Bile duct obstruction	Drugs (cascara)
Brownish black	Methemoglobin, melanin	Drugs (levodopa)
Dark brown or black	Acute glomerulonephritis	Drugs (nitrofurantoin, chlorpromazine, iron preparations)

sample was brought back to room temperature). You will examine these physical characteristics:

- Color and turbidity
- Volume
- Odor
- Specific gravity

Color and Turbidity Normal urine ranges from pale yellow (straw-colored) to dark amber. The color, which comes from a yellow pigment called *urochrome,* depends on food and fluid intake, medications (including vitamin supplements), and waste products present in the urine. In general, a pale color indicates dilute urine and a dark color indicates concentrated urine.

Assess urine for turbidity, or cloudiness, by noting whether the urine is clear, slightly cloudy, cloudy, or very cloudy. Typically, urine is clear, although cloudy urine does not always indicate an abnormal condition.

The color of urine and any turbidity present can reveal medical conditions that require treatment. Table 47-4 provides more information on variations in urine color and turbidity and the possible causes or sources of these variations. Both pathologic (resulting from disease) and nonpathologic causes are noted.

Volume Normal urine volume, or output, varies according to the patient's age. Normal adult urine volume is 600 to 1,800 milliliters per 24 hours (average of 1,250 milliliters per 24 hours). Infants and children have smaller total urine volumes, although they produce more urine per unit of body weight. Urine volume is typically measured on a timed specimen (such as a 24-hour urine specimen) rather than a random specimen.

Oliguria, insufficient production (or volume) of urine, occurs in conditions such as dehydration, decreased fluid intake, shock, and renal disease. The absence of urine production is called **anuria.** Renal or urethral obstruction and renal failure can cause anuria.

Odor Although urine odor is not typically recorded or considered a significant indicator of disease, it can provide clues about the body's condition. The odor of normal, freshly voided urine is distinct but not unpleasant and is sometimes characterized as aromatic. After urine has been standing for a while, bacteria in the specimen decompose the urea, which causes an odor similar to ammonia.

Diseases, the presence of bacteria, and particular foods (such as asparagus and garlic) can cause changes in urine odor. For example, in the presence of urinary tract infections, urine is foul-smelling, and in patients with uncontrolled diabetes, the smell is characterized as fruity (because of the presence of ketones). Phenylketonuria, a congenital metabolic disease, produces a strange, "mousy" or "musty" odor in an infant's wet diaper.

Specific Gravity Urine specific gravity is a measure of the concentration or amount of substances dissolved in urine. Because the kidneys remove metabolic wastes and other substances from the blood, the specific gravity of the urine they produce is an indicator of the body's water balance and/or kidney function. The physician's office laboratory uses one of these two methods to determine specific gravity:

1. Refractometer
2. Reagent strip (dipstick)

Specific gravity is a relative measure that is always compared to a standard. The standard for liquids is distilled water, which contains no dissolved substances.

$$\text{Specific gravity} = \frac{\text{Weight of sample}}{\text{Weight of distilled water}}$$

The specific gravity of distilled water is 1.000. You use special equipment to test for specific gravity (Figure 47-4).

The normal range of urine specific gravity is 1.002 to 1.028. Specific gravity fluctuates throughout the day in response to fluid intake. For example, a first morning urine specimen normally has a higher specific gravity than a specimen provided later in the day. An increase in urine specific gravity may indicate that the kidneys cannot properly dilute the urine. The urine then becomes more concentrated, causing it to darken. Increased specific gravity may indicate conditions such as a urinary tract infection, dehydration (for example, from fever, vomiting, or diarrhea), adrenal insufficiency, hepatic disease, or congestive heart failure.

A decrease in the specific gravity of urine causes a lighter than normal urine color, may indicate that the kidneys cannot properly concentrate the urine, and may suggest conditions such as overhydration (excess fluid in the body), diabetes insipidus, chronic renal disease, or systemic lupus erythematosus.

Refractometer Measurement A **refractometer** is an optical instrument that measures the refraction, or bending, of light as it passes through a liquid. The degree of refraction, or refractive index, is proportional to the amount of dissolved material in the liquid. You must calibrate a refractometer each day with distilled water by setting the instrument at 1.000 with the set screw. Two standard solutions (solutions of known specific gravity) also are used to ensure accuracy. Advantages of using a refractometer to measure urine specific gravity are that the process takes little time and requires little urine. Only a drop of urine is used for this determination. Procedure 47-4, at the end of this chapter, describes how to measure specific gravity with a refractometer.

Reagent Strip Measurement You may use special reagent strips, or dipsticks, to test for specific gravity. Test

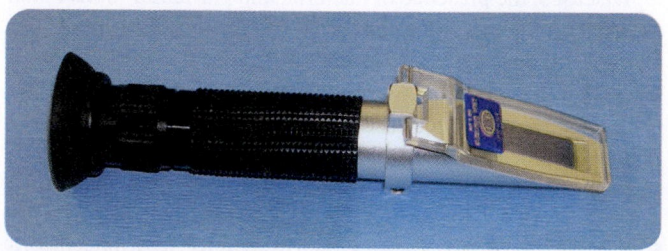

FIGURE 47-4 Specific gravity is commonly determined using a refractometer or reagent strips.
© Leesa Whicker

pads along these plastic strips contain chemicals that react with substances in the urine and change color in precise ways. The reagent strip container includes a color chart for interpreting color changes on the test pads. When you evaluate urine specific gravity in this way, keep in mind that this type of test depends on precisely timed intervals identified by the manufacturer. Follow all directions exactly. Procedure 47-5, at the end of this chapter, describes how to perform a reagent strip test.

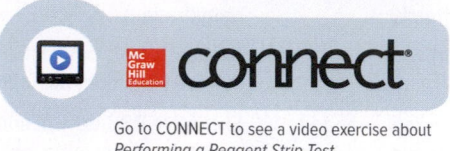

Go to CONNECT to see a video exercise about *Performing a Reagent Strip Test.*

Chemical Testing of Urine Specimens

As a medical assistant, you may be asked to perform chemical tests on urine. Prior to performing chemical tests, always check for proper identification on the urine specimen to be tested. Chemical testing is usually done with reagent strips. It also can be performed with certain automated machines that use photometry.

The licensed practitioner orders chemical testing of urine to determine the status of body processes such as carbohydrate metabolism, liver or kidney function, or acid-base balance. Other reasons for chemical testing include determining the presence of drugs, toxic environmental substances, or infections.

Testing with Reagent Strips As already described in the discussion of specific gravity, reagents (on plastic strips) are chemicals that react with a particular substance in urine and change color in precise ways. These changes indicate the presence of that substance and its amount or concentration in the urine specimen. For example, when a reagent strip is used to test for ketones, the reacted color on the strip will correspond either to a specific concentration of ketone bodies, such as acetoacetic acid, or to the absence of ketones.

Reagent strips are used to test urine for a number of substances. In addition to ketones, reagent strips test for nitrite, pH, blood, bilirubin, glucose, specific gravity, protein, and leukocytes.

There are numerous trade names for urine reagent strips (for example, Multistix® and Chemstrip®). Because not all reagents are reactive for the same chemicals, you must choose the appropriate strip according to the chemical test requested. All reagent strips are used once and discarded.

Follow the exact directions that come with the reagent strips to ensure accurate results. For quality assurance, take these basic precautions: Keep strips in tightly closed containers in a cool, dry area. Never remove them from the container until immediately before testing. Never touch the pads on the strip with your fingers or gloved hands. Examine strips for discoloration before use; discard discolored strips. Check the expiration date on the bottle; do not use strips that have expired. Use strips within 6 months of opening the container. Every time you open a new supply of reagents, run control samples to check for proper operation. Write the date opened on the bottle.

Although the process is essentially the same for all reagent strip tests, there are variations in time intervals before reading results. Some reagent strips are designed to test for several substances at once. The basic procedure for using reagent strips for chemical tests can be found in Procedure 47-5 at the end of this chapter. In some cases, if the reagent strip test is positive, a confirmatory test is performed to ensure the accuracy of the results.

Ketone Bodies Ketone bodies (or ketones) are produced by the liver from fatty acids during fat metabolism. They include acetone, acetoacetic acid, and betahydroxybutyric acid. Only the first two substances can be determined using a reagent strip test. Normally, there are no ketones in urine. The presence of ketones in the urine may indicate that a patient is following a low-carbohydrate diet, or it may indicate that the patient has a condition such as starvation, excessive vomiting, or diabetes mellitus. Because ketones evaporate at room temperature, be sure to test urine immediately or cover the specimen tightly and refrigerate it until testing can be done.

pH **Urinary pH** is a measure of the urine's degree of acidity or alkalinity. Determination of pH can provide information about a patient's metabolic status and diet, the medications being taken, and several conditions. The normal pH of freshly voided urine ranges from 4.5 to 8.0. The average urine pH is 6.0, which is slightly acidic. A pH of 7.0 is neutral, a lower pH is acidic, and a higher one is alkaline. Patients with excessively alkaline urine may have conditions such as urinary tract infection or metabolic or respiratory alkalosis. Those with excessively acidic urine may have conditions such as phenylketonuria or acidosis. Reagent strip tests on both urine and blood are used to measure pH in the body. (See the *Collecting, Processing, and Testing Blood Specimens* chapter for information on blood tests for pH.)

Blood A patient who has blood in the urine may be menstruating, have a urinary tract infection, or have trauma or bleeding in the kidneys. To test for blood in urine, use a reagent strip that reacts with hemoglobin. There are two indicators on the strip: One is for nonhemolyzed blood, the other for hemolyzed blood.

Colors on the strip range from orange through green to dark blue and may indicate **hematuria** (the presence of blood in the urine) caused by cystitis; kidney stones; menstruation; or ureteral, bladder, or urethral irritation. The presence of free hemoglobin in the urine is known as *hemoglobinuria,* a rare condition caused by transfusion reactions, malaria, drug reactions, snakebites, or severe burns. Injured or damaged muscle tissue—as occurs in crushing injuries, myocardial infarction, muscular dystrophy, or contact sports injuries—can cause *myoglobinuria* (the presence of myoglobin in the urine). Reagent strip testing does not distinguish between these two conditions.

Bilirubin and Urobilinogen When hemoglobin breaks down, it converts into conjugated bilirubin in the liver and then to urobilinogen in the intestines. Presence of the bile pigment bilirubin in the urine (*bilirubinuria*) is one of the first signs of liver disease or conditions that involve the liver. When bilirubin is present, urine turns yellow-brown to greenish orange. You usually use a reagent strip to test for bilirubin. If the reagent strip test is positive, a confirmatory test called an Ictotest® is usually performed. The Ictotest® is a reagent tablet test that is more sensitive than the reagent strip test.

Although **urobilinogen** is normally present in the urine in small amounts, elevated levels may indicate increased red blood cell destruction or liver disease. Lack of urobilinogen in the urine may suggest total bile duct obstruction, as a result of which urobilinogen is not formed in the intestines or reabsorbed in the circulation. To test for urobilinogen, you use reagent strips.

Testing for either bilirubin or urobilinogen must be performed on a fresh urine specimen. Bilirubin decomposes rapidly in bright light to form biliverdin, which is not detected by the reagent strip test for bilirubin. Urobilinogen breaks down to urobilin on standing.

Glucose Glucose is normally present in urine, but only in small quantities not detectable by the reagent strip test for glucose. **Glycosuria** (the presence of significant glucose in the urine) is common in patients with diabetes. Blood is more commonly tested for glucose than urine is, because reagent strip tests may show false-negative results when used for testing urine.

Protein Although a small amount of protein is excreted in the urine every day, an excess of protein in the urine (**proteinuria**) usually indicates renal disease. Proteinuria is also common in pregnant patients and after heavy exercise.

Nitrites Bacteria in urine makes an enzyme that changes urine nitrates to nitrites. If nitrites are found in the urine, it suggests a bacterial infection of the urinary tract. The test is not definitive, however. If an insufficient number of bacteria are present in the urine or if the urine has not incubated long enough in the bladder for a reaction to take place, the nitrite test result may be falsely negative. The best urine specimen to test for nitrites is the first morning specimen.

When testing for urinary nitrites, you must test the urine immediately or refrigerate the specimen. Bacteria can multiply in a specimen allowed to sit at room temperature, causing a false-positive test result. Bacteria also can further metabolize the nitrites already produced, causing a false-negative result.

Leukocytes Leukocytes (white blood cells) appear in the urine in urinary tract or renal infections. Use strip tests for leukocyte esterase, a chemical seen when leukocytes are present, to test for leukocytes.

Other Types of Chemical Testing Other types of chemical tests—such as those that test for electrolytes and osmolality—may be performed on urine specimens. Because these tests are performed in an outside laboratory rather than in a physician's office laboratory, you do not need to know the steps in each procedure.

Phenylketones The presence of phenylketones in a patient's urine indicates phenylketonuria (PKU), a genetically inherited disorder in which the body cannot properly metabolize the nutrient phenylalanine. This rare disorder causes phenylalanine to build up in the body, resulting in mental retardation. PKU can be treated successfully by limiting the dietary intake of phenylalanine, which makes up 5% of all natural protein, from early infancy. Although urine can be tested for the presence of phenylketones, blood testing is routine for newborns before discharge, at least 24 hours after birth.

Pregnancy Tests Pregnancy testing is based on detecting the hormone—called *human chorionic gonadotropin, or HCG*—secreted by the placenta. HCG levels vary throughout pregnancy: They usually peak at about 8 weeks, drop to lower levels in the second trimester, and then rise to detectable levels in the last trimester. Many commercial pregnancy tests are manufactured for use both in the clinical setting and at home. These tests are sensitive, are easy to perform and interpret, and give quick results. Most tests are now designed as an enzyme immunoassay (EIA) test, which involves an antigen, an antibody specific for the antigen, and a second antibody conjugated to an enzyme. Newer technologies called *membrane EIAs* have been developed; in these tests, most of the reagents are incorporated into an absorbent membrane in a plastic case. A sample of either urine or serum is added through a chamber window, where it migrates through the membrane and combines with the reagents to produce a reaction. Although the technology used in the design of these tests is quite complex, the test itself is easy to set up and interpret (see Procedure 47-6 at the end of this chapter). The tests are all designed with a control feature incorporated into the reagent pack for quality assurance of the test results.

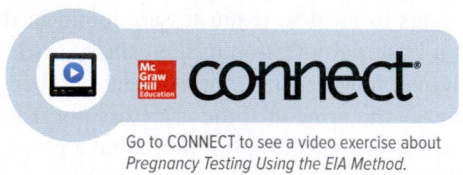

Go to CONNECT to see a video exercise about *Pregnancy Testing Using the EIA Method.*

Urine Tests for the Presence of STIs In response to increasing numbers of sexually transmitted infections, the CDC recommends that all sexually active females between the ages of 15 and 25 be screened annually for chlamydia. To accomplish this, several tests called *nucleic acid amplification tests (NAATs)* have recently been developed. These tests utilize urine samples to detect the presence of nucleic acid. Patients infected with either *Chlamydia trachomatis* or *Neisseria gonorrhoeae* will have nucleic acid in their urine. By amplifying nucleic acids specific to chlamydia and gonorrhea, the test can detect the presence of very small numbers of bacteria.

These tests have several advantages:

- Sample collection is noninvasive and the sample is easily collected.
- The tests are highly specific.
- The tests are highly sensitive. As little as one copy of bacterial nucleic acid can be detected in a urine specimen.
- Organisms do not have to be living to be detected.
- The tests are good screening tools for asymptomatic patients.

The tests also have some disadvantages:

- The tests are expensive.
- No living organisms remain for use in a follow-up culture, so positive tests must be confirmed by culture from an endocervical or urethral swab.

Microscopic Examination of Urine Specimens

A microscopic examination of urine sediment is typically done by the licensed practitioner to view elements only visible with a microscope. You will use a centrifuge to obtain sediment for analysis. A centrifuge spins test tubes containing fluid at speeds that cause heavier substances in the fluid to settle to the bottom of the tubes.

The substances in urine that form sediment (precipitate) when urine is centrifuged include cells, casts, crystals, yeast, bacteria, and parasites. These elements are categorized and counted during microscopic examination. You may use the KOVA System®, manufactured by Hycor Biomedical, Irvine, California, to prepare urine sediment for microscopic examination. When you use the KOVA System®, the sediment is evenly distributed to four calibrated chambers before the microscopic elements are counted. Procedure 47-7, at the end of this chapter, describes how to process a urine specimen for microscopic examination of sediment.

Cells High-power magnification is used to classify and count cells. Three types of cells may be found in urine (Figure 47-5):

- Epithelial cells
- White blood cells
- Red blood cells

Epithelial Cells Epithelial cells are classified as renal, transitional, or squamous. Renal epithelial cells can be round to oval and have a large, oval, and sometimes eccentric nucleus. Although a few of these cells appear normally in urine, several may indicate tubular damage in the kidneys. Damage in the renal tubules causes epithelial cells to die and slough off, or shed. These shed cells can then be seen in a urine sample.

Transitional epithelial cells line the urinary tract from the renal pelvis (the beginning of the ureter) to the upper portion of the urethra. They can be round to oval and may have a tail and, occasionally, two nuclei. Like the renal epithelial cell, a few appear normally in urine, but several may indicate tubular damage.

Squamous epithelial cells—large, flat, irregular cells with a small, round, centrally located nucleus—line the genitourinary tract's lower portion. They often occur in sheets or clumps and can be easily recognized under low-power magnification.

White Blood Cells White blood cells (WBCs) are larger than red blood cells, have a granular appearance, and usually contain a multilobed nucleus. They are typically found in large numbers in the urine (greater than the normal zero to eight per high-power field) if inflammation is present or if the specimen was contaminated during collection.

Red Blood Cells Red blood cells (RBCs) are typically pale, round, nongranular, and flat or biconcave. They have no nucleus and enter the urinary tract during inflammation or injury. From zero to three RBCs per high-power field in urine are normal. However, numerous RBCs may indicate a variety of problems, including urinary infection, obstruction, inflammation, trauma, or tumor.

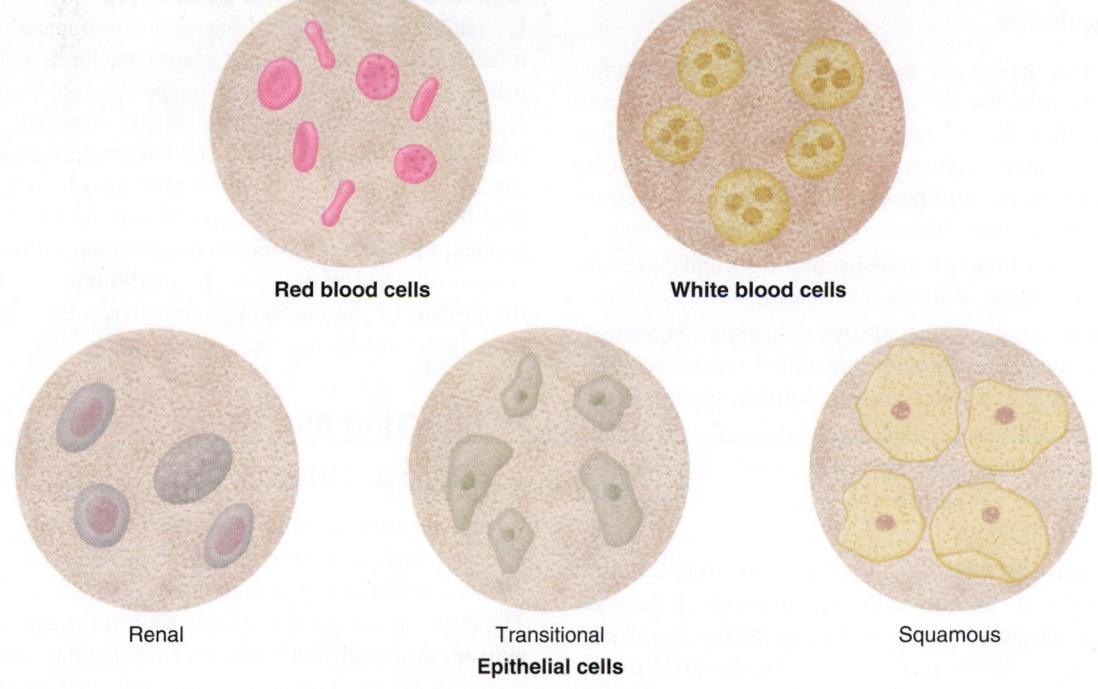

FIGURE 47-5 Cells that may be seen in urine during microscopic analysis.

Red blood cells

White blood cells

Renal

Transitional

Epithelial cells

Squamous

Casts Casts—cylinder-shaped elements with flat or rounded ends—form when protein from the breakdown of cells accumulates and precipitates in the kidney tubules and is washed into the urine. The protein then assumes the size and shape of the tubules. Think of a clogged drain in your bathroom sink. The drain may start out just slow at first but, after a while, very little water will pass through. If you remove the drain pipe, you will find that the material plugging up the drain has taken on the shape of the pipe. It works the same in the kidney tubules, but with different materials. Casts differ in composition and size (Figure 47-6). Classified according to their appearance and composition, casts can indicate renal

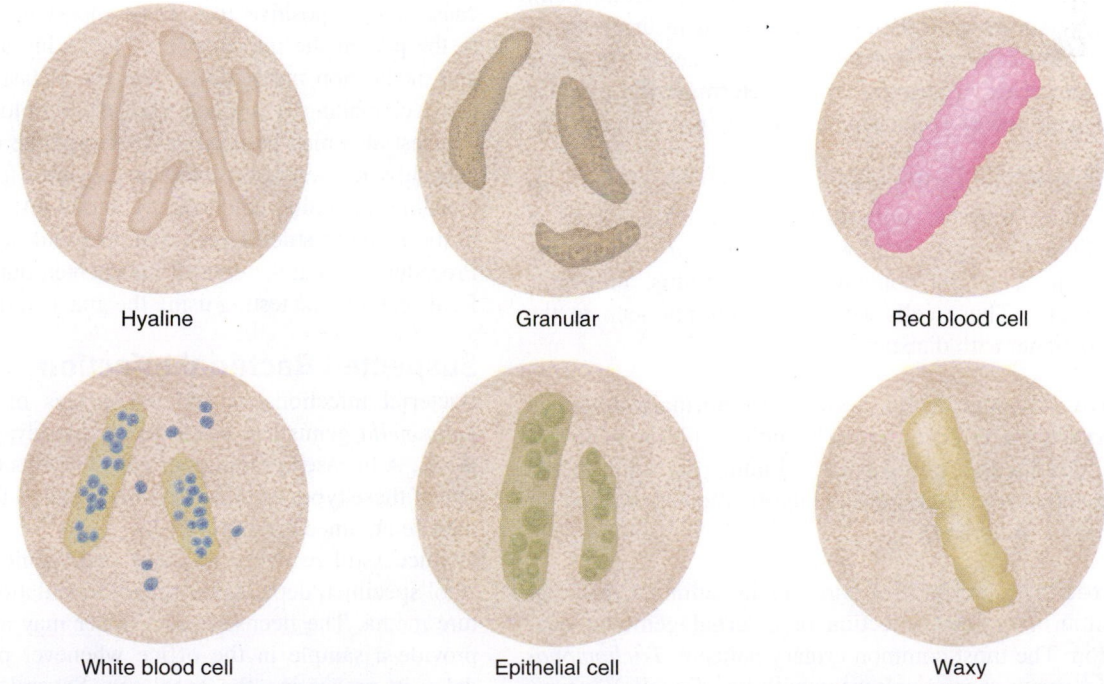

Hyaline

Granular

Red blood cell

White blood cell

Epithelial cell

Waxy

FIGURE 47-6 Casts, which are shaped like cylinders with flat or rounded ends, are formed when protein accumulates in the kidney tubules and is washed into the urine.

pathologic conditions or can be caused by strenuous exercise. Types of casts include

- Hyaline casts, which are pale, transparent, and cylinder-shaped with rounded ends and parallel sides. Composed of protein, they form because of diminished urine flow through individual nephrons. They are present in patients with kidney disease or in people who have exercised strenuously. A few hyaline casts observed in the urine is normal.
- Granular casts, which resemble hyaline casts and can result from kidney disease or strenuous exercise.
- Red blood cell casts, which always indicate an abnormality and are hyaline casts with embedded red blood cells. Because of the RBCs, these casts sometimes appear brown.
- White blood cell casts, which are hyaline casts with leukocytes. These casts typically have a multilobed nucleus and may indicate pyelonephritis—an inflammation of the kidney and renal pelvis.
- Epithelial cell casts, which contain embedded renal tubular epithelial cells and indicate excessive kidney damage. Causes include shock, renal ischemia, heavy-metal poisoning, certain allergic reactions, and nephrotoxic drugs. These casts are often confused with white blood cell casts.
- Waxy casts, which are rare, yellow, glassy, brittle, smooth, and homogeneous structures with cracks or fissures and squared or broken ends. These casts occur with severe renal disease.

Crystals Crystals, naturally produced solids of definite form, are commonly seen in urine specimens, especially those permitted to cool. They usually do not indicate a significant disorder, except when found in large numbers in patients with kidney stones and in a few pathologic conditions (such as hypercalcemia and some inborn errors of metabolism). Figure 47-7 shows crystals commonly found in urine specimens. Because different substances tend to crystallize in acidic and alkaline urine, it is important to determine the pH of a patient's urine before you try to identify any present crystals.

Yeast Cells Yeast cells, which are usually oval and may show budding, may be confused with RBCs. Yeast cells in urine sediment are associated with genitourinary tract infection, external genitalia contamination, vaginitis, urethritis, and prostatitis. These cells are also commonly seen in the urine of patients with diabetes.

Bacteria Although a few bacteria are normally found in urine, urinary tract infection may be indicated if the urine has bacteria along with a putrid odor and numerous white blood cells. Bacteria under high-power magnification appear rod- or cocci-shaped (spherical).

Parasites The presence of parasites in sediment may signal genitourinary tract infection or external genitalia contamination. The most common urinary parasite, *Trichomonas vaginalis* (a pear-shaped protozoan with four flagella), is typically found in vaginal disorders but also may appear in males. When a urine specimen is cooled, *Trichomonas* organisms die.

Urine Culture and Sensitivity

If a patient is suspected of having a complicated urinary tract infection, or if a urinalysis shows bacteria in the patient's urine, a **urine culture** may be performed. For this test, a clean-catch urine specimen is usually required. The urine is placed on a growth medium, and bacteria are allowed to grow for 24 to 48 hours. Any large growths of bacteria are then identified. A sensitivity or susceptibility test may then be performed, in which the bacteria are cultured in the presence of several different antibiotics. The antibiotic that best inhibits the growth of the bacteria is considered the best choice for treating the infection.

▶ Collecting and Processing Stool Specimens   LO 47.4

If the licensed practitioner suspects that the patient has certain diseases, such as cancer or colitis, or bacterial, protozoal, or parasitic infections, you may need to obtain stool specimens. The collection technique varies with the suspected microorganism. Although both you and the patient may be embarrassed to discuss instructions for collecting stool specimens, do not let this interfere with proper specimen collection. For more information about stool sample collection, see the feature *Educating the Patient:* Collecting a Stool Sample.

Screening for Colorectal Cancer

The **fecal occult blood test (FOBT)** is a test for hidden (occult) blood in the stool. The presence of blood in the stool may indicate colorectal cancer, though other diseases and disorders, such as hemorrhoids and gastric ulcers, also may cause blood in the stool. Some food—such as broccoli and beets—and drugs—such as aspirin and ibuprofen—may cause a false-positive test. It is important that you explain to the patient the importance of following all pretest dietary and medication instructions. The test is fast, easy, and inexpensive, making it a good choice for colorectal screening. The test also may be used to determine the cause of anemia. A positive test warrants further investigation for the cause of the bleeding, including colonoscopy, blood tests, and other diagnostic imaging studies such as upper endoscopy or CT scan. Procedure 47-8 at the end of this chapter, outlines the steps in fecal occult blood testing using the guaiac testing method.

Suspected Bacterial Infection

Bacterial infections caused by species of the *Shigella* or *Salmonella* genus can cause loose, bloody, or mucus-tinged stools. A licensed practitioner who suspects that a patient has one of these types of infections may request that a stool specimen be obtained for culture.

Successful recovery of these pathogenic bacteria from a stool specimen depends on timely inoculation of special culture media. The licensed practitioner may ask the patient to provide a sample in the office whenever possible to avoid delay in processing the specimen. Several types of culture media promote the growth of intestinal pathogens while suppressing the growth of other microorganisms.

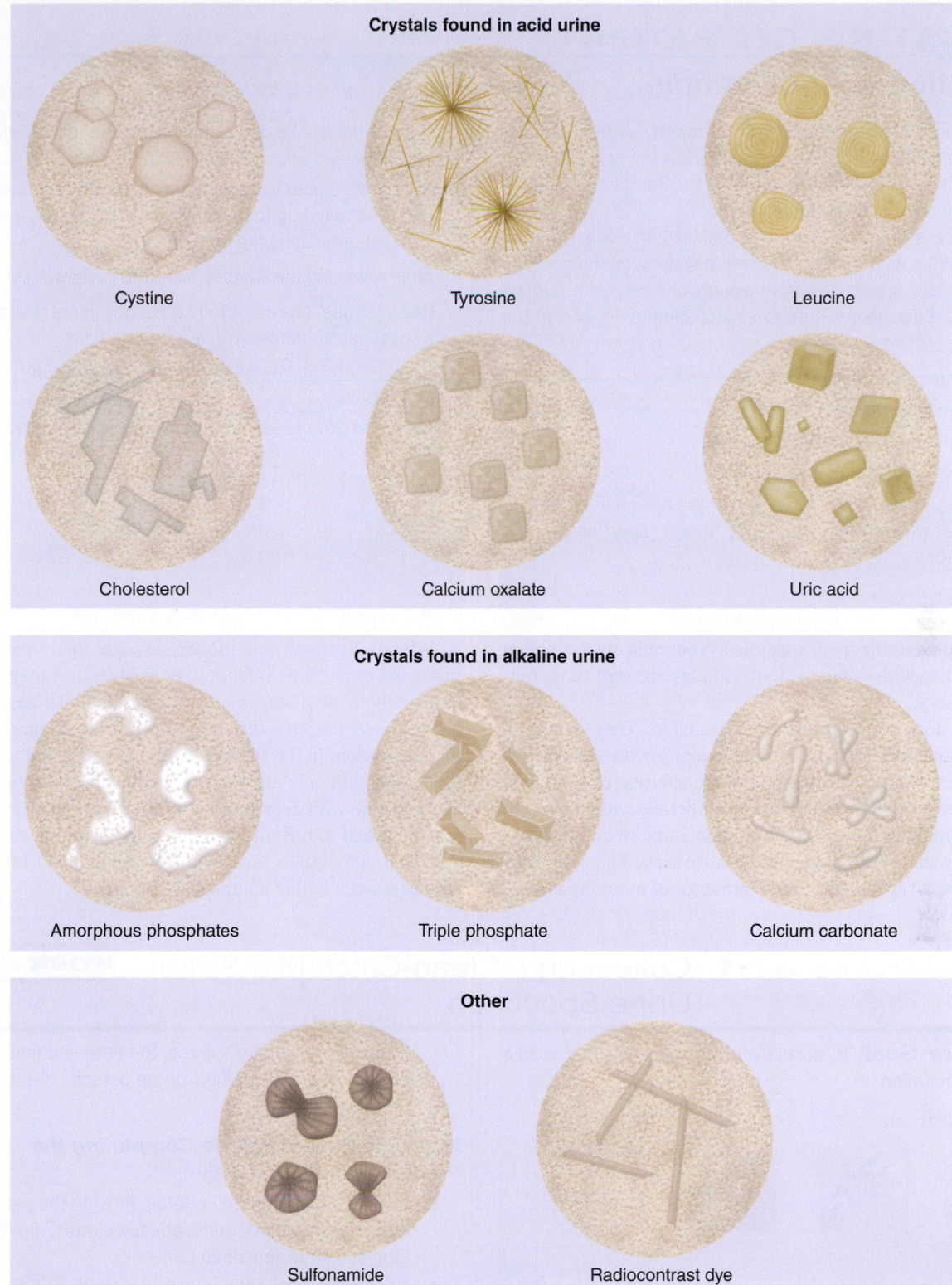

Crystals found in acid urine

Cystine

Tyrosine

Leucine

Cholesterol

Calcium oxalate

Uric acid

Crystals found in alkaline urine

Amorphous phosphates

Triple phosphate

Calcium carbonate

Other

Sulfonamide

Radiocontrast dye

FIGURE 47-7 Common urine crystals.

Suspected Protozoal or Parasitic Infection

In cases of a suspected protozoal or parasitic infection, the licensed practitioner may request an **O&P specimen,** short for *ova and parasites specimen.* This type of stool sample is examined for the presence of certain forms of protozoans or parasites, including their eggs (ova).

When a practitioner requests an O&P test, obtain both a fresh and a preserved stool specimen. A fresh specimen is examined both macroscopically and microscopically for the presence of microorganisms. A preserved specimen is also necessary because certain forms of these organisms are destroyed within a short time after leaving the body and may

Collecting a Stool Sample

Patients must collect stool specimens properly so that they are not contaminated with urine or water from the toilet, both of which can lead to inaccurate results. If the sample is contaminated, it will have to be collected again.

There are a number of ways a patient can collect a stool specimen. What works for one patient may not work for another. Obtaining stool specimens from young children also can be challenging. Educate patients to collect samples in one of the following ways:

- On a clean paper plate
- In a clean waxed-paper carton
- In a clean plastic or glass container
- On collection tissue that you provide
- On plastic wrap draped loosely over the back half of the toilet seat with enough material to form a collection pocket in the middle

- In a plastic hat-like device placed on the toilet under the seat or placed underneath a child
- In a child's diaper lined with plastic positioned toward the back and rolled up to make a dam, which helps keep urine from contaminating the sample

After collecting the sample, have the patient

- Use a tongue depressor to place a portion of the sample in a specimen container with a tight-fitting lid.
- Transport the specimen to the office or laboratory as soon as possible.
- Refrigerate the specimen if transport will be delayed.

---

not be detected in the fresh specimen. You must always obtain a preserved specimen when stool samples are sent to an outside laboratory.

Special stool collection kits are available. They contain a specimen container for a fresh sample along with vials of two types of preservatives: formalin (a dilute solution of formaldehyde) and polyvinyl alcohol (PVA). Instruct the patient to place the stool sample in the specimen container and to mix portions of the specimen in each of the preservative vials. The laboratory will examine all specimens for the presence of microorganisms.

When a licensed practitioner suspects that a patient has a protozoal or parasitic infection, he will request that a series of at least three stool specimens be examined. Three specimens are required because different forms of the microorganism may be present in the stool at different times, and some could be missed with only one sample. Because certain medications can interfere with detecting these microorganisms, the patient may be asked to refrain from using medications such as antidiarrheal compounds, antacids, and mineral oil laxatives for at least a week before samples are obtained.

PROCEDURE 47-1 Collecting a Clean-Catch Mid-Stream Urine Specimen   WORK // DOC

Procedure Goal: To collect a urine specimen that is free from contamination

OSHA Guidelines:

  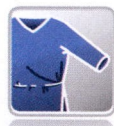

Materials: Dry, sterile urine container with lid; label; written instructions (if the patient is to perform procedure independently); and antiseptic towelettes, laboratory requisition form, patient chart/progress note

Method:

1. Confirm the patient's identity and be sure all forms are correctly completed.
2. Label the sterile urine specimen container with the patient's name, ID number, and date of birth; the

licensed practitioner's name; the date and time of collection; and the initials of the person collecting the specimen.

When the Patient Will Be Completing the Procedure Independently

3. Explain the procedure in detail. Provide the patient with written instructions, antiseptic towelettes, and the labeled sterile specimen container.
4. Confirm that the patient understands the instructions, especially not to touch the inside of the specimen container and to refrigerate the specimen until bringing it to the licensed practitioner's office.

    RATIONALE: *Touching the inside of the container will introduce microorganisms into the container and can interfere with the test results. The specimen should be refrigerated to keep bacteria from growing and causing a false-positive result.*

When You Are Assisting a Patient

3. Explain the procedure and how you will be assisting in the collection.

4. Wash your hands and don exam gloves.

When You Are Assisting in the Collection for Female Patients

5. Remove the lid from the specimen container and place the lid upside down on a flat surface.

6. Use three antiseptic towelettes to clean the perineal area by spreading the labia and wiping from front to back. Wipe with the first towelette on one side and discard it. Wipe with the second towelette on the other side and discard it. Wipe with the third towelette down the middle and discard it. To remove soap residue that could cause a higher pH and affect chemical test results, rinse the area once from front to back with water.

   RATIONALE: *The area must be thoroughly cleaned so that microorganisms from the vulva do not contaminate the specimen.*

7. Keeping the patient's labia spread to avoid contamination, tell her to urinate into the toilet. After she has expressed a small amount of urine, instruct her to stop the flow.

   RATIONALE: *So that microorganisms are washed away from the urethral opening.*

8. Position the specimen container close to but not touching the patient.

9. Tell the patient to start urinating again. Collect the necessary amount of urine in the container. (If the patient cannot stop her urine flow, move the container into the urine flow and collect the specimen anyway.)

10. Allow the patient to finish urinating. Place the lid back on the collection container.

11. Remove the gloves and wash your hands.

12. Complete the test request slip and record the collection in the patient's chart.

When You Are Assisting in the Collection for Male Patients

5. Remove the lid from the specimen container and place the lid upside down on a flat surface.

6. If the patient is circumcised, use an antiseptic towelette to clean the head of the penis. Wipe with a second towelette directly across the urethral opening. If the patient is uncircumcised, retract the foreskin before cleaning the penis. To remove soap residue that could cause a higher pH and affect chemical test results, rinse the area once from front to back with water.

   RATIONALE: *The area must be thoroughly cleaned so that microorganisms from the head of the penis do not contaminate the specimen.*

7. Keeping an uncircumcised patient's foreskin retracted, tell the patient to urinate into the toilet. After he has expressed a small amount of urine, instruct him to stop the flow.

   RATIONALE: *So that microorganisms are washed away from the urethral opening.*

8. Position the specimen container close to but not touching the patient.

9. Tell the patient to start urinating again. Collect the necessary amount of urine in the container. (If the patient cannot stop his urine flow, move the container into the urine flow and collect the specimen anyway.)

10. Allow the patient to finish urinating. Place the lid back on the collection container.

11. Remove the gloves and wash your hands.

12. Complete the laboratory requisition form and record the collection in the patient's chart/progress note.

PROCEDURE 47-2 Collecting a 24-Hour Urine Specimen WORK // DOC

Procedure Goal: To collect a urine specimen that is free from contaminants over a 24-hour period

OSHA Guidelines:

Materials: Urine collection container (disposable urinal or collection hat), sterile urine storage containers, written instructions, laboratory requisition form, and patient chart/progress note

Method:

1. Review the laboratory requisition form and gather the supplies.

2. Confirm the patient's identity, introduce yourself, and check that all forms are completed correctly.

3. Label the sterile urine specimen storage containers with the patient's name, ID number, and date of birth and the licensed practitioner's name.

4. Explain that the urine specimen storage container may have a preservative in it. Tell the patient what to do if he gets the preservative on his skin. (Usually, flushing with cold water is sufficient; follow the manufacturer's provided instructions.)

5. Give the patient the following instructions:

   a. At the start of the observation period (usually early in the morning), void and discard the first urine specimen. This will start the collection period. Write the start date and time on the urine specimen storage containers.

   RATIONALE: *So that only the urine produced in a 24-hour period is collected.*

b. Do not discard the preservative in the urine specimen storage container.

c. For the next 24 hours, each time you void, collect the entire specimen in the provided specimen collection container.

d. Carefully transfer the entire specimen in the urine storage container, being careful not to spill any urine. If the you spill urine or accidently urinate in the toilet, call to reschedule the test.

RATIONALE: *All urine must be collected so that an accurate measure of urine components may be obtained.*

e. Keep the specimen covered and in the refrigerator or in a cooler when not in use.

f. Twenty-four hours after you begin the test, void once more and transfer to the specimen storage container. Write the end date and time on the container.

g. As quickly as possible, bring the specimen back to the office or deliver it to the laboratory if instructed to do so. Keep the specimen cool during transport.

6. When the patient returns the urine specimen, wash your hands, don gloves, and then be sure to do the following:

a. Check that the container lid is secure.

b. Clean the outside of the container with a tissue or gauze pad if necessary.

c. Check that the start and end dates and times are recorded on the container.

d. Note the volume of the collected specimen.

e. Review the procedure with the patient to make sure the specimen was properly collected and stored during the collection period.

f. Complete the necessary laboratory requisition forms.

g. Notify the lab that the specimen is ready for transport.

h. Keep the specimen cold until it is transported to the lab.

7. Remove the gloves and wash your hands.

8. Document the specimen collection, including volume, dates and times, and lab tests requested.

PROCEDURE 47-3   Establishing Chain of Custody for a Urine Specimen

WORK // DOC

Procedure Goal: To collect a urine specimen for drug testing, maintaining a chain of custody

OSHA Guidelines:

  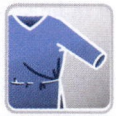

Materials: Dry, sterile urine container with lid; chain-of-custody form (CCF); and two additional specimen containers

Method:

1. Positively identify the patient. (Complete the top part of the CCF with the drug testing laboratory's name and address, the requesting company's name and address, and the patient's Social Security number. Make a note on the form if the patient refuses to give her Social Security number.) Ensure that the number on the printed label matches the number at the top of the form.

2. Ensure that the patient removes any outer clothing and empties her pockets, displaying all items.
   RATIONALE: *So that the patient does not bring anything into the room to adulterate the specimen, resulting in a false-negative result*

3. Instruct the patient to wash and dry her hands.

4. Instruct the patient that no water is to be running while the specimen is being collected. Tape the faucet handles in the *off* position and add bluing agent to the toilet.
   RATIONALE: *So that the patient cannot warm a specimen brought in from another source and has no water available to dilute the specimen.*

5. Instruct the patient to provide the specimen as soon as it is collected so that you can record the specimen's temperature.

6. Remain by the door of the restroom.

7. Measure and record the urine specimen's temperature within 4 minutes of collection. Make a note if its temperature is out of the acceptable range.
   RATIONALE: *To determine that the patient voided the specimen and did not bring it from an outside source.*

8. Examine the specimen for signs of adulteration (unusual color or odor).

9. *In the presence of the patient,* check the "single specimen" or "split specimen" box. The patient should witness you transferring the specimen into the transport specimen bottle(s), capping the bottle(s), and affixing the label on the bottle(s).
   RATIONALE: *To maintain the chain of custody.*

10. The patient should initial the specimen bottle label(s) *after* it is placed on the bottle(s).
    RATIONALE: *To maintain the chain of custody.*

11. Complete any additional information requested on the form, including the authorization for drug screening. This information will include the following:
    - Patient's daytime telephone number
    - Patient's evening telephone number
    - Test requested
    - Patient's name
    - Patient's signature
    - Date

12. Sign the CCF; print your full name and note the date and time of the collection and the name of the courier service.

13. Give the patient a copy of the CCF.

14. Place the specimen in a leakproof bag with the appropriate copy of the form.

15. Release the specimen to the courier service.

16. Distribute additional copies as required.

PROCEDURE 47-4 Measuring Specific Gravity with a Refractometer

Procedure Goal: To measure the specific gravity of a urine specimen with a refractometer

OSHA Guidelines:

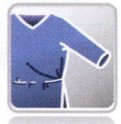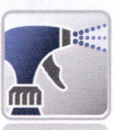

Materials: Urine specimen, refractometer, dropper, laboratory report form, and patient chart/progress note

Method:

1. Wash your hands and don exam gloves.

2. Check the specimen for proper labeling and examine it to make sure there is no visible contamination and that no more than 1 hour has passed since collection (or since the specimen was removed from the refrigerator and brought back to room temperature).

3. Swirl the specimen.
   RATIONALE: To mix the specimen thoroughly.

4. Confirm that the refractometer has been calibrated that day. If not, you must calibrate it with distilled water. You also must use two standard solutions as controls to check the refractometer's accuracy. Follow Steps 6 through 11, using each of the three samples in place of the specimen. Clean the refractometer and the dropper after each use and record the calibration values in the quality control log.
   RATIONALE: To ensure that the refractometer is standardized prior to testing the specimen.

5. Open the hinged lid of the refractometer.

6. Draw up a small amount of the specimen into the dropper.

7. Place one drop of the specimen under the cover.

8. Close the lid.

9. Turn on the light and look into the refractometer's eyepiece. As the light passes through the specimen, the refractometer measures the refraction of the light and displays the refractive index on a scale on the right, with corresponding specific gravity values on the left.

10. Read the specific gravity value at the line where light and dark meet.

11. Record the value on the laboratory report form.

12. Sanitize and disinfect the refractometer and the dropper. Put them away when they are dry.

13. Clean and disinfect the work area.

14. Remove the gloves and wash your hands.

15. Record the value in the patient's chart/progress note.

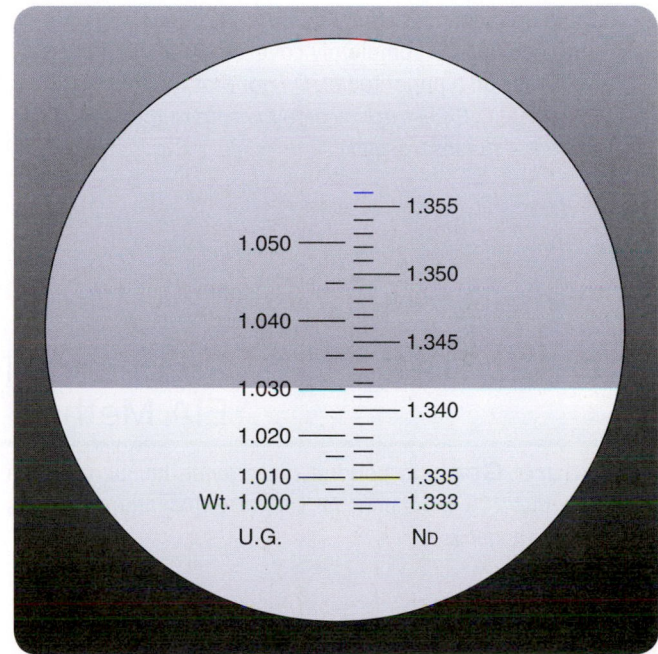

FIGURE Procedure 47-4 Step 9 A refractometer uses light refraction to measure specific gravity.

PROCEDURE 47-5 Performing a Reagent Strip Test

Procedure Goal: To perform chemical testing on urine specimens to screen for the presence of various elements, including leukocytes, nitrites, urobilinogen, protein, pH, blood, specific gravity, ketones, bilirubin, and glucose

OSHA Guidelines:

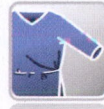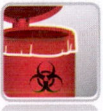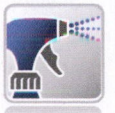

Materials: Urine specimen, laboratory report form, pipette or urinalysis transfer straw, reagent strips, paper towel, timer, and patient chart/progress note

Method:

1. Wash your hands and don personal protective equipment.
2. Check the specimen for proper labeling and examine it to make sure there is no visible contamination. Perform the test as soon as possible after collection. Refrigerate the specimen if testing will take place more than 1 hour later. Bring the refrigerated specimen back to room temperature prior to testing.
3. Check the expiration date on the reagent strip container and check the strip for damaged or discolored pads.
   RATIONALE: *To ensure that the reagent strip is still valid.*
4. Swirl the specimen.
   RATIONALE: *To mix the specimen thoroughly.*
5. Remove a small amount (aliquot) of the urine with a pipette or a urinalysis transfer straw and place it into a labeled secondary container.
   RATIONALE: *In the event that a urine culture is needed, the entire sample is not contaminated by chemicals on the reagent pads. These chemicals could interfere with a urine culture test.*

   Dip a urine strip into the aliquoted specimen, making sure each pad is completely covered. Briefly tap the strip sideways on a paper towel. *Do not blot* the test pads.
   RATIONALE: *Excess urine could migrate to the other pads and alter the test results.*

6. Read each test pad against the chart on the bottle at the designated time.
   Note: It is important to read each pad at the appropriate time. Most reagent strip results are invalid after 2 minutes.

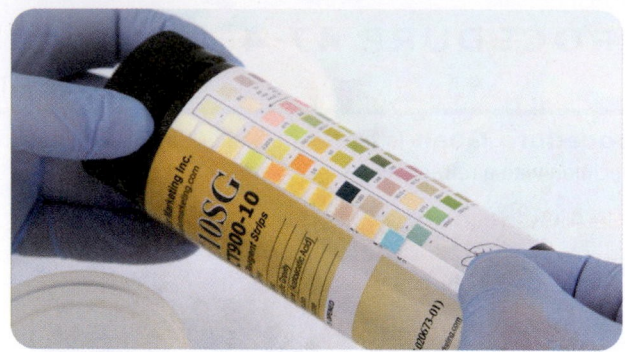

FIGURE Procedure 47-5 Step 6 Read the reagent strip by the time indicated in the manufacturer's instructions.
© McGraw-Hill Education

   RATIONALE: *Test pads read at inappropriate times will yield inaccurate results.*
7. Record the values on the laboratory report form.
8. Discard the used disposable supplies.
9. Clean and disinfect the work area.
10. Remove your gloves and wash your hands.
11. Record the result in the patient's chart/progress note.

PROCEDURE 47-6 Pregnancy Testing Using the EIA Method

WORK // DOC

Procedure Goal: To perform the enzyme immunoassay in order to detect HCG in the urine (or serum) and to interpret results as positive or negative

OSHA Guidelines:

 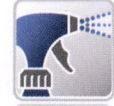

Materials: Gloves, urine specimen, urinalysis transfer straw, timing device, surface disinfectant, pregnancy control solutions, pregnancy test kits, quality control log, and patient chart/progress note

Method:

1. Wash your hands and don exam gloves.
2. Gather the necessary supplies and equipment.
3. If materials have been refrigerated, allow all materials to reach room temperature prior to conducting the testing.
4. Label the test chamber with the patient's name or identification number; label one test chamber for a negative and positive control.
5. Apply the urine (or serum) to the test chamber per the manufacturer's instructions. A urine transfer straw may be used.
   RATIONALE: *Different tests may have slightly different instructions.*
6. At the appropriate time, read and interpret the results.
   RATIONALE: *Most tests are invalid after 10 minutes.*

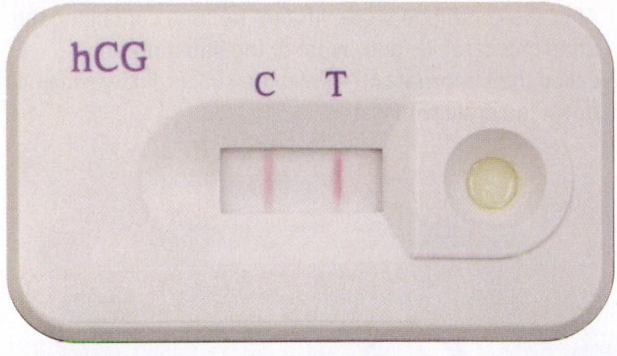

(a)

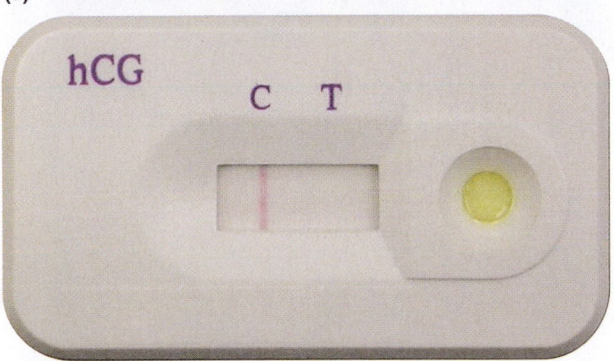

(b)

FIGURE Procedure 47-6 Step 6   A positive pregnancy test (a) and a negative pregnancy test (b). Note that if the line does not appear in the C (Control) area, the test is invalid.

© Leesa Whicker

7. Document the patient's results in the patient chart/progress note: document the quality control results in the appropriate quality control log book.
8. Dispose of used reagents in a biohazard container.
9. Clean the work area with a disinfectant solution.
10. Remove your gloves and wash your hands.

PROCEDURE 47-7   Processing a Urine Specimen for Microscopic Examination of Sediment

WORK // DOC

Procedure Goal: To prepare a slide for microscopic examination of urine sediment

OSHA Guidelines:

  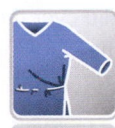

Materials: Fresh urine specimen, two glass or plastic test tubes, water, centrifuge, tapered pipette or urinalysis transfer straw, glass slide with coverslip, microscope with light source, laboratory report form, and patient chart/progress note

Method:

1. Wash your hands and don exam gloves.
2. Check the specimen for proper labeling and examine it to make sure there is no visible contamination and that no more than 1 hour has passed since collection (or since the specimen was removed from the refrigerator and brought back to room temperature).
3. Swirl the urine specimen.
   RATIONALE: *To mix the specimen thoroughly.*
4. Use a urinalysis transfer straw to place approximately 10 mL of urine into a labeled test tube. Pour 10 mL of plain water into the balance tube.

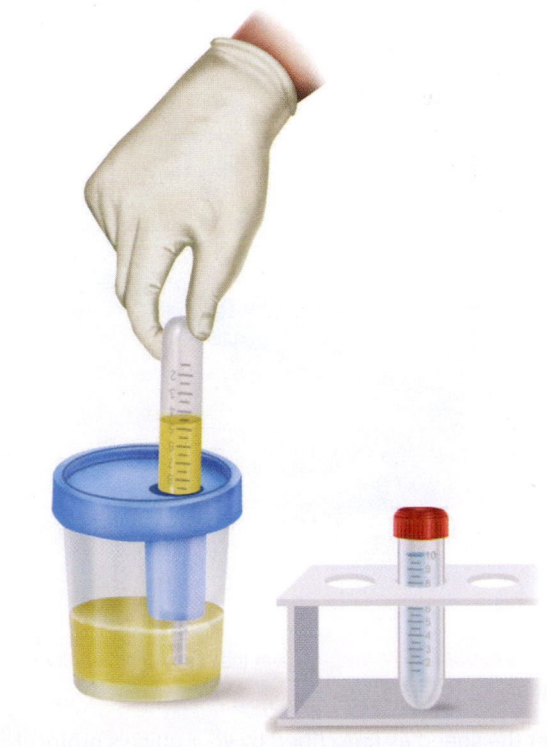

FIGURE Procedure 47-7 Step 4   Fill one test tube with approximately 10 mL of urine and the other with 10 mL of water.

5. Balance the centrifuge by placing the test tubes on opposite sides of the centrifuge.
   RATIONALE: *An unbalanced tube could cause the centrifuge to "walk" or wobble off the table.*

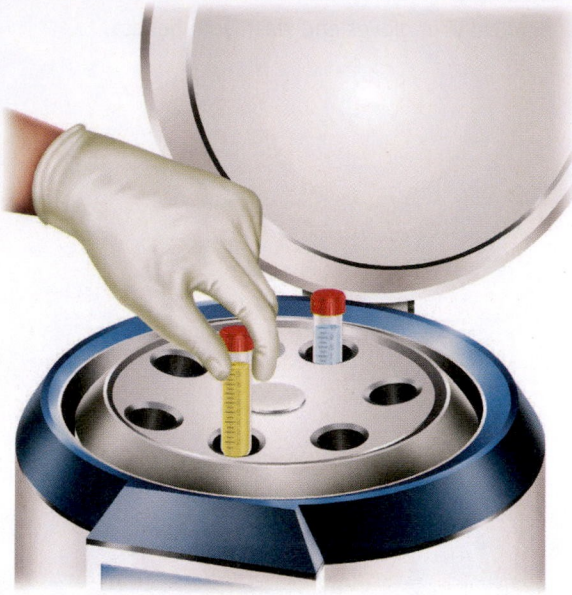

FIGURE Procedure 47-7 Step 5   The centrifuge must be balanced by placing one test tube on each side.

6. Make sure the lid is secure and set the centrifuge timer for 5 to 10 minutes.
   RATIONALE: *Spinning the urine will force the solids (cells, casts, and crystals) to the bottom of the tube.*

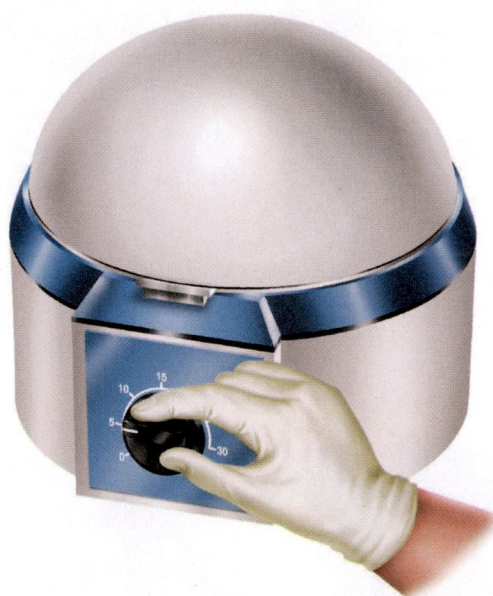

FIGURE Procedure 47-7 Step 6   Set the centrifuge timer for 5 to 10 minutes.

7. Set the speed as prescribed by your office's protocol (usually 1,500 to 2,000 revolutions per minute) and start the centrifuge.

8. After the centrifuge stops, lift out the tube containing the urine and carefully pour most of the liquid portion—called the **supernatant**—down the sink drain, washing it down the drain with water.

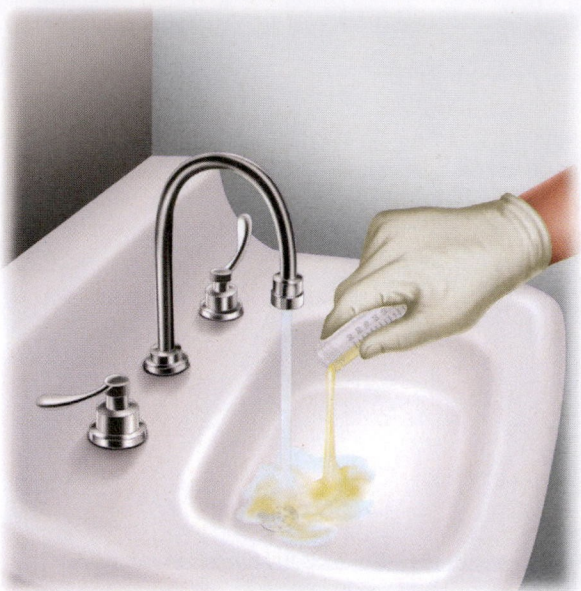

FIGURE Procedure 47-7 Step 8   Make sure you do not lose any sediment when you pour off the urine.

9. A few drops of urine should remain in the bottom of the test tube with any sediment. Mix the urine and sediment together by gently tapping the bottom of the tube on the palm of your hand.
   RATIONALE: *To resuspend the solid material.*

10. Use the tapered pipette or transfer straw to obtain a drop or two of urine sediment. Place the drops in the center of a clean labeled glass slide.

11. Place the coverslip over the specimen, allow it to settle, and place it on the stage of the microscope.

12. Correctly focus the microscope as directed in the *Microbiology and Disease* chapter.
    Note: Most medical assistants are trained to perform this procedure only up to this point. After this, the licensed practitioner usually examines the specimen. You may, however, be asked to clean the items after the examination is completed. The remaining steps are provided for your information.

13. Use a dim light and view the slide under the low-power objective. Observe the slide for casts (found mainly around the coverslip's edges) and count the casts viewed.

14. Switch to the high-power objective. Identify the casts. Identify any epithelial cells, mucus, protozoans, yeasts, and crystals. Adjust the slide position so that you can view and count the cells, protozoans, yeasts, and crystals from at least 10 different fields. Turn off the light after the examination is completed.

15. Record the observations on the laboratory report form.

16. Properly dispose of used disposable materials.

17. Sanitize and disinfect nondisposable items; put them away when they are dry.

18. Clean and disinfect the work area.

19. Remove the gloves and wash your hands.

20. Record the observations in the patient's chart/progress note.

PROCEDURE 47-8 Fecal Occult Blood Testing Using the Guaiac Testing Method

Procedure Goal: To test for the presence of blood in a fecal sample

OSHA Guidelines:

Materials: Fecal occult blood testing cards or slides, fecal collection spoon or other device, written patient instructions, testing reagents, and patient chart/progress note

Method:

1. Confirm the patient's identity and ensure that all forms are completed correctly.

2. Label the occult blood testing card or slide with the patient's name and date of birth. Give the patient the test card or slide and collecting spoon or applicator.

3. Give the patient pretest and collection instructions:

   a. Do not collect a sample if you are menstruating or if visible blood is seen in the feces or toilet.

   b. For 3 days prior to collecting the sample, avoid red meats (beef, veal, and lamb); horseradish; vitamin C supplements; certain fruits and vegetables, such as cabbage, cucumbers, broccoli, carrots, beets, radishes, mushrooms, and citrus fruits; aspirin or other nonsteroidal anti-inflammatory drugs; and other medications, including corticosteroids. (Consult the specific test instructions for dietary and medication restrictions, because these may vary from test to test.)

   RATIONALE: *Some foods and medications may cause a false-positive or a false-negative test result.*

   c. Collect the samples (depending on the specific test) on 2 or 3 different days.

   d. Collect the specimen before it comes into contact with the toilet water. (The patient may use a clean container or a specimen collection hat.)

   RATIONALE: *Chemicals in the toilet could interfere with the test.*

   e. Place a small amount of fecal material on each slide or test card window with the applicator. The sample should be thinly smeared in the sample area.

   f. Close the card window or place the slide in the provided container and write the collection date on the card or slide.

   g. Return the card or slide to the office.

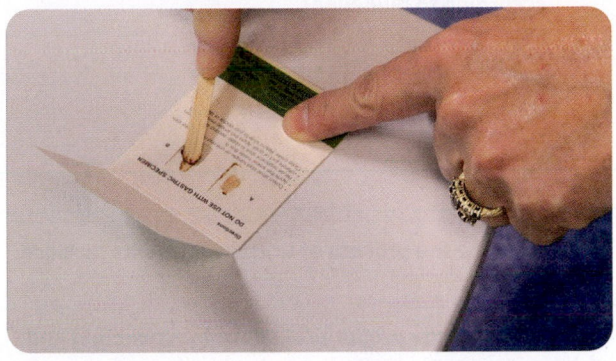

FIGURE Procedure 47-8 Step 3e   The patient should apply a thin smear of fecal material on each window of the test card.
© McGraw-Hill Education

Processing the Test

4. Wash your hands and don gloves.

5. Open the back of the card. Add the recommended amount of developing reagent directly over the smeared area on the back side of the paper and over the positive and negative controls, if present, on the card.

   RATIONALE: *To ensure that the test is working correctly.*

6. Read the test results at the appropriate time according to the manufacturer's instructions (usually within 60 seconds). There will be a blue color on the guaiac paper if blood is present.

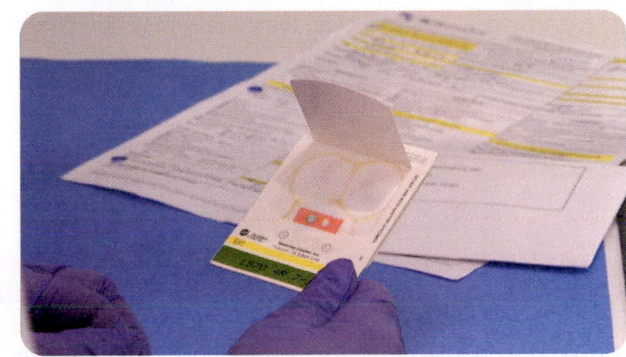

FIGURE Procedure 47-8 Step 6   Read the card by the time indicated in the manufacturer's instructions.
© McGraw-Hill Education

7. Dispose of the testing card according to OSHA regulations.

8. Remove your gloves and wash your hands.

9. Document the results in the patient's chart.

LEARNING OUTCOMES	KEY POINTS
47.1 Discuss the role of the medical assistant in collecting, processing, and testing urine and stool samples.	Your role as a medical assistant includes collecting, processing, and testing urine samples and processing and testing stool samples. You also will be responsible for teaching patients proper collection methods for urine and stool samples.
47.2 Carry out procedures for collecting urine specimens according to guidelines.	The general guidelines for collecting a urine specimen include following the procedure specified for the urine test that will be performed; using the type of specimen container indicated by the laboratory; properly labeling the specimen container; explaining the procedure to the patient when assisting in the collection process; washing your hands before and after the procedure and wearing gloves during the procedure; and completing all necessary paperwork.
47.3 Describe the process of urinalysis and its purpose.	Urinalysis is the evaluation of urine by various types of testing methods to obtain information about body health and disease.
47.4 Carry out the proper procedure for collecting and processing a stool sample for fecal occult blood testing.	The general guidelines for collecting a stool specimen include instructing the patient about the need to follow all collection procedures, including when to collect, how to collect, and how to return the specimen to the office; following the testing procedure for fecal occult blood testing; using standard precautions when performing the test; and documenting the test and results in the patient's chart.

CASE STUDY CRITICAL THINKING

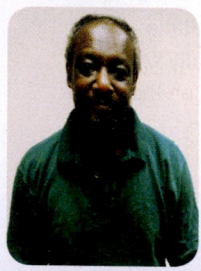

© McGraw-Hill Education

Recall Ken Washington from the beginning of the chapter. Now that you have completed the chapter, answer the following questions regarding his case.

1. What instructions will you give Ken in collecting the urine sample for reagent testing?

2. What tests are included in a reagent test?

3. Describe the instructions you will need to give Ken regarding his 24-hour urine collection.

EXAM PREPARATION QUESTIONS

1. (LO 47.2) Which of the following catheters is used after plastic repair of the ureter?
   a. Indwelling
   b. Urinary
   c. Drainage
   d. Splinting
   e. Permanent

2. (LO 47.3) The average adult urinary output is
   a. 650 mL
   b. 1,000 mL
   c. 1,250 mL
   d. 1,500 mL
   e. 2,000 mL

3. (LO 47.3) A urine sample that is turbid is said to be
   a. Cloudy
   b. Clear
   c. Odorous
   d. Dark
   e. Dilute

4. (LO 47.3) What is the specific gravity of distilled water?
   a. 0.00
   b. 1.000
   c. 1.001
   d. 1.010
   e. 1.100

5. (LO 47.3) Which of the following is (are) normally found in a urine sample?
   a. Cholesterol
   b. Tyrosine
   c. Ketone bodies
   d. Amorphous phosphates
   e. Glucose

6. (LO 47.4) A test for the presence of hidden blood in a stool sample is which of the following?
   a. SGOT
   b. FOBT
   c. Bilirubin
   d. EIA
   e. Urobilinogen

7. (LO 47.3) Calcium carbonate, calcium oxalate, and triple phosphate are types of which kind of structure sometimes present in urine?
   a. Casts
   b. Blood cell components
   c. Bence Jones proteins
   d. Vitamins
   e. Crystals

8. (LO 47.3) Which of the following is a chemical component of urine?
   a. Color
   b. Volume
   c. Blood
   d. Ketones
   e. Clarity

9. (LO 47.2) The most common type of urine sample is
   a. First morning
   b. 24-hour
   c. Timed
   d. Random
   e. Mid-stream

10. (LO 47.3) The term meaning insufficient production of urine is
   a. Anuria
   b. Oliguria
   c. Polyuria
   d. Proteinuria
   e. Hematuria

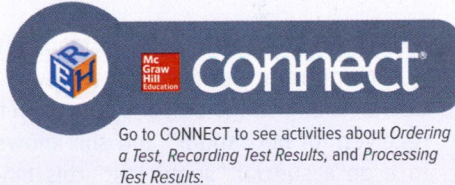

Go to CONNECT to see activities about *Ordering a Test*, *Recording Test Results*, and *Processing Test Results*.

S O F T   S K I L L S   S U C C E S S

The licensed practitioner has ordered a test of stool for blood on a patient. The patient is given a home testing kit, and he will need to take three samples of stool, one on each of 3 separate days. You are teaching the patient about the procedure when, in a rough and hostile voice, he states, "There is no way I am going to collect my own s***! You can tell that doctor to forget it!" What should you do?

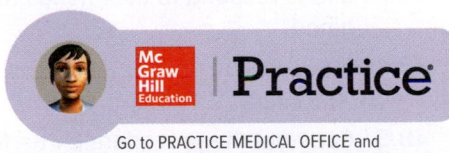

Go to PRACTICE MEDICAL OFFICE and complete the module Clinical - Interactions.

Collecting, Processing, and Testing Blood Specimens

48

CASE STUDY

<table>
<tr><td rowspan="5">PATIENT INFORMATION</td><td>Patient Name</td><td>DOB</td><td>Allergies</td></tr>
<tr><td>Sylvia Gonzales</td><td>9/1/19XX</td><td>PCN</td></tr>
<tr><td>Attending</td><td>MRN</td><td>Other Information</td></tr>
<tr><td>Alexis N.
Whalen, MD</td><td>341-73-792</td><td>Vital Signs:
BP 136/86,
T 97.6, P 92, R 20</td></tr>
</table>

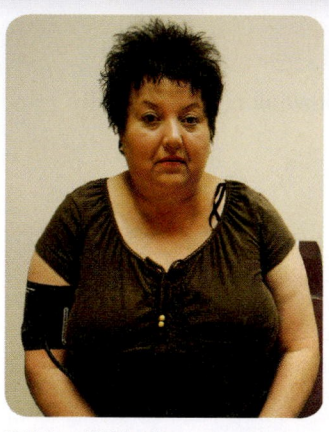

© McGraw-Hill Education

Sylvia Gonzales, a 51-year-old female, is at the office for a 3-month return check for her newly diagnosed Type 2 diabetes. She states that she has taken the medication she received for her "sugar" and she knows the doctor wants to a do a special "sugar test" this time. Her medication list includes Januvia® 100 mg daily. The physician has ordered a fasting blood sugar (FBS), electrolytes, and a CBC. You will need to collect a venipuncture blood specimen to send the lab. During the exam Sylvia states she is feeling lightheaded, so the licensed practitioner asks you to perform a waived blood sugar and hemoglobin A1C immediately.

Keep Sylvia in mind as you study this chapter. There will be questions at the end of the chapter based on the case study. The information in the chapter will help you answer these questions.

McGraw-Hill Education ACTIVSim

LEARNING OUTCOMES

After completing Chapter 48, you will be able to:

48.1 Discuss the role of the medical assistant when collecting, processing, and testing blood specimens.

48.2 Describe the equipment needed to collect a blood specimen.

48.3 Summarize ways to communicate with patients and to respond to their needs when collecting blood.

48.4 Carry out the procedure for collecting a blood specimen.

48.5 Carry out the procedure for performing blood tests.

KEY TERMS

anticoagulants
automatic puncturing devices
buffy coat
butterfly system
capillary puncture
complete blood (cell) count (CBC)
ethylenediaminetetraacetic acid (EDTA)
erythrocyte sedimentation rate (ESR)
formed elements
hematoma

hemolysis
lancet
micropipette
morphology
packed red blood cells
phlebotomy
requisition
serum separators
tourniquet
venipuncture
venoscope
whole blood

CAAHEP

I.C.10 Identify CLIA waived tests associated with common diseases

I.C.12 Identify quality assurance practices in healthcare

I.P.2. Perform:
(b) venipuncture
(c) capillary puncture

I.P.8 Instruct and prepare a patient for a procedure or a treatment

I.P.10 Perform a quality control measure

I.P.11 Obtain specimens and perform:
(a) CLIA waived hematology
(b) CLIA waived chemistry test
(d) CLIA waived immunology test

I.A.3 Show awareness of a patient's concerns related to the procedure being performed

II.P.2 Differentiate between normal and abnormal test results

II.P.3 Maintain laboratory test results using flow sheets

II.A.1 Reassure a patient of the accuracy of the test results

III.P.2 Select appropriate barrier/personal protective equipment (PPE)

III.A.1 Recognize the implications for failure to comply with Centers for Disease Control (CDC) regulations in healthcare settings

X.P.3 Document patient care accurately in the medical record

ABHES

3. Medical Terminology
d. Define and use acceptable medical abbreviations when appropriate and acceptable

9. Medical Office Clinical Procedures
a. Practice standard precautions and perform disinfection/sterilization techniques
j. Make adaptations with patients with special needs

10. Medical Laboratory Procedures
a. Practice quality control
b. Perform selected CLIA-waived tests that assist with diagnosis and treatment
(2) Hematology testing
(3) Chemistry testing
(4) Immunology testing
c. Dispose of biohazardous materials
d. Collect, label, and process specimens
(1) Perform venipuncture
(2) Perform capillary puncture

▶ Introduction

In many healthcare settings, the medical assistant is responsible for collecting blood specimens from patients and sometimes performing waived testing. In this chapter, you will be introduced to venipuncture and capillary collection procedures and you will learn the appropriate supplies and equipment needed to perform these procedures. You also will learn techniques for dealing with different types of patients and how to obtain blood specimens efficiently and effectively. Additionally, you will receive instruction on the performance and screening of common blood tests.

▶ The Role of the Medical Assistant LO 48.1

The examination of blood can provide extensive information about a patient's condition. You may be asked to collect and process blood specimens for examination in your work as a medical assistant. A basic understanding of the anatomy and physiology of the circulatory system will help you properly perform these tasks. You also will need a working knowledge of the functions of blood and the kinds of cells that make up blood tissue. (See the chapters *The Cardiovascular System* and *The Blood* for more information.)

You will use several techniques to obtain blood specimens. **Phlebotomy** is the withdrawal of blood from a vein. This is done using a procedure called **venipuncture:** the puncture of a vein with a needle for the purpose of drawing blood. Phlebotomists receive special training in phlebotomy; drawing blood is the main task in their work. Smaller blood specimens may be obtained by using a small, disposable instrument to pierce the surface of the skin and collect blood from the capillaries there. This is known as **capillary puncture.** It is sometimes referred to as *dermal puncture,* since the puncture is made through the dermis of the skin. You must be able to perform such procedures accurately so that the specimen is appropriate for the ordered tests. You also must be skilled in putting the patient at ease during this procedure. Your reassuring manner, ability to handle technical problems, and careful preparation for answering many kinds of questions will be important to your success in this area.

In addition to your many duties as a medical assistant, you must understand how to process blood specimens and conduct various blood tests, particularly if you work in a laboratory. You also must be able to complete the necessary paperwork to ensure that test results are handled efficiently and accurately. All these skills are essential, regardless of whether you collect blood specimens in a physician's office laboratory (POL), hospital, or laboratory drawing station.

▶ Preparation for Collecting Blood Specimens

LO 48.2

Following the steps in the standard process for drawing blood specimens will enable you to perform the procedure smoothly, accurately, and safely while ensuring properly completed documentation.

Reading and Interpreting the Test Order

The first steps in preparing to draw blood for testing are to review the written testing request and to assemble the equipment and supplies. The patient should arrive with a laboratory **requisition** form and/or the patient's EHR will reflect the licensed practitioner's order for the laboratory tests.

Your first step is to review this blood-collection order to determine what tests will be run. See Figure 48-1. Many tests require expedited or special handling to ensure accurate results.

Your office will have specific collection procedures for each type of test. If you will be sending the blood specimen to a reference laboratory for testing, make sure you know its requirements. The cost of reprocessing a test far surpasses the extra time needed to be sure of the process requirements.

When reviewing the test order, you will need to know the meaning of abbreviations in order to understand the requisition and to collect the correct amount of blood using the correct technique. See Table 48-1. If you are ever in doubt and the resources in your facility do not provide the answers, you should ask your supervisor or supervising practitioner.

Equipment for Drawing Blood

Specific blood-drawing equipment and collection devices vary with the type of test. Make sure you have the appropriate equipment to collect all necessary specimens if more than one test is ordered. All specimen-collection tubes, slides, and other containers should be labeled immediately after collection with the patient's name, the date and time of collection, the initials of the person collecting the specimen, and other information as required by the test procedure or your office (see Figure 48-2a). Some offices use an identification code for each patient.

Alcohol wipes, sterile gauze, and adhesive bandages are standard supplies for procedures during which blood is drawn from a vein or capillaries. However, alcohol can cause inaccurate results for certain tests, so for these tests, povidone-iodine or benzalkonium chloride may be used to clean the puncture site. You will need a **tourniquet** (a flat, broad length of vinyl or rubber or a piece of fabric with a Velcro® closure) for venipuncture (see Figure 48-2b).

All blood collection requires the use of a needle or other sharps device. Recall from the chapter *Infection Control Practices* that you must follow safe injection practices and use safety-engineered devices. In addition, personal protective equipment (PPE) must be used. See the *Caution: Handle with Care* feature Phlebotomy and Personal Protective Equipment.

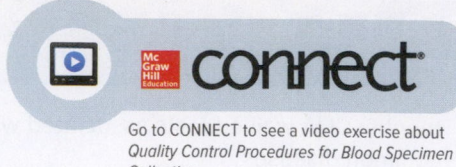

Go to CONNECT to see a video exercise about *Quality Control Procedures for Blood Specimen Collection.*

Venipuncture requires puncturing a vein with a needle and collecting blood into either a tube or in some cases a syringe. Capillary puncture requires a superficial puncture of the skin with a sharp point. Capillary puncture releases a smaller amount of blood.

Various instruments are used to perform venipuncture and capillary puncture. See Figure 48-3. Be familiar with and practice using the devices so that your technique is smooth, steady, and competent.

Evacuated Systems Evacuated systems—the most common is the Vacutainer® system (manufactured by Becton Dickinson—use a double-pointed needle, a plastic needle holder/adapter, and collection tubes (Figure 48-4). The collection tubes are sealed to create a slight vacuum and are called evacuated tubes. You insert the covered inner point of the needle into one end of the holder/adapter and the first collection tube into the other end.

An evacuated system has several advantages over other methods of blood collection. It is easy to collect several specimens from one venipuncture site using the interchangeable collection tubes, which are calibrated by vacuum to collect the exact amount of blood required. Some collection tubes are prepared with additives needed to correctly process the blood specimen for testing, such as anticoagulants. Finally, because there is no need to transfer blood from a collection syringe to a specimen tube, the potential for exposure to contaminated blood is reduced.

Butterfly Systems You may use a **butterfly system,** or winged infusion set, when you work with patients who have small or fragile veins. Flexible wings attached to the needle simplify needle insertion. A length of flexible tubing (either 5 or 12 inches, approximately) connects the needle to the collection device. The inserted needle remains completely undisturbed while the collection device is manipulated. Because it is motionless, the needle causes less trauma to the vein and surrounding tissue than other venipuncture systems. A butterfly system also generally uses a smaller needle (23-gauge) than other venipuncture techniques and can be used with an evacuated collection tube or a syringe (Figure 48-5).

Needle and Syringe Systems When a patient has small or fragile veins, the vacuum created when the collection tube is pressed over the needle point can cause the veins to collapse. Although it is the least desirable method of collection, you may need to collect blood using a sterile needle and syringe assembly when an evacuated system is not suitable, such as when the patient is difficult to stick. You can use a smaller needle—no smaller than 23-gauge to

Laboratory Requisition

BWW
BWW Medical Associates, PC
305 Main Street, Port Snead YZ 12345-9876
Tel: 555-654-3210, Fax: 555-987-6543
Web: BWWAssociates.com

Laboratory Name and Address

_____

_____

_____

Requesting Provider
Paul F. Buckwalter, MD
Alexis N. Whalen, MD
Elizabeth H. Williams, MD

Please Indicate Bill Type Below
Attach Copy of Insurance Card

Patient Data (Please Print)

Last Name **Gonzales**	First Name **Sylvia**	Maiden Name
Address **84 Denham Blvd, Bldg. 2**		Apt No. **21C**
City **Sneadsville**	State **VZ**	Zip **12345-9876**
SS# **101-01-0000**	Phone # **123-555-8901**	

Date of Birth (Month, Day, Year) **09 01 19XX** [ ] Male [X] Female
Date Collected: _____ Time Collected: ___:___ a.m. / p.m.

Physician 1 **Alexis N. Whalen, MD**   Physician 2

Billing Information (Please Print Clearly)

Please Bill to: [ ] Dr. Account (Client) [X] Patient Self Pay [ ] Insurance Co

Responsible Party (Last, First) **Gonzales, Sylvia** Relationship to Subscriber [X] Self [ ] Child [ ] Spouse [ ] Other

Primary Insurance Co. Name   [ ] HMO   [ ] PPO

Insurance Policy #   Insurance Group #

Primary Insurance Co: Address (Street, City, State, Zip)

Insured Date of Birth   Insured SS#

PLEASE PROVIDE MANDATORY ICD 10 CODE BELOW

1. **E11.9**   2.   3.   4.   5.

CALL TEST RESULTS TO:
Test: **CBC, Lytes FBS**
To: **Alexis N. Whalen, MD**
Phone: (**555**) **654-3210**

FAX RESULTS TO:
To:
Fax: (   )

[ ] Veni   Tech Code   Tubes Received

Please (X) desired Panel(s)/Profile(s)/Tests. See back of requisition for profile components.

PANELS/PROFILES	
Hepatitis Panel, Acute	2S
Basic Metabolic Panel	MT
Comp Metabolic Panel	MT
X Electrolyte Panel (Lytes)	MT
Hepatic Function Panel	MT
General Health Panel	MTL
Lipid Panel	MT
Obstetric Panel AMH	P2SL
Renal Panel	MT

MICROBIOLOGY	
Source of Specimen:	
Culture, Anaerobe	
Chlamydia/GC Amp Probe	
Culture, Ear	
Culture, Eye	
Leukocytes Stool	
Culture, Fungal	
Culture, Genital	
Culture, Herpes	
Occult Blood Screen	
Ova & Parasites	
Rapid Strep Throat	
Culture, Stool	
Culture, GROUP A BetaStrep Screen	
Culture GROUP B Screen	
Culture, Throat	
Culture, Urine	
Culture, Wound / Abscess	
Culture, Viral	
C. Difficile Toxin A&B AMH	

INDIVIDUAL TESTS	
ABO Group/RH	P
Acid Phosphatase, Prostatic	S
Albumin	MT
Alkaline Phosphatase	MT
Amylase	MT
Antinuclear Antibodies (ANA Send)	S
HCG, Beta Quant	MT
Bilirubin T / D Neonate	A
Bilirubin T / D Adult	MT
BNP Screen	L
BUN	MT
CA-125	S
CA-125 to Dianon	S
CRP	MT
CRP Cardio	MT
Calcium	MT
Carbamazepine/Tegretol	R
X CBC & PLT w/o Diff	L
CBC & PLT w Diff	L
Carcino Embryonic Antigen (CEA)	S
Cholesterol Total	MT
Cortisol Level	MT
Creatine Kinase, Total (CK)	MT
CPK total w CKMB	MT
Creatinine Clearance	U
Creatinine	MT
D Dimer Quant	B
DNA AB Double Strand	S
Digoxin Level	R

INDIVIDUAL TESTS (cont.)	
Drug Screen Urine	U
Drug Screen Urine c Confirm	U
Estradiol Level	MT
Ferritin Level	MT
Fetal Fibronectin (FFN)	SWAB
Folic Acid (PROTECT)	MT
Follicle Stimulating Hormone	MT
GGT (Gamma Glut Trans)	MT
Glucose	MT
X Glucose Fasting	MT
Glucose Challenge 1° Preg	MT
Glycosylated Hemoglobin (HA1C)	L
Hepatitis B Surface AG	S
Hepatitis B Surface AB	S
Hepatitis C Antibody	S
Herpes Simplex 1 & 2 IgG AB	S
Herpes Simplex 1 & 2 IgM AB	S
HIV I & II Abs	S
Homocysteine	L
Iron/TIBC	MT
Lactate Dehydrogenase (LDH)	MT
Lipase	MT
Lithium	R
Luteinizing Hormone	MT
Microalbumin Random/24 Hr.	U
Magnesium	MT
MONO test heterophile	S
Phenobarbital	R
Phenytoin/Dilantin	R
Phosphorous	MT
Potassium	MT
Progesterone	S
Prolactin	MT
PSA Free and Total	S
PSA Screen (Medicare)	S
PSA Diagnostic	S
Prothrombin Time	B
aPTT	B
PTH Intact	S
Reticulocyte Count	L
Rheumatoid Factor (RF)	MT
RPR QUAL	S
Rubella, IgG	S
ESR (Sed Rate)	L
SGOT (AST)	MT

SGPT (ALT)	MT
Testosterone	S
Testosterone Free & Total	S
TSH	MT
Total T3	MT
T3 Uptake	S
Free T3	MT
Free Thyroxine (FT4)	MT
Total T4	S
Free Thyroxine index (FTI)	S
Thyroid Antibodies	S
Troponin/Quant	MT
Triglycerides	MT
Uric Acid	MT
Urinalysis	U
Valproic Acid / Depakote	R
Vitamin B12 (PROTECT)	MT
Vitamin D 25 Hydroxy	S

ADDITIONAL ORDERS

(a) A physician's office staff may use a written laboratory requisition form to order tests for patients.

FIGURE 48-1   All required patient, specimen, and billing information must be included on a laboratory requisition form.

(continued)

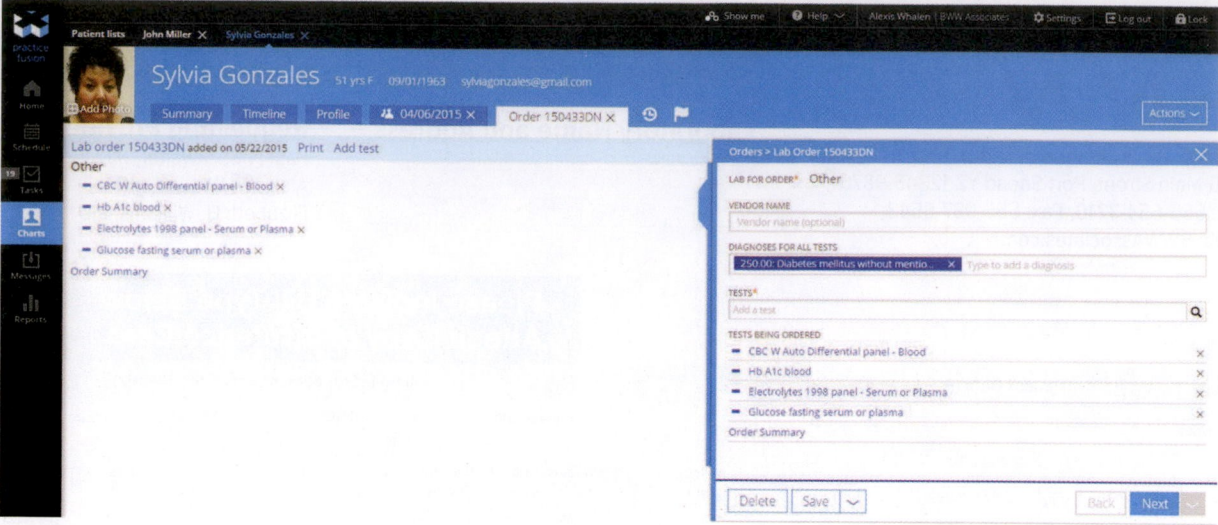

(b) The patient's electronic health record will include the laboratory tests that are ordered.

FIGURE 48-1 The laboratory requisition and/or the EHR order must be reviewed before any specimen is collected.

© Practice Fusion®

TABLE 48-1	**Abbreviations Routinely Used in Blood Tests**		
Abbreviation	**Meaning**	**Abbreviation**	**Meaning**
Ab	Antibody	BT	Bleeding time
ABO	Classification system for four blood groups	BUN	Blood urea nitrogen
AcAc	Acetoacetate	Ca; Ca++	Calcium
ACE	Angiotensin-converting enzyme	CA	Cancer antigen
ACT	Activated coagulation time	CBC	Complete blood (cell) count
ACTH	Adrenocorticotropic hormone	CEA	Carcinoembryonic antigen
ADH	Antidiuretic hormone	CHS	Cholinesterase test
AFB	Acid-fast bacillus	CMV	Cytomegalovirus
AFP	Alpha-fetoprotein	CO	Carbon monoxide
Ag	Antigen	CO_2	Carbon dioxide
AG	Anion gap	COHb	Carboxyhemoglobin
A/G R	Albumin-globulin ratio	CPK	Creatine phosphokinase
ALB	Albumin	CRCL	Creatinine clearance
ALP; alk phos	Alkaline phosphatase	Cre	Creatinine
ALT	Alanine aminotransferase	DHEA-SO4	Dehydroepiandrosterone sulfate
ANA	Antinuclear antibody	Dif, Diff	Differential (blood cell count)
APAP	Acetominophen	EBNA-IgG	Epstein-Barr virus nuclear antigen
APTT	Activated partial thromboplastin time	EBV	Epstein-Barr virus
ASA	Acetylsalicylic acid (aspirin)	EDTA	Ethylenediaminetetraacetic acid
AST	Aspartate aminotransferase	ELP	Electrophoresis, protein
AT-III	Antithrombin III	Eos	Eosinophil
B	Blood (whole blood)	Eq	Equivalent
Baso	Basophil	ESR	Erythrocyte sedimentation rate
BCA; BRCA	Breast cancer antigen	ETOH	Alcohol
BJP	Bence Jones protein	FBS	Fasting blood sugar

(continued)

TABLE 48-1

Abbreviation	Meaning	Abbreviation	Meaning
Free T$_4$	Free thyroxine	MPV	Mean platelet volume
FSH	Follicle-stimulating hormone (follitropin)	msAFP	Maternal serum alpha-fetoprotein
FTI	Free thyroxine index	NE	Norepinephrine
GFR	Glomerular filtration rate	OGTT	Oral glucose tolerance test
GH	Growth hormone	P	Plasma
GHRH	Growth hormone-releasing hormone	PBG	Porphobilinogen
GnRH	Gonadotropin-releasing hormone	PCT	Prothrombin consumption time
GTT	Glucose tolerance test	PCV	Packed cell volume (hematocrit)
HA	Hemagglutination	Pi	Inorganic phosphate
HA1C, HgbA1c	Glycosylated hemoglobin	PKU	Phenylketonuria
HAI	Hemagglutination inhibition test	PLT	Platelet
HAV	Hepatitis A virus	PMN	Polymorphonuclear (leukocyte; neutrophil)
Hb; Hgb	Hemoglobin	PRL	Prolactin
HbCO	Carboxyhemoglobin	PSA	Prostate-specific antigen
HBV	Hepatitis B virus	PT	Prothrombin time
HCG; hCG	Human chorionic gonadotropin	PTH	Parathyroid hormone
Hct	Hematocrit	PTT	Partial thromboplastin time
HCV	Hepatitis C virus	PZP	Pregnancy zone protein
HDL	High-density lipoprotein	RAIU	Thyroid uptake of radioactive iodine
HDV	Hepatitis delta virus	RBC	Red blood cell; red blood (cell) count
HGH; hGH	Human growth hormone	RBP	Retinol-binding protein
HIV	Human immunodeficiency virus	RDW	Red cell distribution of width
HLA	Human leukocyte antigen	Retic	Reticulocyte
HPV	Human papillomavirus	RF	Rheumatoid factor; relative fluorescence unit
HSV	Herpes simplex virus	Rh	Rhesus factor
HTLV	Human T-cell lymphotrophic virus	RIA	Radioimmunoassay
Ig	Immunoglobulin	rT$_3$ or REVT$_3$	Reverse triiodothyronine
IgE	Immunoglobulin E	S	Serum
INH	Inhibitor	Segs	Segmented polymorphonuclear leukocyte
IV	Intravenous	SPE	Serum protein electrophoresis
L	Liver	T$_3$	Triiodothyronine
LD; LDH	Lactate dehydrogenase	T$_4$	Thyroxine
LDL	Low-density lipoprotein	TBG	Thyroxine-binding globulin
LH	Luteinizing hormone	TBV	Total blood volume
LMWH	Low-molecular-weight heparin	TG	Triglyceride
Lytes	Electrolytes	TRH	Thyrotropin-releasing hormone
MCH	Mean corpuscular hemoglobin	TSH	Thyroid-stimulating hormone
MCHC	Mean corpuscular hemoglobin concentration	VDRL	Venereal Disease Research Laboratory (test for syphilis)
MCV	Mean corpuscular volume	VLDL	Very low-density lipoprotein
MHb	Methemoglobin	WB	Western blot
MONO	Monocyte	WBC	White blood cell; white blood (cell) count

Source: http://labtestsonline.org/.

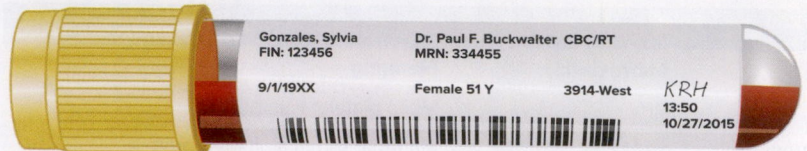

(a) Specimen collection tubes must be labeled with all required information immediately after collection.

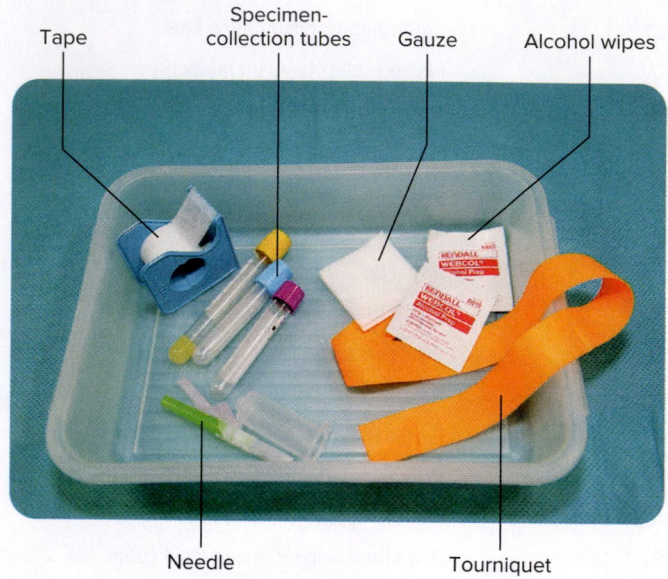

Tape — Specimen-collection tubes — Gauze — Alcohol wipes

Needle — Tourniquet

(b) Common blood collection equipment.

FIGURE 48-2 A variety of equipment is needed to perform routine blood collection.

© McGraw-Hill Education. Sandra Mesrine, photographer

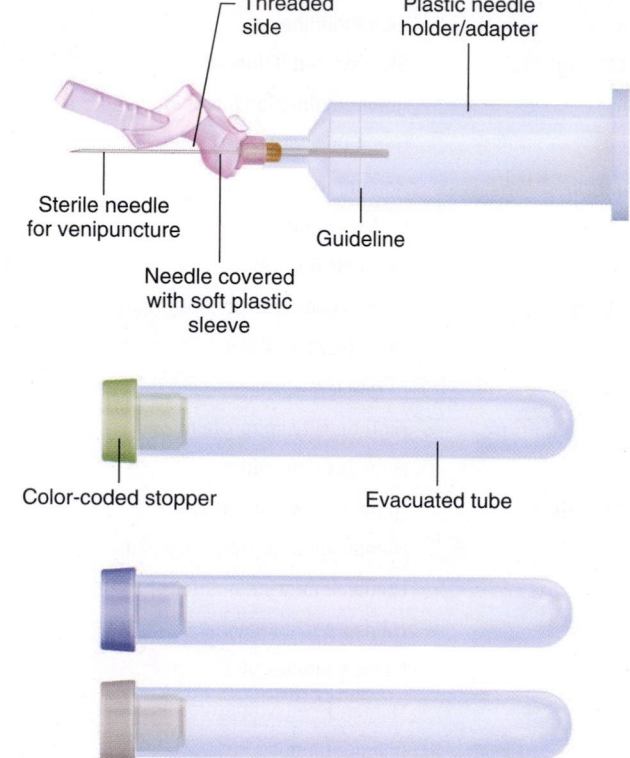

Threaded side — Plastic needle holder/adapter

Sterile needle for venipuncture — Needle covered with soft plastic sleeve — Guideline

Color-coded stopper — Evacuated tube

FIGURE 48-4 The Vacutainer® system uses interchangeable collection tubes that allow you to draw several blood specimens from the same venipuncture site.

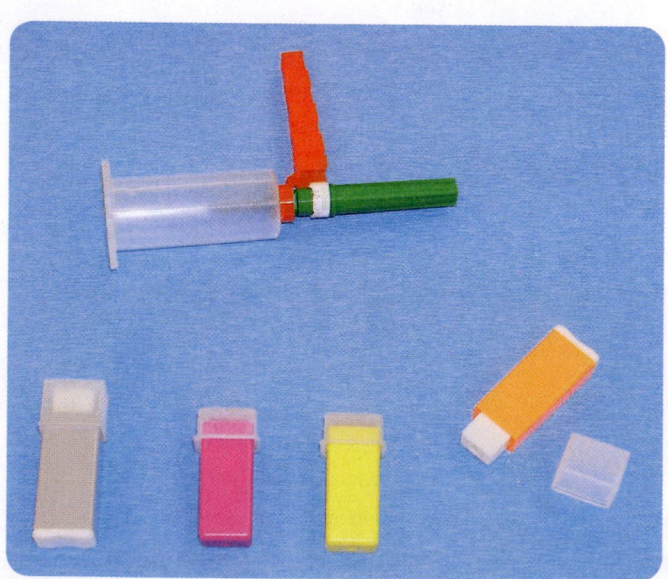

FIGURE 48-3 Various venipuncture and capillary puncture safety devices.

© Leesa Whicker

avoid hemolyzing the blood—and control the vacuum in the syringe by pulling the plunger back slowly. Other aspects of the procedure are essentially the same, except that the blood specimen is collected in the syringe and must immediately be transferred to a collection tube.

Collection Tubes No matter which method is used to collect blood, the specimens must immediately be mixed with the appropriate additives in the correct collection tubes before they are transported to the laboratory for testing. The tube stoppers are different colors, each color identifying the type of additives (if any) a collection tube contains (Figure 48-6).

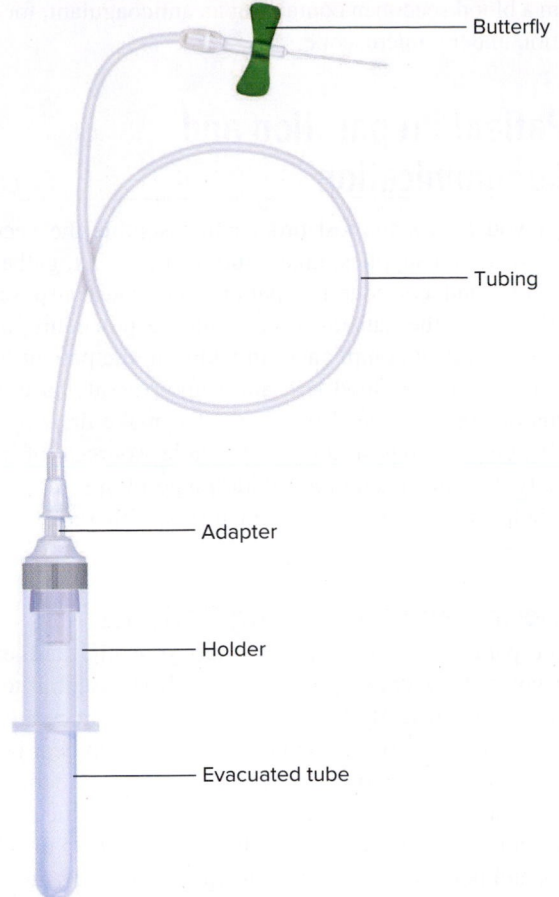

Butterfly

Tubing

Adapter

Holder

Evacuated tube

FIGURE 48-5 Once inserted, the needle of a butterfly system remains undisturbed during specimen collection.

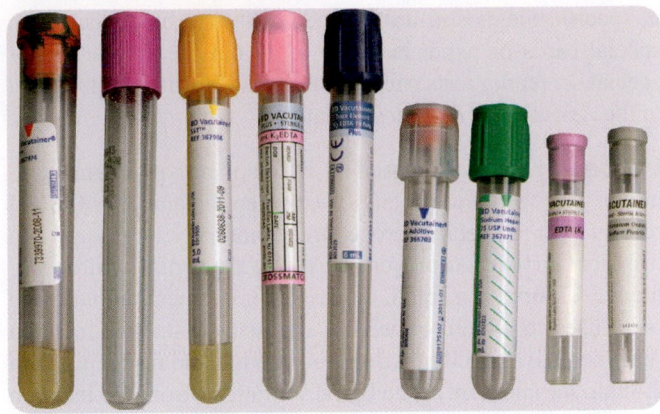

FIGURE 48-6 Special color-coded stoppers on collection tubes indicate which additives are present and, therefore, which types of laboratory tests may be performed on each blood specimen.
© Lillian Mundt

Additives include anticoagulants, such as **ethylenediamine-tetraacetic acid (EDTA),** and other materials that help preserve or process a specimen for particular types of testing. When you collect a blood specimen, double-check that you are using the appropriate collection tubes for the tests ordered. You also must fill the tubes in a specific order to preserve the integrity of each blood specimen by preventing carryover of tube additives from one tube to the next. Each laboratory requires a specific order of draw for collection tubes. The National Committee for Clinical Laboratory Standards also publishes its recommended order of draw. Table 48-2 identifies collection tube stopper colors, additives present in the tubes, and types of tests, in a typical order of draw.

Capillary Puncture Blood from a capillary puncture may be collected in small, calibrated glass tubes; collected on glass microscope slides; or applied directly to reagent strips (or dipsticks), which are specially treated paper or plastic strips used

These additives must be compatible with the laboratory process the specimen will undergo. Each laboratory may choose which tubes to use for a particular test.

TABLE 48-2	Blood-Collection Tubes		
Stopper Color		**Additive**	**Test Types**
Yellow	⬤	Sodium polyanetholsulfonate	Blood cultures
Light blue	⬤	Sodium citrate	Coagulation studies
Red	⬤	None	Blood chemistries, HIV/AIDS antibody, viral studies, and serologic tests
Gold or red/gray	⬤ ⬤	Clot activator Silicone serum separator	Tests requiring blood serum, routine blood donor screening, and infectious disease testing
Green	⬤	Heparin	Electrolyte studies and arterial blood gases
Lavender	⬤	Ethylenediaminetetraacetic acid (EDTA) (anticoagulant)	Hematology and blood chemistries
Gray	⬤	Potassium oxalate or sodium fluoride (anticoagulant)	Blood glucose

Note: Tubes are listed in the order they should be collected (order of draw).

in specific diagnostic tests. Blood also may be collected on special cards or paper and sent to an outside laboratory for special screening tests such as PKU. PKU testing is discussed in the *Assisting in Pediatrics* chapter.

Lancets Lancets are used in the capillary puncture technique. This technique is employed when the amount of blood required for a specific procedure is not very large or when technical difficulties prevent the use of the venipuncture technique. A **lancet** is a small, disposable instrument with a sharp point used to puncture the skin and make a shallow incision (between 2.0 and 3.0 mm deep for an adult and no deeper than 2.4 mm for an infant). The blood welling up from the incision is then collected.

Automatic Puncturing Devices **Automatic puncturing devices** are loaded with a lancet. Because the depth to which they puncture the skin is mechanically controlled, they are more accurate and comfortable than the traditional lancet method. These spring-loaded devices have disposable platforms that rest on the finger. Different platforms are used, depending on the desired depth of the puncture. Both the lancet and the platform should be discarded after use. Pen-like devices also can hold a lancet inside. This device is held against the skin and activated by pushing a button. The advantages of these devices are that they are easy to use, the puncture depth can be easily adjusted, and there is an automatic ejection button for lancet disposal. Some companies also manufacture completely disposable devices, which come individually wrapped and are used only once.

Micropipettes A pipette is a calibrated glass tube for measuring fluids. A **micropipette** is a small pipette that holds a small, precise volume of fluid. You will use micropipettes to collect capillary blood for some tests. Capillary tubes, with a single calibration mark, are also used to collect capillary blood for certain tests.

Microtainer® Tubes Microtainer® tubes (manufactured by Becton Dickinson Vacutainer® Systems) are small plastic tubes with a wide-mouthed collector, similar to a funnel, that allows blood to flow quickly and freely into the tube. Like collection tubes in an evacuated system, Microtainer® tubes have different colored tops indicating the additives, if any, they contain.

Reagent Products Several common tests do not require processing of blood specimens. For these tests, you may apply droplets of freshly collected blood to chemically treated paper or plastic reagent strips (dipsticks) or add freshly collected blood droplets to small containers holding chemicals that react in the presence of specific substances or microorganisms. Some of the blood tests performed in this way detect blood glucose levels, sickle cell anemia, infectious mononucleosis, and rheumatoid arthritis.

Smear Slides You may need to apply a drop of freshly collected blood to a prepared microscope slide for some tests. More commonly, a smear slide is prepared in the laboratory from a blood specimen containing an anticoagulant, for examination under a microscope.

▶ Patient Preparation and Communication

LO 48.3

After you review the test order and assemble the necessary equipment and supplies, take a moment to relax, gather your thoughts, and consider the patient and your purpose. You need to greet the patient and explain the procedure, as well as ensure patient compliance. In addition, the patient may be anxious about the blood test, and some patients have special needs or present special problems that make drawing blood challenging. Being aware of possible sources of patient anxiety and understanding a wide range of special concerns can help you respond to patient needs with sensitivity and competence.

Greeting and Identifying Patients

Greet patients pleasantly, introduce yourself, and explain that you will be drawing some blood. It is essential to identify patients correctly before you begin the procedure. Ask patients to state their full name and be sure you hear both the first and last names correctly. Verify that the name the patient gives is the name on the order. In most facilities, the phlebotomist should ask for a date of birth and verify the patient ID or chart number against the order to further identify the patient as mandated by The Joint Commission (TJC).

Confirming Pretest Preparation

The presence and level of certain substances in blood are affected by food and fluid intake or by other daily life activities. Some tests require the patient to follow certain pretest restrictions to minimize the influence of the restricted food on the blood, or to stress the body to see how it responds, as indicated by the blood.

Fasting is the most common requirement for pretest preparation. For example, a lipid profile, which measures cholesterol, triglycerides, HDL, LDL, and VLDL, requires fasting. A fasting blood sugar (FBS) requires fasting, as do other types of glucose testing. For example, the glucose tolerance test measures a patient's ability to metabolize carbohydrates and is used to detect hypoglycemia and diabetes mellitus. The patient must eat a high-carbohydrate diet for 3 days before the test and fast for 8 to 12 hours before the appointment.

Before you draw blood for any test, determine whether the patient has complied with pretest instructions. If the patient has not complied, explain that the test cannot be performed. Make a note on the order and report the information to the licensed practitioner or your supervisor.

Explaining the Procedure and Safety Precautions

Explain to the patient the procedure you will use to obtain the blood specimen for testing. Be clear and brief when you describe what you will do; too much detail leaves some patients queasy. Explain the need for each of the preventive measures, such as the use of PPE, in language the patient can understand. Assure the patient that these measures protect against exposure to infection.

Establishing a Chain of Custody

You will need to follow specific guidelines to establish a chain of custody for blood specimens drawn for drug and alcohol analysis. Because donating a specimen for drug and alcohol testing is potentially self-incriminating, the patient must sign a consent form for the testing. The *Collecting, Processing, and Testing Urine and Stool Specimens* chapter explains general chain-of-custody procedures.

Patient Fears and Concerns

Some patients express their fears or concerns directly. Other patients ask questions that highlight their fears. Providing more information or a complete understanding is reassuring to many patients. For others, the information serves only to confuse, overwhelm, or create more fear. You must decide how much information to give each patient and be prepared to answer questions.

Patients sometimes ask questions that are not appropriate for you to answer. A patient may ask you about his prognosis, medical condition, blood type, or other medical information. It is not appropriate for you to discuss these topics with the patient. Encourage the patient to discuss these issues with the licensed practitioner. Some commonly expressed fears and concerns to which you should respond, however, are covered in the following paragraphs.

Pain The question medical assistants performing phlebotomy probably hear most often is "Will this hurt"? Never lie to a patient who asks this question. Inform the patient that he will feel a stick just as the lancet or point of the needle is inserted but that this pain goes away almost immediately. Tell a patient who seems particularly nervous to take a deep breath and let it out slowly. Also suggest that the patient focus on something else in the room or close his eyes and relax during the procedure.

A patient may express concern and report a previous unpleasant experience with blood testing. Listen to the patient's concerns. Describe what you will do to reduce discomfort and what the patient can do to be more at ease. Let the patient know you will help him sit comfortably or lie down while the blood specimen is being obtained. Tell the patient to let you know if he begins to feel light-headed. You might also ask the patient whether one arm is better to use than the other. Many patients have had blood drawn before and can tell you which sites were successful. Consulting the patient helps the patient feel more in control and provides you with important information.

CAUTION: HANDLE WITH CARE

Phlebotomy and Personal Protective Equipment

The Centers for Disease Control and Prevention (CDC) has classified all phlebotomy procedures as a risk for exposure to contaminated blood or blood products. You must use appropriate personal protective equipment (PPE) during all phlebotomy procedures. Remember, it is up to you to protect yourself and the patient.

Gloves

Gloves—which protect against spills and splashing of contaminated blood—are the first line of defense during a phlebotomy procedure. Wash your hands and don clean exam gloves that fit snugly before you work with each patient. Remove the gloves, dispose of them in a biohazardous waste container, and wash your hands after working with each patient.

Garments

Garments such as laboratory coats and aprons can protect your clothing from spills and splashes and provide a measure of protection from contaminated materials. Some garments are designed to resist penetration by blood or blood products. You may find it necessary to wear such garments when drawing blood or performing blood tests.

Masks and Protective Eyewear

Mucous membranes are especially vulnerable to invasion by infectious agents. Use masks and protective eyewear to help safeguard mucous membranes in your mouth, nose, and eyes from infection.

Masks help protect your mouth and nose from splashes or sprays of blood or blood products. You cannot predict when exposure to blood may occur. Accidental puncture of an artery during a phlebotomy procedure could result in a spray of blood, or blood may spray or splash accidentally during testing protocols. Most medical assistants do not routinely wear masks for phlebotomy procedures once they have achieved proficiency in performing them. Goggles can also protect your eyes from splashing and spraying during blood drawing or testing.

Clear plastic face shields combine the protection of masks and goggles and are often used during major surgical procedures. You may use a face shield if you do extensive testing on blood specimens, but face shields are not usually worn when drawing blood.

PPE works two ways: It protects you from a patient's contaminated blood and it protects the patient from infectious agents you may be carrying. By using PPE correctly, you will make your workplace a safer place for you and the patients.

Scars Some patients may express fear of getting a bruise or scar from a blood collection procedure. Explain that some bruising is possible but that it will fade within a few days. Most bruising is caused by a hematoma, which occurs when blood leaks out of the vein and collects under the skin. Hematomas can be prevented by releasing the tourniquet before withdrawing the needle and applying proper pressure over the puncture site after the needle has been withdrawn. Bruising is common with fair-skinned patients. Scars, on the other hand, are unlikely.

Serious Diagnosis Patient fears are not always rational. One fear patients express is that the more tubes of blood you require, the more serious their condition must be. Patients also may fear that a blood test is being done to help the practitioner diagnose an extremely serious disease.

You can help relieve a patient's fears by explaining that a blood test is one of the best ways to obtain an overall picture of health (emphasize health, not disease). Note that blood tests show what is normal about the blood as well as any abnormalities. You might also explain that several specimens are being taken because the blood used in blood tests is processed in different ways; the blood collected for one test cannot be used in another.

Blood testing also may be done to determine how well and at what levels medications are acting in the blood. Explain that the practitioner may want to see how much medication is in the blood to better manage the prescribed dosage. When a patient needs repeated tests for drug levels, explain that the tests show how the body is using the medication.

Contracting a Disease from the Procedure Probably the greatest fear of patients undergoing blood tests is contracting HIV/AIDS or hepatitis B virus (HBV). Although many people are now well informed about how HIV/AIDS and other serious diseases are contracted, it is understandable for a patient to worry about bloodborne pathogens. Do not dismiss the patient's concerns and do not downplay the importance of following standard precautions.

Explain the precautions you will take to prevent the spread of infection. Allow the patient to see you wash your hands and put on new gloves before you begin to take the blood specimen. Stress that the needle is sterile. Explain that you have not touched the needle and that it will be discarded when you finish. Let the patient see you put the needle in the sharps container.

Use this opportunity to educate the patient about the transmission of HIV/AIDS. Emphasize that HIV/AIDS, and other infections transmitted by blood, can be transmitted only when there is direct contact with contaminated blood or other body fluids. Explain that your gloves protect both you and the patient by providing a barrier to infection transmission from one person to another. Explain that your other protective equipment, such as goggles or a mask, also helps prevent the spread of infection.

Special Considerations

As you collect blood specimens, you will encounter a variety of patients, some of whom have special needs. You will find yourself in many different situations, some of them problematic. Some special needs and problematic situations are fairly common, and you must be prepared to deal with them.

Patients at Risk for Uncontrolled Bleeding Patients who have hemophilia or are taking blood-thinning medications are at risk for uncontrolled bleeding at the collection site. (Hemophilia is a disorder in which the blood does not coagulate at a wound or puncture site.) Be especially careful and alert as you follow the standard procedures for collecting a blood specimen. In addition, hold several gauze squares over the puncture site for at least 5 minutes to make sure bleeding has stopped completely. If uncontrolled bleeding does occur, call the licensed practitioner immediately.

Difficult Patients You may encounter a particular challenge in working with a patient either because of technical problems or because of personality issues. Being prepared for these situations is the best method for coping with them.

The Difficult Venipuncture There will be times when you simply cannot get a good blood specimen. If your first attempt at drawing blood fails, try again at another site. Give the patient (and yourself) a short break and make an attempt on the other arm, for instance. Sometimes the veins in one arm are easier to work with than the veins in the other arm. Some facilities may have available an instrument, such as a **venoscope,** to visualize the vein. The battery-operated venoscope uses light-emitting diode (LED) lights to illuminate the subcutaneous tissue and highlight the veins, making the veins easier to locate. If you cannot get a good specimen on the second try, stop. Ask for assistance from your supervisor or the licensed practitioner.

Fainting Patients It is impossible to predict which patients will have a reaction to a blood-drawing procedure. Generally, however, an ill patient is more likely to experience a reaction than a well patient. The best way to deal with this potential problem is to position every patient so that, if fainting does occur, no injury will result. Have patients sit in a special venipuncture chair (Figure 48-7), designed to help prevent patients from sliding to the floor in the event of fainting. If your office is not equipped with a venipuncture chair, have patients lie down on an examining table. A patient who has a history of fainting or feels ill should lie down with feet elevated or knees drawn up while you complete the procedure. Sometimes just talking with the patient, asking her simple questions, will help keep her from fainting.

If a patient does faint and the needle is still in the vein, release the tourniquet and withdraw the needle quickly and steadily. Apply pressure to the site. Most people revive promptly and no other action is required. Do not leave the patient alone. Notify the licensed practitioner that the patient has fainted and ask the practitioner whether you should continue with the procedure.

If there is a more severe reaction, notify the appropriate staff member and remain with the patient. If the patient is in a chair and begins to slide out, raise the safety arm and gently

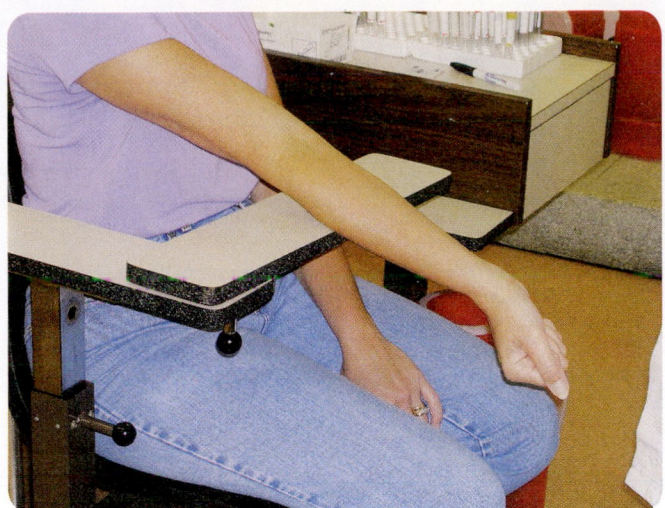

FIGURE 48-7 Venipuncture chairs are designed to make blood drawing easier and to prevent patients from falling if they should faint.
© Leesa Whicker

lower the patient to the floor. Protect the patient's head at all times and make sure the patient is breathing. The licensed practitioner should examine the patient before the patient is moved. Follow the practitioner's instructions.

When the patient begins to recover, assist the patient into a sitting position and then to a chair or couch. The patient should rest until feeling strong enough to walk—usually about 15 minutes. When the patient feels steady, take the patient to another area of the office, such as the patient reception area. At this point, another staff member usually becomes responsible for the patient's care and determines when it is safe for the patient to leave.

Angry or Violent Patients Some patients are extremely resistant to having blood drawn. Although their objections may seem illogical, remember, people often do not think as clearly in moments of high emotion as they normally do.

Encourage a patient who is mildly upset and wants to argue about the need for the blood test to let you take the specimen and then discuss the situation with the licensed practitioner. If you convince the patient to submit to the test, complete the procedure quickly and accurately. Avoid arguing with the patient.

Do not force the issue with a patient who becomes violent or refuses outright to submit to the procedure. A patient does have the right to refuse testing or treatment. Under no circumstances should you attempt to physically force a patient to give a blood specimen. Never endanger yourself, other patients, or your colleagues by refusing to back down from an angry or violent patient. Report the problem to the appropriate staff, make a note on the order, and follow other established procedures as determined by your facility.

▶ Performing Blood Collection LO 48.4

Venipuncture

Some states permit medical assistants to obtain blood specimens. Your office will clarify which phlebotomy-related duties, if any, you may perform. If your duties include

collecting blood specimens, you will obtain them through either venipuncture or capillary puncture. You must understand when these techniques are used and know how to perform them. Procedure 48-1, at the end of this chapter, details quality control procedures for collecting blood specimens.

The most common sites for venipuncture are the median cubital and cephalic veins of the forearm. Other sites may be used if a primary site is unavailable. Figure 48-8 shows the veins in the antecubital fossa (the small depression inside the bend of the elbow) and the forearm.

In order to locate the correct site and perform the venipuncture, you will need to apply a tourniquet. The tourniquet is applied to the arm 3 to 4 inches above the venipuncture site. Follow the steps shown in Figure 48-9 for proper application of the tourniquet. Procedure 48-2, at the end of this chapter, provides step-by-step instructions for performing the venipuncture using an evacuated system.

Capillary Puncture

Capillary puncture requires a superficial puncture of the skin with either a lancet or an automatic puncture device. Capillary puncture in adults and children is usually performed on the great (middle) finger or the ring finger. Use the patient's nondominant hand for this procedure if possible. The puncture should be made slightly off-center on the pad of the fingertip, because the pad's center is usually more sensitive. Capillary puncture in infants is usually performed on one of the outer edges of the underside of the heel (Figure 48-10). An alternate site for both children and adults is the lower part of the earlobe, unless the patient's ear is pierced. Procedure 48-3, at the end of this chapter, explains how to perform a capillary puncture and collect a sample of capillary blood.

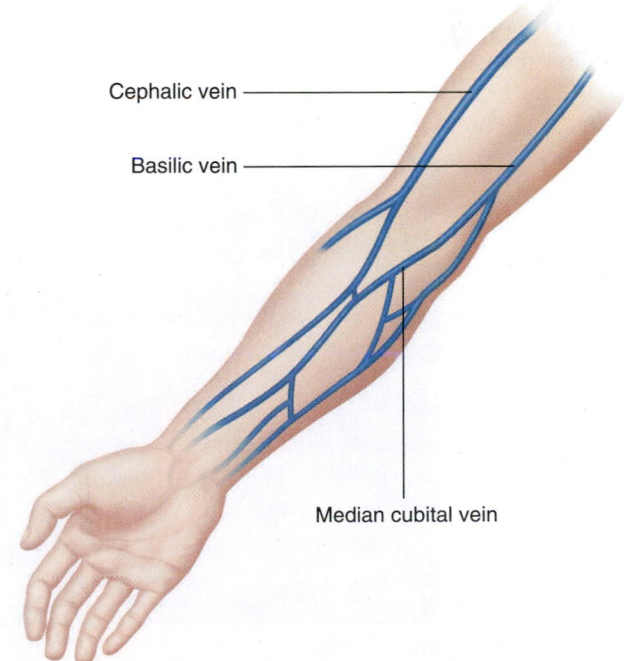

FIGURE 48-8 Veins commonly used for venipuncture include the cephalic vein, the basilic vein, and the median cubital vein.

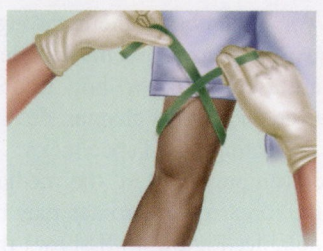 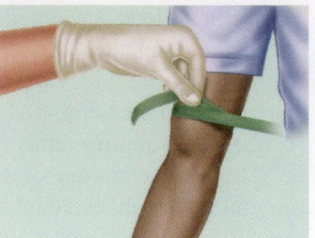 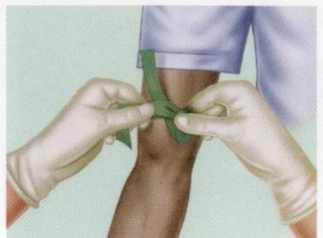 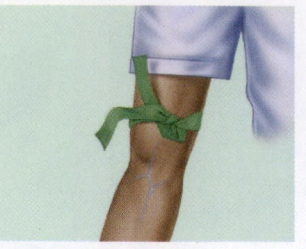

(a) Position the tourniquet under the arm while grasping the ends above the arm and venipuncture area. The tourniquet should be 3 to 4 inches above the site.

(b) Cross the left end over the right end and apply a small amount of tension to the tourniquet.

(c) Using the right middle finger or index finger, tuck the left end under the right end.

(d) A loose end of the tourniquet will be pointing toward the shoulder and the loop will be pointed toward the hand.

FIGURE 48-9   Follow these steps for proper tourniquet application.

Blood Cultures

Blood culture specimens are collected to test for the presence of bacteria in the blood. When collecting blood for a culture, it is important that no skin organisms contaminate the specimen. Skin organisms such as staphylococci and streptococci can cause a false-positive blood culture test result. For this reason, proper aseptic technique is essential. Pay special attention to keeping the collection bottle, syringe, and needle sterile and properly cleansing the skin. If you are drawing additional specimens for other tests, always draw the blood culture first. This eliminates the possibility of contaminating the culture with additives from other tubes. When collecting a blood culture specimen, you should follow these steps:

1. Select the appropriate site for venipuncture.
2. Cleanse the skin with isopropyl alcohol.
3. Cleanse the skin again with an iodine or chlorhexidine solution applied in an outward, circular pattern (cleansing from inside to outside).
4. Allow the iodine solution to air-dry.
5. Remove the plastic top from the collection bottle and wipe with a sterile alcohol pad.
6. Allow the alcohol to air-dry.
7. Draw the blood from the selected site.
8. Properly label the specimens.

Separate blood specimens are put into two collection bottles, one for aerobic and one for anaerobic culture. You may be asked to draw a second set of specimens from another vein. Use the same technique for each specimen, and make sure all specimens are properly identified.

Venipuncture Complications

Venipuncture is, in general, a safe procedure. Most of the complications you encounter are mild and more of a nuisance than anything. Venipuncture can have some serious complications, but they are rare. You must be aware of possible complications and ways to avoid them, and you should understand how to deal with them if they occur. Some of the more serious complications you may encounter are

- **Hematoma.** A collection of blood will sometimes form under the skin. This is especially a problem in patients who

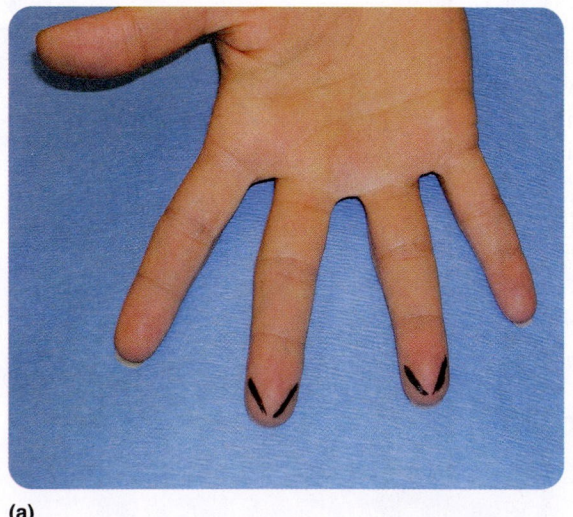 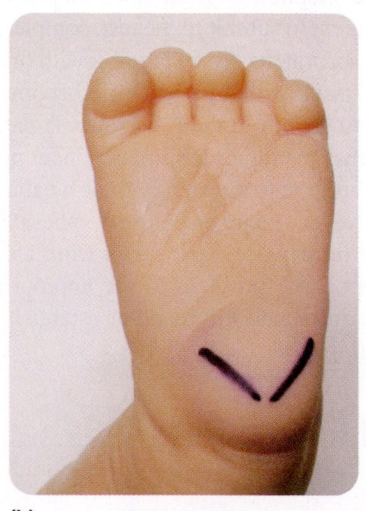

(a)   **(b)**

FIGURE 48-10   Capillary puncture sites for (a) an adult and (b) an infant.
© Leesa Whicker

have bleeding disorders, are elderly, or are taking anticoagulants. To avoid hematomas, hold the needle as still as possible while filling and changing the tubes. You may need to use a butterfly collection device. Hold pressure on the venipuncture site as soon as you remove the needle. Have the patient elevate her arm but not bend the elbow. If a hematoma does form, apply extra gauze to the puncture site and wrap with stretch bandage. Watch the patient and alert the licensed practitioner if necessary.

- *Latex allergy.* Some patients have an allergy to latex. Make sure you ask the patient if he has any allergies before you begin the procedure. If the patient has a latex allergy, make sure you use nonlatex gloves, tourniquet, and bandages. If the patient has an unexpected allergic reaction to latex, alert the licensed practitioner and follow her instructions.

- *Nerve injury.* It is essential that you know the anatomy of the antecubital fossa so that you can accurately locate the proper veins for venipuncture. Inserting a needle into a nerve can cause nerve damage. Permanent sensory and/or motor damage to the arm and hand can occur if the venipuncture is done incorrectly. If you suspect you have stuck the patient's nerve, withdraw the needle immediately and alert the licensed practitioner.

- *Infections.* Though quite rare, infections after venipuncture do occur and can be very serious. Use only approved single-use venipuncture equipment. Cleanse the venipuncture site well before the procedure. An infection at the venipuncture site may not be evident for several days after the procedure. If the patient calls, complaining of redness, heat, or drainage at the site, have her return to the office to see the licensed practitioner. A more serious blood infection (sepsis) may at first seem like the patient has the flu, as fever and chills are the first symptoms. A patient with a blood infection can go into shock if left untreated. If you suspect that the patient has a blood infection, have her see the licensed practitioner immediately.

▶ Performing Common Blood Tests LO 48.5

Many blood tests are routinely ordered as part of a complete general exam to determine a patient's overall health. The results of individual tests can provide information that aids in the diagnosis of specific conditions, diseases, and disorders, as noted in Table 48-3.

The number of blood tests routinely performed in POLs has declined since the implementation of Clinical Laboratory

TABLE 48-3 Common Blood Tests and the Conditions They Help Identify

Substance Identified or Quantified	Stopper Color and Additive	Part of Blood Tested	Indication, Disease, or Disorder
Alanine aminotransferase (ALT)	Clot activator Silicone serum separator	Serum	Liver disorders
Alpha-fetoprotein (AFP)	Clot activator Silicone serum separator	Fetal serum	Fetal liver and gastrointestinal tract status, and hepatitis
Amylase	Clot activator Silicone serum separator	Serum	Drug toxicity and parotid or pancreas disorders
Angiotensin-converting enzyme (ACE)	Clot activator Silicone serum separator	Serum	Lung cancer, sarcoidosis, and acute or chronic bronchitis
Antidiuretic hormone (ADH)	EDTA	Plasma	Syndrome of inappropriate ADH, Guillain-Barré syndrome, and brain tumor

(continued)

TABLE 48-3   Common Blood Tests and the Conditions They Help Identify

Substance Identified or Quantified	Stopper Color and Additive	Part of Blood Tested	Indication, Disease, or Disorder
Aspartate aminotransferase (AST)	Clot activator Silicone serum separator	Serum	Liver disease (including viral hepatitis), infectious mononucleosis, and damaged heart or skeletal muscle
Bilirubin	Clot activator Silicone serum separator	Serum	Liver disease, fructose intolerance, and hypothyroidism
Blood urea nitrogen (BUN)	Clot activator Silicone serum separator	Serum	Kidney disorders
Calcium, total (fasting)	Clot activator Silicone serum separator	Serum	Hyperparathyroidism and malignant disease with bone involvement
Cancer antigens (numbers 125, 15-3, 549, 72-4), tumor-associated glycoprotein (TAG)	Clot activator Silicone serum separator	Serum	Specific cancers identified, depending on antigen tested
Carbon dioxide, total	Clot activator Silicone serum separator	Venous serum	Acidosis or alkalosis (acid-base balance)
Cholesterol, total	Clot activator Silicone serum separator	Serum	Hyperlipoproteinemia, coronary artery disease, and atherosclerosis
Creatine kinase (CK)	Clot activator Silicone serum separator	Serum	Muscular dystrophies, Reye's syndrome, heart disease, shock, and some neoplasms
Erythrocyte count (RBC)	EDTA	Whole blood	Anemia
Erythrocyte sedimentation rate (ESR)	EDTA	Whole blood	Inflammation, infectious diseases, malignant neoplasms, and sickle cell anemia
Glucose (fasting)	Potassium oxalate or sodium fluoride	Whole blood	Pancreatic function and ability of intravenous insulin to offset diet in diabetes mellitus

(continued)

TABLE 48-3 Common Blood Tests and the Conditions They Help Identify

Substance Identified or Quantified	Stopper Color and Additive	Part of Blood Tested	Indication, Disease, or Disorder
Glucose (fasting—tolerance test)	Potassium oxalate or sodium fluoride	Serum	Diabetes mellitus and hypoglycemia
Lactate dehydrogenase (LD)	Clot activator Silicone serum separator	Serum	Anemia, viral hepatitis, shock, hypoxia, and hyperthermia
Leukocyte count (WBC)	EDTA	Whole blood	Leukemia, infection, and leukocytosis
Phenylalanine	Heparin or newborn screening card	Plasma	Hyperphenylalaninemia, obesity, and phenylketonuria
Potassium (K^+) and sodium (Na^+)	Clot activator Silicone serum separator	Serum	Fluid-electrolyte balance
Prostate-specific antigen (PSA)	Clot activator Silicone serum separator	Serum	Prostate cancer and BPH
Sickle cells	EDTA	Whole blood	Sickle cell anemia
Thyroid-stimulating hormone (TSH), triiodothyronine (T_3), thyroxine (T_4)	Clot activator Silicone serum separator	Serum	Thyroid function
Uric acid	Clot activator Silicone serum separator	Serum	Gout and leukemia

Note: Different laboratories may have different testing protocols and may require other tube tops than those represented in this table. Consult your laboratory procedures manual for additional information regarding required collection tubes.

Improvement Amendments of 1988 (CLIA '88) regulations. Many POLs now perform only waived tests. Each POL is different, however, and regulations do change. Check with your employer about what tests your office performs regularly. You should be familiar with a wide range of tests and the steps involved with each, even if you do not anticipate performing them.

Given that some testing can occur in the POL, you may encounter several chemical substances while performing your responsibilities in the laboratory. Chemicals you might encounter in laboratory work include the following:

- **Anticoagulants,** which cause the blood to remain in a liquid, uncoagulated state
- **Serum separators,** which form a gel-like barrier between serum and the clot in a coagulated blood specimen
- Stains, which color specific types of cells, making microscopic studies easier to complete

Anticoagulants or serum separators are already present in blood-collection tubes and do not need to be added to the specimen.

You must be absolutely clear about which chemicals are used for which tests and the precise amounts involved. It is also important to understand the purpose of blood tests so that you can educate patients. You must, in addition, know the range of normal test values so that you can be aware of potential problems and note them for the licensed practitioner's attention. Table 48-4 shows the normal ranges for a variety of blood tests.

TABLE 48-4 Normal Ranges for Blood Tests

Blood Test	Stopper Color and Additive*	Blood Component Tested	Normal Range**
Blood Counts			
Red blood cells (erythrocytes)	EDTA	Whole blood	$4.7–6.1 \times 10^6$ cells/mcL
Men		Whole blood	$4.2–5.4 \times 10^6$ cells/mcL
Women			
White blood cells (leukocytes)	EDTA	Whole blood	$4.5–11.0 \times 10^3$ cells/mcL
Platelets		Whole blood	$150–400 \times 10^3$ cells/mcL
Differential			
Neutrophils		Whole blood	40%–60%
Eosinophils		Whole blood	1%–4%
Basophils		Whole blood	0.5%–1%
Lymphocytes		Whole blood	20%–40%
Monocytes		Whole blood	2%–8%
Hematocrit (Hct)	EDTA	Whole blood	
Men			40.7%–50.3%
Women			36.1–44.3%
Hemoglobin (Hb, Hgb)	EDTA	Whole blood	
Men			13.8–17.2 g/dL
Women			12.1–15.1 g/dL
Erythrocyte Sedimentation Rate (ESR)			
Wintrobe	EDTA	Whole blood	
Men			0–5 mm/hour
Women			0–15 mm/hour
Westergren	EDTA	Whole blood	
Men			0–15 mm/hour
Women			0–20 mm/hour
Coagulation Tests			
Prothrombin time (PT)	Sodium citrate	Plasma	11–15 seconds
Bleeding time	Sodium citrate	Whole blood	2–7 minutes
Electrolytes			
Bicarbonate (HCO_3^-)	Clot activator	Arterial plasma	21–28 mEq/L
	Silicone serum	Venous plasma	27–29 mEq/L
Calcium (Ca^{++})	separator	Serum	8.6–10.0 mEq/L
Chloride (Cl^-)	Heparin	Serum, plasma	98–108 mEq/L
Potassium (K^+)		Serum	3.5–5.1 mEq/L
Sodium (Na^+)		Serum	136–145 mEq/L

(continued)

TABLE 48-4   Normal Ranges for Blood Tests

Blood Test	Stopper Color and Additive*	Blood Component Tested	Normal Range**
Chemical and Serologic Tests			
Alanine aminotransferase (ALT)	Clot activator Silicone serum separator	Serum	
Men			10–40 U/L
Women			7–35 U/L
Alpha-fetoprotein (AFP)	Clot activator Silicone serum separator	Serum	
Fetal, first trimester			20–400 mg/dL
Adult			<15 ng/mL
Aspartate aminotransferase (AST, formerly SGOT)	Clot activator Silicone serum separator	Serum	
Men			11–26 U/L
Women			10–20 U/L
Bilirubin, total direct	Clot activator Silicone serum separatorr	Serum	0.3–1.2 mg/dL
Blood urea nitrogen (BUN)	Clot activator Silicone serum separator	Serum, plasma	6–20 mg/dL
Carcinoembryonic antigen (CEA)	Clot activator Silicone serum separator	Serum	<5.0 ng/mL
Cholesterol, total	Clot activator Silicone serum separator	Serum, plasma	
Men			158–277 mg/dL
Women			162–285 mg/dL
High-density lipoproteins (HDLs)	Clot activator Silicone serum separator	Serum, plasma	
Men			28–63 mg/dL
Women			37–92 mg/dL
Low-density lipoproteins (LDLs)	Clot activator Silicone serum separator	Serum, plasma	
Men			89–197 mg/dL
Women			88–201 mg/dL
Creatine kinase (CK)	EDTA	Serum, plasma	
Men			38–174 U/L
Women			26–140 U/L
Creatinine	Clot activator Silicone serum separator	Serum, plasma	
Men			0.9–1.3 mg/dL
Women			0.6–1.2 mg/dL

(continued)

TABLE 48-4   Normal Ranges for Blood Tests

Blood Test	Stopper Color and Additive*	Blood Component Tested	Normal Range**
Cytomegalovirus (CMV)	Clot activator / Silicone serum separator	Serum	None
Epstein-Barr virus (EBV)	Clot activator / Silicone serum separator	Whole blood	None
Fibrinogen	Sodium citrate	Plasma	200–400 mg/dL
Glucose (fasting blood sugar, FBS)	Potassium oxalate or sodium fluoride	Serum	74–120 mg/dL
Group A beta-hemolytic streptococci	Clot activator / Silicone serum separator	Serum	None
Human immunodeficiency virus (HIV) antibodies	EDTA	Serum, plasma	None
Insulin	Clot activator / Silicone serum separator	Serum	<17 micro U/mL

Iron, total
  Men
  Women
	Clot activator / Silicone serum separator	Serum	
			65–175 micrograms/dL
			50–170 micrograms/dL

Lactate dehydrogenase (LD)	Clot activator / Silicone serum separator	Serum, plasma	140–280 U/L
pH	Clot activator / Silicone serum separator	Arterial blood Venous blood	7.35–7.45 7.32–7.43

(continued)

TABLE 48-4 Normal Ranges for Blood Tests

Blood Test	Stopper Color and Additive*		Blood Component Tested	Normal Range**
Proteins		Clot activator	Serum	
Total				6.2–8.0 g/dL
Albumin		Silicone serum separator		3.4–4.8 g/dL
Uric acid		Clot activator	Serum	
Men				4.4–7.6 mg/dL
Women		Silicone serum separator		2.3–6.6 mg/dL

*Different laboratories may have different testing protocols and may require other tube tops than those represented in this table. Consult your laboratory procedures manual for additional information regarding required collection tubes.

**Reference ranges for normal values may be slightly different in different labs. Consult the reference ranges provided by your individual lab for each test.

Hematologic Tests

Hematologic tests—including blood cell counts, morphologic studies, coagulation tests, and the nonautomated erythrocyte sedimentation rate test—are commonly performed in routine blood testing. These tests can be performed on venous or capillary whole blood specimens.

Blood Counts **Whole blood** contains **formed elements** (RBCs, WBCs, and platelets) and a fluid portion (plasma). The total number of blood cells and the percentage of the whole specimen each type represents can tell the licensed practitioner a great deal about a patient's condition. A practitioner can order an individual test or a **complete blood (cell) count (CBC),** which includes the following tests:

- Red blood (cell) count—the total number of RBCs in a specimen and the red cell morphology
- White blood (cell) count—the total number of WBCs in a specimen
- Differential WBC count—the percentage of each type of WBC (basophils, eosinophils, neutrophils, lymphocytes, and monocytes) in the first 100 leukocytes of a specimen
- Platelet count (automated)—the number of platelets in a specimen, or a platelet estimate, which indicates whether the amount of platelets is adequate
- Hematocrit determination—identifies how much of a specimen's volume (expressed as a percentage) is made up of RBCs after the specimen has spun in a centrifuge
- Hemoglobin determination—measures the amount of hemoglobin by weight per volume in the specimen

Most POLs use automated equipment for performing blood cell counts. Automated equipment performs a differential by counting and classifying all of the WBCs in the sample. You

may need to understand how to perform blood counts manually. All manual counts are estimates. The types of blood cell counts differ in specimen preparation and in the equipment and methods used. Check your state regulations and office policy to find out if you are allowed to perform differential blood counts.

Differential Cell Counts A medical assistant may be trained to prepare a blood smear slide and stain the smear for a manual differential cell count. Procedure 48-4, at the end of this chapter, details preparation of a blood smear slide. When you carry out this process correctly, there will be a region of the slide where blood cells are dense but lie in a single plane (not stacked or bunched together). This is the region where the cells are counted.

A polychromatic (multicolored) stain like Wright's stain simplifies a differential cell count. The blue and red-orange dyes (methylene blue and eosin, respectively) stain cell structures in ways that identify each of the five WBC types. The staining characteristics of each WBC type are

- Neutrophils—dark purple nucleus and pale pink cytoplasm containing fine pink or lavender granules.
- Basophils—purple nucleus and light purple cytoplasm containing large, blue-black granules.
- Eosinophils—purple nucleus and bright orange granules in pink cytoplasm.
- Lymphocytes—large, dark purple nucleus surrounded by a small amount of blue cytoplasm.
- Monocytes—the largest WBC, has gray-blue cytoplasm.

There are several types of blood staining kits. Follow the manufacturer's instructions when performing this procedure.

Figure 48-11 shows the zigzag pattern for counting leukocytes visible in the field when using the microscope's

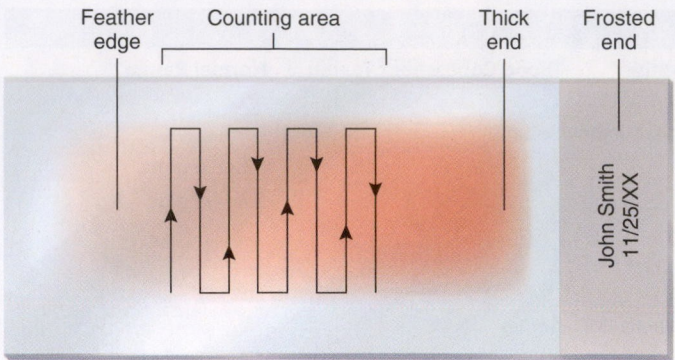

FIGURE 48-11 Follow this pattern when counting leukocytes visible in the field under the oil-immersion objective of the microscope.

oil-immersion objective. A total of 100 leukocytes are counted and recorded on a differential counter. Each cell type is expressed as a percentage of the 100 leukocytes counted. The platelet count is averaged in 10 to 15 fields.

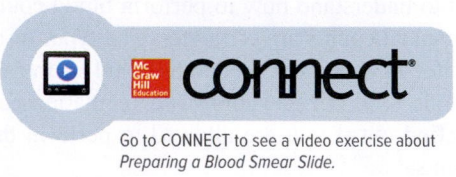

Go to CONNECT to see a video exercise about *Preparing a Blood Smear Slide.*

Hematocrit You measure a patient's hematocrit percentage by collecting a small specimen of the patient's blood in a microhematocrit tube, sealing the tube, and spinning it in a centrifuge. This process is described in Procedure 48-5 at the end of this chapter. During this process, heavier RBCs move to one end of the tube and lighter plasma moves to the other end. Between the RBCs, or **packed red blood cells,** and the plasma is the buffy coat (Figure 48-12). The **buffy coat** contains the WBCs and platelets.

Always run two specimens of the patient's blood. After removing each specimen from the centrifuge, compare the column of packed RBCs with a standard hematocrit gauge. Read on the gauge the percentage of total blood volume represented by the RBCs. The specimens should be within 2% of each other. If they are not, repeat the test. Average the readings of the two patient specimens.

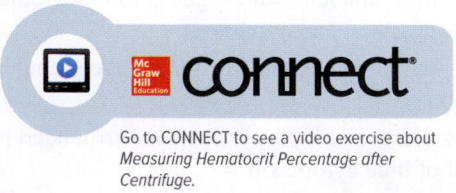

Go to CONNECT to see a video exercise about *Measuring Hematocrit Percentage after Centrifuge.*

Automated Hematocrit Readers You also may use a handheld device to obtain hematocrit readings. Devices such as the UltraCrit® are CLIA-waived testing devices for rapid and accurate measurement of hematocrit. The test may be completed on venous or capillary blood and results are obtained in less than 1 minute. These devices are often used by blood banks to rapidly screen donors for eligibility to donate.

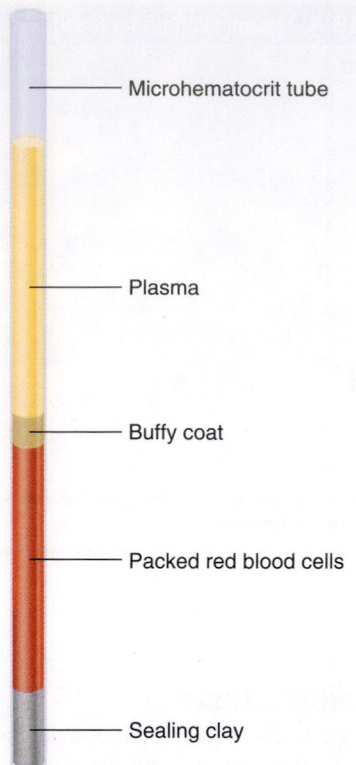

FIGURE 48-12 Blood in a centrifuged capillary tube separates into packed red blood cells, the buffy coat, and plasma.

Hemoglobin Hemoglobin resides within the RBCs. You will determine the concentration of hemoglobin in the blood by lysing (rupturing) the RBCs (**hemolysis**) and evaluating the color of the specimen. This procedure may be done with a hemoglobinometer—a handheld device that makes color evaluation less subjective (open for interpretation) than older methods of visually matching with color samples. Older testing methods had to be read by the human eye, leaving test interpretation up to the individual eye. Any change in color perception by the person reading the test could affect the test result reading. Blood specimens mixed with a reagent, such as Drabkin's reagent, undergo a color reaction that can be quantified by reading color intensity in a photoelectric colorimeter (an instrument that uses light to read color).

Several automated hemoglobin analyzers are now included on the CLIA '88 waived list. These analyzers measure the amount of hemoglobin in a whole blood sample using a photometer (an instrument used to measure absorbed light). The blood sample can be obtained from either a finger stick or venous blood. Examples of automated hemoglobin analyzers are HemoCue HB 301 Analyzer® (HemoCue AB) and the HemoPoint H2 Hemoglobin Measurement System® (Stanbio Laboratory). Follow the manufacturer's instructions when performing these tests.

Morphologic Studies Morphology is the study of the shape or form of objects, which is often performed just after the differential count and platelet estimate on the same blood smear slide. A morphologic study of a blood specimen can provide important information about a patient's condition. It examines a blood smear specimen and records the appearance and shape of cells for abnormal size, shape, or content and abnormal cell organization. Morphologic studies require special training and are not routinely done by medical assistants.

Coagulation Tests A physician may order coagulation tests to identify potential bleeding problems before surgical procedures or to monitor therapeutic drug levels when a patient is receiving anticoagulant medications such as heparin or warfarin (Coumadin®). Coagulation studies include the prothrombin time (PT) and partial thromboplastin time (PTT) tests. These tests are usually performed using automated devices such as the Coaguchek XS System™ (Roche Diagnostics) or the Alere INRatio System™ (Alere). These systems monitor the changing pattern of light transmission through the specimen as coagulation occurs and calculate the INR (International Normalized Ratio). The INR—used to evaluate patients who are taking blood thinners such as warfarin—measures the amount of time it takes for the test specimen to clot and compares it to a reference average. The World Health Organization (WHO) developed the INR method so that specimens from different labs can be compared. Medical assistants sometimes perform these studies.

Erythrocyte Sedimentation Rate The **erythrocyte sedimentation rate (ESR)** is the rate at which red blood cells (RBCs) settle in whole blood. What is actually measured is the distance, in millimeters, that they fall in 1 hour when allowed to settle in a calibrated tube. The ESR screens for the presence of any inflammatory process and does not diagnose any one condition. When inflammation is present, plasma proteins, such as albumin and globulin, are increased. An increase in these substances causes red blood cells to come closer together, which may result in the red blood cells sticking together. Several cells sticking together settle faster than a single RBC does. This results in an elevated sedimentation rate. See Figure 48-13 and these general guidelines:

- Use only a fresh sample of blood.
- Draw the blood into a tube with anticoagulant additives.
- Temperature, either too hot or too cold, will affect the test. Maintain laboratory temperatures near 70°F.
- Precisely position the specimen tubes vertically in the rack. They must not be leaning.
- Avoid vibrating or bumping the rack during the test.
- Avoid introducing bubbles into the specimen when transferring blood into the tube.
- Carefully watch the time and read the results at exactly 1 hour.

Chemical Tests

Blood chemistry analysis examines several dozen chemicals found in human blood. Tables 48-3 and 48-4 include many of these chemical tests. Highly detailed studies are rarely performed in the POL because they require expensive, sophisticated equipment and techniques. Complex testing is also subject to strict CLIA '88 regulations that increase the administrative work and the need for more highly trained personnel. So these types of tests are commonly performed at an

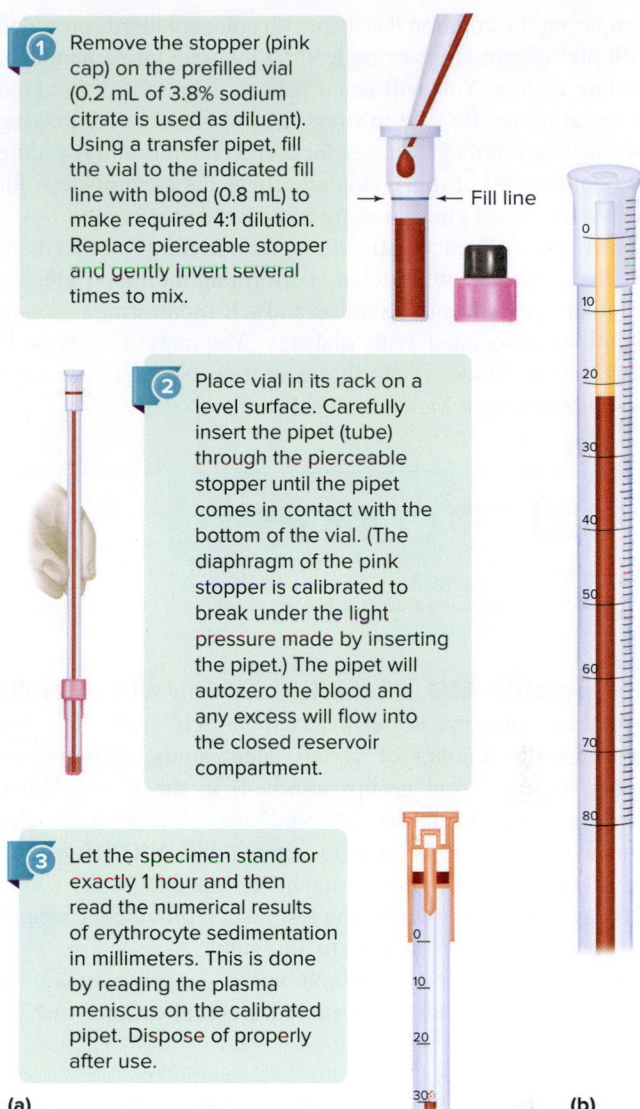

1 Remove the stopper (pink cap) on the prefilled vial (0.2 mL of 3.8% sodium citrate is used as diluent). Using a transfer pipet, fill the vial to the indicated fill line with blood (0.8 mL) to make required 4:1 dilution. Replace pierceable stopper and gently invert several times to mix.

← Fill line →

2 Place vial in its rack on a level surface. Carefully insert the pipet (tube) through the pierceable stopper until the pipet comes in contact with the bottom of the vial. (The diaphragm of the pink stopper is calibrated to break under the light pressure made by inserting the pipet.) The pipet will autozero the blood and any excess will flow into the closed reservoir compartment.

3 Let the specimen stand for exactly 1 hour and then read the numerical results of erythrocyte sedimentation in millimeters. This is done by reading the plasma meniscus on the calibrated pipet. Dispose of properly after use.

(a)   (b)

FIGURE 48-13 Erythrocyte sedimentation rate. (a) An example of one manufacturer's method for Westergren erythrocyte sedimentation rate (Sediplast ESR system). (b) An example of an erythrocyte sedimentation after 1 hour. The reading in this example is 22 millimeters.

independent reference laboratory. Automated equipment for analyzing blood chemistry, however, is becoming more available, less expensive, and simpler to operate than it was in the past. New waived tests for an increasing array of chemicals in the blood are developed each year, making it more likely that you may use automated equipment to perform some blood chemistry tests. Keeping abreast of new developments will help prepare you for possible changes in your laboratory duties.

Blood Glucose Monitoring One of the blood chemistry tests routinely conducted in the POL is blood glucose monitoring, which is often performed by a medical assistant or by a patient. Glucose monitoring systems require sterile lancets to perform a capillary puncture. You will collect the blood on reagent strips that change color in accordance with glucose levels present in the blood. The level is determined either by comparing the color on the strip with color standards provided with the reagent strips or by feeding the strip into a handheld reading device. You will teach patients to perform this kind of test at home. Be sure to stress the importance of following the manufacturer's guidelines for correct operation. Procedure 48-6, at the end of this chapter, outlines the general steps for measuring blood glucose using a handheld glucometer.

You also will teach patients and their families how to manage diabetes. This will include performing the blood glucose test, managing diet and exercise, and self-monitoring for complications associated with diabetes. You may also provide additional resources for further education. See the *Educating the Patient* feature Managing Diabetes.

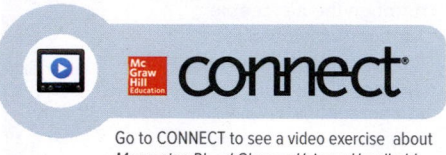

Go to CONNECT to see a video exercise about *Measuring Blood Glucose Using a Handheld Glucometer.*

Hemoglobin A1C Another test used to monitor the health of diabetic patients is the hemoglobin A1C test. This test measures the amount of glycosylated hemoglobin (hemoglobin with glycosal groups attached) in the blood. When blood glucose levels are elevated, the glucose molecules bind with hemoglobin to form hemoglobin A1C (HgbA1c). Once HgbA1c is formed, it remains for the RBC's life (90 to 120 days). For this reason, the test results provide an idea of the average blood sugar for 2 to 3 months.

Large fluctuations in blood sugar are problematic in patients with diabetes and can cause complications such as eye disease, stroke, renal failure, and cardiovascular disease. The HgbA1c test gives the physician a good overall picture of the patient's compliance with and the effectiveness of diabetes treatment.

Several options for performing this test include

- Sending it to an outside reference laboratory. Results are available in 1 to 7 days.

- Performing it in the office laboratory if the necessary equipment is available. Results are usually available in less than 10 minutes.

- Taking the test at home. Several home tests are available, allowing patients to monitor their own HgbA1c levels and therefore, the efficiency of their diabetes treatment.

Testing of HgbA1c should always be done in conjunction with routine blood glucose monitoring. Daily monitoring of blood glucose helps the patient with insulin therapy and diet maintenance. HgbA1c monitoring is important in assessing the patient's overall glucose levels. The advantages of this testing include

- No pretesting preparation. The test may be done without regard to meals.

- Better overall assessment of long-term blood glucose control. Blood glucose testing gives information about glucose levels at one point in time. HgbA1c gives information over a period of 2 to 3 months.

Patients should have their HgbA1c levels checked two to four times per year. The target range for HgbA1c levels is less than 7%. Patients whose HgbA1c levels exceed 8% are at a greater risk for diabetes-associated complications.

EDUCATING THE PATIENT
Managing Diabetes

Diabetes affects an estimated 9% of the US population, with more than 1 million newly diagnosed cases each year. In order to reduce the complications associated with diabetes, patients need to maintain stable blood sugar. Proper patient education and medical care will help patients achieve this goal. As a medical assistant, you can assist patients and their families by providing them with the following information about diabetes:

1. The risks and consequences associated with uncontrolled blood sugar. Patients whose blood sugar is unstable are at greater risk of developing the following conditions:
   - Loss of vision
   - Kidney failure
   - Heart disease
   - Nerve damage
   - Stroke
2. The patient's type of diabetes. Patients need to know the type of diabetes they have so that they can understand the type of treatment prescribed. The types of diabetes are

- Type 1 diabetes—an autoimmune disorder characterized by the body's inability to make enough insulin. Insulin is required for glucose utilization. Patients with Type 1 diabetes will need to take insulin daily.

- Type 2 diabetes—the most common type of diabetes. Insulin is still being produced at normal levels but can no longer be utilized by the body's cells. This causes a buildup of unused glucose in the blood. This type of diabetes is often controlled with careful diet management and increased exercise. A number of oral medications also can be used.

- Gestational diabetes—develops only during pregnancy. This type of diabetes is generally managed through proper diet and exercise. Careful monitoring is important to reduce the risk of fetal complications. Women who have had gestational diabetes have an increased risk of developing Type 2 diabetes.

3. Maintaining proper diet and exercise, including
   - Making proper food choices.

- Keeping a food diary.
- Reading food labels.
- Choosing proper food exchanges.
- Creating and implementing a routine exercise program.

4. Routine self-monitoring of blood sugar and hemoglobin A1C levels. Information should include
   - The types of blood glucose monitors available. Figure 48-14 illustrates one type—a glucometer.
   - Instructions on obtaining monitoring supplies.
   - The number of times and the specific intervals at which blood sugar should be checked, based on individual needs and the physician's recommendations.
   - Instructions on performing blood glucose testing.
   - Guidelines on how to maintain a chart of blood glucose levels, including the time of day, associated meals and activities, and actual blood sugar values.
   - Hemoglobin A1C monitoring. The patient should understand what hemoglobin A1C is and why it is important to monitor these values.
   - Normal (target) values for blood glucose and hemoglobin A1C:
     - Blood glucose levels should remain between 70 and 130 mg/dL before meals and less than 180 mg/dL for 1 to 2 hours after meals. Target ranges may be different for each patient. Consult with the licensed practitioner about individual blood glucose levels.
     - Hemoglobin A1C is a test that shows the average amount of glucose in the blood over a 3-month period. Ideally, this value should be less than 7%.

5. Symptoms of uncontrolled blood sugar. Patients need to be aware of the symptoms of both high and low blood sugar—both require immediate attention. Patients should test their blood sugar if any of the following occur:
   - Nausea, vomiting, or abdominal pain
   - Feeling tired all the time
   - Excessive thirst or dry mouth
   - Flushed skin
   - Confusion or difficulty thinking

6. Self-screening for diabetes complications. Patients should be aware of the complications associated with diabetes and how to recognize them, and patients should be instructed to do the following:

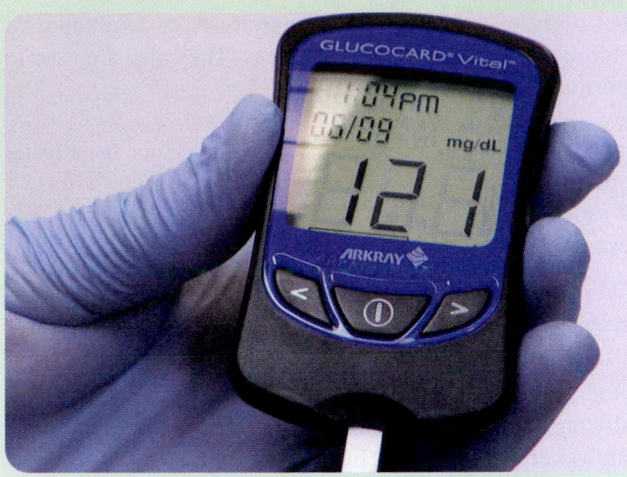

FIGURE 48-14 A handheld glucometer is an important tool in helping patients manage diabetes.
© McGraw-Hill Education

- Perform a daily foot inspection for sores
- Recognize changes in vision
- Recognize the symptoms of kidney failure, which include nausea, vomiting, yellow skin, and swelling of the hands and feet
- Recognize early signs of nerve damage, which include numbness and tingling of the arms, hands, feet, or legs; dizziness; double vision; and drooping of the eyelid or lip

7. Additional sources of information. Encourage patients to continue their education about diabetes. Providing patients with additional information encourages them to take an active role in controlling their diabetes. The following are additional information sources:

- American Association of Diabetes Educators 1-800-338-DMED
- American Diabetes Association 1-800-DIABETES
- American Dietetic Association 1-800-366-1665
- Centers for Disease Control and Prevention Diabetes Public Health Resource 1-800-CDC-INFO (232-4636)
- Juvenile Diabetes Research Foundation International 1-800-223-1138
- National Institute of Diabetes and Digestive and Kidney Diseases: National Diabetes Information Clearinghouse 1-800-860-8747

Cholesterol Tests Blood cholesterol tests are performed on a routine basis in the POL. Several automated devices can be used for metabolic chemistry testing both in the POL and at home. These analyzers test a variety of blood chemicals, including glucose, total cholesterol, HDL cholesterol, and triglycerides. The sample required is minimal and can be obtained with a capillary puncture.

FDA-approved waived tests include the following:

- Polymer Technology Systems CardioChek™ Analyzer (Polymer Technology Systems, Inc.)

- SpotChem™ HDL, Total Cholesterol, and Triglyceride (Arkray, Inc.)
- Piccolo® Lipid Panel Plus Reagent Disc (Abaxis, Inc.)

Serologic Tests

Serologic tests detect the presence of specific substances in a blood specimen. The terms *serologic test* and *immunoassay* refer to the introduction of an antigen or antibody into the specimen and the detection of a specific reaction to the antigen or antibody. Serologic testing methods can be used to detect disease antibodies, drugs, hormones, and vitamins in the blood and to determine blood types. They also are used to test urine and other body fluids.

Immunoassays Although medical assistants usually do not perform immunoassays, you should be familiar with several immunoassay methods that have common applications. These methods include

- Western blot, in which antigens are blotted onto special filter paper for examination. Western blot tests are generally used to confirm HIV infection diagnosis.
- Radioimmunoassay (RIA), in which radioisotopes are used to "tag" antibodies. RIA tests are extremely sensitive and are generally performed in a reference laboratory.
- Enzyme-linked immunosorbent assay (ELISA), in which enzyme-labeled antigens and substances that can absorb antigens generate reactions to specific antibodies. These reactions are identified through visual or photoelectric color detection. HIV infection is diagnosed using an ELISA test.
- Immunofluorescent antibody (IFA) test, in which dye, visible when the specimen is examined under a fluorescent microscope, colors specific antibodies.

Rapid Screening Tests Several serologic tests have been developed for quick processing. Some, such as early pregnancy tests performed on urine, are available for home use. There are also rapid screening tests for detecting antibodies to certain infections:

- Infectious mononucleosis
  - LifeSign Status Mono (Princeton Boimeditech Corp.)
  - BioStar Acceava Mono II (Acon Laboratories, Inc.)
- HIV
  - Clearview HIV—Stat-Pak (Chembio Diagnostic Systems, Inc.)
  - Uni-gold Recombigen HIV Test (Trinity Biotech plc)
- *Helicobacter pylori*
  - Rapid Response *H. pylori* Rapid Test Device (Acon Laboratories, Inc.)
  - Beckman Coulter ICON HP Test (Princeton Biomedtech Corp.)

When you use tests of these types or explain their use to a patient, keep in mind that the manufacturer's guidelines must be carefully followed to ensure accurate results. Procedure 48-7, at the end of this chapter, outlines the steps for performing a rapid mononucleosis test.

PROCEDURE 48-1 Quality Control Procedures for Blood Specimen Collection WORK // DOC

Procedure Goal: To follow proper quality control procedures when collecting a blood specimen

OSHA Guidelines:

   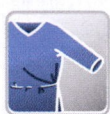
  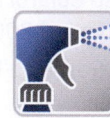

Materials: Necessary sterile equipment, specimen-collection container, paperwork related to the type of blood test the specimen is being drawn for, requisition form (chemistry request form), marker, and proper packing materials for transport

Method:

1. Review the request form for the test ordered, verify the procedure, prepare the necessary equipment and paperwork, and prepare the work area.

2. Identify the patient and confirm the patient's identification. Ask the patient to spell her name. Explain the procedure to be performed and make sure the patient understands it, even if she has had it done before.

3. Confirm that the patient has followed any pretest preparation requirements such as fasting, taking any necessary medication, or stopping a medication. For example, if a fasting specimen is being taken, the patient should not have eaten anything after midnight of the day before. Some practitioners' offices will let the patient drink water or black coffee, however. It often depends on the type of specimen being taken.
   RATIONALE: *The test may be invalid if the patient did not follow the pretest instructions.*

4. Collect the specimen properly. Collect it at the right time intervals if that applies. Use sterile equipment and proper technique.

5. Use the correct specimen-collection containers and the right preservatives, if required. For example, blood collected into a test tube with additives should be mixed immediately.
   RATIONALE: *To prevent clotting.*

6. Immediately label the specimens. The label should include the patient name, the date and time of collection, the test name, and the name of the person collecting the specimen. Do not label the containers before collecting the specimen.
   RATIONALE: *To keep from wasting tubes if there is a problem drawing the blood.*

7. Follow correct procedures for disposing of hazardous specimen waste and decontaminating the work area.

Used needles, for instance, should immediately be placed in a biohazard sharps container.

8. Thank the patient. Keep the patient in the office if any follow-up observation is necessary.

9. If the specimen is to be transported to an outside laboratory, prepare it for transport in the proper container for that type of specimen, according to OSHA regulations. Place the container in a clear plastic bag with a zip closure and dual pockets with the international biohazard label imprinted in red or orange. The requisition form should be placed in the bag's outside pocket. This ensures protection from contamination if the specimen leaks. Have a courier pick up the specimen and place it in an appropriate carrier (such as an insulated cooler) with the biohazard label. Place specimens to be sent by mail in appropriate plastic containers, and then place the containers inside a heavy-duty plastic container with a screw-down, nonleaking lid. Then place this container in either a heavy-duty cardboard box or a nylon bag. The words *Human Specimen* or *Body Fluids* should be imprinted on the box or bag. Seal with a strong tape strip.
RATIONALE: *To protect the courier and anyone else who handles the package from exposure to bloodborne pathogens.*

PROCEDURE 48-2 Performing Venipuncture Using an Evacuated System

WORK // DOC

Procedure Goal: To collect a venous blood specimen using an evacuated system

OSHA Guidelines:

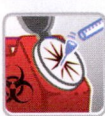 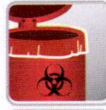 

Materials: Patient chart/progress note, requisition form, blood collection components (safety needle, needle holder/adapter, collection tubes), antiseptic and cotton balls or antiseptic wipes, tourniquet, sterile gauze squares, and sterile adhesive bandages

Method:

1. Review the laboratory requisition form and make sure you have the necessary supplies.
2. Greet the patient, confirm the patient's identity, and introduce yourself.
3. Explain the purpose of the procedure and confirm that the patient has followed the pretest instructions.
   RATIONALE: *To ensure that the test will be valid.*
4. Make sure the patient is sitting in a venipuncture chair or is lying down.
5. Wash your hands. Don exam gloves.
6. Prepare the safety needle holder/adapter assembly by inserting the threaded side of the needle into the adapter and twisting the adapter in a clockwise direction. Push the first collection tube into the other end of the needle holder/adapter until the outer edge of the collection tube stopper meets the guideline.

RATIONALE: *So that the tube is stabilized but not completely punctured.*

7. Ask the patient whether one arm is better than the other for the venipuncture. The chosen arm should be positioned slightly downward.

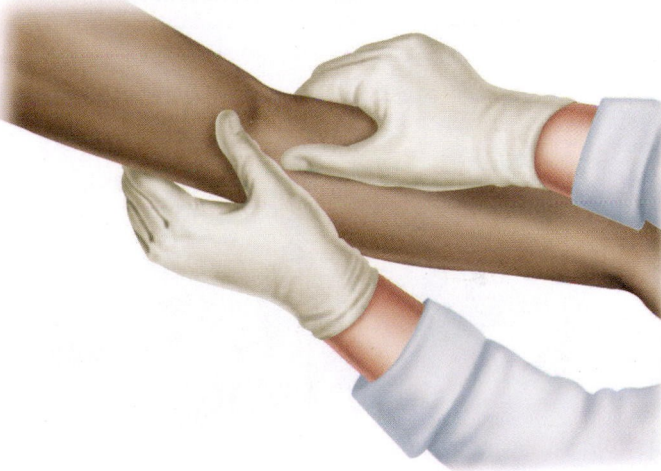

FIGURE Procedure 48-2 Step 7   The patient's arm should be positioned slightly downward for a venipuncture.

8. Apply the tourniquet to the patient's upper arm midway between the elbow and the shoulder. Wrap the tourniquet around the patient's arm and cross the ends. Holding one end of the tourniquet against the patient's arm, stretch the other end to apply pressure against the patient's skin. Pull a loop of the stretched end under the end held tightly against the patient's skin, as shown in the figure on the next page. The tourniquet should be tight enough to cause the veins to stand out but should not stop the flow of blood. You should still be able to feel the patient's radial pulse.
   RATIONALE: *To make the veins in the forearm stand out more prominently.*

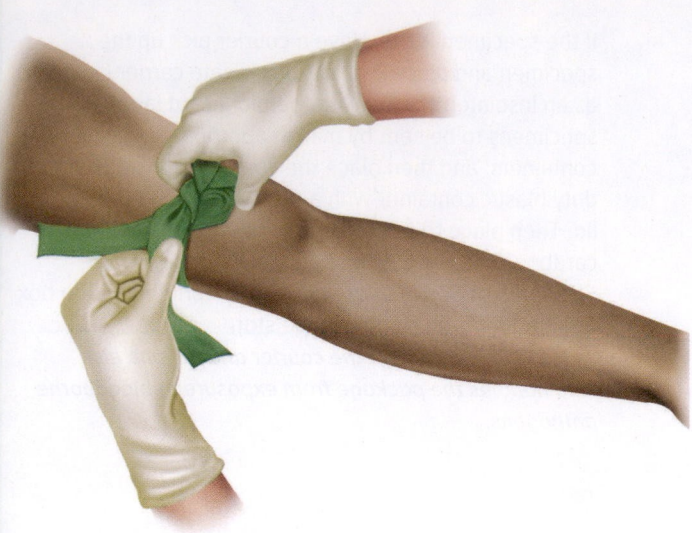

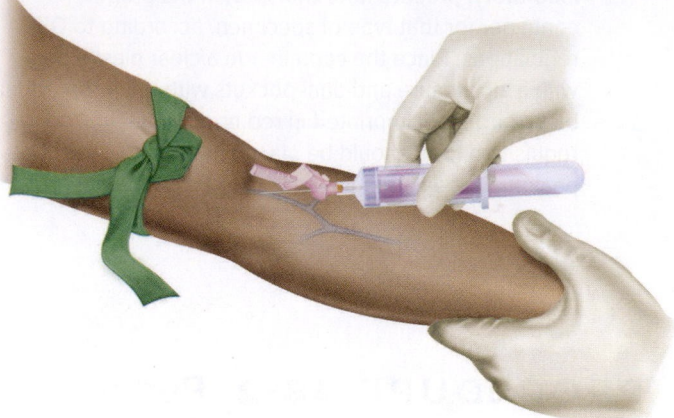

as the needle tip penetrates the vein wall. Penetrate to a depth of ¼ to ½ inch. Grasp the holder/adapter between your index and great (middle) fingers. Using your thumb, seat the collection tube firmly into place over the needle

FIGURE Procedure 48-2 Step 8   Applying a tourniquet makes it easier to find a patient's vein when you are drawing blood.

9. Palpate the proposed site and use your index finger to locate the vein, as shown in the figure. The vein will feel like a small tube with some elasticity. If you feel a pulsing beat, you have located an artery. Do not draw blood from an artery. If you cannot locate the vein within 1 minute, release the tourniquet and allow blood to flow freely for 1 to 2 minutes. Then reapply the tourniquet and try again to locate the vein.

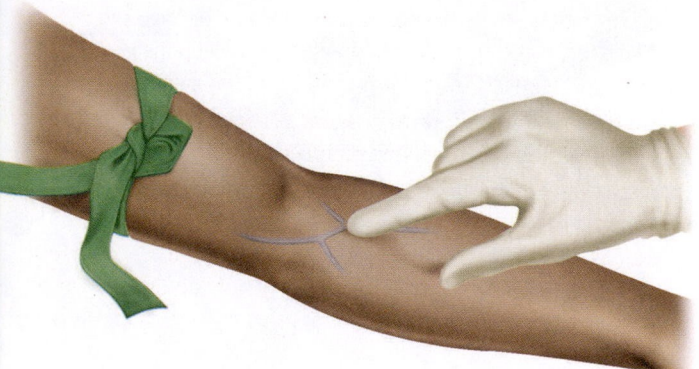

FIGURE Procedure 48-2 Step 9   Use your index finger to locate the vein.

10. After locating the vein, clean the area with an antiseptic wipe. Use a circular motion to clean the area, starting at the center and working outward. Allow the site to air-dry.
    RATIONALE: *The alcohol could interfere with some of the tests and takes 30 seconds to kill the bacteria.*

11. Remove the plastic cap from the outer point of the needle cover and ask the patient to tighten the fist. Hold the patient's skin taut below the insertion site.
    RATIONALE: *To anchor the vein so that it does not roll.*

12. With a steady and quick motion, insert the needle—held at a 15-degree angle, bevel side up, and aligned parallel to the vein—into the vein. You will feel a slight resistance

FIGURE Procedure 48-2 Step 12   When performing venipuncture, hold the needle at a 15-degree angle.

point, puncturing the rubber stopper. Blood will begin to flow into the collection tube.

13. Fill each tube until the blood stops running to ensure the correct proportion of blood to additives. Switch tubes as needed by pulling one tube out of the adapter and inserting the next in a smooth and steady motion. (The soft plastic cover on the inner point of the needle retracts as each tube is inserted and recovers the needle point as each tube is removed.)

14. Once blood is flowing steadily in the last tube, ask the patient to release the fist and untie the tourniquet by pulling the end of the tucked-in loop. The tourniquet should, in general, be left on no longer than 1 minute.
    RATIONALE: *Longer periods may cause hemoconcentration, an increase in the blood-cell-to-plasma ratio, and invalidate test results.*

    You must remove the tourniquet before you withdraw the needle from the vein.
    RATIONALE: *Removing the tourniquet releases pressure on the vein.*

15. Remove the last tube, then withdraw the needle in a smooth and steady motion, while placing a sterile gauze square over the insertion site. Immediately activate the safety device on the needle if it is not self-activating. Properly dispose of the needle immediately. Instruct the patient to hold the gauze pad in place with slight pressure. The patient should keep the arm straight and slightly elevated for several minutes.
    RATIONALE: *To reduce the possibility of a hematoma.*

16. If the collection tubes contain additives, you will need to invert them slowly several times.
    RATIONALE: *To mix the chemical agent and the blood specimen.*

17. Label specimens and complete the paperwork.

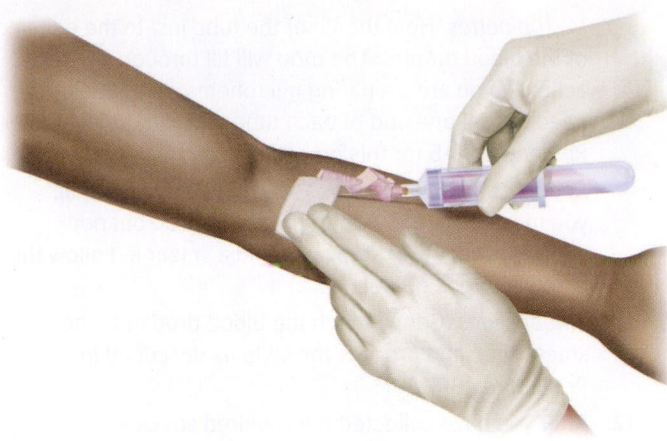

18. Check the patient's condition and the puncture site for bleeding. Replace the sterile gauze square with a pressure dressing.

19. Properly dispose of used supplies and disposable instruments and disinfect the work area.

20. Remove the gloves and wash your hands.

21. Instruct the patient about when to remove the pressure dressing.

22. Document the procedure in the patient's chart/progress note.

FIGURE Procedure 48-2 Step 15 Place a sterile gauze square over the insertion site as you withdraw the needle.

PROCEDURE 48-3 Performing Capillary Puncture

Procedure Goal: To collect a capillary blood specimen using the finger puncture method

OSHA Guidelines:

  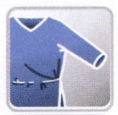 

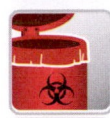 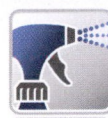

Materials: Patient chart/progress note, laboratory requisition form, capillary puncture device (safety lancet or automatic puncture device such as an Autolet® or Glucolet®), antiseptic and cotton balls or antiseptic wipes, sterile gauze squares, sterile adhesive bandages, reagent strips, micropipettes, and smear slides

Method:

1. Review the laboratory requisition form and make sure you have the necessary supplies.

2. Greet the patient, confirm the patient's identity, and introduce yourself.

3. Explain the purpose of the procedure and confirm that the patient has followed the pretest instructions, if indicated.
   RATIONALE: *The test may be invalid if the patient did not follow the pretest instructions.*

4. Make sure the patient is sitting in the venipuncture chair or is lying down.

5. Wash your hands. Don exam gloves.

6. Examine the patient's hands to determine which finger to use for the procedure. Avoid fingers that are swollen, bruised, scarred, or calloused. Generally, the ring and

great (middle) fingers are the best choices. If you notice that the patient's hands are cold, you may want to warm them between your own, have the patient put them in a warm basin of water or under warm running water, or wrap them in a warm cloth.
   RATIONALE: *Warming the patient's hands improves circulation.*

7. Prepare the patient's finger with a gentle "massaging" or rubbing motion toward the fingertip. Keep the patient's hand below heart level so that gravity helps the blood flow.

8. Clean the area with an antiseptic wipe or a cotton ball moistened with antiseptic. Allow the site to air-dry.
   RATIONALE: *The alcohol may interfere with some tests.*

9. Hold the patient's finger between your thumb and forefinger. Hold the safety lancet or automatic puncture device at a right angle to the patient's fingerprint, as shown in the figure below. Puncture the skin on the pad

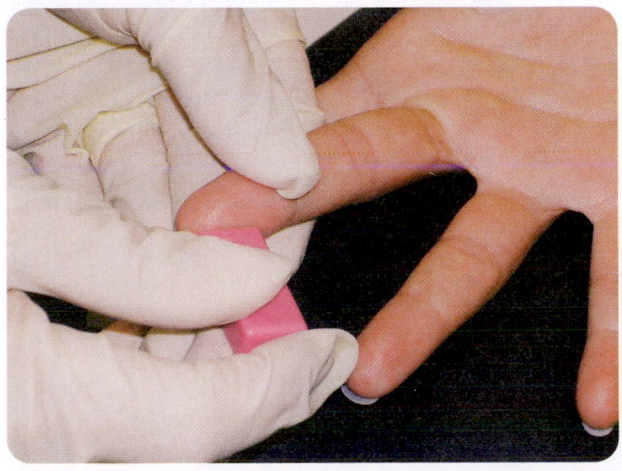

FIGURE Procedure 48-3 Step 9 Hold the lancet or automatic puncture device at a right angle to the patient's fingerprint.
© Leesa Whicker

of the fingertip with a quick, sharp motion. The depth to which you puncture the skin is generally determined by the length of the lancet point. Most automatic puncturing devices are designed to penetrate to the correct depth.

10. Allow a drop of blood to form at the end of the patient's finger. If the blood droplet is slow in forming, apply steady pressure. Avoid milking the patient's finger. **RATIONALE:** *It dilutes the blood specimen with tissue fluid and causes hemolysis.*

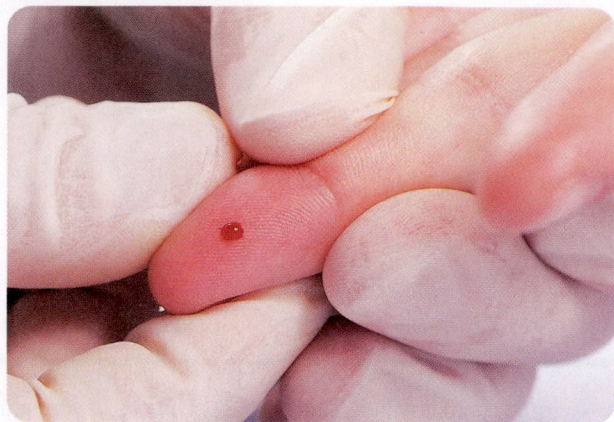

FIGURE Procedure 48-3 Step 10   Apply steady pressure to the patient's finger, but do not milk it.
© Terry Wild

11. Wipe away the first droplet of blood. (This droplet is usually contaminated with tissue fluids released when the skin is punctured.) Then fill the collection devices, as described.

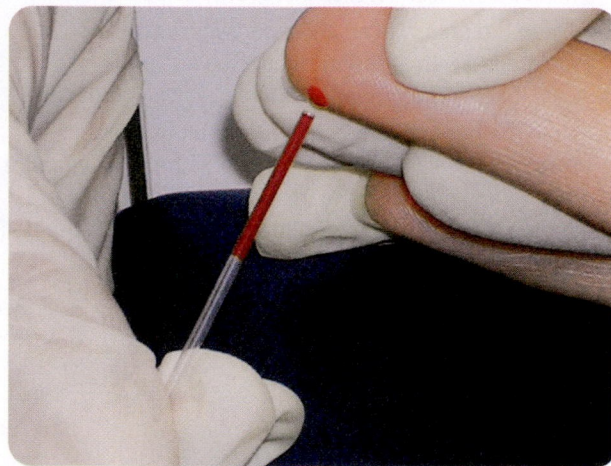

FIGURE Procedure 48-3 Step 11   Touch the tube to the drop of blood to fill it.
© Leesa Whicker

Micropipettes: Hold the tip of the tube just to the edge of the blood droplet. The tube will fill through capillary action. If you are preparing microhematocrit tubes, you need to seal one end of each tube with clay sealant. (See Procedure 48-5 for this process.)

Reagent strips: With some reagent strips (dipsticks), you must touch the strip to the blood drop but not smear it; with other strips, you must smear it. Follow the manufacturer's guidelines.

Smear slides: Gently touch the blood droplet to the smear slide and process the slide as described in Procedure 48-4.

12. After you have collected the required specimens, dispose of the lancet immediately. Then wipe the patient's finger with a sterile gauze square. Instruct the patient to apply pressure to stop the bleeding.

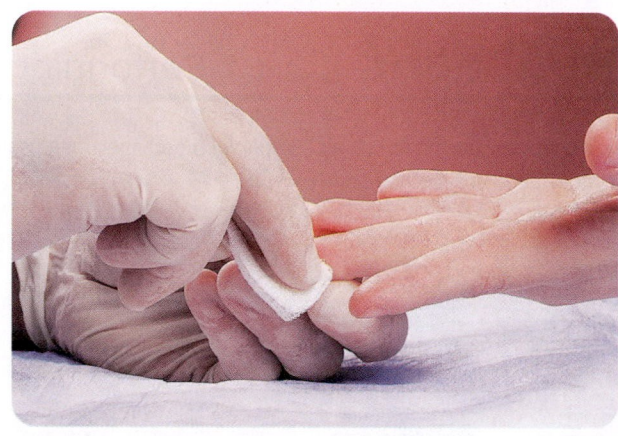

FIGURE Procedure 48-3 Step 12   Use a sterile gauze square to wipe remaining blood from the patient's finger.
© Terry Wild

13. Label specimens and complete the paperwork. Some tests, such as glucose monitoring, must be completed immediately.

14. Check the puncture site for bleeding. If necessary, replace the sterile gauze square with a sterile adhesive bandage.

15. Properly dispose of used supplies and disposable instruments and disinfect the work area.

16. Remove the gloves and wash your hands.

17. Instruct the patient about care of the puncture site.

18. Document the procedure in the patient's chart/progress note. (If the test has been completed, include the results.)

PROCEDURE 48-4 Preparing a Blood Smear Slide

Procedure Goal: To prepare a blood specimen to be used in a morphologic or other study

OSHA Guidelines:

  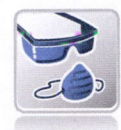 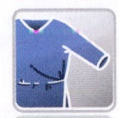
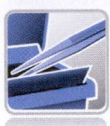 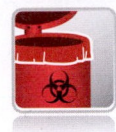 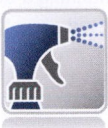

Materials: Blood specimen (from either a capillary puncture or a specimen tube containing anticoagulated blood), capillary tubes, sterile gauze squares, slide with frosted end, and wooden applicator sticks

Method:

1. Wash your hands and don exam gloves.

2. If using blood from a capillary puncture, follow the steps in Procedure 48-3 to express a drop of blood from the patient's finger. If using a venous specimen, check the specimen for proper labeling, carefully uncap the specimen tube, and use wooden applicator sticks to remove any coagulated blood from the inside rim of the tube. You may use a safety transfer device if available.

   RATIONALE: *Uncapping the specimen tube puts you at risk of exposure to bloodborne pathogens. The blood can spray or splatter or the tube could break. The safety device decreases the likelihood of exposure.*

3. Touch the tip of the capillary tube to the blood specimen from either the patient's finger or the specimen tube. The tube will take up the correct amount through capillary action.

4. Pull the capillary tube away from the specimen, holding it carefully to prevent spillage. Wipe the outside of the capillary tube with a sterile gauze square.

   RATIONALE: *To remove excess blood.*

5. With the slide on the work surface, hold the capillary tube in one hand and the frosted end of the slide against the work surface with the other.

6. Apply a drop of blood to the slide, about ¾ inch from the frosted end, as shown in the figure at the top of the next column. Place the capillary tube in the sharps container.

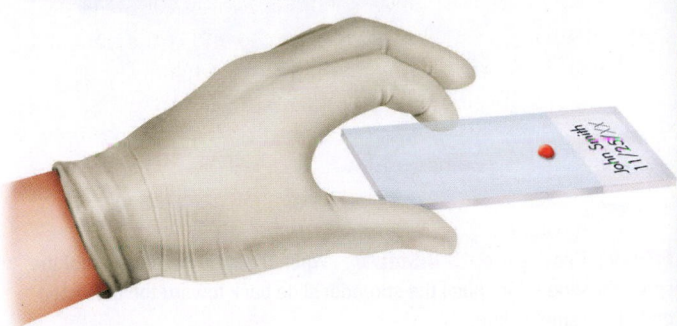

FIGURE Procedure 48-4 Step 6 Apply a drop of blood to the slide about ¾ inch from the frosted end.

7. Pick up the spreader slide with your dominant hand. Hold the slide at approximately a 30- to 35-degree angle. Place the edge of the spreader slide on the smear slide close to the unfrosted end. Pull the spreader slide toward the frosted end until the spreader slide touches the blood drop. Capillary action will spread the droplet along the edge of the spreader slide.

   RATIONALE: *So that the specimen can be thinly spread on the slide.*

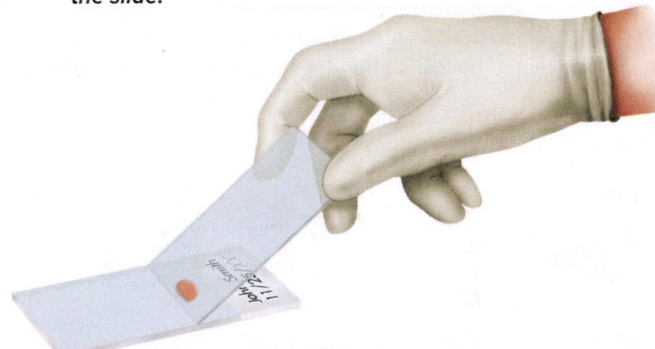

FIGURE Procedure 48-4 Step 7 Hold the spreader slide at a 30- to 35-degree angle. Pull the spreader slide toward the frosted end until it touches the drop of blood.

8. As soon as the drop spreads out to cover most of the spreader slide edge, push the spreader slide back toward the unfrosted end of the smear slide, pulling the specimen across the slide behind it, as shown in in the figure on the next page. Maintain the 30- to 35-degree angle.

9. Continue pushing until the spreader slide comes off the end, still maintaining the angle, as shown in the figure on the next page. The resulting smear should be approximately 1½ inches long, preferably with a margin of

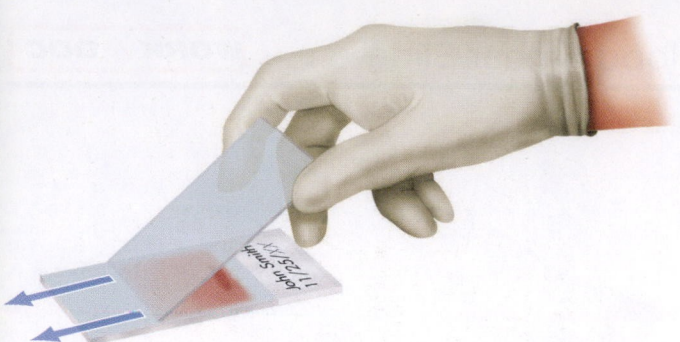

FIGURE Procedure 48-4 Step 8   When the drop covers most of the spreader slide edge, push the spreader slide back toward the unfrosted end of the smear slide.

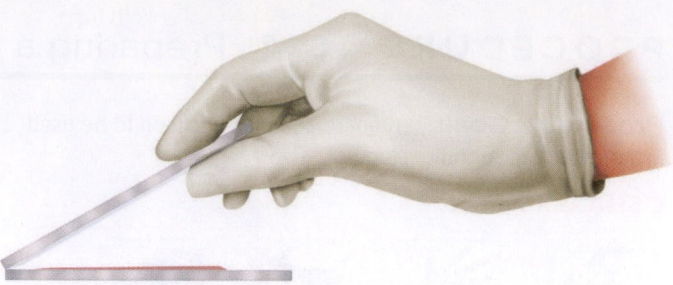

FIGURE Procedure 48-4 Step 9   Push the spreader slide off the end of the smear slide, maintaining a 30- to 35-degree angle. The smear should be thicker on the frosted end of the slide.

empty slide on all sides. The smear should be thicker on the frosted end of the slide.

10. Properly label the slide, allow it to dry, and follow the manufacturer's directions for staining it for the required tests.

11. Properly dispose of used supplies and disinfect the work area.

12. Remove the gloves and wash your hands.

PROCEDURE 48-5   Measuring Hematocrit Percentage After Centrifuge

WORK // DOC

Procedure Goal: To identify the percentage of a blood specimen represented by RBCs after the specimen has been spun in a centrifuge

OSHA Guidelines:

   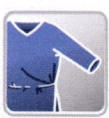

 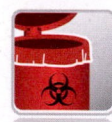 

Materials: Blood specimen (from either a capillary puncture or a specimen tube containing anticoagulated blood), microhematocrit tube, sealant tray containing sealing clay, centrifuge, hematocrit gauge, wooden applicator sticks, gauze squares, patient chart/progress note, and laboratory report form

Method:

1. Wash your hands and don exam gloves.

2. If using blood from a capillary puncture, follow the steps in Procedure 48-3 to express a drop of blood from the patient's finger. If using a venous blood specimen, check the specimen for proper labeling, carefully uncap the specimen tube, and use wooden applicator sticks to remove any coagulated blood from the inside rim of the tube. Alternately, use a safety transfer device if available. **RATIONALE: *The safety device decreases the likelihood of exposure to bloodborne pathogens.***

3. Touch the tip of one of the microhematocrit tubes to the blood specimen, as shown in the figure below. The tube will take up the correct amount through capillary action.

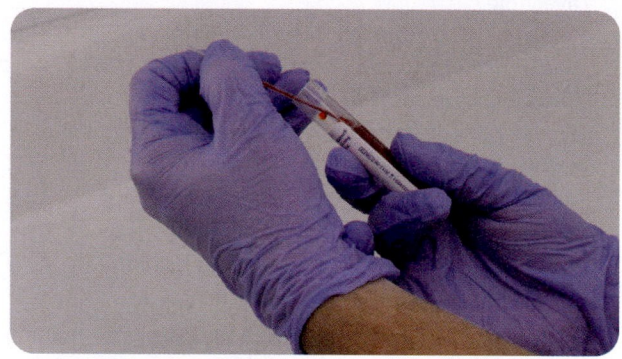

FIGURE Procedure 48-5 Step 3   Touch the tip of one of the microhematocrit tubes to the blood specimen.
© McGraw-Hill Education

4. Pull the microhematocrit tube away from the specimen, holding it carefully to prevent spillage. Wipe the outside of the microhematocrit tube with a gauze square. **RATIONALE: *To remove excess blood so that it is not splashed or splattered on the inside of the centrifuge.***

5. Hold the microhematocrit tube in one hand and press the other end of the tube gently into the clay in the sealant tray. You may need to place a gloved finger over the other end of the tube to prevent leakage. The clay plug must completely seal the end of the tube.

RATIONALE: *The tube must be sealed to prevent the specimen from being forced out of the tube during the spinning process.*

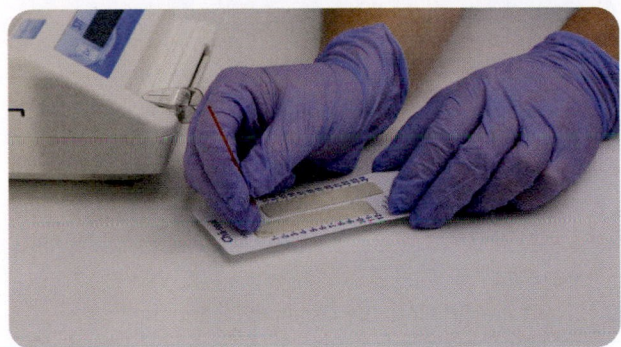

FIGURE Procedure 48-5 Step 5   Press the end of the tube into the clay in the sealant tray.
© McGraw-Hill Education

6. Repeat the process to fill another microhematocrit tube. Tubes must be processed in pairs.
   RATIONALE: *To maintain a balance in the centrifuge.*

7. Place the tubes in the centrifuge, with the sealed ends pointing outward. If you are processing more than one specimen, record the position identification number in the patient's chart to track the specimen.

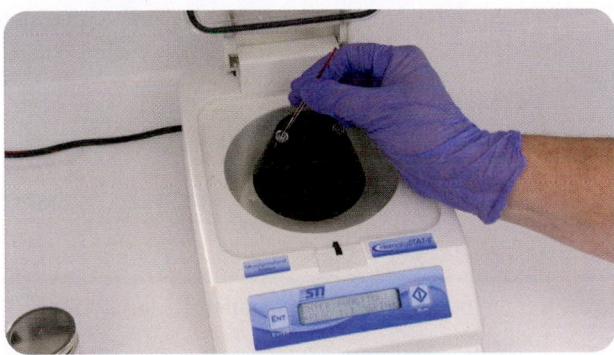

FIGURE Procedure 48-5 Step 7   Be sure to place the tubes in the centrifuge so that the sealed ends are pointing outward or downward.
© McGraw-Hill Education

8. Seal the centrifuge chamber.

9. Run the centrifuge for the required time, usually between 3 and 5 minutes. Allow the centrifuge to come to a complete stop before unsealing it.

10. Determine the hematocrit percentage by comparing the column of packed RBCs in the microhematocrit tubes with the hematocrit gauge, as shown in the figure in the right-hand column. Position each tube so that the boundary between sealing clay and RBCs is at zero on the gauge. Some centrifuges are equipped with gauges, but others require separate handheld gauges.

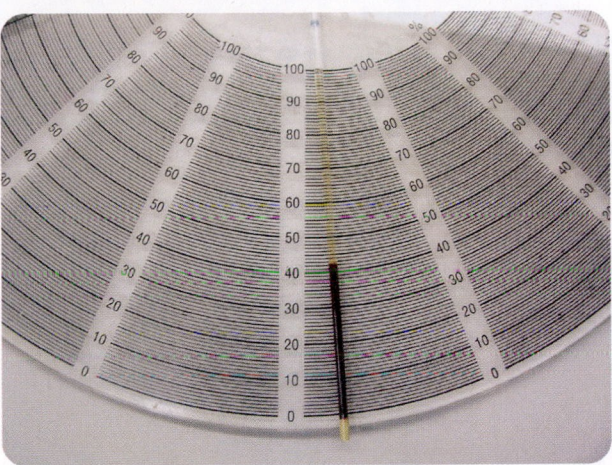

(a)

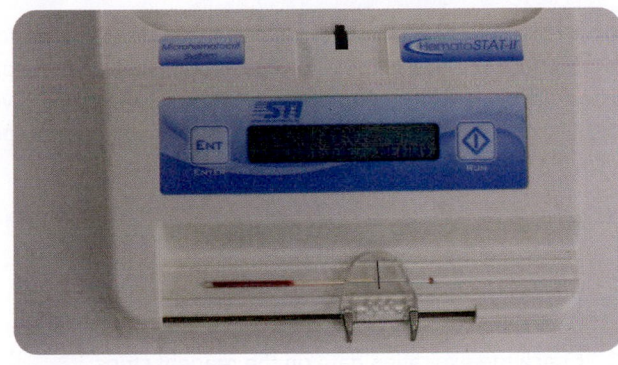

(b)

FIGURE Procedure 48-5 Step 10   Read the column of packed red blood cells using the microhematocrit gauge (a) or reader (b) to determine the hematocrit percentage.
(a) © Total Care Programming, Inc.; (b) © McGraw-Hill Education

11. Record the percentage value on the gauge that corresponds to the top of the column of RBCs for each tube. Compare the two results. They should not vary by more than 2%. If you record a greater variance, at least one of the tubes was filled incorrectly and you must repeat the test.

12. Calculate the average result by adding the two tube figures and dividing that number by 2.

13. Properly dispose of used supplies and clean and disinfect the equipment and the area.

14. Remove the gloves and wash your hands.

15. Record the test result in the patient's chart/progress note and/or the laboratory report form as required. Be sure to identify abnormal results.

PROCEDURE 48-6 Measuring Blood Glucose Using a Handheld Glucometer

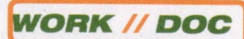

Procedure Goal: To measure the amount of glucose present in a blood specimen

OSHA Guidelines:

   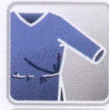

 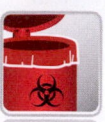 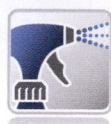

Materials: Safety-engineered capillary puncture device (automatic puncture device or other safety lancet), antiseptic and cotton balls or antiseptic wipes, sterile gauze squares, sterile adhesive bandages, handheld glucometer, reagent strips appropriate for the device, patient's chart/progress note, and quality control log

Method:

1. Wash your hands and don exam gloves.
2. Review the manufacturer's instructions for the specific device used.
3. Check the expiration date on the reagent strips.
   RATIONALE: *To make sure they are not outdated.*

4. Code the meter to the reagent strips if required.
   RATIONALE: *Some machines will need to be coded to account for small differences in the strips that occur during the manufacturing process.*
5. Turn the device on according to the manufacturer's instructions.
6. Perform the required quality control procedures.
   RATIONALE: *To ensure that the machine is working as expected.*
7. Insert the strip into the meter, following the manufacturer's instructions.
8. Perform a capillary puncture, following the steps outlined in Procedure 48-3.
9. Touch the drop of blood to the reagent strip, allowing it to be taken up by the strip.
10. Read the digital result after the required amount of time.
11. Discard the reagent strip and used supplies according to OSHA standards.
12. Record the time of the test and the result on the laboratory slip.
13. Disinfect the equipment and area.
14. Remove the gloves and wash your hands.
15. Document the test results in the patient's chart/progress note. Record the quality control tests in the quality control log.

PROCEDURE 48-7 Performing a Rapid Infectious Mononucleosis Test

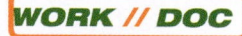

Procedure Goal: To determine the presence of antibodies associated with infectious mononucleosis using whole blood, serum, or plasma

OSHA Guidelines:

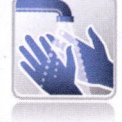   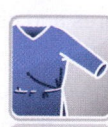

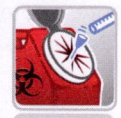  

Materials: Infectious mononucleosis test kit, patient blood specimen, and a watch or timer, patient's chart/progress note, and/or laboratory report form, quality control log

Method:

1. Review the laboratory requisition form and gather the necessary supplies.

2. Greet the patient, confirm the patient's identity, and introduce yourself.
3. Explain the procedure.
4. Wash your hands and don required PPE.
5. Obtain a specimen of the patient's blood using appropriate venipuncture technique.
6. Process the blood specimen to obtain whole blood, plasma, or serum as required by the testing procedure.
7. Open the test kit and check the expiration date.
8. Run the recommended controls according to the manufacturer's instructions and record in the quality control log.
   RATIONALE: *To ensure that the test is working correctly.*
9. Place the required amount of blood, serum, or plasma onto the testing device, following the manufacturer's instructions.
10. Add testing reagent or reagents to the testing device, according to the manufacturer's instructions.
11. Wait the required amount of time. Do not go over the recommended time.

RATIONALE: *Reading the test too early can result in a false negative, and reading the test too long after the recommended time can result in a false positive.*

12. Read the results and record them in the patient's chart/ progress note and/or the laboratory report form.

13. Discard the testing supplies according to OSHA regulations.

14. Disinfect the work area.

15. Remove your PPE and wash your hands.

SUMMARY OF LEARNING OUTCOMES

LEARNING OUTCOMES	KEY POINTS
48.1 Discuss the role of the medical assistant when collecting, processing, and testing blood specimens.	As a medical assistant, you will collect and process blood specimens for examination, make sure the test results are handled efficiently and accurately, and complete the necessary paperwork before and after each test.
48.2 Describe the steps and equipment needed to collect a blood specimen.	Preparation for collecting blood specimens includes reading and interpreting the test order and collecting the necessary equipment for the type of specimen to be collected. General equipment includes alcohol wipes, sterile gauze, and adhesive bandages. For venipuncture, you will need a tourniquet, specimen-collection tubes, and a needle system such as Vacutainer®. For capillary puncture, you will need a puncture device and capillary tubes.
48.3 Summarize ways to communicate with patients and respond to their needs when collecting blood.	Patients are often concerned about pain, bruising, and scarring when having blood drawn. They are sometimes afraid they may have a serious disease, especially if large amounts of blood are drawn. Good communication by the medical assistant is the key to easing these fears. There are always patients who will have special needs, including children, the elderly, patients who have bleeding disorders, and difficult patients. Each patient will present a special set of challenges and should be treated with the utmost care and concern.
48.4 Carry out the procedure for collecting a blood specimen.	Blood is collected by one of two means: venipuncture and capillary puncture. Venipuncture is the process of obtaining a blood specimen from a vein. Capillary puncture is the process of obtaining blood from a superficial skin puncture. When collecting blood specimens, it is essential that you confirm the patient's identity before the specimen is collected, cleanse the skin prior to collection, follow standard precautions, collect the specimen needed in the appropriate tube or container, and ensure the patient's safety at all times.
48.5 Carry out the procedure for performing blood tests.	Hematologic, chemical, and serologic tests require special care when performing them. The medical assistant should review the manufacturer's instructions carefully for important information about correctly performing each test.

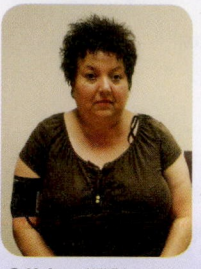

© McGraw-Hill Education

Recall Sylvia Gonzales from the beginning of the chapter. Now that you have completed the chapter, answer the following questions regarding her case.

1. What blood tube(s) would you fill to collect a specimen for the CBC and lytes? Which tube would you fill first?

2. Compare a fasting blood sugar test to a hemoglobin A1C test.

3. What steps will you take to perform a dermal puncture?

4. If Sylvia tells you that she ate breakfast before coming in for the test, what should you do?

EXAM PREPARATION QUESTIONS

1. (LO 48.4) The small depression inside the bend of the elbow is the
   a. Cephalic space
   b. Median cubital depression
   c. Basillic area
   d. Axillary depression
   e. Antecubital fossa

2. (LO 48.5) The rupturing of erythrocytes is known as
   a. Hemolysis
   b. Hemoglobin
   c. Hematopoiesis
   d. Hemorrhage
   e. Erythrocytosis

3. (LO 48.2) A lavender-topped venipuncture collection tube contains which of the following?
   a. Sodium citrate
   b. Heparin
   c. EDTA
   d. SST
   e. Potassium oxalate

4. (LO 48.5) What is contained within the buffy coat?
   a. Plasma
   b. White blood cells
   c. Red blood cells
   d. Fibrinogen
   e. Serum

5. (LO 48.5) Which of the following tests gives the licensed practitioner an overall picture of a patient's compliance with diabetes diet and treatment?
   a. Blood glucose
   b. Hemoglobin A1C
   c. Cholesterol
   d. CBC
   e. Fasting blood sugar

6. (LO 48.2) A flat, broad length of vinyl or rubber used to apply pressure to the forearm so that the underlying veins stick out is a
   a. Drain
   b. Velcro® closure
   c. Butterfly
   d. Tubing
   e. Tourniquet

7. (LO 48.3) A patient arrives at the clinic for a FBS. He tells you he just ate his breakfast. What is your best course of action?
   a. Draw the blood immediately
   b. Tell the patient to come back later in the day
   c. Ask another medical assistant to assist you with the test
   d. Do not draw a fasting blood sugar, since the patient is not fasting
   e. Encourage the patient to drink a lot of water before you draw the blood

8. (LO 48.5) Which of the following keeps blood from clotting?
   a. Serum separator
   b. Anticoagulant
   c. Antibody
   d. Silicone
   e. Clot activator

9. (LO 48.5) Which of the following tests is *most* likely used to test for inflammation, infectious diseases, and malignant neoplasms?
   a. Erythrocyte sedimentation rate
   b. RBC count
   c. AST
   d. Amylase
   e. FBS

10. (LO 48.2) Which of the following represents the correct "order of draw" from first venipuncture collection tube to last?
    a. Gold, light blue, green, lavender, yellow
    b. Light blue, green, gold, yellow, lavender
    c. Yellow, light blue, gold, green, lavender
    d. Green, yellow, lavender, gold, light blue
    e. Yellow, lavender, gold, light blue, green

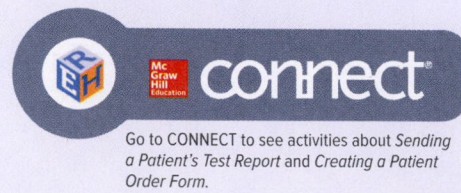

Go to CONNECT to see activities about *Sending a Patient's Test Report* and *Creating a Patient Order Form.*

You are asked to collect a capillary blood specimen on a 3-year-old child. He is crying and kicking. How should you handle this situation?

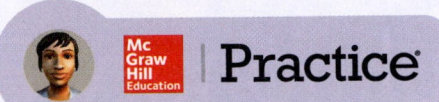

Electrocardiography and Pulmonary Function Testing

CASE STUDY

PATIENT INFORMATION			
Patient Name	**DOB**	**Allergies**	
John Miller	2/5/19XX	Bee stings	
Attending	**MRN**	**Other Information**	
Paul F. Buckwalter, MD	082-09-981	PFT scheduled for next week.	

John Miller, a 65-year-old male, arrives at the clinic complaining of his shoes not fitting and feeling like he cannot take a deep breath. During the patient interview, he also states that he is having intermittent pain in his chest. He is taking glyburide 2.5 mg daily, captopril 25 mg twice a day, and HCTZ 25 mg daily. He has not taken the HCTZ for 2 weeks and is

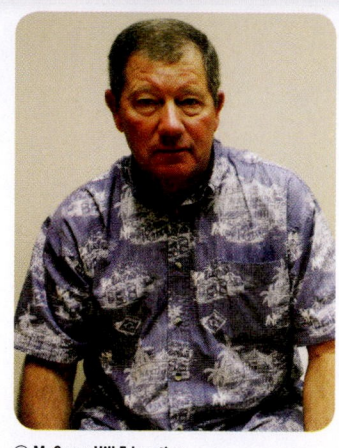

© McGraw-Hill Education

hoping to get this medication refilled. The physician wants to evaluate his congestive heart failure. He orders an ECG and a stress echocardiogram. The patient has not previously had a stress echocardiogram and you need to explain it to him before the test begins.

Keep John in mind as you study this chapter. There will be questions at the end of the chapter based on the case study. The information in the chapter will help you answer these questions.

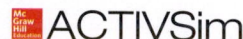 ACTIVSim

LEARNING OUTCOMES

After completing Chapter 49, you will be able to:

49.1 Discuss the medical assistant's role in electrocardiography and pulmonary function testing.

49.2 Explain the basic principles of electrocardiography and how it relates to the conduction system of the heart.

49.3 Identify the components of an electrocardiograph and what each does.

49.4 Carry out the steps necessary to obtain an ECG.

49.5 Summarize exercise electrocardiography and echocardiography.

49.6 Explain the procedure of Holter monitoring.

49.7 Carry out the various types of pulmonary function tests.

49.8 Describe the procedure for performing pulse oximetry testing.

KEY TERMS

artifact
calibration syringe
cardiac cycle
deflection
depolarization
dysrhythmia
echocardiography
electrocardiogram (ECG)
electrocardiograph
electrocardiography
electrode
forced vital capacity (FVC)
Holter monitor

hypoxemia
lead
peak expiratory flow rate (PEFR)
polarity
pulmonary function test (PFT)
repolarization
rhythm strip
sleep apnea
spirometer
spirometry
stress test

CAAHEP

I.C.9 Analyze pathology for each body system including:
(a) diagnostic measures
(b) treatment modalities

I.P.2 Perform:
(a) electrocardiography
(d) pulmonary function testing

I.P.3 Perform patient screening using established protocols

I.A.3 Show awareness of a patient's concerns related to the procedure being performed

ABHES

2. Anatomy and Physiology
c. Identify diagnostic and treatment modalities as they relate to each body system

9. Clinical Procedures
a. Practice standard precautions and perform disinfection/sterilization techniques

e. Perform specialty procedures including but not limited to minor surgery, cardiac, respiratory, OB-GYN, neurological, gastroenterology

▶ Introduction

It is not uncommon for patients to have cardiovascular or respiratory problems when they consult their licensed practitioner. As a medical assistant, you may be responsible for performing screening and/or diagnostic testing in the physician's office. To correctly perform cardiac and respiratory testing, you need to review the anatomy and physiology of the heart and the respiratory system. (Refer to the chapters *The Cardiovascular System* and *The Respiratory System.*) This chapter introduces you to the electrocardiograph instrument and how to administer an electrocardiogram. You also will learn how to apply electrocardiograph electrodes and wires, operate the instrument, and troubleshoot problems that can occur while recording the heart's electrical activity. Because many physicians perform more complex cardiac diagnostic testing, you also will learn about Holter monitors and stress testing. Pulmonary function testing is a procedure performed in physicians' offices, and this chapter introduces you to the basics of performing respiratory procedures such as spirometry, peak flow, and pulse oximetry.

▶ The Medical Assistant's Role in Electrocardiography and Pulmonary Function Testing   LO 49.1

Electrocardiography and pulmonary function testing are two procedures you may be required to perform in a medical office. **Electrocardiography** is the process by which a graphic pattern is created from the electrical impulses generated within the heart as it pumps. It is often performed to evaluate symptoms of heart disease, to detect abnormal heart rhythms, to evaluate a patient's progress after a myocardial infarction (MI), or to check the effectiveness or side effects of certain medications. Electrocardiography is sometimes performed as part of a general examination.

Pulmonary function tests (PFTs) measure and evaluate a patient's lung capacity and volume. Such tests are commonly performed when a person suffers from shortness of breath, but they also may be performed as part of a general examination. Pulmonary function tests can help detect and diagnose pulmonary problems. They also are used to monitor certain respiratory disorders and to evaluate the effectiveness of treatment.

▶ Basic Principles of Electrocardiography   LO 49.2

Weak or strong, fast or slow, each heartbeat produces an electrical current that can be measured with an electrocardiograph. Measuring and recording each heartbeat gives the doctor a "picture" of how the heart's electrical system is working. Understanding the basics of the conduction system and how it appears on an ECG tracing is essential when performing electrocardiography.

Conduction and Electrocardiography

Electrocardiography records the transmission, magnitude, and duration of the heart's various electrical impulses. Before you can understand how electrocardiography works, you must understand **polarity,** the condition of having two separate poles, one of which is positive and the other negative. Similar to a bar magnet with one end north and one south, a resting cardiac cell is polarized; that is, it has a negative charge inside and a positive charge outside. When the cardiac cell loses its polarity (a natural occurrence), depolarization occurs. **Depolarization** is the electrical impulse that initiates a chain reaction resulting in contraction. This wave of depolarization flows from the SA node to the ventricles and can be detected by **electrodes,** or electrical impulse sensors, placed on specific areas on the surface of the body. During electrocardiography, electrodes detect and record the heart's electrical activity, including disturbances or disruptions in its rhythm.

Depolarization is always followed by a period of electrical recovery called **repolarization,** when polarity is restored. Following repolarization, the heart returns to a resting, polarized state. The electrical cycle is then repeated, leading to another **cardiac cycle**—sequence of contraction and relaxation. See Table 49-1 and Figure 49-1.

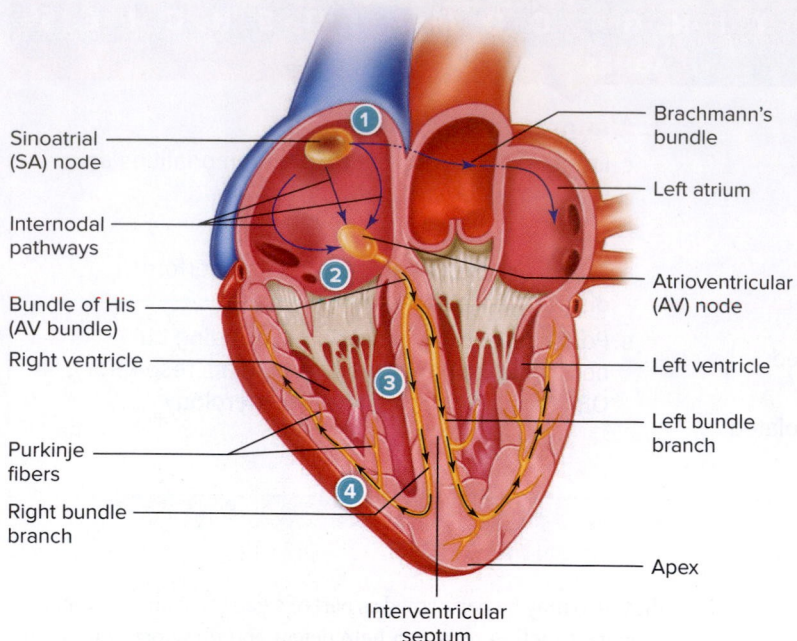

Sinoatrial (SA) node

Internodal pathways

Bundle of His (AV bundle)

Right ventricle

Purkinje fibers

Right bundle branch

Brachmann's bundle

Left atrium

Atrioventricular (AV) node

Left ventricle

Left bundle branch

Apex

Interventricular septum

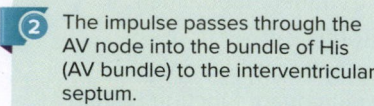

1 The heartbeat originates in the sinoatrial (SA) node; it travels across the wall of the atrium through the internodal pathways to the atrioventricular (AV) node and Bachmann's bundle to the left atrium.

2 The impulse passes through the AV node into the bundle of His (AV bundle) to the interventricular septum.

3 The impulse is divided between the right and left bundle branches and travels to the apex of the heart through the interventricular septum via the bundle branches.

4 The Purkinje fibers carry the impulse throughout the right and left ventricles, causing them to contract.

FIGURE 49-1   Conduction pathways.

TABLE 49-1	Parts of the Conduction System
Part	**Function**
Sinoatrial (SA) node (pacemaker)	Electrical impulses occur at a rate of 60 to 100 beats per minute, initiating the heartbeat with an electrical impulse that causes depolarization
Atrioventricular (AV) node	Delays the electrical impulse to allow for the atria to complete their contraction and ventricles to fill before the next contraction; also serves as a secondary pacemaker if the SA node fails
Bundle of His (AV bundle)	Conducts electrical impulses from the atria to the ventricles
Bundle branches	Conduct impulses down both sides of the interventricular septum
Purkinje fibers (network)	Distribute the electrical impulses throughout the right and left ventricles

The Basic Pattern of the Electrocardiogram

The waves of electrical impulses responsible for the cardiac cycle produce a series of waves and lines on an **electrocardiogram** (abbreviated **ECG** or **EKG**), which is the tracing made by an **electrocardiograph**, an instrument that measures and displays these impulses (Figure 49-2). These peaks and valleys, called waves or **deflections**, are labeled with the letters P, Q, R, S, T, and U. Each letter represents a specific part of the pattern, as explained in Table 49-2. The recognition of abnormalities in the size of the waves or the various time intervals can aid in the diagnosis of certain types of heart problems.

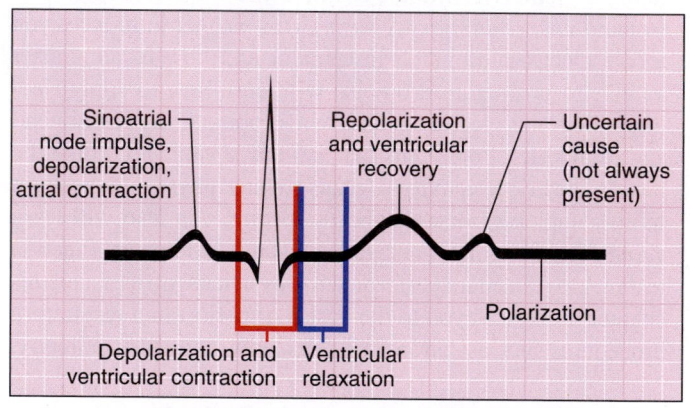

Sinoatrial node impulse, depolarization, atrial contraction

Repolarization and ventricular recovery

Uncertain cause (not always present)

Depolarization and ventricular contraction

Ventricular relaxation

Polarization

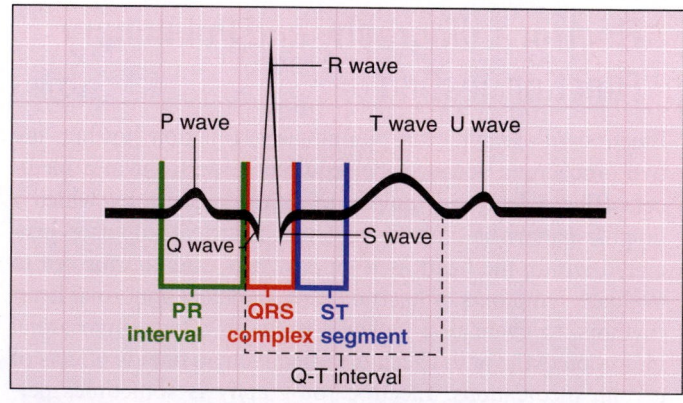

R wave

P wave

T wave   U wave

Q wave

S wave

PR interval

QRS complex

ST segment

Q-T interval

FIGURE 49-2   This ECG tracing shows the pattern of one cardiac cycle in a normal heart. These specific electrical impulses (top) represent the cycle of cardiac contraction and relaxation. The waves and lines (bottom) represent specific parts of the pattern.

Component	Appearance	Heart Activity
P wave	Upward, small curve	Atrial depolarization with resulting atrial contraction
QRS complex	Q, R, and S waves	Ventricular depolarization and resulting ventricular contraction (larger than the P wave); atrial repolarization occurs (not seen)
T wave	Small, upward-sloping curve	Ventricular repolarization
U wave	Small, upward curve	Repolarization of the bundle of His and Purkinje fibers (not always seen); may be seen in instances of electrolyte imbalance
PR interval	P wave and baseline prior to QRS complex	Beginning of atrial depolarization to the beginning of ventricular depolarization
QT interval	QRS complex, ST segment, and T wave	Period of time from the start of ventricular depolarization to the end of ventricular repolarization
ST segment	End of QRS complex to the beginning of T wave	Time between ventricular depolarization and the beginning of ventricular repolarization

TABLE 49-2   ECG Components

▶ The Electrocardiograph   LO 49.3

Each type of electrocardiograph works in the same way. The electrical impulses produced by the heart can be detected through the skin; these impulses are measured, amplified, and recorded on the ECG. Detection begins with electrodes that conduct and transmit the electrical impulses to the electrocardiograph through insulated wires. An amplifier increases the signal, making the heartbeat visible. The impulses received through various combinations of electrodes constitute different **leads,** or views of the electrical activity of the heart, that are recorded on the ECG. Keep in mind that the term *lead* is used to refer to both the view of the heart on the ECG tracing and the physical location where the electrode is placed on the patient.

Types of Electrocardiographs

Several types of electrocardiographs are in use today. The typical ECG machine sits on a small cart that can be pushed to the person requiring the ECG. The most common machine is a 12-lead electrocardiograph, which records the electrical activity of the heart simultaneously from 12 different views. See Figure 49-3. A single-channel electrocardiograph records the electrical activity of one lead and produces a long, thin strip of ECG paper. This strip, or tracing, is sometimes called

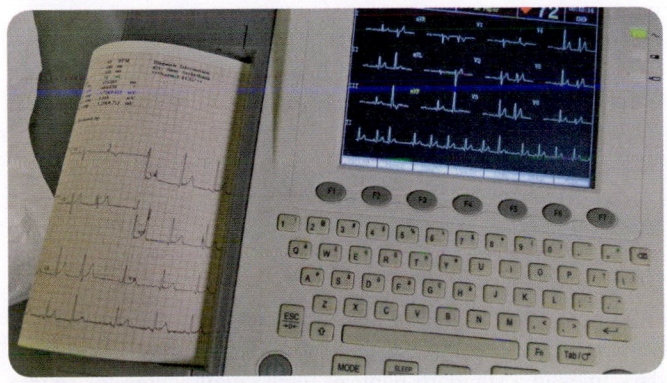

FIGURE 49-3   A typical ECG machine records three, four, or six leads at a time on a large sheet of graph paper.
© McGraw-Hill Education

a **rhythm strip.** When ECG tracings are evaluated, discussed later in this chapter, a single lead tracing is either in print or electronic. The multichannel ECG produces a full sheet of paper with all 12 leads. The actual recording time is about 10 seconds. Some models of multichannel ECGs provide a diagnosis or an interpretation of the electrocardiogram. The interpretive option can be turned on or off. Even though the interpretive electrocardiograph can provide a diagnosis, the physician will review the tracing and confirm the diagnosis before treatment is ordered. Larger medical facilities may use an electronic health records (EHR) software program so that electrocardiograms can be inserted into the patient medical record and transmitted to specialists to interpret. Electrocardiograms can be transmitted electronically, by fax or telephone, depending on the software and model of the electrocardiograph (see Figure 49-4).

Electrodes

Disposable electrodes are attached to the patient's skin during electrocardiography (Figure 49-5). Because the skin does not conduct electricity well, an electrolyte (a substance that enhances transmission of electric current) is needed with each electrode. Disposable electrodes come with an electrolyte preparation in place.

When performing routine electrocardiography, you place electrodes on 10 areas of the body: 1 each on the right arm (RA), left arm (LA), right leg (RL), and left leg (LL) and 6 on specific locations on the chest wall. The right leg is designated as the ground. These 10 electrodes are used to evaluate 12 different pathways of the heart's electrical activity (leads). This is why it is called a 12-lead ECG. Evaluating different leads—the electrical activity measured through various combinations of electrodes—enables the physician to pinpoint the origin of certain problems such as dysrhythmias and heart block.

Leads

Each lead provides an image, or view, of the heart's electrical activity from a different angle. Together, the images give the doctor a full picture of electrical activity moving up and down, left and right, and forward and backward through

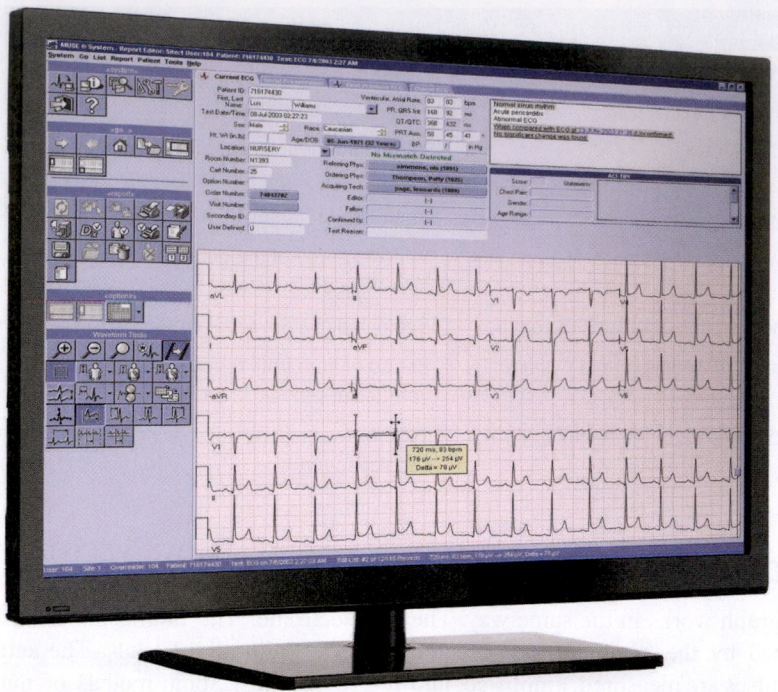

FIGURE 49-4 The electronically stored ECG retrieved by the MUSE Cardiology Information System by GE Healthcare looks just like the printed record.

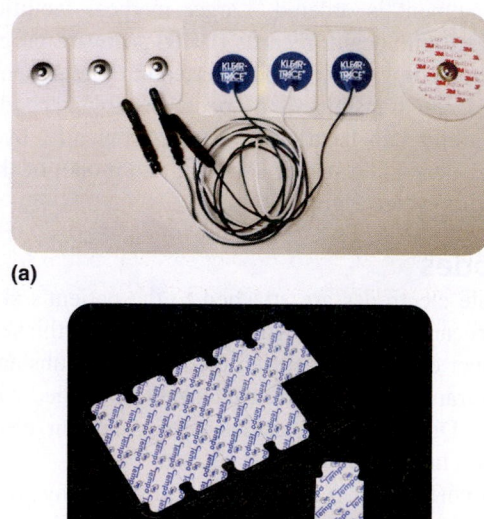

(a)

(b)

FIGURE 49-5 (a) Disposable electrodes come in various shapes and sizes. (b) Standard resting tab electrodes are inexpensive, disposable, and easy to use for a routine ECG.

the heart. Monitoring the electrodes on the arms and legs in two different ways produces six leads that record electrical impulses that move up and down and left and right. The electrodes placed on the chest provide six more leads, showing electrical activity moving forward and backward (from the front of the body toward the back and vice versa). Each lead is given a specific designation and code. See Table 49-3.

Limb Leads Of the six leads that directly monitor electrodes on the arms and legs, three are standard and three are augmented. Each of the standard leads monitors two limb electrodes, recording electrical activity between them. These leads are also called *bipolar leads* because they monitor two electrodes. The augmented leads monitor one limb electrode and a point midway between two other limb electrodes, recording electrical activity between the monitored electrode and the midway point. Because they directly monitor only one electrode, augmented leads are also called *unipolar leads.* The electrical activity recorded by these leads is very slight, requiring the machine to augment (amplify) the tracings to produce readable waves and lines on the ECG paper. The standard limb leads appear on the ECG as I, II, and III, and the augmented limb leads appear as aVF (augmented vector-foot), aVR (augmented vector-right), and aVL (augmented vector-left).

Precordial Leads The six precordial, or chest, leads are unipolar leads. The electrodes are placed across the chest in a precise, specific pattern. Each precordial lead monitors one electrode and a point within the heart. The precordial leads are each designated by a letter and a number: V_1 through V_6.

ECG Paper

ECG paper is provided in a long, continuous roll or pad. It is both heat- and pressure-sensitive and is marked with light and dark lines in a standard pattern. Each small square, or square area delineated by dots, measures 1 mm by 1 mm. Each large square measures 5 mm by 5 mm.

TABLE 49-3 ECG Lead Designations

Lead	Electrodes and Points Monitored
Standard limb	
I	RA and LA
II	RA and LL
III	LA and LL
Augmented limb	
aVR	RA and (LA and LL)
aVL	LA and (RA and LL)
aVF	LL and (RA and LA)
Precordial	
V$_1$	V$_1$ and (LA – RA – LL)*
V$_2$	V$_2$ and (LA – RA – LL)*
V$_3$	V$_3$ and (LA – RA – LL)*
V$_4$	V$_4$ and (LA – RA – LL)*
V$_5$	V$_5$ and (LA – RA – LL)*
V$_6$	V$_6$ and (LA – RA – LL)*

*The point within the heart is identified by averaging the readings from the electrodes.

The vertical, or short, axis of the paper records the voltage, or strength of the impulse; the horizontal axis measures time. Normally, the paper moves through the machine at a speed of 25 mm per second. This means the distance across 1 small square represents 0.04 second. The distance across 1 large square represents 0.2 second. The distance across 5 large squares represents 1.0 second. In 1 minute (60 seconds), the paper advances 300 large squares, or 1,500 mm (150 cm).

Each electrocardiograph is standardized before use so that 1 small square represents 0.1 millivolt (mV). One large square represents 0.5 mV, and 2 large squares represent 1.0 mV. See Figure 49-6.

Electrocardiograph Controls

The location of certain knobs and buttons on an electrocardiograph varies from model to model. However, certain features are common to most machines, including the on/off switch, standardization control, speed selector, sensitivity control, lead selector, centering control, and line control.

On/Off Switch The on/off switch turns the machine on and off. Most machines have an indicator light that signals when the power is on.

Standardization Control Before you obtain an ECG, you must correctly standardize the machine. The standardization control uses a 1-mV impulse to produce a standardization mark on the ECG paper. When you press the standardization control, the stylus should move up 10 small squares, or 10 mm (1 cm) and remain there for 0.08 second (2 small squares, or 2 mm). If it does not, the instrument must be adjusted before you use it. Most newer machines standardize automatically; check the manufacturer's instructions to ensure standardization.

Speed Selector The paper is normally set to run at 25 mm per second for adults. When you run an ECG on infants and children or on adults with a rapid heartbeat, the deflections may appear too close together. In these cases, you may need to adjust the speed to 50 mm per second to separate the peaks and create a tracing that is easier to read. If you must set the speed at 50 mm per second, note it on the strip. Otherwise, a speed of 25 mm per second is assumed. In any case, do not change the speed selection unless the doctor directs you to do so.

Sensitivity Control The sensitivity control—normally set on 1—adjusts the height of the standardization mark and the tracing. When an ECG tracing's height is too high to fit completely on the paper, however, adjust this control to ½ to reduce the size of both the standardization mark and the tracing by half. For tracings that have very low peaks, set this

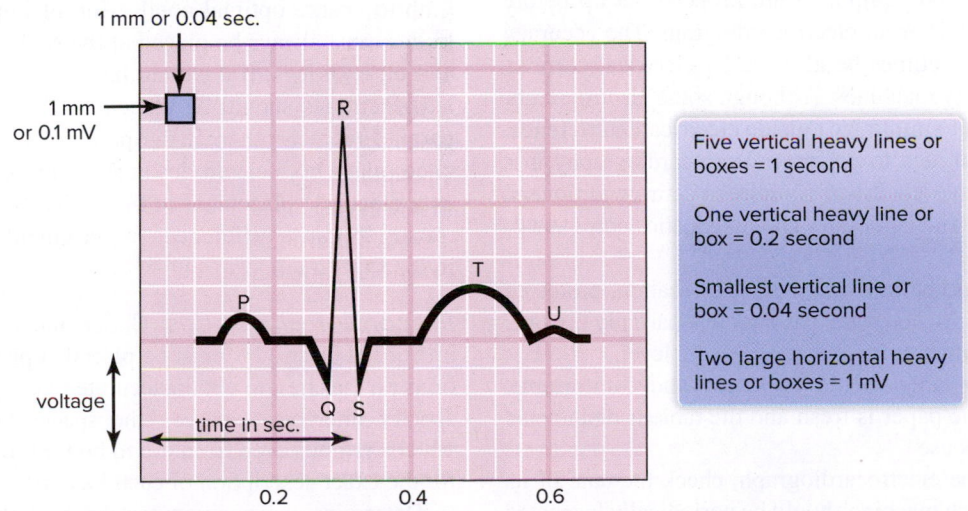

Five vertical heavy lines or boxes = 1 second

One vertical heavy line or box = 0.2 second

Smallest vertical line or box = 0.04 second

Two large horizontal heavy lines or boxes = 1 mV

FIGURE 49-6 The ECG paper is standardized and includes heavy lines that allow measurement of both time and voltage. Note that each small box is either 0.1 mV in voltage or 0.04 second in time.

Mundt, Lillian

control on 2 to double the standardization mark and the height of the tracing. Note this change on the ECG. Digital machines standardize the wave output height (gain) automatically and a standardization mark may be seen on the tracing.

Lead Selector Most electrocardiographs have a setting that enables a standard 12-lead tracing to run automatically. All machines have a lead selector that allows you to run each lead individually, in case you need to repeat a strip containing **artifacts,** which are erroneous marks or defects on the tracking.

Centering Control The centering control allows you to adjust the position of the stylus, which must be centered on the paper. Centering the stylus simplifies the process of measuring wave heights for the person who interprets the ECG.

Line Control Another control allows you to adjust the temperature of the stylus. A higher temperature results in a heavier line, whereas a lower temperature results in a lighter, thinner line. The line should be clear without being so dark that it bleeds or smears on the ECG paper. Newer ECG machines do not have a temperature control but may have an adjustment to change the line. Check the manufacturer's directions.

▶ Performing an ECG
LO 49.4

You must obtain a good-quality tracing when performing electrocardiography. To do so, you must be able to recognize an artifact or a generally defective ECG tracing when you see one. Proper technique is also essential to help you obtain the best-quality tracing. The following sections guide you through the general process; however, you must be familiar with the equipment you will be using. The steps in obtaining a standard 12-lead ECG are listed in Procedure 49-1 at the end of this chapter.

Preparing the Room and Equipment

Be sure the room and equipment are properly set up before you begin to administer an electrocardiogram. The accuracy of an ECG can sometimes be affected by electrical currents emitted from nearby machines. Although some electrocardiographs have filters to minimize outside electrical interference, it is always a good idea to perform electrocardiography in a room where all other electrical equipment—air conditioners, refrigerators, fans, and laboratory and diagnostic equipment—is turned off.

The room should be in a quiet, private location, protected from interruptions. Because the patient must partially disrobe, adjust the room temperature to a comfortable level.

The examining table should be sturdy and comfortable. Make sure the table paper is fresh and the table is disinfected after each patient's use.

Before using the electrocardiograph, check the date of its last inspection. Each machine should be periodically inspected and certified safe to use for a specific period of time. Using a machine only within this time period helps ensure both your and the patient's safety. It is good practice to check the

ECG paper and ECG electrodes prior to preparing the patient, restocking these supplies if necessary, as this will save time for you and the physician.

Preparing the Patient

Introduce yourself to the patient, explain the procedure, and answer any questions the patient has. Keep in mind, some patients are apprehensive about undergoing electrocardiography. Anxiety often stems from the fear of receiving an electric shock from the machine. See the *Caution: Handle with Care* section for ways to allay a patient's anxiety about having an ECG.

Applying the Electrodes and the Connecting Wires

You must prepare the patient's skin before applying the electrodes. Proper contact between an electrode and the skin allows for proper conduction of the impulses. Depending on your office policy, you may be required to trim chest or leg hair if it is dense to ensure proper contact. This should be done with scissors. Shaving is not allowed because of the risk of infection or bleeding.

Electrodes Apply disposable electrodes by simply removing the adhesive backing and pressing the electrode firmly into place on the skin. You must position electrodes at 10 locations on the body (Figure 49-7). This includes 4 limb electrodes and 6 chest electrodes.

Limb Electrodes Limb electrodes are most commonly placed on the inside of the fleshy part of the calf muscle and on the outside of the upper arm. Sometimes they are placed on the thigh, on the abdomen, and above the wrist. Follow office policy on limb placement, but remember, a consistent technique will ensure that all ECGs will be standardized, even with different equipment models. It is generally better to place arm electrodes on the upper arm because this reduces the amount of artifact caused by arm movement. Attach the electrodes to a smooth and fleshy part of each limb to ensure optimal conduction of impulses. Limb electrodes must always be placed at the same level on both arms and on both legs. If a patient has had a leg amputated, both leg electrodes should be placed on the thighs or abdomen, parallel to each other. If the patient has had an arm amputated, place both electrodes at shoulder level. Note the alternate electrode placement in the patient's chart and the ECG tracing, because differences in placement can cause changes in the ECG tracing.

Precordial Electrodes Unlike the limb electrodes, the precordial electrodes must be placed at precise, specific locations on the chest to obtain accurate readings. These locations specify intercostal spaces—the spaces between the ribs—which are numbered from top to bottom. Refer to Figure 49-8 for the exact description of each location.

Determine the position for the first precordial electrode (V_1) by counting to the fourth intercostal space to the right of the sternum (breastbone). The V_1 electrode should be placed over this space, directly adjacent to the sternum. After you

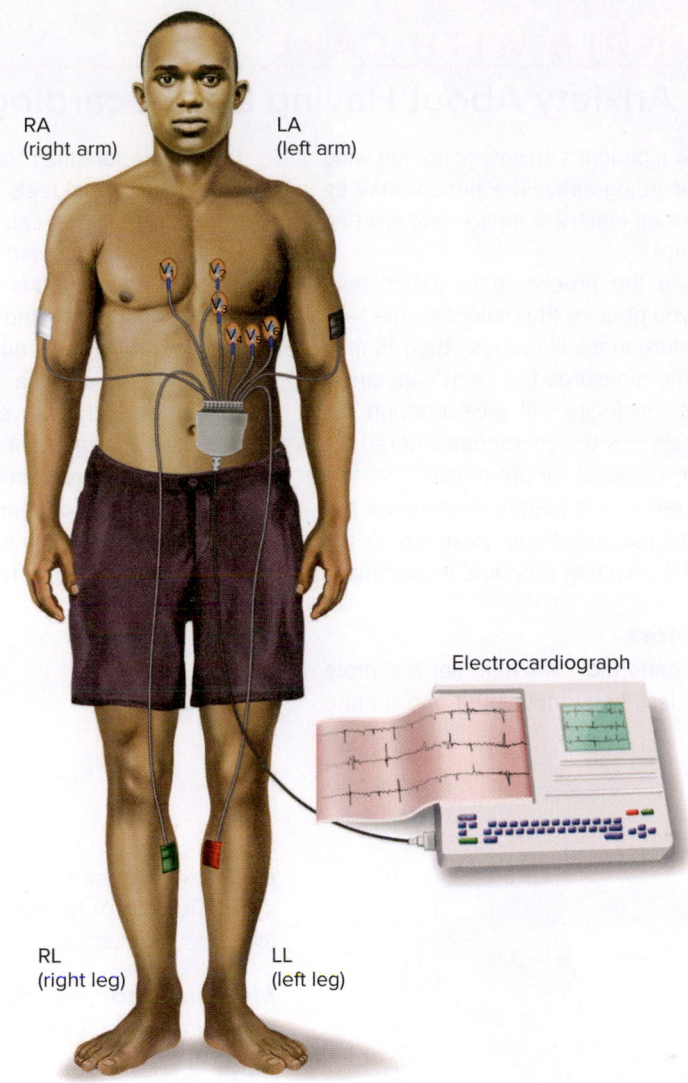

FIGURE 49-7 There are 10 electrode positions for electrocardiography.

have this electrode in place, use it as a guide to position the other electrodes.

Place the V_2 electrode in the fourth intercostal space to the left of the sternum in the same manner. Note that the V_1 and V_2 positions may not line up exactly; one may be higher than the other. Perfect symmetry is rare in the human body.

Next, place the V_4 electrode in the fifth intercostal space, where it intersects an imaginary line drawn straight down from the middle of the clavicle (midclavicular line). When the V_4 electrode is in place, place the V_3 electrode midway between V_2 and V_4 in the fifth intercostal space.

Place the V_6 electrode in the fifth intercostal space directly below the middle of the armpit (midaxillary line). Place the last electrode (V_5) in the fifth intercostal space midway between V_4 and V_6.

Attaching the Wires After placing the electrodes, attach the wires that connect the electrodes to the electrocardiograph. Numbers and letters on the wires correspond to numbers and letters for the electrodes. For example, RA stands for right arm, LL stands for left leg, and so on. The precordial electrode wires are labeled V_1 through V_6. Connect the limb wires first, then the precordial wires, in the sequence already described. Some wires are also color-coded.

Connect the wires to the electrodes using the clips or snaps on the end of the wires. Wires should follow the patient's body contours and lie flat against the body. Drape the wires over the patient to avoid putting tension on the electrodes, which could cause interference. You also may bundle the wires together to form a single cable.

Operating the Electrocardiograph

Before running the ECG, remind the patient to remain as still as possible and not to talk.

Preparing the Electrocardiograph Enter patient identifying information into the ECG machine's LCD display. If the machine does not allow data entry, write the information on the tracing report once completed.

Standardization may be necessary; however, digital ECG machines standardize the wave output heights automatically. These calibration marks can be seen at the beginning or end

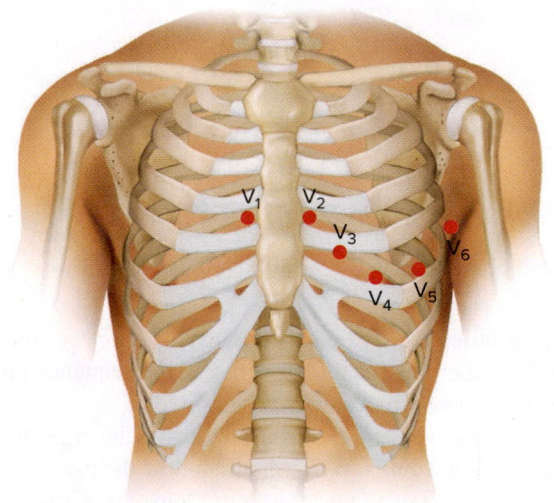

V_1 Fourth intercostal space (between the ribs), to the right of the sternum (breastbone)
V_2 Fourth intercostal space, to the left of the sternum
V_4 Fifth intercostal space, on the left midclavicular line
V_3 Fifth intercostal space, midway between V_2 and V_4
V_6 Fifth intercostal space, on the left midaxillary line
V_5 Fifth intercostal space, midway between V_4 and V_6

FIGURE 49-8 Six precordial electrodes are arranged in specific positions on the chest. Notice that electrode V_4 must be positioned before V_3 and V_6 before V_5.

of a 12-lead tracing. See Figure 49-9. For manual standardization, check the manufacturer's instructions.

Running the ECG You can now run the ECG. On most machines, turning the lead selector to the automatic mode produces a standard 12-lead strip. Because each lead provides a specific view of the heart's electrical activity, each of the 12 leads has a characteristic tracing (Figure 49-9).

Multiple-Channel Electrocardiographs Some electrocardiographs have multiple channels that can record three, four, or six leads simultaneously (Figure 49-10). Electrode placement is the same as for single-channel electrocardiographs.

Checking the ECG Tracing After running the 12 leads and before disconnecting the patient from the machine, check all tracings to make sure they are clear and free of artifacts. If any of the leads do not appear on a tracing, it may mean a wire has come loose. In this case, reconnect the wire and repeat the tracing. Repeat any unclear tracings.

Also, check that all tracings are contained within the paper's boundaries and that no waves peak above its edges. Increase or decrease the sensitivity setting to adjust the size of the peaks.

If the peaks in a tracing are too close together, increase the paper speed to 50 mm per second. Increasing the speed separates the peaks and makes the tracing easier to read.

Make a note on the ECG tracing whenever it is necessary to adjust sensitivity or speed settings. This information is vital to the interpretation of the test.

Troubleshooting: Artifacts and Other Problems

To ensure high-quality tracings, it is essential to recognize artifacts and identify sources of interference. You also must know how to correct them.

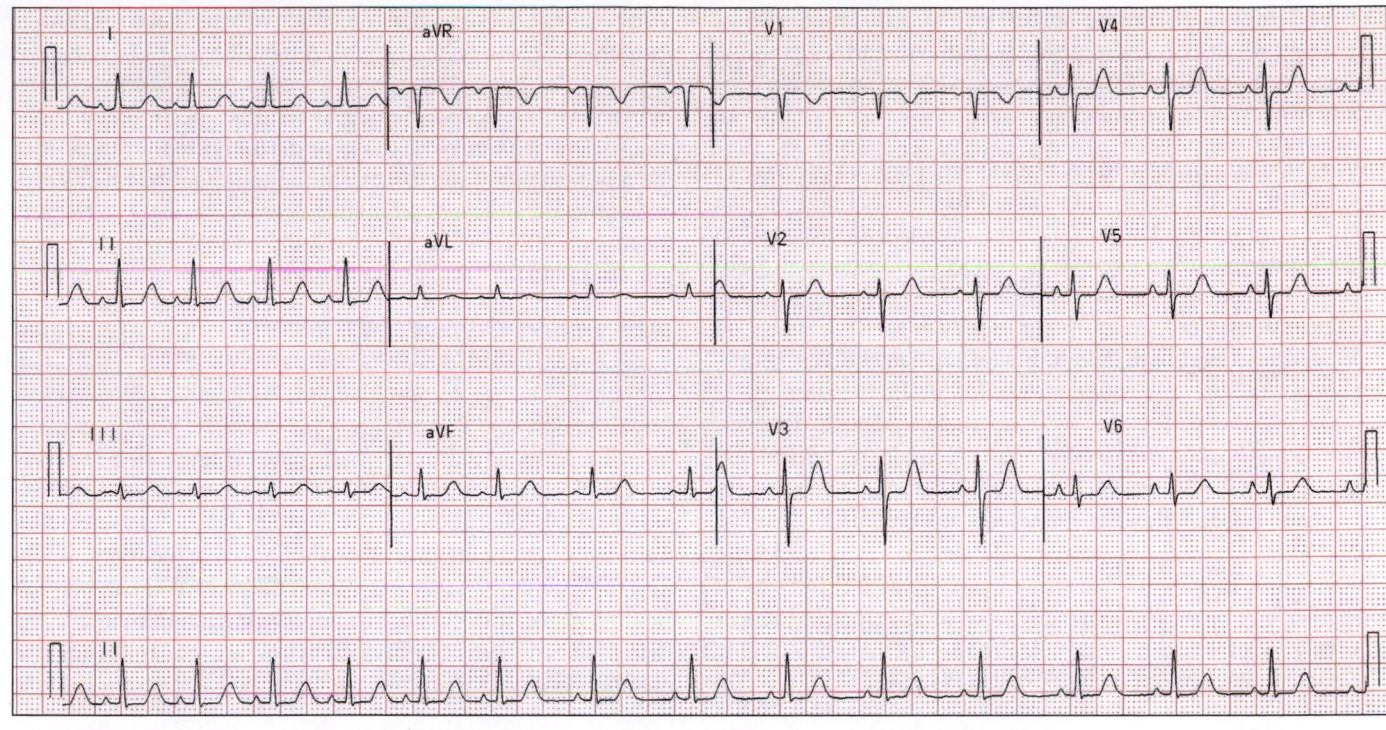

FIGURE 49-9 The tracing from each lead will differ. The long tracing of a single lead along the bottom is the rhythm strip.

Artifacts Improper technique, poor conduction, outside interference, and improper handling of a tracing can cause artifacts. If artifacts are present on an ECG tracing, the licensed practitioner may not be able to make an accurate diagnosis of the patient's condition.

There are several types of artifacts. Among the common ones you may see are a wandering baseline or a flat line. Recognizing the presence of an artifact in the baseline during setup allows you to correct the problem before the tracing is recorded. You also may see marks that are not characteristic

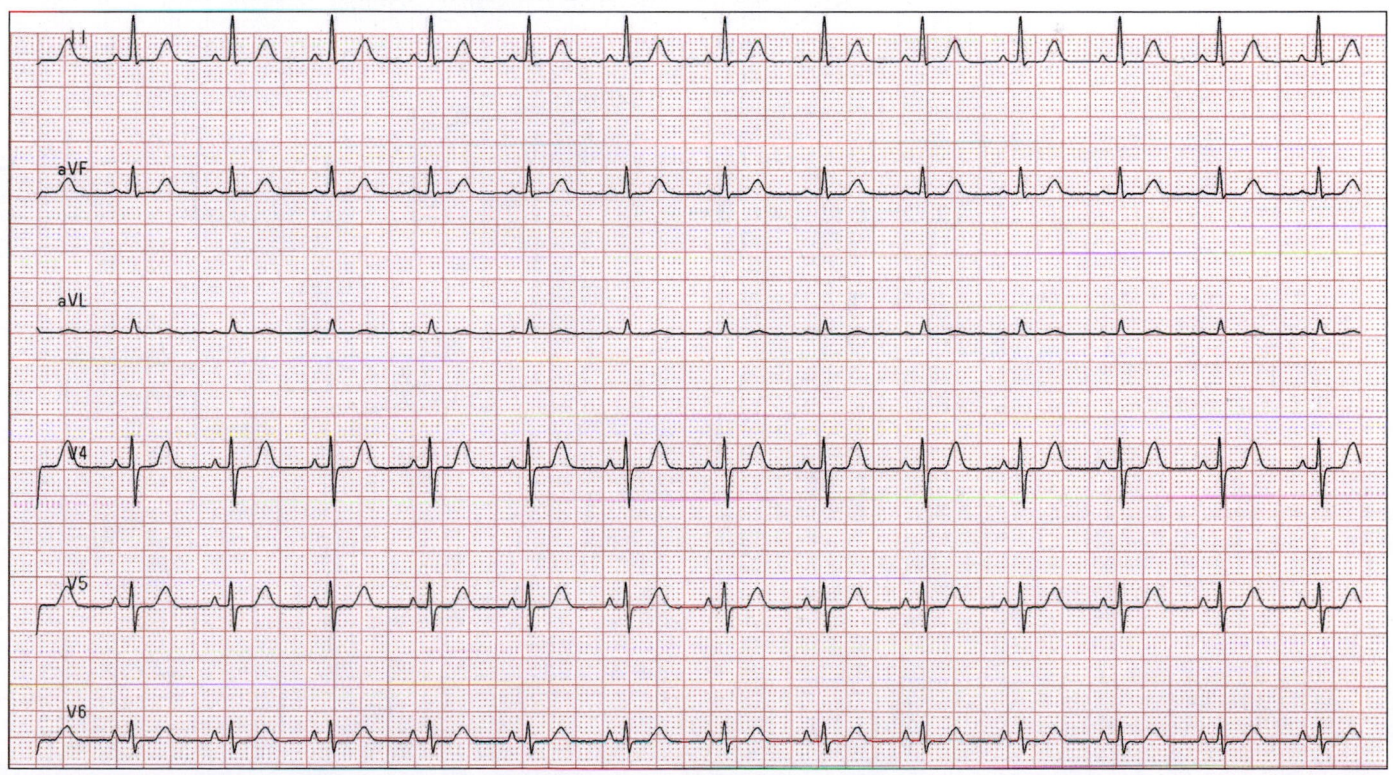

FIGURE 49-10 Some electrocardiographs allow you to run six leads at the same time.

of a tracing; large, erratic spikes; or uniform, small spikes. Table 49-4 outlines these artifacts and summarizes possible causes and solutions. Follow these guidelines to correct artifacts when recording an ECG.

Wandering Baseline A wandering baseline, shown in Figure 49-11, is identified by a shift in the baseline from the center position for that lead. Causes include somatic interference (muscle movement) and a variety of mechanical problems. Mechanical problems may include improper application of electrodes (too loose or incorrectly placed), tension on electrodes caused by a dangling wire, inadequate skin preparation, or the presence of creams or lotions on the skin.

Having the patient lie still can reduce somatic interference. Proper skin preparation and electrode placement are also essential. When the electrocardiography appointment is made, instruct the patient to use no creams or lotions, deodorant, perfume, or powder. Be sure to include specific instructions in patient education materials and ask the patient whether any of these substances were used before the procedure. If so, clean each area of electrode placement thoroughly with alcohol to avoid conduction disturbances.

Flat Line A flat line on one of the lead's tracings (Figure 49-12) is typically caused by a loose or disconnected wire. If flat lines occur on more than one lead, two of the wires may have been switched. If flat lines occur on all leads, the patient cable may be loose or disconnected, or there may be a break (short) somewhere in the unit. On the other hand, a flat line on all leads can indicate cardiac arrest. If a flat line occurs on all leads, always check the patient's pulse and respiration first.

Alternating Current (AC) Interference AC interference occurs when the electrocardiograph picks up a small amount of electric current given off by another piece of electrical equipment. The tracing's line will be jagged, consisting of a series of uniform, small spikes (Figure 49-13). Many newer electrocardiographs have filters to reduce or eliminate most of this interference, and it often can be eliminated by turning off or unplugging other appliances in the room. Keeping the examining table away from the wall also can help, as wiring in the wall can contribute to AC interference. If the wires are crossed and the lead wires are not following the patient's body contour, this can cause AC interference. Make

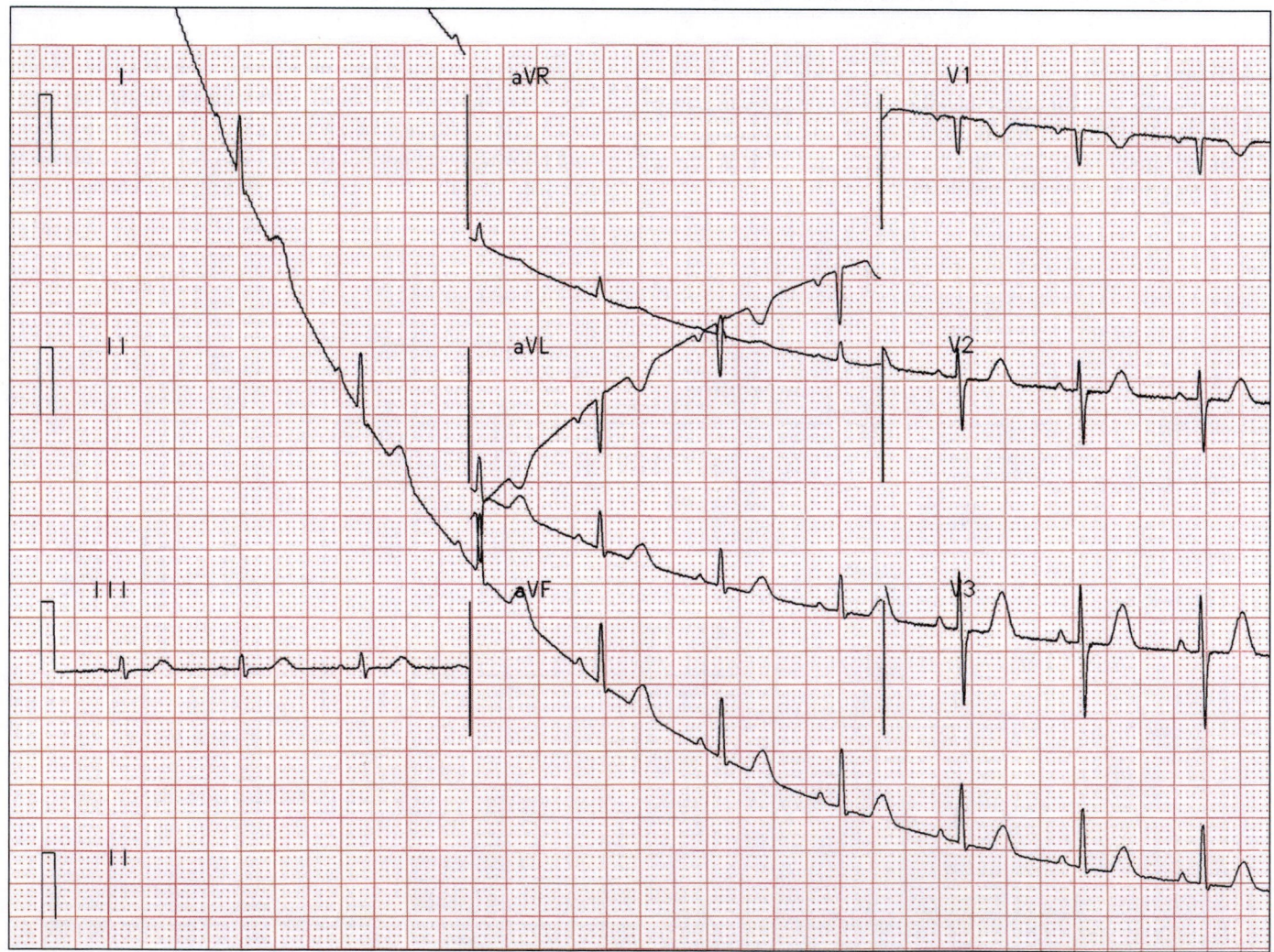

FIGURE 49-11 A wandering baseline may be caused by somatic interference or a mechanical problem.

TABLE 49-4 Correcting ECG Artifacts

Problem	Possible Causes	Solutions
Wandering baseline	Poor skin preparation	Repeat skin preparation and lead placement.
	Loose electrode	Reapply electrode.
	Improper electrode placement	Reapply electrode.
	Somatic interference	Help patient relax and be comfortable.
	Pickup of breathing movement	Reposition electrode.
	Tension on electrode	Drape wires over patient.
Flat line	Detached/loose wire or cable	Reattach wires or cable.
	Crossed wires	Check/switch wires.
	Short circuit in wires	Check/replace broken equipment.
	Cardiac arrest	Check pulse/respiration; begin CPR.
Marks not part of tracing	Careless handling	Handle carefully.
	Use of paper clips	Use a rubber band.
	Wet hands	Ensure that hands are dry.
Uniform, small spikes	AC interference	Turn off/unplug other electrical equipment; remove patient's watch.
	Improper electrode placement	Reapply electrode.
	Inadequate grounding	Check and apply proper grounding.
	Dirty electrode	Clean and reapply electrode.
Large, erratic spikes	Somatic interference	Help patient relax and be comfortable.
	Loose/dry electrode	Reapply electrode.

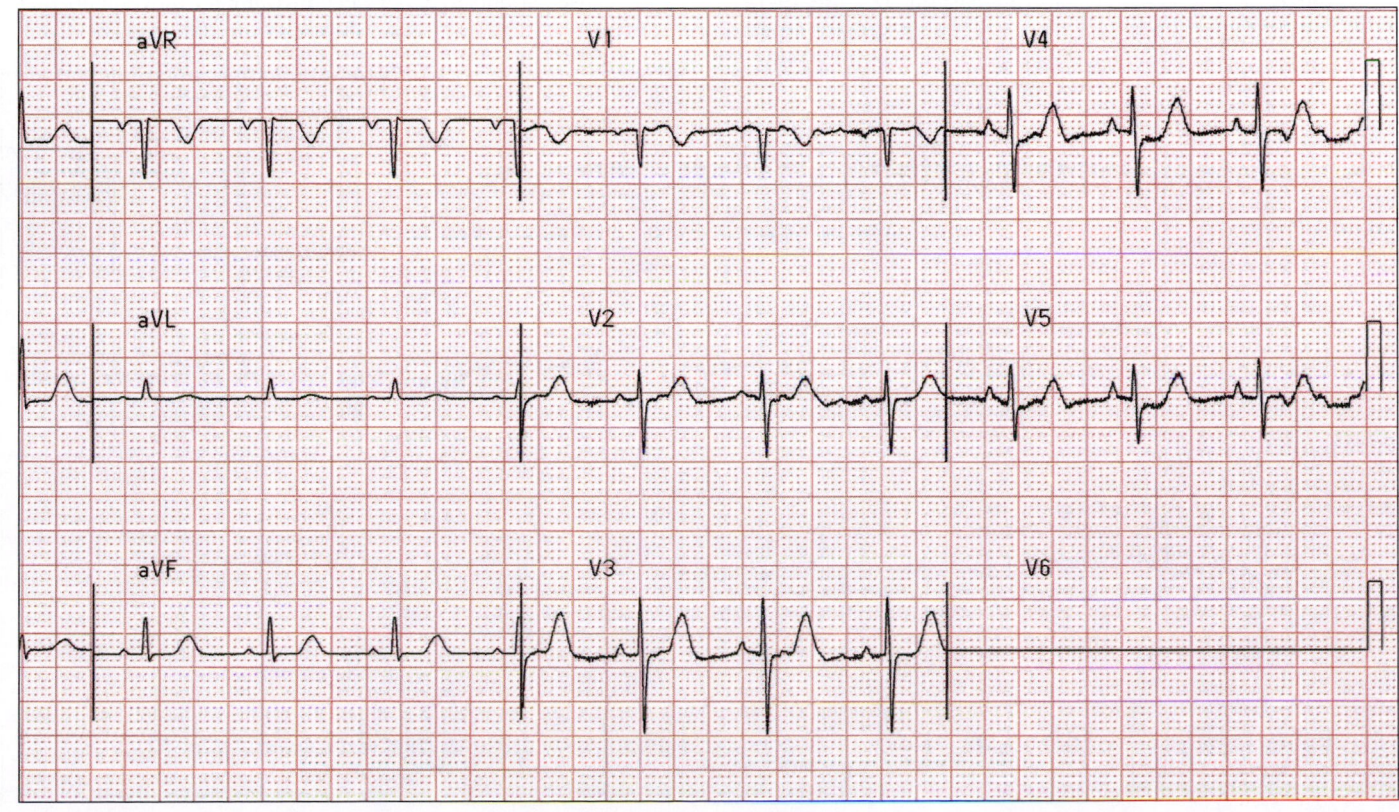

FIGURE 49-12   A flat line on one of the leads is caused by a loose or disconnected wire.

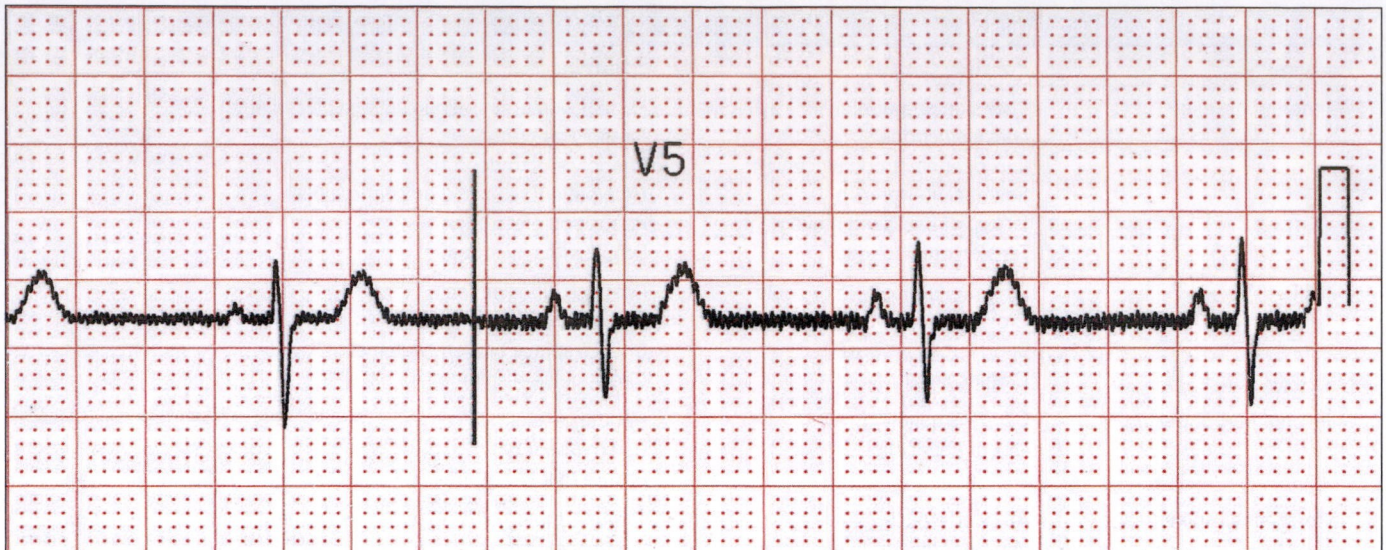

FIGURE 49-13 This type of artifact is caused by AC interference.

sure the ECG cable is not underneath the examination table. If these remedies do not work, check to see whether the electrodes are dirty or attached improperly or whether the machine is incorrectly grounded.

Somatic Interference Muscle movement—tensing of voluntary muscles, shifting of body position, tremors, or even talking (which requires muscular contractions that generate electrical impulses)—causes somatic interference. A sensitive electrocardiograph detects these impulses, possibly resulting in large, erratic spikes and a shifting baseline (Figure 49-14).

Eliminate this type of interference by reminding the patient to remain still and to refrain from talking. To reduce the chance of the patient shivering, shifting, and moving, be sure the room temperature is comfortable for the patient.

Placing the limb electrodes closer to the body's trunk—on the upper arms, close to the shoulder, and on the upper thighs—can reduce interference. Reducing patient anxiety by explaining the procedure also can help reduce somatic interference.

Certain nervous system disorders, such as Parkinson's disease, cause patients to experience involuntary movements that

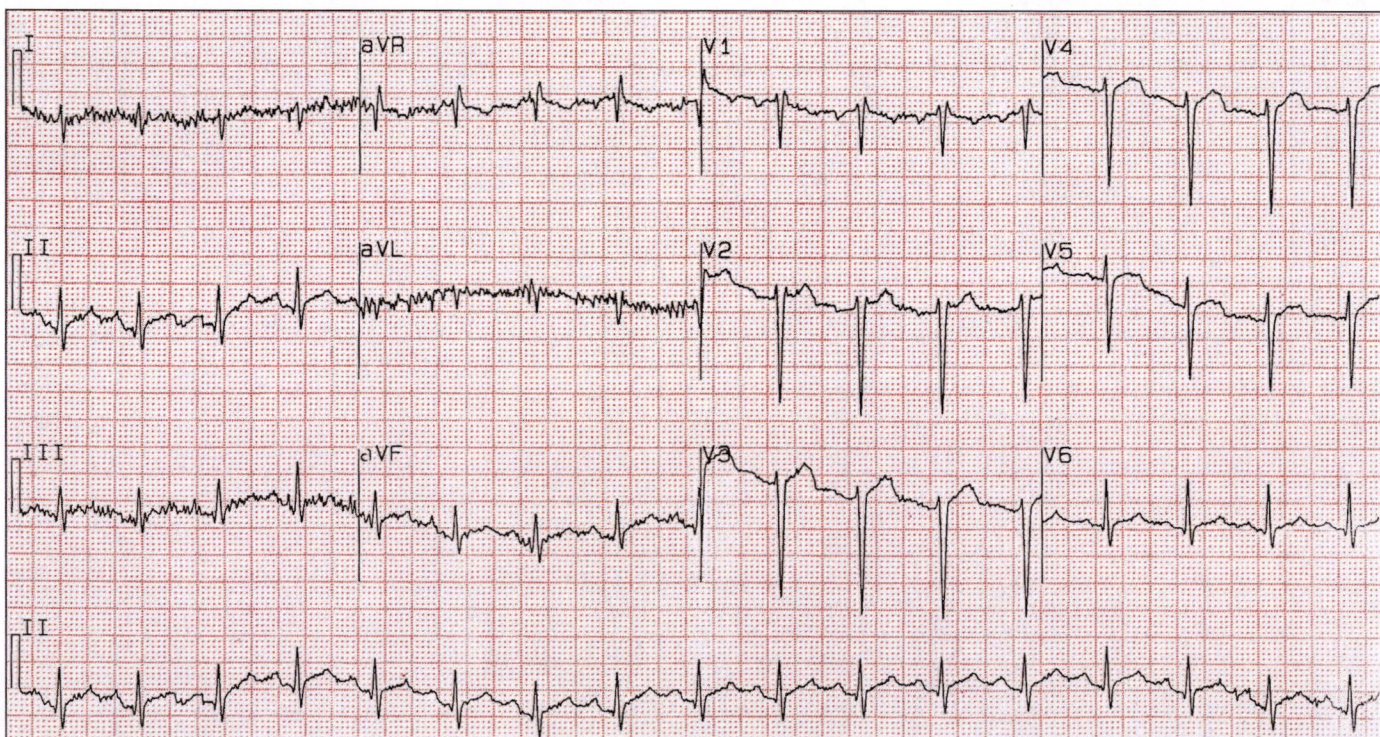

FIGURE 49-14 The somatic interference in this ECG was caused by patient tremors.

can cause interference. So, although placing the limb electrodes closer to the body's trunk is often helpful, it may be necessary to interrupt the tracing until the tremors subside.

Identifying the Source of Interference Frequently, interference is caused by one of the limb electrodes. The source of interference on an ECG can be identified by checking the ECG tracings obtained on leads I, II, and III. If there is a problem with a particular limb electrode, the interference will be prominent in two leads.

Use these guidelines:

- If there is interference in leads I and II on the tracing, check the right arm electrode.
- If there is interference in leads I and III, check the left arm electrode.
- If there is interference in leads II and III, check the left leg electrode.

If the cause of the artifact or the source of interference cannot be determined, stop the machine and notify your supervisor or the physician. Do not disconnect the patient from the electrocardiograph.

Completing the Procedure

When you are sure the quality of all ECG tracings is acceptable, disconnect the patient from the machine. Remove the tracing and label if necessary; then disconnect the wires from the electrodes and remove the electrodes from the patient. Wipe excess electrolyte from the patient's skin with a moist towel if needed. Assist the patient to a sitting position, allowing a moment's rest before assisting the patient from the table. Help the patient dress if necessary, or allow the patient privacy to dress. Remove disposable paper covers from the table and pillows, clean surfaces according to OSHA guidelines, and discard all disposable materials in a biohazardous waste container.

Interpreting the ECG Although you are not responsible for interpreting an ECG as a medical assistant, knowing something about how ECGs are interpreted may allow you to recognize an urgent problem. Some of the features assessed by an ECG include heart rhythm, heart rate, the length and position of intervals and segments, and wave changes. A series of ECGs is often taken before a physician makes a diagnosis. The tracings are compared for changes in a patient's condition, progress, or response to a specific medication.

Heart Rhythm The ECG is the best way to assess heart rhythm—the regularity of the heartbeat. A normal heart rhythm is indicated on the ECG by regularly spaced complexes. In regularly spaced complexes, the distance between one P wave and the next P wave—or one R wave and the next R wave—is consistent. The physician assesses the patient's rhythm by viewing the rhythm strip you obtain from lead II.

Heart Rate The heart rate can easily be determined by counting the number of QRS complexes in a 6-second strip of the tracing (30 large squares at 25 mm per second) and multiplying by 10. Heart rate irregularities may result from conduction abnormalities or reactions to certain drugs.

Intervals and Segments Variations in the length and position of the intervals and segments can indicate many heart conditions, including conduction disturbances and myocardial infarction. For example, following a myocardial infarction, the ST segment will be elevated in the tracing for a period of time. Thus, the ECG can be used to determine not only the occurrence of a myocardial infarction but also whether it occurred recently. Electrolyte disturbances in the blood and drug reactions also can affect intervals and segments.

Wave Changes The direction of certain waves may vary, depending on which lead is being viewed. Normally, each wave should have a similar appearance in each of the leads. Changes in the height, width, or direction of a wave may indicate a problem. During the early stages of a myocardial infarction, for example, the T wave forms a large peak. Not long afterward, the T wave inverts and appears below the baseline.

Cardiac Dysrhythmias Irregularities in heart rhythm are called **dysrhythmias,** also known as *arrhythmias.* Although some dysrhythmias do not cause problems, many of them can be dangerous, so it is important to detect these irregularities with an ECG.

Ventricular Fibrillation (V-fib) Ventricular fibrillation, commonly referred to as *v-fib,* is a life-threatening heart condition in which the ventricles of the heart appear to "quiver" and there is no cardiac output. The patient will quickly lose consciousness, and cardioversion (defibrillation) must be used to stop the dysrhythmia. Ventricular fibrillation is seen in patients experiencing a myocardial infarction. The tracing is often described as a "saw tooth" image (Figure 49-15).

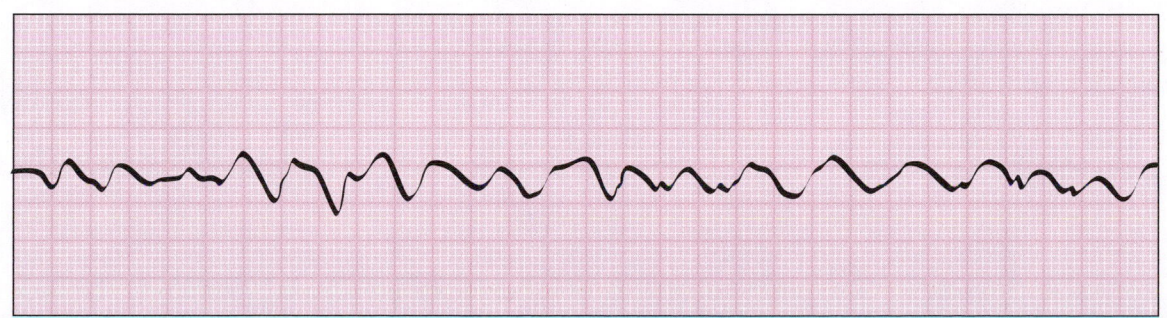

FIGURE 49-15 Ventricular fibrillation resembles and is sometimes referred to as a "saw tooth" pattern.

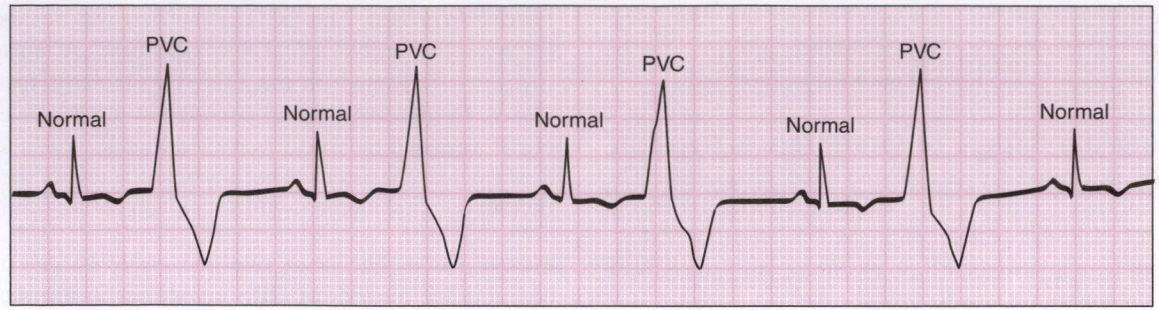

FIGURE 49-16   This rhythm strip compares a normal deflection to a premature ventricular contraction (PVC).

Premature Ventricular Contractions (PVCs) Premature ventricular contractions (PVCs) are premature heartbeats that originate from the heart's ventricles. A PVC is identified as a beat that occurs early in the cycle, followed by a pause before the next cycle (Figure 49-16). PVCs are premature because they occur before the regular heartbeat. These heartbeats are the result of an irritability of the heart muscle in the ventricles and can be caused by myocardial infarctions, electrolyte imbalances, lack of oxygen, or certain medications. A PVC appears on the ECG as having no P wave, a wide QRS complex, and T waves that deflect in the opposite direction from the R wave.

Atrial Fibrillation Atrial dysrhythmias occur because of electrical disturbances in the atria and/or the AV node, which lead to fast heartbeats (tachycardia). Atrial fibrillation is a common atrial dysrhythmia that causes speedy, multiple electrical signals that fire rapidly from different areas in the atria rather than from the SA node. Causes of atrial fibrillation include myocardial infarction; hypertension; heart failure; mitral valve diseases, such as MVP; overactive thyroid; pulmonary embolisms (blood clots); excessive alcohol consumption; emphysema; and pericarditis. Atrial fibrillation is seen on the ECG as small, irregular, uncoordinated complexes that are difficult to interpret because the P waves cannot be identified (Figure 49-17).

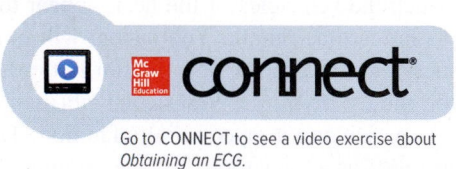

Go to CONNECT to see a video exercise about *Obtaining an ECG.*

▶ Exercise Electrocardiography (Stress Testing) and Echocardiography   LO 49.5

The resting ECG does not always provide a doctor with enough information to diagnose a problem. A licensed practitioner can use several additional tests for diagnosing heart diseases and disorders. Exercise electrocardiography, more commonly known as a **stress test,** assesses the heart's conduction system during exercise, when the demand for oxygen increases. This test measures a patient's response to a constant or increasing workload. **Echocardiography** uses ultrasound to view the heart in motion. This can be done at rest or after strenuous activity such as riding a bike or walking on a treadmill.

Exercise Electrocardiography

A stress test may be performed on a patient who has had surgery or a myocardial infarction to determine how the heart is functioning. It is sometimes used to screen a patient for heart disease and to determine a patient's ability to undertake an exercise program.

During the procedure, the patient is required to walk on a treadmill, pedal a stationary bicycle, or walk on a stair-stepping ergonometer while ECG readings are taken (Figure 49-18). An ergonometer measures work performed. You are responsible for preparing the patient for electrocardiography and monitoring blood pressure throughout the procedure. The test continues until the patient reaches a target heart rate, experiences chest pain or fatigue, or develops complications, such as tachycardia or dysrhythmia.

A patient who undergoes stress testing is often suspected of having a heart problem or is recovering from a myocardial

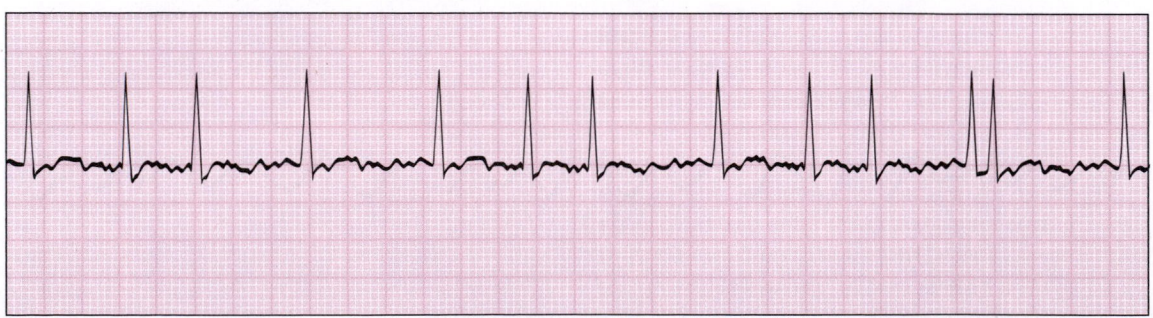

FIGURE 49-17   Atrial fibrillation.

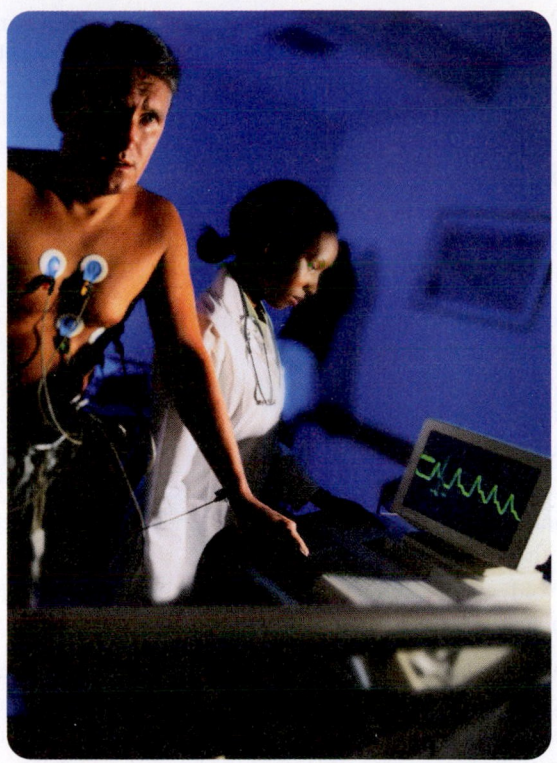

FIGURE 49-18 During a stress test, the patient exercises on special equipment to see how well the heart handles increased physical demands.
© Stockbyte/Getty Images RF

infarction or surgery. Consequently, there may be a risk of cardiac distress, myocardial infarction, or cardiac arrest during testing. Because of the risks, the patient must sign an informed consent form before the procedure and a physician must monitor the patient throughout the test. Emergency medication and equipment, such as a defibrillator, must always be present in the room. Because of the potential risk, patients may be apprehensive about the test. As a medical assistant, you can be instrumental in helping them feel comfortable about undergoing the procedure and in making the procedure as safe as possible for them. See the *Caution: Handle with Care* section for ways to help a patient safely undergo stress testing.

Echocardiography

The ability to view the moving heart is essential to understanding how the structures within the heart are functioning. An echocardiogram produces a video image of the working heart valves and chambers and shows how well blood moves through these structures. There are several types of echocardiograms:

- Transthoracic—the ultrasound transducer is moved around on the chest and or abdomen to produce heart images.

- Transesophageal—the transducer is passed into the esophagus, where it produces clearer images of the heart because it is closer to the heart and the sound waves do not have to penetrate the ribs.

- Doppler—uses a special type of ultrasound to look at blood flow through the heart. The direction and speed of blood flow through the heart are assessed with this type of test, giving the physician information about coronary artery blockage and heart valve damage.

- Stress echo—echocardiography is done before and after exercise or injection of a drug that makes the heart work faster and harder. This is usually done in conjunction with an electrocardiogram to assess how well the heart responds to increased demand.

Pretest Preparation There is usually no special pretest preparation for transthoracic and doppler echocardiography. The patient should not eat a heavy meal prior to a stress

CAUTION: HANDLE WITH CARE

Ensuring Patient Safety During Stress Testing

Although some risk is involved in exercise electrocardiography, the risk of having a myocardial infarction during a stress test is less than 1 in 500. The risk of death is less than 1 in 10,000. Patients are sometimes apprehensive about the procedure, especially patients who have recently had a myocardial infarction. You can help educate patients to reduce their apprehension and prepare them for stress tests. Assist during the procedure using these techniques:

- Ask patients to wear comfortable shoes and clothes so that they will be more comfortable during the exercise portion of the text.

- Inform the patient of the symptoms he can expect during the test—including fatigue, slight breathlessness, an increased heart rate, and increased perspiration—so that the patient will be better able to cope with the test.

- Explain that advance notice of adjustments or changes during the test, such as an increased workload, will be given.

- Assure the patient that there are few risks associated with the test and that the test can be stopped if he experiences chest pain or extreme fatigue.

- Tell the patient that both you and the physician will be monitoring his vital signs during and after the procedure and that all safety precautions will be taken.

- Explain the presence of the safety equipment—for example, the crash cart with medication, equipment, and supplies in the remote chance that an emergency occurs.

- Encourage the patient to report any symptoms during the test. Even symptoms that are not cardiac-related should be reported.

- Observe the patient for signs of distress, and inform the physician immediately if such symptoms appear.

echo. Since patients having transesophageal echocardiography receive a sedative and the transducer is passed into the esophagus, they should not eat for at least 6 hours prior to the test. Make sure you carefully explain all pretest instructions verbally and in writing and give the patient an opportunity to ask any questions. Reassure the patient of the limited risk during the procedure. Finally, have the patient sign a consent form prior to having the echocardiogram.

▶ Ambulatory Electrocardiography (Holter Monitoring)   LO 49.6

Patients who experience intermittent chest pain or discomfort may have a normal resting ECG and a normal stress test. When this is the case, the electrical activity of the patient's heart can be monitored over a 24-hour period of normal activity to help diagnose the problem. A Holter monitor is used for this purpose.

Function of the Holter Monitor

A **Holter monitor** is an electrocardiography device that includes a microchip or small cassette recorder and is worn around a patient's waist or on a shoulder strap to record the heart's electrical activity. The monitor is connected to electrodes on the patient's chest (Figure 49-19). During the testing period, the patient is asked to perform usual daily activities and to keep a written log of activities undertaken and of stress or symptoms experienced. To aid in the diagnosis, some monitors allow patients to press an event button to mark the area on the recording whenever symptoms appear.

The patient returns to the office at the end of the 24-hour test period to have the monitor and electrodes removed. The recording is analyzed by a computer in the office or at a reference laboratory and a printout of the results is prepared. When the tracing has been evaluated, the doctor can correlate cardiac irregularities, such as dysrhythmias or ST segment changes, with the activities and symptoms listed in the patient's diary.

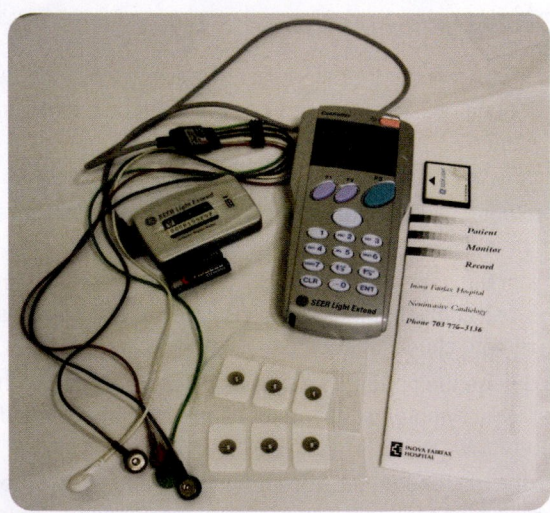

FIGURE 49-19   The Holter monitor is used to determine electrical activity of a patient's heart over a 24-hour period. This Burdick Vision Holter is one type of monitor.

© Total Care Programming, Inc

In addition to its role as a diagnostic tool, Holter monitoring can be used to evaluate the status of a patient who is recovering from a myocardial infarction. It can indicate progress or the need to change therapy or the rehabilitation plan.

Patient Education

It is an essential that the patient continue normal activities during Holter monitoring. Give the patient the following additional instructions:

- Record all activities, emotional upsets, physical symptoms, and medications taken.
- Wear loose-fitting clothing that opens in the front while wearing the monitor.
- Avoid going near magnets, metal detectors, and high-voltage areas and avoid using electric blankets during the monitoring period. These devices and areas can interfere with the recording.
- Avoid getting the monitor wet. Do not take a bath or shower. A sponge bath is permissible.

Show the patient how to check the monitor to make sure it is working properly. This step is particularly important if any of the electrodes seem loose. Instruct the patient to inform the office if there are any problems.

Connecting the Patient

Holter monitors have either three or five electrodes, depending on the unit. As with a resting ECG, correct placement of the electrodes is necessary for accurate readings. Before connecting the patient to the Holter monitor, make sure he has signed an informed consent form and explain that you need to attach electrodes to the patient's skin.

Because the electrodes must stay in place for 24 hours, you may need to clip the hair in the areas where the electrodes are attached to permit optimum adherence. The wires may be connected to the electrodes before they are attached to minimize patient discomfort.

After the electrodes and wires are attached and the monitor is in place, tape the wires to the patient's chest to eliminate tension on the wires or electrodes. Be sure that the unit has a fresh battery, that a cassette tape or other data storage device has been inserted if necessary, and that the unit is turned on. The steps in performing Holter monitoring are outlined in Procedure 49-2 at the end of this chapter.

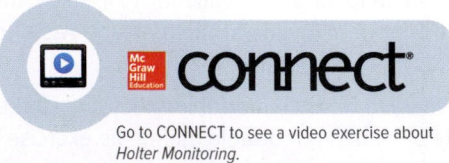

Go to CONNECT to see a video exercise about *Holter Monitoring.*

▶ Pulmonary Function Testing   LO 49.7

Pulmonary function tests (PFTs) help the doctor evaluate ventilatory function of the lungs and chest wall. They evaluate lung volume and capacity and are commonly used to evaluate shortness of breath and to help detect and classify pulmonary disorders. They also may be performed as part of a general examination. PFTs are used to monitor conditions such as asthma, certain allergies, cystic fibrosis, and chronic obstructive pulmonary disease (COPD), a chronic lung disorder. The tests are also used to evaluate the effectiveness of particular treatments on a patient's lung function.

Spirometry

Spirometry is a test used to measure breathing capacity. An instrument called a **spirometer** measures the air taken in by and expelled from the lungs. Several different measurements related to lung volume and capacity can be made with a spirometer. Some of these measurements are made directly by the spirometer; others are calculated. For more information about lung volumes and capacities, see the chapter *The Respiratory System*.

Forced Vital Capacity

Many measurements can be obtained during one particular maneuver—obtaining the **forced vital capacity (FVC),** the greatest volume of air that can be expelled when a person performs rapid, forced expiration. To obtain the FVC, ask the patient to take as deep a breath as possible and to exhale into the spirometer as quickly and completely as possible. You can determine the lung's ability to function by taking into account the volume of air expelled and the time it takes to perform this maneuver.

Types of Spirometers

Many models of computerized spirometers are used in physicians' offices. Each consists of a mouthpiece or a mouthpiece and a tube to carry air to the machine, a mechanism to measure the volume or flow of air, and a means of calculating and printing the results.

Computerized spirometers measure air volume and airflow, perform various calculations, and print a graphic representation of the information. Figure 49-20 shows a computerized spirometer.

Performing Spirometry

The technique for performing pulmonary function testing is similar for all types of spirometers. Successful spirometry depends on proper patient preparation and consistent

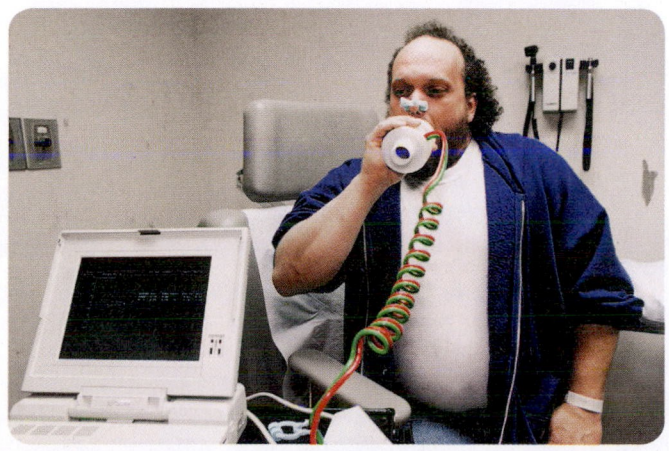

FIGURE 49-20 This computerized spirometer measures air volume and airflow.
© Getty Images

technique in performing the procedure and analyzing the results. The steps involved in measuring forced vital capacity using a spirometer are described in detail here and outlined in Procedure 49-3 at the end of this chapter.

Patient Preparation Certain conditions and activities affect the accuracy of pulmonary function tests. Patients should be made aware of these conditions prior to scheduling to ensure accuracy:

- Viral infection or acute illness within the previous 2 to 3 weeks
- Serious medical condition, such as a recent myocardial infarction
- Recent use of a prescribed medication if the test order calls for spirometry before and after prescribed medication
- Use of a sedative or opioid substance before the test
- Smoking or eating a heavy meal within 1 hour of taking the test

Review the conditions and activities with patients again on the day of the test to ensure that none apply. If there are no contraindications, weigh and measure patients. Use simple terms to explain the procedure and its purpose. Have them loosen tight clothing so that they will be comfortable and their breathing will not be restricted in any way. The procedure is performed with patients sitting down. Make sure their legs are not crossed and that both feet are flat on the floor.

Explain that they need to wear a nose clip or hold the nose tightly closed to be sure they will inhale and exhale through the mouth. The mouthpiece of the unit may be a disposable cardboard tube or a reusable rubber one that can be disinfected after use. If disposable mouthpieces are used, instruct patients to avoid biting down on them, as that will obstruct airflow. Be sure patients form a tight seal around the mouthpiece with their lips. Dentures normally help maintain a tight seal; however, they should be removed if they hinder the process.

Proper Positioning Instruct patients to keep their chin and neck in the correct position during the procedure. The chin should be slightly elevated and the neck slightly extended. Bending the chin to the chest tends to restrict airflow and should be avoided (Figure 49-21). Some bending at the waist is acceptable.

Explaining and Demonstrating the Procedure Tell patients to take the deepest breath possible, insert the mouthpiece into the mouth, form a tight seal, and then blow into the mouthpiece as hard and as fast as possible to completely exhale. Tell them to exhale as long as they can to force air from the lungs. Remind them that the initial force of their exhalation must be strong to get a valid reading. Demonstrate the procedure to show how to do the test correctly.

Performing the Maneuver You can improve patients' performance during the maneuver by actively and forcefully coaching them. Urge patients to blow hard and to continue blowing. After a maneuver, give them feedback on their performance and indicate corrective actions they can take to improve the next maneuver.

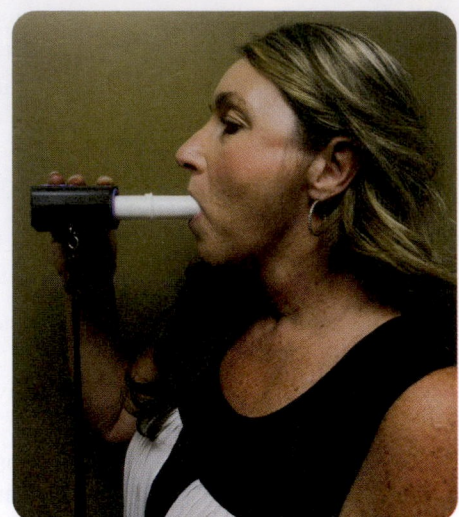

(a) Correct position

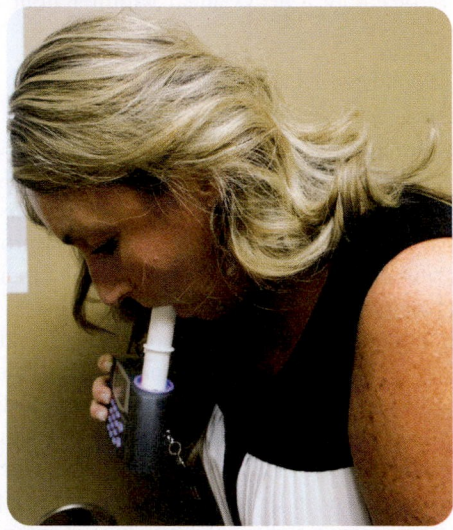

(b) Incorrect position

FIGURE 49-21 During a pulmonary function test, the patient must maintain the proper position. (a) The chin should be slightly elevated and the neck slightly extended. (b) The chin should not approach the chest.
© McGraw-Hill Education. David Moyer, photographer

Some spirometers indicate whether a particular maneuver was of adequate force and duration to be measured. However, adequate force does not indicate that the maneuver was acceptable. An acceptable maneuver must have the following five features:

1. No coughing, particularly during the first second
2. A quick and forceful start
3. An adequate length of time (a minimum of 6 seconds)
4. A consistent and fast flow with no variability
5. Consistency with other maneuvers

Spirometry tracings plot volume and time. You will need to obtain three acceptable maneuvers, which may require more than three attempts. Observe the patient for signs of breathing difficulty, dizziness, light-headedness, or changes in pulse and blood pressure. If necessary, allow the patient to rest briefly before continuing. Notify the physician immediately if symptoms are severe.

Determining the Effectiveness of Medication Spirometry is often used to determine the effectiveness of certain medications a patient is taking. You will perform two sets of maneuvers if this determination is required. Instruct the patient to refrain from taking the prescribed medication on the day of the test. Before performing the test, confirm that the patient has followed this instruction. Conduct the first set of maneuvers, ensuring that they are acceptable. After obtaining the results, instruct the patient to take the prescribed medication. Allow the medication to take effect, and then perform a second set of maneuvers. Comparing the two sets of readings shows whether the medication has effectively improved the patient's lung function. Some computerized spirometers can graph both sets of readings together to simplify the comparison (Figure 49-22).

Special Considerations On occasion, you may have to deal with an uncooperative patient, one who cannot understand or follow directions, or one who cannot perform the procedure. In these situations, patience and skill are essential for obtaining an acceptable spirometry tracing.

The doctor may be able to convince an uncooperative patient to perform the maneuver. You can help by taking a nonsense approach, perhaps stating that the doctor needs these test results to help the patient. Patients who cannot understand or follow directions—the very young, the very old, those who have limited proficiency in English, or those with a hearing impairment—may need extra attention and patience to obtain acceptable results. Explain the procedure in simple terms and repeat instructions as necessary. If, after eight attempts, the

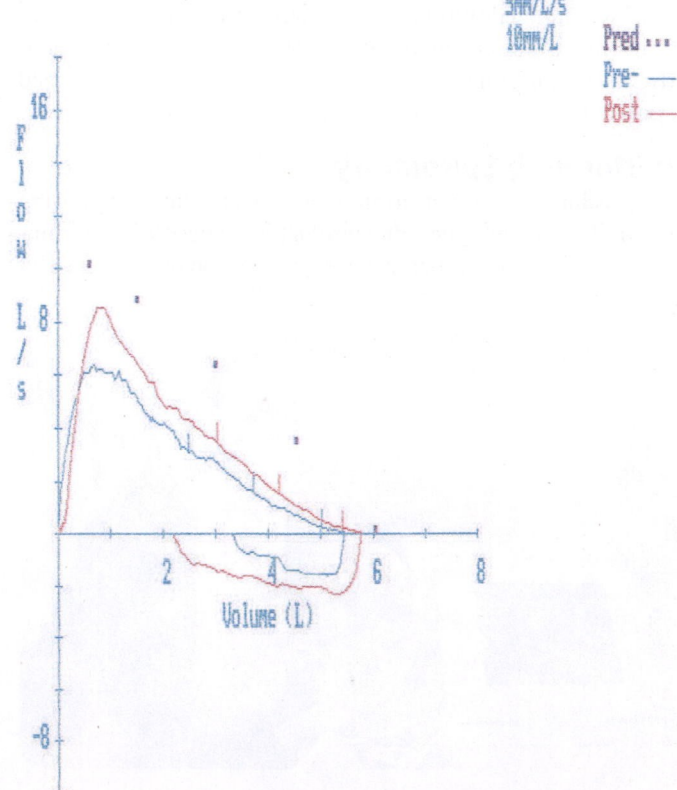

FIGURE 49-22 These spirometry tracings show air volume per second before and after use of a medication.

patient is unable to perform the procedure, stop and report the situation to the doctor.

The Importance of Calibration Spirometers should be calibrated each day they are used to ensure accurate readings. You may be responsible for this procedure, which requires the use of a standardized measuring instrument called a **calibration syringe** (Figure 49-23). When the plunger is pulled back, this syringe contains a fixed volume of air. Connect the syringe to the patient tubing (this tubing runs from the mouthpiece to the machine) and depress the plunger to inject the entire volume of air. The spirometer reading should be within 3% of the stated volume. Keep a calibration logbook for each spirometer.

While calibrating the spirometer, you can detect leaks by checking the volume/time graph. The volume should remain at a steady reading; if it declines with time, a leak exists in the system.

Infection Control After a patient completes the pulmonary function test, you must clean the spirometer and other pulmonary function devices thoroughly to prevent transmission of microorganisms. If disposable mouthpieces, nose clips, and patient tubing are used, discard them in a biohazardous waste container. If reusable mouthpieces, nose clips, and tubing are used, clean and disinfect them between patients. Most important, wash your hands thoroughly before and after performing a pulmonary function test.

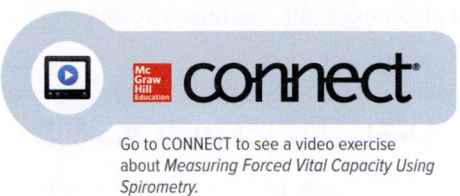

Go to CONNECT to see a video exercise about *Measuring Forced Vital Capacity Using Spirometry.*

Peak Expiratory Flow Rate (PEFR)

A **peak expiratory flow rate (PEFR)** is a measurement taken to determine the amount of air that can be quickly forced from the lungs. A peak flow meter—a small, handheld device that can be used in the medical office or the patient's home (Figure 49-24)—is often used to obtain a PEFR. Patients who suffer from asthma are commonly asked to monitor their asthma by using a peak flow meter and recording their results. During an asthma flare-up, the large airways of the lungs begin to narrow, which slows the speed of air leaving the lungs. A peak flow meter, when used properly, can reveal narrowing of the airways in advance of an asthma attack. Peak flow meters can help determine

- When to seek emergency medical care.
- The effectiveness of an asthma management treatment plan.
- When to stop or add medication as directed by a physician.
- Asthma triggers, such as stress or exercise.

Procedure 49-4, at the end of this chapter, explains the procedure for obtaining a peak expiratory rate using a peak flow meter.

Peak Flow Zones After obtaining a peak expiratory flow rate, the type of patient care given will be determined based on the individual's results. The physician will instruct the patient about the peak flow zones and how to respond to each zone. Peak flow zones are different for each patient and will be determined by the physician. The three peak flow zones are green, yellow, and red. These three color zones can be seen in Figure 49-24.

Green Zone The green zone indicates good control of asthma, with peak flow rates of 80% to 100% of the highest peak flow rate. Measurements in this zone indicate that air moves well through the large airways and the patient's usual activities can be continued.

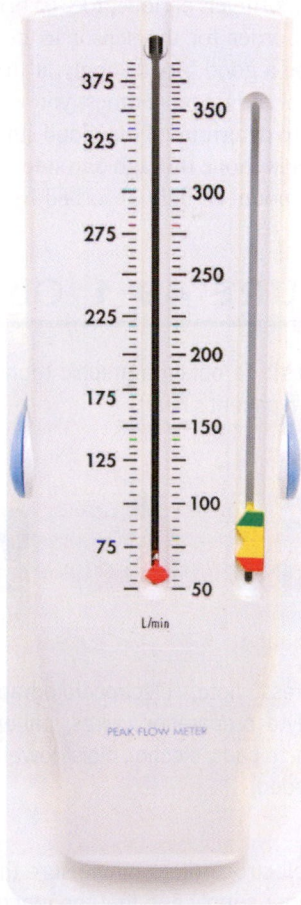

FIGURE 49-24 Peak expiratory flow meter markings will determine the patient's treatment based on accurate readings.
© andres balcazar/Getty Images RF

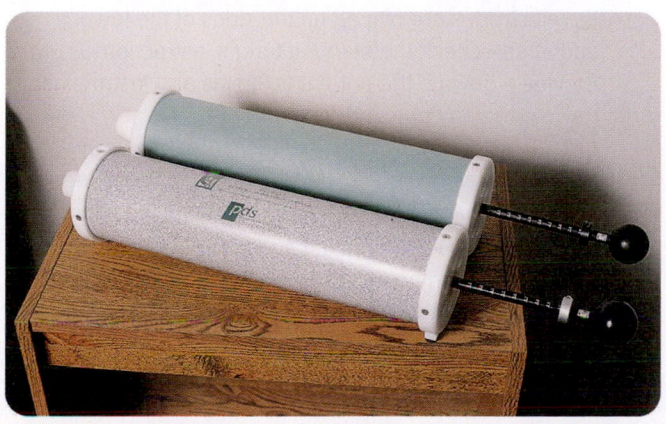

FIGURE 49-23 A calibration syringe delivers a fixed volume of air.
© Cliff Moore

Yellow Zone Peak flow rates in the yellow zone range from 50% to 80% of the highest peak flow rate. Measurements in this zone indicate that the large airways are beginning to narrow and medication is needed. Patient symptoms include tiredness and tightening of the chest.

Red Zone Peak flow rates in the red zone are less than 50% of the highest or best personal reading recorded. Narrowing of the largest airways has occurred and is considered a medical emergency. Medical treatment should be sought immediately. Patients are usually directed to take a bronchodilator or other medication that will open the airway and call their physician. Symptoms include wheezing, shortness of breath, and trouble walking and talking.

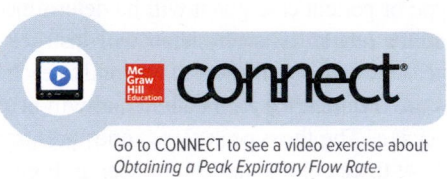

Go to CONNECT to see a video exercise about *Obtaining a Peak Expiratory Flow Rate.*

▶ Pulse Oximetry

LO 49.8

Pulse oximetry is a noninvasive test that measures the saturation of oxygen in a patient's arterial blood. The pulse oximeter includes a sensor and a monitoring device. The sensor is placed on a patient's finger, earlobe, toe, or bridge of the nose (Figure 49-25). In order for the sensor to detect the oxygen level, there must be a good blood supply at the site where the sensor is placed. For the fingers or toes, you will need to check the capillary refill to determine if the blood supply is adequate. A red infrared light is shone through one side of the appendage to the other. The amount of light absorbed by the hemoglobin

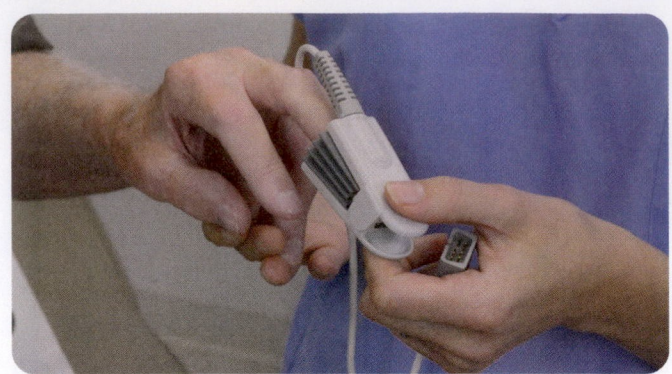

FIGURE 49-25 A pulse oximeter is a portable, handheld device used by many medical facilities.
© McGraw-Hill Education

in the blood is detected by the pulse oximeter. Any reading less than 95% indicates **hypoxemia** (low blood oxygen). Pulse oximetry is performed on patients with pulmonary or cardiac conditions and during postoperative patient observation. It is also used to help diagnose **sleep apnea,** a condition characterized by pauses in breathing during sleep. The pauses are often long enough to cause a drop in blood oxygen levels. Some medications after surgery can slow breathing rates and it is important that patient blood oxygen levels be carefully monitored. Procedure 49-5, at the end of this chapter, explains the process of obtaining a pulse oximetry reading.

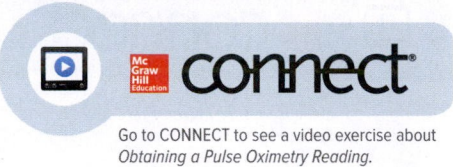

Go to CONNECT to see a video exercise about *Obtaining a Pulse Oximetry Reading.*

PROCEDURE 49-1 Obtaining an ECG

WORK // DOC

Procedure Goal: To obtain a graphic representation of the electrical activity of a patient's heart

OSHA Guidelines:

 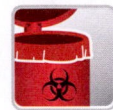 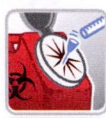 

Materials:
Patient chart/progress note, electrocardiograph, ECG paper, electrodes, electrolyte preparation, wires, patient gown, drape, blanket, pillows, gauze pads, alcohol, moist towel, and scissors for trimming hair (if needed)

Method:

1. Turn on the electrocardiograph. Ensure that there is an adequate paper supply and that the machine inspection is up to date.

2. Identify the patient, introduce yourself, and explain the procedure.

3. Wash your hands.

4. Ask the patient to disrobe from the waist up and remove jewelry, socks or stockings, bra, and shoes. If the electrodes will be placed on the patient's legs, have the patient roll up his or her pant legs. Sometimes the electrodes are placed on the sides of the lower abdomen—check the manufacturer's instructions. Provide a gown if the patient is female and instruct her to wear the gown with the opening in front.
   RATIONALE: *Making sure the patient knows exactly what clothing to remove and the correct way to put on the gown will make the process more efficient.*

5. Assist the patient onto the table and into a supine position. Cover the patient with a drape (and a blanket if the room is cool). If the patient experiences difficulty breathing or cannot tolerate lying flat, use a Fowler's or semi-Fowler's position, adjusting with pillows under the head and knees for comfort if needed.

6. Tell the patient to rest quietly and breathe normally. Explain the importance of lying still to prevent false readings.

7. Wash the patient's skin, using gauze pads moistened with alcohol. If needed, rub it vigorously with dry gauze pads to promote better contact of the electrodes.
   RATIONALE: *If a patient has applied lotion in the areas where electrodes are placed, it may cause conduction problems.*

8. If the patient's leg or chest hair is dense, use a small pair of scissors to closely trim the hair where you will attach the electrode. (Shaving is not allowed because of the risk of bleeding and infection.)

9. Apply electrodes to fleshy portions of the limbs, making sure the electrodes on one arm and leg are placed similarly to those on the other arm and leg. Attach electrodes to areas that are not bony or muscular. The arm lead tabs on the electrode point downward and the electrode tabs for the leg leads point upward. Peel off the backings of the disposable electrodes and press them into place.
   RATIONALE: *Using the correct tab position will reduce tension on the limb wires. Artifacts can occur when electrodes are placed on bones and muscles.*

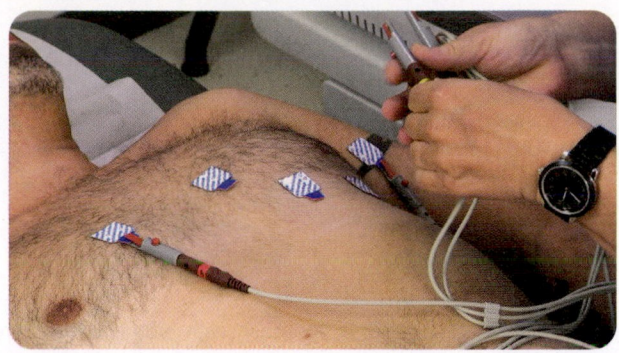

FIGURE Procedure 49-1 Step 12 Attach wires and cables, draping wires over the patient to avoid tension, which can result in artifacts.
© McGraw-Hill Education

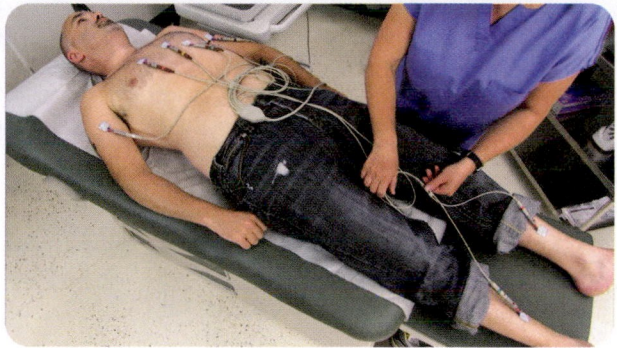

FIGURE Procedure 49-1 Step 9 Place electrodes at the specified locations on the chest, arms, and legs.
© McGraw-Hill Education

10. Apply the precordial electrodes at specified locations on the chest. If you are unsure of the placement, check a reliable reference. Precordial electrode tabs point downward.

11. Attach wires and cables, making sure all wire tips follow the patient's body contours.

12. Check all electrodes and wires for proper placement and connection; drape wires over the patient to avoid creating tension on the electrodes, which could result in artifacts.

13. Enter the patient data into the electrocardiograph. Press the on, run, or record button. If standardization is needed, check the manufacturer's instructions.

14. Remind the patient to lie quietly, and run the ECG.

15. Check tracings for artifacts.

16. Correct problems and repeat any tracings that are not clear.

17. Disconnect the patient from the machine.

18. Remove the tracing from the machine and label it with the patient's name, the date, and your initials if these do not print out with the tracing.

19. Disconnect the wires from the electrodes and remove the electrodes from the patient.

20. Clean the patient's skin with a moist towel.

21. Assist the patient into a sitting position.

22. Allow a moment for rest and then assist the patient from the table.
    RATIONALE: *Some patients may experience postural hypotension after lying and may feel dizzy.*

23. Assist the patient in dressing if necessary, or allow the patient privacy to dress.

24. Wash your hands.

25. Record the procedure in the patient's chart/progress note.

26. Properly dispose of used materials and disposable electrodes.

27. Clean and disinfect the equipment and the room according to OSHA guidelines.

PROCEDURE 49-2 Holter Monitoring

WORK // DOC

Procedure Goal: To monitor the electrical activity of a patient's heart over a 24-hour period to detect cardiac abnormalities that may go undetected during routine electrocardiography or stress testing

OSHA Guidelines:

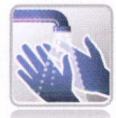 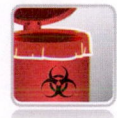 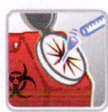

Materials: Patient chart/progress note, Holter monitor, battery, microchip or small cassette, patient diary or log, alcohol, gauze pads, scissors, disposable electrodes, hypoallergenic tape, drape, and electrocardiograph

Method:

1. Identify the patient, introduce yourself, and explain the procedure.

2. Ask the patient to remove clothing from the waist up; provide a drape if necessary.

3. Wash your hands and assemble the equipment.

4. Assist the patient into a comfortable position (sitting or supine).

5. If the patient's body hair is particularly dense, don examination gloves and trim the areas where the electrodes will be attached.
   RATIONALE: *Trimming the area will ensure that the electrodes will stay secure during the 24-hour period.*

6. Clean the electrode sites with alcohol and gauze.

7. Rub each electrode site vigorously with a dry gauze square.
   RATIONALE: *To help electrodes adhere to the skin.*

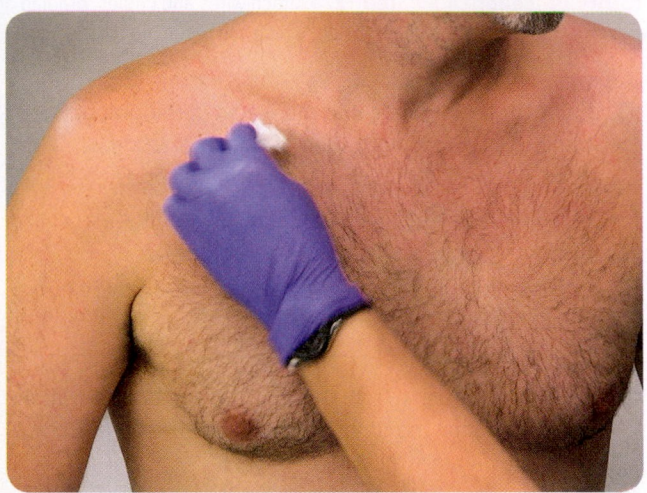

FIGURE Procedure 49-2 Step 7 Rub each electrode site vigorously to ensure that the electrodes adhere and stay in place during the monitoring.
© McGraw-Hill Education

8. Attach wires to the electrodes and peel off the paper backing on the electrodes. Apply electrodes at locations as indicated by the manufacturer's instructions. Press firmly to ensure that each electrode is making good contact with the skin.
   RATIONALE: *Good skin contact is essential to obtain an accurate reading.*

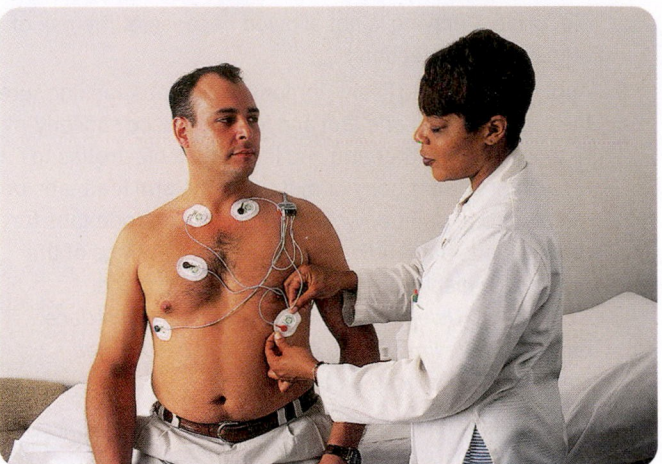

FIGURE Procedure 49-2 Step 8 Correctly connecting the patient to the Holter monitor is essential. Check the manufacturer's instructions for the monitor you are using.
© David Kelly Crow

9. Attach the patient cable.

10. Insert a fresh battery, and position the unit.

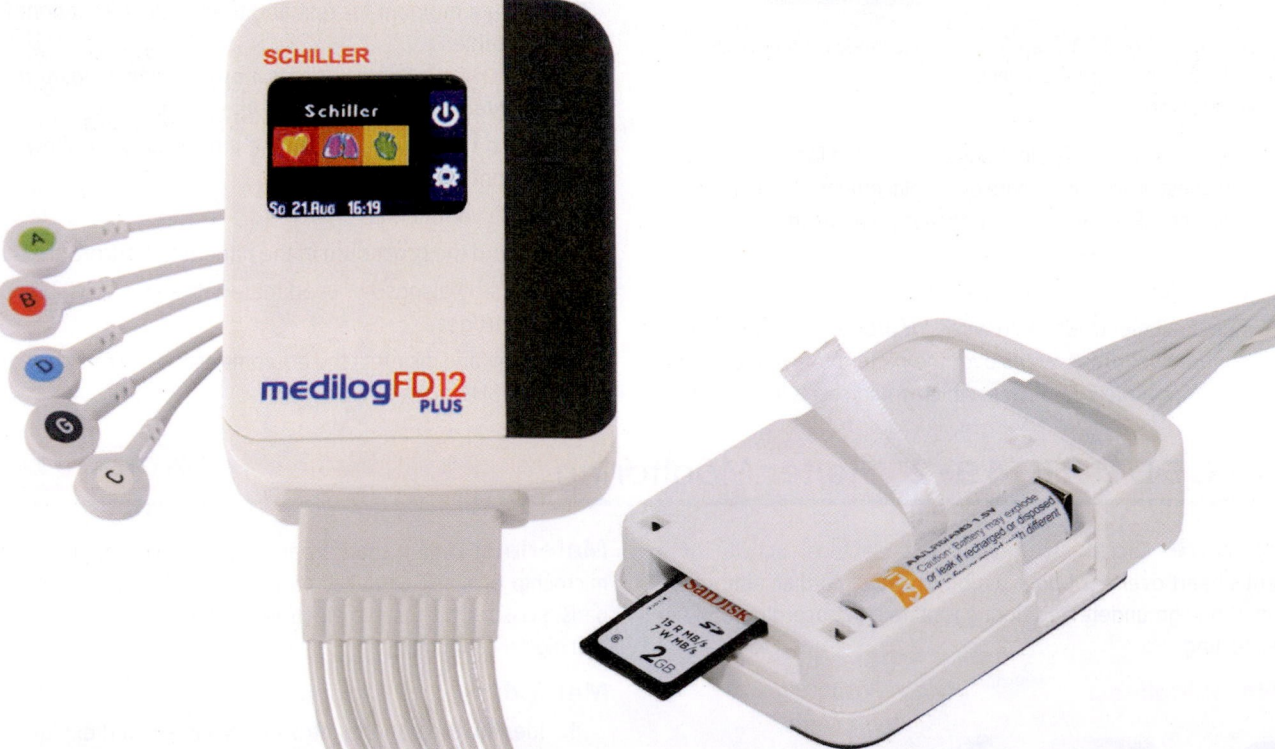

FIGURE Procedure 49-2 Step 10 Make sure that the monitor has a microchip or other type of data storage and a fresh battery.
© 2014 SCHILLER AG

11. Tape wires, cable, and electrodes as necessary to avoid tension on the wires as the patient moves.

12. Insert the microchip or cassette, and turn on the unit.

13. Ensure that the unit is on and indicate the start time in the patient's chart.
    RATIONALE: *If the unit is not running, results will not be recorded and the test will have to be repeated.*

14. Instruct the patient on proper use of the monitor and how to enter information in the diary. Caution the patient not to alter any diary entries; it is crucial to know what the patient is doing at all times.

15. Schedule the patient's return visit for the same time on the following day.

16. On the following day, remove the electrodes, discard them, and clean the electrode sites.

17. Wash your hands.

18. Transfer the data from the monitor to the patient's chart according to office procedure and the manufacturer's directions.

19. Document the procedure (refer to Progress Note).

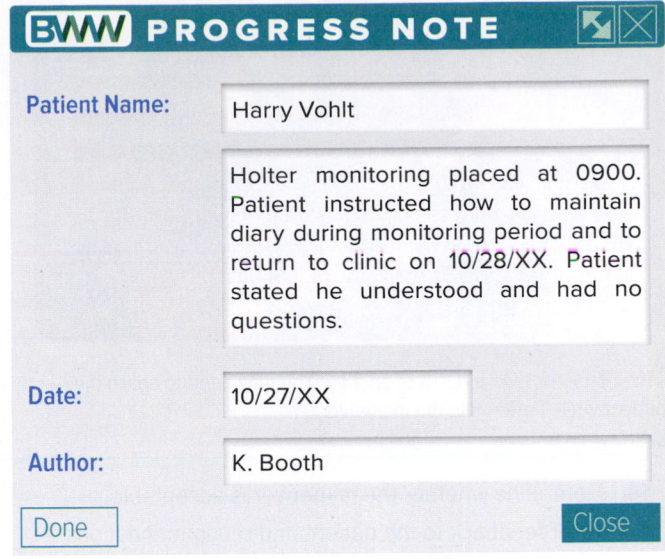

BWW PROGRESS NOTE

Patient Name: Harry Vohlt

Holter monitoring placed at 0900. Patient instructed how to maintain diary during monitoring period and to return to clinic on 10/28/XX. Patient stated he understood and had no questions.

Date: 10/27/XX

Author: K. Booth

Done   Close

PROCEDURE 49-3 Measuring Forced Vital Capacity Using Spirometry

WORK // DOC

Procedure Goal: To determine a patient's forced vital capacity using a volume-displacing spirometer

OSHA Guidelines:

  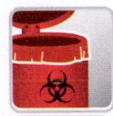 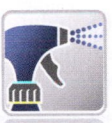

Materials: Patient chart/progress note, adult scale with height bar, spirometer, patient tubing (tubing that runs from the mouthpiece to the machine), mouthpiece, nose clip, and disinfectant

Method:

1. Prepare the equipment. Ensure that the paper supply in the machine is adequate.

2. Calibrate the machine as necessary.

3. Identify the patient and introduce yourself.

4. Check the patient's chart to see whether there are special instructions to follow.

5. Ask whether the patient has followed instructions.

6. Wash your hands and don examination gloves.

7. Measure and record the patient's height and weight.

8. Explain the proper positioning.

9. Explain the procedure.

10. Demonstrate the procedure.
    RATIONALE: *Explanations and demonstrations are effective patient teaching methods.*

11. Turn on the spirometer and enter applicable patient data and the number of tests to be performed.

12. Ensure that the patient has loosened any tight clothing, is comfortable, and is in the proper position. Apply the nose clip.

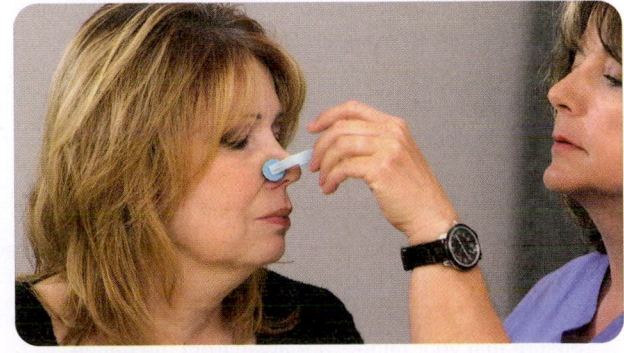

FIGURE Procedure 49-3 Step 12 The nose clip is applied over the fleshy part of the nose.
© McGraw-Hill Education

13. Have the patient perform the first maneuver, coaching when necessary.

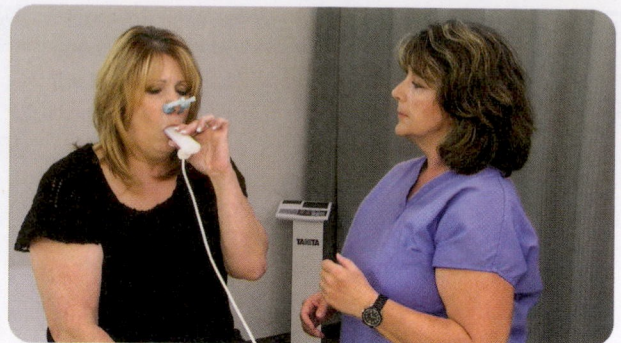

FIGURE Procedure 49-3 Step 13   You may need to coach the patient while performing the maneuver.
© McGraw-Hill Education

14. Determine whether the maneuver is acceptable.

15. Offer feedback to the patient and recommendations for improvement if necessary.

16. Have the patient perform additional maneuvers until three acceptable maneuvers are obtained.

17. Record the procedure in the patient's chart and place the chart and the test results on the physician's desk for interpretation.

18. Ask the patient to remain until the physician reviews the results.
    RATIONALE: *The physician may want to speak with the patient regarding results or may want to order additional testing.*

19. Properly dispose of used materials and disposable instruments.

20. Sanitize and disinfect patient tubing, reusable mouthpiece, and nose clip.

21. Clean and disinfect the equipment and room according to OSHA guidelines.

PROCEDURE 49-4   Obtaining a Peak Expiratory Flow Rate

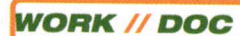

Procedure Goal: To determine a patient's peak expiratory flow rate

OSHA Guidelines:

  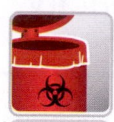 

Materials: Patient chart/progress note, peak flow meter, and a disposable mouthpiece

Method:

1. Assemble all necessary equipment and supplies for the test.

2. Wash your hands and identify the patient.

3. Explain and demonstrate the procedure to the patient.
   RATIONALE: *Patient education and understanding are crucial for getting accurate test results.*

4. Position the patient in a sitting or standing position with good posture. Make sure any chewing gum or food is removed from the patient's mouth.

5. Set the indicator to zero.
   RATIONALE: *Helps to ensure accurate results*

6. Ensure that the disposable mouthpiece is securely placed onto the peak flow meter.

7. Hold the peak flow meter with the gauge uppermost and ensure that your fingers are away from the gauge.

8. Instruct the patient to take as deep a breath as possible.

9. Instruct the patient to place the mouthpiece into his mouth and close his lips tightly around the mouthpiece, sealing his lips around it.

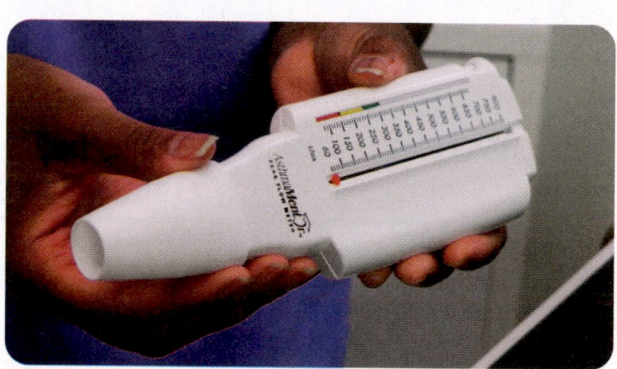

FIGURE Procedure 49-4 Step 6   A disposable mouthpiece is securely fastened to the peak flow meter.
© McGraw-Hill Education

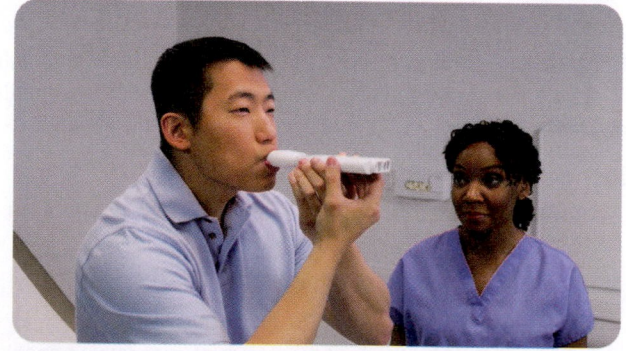

FIGURE Procedure 49-4 Step 9   Have the patient close his lips tightly around the mouthpiece so that no air escapes.
© McGraw-Hill Education

10. Instruct the patient to blow out as fast and as hard as possible.
    RATIONALE: *A fast blast is better than a slow blow.*

11. Observe the reading where the arrowhead is on the indicator.

12. Reset the indicator to zero and repeat the procedure two times, for a total of three readings. You will know the technique is correct if the reading results are close. If coughing occurs during the procedure, repeat the step.

13. Document the readings in the patient's chart. The highest reading will be the peak flow rate.

RATIONALE: *The highest reading represents the personal best reading for the patient, and future measurements are based on this result. Do not average the results.*

14. Dispose of the mouthpiece in a biohazardous waste container.

15. Disinfect or dispose of the peak flow meter per office policy.

16. Wash your hands.

PROCEDURE 49-5 Obtaining a Pulse Oximetry Reading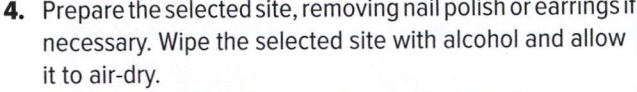

Procedure Goal: To obtain a pulse oximetry reading

OSHA Guidelines:

  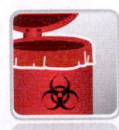 

Materials: Pulse oximeter, patient chart/progress note

Method:

1. Assemble all the necessary equipment and supplies.

2. Wash your hands and correctly identify the patient.

3. Select the appropriate site to apply the sensor by assessing the capillary refill in the patient's toe or finger. This is done by applying pressure to the nail bed until it turns white, then releasing the pressure and watching for the return of blood flow. The pink color should return in less than 2 seconds.
   RATIONALE: *If the patient has poor circulation in his fingers or toes, use the bridge of his nose or an earlobe.*

4. Prepare the selected site, removing nail polish or earrings if necessary. Wipe the selected site with alcohol and allow it to air-dry.
   RATIONALE: *Nail polish can alter the test results.*

5. Attach the sensor to the site (if a finger is used, place the finger in the clip).

6. Instruct the patient to breathe normally.

7. Attach the sensor cable to the oximeter. Turn on the oximeter and listen to the tone.

8. Set the alarm limits for high and low oxygen saturations and high and low pulse rates, as directed by the physician's order, and turn on the oximeter.

9. Read the saturation level and document it in the patient's chart. Report to the physician readings that are less than 95%. Manually check the patient's pulse and compare it to the pulse oximeter. Document all the readings and the application site in the patient's chart/progress note.

10. Wash your hands.

11. Rotate the patient's finger sites every 4 hours if using a pulse oximeter long-term.

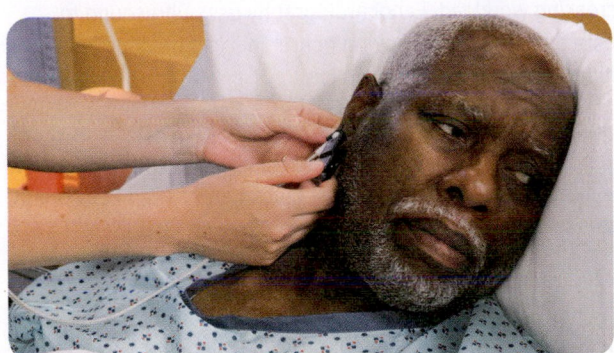

FIGURE Procedure 49-5 Step 3   The earlobe and bridge of the nose are alternative sites for placement of the sensor during pulse oximetry.
© McGraw-Hill Education

LEARNING OUTCOMES	KEY POINTS
49.1 Discuss the medical assistant's role in electrocardiography and pulmonary function testing.	As a medical assistant, you will be responsible for preparing the patient for ECG and pulmonary function tests, maintaining the equipment used for these tests, and performing them.
49.2 Explain the basic principles of electrocardiography and how it relates to the conduction system of the heart.	The heart's conduction system is responsible for the electrical pathway that occurs during a heartbeat. The pathway begins with the SA node, travels through the AV node, the bundle of His, the right and left bundle branches, and ends with the Purkinje fibers. This electrical energy pathway is measured with an electocardiograph and a tracing of the impulses is produced. The electrical impulses are represented in wave forms or deflections. Each deflection is labeled by letters PQRSTU and represents a part of the pattern.
49.3 Identify the components of an electrocardiograph and what each does.	The electrocardiograph consists of the following components: electrodes, which detect and conduct electrical impulses to the electrocardiograph; amplifier, which increases the signal, making the heartbeat visible; leads, combinations of electrodes with each providing different views of the electrical activity of the heart; LCD display and/or ECG paper, where the tracing of the electrical activity is viewed and recorded; and various controls that allow you to input the patient information and change such things as the speed of the tracing.
49.4 Carry out the steps necessary to obtain an ECG.	The steps in obtaining an accurate ECG include preparing the room and equipment, identifying the patient, properly placing the limb and chest electrodes, attaching the lead wires, entering the patient data into the ECG machine, running the tracing, checking the tracing for artifacts, disconnecting the patient from the lead wires and removing the electrodes, and assisting the patient as required.
49.5 Summarize exercise electrocardiography and echocardiography.	Exercise electrocardiography is referred to as *stress testing*. This measures the efficiency of the heart during constant or increasing workload. Echocardiography uses ultrasound to create a picture of the moving heart. This can be done while the patient is resting or after exercise.
49.6 Explain the procedure of Holter monitoring.	A Holter monitor is used to measure the heart's activity over an extended period, usually 24 hours. This is used when the patient has intermittent chest pain or discomfort and a normal ECG and stress test do not identify the cause.
49.7 Carry out the various types of pulmonary function tests.	Forced vital capacity is the measurement of the greatest volume of air expelled when a patient performs a rapid, forced expiration. The lung's ability to function is measured by the volume of air expelled and the time taken to perform the maneuver. Accurate spirometry testing includes positioning the patient properly, coaching the patient during the procedure, obtaining three acceptable maneuvers, and recording the results in the patient's chart. A peak expiratory flow rate is obtained by having the patient sit or stand using good posture, take in as deep a breath as possible, and blow out through the peak flow meter as fast and as hard as possible three times. The highest reading of the three is the peak flow rate and should be recorded in the patient's chart.

LEARNING OUTCOMES	KEY POINTS
49.8 Describe the procedure for performing pulse oximetry testing.	Pulse oximetry testing is performed by applying the pulse oximeter to the patient's finger or toe, attaching the sensor cable to the oximeter, turning the oximeter on, setting the alarm limits for high and low oxygen saturations, and reading the patient's oxygen saturation levels. The oxygen saturation levels should be recorded in the patient's chart.

CASE STUDY CRITICAL THINKING

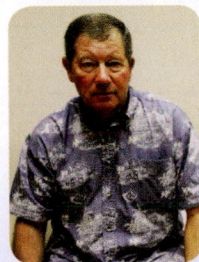

© McGraw-Hill Education

Recall John Miller from the beginning of the chapter. Now that you have completed the chapter, answer the following questions regarding his case.

1. Explain to John the difference between an ECG and an echocardiogram.

2. John expresses concern about having a heart attack during the procedure. How can you alleviate his fear?

3. You must perform an ECG on this patient. Describe the steps in the procedure.

EXAM PREPARATION QUESTIONS

1. (LO 49.2) Which of the following initiates the heartbeat?
   a. AV node
   b. SA node
   c. Bundle of His
   d. Purkinje fibers
   e. Bundle branch

2. (LO 49.4) The ECG tracing is showing somatic interference. What can be done?
   a. Turn off or unplug appliances in the room
   b. Remove oil from the patient's skin
   c. Connect a loose wire
   d. Remind the patient to remain still
   e. Reschedule the test

3. (LO 49.8) What does a pulse oximeter measure?
   a. Oxygen saturation of the blood
   b. Oxygen saturation of the skin
   c. Electrical activity of the heart
   d. Forced vital capacity
   e. Lung capacity

4. (LO 49.7) When obtaining a peak flow rate, you should _____ the _____ readings.
   a. Average, two
   b. Average, three
   c. Add, two
   d. Document, three
   e. Document, two

5. (LO 49.4) Which of the following irregularities on an ECG would be considered the *most* severe?
   a. PVC
   b. V-fib
   c. A-fib
   d. AC interference
   e. Tachycardia

6. (LO 49.3) The precordial ECG leads are also called
   a. AVR leads
   b. Ground leads
   c. Chest leads
   d. Augmented leads
   e. Limb leads

7. (LO 49.6) Which of the following should a patient do when wearing a Holter monitor?
   a. Avoid normal daily activities and focus on relaxing during the monitoring
   b. Bathe and/or shower as usual because the monitor will not be affected
   c. Wear a tight-fitting shirt to hold the electrodes and monitor in place
   d. Return the Holter monitor through the mail to avoid a return visit
   e. Inform the office if the monitor is not working properly

8. (LO 49.4) Turning off unnecessary electrical equipment in the room when performing an ECG is helpful in reducing which type of artifact?

a. Extraneous marks
b. Flat line
c. Somatic interference
d. AC interference
e. Wandering baseline

9. (LO 49.8) Low blood oxygen is known as

a. Hypoxemia
b. Sleep apnea
c. Hyperpnea
d. Oximetry
e. COPD

10. (LO 49.7) The greatest volume of air that can be expelled when a person performs rapid, forced expiration is

a. Peak expiratory flow
b. Total lung capacity
c. Maximum voluntary ventilation
d. Forced vital capacity
e. Tidal volume

SOFT SKILLS SUCCESS

1. Andrea Hochradel arrives to have her Holter monitor removed. She sits down in the exam room, takes the monitor and all the electrodes and wires out of her purse, and plops them on the table. What should you do?

2. John Miller arrives for a pulmonary function test and he has just finished a cigarette. How should you handle this situation?

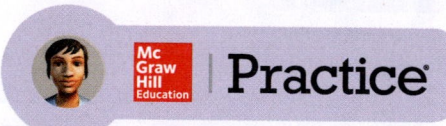

Go to PRACTICE MEDICAL OFFICE and complete the module Clinical—Work Task Proficiencies.

Diagnostic Imaging

CASE STUDY

Patient Name	DOB	Allergies
Raja Lautu	2/23/19XX	Benzalkonium chloride

Attending	MRN	Other Information
Elizabeth H. Williams, MD	224-86-564	Schedule DXA prior to starting brachytherapy.

Raja Lautu, a 42-year-old woman, has arrived at the office for her annual gynecologic physical. After her physical exam, she is scheduled for her annual digital mammogram. The digital mammogram results reveal a small, abnormal density close to the chest wall on the right breast. Stereotactic fine-needle breast biopsy reveals a grade II infiltrating ductal carcinoma (IDC). Dr. Williams refers Raja to a radiation oncologist for treatment. She will most likely be treated with brachytherapy.

Keep Raja in mind as you study this chapter. There will be questions at the end of the chapter based on the case study. The information in the chapter will help you answer these questions.

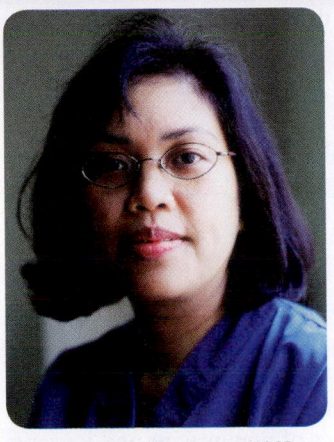

© ERproductions Ltd/Blend Images LLC RF

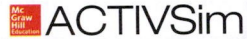

LEARNING OUTCOMES

After completing Chapter 50, you will be able to:

50.1 Explain what X-rays are and how they are used for diagnostic and therapeutic purposes.

50.2 Compare invasive and noninvasive diagnostic procedures.

50.3 Carry out the medical assistant's role in X-ray and diagnostic radiology testing.

50.4 Discuss common diagnostic imaging procedures.

50.5 Describe different types of radiation therapy and how they are used.

50.6 Explain the risks and safety precautions associated with radiology work.

50.7 Relate the advances in medical imaging to EHR.

KEY TERMS

arthrography

barium enema

barium swallow

brachytherapy

cholangiography

contrast medium

diagnostic radiology

dual-energy X-ray absorptiometry (DXA)

intravenous pyelography (IVP)

invasive

KUB radiography

mammography

MUGA scan (nuclear ventriculography)

myelography

noninvasive

nuclear medicine

PET

radiation therapy

retrograde pyelography

SPECT

teletherapy

I.C.9 Analyze pathology for each body system including:
(a) diagnostic measures
(b) treatment modalities

I.P.8 Instruct and prepare a patient for a procedure or a treatment

V.A.4 Explain to a patient the rationale for performance of a procedure

2. Anatomy and Physiology
c. Identify diagnostic and treatment modalities as they relate to each body system

8. Administrative Procedures
e. Maintain inventory of equipment and supplies
(1) Perform routine maintenance of administrative equipment

9. Clinical Procedures
a. Practice standard precautions and perform disinfection/sterilization techniques

▶ Introduction

Diagnostic radiology has evolved immensely since the discovery of the simple X-ray beam, which has become a valuable screening and clinical diagnostic tool for physicians. In this chapter, you will learn the basics of noninvasive and invasive radiology along with your role as a medical assistant in this testing. Safety issues for the administration of radiologic testing are discussed, as are the proper handling and storage of the films. In addition, you will learn about preparing and instructing patients for the more common radiology procedures.

▶ Brief History of the X-ray   LO 50.1

In 1895, Wilhelm Konrad Roentgen (1845–1923) discovered the X-ray, or roentgen ray, a type of electromagnetic wave. It has a high energy level, traveling at the speed of light (186,000 miles per second), and an extremely short wavelength (one-billionth of an inch) that can penetrate solid objects. X-rays react with photographic film to produce a permanent record (X-ray, or radiograph). The X-ray image is lightest where the film is struck by the least X-ray energy. Differences in tissue densities produce the X-ray image, with the most dense—such as bone—being lightest and the least dense—such as air in the lungs— being darkest on the film.

Today, X-rays and radioactive substances have both diagnostic—such as a wrist X-ray to diagnose a fracture—and therapeutic—such as radiation treatment for cancerous tumors—uses. Radiologic technologists are trained medical personnel, certified to perform certain radiologic procedures upon completion of a 2- to 4-year radiology curriculum. Some radiologic technologists receive further training in radiology subspecialties, such as ultrasound, mammography, magnetic resonance imaging, and nuclear medicine. Radiographers, sonographers, radiation therapists, and nuclear medicine technologists are all radiologic technologists. Invasive radiologic procedures and procedures requiring a high degree of expertise are nearly always performed by a radiologist—a physician who specializes in radiology. A radiologist is also the physician who interprets the films for other physicians. Other specialists who perform radiologic procedures, either alone or with a radiologist's assistance, include cardiologists, orthopedists, obstetricians, and oncologists.

▶ Diagnostic Radiology   LO 50.2

Diagnostic radiology is the use of X-ray technology for diagnostic purposes. Radiologic tests sometimes use contrast media as well as special techniques or instruments for viewing internal body structures and functions. A **contrast medium** is a substance that makes internal organs denser and blocks the passage of X-rays to the photographic film. Introducing contrast media into certain structures or areas of the body can provide a clearer image of organs and tissues and an indication of how well they are functioning. Contrast media include gases (air, oxygen, or carbon dioxide); heavy metal salts (barium sulfate or bismuth carbonate); paramagnetic compounds (substances that are attracted to a magnetic field), which are used for MRI contrast (gadolinium); and iodine compounds. They can be administered orally, parenterally (for example, intravenously), or by routes that introduce them into an organ or a body cavity (for example, by insertion). Types of diagnostic imaging include X-rays, computed tomography (CT), nuclear medicine, magnetic resonance imaging (MRI), and ultrasound.

Invasive Procedures

Diagnostic tests can be invasive or noninvasive. An **invasive** procedure, such as angiography, requires a radiologist to insert a catheter, wire, or other testing device into a patient's blood vessel or organ through the skin or a body orifice. All invasive tests require surgical aseptic technique. Some procedures, including angiography, are performed in a hospital or same-day surgical facility. The patient may need general anesthesia for some procedures. The anesthetist must closely monitor the patient, who is under anesthesia during and after the test, for life-threatening complications such as anaphylaxis.

Noninvasive Procedures

Noninvasive procedures, such as standard X-rays or ultrasonography, use other technologies to view internal structures.

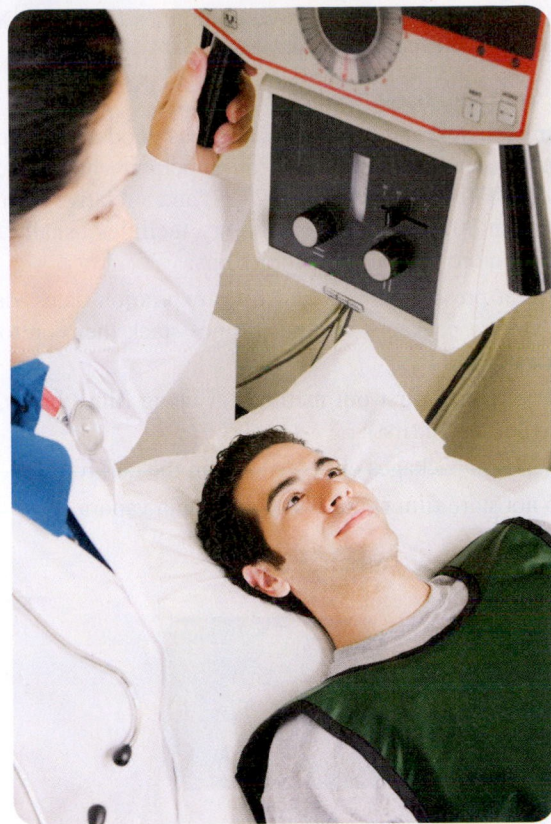

FIGURE 50-1 A standard X-ray is one of the most frequently performed radiologic tests.
© Steve Hix/Fuse/Getty Images RF

They do not require inserting devices, breaking the skin, or monitoring at the degree needed with invasive procedures.

The most familiar equipment used for diagnostic imaging is the conventional X-ray machine, as shown in Figure 50-1. This machine consists of a table, an X-ray tube, a control panel, and a high-voltage generator. The image produced by a conventional X-ray may be developed on standard X-ray film or captured digitally. Digital radiography is discussed later in the chapter. Other equipment used for diagnostic radiology includes instruments specifically designed for the test. Examples are a mammography unit, a scanner for CT, and a transducer for ultrasound.

▶ The Medical Assistant's Role in Diagnostic Radiology   LO 50.3

As a medical assistant, you may work with diagnostic radiology in a radiology facility or in a medical office. Your duties in a radiology facility will include assisting a radiologic technologist or a radiologist in performing diagnostic radiologic procedures. Depending on the scope of practice in your state, you may be allowed to learn how to operate certain X-ray equipment. Even if you are not allowed to assist with an X-ray procedure or to operate X-ray equipment, you will probably provide preprocedure and postprocedure patient care. Your duties in an orthopedic office may include assisting a radiologic technologist in performing X-ray procedures. In an obstetric practice, you might assist a physician in performing an ultrasound examination of a pregnant woman. Even if you work in a medical office that does not perform radiologic testing, you must still provide a certain amount of preprocedure care and education. In order to properly explain a test to a patient and to assist a radiologic technologist or radiologist in performing a test, you must have a basic understanding of X-ray technology. You also may need in-service training to ensure accuracy and patient safety for some procedures. See the *Educating the Patient* feature Providing Patient Instruction for Radiologic Procedures.

Preprocedure Care

Preprocedure care varies somewhat, depending on the test. In general, however, you may do the following:

- Schedule the patient's appointment, if necessary. Inform the patient of the location, date, and time of the procedure.

- Provide preparation instructions. Advise the patient about dietary restrictions or requirements (such as fasting or drinking liquids) as well as medication requirements (such as taking a laxative). Always check with the radiology facility for specific requirements and be sure the patient receives this information.

- Explain the procedure to the patient briefly and clearly. Use proper terminology and nontechnical language. Reinforce the doctor's reason for requesting the procedure and provide any available written information about the test. Inform the patient about the length of the examination, possible side effects or safety precautions and warnings, and injections or uncomfortable steps. Check for clarity and understanding by using the mirroring communication technique when communicating with the patient. You must ensure that the patient understands the preprocedure directions.

- Ask pertinent questions. Obtain a medication history from the patient, because current medications could interfere with some procedures. If the patient is a woman of childbearing age, ask whether she is pregnant or if there is any chance she could be pregnant. Report the answers to the physician in a medical office or to the radiologic technologist in a radiology facility.

Care During and After the Procedure

If you work in a radiology facility, your responsibilities include preparing and guiding the patient through the procedure. You also may assist the radiologic technologist or the radiologist in performing the procedure by placing, removing, and developing film in the X-ray machine. Procedure 50-1, at the end of this chapter, describes the general process of assisting with a radiologic procedure.

You may care for a patient and assist the radiologic technologist or radiologist during a wide variety of X-ray and other diagnostic imaging tests. While requirements of different procedures vary, you will probably be asked to perform many of the duties described in Procedure 50-1. Although you are unlikely to position the patient, you should know that the position relative to the X-ray source determines the path of the X-rays and the resulting images. Figure 50-2 illustrates common X-ray pathways and the images produced.

Verifying Insurance for Radiologic Procedures

Managed care health insurance plans are the most common type of insurance you will encounter in the office. Patients with HMOs are often required to use the services of certain radiology facilities. Because managed care plans often have facilities with which they are contracted, be sure the patient is sent to a radiology facility that is contracted with his or her health insurance. If needed, verify and complete the necessary referrals for all radiology testing. Make insurance verification a regular step in preprocedure care.

Storing and Filing X-rays

Many X-rays are now stored digitally, but there may be some instances where an actual X-ray film is produced. In this case, you may be responsible for storing X-ray films if you work in a radiology facility. Follow these guidelines for proper X-ray storage:

- Keep fresh film on hand at all times.
- Maintain new and exposed films in as good a condition as possible by keeping them at a temperature between 50°F and 70°F (between 10°C and 20°C) and a relative humidity between 30% and 50%. Radiology facilities usually have one or more special rooms for films.
- Prevent pressure marks and keep expiration dates visible by storing packages on end; do not stack them on top of each other.
- Use a first-in, first-out method for using film (that is, use the oldest film first).
- Open film packages or boxes only in the darkroom.
- Do not store film near acid or ammonia vapors.

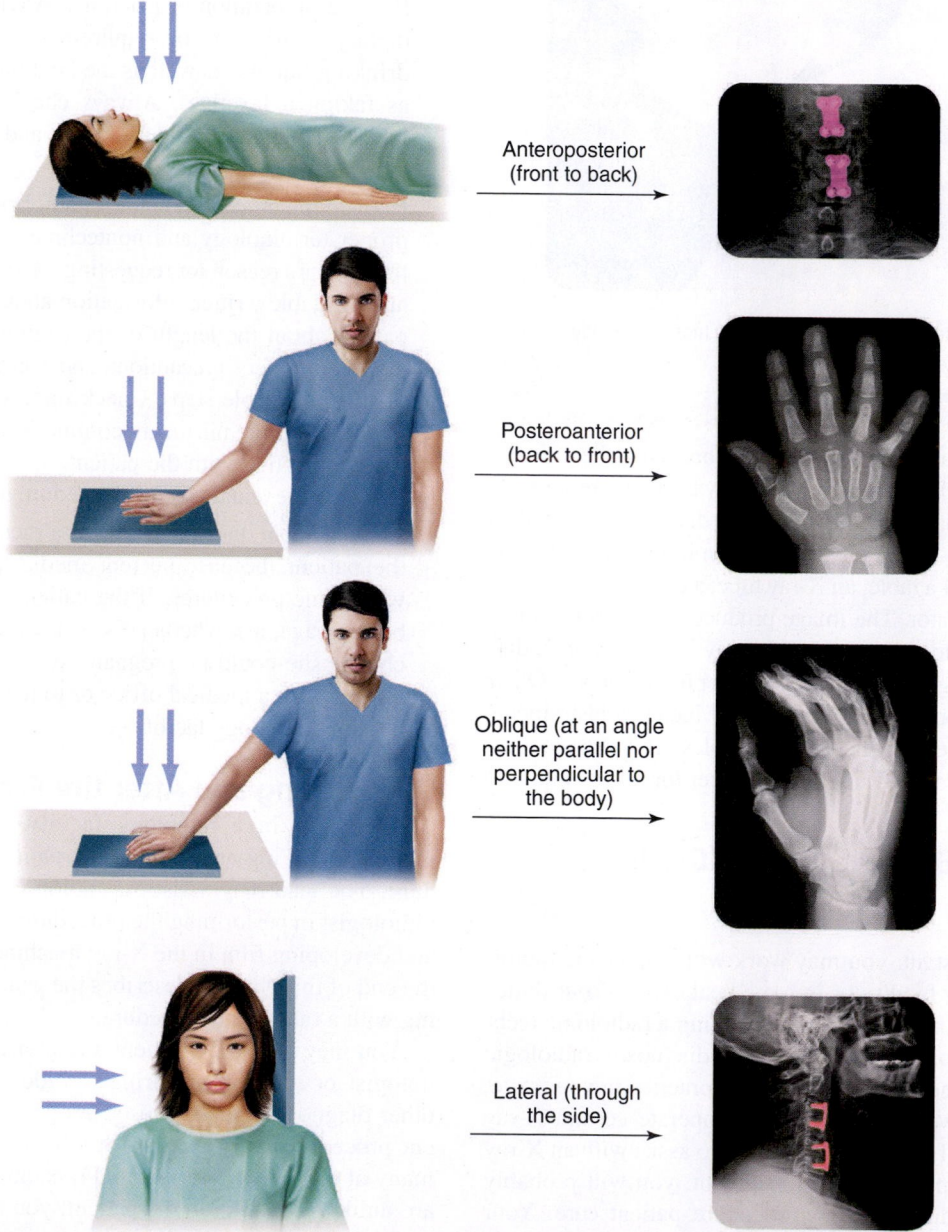

Anteroposterior (front to back)

Posteroanterior (back to front)

Oblique (at an angle neither parallel nor perpendicular to the body)

Lateral (through the side)

FIGURE 50-2 These are X-ray pathways and resulting projections for the most common types of X-rays. (Images are for instruction only. Patients should have protective lead shields during X-ray procedures.)

You also will be responsible for providing accurate record-keeping of X-rays. See Procedure 50-2, at the end of this chapter, for guidelines on documentation and filing techniques.

Remember, X-ray films are the property of the radiology facility or the doctor's office where they are taken. Although the films may be sent (or taken by the patient) to a hospital or another doctor for consultation, they should be returned to the original facility (for example, the radiologist's office). In some facilities, the images are stored on the computer and the patient receives an electronic copy to take to another doctor or medical facility. The information, however, is the patient's property, so the patient need not return reports.

▶ Common Diagnostic Radiologic Tests   LO 50.4

A variety of radiologic imaging tests are available. Table 50-1 identifies some of the most frequently ordered tests and the disorders they are used to diagnose.

Contrast Media in Diagnostic Tests

Various procedures involve the use of contrast media to see body structures and observe their function. These procedures include angiography, arthrography, barium enema, barium swallow, cholangiography, cholecystography, cystography, fluoroscopy, hepatobiliary (HIDA) scan, intravenous pyelography, magnetic resonance imaging (sometimes), myelography, nuclear medicine studies, and retrograde pyelography.

As mentioned, contrast media can be administered by mouth, by needle or catheter into a blood vessel, or by a route that introduces the medium into an organ or a body cavity (for example, into the colon). A contrast medium can cause adverse effects in some patients. Common adverse effects with oral agents include mild and transient abdominal cramping, constipation, nausea, vomiting, diarrhea, skin rashes, itching, heartburn, dizziness, and headache. Intravenous agents cause some of the same adverse effects, as well as localized injection-site reactions and more serious reactions such as anaphylaxis.

Because many contrast media contain iodine, a common allergen, patients should be questioned about known allergies to iodine or shellfish, which contain iodine, before procedures involving the use of contrast media. All patients should be observed during such procedures for signs of allergic reaction.

Fluoroscopy

X-rays can cause certain chemicals to fluoresce, or emit visible light. When X-rays penetrate a body structure and are directed onto a fluorescent screen, they produce an image the radiologist can view either directly or through special glasses. Usually, a radiologist, rather than a radiology technician or medical assistant, performs fluoroscopic procedures.

Many diagnostic procedures involve fluoroscopy, which allows viewing of internal organ movement or the movement of a contrast medium, such as barium sulfate, while the contrast medium travels through the alimentary canal. Fluoroscopy also guides the radiologist in locating a precise internal area that needs to be recorded on film or digitally.

Fluoroscopic images are sometimes photographed for further study. Photofluorography is a series of these photographs that records the body's internal movements over time. Cinefluorography is a motion picture of the internal movements of the body.

Hysterosalpingography

Hysterosalpingography, also called uterosalpingography, is a radiologic examination of a women's uterus and fallopian tubes using fluoroscopy. This procedure is used to examine women who have difficulty becoming pregnant. It is sometimes ordered as part of a fertility exam or when the woman has a history of miscarriages that result from congenital abnormalities of the uterus. It is also used to determine the presence and severity of tumor masses or adhesions, uterine fibroids, and fallopian tube adhesions or obstructions. A hysterosalpingogram (Figure 50-3) assists the radiologist in evaluating the shape and structure of the uterus, the openness (patency) of the fallopian tubes, and any scarring within the fallopian tubes and peritoneal cavity. Hysterosalpingography is usually performed on an outpatient basis.

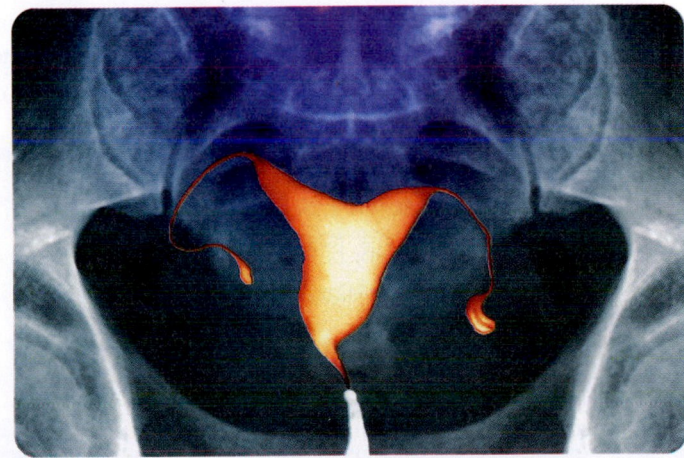

FIGURE 50-3   A hystersalpingogram of the uterus and fallopian tubes.
© ISM/Phototake

TABLE 50-1 Common Radiologic Tests and Disorders Diagnosed

Test	Disorders Diagnosed/Treated
Angiography	
Cardiovascular	Status of blood flow, collateral circulation, malformed vessels, aneurysms, narrowing or blockages of vessels, and presence of hemorrhage
Cerebral	Aneurysm, hemorrhage, evidence of cerebrovascular accident, and arteriosclerosis
Gastrointestinal (GI)	Upper gastrointestinal bleeding
Pulmonary	Pulmonary emboli (especially when lung scan is inconclusive) and evaluation of pulmonary circulation in some heart conditions before surgery
Renal	Abnormalities of blood vessels in urinary system
Arthrography	Joint conditions
Barium enema (lower GI series)	Obstructions, ulcers, polyps, diverticulosis, tumor, and motility problems of colon or rectum
Barium swallow (upper GI series)	Obstructions, ulcers, polyps, diverticulosis, tumor, and motility problems of esophagus, stomach, duodenum, and small intestine
Cholangiography	Gallstones, gallbladder, or common bile duct stones or obstructions and ability of gallbladder to concentrate and store dye
Computed tomography (CT)	Aortic and heart aneurysms, disorders of liver and biliary systems, renal and pulmonary tumors, brain abnormalities (tumors, blood clots, evidence of cerebrovascular accident, outlines of brain ventricles), GI tract lesions, GI disorders (acute pseudocyst of pancreas, abdominal abscesses, biliary obstruction), breast diseases and disorders, spinal disorders, and to guide biopsy procedures
Fluoroscopy	Structure, process, and function of organs in motion to detect abnormalities
HIDA (hepatobiliary) scan	Diagnosis of structural and functional problems with the liver, gallbladder, and bile ducts
Intravenous pyelography (IVP) (excretory urography)	Urinary system abnormalities, including renal pelvis, ureters, and bladder (for example, kidney stones); abnormal size, shape, or structure of kidneys, ureters, or bladder; space-occupying lesions; pyelonephrosis; hydronephrosis; and trauma to the urinary system
KUB (kidneys, ureters, bladder) radiography	Size, shape, and position of urinary organs; urinary system diseases or disorders; and kidney stones
Magnetic resonance imaging (MRI)	Cancerous tissue, atherosclerotic tissue, blood clots, tumors, and deformities, particularly of the heart valves, brain, spine, and joints
Mammography	Breast tumors and lesions
Myelography	Irregularities or compression of spinal cord
Nuclear medicine (radionuclide imaging)	Abnormal function (defects), lesions, or disorders of bone, brain, lungs, kidneys, liver, pancreas, thyroid, and spleen
Radiation therapy	Treatment of cancer
Retrograde pyelogram	Obstruction of ureters, bladder, or urethra (including tumors, stones, strictures, or blood clots) and perinephritic abscess
Ultrasound	Abnormalities of gallbladder, liver, spleen, heart, kidneys, gonads, blood vessels, lymphatic system, and fetal conditions (including number of fetuses; age and sex of fetus; fetal development, position, and deformities)

Angiography

Angiography is a test used to diagnose abnormalities in blood vessels, including the following:

- Aneurysm—a widening or ballooning of an artery
- Atherosclerotic disease—fatty plaques on the walls of arteries
- Arteriovenous malformations (AVM)—abnormal connections between arteries and veins
- Arterial stenosis—narrowing of an artery

The test is done in one of three ways:

- Catheter angiography with X-rays
- CT angiography
- MRI angiography

Catheter angiography requires a physician (usually a radiologist) to insert a catheter into the patient's vein (venography) or artery (arteriography). The physician first guides the catheter tip to the vessel being examined, then injects a contrast medium through the catheter and takes a series of X-rays to assess the vessel's blood flow and condition (Figure 50-4). The test—used to evaluate the heart vessels (coronary angiography), the brain (cerebral angiography), or the femoral, brachial, or carotid artery—may be performed jointly by a radiologist and a vascular surgeon or other specialist.

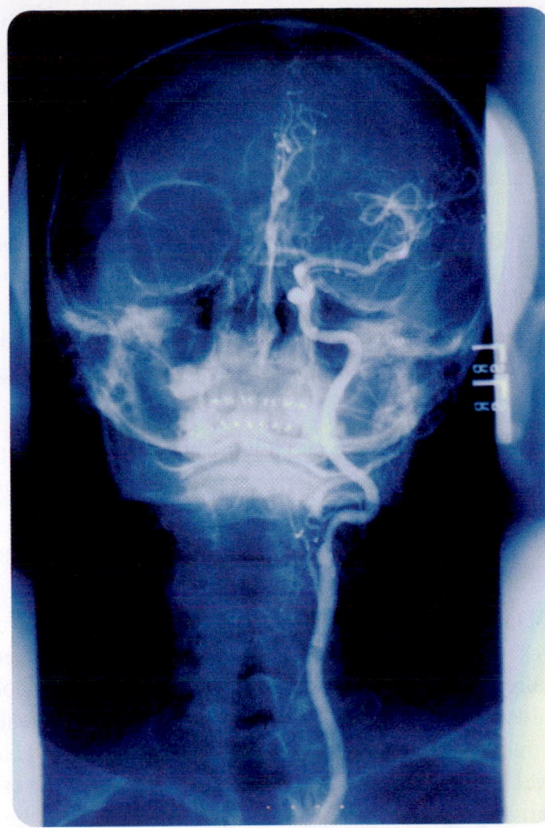

FIGURE 50-4 Carotid angiogram: an intra-arterial catheter is inserted and a contrast medium is injected to create an image of the arteries.
© Royalty-Free/CORBIS

Because this procedure requires insertion of a catheter into a blood vessel and the use of local anesthesia, the patient is admitted to a hospital or same-day surgical facility. The physician who performs the examination provides the patient with instructions immediately before the procedure. You will, however, schedule the procedure, and you can encourage the patient to ask questions. Radiology facilities usually have information sheets for each procedure. If the patient has questions you cannot answer or if you have any doubt about preprocedure instructions, check with your supervisor.

CT and MRI angiography (MRA) may be performed with or without contrast medium. The contrast medium is injected into a vein, usually in the arm, and images are made using computer programs that produce detailed images of blood vessels. Because CT and MRI angiography are less invasive than catheter angiography, they are usually performed on an outpatient basis. CT and MRI are discussed in more detail later in the chapter.

Arthrography

Arthrography is performed by a radiologist, who uses a contrast medium and fluoroscopy to help diagnose abnormalities or injuries in the cartilage, tendons, or ligaments of the joints—usually the knee or shoulder. Although MRI is used more often to evaluate soft-tissue injuries in joints, arthrography can provide an image while the patient moves the joint. When preparing patients for arthrography or assisting with the procedure, follow these guidelines:

- Describe the procedure to patients and inform them the examination will take about 1 hour. Ask patients about possible allergies to contrast media, iodine, or shellfish. If they have any of these allergies, inform the radiologist immediately.

- Explain to patients that no special preprocedure preparations are necessary.

- Tell patients the doctor will first inject a local anesthetic to numb the area being examined. Then the doctor will inject the contrast medium (dye, air, or both) into the joint and will use a fluoroscope to evaluate the joint's function. Inform patients who are having a knee examined that the doctor may ask them to walk a few steps to spread the contrast medium.

- After the test is completed, advise patients that for 1 or 2 days they may experience some pain or swelling, particularly if the joint is exercised. Tell them to rest and avoid putting strain on the joint.

Barium Enema (Lower GI Series)

A **barium enema** is performed by a radiologist, who instills barium sulfate through the anus into the rectum and then into the colon, to help diagnose and evaluate obstructions, ulcers, polyps, diverticulosis, tumors, or motility problems of the colon or rectum. This procedure is called a *lower GI (gastrointestinal) series*—a series of X-rays of the colon and rectum. The two types of barium enema techniques are single-contrast, in which only barium is instilled into the colon, and double-contrast, in which air is forced into the colon to distend or inflate the tissue. The air may be added while the barium is present, after it has been expelled, or both. The double-contrast technique makes structures more visible by fluoroscopy and allows identification of small lesions. The digestive tract must be totally empty, requiring the patient to thoroughly cleanse the tract with a series of preparatory steps and to have nothing by mouth for 8 hours before the test, except for one cup of clear liquid on the morning of the test. In most facilities, a radiologic technologist assists with a barium enema, but you may assist the patient before and after the procedure. If you do assist with a barium enema, you will have various responsibilities before, during, and after the procedure.

Before the Procedure Schedule the patient's appointment in the morning so that he can sleep through most of the period during which his digestive tract must be empty and thus avoid experiencing hunger unnecessarily. Include the following items when you instruct a patient about the preparation for a barium enema:

- Describe the procedure and tell the patient the examination will take 1 to 2 hours.

- Ask about possible allergies to contrast media, iodine, or shellfish and report such allergies to the radiologist.

- Explain the importance of following the preparation instructions so that the colon and rectum are free of residual material. Residual material in the colon or rectum could cause blockages or shadows, resulting in an inaccurate test.

- Preprocedure preparation on the day before the examination includes following a clear liquid diet beginning in the morning (coffee, tea, carbonated beverages, clear gelatin, strained fruit juice, bouillon, or clear broths; milk is not permitted) and taking prescribed amounts of electrolyte solution or other laxative preparations and fluids on a specified schedule.
- Tell the patient he may have one cup of coffee, tea, or water on the morning of the examination.

During the Procedure Follow these steps when assisting during a barium enema:

1. Have the patient undress and put on a gown.
2. Tell the patient to expect some discomfort during the examination, as well as frequent side-to-side turning.
3. Have the patient lie on his side. The radiologist inserts the enema tip, designed to help the patient hold the liquid, into the rectum and instills the barium sulfate into the colon. If the patient experiences cramping or the urge to defecate during instillation of the barium, instruct him to relax the abdominal muscles by breathing slowly and deeply through the mouth.
4. Instruct the patient to remain still and hold his breath when X-rays are taken. Using a fluoroscope, the doctor observes the barium as it flows through the lower bowel and periodically takes X-rays while the patient is placed in various positions. You may be asked to assist with placing the patient in these positions.
5. If a double-contrast study is being performed, tell the patient that air will be introduced into the colon to expand the colon tissue. Explain that the combination of air and barium provides a clearer view of structures than only one contrast medium would provide and allows possible identification of small lesions if they are present.
6. When the doctor has completed the barium portion of the examination, including X-rays with both barium and air, tell the patient to use the toilet and expel as much barium as possible. Explain that if enough barium is expelled, the doctor may take a final X-ray of the empty colon.
7. Have the patient wait to dress until the doctor tells you that no additional X-rays are needed.

After the Procedure After the radiologist has completed the barium enema, instruct the patient in postprocedure care. Tell the patient the following:

- He may now have a regular meal.
- The residual barium may make his stools appear whitish or lighter than usual, but this is normal.
- The barium may cause constipation, so he should drink extra water to help relieve constipation and to eliminate the remaining barium sulfate. The physician may order a laxative to be taken if constipation is not relieved within 1 or 2 days.

Barium Swallow (Upper GI Series)

A **barium swallow** involves oral administration of a barium sulfate drink to help diagnose and evaluate obstructions,

ulcers, polyps, diverticulosis, tumors, or motility problems of the esophagus, stomach, duodenum, and small intestine. This test is called an *upper GI series*. In preparation for this test, the patient can have nothing by mouth for at least 8 hours before the test. You will have various responsibilities before, during, and after the procedure.

Before the Procedure Schedule the patient's appointment in the morning so that she can sleep through most of the period during which her digestive tract is empty and thus avoid experiencing hunger unnecessarily. When instructing a patient about the preparation for an upper GI series, include the following items:

- Describe the procedure and tell the patient the examination will take about 1 hour. If X-rays of the small bowel are needed, the test may take several hours.
- Ask about possible allergies to contrast media, iodine, or shellfish and report such allergies to the radiologist.
- Explain the importance of following the preparation instructions so that the stomach is empty. Preprocedure requirements include having nothing by mouth (food or liquids) after midnight the night before and no breakfast the morning of the examination. If the patient's small bowel is to be evaluated, also tell her to take the prescribed laxative preparation between 2:00 and 4:00 p.m. the day before the examination.
- Instruct the patient not to swallow water when brushing her teeth or rinsing her mouth and, if applicable, to stop smoking because nicotine stimulates gastric secretions and can affect the test results.

During the Procedure When assisting during an upper GI series, take the following steps:

1. Have the patient undress and put on a gown.
2. Explain that she will be drinking a barium sulfate drink that tastes chalky and resembles a milk shake.
3. Have the patient stand and drink part of the barium.
4. The radiologist will use a fluoroscope to observe the flow of the barium and to assess the functioning of the esophagus, stomach, duodenum, and small intestine as the barium passes through the structures. (The doctor will then direct the patient to drink additional barium and continue to observe the function of the various structures.)
5. Place the patient on the X-ray table and move her into different positions (if medical assistants are permitted to do so in your state), as instructed by the doctor, to allow X-rays to be taken of the upper digestive tract. Instruct the patient to remain still and hold her breath when X-rays are taken.

After the Procedure After the physician completes the upper GI series, instruct the patient in postprocedure care. Give the patient the following information:

- She may now have a regular meal.
- Her stools may appear whitish or lighter than usual as the barium is eliminated, but this is normal.

- Sometimes, another examination is required after 24 hours to determine whether the barium has moved into the large intestine. If this test is indicated, tell the patient to follow a clear liquid diet (coffee, tea, carbonated beverages, clear gelatin, strained fruit juices, bouillon, or clear broths; milk is not permitted) and to return in 24 hours.

Cholangiography

Cholangiography is performed by a radiologist to evaluate the function of the bile ducts. It involves injection of the contrast medium directly into the common bile duct (during gallbladder surgery) or through a T tube (after gallbladder surgery or during radiologic testing). X-rays or MRIs are taken immediately after injection. Instruct the patient as follows:

- Describe the procedure to the patient and tell him the examination will take about 2 to 3 hours. Ask the patient about possible allergies to contrast media, iodine, or shellfish and report them to the radiologist.
- Explain the preparation instructions. Tell the patient to eat a light evening meal the night before the examination, to take a laxative (as prescribed by the doctor), and to have no food or liquids after midnight. He also should have no solid food the morning of the examination.

Computed Tomography (CT)

Computed tomography (CT) scans are produced by a specialized X-ray camera that rotates completely around the patient and a computer that compiles one cross-sectional view from each rotation of the camera. The patient is lying on a table that gradually moves through the doughnut-shaped machine containing the rotating camera. Cross-sectional images can be reconfigured by a computer program into different planes (frontal, transverse, and sagittal), creating images that give different views of the same area. The images can also be combined to create three-dimensional images.

CT scans are used to diagnose abnormalities in almost all body structures, including the head, kidneys, heart, chest, liver, biliary tract, pancreas, GI tract, spine, pelvis, bones, and breast. Abnormalities and disorders that can be detected using CT scans include the following:

- Cancer
- Injuries from trauma
- Spinal injury
- Pulmonary embolism (blood clot in the vessels of the lung)
- Aortic aneurysm
- Skeletal injuries and abnormalities

When preparing the patient for a CT scan,

- Ask the patient about possible allergies to contrast media, iodine, or shellfish and report them to the radiologist.
- Tell the patient he will be placed on a table that moves through the scanner but he will be able to see around the room during the test.
- Inform the patient that the procedure will last about 45 to 90 minutes and that he must lie still while the scans are taken.

- If a contrast medium will be used, advise the patient that it will be injected into a vein in the arm or on the back of the hand (except with a CT scan of the spine) to enhance detail of the structure being evaluated.
- If the patient is having a CT scan of the head, chest, abdomen, or pelvis, instruct him not to eat anything for 4 hours or drink any liquids for 2 hours before the examination. Explain that he may experience mild nausea after injection of the contrast medium if the stomach is too full.
- Tell the patient to remove metallic objects that could interfere with the path of the X-rays. Also, ask if the patient has skin staples or metallic prostheses that could interfere.
- Inform the patient that a written report of the results should be available within 24 hours of the test and that a report will be sent to his primary care physician (or the referring physician).

Intravenous Pyelography

Also known as *excretory urography*, **intravenous pyelography (IVP)** is performed by a radiologist who injects a contrast medium into a vein. The doctor then takes a series of X-rays as the contrast medium travels through the kidneys, ureters, and bladder. IVP is used to evaluate urinary system abnormalities or trauma to the urinary system. In most facilities, a radiologic technologist assists with IVP, but you may assist the patient before the procedure. If you assist with IVP, you will have several responsibilities both before and during the procedure.

Before the Procedure Schedule the patient's appointment in the morning so that she can sleep through most of the period during which her digestive tract is empty and thus avoid experiencing hunger unnecessarily. When instructing a patient about the preparation for an IVP, include the following information:

- Describe the procedure and tell the patient the examination will take about 1½ hours.
- Ask the patient about possible allergies to contrast media, iodine, or shellfish and report such allergies to the radiologist.
- Explain the importance of adhering to the preparation instructions so that the bowel is free of any material that could obstruct the view of the urinary organs.
- Tell the patient to follow a liquid diet (coffee, tea, carbonated beverages, clear gelatin, strained fruit juice, bouillon, or clear broths, but no milk) the day before the examination. The patient may be given a laxative preparation to take the night before the examination.
- No food or liquids are allowed after midnight and no breakfast the morning of the examination. Some physicians also order an enema to be taken about 2 hours before the examination.

During and After the Procedure When assisting during an IVP, you will generally proceed in this manner:

1. Have the patient undress and put on a gown.
2. Explain that a contrast medium will be injected into her vein (usually in the arm). Instruct her to inform the physician if she notices shortness of breath or itching after injection of the dye because this can indicate an allergic reaction.

3. Have the patient lie on the X-ray table and move her into different positions, as instructed by the physician, to allow X-rays to be taken of the urinary tract as the contrast medium is excreted. Instruct the patient to remain still and hold her breath when X-rays are taken.

4. Note that some physicians place a compression device on the abdomen, which helps hold the contrast medium in the kidneys and ureters by exerting moderate pressure.

5. After the physician takes the series of X-rays to evaluate urinary system function, ask the patient to urinate, and explain that a final X-ray will be taken.

6. Inform the patient that she may resume a normal diet after the test and that the contrast medium will be eliminated in the urine.

Retrograde Pyelography

Retrograde pyelography is similar to the IVP, except that the doctor injects the contrast medium through a urethral catheter. This procedure, which evaluates function of the ureters, bladder, and urethra, is often used for patients with poor kidney function. Follow the same preparation and assistance instructions as for the IVP.

Kidneys, Ureters, and Bladder (KUB) Radiography

Also called a *flat plate of the abdomen*, **KUB radiography** is an X-ray of the abdomen used to assess the size, shape, and position of the urinary organs; to evaluate urinary system diseases or disorders; and to determine the presence of kidney stones. It also can be helpful in determining the position of an intrauterine device (IUD) or in locating foreign bodies in the digestive tract. No patient preparation is required. A radiologic technologist takes a KUB X-ray; thus, you follow the guidelines you would use for a patient having any type of standard, noninvasive X-ray.

Magnetic Resonance Imaging (MRI)

Magnetic resonance imaging (MRI) uses a strong magnetic field and radio frequency signals in combination with a computer to allow the physician to examine internal structures and soft tissues. The combination of nonionizing (radio frequency) radiation and a magnetic field allows the MRI scanner to produce images based primarily on the water content of tissues, making MRI a useful imaging tool for soft tissues. Because no ionizing radiation (X-ray) is used to produce the image, the risk of harmful effects to the patient is very low. The test may be performed with or without contrast. You will be responsible for preparing the patient for an MRI and assisting with the procedure.

Before the Procedure When instructing a patient about preparing for an MRI, include the following steps:

- If a contrast medium is going to be used, ask the patient and inform the radiologist about possible allergies to contrast media, iodine, or shellfish.
- Screen the patient to determine whether any internal metallic materials are present. (This is especially important

because a strong magnetic field is involved in creating the image.) Ask about a pacemaker, brain or aneurysm clips, brain or heart surgery, shunts and heart valves, other surgeries, and shrapnel or metal fragments (particularly in an eye).

- Ask the patient whether he is or has been a metalworker. If so, he may carry metal slivers, chips, or filings under his nails or skin.
- Instruct women not to wear eye makeup the day of the examination, as it often contains metallic ingredients.
- Describe the procedure to the patient and explain that the examination will take between 45 minutes and 2 hours.
- Inform the patient that he may wear street clothing during the test but to avoid wearing clothing with metallic thread, metal stays or grippers, or thick elastic. Tell the patient that depending upon the location to be examined he could be asked to undress and put on a gown.
- Tell the patient he does not need to fast before the examination or follow any preprocedure diet, unless he is having an MRI of the pelvis. In that case, instruct him to have no solid food for 6 hours and no liquids for 4 hours before the examination. Inform the patient that he may take prescription medications.
- Explain that he will not be required to drink an oral contrast preparation but should avoid caffeine for 4 hours before the examination. Tell the patient he will probably have no side effects from the examination but that some nausea may occur as a result of the contrast medium.

During and After the Procedure When assisting during an MRI, you will need to follow these specific steps:

1. Have the patient lie on the padded table.

2. Explain that the table will be placed inside a long, narrow tube about 22 inches in diameter and that he will hear a loud knocking noise as the machine scans. Offer the patient hearing protection devices (ear plugs or headphones) during the test. Warn the patient to remain still to avoid blurring the image and the consequent need for a retake. Note that physicians may order sedation for patients who are claustrophobic or cannot lie still for a long period (Figure 50-5).

3. Advise the patient that although the technician will not be in the scanning room during the examination, she will maintain contact with a camera and a microphone. The patient may speak to the technician at any time in case of a problem, but he is encouraged to be still for each series.

4. Inform the patient that his primary care physician or referring doctor should have a preliminary report of test results within about 24 hours.

Mammography

Mammography, the X-ray exam of the internal breast tissues, helps in diagnosing breast abnormalities (Figure 50-6). A specially trained radiologic technologist takes mammograms.

You will have several responsibilities during both setup and patient care before and after mammography. However,

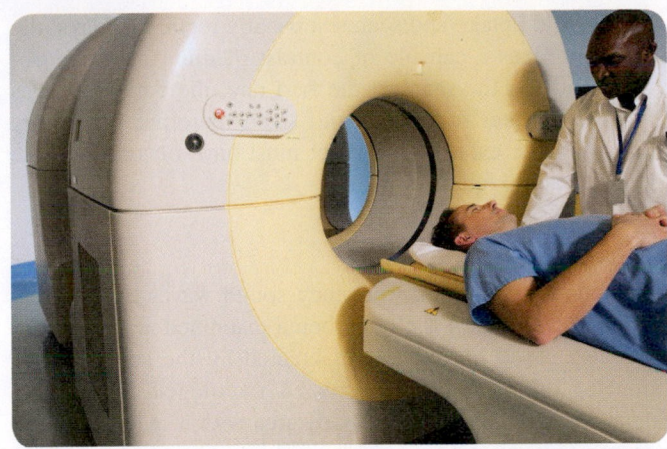

FIGURE 50-5 A patient who is claustrophobic or unable to lie still may require sedation during an MRI.
© UpperCut Images/SuperStock RF

a medical assistant does not assist during mammography in most states. Instead, you will prepare the patient for the procedure and ease her fears. For more information regarding patient education before a mammogram, see the *Assisting in Reproductive and Urinary Specialties* chapter.

Stereotactic Breast Biopsy

When a mammogram reveals an abnormality in the breast tissue, the physician may want a biopsy to determine if it is malignant. Because so many abnormalities revealed by mammography are benign and present no health risk, physicians now perform *stereotactic breast biopsies,* which are less painful and less invasive than conventional excisional biopsies. The procedure is performed by a physician and a radiologic technologist and is similar to mammography, except that the patient is usually lying face down or sitting rather than

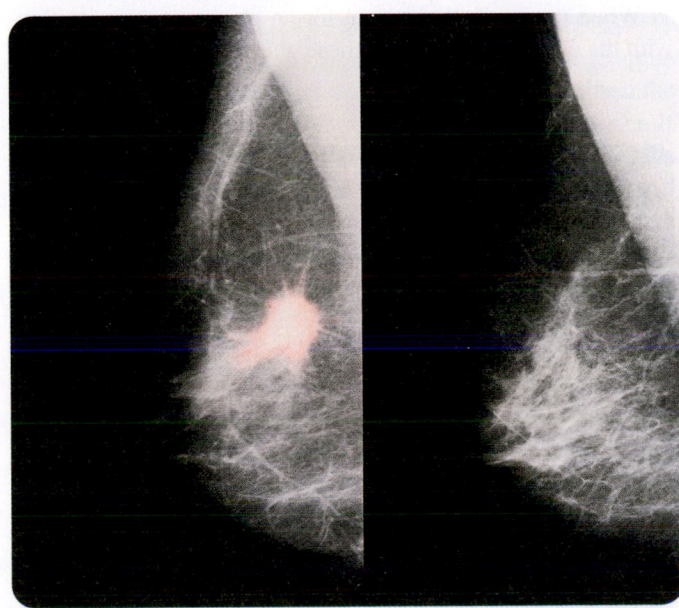

FIGURE 50-6 Mammograms can reveal the presence of tumors that are not detected by other means. The mammogram on the right indicates normal breast tissue, whereas the one on the left suggests a malignancy.
© UHB Trust/Stone/Getty Images

standing. The breast is compressed with a compression paddle to confirm that the area of the breast with the lesion is correctly centered in the paddle window. X-rays are taken of the breast from two different angles. A computer is used to help determine the exact positioning of the biopsy needle and the physician uses a needle to take a small sample of tissue for examination by a pathologist. The attending physician later contacts the patient with the test results.

Myelography

Although MRI is used more often to evaluate the spinal cord and spinal nerves, **myelography** is a kind of fluoroscopy of the spinal cord used when MRI is not practical—if a patient has a pacemaker or other medical device that prevents the patient from undergoing MRI. The physician performs a lumbar puncture, removes some cerebrospinal fluid (CSF), and instills a contrast medium to evaluate spinal abnormalities, such as compression of the spinal cord. Sometimes the physician performs pneumoencephalography, which involves instilling air after removal of the CSF to allow viewing of the cerebral cavities.

The physician who performs myelography or pneumoencephalography must be skilled in performing lumbar puncture—most likely a radiologist, neurologist, neuro-surgeon, or anesthetist. A radiologic technologist is typically the only other person present for the test. Although myelography is not used as frequently as it was before the invention of CT and MRI, it is still performed when these newer techniques do not provide enough information about the spinal canal. Myelography may be reserved for cases in which the clinical findings are unusual or the scanning results uncertain.

Nuclear Medicine

Also known as *radionuclide imaging,* **nuclear medicine** involves the use of radionuclides, or radioisotopes (radioactive elements or their compounds). The radionuclides are administered orally, intravenously, or through routes that introduce them into organs or body cavities. The purpose is to evaluate the bone, brain, lungs, kidneys, liver, pancreas, thyroid, or spleen. Sometimes, the entire body is scanned for "hot spots," or places where the radioisotope is concentrated.

For common nuclear medicine scans, the technician uses a scanner called a *gamma camera.* This scanner detects radiation from the radioisotope and converts it into an image (called a *scintiscan* or *scintigram*) to be photographed or displayed on a screen (see Figure 50-7). Some images are produced immediately, whereas others take up to several days. Radionuclide imaging exposes patients to lower doses of radiation than some radiologic techniques because the amount of ionizing radiation in the isotope is less than that emitted from X-ray cameras. Other nuclear medicine procedures include single photon emission computed tomography (SPECT), positron emission tomography (PET), and MUGA (multiple gated acquisition) scan.

- **SPECT** is often used to locate and determine the extent of brain damage from a stroke. The gamma camera detects signals induced by gamma radiation and a computer converts these signals into either two- or three-dimensional images that are displayed on a screen.

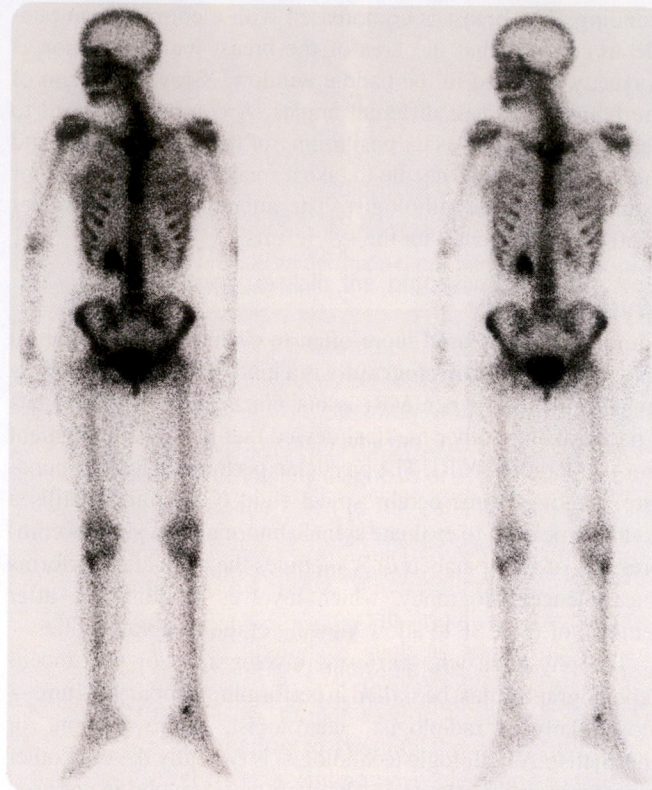

FIGURE 50-7 This bone scan shows the uptake of the radioactive contrast medium.

© Jim Wehtje/Getty Images RF

- **PET** entails injecting isotopes combined with other substances involved in metabolic activity, like glucose. These special isotopes emit positrons, which a computer processes and displays on a screen. PET is especially useful for diagnosing brain-related conditions like epilepsy, mental illnesses, and Parkinson's disease.

- **MUGA scan (nuclear ventriculography)**—evaluates the condition of the heart's myocardium. It can be done while the patient is at rest or in stress (exercise) and involves the injection of radioisotopes that concentrate in the myocardium. The gamma camera allows the physician to measure ventricular contractions to evaluate the patient's heart wall.

When preparing a patient for a nuclear medicine procedure, describe the procedure and explain how long it will take. Also, explain any preparation requirements and other special instructions and tell the patient she will need to wait the required length of time for the uptake of the radioisotope. Length of examination and requirements for common scans are as follows:

- A bone scan lasts about 1 hour; it is done 2 to 3 hours after a 15-minute injection; the patient drinks 1 quart of liquid between the injection and the scan; a normal diet is permitted.

- A liver/spleen or lung scan lasts approximately 1 hour; there are no dietary restrictions.

- A kidney scan lasts about 2 hours; there are no dietary restrictions.

- A thyroid uptake and scan test usually requires 2 days; the patient takes a capsule of contrast medium in the morning and has the scan on the first day; the patient returns 24 hours later for the second scan; there are no dietary restrictions, except the patient must have no fish because of its natural iodine content.

Ultrasound

Ultrasound directs high-frequency sound waves through the skin over the area of the body being examined and produces an image based on the echoes created by the sound waves bouncing off of body structures. A radiologist or an ultrasound sonographer coats the body area with a special gel and passes a transducer (instrument similar to a microphone) over the area. As the transducer passes back and forth, it picks up echoes from the sound waves, which a computer converts into an image—sometimes called a sonogram—on a screen. Ultrasound is used to detect abnormalities in the gallbladder, liver, spleen, heart, and kidneys. It is also safe to use in obstetrics to evaluate the developing fetus or to detect multiple fetuses because it does not expose the patient (or the fetus) to radiation (Figure 50-8). In this case, the obstetrician may perform the test in the office.

One form of ultrasound—Doppler echocardiography—involves sound waves that echo against the flow of blood through vessels. Doppler echocardiography is usually performed by a cardiologist to determine whether blood flow is laminar (normal) or turbulent (disturbed).

Echocardiography, a type of ultrasound test, is used to study the structure and function of the heart. The test is usually performed while the patient is resting and again after exercising on a treadmill or bicycle. Images of the heart before and after exercise help the physician diagnose abnormalities of the structure and function of the heart and heart valves.

When preparing the patient for an ultrasound or assisting with the examination, follow these guidelines:

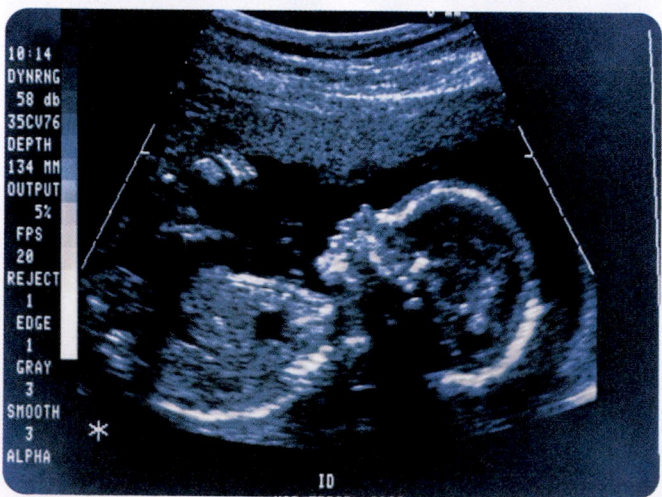

FIGURE 50-8 Ultrasound is commonly used to evaluate the health of a developing fetus.

© UHB Trust/Stone/Getty Images

- Describe the procedure to the patient and inform her that the examination will take about 1½ to 2 hours, depending on the type of ultrasound. For example, a cardiac ultrasound takes about 1½ hours; pelvic, 1 to 2 hours; and abdominal, ½ to 1 hour.

- Explain the preparation requirements, which vary according to the type of ultrasound. Tell a patient who is having a gallbladder or liver ultrasound not to eat for several hours before the test. Tell a pregnant patient to drink the prescribed amount of water 1 hour before the examination and not to void. Advise a patient having a pelvic ultrasound to take the prescribed laxative (if indicated), drink three to four glasses of water within 1 hour, and not to void within 1 hour of the test. If the patient is having an abdominal ultrasound, instruct her to take a laxative the night before the examination and not to have any food or fluids for 8 hours before the test.

- Advise the patient to wear loose, easy-to-remove clothing.

Dual-Energy X-ray Absorptiometry (DXA)

Dual-energy X-ray absorptiometry (DXA), often called bone densitometry, is a screening test that uses small doses of X-rays to determine the mineral density of a person's bones. The test may be used to diagnose osteoporosis or to monitor treatment of osteoporosis or other conditions that cause bone loss after diagnosis. Patients who take medications known to cause bone loss, such as Dilantin®, corticosteroids, and some barbiturates, should be screened for bone loss using DXA. Bone densitometry is also recommended for people with the following conditions:

- Postmenopausal women
- Smokers
- Hyperthyroidism
- Hyperparathyroidism
- Type 1 diabetes
- Kidney disease
- Recurrent fractures

During the test, the patient will lie on a padded table while very low-dose radiation is generated below the table and detected with a specialized arm that passes over the patient. The patient must lie very still while the test is being performed. DXA is usually completed within 30 minutes.

When instructing patients preparing for a DXA, tell them to wear loose-fitting clothing that does not have zippers, metal buttons, or belts. Patients will be asked to remove wallets, keys, or jewelry in the area being scanned. Tell patients they should avoid taking calcium supplements 24 hours before the test. A patient who has recently had X-rays or CT scans using a contrast medium such as barium may need to wait 2 weeks after the contrast before having a DXA scan.

The test is most often read by a radiologist; however, rheumatologists and endocrinologists can also read DXA scans. The report includes two results: the T score and the Z score. The T score is a measure of the amount of bone the person has compared to that of young adults. This number is used to assess risk of bone fractures. The Z score is the amount of bone the patient has compared to people of the same race, gender, age, and size. If the Z score test is high or low, additional medical tests for other underlying conditions, such as hyperparathyroidism, may be needed.

▶ Common Therapeutic Uses of Radiation

LO 50.5

Used therapeutically, radiology is called **radiation therapy,** which is used to treat cancer by preventing cellular reproduction. The two types of radiation therapy are teletherapy and brachytherapy. **Teletherapy,** also called external beam radiotherapy, is the most common form of radiation therapy and is done on an outpatient basis. It allows deep penetration of tissues and is used primarily for deep tumors. The patient experiences minimal side effects, which may include a "sunburn" effect at the treatment site, mild swelling and tenderness, and sometimes mild fatigue. Generally, the superficial tissues are not permanently damaged.

Stereotactic radiosurgery is a type of teletherapy that uses CT or MRI scanning in conjunction with radiation to treat brain tumors, acoustic neuromas, and arteriovenous malformations—defects in connections between arteries and veins—deep in the brain. In some cases, liver, prostate, and lung tumors are also treated with stereotactic radiosurgery. This method allows for very precise delivery of radiation to areas of the brain or other organs that are normally inaccessible with traditional surgical techniques, helping spare precious healthy tissue while still treating the tumor.

For a patient having stereotactic radiosurgery for brain tumors, first a neurosurgeon temporarily fastens a stereotactic frame to the patient's head using local anesthesia. The frame helps guide the physician to precisely locate the treatment. A CT or MRI scan is then performed to locate the tumor or malformation. Once the frame is in place and the imaging scan is complete, a radiation oncologist and a neurosurgeon plan the patient's treatment. The patient undergoes treatment based on this plan, has the stereotactic frame removed, and, in most cases, can go home the same day.

Localized cancers are treated with **brachytherapy.** In this technique, the radiologist places temporary radioactive implants close to or directly into cancerous tissue. This technique limits radiation exposure to healthy tissue, targeting only the area where the tumor is located. During brachytherapy, both the staff and the patient are subject to radiation exposure, so radiation safety precautions must be closely followed. When preparing the patient for radiation therapy, follow these guidelines:

- Describe the procedure and explain how long it will take, as determined by the radiologist and oncologist according to the patient's diagnosis and condition.

- Encourage patients to tell the physician about all medications, vitamins, or supplements they are taking.

- Inform the patient that the radiologist or oncologist will explain the treatment's possible side effects. Common side effects include nausea, vomiting, hair loss, ulceration of mucous membranes, weakness, and malaise. Other possible effects include localized burns on tissue and damage to organs in the treatment path. Encourage the patient to discuss with the doctor (or the oncology nurse specialist) measures to relieve or minimize stress and discomfort.

- Advise the patient to immediately report any other symptoms to the doctor.
- Encourage the patient to get plenty of rest, eat a balanced diet, and drink plenty of fluids.

▶ Radiation Safety and Dose   LO 50.6

For many years after the X-ray's discovery, the seriousness of radiation hazards was not addressed. In the 1920s, the government of Great Britain took the first steps to limit X-ray exposure. Since World War II, studies have been performed, mostly on the effects of high-dose radiation.

Other studies on the effects of background radiation and nonradiologic versus radiologic (X-ray-related) risks have enabled scientists to assess diagnostic X-ray risks. Results from these studies show the risk of excess radiation from routine X-rays to be minimal.

Reducing Patient Exposure

Advances in diagnostic imaging technology, and limits to radiation exposure, have helped reduce the dose of radiation to which a patient is exposed during a diagnostic procedure. Another way to reduce excessive radiation exposure risk lies with the physician, who must assess the benefit-to-risk ratio when recommending a diagnostic radiology procedure. Because radiation has a cumulative effect, the physician must have valid medical reasons for ordering the test, particularly if the patient has recently had other X-rays. Some types of X-rays, such as mammograms, should be repeated regularly, however, because of their potential to prevent or promote treatment of life-threatening disorders.

According to a 1993 report by the National Council on Radiation Protection and Measurements (NCRP), titled *Limitation of Exposure to Ionizing Radiation,* one of the earliest pieces of legislation in the United States to limit occupational radiation exposure was enacted in the 1930s. The first legislation to limit public exposure, however, was not enacted until the 1950s. The 1993 NCRP report set guidelines for protection from radiation in and out of the workplace. The two primary objectives outlined in the report are to prevent serious general tissue damage from radiation by limiting radiation dose to levels below known thresholds for such damage and to reduce the risk of cancer and genetic effects to a level balanced by potential benefits to the individual and society.

Because radiation exposure always poses some degree of risk, the NCRP recommends that any activity involving radiation exposure be justified, or balanced against the expected benefits to society. Furthermore, the NCRP recommends the cost, or detriment, to society from such activities be kept *as low as reasonably achievable* (ALARA) and that individual dose limits be applied to ensure that justification and ALARA principles do not result in unacceptable risk levels for individuals or groups.

The NCRP has developed detailed lists on radiation doses to achieve the primary objectives stated in the report. Separate specific limits exist for occupational and public exposure.

Safety Precautions

Understanding and following standard safety precautions are crucial for protection from radiation exposure and are essential to the health and safety of both medical personnel and patients.

Personnel Safety If you work in a medical facility that performs radiologic tests, you are at risk for excessive radiation exposure. To protect yourself from exposure, you must adhere to the following guidelines:

- You (and other members of the medical staff) must always wear a radiation exposure badge, or dosimeter, which is a sensitized piece of film in a holder (Figure 50-9). You must have the badge checked regularly by specially qualified personnel, who measure the degree of radiation uptake on the film to determine the amount of radiation to which you have been exposed.
- Make sure all equipment is in good working order and is checked routinely for radiation leakage and any other problems.
- Be aware that the technician and any other staff members present when equipment is operating should always wear a garment that contains a lead shield.

Patient Safety You must follow all rules governing patient safety from radiation exposure. The *Educating the Patient* section explains safety measures and information that help protect a patient from exposure to unnecessary radiation.

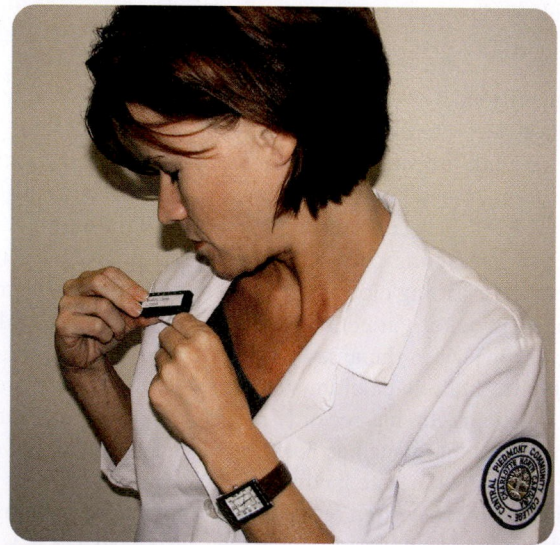

FIGURE 50-9   A radiation exposure badge contains a film that registers the levels of radiation to which a medical staff member is exposed at work.
© Total Care Programming, Inc.

EDUCATING THE PATIENT

Safety with X-rays

You are responsible for teaching the patient about X-ray safety. In this role, you will need to obtain pertinent patient history data, answer questions, and provide basic information on X-rays, possible side effects, and other important guidelines. Consider the following points when teaching the patient about X-ray safety.

Patient History

- Ask the patient about X-rays received in the past, including how many and what type, and about the possibility of exposure to radiation in the home, school, or workplace. Explain that the effects of radiation exposure are cumulative; that is, the effects are related to total exposure over the lifetime as well as to exposure from each procedure.

- Ask a female patient about the possibility of pregnancy. Use the 10-day rule—take an X-ray only within 10 days of the last menstrual period to avoid taking an X-ray of a patient who is unknowingly pregnant. If the patient knows she is pregnant, do not schedule an X-ray unless approved by the radiologist.

- Inform the patient about possible radiation exposure side effects, which include fetal abnormality or genetic mutation in a fetus (when a patient is pregnant) and the depression of bone marrow activity, which decreases the production of red blood cells and white blood cells.

Patient Questions

- Always answer questions in simple, easy-to-understand language; make explanations brief and clear. Do not use complex medical terms; however, do include proper terminology. Offer written information about the test, if available.

- Answer fully any questions about examinations, including descriptions of procedures; the doctor's reason for ordering them; their length, side effects, injections, or other uncomfortable aspects; preprocedure requirements; cost and insurance issues; and availability of test results.

- Help reduce the patient's fear or anxiety surrounding the scheduled test and help her feel comfortable and informed about the procedure.

General X-ray Information

- Be aware of the most current guidelines established by the American College of Radiology. Always keep up with new studies on radiation exposure risks.

- Encourage the patient to ask questions about the need for X-rays ordered by the doctor and risks associated with those X-rays.

- If the patient's employer requires annual X-rays or a potential employer asks for preemployment X-rays, advise the patient to question the necessity of these tests. Suggest that the patient find out whether the doctor has submittable X-rays on file.

- Advise the patient to discuss testing options with the doctor. For instance, if the doctor orders fluoroscopy, the patient might ask whether standard X-rays can be taken instead, as fluoroscopy, and often mobile X-ray exams, usually carry a higher radiation exposure risk than standard X-rays. Advise the patient to ask questions about X-ray safety standards in the office or hospital in which the tests are to take place.

- Tell the patient to avoid dental X-rays performed with wide-beamed plastic cones; narrow-beamed cones are more exact and less dangerous. In addition, educate the patient about the opinions of the American Dental Association and the National Conference of Dental Radiology, both of which believe X-rays should not be performed solely for insurance claim purposes. Advise the patient to always ask for a lead apron over organs not being studied. Tell the patient to avoid retakes of X-rays because of blurriness or shadows (which are caused by movements or breathing) by remaining still when instructed to do so during X-ray exams.

- Explain the importance of X-rays in proper diagnosis of disorders. Inform the patient about the constant improvements in equipment and X-ray procedures and the much lower doses of radiation now used in these procedures.

- Advise the patient to keep a family record of X-ray exams.

- Educate a female patient without breast disease on the correct schedule for mammography exams. The patient should have a baseline mammogram between ages 35 and 40; a mammogram every 1 to 2 years between ages 40 and 49; and an annual mammogram after age 50.

- Also, tell the patient to see a doctor immediately if she notices a breast mass, lump, or nipple discharge.

▶ Electronic Medicine   LO 50.7

Recent major advances in telemedicine technology, including rapid video and computer-based communications of medical information, enable physicians to "examine" a patient in another city or country, view highly detailed medical images, consult with specialists in other cities, and supervise complex medical procedures. In addition, healthcare personnel, including medical assistants, can participate in interactive teaching conferences by means of closed-circuit television.

In some cities, emergency medical technicians (EMTs) can transmit an electrocardiogram (ECG) electronically to an emergency room physician to obtain life-saving directives from the physician. These directives may involve administration of drugs or other measures the EMTs would not be permitted to perform without a physician's order. Similarly, cardiologists monitor some patients by the transmission of daily ECGs through telephone lines to the cardiologist's office.

Digital Imaging and the EHR

With the emergence of electronic health records (EHR), technology in healthcare is expanding rapidly. However, no department is affected more than radiology because it is the only completely technology-driven specialty. Digital radiology (DR) devices are integrated with the EHR system to provide quality images and rapid access and to eliminate the time and equipment associated with film processing and development (Figure 50-10).

Digital Radiography

Conventional, film-based radiography is quickly being replaced by digital imaging techniques. Digital radiography uses a digital reader to "capture" or digitize the X-ray image instead of exposing traditional film (Figure 50-11). Using digital radiography has several advantages, including:

- Better image consistency and quality
- Faster results
- Decreased radiation to patient
- Easier X-ray file sharing
- Simpler storage
- Environmentally safer (producing the image requires no chemicals)

Digital Imaging and Communications (DICOM)

in Medicine Digital Imaging and Communications is a communications protocol or standard for handling, storing,

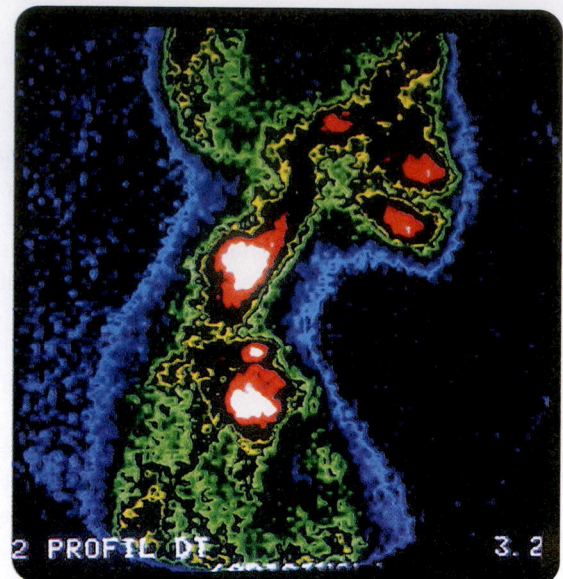

FIGURE 50-11 A digital bone scan of the neck and skull showing malignant tumors.
© SPL/Science Source

printing, and transmitting information in medical imaging. DICOM was designed as part of the Integrating the Healthcare Enterprise (IHE) initiative that makes it easier for medical systems to share information. A Picture Archive and Communication System (PAC) is the digital storage area where digital images are sent and stored for diagnostic viewing and electronic image storage and distribution.

Advances in Radiology

As radiology continues to experience technological changes, more advances are occurring to enhance digital imaging quality. Some major advances include 3D/4D ultrasound, which provides "live-action" images that allow physicians to observe fetal movement, study body organs, and guide needle biopsies (Figure 50-12).

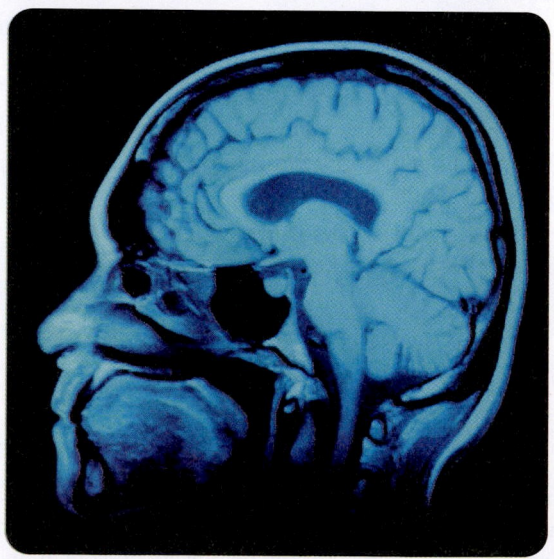

FIGURE 50-10 A digital sagittal MRI image of the brain.
© Royalty-Free/CORBIS

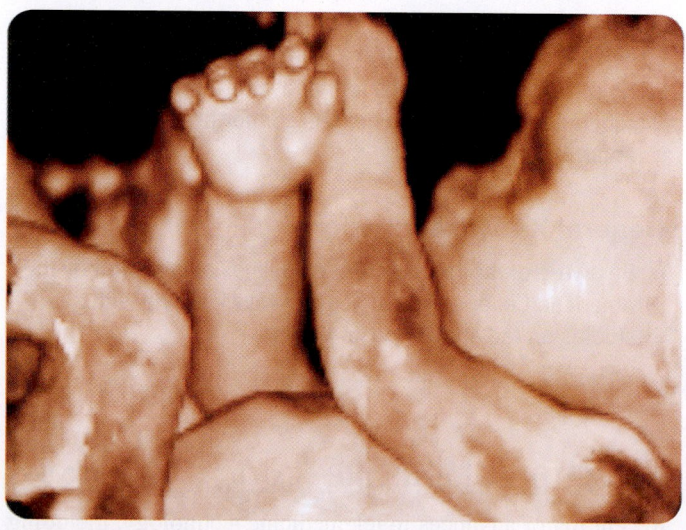

FIGURE 50-12 A 3D ultrasound shows the fetus in great detail.
© SPL/Science Source

PROCEDURE 50-1 Assisting with an X-ray Examination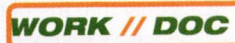

Procedure Goal: To assist with a radiologic procedure under the supervision of a radiologic technologist

OSHA Guidelines: This procedure does not involve exposure to blood, body fluids, or tissue. You must wear a radiation exposure badge (dosimeter), however, and will be required to wear a garment containing a lead or approved nonlead shield if you remain in the room during the operation of X-ray equipment.

Materials: Patient chart/progress note, X-ray examination order, X-ray machine, X-ray film and holder, X-ray film developer, drape, and patient shield

Method:

1. Check the X-ray examination order and equipment needed.

2. Identify the patient and introduce yourself.

3. Determine whether the patient has complied with the preprocedure instructions. Do not depend on the patient to inform you, but ask the patient if and how he prepped for the procedure.
   RATIONALE: *If a patient has not been compliant with preprocedural directions, then the test ordered may not be as effective as it should and will need to be rescheduled.*

4. Explain the procedure and the purpose of the examination to the patient.

5. Instruct the patient to remove clothing and all metals (including jewelry) as needed, according to the body area to be examined, and to put on a gown. Explain that metals may interfere with the image. Ask whether the patient has any surgical metal or a pacemaker and report this information to the radiologic technologist. Leave the room to ensure patient privacy.

Note: Steps 6 through 11 are nearly always performed by a radiologic technologist.

6. Position the patient according to the X-ray view ordered.

7. Drape the patient and place the patient shield appropriately.

8. Instruct the patient about the need to remain still and to hold the breath when requested.

9. Leave the room or stand behind a lead shield during the exposure.

10. Ask the patient to assume a comfortable position while the films are developed. Explain that X-rays sometimes must be repeated.

11. Develop the films.

12. Determine if the X-ray films are satisfactory by allowing the radiologist to review the films.
    RATIONALE: *The radiologist may want another film or view.*

13. Instruct the patient to dress and tell the patient when to contact the physician's office for the results.

14. Label the dry, finished X-ray films; place them in a properly labeled envelope; and file them according to your office's policies.

15. Record the X-ray examination, along with the final written findings, in the patient's chart (refer to Progress Note).

BWW PROGRESS NOTE	
Patient Name:	Harry Smitts
Date:	AP and lateral chest X-rays completed. Report added to medical record.
Author:	
	11/17/XX
	K. Booth
Done	Close

PROCEDURE 50-2 Documentation and Filing Techniques for X-rays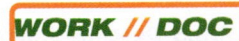

Procedure Goal: To document X-ray information and file X-ray films properly

OSHA Guidelines: This procedure does not involve exposure to blood, body fluids, or tissues.

Materials: X-ray film(s), patient X-ray record card or book, label, film-filing envelopes, film-filing cabinet, inserts, and a marking pen

Method:

1. Document the patient's X-ray information on the patient record card or in the record book. Include the patient's name, the date, the type of X-ray, and the number of X-rays taken.

		X-RAY EXAMINATIONS RECORD			
Patient	**Date**	**Type X-Ray**	**No. Taken**	**Referring Doctor**	**Comments**
Jill Cabot	2/16	Chest	4	Wapnir	
M. C. Gaines	2/16	Right knee	8	Wright	
J. Hale	2/19	Right wrist	6	McCarthy	
L. Becker	2/23	Left hip	4	Wright	
R. Bell	2/24	Chest	4	Wapnir	
Donna Lin	2/24	Sinuses	6	Harris	
Jon Carey	2/26	Right hand	2	Cohen	

FIGURE Procedure 50-2 Step 1   Keeping accurate records of patient X-ray information is an important duty of the medical assistant.

2. Verify that the film is properly labeled with the referring doctor's name, the date, and the patient's name. To note corrections or unusual positions or to identify a film that does not include labeling, attach the appropriate label and complete the necessary information. Some facilities also record the name of the radiologist who interpreted the X-ray.

   RATIONALE: *To reduce the likelihood of misidentifying a patient's X-ray.*

3. Place the processed film in a film-filing envelope. File the envelope alphabetically or chronologically (or according to your office's protocol) in the filing cabinet.

4. If you remove an envelope for any reason, put an insert or an "out card" in its place until it is returned to the cabinet.

   RATIONALE: *Proper filing techniques save time and prevent litigation.*

SUMMARY OF LEARNING OUTCOMES

LEARNING OUTCOMES	KEY POINTS
50.1 Explain what X-rays are and how they are used for diagnostic and therapeutic purposes.	An X-ray is a high-energy electromagnetic wave that travels at the speed of light and can penetrate solid objects. X-rays can be used for diagnosis by producing images of internal body structures. Therapeutically, X-rays are used to treat cancer by preventing cellular reproduction.
50.2 Compare invasive and noninvasive diagnostic procedures.	Invasive procedures require a radiologist to insert a catheter, wire, or other testing device into a patient's blood vessel or organ through the skin or a body orifice. Noninvasive diagnostic procedures do not require inserting devices, breaking the skin, or monitoring at the degree needed with invasive procedures.
50.3 Carry out the medical assistant's role in X-ray and diagnostic radiology testing.	A medical assistant can work directly with a radiology facility to assist the radiologist or technicians in performing diagnostic procedures. Providing preprocedure and postprocedure care are duties a medical assistant can perform in a medical or radiology facility.
50.4 Discuss common diagnostic imaging procedures.	Numerous diagnostic imaging procedures are used in medicine today, including angiography, fluoroscopy, MRI, CT, arthrography, IVP, KUB, mammography, stereotactic breast biopsy, upper and lower GI series, ultrasound, and bone densitometry.
50.5 Describe different types of radiation therapy and how they are used.	The two basic types of radiation therapy are teletherapy and brachytherapy. Teletherapy is also called external beam radiotherapy because an external beam of radiation is used to penetrate deep tumors. Brachytherapy uses temporary radioactive implants positioned close to or directly into cancerous tissue to treat the tumor and spare healthy tissue.
50.6 Explain the risks and safety precautions associated with radiology work.	The greatest risk associated with a radiology facility is the potential for radiation exposure to patients and healthcare workers. To eliminate this risk, certain safety precautions should be followed. These include careful evaluation by the physician to determine the medical necessity of radiology testing, avoidance of X-rays altogether if a patient is pregnant, and the requirement that all personnel who work in a radiology facility wear a dosimeter.

LEARNING OUTCOMES	KEY POINTS
50.7 **Relate the advances in medical imaging to EHR.**	Major advances in telemedicine technology, including rapid video and computer-based communications of medical information, enable physicians to "examine" a patient in another city or country, view highly detailed medical images, consult with specialists in other cities, and supervise complex medical procedures. Sharing records, including actual radiographic images, between facilities is easier with the advent of digital radiographic procedures and the electronic health record.

C A S E   S T U D Y   C R I T I C A L   T H I N K I N G

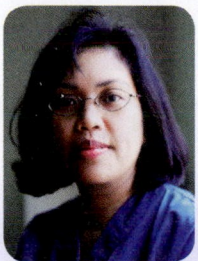

© ERproductions Ltd/Blend Images LLC RF

Recall Raja Lautu from the beginning of the chapter. Now that you have read the chapter, answer the following questions regarding her case.

1. What is the difference between brachytherapy and teletherapy?

2. What should you tell Raja to help prepare her for her radiation treatment?

3. What are the advantages of brachytherapy?

4. What instructions will you give Raja to prepare for her screening DXA test?

5. Why should the DXA be completed before the brachytherapy?

E X A M   P R E P A R A T I O N   Q U E S T I O N S

1. (LO 50.3) Which of the following would the medical assistant *least* likely perform?
   a. Performing stereotactic breast imaging
   b. Filing X-rays
   c. Providing preprocedure instruction for a mammogram
   d. Advising the patient to report symptoms after radiation treatment
   e. Assisting with an ultrasound

2. (LO 50.6) A dosimeter is used to
   a. Prevent radiation exposure
   b. Measure radiation exposure
   c. Measure the dose of medicine given during radiation treatments
   d. Monitor fluctuations in radiation exposure
   e. Determine how much radiation is needed to obtain an image

3. (LO 50.2) Which of the following is considered invasive?
   a. Chest X-ray
   b. Mammogram
   c. MRI
   d. Fluoroscopy
   e. Angiogram

4. (LO 50.4) What organs are evaluated with a KUB?
   a. Kidneys, ureters, bladder
   b. Kidneys, urethra, bladder
   c. Kidneys, ureters, bowels
   d. Kidneys, urethra, bowels
   e. Kidneys and urethra for blood

5. (LO 50.3) Which step in the X-ray procedure would *most* likely be performed by a medical assistant?
   a. Develop the films
   b. Evaluate the films
   c. Label the films
   d. Position the patient
   e. Set up the X-ray machine

6. (LO 50.2) A substance that makes internal organs denser and blocks the passage of X-rays to the photographic film is a
   a. Shielding material
   b. Dosimeter
   c. Radiolucent medication
   d. Digital reader
   e. Contrast medium

7. (LO 50.4) Which of the following is used to detect osteoporosis?
   a. Angiography
   b. DXA
   c. MUGA scan
   d. Lower GI series
   e. IVP

8. (LO 50.4) Hysterosalpingography is used to determine which of the following?
   a. Position of the kidneys
   b. Presence of gallstones
   c. Liver abscess
   d. Patency of the fallopian tubes
   e. Development of the fetus

9. (LO 50.5) Which of the following is used to treat tumors deep in the brain while sparing healthy tissue?
   a. Stereotactic radiosurgery
   b. Chemotherapy
   c. MRI
   d. Cerebral angiography
   e. Paramagnetic contrast

10. (LO 50.1) Wilhelm Konrad Roentgen is credited with discovering
   a. X-rays
   b. Photographic film
   c. Radiation therapy
   d. Magnetic resonance imaging
   e. SPECT scanning

SOFT SKILLS SUCCESS

Recall Raja Lautu from the case study at the beginning of the chapter. While reviewing the patient preparation information for the DXA scan with Raja, you notice she is distracted and looks worried. After you complete the instructions, you ask if she has any questions. Raja tells you that she doesn't understand why she is having the DXA before her brachytherapy and wants to know why she can't wait until they start the treatment for her breast cancer. What should you tell Raja about the timing of the DXA?

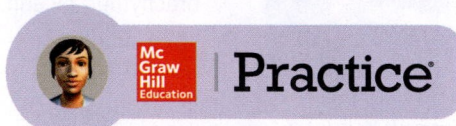

Go to PRACTICE MEDICAL OFFICE and complete the module Clinical - Interactions.

Principles of Pharmacology

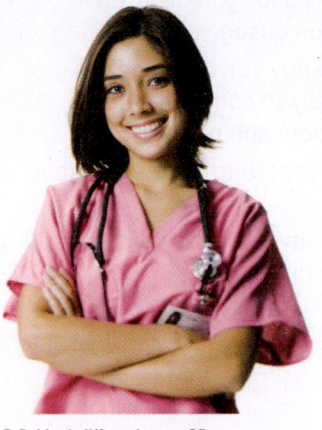

© Rubberball/Getty Images RF

to the samples and office medications, but the area is very disorganized. Kaylyn's first task will be to organize and implement an inventory system for the drugs. Kaylyn is concerned about her abilities because she has only been working for BWW Associates for a couple of months.

Keep Kaylyn Haddix, RMA (AMT), in mind as you study the chapter.

There will be questions at the end of the chapter based on the case study. The information in the chapter will help you answer these questions.

LEARNING OUTCOMES

After completing Chapter 51, you will be able to:

51.1 Identify the medical assistant's role in pharmacology.

51.2 Recognize the five categories of pharmacology and their importance to medication administration.

51.3 Differentiate the major drug categories, drug names, and their actions.

51.4 Classify over-the-counter (OTC), prescription, and herbal drugs.

51.5 Use credible sources to obtain drug information.

51.6 Carry out the procedure for registering or renewing a physician with the Drug Enforcement Administration (DEA) for permission to administer, dispense, and prescribe controlled drugs.

51.7 Identify the parts of a prescription, including commonly used abbreviations and symbols.

51.8 Discuss nonpharmacologic treatments for pain.

51.9 Describe how vaccines work in the immune system.

KEY TERMS

administer	opioid
adverse effects	package insert
controlled substance	pharmacodynamics
dispense	pharmacognosy
efficacy	pharmacokinetics
e-prescribing	pharmacology
generic name	pharmacotherapeutics
indication	prescribe
labeling	side effects
magnetic therapy	toxicology
narcotic	trade name

I.C.11 Identify the classifications of medications including:
- (a) indications for use
- (b) desired effects
- (c) side effects
- (d) adverse reactions

II.C.5 Identify abbreviations and symbols used in calculating medication dosages

V.P.3 Use medical terminology correctly and pronounced accurately to communicate information to providers and patients

X.P.5 Perform compliance reporting based on public health statutes

X.P.6 Report an illegal activity in the healthcare setting following the proper protocol

3. Medical Terminology
- d. Define and use medical abbreviations when appropriate and acceptable

4. Medical Law and Ethics
- f. Comply with federal, state, and local health laws and regulations as they relate to healthcare settings

6. Pharmacology
- a. Identify drug classification, usual dose, side effects, and contraindications of the top most commonly used medications
- c. Prescriptions
  - (1) Identify parts of prescriptions
  - (2) Identify appropriate abbreviations that are accepted in prescription writing
  - (3) Comply with legal aspects of creating prescriptions, including federal and state laws
- d. Properly utilize Physician's Desk Reference (PDR), drug handbook and other drug references to identify a drug's classification, usual dosage, usual side effects, and contraindications
- e. Comply with federal, state, and local health laws and regulations

7. Records Management
- a. Perform basic keyboarding skills (i.e. Microsoft Word, etc.)

8. Administrative Procedures
- a. Gather and process documents

▶ Introduction

Pharmacology—the science of drugs—is a great responsibility of allied health professionals. Medication mistakes can injure or even cause the death of a patient. Before you administer drugs, it is important to begin with a good working knowledge of the foundations of pharmacology, including how medications work, how they should be taken, and what problems can occur when they are taken. This chapter provides an overview of the role of drugs in ambulatory healthcare facilities.

▶ The Medical Assistant's Role in Pharmacology
LO 51.1

As a medical assistant, you will be expected to have a basic knowledge of medications. This includes knowledge of prescription drugs and over-the-counter (OTC) drugs. Prescription drugs require a licensed practitioner's written order to authorize the dispensing (and, sometimes, administering) of drugs to a patient. OTC drugs—available in pharmacies and supermarkets—are purchased by people to treat themselves for ailments ranging from arthritis to colds to stomach ulcers. As a medical assistant you will need to

- Ensure that the licensed practitioner is aware of all medications a patient is taking, both prescription and OTC, as well as vitamins and herbal remedies.
- Ask each patient about alcohol and recreational drug use (both past and present).
- Assist in managing and renewing medication prescriptions.
- Educate the patient, using guidelines provided by the licensed practitioner, about the purpose of a drug and how to take the drug for maximum effectiveness and minimum side effects.

As your state and scope of practice permit, you also may be asked to enter medication orders and give drugs to a patient. Safe and effective drug therapy requires additional knowledge and special skills. To handle these important functions, you must understand pharmacologic principles and sources of drug

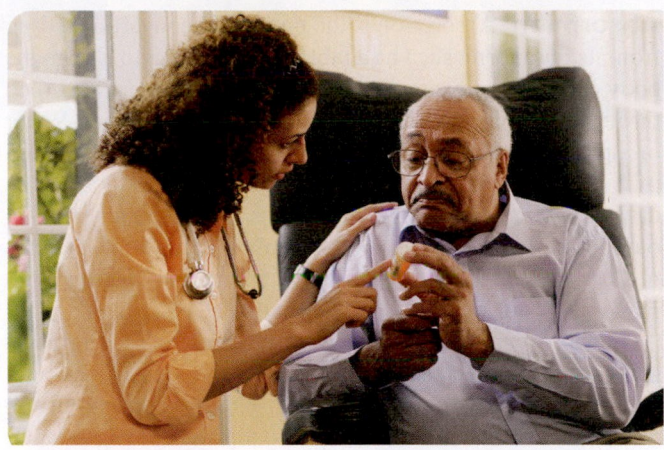

FIGURE 51-1 A medical assistant may need to be prepared to answer the patient's questions about a drug the doctor is prescribing.
© Fuse/Getty Images

information, be able to read prescriptions accurately, and be prepared to answer basic patient questions (Figure 51-1). You also must adhere to legal requirements and keep accurate records. Additionally, the Centers for Medicare and Medicaid Services (CMS) ruled in September 2012 that credentialed medical assistants may enter medication orders into a computerized order entry system. This is another excellent reason to become a credentialed medical assistant once you complete your program.

▶ Pharmacology
LO 51.2

A drug is a chemical compound used to prevent, diagnose, or treat a disease or other abnormal condition. The study of drugs is called **pharmacology**. A specialist in pharmacology is called a *pharmacologist*. Included in pharmacology are

- **Pharmacognosy** (the study of characteristics of natural drugs and their sources).
- **Pharmacodynamics** (the study of what drugs do to the body).
- **Pharmacokinetics** (the study of what the body does to drugs).
- **Pharmacotherapeutics** (the study of how drugs are used to treat disease).
- **Toxicology** (the study of poisons or poisonous effects of drugs).

According to the Department of Justice's Drug Enforcement Administration (DEA) guidelines, a doctor **prescribes** a drug when he gives a patient a prescription to be filled by a pharmacy. To **administer** a drug is to give it directly by injection, by mouth, or by any other route that introduces the drug into a patient's body. A healthcare professional **dispenses** a drug by distributing it, in a properly labeled container, to a patient who is directed to use it.

Sources of Drugs (Pharmacognosy)
Many drugs originate as natural products. Other drugs are developed in the chemical laboratory, as chemists seek to improve existing drugs.

Natural Products Most often, drugs originate as substances from natural products, such as plants, animals, minerals, bacteria, or fungi. For hundreds of years, drugs have been made from seeds, bulbs, roots, stems, buds, leaves, and other parts of plants. Two examples of plant-derived drugs are digitoxin, which comes from the foxglove plant (see Figure 51-2), and quinine, which comes from cinchona tree bark. Digitoxin is used to treat heart failure and abnormal heartbeats. Quinine is used to treat malaria.

Animals also are used as a source of drugs. Certain animal substances have been shown to be compatible with human physiology. Some examples of animal substances used as drugs are glandular substances, such as thyroid hormones; fats and oils, such as cod-liver oil; enzymes, such as pancreatin and pepsin; and antiserums and antitoxins for vaccines.

Mineral sources yield various substances that can be used as they occur naturally or mixed with other substances. Two drugs derived from mineral sources are potassium chloride and mineral oil. Simple organisms, such as bacteria and fungi, produce substances that are used to make certain antibiotics, such as cephalosporins and penicillins (see Figure 51-3).

Chemical Development A chemist conducts investigations that lead to the synthesis (creation) of drugs based on a natural substance's chemical properties. Some drugs are synthesized by strictly chemical methods. Others are created by manipulating genetic information in a host organism. For example, human insulin is produced by these means, also known as *recombinant deoxyribonucleic acid (DNA)* techniques.

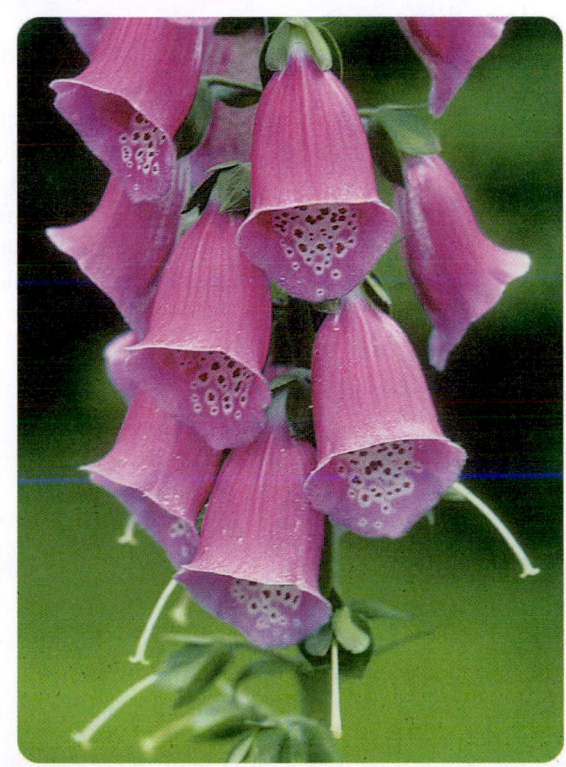

FIGURE 51-2 The foxglove plant, shown here, is the natural source for the medication digitoxin.
© Stephen P. Lynch

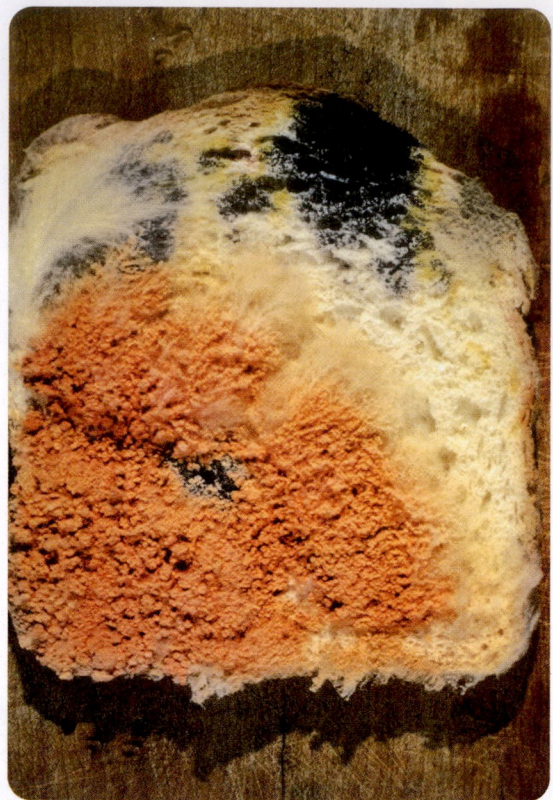

FIGURE 51-3 Bacteria, fungi, and yeasts are natural sources of antibiotics.
© Phototake

Pharmacodynamics

Pharmacodynamics is the study of the mechanism of action, or how the drug works to produce a therapeutic effect. Drugs are placed in categories based on their mechanism of action. Pharmacodynamics includes the interaction between the drug and target cells or tissues and the body's response to that interaction. For example, when a patient with diabetes takes insulin, the drug acts by allowing the movement of glucose across cell membranes. This movement makes the glucose available to cells to use as an energy source. The end result is a decrease in the blood glucose level.

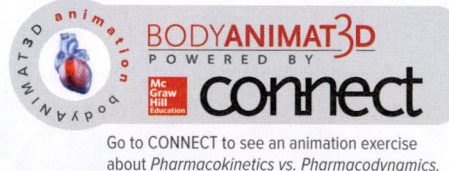

Go to CONNECT to see an animation exercise about *Pharmacokinetics vs. Pharmacodynamics.*

Pharmacokinetics

Pharmacokinetics is what the body does to a drug—that is, how the body absorbs, distributes, metabolizes, and excretes the drug. It is important to understand these processes so that you will be able to explain to patients the reasons for taking a particular drug with food or for drinking plenty of water while taking a drug. These four processes can be remembered by using the acronym ADME: **A**bsorption–**D**istribution–**M**etabolism–**E**xcretion.

Absorption Absorption is the process of converting a drug from its dose form, such as a tablet or capsule, into a form the body can use. For example, tablets and capsules are absorbed through the stomach or intestines into the bloodstream. Water or a particular food may either hinder or assist the absorption of a specific drug through the stomach or intestines. Some drugs may irritate the digestive organs if they are taken without food or water. Because of such possible reactions, patients must precisely follow instructions for taking a drug with plenty of water, with food, or without food.

Injected drugs are absorbed through the skin (intradermally), through the tissue just beneath the skin (subcutaneously), or through muscle (intramuscularly), depending on the method of injection. Absorption allows the drug to enter the bloodstream and pass into tissues. The extent and rate of drug absorption depend on several factors, including the route of administration. When the drug is administered by mouth, for example, coatings on tablets or capsules and the amount and type of food consumed with the drug may affect absorption. Drugs administered intravenously do not require absorption; they are directly available to target cells from the bloodstream.

Distribution Distribution is the process of transporting a drug from its administration site, such as the muscle of an injection site, to its site of action. Distribution also pertains to the length of time a drug takes to achieve maximum or peak plasma levels—that is, the length of time between dosing and availability in the bloodstream.

Metabolism Drug metabolism is the process by which drug molecules are transformed into simpler products called *metabolites.* This transformation usually occurs in the liver, where enzymes break down the drug. Some drugs, however, are metabolized in the kidneys. Metabolism can be affected by disease, a patient's age or genetic makeup, a drug's characteristics, and other factors. When drugs metabolized in the liver are prescribed for either children or the elderly, the dose is likely to be lower than that prescribed for young adults. Metabolism in children and the elderly is different from metabolism in other patients; the drugs may remain in the body longer and possibly reach harmful levels. The same concern holds true for any patient with impaired liver or kidney function if prescribed drugs are metabolized in the affected organ.

Excretion *Excretion* describes the manner in which a drug is eliminated from the body. Most drugs are eliminated in urine. Drugs also may be excreted in feces, perspiration, saliva, bile, exhaled air, and breast milk.

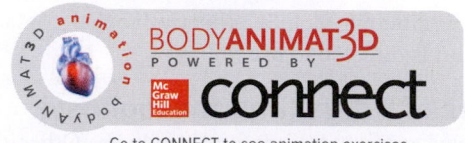

Go to CONNECT to see animation exercises about *Medication Absorption, Medication Distribution, Medication Metabolism,* and *Medication Excretion.*

Pharmacotherapeutics

Pharmacotherapeutics is the study of how drugs are used to treat disease. This area of pharmacology is sometimes called *clinical pharmacology*. Pharmacotherapeutics includes topics such as drug categories, drug indications and labeling, safety, **efficacy** (therapeutic value), and kinds of therapy.

Indications and Labeling An **indication** is the purpose or reason for using a drug. The Food and Drug Administration (FDA) must approve indications before they can become part of a drug's **labeling.** The FDA is an agency of the Department of Health and Human Services. It regulates the manufacture and distribution of every drug used in the United States. Labeling also includes the form of the drug, such as tablet or liquid. Regardless of category, some drugs may be used to treat several different conditions. Multiple uses are possible if the drug affects several body systems at once or if the drug's primary effect produces significant secondary effects in other body systems.

When a drug is used for multiple indications, one or more indications might not be in its labeling. Off-label prescribing is legal. For example, Benadryl® (diphenhydramine) is an antihistamine used to treat allergic symptoms in both children and adults. Because it tends to make a patient sleepy but is safe for children, a pediatrician may use a low dose of Benadryl® as a temporary sedative for a young child. Its use as a sedative, however, is not part of the labeling for Benadryl®.

Another example of a drug with multiple uses is minoxidil. As a trade-name tablet, it is known as the antihypertensive Loniten; as a trade-name topical solution, it is known as the hair-growth stimulant Rogaine®. In the case of minoxidil, both indications are approved, but the tablet labeling is for hypertension and the topical solution labeling is for hair growth. It is important to be aware of these labeling considerations when dealing with questions from patients. Never assume a drug is appropriate for only one use or administered in only one form. Always consult the licensed practitioner or other approved source of drug information before answering a patient's question.

Safety The safety of a drug is determined by how many and what kinds of adverse reactions are associated with it. Adverse reactions include both side effects and adverse effects. **Side effects** are unintended but fairly mild and common effects of a medication. For example, patients may experience constipation as a side effect of taking codeine for pain. Side effects generally are not severe enough to warrant stopping a medication. Some side effects are common, whereas others are rare. **Adverse effects** are potentially more harmful, but less common, effects. For example, reported adverse effects of Benadryl® include confusion and disturbed coordination. A patient experiencing these effects may be told to stop taking Benadryl® because the adverse effects outweigh the benefit of taking the medication. An adverse effect may require immediate attention.

It is not uncommon for a patient to call the physician's office with complaints of new symptoms soon after beginning therapy with a drug. Be alert for such complaints because they might be signs of an adverse reaction to the drug or an interaction with another medication. These calls should be brought to the attention of the licensed practitioner.

Efficacy A patient may complain that a newly prescribed drug is not doing what the doctor said it would. There are a variety of possible explanations for such a complaint, including

- The drug is working adequately, but the patient does not understand how it works.
- The dosage (size, frequency, and number of doses) needs to be adjusted.
- The patient is not taking the medication according to the directions.
- The drug has not yet reached a therapeutic level in the bloodstream.
- The wrong drug was prescribed, or the wrong drug was dispensed by the pharmacy (this is rare, but possible).
- Some drugs work better in some patients than in others; not every drug is for everyone (this is particularly true of antihistamines).
- Some forms of a drug work better than others, such as tablets versus injection.
- The generic drug does not work, but the trade-name drug does. A generic drug may not work because it is made with additional or different inert (not active) ingredients. These inert ingredients could interfere with the drug's active ingredient or could change the patient's response to the medication.

Kinds of Therapy Depending on a patient's condition, the licensed practitioner may use drugs for any of the following kinds of therapy:

- Acute: drug is prescribed to improve a life-threatening or serious condition, such as epinephrine for severe allergic reaction
- Empiric: drug is prescribed according to experience or observation until blood or other tests prove another therapy to be appropriate, such as penicillin for suspected strep throat
- Maintenance: drug is prescribed to maintain health or protect against exacerbations of a condition, especially in chronic disease, such as an anti-inflammatory medication for inflammatory bowel disease
- Palliative: drug is prescribed to reduce the severity of symptoms of a condition such as its accompanying pain. For example, morphine is given to reduce the pain caused by cancer
- Prophylactic: drug is prescribed to prevent a disease or condition, such as immunizations or birth control drugs
- Replacement: drug is prescribed to provide chemicals otherwise missing in a patient, such as hormone replacement therapy for a woman in menopause
- Supportive: drug is prescribed for a condition other than the primary disease until that disease resolves, such as a corticosteroid for severe allergic reactions
- Supplemental: drug or nutrients are prescribed to avoid deficiency, such as iron for a woman who is pregnant

Toxicology

Toxicology is the study of the poisonous effects, or toxicity, of drugs, including adverse effects and drug interactions. In addition to immediate toxic effects that can occur when drugs are administered, you must be aware of some possible toxic effects that may not be apparent right away:

- An adverse effect on a fetus when the drug crosses the placenta
- An adverse effect on infants when the drug passes easily into breast milk
- Adverse reactions reported in clinical trials, such as headache, drowsiness, gastric upset, or other effects
- An adverse effect in immunocompromised patients who are unable to metabolize a drug normally
- An adverse effect in pediatric or elderly patients or in patients with hypertension, diabetes mellitus, or other serious chronic conditions
- An adverse drug interaction when the drug is taken with another drug or food that is incompatible
- A carcinogenic (cancer-causing) effect in some patients

Adverse reactions are nearly always encountered during the clinical trials of a drug, and there will be mention of these reactions under that heading in the package insert or in accepted drug reference works. In the reports of clinical trials, the drug company must report all adverse reactions noted during testing. As a result, all of the adverse reactions that, at least theoretically, could be caused by the drug are included.

In dealing with patients who are about to begin drug therapy, use discretion when mentioning specific adverse reactions associated with drugs. The patient must be informed; however, you do not want to cause undue alarm or discourage patients from taking the needed medication. Always ask patients if they have any questions and have the licensed practitioner answer patients' drug-related questions. Because patients will receive lists of possible adverse reactions from the pharmacist, encourage them to discuss concerns with the pharmacist or to call the practitioner's office. Also encourage patients to inform the practitioner of adverse reactions they experience after beginning drug therapy.

▶ Drug Names and Categories   LO 51.3

One drug may have several different names, including the drug's **generic name** (official, nonproprietary name), chemical name, and **trade name** (brand, or proprietary name). For instance, the trade-name cholesterol-lowering drug prescribed by authorized prescribers as Mevacor® or Altoprev® is also identified by the following names:

- Lovastatin (generic name)
- 2-methyl-1S,2,3R,7S,8S,8aR-hexahydro-3,7-dimethyl-8-[2-[2(2R,4R)-tetrahydro-4-hydroxy-6-oxo-2H-pyran-2-yl] ethyl-1-naphthalenyl ester, butanoic acid (chemical name)

As a medical assistant, you will probably need to use only generic and trade names. In general, think of the generic name of a drug as a simple form of its chemical name. For each new drug

marketed by a manufacturer, the United States Adopted Names (USAN) Council selects a generic name. This name is nonproprietary, meaning it does not belong to any one manufacturer. A generic name is also considered a drug's official name, which is listed in the *United States Pharmacopeia/National Formulary.*

A drug's manufacturer selects the drug's trade name, which is protected by copyright and is the property of the manufacturer. When a new drug enters the market, its manufacturer has a patent on that drug, which means that no other manufacturer can make or sell the drug for 17 years. When the patent runs out, any manufacturer can sell the drug under the generic name or a different trade name. The original manufacturer, however, is the only one allowed to use the drug's original trade name. For example, the antibiotic amoxicillin has two trade names, Amoxil® and Prevpac®. A different manufacturer owns each of these names.

A licensed practitioner may prescribe a drug by its generic or trade name. Because generic drugs are usually less expensive, most practitioners try to prescribe them if possible. Many states allow pharmacists to substitute a generic drug for a trade-name drug unless the practitioner specifies otherwise. In fact, most health insurance prescription plans require the substitution of generic drugs for trade-name drugs (unless otherwise specified by a licensed practitioner). Frequently, they also require the pharmacy to charge a higher copay amount for trade-name drugs than for generic drugs. Some prescription plans offer a mail-in pharmacy, through which a patient can obtain generic drugs with a reduced copayment or without any copayment.

Drugs are categorized by their action on the body, general therapeutic effect, or body system affected. Table 51-1 lists a variety of drug categories, their actions, and common drugs, including drugs from the top 200 drugs most commonly prescribed in the year 2014.

▶ FDA Regulation and Drugs   LO 51.4

The Food and Drug Administration (FDA) requires that drug manufacturers perform clinical tests on new drugs before humans use the drugs. These tests include toxicity tests in laboratory animals, followed by clinical studies (clinical trials) in controlled groups of volunteers. Some volunteers are patients; others are healthy subjects. Clinical tests are designed to consider the ratio of benefits to the risk of adverse reactions. If the clinical tests prove the drug is safe and effective, the FDA approves it for marketing. The manufacturer must continue to demonstrate the drug's safety and efficacy and must submit reports whenever it discovers unexpected adverse reactions. The FDA can withdraw a drug from the market at any time if evidence suggests it is no longer safe or effective. This is known as a *recall.*

The FDA also regulates drug manufacturing. It ensures that drugs shipped between states have the proper identity, strength, purity, and quality. Each manufacturer must consistently identify each drug by a particular color, form, shape, size, and label. It must produce every dose at the same tested strength, using the exact formula approved by the FDA. The manufacturer also must use high-quality, contaminant-free ingredients. The FDA regulates all drugs, including over-the-counter, prescription, and even complementary and alternative medicine (CAM). See *Points on Practice:* The FDA and CAM Therapies. To

TABLE 51-1 Drug Categories and Actions for Commonly Prescribed Drugs

Drug Category	Action of Drug	Examples* Generic Name (Trade Name)
Analgesic	Relieves mild to severe pain	Acetaminophen (Tylenol®); acetylsalicylic acid, or aspirin; morphine sulfate (MS Contin®)*; oxycodone HCl (Oxycontin®)*
Anesthetic	Prevents sensation of pain (generally, locally, or topically)	Lidocaine HCl (Xylocaine®, Lidoderm®)*; tetracaine HCl (Pontocaine®)
Antacid/antiulcer	Neutralizes stomach acid	Calcium carbonate (Tums®); esomeprazole (Nexium®)*; lansoprazole (Prevacid®); pantoprazole sodium (Protonix®)*
Anthelmintic	Kills, paralyzes, or inhibits the growth of parasitic worms	Mebendazole (Vermox®); pyrantel pamoate (Combantrin®, Antiminth®)
Antidysrythmic (antiarrhythmic)	Normalizes heartbeat in cases of certain cardiac arrhythmias	Disopyramide phosphate (Norpace®); propafenone HCl (Rythmol®); propranolol HCl (Inderal®)
Antiasthmatic	Treats or prevents asthma attacks	Montelukast (Singulair®)*; fluticasone propionate/salmeterol (Advair Diskus®)*; albuterol (ProAir HFA®)*
Antibiotics (antibacterial)	Kills bacterial microorganisms or inhibits their growth	Amoxicillin (Amoxil®)*; azithromycin (Zithromax®)*; cefprozil (Cefzil®); ciprofloxacin (Cipro®)*; clarithromycin (Biaxin® XL); clindamycin (Cleocin®)*
Anticholinergic	Blocks parasympathetic nerve impulses	Atropine sulfate (Isopto® Atropine); dicyclomine HCl (Bentyl®); ipratropium (Atrovent®)
Anticoagulant	Prevents blood from clotting	Enoxaparin sodium (Lovenox®); heparin sodium (Hep-Lock®); warfarin sodium (Coumadin®)*
Anticonvulsant	Relieves or controls seizures (convulsions)	Clonazepam (Klonopin®)*; divalproex (Depakote®); phenobarbital sodium (Luminol® Sodium); phenytoin (Dilantin®)
Antidepressant (four types)	Relieves depression	
Tricyclic		Amitriptyline HCl (Elavil); doxepin HCl (Sinequan®)
Monoamine oxidase inhibitor (MAOI)		Phenelzine sulfate (Nardil®); tranylcypromine sulfate (Parnate®)
Selective serotonin reuptake inhibitor (SSRI)		Escitalopram (Lexapro®)*; fluoxetine HCl (Prozac®); paroxetine (Paxil®)*; sertraline HCl (Zoloft®)*
Serotonin-norepinephrine reuptake inhibitor (SNRI)		Venlafaxine HCl (Effexor XR®)*; duloxetine HCl (Cymbalta®)*
Antidiabetic	Treats diabetes by reducing glucose	Metformin (Glucophage®)*; glipizide (Glucotrol®) pioglitazone HCl (Actos®)*; insulin glargine (Lantus®)*
Antidiarrheal	Relieves diarrhea	Bismuth subsalicylate (Pepto-Bismol®); kaolin and pectin mixtures (Kaopectate®); loperamide HCl (Imodium®)
Antiemetic	Prevents or relieves nausea and vomiting	Prochlorperazine (Compazine®); promethazine (Phenergan®); trimethobenzamide HCl (Tigan®)
Antifungal	Kills or inhibits growth of fungi	Amphotericin B (Fungizone®); fluconazole (Diflucan®)*; nystatin (Mycostatin®); terbinafine (Lamisil®)
Antihistamine	Counteracts effects of histamine and relieves allergic symptoms	Cetirizine HCl (Zyrtec®); diphenhydramine HCl (Benadryl®); fexofenadine (Allegra®); desloratadine (Clarinex®)
Antihypertensive	Reduces blood pressure	Amlodipine (Norvasc®)*; diltiazem HCl (Cartia XL®); quinapril (Prinivil®); metoprolol succinate (Toprol-XL®)*; valsartan (Diovan®)*
Anti-inflammatory (two types)	Reduces inflammation	
Nonsteroidal (NSAIDs)		Naproxen (Aleve)*; colchicine* (Colcrys®); ibuprofen (Motrin®, Advil®)*; celecoxib (Celebrex®)*
Steroids		Dexamethasone (Decadron®); methylprednisolone (Medrol®)*; prednisone (Deltasone™)*; triamcinolone (Kenalog®)*

(Continued)

TABLE 51-1 Drug Categories and Actions for Commonly Prescribed Drugs

Drug Category	Action of Drug	Examples* Generic Name (Trade Name)
Antilipemic (antilipidemic)	Lowers blood lipids such as triglycerides	Gemfibrozil (Lopid®); atorvastatin (Lipitor®)*; fenofibrate (TriCor®)*; ezetimibe/simvastatin (Vytorin®)*; ezetimibe (Zetia®)*; rosuvastatin (Crestor®)*
Antineoplastic	Prevents or inhibits the growth of cancer	Bleomycin sulfate (Blenoxane®); dactinomycin (Cosmegen®); paclitaxel (Taxol®); tamoxifen citrate (Nolvadex®)
Antipsychotic	Controls psychotic symptoms	Chlorpromazine HCl (Thorazine®); clozapine (Clozaril®); haloperidol (Haldol®); risperidone (Risperdal®)*; thioridazine HCl (Mellaril®)
Antipyretic	Reduces fever	Acetaminophen (Tylenol®); acetylsalicyclic acid, or aspirin
Antiseptic	Inhibits growth of microorganisms	Isopropyl alcohol; 70% povidone-iodine (Betadine®); chlorhexidine gluconate (PerioChip®)
Antitussive	Inhibits cough reflex	Codeine; dextromethorphan hydrobromide (component of Robitussin® DM)
Bronchodilator	Dilates bronchi (airways in the lungs)	Albuterol (Proventil®)*; epinephrine (Epinephrine Mist); salmeterol (Serevent®); tiotropium bromide (Spiriva®)*
Cathartic (laxative)	Induces defecation, alleviates constipation	Bisacodyl (Dulcolax®); casanthranol (Peri-Colace®); magnesium hydroxide (Milk of Magnesia®)
Contraceptive	Reduces risk of pregnancy	Ethinyl estradiol and norgestimate (Ortho Tri-Cyclen®); norethindrone and ethinyl estradiol (Loestrin® 24 Fe)* norgestrel (Ovrette®)
Decongestant	Relieves nasal swelling and congestion	Oxymetazoline HCl (Afrin®); phenylephrine HCl (Neo-Synephrine®); pseudoephedrine HCl (Sudafed®)
Diuretic	Increases urine output, reduces blood pressure and cardiac output	Bumetanide (Bumex®); furosemide (Lasix®)*; hydrochlorothiazide (HydroDIURIL®)*; mannitol (Osmitrol®); spironolactone (Aldactone®)
Expectorant	Liquefies mucus in bronchi; allows expectoration of sputum, mucus, and phlegm	Guaifenesin (Mucinex®)
Hemostatic	Controls or stops bleeding by promoting coagulation	Aminocaproic acid (Amicar®); phytonadione or vitamin K_1 (Mephyton®); thrombin (Thrombogen)
Hormone replacement	Replaces or resolves hormone deficiency	Insulin (Humulin®) for pancreatic deficiency; levothyroxine sodium (Synthroid®)* for thyroid deficiency; conjugated estrogens (Premarin Tabs®)*
Hypnotic (sleep-inducing) or sedative	Induces sleep or relaxation (depending on drug potency and dosage)	Chloral hydrate (Noctec®); secobarbital sodium (Seconal® Sodium); zolpidem (Ambien®)*
Muscle relaxant	Relaxes skeletal muscles	Carisoprodol (Rela or Soma®); cyclobenzaprine HCl (Flexeril®)*
Mydriatic	Constricts vessels of eye or nasal passage, raises blood pressure, dilates pupil of eye in ophthalmic preparations	Atropine sulfate (Atropisol) for ophthalmic use; phenylephrine HCl (Alcon Efrin) for ophthalmic use or (Neo-Synephrine®) for nasal use
Stimulant (central nervous system)	Increases activity of brain and other organs, decreases appetite	Amphetamine sulfate (Benzedrine); caffeine (No-Doz®); also a component of many analgesic formulations and coffee
Vasoconstrictor	Constricts blood vessels, increases blood pressure	Dopamine HCl (Intropin); norepinephrine bitartrate (Levophed®)
Vasodilator	Dilates blood vessels, decreases blood pressure	Enalopril (Vasotec®); lisinopril (Prinivil®)*; nitroglycerin (Nitrostat®, NitroQuick®)

*Indicates top 200 commonly prescribed drugs in the year 2014.

Sources: RXList, http://www.rxlist.com.

help regulate the safety of drugs, the FDA has a program called MedWatch for voluntary reporting of adverse events noted during clinical care. An adverse event is any undesirable experience for a patient associated with the use of a medical product. Reporting of these events is done on the FDA site at http://www.fda.gov/Safety/MedWatch/default.htm.

Over-the-Counter Drugs

A nonprescription, or over-the-counter (OTC), drug is one the FDA has approved for use without a licensed healthcare practitioner's supervision. The consumer must follow the manufacturer's directions to use the drug safely. Some drugs, such as aspirin and vitamin supplements, have been OTC drugs for many years. The number of prescription drugs granted OTC status is increasing. Although OTC drugs are safe when used as directed on the package, patient education contributes significantly to their safe use.

Prescription Drugs

A prescription drug is one that can be used only by order of a licensed practitioner. It must be dispensed by a licensed healthcare professional, such as a pharmacist, physician, podiatrist, or licensed midwife. Some prescription drugs are available at much lower strengths as OTC medications.

Pregnancy Categories

Because clinical trials are not typically done on pregnant women, most of the data about the effect of medications on pregnant women are obtained after FDA approval. Drugs can cause defects to the fetus if taken during pregnancy. Prior to June 2015, drugs were labeled as a category A, B, C, D, or X based on the degree to which information has ruled out risk to the fetus. In June 2015, more comprehensive labeling requirements were set for three categories: Pregnancy, Lactation, and Females and Males of Reproductive Potential. The new

---

POINTS ON PRACTICE
The FDA and CAM Therapies

Complementary and alternative medicine (CAM) such as dietary supplements, herbal products, and other natural but as yet scientifically unproven therapies are increasing in use. Many licensed practitioners prescribe these therapies and even more patients take them on their own with positive effects.

There is one important difference between dietary supplements and medications. Medications must earn FDA approval prior to being marketed and sold. Drug manufacturers must provide scientific documentation of the effectiveness of a drug before it can be marketed. On the other hand, manufacturers of dietary supplements do not have to provide evidence of effectiveness or safety. Of course, they are not permitted to market or sell a product that is proven unsafe. However, once a supplement is marketed, the FDA must prove that the product is not safe to have it taken from the market. Additionally, dietary supplements are not standardized between batches or among manufacturers. Standardization is a process that ensures the consistency and quality of each batch of supplement produced. Thus, the amount and quality of a dietary supplement may differ between batches produced by one manufacturer or between the same supplement made by two different manufacturers. FDA-approved medications must be standardized and will always be consistent between batches and manufacturers.

The FDA does require that certain information appear on dietary supplement labels. Dietary supplements may include claims on their labels that describe the effect of a substance in maintaining the body's normal structure or function. For example, a label might state "Promotes healthy joints and bones." The FDA does not review or authorize this claim, so the manufacturer is also required to place a disclaimer on the product. This disclaimer is a statement indicating that the claims have not been evaluated by the FDA—for example, "This statement has not been evaluated by the Food and Drug

Administration. This product is not intended to diagnose, treat, cure, or prevent disease." Figure 51-4 shows an example of a label that meets the FDA's labeling requirements.

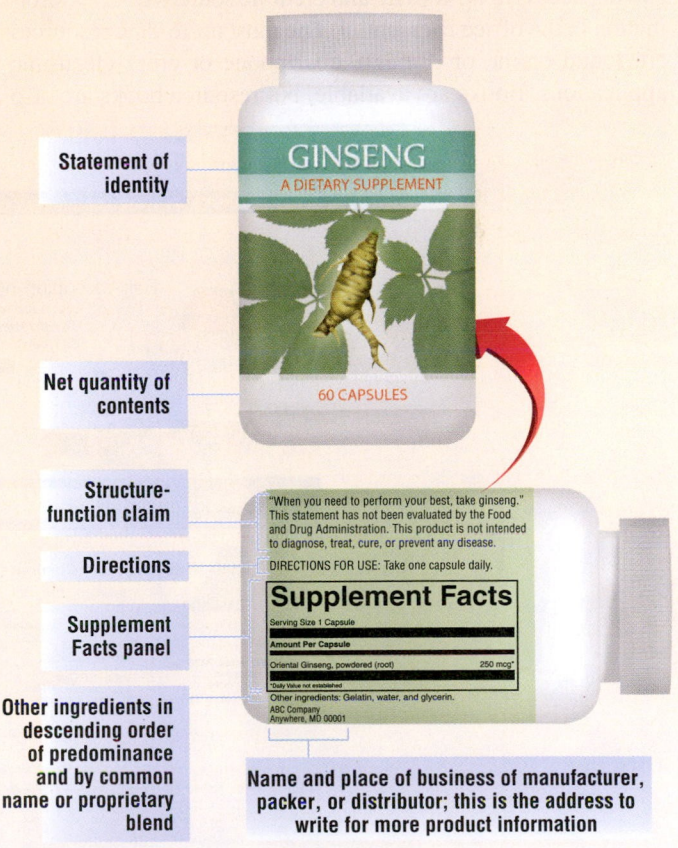

Anatomy of the Requirements for Dietary Supplement Labels (Effective March 1999)

FIGURE 51-4 The Food and Drug Administration provides specific guidelines for the information to be included on a dietary supplement label.

TABLE 51-2   Pregnancy and Lactation Drug Label Requirements (June 2015)

The FDA requires the following information on prescription drug labels to assist the prescriber and the patient in determining the risks and benefits of each.

Category	Label Requirements
Pregnancy (Includes Labor and Delivery)	• Pregnancy/fetal risk summary
	• Clinical considerations and data
	• Inadvertent exposure considerations
	• Prescribing decisions for pregnant patients
	• Information for the pregnancy exposure registry when available
Lactation (Includes Nursing Mothers)	• Information about the amount of drug in the breast milk
	• Information about potential effects of the drug on the breastfed infant
Females and Males of Reproductive Potential	• Need for pregnancy testing when taking the drug
	• Contraception recommendations
	• Information about infertility as it relates to the drug

labeling requirement starts for all medications submitted to the FDA after June 30, 2015, and the old labeling will be phased out. The new labels include pregnancy exposure registries that collect and maintain data on the effects of medications used by pregnant women. The new rule dictates what must be included on the drug label based on the three categories. See Table 51-2.

▶ Sources of Drug Information   LO 51.5

Having access to up-to-date and credible sources of drug information in the office is essential. The most up-to-date resources are found online or through smartphone or other electronic applications. Books are available, but resource books are also available online. *Physicians' Desk Reference*® (Figure 51-5), *United States Pharmacopeia/National Formulary, American Hospital Formulary Service* (*AHFS*®), and Epocrates® are credible sources of drug information. Package inserts and drug labels are also valuable drug information sources.

Physicians' Desk Reference® (PDR)

The *Physicians' Desk Reference*®, or *PDR*, is published annually, along with supplements twice a year. It is sent free to doctors' offices and sold through bookstores. PDR Network, the company that publishes the *PDR*, also publishes separate editions for generic, nonprescription, and ophthalmologic drugs, as well as a guide to drug interactions, adverse effects, and

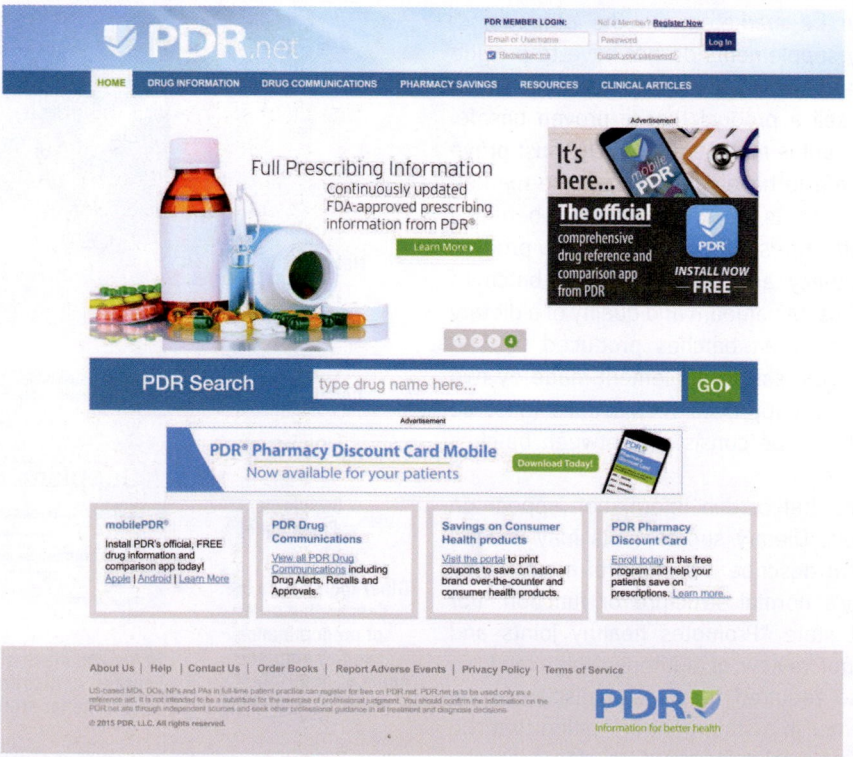

FIGURE 51-5   PDR.net® is a complete and current resource for drug information which includes all the information found in the PDR.
Physicians' Desk Reference. 70th ed. Montvale, NJ: PDR, LLC; 2015:100–105

indications. It is also available online. The *PDR* presents information provided by pharmaceutical companies about more than 2,500 prescription drugs. It has the following sections:

- Section 1—manufacturer's index (color-coded white), which includes the pharmaceutical company's name, address, emergency telephone number, and available products
- Section 2—brand- and generic-name index (color-coded pink)
- Section 3—product category index (color-coded blue)
- Section 4—product identification guide with full-color photos of more than 2,400 medications
- Section 5—product information
- Section 6—diagnostic product information

The product information section is divided according to manufacturer, and the drugs are then grouped alphabetically within each manufacturer's subsection. The information is provided for the *PDR* by the manufacturer and is either the drug package insert or a similar document.

After the large product information section, various smaller other sections are provided, which include diagnostic product information, state drug information centers, ratings for drug use in pregnancy, a state DEA directory, state-aided drug-assistance programs, patient assistance programs, drugs that should not be crushed, dosing instructions in Spanish, and the system for reporting adverse reactions to medications. All of these plus the *PDR* Internet site and *PDR* electronic library that come with the *PDR* are important resources for drug information.

United States Pharmacopeia/ National Formulary

The *United States Pharmacopeia/National Formulary*, or *USP-NF*, is the official source of drug standards in the United States, published about every 5 years. It is the official public standards-setting authority for all prescription medications, OTC drugs, dietary supplements, and other healthcare products. By law, every product sold under a name listed in the *USP-NF* must meet the USP's strict standards.

The *USP-NF* describes each product approved by the federal government and lists its standards for purity, composition, and strength as well as its uses, dosages, and storage. The NF portion of the book provides the chemical formulas of the drugs. The *USP-NF* is available online.

American Hospital Formulary Service (AHFS®)

The American Society of Hospital Pharmacists in Bethesda, Maryland, publishes *American Hospital Formulary Service Drug Information®*, or *AHSF DI*. It sells the two-volume set by subscription and provides four to six supplements each year. The *AHFS®* lists generic names and is divided into sections based on drug actions. The *AHFS®* is also available online.

Epocrates®

Epocrates® is a software program that can be loaded onto a smartphone or other personal digital assistant. Epocrates® includes more than 3,300 brand and generic drugs, alternative medicines, a drug-drug interaction checker, an IV compatibility checker, health insurance Medicare Part D formularies, and an infectious disease treatment guide.

Package Insert

The **package insert** for each drug describes the drug: its purpose and effects (clinical pharmacology), indications, contraindications (conditions under which the drug should not be administered), warnings, precautions, adverse reactions, drug abuse and dependence, overdosage, and dosage and administration, as well as how the drug is supplied (for example, tablets in different doses, or liquid). The package insert, whether part of the *PDR* or found in the medication package, is a valuable resource for drug information. See Figure 51-6.

Drug Labels

To prepare and administer drugs, you must understand information that appears on drug labels, including the drug name, form, dosage strength, total amount in the container, route of administration, warnings, storage requirements, and manufacturing information. See Figure 51-7. By law, the generic name, as listed in the *USP-NF*, must appear on the drug's label. The drug label also may include the trade (brand) name used to market the drug. The trade name is typically indicated by the registered trademark symbol®. The form of the drug is included, such as tablet, capsule, or liquid for oral administration. In some cases, a drug may be a combination drug, meaning more than one drug is in each tablet, capsule, or amount of liquid. Drug labels also include information about the amount of the drug present.

On the label, the dosage strength is stated as the amount of drug per dosage unit. In most cases, the amount of the drug is listed in grams (g), milligrams (mg), or micrograms (mcg), or if it is a liquid, in milliliters (mL). If a container holds more than one dose of medication, then the total number or volume of medication is listed on the label.

The label also should include the route of administration, especially if it is a liquid. Warnings, such as "May be habit forming," are included, as well as storage information. Storage information indicates the specific conditions under which a medication must be stored. The manufacturer's information is always included. Information about how to mix or reconstitute a medication also may be found on the label.

▶ Controlled Substances LO 51.6

A **controlled substance** is a drug or drug product categorized as potentially dangerous and addictive. The greater the potential for abuse, the more severe the limitations on prescribing it. Federal laws strictly regulate use of these controlled drugs. States, municipalities, and institutions must adhere to these laws but may also impose their own regulations, as long as they are at least as strict as the federal laws.

Comprehensive Drug Abuse Prevention and Control Act

The Comprehensive Drug Abuse Prevention and Control Act, also known as the Controlled Substances Act (CSA) of 1970,

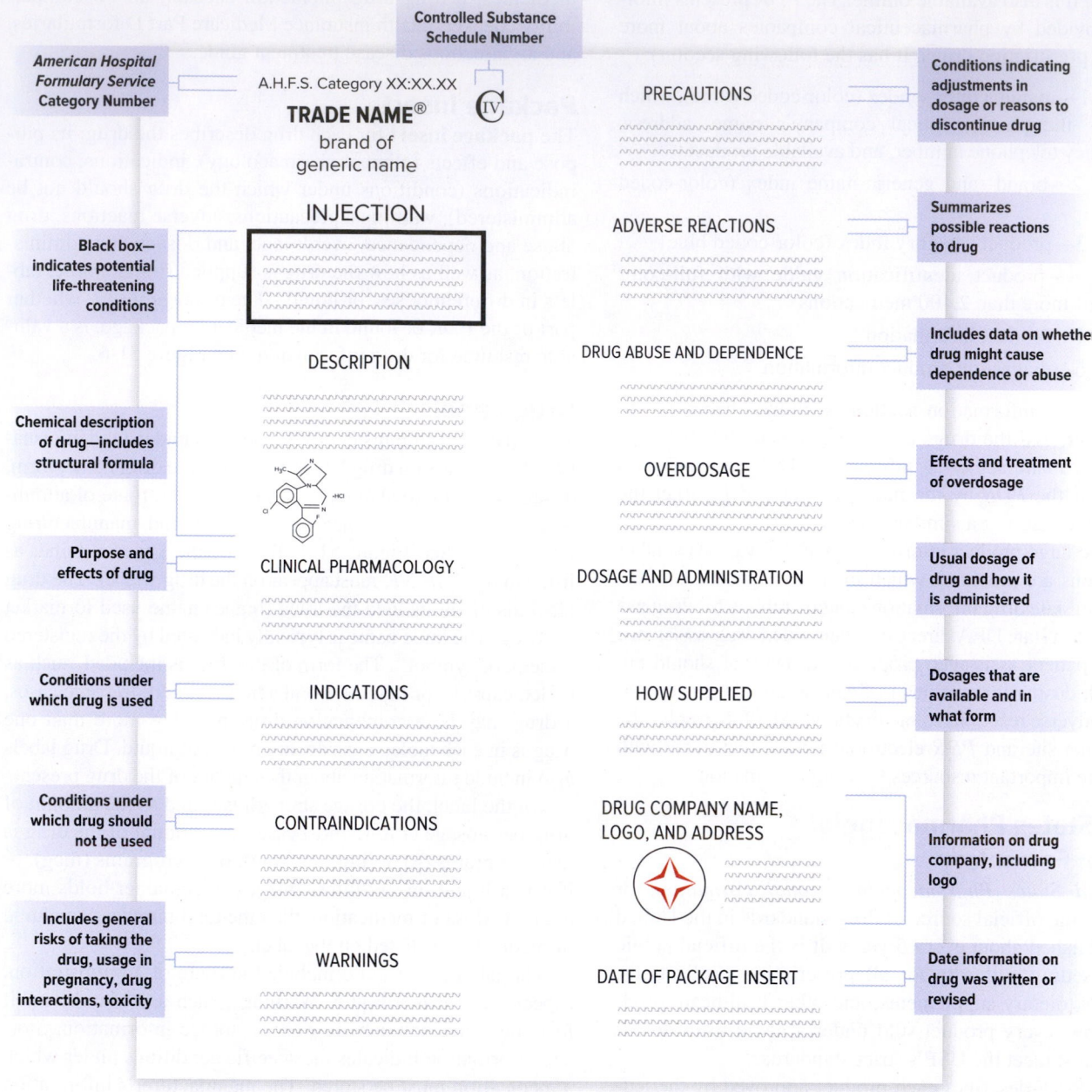

FIGURE 51-6 Use the package insert to become familiar with a drug's indications, contraindications, dosage, and potential adverse reactions.

is the federal law that created the DEA and strengthened drug enforcement authority. The CSA designates five schedules, according to degree of potential for a substance to be abused or used for a nontherapeutic effect. Schedule I drugs do not have a medical use and cannot be prescribed in the United States. Schedule II drugs include **opioids,** which are natural or synthetic drugs that produce opium-like effects. Examples of Schedule II drugs include codeine, morphine, and meperidine (Demerol®). Government agencies use the popular term **narcotics** for opioids. Prescription requirements are the strictest for Schedule II drugs. Schedule III through V drugs have reduced prescription requirements and are progressively less addictive the larger the schedule number.

Sometimes the DEA reclassifies drugs. For example, a Schedule III drug may eventually be found to be less addictive than originally determined and therefore reclassified as a Schedule IV drug. The five schedules, their prescription and legal requirements, and examples of substances in each are outlined in Table 51-3.

Controlled Substance Labeling
The CSA also set up a labeling system to identify controlled substances. An example of this label is shown in Figure 51-8. The large C means the drug is a controlled substance and the Roman numeral inside the C corresponds to the drug's DEA schedule.

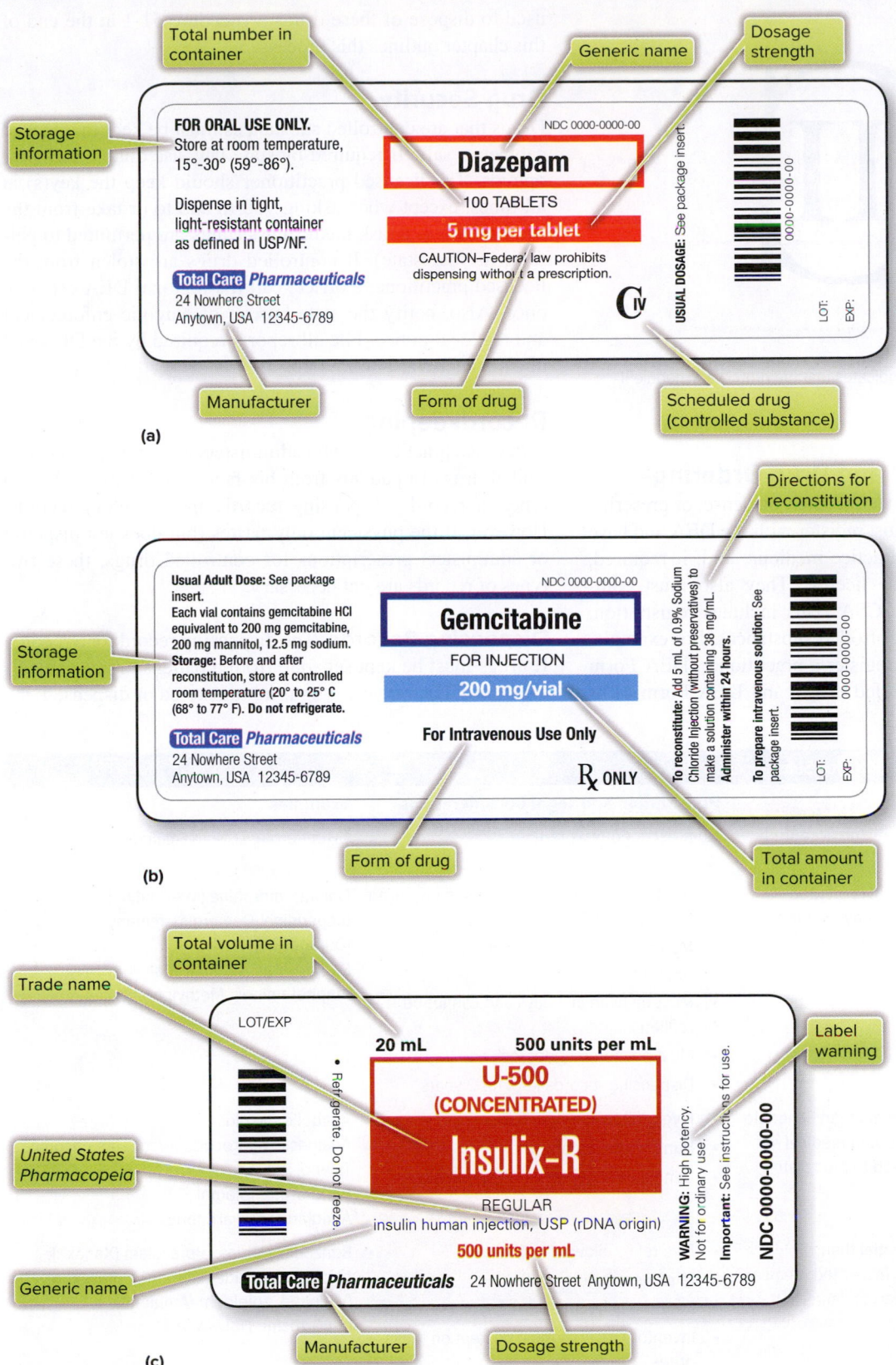

Storage information → FOR ORAL USE ONLY. Store at room temperature, 15°-30° (59°-86°).

Dispense in tight, light-resistant container as defined in USP/NF.

Total Care *Pharmaceuticals*
24 Nowhere Street
Anytown, USA 12345-6789

Total number in container

Generic name

Dosage strength

NDC 0000-0000-00

Diazepam

100 TABLETS

5 mg per tablet

CAUTION—Federal law prohibits dispensing without a prescription.

C IV

USUAL DOSAGE: See package insert.

0000-0000-00

LOT: EXP:

Storage information ← **Manufacturer** ← **Form of drug** ← **Scheduled drug (controlled substance)**

(a)

Storage information

Usual Adult Dose: See package insert.
Each vial contains gemcitabine HCl equivalent to 200 mg gemcitabine, 200 mg mannitol, 12.5 mg sodium. **Storage:** Before and after reconstitution, store at controlled room temperature (20° to 25° C (68° to 77° F). Do not refrigerate.

Total Care *Pharmaceuticals*
24 Nowhere Street
Anytown, USA 12345-6789

NDC 0000-0000-00

Gemcitabine

FOR INJECTION

200 mg/vial

For Intravenous Use Only

Rx ONLY

To reconstitute: Add 5 mL of 0.9% Sodium Chloride Injection (without preservatives) to make a solution containing 38 mg/mL. **Administer within 24 hours.**

To prepare intravenous solution: See package insert.

0000-0000-00

LOT: EXP:

Directions for reconstitution

Form of drug — **Total amount in container**

(b)

Trade name

Total volume in container

LOT/EXP

20 mL   500 units per mL

U-500 (CONCENTRATED)

Insulix-R

REGULAR
insulin human injection, USP (rDNA origin)

500 units per mL

Total Care *Pharmaceuticals*   24 Nowhere Street Anytown, USA 12345-6789

• Refrigerate. Do not freeze.

WARNING: High potency. Not for ordinary use.

Important: See instructions for use.

NDC 0000-0000-00

Label warning

United States Pharmacopeia

Generic name

Manufacturer — **Dosage strength**

(c)

FIGURE 51-7 (a) Check the medication label carefully. (b) Always read reconstitution instructions and storage information. (c) Note any warnings on the label.

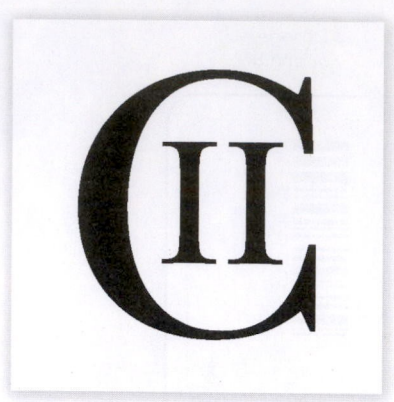

FIGURE 51-8 This symbol indicates that the drug is a Schedule II controlled substance.

Doctor Registration and Drug Ordering

Authorized prescribers who administer, dispense, or prescribe any controlled substance must register with the DEA and have a current state license to practice medicine and, if required, a state-controlled substance license. They also must comply with all aspects of the CSA. This includes registration, renewal, and ordering of controlled substances. For example, DEA Form 224 is used to register a practitioner, DEA Form 222 is used to order scheduled drugs, and DEA Form 41 is used to dispose of these drugs. Procedure 51-1 at the end of this chapter outlines this process.

Drug Security

Drugs that are controlled substances must be kept in a locked cabinet or safe. If required by state law, use double locks for opioids. The licensed practitioner should keep the key(s) at all times, except when asking you to add to or take from the stock (if this is a task medical assistants are permitted to perform in your state). If controlled drugs are stolen from the licensed practitioner's office, call the regional DEA office at once. Also, notify the state bureau of narcotic enforcement and the local police. File all reports required by the DEA and other agencies as a follow-up.

Recordkeeping

A licensed practitioner who administers and/or dispenses controlled drugs to patients from his facility must maintain two types of records: dispensing records and inventory records. However, if the physician only writes (but does not dispense or administer) prescriptions for controlled drugs, these two types of records are not necessary.

Dispensing Records The dispensing record for Schedule II drugs must be kept separate from a patient's regular medical record. Each time a drug is administered or dispensed, the

TABLE 51-3	Schedule of Controlled Substances		
Schedule	**Description**	**Prescription and Legal Considerations**	**Examples**
I	High abuse potential (no accepted medical use)	No prescriptions written	GHB, heroin, LSD, mescaline
II	High abuse potential (accepted medical use; abuse may lead to dependence)	• Must be written by DEA-licensed physician and include DEA number • Multiple and/or special forms may be required • Must be filled in 7 days and cannot be refilled • Must be stored under lock and key • Dispensing records kept for 2 years	Opioids: morphine (MS-Contin®), meperidine (Demerol®), fentanyl (Duragesic®) Barbiturates: secobarbital Amphetamines: Methylphenidate (Ritalin®)
III	Lower abuse potential than Schedule I and II drugs (accepted medical use; abuse may lead to moderate dependence)	• Five refills allowed in 6 months • Handwritten by physician • Can be telephoned by physician only	Anabolic steroids Analgesic: hydrocodone/codeine (Vicodin®, Tylenol 3®) Barbiturate: talbutal Antidiarrheal: Paregoric
IV	Lower abuse potential than Schedule III drugs (accepted medical use; abuse may lead to limited dependence)	• Five refills allowed in 6 months • Must be signed by physician • Refills may be authorized over the phone • Inventory records must be kept on these drugs	Benzodiazepines: alprazolam (Xanax®), chloridiazepoxide (Librium®), diazepam (Valium®), zolpidem (Ambien®), pentazocine (Talwin®)
V	Lower abuse potential than Schedule IV drugs (accepted medical use; very limited physical dependence)	• Inventory records must be kept on these drugs • Five refills allowed in 6 months • Must be signed by physician • Refills may be authorized over the phone	Antitussive and antidiarrheals that combine small amounts of opioids, including Lomotil®, Kaolin, and Robitussin AC®

Source: US Department of Justice, Drug Enforcement Administration, Office of Diversion Control, http://www.deadiversion.usdoj.gov.

licensed practitioner must note the date, the patient's name and address, the drug, and the quantity dispensed. The dispensing record for drugs on Schedules III through V must include the same information. The record for these drugs may be kept in the patient's medical record unless the physician charges for the drugs dispensed. All dispensing records must be kept for 2 years and are subject to inspection by the DEA.

Inventory Records A licensed practitioner who regularly dispenses controlled drugs also must keep inventory records of all stock on hand. This regulation applies to all scheduled drugs. To take an inventory, count the amount of each drug on hand. Compare this amount with the amount of the drug ordered and the amount dispensed to patients. The controlled drug inventory must be repeated every 2 years. You must include copies of invoices from drug suppliers in the inventory record. All Schedule II drug inventories and records must be kept separate from other records.

Inventories and records of other controlled drugs must be separate or easily retrievable from ordinary business and professional records. All records on controlled drugs must be retained for 2 years and made available for inspection and copying by DEA officials if requested.

Disposing of Drugs If the doctor asks you to dispose of any outdated, noncontrolled drugs, you will most likely use the disposal company that takes your biohazardous waste. The DEA does not allow businesses to flush any medications, and medications should not be placed in the trash. In some cases, you may work with a larger healthcare facility or pharmacy to ensure proper disposal so that medications do not pollute the environment or end up in the trash, where someone may take them.

If the licensed practitioner needs to dispose of controlled drugs, such as expired samples, obtain DEA Form 41, called Registrants Inventory of Drugs Surrendered, which is available from the nearest DEA office or the Internet. Complete the form in quadruplicate, have the doctor sign it, and call the DEA to obtain instructions for disposal of the drugs. If you must ship them, use registered mail. After the drugs have been destroyed, the DEA will issue the licensed practitioner a receipt, which you should keep in a safe place. If practitioners terminate their medical practice, they must return their DEA registration certificate and any unused copies of DEA Form 222, which is used for ordering scheduled medications, to the nearest DEA office. To prevent unauthorized use, write the word VOID across the front of these forms. Regional DEA offices will tell the practitioner how to dispose of any remaining controlled drugs.

▶ Prescriptions
LO 51.7

Any drug not available over the counter requires a prescription. As a medical assistant, you should be able to interpret a prescription in order to discuss it with the patient, authorized prescriber, or pharmacist. You must become familiar with the prescriber's style of writing or the electronic prescription process at your facility.

Interpreting a Prescription

Prescriptions for new or refilled medications are completed or approved by the licensed practitioner. A prescription has specific parts that must be present before it can be filled or refilled (Figure 51-9).

The basic components of a prescription are

1. *Prescriber information:* Name, address, telephone number, and other information identifying the prescriber.
2. *Patient information:* Patient's full name, date of birth, address, and other information to identify the patient.
3. *Medication prescribed:* Includes generic or brand name, strength, and quantity. This is sometimes called the inscription and is found after the *Rx.*
4. *Subscription:* Instructions to the pharmacist dispensing the medication. This may include generic substitution and refill authorization.
5. *Signa:* Also known as the transcription; refers to patient instructions. These instructions generally follow the abbreviation *Sig,* which means "mark."
6. *Signature:* Prescriber's signature for handwritten prescriptions. The prescriber's signature must be in ink, but it cannot be a stamped signature. A digital signature is used if it is secure; otherwise, the prescription must be printed and then signed or otherwise authorized. The prescriber must also include the date the prescription was generated.
7. *DEA number:* This is required for prescriptions of Schedules II, III, IV, and V medications only.

Many terms and abbreviations are used in prescriptions. See Table 51-4 for some examples. Abbreviations for drug names should not be used, because there are similar abbreviations for multiple drugs. Recall from the *Patient Interview and History* chapter that there are many abbreviations that should not be used. These are known as the "Do Not Use" abbreviations, as identified by The Joint Commission (http://www.jointcommission.org), and "Error Prone," as identified by the Institute for Safe Medical Practices (http://www.ismp.org).

A medical assistant must be able to interpret a prescription with accuracy. Refer to Procedure 51-2 at the end of this chapter.

Managing Prescriptions Prescriptions may be printed or handwritten on a prescription blank. They also may be entered electronically and printed, or entered electronically and transmitted directly to a pharmacy. When the information is entered electronically and transmitted directly, this is known as **e-prescribing.** With e-prescribing, the medication information is received at the pharmacy; the actual prescription is never in the patient's hands. This is the most secure and efficient way for prescriptions to be completed. See *Points on Practice:* E-prescribing.

In rare cases, preprinted prescription blanks are used that include the licensed practitioner's name, address, telephone number, state license number, and DEA registration number plus blank space for writing the patient's name and address, the date, and other information. To prevent unauthorized use

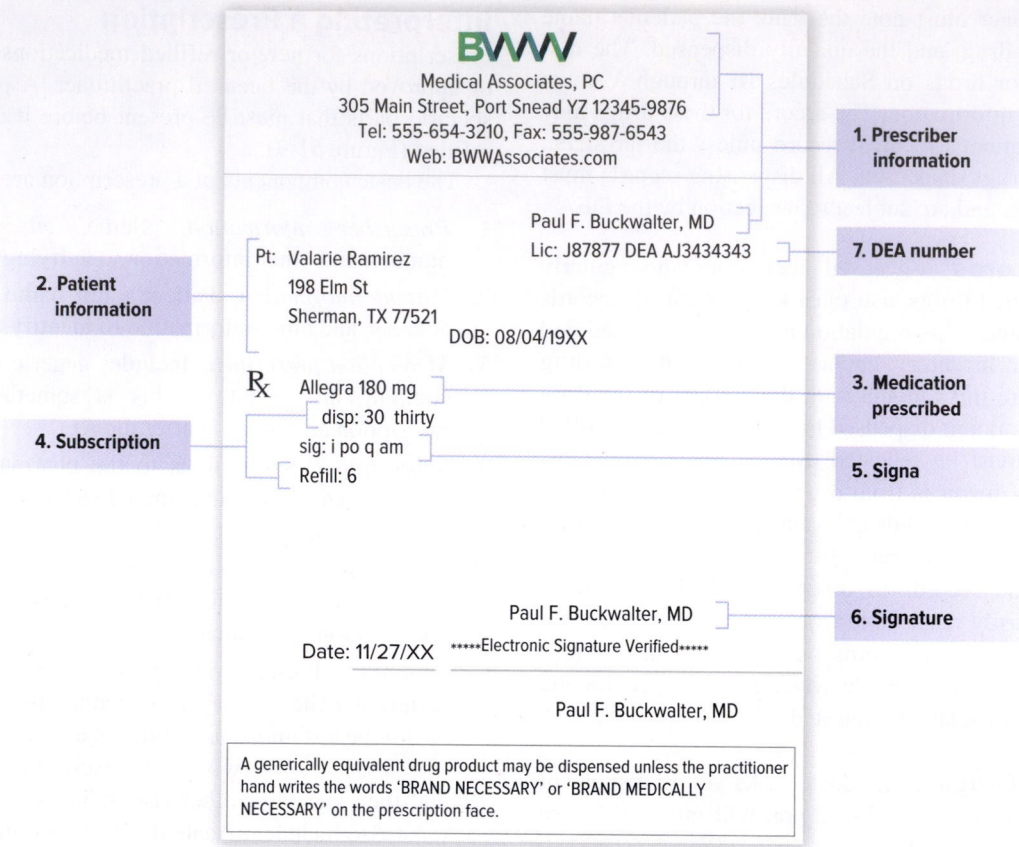

FIGURE 51-9 Parts of a prescription.

of prescription blanks, never leave them unattended. Most frequently, prescriptions are entered into an EHR, then printed and signed for patients to take with them to the pharmacy. If something about a prescription arouses suspicion, the pharmacist who receives a prescription may call the licensed practitioner's office to verify it. You should be able to check the patient's records and tell the pharmacist whether the practitioner wrote a prescription for that patient. If the prescription is a forgery, notify the licensed practitioner and, if she gives you authorization, notify the DEA.

Telephone Prescriptions If requested by the licensed practitioner, you may telephone a new or renewal prescription to the patient's pharmacy. You may not, however, telephone a prescription for a Schedule II drug. In an emergency situation, when a patient needs a drug immediately and no alternative

TABLE 51-4 Abbreviations Used in Prescriptions

Abbreviation	Meaning	Abbreviation	Meaning
ā	Before	min	Minute, minimum
aa	Of each	mL	Milliliters
ac	Before meals	mm	Millimeters
AM	Morning	neb	Nebulizer
amp	Ampule	noct	Night
apl	Applicatorful	NPO	Nothing by mouth
aq	Water	nr	No refills
bid	Twice daily	oz	Ounce
c̄	With	pc	After meals
cap	Capsule	per	By means of; through
cd	Cycle day (menstrual cycle)	PM	Evening or nighttime
cmpd	Compound	po, PO	By mouth
cr	Cream	PR, pr	Rectally
d	Daily or day	q	Every
DAW	Dispense as written (no generic)	qam	Every morning
disp	Dispense	q4h	Every 4 hours
ds	Double strength	qid	Four times daily
dx	Diagnosis	qs	Sufficient amount
elix	Elixir	r, rec	Rectally
eq	Equivalent	rept	Repeat
g, gm	Gram	rf	Refill(s)
gen	Generic	s̄	Without
gr	Grain (60 to 65 mg)	stat	Immediately
gtt	Drop(s)	subcut, subQ	Subcutaneously
h, hr	Hour	sup	Suppository
H₂O	Water	susp	Suspension
IM	Intramuscularly	sx	Symptoms
inj	Inject, injection	syr	Syrup
IV	Intravenously	tab	Tablet(s)
kg	Kilogram	tbsp	Tablespoon
L	Liter	tsp	Teaspoon
liq	Liquid	tx	Treatment
lot	Lotion	ud, utd	As directed
MDI	Metered dose inhaler	ung	Ointment
mEq	Milliequivalent	vag	Vaginally, into vagina
mg	Milligram(s)	YO	Years old

is available, the physician may telephone a prescription for a Schedule II drug. The amount must be limited to the period of emergency, and a written prescription must be sent to the pharmacist within 72 hours. The pharmacist must notify the DEA if a written prescription does not arrive within the specified time.

Patient requests for prescription renewals occur daily. The renewal requests may be called in to the receptionist or left on a designated phone or mail system. It is the medical assistant's responsibility, if asked, to handle the prescription renewals/refills in an appropriate manner.

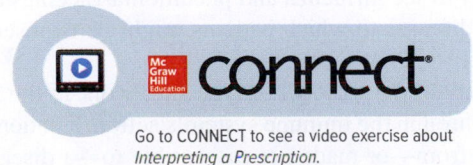

Go to CONNECT to see a video exercise about *Interpreting a Prescription.*

▶ Nonpharmacologic Pain Management
LO 51.8

Because of drug interactions, adverse reactions, or the risk of dependence, many patients either prefer not to or should not take drugs to relieve chronic pain. The overuse and abuse of pain medications can be a problem. Pain frequently motivates these patients to use complementary and alternative medicine (CAM). The following are some examples:

- Chiropractors use spinal adjustments to treat chronic back or neck pain.
- Massage is used to treat headache or arthritis and to promote healing through relaxation.
- An acupuncture procedure in which very small amounts of electrical current are applied through needles has been used successfully to block the pain of surgery without anesthesia.
- Yoga uses postures to exercise the spine and stimulate the lymphatic system, helping to remove from the body toxins that may cause pain and stiffness in muscles and joints.
- Meditation is said to balance a person's physical, emotional, and mental states and is used as an aid in treating stress, anxiety, and pain.
- Hypnotism may be used to help patients overcome pain caused by stress-induced migraine headaches.
- Glucosamine chondroitin, a dietary supplement, is taken to treat osteoarthritis by reducing pain and slowing down joint cartilage damage.
- **Magnetic therapy** involves the use of magnets of varying sizes and strengths placed on the body to relieve pain or treat disease.
- Biofeedback can help a patient learn to evoke relaxation, which helps block pain perception.

CAM approaches and therapies have become more common in recent years. Some physicians and patients are seeking agents and treatments to manage health problems, such as chronic pain, that are less expensive, have fewer side effects, and are more accessible than traditional medical interventions. Pain clinics that use multiple pain management techniques are common.

▶ Vaccines
LO 51.9

A vaccine is a preparation made from microorganisms and administered to a person to produce reduced sensitivity to, or increased immunity to, an infectious disease. Vaccines are stored with the office supply of drugs and require similar handling. If you work in a pediatrician's office, you will handle the vaccines for childhood diseases. In an adult practice, you can expect to see influenza and pneumonia vaccines and vaccines for diseases to which patients might be exposed in foreign travel.

It is important to know how vaccines work in the immune system. Through the immune system's action, a patient can be protected from—or made not susceptible to—a disease. This immunity results from the formation of antibodies that destroy or alter disease-causing agents. You can review information about immunity discussed in the chapter *The Lymphatic and Immune Systems.*

Antibody Formation

Antigens are foreign substances—bacteria, viruses, and other organisms—that can enter the human body in spite of its natural defenses. In response to an invasion by antigens, the body's specialized white blood cells (lymphocytes) produce antibodies. These antibodies are specific to the invading antigens and combine with the antigens to neutralize them. This action arrests or prevents the reaction or disease that the antigens would otherwise cause. Toxins, pollens, and drugs also can be antigens if the body reacts to them by forming antibodies. (Allergens are antigens that induce an allergic reaction.)

Vaccines contain organisms that have been killed or attenuated (weakened) in a laboratory. Because the organisms have been weakened, they stimulate antibody formation but do not overpower the body and cause disease. They may, however, still be strong enough to cause a fever and slight inflammation at the injection site. Some vaccines, such as those for influenza, may even produce some of the lesser effects of the disease against which they provide protection.

Immunizations made from organisms are called *vaccines.* Those made from the toxins of organisms are called *toxoids.* Some immunizations, such as the polio vaccine, last a lifetime. Others, such as tetanus toxoid, do not. In the latter case, booster immunizations must be used to stimulate the lymphocytes to produce antibodies again.

Immunizations

The Advisory Committee on Immunization Practices, the American Academy of Pediatrics, and the American Academy of Family Physicians jointly publish immunization schedules (see the *Assisting in Pediatrics* chapter). These schedules cover children from infancy through 18 years of age. Just as children receive immunizations before exposure to disease, adults may receive immunizations for influenza, pneumonia, or other diseases, including those to which an adult could be exposed during travel. Figure 51-10 displays the adult immunization schedules based on age and on health condition.

Patients are sometimes immunized after exposure. For example, if patients have been exposed to a serious disease and there is too little time for them to produce antibodies, they may receive an antiserum containing antibodies to the disease-carrying organism. These immunizations are made from human or animal serum. If bacterial toxins (rather than bacteria) cause the disease, the patient may receive an antitoxin.

Antiserums and antitoxins must be used cautiously and are usually reserved for life-threatening infectious diseases. Because patients can be allergic to substances in animal antiserums and antitoxins, human serums are usually preferred. An example of a postexposure immunization is one given to a patient who has been exposed to hepatitis B virus (HBV). This patient should be given the antiserum hepatitis B immune globulin (HBV-Ig) within 7 days after exposure and again

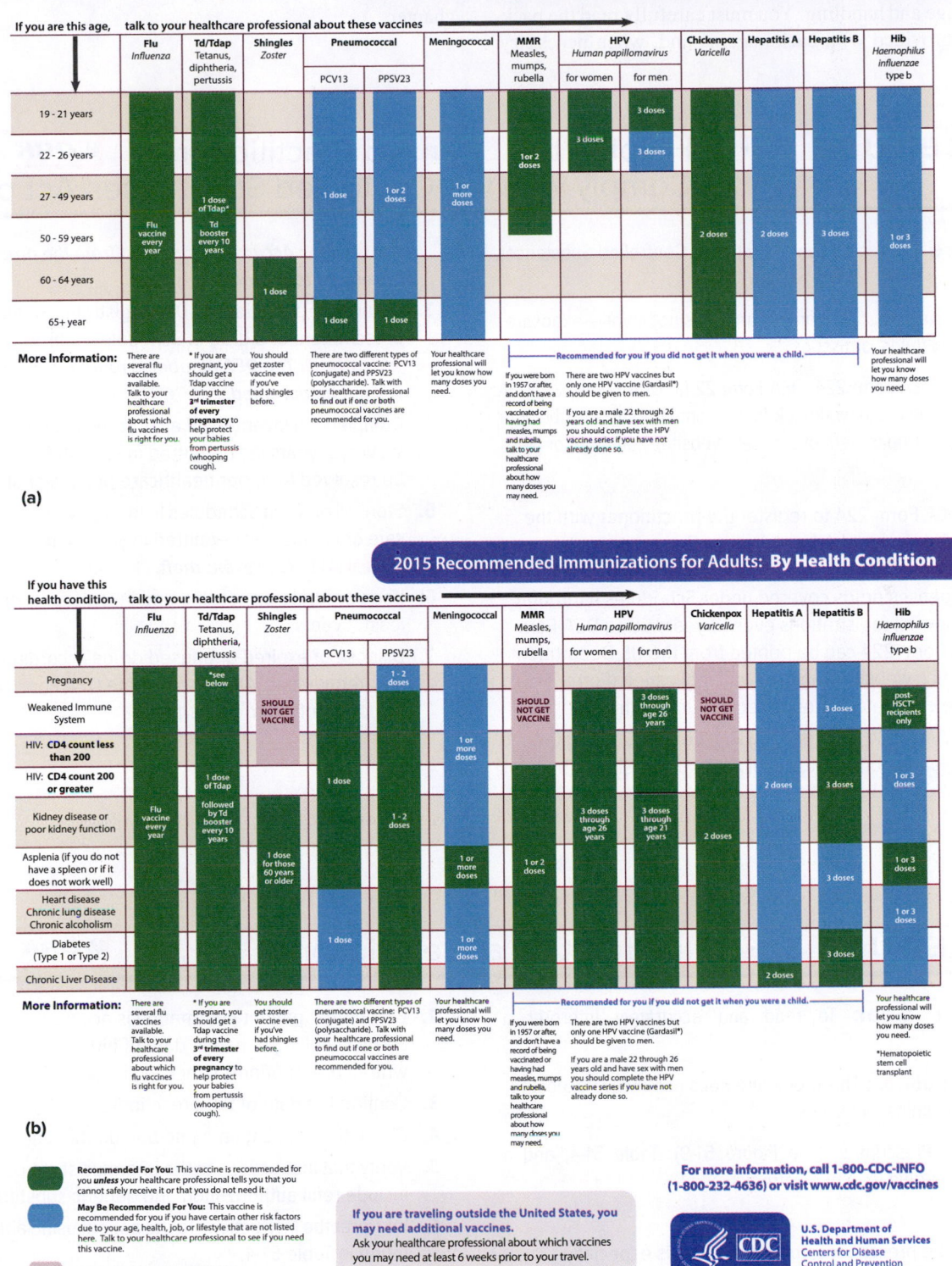

FIGURE 51-10 Adult immunization schedule (a) by age and (b) by health condition.

28 to 30 days later. Because HBV-Ig is made from human serum, it causes relatively few adverse reactions. Another example is a patient who may have been exposed to tetanus (lockjaw) organisms as the result of an injury such as a puncture wound. This patient may receive tetanus immune globulin (T-Ig, a human product) or tetanus antitoxin. Because tetanus antitoxin is made from horse serum, it may cause serious reactions in patients who are allergic to horses or horsehair.

For every vaccine in your medical office, you must be familiar with the indications, contraindications, dosages, administration routes, potential adverse reactions, and methods of storage and handling. You must carefully read the package insert provided with each vaccine and, when necessary, consult drug reference books for further information. Knowledge of correct administration techniques is required and will be discussed in the *Medication Administration* chapter.

PROCEDURE 51-1 Helping the Licensed Practitioner Comply with the Controlled Substances Act of 1970

WORK // DOC

Procedure Goal: To comply with the Controlled Substances Act of 1970

OSHA Guidelines: This procedure does not involve exposure to blood, body fluids, or tissues.

Materials: DEA Form 224, DEA Form 224a, DEA Form 222, DEA Form 41 (available in the workbook that accompanies this textbook or online at the US Department of Justice's website), computer or pen

Method:

1. Use DEA Form 224 to register the practitioner with the Drug Enforcement Administration. Be sure to register each office location at which the practitioner administers or dispenses drugs covered under Schedules II through V. Renew all registrations every 3 years using DEA Form 224a. Form 224 can be printed from the US Department of Justice website. The renewal application (Form 224a) can be completed through registration at this site.

2. Order Schedule II drugs using DEA Form 222, as instructed by the practitioner. (Stocks of these drugs should be kept to a minimum.)

RATIONALE: *Accurate instruction from the practitioner is necessary to ensure safety.*

3. Include the practitioner's DEA registration number on every prescription for a drug in Schedules II through V.
   RATIONALE: *The DEA number is required or prescriptions will not be accepted.*

4. Complete an inventory of all drugs in Schedules II through V every 2 years (as permitted in your state; this task may be reserved for other healthcare professionals).

5. Store all drugs in Schedules II through V in a secure, locked safe or cabinet (as permitted in your state).
   RATIONALE: *To prevent theft.*

6. Keep accurate dispensing and inventory records for at least 2 years.

7. Dispose of expired or unused drugs according to the DEA regulations. Always complete DEA Form 41 when disposing of controlled drugs.

PROCEDURE 51-2 Interpreting a Prescription

WORK // DOC

Procedure Goal: To read and accurately interpret a prescription

OSHA Guidelines: This procedure does not involve exposure to blood, body fluids, or tissues.

Materials: Prescription (use Figure 51-9), Table 51-4, and a method of recording (pen or electronic)

Method:

1. Verify the prescriber information. This is especially important in a multiphysician practice or electronic health record.

2. Ensure that patient information is accurate, including correct spelling of name, date of birth, and address. For written prescriptions, check legibility.

3. Confirm the date of the prescription.

4. Check the medication name and double-check spelling.

5. Verify that instructions to the pharmacist are complete and include refill authorization and generic substitution.

6. Interpret the instructions to the patient using abbreviations found in Table 51-4.

7. Make sure that the prescription is signed in ink for handwritten prescriptions and digitally for electronic prescriptions.

LEARNING OUTCOMES	KEY POINTS
51.1 Identify the medical assistant's role in pharmacology.	The role of the medical assistant in pharmacology includes being attentive to ensure that the licensed practitioner is aware of all medications, both prescription and OTC, that a patient is taking; asking each patient about alcohol and recreational drug use (both past and present), as well as herbal remedies; assisting in managing and renewing medication prescriptions; and educating the patient, using guidelines provided by the licensed practitioner, about the purpose of a drug and how to take the drug for maximum effectiveness and minimum adverse reactions.
51.2 Recognize the five categories of pharmacology and their importance to medication administration.	The five categories of pharmacology are pharmacognosy, pharmacokinetics, pharmacodynamics, pharmacotherapeutics, and toxicology. It is important to understand each of these in order to carry out the medical assistant's role in pharmacology.
51.3 Differentiate the major drug categories, drug names, and their actions.	Drug categories are sometimes named based on their action; for example, anticonvulsants are used to treat convulsions (seizures). The major drug categories and their actions are outlined in Table 51-1.
51.4 Classify over-the-counter (OTC), prescription, and herbal drugs.	Nonprescription drugs, including herbal and OTC drugs, can be obtained without a licensed practitioner's order. For prescription drugs, patients must have an authorized prescriber's written (or oral) order.
51.5 Use credible sources to obtain drug information.	Credible sources for drug information are the *Physicians' Desk Reference® (PDR), United States Pharmacopeia/National Formulary,* and *American Hospital Formulary Service (AHFS®).* You also may access medication information from package inserts, drug labels, and reliable Internet sites.
51.6 Carry out the procedure for registering or renewing a physician with the **Drug Enforcement Administration (DEA)** for permission to administer, dispense, and prescribe controlled drugs.	The medical assistant should assist the licensed practitioner with registration, renewal, and ordering of controlled substances, as outlined in the Controlled Substances Act of 1970 and Procedure 51-1.
51.7 Identify the parts of a prescription, including commonly used abbreviations and symbols.	A prescription must be complete to be filled. The medical assistant must be able to interpret a prescription in order to manage new and refilled medications. Procedure 51-2 and Table 51-4 will assist the medical assistant in performing these tasks.
51.8 Discuss nonpharmacologic treatments for pain.	Multiple nonpharmacologic methods are used to treat pain, including CAM therapies such as massage, yoga, biofeedback, chiropractic, acupuncture, magnetic therapy, hypnotism, and glucosamine chondroitin.
51.9 Describe how vaccines work in the immune system.	Immunizations usually contain killed or weakened organisms. When given, they stimulate the body to build up a resistance to the organism. They are used to provide immunity against specific diseases.

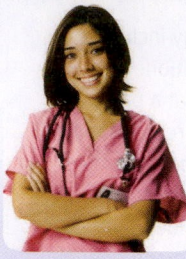

© Rubberball/Getty Images RF

Recall Kaylyn Haddix, RMA (AMT), from the beginning of the chapter. Now that you have completed the chapter, answer the following questions regarding her case.

1. Detail the steps Kaylyn should take to design and implement an inventory system.

2. What are some credible sources of drug information Kaylyn can use to complete her task?

3. Why is Kaylyn's attention to detail a critical skill for managing the office sample drug inventory and office medications?

EXAM PREPARATION QUESTIONS

1. (LO 51.3) Which drug may prevent an asthma attack?
   a. ProAir HFA®
   b. Elavil®
   c. Lovenox®
   d. Levaquin®
   e. Lipitor®

2. (LO 51.5) Which source of medication information is divided into six major sections?
   a. *American Hospital Formulary Service (AHFS®)*
   b. *United States Pharmacopeia/National Formulary*
   c. *Physicians' Desk Reference® (PDR)*
   d. Epocrates®
   e. RXList.com

3. (LO 51.6) Which of the following medications has the highest potential for addiction?
   a. Lomotil®
   b. Vicodin®
   c. Valium®
   d. Demerol®
   e. Ambien®

4. (LO 51.6) What method is used for disposing of controlled drugs?
   a. Discard drugs; then complete DEA Form 41
   b. Use the disposal company that takes your biohazardous waste
   c. Turn drugs over to a larger healthcare facility
   d. Complete DEA Form 41 and call the DEA for disposal instructions
   e. Complete DEA Form 222; then dispose of drugs with biohazardous waste

5. (LO 51.4) An example of an OTC medication is
   a. Glucophage®
   b. Lasix®
   c. Coumadin®
   d. Lipitor®
   e. Prevacid®

6. (LO 51.7) The *Sig* line of a prescription reads "i tab po bid" What does it mean?
   a. Take 1 tablet by mouth twice a day
   b. The order is not accurate and cannot be used
   c. Take 1 tablet by mouth daily
   d. Take ½ tablet daily
   e. Take daily 1 tablet

7. (LO 51.8) A patient would like to know more about non-pharmacologic treatments for pain. Which of the following would you *least* likely discuss with this patient?
   a. Massage therapy
   b. Biofeedback therapy
   c. Acupuncture
   d. Glucosamine chondroitin
   e. Opioids

8. (LO 51.1) Which of the following would *least* likely be the medical assistant's role?
   a. Make sure the licensed practitioner is aware of all medications a patient is taking
   b. Ask each patient about alcohol and recreational drug use
   c. Prescribe and dispense certain medications
   d. Manage and renew medication prescriptions
   e. Educate the patient according to licensed practitioner guidelines

9. (LO 51.9) Which of the following is made from microorganisms and administered to a person to produce reduced sensitivity to an infectious disease?
   a. Controlled substance
   b. Immunity
   c. Vaccine
   d. Antibiotic
   e. Pharmaceutical

10. (LO 51.2) Which of the following is the category of pharmacology that is also called *clinical pharmacology?*
   a. Pharmacodynamics
   b. Pharmacognosy
   c. Pharmacokinetics
   d. Pharmacotherapeutics
   e. Toxicology

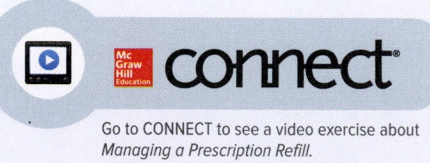

Go to CONNECT to see a video exercise about *Managing a Prescription Refill.*

Recall Kaylyn Haddix from the case study at the beginning of the chapter. Once Kaylyn finished her organization of the drugs at BWW, she received compliments from Malik, and he even gave her a small raise. She was so excited that at dinner one night with a group of friends she mentioned how she had organized the drug inventory at work and that she had gotten a raise. Someone at the table said, "Hey, can you get me some drugs?" Later, the same person, whom Kaylyn did not know very well, asked what kind of drugs she was working with and explained how she had a lot of trouble getting enough medication for her back pain. What should Kaylyn say or do in this situation?

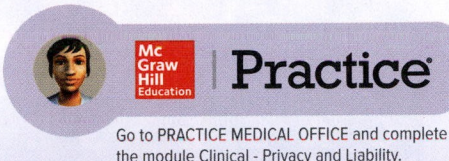

Go to PRACTICE MEDICAL OFFICE and complete the module Clinical - Privacy and Liability.

Dosage Calculations

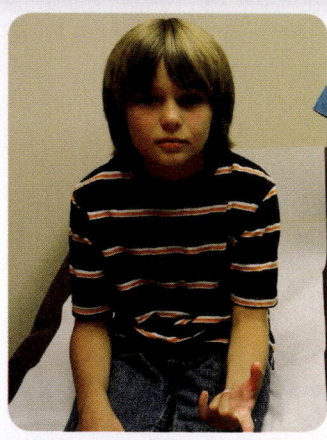
LEARNING OUTCOMES

After completing Chapter 52, you will be able to:

52.1 Explain the role of the medical assistant to ensure safe dosage calculations.

52.2 Identify systems of measurements and their common uses.

52.3 Convert among systems of measurements.

52.4 Execute dosage calculations accurately.

52.5 Calculate dosages based on body weight and body surface area.

KEY TERMS

amount to administer (*A*)

apothecary system

body surface area (BSA)

desired dose (*D*)

dose on hand (*H*)

formula method

household system

metric system

nomogram

proportion method

proportions

quantity (*Q*)

volume

weight

CAAHEP

ABHES

II.C.1 Demonstrate knowledge of basic math computations

II.C.2 Apply mathematical computations to solve equations

II.C.3 Define basic units of measurement in:
  (a) the metric system
  (b) the household system

II.C.4 Convert among measurement systems

II.C.5 Identify abbreviations and symbols used in calculating medication dosages

II.P.1 Calculate proper dosages of medication for administration

6. Pharmacology
  b. Demonstrate accurate occupational math and metric conversions for proper medication administration

9. Clinical Procedures
  j. Make adaptations with patients with special needs

▶ Introduction

Depending on the facility and state where you work as a medical assistant, you may be called on to administer medications. All aspects of this skill require close attention to detail for the safety of the patient. Before you administer a drug, you may need to calculate the dose prescribed by the licensed practitioner. You should also be familiar with the equipment you will be using. You must execute all dosage calculations carefully and accurately in order to prevent medication errors. To do so, you must perform basic math, understand various systems of measurement, and be able to convert from one measurement system to another or within a system. You also may need to know calculations for special patient populations. This chapter will provide the basics of safe dosage calculations. Remember to check the scope of practice in your state and at your place of employment before working with dosages.

▶ Ensuring Safe Dosage Calculations LO 52.1

In order to calculate dosages, you must understand and be able to perform basic math accurately. Whether you are using a calculator or doing it by hand, accuracy is key. Remember that a minor mistake in basic math can mean major errors in the patient's medication. When you perform any calculation, think about the answer you obtain and determine if it is reasonable.

Consider this example: While performing a calculation, a medical assistant adds the following numbers: 21¾, 12½, and 1½. He calculates an answer of 49¼. Before he accepts this answer as correct, however, he asks himself, "Is this reasonable?" In order to answer this question, he does a quick estimation. First, he adds the whole numbers from each of the mixed numbers in the problem: 21 + 12 + 1 = 34. Then he rounds each mixed number up to a whole number and

adds them: 22 + 13 + 2 = 37. He recognizes that the correct answer to the problem must be between 34 and 37, so his original answer is incorrect. He probably entered one of the numbers into his calculator incorrectly. When he repeats the original calculation, he now comes up with an answer of 35¾. This is between the values that he expected based on his estimate, so it is a reasonable answer to the problem.

Think about the example. When performing calculations, there are many steps in which an error might be made. In this case, a number had been entered incorrectly into a calculator. While errors like this can happen to anyone, they can usually be detected by performing a quick check to see if the answer

POINTS ON PRACTICE
Math Review

Recall the following math rules while performing dosage calculations.

1. Order of operations: When solving a math problem, first divide or multiply from left to right; then add or subtract from left to right. For example, for the equation $\frac{650}{325} \times 3 = x$, you would need to divide 650 by 325 first. This equals 2.

   $x = 2 \times 3$

   Multiply second: $= 6$.

2. Proportions: Proportions are two fractions that are equal to each other. When 3 of the 4 values in a proportion are known, the unknown value can be calculated. Proportions using fractions are solved by cross multiplying. For example, to solve for the unknown in $\frac{2}{3} = \frac{x}{12}$, cross multiply ($3 \times x = 2 \times 12$) and then solve for the unknown ($3 \times x = 24$; divide both sides by 3; $x = 8$).

CAUTION: HANDLE WITH CARE

Working with Decimals

Consider the following when working with decimals to prevent errors in dosage calculations.

1. Writing decimals

- Write the whole-number part of the decimal to the left of the decimal point.
- Write the decimal fraction part to the right of the decimal point. Decimal fractions are equivalent to fractions that have denominators of 10, 100, 1,000, and so forth.
- Use zero as a placeholder to the right of the decimal point just as you use zero for whole numbers. The decimal number 1.203 represents 1 ones, 2 tenths, 0 hundredths, and 3 thousandths.

2. Using zeros

- Always write a zero to the left of the decimal point when the decimal number has no whole-number part. Using the zero makes the decimal point more noticeable.

- Never place a zero after the last nonzero digit to the right of the decimal point when working with medication dosages. These "trailing zeros" can be misinterpreted and cause medication errors.

3. Rounding decimals

- Underline the place value to which you want to round.
- Look at the digit to the right of this target place value. If this digit is 4 or less, do not change the digit in the target place value. If this digit is 5 or more, round the digit in the target place value up one unit. For example, to round 2.7384 to the hundredths place, underline the 3, which is in the hundredths place. The digit to the right of the 3 is 8, which is greater than 5, so you round the number up to 2.74.
- Drop all digits to the right of the target place value.

---

is reasonable. You should develop the habit of asking yourself the same question *every time you perform a calculation.* When performing a calculation, analyze the problem and try to estimate a reasonable range for the answer. This critical thinking skill can help you to detect errors and should become a part of every calculation you perform.

Safe dosage calculations also depend on your understanding of basic math calculations. Refer to the *Points on Practice feature:* Math Review for a quick refresher on some important math concepts.

▶ Measurement Systems   LO 52.2

The three systems of measurement used in the United States for pharmacology and drug administration are the metric, apothecary, and household systems. Metric is the most commonly used system. Although apothecary and household systems are rarely used, you may need a basic knowledge of these systems.

To understand drug measurement, focus primarily on remembering the basic unit of volume and weight. **Volume** refers to the amount of space a drug occupies. **Weight** refers to its heaviness. Length, which is also a basic unit, is discussed in the *Vital Signs and Measurements* chapter.

Metric System

Like the decimal system, the **metric system** is based on multiples of 10. The greater your confidence working with decimals, the more comfortable you will be working with metric units. See the *Caution: Handle with Care* feature Working with Decimals. The basic units of volume and weight in the decimal-based metric system are liters (L) to measure volume and grams (g) to measure weight. Prefixes are added to these basic units of measurement to indicate multiples, such as kilogram (kg), or fractions, such as milliliter (mL) or microgram (mcg). Common metric units and equivalents are presented in Table 52-1. Note that a cubic centimeter (cc) is the amount of space occupied by 1 mL. Although these two measurements are equal, the accepted medical abbreviation is mL. Do not use the abbreviation "cc," even though you may sometimes see it in practice. Additionally, note that the abbreviation for liters is a capital L instead of a small l. The small l can be confused with the numeral 1.

Apothecary and Household Systems

Although the metric system is preferred for dosage calculations, as a medical assistant you should have basic knowledge of the much older apothecary system, as well as the commonly known **household system.** The **apothecary system** uses units such as fluid ounces, fluid drams, pints, and quarts for volume,

---

TABLE 52-1	Common Metric Units				
Prefix	**Kilo-**	**Base Unit**	**Centi-**	**Milli-**	**Micro-**
Value	× 1,000	—	÷ 100	÷ 1,000	÷ 1,000,000
Weight	kilogram (kg) 1,000 g	gram (g) 1 g	centigram (cg) 0.01 g	milligram (mg) 0.001 g	microgram (mcg) 0.000001 g
Volume	kiloliter (kL) 1,000 L	liter (L) 1 L	centiliter (cL) 0.01 L	milliliter (mL) 0.001 L	microliter (mcL) 0.000001 L

TABLE 52-2 Apothecary Units and Equivalents

Apothecary Units	Equivalents
Measures of Volume	
8 fluid drams (fl dr) =	1 fluid ounce (fl oz)
16 fl oz =	1 pint (pt)
2 pt =	1 quart (qt)
4 qt =	1 gallon (gal)
Measures of Weight	
60 gr =	1 dram (dr)
8 dr =	1 ounce (oz)
16 oz =	1 pound (lb)

TABLE 52-3 Household Units and Equivalents

Household Units	Equivalents
Measures of Volume	
60 drops* (gtt) =	1 teaspoon (tsp)
3 tsp =	1 tablespoon (tbsp)
6 tsp =	1 ounce (oz) or 2 tbsp
8 fl oz =	1 cup (c)
2 c =	1 pint (pt)
4 c =	1 quart (qt) or 2 pt

*Droppers may vary.

and drams, ounces, and pounds for weight. The only household units used for measurement are units of volume. They include drops, teaspoons, tablespoons, ounces, cups, pints, quarts, and gallons. Keep in mind that similar units of measurement in both the apothecary and the household systems are equal: An apothecary ounce equals a household ounce. Apothecary and household units and equivalents you may come across in practice are outlined in Table 52-2 and Table 52-3.

▶ Conversions Within and Between Measurement Systems   LO 52.3

Frequently, you will need to convert units of measure within or between systems of measurement. Most commonly, you will convert within the metric system. For example, you may need to determine how many milligrams of medication to give a patient when the medication only comes in grams. Sometimes you may need to convert from one measurement system to another. For example, a patient may need to take 5 milliliters of medication and the only measuring device she has is a teaspoon.

Converting Within the Metric System

Converting one metric unit of measurement to another is similar to multiplying and dividing decimal numbers. When you convert a quantity from one unit of metric measurement to another, you should follow these rules:

1. Move the decimal point to the right when you convert from a larger to a smaller unit. This is dividing.

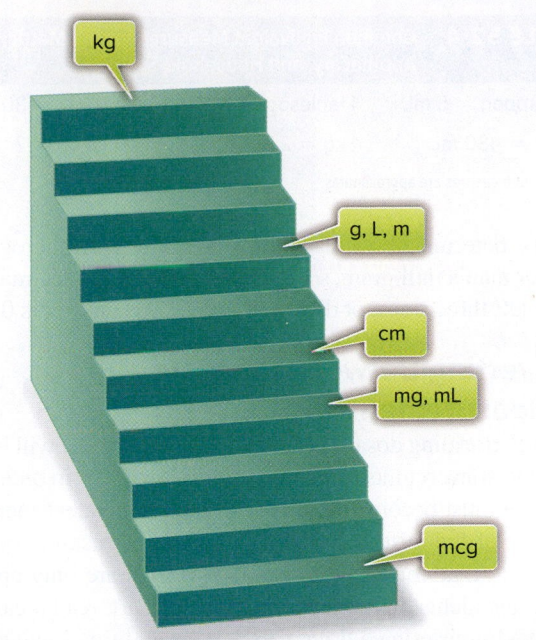

FIGURE 52-1 Use the metric steps to convert between units in the metric system.

2. Move the decimal point to the left when you convert from a smaller to a larger unit. This is multiplying.

Use Table 52-1 and Figure 52-1 to help determine both the direction and the number of places to move the decimal point when you convert between units of metric measurement. For example, milliliter is three decimal places to the right of liter, the basic unit. To convert a quantity from liters (larger) to milliliters (smaller), move the decimal point three places to the right, or three steps down the stairs shown in Figure 52-1. Similarly, to convert a quantity from grams (smaller) to kilograms (larger), move the decimal point three places to the left, or three steps up the stairs.

Let's try these examples.

Example A You need to change the patient's weight from grams to kilograms to determine how much medication should be given based on the patient's weight. An infant weighs 9,600 grams (g). How many kilograms (kg) does she weigh? A gram is smaller than a kilogram, so you need to move the decimal point to the left three steps, or divide by 1,000.

9.600 g ÷ 1,000 = 9.6 kg

Example B The physician orders a patient to have a 1-gram dose of amoxicillin. The medication is supplied in 1,000-mg tablets. You will need to determine how many milligrams are in a gram. A gram is larger than a milligram, so you need to move the decimal point to the right three steps, or multiply by 1,000.

1.000. gram × 1,000 = 1,000 mg

Your Turn A patient takes a daily dose of Synthroid® 100 mcg (micrograms). How many mg (milligrams) does he take?

*Equivalent measures are approximates.

First determine how many mg are in a mcg. A microgram is smaller than a milligram, so you need to move the decimal point to the left three steps, or divide by 1,000. The answer is 0.1 mg.

Converting Between Systems of Measurement

When performing dosage calculations, sometimes it will be necessary to convert units from one system to another. In order to do this, you must become familiar with their equivalent measures. Because of the difference in basic units of measure, you must remember that conversions between systems are only approximate equivalents. If you use a conversion chart, read it carefully before administering a drug. Check it several times and place a ruler under the line you are reading to be absolutely sure you are reading the chart properly. Table 52-4 provides equivalent measures for the metric, apothecary, and household systems.

In some cases, you may need to convert between systems of measurement by doing a calculation. You can use the **proportion method** to calculate these conversions. Let's try these examples.

Example A Suppose the licensed practitioner orders 10 milliliters (mL) of Benadryl® elixir. However, there is only a teaspoon (tsp) available to measure the dose. To make this conversion, follow these steps.

1. Set up a fraction with the ordered dose on the top and the unknown amount on the bottom:

$$\frac{10 \text{ mL}}{x}$$

2. Next set up a fraction with the standard equivalent. See Table 52-4. Make sure that for this fraction you use units of measure on the top and the bottom that match the units of measure on the top and the bottom of the first fraction:

$$\frac{5 \text{ mL}}{1 \text{ tsp}}$$

3. Then set up a proportion with both fractions:

$$\frac{10 \text{ mL}}{x} = \frac{5 \text{ mL}}{1 \text{ tsp}}$$

4. Now cross multiply. Multiply the bottom left number by the top right number, and multiply the top left number by the bottom right number:

$$x \times 5 \text{ mL} = 10 \text{ mL} \times 1 \text{ tsp}$$

5. To solve for x, divide both sides of the equation by 5 mL; then do the arithmetic, canceling out like terms in the top and bottom of each fraction:

$$\frac{x \times 5 \text{ mL}}{5 \text{ mL}} = \frac{10 \text{ mL} \times 1 \text{ tsp}}{5 \text{ mL}}$$

$$x = 2 \text{ tsp}$$

Example B Suppose the medication is ordered based on the patient's weight in kilograms. You know the patient's weight is 168 lb. To make this conversion, follow these steps:

1. Set up a fraction with the weight in pounds on top and the unknown weight in kilograms on the bottom:

$$\frac{168 \text{ lb}}{x \text{ kg}}$$

2. Next set up a fraction with the standard equivalent. See Table 52-4. Make sure that for this fraction you use units of measure on the top and the bottom that match the units of measure on the top and the bottom of the first fraction:

$$\frac{2.2 \text{ lb}}{1 \text{ kg}}$$

3. Then set up a proportion with both fractions:

$$\frac{168 \text{ lb}}{x \text{ kg}} = \frac{2.2 \text{ lb}}{1 \text{ kg}}$$

4. Now cross multiply. Multiply the bottom left number by the top right number, and multiply the top left number by the bottom right number:

$$x \times 2.2 \text{ lb} = 168 \text{ lb} \times 1 \text{ kg}$$

5. To solve for x, divide both sides of the equation by 2.2 lb; then do the arithmetic, canceling out like terms in the top and bottom of each fraction and then dividing 168 by 2.2:

$$\frac{x \times 2.2 \text{ lb}}{2.2 \text{ lb}} = \frac{168 \text{ lb} \times 1 \text{ kg}}{2.2 \text{ lb}}$$

$$x = 76.36 \text{ kg}$$

Your Turn You need to prepare a solution for the licensed practitioner to clean a wound. He asks for 3½ fluid ounces (fl oz) of saline to be placed in sterile bowl. Your container of saline is marked in milliliters (mL). Use these steps to make the conversion:

1. Set up a fraction with the ordered dose on the top and the unknown amount on the bottom.

2. Next, set up a fraction with the standard equivalent. See Table 52-4. Make sure that for this fraction you use units of measure on the top and the bottom that match the units of measure on the top and the bottom of the first fraction.

3. Then set up a proportion with both fractions.

4. Now cross multiply. Multiply the bottom left number by the top right number, and multiply the top left number by the bottom right number.

5. To solve for x, cancel out like terms in the top and bottom of each fraction, then do the arithmetic.

If you followed each step correctly, you find that you need 105 mL of saline.

▶ Dosage Calculations   LO 52.4

As a medical assistant, you may be called on to calculate medication doses. Remember to follow your scope of practice. You may be able to calculate these using either the proportion method or a **formula method.** No matter which method you use, you must be aware that the patient's health or life can depend on your calculations. Always take the time to check and recheck your arithmetic. If you have a question or you are not sure about your calculations, check them again and then have a coworker check. If you are not 100% sure you know how to do dosage calculations correctly, consider buying and using a dosage calculation workbook or searching the Internet for extra practice.

Proportion Method for Dosage Calculations

The proportion method described earlier in the chapter for unit conversion also can be used to perform dosage calculations. Let's try some examples.

Example A Suppose the doctor orders 500 mg of ampicillin, but each tablet contains only 250 mg. To calculate how to provide this dose, follow these steps:

1. Set up a fraction with the amount of the drug ordered over the unknown (in this case, the number of tablets).

$$\frac{500 \text{ mg}}{x \text{ tab}}$$

2. Next, set up a fraction with the amount of drug in a single tablet (dose on hand) over 1 tablet (dosage unit).

$$\frac{250 \text{ mg}}{1 \text{ tab}}$$

3. Now set up the proportion with both fractions, making sure the same units of measure are on the top and bottom of each side of the proportion.

$$\frac{500 \text{ mg}}{x \text{ tab}} = \frac{250 \text{ mg}}{1 \text{ tab}}$$

4. Cross multiply. Multiply the bottom left number by the top right number, and multiply the top left number by the bottom right number:

$$x \text{ tab} \times 250 \text{ mg} = 500 \text{ mg} \times 1 \text{ tab}$$

5. To solve for x, divide both sides of the equation by 250 mg; then do the arithmetic, canceling out like terms in the top and bottom of each fraction:

$$\frac{x \times 250 \text{ mg}}{250 \text{ mg}} = \frac{500 \text{ mg} \times 1 \text{ tab}}{250 \text{ mg}}$$
$$x = \frac{500 \text{ tab}}{250}$$
$$x = 2 \text{ tab}$$

The patient will receive 2 tablets.

Example B The doctor orders 30 mg of Adalat®, but each capsule (cap) contains only 10 mg. To calculate the prescribed drug dose using the proportion method, you would follow these steps:

1. Set up a fraction with the amount of the drug ordered over the unknown amount (in this case, the number of capsules).

$$\frac{30 \text{ mg}}{x \text{ cap}}$$

2. Next set up a fraction with the amount of drug in a single capsule (dose on hand) over 1 capsule (dosage unit).

$$\frac{10 \text{ mg}}{1 \text{ cap}}$$

3. Now set up the proportion using both fractions, making sure the same units of measure are on the top and bottom of each side of the proportion.

$$\frac{30 \text{ mg}}{x \text{ cap}} = \frac{10 \text{ mg}}{1 \text{ cap}}$$

4. Cross multiply. Multiply the bottom left number by the top right number, and multiply the top left number by the bottom right number:

$$x \text{ cap} \times 10 \text{ mg} = 30 \text{ mg} \times 1 \text{ cap}$$

5. To solve for x, divide both sides of the equation by 10 mg; then do the arithmetic, canceling out like terms in the top and bottom of each fraction:

$$\frac{x \times 10 \text{ mg}}{10 \text{ mg}} = \frac{30 \text{ mg} \times 1 \text{ cap}}{10 \text{ mg}}$$
$$x = \frac{30 \text{ cap}}{10}$$
$$x = 3 \text{ cap}$$

The patient will receive 3 capsules.

Example C Now let's try a liquid medication. The licensed practitioner wants a patient to have 375 mg of valproic acid. You have on hand a bottle of valproic acid oral solution. See the label in Figure 52-2. Follow these steps:

1. Set up a fraction with the amount of the drug ordered over the unknown amount (in this case, the amount of liquid in mL).

$$\frac{375 \text{ mg}}{x \text{ mL}}$$

2. Next set up a fraction with the amount of drug in a single dose (dose on hand) over the number of mL in a single dose (dosage unit).

$$\frac{250 \text{ mg}}{5 \text{ mL}}$$

3. Now set up the proportion using both fractions, making sure the same units of measure are on the top and bottom of each side of the proportion.

$$\frac{375 \text{ mg}}{x \text{ mL}} = \frac{250 \text{ mg}}{5 \text{ mL}}$$

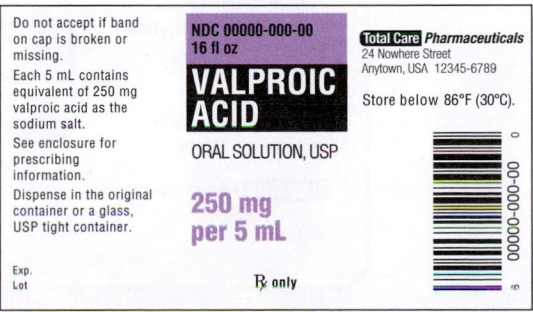

FIGURE 52-2 Valproic acid oral solution.

4. Cross multiply. Multiply the bottom left number by the top right number, and multiply the top left number by the bottom right number:

$$x \times 250 \text{ mg} = 375 \text{ mg} \times 5 \text{ mL}$$

5. To solve for x, divide both sides of the equation by 250 mg; then do the arithmetic, canceling out like terms in the top and bottom of each fraction and then multiplying 375×5 and dividing by 250:

$$\frac{x \times \cancel{250 \text{ mg}}}{\cancel{250 \text{ mg}}} = \frac{375 \text{ mg} \times 5 \text{ mL}}{250 \text{ mg}}$$

$$x = \frac{375 \times 5 \text{ mL}}{250}$$

$$x = 7.5 \text{ mL}$$

The patient will receive 7.5 mL of medication.

Your Turn The physician has ordered diazepam 4 mg by mouth. You have on hand the bottle of diazepam shown in Figure 52-3. Follow the steps below to determine how much medicine the patient should receive.

1. Set up a fraction with the amount of the drug ordered over the unknown (in this case, the number of tablets).

2. Next, set up a fraction with the amount of drug in a single tablet (dose on hand) over 1 tablet (dosage unit).

3. Now set up the proportion with both fractions, making sure the same units of measure are on the top and bottom of each side of the proportion.

4. Cross multiply. Multiply the bottom left number by the top right number, and multiply the top left number by the bottom right number.

5. To solve for x, cancel out like terms in the top and bottom of each fraction, then do the arithmetic.

If you did the problem correctly, you will discover that the patient needs 2 tablets.

Formula Method for Dosage Calculations

In some instances, you can use a basic formula to calculate drugs that have the same units as the dose ordered—such as milligrams and milligrams—and therefore do not require a conversion. When you use the formula method, you substitute the correct numbers for what each of the letters represents. The basic formula that you would use looks like this:

$$A = \frac{D}{H} \times Q$$

Using this formula, you will need to know the following:

A = **Amount to administer** (the amount of medication the patient will receive)

D = **Desired dose** (the amount of medication the licensed practitioner has ordered the patient to take)

H = **Dose on hand** (the amount of medication in each unit of the drug—for example, the number of mcg, mg, or g in each unit dose)

Q = **Quantity** of the dose on hand or dosage unit—for example, a pill or an amount of liquid

Let's try some examples.

Example A Suppose that the licensed practitioner orders acetaminophen 650 milligrams (mg). This is the desired dose (D). However, all that the office has on hand are 325 mg Tylenol® tablets. The dose on hand (H) is 325 mg, and the quantity (Q) or dosage unit is 1 tablet, because the dose on hand (325 mg) is given per tablet. Follow these steps to perform the calculation:

1. Use the formula, inserting each number, and label all the parts:

$$A = \frac{D}{H} \times Q$$

$$A = \frac{650 \text{ mg}}{325 \text{ mg}} \times 1 \text{ tablet}$$

2. Cancel and solve:

$$A = \frac{650 \cancel{\text{ mg}}}{325 \cancel{\text{ mg}}} \times 1 \text{ tablet}$$

$$A = \frac{650}{325} \times 1 \text{ tab}$$

$$A = 2 \text{ tablets}$$

Two tablets need to be given to the patient. See the *Medication Administration* chapter for the correct procedure for administering a medication.

Example B Now let's say the licensed practitioner asks you to administer 10 mg of Compazine® by injection. The desired dose (D) is 10 mg. According to the Compazine®

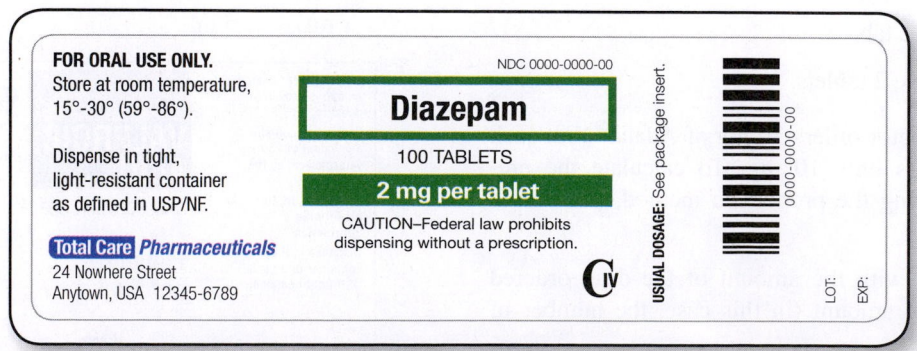

FIGURE 52-3 Diazepam tablets.

label, the liquid contains 5 mg/mL, which means there are 5 mg of Compazine® in every 1 mL of liquid, so 5 mg is the dose on hand (*H*) and 1 mL is the quantity (*Q*) or dosage unit. Always read the label carefully to determine the dose on hand and the quantity or dosage unit. See the *Caution: Handle with Care* feature Preventing Errors During Dosage Calculations. Follow the same steps to perform the calculation:

1. Use the formula, inserting each number in the correct place, and label all the parts:

$$A = \frac{D}{H} \times Q$$

$$A = \frac{10 \text{ mg}}{5 \text{ mg}} \times 1 \text{ mL}$$

2. Cancel and solve:

$$A = \frac{10 \text{ mg}}{5 \text{ mg}} \times 1 \text{ mL}$$

$$A = \frac{10}{5} \times 1 \text{ mL}$$

$$A = 2 \text{ mL}$$

The amount to administer to the patient is 2 mL. See the *Medication Administration* chapter for the correct procedure for administering a medication.

Example C The licensed practitioner wants a pediatric patient to have 200 mg of clarithromycin. The label of the only bottle you have on hand is pictured in Figure 52-4.

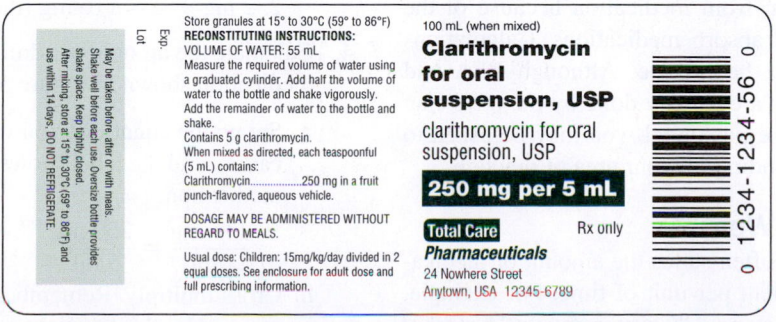

FIGURE 52-4 Clarithromycin for oral suspension.

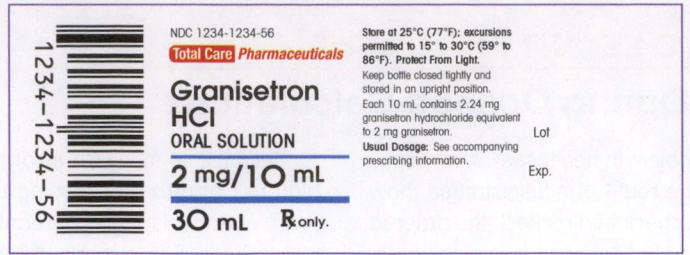

FIGURE 52-5 Granisetron hydrochloride oral solution.

1. Use the formula, inserting each number, and label all the parts:

$$A = \frac{D}{H} \times Q$$

$$A = \frac{200 \text{ mg}}{250 \text{ mg}} \times 5 \text{ mL}$$

2. Cancel and solve:

$$A = \frac{200 \cancel{\text{ mg}}}{250 \cancel{\text{ mg}}} \times 5 \text{ mL}$$

$$A = \frac{200}{250} \times 5 \text{ mL}$$

$$A = 4 \text{ mL}$$

The patient should receive 4 mL of oral suspension. See the *Medication Administration* chapter for the correct procedure for administering an oral medication.

Your Turn The licensed practitioner orders 1.5 mg of granisetron hydrochloride oral solution. You have on hand the medication shown in Figure 52-5. How much medication should the patient receive?

1. Use the formula, inserting each number, and label all the parts.
2. Cancel units and solve.

The patient should receive 7.5 mL of medication. See the *Medication Administration* chapter for the correct procedure for administering an oral medication.

▶ Body Weight and Body Surface Area Calculations
LO 52.5

In certain cases, a drug dose is determined based on the **body surface area (BSA)** or the weight of the patient. This is more common with pediatric and geriatric patients. These patients are at greater risk of harm from medication because of the way they break down and absorb medications. Calculations for these individuals must be precise. Although BSA and weight dosage calculations are usually done by the physician or other licensed healthcare personnel, you may be asked to perform calculations, depending on your area of practice.

Dosages Based on Weight

An order based on weight often states the amount of medication per weight of the patient per unit of time. For example, an order for a 34 lb child may read "Clarithromycin 15 mg/kg/day po q12h." This means that over the course of a day, the

patient should receive 15 mg of medication for every kilogram (kg) he or she weighs. A portion of this total amount is to be given every 12 hours, or 2 times during a 24-hour period. You will need to calculate the patient's weight in kilograms, the total medication to administer in 24 hours, and the amount of medication to administer in each dose. Use these steps:

1. Calculate the weight in kilograms using the proportion method. For accuracy, round the results to the nearest hundredth.
   a. Set up the proportion. Recall from Table 52-4 that 2.2 lb = 1 kg.

   $$\frac{34 \text{ lb}}{x \text{ kg}} = \frac{2.2 \text{ lb}}{1 \text{ kg}}$$

   b. Cross multiply. Remember to multiply the bottom left number by the top right number, and multiply the top left number by the bottom right number.

   $$x \text{ kg} \times 2.2 \text{ lb} = 34 \text{ lb} \times 1 \text{ kg}$$

   c. Solve for x (the unknown).

   $$x = \frac{34}{2.2} \text{ kg}$$

   $$x = 15.45$$

2. Calculate the desired dose (D) for 24 hours by multiplying the dose ordered by the weight in kilograms. (Round your answer to the nearest milligram.)

   $$15 \text{ mg} \times 15.45 \text{ kg} = \text{desired dose } (D) \text{ for 24 hours}$$

   231.75 mg, rounded to 232 mg = D (for 24 hours)

3. Calculate the amount of medication to administer in each dose. To do this, divide the amount to be administered in 24 hours by the number of times the medication will be administered in 24 hours. In this case, the medication is to be given two times in 24 hours.

   $$232 \text{ mg} \div 2 = 116 \text{ mg (the desired dose for one dose)}$$

4. Calculate the amount to administer. On hand you have the medication shown in Figure 52-6.

   a. Set up the equation. You want to give 116 mg of medication, and the label shows there are 250 mg in 5 mL of medication.

   $$\frac{116 \text{ mg}}{x \text{ mL}} = \frac{250 \text{ mg}}{5 \text{ mL}}$$

   b. Cross multiply. Remember to multiply the bottom left number by the top right number, and multiply the top left number by the bottom right number.

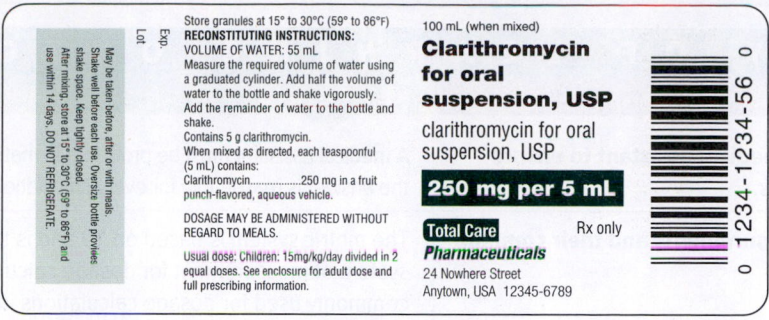

FIGURE 52-6 Clarithromycin for oral suspension.

$$x \text{ mL} \times 250 \text{ mg} = 116 \text{ mg} \times 5 \text{ mL}$$

  c. Solve for x to determine the amount of liquid medication to administer to this patient.

$$x \text{ mL} = 116 \times \frac{5}{250}$$

$$\text{mL} = 2.32$$

$$\text{mL} = 2.3 \text{ (rounded to the nearest tenth)}$$

Now that you have determined the amount, refer to the *Medication Administration* chapter before you give the medication to the patient.

Dosages Based on Body Surface Area

The total surface area of the body or body surface area (BSA) is measured in square meters (m^2). A person's BSA is used to calculate very precise medication dosages. Pediatric patients, as well as burn victims and patients undergoing chemotherapy or radiation therapy, may need BSA dosage calculations. A complex formula or a nomogram, as shown in Figure 52-7, may be used to determine the BSA. A **nomogram** is a set of scales arranged so that a ruler aligned with two of the values shows the corresponding value on the third scale. Aligning the ruler with a person's height and weight shows the body surface area. In this case, the child is 89 cm tall and weighs 13.9 kg. The line drawn between these values in the first and third columns crosses the second column at approximately 0.57, so the child's BSA is 0.57 m^2. For a medication ordered as 30 mcg/m^2, this patient would receive 30 mcg $\times$ 0.57 = 17.1 mcg of the medication.

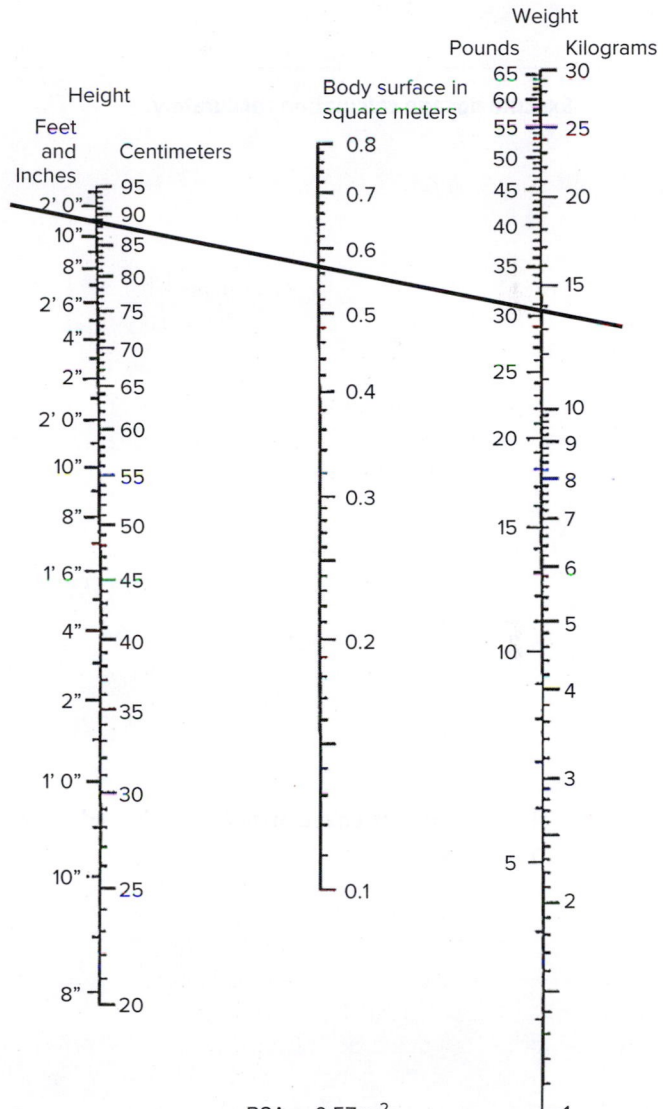

FIGURE 52-7 A nomogram is used to determine the BSA in order to calculate a medication dose.

SUMMARY OF LEARNING OUTCOMES

LEARNING OUTCOMES	KEY POINTS
52.1 Explain the role of the medical assistant to ensure safe dosage calculations.	A medical assistant must be proficient in math and determine whether the answer is reasonable for every calculation he or she performs.
52.2 Identify systems of measurements and their common uses.	The metric system is based on 10 and is the most common system of measurement for dosage calculations. Metric units commonly used for dosage calculations include g, mg, mcg, and mL. The apothecary and household systems have some equal measures, but they are used rarely.
52.3 Convert among systems of measurements.	To convert among systems of measurements, you can refer to a conversion chart or perform a proportion method calculation. Keep in mind that measurements between the metric and the apothecary and household systems are only approximations.
52.4 Execute dosage calculations accurately.	Use the proportion method or formula method to perform dosage calculations. *Proportion Method* 1. Set up a fraction with the amount of the drug ordered over the unknown amount. 2. Set up a fraction with the amount of drug in a single dose (dose on hand) over the dosage unit. 3. Set up the proportion using both fractions, making sure the same units of measure are on the top and bottom of each side of the proportion. 4. Cross multiply. 5. To solve for *x*, do the arithmetic; then cancel out like terms in the top and bottom of each fraction. *Formula Method* $A = \dfrac{D}{H} \times Q$ A = Amount to administer (the amount of medication the patient will receive) D = Desired dose (the amount of medication the licensed practitioner has ordered the patient to take) H = Dose on hand (the amount of medication in each unit of the drug) Q = Quantity of the dose on hand or dosage unit
52.5 Calculate dosages based on body weight and body surface area.	Dosages based on body weight and BSA are used when precise amounts of medication must be administered. Body weight calculations are usually ordered in mg/kg/day. BSA calculations use special formulas or a nomogram.

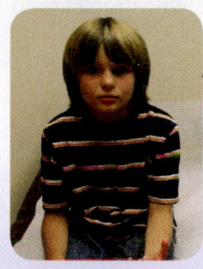

Recall Chris Matthews from the beginning of the chapter. Now that you have completed the chapter, answer the following questions.

1. The physician ordered amoxicillin 50 mg/kg/day po q8h. What is Chris's weight in kilograms?

2. The medication on hand is amoxicillin oral suspension 200 mg per 5 mL. How much medication, in milliliters, should Chris receive for each dose?

3. Name at least three things you can do to ensure that Chris receives a safe and accurate dose of medication.

EXAM PREPARATION QUESTIONS

There may be more than one correct answer. Circle the *best* answer.

1. (LO 52.1) As a medical assistant, how can you *best* ensure safe dosage calculations?
   a. Use a calculator for every calculation
   b. Check with a coworker for every calculation you perform
   c. Do not use the unit of measurement when performing calculations
   d. Use a trailing zero after the decimal point for whole numbers
   e. Check your calculation by determining if the results are reasonable

2. (LO 52.2) What do the following metric prefixes represent in comparison to the base unit: kilo; milli; micro?
   a. $\times$ 1,000; $\div$ 100; $\div$ 1,000,000
   b. $\times$ 100; $\div$ 1,000; $\div$ 1,000,000
   c. $\div$ 1,000,000; $\times$ 1,000; $\div$ 1,000
   d. $\times$ 1,000; $\div$ 1,000; $\div$ 1,000,000
   e. $\div$ 1,000; $\times$ 1,000; $\div$ 1,000,000

3. (LO 52.4) How much medication should be given if the physician ordered Keflex® 500 mg and you have on hand Keflex® 250 mg per 5 mL?
   a. 5 mL
   b. 250 mg
   c. 250 mL
   d. 10 mL
   e. 125 mL

4. (LO 52.4) How much medication would be in the syringe if the physician ordered Decadron® 6 mg IM now and you have on hand Decadron® 4 mg per mL?
   a. 1.5 mg
   b. 1.5 mL
   c. 4 mL
   d. 1 mL
   e. 3 mL

5. (LO 52.4) The doctor orders 5 mg of glyburide, but each tablet contains only 1.25 mg. How many tablets should the patient take?
   a. 3
   b. 1.25
   c. 5
   d. 1
   e. 4

6. (LO 52.5) The physician has ordered gemcitabine 400 mg/m^2 IV for a patient whose BSA is 0.47 m^2. You have on hand a 200 mg vial of gemcitabine for injection that contains 38 mg per mL. How much medication should this patient receive?
   a. 94 mg
   b. 17.9 mL
   c. 200 mg
   d. 5 mL
   e. 10.5 mL

7. (LO 52.3) The licensed practitioner orders Ceclor® 0.375 g PO bid. You have on hand Ceclor® oral suspension 187 mg per 5 mL. How many mg of Ceclor® are ordered?
   a. 187
   b. 5
   c. 0.375
   d. 375
   e. 0.187

8. (LO 52.4) The licensed practitioner orders Ceclor® 0.375 g PO bid. You have on hand Ceclor® oral suspension 187 mg per 5 mL. How many mL of Ceclor® do you need to administer?
   a. 10
   b. 5
   c. 187
   d. 2.5
   e. 0.375

9. (LO 52.4) The physician wants you to give the patient an IM injection of 135 mg of ceftriaxone. You have on hand the medication pictured here. How many mL of medication would you inject?

a. 2 mL
b. 135 mcg
c. 0.11 mL
d. 1,000 mg
e. 1.35 mL

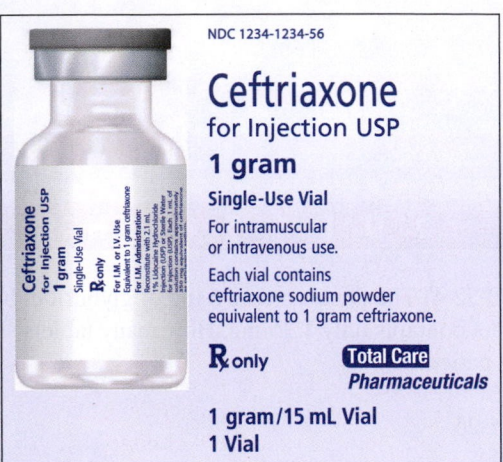

10. (LO 52.5) A 5-year-old child weighs 44 lb. The licensed practitioner orders him to receive Zinacef® 50 mg/kg/day IM q6h. How many milligrams of medication should the child receive in one dose?

a. 1,000 mg
b. 167 mg
c. 20 kg
d. 250 mg
e. 50 mg

SOFT SKILLS SUCCESS

1. The patient says she is here for a B_{12} injection and the order reads "Cyanocobalamin 500 mcg IM now." You have never given cyanocobalamin or a B_{12} injection before. What should you do?

2. Using the order in question 1, you find a vial of cyanocobalamin that is 1,000 mcg/mL and give the patient a 1 mL injection in the deltoid muscle of her left arm. When you get ready to chart the medication, you realize you should have given only 0.5 mL of the medication. What should you do now?

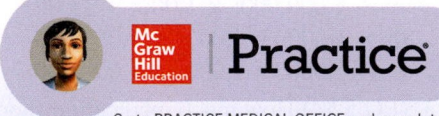

Go to PRACTICE MEDICAL OFFICE and complete the module Clinical - Privacy and Liability.

Medication Administration

CASE STUDY

PATIENT INFORMATION		
Patient Name John Miller	**DOB** 12/5/19XX	**Allergies** Bee stings
Attending Paul F. Buckwalter, MD	**MRN** 082-09-981	**Other Information** Seeing physical therapist 3X a week for injury.

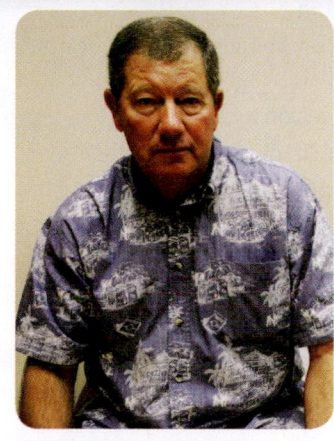

© McGraw-Hill Education

John Miller, a 65-year-old patient, has arrived at the clinic for a return-to-work visit. He has a history of hypertension, diabetes Type 2, myocardial infarction (MI) 4 years ago, and congestive heart failure (CHF). He has been taking glyburide 2.5 mg daily, captopril 25 mg twice a day, and HCTZ 25 mg daily. He is here for a blood pressure check and the physician wants to evaluate the medications he just started 3 months ago. He also is scheduled for a pneumococcal immunization. As you read through this chapter, think about what the medical assistant should do next and why.

Keep John Miller in mind as you study this chapter. There will be questions at the end of the chapter based on the case study. The information in the chapter will help you answer these questions.

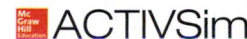 ACTIVSim

LEARNING OUTCOMES

After completing Chapter 53, you will be able to:

53.1 Describe rules and responsibilities regarding drug administration and the initial preparation for drug administration.

53.2 List the rights of drug administration.

53.3 Recognize the correct equipment to use for administering medications.

53.4 Carry out the procedures for administering oral medications.

53.5 Carry out procedures for administering parenteral medications by injection.

53.6 Carry out procedures for administering parenteral medications by other routes.

53.7 Relate special considerations required for medication administration to pediatric, pregnant, breast-feeding, and geriatric patients.

53.8 Outline patient education information related to medications.

53.9 Implement accurate and complete documentation of medications.

KEY TERMS

buccal	ointment
calibrated spoon	scored
diluent	solution
douche	subcutaneous (subcut)
infusion	sublingual
intradermal (ID)	transdermal
intramuscular (IM)	triple check
intravenous (IV)	Z-track method

I.P.4 Verify the rules of medication administration:
    (a) right patient
    (b) right medication
    (c) right dose
    (d) right route
    (e) right time
    (f) right documentation

I.P.5 Select proper sites for administering parenteral medication

I.P.6 Administer oral medications

I.P.7 Administer parenteral (excluding IV) medications

II.C.5 Identify both abbreviations and symbols used in calculating medication dosages

II.P.1 Prepare proper dosages of medication for administration

V.P.4 Coach patients regarding:
    (b) health maintenance
    (c) disease prevention
    (d) treatment plan

X.C.11 Describe the process in compliance reporting:
    (a) unsafe activities
    (b) errors in patient care
    (d) incident reports

X.P.3 Document patient care accurately in the medical record

X.P.6 Report an illegal activity in the healthcare setting following proper protocol

2. Anatomy and Physiology
    c. Identify diagnostic and treatment modalities as they relate to each body system

6. Pharmacology
    a. Identify drug classification, usual dose, side effects, and contraindications of the top most commonly used medications
    d. Properly utilize Physicians' Desk Reference (PDR), drug handbook and other drug references to identify a drug's classification, usual dosage, usual side effects, and contraindications

9. Medical Office Clinical Procedures
    f. Prepare and administer oral and parenteral medications and monitor intravenous (IV) infusions

▶ Introduction

Drug administration is one of the most important and most dangerous duties for a medical assistant. By following the procedures for proper drug administration, you can help restore patients to health. If you calculate dosages inaccurately, measure drugs incorrectly, or administer drugs improperly, patients' medications may have no therapeutic effect, may worsen their disease or abnormal condition, or may even cause them to die.

To administer drugs safely and effectively to all patient groups, including pediatric, pregnant, and elderly patients, you must know and understand the principles of pharmacology (see the *Principles of Pharmacology* chapter) and how to perform dosage calculations (see the *Dosage Calculations* chapter). This chapter prepares you to understand the fundamentals of drug administration, including

- Rules and responsibilities of drug administration.
- Rights of drug administration.
- Routes of medication administration.
- Techniques needed to administer drugs.
- Special patient considerations.
- Patient education.

Your role may vary depending on the state and practice where you are employed. Many states have medical practice acts that define the exact duties of medical assistants in drug administration. For example, an act may specify which drugs you are allowed to administer and by which routes. Because state laws vary, you need to research the scope of practice for medical assistants in the state where you will work.

▶ Preparing to Administer a Drug   LO 53.1

To administer drugs, you should know the uses, contraindications, interactions, and adverse effects of common drugs. You should be familiar with the medications frequently prescribed in your practice. Furthermore, to be able to assume a role in patient education, you must be comfortable with all aspects of drug administration so that you can instruct patients about the drugs prescribed to them.

Although the physician gives the order to administer a drug, the medical assistant has a lot of responsibility before a medication can be administered. As a medical assistant, you will often interview the patient. You must be alert to—and inform the licensed practitioner of—any change in the patient's condition that could affect drug therapy. Some preparation tasks are related to the drugs and drug allergies, administration site, patient condition, and patient consent.

Drugs and Drug Allergies

Before any medication is given, the physician should be aware of the medications the patient is currently taking. As you learned in the *Principles of Pharmacology* chapter, some medications, including herbal medications, can interact in a negative way, so the physician needs to know everything the patient is taking before ordering a medication. The medical assistant is responsible for ensuring that a complete and accurate medication list is maintained on the patient's chart. This medication list must be updated every time the patient comes for an appointment. See Figure 53-1. While asking about medications, you also must ask the patient about any drug allergies. Even though you may see a patient on a regular basis, be in the habit of asking about drugs and drug allergies at every patient visit. Patients often see other physicians or specialists, who may have prescribed different medications. A patient could have had a drug reaction to a medication prescribed by another physician. If applicable, document in the patient chart "NKDA," or "no known drug allergies."

Administration Site

Drugs may be administered for either local or systemic effects. Generally, drugs that have local effects are applied directly to the skin, tissues, or mucous membranes. Drugs that produce systemic effects are administered by routes that allow the drug to be absorbed and distributed in the bloodstream throughout the body. These various routes are discussed in the Drug Routes and Equipment section of this chapter. Before you administer a drug, you must check the site of administration. For example, if you are asked to give an oral medication, you must make sure the patient can take the medication. You may ask if the patient is nauseated, can swallow a pill, or has had anything to eat or drink, depending on the medication.

For an injection, you must locate and inspect the injection site. Find the appropriate injection site by using anatomical landmarks. Inspect the skin by checking for the following conditions, which may eliminate the site:

- Moles
- Scars
- Birthmarks
- Traumatic injury
- Redness
- Rash
- Edema
- Cyanosis
- Burns
- Tattoos
- Site of a mastectomy
- Paralyzed areas
- Warts

If you are unsure about any of these conditions, inform the physician.

Patient Condition

Before administering a medication, observe the patient for any condition that might interfere with the medication you will be administering. For example, a patient who is nauseated or vomiting may not be able to swallow a pill. In addition, review the patient's drug list to ensure that any medications already being taken will not interfere with the ordered drug or route of administration. Double-check the order and ensure that it is appropriate for the patient's age and weight.

Patient Consent Form

Many physicians require that a patient sign a consent form before receiving an injection. A consent is necessary for vaccines, for example. This form provides general information regarding the medication or vaccine and lists the possible side effects or adverse effects. If a consent form is needed, make sure that the patient signs the form and that you have answered any questions prior to giving the injection.

General Rules for Drug Administration

No matter what drug or administration route is ordered, follow these general rules when administering drugs.

- Give only the drugs the physician has ordered. Written orders are preferable, but oral orders are appropriate for emergencies. If you are unfamiliar with any aspect of a drug the physician orders, consult a credible drug reference.
- Wash your hands before handling the drug. Prepare the drug in a well-lit area, away from distractions. Focus only on the task at hand.
- Perform a **triple check** by checking the medication three times. Check the medication three times even if the dose is prepackaged, labeled, and ready to be administered.

> *1st check*—when you take it from the storage container and match it to the medication administration record (MAR)
>
> *2nd check*—when you prepare it
>
> *3rd check*—before you close the storage container or just before you administer the medication to the patient

- Calculate the dose if necessary. See the *Dosage Calculations* chapter. Remember, if you are unsure of your computation, ask another medical assistant or a licensed practitioner to check it.
- Avoid leaving a prepared drug unattended and never administer a drug that someone else has prepared.
- Ask the patient to state his name and date of birth to ensure correct identification. Double-check with the patient about possible drug allergies. Do not rely on documentation in his chart; he may have developed a new allergy that has not yet been added to the record.
- Be sure the physician is in the office when you administer a drug or vaccine. If the patient develops an anaphylactic reaction (sudden, severe allergic reaction) to the drug or vaccine, the physician must administer epinephrine.

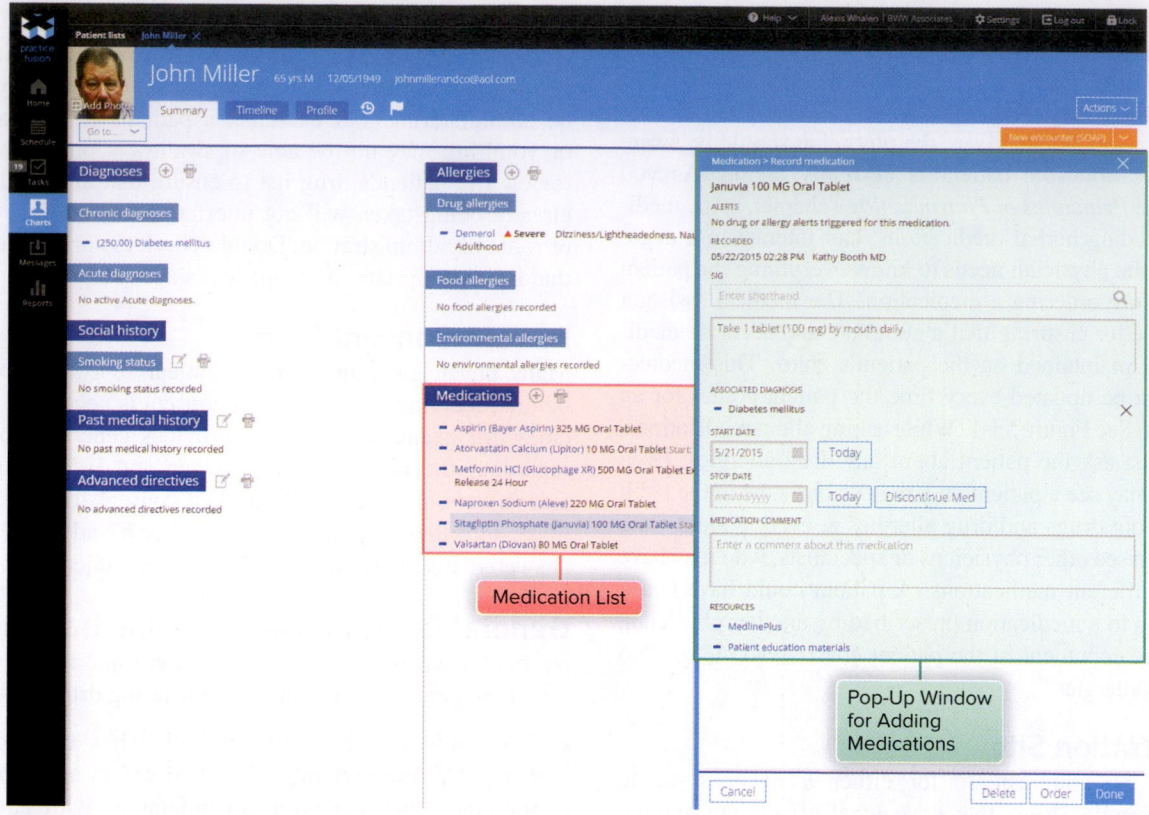

(a)

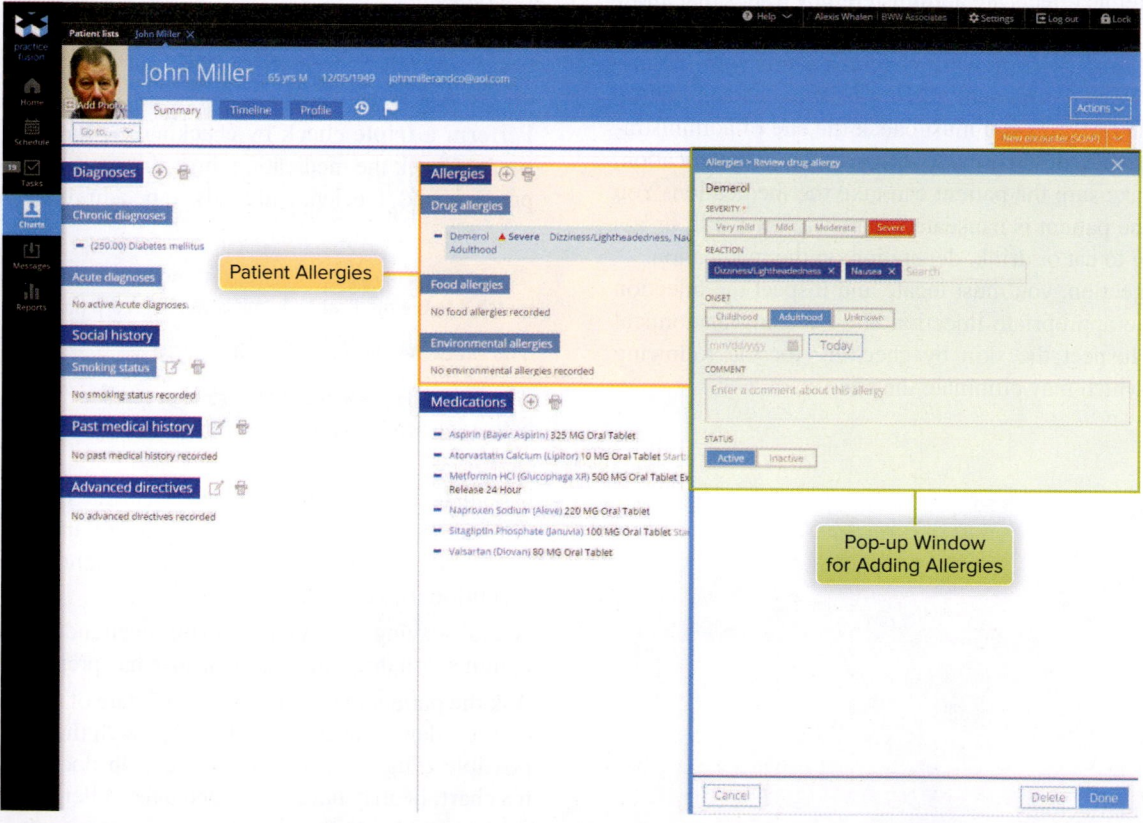

(b)

FIGURE 53-1 (a) Each time a patient visits the clinic, update the medication list as needed. (b) Be certain to ask about allergies and record these in the allergy window in the electronic health record.

© Practice Fusion®

Handling Medication Errors

Medication errors are a serious, yet inevitable, problem. Great care should always be taken to prevent them. However, if an error does occur, no matter the cause, it must be reported. Immediately tell the licensed practitioner. Not reporting an error is unethical and in some cases illegal, especially if a serious consequence occurs. Most facilities require that an incident report be completed. This form documents the error. It is completed and then signed by everyone involved, as well as your supervisor. Errors also are reported online through an online program developed by the US Pharmacopeia and the Institute for Safe Medical Practices. Reporting errors at these sites provides information to assist in the prevention of errors.

- After administering the drug, ask the patient to remain in the facility for 10 to 20 minutes so that you can observe the patient for any unexpected effects, such as anaphylaxis. See the *Emergency Preparedness* chapter.

- Give the patient specific instructions about the effects of the drug as well as general information about drug use.

- If the patient refuses to take the drug, discard it according to your facility policy. Do not flush it down the toilet or return it to the original container. Be sure to document the refusal in the patient's record and tell the physician.

- If you make an error in drug administration, tell the physician immediately. See the *Caution: Handle with Care* feature Handling Medication Errors.

- Document the drug and dose immediately after administration; never document administration before giving medicine.

▶ Rights of Medication Administration

LO 53.2

The rights of medication administration are a set of safety checks the medical assistant must follow to prevent errors and ensure patient safety when administering medications (see

TABLE 53-1	The Rights of Medication Administration
Basic Rights	**Additional Rights**
1. Right patient	7. Right reason
2. Right drug	8. Right to know
3. Right dose	9. Right to refuse
4. Right route	10. Right technique
5. Right time	
6. Right documentation	

Table 53-1). The basic rights of medication administration are the following: right patient, right drug, right dose, right route, right time, and right documentation. Additional rights include right reason, right to know, right to refuse, and right technique. A violation of any of the rights constitutes a medication error.

Right Patient

Always check the name and date of birth on the order for a drug or vaccine in the patient's chart, then compare to the name and date of birth that the patient tells you. Do not call the patient by name because a forgetful or confused patient might answer to any name. Have an attending caregiver or family member state the name and date of birth if the patient is unable.

Right Drug

Carefully compare the name of the prescribed drug or vaccine in the patient's chart with the label on the drug container. As you check the drug name on the label, look at the expiration date. Never use a drug that has passed this date (Figure 53-2). If you are unfamiliar with the drug, look it up in a credible drug reference. Also, never prepare a drug from a container with a damaged or handwritten label. Always perform the triple check every time you prepare a medication.

Right Dose

Compare the dose on the order in the patient's chart with the dose you prepare. To obtain the right dose, read the label closely and calculate accurately. Do not confuse the dose contained in one tablet with the number of tablets in the container.

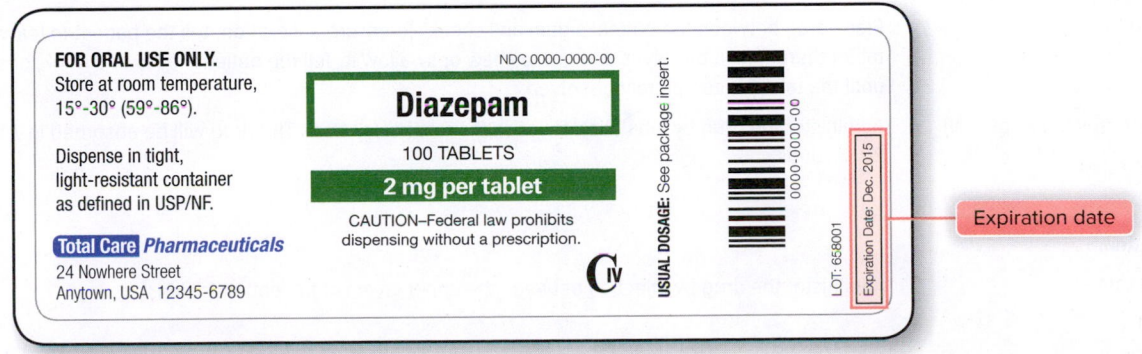

FIGURE 53-2 Check the label for the expiration date before administering a drug.
© McGraw-Hill Education

Right Route

Double-check to make sure the administration route you are preparing to use matches the route the licensed practitioner ordered. Also check that the medication you are using can be administered by the route ordered. For example, do not confuse ear (otic) drops with eye (optic) drops. Check that the patient can receive the drug by this route and that the route seems appropriate. For example, if the patient has an injury at the specified injection site, consult the licensed practitioner for a possible alternative site or a different route.

Right Time

Be sure to give the drug at the right time. If it must be given after meals, make sure the patient has eaten recently. For certain drugs, you must ensure that it is the correct time of day and the correct time in a series of doses. For example, timing is crucial with allergy shots because of possible reactions.

Right Documentation

Document the procedure immediately after administering the drug or vaccine to the patient. Do not wait until later and do not document before administration. Be sure to include the date, time, drug or vaccine name, lot number, dose, administration route, patient reaction, and patient education about the drug, as well as your first initial and last name. If the drug is a controlled substance, also document it on the controlled substance inventory record. Always double-check your entry for computer documentation before submitting. Use neat handwriting for written documentation.

Right Reason

The person who administers the medication should know the reason the medication is being given.

Right to Know

All patients have the right to be educated about the medications they are receiving. This should include the reason, the effect, and the side effects of medications.

Right to Refuse

Every patient has the right to refuse a medication. If a patient does refuse a medication or vaccine, you should report this to the physician who ordered the medication. A refusal of medication by a patient should be documented in the patient's medical record.

Right Technique

Always use the proper administration technique. If you have not given a drug or vaccine by the ordered route recently, review the technique before administering the drug.

▶ Drug Routes and Equipment   LO 53.3

The physician may ask you to administer drugs by one of the routes outlined in Table 53-2. Most patients take a prescription to a pharmacy to be filled and then take oral drugs at home, so you may not need to administer these drugs in the office very often. However, you are likely to be asked to

- Place drugs in the patient's mouth between the cheek and gum or under the tongue.
- Administer or teach a parent to administer a medication using a dropper, a medicine cup, an oral syringe, or a calibrated syringe. A **calibrated spoon** has markings (calibrations) that allow you to measure a dose. An oral syringe also has calibrations and a soft, flexible tip. See Figure 53-3.
- Administer a drug by any means other than by mouth (if permitted by your scope of practice and state laws). This would require the use of a syringe and safety-engineered needles, which are discussed later in the chapter.
- Demonstrate how to use an inhaler.
- Apply topical drugs (those applied to the skin).
- Administer or assist in administering drugs into the urethra, vagina, or rectum.
- Administer medications to the eye or ear, as discussed in the *Assisting with Eye and Ear Care* chapter.

These duties require you to master a variety of techniques to give drugs safely by any route.

TABLE 53-2	Routes and Methods of Drug Administration
Route and Drug Forms	**Method**
Buccal route Tablets	Place drug between the patient's gum and cheek. To ensure absorption, tell the patient to leave the tablet there until it dissolves and not to chew or swallow it. Tell the patient not to eat, drink, or smoke until the tablet is completely dissolved.

Inhalation therapy (nasal or oral)
 	
    Aerosols
 	
    Sprays
 	
    Mists or steam
	Administer the drug by inhalation to reach the respiratory tract. The drug will be absorbed in 7 to 20 seconds.

Intradermal route
 	
    Solutions
 	
    Powders for reconstitution
	Administer the drug by injection between the upper layers of the patient's skin.

(Continued)

TABLE 53-2 Routes and Methods of Drug Administration

Route and Drug Forms	Method
Intramuscular route Solutions Powders for reconstitution	Administer the drug by injection into the muscle. The drug will be absorbed in 3 to 5 minutes.
Intravenous route Solutions (often in bags of 250, 500, or 1,000 mL) Powders for reconstitution Blood and blood products	Administer the drug by injection or infusion into a vein. The drug will be absorbed in 15 to 30 seconds.
Ophthalmic (eye) or otic (ear) route Solutions Ointments	Apply the drug, usually as drops, in the patient's eye or ear.
Oral route Tablets Capsules Liquids Lozenges	Give the drug to the patient to swallow. The drug will be absorbed in 20 minutes to 3 hours, depending on food and drug ingestion.
Rectal route Suppositories Solutions	Insert a suppository into the patient's rectum. Administer a solution as an enema, using a tube and nozzle.
Subcutaneous route Solutions Powders for reconstitution	Administer the drug by injection into the subcutaneous layer of skin. The drug will be absorbed in 3 to 5 minutes.
Sublingual route Tablets Sprays	Place the drug under the patient's tongue. To ensure absorption, tell the patient to leave the tablet there until it dissolves and not to chew or swallow it. Tell the patient not to eat, drink, or smoke until the tablet is completely dissolved.
Topical route Ointments Lotions Creams Tinctures Powders Sprays Solutions	Apply the drug to the patient's skin or rub it into the skin.
Transdermal route Patches	Apply the drug to a clean, dry, nonhairy area of the patient's skin.
Urethral route Solutions	Administer the drug by instilling it in the patient's bladder, using a catheter.
Vaginal route Solutions Suppositories Ointments Foams Creams	Administer a solution as a douche, using a tube and nozzle. Administer other forms by inserting them into the vagina with an applicator.

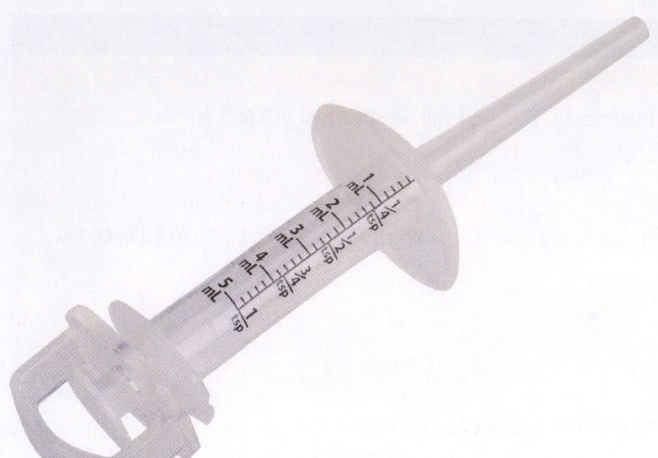

(a) Oral syringe

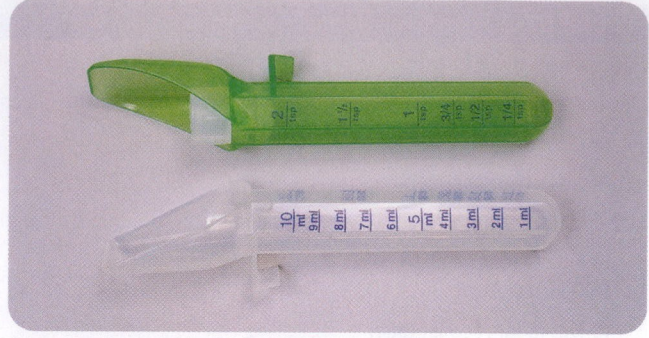

(b) Calibrated spoons

FIGURE 53-3 (a) Oral syringes and (b) calibrated spoons have markings, so that liquid medications given by mouth can be measured accurately.
(a) Apothercary Products LLC; (b) © Total Care Programming, Inc.

▶ Medications by Mouth   LO 53.4

Medications that are put in the mouth are usually swallowed. This is called *oral administration*. Medications that are not meant to be swallowed also may be placed in the mouth. These methods include buccal and sublingual administration.

Oral Administration

Drugs that are swallowed are absorbed relatively slowly as they travel along the gastrointestinal (GI) tract. Drugs for oral administration include tablets, capsules, lozenges, and liquids. One special type of tablet you should be aware of is a **scored** tablet. See Figure 53-4. This medication can be broken into pieces along a scored (indented) line on the tablet.

Oral administration is contraindicated in patients who have severe nausea, are comatose, or cannot swallow. Certain drugs are ineffective when administered orally because the digestive process changes them chemically to an ineffective form or does not deliver them to the bloodstream quickly enough.

Many drugs, however, are most effective when given orally. These include antibiotics, vitamins, throat lozenges, and cough syrups. Although these drugs are familiar to most people, as a medical assistant, you must follow certain steps to ensure that the patient understands the drug and that the drug is administered safely and effectively. The steps for oral administration are outlined in Procedure 53-1 at the end of this chapter.

Buccal and Sublingual Administration

Although **buccal** and **sublingual** drugs are placed in the mouth, they do not continue along the GI tract. Instead, they dissolve and are absorbed in the buccal area (between the cheek and gum) or the sublingual area (under the tongue), where they are placed. The medication is absorbed through tissue that is rich in capillaries and the drug enters the bloodstream directly. Because the drug does not pass into the stomach or intestines before absorption, it produces a therapeutic effect more quickly than do oral drugs.

Specially formulated tablets may be given by the buccal or sublingual routes. When you administer buccal or sublingual medications, your role usually includes teaching the patient how to administer these medications at home. See Procedure 53-2 at the end of this chapter.

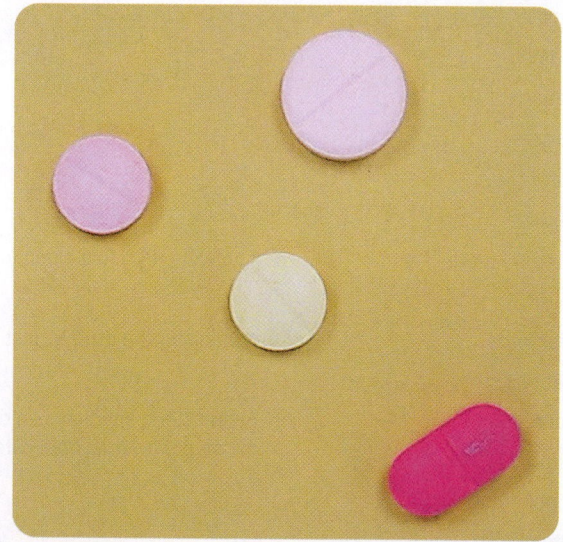

FIGURE 53-4 Unscored tablets should never be broken. Scored tablets, like the ones shown here, can be broken only along the scored line.
© Total Care Programming Inc.

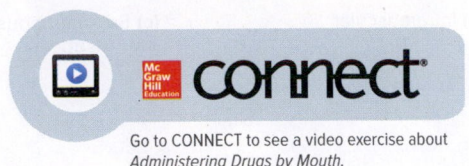

Go to CONNECT to see a video exercise about *Administering Drugs by Mouth.*

▶ Medications by Injection
LO 53.5

Medications given by injection are called *parenteral medications.* Parenteral administration is the administration of a substance such as a drug by muscle, vein, or any means other than through the GI tract. Although the parenteral route offers the advantage of rapid drug action, it has several potential drawbacks. Parenteral administration poses more safety risks for the patient because, after the drug has been injected, it cannot be retrieved.

Parenteral administration also increases your risk of potential exposure to bloodborne pathogens when you perform injections and dispose of used needles. To minimize risks, follow standard precautions during injections. Also adhere to Occupational Safety and Health Administration (OSHA) and Environmental Protection Agency (EPA) regulations for disposing of contaminated needles and other sharp items. Offices must provide a rigid, puncture-proof container for collecting disposable sharp instruments. This container must be self-sealing and must have a lock-tight cap and a safety neck.

After using a needle, lancet, or syringe, engage the safety mechanism; then immediately place it in the sharps container. See Figure 53-5. To avoid puncturing yourself, always ensure that the safety mechanism is engaged and do not force the needle, lancet, or syringe into the container. If you do accidentally stick yourself, follow OSHA guidelines. Wash the area with soap and water, report the incident to your supervisor, and seek medical treatment.

Never let a sharps container become full. When the container is two-thirds full, seal it and follow your office procedure for container disposal. Before giving an injection, be aware of all injection safety practices, as discussed in the *Infection Control Practices* chapter.

Needles

When you administer a parenteral drug, you must select the appropriate needle, syringe, and drug form to use on the basis of the type of injection. The following are methods of injection:

- Intradermal (ID), or within (between) the upper layers of the skin
- Subcutaneous (subcut), or beneath the skin
- Intramuscular (IM), or within a muscle
- Intravenous (IV), or directly into a vein

See Figure 53-6.

Needles consist of a hub, hilt, shaft, lumen, point, and bevel (Figure 53-7). The hub of the needle fits onto the syringe. The needle tip is beveled (sloped at the opening). The bevel helps the needle cut through the skin with minimum trauma.

Needles are available in various gauges (inside diameters) and lengths (Figure 53-8). A needle's gauge is expressed

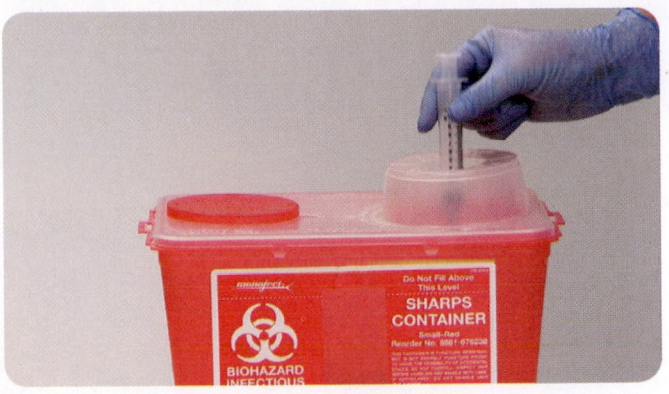

FIGURE 53-5 To prevent needlestick injuries, engage the safety mechanism and place all needles in a sharps container like this one immediately.
© McGraw-Hill Education

with numbers. The smaller the number, the larger the gauge. For example, a 25-gauge needle is smaller than an 18-gauge needle. Use the right gauge for the type of injection and the viscosity (thickness) of the drug to be administered.

When selecting a needle, consider its length. It must be long enough to penetrate the appropriate layers of tissue, but not so long as to go too deep. Choose the correct needle length on the basis of the type of injection as well as the patient's size, amount of fatty tissue, and injection site. Table 53-3 lists the approximate ranges of needle gauge and length that are typically used for intradermal, subcutaneous, and intramuscular injections. Always use the smallest allowable needle that will work for the patient, medication, and injection site. For example, you will rarely use an 18-gauge needle for an IM injection. One exception is if you are injecting viscous (thick) medication into a large muscle on a large patient.

Syringes

Syringes have two basic parts: a barrel and a plunger. The barrel is the calibrated cylinder that holds the drug. The plunger forces the drug through the barrel and out the needle. The syringe may be packaged with the needle attached and a guardcap over the needle, or the syringe and needle may be packaged separately. All syringes must include a needlestick prevention safety device. See Figure 53-9.

Syringes come in many sizes and are calibrated according to how the syringe will be used. For example, the common 3-mL syringe is divided into tenths of a milliliter. It is used to measure most drugs. A tuberculin (TB) syringe holds 1 mL and is calibrated in hundredths of a milliliter. Insulin syringes are calibrated in units (U), commonly either 50 U or 100 U (Figure 53-10). Unlike other syringes, insulin syringes have permanently attached needles and no dead space (fluid remaining in the needle or syringe after the plunger is depressed fully). These differences help the patient self-administer the correct amount of insulin.

Forms of Packaging for Parenteral Drugs

Parenteral drugs are supplied in the forms shown in Figure 53-11. They include cartridges, ampules, and vials.

MEDICATION ADMINISTRATION   1129

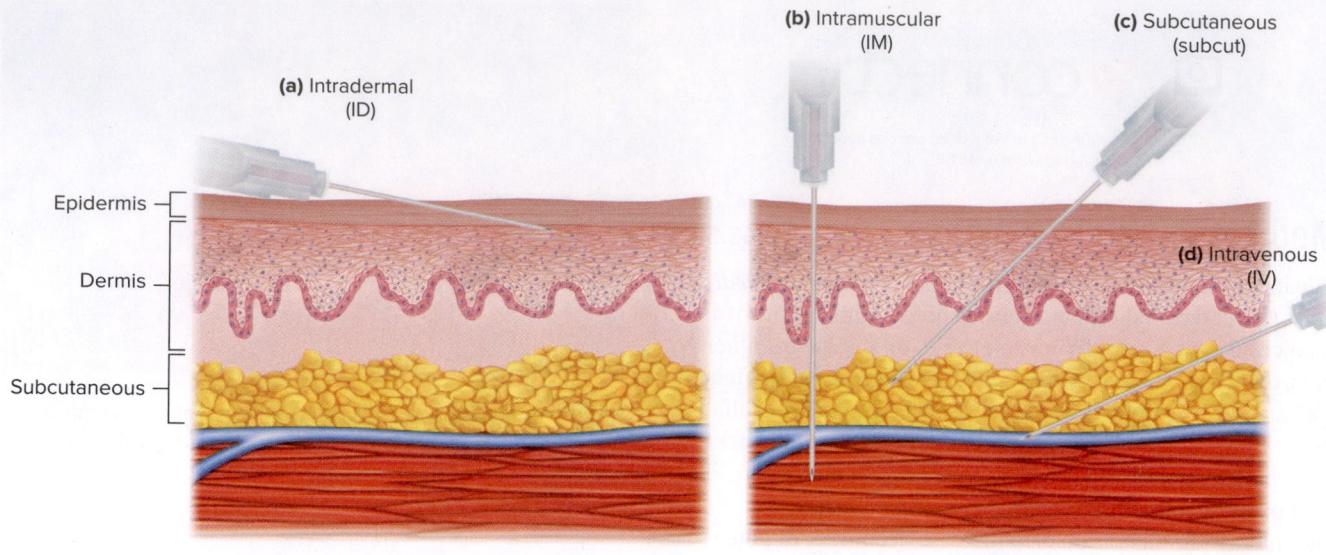

FIGURE 53-6 Injection needles are placed into separate areas under the skin: (a) intradermal (ID), (b) intramuscular (IM), (c) subcutaneous (subcut), or (d) intravenous (IV).

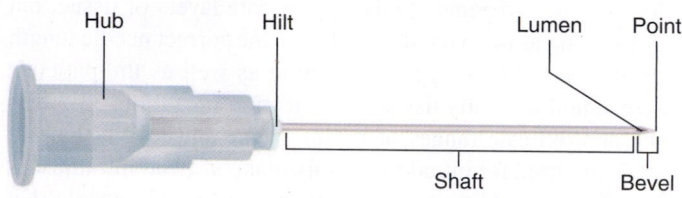

FIGURE 53-7 Understanding the parts of a needle will help you use it correctly.

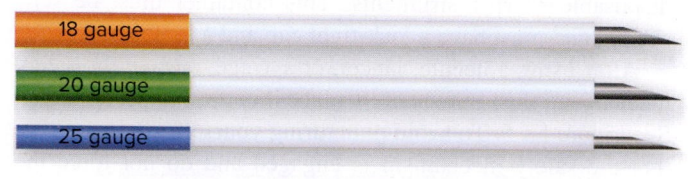

(a)

- A cartridge is a small barrel prefilled with a sterile drug. It slips into a reusable syringe assembly.

- An ampule is a small glass or plastic container that is sealed to keep its contents sterile. It must be opened and used with care, as described in Procedure 53-3 at the end of this chapter.

- A vial is a small bottle with a rubber diaphragm that can be punctured by needle. A vial contains a liquid or powder, which must first be reconstituted with a **diluent** (liquid used to dissolve and dilute a drug), as described in Procedure 53-4 at the end of this chapter. It may contain a single or multiple doses. This procedure requires two needles and syringe sets—one for inserting the diluent into the vial and another to draw and administer the reconstituted drug—to avoid using a contaminated needle. The first needle is considered contaminated when you set it down to mix the diluent and the drug.

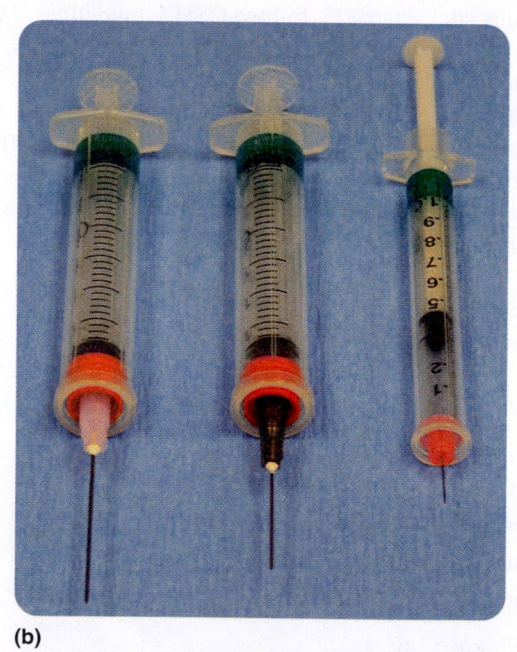

(b)

FIGURE 53-8 (a) The gauge of the needle relates to the diameter. The larger the number, the smaller the needle diameter. (b) Always choose a needle with a length and gauge appropriate to the type of injection, the drug being injected, and the patient receiving the injection.

© Total Care Programming Inc.

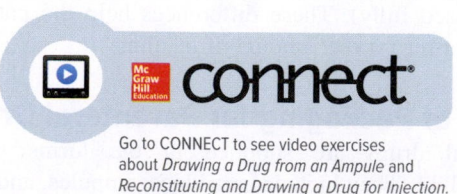

Go to CONNECT to see video exercises about *Drawing a Drug from an Ampule* and *Reconstituting and Drawing a Drug for Injection.*

TABLE 53-3   Suggested Needle Gauge, Length, Injection Amount, and Location

Type	Age	Needle Size	Needle Length	Maximum Injection Amount	Location
Intradermal (ID)					
ID	All ages	25 to 26 gauge	⅜ to ½ inch	0.1 mL	Interior aspect of forearm (most common)
Subcutaneous (Subcut)					
Subcut	1 to 12 months	23 to 27 gauge	⅝ inch	1 mL	Fatty tissue over anterior lateral thigh muscle
Subcut	> 12 months to adult	23 to 27 gauge	½ to ¾ inch; ⅝ is most common	1 mL	Fatty tissue over anterior lateral thigh muscle or over triceps
Intramuscular (IM)					
IM	1 to 28 days	18 to 23 gauge	⅝ inch	1 mL	Anterolateral thigh muscle
IM	1 to 12 months	18 to 23 gauge	1 inch	1 mL	Anterolateral thigh muscle
IM	1 to 2 years	18 to 23 gauge	1 to 1¼ inch; ⅝ to 1 inch	1 mL	Anterolateral thigh muscle Deltoid muscle of arm
IM	3 to 18 years	18 to 23 gauge	⅝ to 1 inch; 1 to 1¼ inch	2 mL	Deltoid muscle of arm Anterolateral thigh muscle
IM	All adults ≥ 19 years < 130 lb	18 to 23 gauge	⅝ to 1 inch	3 mL	Deltoid muscle of arm
IM	All adults ≥ 19 years Female 130 to 200 lb Male 130 to 260 lb	18 to 23 gauge	1 to 1½ inch	3 mL	Deltoid muscle of arm
IM	Male adults ≥ 19 years Female 200 + lb Male 260 + lb	18 to 23 gauge	1½ inch	3 mL	Deltoid muscle of arm

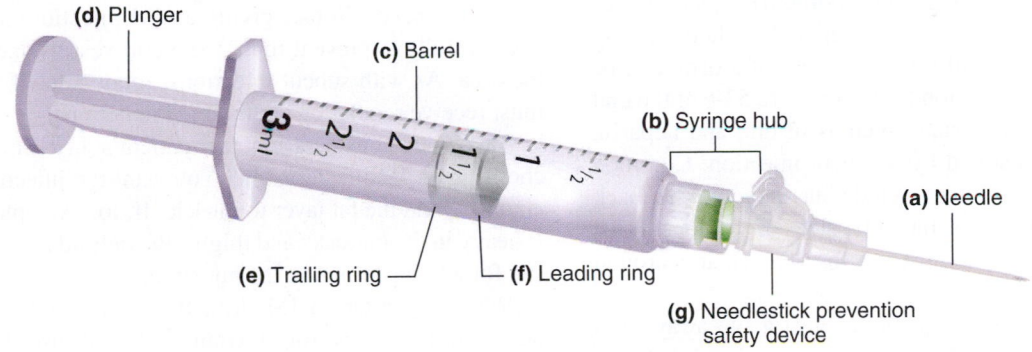

FIGURE 53-9   The parts of a standard syringe include (a) the needle; (b) the syringe hub; (c) the barrel that contains the liquid; (d) the plunger; (e) the trailing ring; (f) the plunger tip, also called the leading ring; and (g) the needlestick prevention safety device.

Methods of Injection

Injections are the most common method of drug administration in a medical office. You need to be knowledgeable about all injection methods: intradermal, subcutaneous, intramuscular, and intravenous.

Intradermal An **intradermal (ID)** injection is administered between the upper layers of skin at an angle almost parallel to the skin, as described in Procedure 53-5 at the end of this chapter. Common sites for intradermal injections are the forearm and back. Intradermal injections are usually used to administer a skin test, such as an allergy test or a TB test. When choosing an injection site on patients, avoid scarred, blemished, or hairy areas because those features interfere with your ability to interpret test results on the skin.

The drug is injected under the top skin layer and a little bubble, or wheal, is raised. If the body reacts to the drug, erythema (redness) and induration (hardening) occur. This reaction generally takes place 15 to 20 minutes after an allergy test and from 48 to 72 hours after a TB test.

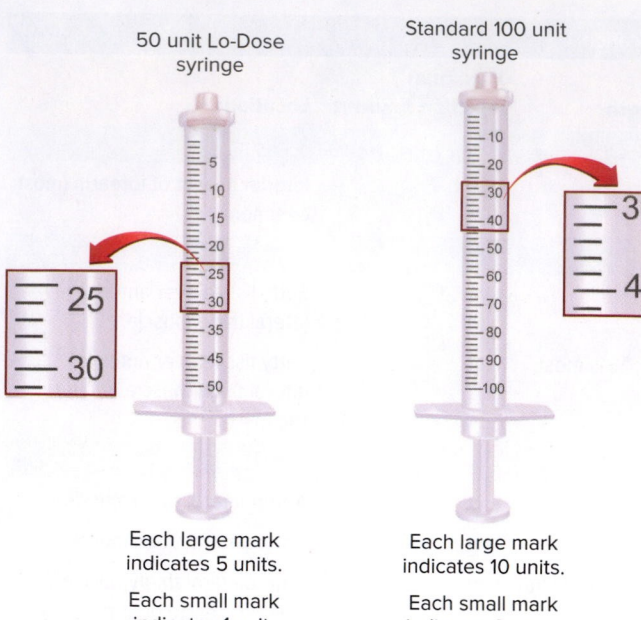

50 unit Lo-Dose syringe

Standard 100 unit syringe

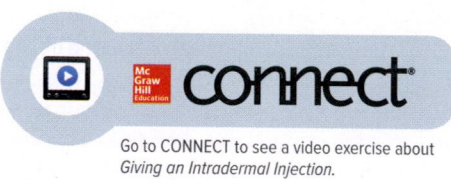

Each large mark indicates 5 units.

Each small mark indicates 1 unit.

Each large mark indicates 10 units.

Each small mark indicates 2 units.

FIGURE 53-10 Always check the calibrations of insulin syringes carefully because the marks on syringes of different sizes use different scales.

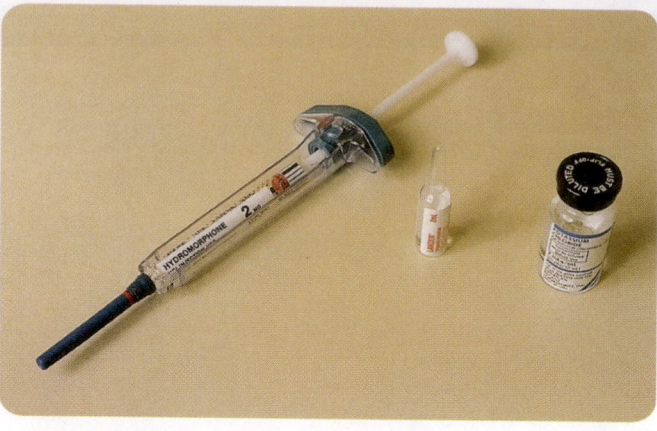

FIGURE 53-11 Injectable drugs come in a cartridge (left), an ampule (center), or a vial (right).
© Cliff Moore

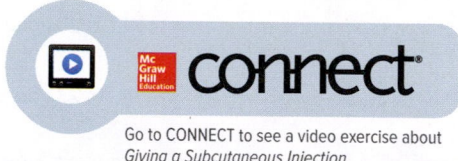

Go to CONNECT to see a video exercise about *Giving a Subcutaneous Injection.*

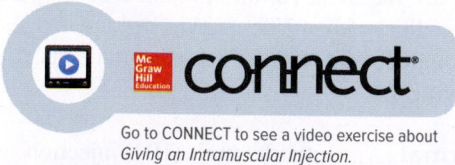

Go to CONNECT to see a video exercise about *Giving an Intradermal Injection.*

Subcutaneous A **subcutaneous (subcut)** injection provides a slow, sustained release of a drug and a relatively long duration of action. Generally, 1 mL or less of a drug can be delivered by a subcut injection (see Procedure 53-6 at the end of this chapter). Various drugs, such as insulin and heparin, are commonly administered by a subcut injection. Common subcutaneous injection sites include an area on the back between the shoulder blades, the outer sides of the upper arms and thighs, and the abdomen (except for a 2-inch area around the umbilicus).

To prepare for a subcut injection, select a site away from bones and blood vessels. Do not use an area that is edematous (swollen), scarred, or hardened or one that has a large amount of fat because these areas may not have the capillary network needed for absorption. When patients need regular subcut injections, remember to rotate injection sites systematically. Begin the rotation pattern by giving injections in rows in the same area of the body (such as the abdomen). After all those sites have been used once, proceed to the next area on the body (such as the right leg) and follow a similar pattern there. Rotating sites promotes drug absorption and prevents hard subcutaneous lumps from forming. At the injection site, ensure that you can pinch at least a 1-inch skinfold for the injection. If a patient is frail, dehydrated, or thin, you may need to use a site other than the back or abdomen to provide the necessary fold of skin.

Intramuscular When a patient requires rapid drug absorption, you may be asked to administer an **intramuscular (IM)** injection, as described in Procedure 53-7 at the end of this chapter. An IM injection usually irritates a patient's tissues less than a subcut injection and allows administration of a larger amount of drug.

Common IM injection sites include the ventrogluteal, vastus lateralis, and deltoid muscles, illustrated in Figure 53-12. The dorsogluteal is used less because of the chance of hitting the sciatic nerve. Before giving an IM injection, identify the site carefully to prevent injury to blood vessels and nerves in the area. As with subcut injections, rotate sites if the patient must receive regular or multiple IM injections.

Take into consideration the patient's layer of fat when choosing an IM injection site. You want the injection to penetrate beyond the fat layer to muscle. If, for example, a patient is heavy in the buttocks and thighs, the deltoid may be the best site for administering an IM injection.

When injecting an IM drug that can irritate subcutaneous tissues, such as iron dextran (Imferon), use the **Z-track method,** illustrated in Figure 53-13. To do this, pull the skin and subcutaneous tissue to the side before inserting the needle at the site. After the drug is injected, release the tissue. This technique creates a zigzag path in the tissue layers, which prevents the drug from leaking into the subcutaneous tissue and causing irritation.

Go to CONNECT to see a video exercise about *Giving an Intramuscular Injection.*

Intravenous Although **intravenous (IV)** injections are not commonly performed in a medical office or by medical

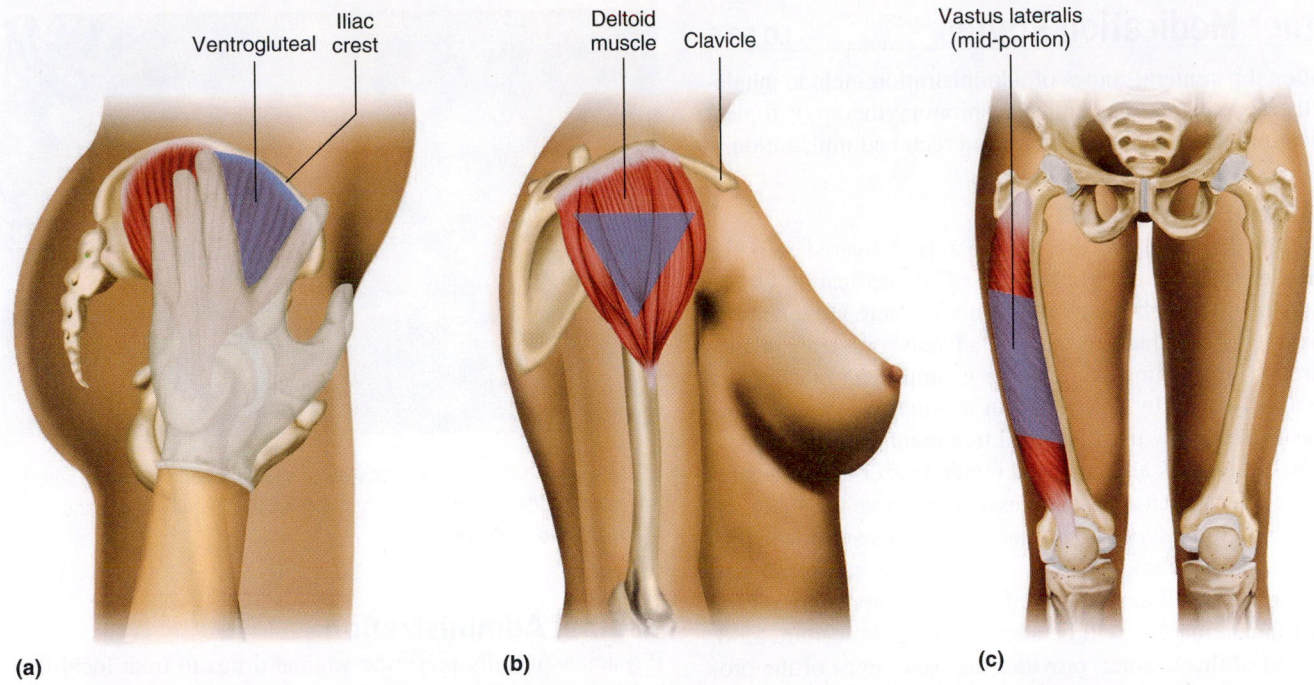

FIGURE 53-12   For intramuscular injection in an adult, use (a) the ventrogluteal site, (b) the deltoid site, or (c) the vastus lateralis site.

assistants, certain drugs may be administered this way. Drugs also may be mixed and dissolved into a **solution** (a homogeneous mixture of a solid, liquid, or gaseous substance in a liquid) and given by IV **infusion** (slow drip) into a vein. Examples of IV drugs include powerful antibiotics, chemotherapeutic drugs, emergency drugs, and electrolytes. Because these drugs are introduced directly into the bloodstream, they produce an almost immediate effect. They also can cause sudden adverse reactions.

Although in most cases a licensed practitioner must administer an IV drug, you may assist by laying out supplies and equipment. When assisting with any intravenous medications, gather the ordered drug and a tourniquet, bedsaver pad, gloves, iodine and alcohol swabs, venipuncture device, tape, and gauze pad, as ordered. Obtain other supplies and equipment depending on the specific type of infusion or injection being administered.

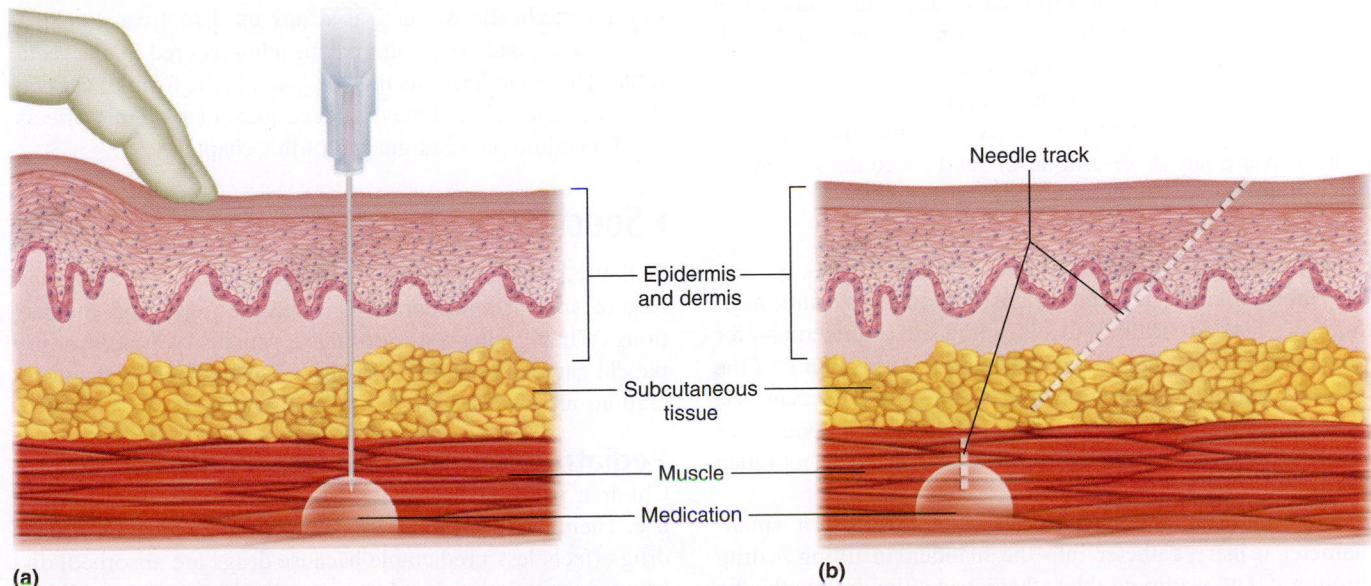

FIGURE 53-13   Use the Z-track method for IM injection of irritating solutions. (a) Pull the skin to one side before inserting the needle. (b) After injecting the drug, release the skin to seal off the needle track.

▶ Other Medication Routes

LO 53.6

Additional parenteral routes of administration include inhalation therapy (sometimes called respiratory therapy); topical application; and urethral, vaginal, and rectal administration.

Inhalation Therapies

Inhalation therapy is medication that is delivered into the respiratory system during inhalation. This medication can be administered through the mouth or nose. There are a number of disorders for which the physician may order an inhaler or aerosol form of medication. For example, an oral inhaler is frequently used by patients with asthma, whereas a nasal inhaler is frequently used for local treatment of nasal congestion. Nasal inhalers also are used to administer medicines for systemic effect, such as a vasopressin derivative for nocturnal bedwetting. Some types of influenza vaccines are now delivered by nasal inhalation. Always read the inserts for inhaled drugs for a detailed description of the exact procedure for the type of inhalation you will be administering. Procedure 53-8, at the end of this chapter, provides the basic steps of the procedure, as well as needed patient education.

Topical Application

Topical application is the direct application of a drug on the skin. Topical drugs can take the form of creams, lotions, **ointments** (salves), tinctures, powders, sprays, and solutions, which are used for their local effects. They include antibacterial and antifungal drugs, as well as corticosteroids.

To apply a cream, lotion, or ointment, use long, even strokes with a cotton-tipped applicator and/or a gloved finger when rubbing it into the skin. Follow the direction of the hair growth to avoid irritating the hair follicles and skin. To apply a powder, shake it on but do not rub it in.

A specialized type of topical administration that produces a systemic effect is the **transdermal** system (or patch). See Figure 53-14. A drug administered through the transdermal patch is absorbed through the skin directly into the bloodstream. The patch slowly and evenly releases a systemic drug, such as scopolamine, nitroglycerin, estrogen, or fentanyl, through the skin. The patient receives a timed-release dose, usually over a day or several days. See Procedure 53-9 at the end of this chapter.

Urethral Administration

The urethral route is used when antibiotic and antifungal drugs are needed locally—that is, at the site of infection—for some urinary tract infections. Depending on the nature of the infection and the duration of drug action, the physician or a nurse may instill liquid drugs only one time or several times a day for a week. Urethral administration is used in both men and women.

Urethral drug administration requires passing a small-diameter urinary catheter into the bladder, instilling a drug through it, and clamping the catheter to let the drug bathe the urinary bladder walls. See Procedure 53-10 at the end of this chapter.

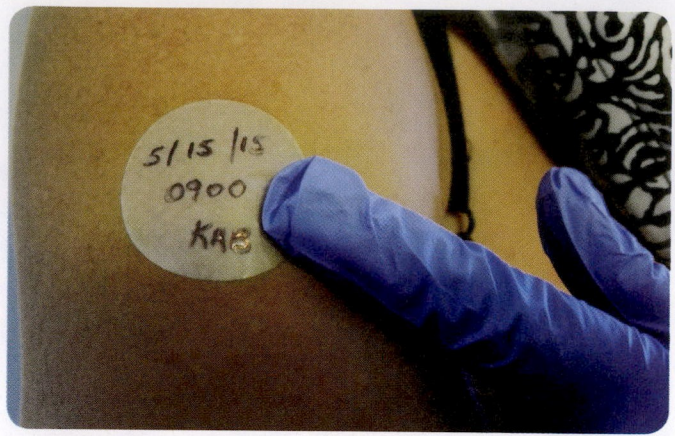

FIGURE 53-14   A transdermal patch should include the date, time, and initials added to the patch when applied by a medical assistant.
© Total Care Programming, Inc.

Vaginal Administration

Physicians usually prescribe vaginal drugs to treat local fungal infections. The drugs also may be used for local bacterial infections. They are usually packaged as suppositories (the most common form), solutions, creams, ointments, and foams. The liquid form of vaginal medication is administered by performing a **douche** (vaginal irrigation). This process is similar to giving a urethral drug, but it requires a special irrigating nozzle. Patients frequently ask about administering vaginal medications, and they usually administer such medications at home. Therefore, you must be prepared to provide detailed patient education for this route of administration. The physician may ask you to administer the first dose as a means of teaching a patient the method to use at home, or you may be asked to administer a one-time-only dose. See Procedure 53-11 at the end of this chapter.

Rectal Administration

Certain medications, such as drugs used to treat constipation, nausea, and vomiting, may be administered by the rectal route. These medications may be given in the form of suppositories or enemas and may produce local or systemic effects. See Procedure 53-12 at the end of this chapter.

▶ Special Considerations

LO 53.7

Pediatric, pregnant, breast-feeding, and geriatric patients require special considerations when administering medications. When giving a drug to these patients, you must adjust patient care and technique as needed. Note: Geriatric considerations are discussed in the *Assisting in Geriatrics* chapter.

Pediatric Patients

Children pose special challenges in drug administration and use. Their physiology and immature body systems may make drug effects less predictable because drugs are absorbed, distributed, metabolized, and excreted differently in children than in adults. Therefore, plan to observe a pediatric patient closely for adverse effects and interactions.

A child's small size increases the risk of overdose and toxicity. These factors require dosage adjustments and careful measurement of small doses. To help administer drugs safely to pediatric patients, always check your calculations for providing a prescribed dose, and then ask a licensed practitioner to double-check them.

Administration sites and techniques for a child may differ from those for an adult. For example, fewer IM injection sites can be used for a young child. Also, the technique for eardrop administration varies slightly (see the *Assisting with Eye and Ear Care* chapter).

When dealing with an infant or a young child, teach the parents—not the patient—about the drug. With an older child, include parents and patient in the teaching session. Be sure to use age-appropriate language when speaking to children.

Patience and sensitivity are important when working with pediatric patients. The first memorable exposure to an office visit may often determine how the child will react to physician visits for years to come. Infants and children can sense when you are irritated or annoyed. Pay close attention to your nonverbal communication as well as your verbal communication. New mothers are often apprehensive about invasive procedures when it concerns their children and this apprehension is often reflected in the child. Empathy and compassion are needed to ensure that the office visit is a pleasant one.

Administering medications to a pediatric patient may become a challenge if the child is not cooperative. It is important to ensure that the child receives the full dose as ordered.

Oral Medications When administering oral medications to infants and small children, follow these guidelines:

- Use a pediatric calibrated dropper to measure the ordered dose. See Figure 53-15.
- Administer the medication to the side of the tongue; this method prevents the child from spitting out the medication.
- Hold the child until you are sure the medication has been swallowed. In some cases, you may gently hold the child's mouth closed to ensure that the medication is swallowed.
- If a small amount dribbles from the mouth, do not attempt to give more medication to the child.
- If the child vomits within 5 minutes and you can see the medication in the vomit, you should readminister the medication after the child is calm. If you are unsure of readministering medication, consult with the physician.
- If the medication comes only in tablet form and the child is unable to swallow a tablet or capsule, check a creditable drug reference to see if the medication can be crushed and given with food, such as applesauce.

Injections Stress and anxiety will differ from child to child. When giving injections to pediatric patients, the following steps will help ensure a smooth procedure:

- Distract the patient. Talk to the child while giving the injection. Don't ask permission. Often the injection is performed and over before the child realizes it.

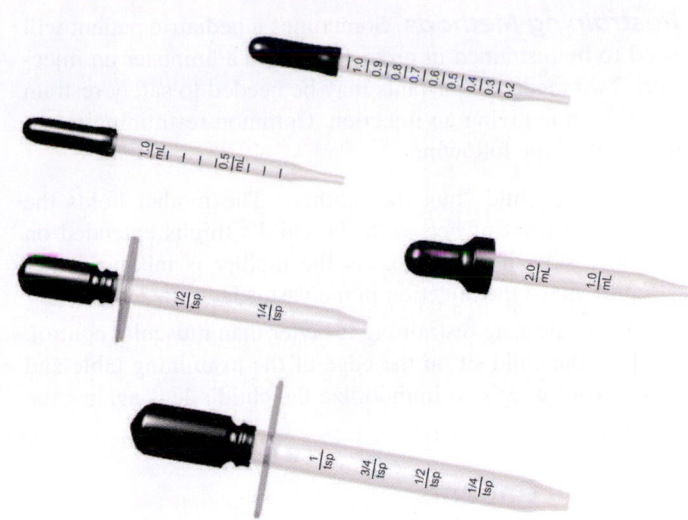

FIGURE 53-15 Pediatric droppers come in various sizes with different calibration marks.

- Use an anesthetic topical agent prior to the injection. This can be applied in the office or at home before the patient arrives in the office.
- Try not to allow the child to see the syringe before giving the injection.
- Be swift. Do not allow a lot of time to pass before giving the injection—the faster the better.
- Praise the child. Say things that promote maturity and self-esteem.

Pediatric Injection Sites Pediatric patients have less muscle development than adults do, which limits the sites for intramuscular injections. The deltoid muscle is not developed enough for an injection and can be painful for the child. The sciatic nerve is larger in children; dorsogluteal injections are therefore not recommended because of the danger of hitting the sciatic nerve.

The vastus lateralis and ventrogluteal sites are recommended for infants and children. The vastus lateralis site is good because it is a large and thick muscle that is developed before the child begins to walk. It is also the most desirable site for infants and children because it is not near major nerves and blood vessels. For a child who has been walking for about a year, you can use the ventrogluteal or dorsogluteal site. For an older, well-developed child, use any adult site. The vastus lateralis site is an easier site if you need to incorporate restraining methods.

The most common injections given to pediatric patients are vaccines. Most vaccines are given intramuscularly with a 25-gauge, ⅝-inch needle. The gauge and length vary based on the size of the patient. Use the shortest needle that will allow you to reach muscle, usually ⅝ to 1 inch.

In many cases, pediatric patients require more than one vaccine injection in a single limb (vastus lateralis). When this is the case, the injections should be at least 1 inch apart on the site, and the specific location of each vaccine should be documented.

Restraining Methods Sometimes a pediatric patient will need to be restrained in order for you to administer an injection. Two medical assistants may be needed to safely restrain a child while giving an injection. Common restraining methods include the following:

- Have the child "hug the mother." The mother holds the child in front of her, with the child's thighs extended on either side of her torso. As the mother is talking to her child, make the injection in the vastus lateralis.
- Weight-bearing restraining is better than muscular control. Have the child sit on the edge of the examining table and use your weight to immobilize the child's legs against the table.

Pregnant Patients

When dealing with pregnant patients, remember that you are caring for two patients at once: the mother and her fetus. When you give the mother a drug, you also may be giving it to the fetus. Some drugs can cause physical defects in the fetus if the mother takes them during pregnancy (especially in the first trimester). It is extremely important to double-check the drug in a credible drug reference for toxicology or pregnancy warnings. After administering the drug, assess the patient carefully for therapeutic and adverse effects of the drug. If the physician orders a drug for a pregnant patient, double-check the order against the pregnancy drug risk categories discussed in the *Principles of Pharmacology* chapter. If it is a high-risk drug, check with the physician before administering the drug.

Patients Who Are Breast-Feeding

Some drugs are excreted in breast milk and can thus be ingested by a breast-feeding infant. This ingestion can be dangerous because infants have immature body systems and cannot metabolize and excrete drugs that are safe for the mother. Some drugs, such as sedatives, diuretics, and hormones, can reduce the mother's flow of breast milk.

Whenever a drug is ordered for a patient who is breast-feeding, check a drug reference to see whether the drug is contraindicated during lactation. If so, consult the licensed practitioner. If not, teach the mother to recognize signs of adverse drug effects in her infant. If a mother must take a drug that affects lactation, advise her to supplement breast-feedings with infant formula.

▶ Patient Education About Medications
LO 53.8

As a medical assistant, you have an important role in patient instruction about medications. This role may vary depending on your state, training, or place of employment, but the importance of drug education should not be underestimated. Specific instructions should be given about all the drugs a patient is taking, whether prescription or over-the-counter (OTC). Patients also should know how to take and record their medications safely and correctly.

Over-the-Counter Drugs

Even though patients can obtain OTC drugs without a prescription, they need to know several important facts to use them safely. Patients should not treat themselves with OTC drugs as a way to avoid medical care. For example, OTC drugs are available to treat recurrent yeast infections. Nonetheless, a patient should consult a licensed practitioner the first time she develops an infection.

Patients also should know that OTC drugs may not produce enough therapeutic benefit in some cases or be dangerous when used in combination with other substances. For example, a combination of the OTC medication acetaminophen (Tylenol®) and alcohol can cause liver damage. In addition, some OTC drugs may even mask symptoms or aggravate a problem.

Many OTC drugs contain more than one active ingredient. These extra ingredients, such as aspirin, acetaminophen, or caffeine, can cause allergic reactions or other undesirable effects. Excess caffeine can cause elevated heart rates. Too much acetaminophen (Tylenol®)—over 4 grams in 24 hours—can inadvertently be taken, causing severe liver damage.

Prescription Drugs

Before patients begin drug therapy, they should be informed of certain considerations (such as when and how to take the drug) and drug safety precautions. First you must check a credible drug information resource about any drug with which you are not familiar.

As part of your patient education, provide instructions orally and, if possible, in writing. For commonly prescribed medications, you can obtain preprinted information sheets or create one using an electronic health record (EHR) program. Most pharmacies now routinely provide these with each dispensed drug. See Figure 53-16.

An important aspect of this kind of information is teaching the patient how to read a prescription drug label. Instruct the patient to be particularly alert for special instructions and warning labels, such as those shown in Figure 53-17.

Interactions

Interactions may occur between two prescription or nonprescription drugs or between a drug and food and may cause serious effects. The greater the number of drugs the patient takes, including over-the-counter medications or supplements, the greater the chance of a drug interaction.

Drug-Drug Interactions When two drugs are taken at the same time, there are several possible interactions. In some cases, the effects of both drugs are increased, causing either a toxic or beneficial effect. For example, when alcohol is combined with diazepam (Valium®), there is a potential toxic effect of severe central nervous system depression because one drug intensifies the effect of the other. An example of a beneficial effect is the combination of acetaminophen and codeine, which increases the activity of both drugs, allowing the physician to prescribe a lower dose of each. In fact, this combination of drugs is available in one tablet (Tylenol® with codeine).

In other cases, the effects of both drugs are decreased, or one drug cancels out the effect of the other. For example,

BWW Medical Associates, PC
305 Main Street
Port Snead, YZ 12345-9876

Patient Name: Mohammad Nassar

RX#: 711428172

Drug: Albuterol Inhalation Aerosol

COMMON USES:

To treat asthma, bronchitis, and other lung diseases.

HOW SHOULD I USE IT?

Follow your doctor's and/or the package instructions. Shake well before each use. Rinse mouth after each inhalation to avoid dryness. If breathing has not improved in 20 minutes, call the doctor.

ARE THERE ANY SIDE EFFECTS?

Very unlikely, but report: Flushing, trembling, headache, nausea, vomiting, rapid heartbeat, chest pain, weakness, dizziness.

HOW DO I STORE THIS?

Store at room temperature away from moisture and sunlight. Do not puncture. Do not store in the bathroom. Rinse and clean inhaler regularly as described in package instructions.

FIGURE 53-16 Drug information sheets, like this one, are important for consumers to understand the medications they are taking.

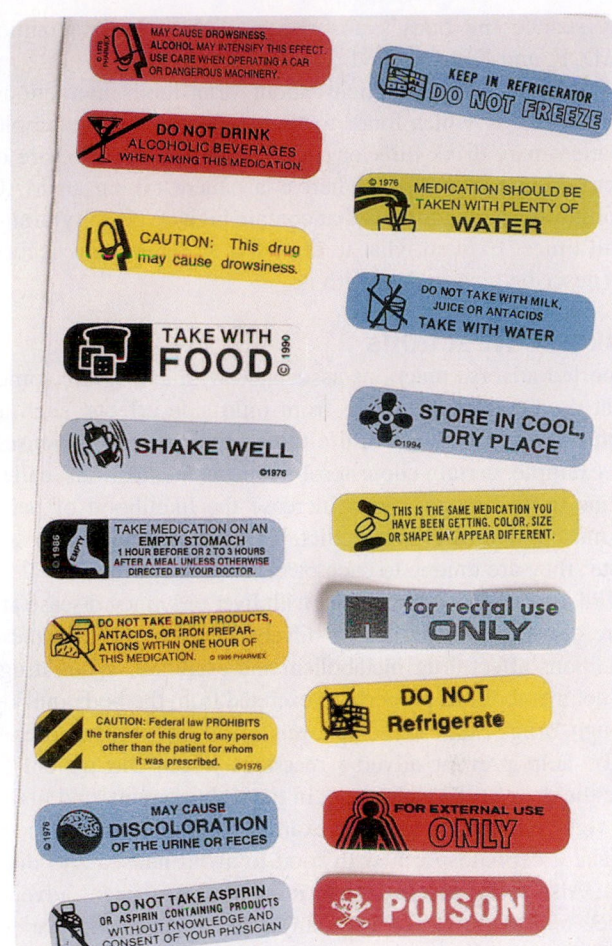

FIGURE 53-17 Teach the patient to heed warning labels and instructions on drug bottles.
© Cliff Moore

combining propranolol (Inderal®) with albuterol (Proventil®) causes each drug to lose its effectiveness.

In still other cases, the effect of one of the drugs is increased by the other. For example, the effect of digoxin (Lanoxin®) is increased by the presence of furosemide (Lasix®), but the furosemide still works at the same degree of effectiveness as when administered alone.

Drug interactions can lead to adverse reactions. For example, a patient who takes the prescription blood modifier (anticoagulant) warfarin (Coumadin®) to prevent blood clots must avoid taking aspirin for pain relief. Taking these drugs together increases the risk of uncontrolled bleeding.

To help prevent unintentional drug interactions, thoroughly check the patient's medication use. Be sure to ask about medications prescribed by specialists as well as OTC drugs and supplements. Question the patient about past and present use of alcohol and recreational drugs as well as herbal remedies. Update the chart as needed. If you detect a potential for drug interactions, notify the physician. Drug interaction checkers are available online.

Also teach patients about possible drug interactions and how to avoid or minimize them. For example, patients may need to take certain drugs at least 4 hours apart. As an example, the hormone replacement drug Synthroid® and calcium should not be taken together. Instruct patients to call the office if they think their drugs are interacting adversely.

Drug-Food Interactions Interactions between a drug and food can alter a drug's therapeutic effect. For example, taking tetracycline with milk can reduce the drug's effectiveness because of decreased absorption from the GI tract. The drug-food interaction between a monoamine oxidase (MAO) inhibitor (such as Parnate®, an antidepressant drug) and aged cheese or meat or other foods containing high levels of tyramine can produce a toxic effect. This interaction can cause a dangerous hypertensive crisis in which the patient's blood pressure rises quickly to dangerous levels, possibly leading to stroke and death.

A food that may interact with drugs is grapefruit and grapefruit juice. Interactions with some heart or blood pressure medications, such as nifedipine, might cause irregularities in heartbeat, called dysrhythmia.

Some drug-food interactions can affect the body's use of nutrients. For example, the cholesterol-lowering drugs cholestyramine resin (Locholest®) and colestipol HCl (Colestid®)

may reduce the body's absorption of fat-soluble vitamins (A, D, E, and K) from food.

When teaching a patient about drug-food interactions, specify exactly which foods to avoid and when. For example, a patient may drink milk or eat food several hours before or after taking tetracycline, whereas a patient taking an MAO inhibitor must avoid foods that contain high levels of tyramine at all times. Explain what to expect if an interaction occurs, and describe how to deal with it.

Adverse Reactions

Reported adverse reactions associated with a drug are somewhat predictable and range from mild side effects, such as stomach upset, to severe or life-threatening allergic responses. For example, certain cholesterol-lowering medications, called statins (e.g., Lipitor®), can increase the likelihood of painful muscle disorders. Unpredictable adverse effects also can occur; they are unique to each patient.

Elderly patients and patients with liver or kidney disease are more susceptible than others to adverse reactions, because these conditions affect drug metabolism and excretion. When drugs are not metabolized properly or excreted from the body quickly enough, drugs can reach toxic levels, even with normal doses.

To help prevent adverse reactions, teach the patient to take the drug at the right time, in the right amount, and under the right circumstances. For example, the patient may need to take a cephalosporin with food to avoid nausea and diarrhea. Also teach the patient to recognize significant adverse effects and to call the office if any of them occur. The patient also should report any change in overall health because that change could be drug-related.

Tell patients to inform each of their doctors of any adverse reactions (including allergic reactions) they have had to drugs. Previous adverse reactions may prompt a doctor to adjust a dosage or select a different drug. A history of drug allergies may contraindicate the use of a particular drug.

Complete Medication List

Patients must inform the doctor of all substances they use regularly or periodically. This includes prescription and OTC drugs, plus herbals and supplements. It also includes past and present use of alcohol and recreational drugs. When patients have more than one doctor, tell them to inform each doctor about all medications they are taking. Encourage them to keep up-to-date medication lists with dosages (some patients keep this information on their home computers). This information can help patients and healthcare professionals prevent and monitor for drug interactions. The list should be kept on the patient chart and updated with every visit to the physician's office.

Patient Compliance

To help ensure that patients comply with instructions, confirm that they completely understand the name, dosage, and purpose of each drug prescribed for them. If patients must take more than one drug at a time, be sure they know the correct and relevant information for each one. In addition, cover each of the following points when educating patients about drugs:

- Explain how and when to take each drug to ensure its safety and effectiveness. Some drugs should be taken with food to minimize gastrointestinal irritation. Others should be taken on an empty stomach for proper absorption and metabolism. Some drugs must be taken once a day in the morning; others should be taken three or four times a day. If patients' medication schedules are complex, suggest that they create an alarm, chart, calendar, or diary to remind them of what drug to take and when, or create a schedule for them.

- Tell patients how long to take each drug. In the case of antibiotics, advise them to take the entire course of the drug as scheduled, even if they feel better before finishing it. In the case of medicines prescribed for chronic disease, advise patients that they will need to continue taking the medication unless the doctor tells them to stop. Be aware that some drugs, such as prednisone, must be tapered off slowly to prevent adverse reactions.

- Explain how to identify possible adverse reactions of each drug and safety measures related to adverse reactions. For example, instruct patients to avoid certain activities, such as driving or operating machinery, while taking a drug that causes drowsiness. If appropriate, inform patients that misuse of the drug may lead to dependence, and mention the dangers of drug dependence.

- Tell patients not to save medications that are over 1 year old or share them with anyone else. Old medications and those taken by people other than the patient for whom they were prescribed can cause severe, unexpected adverse effects. Advise patients to check the expiration date on all drugs and to discard them by wrapping in a tightly sealed container and placing in the trash. Flushing is not recommended due to possible water contamination. Some pharmacies will dispose of medications for patients.

- Suggest that patients avoid alcohol when taking certain drugs. Alcohol interacts with some drugs, causing adverse reactions such as lethargy, confusion, or coma.

- Tell patients to ask their pharmacists where to store each medication. Some drugs must be refrigerated. Others should be kept in a dry, cool area. Drugs should not usually be kept in a hot, damp place, such as a bathroom. They must always be kept out of the reach of children.

- Tell patients to take their drugs in a well-lit area so that they can read each drug label carefully before taking each dose. They should never assume that they are taking the right medication without reading the label on the container. If patients have poor vision, print the name of the drug and the dosage schedule clearly on a separate piece of paper or card to attach to the medication container.

- Instruct patients to call the licensed practitioner if they have any questions about their drug therapy.

▶ Charting Medications   LO 53.9

Whenever a patient receives some form of treatment, such as medication, a record is kept of that treatment. Special problems or circumstances are also recorded, such as new symptoms, the patient's own statements, and how the patient tolerated the medications or treatment. Most charting in the physician's office is documented on a progress note or a medication administration record (MAR). These documents are essential to serve as communication tools for all health-care members who are connected to that patient. The medical record is considered a legal document and is taken as proof that medication or treatment was administered to the patient.

All chart entries must be factual, accurate, complete, current, organized, and confidential. Avoid using words or statements that can be interpreted as your opinion. For example, if a patient gags and spits up cough syrup you have just administered, you would not write that the patient did not like the taste of the medication; you would simply state "patient experienced difficulty in swallowing medication and expelled medication." Avoid terms such as *appear* and *seems*, which can lead you to draw assumptions without objective data to support them. Be specific. Chart what the patient said or did, not what you think. Use abbreviations when appropriate because they allow you to say a great deal in a small space.

Below you can see an EHR medicine charting example or progress note for Valarie Ramirez.

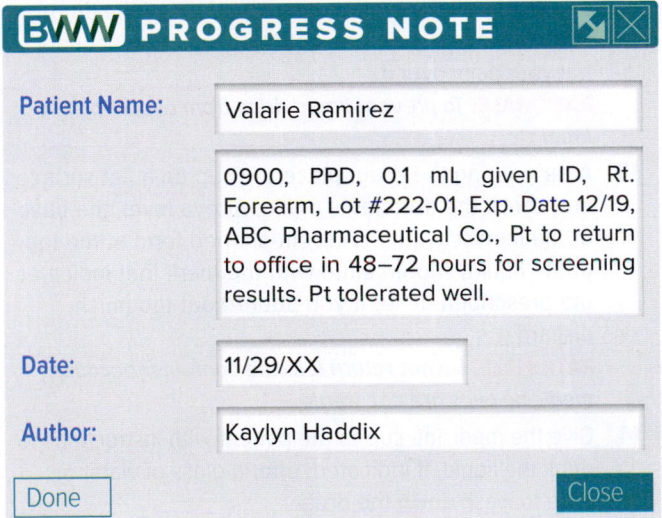

BWW PROGRESS NOTE

Patient Name: Valarie Ramirez

0900, PPD, 0.1 mL given ID, Rt. Forearm, Lot #222-01, Exp. Date 12/19, ABC Pharmaceutical Co., Pt to return to office in 48–72 hours for screening results. Pt tolerated well.

Date: 11/29/XX

Author: Kaylyn Haddix

Done   Close

Review your office's medical records to keep consistent with the charting methods used in them. Follow these simple rules:

- Before you begin, make sure you have the right chart and the right location in the chart.
- Chart medications directly from the physician order.
- Be specific. Do not write "Gave Demerol for pain in the evening." Instead, write, "(Date/Time), Demerol 100 mg given IM in right upper outer quadrant of gluteus maximus for c/o sharp pain, rated 7 on a scale of 10, in left arm, lot number, expiration date, initials."
- If using paper charts, do not leave gaps or skip lines. If an entry does not fill a complete line, draw a straight line to fill the gap. Put your signature or first initial and last name and title at the right side directly after the note.
- If you make an error, do not erase it. Draw a line through the mistake. The mistake should still be visible, so do not black it out. Initial it and then rechart the information correctly. Follow the specific procedure for making corrections in an electronic health record.
- Never use ditto marks.
- Write neatly in longhand or carefully enter into the electronic chart and check your note before submitting it. Ensure that your spelling is accurate.
- Use abbreviations and correct symbols. Most facilities have an approved abbreviation list to use as a reference.
- If you are unsure about charting, check with your supervising licensed practitioner.

PROCEDURE 53-1 Administering Oral Drugs

WORK // DOC

Procedure Goal: To safely administer an oral drug to a patient

OSHA Guidelines: This procedure does not involve exposure to blood, body fluids, or tissues.

Materials: Patient chart/progress note, drug order (in patient chart), container of oral drug, small paper cup (for tablets, capsules, or caplets) or plastic calibrated medicine cup (for liquids), glass of water or juice, straw (optional), package insert or drug information sheet

Method:

1. Identify the patient and wash your hands.
2. Select the ordered drug (tablet, capsule, or liquid).
3. Check the rights, comparing information against the drug order.
   RATIONALE: *To ensure necessary accuracy.*
4. If you are unfamiliar with the drug, check a drug reference, read the package insert, or speak with the physician. Determine whether the drug may be taken with or followed by water or juice.

5. Ask the patient about any drug or food allergies. If the patient is not allergic to the ordered drug or other ingredients used to prepare it, proceed.
   RATIONALE: *To prevent a reaction to the medication.*

6. Perform any calculations needed to provide the prescribed dose. If you are unsure of your calculations, check them with a coworker or the licensed practitioner.

Giving Tablets or Capsules

7. Open the container and tap the correct number into the cap. Do not touch the inside of the cap because it is sterile. If you pour out too many tablets or capsules and you have not touched them, tap the excess back into the container.

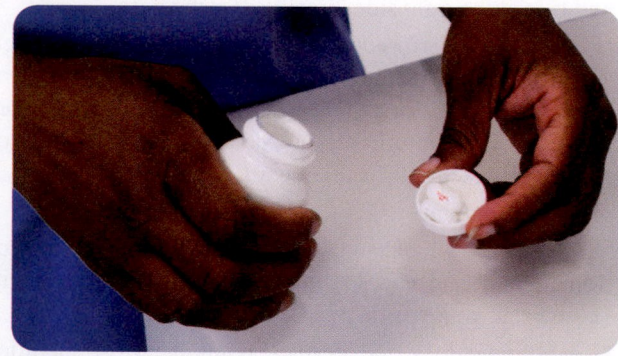

FIGURE Procedure 53-1 Step 7   Tap tablets gently into the cap.
© McGraw-Hill Education

8. Tap the tablets or capsules from the cap into the paper cup.

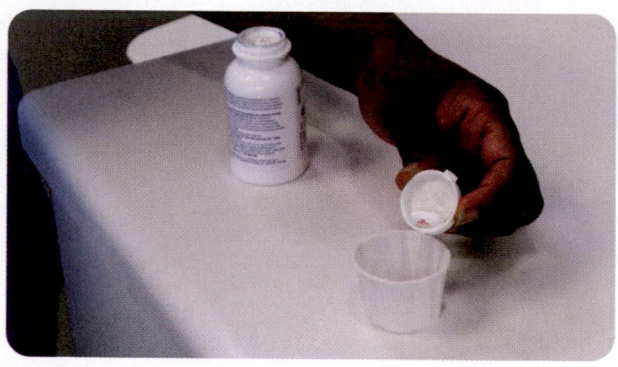

FIGURE Procedure 53-1 Step 8   Tap tablets from the cap into the paper cup.
© McGraw-Hill Education

9. Recap the container immediately.
   RATIONALE: *Recapping immediately protects the medication from exposure to air, which can break down the medication.*

10. Give the patient the cup along with a glass of water or juice. If the patient finds it easier to drink with a straw, unwrap the straw and place it in the fluid. If patients have difficulty swallowing pills, have them drink some water or juice before putting the pills in the mouth.

RATIONALE: *Additional fluid makes the pills float in the mouth and allows patients to swallow more easily.*

Giving a Liquid Drug

11. If the liquid is a suspension, shake it well.

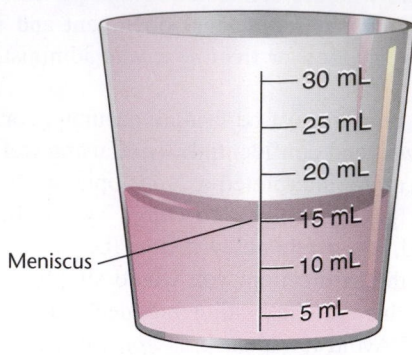

FIGURE Procedure 53-1 Step 11   Looking at eye level, find the base of the meniscus, which is the crescent-shaped form at the top of the liquid, for the correct measure.

12. Locate the mark on the medicine cup for the prescribed dose. Keeping your thumbnail on the mark, hold the cup at eye level and pour the correct amount of the drug. Keep the label side of the bottle on top as you pour or put your palm over it.
   RATIONALE: *To prevent liquid drips from obscuring the label.*

13. After pouring the drug, place the cup on a flat surface and check the drug level again. At eye level, the base of the meniscus (the crescent-shaped form at the top of the liquid) should align with the mark that indicates the prescribed dose. If you poured out too much, discard it.
   RATIONALE: *Do not return it to the container because medicine cups are not sterile.*

14. Give the medicine cup to the patient with instructions to drink the liquid. If indicated, offer a glass of water or juice to wash down the drug.

After You Have Given an Oral Drug

15. Wash your hands.

16. Give the patient an information sheet about the drug. Discuss the information with the patient and answer any questions. If the patient has questions you cannot answer, refer her to the licensed practitioner.

17. Document the drug administration in the patient's chart with date, time, drug name, dosage, expiration date, lot number, manufacturer, route, site, significant patient reactions, and any patient education.

PROCEDURE 53-2 Administering Buccal or Sublingual Drugs

Procedure Goal: To safely administer a buccal or sublingual drug to a patient

OSHA Guidelines: This procedure does not involve exposure to blood, body fluids, or tissues.

Materials: Patient chart/progress note, drug order (in patient chart), container of buccal or sublingual drug, small paper cup, package insert or drug information sheet

Method:

1. Identify the patient and wash your hands.

2. Select the ordered drug.

3. Check the rights, comparing information against the drug order.
   RATIONALE: *To ensure necessary accuracy.*

4. If you are unfamiliar with the drug, check the *PDR* or other credible drug reference, read the package insert, or speak with the licensed practitioner.

5. Ask the patient about any drug or food allergies. If the patient is not allergic to the ordered drug or other ingredients used to prepare it, proceed.
   RATIONALE: *To prevent a reaction to the medication.*

6. Perform any calculations needed to provide the prescribed dose. If you are unsure of your calculations, check them with a coworker or the licensed practitioner.

7. Open the container and tap the correct number into the cap. Do not touch the inside of the cap because it is sterile. If you pour out too many tablets or capsules and you have not touched them, tap the excess back into the container.

8. Tap the tablets or capsules from the cap into the paper cup.

9. Recap the container immediately.
   RATIONALE: *Recapping immediately protects the medication from exposure to air, which can break down the medication.*

Giving Buccal Medication

10. For a *buccal* drug, provide patient instruction, including
    - Do not chew or swallow the tablet.
    - Place the medication between the cheek and gum until it dissolves.
    RATIONALE: *This area is rich in blood supply to promote rapid absorption of the drug.*
    - Do not eat, drink, or smoke until the tablet is completely dissolved.
    RATIONALE: *Food and fluids wash the drug into the gastrointestinal (GI) tract, slowing absorption or allowing gastric juices to destroy it. Smoking increases salivation, causing impaired absorption of the drug.*

Giving a Sublingual Drug

11. For a *sublingual* drug, provide patient instruction, including
    - Do not chew or swallow the tablet.

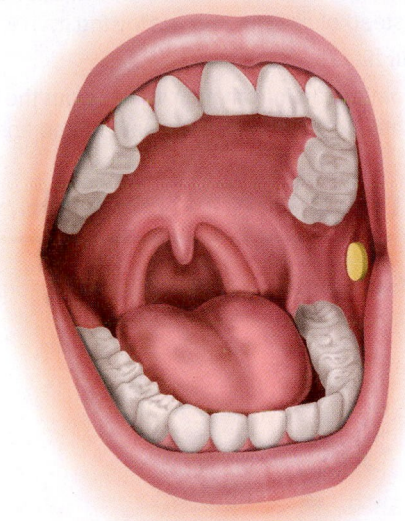

FIGURE Procedure 53-2 Step 10   Place a buccal drug between the cheek and gum.

- Place the medication under the tongue until it dissolves.
RATIONALE: *The capillaries in this area promote rapid absorption of the drug.*

- Do not eat, drink, or smoke until the tablet is completely dissolved.
RATIONALE: *Food and fluids wash the drug into the GI tract, slowing absorption or allowing gastric juices to destroy it. Smoking increases salivation, causing impaired absorption of the drug.*

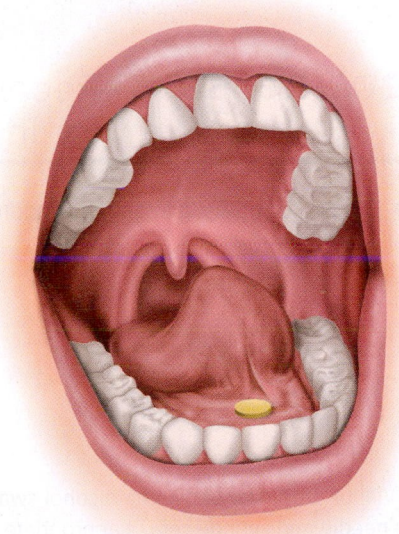

FIGURE Procedure 53-2 Step 11   Place a sublingual drug under the tongue.

After You Have Given a Buccal or Sublingual Medication

12. Remain with the patient until the tablet dissolves to monitor for possible adverse reactions and to ensure that the patient has allowed the tablet to dissolve in the mouth instead of chewing or swallowing it.

13. Wash your hands.

14. Give the patient an information sheet about the drug. Discuss the information with the patient and answer

any questions. If the patient has questions you cannot answer, refer her to the licensed practitioner.

15. Document the drug administration in the patient's chart with date, time, drug name, dosage, expiration date, lot number, manufacturer, route, site, significant patient reactions, and any patient education.

PROCEDURE 53-3 Drawing a Drug from an Ampule

Procedure Goal: To safely open an ampule and draw a drug, using sterile technique

OSHA Guidelines:

Materials:
Ampule of drug, alcohol swab, 2 × 2 gauze square, small file (provided by the drug manufacturer), sterile filtered needle, sterile needle, and a syringe of the appropriate size

Method:

1. Wash your hands and put on exam gloves.

2. Gently tap the top of the ampule with your forefinger to settle the liquid to the bottom of the ampule.

3. Wipe the ampule's neck with an alcohol swab.

4. Wrap the 2 × 2 gauze square around the ampule's neck; then snap the neck away from you. If it does not snap easily, score the neck with the small file and snap it again.

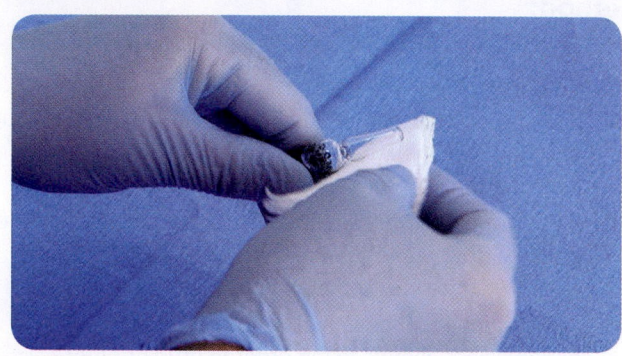

FIGURE Procedure 53-3 Step 4   To prevent possible injury, wrap the neck of the ampule with gauze before snapping.
© McGraw-Hill Education

5. Insert the filtered needle into the ampule without touching the side of the ampule.
   RATIONALE: *A filtered needle will prevent contamination of the medication.*

6. Pull back on the plunger to aspirate (remove by vacuum or suction) the liquid completely into the syringe.

7. Replace with the regular needle and push the plunger on the syringe until the medication just reaches the tip of the needle. The drug is now ready for injection.

PROCEDURE 53-4 Reconstituting and Drawing a Drug for Injection

Procedure Goal: To reconstitute and draw a drug for injection, using sterile technique

OSHA Guidelines:

Materials: Vial of drug, vial of diluent, alcohol swabs, two disposable sterile needle and syringe sets of appropriate size, sharps container

Method:

1. Wash your hands and put on exam gloves.

2. Place the drug vial and diluent vial on the countertop. Wipe each rubber diaphragm with a fresh alcohol swab.

3. Loosen the cap from the needle and the guard from the syringe. Pull the plunger back to the mark that equals the amount of diluent needed to reconstitute the drug ordered.
   RATIONALE: *This action aspirates air into the syringe.*

4. Puncture the diaphragm of the vial of diluent with the needle and inject the air into the diluent.
   RATIONALE: *This action creates positive pressure that lets you draw the diluent easily. If you do not add air, a vacuum forms, making it difficult to draw the diluent.*

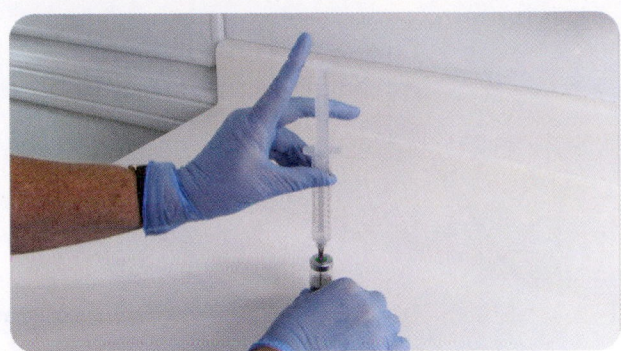

FIGURE Procedure 53-4 Step 4 Injecting air into the diluent.
© McGraw-Hill Education

solution may be clear or cloudy when completely mixed (depending on the drug).

8. Remove the cap and guard from the second needle and syringe.
9. Pull back the plunger to the mark that reflects the amount of drug ordered. Inject the air into the drug vial.
10. Invert the vial and aspirate the proper amount of the drug into the syringe. The drug is now ready for injection.

5. Invert the vial and aspirate the diluent.
6. Remove the needle from the diluent vial, inject the diluent into the drug vial, and withdraw the needle. Properly dispose of this needle and syringe.
7. Roll the vial between your hands to mix the drug and diluent thoroughly. Do not shake the vial unless so directed on the drug label. When completely mixed, the solution in the vial should have no flakes. The

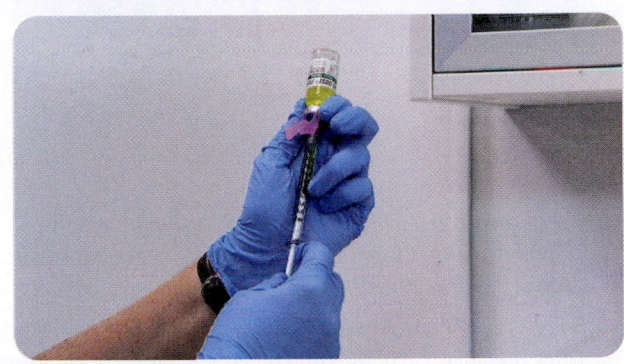

FIGURE Procedure 53-4 Step 10 Aspirating the drug into the syringe.
© McGraw-Hill Education

PROCEDURE 53-5 Giving an Intradermal (ID) Injection WORK // DOC

Procedure Goal: To administer an intradermal injection safely and effectively, using sterile technique

OSHA Guidelines:

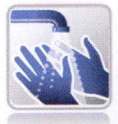   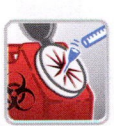

Materials: Patient chart/progress note, drug order (in patient chart), alcohol swab, disposable needle and syringe of the appropriate size filled with the ordered dose of drug, sharps container

Method:
1. Identify the patient. Wash your hands and put on exam gloves.
2. Check the rights, comparing information against the drug order.
   RATIONALE: *To ensure necessary accuracy.*
3. Ask the patient about any drug or food allergies. If the patient is not allergic to the ordered drug or other ingredients used to prepare it, proceed.
4. Identify the injection site on the patient's forearm. To do so, rest the patient's arm on a table with the palm up. Measure two to three finger-widths below the antecubital space and a hand-width above the wrist. The space between is available for the injection.
5. Prepare the skin with the alcohol swab, moving in a circle from the center out.

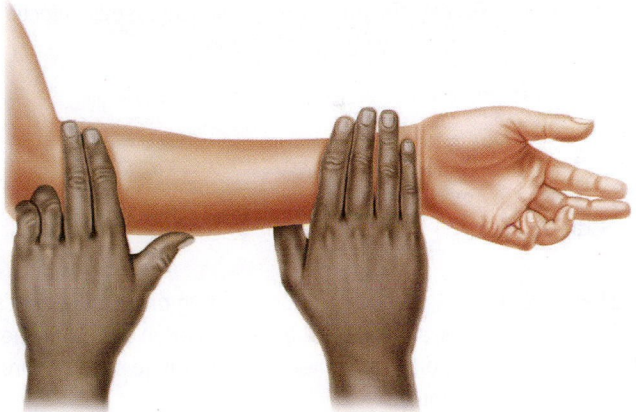

FIGURE Procedure 53-5 Step 4 This space is available for intradermal injection sites.

6. Let the skin dry before giving the injection.
   RATIONALE: *To prevent you from introducing antiseptic under the skin, which could cause irritation and falsify intradermal test results.*
7. Hold the patient's forearm and stretch the skin taut with one hand.
8. With the other hand, place the needle—bevel up—almost flat against the patient's skin. Press the needle against the skin and insert it.

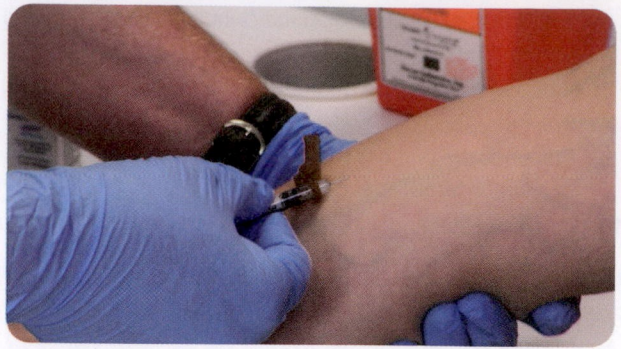

FIGURE Procedure 53-5 Step 8   Inserting the needle for an intradermal injection.
© McGraw-Hill Education

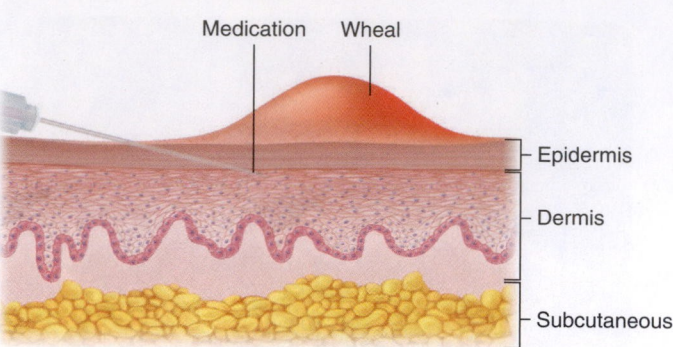

FIGURE Procedure 53-5 Step 9   Medication collects under the skin, forming a wheal, during an intradermal injection.

9. Inject the drug slowly and gently. You should see the needle through the skin and feel resistance. As the drug enters the upper layer of skin, a wheal (raised area of the skin) will form.

10. After the full dose of the drug has been injected, withdraw the needle. Properly dispose of used materials and the needle and syringe immediately.

11. Remove the gloves and wash your hands.

12. Stay with the patient to monitor for unexpected reactions.

13. Document the injection in the patient's chart with date, time, drug name, dosage, expiration date, lot number, manufacturer, route, site, significant patient reactions, and any patient education.

PROCEDURE 53-6   Giving a Subcutaneous (Subcut) Injection

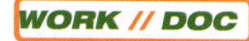

Procedure Goal: To administer a subcutaneous injection safely and effectively, using sterile technique

OSHA Guidelines:

  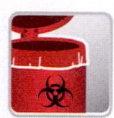 

Materials: Patient chart/progress note, drug order (in patient's chart), alcohol swabs, sterile 2 × 2 gauze or cotton ball, container of the ordered drug, disposable needle and syringe of the appropriate size, sharps container

Method:

1. Identify the patient. Wash your hands and put on exam gloves.

2. Check the rights, comparing information against the drug order.
   RATIONALE: *To ensure necessary accuracy.*

3. Ask the patient about any drug or food allergies. If the patient is not allergic to the ordered drug or other ingredients used to prepare it, proceed.

4. Prepare the drug and draw it up to the mark on the syringe that matches the ordered dose.

5. Choose a site and clean it with an alcohol swab, moving in a circle from the center out. Let the area dry.

6. Pinch the skin firmly to lift the subcutaneous tissue.

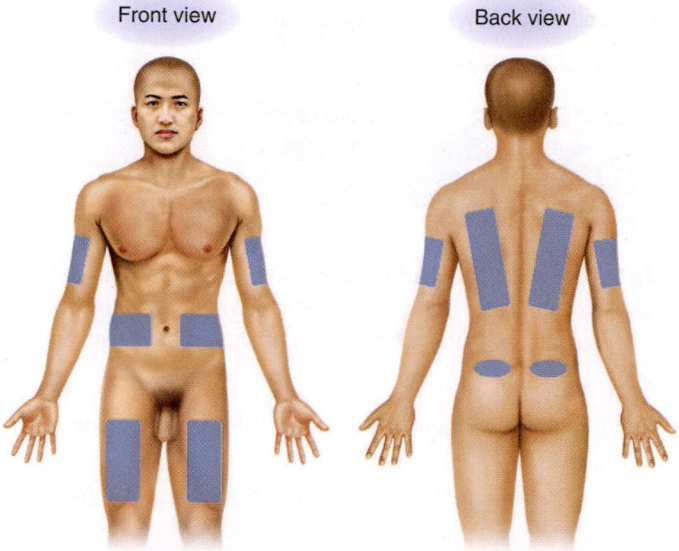

FIGURE Procedure 53-6 Step 5   Many sites are available for subcutaneous injection.

7. Position the needle—bevel up—at a 45- to 90-degree angle to the skin.
   RATIONALE: *The angle of the needle helps ensure that the medication is administered into the correct location. A 90-degree angle is used when you can pinch at least 2 inches. A 45-degree angle is used when you can only pinch 1 inch of skin.*

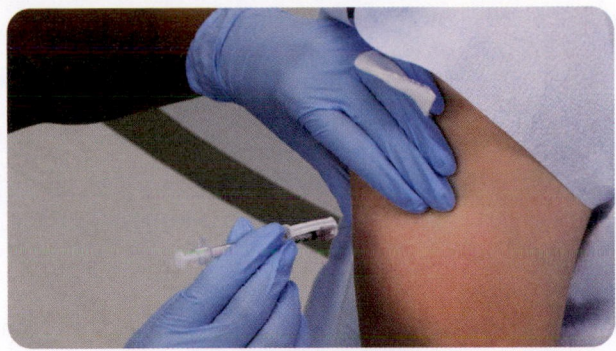

(a)

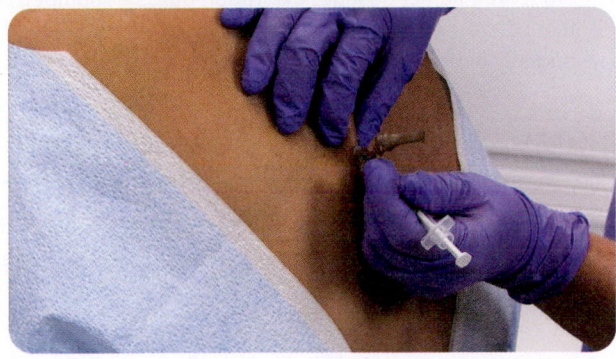

(b)

FIGURE Procedure 53-6 Step 7   Positioning the needle for subcutaneous injection using your dominant hand: (a) 90-degree angle (right hand dominant); (b) 45-degree angle (left hand dominant).
© McGraw-Hill Education

8. Insert the needle in one quick motion using your dominant hand; then release the skin and inject the drug slowly. With some medications, you will check the placement of the needle by pulling back on the plunger before injecting. If blood is seen in the hub, you should withdraw the needle and start with a fresh needle and syringe. If no blood is seen, inject the medication slowly.

9. After the full dose of the drug has been injected, place a 2 × 2 gauze over the site and withdraw the needle at the same angle you inserted it. You can hold this gauze in your non-dominant hand as shown in Figure 53-6 Step 7(a).

10. Apply pressure at the puncture site with the gauze or cotton ball.

11. Massage the site gently to help distribute the drug, if indicated. Do not massage insulin, heparin, or other anticoagulant medications.
    RATIONALE: *Massaging a site for heparin can cause bruising.*

12. Properly dispose of the used materials and the needle and syringe.

13. Remove the gloves and wash your hands.

14. Stay with the patient to monitor for unexpected reactions.

15. Document the injection in the patient's chart with date, time, drug name, dosage, expiration date, lot number, manufacturer, route, site, significant patient reactions, and any patient education.

PROCEDURE 53-7   Giving an Intramuscular (IM) Injection   *WORK // DOC*

Procedure Goal: To administer an intramuscular injection safely and effectively, using sterile technique

OSHA Guidelines:

  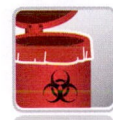 

Materials: Patient chart/progress note, drug order (in patient's chart), alcohol swabs, sterile 2 × 2 gauze or cotton ball, container of the ordered drug, disposable needle and syringe of the appropriate size, sharps container

Method:

1. Identify the patient. Wash your hands and put on exam gloves.

2. Check the rights, comparing information against the drug order.
   RATIONALE: *To ensure necessary accuracy.*

3. Ask the patient about any drug or food allergies. If the patient is not allergic to the ordered drug or other ingredients used to prepare it, proceed.

4. Prepare the drug and draw it up to the mark on the syringe that matches the ordered dose.

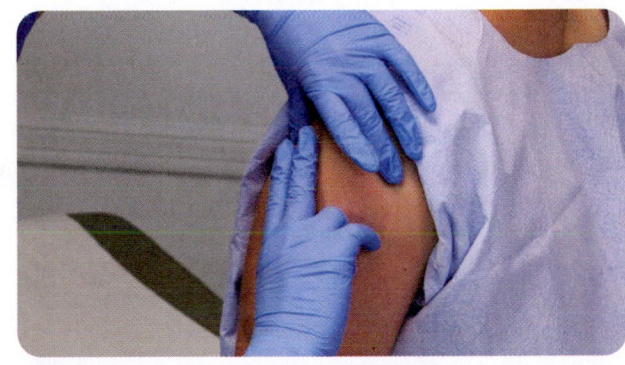

FIGURE Procedure 53-7 Step 5   Gently tap the site to stimulate the nerve endings.
© McGraw-Hill Education

5. Choose a site and gently tap it. Tapping stimulates the nerve endings and reduces pain caused by the needle insertion.

6. Clean the site with an alcohol swab, moving in a circle from the center out. Let the site dry.

7. Stretch the skin taut over the injection site between the thumb and forefinger. For pediatric and geriatric patients, you can grasp the tissue and "bunch up" the muscle. For a Z-track, stretch and hold the skin and fat laterally.

8. Hold the needle and syringe at a 90-degree angle to the skin; then insert the needle with a quick, dart-like thrust.
   RATIONALE: *The angle of the needle helps ensure that the medication is administered into the correct location.*

9. Release the skin and aspirate by pulling back slightly on the plunger to check the needle placement. If pulling back on the plunger produces blood, placement is incorrect and you must draw up new medication again with a fresh needle and syringe. If pulling back on the plunger produces no blood, placement is correct. Inject the drug slowly.
   RATIONALE: *Injecting an intramuscular drug into the bloodstream can cause severe adverse effects for the patient.*

10. After the full dose of the drug has been injected, place a 2 × 2 gauze over the site which is held in your non-dominant hand during the injection; then quickly remove the needle at a 90-degree angle.

11. Use the 2 × 2 gauze to apply pressure to the site and massage it, if indicated.

12. Properly dispose of used materials and the needle and syringe.

13. Remove the gloves and wash your hands.

14. Stay with the patient to monitor for unexpected reactions.

15. Document the injection in the patient's chart with date, time, drug name, dosage, expiration date, lot number, manufacturer, route, site, significant patient reactions, and any patient education.

PROCEDURE 53-8 Administering Inhalation Therapy

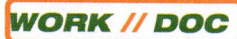

Procedure Goal: To administer inhalation therapy safely and effectively

OSHA Guidelines: This procedure does not involve exposure to blood, body fluids, or tissues.

Materials: Patient chart/progress note, drug order (in patient's chart), container of the ordered drug, tissues, package insert or patient education sheet about medication

Method:

1. Identify the patient. Wash your hands.

2. Check the rights, comparing information against the drug order. Make sure you have the correct type of inhaler based on the order (oral or nasal).
   RATIONALE: *To ensure necessary accuracy.*

3. Ask the patient about any drug or food allergies. If the patient is not allergic to the ordered drug or other ingredients used to prepare it, proceed.

4. Prepare the container of medication as directed. Use the package insert and show the directions to the patient.

5. Shake the container as directed and stress this step to the patient.
   RATIONALE: *The drug must be evenly distributed in the inhaler to ensure its effectiveness.*

Nasal Inhaler

6. Instruct the patient to
   - Blow your nose to clear the nostrils.
   - Tilt the head back and, with one hand, place the inhaler tip about ½ inch into the nostril.
   - Point the tip straight up toward the inner corner of the eye.
   RATIONALE: *Angling the inhaler downward makes the drug run down the back of the throat, causing a burning sensation.*
   - Use the opposite hand to block the other nostril.
   - Inhale gently while quickly and firmly squeezing the inhaler.

   - Remove the inhaler tip and exhale through the mouth.
   - Shake the inhaler and repeat the process in the other nostril.
   - Keep your head tilted back and do not blow your nose for several minutes (if indicated in the package insert).

Oral Inhaler

7. Instruct the patient to
   - Warm the canister by rolling it between the palms of your hands.
   - Uncap the mouthpiece and assemble the inhaler as directed on the package insert.
   - Hold your mouth open and place the canister in your mouth or about 1 inch from your mouth. Check the package insert for the proper placement.
   - Exhale normally and inhale through the canister as you depress it. The medication must be inhaled.
   - Breathe in until your lungs are full and hold your breath for 10 seconds.
   - Breathe out normally.

After You Have Given an Inhalation Medication

8. Remain with the patient to monitor for changes and possible adverse reaction.

9. Recap and secure the medication container. Instruct the patient in this procedure.

10. Wash your hands.

11. Give the patient an information sheet about the drug. Discuss the information with the patient and answer any questions. If the patient has questions you cannot answer, refer her to the licensed practitioner.

12. Document the drug administration in the patient's chart with date, time, drug name, dosage, expiration date, lot number, manufacturer, route, site, significant patient reactions, and any patient education.

Procedure Goal: To safely administer a transdermal patch drug to and remove it from a patient

OSHA Guidelines: This procedure does not involve exposure to blood, body fluids, or tissues.

Materials: Patient chart/progress note, drug order (in patient chart), transdermal patch medication, gloves, package insert or drug information sheet

Method:

1. Identify the patient, wash your hands, and put on gloves.
   RATIONALE: *Gloves prevent the medication from being absorbed through your skin.*

2. Select the ordered transdermal patch and check the rights, comparing information against the drug order.
   RATIONALE: *To ensure necessary accuracy.*

3. Ask the patient about any drug or food allergies. If the patient is not allergic to the ordered drug or other ingredients used to prepare it, proceed.
   RATIONALE: *To prevent a reaction to the medication.*

4. If you are unfamiliar with the drug, check the *PDR* or other credible drug reference, read the package insert, or speak with the licensed practitioner. The package insert is extremely detailed for transdermal medications and should be used when applying the medication and/or doing patient teaching.

5. Perform any calculations needed to provide the prescribed dose. If you are unsure of your calculations, check them with a coworker or the licensed practitioner.

Applying the Transdermal Medication

6. Remove the patch from its pouch. The plastic backing is easily peeled off once the patch is removed from the pouch. For patches without a protective pouch, bend the sides of the transdermal unit back and forth until the clear plastic backing snaps down the middle.

7. For either type of patch, demonstrate how to peel off the clear plastic backing to expose the sticky side of the patch.

8. Apply the patch to a reasonably hair-free site, such as the abdomen. Note that estrogen patches are usually placed on the hip.

9. Instruct the patient on how to apply the patch. Tell the patient that if she is applying the patch, she does not have to wear gloves, but if a caregiver or any other third party applies the patch, that person must wear gloves to avoid absorbing the medication through the skin. Advise the patient to avoid using the extremities below the knee or elbow, skinfolds, scar tissue, or burned or irritated areas.
   RATIONALE: *These areas do not absorb the medication as well because of the reduced blood supply.*

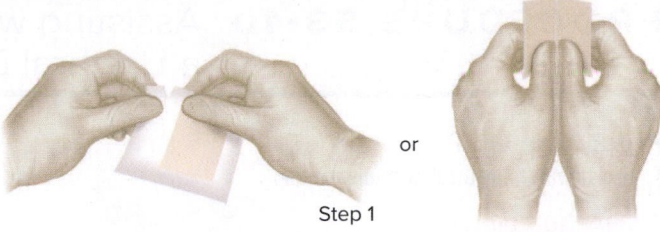

or

Step 1

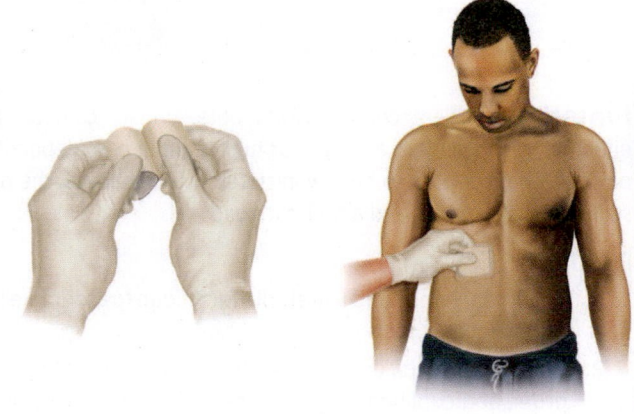

Step 2   Step 3

FIGURE Procedure 53-9 Steps 6–8 To apply a transdermal patch, first (1) either remove it from the pouch or bend the sides back and forth until the backing snaps; then (2) peel the backing off the patch and (3) apply the patch, sticky side down, to a clean, relatively hairless site.

Removing the Transdermal Patch

10. Gently lift and slowly peel the patch back from the skin. Wash the area with soap and dry it with a towel. Instruct the patient on this technique.

11. Explain to the patient that the skin may appear red and warm, which is normal. Reassure the patient that the redness will disappear. In some cases, lotion may be applied to the skin if it feels dry.

12. Instruct the patient to notify the licensed practitioner if the redness does not disappear in several days or if a rash develops.

13. *Never* apply a new patch to the site just used. It is best to allow each site to rest between applications. Some transdermal systems call for waiting 7 days before using a site again. Be sure to check the package directions regarding site rotation.

After You Have Applied and/or Removed the Transdermal Patch

14. Wash your hands and instruct the patient to do the same after applying or removing a transdermal system at home.

15. Give the patient an information sheet about the drug. Discuss the information with the patient and answer any questions. If the patient has questions you cannot answer, refer her to the licensed practitioner.

16. Document the drug administration in the patient's chart with date, time, drug name, dosage, expiration date, lot number, manufacturer, route, site, significant patient reactions, and any patient education.

PROCEDURE 53-10 Assisting with Administration of a Urethral Drug

WORK // DOC

Procedure Goal:
To assist with a urethral administration

OSHA Guidelines:

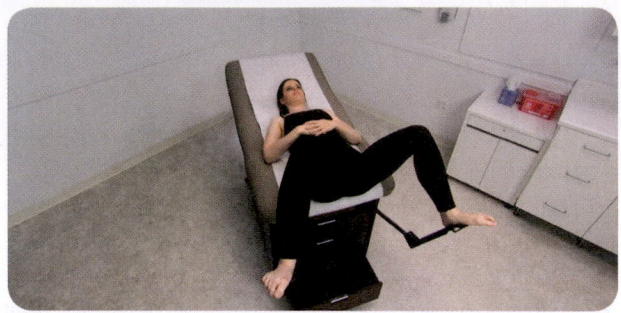

FIGURE Procedure 53-10 Step 4   Use the stirrups to place the patient in the lithotomy position. Clothing should be removed and a drape applied.
© McGraw-Hill Education

Materials: Patient chart/progress note, urinary catheter kit, either a syringe without a needle or tubing and a bag (depending on the amount of drug to be administered), sterile gloves, the prescribed drug, a drape, and a bedsaver pad

Method:

1. Wash your hands and use sterile technique to assemble the equipment.

2. Check the rights, comparing information against the drug order, and explain the procedure and the drug order to the patient.
RATIONALE: *To ensure necessary accuracy.*

3. Ask the patient about any drug or food allergies. If the patient is not allergic to the ordered drug or other ingredients used to prepare it, proceed.

4. Assist the patient into the lithotomy position and drape her to preserve her modesty while exposing the vulva.

5. Place a bedsaver pad under the buttocks.

6. Open the catheter kit.

7. Put on sterile gloves.

8. Cleanse the vulva as you would to perform catheterization, using the materials in the kit. As you sweep down with the antiseptic swab, watch for the urethral opening to "wink."
RATIONALE: *The wink is where the cleanser stimulates and fills the opening of the urethra, making it look like a*

winking eye. Finding the wink helps you accurately locate the urethral opening.

9. The physician or nurse will insert the lubricated catheter. Tell the patient that she should feel pressure, not pain, and that the physician or nurse is going to attach the syringe to the catheter and insert the drug (or attach the tubing and bag to the catheter and let the drug run in by gravity).

10. After instilling the drug, the physician or nurse will clamp the catheter and leave the drug in place for the ordered amount of time.

11. Stay with the patient not only to ensure that she remains still but also to reassure her that the full feeling in the bladder is normal. She also may say she feels the need to urinate. Advise her that this feeling, too, is normal and is caused by the catheter.

12. When the time is up, unclamp the catheter, gently remove it, and allow the patient to urinate. Assist the patient as needed.

13. While the patient is dressing, immediately document the drug instillation with date, time, drug, dose, route, and any significant patient reactions.

PROCEDURE 53-11 Administering a Vaginal Medication

WORK // DOC

Procedure Goal: To safely administer a vaginal medication with patient instruction

OSHA Guidelines:

  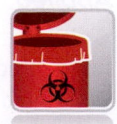 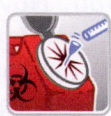

Materials: Patient chart/progress note, prescription or drug order in the patient's chart, a cloth or paper drape, a bedsaver pad, gloves, cotton balls, water-soluble lubricant, and the prescribed drug

Method:

1. Wash your hands.

2. Check the rights, comparing information against the drug order, and explain the procedure and the drug order to the patient.
RATIONALE: *To ensure necessary accuracy.*

3. Ask the patient about any drug or food allergies. If the patient is not allergic to the ordered drug or other ingredients used to prepare it, proceed.

4. Give the patient the opportunity to empty her bladder before beginning.

5. Assist the patient into the lithotomy position and drape her.
   RATIONALE: *To preserve her modesty while exposing the vulva.*

6. Place a bedsaver pad under the buttocks.

7. Put on gloves.

8. Cleanse the perineum with soap and water, using one cotton ball per stroke, and cleanse the center last, while spreading the labia.
   RATIONALE: *This technique prevents contamination of areas already cleaned.*

9. Lubricate the vaginal suppository applicator in lubricant spread on a paper towel. For vaginal drugs in the form of creams, ointments, gels, and tablets, use the appropriate applicator, preparing it according to the package insert.

10. While spreading the labia with one hand, insert the applicator with the other (the applicator should be about 2 inches into the vagina and angled toward the sacrum).

11. Release the labia and push the applicator's plunger to release the suppository into the vagina.

12. Remove the applicator and wipe any excess lubricant off the patient.

13. Help her to a sitting position and assist with dressing if needed.

14. Document the administration with date, time, drug, dose, route, and any significant patient reactions.

PROCEDURE 53-12 Administering a Rectal Medication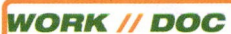

Procedure Goal: To safely administer a rectal medication

OSHA Guidelines:

   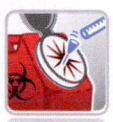

Materials: Patient chart/progress note, prescription or drug order in the patient's chart, a cloth or paper drape, a bedsaver pad, gloves, water-soluble lubricant, and the prescribed drug

Method:

1. Check the rights, comparing information against the drug order.
   RATIONALE: *To ensure necessary accuracy.*

2. Explain the procedure and the drug order to the patient.

3. Ask the patient about any drug or food allergies. If the patient is not allergic to the ordered drug or other ingredients used to prepare it, proceed.

4. Give the patient the opportunity to empty the bladder before beginning.

5. With the patient in a gown, help the patient into Sims' position and use a drape to prevent exposing the patient. Place a bedsaver pad under the patient.

6. Lift the patient's gown to expose the anus.

7. Wash your hands, put on gloves, and prepare the medication.

Administering a Suppository

8. Lubricate the tapered end of the suppository with about 1 tsp of lubricant.

9. While spreading the patient's buttocks with one hand, insert the suppository—tapered end first—into the anus with the other hand.

10. Gently advance the suppository past the sphincter with your index finger. Before it passes the sphincter, the suppository may feel as if it is being pushed back out of the anus. When it passes the sphincter, it seems to disappear.

11. Use tissues to remove excess lubricant from the area.

12. Remove your gloves and ask the patient to lie quietly and retain the suppository for at least 20 minutes. When the treatment is completed, help the patient to a sitting, then standing, position.
    RATIONALE: *To ensure the maximum effectiveness of the medication.*

Administering a Retention Enema

13. Place the tip of a syringe into a rectal tube. Let a little rectal solution flow through the syringe and tube. While holding the tip up, clamp the tubing.

14. Lubricate the end of the tube, spread the patient's buttocks, and slide the tube into the rectum about 4 inches.

15. Slowly pour the rectal solution into the syringe, release the clamp, and let gravity move the solution into the patient. When you have administered the ordered amount of solution, clamp the tube and then remove it.

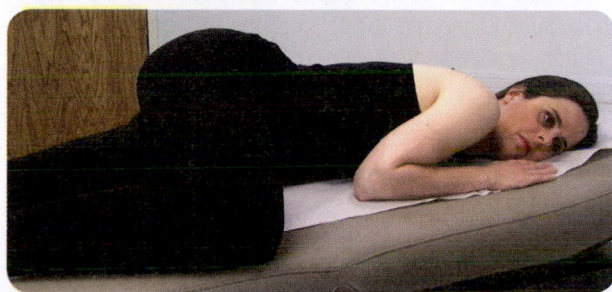

FIGURE Procedure 53-12 Step 5   Place the patient into Sims' position. The patient should be in a gown with a drape in place.
© McGraw-Hill Education

16. Using tissues, apply pressure over the anus for 20 seconds to stifle the patient's urge to defecate, and then wipe any excess lubricant or solution from the area. Remove your gloves and encourage the patient to retain the enema for the time ordered.
    RATIONALE: *To ensure the maximum effectiveness of the medication.*

17. When the time has passed, put on gloves and help the patient use a bedpan or direct the patient to a toilet to expel the solution.

After the Administration Is Complete

18. Remove your gloves and wash your hands.

19. Immediately document the drug administration with date, time, drug, dose, route, and any significant patient reactions.

SUMMARY OF LEARNING OUTCOMES

LEARNING OUTCOMES	KEY POINTS
53.1 Describe the rules and responsibilities regarding drug administration and the initial preparation for drug administration.	Before administering a medication, you should check the patient for allergies and evaluate any drug-drug interactions. You should check all injection sites for abnormalities such as scars, bruises, burns, rash, edema, moles, birthmarks, traumatic injuries, redness, cyanosis, tattoos, warts, site of a mastectomy, and paralyzed areas. Additionally, you should be aware of the patient's condition and have the patient sign a consent form if necessary.
53.2 List the rights of drug administration.	The rights of drug administration include the right patient, right drug, right dose, right route, right time, right documentation, right reason, right to know, right to refuse, and right technique.
53.3 Recognize the correct equipment to use for administering medications.	Drugs may be administered for either local or systemic effects. Generally, drugs that have local effects are applied directly to the skin, tissues, or mucous membranes. Drugs that produce systemic effects are administered by routes that allow the drug to be absorbed and distributed in the bloodstream throughout the body. Table 53-2 outlines the many drug administration routes.
53.4 Carry out the procedures for administering oral medications.	Oral medications typically are swallowed and absorbed through the digestive tract. Sublingual medications go under the tongue, and buccal medications go between the cheek and gum.
53.5 Carry out procedures for administering parenteral medications by injection.	The three most common injection routes are ID, subcut, and IM. IV is less frequently used in a medical office. All injections are given using aseptic technique. Intradermal (ID) injections are administered between the upper layers of skin and create a wheal. Subcutaneous (subcut) injections are administered just under the skin, and intramuscular (IM) injections are administered into a muscle.
53.6 Carry out procedures for administering parenteral medications by other routes.	Other medication routes include inhalants (respiratory), topical (including transdermal), urethral, vaginal, and rectal.

LEARNING OUTCOMES	KEY POINTS
53.7 **Relate special considerations required for medication administration to pediatric, pregnant, breast-feeding, and geriatric patients.**	Certain special considerations must be made when caring for pediatric, pregnant, and breast-feeding patients. Pediatric patients require extreme care when calculating doses due to the differences in how their bodies absorb, metabolize, eliminate, and distribute the medications. Treat pediatric patients with special care and communication to make the experience as positive as possible. Restraining may be necessary. Checking medications given to pregnant and breast-feeding patients for possible adverse effects is essential. Geriatric considerations are discussed in the *Assisting in Geriatrics* chapter.
53.8 **Outline patient education information related to medications.**	Patients should be educated about why, when, and how they should take medications. This includes instruction to ensure patient compliance regarding nonprescription and prescription drugs as well as herbal remedies and supplements. Patients also should be instructed about the dangers of medication combinations, the importance of reporting an adverse effect, and the maintenance of a complete medication list.
53.9 **Implement accurate and complete documentation of medications.**	Documentation of medication administered should occur immediately after the medication is given and should include name, date, time, medication administered, dose, route, location, lot number, and how the patient tolerated it.

CASE STUDY CRITICAL THINKING

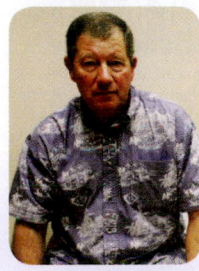

© McGraw-Hill Education

Recall John Miller from the beginning of the chapter. Now that you have completed this chapter, answer the following questions regarding his case.

1. What questions do you need to ask Mr. Miller during his initial interview regarding his medications?

2. When you get ready to administer the pneumococcal immunization, Mr. Miller states that he had a bad reaction the last time he received a shot. What should you do?

3. If the site of the injection from his last visit was just irritated due to the medication, what could be done to reduce the irritation for his next IM injection?

EXAM PREPARATION QUESTIONS

1. (LO 53.3) Which of the following would you expect to be absorbed in the *least* amount of time?
   a. 200 mL of D5W IV
   b. 5 mL of Compazine® IM
   c. 325 mg of ASA orally
   d. ii puffs of albuterol by oral inhalation
   e. PPD subcut injection

2. (LO 53.2) Which of the following is *not* a basic right of medication administration?
   a. Right dose
   b. Right drug
   c. Right to refuse
   d. Right patient
   e. Right time

3. (LO 53.8) Which of the following patients has the greatest risk of overdose and toxicity from a medication?
   a. A 35-year-old woman
   b. A 6-year-child with the flu
   c. A 50-year-old male with hypertension
   d. A 16-year-old Hispanic girl with mononucleosis
   e. A 25-year-old man with diabetes

4. (LO 53.1) When performing a triple check, which of the following would you *least* likely do?
   a. *1st check*—when you take it from the storage container and match it to the MAR
   b. *2nd check*—when you prepare it
   c. *3rd check*—before you close the storage container
   d. *3rd check*—just after you administer the drug
   e. *3rd check*—just before you administer the drug

5. (LO 53.4) A patient is taking a nitroglycerin tablet under his tongue. What route of administration is this?
   a. Urethral
   b. Topical
   c. Inhalant
   d. Sublingual
   e. Buccal

6. (LO 53.5) You are injecting a medication ID; what would *best* let you know that you have done it correctly?
   a. The patient does not have pain
   b. There is a wheal on the skin at the site
   c. The angle of the needle is at 90 degrees
   d. The medication went into a muscle
   e. The medication went under the skin

7. (LO 53.6) You are administering a suppository. What route of administration are you performing?
   a. Oral
   b. Vaginal
   c. Respiratory
   d. IV
   e. Topical

8. (LO 53.7) An infant needs an immunization subcut. What site and what needle would be your *best* choice?
   a. Vastus lateralis, 20 gauge, ⅝ inch
   b. Vastus lateralis, 25 gauge, 1½ inch
   c. Ventrogluteal, 25 gauge, ⅝ inch
   d. Dorsogluteal, 23 gauge, 1 inch
   e. Vastus lateralis, 25 gauge, ⅝ inch

9. (LO 53.8) Which of the following would be done to improve patient compliance?
   a. Have patients with multiple meds create an alarm, calendar, or chart
   b. Remind patients taking antibiotics to stop once they are feeling better
   c. To avoid waste, encourage patients to share medication if they have too much
   d. Dispose of expired drugs 1 year after the expiration date on the medication
   e. Encourage anxious patients to have at least three servings of alcohol each day

10. (LO 53.9) Which of the following is the most complete medication documentation?
    a. Gave Demerol® for pain at 2 pm
    b. Demerol® 100 mg IM in deltoid
    c. 4/12/XX Demerol® IM in left deltoid
    d. 4/12/XX Phenergan® 200 mg PO for nausea
    e. Phenergan® PO for nausea—Kaylyn R. Haddix RMA(AMT)

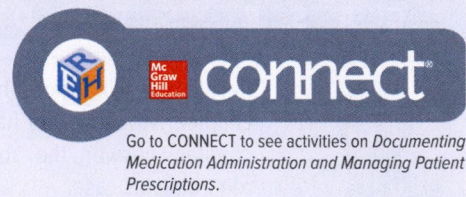

Go to CONNECT to see activities on *Documenting Medication Administration and Managing Patient Prescriptions.*

SOFT SKILLS SUCCESS

While working at BWW Associates with a medical assisting student from a local school, you enter an examination room with a patient and notice there is a small needle and syringe with medication in it on the tray table. You know that it was the medical assisting student's responsibility to clean the room between patients. What should you do?

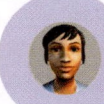

Go to PRACTICE MEDICAL OFFICE and complete the module Clinical – Office Operations.

Physical Therapy and Rehabilitation

CASE STUDY

PATIENT INFORMATION

Patient Name	DOB	Allergies
Chris Matthews	11/19/20XX	NKA

Attending	MRN	Other Information
Alexis N. Whalen, MD	324-95-786	AP and lateral X-ray right ankle show no signs of fractures.

Chris Matthews is an 8-year-old male patient who arrives at the office with a swollen right ankle. Chris was climbing a tree this morning and jumped from a lower limb to the ground. When he landed, he felt his ankle "turn over" and he could not stand up. Chris's mother tells you that she thinks it was about 6 feet from the limb to the ground. She also tells you that she put ice on Chris's ankle after she brought him into the house but his ankle just kept swelling and Chris still cannot walk. She says that his ankle is badly bruised. Mrs. Matthews is very distraught and asks that Chris be seen immediately. You speak with Dr. Whalen, and she asks you to take Chris to the X-ray department for X-rays. Dr. Whalen examines Chris and reads the X-rays. She wraps Chris's ankle and tells you Chris has a badly sprained ankle and will need crutches for a few weeks using a non-weight-bearing gait.

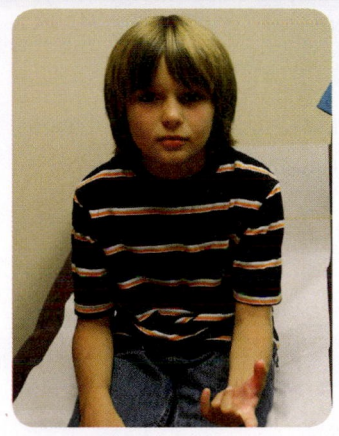

© McGraw-Hill Education

Keep Chris in mind as you study this chapter. There will be questions at the end of the chapter based on the case study. The information in the chapter will help you answer these questions.

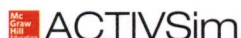

LEARNING OUTCOMES

After completing Chapter 54, you will be able to:

54.1 Discuss the general principles of physical therapy.

54.2 Relate various cold and heat therapies to their benefits and contraindications.

54.3 Recall hydrotherapy methods.

54.4 Name several methods of exercise therapy.

54.5 Describe the types of massage used in rehabilitation therapy.

54.6 Compare different methods of traction.

54.7 Carry out the procedure for teaching a patient to use a cane, a walker, crutches, and a wheelchair.

54.8 Model the steps you should take when referring a patient to a physical therapist.

KEY TERMS

cryotherapy

diathermy

erythema

fluidotherapy

gait

goniometer

hydrotherapy

mobility aid

physical therapy

posture

range of motion (ROM)

therapeutic team

thermotherapy

traction

M E D I C A L   A S S I S T I N G   C O M P E T E N C I E S

CAAHEP

I.P.8	Instruct and prepare a patient for a procedure or a treatment
I.P.9	Assist provider with a patient exam
I.A.1	Incorporate critical thinking skills when performing patient assessment
I.A.2	Incorporate critical thinking skills when performing patient care
V.C.6	Define coaching a patient as it relates to: (c) compliance with treatment plan (e) adaptations relevant to individual patient needs
V.P.4	Coach patients regarding: (d) treatment plan
XII.C.7	Identify principles of: (a) body mechanics (b) ergonomics

ABHES

2. Anatomy and Physiology

c. Identify diagnostic and treatment modalities as they relate to each body system

9. Clinical Procedures

d. Assist provider with specialty examination including cardiac, respiratory, OB-GYN, neurological, gastroenterology procedures

e. Perform specialty procedures including but not limited to minor surgery, cardiac, respiratory, OB-GYN, neurological, gastroenterology

j. Make adaptations with patients with special needs

▶ Introduction

Applying cold and heat therapy and assisting patients with ambulation (walking around) are common responsibilities of a medical assistant. These activities are part of the physical therapy field. For a full program of physical therapy, a physician generally refers a patient to a licensed physical therapist. However, a physician may request that you assist with some forms of physical therapy, including

- Applying cold and heat.
- Teaching basic exercises.
- Demonstrating how to use a cane, a walker, and crutches.
- Demonstrating how to use a wheelchair.
- Discussing with the patient specific therapies for use at home.

▶ General Principles of Physical Therapy

LO 54.1

Physical therapy is a medical specialty for the treatment of musculoskeletal, nervous, and cardiopulmonary disorders. A physical therapist uses a variety of treatments, including cold, heat, water, exercise, massage, and traction. Some physical therapy regimens combine two or more treatments. Exercising in a pool, for example, combines the use of water and exercise. In addition, the physical therapist actively promotes patient education and rehabilitation programs.

Physical therapy benefits patients in several ways. It restores and improves muscle function, builds strength, increases joint mobility, relieves pain, and increases circulation. Physical therapy is used to treat various disorders, including arthritis, stroke, lower back pain, muscle spasms, muscle injuries or diseases, pressure sores, skin disorders, and burns.

Assisting Within a Therapeutic Team

Many people who require physical therapy are recovering from traumatic injuries or dealing with chronic illnesses, so they may be receiving therapeutic attention from several specialists. Physicians, nurses, medical assistants, and other specialists who work with patients dealing with chronic illness or recovery from major injuries make up a **therapeutic team.** When you work with such patients, your responsibilities may include

- Coordinating the patient's schedule of sessions with different specialists.
- Making referrals, as directed by the physician.
- Explaining a specialist's treatment approach to the patient.
- Communicating the physician's findings to the specialist.
- Documenting the specialist's treatments and findings for the physician.
- Reinforcing the specialist's instructions for the patient.
- Answering the patient's questions.

To fulfill these responsibilities, you must have a working knowledge of therapy techniques. If, for example, the physician refers a patient to an art therapist, you would set up an art therapy appointment and explain in general terms what the patient can expect. The *Educating the Patient* feature offers basic information about various specialized therapies.

Besides learning the basic information you need to know about physical therapy, you will want to keep up-to-date on emerging techniques. You may want to become proficient in some of these new techniques. By expanding your knowledge and skills, you increase your value as a member of the therapeutic team.

Assisting with Patient Assessment

Before the doctor prescribes physical therapy, she assesses the patient's physical abilities and condition. She inspects and palpates the patient's joints and muscles and tests the patient's

Specialized Therapies and Their Benefits

Healthcare professionals recognize the contribution of specialized therapies to a patient's recovery. Because many people do not know about these specialized therapies, you may be called on to explain them to patients. You can educate patients about potential benefits of art therapy or other specialized therapies. When specialized therapies are ordered, patients will be more at ease if they know what to expect. You can help when necessary by explaining the following types of therapies and their advantages.

- In art therapy, patients learn to express themselves visually through drawing, painting, and sculpture. Art therapy aids both physical and mental healing, provides a recreational outlet, improves mobility and fine motor coordination, provides an outlet for expressing fears or other emotions patients may be unaware of or unable or unwilling to express verbally, helps relieve anxiety, allows patients to focus on something other than their physical condition, and encourages patients to take better care of themselves. To aid in the art therapy process, encourage patients to relax and give this approach time to work. Although the benefits of art therapy may be evident immediately, they are just as likely to be perceived only after the course of therapy is well under way.

- In music therapy, patients listen to and create music to help them relax and alleviate anxiety. This therapy is often used with surgical patients and patients with chronic pain.
- In dance therapy, patients participate in dance to improve balance, flexibility, strength, and quality of life.
- In writing therapy, patients express themselves through a chosen form of writing, such as composing poetry or keeping a journal.
- In crafts therapy, patients express themselves by using a variety of media to create handiworks.
- In pet therapy, patients play with, groom, or walk a pet. Pets provide companionship and the opportunity to nurture.
- In aquatic therapy, patients swim in a therapeutic pool equipped with a ramp and a lift so that it is accessible to all. Many patients who cannot walk on land can move their legs remarkably well in water.
- In horticultural therapy, patients work with plants and flowers to bring beauty into their daily lives and to help improve their balance, strength, memory, and socialization skills.
- In equestrian therapy, patients ride horses to develop strength, coordination, and muscle tone and to improve balance.

---

joint mobility, muscle strength, gait, and posture. You will typically assist with these tests. In some cases, the doctor may direct you to perform them.

Joint Mobility Testing People usually assume their joints are mobile until stiffness or injury limits them. When a patient complains of these difficulties, the doctor may ask you to assist in testing range of motion. **Range of motion (ROM)** is the degree to which a joint is able to move, measured in degrees with a protractor device called a universal **goniometer** (Figure 54-1). The measurement of joint mobility, known as *goniometry*, is a noninvasive test frequently performed in doctors' offices, requiring the patient to move each major joint in various ways. The specific movements evaluated are described in Figure 54-2. Review the chapter *The Muscular System* for more information about body movement. The doctor may ask you to assist with goniometry and, after special training, you may be asked to perform it. When performing goniometry, you measure the joints from the head to the feet, comparing each joint measurement with a standard measurement (in degrees of movement) for that joint.

Muscle Strength Testing The physician tests muscle strength to determine the amount of force the patient is able to exert with a muscle or group of muscles. This test—usually done at the same time as ROM testing—may be performed by the physician with your assistance or, once you

have had special training, the physician may ask you to perform it yourself.

Like the ROM test, the muscle strength test is usually done from head to foot. The patient is asked to resist the pressure that you or the physician applies to each muscle or group of muscles (usually near a joint). Strength is rated on a five-point scale.

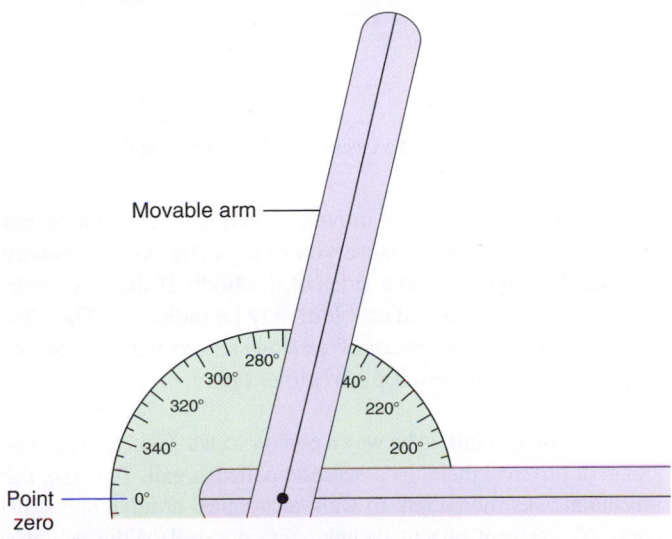

FIGURE 54-1 A universal goniometer is a protractor with a movable pointer that measures degrees of joint movement.

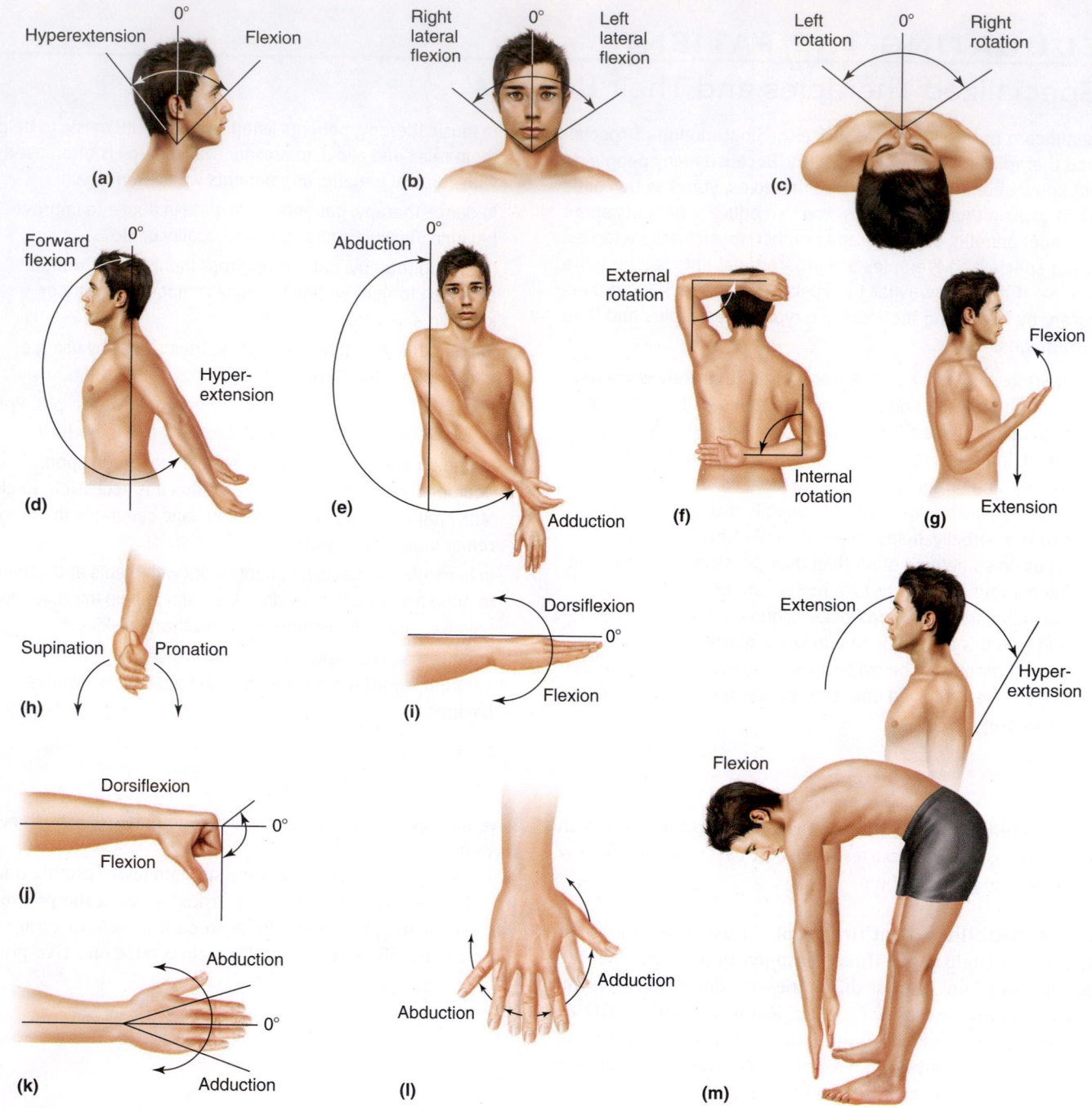

FIGURE 54-2 When you measure joint ROM, begin at the head and work down to the feet.

(continued)

Typically, a patient can move a joint a certain distance and can easily resist the pressure you apply. The patient usually has equal strength on both sides of the body. If there is weakness, however, a medical problem may be indicated. The physician must be made aware of weaknesses so that he can use this information to develop a treatment plan.

Gait Testing Gait is the way a person walks. Generally, a physician or physical therapist assesses a patient's gait. To do so, the physician asks the patient to walk away, turn around, and walk back. Assessment of gait includes an appraisal of the patient's length of stride, balance, coordination, direction of knees (inward or outward), and direction of feet (inward or outward).

Posture Testing Posture is body position and alignment. The doctor assesses posture by looking at the patient's spinal curve from the sides, back, and front. Normally, the thoracic spine has a convex (outward) curve and the lumbar spine has a concave (inward) curve. The doctor also notes the symmetry of alignment of the shoulders, knees, and hips.

To assess alignment and degree of straightness of the spine, the doctor asks the patient to bend at the waist and let the arms dangle freely. To assess knee position, the doctor asks the patient to stand with both feet together to determine whether the knees are at the same height, facing forward, and symmetrical.

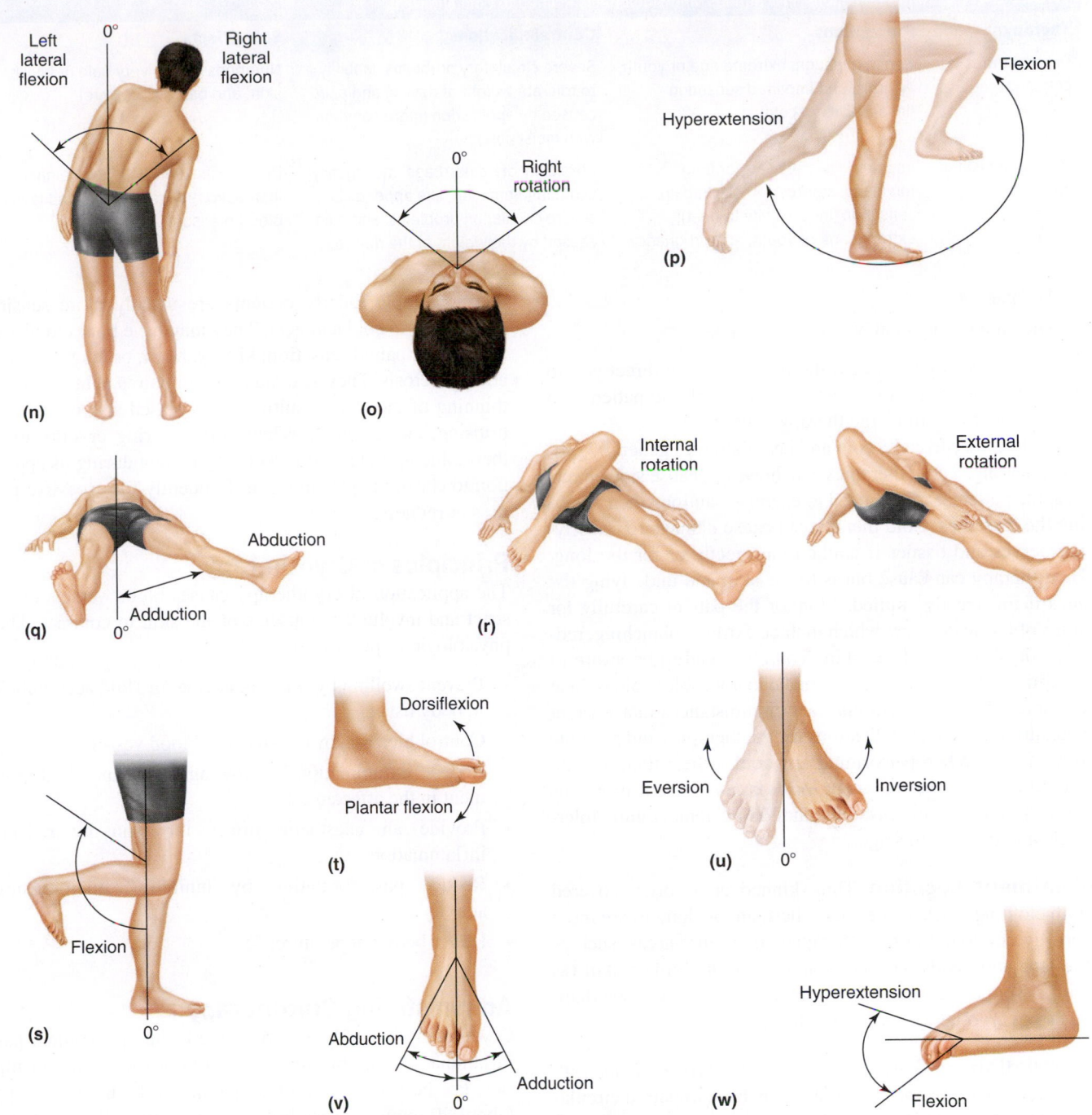

FIGURE 54-2 When you measure joint ROM, begin at the head and work down to the feet.

▶ Cryotherapy and Thermotherapy LO 54.2

Applying cold to a patient's body for therapeutic reasons is called **cryotherapy.** This type of therapy can be administered in a number of ways. Treatments may be dry or wet, and they may be chemical or natural. Examples of dry cold applications are ice bags and ice packs. Wet cold applications include cold compresses and ice massage.

Applying heat to a patient's body for therapeutic reasons is called **thermotherapy.** As with cryotherapy, thermotherapy can be administered in a variety of ways. Examples of devices

used in dry heat treatments are electric heating pads, hot-water bottles, and heat lamps. Moist heat treatments include hot soaks and the use of hot compresses and hot packs.

Factors Affecting the Use of Cryotherapy and Thermotherapy

A healthcare practitioner takes several things into consideration before choosing a cold or heat therapy for a patient:

- The purpose of the therapy
- The location and condition of the affected area

TABLE 54-1 Contraindications, Precautions, and Side Effects Related to Cold and Heat

Therapy	Precautions	Contraindications	Side Effects
Dry and moist cold applications	Poor circulation, extreme age or youth, arthritis, and impaired sensation (insensitivity to cold)	Severe circulatory problems, inability to tolerate weight of device, and pain caused by application (more common with moist cold)	Numbness, pain, very pale or bluish skin, and blood clots (rare)
Dry and moist hot applications	Impaired kidney, heart, or lung functions; atherosclerosis; impaired sensation (insensitivity to heat); extreme age or youth; and pregnancy	Possibility of hemorrhage, malignancy; acute inflammation, like appendicitis; severe circulation problems; and pain caused by the weight of the device	Burns (especially with heat lamps), increased respiratory rate, and lowered blood pressure

- The patient's age
- The patient's general health

After choosing a therapy, the physician may direct you to apply the cold or heat treatment and to teach the patient and family how to continue the therapy at home.

Performed correctly, cold and heat therapies generally promote healing. These therapies can, however, cause side effects in some patients, so you need to exercise caution when applying the therapies. Cold therapy can cause damage to underlying nerves and tissues if applied incorrectly or for too long. Heat therapy can cause burns to the skin and underlying tissues if incorrectly applied. Monitor the patient carefully for signs of tissue damage, which include extreme blanching, redness, or blistering of the skin. You also need to be aware of conditions that contraindicate (make inadvisable) cold or heat therapies. Table 54-1 summarizes circumstances that warrant precautions or contraindications for the therapies and possible side effects. When performing any cold or heat therapy, you should consider the treatment location, any patient problems with circulation or sensation, individual temperature tolerance, and the patient's age.

Treatment Location Thin-skinned areas often covered with clothing (such as the back, chest, and abdomen) are more sensitive to cold and heat therapies than other areas, such as the face and hands. Use caution around any broken skin (as with a wound) because it is susceptible to further tissue damage from cryotherapy or thermotherapy.

Circulation or Sensation Impairment Patients with diabetes or cardiovascular disease may have impaired circulation or sensory perception. These impairments may prevent such patients from sensing that a treatment is too cold or too hot. These patients require close monitoring during cryotherapy or thermotherapy. Carefully observe their skin to determine the treatment's therapeutic effect.

Temperature Tolerance Tolerance of temperature extremes varies greatly from person to person. Some people are unusually sensitive to cold or to heat. Listen carefully to patients for any indication of temperature intolerance during treatment. Cases of intolerance should be reported to the physician, who may decide to change the treatment.

Elderly Patients' Sensitivity to Cold and Heat Age is an important consideration when using cryotherapy and thermotherapy. Elderly patients are usually more sensitive than others to cold and heat. They may have poor circulation; arthritis; impaired sensation; kidney, heart, or lung disease; or atherosclerosis. They also may have impaired skin integrity—thinning of the skin, resulting in increased risk of skin tear, bruising, and burning. When administering cryotherapy or thermotherapy, stay with an elderly patient during its application to check the patient's skin frequently for excessive paleness or redness.

Principles of Cryotherapy

The application of cryotherapy causes blood vessels to constrict and involuntary muscles of the skin to contract. These physiologic responses can:

- Prevent swelling by limiting edema, or fluid accumulation in body tissue.
- Control bleeding by constricting blood vessels.
- Reduce inflammation by slowing blood and fluid movement in the affected area.
- Provide an anesthetic effect for pain by reducing inflammation.
- Reduce pus formation by inhibiting microorganism activity.
- Lower body temperature.

Administering Cryotherapy

Cryotherapy is highly effective in alleviating swelling, pain, inflammation, and bleeding caused by various types of injuries. For best results, cryotherapy should be used frequently (about 20 minutes every hour) for the first 48 hours after an injury. As cold is applied, the skin becomes cool and pale because blood vessels constrict, decreasing the blood supply to the area. The decreased blood supply also reduces tissue metabolism, oxygen use, and waste accumulation.

Dry Cold Applications Dry cold applications include ice bags, ice collars, and chemical ice packs. An ice bag is a rubber or plastic bag with a locking lid. An ice collar is a rubber or plastic kidney-shaped bag curved to fit around the back of the neck. A chemical ice pack is usually a flat plastic bag containing a semifluid chemical (Figure 54-3). Ice packs come in various sizes and types; some are disposable and others can be stored in a freezer and reused. The chemical prevents them from freezing solid, allowing them to be molded to the area to

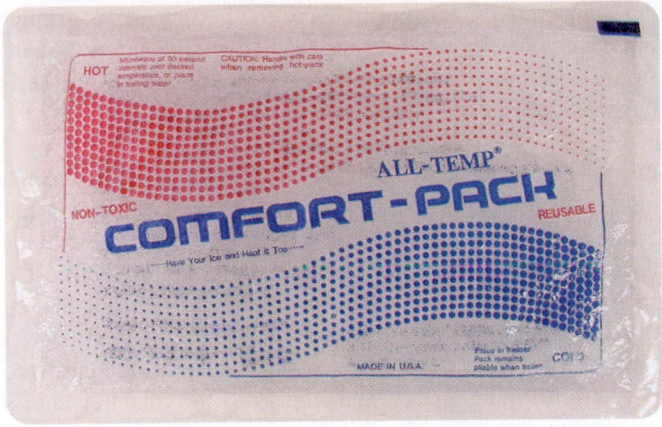

FIGURE 54-3 This chemical pack can be frozen, boiled, or microwaved for cold and heat therapy.
© Total Care Programming, Inc.

be treated. Chemical ice packs may require squeezing or shaking to activate the cooling action. Most packs remain cold for 30 to 60 minutes. Some ice packs come with a soft covering; others must be wrapped in a cloth before they are applied to the skin.

Wet Cold Applications Wet cold applications include cold compresses and ice massage. A cold compress is a cloth or gauze pad moistened with ice water. It may be used to treat the pain associated with a toothache, tooth extraction, eye injury, or headache. The ice used in ice massage may be a cube wrapped in a plastic bag or water frozen in a paper cup. The combination of the cold temperature and the motion of the massage can provide therapeutic relief for the localized pain resulting from a sprain or strain. Although cold causes muscles to contract, the pain-relieving effect can help a patient relax. The procedure for administering cryotherapy is outlined in Procedure 54-1 at the end of this chapter.

Principles of Thermotherapy

The application of thermotherapy causes blood vessels to dilate (expand), which increases the blood supply to the area. Increased blood supply brings about an increased tissue metabolism that carries oxygen and nutrients to the cells of the area being treated. Increased metabolism carries toxins and wastes away from the cells. During thermotherapy, the treated skin becomes warm and develops **erythema** (redness) as the capillaries in the skin's deep layers fill with blood. These physiologic responses can have the following results:

- Relief of pain and congestion
- Reduction of muscle spasms
- Muscle relaxation
- Reduction of inflammation
- Reduction of swelling by increasing the fluid absorption from the tissues

Administering Thermotherapy

Thermotherapy is highly effective in relieving pain, congestion, muscle spasms, and inflammation and promoting muscle

relaxation. However, if heat is applied for too long, it may increase skin secretions that soften the skin and lower its resistance to infection. Heat that is too extreme can burn the skin or increase edema. Always monitor patients receiving thermotherapy, particularly children and elderly patients. The three basic types of thermotherapy are dry heat, moist heat, and diathermy. The general principles for administering the following types of thermotherapy are outlined in Procedure 54-2 at the end of this chapter.

Dry Heat Therapies Several types of dry heat therapy are available. They include the use of chemical hot packs, heating pads, hot-water bottles, heat lamps with infrared or ultraviolet bulbs, and fluidotherapy.

Chemical Hot Pack A chemical hot pack is a disposable, flexible pack of chemicals that becomes hot when you activate it by kneading or slapping it. After activating the pack, cover it with a cloth and place it on the patient's skin in the area being treated. Chemical hot packs are pliable and conform to body contours. For best results, follow the manufacturer's directions.

Heating Pad A heating pad is a flat pad with electrical coils between layers of soft fabric. When turned on, the coils provide localized heat. The physician should specify the heating pad temperature (low, medium, or high) and the length of time the pad should be applied.

Before applying a heating pad, cover it with a pillowcase or towel, check to be sure the cord is not frayed, and plug it into an electrical outlet. Make sure the patient's skin is dry. Then turn on the pad and set the temperature selector switch to the specified temperature. The patient should never lie on top of a heating pad, as burns could result.

Hot-Water Bottle A hot-water bottle is a flat, flexible, plastic or rubber bottle with a stopper. Fill the bottle with hot water, using a thermometer to make sure the water temperature does not exceed 125°F. For children under the age of 2 years and for elderly patients, the temperature should range from 105°F to 115°F. For older children, a safe temperature is 115°F to 125°F. Fill the bottle halfway; then compress it to expel air. The half-filled bottle can conform to the area to be treated. A half-filled bottle is also lighter than a full one, so it is more comfortable for the patient. Cover the bottle with a cloth or pillowcase before you apply it.

After you apply the hot-water bottle, check with the patient to make sure the temperature is not too hot. Check the temperature frequently and replace the hot water as needed. Each time you remove the bottle, check the patient's skin to make sure it is merely warm to the touch.

Heat Lamp A heat lamp uses an infrared or ultraviolet bulb to provide heat. When the lamp is turned on, infrared rays heat and penetrate the skin's surface to a depth of 3 to 5 millimeters. To avoid burning the skin, place an infrared heat lamp 2 to 4 feet from the area being treated. Treatment usually lasts for 20 to 30 minutes or as directed by the physician.

Although ultraviolet rays produce little heat, they can burn the skin and damage the eyes. Ultraviolet rays are used to kill bacteria and promote vitamin D formation. They stimulate epithelial cells and cause blood vessels to overfill, increasing the skin's defenses against bacterial infections. Ultraviolet lamps are used to treat psoriasis, pressure sores, and wound infections.

Before recommending the use of an ultraviolet lamp, the physician assesses the patient's sensitivity and determines the treatment duration, which usually ranges from 30 seconds to a few minutes. The duration is usually increased in 10-second intervals. Because ultraviolet rays can burn the skin, monitor the patient closely. Do not leave the room during treatment. Both you and the patient must wear goggles to protect the eyes.

Fluidotherapy **Fluidotherapy** is a technique for stimulating healing, particularly in the hands and feet. The patient places the affected body part in a container of glass beads or other fine, granular particles that are heated and agitated with hot air. Although the therapy is dry, its effect is similar to that of a therapy using water.

Moist Heat Applications Moist heat is often used to increase circulation and decrease pain to specific body areas, especially muscles and tendons. Moist heat applications include hot soak, hot compress, hot pack, and paraffin bath.

Hot Soak With hot-soak therapy, the patient places the affected body part—usually an arm or a leg—in a container of plain or medicated water that has been heated to no more than 110°F. A hot soak should last about 15 minutes.

Hot Compress A compress is a piece of gauze or cloth suitable for covering a small area. After soaking the compress in hot water, wring it out and apply it to the area to be treated. Keep the compress warm either by placing a hot-water bottle on top of it or by frequently rewarming the compress in hot water.

Hot Pack A hot pack is a large canvas bag filled with a heat-retaining gel that is used on a large body area. Like a hot compress, a hot pack retains heat after being placed in hot water.

Paraffin Bath A paraffin bath is a receptacle of heated wax and mineral oil. It is used to reduce pain, muscle spasms, and stiffness in patients with arthritis and similar disorders. The patient's affected area should first be washed. Then it is dipped repeatedly into the mixture until the area is covered with a thick coat of wax. The wax remains on the area for about 30 minutes and then is peeled off. Particularly useful for joints, especially the hands and feet, the paraffin bath has the added benefit of leaving the skin warm, flexible, and soft. Some erythema may result.

Alternating Hot and Cold Packs A physician may order application of a hot pack followed by a cold pack. This increases circulation to the area by dilating and constricting the blood vessels. Be sure to apply the hot pack first. Applying the cold pack first can numb the skin and keep the patient from recognizing a hot pack is too hot. This can result in serious skin burns.

Diathermy **Diathermy** is a type of heat therapy in which a machine produces high-frequency electromagnetic waves that create deep heat penetration in muscle tissue. The heat helps decrease joint stiffness, dilate blood vessels, relieve muscle spasms, and reduce discomfort from sprains and strains. Three types of diathermy are ultrasound, shortwave, and microwave. Equipment for these therapies is continually being improved. Be sure to familiarize yourself with the manufacturer's instructions regarding the specific equipment in your office.

Ultrasound Ultrasound is the most common type of diathermy, used to treat sprains, strains, and other acute ailments. It projects high-frequency sound waves that are converted to heat in muscle tissue.

Ultrasound diathermy may be administered by rubbing a gel-covered transducer over the skin in circular patterns. It also may be administered to a body part under water. Do not use ultrasound in areas where bones are near the skin's surface, as this could cause bone damage.

Shortwave Shortwave diathermy uses radio waves that travel through the body between two condenser plates and are converted to heat in the tissues. This type of diathermy is used to treat acute, subacute, and chronic inflammation. Treatment typically ranges from 20 to 30 minutes. Do not use shortwave diathermy on a patient who has a pacemaker.

Microwave Microwave diathermy uses microwaves to provide heat deep in body tissues. Contraindications include use on patients with pacemakers, use in combination with wet dressings, and use in high dosages on patients with swollen tissue. Also, never use microwave diathermy near metal implants because the reaction between metal and microwaves could cause burns.

▶ Hydrotherapy LO 54.3

Hydrotherapy is the use of water to treat physical problems. It is typically performed in the physical therapy department of a hospital, in an outpatient clinic, or at home. Common forms of hydrotherapy include the use of whirlpools and contrast baths and underwater exercises.

Whirlpools

Whirlpools are tanks in which water is agitated by jets of air under pressure. Whirlpools vary in size from small (capable of accommodating only one body part) to very large (capable of accommodating a wheelchair or full-body submersion). The agitated water's action in a whirlpool generates a hydromassage, which relaxes muscles and increases circulation. Whirlpools also are used to cleanse and debride (remove foreign matter and dead tissue from) the skin of patients with wounds, ulcers, or burns.

Contrast Baths

Contrast baths are separate baths, one filled with hot water and the other with cold water. The patient alternately moves the treated body part quickly from one bath to the other. This treatment induces relaxation, stimulates improved circulation (which speeds up healing), and results in greater mobility.

Underwater Exercises

Underwater exercises—prescribed for patients with joint injuries, burns, and arthritis—are usually performed in a warm swimming pool. Because the water's buoyancy takes pressure off the joints, these exercises are particularly useful for patients with painful or limited movement. Combined with the movement of the water around the body, the exercises promote relaxation and increased circulation.

▶ Exercise Therapy   LO 54.4

For many patients, exercise is as important as medications or other treatments and offers both preventive and therapeutic benefits. As a patient ages, exercise helps promote flexibility, mobility, muscle tone, and strength. Exercise is a primary treatment for fractures, arthritis, and some respiratory disorders; it can minimize symptoms or help slow disease progression. For patients who have had surgery, stroke, burns, or amputation, regular exercise therapy can help prevent problems caused by inactivity.

A doctor orders exercise therapy for many reasons. Exercise improves or restores general health and is especially therapeutic when a patient is weak from illness. Explain to patients that exercise will help them to:

- Improve muscle tone and strength.
- Regain ROM after an injury.
- Prevent ROM from diminishing in chronic conditions.
- Prevent or correct physical deformities.
- Promote neuromuscular coordination.
- Improve circulation.
- Relieve stress.
- Lower cholesterol levels.
- Aid in the resumption of normal daily activities.

Commonly used for treating sports injuries, exercise therapy for injured athletes is described in the *Educating the Patient* feature. This type of therapy focuses primarily on regaining muscle strength and flexibility in the injured area.

Role of the Medical Assistant

As a medical assistant, you may have several roles in exercise therapy. As an information resource for the patient and family, you must understand various types of exercise programs and the patient's specific treatment plan. You also may serve as a source of support and encouragement when exercise programs are long and difficult. You may, for example, assist with ROM exercises and teach the patient and family how to perform them at home.

When teaching patients about exercises, give them illustrations of the exercises. Include with each illustration written instructions on the number of times to perform the exercise, as prescribed by the doctor.

After demonstrating each exercise, have patients perform it while you watch and give direction. Patients are more likely to perform exercises properly at home if they can perform them correctly in your presence. It is also helpful for patients' caregivers or family members to watch and perform the exercises to become familiar with them.

Types of Exercise

There are various types of exercise in a therapeutic program; however, before a patient begins an exercise program, the doctor must evaluate the patient's heart and lung function and overall physical condition. The doctor adjusts the level of exercise accordingly and may prescribe other forms of physical therapy, such as cryotherapy, thermotherapy, or hydrotherapy. Careful preparation by the doctor and patient before beginning an exercise therapy program helps prevent injuries. Some measures to prevent and treat common exercise therapy problems are outlined in Table 54-2.

Types of exercises in therapeutic programs include active mobility, passive mobility, aided mobility, active resistance, isometric, and ROM.

Active Mobility Exercises Active mobility exercises are exercises the patient performs without assistance to increase muscle strength and function. They often require equipment such as a stationary bicycle or a treadmill.

Passive Mobility Exercises In passive mobility exercises, the physical therapist or a machine moves a patient's body part. The patient does not actively assist in these exercises. Patients who require passive mobility exercises may have neuromuscular disability or weakness. These exercises can help retain patients' ROM and improve their circulation.

TABLE 54-2	Preventing and Treating Common Problems of Exercise Therapy	
Problem	**Prevention Methods**	**Treatment**
Muscle strain	Beginning with gentle warm-up exercises	Rest and application of heat followed by ice
Muscle aches	Keeping track of the number of repetitions and amount of weight (resistance), if used; increasing the number of repetitions or amount of weight slowly	Rest and soaking in hot bath to relieve aches
Impatience with slowness of progress	Discussing expectations with patient; setting realistic goals with patient; stressing necessity of avoiding recurrent injury, which would prolong recovery	Creation of goal sheet, noting small successes as therapy progresses

The risk of injury is associated with most sports, but some sports carry a greater risk of serious injury. Many sports-related injuries affect joints in the neck, shoulders, elbows, wrists, hands, knees, ankles, or feet.

You may be called on to educate injured athletes and to start them on the road to recovery. To do so, you need to understand the mind of the athlete. Why do many athletes get injured in the first place? Here are some reasons:

- The sport they participate in has a high injury rate.
- They return to a sport before their injuries are completely healed.
- They become impatient with a physical therapy regimen.
- They do not work at gradual muscle strengthening.

When does your job begin? After diagnosing the injury, the physician will probably refer the athlete to a sports medicine center or other physical therapy setting, where an individualized program will be set up. As a medical assistant, you will often be responsible for counseling an athlete about the physical therapy program she will be entering. Here are some basic rules you can communicate:

- Follow the physical therapy regimen set up by the physician or physical therapist—even if it is tedious or time-consuming.
- Use only the equipment specified by the therapist: free weights, weight-training equipment, stationary bike, other aerobic equipment, or swimming pool. The physical therapist recommends the designated equipment based

on the type of injury. Using other equipment could cause further injury or interfere with healing.

- Do not rush the therapy in an attempt to recover more quickly.
- Work slowly to strengthen muscles and improve flexibility.
- Continue exercises at home as instructed.
- Be patient.

Explain to the athlete how the physical therapy program will be presented. Knowing what to expect from the physical therapist can improve the athlete's compliance. Here are some explanations you might offer:

- The therapist will demonstrate exercises and then watch you perform them.
- The therapist may increase the number of repetitions or the amount of resistance (weight) but probably not both at the same time.
- The therapist will provide handouts illustrating the exercises, along with instructions on how to perform them.
- The therapist may provide an activity log to help you chart your progress.

An athlete who is impatient with a physical therapy regimen and returns to a sport before an injury has completely healed has an increased risk of repeated injury. Impress on the athlete the importance of the physical therapy process. Emphasize the need for gradual strengthening and healing over a period of time. To help the athlete in the long run, focus on recovery from injury and on the need to prevent recurrent injury.

Aided Mobility Exercises Aided mobility exercises are self-directed exercises. The patient performs them with the aid of a device such as an exercise machine or a therapy pool. Aided mobility exercises help retain or increase patients' ROM.

Active Resistance Exercises In active resistance exercises, the patient works against resistance (counter-pressure) to increase muscle strength. Resistance is provided manually by the therapist or mechanically by an exercise machine.

Isometric Exercises During isometric exercises, the patient relaxes and then contracts the muscles of a body part while in a fixed position. Isometric exercises can maintain the patient's muscle strength when a joint is temporarily or permanently immobilized.

ROM Exercises ROM exercises move each joint through its full range of motion. These exercises should be done slowly and gently. Doing them too quickly or too soon after an injury can cause pain, fracture, or bleeding into the joint. For this reason, a physical therapist assesses the patient and determines a recommended regimen of ROM exercises. You

may be asked to educate the patient and caregiver or family about the regimen.

ROM exercises are typically prescribed after a joint injury. The physical therapist may recommend that the joint be moved in its full range of motion three times, twice a day. ROM exercises are also recommended for elderly people, to improve circulation and muscle function. The therapist will prescribe one of three types of ROM exercises for patients:

1. Active range-of-motion exercises: performed by the patient without assistance
2. Assisted range-of-motion exercises: performed by the patient with the help of another person or a machine
3. Passive range-of-motion exercises: performed by another person or a machine

ROM exercises do not build muscle strength but do improve flexibility and mobility. Typical ROM exercises are illustrated in Figure 54-4.

Electrical Stimulation

Electrical stimulation helps prevent atrophy in muscles that cannot move voluntarily by causing the muscles to contract

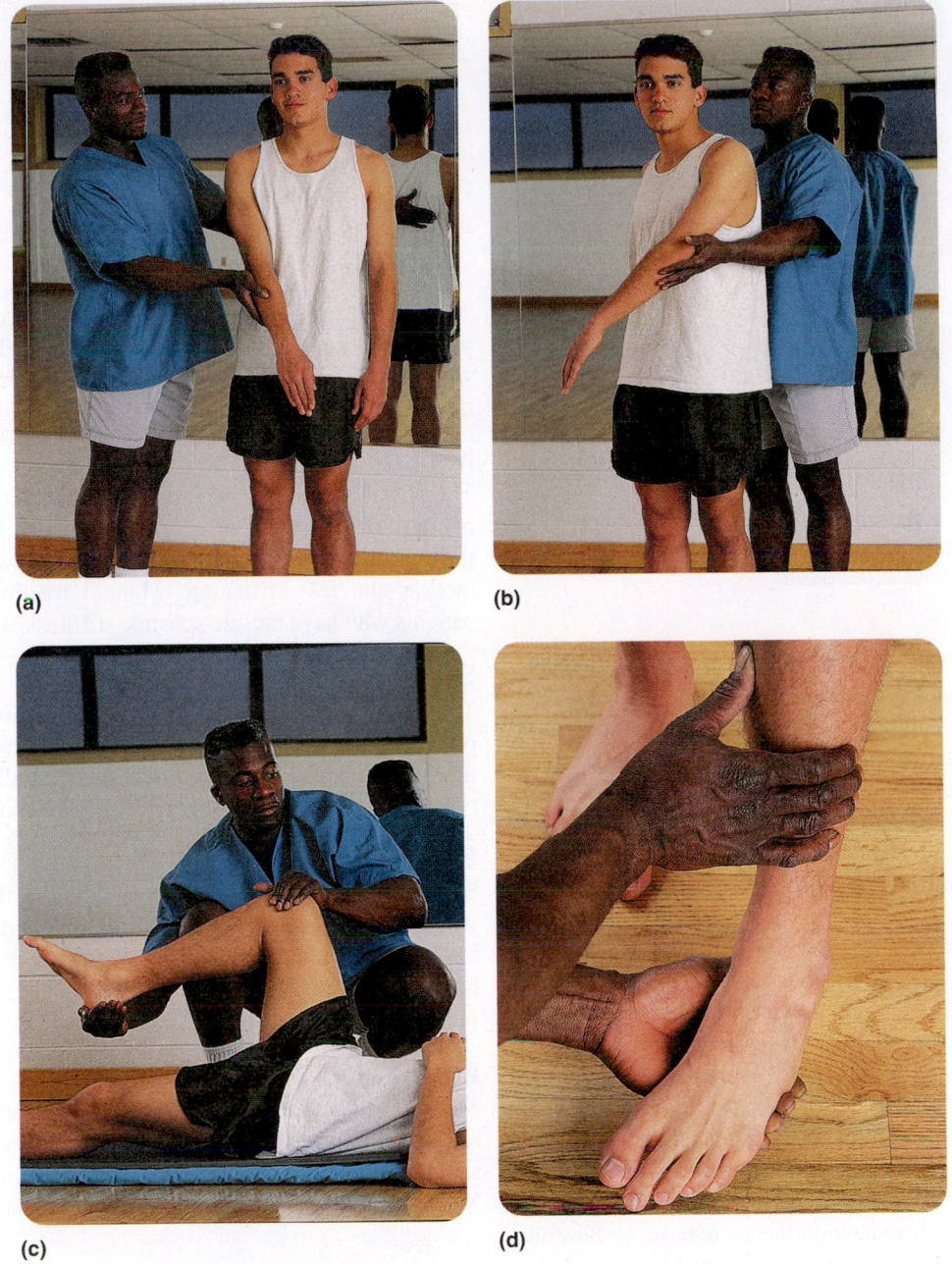

FIGURE 54-4   A medical assistant helps a patient perform typical ROM exercises: (a) shoulder abduction, (b) back rotation, (c) hip flexion, and (d) toe abduction.
© David Kelly Crow

involuntarily (on impulse) and relax. Electrical stimulators deliver controlled amounts of low-voltage electric current to motor and sensory nerves to stimulate muscles. Frequent and regular electrical stimulation also aids in healing injured joints and in revitalizing muscles.

Electrical stimulation can help retrain a patient to use injured muscles by creating a perceivable connection between the stimulus (muscle movement) and the area of the brain that controls those muscles. If a limb does not function because of injury or disease, this therapy can give the patient hope that injured muscles are not dead. Hope often encourages a patient to work harder and to cooperate in the physical therapy regimen, which can be long and arduous.

Wearable electrical stimulation units are being developed for people with spinal cord injuries to help them retrain affected muscles.

▶ Massage   LO 54.5

The practice of massage uses pressure, kneading, stroking, vibration, and tapping to positively affect patients' health and well-being. Massage helps the patient relax and counteracts the effects of stress. During massage, the heart rate and blood pressure are lowered and blood circulation and lymph flow are increased. Massage helps reduce pain caused by tight muscles and helps relax muscle spasms.

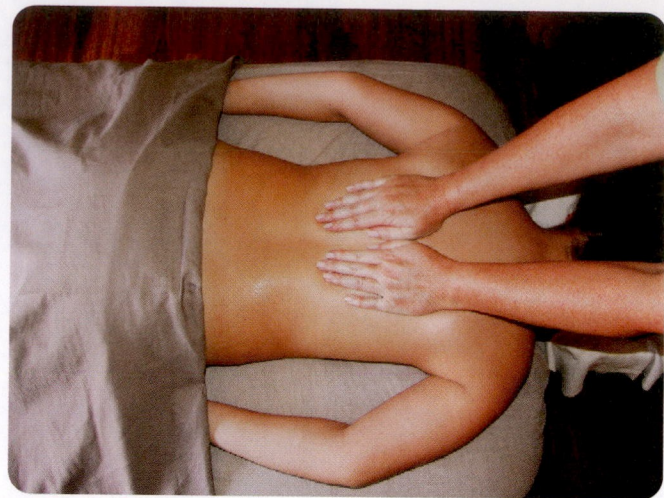

FIGURE 54-5 Swedish massage uses kneading, pressure, stroking, and human touch to alleviate pain and promote healing through relaxation.
© McGraw-Hill Education/Shaana Pritchard, photographer

Massage benefits the mind as well as the body: It helps improve concentration, promotes restful sleep, and helps the mind relax. Many patients find they handle daily stresses better when they have regular massage. People who get massages on a regular basis find they become ill less often and less severely and they feel less stressed and tense. Some patients notice their muscles beginning to tighten and are aware that if they get a massage, it will decrease muscle tension before it becomes severe.

Swedish Massage

Swedish massage is one of the best known and most frequently taught massage techniques. It stimulates circulation and lymph flow with five basic strokes that manipulate the body's soft tissues. The strokes include pétrissage (kneading), effleurage (stroking), tapotement (percussion), vibration, and friction. Oils and/or lotions are used to reduce friction on the patient's skin. One type of Swedish massage is done on warm muscles immediately after exercise. Another type is a stress-reduction massage that is done with the same basic strokes on patients who have not been exercising (Figure 54-5).

Neuromuscular Massage

Neuromuscular massage is applied to specific muscles and helps release tension and knots, relieve pain and release pressure on nerves, and increase blood flow. Trigger point therapy is one type of neuromuscular massage in which strong finger pressure is applied to trigger points in the muscles.

▶ Traction   LO 54.6

Traction is the pulling of the bones and joints to create a mechanical force that is used to treat fractured bones and dislocated, arthritic, or other diseased joints. It is often performed by a physical therapist using special equipment. The therapist may set up traction in the patient's home and visit regularly to ensure that the equipment is used and maintained properly.

Traction is used to:

- Create and maintain proper bone alignment after a fracture or other injury.
- Reduce or prevent joint stiffening and abnormal muscle shortening.
- Correct deformities.
- Relieve compression of vertebral joints.
- Reduce or relieve muscle spasms.

Although you will not be setting up or performing traction, you should know about its types and uses. This information will prepare you to answer basic questions from patients and family members.

Manual Traction

The physical therapist performs manual traction by using his hands to pull a patient's limb or head gently. Pulling stretches the muscles and separates the joints, allowing for greater motion and less stiffening. Manual traction is used with patients who have muscle spasms, stiffness, and arthritis.

Static Traction

To perform static traction, or weight traction, the therapist places a patient's limb, pelvis, or chin in a harness. The harness is then attached to weights through a pulley system. This type of traction is commonly used to relieve muscle spasms.

Skeletal Traction

Skeletal traction is performed in inpatient facilities on patients whose injuries require long traction time and heavy weights. During surgery, a surgeon inserts pins, wires, or tongs into bones. After surgery, the pins, wires, or tongs are attached to pulleys and weights to provide continuous traction.

Mechanical Traction

Mechanical traction uses a device that intermittently pulls and relaxes a prescribed body part, such as the neck. The therapist sets the time intervals between contractions and relaxations. Mechanical traction is used to promote relaxation.

▶ Mobility Aids   LO 54.7

Mobility aids (also called *mobility assistive devices*) are designed to improve patients' ability to ambulate, or move from one place to another. These include canes, walkers, crutches, and wheelchairs.

The appropriate aid depends on the patient's disability, muscle coordination, strength, and age. The patient may need a device temporarily—perhaps crutches after a sprain—or permanently—such as a wheelchair in the case of permanent paralysis.

Canes

Canes provide support and help patients maintain balance. They come in several styles, including standard, tripod, and quad-base (Figure 54-6), which are all lightweight, are made of wood or aluminum, and have a rubber tip or tips at the bottom. Canes are especially useful for patients with weaknesses

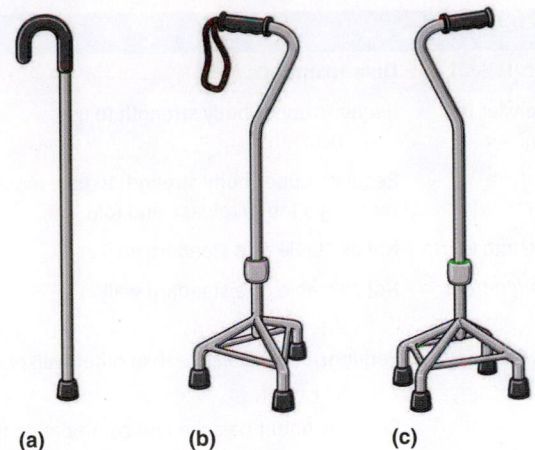

FIGURE 54-6 Shown here are three styles of canes: (a) standard, (b) tripod, and (c) quad-base.

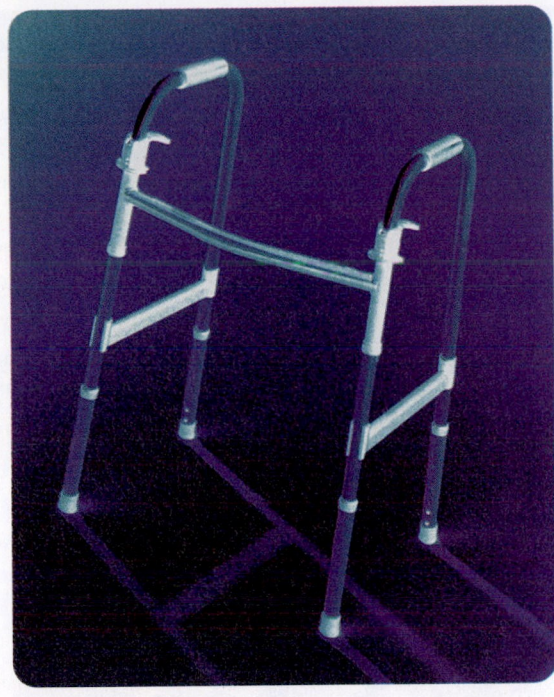

FIGURE 54-7 A standard walker.
© SS36 PhotoDisc/Getty Images RF

on one side of the body (possibly due to a stroke), joint disability, or neuromuscular defects.

A standard cane is best for a patient who needs only a small amount of support. Its curved handle is convenient, allowing the patient to hang it from a pocket or a doorknob. When the patient uses a standard cane, however, the curved handle concentrates most of the patient's weight in one small area of the hand. To avoid stressing the hand in this way, some standard canes have a T-shaped handle, which distributes pressure on the hand more evenly. Tripod canes have three legs, and quad-base canes have four. The multiple legs create a wide base of support, making them more stable than a standard cane. Tripod and quad-base canes can stand alone, freeing up the patient's hands when she sits down. These canes are bulkier and more difficult to pick up and put down than a standard cane, however. Both styles have T-shaped handles.

After determining the most suitable cane for the patient, the physical therapist adjusts the cane's height. When the cane is the correct height, the patient's elbow is flexed at 20 to 25 degrees and the patient stands tall while using the cane (instead of leaning on it for support). The therapist makes sure the handle is the right size for the patient's hand and instructs the patient on how to use the cane. If directed, you may do the teaching or reinforce it, as discussed in Procedure 54-3 at the end of this chapter.

Walkers

A walker is a lightweight, easy-to-use aluminum frame that is open on one side and has four widely placed, adjustable, rubber-tipped legs that can be adjusted to various heights (Figure 54-7). Some models are designed to fold up for storage. To use a walker, the patient stands within the frame and leans on the upper bar, which has a handgrip on each side.

Typically, older patients who are too weak to walk unassisted or who have balance problems use a walker. The walker is designed to give these patients a sense of stability as they ambulate. In tight spaces or in areas with throw rugs, however, a walker may be difficult to manage. A patient who is too weak to pick up the walker may use a walker on wheels. Wheeled walkers have brakes for safety. Patients should never

slide a walker that does not have wheels because the movement could easily result in a fall.

A physical therapist selects a walker that suits the patient's abilities and height. A walker should reach the patient's hipbone. See Table 54-3 for more information about different types of walkers. Although the physical therapist usually trains the patient in the use of a walker, you may be asked to do this, or you may need to reinforce the information presented in Procedure 54-4 at the end of this chapter.

Crutches

Crutches allow a patient to walk without putting weight on the feet or legs by transferring that weight to the arms. Crutches are made of aluminum or wood. Aluminum crutches are lighter and usually more expensive than those made of wood. Pediatric crutches are available for children. The two basic types of crutches are axillary and Lofstrand®. Procedure 54-5, at the end of this chapter, provides the steps for teaching patients how to use crutches.

Axillary crutches reach from the ground to the armpit. Each crutch has a rubber tip on the bottom to prevent slipping. This type of crutch is designed for short-term use by patients with injuries such as a sprained ankle.

Lofstrand®, or Canadian, crutches reach from the ground to the forearm, and each one has a rubber tip on the bottom to prevent slipping. For additional support, this type has a handgrip extension attached at a 90-degree angle and a metal cuff that fits securely around the patient's forearm. Lofstrand® crutches are geared for long-term use by patients with disorders such as paraplegia (Figure 54-8).

Measuring the Patient for Crutches To prevent back pain and nerve injury to the armpits and palms, crutches must

TABLE 54-3   Types of Walkers

Walker	Features	Advantages	Disadvantages
Standard	No wheels, adjustable legs	Very stable on flat surfaces; easier to use than crutches	Requires upper-body strength to use
Standard folding	No wheels, sides fold in	Easy to transport and store	Requires upper-body strength to use, requires pressing a tab to release and fold
Rolling	Front wheels	Requires less upper-body strength to use	Not as stable as a standard walker
Rolling with brakes	Front wheels and brakes	Disengages wheels when weight from upper body is applied	Not as stable as a standard walker
Three-wheel rolling with brakes	Bicycle-style hand brakes	Better maneuverability; folds for transport and storage	Requires better balance than other walkers
Reciprocal	Each side of walker moves alternately	Allows for more natural gait	Requires better balance and coordination than other walkers; catches on some floor surfaces

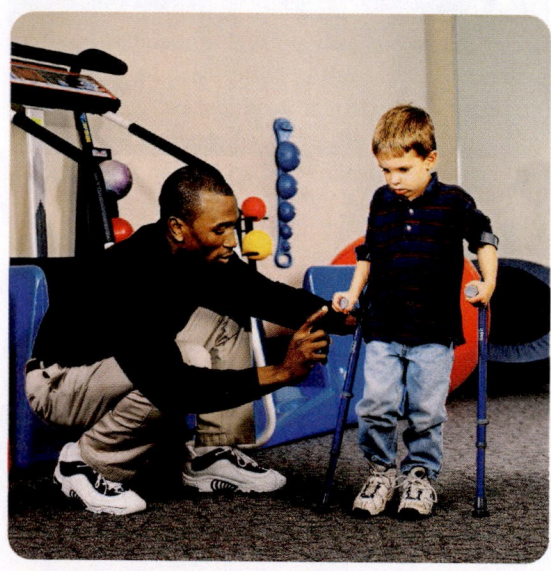

FIGURE 54-8   A child using Lofstrand® crutches.
© Royalty-Free/CORBIS

be measured to fit each patient. Axillary crutches that are too long can put pressure on nerves in the armpit, causing a condition called crutch palsy (muscle weakness in the forearm, wrist, and hand). They also can force the patient's shoulders forward, causing strain on the back and making ambulation difficult. Crutches that are too short force the patient to bend forward during ambulation, causing back pain or imbalance, which can lead to falls.

Before a patient who uses crutches leaves the office, make sure the crutches fit properly and that the patient is comfortable walking with them. To confirm a correct fit, check for the following conditions (see Figure 54-9):

- The patient is wearing the type of shoes he will wear when walking.
- The patient is standing erect with feet slightly apart.
- The crutch tips are positioned 4 to 6 inches in front of the patient's feet and 4 to 6 inches to the side of each foot.
- The axillary supports allow two to three finger-widths between supports and armpits. (Use wing nuts and bolts to adjust crutches.)

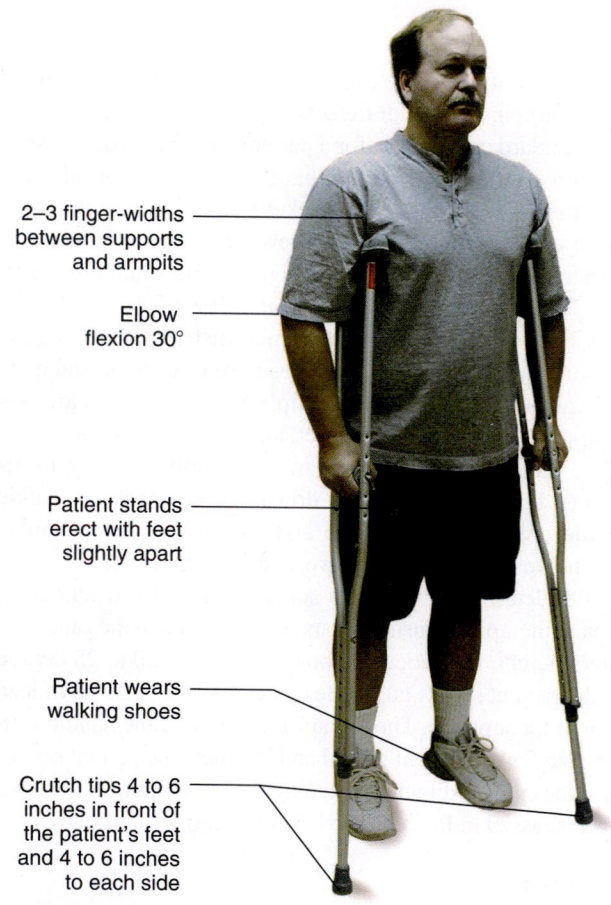

2–3 finger-widths between supports and armpits

Elbow flexion 30°

Patient stands erect with feet slightly apart

Patient wears walking shoes

Crutch tips 4 to 6 inches in front of the patient's feet and 4 to 6 inches to each side

FIGURE 54-9   Use these guidelines when measuring a patient for crutches.
© Total Care Programming, Inc.

- The handgrips are positioned to create 30-degree flexion at the elbows. (Use wing nuts and bolts to adjust; use a goniometer to check flexion.)

Crutch Gaits   To teach a patient how to stand and walk with crutches, you must learn the crutch gaits, or walks. First, show the patient the standing, or tripod, position. To do this, have the patient stand erect and look straight ahead. The patient should place the crutch tips 4 to 6 inches in front of

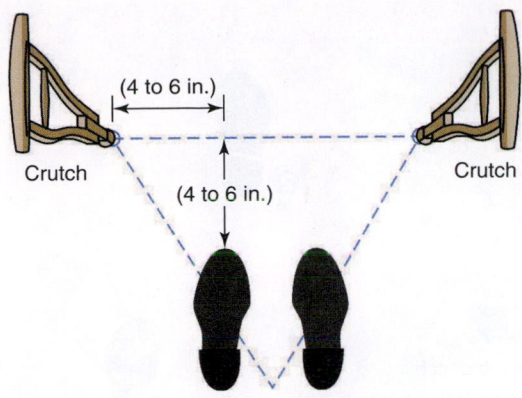

FIGURE 54-10 This is the correct beginning position for the patient's feet and crutches when you are teaching a patient to walk with crutches.

her feet and 4 to 6 inches away from the side of each foot. See Figure 54-10.

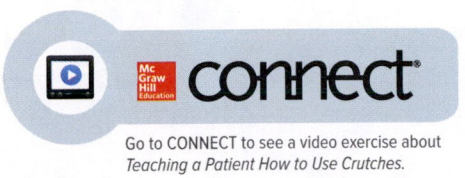

Go to CONNECT to see a video exercise about *Teaching a Patient How to Use Crutches.*

To determine the proper gait for a patient, you will make a preteaching assessment of the patient's muscle coordination and physical condition. In general, instruct a patient to use a slow gait in crowded areas or when feeling tired. The patient can use a faster gait in open places or when feeling more energetic. Using various gaits and speeds enables the patient to exercise different muscle groups and improve overall conditioning.

Four-Point Gait The four-point gait is a slow gait used only when a patient can bear weight on both legs. Because this gait has three points of contact with the ground at all times, it is stable and safe. It is especially useful for patients with leg muscle weakness, spasticity, or poor balance or coordination. To teach this gait, have the patient start in the tripod position. Then outline the following steps, as illustrated in Figure 54-11a:

1. Move the right crutch forward.
2. Move the left foot forward to the level of the left crutch.
3. Move the left crutch forward.
4. Move the right foot forward to level of the right crutch.

Three-Point Gait The three-point gait is used when a patient cannot bear weight on one leg but can bear full weight on the unaffected leg. This gait allows the patient's weight to be carried alternately by the crutches and by the unaffected leg. It is appropriate for amputees, patients with tissue or musculoskeletal trauma (such as a fractured or sprained leg), and those recovering from leg surgery. The patient must have good muscle coordination and arm strength, however. To teach this gait, have the patient start in the tripod position. Then give the patient the following instructions, as illustrated in Figure 54-11b:

1. Move both crutches and the affected leg forward.
2. Move the unaffected leg forward while weight is balanced on both crutches.

Two-Point Gait The two-point gait is faster than the four-point gait and is used by patients who can bear some weight on both feet and have good muscle coordination and balance. To teach this gait, have the patient start in the tripod position. Then outline the following steps, as illustrated in Figure 54-11c:

1. Move the left crutch and the right foot forward at the same time.
2. Move the right crutch and the left foot forward at the same time.

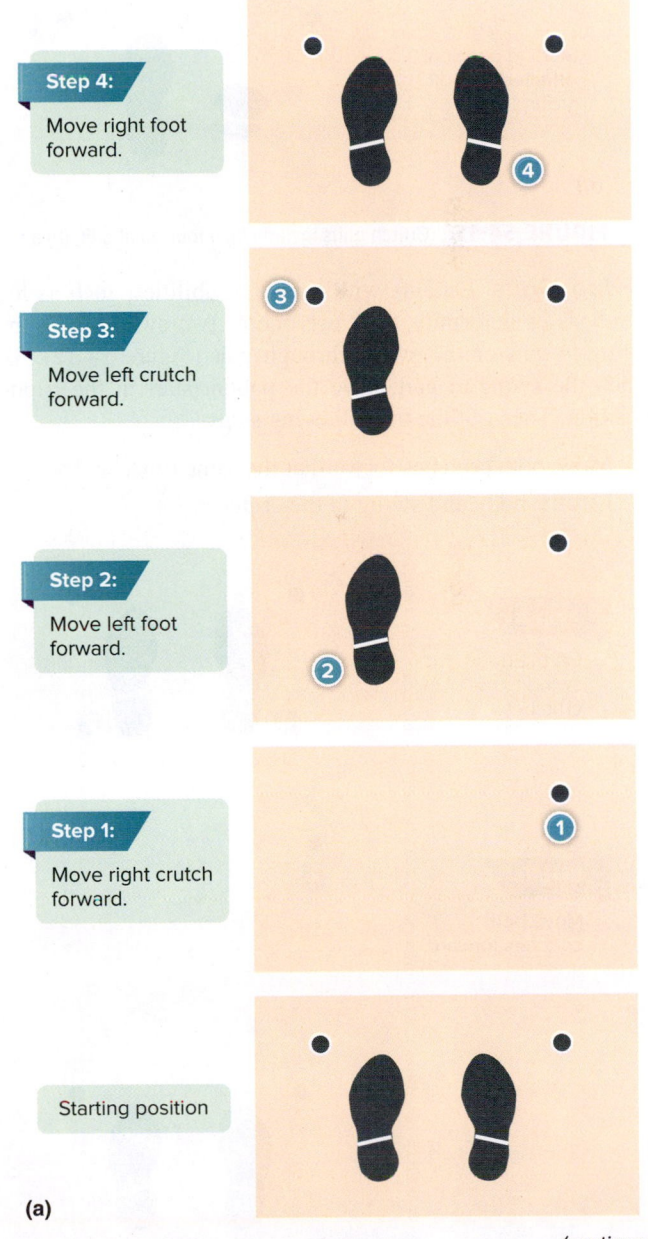

Step 4: Move right foot forward.

Step 3: Move left crutch forward.

Step 2: Move left foot forward.

Step 1: Move right crutch forward.

Starting position

(a)

(continued)

FIGURE 54-11 Crutch gaits include (a) a four-point gait, (b) a three-point gait, and (c) a two-point gait.

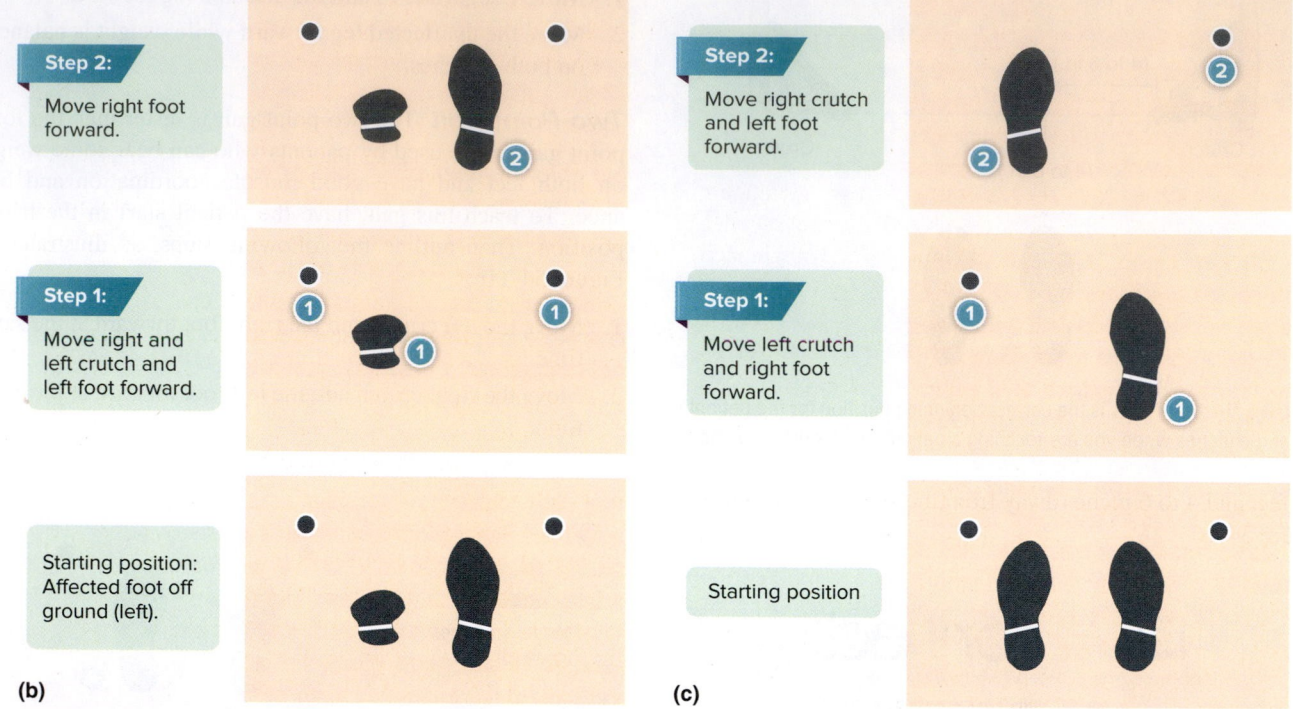

Step 2:
Move right foot forward.

Step 1:
Move right and left crutch and left foot forward.

Starting position: Affected foot off ground (left).

(b)

Step 2:
Move right crutch and left foot forward.

Step 1:
Move left crutch and right foot forward.

Starting position

(c)

FIGURE 54-11 Crutch gaits include (a) a four-point gait, (b) a three-point gait, and (c) a two-point gait.

Swing Gaits Patients with severe disabilities, such as leg paralysis or deformity, may use one of two swing gaits: the swing-to gait or the swing-through gait (Figure 54-12). To teach the swing-to gait, have the patient start in the tripod position. Then outline the following steps:

1. Move both crutches forward at the same time.
2. Lift the body and swing to the crutches.

3. End with the tripod position again.

To teach the swing-through gait, have the patient start in the tripod position. Then review the following steps:

1. Move both crutches forward.
2. Move the body and swing past the crutches.

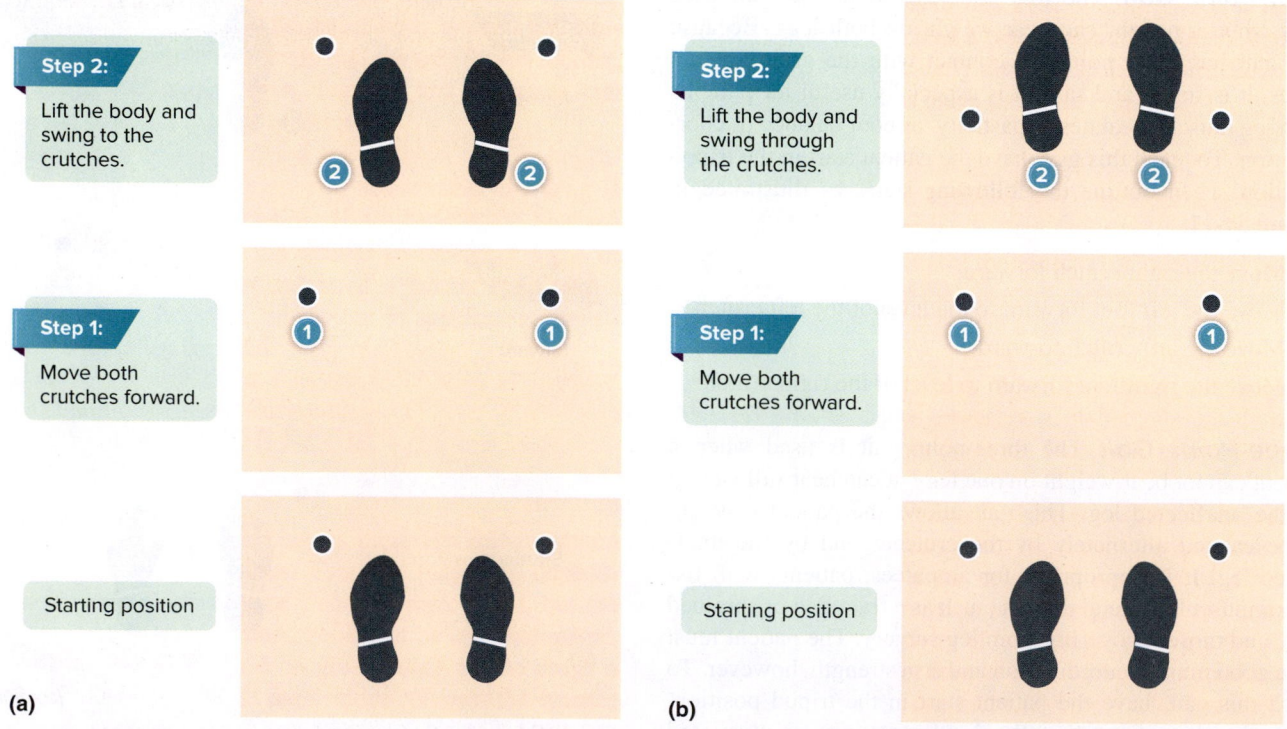

Step 2:
Lift the body and swing to the crutches.

Step 1:
Move both crutches forward.

Starting position

(a)

Step 2:
Lift the body and swing through the crutches.

Step 1:
Move both crutches forward.

Starting position

(b)

FIGURE 54-12 Patients with severe disabilities may walk with crutches using (a) the swing-to gait or (b) the swing-through gait.

Wheelchairs

Wheelchairs range from small, folding models to large, motorized ones. The physical therapist will select an appropriate wheelchair depending on the patient's disability and the length of time the wheelchair will be needed.

When patients come to the medical office in a wheelchair, the doctor may not be able to examine them adequately if they remain in the wheelchair. If this is the case, you will be responsible for transferring the patients from the wheelchair to the examining table and back to the wheelchair after the exam. To ensure their safety and yours, see the *Assisting with a General Physical Examination* chapter for more information about transferring patients from a wheelchair. Here are some reminders on preventing injury:

- Ask for help if the patient is weak, heavy, or unstable.
- Explain to the patient the steps of transfer you will use.
- Before starting the transfer, make sure the wheelchair is in the locked position and the patient is sitting at the front of the wheelchair seat.
- When you lift, use the large muscles in your thighs, which are stronger than your back muscles.
- When lifting, bend from the knees and keep your back straight.
- Count to 3 and enlist the patient's help on the count of 3.

▶ Referral to a Physical Therapist LO 54.8

If the doctor refers the patient to a physical therapist or other specialist, you may be asked to contact the specialist directly or to give the patient a written order and information about contacting the specialist. Keep a file with information about the therapists your office uses. In the file, note the forms and information each therapist requires. If you speak to the therapist, be sure to inform the doctor and to document the referral in the patient's chart. The therapist may be an independent practitioner or may be employed by a hospital, clinic, or home healthcare agency.

In addition to physical therapy, some patients may decide to try alternative therapies, such as acupuncture, chiropractic, or biofeedback training. These therapies are acknowledged by many healthcare professionals and often provide relief for people with chronic pain or other debilitating conditions.

PROCEDURE 54-1 Administering Cryotherapy   WORK // DOC

Procedure Goal: To reduce pain and swelling by safely and effectively administering cryotherapy

OSHA Guidelines:

Materials:
Patient chart/progress note, gloves, cold application materials required as ordered: ice bag, ice collar, chemical cold pack, washcloth or gauze squares, or ice

Method:

1. Double-check the physician's order. Be sure you know where to apply therapy and how long it should remain in place.
2. Identify the patient and explain the procedure and its purpose. Ask if the patient has any questions.
3. Have the patient undress and put on a gown, if required; provide privacy or assistance as needed.
4. Wash your hands and don gloves.
5. Position the patient comfortably and drape appropriately.
   RATIONALE: *The patient should be able to relax during the therapy.*
6. Prepare the therapy as ordered.
   - Ice bag or collar
     a. Prior to use, check the ice bag or collar for leaks.

   b. Fill the ice bag or collar two-thirds full with ice chips or small ice cubes. Compress the container to expel any air and then close it.
   RATIONALE: *Ice will not conform to the patient if there is air in the bag.*
   c. Dry the bag or collar completely and cover it with a towel. This will absorb moisture and provide comfort.
   - Chemical ice pack
     a. Check the pack for leaks.
   RATIONALE: *To avoid the chemicals coming in contact with the patient.*
     b. Shake or squeeze the pack to activate the chemicals, or use a cold chemical pack taken from a refrigerator or freezer.
   RATIONALE: *Pack will not be cold if it is not activated.*
     c. Cover the pack with a towel.
   RATIONALE: *To keep the patient comfortable and avoid cold burn.*
   - Cold compress
     a. Place the washcloth or gauze squares under a stream of running water.
     b. Wring them out.
     c. Rewet at frequent intervals.
7. Place the device on the patient's affected body part. If you are using a compress, place an ice bag on it, if desired, to keep it colder longer.

8. Ask the patient how the device feels.
   RATIONALE: *To prevent cold burn of the skin.*

9. Explain that the cold is of great benefit, although it may be somewhat uncomfortable.

10. Leave the device in place for the length of time ordered by the physician. Periodically check the skin for color, feeling, and pain. If the area becomes excessively pale or blue, numb, or painful, remove the device and have the physician examine the area. For cold application using ice, limit application time to 20 minutes.
    RATIONALE: *To reduce the possibility of cold burn.*

11. Remove the application and observe the area for reduced swelling, redness, and pain. If the patient has a dressing, replace it at this time.

12. Help the patient dress, if needed.

13. Remove equipment and supplies, properly discarding used disposable materials; sanitize, disinfect, and/or sterilize reusable equipment and materials as needed.

14. Remove the gloves and wash your hands.

15. Document the treatment and your observation in the patient's chart. If you teach the patient or the patient's family how to use the device, document your instructions.

PROCEDURE 54-2 Administering Thermotherapy

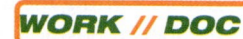

Procedure Goal: To administer thermotherapy safely and effectively

OSHA Guidelines:

 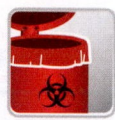 

Materials: Patient chart/progress note, gloves, towels, blanket, heat application materials required for order: chemical hot pack, heating pad, hot-water bottle, heat lamp, container and medication for hot soak, and container and gauze for hot compress

Method

1. Double-check the physician's order. Be sure you know where to apply therapy, the proper temperature for the application, and how long it should remain in place.

2. Identify the patient and explain the procedure and its purpose. Ask if the patient has any questions.

3. Have the patient undress and put on a gown, if required; provide privacy or assistance as needed.

4. Wash your hands and don gloves.

5. Position the patient comfortably and drape appropriately.
   RATIONALE: *The patient should be able to relax during the therapy.*

6. If the patient has a dressing, check the dressing for blood and change as necessary. Alert the physician and ask if treatment should continue.
   RATIONALE: *If the wound is actively bleeding, heat application could cause increased bleeding.*

7. Check the temperature by touch and look for the presence of adverse skin conditions (excessive redness, blistering, or irritation) on all applications before and during the treatment.
   RATIONALE: *To avoid patient burn injuries.*

8. As necessary, reheat devices or solutions to provide therapeutic temperatures and then reapply them.

9. Prepare the therapy as ordered.
   - Chemical hot pack
     a. Check the pack for leaks.
     RATIONALE: *To avoid the chemicals coming in contact with the patient.*
     b. Activate the pack. (Check manufacturer's directions.)
     RATIONALE: *The pack will not get hot if it is not activated.*
     c. Cover the pack with a towel.
   - Heating pad
     a. Turn the heating pad on, selecting the appropriate temperature setting.
     b. Cover the pad with a towel or pillowcase.
     c. Make sure the patient's skin is dry and do not allow the patient to lie on top of the heating pad.
     RATIONALE: *To avoid burns.*
   - Hot-water bottle
     a. Fill the bottle one-half full with hot water of the correct temperature—usually 110°F to 115°F. Use a thermometer. The physician can provide information on the ideal water temperature that should be used, which will depend on the area being treated.
     b. Expel the air and close the bottle.
     RATIONALE: *The bottle should conform to the body part.*
     c. Cover the bottle with a towel or pillowcase.
     RATIONALE: *To avoid burns.*
   - Heat lamp
     a. Place the lamp 2 to 4 feet away from the treatment area. (Check manufacturer's directions.)
     b. Follow the treatment time as ordered.

- Hot soak
  a. Select a container of the appropriate size for the area to be treated.
  b. Fill the container with hot water that is no more than 110°F. Use a thermometer. Add medication to the container if ordered.
- Hot compress
  a. Soak a washcloth or gauze in hot water. Wring it out.
  b. Frequently rewarm the compress to maintain the temperature.

10. Place the device on the patient's affected body part, or place the affected body part in the container. If you are using a compress, place a hot-water bottle on top, if desired, to keep it warm longer.

11. Ask the patient how the device feels. During any heat therapy, remember, dilated blood vessels cause heat loss from the skin and this heat loss may make the patient feel chilled. Be prepared to cover the patient with sheets or blankets.

12. Leave the device in place for the length of time ordered by the physician. Periodically check the skin for redness, blistering, or irritation. If the area becomes excessively red or develops blisters, remove the patient from the heat source and have the physician examine the area.

13. Remove the application and observe the area for inflammation and swelling. Replace the patient's dressing if necessary.

14. Help the patient dress, if needed.

15. Remove equipment and supplies, properly discarding used disposable materials, and sanitize, disinfect, and/or sterilize reusable equipment and materials as needed.

16. Remove the gloves and wash your hands.

17. Document the treatment and your observation in the patient's chart. If you teach the patient or the patient's family how to use the device, document your instructions.

PROCEDURE 54-3 Teaching a Patient How to Use a Cane

Procedure Goal: To teach a patient how to use a cane safely

OSHA Guidelines: This procedure does not involve exposure to blood, body fluids, or tissues.

Materials: A cane suited to the patient's needs

Method:

Standing from a Sitting Position

1. Instruct the patient to slide his buttocks to the edge of the chair.

2. Tell the patient to place his right foot slightly behind and inside the right front leg of the chair and his left foot slightly behind and inside the left front leg of the chair. (This provides him with a wide, stable stance.)

3. Instruct the patient to lean forward and use the armrests or seat of the chair to push upward. Caution the patient not to lean on the cane.

4. Have the patient position the cane for support on the uninjured or strong side of his body, as indicated.

Walking

5. Teach the patient to hold the cane on the uninjured or strong side of her body with the tip(s) of the cane 4 to 6 inches from the side and in front of her strong foot. Remind the patient to make sure the tip is flat on the ground.
   RATIONALE: *To reduce the risk of the patient falling.*

6. Have the patient move the cane forward approximately 8 inches and then move her affected foot forward, parallel to the cane.

7. Next, have the patient move her strong leg forward past the cane and her weak leg.

8. Observe as the patient repeats this process.

Ascending Stairs

9. Instruct the patient to always start with his uninjured or strong leg when going up stairs.

10. Advise the patient to keep the cane on the uninjured or strong side of his body and to use the wall or rail, if available, for support on the weak side. If a rail is not available, the patient may need assistance for safety.

11. After the patient steps on the strong leg, instruct him to bring up his weak leg and then the cane.

12. Remind the patient not to rush.

Descending Stairs

13. Instruct the patient to always start with her weak leg when going down stairs.

14. Advise the patient to keep the cane on the uninjured or strong side of her body and to use the wall or rail, if available, for support on the weak side. If a rail is not available, the patient may need assistance for safety.

15. Have the patient use the uninjured or strong leg and wall or rail to support her body, put the cane on the next step, and bend the strong leg as she lowers the weak leg to the next step.

16. Instruct the patient to step down with the strong leg.

Walking on Snow or Ice

17. Suggest that the patient try a metal ice-gripping cane or a ski pole. These can be dug into the snow or ice to prevent slipping. Instruct the patient to avoid walking on ice unless absolutely necessary.

PROCEDURE 54-4 Teaching a Patient How to Use a Walker

Procedure Goal: To teach a patient how to use a walker safely

OSHA Guidelines: This procedure does not involve exposure to blood, body fluids, or tissues.

Materials: A walker suited to the patient's needs

Method:

Walking

1. Instruct the patient to step into the walker.
2. Tell the patient to place her hands on the handgrips on the sides of the walker.
3. Make sure the patient's feet are far enough apart so that she feels balanced.
   RATIONALE: *A wider base provides for better balance.*
4. Instruct the patient to pick up the walker and move it forward about 6 inches.
5. Have the patient move one foot forward and then the other foot.
6. Instruct the patient to pick up the walker again and move it forward. If the patient is strong enough, explain that she may advance the walker after moving each leg rather than waiting until she has moved both legs.

Sitting

7. Teach the patient to turn his back to the chair or bed.
8. Instruct the patient to take small, careful steps and to back up until he feels the chair or bed at the back of his legs.
9. Instruct the patient to keep the walker in front of himself, let go of the walker, and place both his hands on the arms or seat of the chair or on the bed.
10. Teach the patient to balance himself on his arms while lowering himself slowly to the chair or bed.
11. If the patient has an injured or affected leg, he should keep it forward while bending his unaffected leg and lowering his body to the chair or bed.

Ascending and Descending Stairs

12. If a patient needs to use a walker on stairs, refer him to a physical therapist for additional training.

PROCEDURE 54-5 Teaching a Patient How to Use Crutches

Procedure Goal: To teach a patient how to use crutches safely

OSHA Guidelines: This procedure does not involve exposure to blood, body fluids, or tissues.

Materials: A pair of crutches suited to the patient's needs

Method:

1. Verify the physician's order for the type of crutches and gait to be used.
2. Wash your hands, identify the patient, and explain the procedure.
3. Elderly patients or patients with muscle weakness should be taught muscle strength exercises for their arms.
4. Have the patient stand erect and look straight ahead.
5. Tell the patient to place the crutch tips 4 to 6 inches in front of and 4 to 6 inches to the side of each foot.
6. When instructing a patient to use an axillary crutch, make sure the patient has a 2-inch gap between the axilla and the axillary bar and that each elbow is flexed 25 to 30 degrees.
   RATIONALE: *To reduce the incidence of nerve injury to the axilla.*
7. Teach the patient how to get up from a chair:
   a. Instruct the patient to hold both crutches on his affected or weaker side.

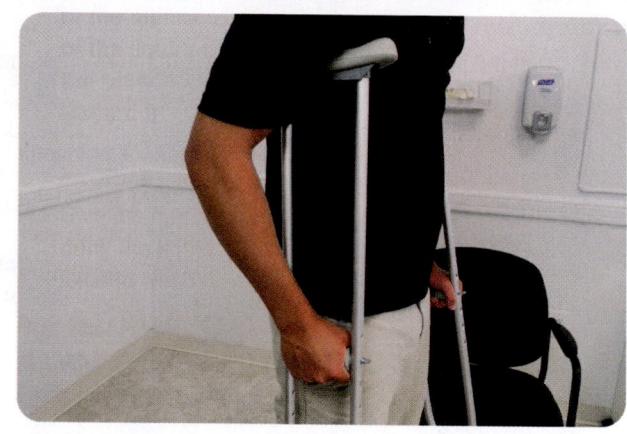

FIGURE Procedure 54-5 Step 6   The patient's elbow should be flexed 25 to 30 degrees.
© McGraw-Hill Education

   b. Have the patient slide to the edge of the chair.
   c. Tell the patient to push down on the arm or seat of the chair on his stronger side and use his strong leg to push up. If indicated, keep the affected leg forward.
   d. Advise the patient to put the crutches under his arms and press down on the handgrips with his hands.
8. Teach the patient the required gait. Which gait the patient will use depends on the patient's muscle strength and coordination. It also depends on the type of crutches, the

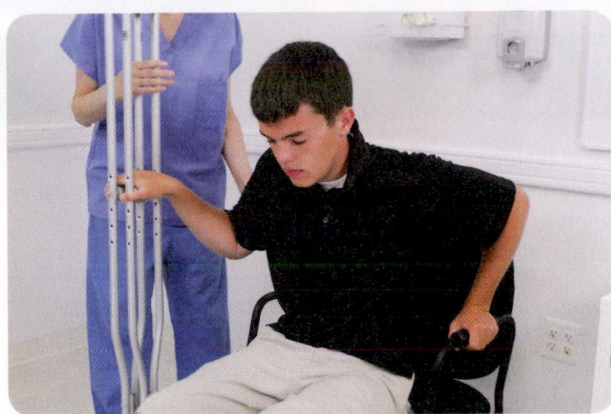

FIGURE Procedure 54-5 Step 7c   The patient should push up from his stronger side.
© McGraw-Hill Education

injury, and the patient's condition. Check the physician's orders, and see Figures 54-11 and 54-12 for examples.

9. Teach the patient how to ascend stairs:
   a. Start the patient close to the bottom step and tell him to push down with his hands.
   b. Instruct the patient to step up on the first step with his good foot.

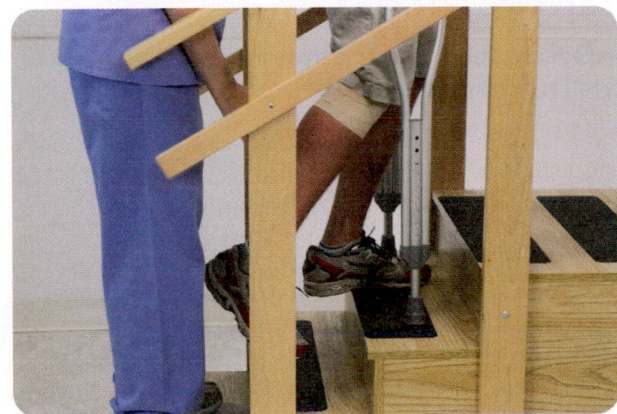

FIGURE Procedure 54-5 Step 9b   The patient should lead with his unaffected leg when ascending stairs.
© McGraw-Hill Education

   c. Tell the patient to lift the crutches to the same step and then lift his other foot. Advise the patient to keep his crutches with his affected limb.
   d. Remind the patient to check his balance before he proceeds to the next step.
10. Teach the patient how to descend stairs:

a. Have the patient start at the edge of the steps.
b. Instruct the patient to bring his crutches and then the affected foot down first. Advise the patient to bend at the hips and knees to prevent leaning forward, which could cause him to fall.

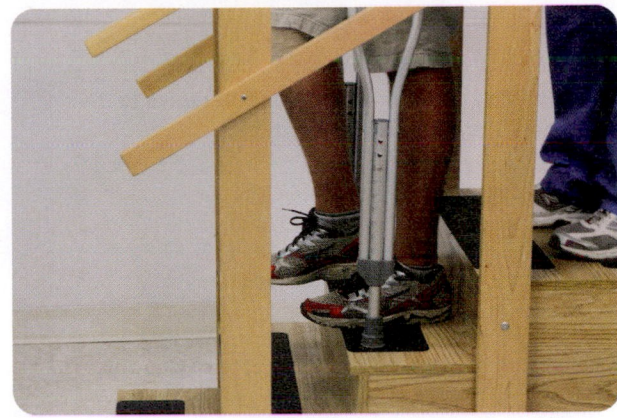

FIGURE Procedure 54-5 Step 10b   The patient should lead with the affected foot when descending stairs.
© McGraw-Hill Education

   c. Tell the patient to bring his unaffected foot to the same step.
   d. Remind the patient to check his balance before he proceeds. In some cases, a handrail may be easier and can be used with both crutches in one hand.
11. Give the patient the following general information related to the use of crutches:
   a. Do not lean on crutches.
   b. Report to the physician any tingling or numbness in the arms, hands, or shoulders.
   c. Support body weight with the hands.
   d. Always stand erect to prevent muscle strain.
   e. Look straight ahead when walking.
   f. Generally, move the crutches not more than 6 inches at a time to maintain good balance.
   g. Check the crutch tips regularly for wear; replace the tips as needed.
   h. Check the crutch tips for wetness; dry the tips if they are wet.
   i. Check all wing nuts and bolts for tightness.
   j. Wear flat, well-fitting, nonskid shoes.
   k. Remove throw rugs and other unsecured articles from traffic areas.
   l. Report any unusual pain in the affected leg.

LEARNING OUTCOMES	KEY POINTS
54.1 Discuss the general principles of physical therapy.	Physical therapy is a medical specialty for the treatment of musculoskeletal, nervous, and cardiopulmonary disorders using a variety of treatments, including cold, heat, water, exercise, massage, and traction.
54.2 Relate various cold and heat therapies to their benefits and contraindications.	There are various types of cold and heat therapies, including dry and wet cold and heat applications. Cold and heat therapy promote healing and increase patient comfort. Contraindications to cold and heat therapies include circulation problems, pain, and hemorrhage.
54.3 Recall hydrotherapy methods.	Various types of hydrotherapy used to treat physical problems include whirlpools, contrast baths, and underwater exercises.
54.4 Name several methods of exercise therapy.	There are several methods of exercise therapy, including active mobility, passive mobility, aided mobility, and active resistance.
54.5 Describe the types of massage used in rehabilitation therapy.	The two major types of massage used in rehabilitation therapy are Swedish and neuromuscular. Swedish massage uses five basic strokes to manipulate soft tissues. Neuromuscular massage is applied to specific muscles and helps release tension and knots, relieve pain and release pressure on nerves, and increase blood flow. Trigger point therapy is commonly used during neuromuscular massage.
54.6 Compare different methods of traction.	The methods of traction used to treat physical problems include manual, static, skeletal, and mechanical.
54.7 Carry out the procedure for teaching a patient to use a cane, a walker, crutches, and a wheelchair.	The various mobility aids include canes, walkers, crutches, and wheelchairs. Specific instructions for each of these aids must be followed to reduce the possibility of patient injury during their use.
54.8 Model the steps you should take when referring a patient to a physical therapist.	You may be asked to contact the specialist directly or to give the patient a written order and information about contacting the specialist. Keep a file with information about the therapists your office uses, noting the forms and information each therapist requires.

CASE STUDY CRITICAL THINKING

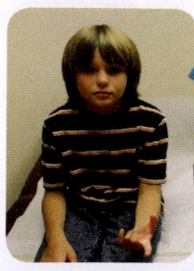

Recall Chris Matthews from the beginning of the chapter. Now that you have completed the chapter, answer the following questions regarding his case.

1. What X-ray views did Dr. Whalen order?
2. What type of crutches would be best to give Chris?
3. What crutch gait will you teach Chris?
4. Dr. Whalen wants Chris to continue cryotherapy for the next 48 hours. What instructions will you give Chris and his mom?

1. (LO 54.1) Which of the following is an example of inversion?
   a. Flexing the foot
   b. Pointing the foot upward
   c. Turning the sole of the foot inward
   d. Rotating the foot back and forth
   e. Turning the sole of the foot downward

2. (LO 54.1) Body position and alignment are known as
   a. Posture
   b. Gait
   c. Range of motion
   d. Flexion
   e. Extension

3. (LO 54.4) Which of the following is a type of exercise whereby the patient relaxes and contracts the muscles of a specific body part without moving the body part?
   a. ROM
   b. Passive mobility
   c. Active resistance
   d. Isometric
   e. Aided mobility

4. (LO 54.6) Another name for weight traction is
   a. Static
   b. Skeletal
   c. Mechanical
   d. Manual
   e. Harness

5. (LO 54.7) Which of the following crutch gaits is the best for someone with leg paralysis?
   a. Two-point
   b. Three-point
   c. Swing-to
   d. Four-point
   e. Crutches are never used by people with leg paralysis

6. (LO 54.2) Which of the following therapies causes blood vessels to constrict?
   a. Neuromuscular massage
   b. Thermotherapy
   c. ROM
   d. Active resistance exercise
   e. Cryotherapy

7. (LO 54.5) In Swedish massage, which of the following strokes is a percussive stroke?
   a. Pétrissage
   b. Effleurage
   c. Vibration
   d. Tapotement
   e. Friction

8. (LO 54.4) Riding a stationary bicycle is an example of a(n)
   a. Active mobility exercise
   b. Isometric exercise
   c. Passive mobility exercise
   d. Active range-of-motion exercise
   e. Aided mobility exercise

9. (LO 54.7) Which of the following crutch gaits is considered the slowest?
   a. Two-point
   b. Swing-through
   c. Three-point
   d. Swing-to
   e. Four-point

10. (LO 54.1) A goniometer is used to measure
    a. Pain
    b. The effectiveness of cold therapy
    c. Range of motion
    d. Muscle contraction
    e. The type of traction needed

Recall Chris Matthews from the case study at the beginning of the chapter. Dr. Whalen asks you to assist with wrapping Chris's ankle. She wants you to hold and stabilize his leg while she applies the elastic wrap. Chris's mom asks you if she will need any help rewrapping Chris's ankle. What should you tell Mrs. Matthews about taking care of Chris's bandage?

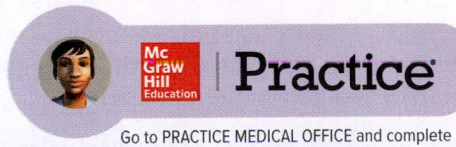

Go to PRACTICE MEDICAL OFFICE and complete the module Clinical - Work Task Proficiencies.

Nutrition and Health

CASE STUDY

PATIENT INFORMATION	Patient Name	DOB	Allergies
	Mohammad Nassar	5/17/20XX	Animal dander
	Attending	**MRN**	**Other Information**
	Elizabeth H. Williams, MD	423-90-687	Current medications: Albuterol 4 mg bid

A 16-year-old male patient is brought to BWW Associates by his parents. As the medical assistant, you take his history and physical, noting that he has a past history of mild asthma. The patient mentions that he is avoiding food because he is being "careful not to eat too many calories" so that he can keep his weight down and have a chance to fight in the lightest

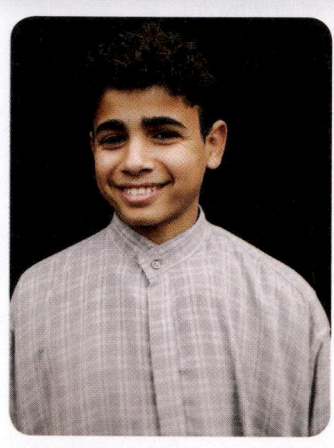

© David Sacks/Getty Images

weight class. He tells you he hopes to get a scholarship for wrestling so that he can attend college next fall. You note that his vital signs are blood pressure 100/60, height 5′ 10″, weight 131 lb, pulse rate 50. He appears dehydrated and exhibits signs of muscle weakness.

Keep Mohammad Nassar in mind as you study the chapter. There will be questions at the end of the chapter based on the case study. The information in the chapter will help you answer these questions.

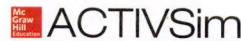

LEARNING OUTCOMES

After completing Chapter 55, you will be able to:

55.1 Relate daily energy requirements to the role of calories.

55.2 Identify nutrients and their role in health.

55.3 Implement a plan for a nutritious, well-balanced diet and healthy lifestyle using the USDA's guidelines.

55.4 Describe methods used to assess a patient's nutritional status.

55.5 Explain reasons that a diet may be modified.

55.6 Identify types of patients who require special diets and the modifications required for each.

55.7 Describe the warning signs, symptoms, and treatment for eating disorders.

55.8 Educate patients about nutritional requirements.

KEY TERMS

amino acid	dehydration
anabolism	fiber
anorexia nervosa	food exchange
antioxidant	gluten
behavior modification	lipid
bulimia nervosa	mineral
calorie	parenteral nutrition
catabolism	protein
celiac disease	saturated fat
cholesterol	unsaturated fat
complex carbohydrate	vitamin

IV.C.1 Describe dietary nutrients including:
- (a) carbohydrates
- (b) fat
- (c) protein
- (d) minerals
- (e) electrolytes
- (f) vitamins
- (g) fiber
- (h) water

IV.C.2 Define the function of dietary supplements

IV.C.3 Identify the special dietary needs for:
- (a) weight control
- (b) diabetes
- (c) cardiovascular disease
- (d) hypertension
- (e) cancer
- (f) lactose sensitivity
- (g) gluten-free
- (h) food allergies

IV.P.1 Instruct a patient according to a patient's special dietary needs

IV.A.1 Show awareness of patient's concerns regarding a dietary change

X.P.3 Document patient care accurately in the medical record

2. Anatomy and Physiology
- b. Describe common diseases, symptoms, and etiologies as they apply to each system
- d. Apply a system of diet and nutrition
  - i. Explain the importance of diet and nutrition
  - ii. Educate patients regarding proper diet and nutrition guidelines
  - iii. Identify categories of patients that require special diets or diet modifications

9. Medical Office Clinical Procedures
- h. Teach self-examination, disease management and health promotion

▶ Introduction

Nutrition is the process of how the body takes in and utilizes food and other sources of nutrients. It is a five-part process that includes ingestion, digestion, absorption, metabolism, and elimination.

You need to know what effect nutrition has on health so that you can help patients meet their dietary requirements. Food is the body's source of nutrients, or substances the body needs to function properly. As you study this chapter, you will learn how the body uses nutrients and the importance of a well-planned diet to health. People need specific types of foods to stay healthy or to regain their health after illness or surgery. People with specific conditions also may need to follow special diets. As a medical assistant, you will work closely with the rest of the healthcare team to ensure that patients understand the role of diet in health and that they adhere to any diet prescribed by their licensed practitioner or dietitian.

▶ Daily Energy Requirements   LO 55.1

The human body requires the nutrients in food for three major purposes:

- To provide energy
- To build, repair, and maintain body tissues
- To regulate body processes

A person's daily energy requirements depend on many factors. To understand the relationship of food to good health, you need to understand how the body uses food.

Metabolism

Food must be broken down before the body can use it. This process is an integral part of metabolism. Metabolism is the sum of all the cellular processes that build, maintain, and supply energy to your body tissues. During metabolism, body chemicals such as carbohydrates, proteins, and fats are built up and broken down, and heat and energy are produced.

Metabolism takes place in two phases. In **anabolism,** substances such as nutrients are changed into more complex substances and used to build body tissues. In **catabolism,** complex substances, including nutrients and body tissues, are broken down into simpler substances and converted into energy. The body uses this energy to maintain and repair itself. Of the energy people get from the food they eat, about 25% is directly used for bodily functions, and the rest becomes heat.

Each person's body requires a minimal amount of nutrients to carry on a basic level of metabolism to live. Each person's daily nutritional requirements vary with age, weight, percentage of body fat, activity level, state of health, and other variables. The body's metabolic rate, or speed of metabolism, also can be affected by many factors, such as pregnancy, malnutrition, and disease.

Calories

The amount of energy a food produces in the body is measured in kilocalories. A kilocalorie, commonly called a **calorie**, is the amount of energy needed to raise the temperature of 1 kilogram of water by 1°C. Foods differ in the number of calories they contain. The more calories in a food, the more available energy it has. Calories also are used to measure the energy the body uses during all activities and metabolic processes.

As mentioned, people's daily nutritional needs differ, depending on variables of age, weight, percentage of body fat, activity level, and state of health. If people eat an excess of calories—more than the body can use—the excess is stored as fat in the body. Conversely, lowering caloric intake causes the body to burn off stored fat for energy.

Depending on the food's weight (in grams) or volume, each food has a value in calories. Therefore, you can count the number of calories a person consumes by monitoring food intake and adding up the calories in each food serving. You can use a food calorie counter, such as those often found in books or software applications, to look up caloric values. A calorie counter tells you, for instance, that 1 cup of cooked carrots contains 50 calories or that 1 cup of cooked corn kernels contains 130 calories. Calories also are listed on the labels of food packages. You can estimate the number of calories a person burns during certain activities by consulting a chart similar to Table 55-1.

TABLE 55-1 Calories Burned per Hour in Selected Activities

Moderate Physical Activity	Approximate Calories/Hr for a 154-lb Person*
Hiking	370
Light gardening/yard work	330
Dancing	330
Golf (walking and carrying clubs)	330
Bicycling (<10 mph)	290
Walking (3.5 mph)	280
Weight lifting (general light workout)	180
Vigorous Physical Activity	**Approximate Calories/Hr for a 154-lb Person***
Running/jogging (5 mph)	590
Bicycling (>10 mph)	590
Swimming (slow freestyle laps)	510
Aerobics	480
Walking (4.5 mph)	460
Heavy yard work (chopping wood)	440
Weight lifting (vigorous effort)	440
Basketball (vigorous)	440

*Calories burned per hour will be higher for people who weigh more than 154 lb (70 kg) and lower for people who weigh less.
Source: US Department of Health and Human Services, US Department of Agriculture, *Dietary Guidelines for Americans 2010,* http://www.healthierus.gov/dietaryguidelines.

▶ Nutrients

The body needs a variety of nutrients for energy, growth, repair, and basic processes. Seven basic food components provide these nutrients and work together to help keep the body healthy:

1. Proteins
2. Carbohydrates
3. Fiber
4. Lipids
5. Vitamins
6. Minerals
7. Water

As the body digests foods that contain these components, it breaks them down so that it can use them. Of the seven components, only proteins, carbohydrates, and lipids contain calories and provide the body with energy. The rest perform a variety of other essential functions.

Proteins

Protein is the most essential nutrient for building and repairing cells and tissues. Therefore, it is especially important for people to get enough protein during illness and healing. Other major functions of protein are to

- Help maintain the body's water balance.
- Assist with antibody production and disease resistance.
- Help maintain body heat.

The optimal level of protein in a healthy person's diet is 10% to 35% of total caloric intake. Eating a variety of lean proteins is best. A deficiency in protein leads to weight loss and fatigue, malnutrition, extremely dry skin, lowered resistance to infection, and interference with normal growth processes.

The body makes protein out of **amino acids,** which are natural organic compounds found in plant and animal foods. Besides being used to build and maintain tissue, protein can be broken down to produce energy, especially if other quick energy sources such as carbohydrates are low. Each gram of protein contains 4 calories. Excess protein is broken down by the body and contributes to fat stores.

Amino acids are found in animal sources such as meats, milk, fish, and eggs, as well as in plant sources such as soy, beans, legumes, nut butters, and some grains (such as wheat germ). Individuals do not need to eat animal products to get all the protein they need in their diet. See Figure 55-1.

Amino acids are classified into three groups:

- *Essential amino acids* cannot be made by the body and must be supplied by food. They do not all need to be eaten at one meal. The balance over the whole day is more important. There are nine essential amino acids.
- *Nonessential amino acids* are made by the body from essential amino acids or in the normal breakdown of proteins. There are four nonessential amino acids.
- *Conditional amino acids* are usually not essential, except in times of illness and stress. There are at least eight conditional amino acids.

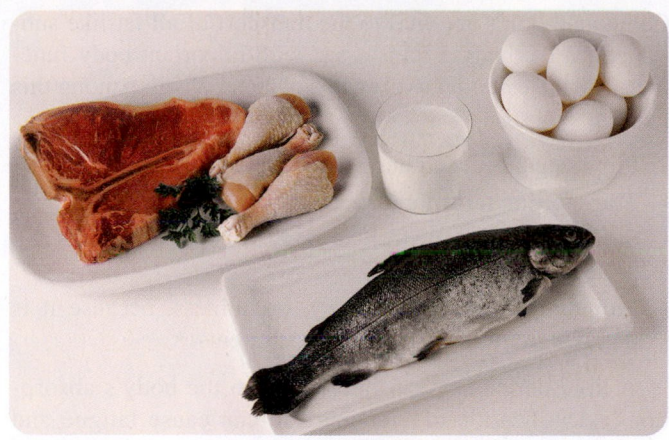

(a)

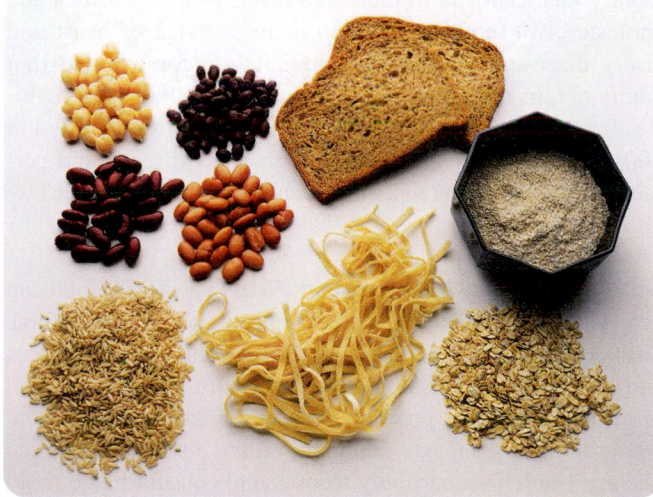

(b)

FIGURE 55-1   Protein foods supply essential, nonessential, and conditional amino acids. (a) Individuals who eat animal products should select lean proteins and have seafood at least once a week. (b) Individuals who do not eat animal products can get protein from these foods.

(a) © McGraw-Hill Education/Jill Braaten, photographer; (b) © Royalty-Free/Corbis

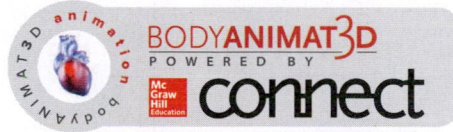

Go to CONNECT to see an animation exercise about *Protein Synthesis.*

Carbohydrates

Carbohydrates in food provide about two-thirds of a person's daily energy needs. Carbohydrates also provide heat and help metabolize fat. Each gram of carbohydrate contains 4 calories. The daily requirement for carbohydrates is 45% to 65% of total caloric intake. Carbohydrate deficiency leads to weight loss, protein loss, and fatigue.

There are two basic types of carbohydrates:

- *Simple carbohydrates* (sugars), found in fruits, some vegetables, milk, and table sugar

- *Complex carbohydrates,* found in grain foods, such as breads, pastas, cereals, and rice; in some fruits and

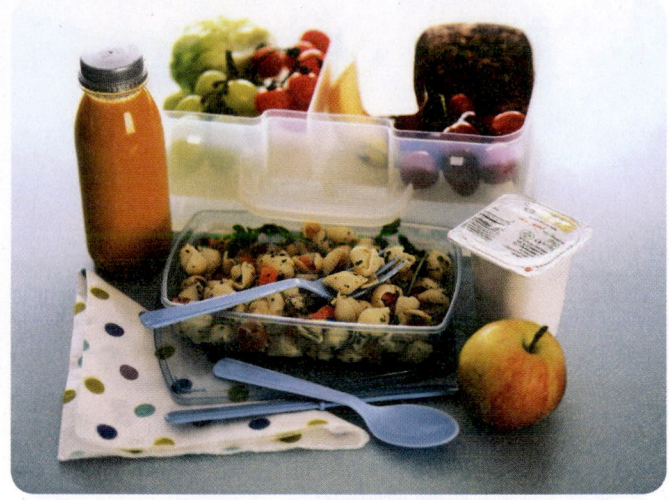

FIGURE 55-2   Healthful sources of carbohydrates are plentiful.
© Sian Invine/Getty Images

vegetables, such as potatoes, corn, broccoli, apples, and pears; and in legumes, such as peas, peanuts, and beans

Simple sugars are small molecules that consist of one or two sugar (saccharide) units. **Complex carbohydrates,** or polysaccharides, are long chains of sugar units. Starch is a type of complex carbohydrate that is a major source of energy from foods of plant origin. Fiber, another type of complex carbohydrate, is discussed in the next section.

Carbohydrates used for immediate fuel are converted to glucose, a simple sugar that cells use for energy. An excess of carbohydrates is either stored in the liver and muscle cells as glycogen (long chains of glucose units—the animal equivalent of starch) or converted into and stored as fat. After the body's carbohydrate reserves are depleted, it starts burning fat. Healthful, nutritive sources of carbohydrates include fruits and vegetables, whole-grain pasta and cereal, and potatoes (Figure 55-2). The American Dietetic Association suggests these sources of carbohydrates with an emphasis on complex carbohydrates such as vegetables, legumes, and whole-grain breads and cereals. Sugary foods such as sweet desserts, candy, and soft drinks also contain carbohydrates, but they are high in calories and low in nutritional value.

Fiber

Fiber is in a separate category, although it is a type of complex carbohydrate. Fiber does not supply energy or heat to the body. It is the tough, stringy part of vegetables and grains. Fiber is not absorbed by the body, but it serves these important digestive functions:

- Increasing and softening the bulk of the stool, thus promoting normal defecation

- Absorbing organic wastes and toxins in the body so that they can be expelled

- Decreasing the rate of carbohydrate breakdown and absorption

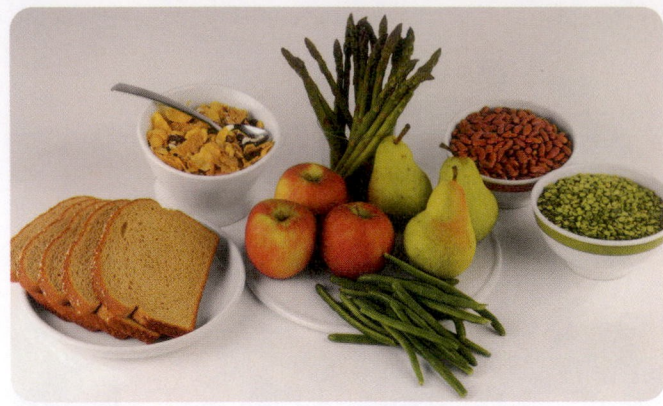

FIGURE 55-3 Dietary fiber serves many functions in the human body and is considered a basic food component.
© McGraw-Hill Education/Jill Braaten, photographer

Therapeutically, fiber can help treat and prevent constipation, hemorrhoids, diverticular disease, and irritable bowel syndrome. It is linked to reduced blood cholesterol levels, reduction of gallstone formation, control of diabetes, and reduction in the risk of certain types of cancer and other diseases. Too little fiber can result in an increased risk of colon cancer, hypercholesterolemia (high blood cholesterol), and increased blood glucose levels after eating. Too much fiber can cause constipation, diarrhea, and other gastrointestinal disorders and can impair mineral absorption.

The recommended amount of fiber for adults is 14 grams for every 1,000 calories you eat per day. So if you eat 2,000 calories each day, you should have 28 grams of fiber. Because fiber works in conjunction with other substances and nutrients, it is advisable to get dietary fiber from a variety of food sources (Figure 55-3). Adequate water intake is especially important for fiber to work properly.

Fiber can be classified as soluble or insoluble. Soluble fiber absorbs fluid and swells when eaten. It slows the absorption of food from the digestive tract, helps control the blood sugar level of diabetics, lowers blood cholesterol levels, and softens and increases the bulk of stools. Soluble fiber is found in foods such as oats, dry beans, barley, and some fruits and vegetables. Insoluble fiber promotes regular bowel movements by contributing to stool bulk. It is found in bran, whole-wheat bread, brown rice, and similar foods.

Lipids

Lipids in the diet include dietary fats and fat-related substances. Fats are a concentrated source of energy that the body can store in large amounts. Each gram of fat contains 9 calories (more than twice the calorie content of proteins and carbohydrates). About 95% of the lipids from plant and animal sources of food are fats. These simple lipids, or triglycerides, consist of glycerol (an alcohol) and three fatty acids. Chemical qualities of the fatty acids in a triglyceride determine the fat's characteristic flavor and texture. About 5% of dietary lipids are compound lipids such as cholesterol. Compound lipids are fat-related substances that are important components of cell membranes, nervous tissue, and some hormones.

Compound lipids are vital to the transport of all fat-like substances in the body. Lipids assist with important body functions and are essential to growth and metabolism. Among this nutrient's jobs are

- Providing a concentrated source of heat and energy.
- Transporting fat-soluble vitamins.
- Storing energy in the form of body fat, which insulates and protects the organs.
- Providing a feeling of satiety, or fullness, because it is digested more slowly than other nutrients.

A lipid deficiency can interfere with the body's absorption and utilization of vitamins and can cause fatigue and dry skin. However, an excess of lipids, particularly some dietary fats, can lead to increased levels of triglycerides and cholesterol in the blood and an increased risk of heart and artery disease and other diseases. It is recommended that adults obtain no more than 20% to 30% of their daily calories from fat sources. Cholesterol intake should be limited to 300 milligrams per day. People with heart disease and certain other diseases or risks may benefit from even lower levels of lipid intake.

Saturated and Unsaturated Fats The fats in food can be classified as either saturated or unsaturated (Figure 55-4). **Saturated fats** are derived primarily from animal sources and are usually solid at room temperature. They are found in meats and animal products such as butter, egg yolks, and whole milk. Coconut oil and palm oil are also saturated fats. Dietary Guidelines currently recommend consuming no more than 10% of total daily calories in the form of saturated fats. However, because research links high blood cholesterol levels with increased risk of heart disease, people who have heart disease or are already at risk for it should reduce their intake to no more than 5% or 6% of daily calories.

Unsaturated fats are usually liquid at room temperature. They include most vegetable oils. Unsaturated fats can be divided into two classes:

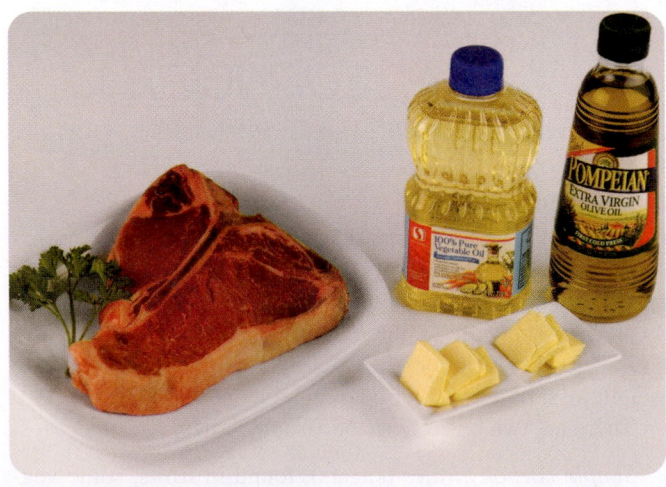

FIGURE 55-4 Foods that contain saturated fats include meat and butter. Most vegetable oils contain unsaturated fats.
© McGraw-Hill Education/Jill Braaten, photographer

- Polyunsaturated fats, such as corn, soya, safflower, and sunflower oils
- Monounsaturated fats, such as peanut, canola, and olive oils

The body needs essential fatty acids (primarily linoleic acid) to build and maintain body tissues. Because the body cannot produce these fatty acids, they must be supplied by food. Saturated fats in butter, egg yolks, and milk, as well as unsaturated fats in corn, canola, sunflower, and safflower oils, are good sources of essential fatty acids.

Trans Fats Also known as trans fatty acids, trans fats are a specific type of fat that is formed when hydrogen is added to vegetable oil through a process called *hydrogenation,* which turns liquid oils into solid fats. Trans fats can be found in vegetable shortenings, some margarines, crackers, candy, cookies, snack foods, fried foods, baked goods, and other processed foods. The US Food and Drug Administration (FDA) recommends that individuals consume as close to zero grams as possible on a daily basis. The FDA currently requires that the amount of trans fat be displayed on all food labels.

Cholesterol Cholesterol is a fat-related substance produced by the liver that also can be obtained through dietary sources. Only animal-based foods contain cholesterol. It is essential to health because it

- Serves as an integral part of cell membranes.
- Provides the structural basis for all steroid hormones and vitamin D.
- Is a component of bile, which aids in digestion.

Lipid Levels in the Blood Lipids, like other nutrients, are carried throughout the body in the bloodstream. When blood lipid levels become excessive, however, they pose certain risks. Licensed practitioners often order blood tests to determine the level of triglycerides and cholesterol in their patients' blood as a measure of overall health. High levels of cholesterol, especially if accompanied by high levels of triglycerides, may indicate an increased risk of heart disease, stroke, and peripheral vascular disease.

Lipids are not soluble in water; fats (or oils) and water do not mix. Because the fluid portion of blood is 90% water, lipids are encased in large molecules that are fat-soluble on the inside and water-soluble on the outside. These large molecules, called lipoproteins, carry lipids such as cholesterol and triglycerides through the bloodstream.

Low-density lipoproteins (LDL) and high-density lipoproteins (HDL) are the two main types of lipoproteins. Cholesterol in blood is identified as HDL or LDL, depending on which type of lipoprotein carries it. High levels of LDL cholesterol in blood are a primary risk factor for heart attacks. High levels of LDL cholesterol occur in people whose diets are high in saturated fats. HDL cholesterol, commonly referred to as good cholesterol, carries excess cholesterol away from arteries and back to the liver for breakdown and elimination. Patients often can reduce elevated cholesterol

TABLE 55-2	Saturated Fat and Cholesterol Content of Various Foods	
Food	**Saturated Fat (g)**	**Cholesterol (mg)**
Cheddar cheese (1 oz)	6.0	30
Mozzarella, part skim (1 oz)	3.1	15
Whole milk (1 c)	5.1	33
Skim milk (1 c)	0.3	4
Butter (1 tbsp)	7.1	31
Mayonnaise (1 tbsp)	1.7	8
Tuna in oil (3 oz)	1.4	55
Tuna in water (3 oz)	0.3	48
Lean ground beef, broiled (3 oz)	6.2	74
Leg of lamb, roasted (3 oz)	5.6	78
Bacon (3 slices)	3.3	16
Chicken breast, roasted (3 oz)	0.9	73

Source: US Department of Agriculture.

levels by increasing exercise and intake of soluble fiber and decreasing the dietary intake of saturated fats. These measures tend to elevate the level of HDL cholesterol in the bloodstream and reduce the level of LDL cholesterol. Table 55-2 lists the saturated fat and cholesterol contents of various foods.

Vitamins

Vitamins are organic substances that are essential for normal body growth and maintenance and resistance to infection. Vitamins also help the body use other nutrients and assist in various body processes.

Most vitamins are absorbed directly through the digestive tract. Some vitamins are water-soluble and others are fat-soluble. Water-soluble vitamins, such as vitamin C and the B vitamins, are not stored by the body and therefore must be replaced every day. Fat-soluble vitamins, such as vitamins A, D, E, and K, are stored for longer periods.

The amounts of vitamins the body needs are relatively small; however, a vitamin deficiency through lack of ingestion or absorption can lead to disease. Some vitamins also can cause health problems if taken in excess. Toxic levels of vitamin A, for example, can produce effects ranging from headache to liver damage. Because the level of vitamin intake is so essential to health, the Food and Nutrition Board of the National Research Council has established recommended dietary allowances (RDAs) for vitamins. For detailed information on specific vitamins, see Table 55-3.

Eating a well-balanced, nutritious diet minimizes the likelihood of vitamin deficiency. Many manufactured foods are also vitamin-fortified. Even so, some people choose to augment their diets with vitamin supplements (Figure 55-5). A licensed practitioner may, in some instances, prescribe vitamin supplements for patients.

TABLE 55-3 Vitamins

Vitamin	Functions	Adult RDA*	Food Sources	Deficiencies and/or Toxicities
Vitamin A (retinol, provitamin, carotene)	Aids in night vision; cell growth and maintenance; normal reproductive function; health of skin, mucous membranes, and intestines	Males: 900 mcg retinol equivalents Females: 700 mcg retinol equivalents	Milk fat; butter; egg yolks; meat; fish liver oil; liver; green, yellow, and orange leafy vegetables; yellow and orange fruits	Deficiency: night blindness; dry, rough skin; risk of internal infection Toxicity: headache, vomiting, joint pain, hair loss, jaundice, liver damage
Vitamin B$_1$ (thiamine)	Aids enzymes in breaking down and using carbohydrates; helps the nerves, muscles, and heart function efficiently	Males: 1.2 mg Females: 1.1 mg	Whole grains, brewer's yeast, organ meats, lean pork, beef, liver, legumes, seeds, nuts	Deficiency: beriberi with appetite loss, digestive problems, muscle weakness and deterioration, nervous disorders, heart failure
Vitamin B$_2$ (riboflavin)	Aids enzymes in metabolism of fats and proteins	Males: 1.3 mg Females: 1.1 mg	Dairy products, organ meats, green leafy vegetables, enriched and fortified grain products	Deficiency: cracks at lip corners, irritations at nasal angles, inflammation of the tongue, seborrheic dermatitis, anemia
Vitamin B$_3$ (niacin)	Aids enzymes in metabolism of carbohydrates and fats	Males: 16 mg Females: 14 mg	Meat, fish, poultry, enriched and fortified grain products	Deficiency: pellagra with dermatitis, diarrhea, inflammation of mucous membranes, dementia Toxicity: dilation of blood vessels; if sustained, abnormal liver function
Vitamin B$_6$ (pyridoxine)	Aids enzymes in synthesis of amino acids	Males: 1.7 mg Females: 1.3–1.5 mg	Chicken, fish, pork, liver, kidney, some vegetables, grains, nuts, legumes	Deficiency: convulsions, dermatitis, anemia Toxicity: loss of muscle coordination, severe sensory neuropathy
Folate/folic acid (compounds)	Works with cobalamins in nucleic acid synthesis and metabolism of amino acids; maintains red blood cells	Males: 400 mcg Females: 400 mcg	Liver, yeast, legumes, green leafy vegetables, some fruits	Deficiency: glossitis, diarrhea, anemia, lethargy; folic acid deficiency during embryonic development may increase the risk of spina bifida
Vitamin B$_{12}$ (cobalamins)	Works with folate in nucleic acid synthesis and metabolism of amino acids; coenzyme in metabolism of fatty acids	2.4 mcg	Seafood, meat, milk, eggs, cheese, brewer's yeast, blackstrap molasses	Deficiency: pernicious anemia, irreversible liver damage
Vitamin C (ascorbic acid)	Coenzyme involved in collagen production, capillary integrity, use of iron in hemoglobin, and synthesis of many hormones; improves absorption of iron; antioxidant	Males: 90 mg Females: 75 mg	Citrus fruits, mangoes, strawberries, green peppers, broccoli, potatoes, green leafy vegetables	Deficiency: scurvy with hemorrhages, loose teeth, poor wound healing Toxicity: stomachache, diarrhea
Vitamin D (calciferol)	Builds bones and teeth; helps maintain calcium-phosphorus balance in blood	5–15 mcg	Egg yolks, butter, liver, fortified milk, margarine, and prepared cereals	Deficiency: rickets in children, osteomalacia in adults Toxicity: excess blood calcium and phosphorus, calcium deposits in soft tissue, bone pain, irreversible kidney and cardiovascular damage
Vitamin E (group)	Aids in formation of red blood cells; maintains cell structure; intracellular antioxidant	15 mg	Vegetable oils, margarine, shortening, wheat germ, nuts, green leafy vegetables	Deficiency: damage to cells, hemolytic anemia
Vitamin K (compounds)	Aids in blood clotting and bone growth	Males: 120 mcg Females: 90 mcg	Green leafy vegetables, milk, dairy products, meat, eggs, cereals, fruits, vegetables	Deficiency: slow blood clotting; hemorrhagic disease in newborns

*RDAs may vary for different age groups.

Source: Adapted from the Institute of Medicine of the National Academies, http://www.iom.edu (accessed April 2012), and Office of Dietary Supplements, National Institutes of Health, http://ods.od.nih.gov (accessed April 2012).

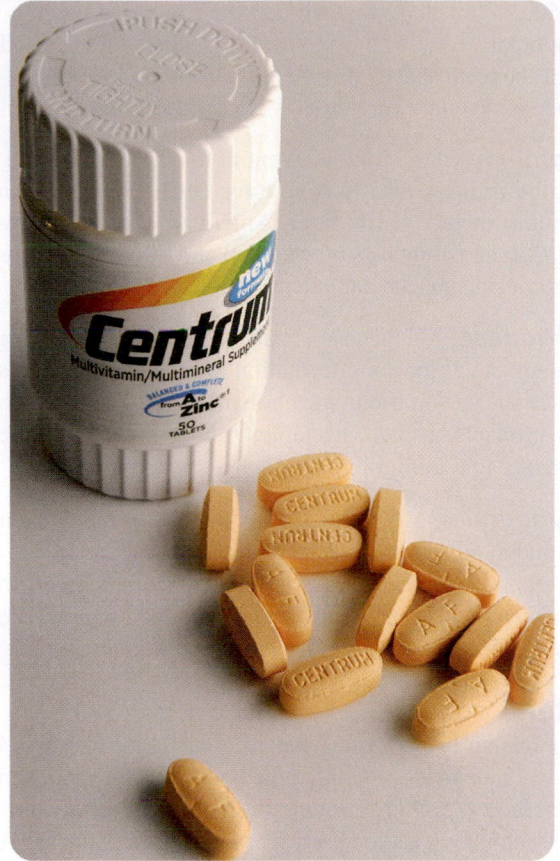

FIGURE 55-5 Some people use supplements to augment their dietary intake of vitamins and minerals.
© McGraw-Hill Education/Jill Braaten, photographer

Minerals

Minerals are natural, inorganic substances the body needs to help build and maintain body tissues and carry on life functions. Minerals are classified according to the relative amounts the body requires:

- Major minerals are those that the body needs in fairly large quantities, including calcium, magnesium, and phosphorus.
- Trace minerals are those that the body needs in tiny amounts, including iron, iodine, zinc, selenium, copper, fluoride, chromium, manganese, and molybdenum.

Most minerals are absorbed in the intestines, and any excess is eliminated. Calcium, iron, and iodine are the minerals in which people are most often deficient.

Minerals with Recommended Dietary Allowances

There are several minerals for which RDAs have been established. These minerals are calcium, iron, iodine, zinc, magnesium, phosphorus, and selenium.

Calcium Calcium builds healthy bones and teeth, aids in blood clotting, and helps nerves and muscles function properly. It is found in dairy products, green leafy vegetables, broccoli, legumes, and the soft bones of sardines and salmon (Figure 55-6).

Calcium deficiency can cause poor bone growth and tooth development in children, osteoporosis in adults,

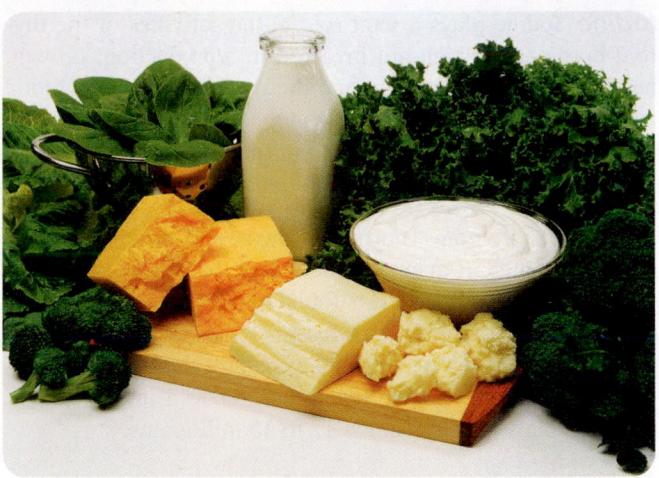

FIGURE 55-6 These foods are excellent sources of calcium, a mineral that is necessary for strong bones and teeth.
© Mitch Hrdlicka/Getty Images RF

and poor blood clotting. The normal requirement is 800 to 1,200 milligrams per day.

Iron Iron, one of the most important nutrients, is essential for the production of red blood cells, which transport oxygen throughout the body. It is also a component of enzymes needed for energy production. Although iron is found in a wide variety of foods, it is the most frequently deficient nutrient in people's diets. Liver, meat, poultry, fish, egg yolks, fortified breads and cereals, dark green vegetables, and dried fruits are good dietary sources of iron (Figure 55-7), although less than 20% of it is usually absorbed.

Iron deficiency can cause anemia, a blood disorder that results in fatigue, weakness, and impaired mental abilities. At toxic levels, iron may increase the risk of coronary heart disease (CHD). The daily requirement is 10 to 15 milligrams.

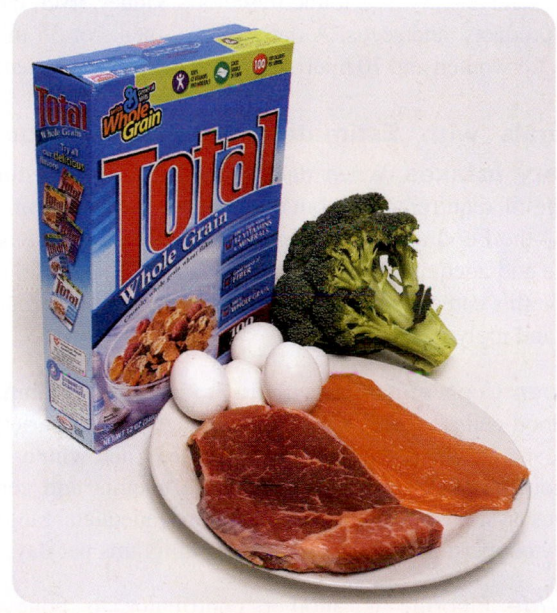

FIGURE 55-7 Iron, a mineral that is needed in small amounts, is found in a wide variety of foods.
© McGraw-Hill Education/John Flournoy, photographer

Iodine Iodine plays a vital role in the activities of the thyroid hormones, which are involved in reproduction, growth, nerve and muscle function, and the production of new blood cells. Deficiency can cause an enlarged thyroid gland, known as *goiter*. Iodine can be obtained in seafood, iodized salt, and seaweed products. The daily requirement is 150 micrograms.

Zinc Zinc promotes normal growth and wound healing and participates in many cell activities that involve proteins, enzymes, and hormones. It is found in liver, lamb, beef, eggs, oysters, and whole-grain breads and cereals, although it is not always easily absorbed. Deficiency can result in growth retardation, impaired taste and smell, and reduced immune function. The daily requirement is 12 to 15 milligrams.

Magnesium Magnesium activates cell enzymes, helps metabolize proteins and carbohydrates, maintains the structural integrity of the heart and other muscles, and aids in muscle contraction. Good sources include green leafy vegetables, nuts, legumes, bananas, and whole-grain products. A deficiency may result from persistent vomiting or diarrhea, kidney disease, general malnutrition, alcoholism, and the use of certain medications. The daily requirement is 280 milligrams for women and 350 milligrams for men.

Phosphorus Phosphorus is involved in bone and tooth formation, chemical reactions in the body, and energy production. It is found in dairy foods, animal foods, fish, cereals, nuts, and legumes. A deficiency of phosphorus can cause gastrointestinal, blood cell, and other disorders. Toxicity is harmful as well, especially in people with kidney disorders. Too much phosphorus in the blood can decrease blood calcium levels and cause bone loss. The daily requirement is 800 milligrams for adults 25 and over.

Selenium Selenium works with vitamin E to aid metabolism, growth, and fertility. It is found in seafood, kidney, liver, meats, grain products, and seeds. A daily dietary intake of 55 micrograms for women and 70 micrograms for men is recommended.

Minerals with Estimated Safe and Adequate Dietary Intakes When data were sufficient to estimate a range of requirements—but insufficient for developing an RDA—the Food and Nutrition Board established a category of safe and adequate intakes for essential nutrients. The minerals in this category are copper, fluoride, chromium, manganese, and molybdenum.

Copper Copper interacts with iron to form hemoglobin and red blood cells. It can be obtained through a wide variety of foods, such as liver, seafood, nuts and seeds, and whole-grain products. Copper deficiency can cause anemia and central nervous system problems. The safe and adequate range of dietary copper for adults is 1.5 to 3.0 milligrams per day.

Fluoride Fluoride is another contributor to bone and tooth formation, and it protects against tooth decay. Many municipal water supplies are fluoridated, and the mineral is contained in saltwater fish, tea, and fluoridated toothpaste.

Fluoride deficiency may predispose people to cavities and osteoporosis. Excess fluoride can cause discoloration and pitting of the teeth as well as other conditions. The range of safe and adequate intake for adults is 1.5 to 4.0 milligrams per day.

Chromium Chromium is essential for the body to use glucose, the primary energy source for cells. Foods containing chromium include calf's liver, American cheese, and wheat germ. A range of intakes between 50 and 200 micrograms per day is considered safe and adequate for adults.

Manganese Manganese is part of several cell enzymes. It is also essential for bone formation and maintenance, insulin production, and nutrient metabolism. It is found in whole-grain products, fruits, vegetables, and tea. A daily dietary intake of 2 to 5 milligrams for adults is recommended.

Molybdenum Molybdenum helps in the metabolism of the mineral sulfur and the production of uric acid. The best sources are legumes, whole grains, milk, and organ meats such as liver and kidneys. The recommended range for dietary intake is 75 to 250 micrograms per day for adults.

Water

Water has no caloric value, but it contributes about 65% of body weight and is essential to the body's normal functioning. In general, water helps provide the body with other nutrients it needs and helps rid the body of what it does not need. Water has many functions, including:

- Helping to maintain the balance of all the fluids in the body.
- Lubricating the body's moving parts.
- Dissolving chemicals and nutrients.
- Aiding in digestion.
- Helping to transport nutrients and secretions throughout the body.
- Flushing out wastes.
- Regulating body temperature through perspiration.

The amount of water in the body directly affects the concentration and distribution of body fluids and all the functions related to them. The body maintains a careful balance between water consumed (in foods and beverages) and water lost (through urination, perspiration, and respiration). In a healthy fluid balance, water input equals water output. Measuring an ill person's level of water intake and output can help determine the best fluid replacement regimen to use.

People obtain most of their water from beverages such as tap water, milk, and fruit juices as well as coffee, tea, and soft drinks. On average, a person needs to drink six to eight glasses of water a day to maintain a healthy water balance. The daily need for water varies with size and age, the temperatures to which the person is exposed, the degree of physical exertion, and the water content of the foods the person eats. Someone who is eating mostly foods with a high water content, such as fruits and vegetables, can drink a little less water than someone who is eating mostly foods with a low water content.

If people get too little water or lose too much water through vomiting, diarrhea, burns, or perspiration, they become dehydrated. Signs and symptoms of **dehydration** include dry lips and mucous membranes, weakness, lethargy, decreased urine output, and increased thirst. Severe dehydration can lead to hypovolemia, a reduction in the volume of blood in the body. Severe hypovolemia can result in inadequate blood pressure, which affects the functioning of the heart, central nervous system, and various organs—a condition known as hypovolemic shock. If dehydration progresses so that water is lost from body cells, death usually occurs within a few days. Patients should know whether they are to drink extra fluids to replace fluids lost in an illness or to help rid the body of waste.

Principal Electrolytes and Other Nutrients of Special Interest

The principal electrolytes are essential to normal body functioning. Other nutrients, such as antioxidants, also merit special mention.

Principal Electrolytes Although the principal electrolytes in the body—sodium, potassium, and chloride—are often excluded from lists of nutrients, they are essential dietary components. Electrolytes play an important role in maintaining body functions, such as normal heart rhythm.

Sodium Sodium (Na) maintains fluid and acid-base balances, assists in the transport of glucose, and maintains normal conditions inside and outside cells. Salt is the main dietary source of sodium, and high salt intakes are normally associated with a diet high in processed foods. Too much sodium can be associated with high blood pressure in salt-sensitive individuals. It is recommended that daily sodium intake be limited to 2.4 grams or less, although many Americans consume far more.

Potassium Potassium (K) is a crucial element in the maintenance of muscle contraction and fluid and electrolyte balance. It contributes to acid-base balance and the transmission of nerve impulses. Its role in fluid balance helps regulate blood pressure. Potassium occurs in unprocessed foods, particularly in fruits such as bananas, raisins, and oranges; many vegetables; and fresh meats (Figure 55-8). The minimum requirement is 1,600 to 2,000 milligrams per day.

Chloride Chloride (Cl) is essential in maintaining fluid and electrolyte balance, and it is a necessary component of hydrochloric acid, secreted into the stomach during digestion of food. Because dietary chloride comes almost entirely from sodium chloride, sources are essentially the same as those of sodium.

Antioxidants **Antioxidants** are chemical agents that fight certain cell-destroying chemical substances called *free radicals.* In fact, antioxidants may help ward off cancer and heart disease by neutralizing free radicals, which are by-products of normal metabolism that also may form as a result of exposure to various damaging factors such as cigarette smoke, alcohol, or X-rays. Antioxidants may be added to foods and cosmetics as preservatives. The nutrients beta-carotene, vitamin C, vitamin E, and selenium are natural antioxidants (Figure 55-9).

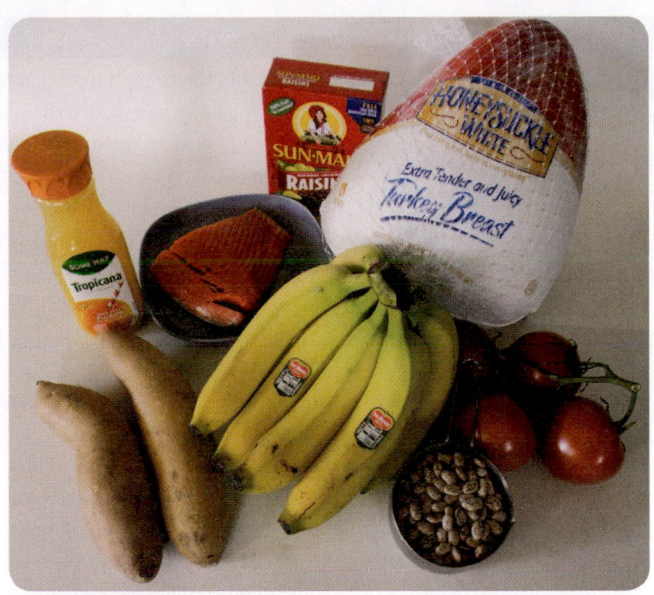

FIGURE 55-8   These foods are good sources of potassium.
© McGraw-Hill Education. David Moyer, photographer.

▶ Dietary Guidelines   LO 55.3

Dietary guidelines exist to help people get proper nutrition, reduce the occurrence of disease, and control their weight. These recommendations are designed to encourage healthy eating habits.

Dietary guidelines suggest the types and quantities of food that people should eat each day. They also may contain recommendations about which types of foods to limit and which types of foods to increase.

USDA Dietary Guidelines for Americans

The US Department of Agriculture (USDA) and the US Department of Health and Human Services updated their *Dietary Guidelines for Americans* in 2015. These guidelines encourage people to eat a balanced diet, limit consumption of less nutritious foods, increase physical activity, and make good nutritional decisions consistently.

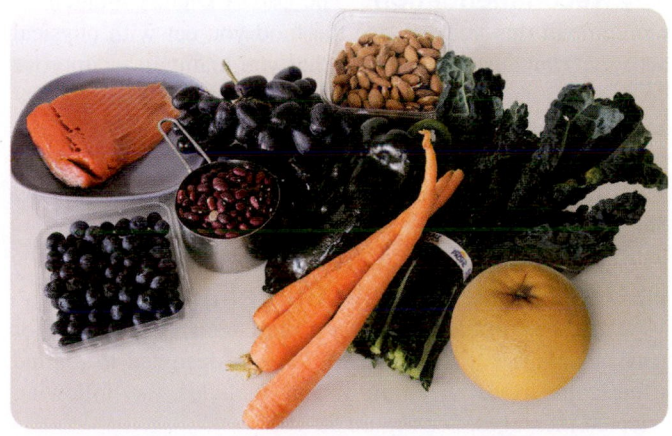

FIGURE 55-9   Antioxidants are substances in food that may offer protection against certain chronic diseases. Foods rich in beta-carotene, vitamin C, vitamin E, and selenium contain antioxidants.
© McGraw-Hill Education. David Moyer, photographer.

TABLE 55-4 USDA Dietary Guidelines Key Recommendations

Balancing calories to manage weight	• Promote healthy weight through improved eating and physical activity behaviors. • Control total calorie intake to manage body weight. For people who are overweight or obese, this will mean consuming fewer calories from foods and beverages. • Maintain appropriate calorie balance during each stage of life: childhood, adolescence, adulthood, pregnancy and breast-feeding, and older age.
Foods and food components to reduce	• Reduce daily sodium intake to less than 2,300 milligrams (mg). Further reduce intake to 1,500 mg among people who are 51 and older and those of any age who are African American or have hypertension, diabetes, or chronic kidney disease. • Consume less than 10% of calories from saturated fatty acids by replacing them with monounsaturated and polyunsaturated fatty acids. • Consume less than 300 mg per day of dietary cholesterol. • Keep trans fatty acid consumption as low as possible by limiting foods that contain synthetic sources of trans fats and by limiting other solid fats. • Reduce the intake of calories from solid fats and added sugars, but do not increase the use of low-calorie sweeteners to reduce sugar intake. • Limit the consumption of foods that contain refined grains, especially refined grain foods that contain solid fats, added sugars, and sodium. • If alcohol is consumed, it should be consumed in moderation (up to one drink per day for women and two drinks per day for men) and only by adults of legal drinking age.
Food and nutrients to increase (within calorie needs)	• Increase vegetable and fruit intake. • Eat a variety of vegetables, especially dark green, red and orange, beans, and peas. • Consume at least half of all grains as whole grains. • Increase intake of fat-free or low-fat milk and milk products. • Choose a variety of protein foods, which include seafood, lean meat and poultry, eggs, beans and peas, soy products, and unsalted nuts and seeds. • Increase the amount and variety of seafood consumed by choosing seafood in place of some meat and poultry. • Replace protein foods that are higher in solid fats with choices that are lower in solid fats and calories and/or are sources of oils. • Use oils to replace solid fats where possible. • Choose foods that provide more potassium, dietary fiber, calcium, and vitamin D, which are nutrients of concern in American diets.
Building healthy eating patterns	• Select an eating pattern that meets nutrient needs at an appropriate calorie level. • Monitor foods and beverages consumed, and their fit within a healthy eating pattern. • Follow food safety recommendations when preparing and eating foods.

Key Recommendations The USDA Dietary Guidelines recommend that you balance the food you eat with physical activity. They also recommend that you maintain or improve your weight to help reduce your chances of high blood pressure, heart disease, stroke, some types of cancer, and diabetes. Specific recommendations are included in Table 55-4. The latest information can be found at http://www.health.gov/dietaryguidelines/.

USDA Choose MyPlate Guidelines

MyPlate is an initiative based on the Dietary Guidelines for Americans discussed earlier. MyPlate is designed to remind Americans to eat healthfully and includes the following selected messages. See Figure 55-10.

Balancing Calories

• Enjoy your food, but eat less.
• Avoid oversized portions.

Foods to Increase

• Make half your plate fruits and vegetables.
• Make at least half your grains whole grains.
• Switch to fat-free or low-fat (1%) milk.

Foods to Reduce

• Compare sodium in foods such as soup, bread, and frozen meals—and choose foods with lower numbers.
• Drink water instead of sugary drinks.

You can educate patients to help them make better food choices by following the latest guidelines and using the Super-Tracker and other tools found at http://www.choosemyplate.gov.

American Cancer Society Nutritional and Physical Activity Guidelines

The American Cancer Society updated its nutritional and physical activity guidelines in 2011 to aid in the prevention of cancer.

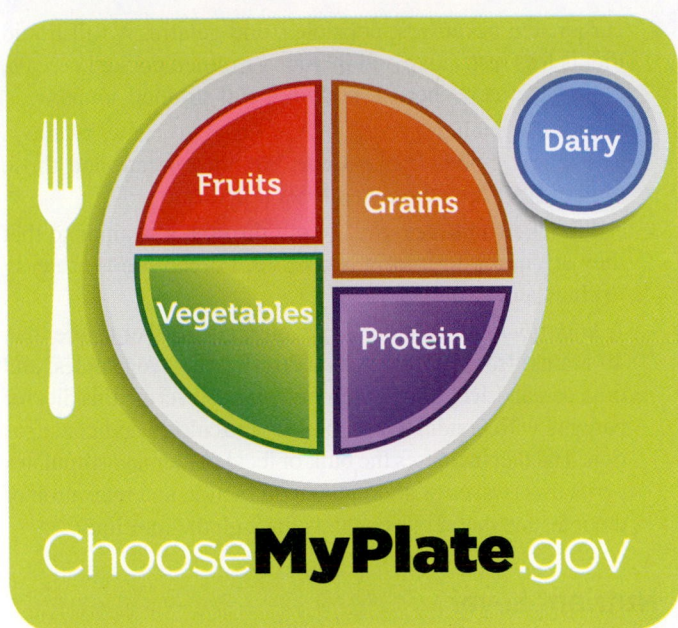

FIGURE 55-10 MyPlate is designed to remind Americans to make healthful food choices.
USDA

A summary of these guidelines is found in Table 55-5. For more information, visit its website at http://www.cancer.org.

Assessing Nutritional Levels   LO 55.4

Licensed practitioners assess a patient's nutritional status by analyzing age, health status, height, weight, type of body frame, body circumference, percentage of body fat, body mass

index, nutritional and exercise patterns, and energy needs. They accomplish this assessment through direct measurement as well as through questionnaires and interviews. During the analysis, practitioners take into account individual factors such as culture, beliefs, lifestyle, and education.

Body mass index (BMI) is a measure of body fat based on height and weight that applies to adult men and women. Body mass index calculators are available online. One example is at the National Heart, Lung, and Blood Institute's website. BMI is discussed in the *Vital Signs and Measurements* chapter.

To measure fat as a percentage of body weight, practitioners may perform a *skinfold test,* measuring the thickness of a fold of skin with a caliper (Figure 55-11). The test indicates the total percentage of fat because about 50% of body fat is just below the skin and the volume of fat below the skin is related to the volume of inner fat. A trained individual must perform this test, which must be precise to be reliable.

The optimal percentage of body fat differs between men and women. For males younger than age 50, it is 10% to 14%; age 50 and older, 12% to 19%. In females younger than age 50, it is 14% to 23%; age 50 and older, 16% to 25%. Aging usually changes the ratio a bit because some muscle tissue is replaced by fat, even if weight remains constant.

▸ Modified Diets   LO 55.5

A person's diet has a significant effect on health, appearance, and recovery from disease. After a licensed practitioner or dietitian has established a patient's nutritional status, any necessary or beneficial dietary adjustments can be instituted. Dietary modification may be used alone or in combination with other therapies to prevent or treat illness.

TABLE 55-5	Summary of the American Cancer Society Guidelines on Nutrition and Physical Activity for Cancer Prevention
Recommendations for Individual Choices	
Achieve and maintain a healthy weight throughout life.	• Be as lean as possible throughout life without being underweight. • Avoid excess weight gain at all ages. For those who are overweight or obese, losing even a small amount of weight has health benefits and is a good place to start. • Get regular physical activity and limit intake of high-calorie foods and drinks as keys to help maintain a healthy weight.
Be a physically active.	• Adults: Get at least 150 minutes of moderate-intensity or 75 minutes of vigorous-intensity activity each week (or a combination of these), preferably spread throughout the week. • Children and teens: Get at least 1 hour of moderate- or vigorous-intensity activity each day, with vigorous activity on at least 3 days each week. • Limit sedentary behavior such as sitting, lying down, watching TV, and other forms of screen-based entertainment. • Doing some physical activity above usual activities, no matter what one's level of activity, can have many health benefits.
Eat a healthy diet, with an emphasis on plant foods.	• Choose foods and drinks in amounts that help you get to and maintain a healthy weight. • Limit how much processed meat and red meat you eat. • Eat at least 2½ cups of vegetables and fruits each day. • Choose whole grains instead of refined grain products.
If you drink alcohol, limit your intake.	• Drink no more than one drink per day for women or two per day for men.

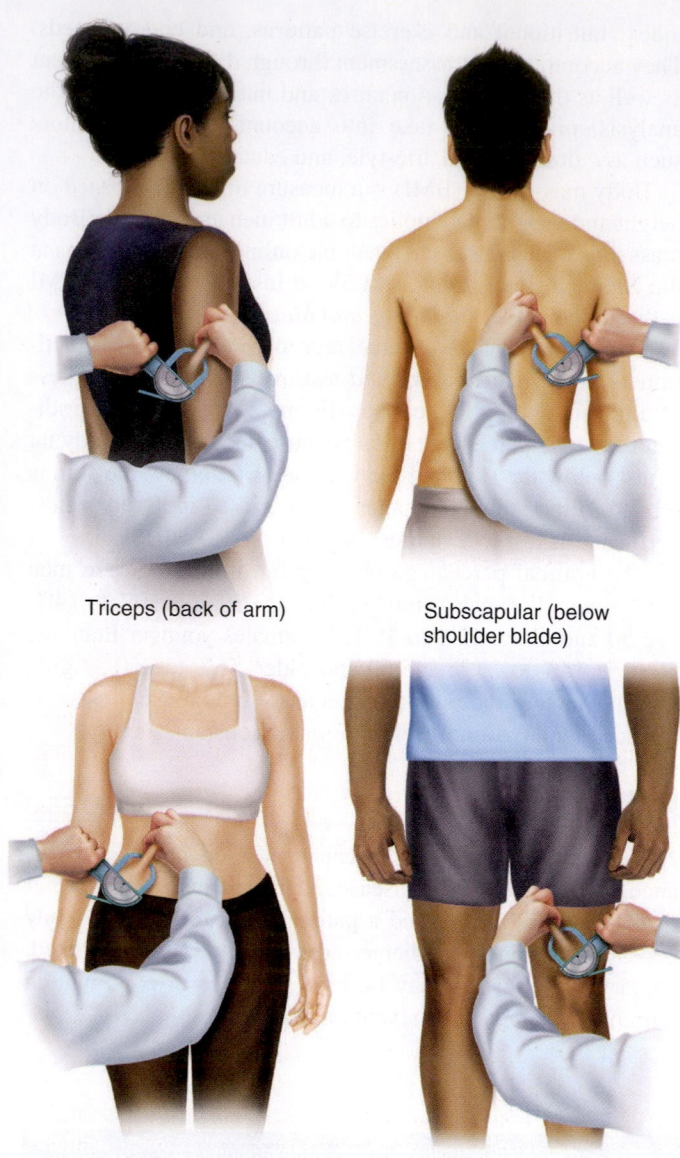

Triceps (back of arm)

Subscapular (below shoulder blade)

Suprailiac (above hipbone)

Thigh (front)

FIGURE 55-11 To estimate an individual's body fat percentage, a professional uses a tool called a caliper to measure the thickness of a fold of skin at one or more points on the body.

Licensed practitioners work with dietitians to determine the best diet therapy to initiate for individual patients. Diet therapy is based on many factors, including particular foods and nutrients associated with different diseases or body states. Specific types of dietary modifications include changes in texture, nutrient level, frequency and timing of meals, and exclusions.

Texture

A patient may need changes in food consistency as a result of swallowing, chewing, or other gastrointestinal problems or to fulfill short-term needs that result from events such as laboratory tests or surgical procedures. The following special diets are based on texture:

- A *clear-liquid diet* consists solely of foods that you can see through, such as tea, broth, noncitrus juices, clear

carbonated beverages, popsicles, and gelatin. A full-liquid diet is less restrictive and includes strained cooked cereals, plain ice cream, sherbet, pudding, and strained soups.

- A *soft diet* includes foods that are easy to chew, swallow, and digest. Foods that patients cannot tolerate and those high in fiber are eliminated from this diet.
- All foods in a *puréed diet* are put through a strainer so that they are in the form of a semisolid. Puréed foods are easy to chew and swallow.
- A *high-fiber diet* contains large amounts of fiber (more than 40 grams) from sources such as fresh fruits, vegetables, and bran cereal. Licensed practitioners may prescribe this diet for patients with conditions such as diverticulosis and constipation. The diet increases the bulk of fecal matter and stimulates peristalsis (waves of alternating contraction and relaxation of the intestine that move contents through the intestine).

Nutrient Level

Licensed practitioners may make nutrient-level modifications in patients' diets before or after surgical or medical procedures or for patients who have specific conditions. Some of these types of diets are discussed in more detail in the next section. The following special diets are based on nutrient levels:

- Practitioners may prescribe *low-sodium diets* for patients who suffer from many disease conditions such as those affecting the cardiovascular or urinary system, liver, pancreas, and gallbladder, including edema and hypertension. The typical American diet contains 2 to 5 grams of sodium daily. Following are sodium-restricted dietary levels:
  - Mild restriction, 2 to 3 grams: reduce salt in cooking, add no salt at the table, and avoid processed foods
  - Moderate restriction, 1 gram per day: add no salt in cooking or at the table and limit high-sodium vegetables, meat, and milk
  - Severe restriction, 500 milligrams per day: greatly limit high-sodium vegetables, meat, milk, and eggs
- Practitioners recommend *low-cholesterol diets* for patients with high blood cholesterol levels. Such diets involve replacing saturated fats with unsaturated fats, using low-fat or nonfat cooking methods, and restricting fatty foods.
- Practitioners may prescribe *reduced-calorie diets* to promote weight loss in patients who are overweight.
- Practitioners may recommend *low-tyramine diets* for patients who have migraine headaches and patients who are taking certain antidepressant drugs. The compound tyramine is found in aged cheeses, red wine, beer, cream, chocolate, and yeast.
- Practitioners may order *high-calorie, high-protein diets* for patients who have infections, are recovering from burns or surgery, or have had weight loss caused by a severe illness. Food intake is increased to provide 3,000 to 5,000 calories per day. Protein usually accounts for the greatest caloric increase in these diets.
- Practitioners may prescribe *high-carbohydrate diets* for patients with kidney diseases and some cardiac conditions.

TABLE 55-6 Food Label Terms and Definitions

Term	Definition
Low calorie	Less than or equal to 40 calories per serving
Reduced calorie	At least 25% fewer calories per serving than the food it replaces
Cholesterol free	Less than or equal to 2 mg cholesterol per serving
Low cholesterol	Less than or equal to 20 mg cholesterol per serving
Reduced cholesterol	At least 25% less cholesterol per serving than the food it replaces
Low fat	Less than or equal to 3 g fat per serving
Reduced fat	At least 25% less fat per serving than the food it replaces
Sodium free	Less than or equal to 5 mg sodium per serving
Very low sodium	Less than or equal to 35 mg sodium per serving
Low sodium	Less than or equal to 140 mg sodium per serving
Reduced sodium	At least 25% less sodium per serving than the food it replaces

Source: US Department of Health and Human Services, Food and Drug Administration.

You can help patients who need to make nutrient-level modifications by teaching them how to read food labels. All packaged foods carry a Nutrition Facts label that contains information on the ingredients, major nutrients, and recommended amounts of key nutrients in daily diets. Procedure 55-1, at the end of this chapter, explains how to educate patients about reading food labels. You also can teach patients how to interpret the terms on food labels (Table 55-6). Understanding marketing terms simplifies the process of buying the right foods to meet special dietary needs.

Frequency and Timing of Meals

A patient's diet also may be modified by adjusting the standard three-meal pattern. The goal may be to eat six small meals rather than three large meals to minimize stress on organs affected by disease conditions—as in patients with an ulcer or a hiatal hernia. Six small meals also may be recommended to help regulate the blood sugar for patients with hypoglycemia, or low blood glucose. In other cases, meals may simply be timed to follow tests or therapeutic procedures.

Exclusion of Certain Foods

Licensed practitioners may order that specific foods be omitted from patients' diets for health reasons.

- In a *bland diet*, specific foods that cause irritation are eliminated, along with caffeine, alcohol, nicotine, aspirin, and some spices. A typical bland diet includes easily digested foods such as mashed potatoes and gelatins. Raw fruits and vegetables, whole-grain foods, and very hot or cold items are among foods to avoid. A practitioner may prescribe this type of diet for a patient with a peptic ulcer, for example. A patient with diverticulosis may be on a bland diet and

be restricted from eating nuts and seeds. In *diverticulosis* small pockets in the large intestine get blocked with food, causing pain and inflammation in the abdomen.

- *Exclusion diets* are prescribed for patients who have food intolerances. These diets eliminate foods that contain the offending substances but still provide the nutrients needed for good health. Intolerance to lactose, the sugar in milk, is fairly common. Intolerance to the amino acid phenylalanine—a condition present at birth—is fairly rare but very serious. Infants born in hospitals in the United States are tested for this intolerance because if these infants were to receive a standard diet, they would develop severe mental disability. People with this condition, known as phenylketonuria (PKU), must be vigilant about checking labels on prepared foods as well as knowledgeable about the phenylalanine content of fresh foods.

Intolerance to **gluten,** a protein substance found naturally in wheat, barley, and rye, can result from several conditions, including celiac disease and non-celiac gluten sensitivity (NCGS). Gluten consumption in non-celiac gluten–sensitive patients can cause intestinal symptoms such as bloating and nausea. Unlike with NCGS, **celiac disease** is an autoimmune reaction to gluten. After eating gluten, the patient with celiac disease experiences damage to the small intestine, which causes reduction in the absorption of nutrients from foods. Patients with gluten intolerance should eat only gluten-free foods. The FDA has established specific guidelines for labeling foods "gluten-free" so that gluten-intolerant individuals can select foods with more confidence that they will not contain gluten.

▶ Patients with Specific Nutritional Needs   LO 55.6

A variety of conditions require special diets or nutrients. In situations such as those that follow, you may need to educate patients about their diets and answer their questions. You may need to provide encouragement and emotional support and teach patients' caregivers how to perform physical tasks, such as holding utensils for patients during meals.

Patients with Allergies

Some patients have food allergies. Usually, specific foods must be eliminated from or restricted in an allergic patient's diet. Procedure 55-2, at the end of this chapter, provides information on discussing with the patient potential dangers of common foods and reactions to those foods.

Some of the most common food allergens are wheat, milk, eggs, shellfish, peanuts, and chocolate. The licensed practitioner may confirm an allergy by eliminating and then reintroducing the patient's suspect foods one by one. The patient's allergy may decrease over time through systematic desensitization by means of allergy shots and other regimens.

If a food that is being eliminated or restricted was a primary source of nutrients for the patient, then the practitioner must adjust the diet to include another source of those nutrients. For example, for a baby who is allergic to milk, the licensed practitioner may recommend a milk-substitute formula.

Regardless of how careful they try to be, patients with food allergies may occasionally ingest a food to which they are allergic. It is a good idea to prepare the patient by explaining how to treat an allergic reaction. For mild reactions, an over-the-counter antihistamine such as Benadryl® may reduce the symptoms. For severe reactions, the patient should be transported to the nearest emergency room or urgent care center, where a licensed practitioner will order a shot of epinephrine. For some patients with severe allergies, the licensed practitioner may prescribe epinephrine in the form of an EpiPen® that the patient can self-administer as a shot immediately when an allergic reaction begins. Researchers are currently experimenting with desensitization methods that may help reduce the severity of a person's reaction to food allergens.

Patients with Anemia

Iron deficiency anemia, the most common type of anemia, is usually caused by chronic blood loss, a lack of iron in the diet, impaired intestinal absorption of iron, or an increased need for iron, as in pregnancy. A patient may need to take iron supplements and ingest more dietary iron as part of the treatment for this disorder. Foods high in iron include liver, egg yolks, dark green vegetables, beans, some dried fruits, and fortified breads and cereals.

Patients with Cancer

Many patients being treated for cancer undergo weight loss resulting both from the cancer and from treatments involving radiation or chemotherapy. To help their bodies fight off the cancer, it is especially important that they get enough protein because protein is needed to regenerate cells to replace the cells destroyed by the cancer and cancer treatments. These patients also may need to increase their intake of B vitamins and vitamins A, C, D, and E to support tissue growth and repair and promote efficient metabolism and use of all nutrients in the diet.

Encourage patients with cancer to follow the diet the licensed practitioner sets for them. Patients may find this difficult because cancer often produces loss of appetite. They also may experience nausea and vomiting. Educate patients and their caregivers about ways to make food more appealing and easier to digest. Consuming small meals at frequent intervals may help. Patients also may follow a liquid diet. Bringing food to room temperature or chilling it slightly may reduce food odors that can trigger nausea. In some cases, especially during cancer treatment, the practitioner will prescribe medications to reduce the nausea and thus increase the patient's appetite.

Patients with Diabetes

A special diet is one of the foundations of treatment for diabetes. Dietary guidelines for patients with diabetes must not only provide them with adequate nutrition but also keep their blood sugar level under control and interact appropriately with medication.

The diet a practitioner or dietitian prescribes for someone with diabetes includes specific numbers of calories, meals per day, amount of carbohydrates, and amounts of other nutrients. As a way to simplify the diet, a system of **food exchanges** is used. All food exchanges in a particular food category provide the same amounts of protein, fat, and carbohydrates.

The list of exchanges is divided into seven categories—nonstarchy vegetables, fruits, starches, meats/meat alternatives, fats, milk, and sweets—and indicates how large a portion of each food in a category is equal to one "exchange" of food in that category. This information tells patients what portions of specific foods are interchangeable and whether they are eating the correct amounts of those foods. The list includes a variety of foods from which patients make their selections. It is important that patients with diabetes not skip a meal because skipping meals disturbs the balance of blood sugar and metabolism. Table 55-7 provides example food exchanges recommended for diabetics. These lists also can be obtained from a registered dietitian or the American Diabetes Association.

Patients with diabetes who are dependent on insulin should eat regular meals at consistent times. Skipping or delaying meals can result in hypoglycemia or an insulin reaction. The healthcare team specifies the proportion of carbohydrates and calories in meals, depending on the type of insulin each patient uses and the timing of injections.

Fiber is also important for patients who have diabetes. Fiber can sometimes prevent a sharp rise in blood glucose after a meal and may reduce the amount of insulin needed. It is therefore recommended that people with diabetes gradually increase their fiber intake until it is at about 45 grams per day.

Patients with Heart Disease

Coronary heart disease that is caused by atherosclerosis usually results from hyperlipidemia, or an excess of lipids in the bloodstream. Left untreated, this condition can lead to angina, heart attack, or stroke.

Patients can significantly lower their risk by reducing their blood cholesterol levels and losing weight if they are overweight. Patients who have coronary heart disease usually must reduce their consumption of fats to a level that provides less than 30% of their total caloric intake. Saturated fats should provide less than 10% of their caloric intake. Patients who have had a heart attack or are at increased risk for a heart attack are also encouraged to increase their consumption of soluble fiber.

As a medical assistant, your role with these patients is to encourage them to follow the nutritional regimen prescribed by the licensed practitioner.

Patients with Hypertension

Hypertension (high blood pressure) is a condition that affects more than 20% of American adults. Nutritional therapy for patients with hypertension involves:

- Restricting sodium intake to 2 to 3 grams per day, especially in salt-sensitive individuals.
- Increasing potassium intake through consumption of fresh fruits and vegetables, especially when taking certain medications.
- Ensuring adequate calcium intake to meet an RDA of 800 milligrams.
- Eliminating or reducing alcohol use.
- Decreasing total fat intake and obtaining no more than 10% of calories from saturated fats.

TABLE 55-7 Diabetic Food Exchange Table

Food Exchange	US Unit	Comments
Starches		
15 g Carb, 3 g Protein, 1 g Fat		• Most starches are a good source of B vitamins.
• English muffin	½	• Choose whole-grain foods such as 100% whole-wheat bread and flour, brown rice, and tortillas for nutrients and fiber.
• Graham crackers (2½-inch squares)	3	
• Bagel, large (4 ounces)	¼ (1 oz)	• Combine beans (starch and meat) with grains (starch) for their complementary proteins and fiber.
• Bread, pumpernickel, rye, white, whole-grain	1 slice (1 oz)	
• Bread, reduced calorie	2 slices (1½ oz)	• Combine grains (starch) with milk (milk exchange) or cheese (meat exchange) to complement proteins.
• Cereal: bran, oats, spoon-size shredded wheat, frosted cereals	½ cup	• Add 1 fat exchange for starchy foods prepared with fat.
• Cereal: unsweetened	¾ cup	
• Grits, cooked	½ cup	
• Tabbouleh, prepared	½ cup	
• Pasta, cooked	⅓ cup	
• Wild rice, cooked	½ cup	
• Corn	½ cup	
• Popcorn, popped	3 cups	
• Potato (large, baked with skin)	¼ (3 oz)	
• Potato, mashed	½ cup	
• Sweet potato	½ cup (4 oz)	
• Squash, acorn, butternut	1 cup	
Add 1 meat exchange for the following starches:		
• Baked beans	⅓ cup	
• Beans, cooked: black, garbanzo, kidney, lima, pinto, navy, white	½ cup	
• Peas, cooked: black-eyed, green	½ cup	
• Refried beans, canned	½ cup	
Vegetables (3–5 exchanges)		
5 g Carb, 2 g Protein		• Choose more dark green leafy and deep yellow vegetables such as spinach, broccoli, carrots, and peppers.
• Raw vegetables	1 cup	
• Cooked vegetables	½ cup	
Fruit (2–4 exchanges)		
15 g Carb		• Choose whole fruits for fiber.
Fresh fruit:		• Choose citrus fruits such as oranges, grapefruits, or tangerines.
• Apple, small (2 inches across)	1 (4 oz)	
• Berries: blackberries, blueberries	¾ cup	
• Grapefruit, large	½	
• Mango, cubed	½ cup	
• Orange, small	1 (6 oz)	
• Strawberries	¼ cup (13½ oz)	
Dried fruit:		
• Apple	4 rings	
• Prunes	3	
• Raisins	2tbsp	

(Continued)

TABLE 55-7   Diabetic Food Exchange Table

Food Exchange	US Unit	Comments
Canned fruit, unsweetened:		
• Applesauce, apricots, cherries, peaches, pears, pineapple, plums	½ cup	
• Grapefruit	¾ cup	
• Mandarin oranges	¾ cup	
Fruit juice, unsweetened:		
• Apple, grapefruit, orange, pineapple	½ cup (4 fl oz)	
Meat & Substitutes (5–7 exchanges)		
7 g Protein, 0–13 g Fat		• Choose leaner meats such as chicken, fish, and lean cuts of meat; add fat exchange for higher-fat meats and substitutes.
• Beef	1 oz	• Remove skin from poultry.
• Cheese	1 oz	• Limit frying or adding fat.
• Cottage cheese	¼ cup	• Have 2 servings of fish per week for omega-3 fatty acid.
• Egg whites	2	
• Egg substitutes	¼ cup	
• Fish, fresh or frozen	1 oz	
• Pork	1 oz	
• Bacon	2 slices	
• Poultry	1 oz	
• Peanut butter	1 tbsp	
• Tofu	½ cup	
Milk (2–3 exchanges)		
12 g Carb, 8 g Protein, 0–8 g Fat		• Choose lower-fat milks; add fat exchange for higher-fat milk.
• Milk	1 cup	
• Soy milk	1 cup	
• Rice drink, low-fat, flavored	1 cup (8 fl oz)	
• Yogurt, low-fat with fruit	⅔ cup (6 oz)	
Fat (use sparingly)		
5 g Fat		• Eat less fat.
• Almonds	6	• Eat less saturated fat, such as animal fat found in fattier meat, cheese, and butter; also eat less hydrogenated fat.
• Coconut, shredded	2 tbsp	• Check Nutrition Facts on food labels; 5 g Fat 5 1 Fat exchange.
• Oil: canola, olive, peanut, corn, safflower, soybean, sunflower	1 tsp	
• Mayonnaise	1 tsp (1 tbsp if reduced-fat)	
• Cream cheese	1 tbsp (1½ tbsp if reduced-fat)	
• Salad dressing	1 tbsp (2 tbsp if reduced-fat)	
• Peanuts	10	
• Avocado	2 tbsp (1 oz)	
• Butter or margarine	1 tsp	

Sources: Diet.com (http://www.diet.com/g/exchange-system), USDA National Agricultural Library (http://fnic.nal.usda.gov/diet-and-disease/diabetes/carbohydrate-counting-and-exchange-lists), and American Diabetes Association (http://www.diabetes.org/food-and-fitness/food/planning-meals/diabetes-meal-plans-and-a-healthy-diet.html) (Accessed October 6, 2015).

Patients with Lactose Sensitivity

Lactose is the sugar contained in human and animal milk. It must be broken down in the body by the enzyme lactase to enable the body to digest dairy products. In people from some parts of the world, lactase is present in the body until age 3 or 4, after which it all but disappears. As a result, after early childhood many people have trouble digesting foods that contain lactose and eliminate these foods from their diets. People who are especially sensitive to dietary lactose are often referred to as *lactose intolerant.*

Chemical preparations can help a person digest lactose. Those preparations may be added to certain foods, such as ice cream, for lactose-sensitive people. If people with a lactose sensitivity choose to avoid dairy products, they need to be sure to obtain protein and calcium from other sources.

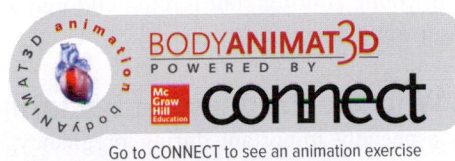

Go to CONNECT to see an animation exercise about *Digestion: Lactose Intolerance.*

Patients Who Are Overweight

More than two-thirds of American adults are overweight or obese. Seventeen percent of children age 2 to 19 are obese. Overweight patients weigh 10% to 20% more than is recommended for their height and gender. Patients who are more than 20% overweight are considered obese. Morbid obesity is when someone is more than 100 pounds overweight. Obesity can lead to medical complications such as elevated blood cholesterol levels, hypertension, diabetes, joint problems, respiratory problems, and heart disease. See *Educating the Patient* to learn more about how to help patients avoid these complications.

Approaches to Weight Loss Weight reduction may be approached with dietary modification alone, but an exercise program is usually included. Behavior modification is also a common element of weight-loss programs. In a weight-loss program, foods should be proportioned in accordance with dietary guidelines and the diet should be appealing and enjoyable. The goal is to have the patient decrease daily caloric intake and increase physical activity at an appropriate rate while remaining comfortable and healthy.

Weight loss will not occur unless patients expend more energy than they consume. Calculators are available online and in smartphone apps that help individuals determine how much they can eat and how much exercise will result in weight loss. Foods that are high in nutrients but low in calories are desirable.

One example of a healthy diet is the Dietary Approaches to Stop Hypertension (DASH) diet. Originally created to help reduce hypertension, the DASH diet is now considered one of the healthiest diets for weight loss as well. It emphasizes "real foods"—foods that do not contain additives. It is a low-sodium, high-fiber diet that emphasizes vegetables and fruits and includes plenty of sources of important minerals and vitamins. Versions are available for both vegetarians and nonvegetarians. Credible organizations, including the American Heart Association, the Mayo Clinic, and the National Heart, Lung, and Blood Institute, have endorsed this method.

The **behavior modification** facet of weight loss includes methods such as keeping a food diary to pinpoint overeating patterns, controlling the stimuli associated with overeating, and providing rewards for successful behavior. Weight-loss behaviors are important to maintain for a lifetime.

You can help overweight patients in their weight-loss efforts by teaching them to

- Eat slowly, because the message that the stomach is full takes 20 minutes to register with the brain.
- Eat five or six small meals daily.
- Be patient—reliable weight loss occurs over time, not immediately.

EDUCATING THE PATIENT
Preventing Obesity

Most organizations recommend the same general steps for preventing obesity: make healthy food and drink choices, get a moderate amount of exercise, and control calories. Many patients have heard this advice many times and may tend to tune it out. To prevent this, try to give patients some new information and tips they may not have heard before.

One method that patients may not be aware of is the need to avoid distractions while eating. Eating in front of the television or while reading a book or newspaper may seem relaxing, but when attention is distracted from eating, people tend to continue to eat even though they may feel full. The body signals when you have had enough to eat, but if your attention is on a good movie or the action in a book, you may not even notice that you are full.

A related tip is to concentrate on the food. By focusing all of the senses on the food being eaten, a person can enjoy and savor the food. This, in turn, can result in being satisfied with a smaller portion, which reduces calorie intake.

Finally, explain to patients the importance of getting sufficient sleep. Although the amount of sleep needed varies with the individual, research has provided evidence that getting a good night's sleep can actually help keep a person at a healthier weight. In general, adults need 7 to 8 hours of sleep per night. The number of hours per night increases as a person's age decreases; adolescents may need up to 9.25 hours per night, while toddlers may need up to 14 hours per night.

Motivation and Education Patients who are trying to lose weight may have trouble with motivation. You may be able to introduce the patient to low-calorie or low-fat recipes, for instance, and positively reinforce the patient's efforts by complimenting small, gradual successes.

Tell patients that fad weight-loss methods can lead to vitamin, mineral, and protein deficiency; serious medical disorders; and even death. Use the following criteria to identify fad diets:

- They promise ease and comfort in weight loss.
- They include only a few foods, such as grapefruit or low-protein foods.
- They require the purchase of a secret ingredient or pill.
- They are often published in a book or magazine.

Truly effective weight-loss regimens usually possess the following qualities:

- They include a variety of foods that contain adequate nutrients.
- They include an activity component.
- They may be safely followed over a long period of time.

An effective program is one in which the patient is able to lose weight (including fat) gradually and constantly, with some plateaus, and then maintain the loss indefinitely afterward. You can help patients with the challenge of maintaining their weight loss by recommending a reputable weight-loss group or support group that will help them make the necessary lifestyle changes and remain motivated.

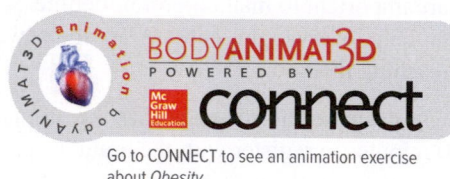

Go to CONNECT to see an animation exercise about *Obesity.*

Pediatric Patients

During the first year of life, an infant experiences the most rapid period of growth and development that occurs during the lifespan. Breast milk is the best food for an infant up to 6 months of age. It contains the right amount of fat, sugar, water, and protein for an infant's growth and development. Breast-feeding saves time and money and helps the mother recover as well as reduces the risk of breast and ovarian cancers. If breast-feeding is not an option, infant formula is recommended by the licensed practitioner. Regular, full-fat cow's milk should not be given to a child until after his or her first birthday.

Solid foods are introduced gradually starting at age 4 to 6 months. Infants should be able to hold their head up while sitting, open their mouth, swallow, and have an interest in food. The following are some basic guidelines for introducing foods to infants and toddlers:

- About 4 to 6 months: iron-fortified, single-grain baby cereal; strained/puréed vegetables and fruit
- 6 to 9 months: strained meats/poultry; mixtures of strained vegetables and fruits; chunky, soft prepared baby foods; egg yolk; yogurt; cottage cheese

- 9 to 12 months: soft, finely chopped foods; soft combination foods such as casseroles; macaroni and cheese; spaghetti; cheese; beans
- Over 12 months: toddler foods; family foods; fiber foods; whole cow's milk

Additional detailed information is available about the nutritional requirements for infants and children at the US Department of Agriculture website, http://www.usda.gov. Parents should be educated about these guidelines during their visits to the pediatrician's office.

The pace of growth is steadier and slower during childhood, with growth spurts throughout. Nutritional needs change to reflect growth, maturation, and increasing activity levels. Vitamin D and calcium are critical to tooth and bone formation, and fluoride strengthens teeth. Hunger regulates food intake in young children, but forcing children to eat can promote eating habits that lead to obesity.

Patients Who Are Pregnant or Lactating

Nutrition is especially important during pregnancy, when it provides for the normal growth and health of the baby as well as the health of the pregnant woman. Licensed practitioners recommend that pregnant women gain a certain amount of weight during each trimester of pregnancy, with a total weight gain of about 25 to 35 pounds. The rate of weight gain should be 2 to 5 pounds in the first trimester and about 1 pound per week after that. Gaining too little or too much weight during pregnancy can result in serious complications. See Figure 55-12.

Here are some nutritional suggestions for pregnant women:

- An additional 10 to 15 grams of protein a day in the form of meat, poultry, fish, eggs, and dairy products
- 1,200 milligrams of calcium a day, preferably in the form of low-fat dairy products such as skim milk

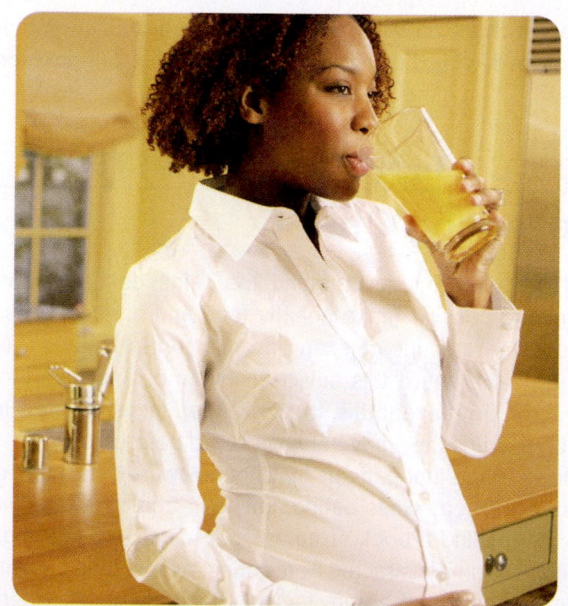

FIGURE 55-12 Pregnant patients should follow special nutritional guidelines to help ensure a healthy baby and mother.
© Brand X Pictures/Jupiterimages RF

- 30 milligrams of iron a day through meat, liver, egg yolks, grains, leafy vegetables, nuts, dried fruits, legumes, and supplements (it is difficult to meet the daily need with food alone)
- Folic acid intake of 400 micrograms a day through leafy vegetables, yeast, and liver as well as supplements
- Adequate fiber intake to prevent the constipation that often accompanies pregnancy

Breast-feeding has specific nutritional and dietary requirements as well, because breast milk is nutrient-rich and the body requires considerable energy and nutrients to produce it. The infant depends on this milk for the extensive growth that takes place during the first months of life. Lactating women need to consume an additional 500 calories and an additional 12 to 19 grams of protein per day as well as 260 to 280 micrograms of folic acid and 1,200 milligrams of calcium.

Patients Requiring Supplements and/or Parenteral Nutrition

When a patient has a loss or lack of appetite or cannot tolerate a normal meal, the licensed practitioner may prescribe a specially formulated food supplement that provides protein, carbohydrates, fat, vitamins, and minerals. A patient who is chronically ill, underweight, or anemic or who has just undergone surgery may take supplements orally or through a tube to the stomach or small intestine. If the supplement is being taken orally, encourage the patient to follow the prescribed directions.

When patients cannot tolerate receiving supplements enterally (by way of the digestive tract), they may be fed parenterally. **Parenteral nutrition** is provided to patients as specially prepared nutrients injected directly into their veins rather than given by mouth. Because a parenteral feeding bypasses the digestive system, the nutrients it contains must already be in a form the body can use as they enter the blood.

Patients Undergoing Drug Therapy

Drugs may change a patient's nutritional status and needs. Long-term drug therapy and the need to take multiple medications make close nutritional monitoring a high priority.

Drug therapy can cause a change in food intake, a change in the body's absorption of a nutrient, or both. Likewise, foods can interfere with the metabolism and action of a drug. For example, laxatives and certain other types of drugs may suppress the appetite. Antihistamines, alcohol, insulin, thyroid hormones, and some other drugs can stimulate appetite. Anesthetics can interfere with taste. Calcium in milk can diminish the absorption of some antibiotics. Be sure to discuss any possible interactions with the licensed practitioner or dietitian before discussing diet and drug regimens with a patient.

▶ Eating Disorders   LO 55.7

Eating disorders, characterized by extremely harmful eating behavior, can lead to health problems. These disorders can damage the body and even cause death. They are most common in adolescent girls and young women, although 10% to 15% of patients with eating disorders are male. Refer to the *Points on Practice* feature to identify the signs and symptoms of common eating disorders.

Anorexia Nervosa

Anorexia nervosa is an eating disorder in which people starve themselves. They fear that if they lose control of eating, they will become grossly overweight. They lose an excessive amount of weight and become malnourished, and women often stop menstruating. The typical patient with anorexia nervosa is a high-achieving, white female in her teens or early 20s. The numbers of children and middle-aged women who suffer from the disorder, however, have been increasing. The cause of anorexia remains unknown, but risk factors include

- Coming from a family that has problems with alcoholism.
- Suffering a childhood trauma, such as sexual abuse (20% to 50% of patients were sexually abused).
- Having a high stress level.
- Suffering from depression.
- Suffering from shame and low self-esteem.
- Having an extreme need to be in control.

It also has been noted that anorexia tends to run in families. The victim of anorexia often uses food as a way to deal with the psychological effects of trauma by numbing the emotions or as a means of getting some measure of control in life. Anorexia can be precipitated by any major life change.

This disorder can be fatal. The first stage of treatment is to restore normal nutrition. Patients may need to be hospitalized and fed intravenously or by nasogastric tube, which enters through the nose and delivers food into the stomach. Hospitalization may be necessary because patients with excessive weight loss may develop cardiac and other medical disorders. These patients also may be at risk for suicide. The hospital stay may eventually provide patients with the structure and support they need to establish healthy eating patterns.

Psychotherapy is essential and involves a combination of one-on-one and group therapy. Therapy groups that are single-sex rather than coed are preferable because of the different gender and peer group issues men and women face. Licensed practitioners may prescribe medication for depression and anxiety. The later stages of treatment include teaching patients and their families about nutrition concepts.

Bulimia

Bulimia nervosa is an eating disorder in which people eat a large quantity of food in a short time (bingeing) and then attempt to counter the effects of bingeing by self-induced vomiting, use of laxatives or diuretics, and/or excessive exercise. People with bulimia may use such behavior to try to gain control of their lives and weight.

Bulimia can be triggered when a slightly overweight person diets but fails to achieve the goal. Episodes are usually frequent, rapid, and uncontrollable. The behavior may occur only during periods of stress.

People with bulimia often diet when not bingeing. Psychologically, they believe their worth depends on being thin.

Behind their cheerful exterior, they usually feel depressed, lonely, ashamed, and empty.

Most bulimics who seek help are in their early 20s and report that they have been bulimic for 4 to 6 years. Because they are more likely to want and seek help, they are slightly easier to treat than anorexics are.

Bulimia is usually not life-threatening, but it can cause the following serious health problems:

- Erosion of tooth enamel
- Enlarged salivary glands
- Lesions in the esophagus
- Stomach spasms
- Chemical and hormonal imbalances

As with anorexia, treatment for bulimia involves a combination of psychotherapy and medication. Dental work, medication for depression and anxiety, nutritional counseling, and support groups may be used. The goal is to establish a healthy weight and good eating patterns as well as to resolve the psychosocial triggers.

Getting Help

Studies show an unsatisfactory rate of recovery from eating disorders; only about half of anorexic patients fully recover. The disorders can become chronic, with periods of remission and relapse. Chronic anorexia can be fatal, and many people who do recover from eating disorders remain preoccupied with food.

If you suspect that a patient has an eating disorder, be alert for the following eating or activity patterns that the patient might mention in conversation:

- Skipping two or more meals a day or limiting caloric intake to 500 or fewer calories a day
- Eating a very large amount of food in an uncontrollable manner over the course of 2 hours
- Eating large quantities of food without being hungry
- Using laxatives, excessive exercise, vomiting, diuretics, or other purges for weight control
- Avoiding social situations because they may interfere with a diet or exercise
- Feeling disgust, depression, and guilt after a binge
- Feeling that food controls life

▶ Patient Education
LO 55.8

Whenever you teach patients about nutrition and diet, you help them take steps to improve their health. In most instances, a licensed practitioner or dietitian gives the patient instructions, which you then reinforce. Patients may feel more comfortable asking you questions about their diet than asking other members of the healthcare team. They may think their concerns are too trivial or simple for the practitioner or dietitian.

Because of your frequent contact with patients, you can play a major role in education. You can teach patients about the role of nutrition in helping to prevent specific medical conditions. You also can teach patients how to be wise consumers when they shop by reading food package labels. You will be better equipped to educate patients and answer their questions if you have a solid knowledge of diet and nutrition and if you stay current with recent research findings. See the

Educating the Patient section for information on the relevance of such research. Before discussing a diet with any patient, be sure you understand the regimen the practitioner or dietitian is recommending as well as how to implement it.

If you are unsure of answers to any patient's questions, always ask the licensed practitioner. Refer patients who have questions about meal patterns and food selections to the registered dietitian, if one is available.

Your Role in Patient Education

When discussing dietary requirements with a patient, keep in mind that the patient is always the focus of nutritional care. Specific factors to take into account include the following:

- Any psychological or lifestyle factors that affect food choices and behaviors. Learn about the patient's dietary likes and dislikes, as well as religious or cultural restrictions, before you suggest the use of specific foods in meeting dietary requirements.
- The patient's age and family circumstances. For example, parents need to know the specifics about an infant's or a child's diet. An elderly person's diet needs to be physically and economically manageable as well as nutritious.
- Diseases and disorders. For example, if the patient has chewing or breathing problems or is nauseous, the licensed practitioner will have to prescribe treatments or medications to address those problems.
- The patient's psychological condition. You can learn a great deal about psychological status through discussion and nonverbal cues. For instance, you might look for signs that the patient is frustrated with the dietary changes or is in denial about a problem. The greater the rapport you develop with a patient, the more you will be able to help.

Remind patients that eating healthfully will help them feel and look better and help their bodies work better. When the licensed practitioner prescribes therapeutic diets, be sure patients are fully aware of the reasons they must follow the diets. Help patients set realistic goals and praise them for even the smallest accomplishments. Offer positive reinforcement for current and new good food habits.

As with all patient education, teaching methods such as role-playing, repetition of concepts, and the use of literature and other media reinforce your discussion. Use printed and audio-visual materials. Patient education sessions can be formal or informal and can take place at any appropriate time and place, such as in the office, over the telephone, or during a treatment or procedure. If possible, let patients decide which arrangements they prefer, or let them know the schedule in advance.

Patients need your support and empathy in working toward diet and nutrition goals, whether preventive or therapeutic. Follow these guidelines for best results when discussing diets with patients:

- Treat each patient as an individual with unique eating habits, knowledge of nutrition, and ability to learn.
- Teach a small amount of material at a time; 15- to 30-minute sessions are better than hour-long ones.

- Keep explanations at the level of the patient's understanding and vocabulary.
- Emphasize the patient's good eating behavior to reinforce it.
- Let the patient play an active role in the learning process— for example, by helping to plan the diet.
- Give the patient a written dietary plan to take home as well as any other helpful materials you have to offer.
- Suggest that the patient contact local support groups to connect with people who are trying to maintain the same kind of diet.

Nutritional education is part of preventive healthcare. Documentation is necessary to ensure payment by managed care and other health insurance providers. Failure to document can jeopardize a patient's insurance coverage. Document all patient education, including the specific topic, the amount of involvement by the patient, what types of materials were used, and if follow-up is planned. The progress note for Hilda Grubber is an example of nutritional documentation.

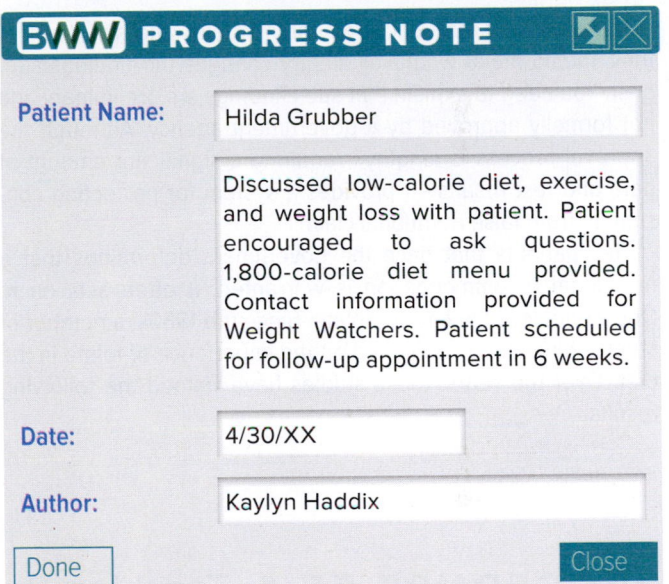

BWW PROGRESS NOTE	
Patient Name:	Hilda Grubber
	Discussed low-calorie diet, exercise, and weight loss with patient. Patient encouraged to ask questions. 1,800-calorie diet menu provided. Contact information provided for Weight Watchers. Patient scheduled for follow-up appointment in 6 weeks.
Date:	4/30/XX
Author:	Kaylyn Haddix
Done	Close

Cultural Considerations

Eating is a personal and social activity, and cultural issues play an especially important part in diet and nutrition. A person's cultural heritage, religious background, family traditions, socioeconomic status, and personal beliefs help determine eating habits and preferences. Culture and lifestyle also help shape food purchasing and serving habits, likes and dislikes, meal timing and frequency, attitudes toward food supplements, and the tendency to snack.

Dietitians and nutritionists who design diets and recipes for patients know that successful diets must take into account cultural and lifestyle factors. You can increase the effectiveness of your patient education if you become familiar with the food habits and beliefs common to your patients' cultural backgrounds. Learn to recognize the eating patterns belonging to different cultures and make a special effort to familiarize yourself with the food preferences of the ethnic groups most commonly represented among the patients in the practice where you work.

Changes in Nutritional Recommendations

In the field of nutrition—as in other scientific fields—research continues to provide people with additional information. You can help answer patients' questions about the potential usefulness of new information by understanding the difference between initial research findings and those evaluated and endorsed by the government. In many cases, information is not officially released or endorsed until the government has studied the facts and determined that they are accurate and concrete enough for public consideration. For example, *initial findings* have suggested the following information:

- Beta-carotene supplements may provide no benefit and may even be harmful.
- Certain fruit-derived flavonoids—pigmented antioxidants— may help halt the growth of cancer cells.
- Vitamin D may reduce the risk of certain cancers.

Patients may read about research studies and ask whether they should make whatever dietary changes the findings suggest. You need to explain that such findings are preliminary and not formally approved by a government agency. Although the approval process is lengthy—requiring a significant amount of data and test results—it provides a system for protecting consumers from false nutritional claims.

Tell patients that once the government determines that a nutritional recommendation is warranted, it often acts on it. One example is the case of folate. Since the 1960s, a number of studies have been conducted on the importance of folate in the diet. Over the years, those studies have yielded the following results:

- Folate offers protection from neural tube defects in unborn babies.
- Folate can reverse certain anemias.
- Folate may reduce the risk of cervical dysplasia.
- Folate appears to lower the likelihood of heart attacks.

As a result of these studies, the Department of Health and Human Services' Food and Drug Administration considered folate to be so important to all people that it approved the addition of folate to flour. Several nutrients have long been added to certain products to improve the products' nutritional value and to increase people's intake of important nutrients lacking in the general diet:

- Vitamin A and vitamin D, added to dairy products
- Iodine, added to salt
- Niacin, added to milled grain products
- Various vitamins and minerals, added to processed cereals

Explain to patients that nutritional recommendations change as scientists learn more about the ways various foods affect the human body and the exact amount of nutrients the body requires. Keep up-to-date on nutrition research so that you can provide patients with the latest information and help them steer clear of unsubstantiated claims.

Organizations such as the American Dietetic Association, American Heart Association, and many others have Internet sites that provide excellent information about diet and nutrition. Websites such as http://www.health.gov are available to you and your patients.

PROCEDURE 55-1 Teaching Patients How to Read Food Labels

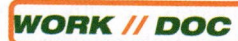

Procedure Goal: To explain how patients can use food labels to plan or follow a diet

OSHA Guidelines: This procedure does not involve exposure to blood, body fluids, or tissues.

Materials: Patient chart/progress note, food labels from products

Method:

1. Identify the patient and introduce yourself.
2. Explain that food labels can be used as a valuable source of information when planning or implementing a prescribed diet.
3. Using a label from a food package, such as the ice-cream label in Figure Procedure 55-1 Step 3, point out the Nutrition Facts section.
4. Describe the various elements on the label.

- Serving size is the basis for the nutrition information provided. One serving of the ice cream is ½ cup. There are 12 servings in the package of ice cream.
  RATIONALE: *Paying close attention to the serving size and how many servings are in a container helps determine how many servings are being consumed.*
- Calories and calories from fat show the proportion of fat calories in the product. One serving of the ice cream contains 140 calories and 60 calories of each serving comes from fat.
- The (%) Daily Value section shows how many grams (g) or milligrams (mg) of a variety of nutrients are contained in one serving. Then the label shows the percentage (%) of the recommended daily intake of each given nutrient (assuming a diet of 2,000 calories a day). The ice cream contains 23% of a person's

recommended daily saturated fat intake and no dietary fiber.

- Recommendations for total amounts of various nutrients for both a 2,000-calorie and a 2,500-calorie diet are shown in chart form on th side of the label. These numbers provide the basis for the daily value percentages.
- Ingredients are listed in order from largest quantity to smallest quantity. In this half-gallon of ice cream, milk, cream, sugar, and skim milk are the most abundant ingredients.

5. Inform the patient that a variety of similar products with significantly different nutritional values are often available. Explain that patients can use nutrition labels to evaluate and compare such similar products. Patients must consider what a product contributes to their diets, not simply what it lacks. To do this, patients must read the entire label. Compared with the regular ice cream, the "light" ice cream contains less fat, fewer carbohydrates, as well as less sodium and cholesterol.

6. Ask the patient to compare two other similar products and determine which would fit in better as part of a healthful, nutritious diet that meets that patient's individual needs.

7. Document the patient education session in the patient's chart, indicate the patient's understanding, and initial the entry (Refer to Progress Note).

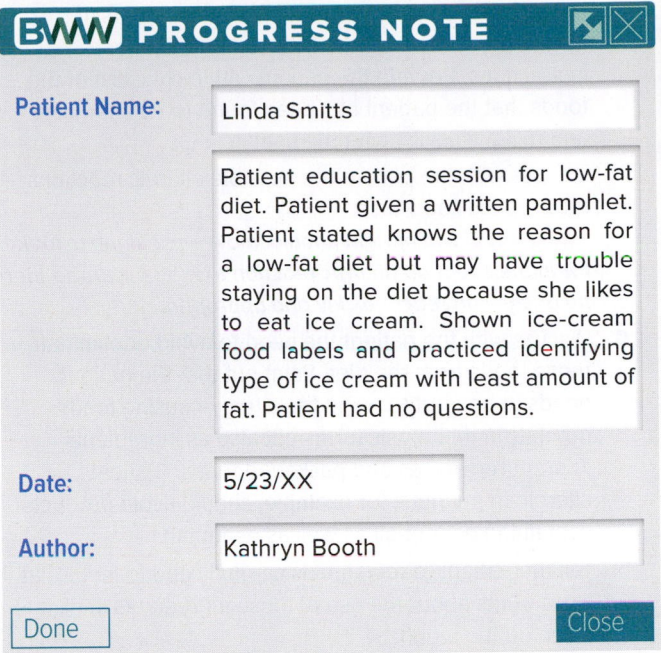

BWW PROGRESS NOTE

Patient Name: Linda Smitts

Patient education session for low-fat diet. Patient given a written pamphlet. Patient stated knows the reason for a low-fat diet but may have trouble staying on the diet because she likes to eat ice cream. Shown ice-cream food labels and practiced identifying type of ice cream with least amount of fat. Patient had no questions.

Date: 5/23/XX

Author: Kathryn Booth

Done   Close

RATIONALE: *Many insurance companies require evidence of preventive health counseling, and documentation is an important aspect of patient insurance coverage.*

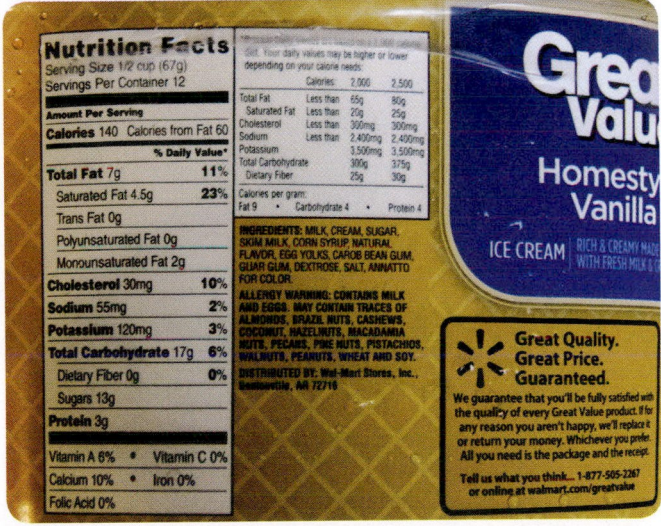

FIGURE Procedure 55-1 Step 3   Food labels are a source of nutrition information. This label provides facts on the nutrients and ingredients contained in this homestyle vanilla ice cream.
© McGraw-Hill Education/Mark Dierker, photographer

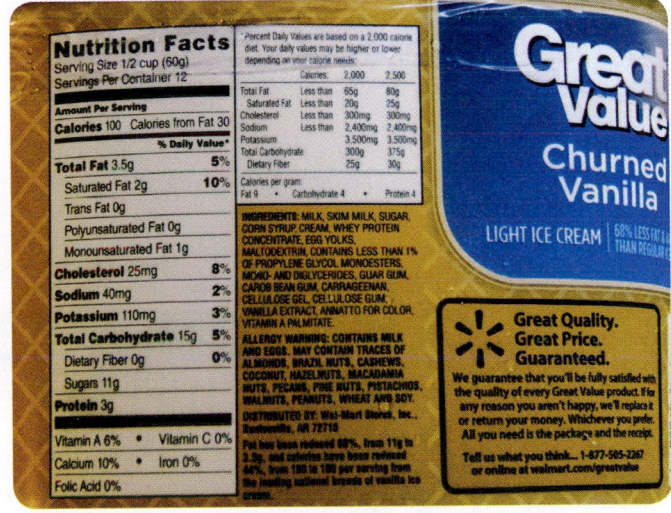

FIGURE Procedure 55-1 Step 5   By reading this label, a patient would learn that this light ice cream contains less sugar, fat, cholesterol, and sodium, and has fewer calories than regular ice cream.
© McGraw-Hill Education/Mark Dierker, photographer

PROCEDURE 55-2 Alerting Patients with Food Allergies to the Dangers of Common Foods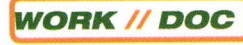

Procedure Goal: To explain how patients can eliminate allergy-causing foods from their diets

OSHA Guidelines: This procedure does not involve exposure to blood, body fluids, or tissues

Materials: Results of the patient's allergy tests, patient's chart/progress note, pen, patient education materials

Method:
1. Identify the patient and introduce yourself.

2. Discuss the results of the patient's allergy tests (if available), reinforcing the licensed practitioner's instructions. Provide the patient with a checklist of the foods that the patient has been found to be allergic to and review this list with the patient.

3. Discuss with the patient the possible allergic reactions those foods can cause.

   RATIONALE: *The patient should know what signs to look for in the event an allergic reaction to food occurs so that he or she can react quickly and appropriately.*

4. Discuss with the patient the need to avoid or eliminate those foods from the diet. Point out that the patient needs to be alert to avoid the allergy-causing foods not only in their basic forms but also as ingredients in prepared dishes and packaged foods. (Patients allergic to peanuts, for example, should avoid products containing peanut oil as well as peanuts.)

5. Tell the patient to read labels carefully and to inquire at restaurants about the use of those ingredients in dishes listed on the menu.

6. With the licensed practitioner's or dietitian's consent, talk with the patient about the possibility of finding adequate substitutes for the foods if they are among the patient's favorites. Also discuss, if necessary, how the patient can obtain the nutrients in those foods from other sources (for example, the need for extra calcium sources if the patient is allergic to dairy products). Provide these explanations to the patient in writing, if appropriate, along with supplementary materials such as recipe pamphlets, a list of resources for obtaining food substitutes, and so on.

7. Discuss with the patient the procedures to follow if the allergy-causing foods are accidentally ingested.

   RATIONALE: *Do not assume a patient will know what to do in the event of an allergic reaction.*

8. Answer the patient's questions and remind the patient that you and the rest of the medical team are available if any questions or problems arise later on.

9. Document the patient education session or interchange in the patient's chart, indicate the patient's understanding, and initial the entry (Refer to Progress Note).

   RATIONALE: *Many insurance companies require evidence of preventive health counseling, and documentation is an important aspect of patient insurance coverage.*

BWW PROGRESS NOTE

Patient Name: Harrison Potts

Patient tested positive for peanut allergy. Explained the dangers of exposure to peanuts as well as products cooked in peanut oils. Instructed to read package and inquire at restaurants before eating foods. Patient restated how to use EpiPen and other emergency actions in case an exposure to peanuts occurs. Education brochure provided to patient.

Date: 8/30/XX

Author: Kathryn Booth

Done   Close

SUMMARY OF LEARNING OUTCOMES

LEARNING OUTCOMES	KEY POINTS
55.1 Relate daily energy requirements to the role of calories.	The body uses food for three major purposes: to provide energy; to build, repair, and maintain body tissues; and to regulate body processes. Calories provide energy for the body. Calories are measured in the foods we eat. We also can estimate the amount of calories used by the body during activity.
55.2 Identify nutrients and their role in health.	The body needs a variety of nutrients for energy, growth, repair, and basic processes. Several food components provide nutrients. These are proteins, carbohydrates, fiber, lipids, vitamins, minerals, and water.
55.3 Implement a plan for a nutritious, well-balanced diet and healthy lifestyle using the USDA's guidelines.	Dietary guidelines suggest the types and quantities of food that people should eat each day. They also may contain the recommendations about which types of foods to limit and which types of foods to increase. MyPlate provides recommendations for eating a variety of nutrients and maintaining physical activity. Using MyPlate recommendations promotes a well-balanced diet and healthy lifestyle.

LEARNING OUTCOMES	KEY POINTS
55.4 Describe methods used to assess a patient's nutritional status.	Calipers are used to perform a skinfold test that determines the percentage of body fat. BMI is the body mass index. Both measurements, along with other factors, may be used to assess a patient's nutritional status.
55.5 Explain reasons that a diet may be modified.	Dietary modifications may be used alone or in combination with other therapies to prevent or treat illness.
55.6 Identify types of patients who require special diets and the modifications required for each.	Patients with allergies, anemia, cancer, diabetes, heart disease, hypertension, lactose sensitivity, or obesity need special diets. In addition pediatric, pregnant, lactating, and debilitated patients as well as those undergoing drug therapy need modifications to their diet.
55.7 Describe the warning signs, symptoms, and treatment for eating disorders.	You should know the signs and symptoms of eating disorders in order to evaluate for these disorders during the patient interview: • Anorexia nervosa—unexplained weight loss, self-starvation, and fear of weight gain • Bulimia nervosa—eating large quantities of food in a short period of time, going to the bathroom immediately after eating, and using laxatives to excess • Binge eating—eating large quantities of food, not followed by purging, and weight gain
55.8 Educate patients about nutritional requirements.	Patients need to be educated about special diets and how to implement dietary changes as instructed by licensed practitioners and dietitians. Knowledge of basic nutritional principles and current nutritional findings is necessary. Documentation is required to help ensure payment by managed care and other health insurance companies.

CASE STUDY CRITICAL THINKING

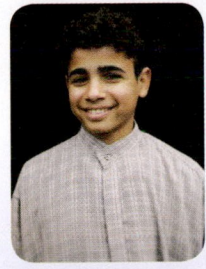

© David Sacks/Getty Images

Recall Mohammad Nassar from the beginning of this chapter. Now that you have completed this chapter, answer the following questions:

1. What is the patient's probable diagnosis?

2. Do you think that the patient's attention to calorie intake is simply, as he says, preparation for wrestling competition?

3. Why is this patient experiencing muscle weakness?

EXAM PREPARATION QUESTIONS

1. (LO 55.6) What is the most highly recommended food for a patient less than 6 months old?
   a. Single-grain baby cereal
   b. Iron-fortified infant formula
   c. Breast milk
   d. Whole milk
   e. Two percent milk

2. (LO 55.5) Which of the following foods should not be given to a patient with lactose sensitivity?
   a. Cheese
   b. Broccoli
   c. Chicken
   d. Eggs
   e. Bananas

3. (LO 55.3) Which of the following is a key recommendation of the USDA Dietary Guidelines?

a. Reduce physical activity to less than 2 days per week
b. Reduce sodium intake to less than 2,300 mg a day
c. Consume no more than three alcoholic beverages a day
d. Consume at least 500 mg of cholesterol a day
e. Avoid oils and use solid fats for cooking

4. (LO 55.2) On average, an adult should drink _____ glasses of water a day.

a. 2 to 8
b. 6 to 8
c. 4 to 10
d. 4 to 6
e. 2 to 6

5. (LO 55.2) Which of the following statements about protein is correct?

a. Protein decreases the rate of carbohydrate breakdown and absorption
b. Protein serves as a constituent of bile, which aids in digestion
c. Protein assists with antibody production and disease resistance
d. Protein provides a concentrated source of heat and energy
e. Protein flushes out wastes

6. (LO 55.4) Which of the following *best* describes the skinfold test?

a. Measures body fat based on height and weight of adult men and women
b. Depends on the amount of water intake over the past 24 hours
c. Pinches the skin with a caliper to determine the weight of a patient
d. Measures fat as a percentage of body weight
e. Requires a formula to be determined

7. (LO 55.1) Which of the following is *not* a part of the process of nutrition?

a. Absorption
b. Elimination
c. Intake
d. Metabolism
e. Indigestion

8. (LO 55.8) Which of the following guidelines would you *least* likely use when educating a patient about nutrition?

a. Treat each patient as an individual with unique eating habits, knowledge of nutrition, and ability to learn
b. Teach an eating plan that you have developed using specific dietary guidelines
c. Teach a small amount of material at a time; 15- to 30-minute sessions are better than hour-long ones
d. Keep explanations at the level of the patient's understanding and vocabulary
e. Emphasize the patient's good eating behavior to reinforce it

9. (LO 55.7) A patient is 5′6″ and weighs 145 lb, which is the same as her last visit 6 months ago. She says she can easily eat at least a dozen donuts for breakfast and her mother is always telling her she is moody. You know you need to report this information to the licensed practitioner because it is possible the patient has

a. Anorexia
b. Lactose intolerance
c. Bulimia
d. Binge eating
e. Hypertension

10. (LO 55.5) Which of the following diets may be prescribed for a patient who has difficulty swallowing?

a. Soft diet
b. Low-cholesterol diet
c. Low-sodium diet
d. High-fiber diet
e. High-carbohydrate diet

SOFT SKILLS SUCCESS

A 14-year-old female has come to the office with a fever of 100.2 and complaining of a sore throat. You check her weight from the previous visit and notice she has lost 20 pounds. Although she appears of normal weight for her size, when you mention she has lost 20 pounds in a disgusted tone she says, "I just wish I could lose a few more. I am so tired of being such a big cow. I really don't think my weight is any of your business!" What should you say to or do for this patient?

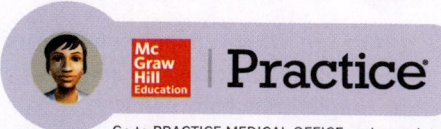

Go to PRACTICE MEDICAL OFFICE and complete the module Admin: Check In - Interactions..

Practice Management

CASE STUDY

PATIENT INFORMATION		
Patient Name Cindy Chen	**DOB** 07/15/19XX	**Allergies** NKA
Attending Alexis N. Whalen, MD	**MRN** 324-86-542	**Other Information** Medication(s): Retrovir®

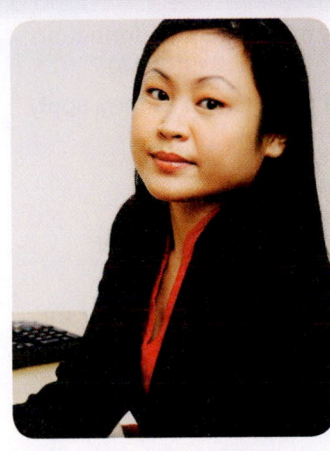

© Red Chopsticks/Getty Images RF

Cindy Chen is a 28-year-old HIV-positive female who is a patient of Dr. Whalen. Since adding Retrovir® to her management, she is again feeling well and has actually gained a few pounds. Cindy has recently completed a phlebotomy course at the local community college—in fact, she did her externship at BWW Medical Associates and did very well.

There is an opening at BWW for a phlebotomist and Cindy has applied for the position. The staff all like Cindy and would like to be part of her "new lease on life."

Keep Cindy in mind as you study the chapter. There will be questions at the end of the chapter based on the case study. The information in the chapter will help you answer these questions.

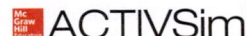

LEARNING OUTCOMES

After completing Chapter 56, you will be able to:

56.1 Explain the basic organizational designs of the medical office and the relationship of the physician and the medical assistant with the practice manager and direct supervisors.

56.2 Describe the responsibilities of the practice manager.

56.3 Summarize the basic human resources functions in practice management.

56.4 Distinguish four of the possible traits of someone with leadership skills and the importance of these skills to the healthcare team.

56.5 Compare risk management and quality assurance in a medical facility.

56.6 Calculate an employee's gross earnings, deductions, and net earnings for a pay period.

56.7 Describe the tax forms commonly used in the medical office and the purpose of the office tax liability account.

KEY TERMS

agenda
budget
chain of command
diversity
employee handbook
Federal Insurance Contributions Act (FICA)
Federal Unemployment Tax Act (FUTA)
Form I-9
Form W-2
Form W-4
grievance process
gross earnings

incident report
labor relations
mediation
midlevel provider
net earnings
organizational chart
policies and procedures (P&P) manual
probationary period
quality assurance (QA)
risk management (RM)
sexual harassment
tax liability account

I.C.12	Identify quality assurance practices in healthcare
V.P.4	Coach patients regarding: (a) office policies
V.A.1	Demonstrate: (a) empathy (b) active listening
X.C.3	Describe components of the Health Information Portability and Accountability Act (HIPAA)
X.C.5	Discuss licensure and certification as they apply to healthcare providers
X.C.7	Define: (i) risk management
X.C.9	List and discuss legal and illegal applicant interview questions
X.P.7	Complete an incident report related to an error in patient care
XI.C.3	Identify the effects of personal morals on professional performance

4. Medical Law and Ethics

   f. Comply with federal, state, and local health laws and regulations as they relate to healthcare settings

8. Medical Office Business Procedures/ Management

   f. Display professionalism through written and verbal communications

11. Career Development

   b. Demonstrate professional behavior

▶ Introduction

In previous chapters, you have explored many of the complex systems, procedures, requirements, and roles required in the modern medical office. Today, it is much more difficult for the practitioner to care for patients and manage the office as he or she may have done in the past. While the healthcare facility's management differs by ownership, size, and other variables (addressed in the *Legal and Ethical Issues* chapter), one person is generally in charge of overseeing the day-to-day operations, working closely with the licensed practitioners to keep the practice running smoothly and its staff working at its professional peak (Figure 56-1). The title of this person has varying names, including *practice* or *office manager, executive,* or *director* and *healthcare administrator*. This chapter discusses this person's position, responsibilities, and relationship with the practitioners and medical assistant. The terms *medical practice manager* and *office manager* represent the role. Employee management functions, including human resources and facility management, also are discussed in this chapter.

▶ Organizational Design   LO 56.1

Every medical office has an organizational design, which may or may not be represented by a formal **organizational chart.** The design and chart show the supervisory structure and reporting relationships between different functions and positions—in other words, who is responsible for whom and for what. In most states, the medical assistant is required to be under the direct supervision of the physician, physician assistant, or nurse practitioner for direct patient care activities. However, the practice manager or that person's designee

is usually responsible for interviewing, hiring, firing, evaluating, and ensuring training and credentialing, which are all considered administrative and not direct patient care

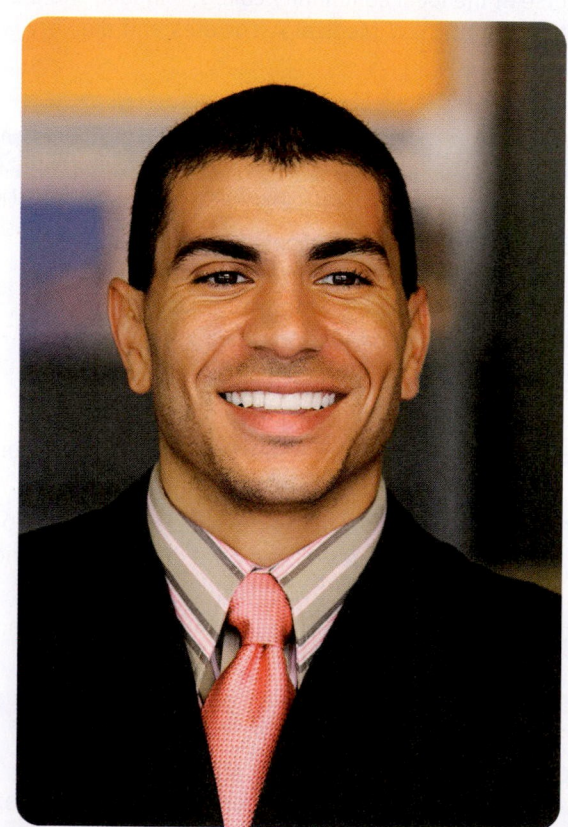

FIGURE 56-1 As the practice manager of BWW Medical Associates, Malik Katahri keeps the practice running smoothly.
© HBSS/Corbis RF

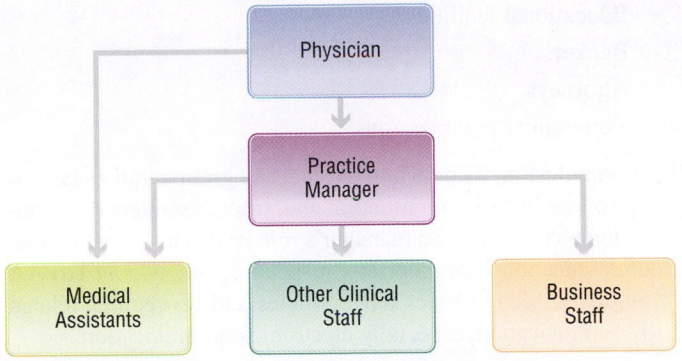

FIGURE 56-2 Practice organizational chart for a physician-owned practice.

functions. Both physician-owned and company-owned medical practices rely on some form of organizational design to function effectively.

Physician-Owned Medical Practice

Figure 56-2 represents a physician-owned practice's simplified organizational chart. As you learned in the *Legal and Ethical Issues* chapter, a physician-owned medical practice sometimes obtains the legal designation of a professional corporation (PC). The owner is usually an individual doctor or a group of physicians. In the organizational chart in Figure 56-2, the placement of the boxes and arrows shows that the physician carries the ultimate responsibility but designates it to the person below him—the practice manager. The practice manager reports to the physician, who also pays her salary. The manager is the physician's employee who oversees the daily operations and the administrative functions of the entire office and staff, including the medical assistants. The arrow from the physician to the medical assistants demonstrates that the physician also has direct responsibility for the medical assistants. As mentioned previously, this responsibility involves direct patient care. Depending on the size of the practice, other supervisory personnel might report to the practice manager. Each supervisor would then have staff reporting directly to him or her. In multispecialty organizations, supervisors might be designated by specialty, such as pediatrics, internal medicine, and cardiology.

Company-Owned Medical Practice

Figure 56-3 represents a simplified organizational chart of a company-owned medical facility. The company may be nonprofit, such as a community health center, or for-profit, such as Cigna HealthCare. The president or chief executive officer (CEO) has the ultimate responsibility. However, again, the practice manager is in charge of the day-to-day operations, with the exception of direct patient care functions. The medical director is in charge of the patient care end of the practice, overseeing the physicians, nurses, **midlevel providers** (physician assistants and nurse practitioners), and medical assistants. The dotted line between the practice manager and the medical director indicates that they are equal in rank and collaborate with each other. The dotted line from the practice manager to the other physicians indicates collaboration. For example, the practice manager may work with the physicians to help obtain documentation of credentials, but the medical director has the majority of the responsibility for the providers, including their schedules and periodic evaluations. The president, the practice manager, the medical director, and other physicians and staff are paid employees of the company. A board of directors is ultimately responsible for the practice, through the CEO, but this board is not involved in the company's daily operations.

The Chain of Command

The term **chain of command** began in the military to demonstrate how each rank is accountable to those directly superior and how authority passes from one link in the chain to the next from bottom to top or top to bottom. For example, in the military, a private is accountable to a sergeant, who is accountable to a lieutenant, and so on. The lieutenant gives an order to the sergeant, who gives it to the private. Each level of the chain has many steps, including the determination of the equipment, training, and strategies needed to carry out the order or mission. The majority of today's businesses, including medical practices, operate using this approach.

It is important to understand the chain of command in your facility and to understand who your supervisor is. Since medical assistants work closely with physicians, the tendency may be to go to the physician with requests such as asking for time off. If the physician is not your supervisor, it is inappropriate

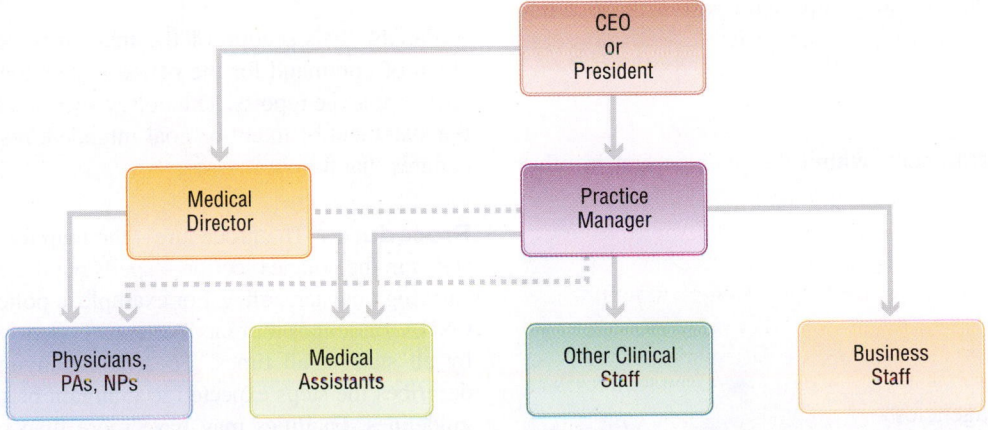

FIGURE 56-3 Practice organizational chart for a company-owned medical practice.

to "go over your supervisor's head" and make the request of the physician, as he may not have the authority to grant your request. It is also inappropriate to go outside the chain of command with a complaint, even if the complaint is about your supervisor. First, address the issue with your supervisor. If this issue is not resolved, then go to the next person in the chain of command, such as the practice manager. Most offices have policies and procedures for handling complaints. Should you seek other employment, that organization will contact your previous supervisor for references. No matter how friendly or informal the medical practice is, stay within the chain of command.

▶ Managing the Medical Practice · LO 56.2

The practice manager's role includes providing communication avenues for all medical team members as well as communicating with members of the community outside the medical practice. The practice manager is also responsible for ensuring that legal, business, health, and safety requirements are in compliance; guaranteeing the adequacy of the technology and physical plant; providing for the practice's financial viability; and monitoring risk management and customer care and satisfaction. Sometimes, the manager is also in charge of multiple satellite offices.

By now, you have probably realized that in today's complex healthcare world, any medical assistant who aspires to become a practice manager will need additional education and training to attain this goal. The information in this chapter will introduce you to the role so that you can begin to understand all aspects of running a medical office and think about all the possibilities that may be open for you once you become a certified medical assistant. Your path will be up to you.

Communication Skills of the Practice Manager

The *Interpersonal Communication* chapter describes general communication techniques used in communication with patients, persons with special needs, and coworkers. The *Written and Electronic Communication* chapter outlines the general practices for producing effective and professional written communication. The practice management position requires exceptional verbal and written communication skills and excellent interpersonal skills. The following are some of the routine individuals and groups with whom the practice manager communicates on a regular basis:

- Staff
- Patients
- Physicians/practitioners (within the practice and in other practices)
- Hospitals
- Insurers
- Vendors
- Employers
- Contractors
- Governmental agencies
- Other regulatory and professional agencies

- Educational facilities
- Bankers
- Attorneys
- Community organizations

Communicating with each individual and group requires knowledge of the business or situation and, often, excellent problem-solving techniques. The manager's role is also to ensure that all communication is appropriate, respectful, timely, and HIPAA compliant. Many offices have policies and procedures related to communication, especially electronic communication.

The Policies and Procedures Manual

The **policies and procedures (P&P) manual** is a key written communication tool in the medical office. Both permanent and temporary employees use this manual, which covers all office policies for administrative and clinical procedures. The practitioner (or practitioners), practice manager, and staff (often including the medical assistant) usually develop this manual as a joint effort. See Figure 56-4.

Policies are rules or guidelines that dictate an office's day-to-day workings. Although individual policies vary from office to office, most medical office manuals describe the following policy areas:

- Office purposes, objectives, and goals as set by the practitioner(s)
- Rules and regulations
- Job descriptions and duties of staff personnel
- Office hours
- Dress code
- Insurance and other benefits
- Vacation, sick leave, family medical leave, and other time away from the office
- Salary and performance evaluations
- Maintenance of equipment and supplies
- Mailings
- Bookkeeping
- Scheduling of appointments and maintenance of patient records
- OSHA guidelines

Policies This section of the manual typically includes the chain of command for the office and/or the person to whom each employee reports. The policy section often also includes the statement of intent or goal intended, resulting in the procedures that follow.

Procedures The procedure—the map for reaching the goal stated in the policies section—spells out the correct manner for carrying out each policy. For example, a policy might state that OSHA guidelines for bloodborne pathogens will be maintained by all staff at all times. The accompanying procedure then describes the steps expected to maintain bloodborne pathogen guidelines. Facilities may have more than one P&P manual, such as one for human resources, one for safety, one for clinical

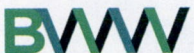

BWW Medical Associates, PC
305 Main Street, Port Snead YZ 12345-9876
Tel: 555-654-3210, Fax: 555-987-6543
Web: BWWAssociates.com

Paul F. Buckwalter, MD
Alexis N. Whalen, MD
Elizabeth H. Williams, MD

POLICY AND PROCEDURE

Subject: Competency of Staff

Date of Issue: Sept. 25, 20XX

Policy # 1001

Effective Date: Oct. 1, 20XX

I. POLICY

It is the policy of BWW Medical Associates, PC that all employees meet the standards of competency as defined by its various policies and the requirements of TJC and other regulatory and credentialing agencies.

II. PURPOSE

The competence of staff members is (a) defined by job descriptions designed by the director; (b) assessed initially during the orientation process; (c) maintained through educational updates; and (d) evaluated periodically in conjunction with the performance appraisal process.

III. IMPLEMENTATION

a. Job Descriptions
i. The office manager will write and/or review each job description annually. Each job description will reflect the educational experience and training needed for the position and include competency-based performance standards.

FIGURE 56-4 Sample policy statement from the BWW Medical Associates policies and procedures manual.

procedures, and one for administrative procedures. The practice manager must stay current with new practices and standards of the community and all applicable professional organizations, updating the office manual as required. In addition, new laws and requirements of governmental agencies such as OSHA and CMS must be monitored and incorporated. Reading the policies and procedure manual(s) is typically part of new employee orientation. Each employee should know the location of the policies and procedures manual; an employee should look here if he or she is unsure about a specific duty or task.

The *clinical procedures* portion of a P&P manual should include instructions regarding the following for each test performed:

- Purpose of the test, clinical application, and usefulness
- Specimen required and collection method; special patient preparation or restrictions
- Reagents, standards, controls, and media used; special supplies
- Instrumentation, including calibration and schedules
- Step-by-step directions

The *administrative procedures* portion of a P&P manual may include instructions regarding the following procedures:

- Appropriate telephone procedures for emergency and non-emergency calls
- Releasing of patient PHI
- Guidelines for submission of "clean" claims for each provider
- Templates for frequently created communications such as normal lab and X-ray results

Licenses, Certifications, and Contracts

The medical practice includes many positions and facets that require federal, state, or local approval. Approvals take the form of a license, certification, or other credential or contract. Some are simple procedures; others are more complicated and expensive. Common responsibilities include ensuring that:

- Physicians and midlevel providers are properly licensed and credentialed with CMS and other payers as required and that the credentialing is up-to-date.
- Physician and midlevel provider DEA forms are up-to-date.
- Medical assistants, phlebotomists, coders, and other personnel are properly trained and certified or credentialed according to federal, state, and professional standards.
- Required licenses to operate the facility, such as local business licenses, are up-to-date.

- Insurance requirements, such as malpractice and liability contracts, are up-to-date and reflect current values.
- Health insurance companies, laboratories, attorneys, and service contracts necessary to conduct business are current.
- The practice is compliant with required reporting to authorities, such as that for reporting communicable diseases.

Depending on the healthcare organization's size, the manager may have other employees involved in carrying out these duties. However, the manager has the ultimate responsibility to guarantee that these tasks are completed in a proper and timely fashion.

Budget and Overall Finances

With the exception of large organizations that have a chief financial officer (CFO), the responsibility for the practice finances is part of the manager's extensive role. A **budget** is created annually and reviewed at least monthly. The budget predicts the expenses and revenues related to operations over a given period of time. First, the manager must know the total expenses. Salaries are usually the biggest budget expense. The manager reviews the healthcare insurance and governmental agencies' patient care contracts and other sources of income. Sometimes the manager must renegotiate the contract if costs have risen. If revenues are lower than expected and costs are higher, the manager must make unpopular budget cuts so that the practice remains profitable and able to continue to provide care for the community it serves.

As the office medical assistant, be mindful that financial responsibility is the role of every employee. Even something as seemingly inconsequential as taking pens home from the office can have an impact on the practice. The immediate thought may be "it's just a pen," but the reality is that you did not purchase the pen—the practice did—and if every member of the staff took "only a pen or two," soon there would not be enough pens in the practice. Part of the ethics and integrity of being in the medical profession is your professional behavior—particularly "when no one is looking."

Managing Petty Cash Another budget function that is often managed by the medical assistant with oversight by the practice manager is the petty cash fund. This fund is used to make small (petty) cash disbursements for minor expenses such as postage-due fees or holiday decorations (Figure 56-5). To avoid writing checks for such small amounts, you may pay for them from the petty cash fund (also known as the revolving fund)—cash kept on hand in the office for small purchases. The practice manager often determines the amount of the petty cash account (usually $50) and the minimum amount of cash to be kept on hand (such as $15).

Starting and Maintaining a Petty Cash Fund To start the fund with $50, write a check to "Petty Cash" or "Cash" for that amount. Enter the check in the miscellaneous column of the monthly disbursements journal (refer to the *Patient Collections and Financial Management* chapter). Then, cash the check. Because this money will be used for small disbursements, be sure to get some of it in pennies, nickels, dimes, quarters, and dollar bills. Put this money in a petty cash box.

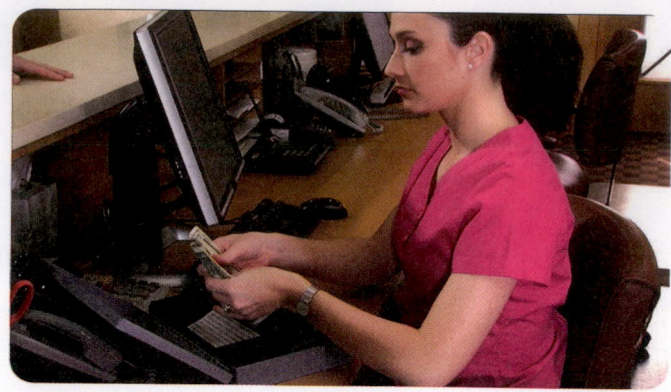

FIGURE 56-5 Managing petty cash is often the task of the medical assistant.
© McGraw-Hill Education

For each payment from the petty cash fund, obtain a receipt or create a petty cash voucher. The voucher should record the transaction number, date, amount paid, purpose of the expense, your signature (as the person issuing the money), and the signature of the person receiving it. Keep the receipt for any item purchased, along with the completed voucher, in the petty cash box to verify expenses later.

Also, document each petty cash withdrawal on a petty cash record form. Include the transaction number, the date, the payee, a brief description, the amount, and the type of expense (such as office expense, auto expense, or miscellaneous expense). If a space is provided, calculate and record the new balance in the petty cash fund.

Replenishing the Petty Cash Fund At the end of the month (or whenever the fund is low), compare the latest petty cash balance, found in the petty cash record or in the petty cash column of the disbursements journal, to the money in the petty cash box. If you have not kept a running balance, total the receipts and vouchers; then count the cash on hand. Subtract the total amount on the receipts and vouchers (for example, $35) from the original balance (for example, $50). The difference ($15) should equal the cash on hand in the petty cash box ($15).

To replenish the account, write a check to "Cash" or "Petty Cash" for the amount spent ($35). Cash the check and add the money to the box, bringing the total back up to the original amount of $50. Record the check for $35 in the disbursements journal. Also, total the receipts and vouchers by expense category. Record those totals in the appropriate columns on the disbursement record.

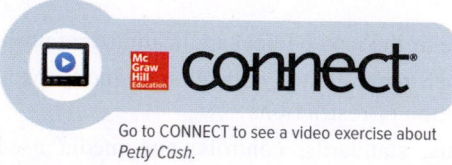

Go to CONNECT to see a video exercise about *Petty Cash.*

Scheduling and Travel

Ensuring that an adequate number of staff members are on duty at all times for the business to function properly is an additional aspect of the practice manager's role. Scheduling is a job that may be delegated to a supervisor or other person, depending on the practice's size, but the practice manager monitors it. When office staff members are absent due to vacation, extended illness, or educational purposes, it may be necessary to rearrange remaining staff member schedules to provide coverage. If practitioners are not available to see patients, the office may be closed during their absence.

Sometimes, practitioners and other staff, including medical assistants, travel for educational purposes with expenses covered by the practice, in which case work-related expenses may be reimbursed if the appropriate receipts are kept and an expense report is completed (Figure 56-6). Procedure 56-1, at the end of this chapter, provides practice in completing a travel expense report.

Other Business Functions

The contemporary medical office relies on technology for communication, appointment scheduling, coding, billing, diagnostic test ordering and reporting, prescription refills, and the electronic health record. The office manager evaluates and purchases the systems that fit the practice's needs and budget, facilitates the installation and staff training, then oversees the ongoing operations through an in-house technical support person or through a service contract. Other managerial functions include ensuring the availability of mailing and shipping services, inventory and supply purchases, and appropriate marketing and public relation strategies, which may include websites, brochures, and community event sponsorship.

BWW Medical Associates, PC
305 Main Street, Port Snead YZ 12345-9876
Tel: 555-654-3210, Fax: 555-987-6543
Web: BWWAssociates.com

Paul F. Buckwalter, MD
Alexis N. Whalen, MD
Elizabeth H. Williams, MD

TRAVEL EXPENSE REPORT
(Travel with estimated expenses must be approved prior to the event)

Applicant's name: _____ Date: _____

Applicant's address: _____

Applicant's cell phone and home phone: _____

Name of activity and type (example: professional meeting, conference; attach Web or brochure information): _____

Purpose of travel: _____

Location of activity: _____

Registration fee	$
Transportation: *indicate major mode of travel	$
Airport shuttle or parking	$
Taxi	$
Lodging (daily rate _____ × _____ number of days)	$
Meals ($30 per day × _____ number of days)	$
Other (explain)	$
Total	$

Did you miss work days: [ ] NO [ ] YES (If "YES" include dates and number of days)

Dates: _____ Number of days: _____

Signature: _____

*If using your own vehicle, mileage is reimbursed at the current rate. Check with your supervisor prior to travel.

This form must be submitted with receipts in 10 working days upon return. Noncompliance may result in denial of reimbursement or if funds were previously awarded, payroll deduction may occur to recover the amount.

For Management Use Only

[ ] Not approved [ ] Approved Amount: _____

Name (print): _____ Date: _____

Signature: _____

FIGURE 56-6 Typical travel expense report to be submitted with appropriate receipts to allow for reimbursement of business-related travel expenses.

Human Resources and Practice Management
LO 56.3

The practice manager's role includes the human resources (HR) component of the medical office. This area of the organization is probably the only one that does not involve the patient directly. If the practice or facility is large, it may have its own human resources coordinator or supervisor who reports to the practice manager. If the practice is smaller, the practice manager often functions as the human resources "department." In the business world, human resources personnel deal with employee-related issues such as hiring, training, benefits, labor relations, and employment termination. Other names for HR include personnel services, personnel department, and people services. Within this section of the chapter, we will follow Miguel A. Perez's experience with the hiring process at BWW Medical Associates.

The Hiring Process

As discussed in the *Legal and Ethical Issues* chapter, federal, state, and local governments regulate many hiring practices, including the Equal Employment Opportunity Commission (EEOC), Fair Labor Standards Act, Equal Pay Act, Age Discrimination in Employment Act, and Americans with Disabilities Act (ADA), as well as the Family Medical Leave Act (FMLA). The FMLA allows employees up to 12 job-protected weeks of unpaid leave for approved medical needs for the employee and certain family members. The EEOC act prevents discrimination. See Figure 56-7. Violations can result in monetary and other penalties. Understanding and staying current with these often complex laws is a major HR role. Table 56-1 outlines some legal versus illegal questions that may be asked during the interview process. Keep in mind, one of the best techniques may be to ask a legal question and then remain quiet. Most people get nervous during silent moments and often end up giving you more information than you asked for.

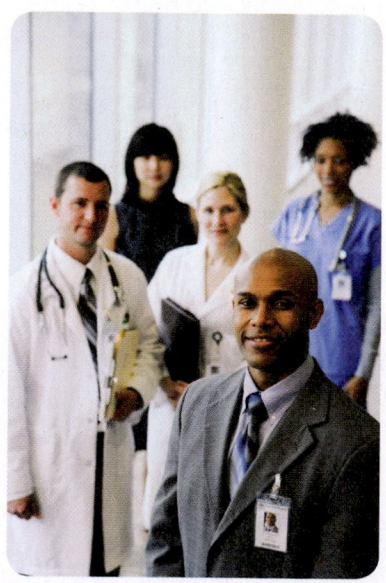

FIGURE 56-7 The EEOC prevents discrimination based on race, color, religion, sex, or national origin.
© Terry Vine/Blend Images RF

In addition to understanding the laws surrounding the hiring process, it is always best to stress competencies such as teamwork, policies and procedures, and cross-training during the interview process and during orientation. Potential employees should understand the qualities that are important to the practice at which they are seeking employment—they need to know if they will be a good fit in the practice and if the practice will be a good fit for them.

Employee orientation is essential in the personnel management phase. During this process, the new hire gets to see and meet important people within the organization. He or she also gets to know what is expected of the position, as well as gain information about company benefits.

The basics of hiring a successful employee are

- Always try to find the most qualified person for the job.
- Scrutinize and check references carefully.
- Have a salary range so that you can negotiate successfully and pay for the most qualified person.
- Discuss policies and procedures (and expectations) early.
- Train properly and retrain when new technology arrives.

When BWW Medical Associates decided to hire an administrative medical assistant, a job description was written that consisted of the following:

- Name of the organization
- Name of the position
- Employment grade
- Summary of the position
- Job responsibilities
- Requirements and qualifications
- Title of the supervisor

One of the job description requirements was that the applicant have a current CMA (AAMA) or RMA (AMT) certification. The next step was to recruit qualified candidates. Miguel A. Perez was a CMA (AAMA) who applied for the position, and his application was one of those selected. He interviewed very well and, after his references were checked, Miguel was offered the position with an appropriate salary. HR maintains a personnel file for every employee. Malik Katahri, the office manager at BWW, initiated an HR file for Miguel.

Orientation and Staff Development

The human resources department provides orientation for new employees and facilitates training and staff development for established employees. Orientation has three overarching sections: the organization, health and safety, and the employee's job. The US Department of Labor (DOL) publishes and provides online copies of the *Employment Law Guide* that addresses many aspects of each of these sections. An **employee handbook** provides a synopsis of the HR policies and procedures. Employee handbooks and HR policies should address **sexual harassment,** which is a violation of federal and some state laws. The legal definition is *unwelcome verbal, visual, or physical conduct of a sexual nature*

TABLE 56-1   Legal Versus Illegal Interview Questions

Topic	Illegal Questions	Legal Questions
Reliability/attendance	Number of children? Who is going to baby-sit? What religion are you? Do you have preschool-age children at home? What is your marital status? Do you have a car?	What hours and days can you work? Are there specific times that you cannot work? Do you have responsibilities other than work that will interfere with specific job requirements such as traveling?
Citizenship/national origin	What is your national origin? Where are your parents from?	Are you legally eligible for employment in the United States?
References	What is your maiden name? What is your father's surname? What are the names of your relatives?	Have you ever worked under a different name?
Arrests/convictions	Have you ever been arrested?	Have you ever been convicted of a crime? If so, when, where, and what was the disposition of the case?
Disability	Do you have any disabilities?	Can you perform the duties of the job you are applying for?
Birth date	What is your date of birth?	If hired, can you furnish proof that you are over age 18?
Emergency contact	What is the name and address of the relative to be notified in case of an emergency?	What is the name and address of the person to be notified in case of an emergency? (Request only after the individual has been employed.)
Credit history	Do you own your own home? Have your wages ever been garnished? Have you ever declared bankruptcy?	Credit references may be used in compliance with the Fair Credit Reporting Act of 1970 and the Consumer Credit Reporting Reform Act of 1996.
Military service	What type of discharge did you receive?	What type of education, training, or work experience did you receive while in the military?
Languages	What is your native language? Inquiry into how applicant acquired the ability to read, write, or speak a foreign language	Inquiry into languages applicant speaks and writes fluently (if the job requires additional languages)
Organizations	List all clubs, societies, and lodges to which you belong. Are you a union member?	Inquiry into applicant's membership in organizations that the applicant considers relevant to his or her ability to perform the job
Race/color	Inquiry about complexion or color of skin Inquiry about coloring	None
W/C	Have you ever filed for workers' compensation? Have you had any prior work injuries?	None
Religion/creed	Inquiry into applicant's religious denomination, religious affiliations, church, parish, pastor, or religious holidays observed	None
Gender	Do you wish to be addressed as Mr., Mrs., Miss, or Ms.?	None
Address	What was your previous address? How long did you reside there? How long have you lived at your current address? Do you own your own home?	None
Education	When did you graduate from high school or college?	Do you have a high school diploma or equivalent? Do you have a university or college degree?
Personal	What color are your eyes, hair? What is your weight?	Only permissible if there is a bona fide occupational qualification

that is severe or pervasive and affects working conditions or creates a hostile work environment. Other topics in a typical employee handbook are found in Table 56-2.

When Miguel began his employment, he, like all new employees, was on a 90-day **probationary period** or *trial period*. During this time frame, the HR department begins to facilitate staff development and training. Miguel, along with other staff members, attended training for the new electronic health record system the practice is implementing. Other training may include new policies and procedures, cultural diversity and sensitivity, CPR certification, new equipment, and wellness topics such as stress management.

TABLE 56-2 Typical Topics Found in an Employee Handbook

Welcome Message	EEOC Statement	Personal Communications
Organization mission statement	Employment application	Personnel records
Orientation	Equipment and facility use	Probationary periods
Attendance policies	Electronic communication and device use	Performance reviews and improvement plans
Benefits	Job descriptions	Safety and security
Disability benefits	Grievance process	Risk management and incident reports
Leaves of absence	On-the-job injuries	Sexual harassment guidelines
Bereavement policies	OSHA	(Non) Smoking policy
Holidays	Overtime policies	Substance abuse
Jury duty	Payroll periods	Subpoenas
Confidentiality and HIPAA	ADA statements	Wage increases and adjustments
Continuing education and tuition reimbursement	Disaster preparedness and emergency response	Schedules, accountability, and time-off requests
Dress code	Drug testing	

The trial period allows both the new employee and the organization an opportunity to decide if they are a "good fit." During the probationary period, the employer may terminate the new employee without cause. Likewise, the employee can also decide to leave the new position with little or no notice.

BWW Medical Associates conducts employee performance reviews at the end of the probationary period and then annually. The performance review typically includes the responsibilities in the job description and a form that includes the professional behaviors discussed throughout this textbook. Salary increases are usually based on the review rating.

Many medical practices also provide tuition reimbursement and reimburse expenses for employees who attend conferences that provide continuing education units so that the employee can maintain the appropriate credentials for his or her position. Copies of all training and staff development activities and certificates are maintained in the employee's personnel file.

Staff Communication

An effective manager ensures convenient, two-way, open, and consistent avenues of communication with the staff, using the following:

- Staff meetings. Staff meetings should be at a consistent time each month when patients are not seen. The time is blocked off in the appointment matrix. The location should allow privacy. An **agenda,** which is a list of meeting topics and the order in which they will be addressed, should be used (Figure 56-8). See Procedure 56-2 at the end of this chapter. Formal minutes (the meeting record) may or may not be kept, but at least meeting notes should be maintained by the practice manager that contain the date and time, who was present and absent, what was discussed, and who was responsible for any follow-up actions. These minutes may be needed for credentialing and licensing agencies or as proof of educational and informational topics addressed and as a tool for staff evaluations.

- E-mail. Most offices have e-mail for each employee or group of employees. E-mail is rapid and convenient but should be read and edited carefully. Staff and management messages should maintain a professional tone and responses provided in a reasonable time.

- Newsletters. Larger practices may have a monthly or quarterly electronic or hard-copy newsletter, which may be the responsibility of the practice manager. The content usually provides information on what is going on in the practice, new policies and procedures or requirements, accomplishments and awards, and internal and community events, often highlighting staff members or departments.

- Bulletin boards. Usually located in the staff lounge, these boards should not contain any confidential or sensitive information, since janitorial staff and others outside the practice may have access.

- Open-door policy. This policy, maintained by many practice managers, gives staff the freedom to come talk any time the manager's office door is open. Staff should be respectful of the manager's time and, if the topic is involved and lengthy, schedule an appointment.

- Suggestion boxes. In some facilities, staff and sometimes patients are encouraged to place ideas in a suggestion box; they can submit the suggestion with a name or anonymously. If the suggestion is implemented, some organizations provide a monetary or other award.

Labor Relations

Labor relations is an HR role referring to issues that arise between employees and management. When most people hear the term *labor relations,* they tend to think of the process of hiring and terminating employees, but other functions relate to labor relations. For instance, overseeing the **grievance process** if an employee feels he or she was unjustly treated comes under the heading of labor relations. HR also may mediate or arrange **mediation** for differences between employees, groups of employees, or employees and management. The mediator's role

BWW Medical Associates, PC: Staff Lounge
Staff Meeting Agenda
October 1, 20XX, 12:00 to 1:30 p.m.

Lunch provided

Introductions	Malik Katahri
Staff News	All
Quality Assurance Report	Kalyn Haddix
Policies and Procedures Update	Malik Katahri
EHR Committee Report	Miguel Perez
Report from AAMA Conference	Miguel Perez

Old Business:

• Extending office hours	Paul Buckwalter, MD
• Upcoming flu shot clinic	Kalyn Haddix

New Business:

• Holiday Party	Malik Katahri
• Volunteers for Flu Preparedness Committee	Alexis Whalen, MD

Other

Adjournment

Next meeting November 3, 20XX, 12:00 to 1:30 p.m.

FIGURE 56-8 Sample of a staff meeting agenda.

is to facilitate communication between the parties, assist them in focusing on the real issues of the disagreement in a nonadversarial manner, and attempt to reach conflict resolution.

▶ Being a Leader   LO 56.4

Think about someone you admire and the reasons you admire that person. Now think of three words that describe that person. It will not be surprising if words such as *confident, honest, responsible,* and *organized* come to mind. These are terms, along with others, that describe leaders. Leaders are people who can influence other people to work toward a common goal, to build a team to accomplish those goals. Do not confuse leadership with supervising. There are many excellent leaders who are not supervisors and probably just as many supervisors who are not effective leaders. Let's look at

why leadership, particularly in the healthcare field, is important and how you can become a leader as a medical assistant.

Becoming a Leader

It may sound strange, but to be a good leader, you must first be a good follower; to learn to lead, you must first understand how to be supervised and have a willingness to follow directions. How can you ask someone to follow your directions if you consistently show an unwillingness to follow your own superior's direction? Other traits of effective leaders are

- A desire to achieve both personal and organizational goals.
- Confidence based on a good understanding of the situation at hand.
- An ability to be a team member and influence other members of the team to accomplish stated goals.
- Excellent communication skills (oral and written).
- An ability and willingness to accommodate change.
- Integrity.
- Willingness, even eagerness, to accept responsibility.
- Realization that goals are best achieved through the efforts of many.
- Giving genuine recognition to others that assist in achieving goals.

Building Your Team Good leaders know that effective teams accomplish goals by capitalizing on each member's strengths. But how do you build a team in a medical office when each healthcare worker's job requires her to focus on her area of expertise so that the office runs smoothly? The key is participation. It is up to the leader to create an atmosphere that values and *encourages* teamwork. To do this, an effective leader

- Ensures that each team member knows her job and performs those tasks to the best of her ability.
- Values each team member and encourages each member's contributions.
- Uses excellent communication skills to build trust between the team members.
- Helps each team member set worthwhile and attainable goals.

Setting Goals Most people say they achieve more when they know what is expected of them. Setting goals allows team members to know and understand those expectations and provides a method to measure their progress and identify areas that require attention. When setting goals, it is important to remember some key points:

- Make goals challenging, but not so much so that the goal is impossible to attain.
- Allow team members to contribute their ideas regarding personal and team goals.
- Make sure that the goal is measurable in some way so that success can be *seen.*
- Make sure to have an action plan to reach the goal. The plan should outline what is to be done, the responsible person, and a time frame for completion of the task.

- The team leader should meet with individuals and teams to evaluate progress. If the goal was met, did it meet expectations? What is working and what needs improving? These evaluations provide the basis for the next goal-setting session.

Diversity and Leadership

We have all heard the sayings "Opposites attract" and "It takes all kinds." Both are true, and respecting differences will make you a better leader. Keep in mind that if you feel that someone is "different," it is very likely that person is thinking the same thing about you! **Diversity** includes differences among people in terms of identity, age, sex, race, physical ability, ethnicity, religious beliefs, values and mores, sexual orientation, and personality. Open communication among people who are different from each other leads to an understanding of and respect for those differences. It does not mean you must agree with all the differences or beliefs, but you will develop a respect and acceptance of the right of people to be "different." The following are some suggestions to help you increase your respect for diversity:

- Communicate openly to increase your awareness of diversity. This will increase your knowledge of similarities and differences among individuals.

- Examine your own feelings. No one is immune to biases, and people tend to stereotype others, which leads to discrimination—the opposite of accepting diversity. What are your biases? Are they hurting your ability to communicate effectively with others? Be honest with yourself.

- Look at each person as an individual and not as part of a group. By communicating with individuals, biases and "walls" begin to come down.

- Learn to value each person's uniqueness. Every person on the team is valuable and has a contribution to make. Be open to each person's insight and contribution.

- Keep in mind that in healthcare you must be open and respectful of diversity in order to provide quality care to each patient. This respect must carry over to all members of the healthcare team.

Think back to the beginning of this section and the person you said you admire. Does he or she possess traits you would like to emulate? Many effective leaders learn from their mentors. They also learn not only from their own successes but also from their failures. Anyone can make a mistake—the trick is to not make the same mistake repeatedly. If you do not like the result of something, change how or what you are doing, and the result will change. There is almost always more than one way to accomplish a task; listen to everyone in the office and try new ideas. When you do, you are on your way to not only being a team member, but also a team leader.

The practice manager's role as a leader in the medical office is not easy but carries the opportunity for many personal and professional rewards. Seeing the healthcare organization provide excellent patient care in a safe, financially sound environment where staff members are happy to come to work is an accomplishment of much pride and satisfaction. To create or sustain this environment, the manager, as in all

positions in healthcare, must stay current in the field by reading appropriate journals and books; attending seminars and courses; maintaining membership in his or her professional organizations; and networking with local, state, and national managers. When you experience your applied training, sometimes called an externship or practicum, think about the practice manager's many jobs.

▶ Risk Management and Quality Assurance
LO 56.5

The term **risk management (RM)** is defined as plans and processes that continually identify, assess, correct, and monitor functions of the medical office to prevent negative outcomes and minimize exposure to risk and consequent liability. Immediately recognizing and addressing potential problems should be everyone's focus. Risk management also identifies opportunities for improvement. A simple example of risk management is the procedure you learned for opening and closing the office, discussed in the *Safety and Patient Reception* chapter.

On the other hand, **quality assurance (QA)** procedures ensure that the services provided in the medical practice meet or exceed requirements and standards. Quality assurance encompasses *utilization review* (UR), which is ensuring that treatment plans and services are appropriate and cost-effective. Determining medical necessity is usually required.

Risk management and quality assurance include almost every aspect of the practice manager's role and are a huge responsibility. The Joint Commission (TJC) and the National Committee on Quality Assurance (NCQA) review the office's RM and QA plans and outcomes during accreditation visits. They look for a problem-solving model that follows each issue to resolution, referred to as *closing the loop*. The following is an example of a typical five-step problem-solving model (Figure 56-9):

1. Identification
2. Assessment

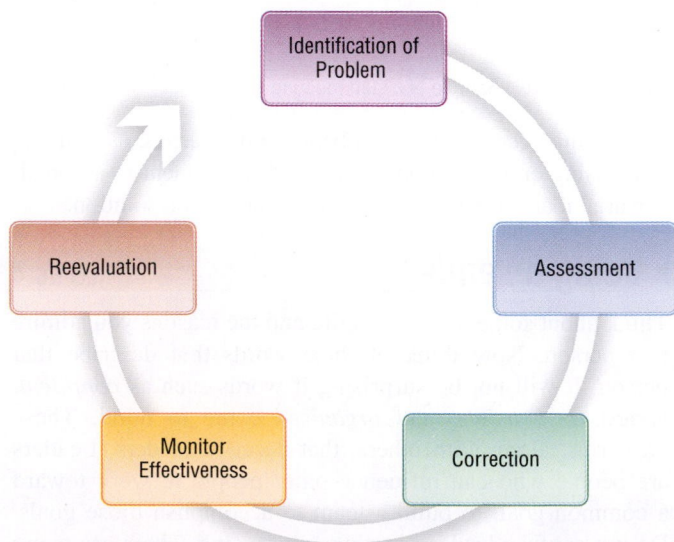

FIGURE 56-9 The problem-solving process.

3. Correction (design and implementation of an improvement plan)
4. Monitoring to ensure effectiveness of the plan
5. Reevaluation

In a simple example of problem solving, Malik, the practice manager at BWW Medical Associates, PC, notices that the carpet in the reception area is torn, and the patients and staff are placed at risk of falling (identification). He examines the tear and the entire carpet (assessment). He places tape over the tear and orders replacement carpeting (correction). The staff members are made aware of the tear and asked to be observant for other tears and similar problems (monitoring of effectiveness). Malik will reevaluate the condition of the carpet at intervals to ensure that it is not a risk for tripping and falling, until the new carpeting is installed.

Incident Reports

An **incident report** (Figure 56-10), or occurrence report, is a form required by a facility when an adverse outcome or event with risk of liability occurs. Refer to Procedure 56-3 at the end of this chapter. A fall caused by torn carpeting, for example, requires an incident report.

BWW Medical Associates, PC
305 Main Street, Port Snead YZ 12345-9876
Tel: 555-654-3210, Fax: 555-987-6543
Web: BWWAssociates.com

Paul F. Buckwalter, MD
Alexis N. Whalen, MD
Elizabeth H. Williams, MD

Incident Report
(Only for Internal Use)

Date/time of incident: _____   Location: _____

Name of injured or at-risk party: _____

Circle one: Patient   Staff Member   Other (complete blank) _____

Address of above party: _____

Phone numbers of above party: home _____ cell _____

Describe the incident (use back of sheet if additional space needed): _____

Describe action(s) taken and by whom: _____

Name(s)/contact information of witnesses: _____

Name(s)/time of all parties notified: _____

Name of person completing report: _____   Date/time: _____

Report submitted to: _____   Date/time: _____

(Submit form to immediate supervisor of area where the incident occurred)

FIGURE 56-10 Typical incident report form.

This report contains only factual information about the incident, no opinions or assumptions. Incident reports are not placed in a patient's medical record, and some institutions prefer that the incident report not be completed in the presence of the injured party. The standard practice is that no copies of an incident report are made, and only the original is maintained in a dedicated risk management file. As part of risk management, the practice manager routinely monitors incident reports and identifies any trends to work on reducing risk. While risk management includes anyone who enters the medical office, quality assurance generally involves the patient and his or her care.

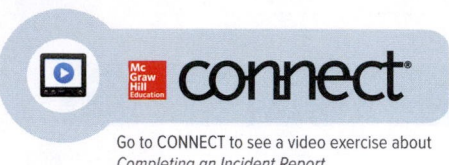

Go to CONNECT to see a video exercise about *Completing an Incident Report*.

▶ Handling Payroll
LO 56.6

As a medical assistant, you may be responsible for handling the office payroll (Table 56-3). If so, your duties may include

- Obtaining tax identification numbers.
- Creating employee payroll information sheets.
- Calculating employees' earnings.
- Subtracting taxes and other deductions.
- Writing paychecks.
- Creating employee earnings records.
- Preparing a payroll register.
- Submitting payroll taxes.

Applying for Tax Identification Numbers

Every employer—whether a single practitioner or a corporate practice—must have an employer identification number (EIN). An EIN is required by law for federal tax accounting purposes. To obtain an EIN, complete Form SS-4 (Application for Employer Identification Number) from http://www.federaltaxid.us and submit it to the Internal Revenue Service (IRS) at http://www.irs.gov. Some states also require employer tax reports, for which the practice must have a state identification number, obtained from the proper state agency.

Creating Employee Payroll Information Sheets

The practice must maintain up-to-date, accurate payroll information about each employee. You should prepare a payroll information sheet with the following information for each employee:

- The employee's name, address, Social Security number, and marital status
- An indication that the employee has completed an Employment Eligibility Verification (**Form I-9**), verifying that the employee is a US citizen, a legally admitted alien, or an alien authorized to work in the United States.
- The employer also must complete a new hire reporting form (NHR) on the employee's behalf and submit it to the applicable state agency before the employee receives her first paycheck. Usually, this form is collected along with the W-4 and I-9 forms. Each state has its own format, but the information gathered is universal. Some states allow electronic submission, while others accept the information via mail. Figure 56-11 shows an example of an NHR form.
- The employee's pay schedule, number of dependents, payroll type, and voluntary deductions

TABLE 56-3	Payroll Duties
Frequency	**Duties**
Upon assuming payroll responsibilities	Apply for an employer identification number (EIN) with Form SS-4 if the physician does not already have an EIN.
When a new employee is hired	Have the employee complete an Employee's Withholding Allowance Certificate (Form W-4) and Employment Eligibility Verification (Form I-9). Record the employee's name and Social Security number from the employee's Social Security card.
Every payday	Withhold federal income tax and state and local income taxes (if any). Withhold the employee's share of FICA taxes (for Social Security and Medicare). Record matching amount for the employer's share. Calculate how much the practice must pay for each employee's federal and state unemployment tax.
Monthly or biweekly (depending on your deposit schedule)	Deposit withheld income taxes, withheld and employer Social Security taxes, and withheld and employer Medicare taxes.
Quarterly (by April 30, July 31, October 31, and January 31)	File Employer's Quarterly Federal Tax Return (Form 941). With the return, pay any taxes that were not deposited earlier. Deposit federal unemployment tax, if over $100.
At least once a year	Have all employees update their W-4 forms.
On or before January 31	Give employees their Wage and Tax Statements (Form W-2), which show total wages and various withheld taxes. File Employer's Annual Federal Unemployment (FUTA) Tax Return (Form 940) with tax amount due.
On or before February 28	File Transmittal of Wage and Tax Statements (Form W-3) along with the government's copies of the W-2 forms.

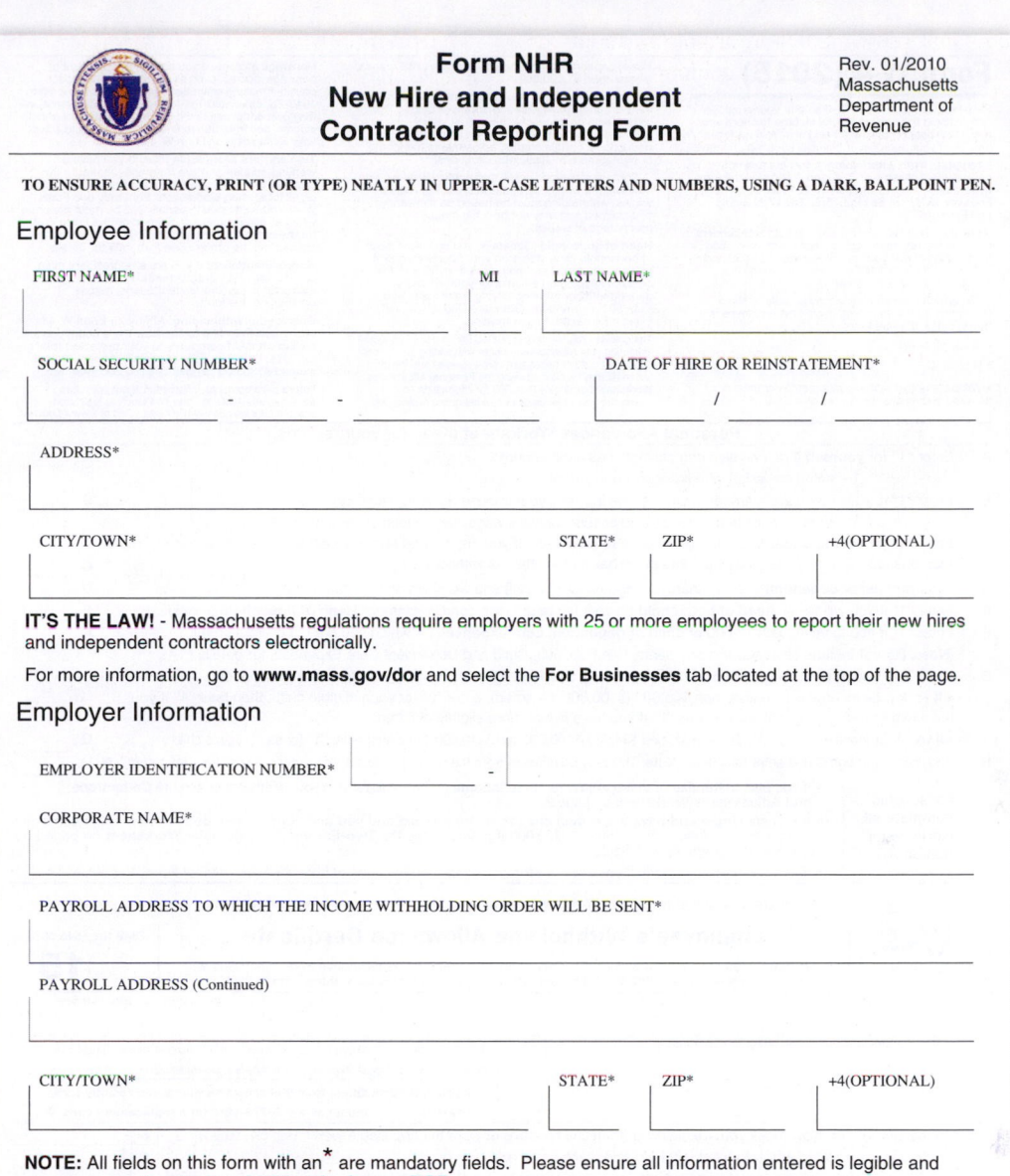

Form NHR
New Hire and Independent
Contractor Reporting Form

Rev. 01/2010
Massachusetts
Department of
Revenue

TO ENSURE ACCURACY, PRINT (OR TYPE) NEATLY IN UPPER-CASE LETTERS AND NUMBERS, USING A DARK, BALLPOINT PEN.

Employee Information

FIRST NAME*   MI   LAST NAME*

SOCIAL SECURITY NUMBER*   DATE OF HIRE OR REINSTATEMENT*

ADDRESS*

CITY/TOWN*   STATE*   ZIP*   +4(OPTIONAL)

IT'S THE LAW! - Massachusetts regulations require employers with 25 or more employees to report their new hires and independent contractors electronically.

For more information, go to **www.mass.gov/dor** and select the **For Businesses** tab located at the top of the page.

Employer Information

EMPLOYER IDENTIFICATION NUMBER*

CORPORATE NAME*

PAYROLL ADDRESS TO WHICH THE INCOME WITHHOLDING ORDER WILL BE SENT*

PAYROLL ADDRESS (Continued)

CITY/TOWN*   STATE*   ZIP*   +4(OPTIONAL)

NOTE: All fields on this form with an * are mandatory fields. Please ensure all information entered is legible and accurate prior to submitting the form to DOR.

Helpful Hint: Once you have completed your employer information, you may copy this form to save time when reporting future new hires and independent contractors.

Send Completed Form NHR to:
Massachusetts Department of Revenue, PO Box 55141, Boston, MA 02205-5141 or,
you may fax the completed form to 617-376-3262.

FIGURE 56-11   New hire and independent contract reporting (NHR) form.

Pay Schedule and Payroll Type On the payroll information sheet, list the employee's *pay schedule,* showing how often the employee is paid. Common pay schedules are weekly, biweekly, and monthly.

List the employee's payroll type—hourly wage, salary, or commission—on the payroll information sheet. An hourly wage is a set amount of money per hour of work. A salary is a set amount of money per pay period, regardless of the number of hours worked. A commission is a percentage of the amount an employee earns for the employer. Salespeople, for example, are often paid by commission.

Number of Dependents Record the number of dependents (people who depend on the employee for financial support who will be claimed by the employee). Dependents include a spouse, children, and other family members.

You can find the number of dependents on the Employee's Withholding Allowance Certificate (**Form W-4**), which should have been completed when the employee was hired (Figure 56-12). Remember, keep the completed W-4 forms in the physician's personnel file and update them annually.

Voluntary Deductions Voluntary deductions are those items not required by law to be deducted from the employee's

Form W-4 (2015)

Purpose. Complete Form W-4 so that your employer can withhold the correct federal income tax from your pay. Consider completing a new Form W-4 each year and when your personal or financial situation changes.

Exemption from withholding. If you are exempt, complete **only** lines 1, 2, 3, 4, and 7 and sign the form to validate it. Your exemption for 2015 expires February 16, 2016. See Pub. 505, Tax Withholding and Estimated Tax.

Note. If another person can claim you as a dependent on his or her tax return, you cannot claim exemption from withholding if your income exceeds $1,050 and includes more than $350 of unearned income (for example, interest and dividends).

Exceptions. An employee may be able to claim exemption from withholding even if the employee is a dependent, if the employee:

• Is age 65 or older,

• Is blind, or

• Will claim adjustments to income; tax credits; or itemized deductions, on his or her tax return.

The exceptions do not apply to supplemental wages greater than $1,000,000.

Basic instructions. If you are not exempt, complete the **Personal Allowances Worksheet** below. The worksheets on page 2 further adjust your withholding allowances based on itemized deductions, certain credits, adjustments to income, or two-earners/multiple jobs situations.

Complete all worksheets that apply. However, you may claim fewer (or zero) allowances. For regular wages, withholding must be based on allowances you claimed and may not be a flat amount or percentage of wages.

Head of household. Generally, you can claim head of household filing status on your tax return only if you are unmarried and pay more than 50% of the costs of keeping up a home for yourself and your dependent(s) or other qualifying individuals. See Pub. 501, Exemptions, Standard Deduction, and Filing Information, for information.

Tax credits. You can take projected tax credits into account in figuring your allowable number of withholding allowances. Credits for child or dependent care expenses and the child tax credit may be claimed using the **Personal Allowances Worksheet** below. See Pub. 505 for information on converting your other credits into withholding allowances.

Nonwage income. If you have a large amount of nonwage income, such as interest or dividends, consider making estimated tax payments using Form 1040-ES, Estimated Tax for Individuals. Otherwise, you may owe additional tax. If you have pension or annuity income, see Pub. 505 to find out if you should adjust your withholding on Form W-4 or W-4P.

Two earners or multiple jobs. If you have a working spouse or more than one job, figure the total number of allowances you are entitled to claim on all jobs using worksheets from only one Form W-4. Your withholding usually will be most accurate when all allowances are claimed on the Form W-4 for the highest paying job and zero allowances are claimed on the others. See Pub. 505 for details.

Nonresident alien. If you are a nonresident alien, see Notice 1392, Supplemental Form W-4 Instructions for Nonresident Aliens, before completing this form.

Check your withholding. After your Form W-4 takes effect, use Pub. 505 to see how the amount you are having withheld compares to your projected total tax for 2015. See Pub. 505, especially if your earnings exceed $130,000 (Single) or $180,000 (Married).

Future developments. Information about any future developments affecting Form W-4 (such as legislation enacted after we release it) will be posted at www.irs.gov/w4.

Personal Allowances Worksheet (Keep for your records.)

A Enter "1" for **yourself** if no one else can claim you as a dependent . . . . **A** _____

B Enter "1" if:
- You are single and have only one job; or
- You are married, have only one job, and your spouse does not work; or
- Your wages from a second job or your spouse's wages (or the total of both) are $1,500 or less.

. . . **B** _____

C Enter "1" for your **spouse**. But, you may choose to enter "-0-" if you are married and have either a working spouse or more than one job. (Entering "-0-" may help you avoid having too little tax withheld.) . . . . **C** _____

D Enter number of **dependents** (other than your spouse or yourself) you will claim on your tax return . . . . **D** _____

E Enter "1" if you will file as **head of household** on your tax return (see conditions under **Head of household** above) . . **E** _____

F Enter "1" if you have at least $2,000 of **child or dependent care expenses** for which you plan to claim a credit . . . **F** _____
(**Note.** Do **not** include child support payments. See Pub. 503, Child and Dependent Care Expenses, for details.)

G **Child Tax Credit** (including additional child tax credit). See Pub. 972, Child Tax Credit, for more information.
- If your total income will be less than $65,000 ($100,000 if married), enter "2" for each eligible child; then **less** "1" if you have two to four eligible children or **less** "2" if you have five or more eligible children.
- If your total income will be between $65,000 and $84,000 ($100,000 and $119,000 if married), enter "1" for each eligible child . . . **G** _____

H Add lines A through G and enter total here. (**Note.** This may be different from the number of exemptions you claim on your tax return.) ▶ **H** _____

For accuracy, complete all worksheets that apply.
- If you plan to **itemize** or **claim adjustments to income** and want to reduce your withholding, see the **Deductions and Adjustments Worksheet** on page 2.
- If you are **single and have more than one job** or are **married and you and your spouse both work** and the combined earnings from all jobs exceed $50,000 ($20,000 if married), see the **Two-Earners/Multiple Jobs Worksheet** on page 2 to avoid having too little tax withheld.
- If **neither** of the above situations applies, **stop here** and enter the number from line H on line 5 of Form W-4 below.

Separate here and give Form W-4 to your employer. Keep the top part for your records.

Form **W-4**
Department of the Treasury
Internal Revenue Service

Employee's Withholding Allowance Certificate

▶ Whether you are entitled to claim a certain number of allowances or exemption from withholding is subject to review by the IRS. Your employer may be required to send a copy of this form to the IRS.

OMB No. 1545-0074

2015

1 Your first name and middle initial	Last name	2 Your social security number

Home address (number and street or rural route)	3 ☐ Single ☐ Married ☐ Married, but withhold at higher Single rate.
City or town, state, and ZIP code	**Note.** If married, but legally separated, or spouse is a nonresident alien, check the "Single" box.

4 If your last name differs from that shown on your social security card, check here. You must call 1-800-772-1213 for a replacement card. ▶ ☐

5	Total number of allowances you are claiming (from line **H** above **or** from the applicable worksheet on page 2)	5	
6	Additional amount, if any, you want withheld from each paycheck	6	$
7	I claim exemption from withholding for 2015, and I certify that I meet **both** of the following conditions for exemption.		

- Last year I had a right to a refund of **all** federal income tax withheld because I had **no** tax liability, **and**
- This year I expect a refund of **all** federal income tax withheld because I expect to have **no** tax liability.

If you meet both conditions, write "Exempt" here . . . . ▶ | 7 |

Under penalties of perjury, I declare that I have examined this certificate and, to the best of my knowledge and belief, it is true, correct, and complete.

Employee's signature
(This form is not valid unless you sign it.) ▶ _____ Date ▶ _____

8 Employer's name and address (Employer: Complete lines 8 and 10 only if sending to the IRS.)	9 Office code (optional)	10 Employer identification number (EIN)

For Privacy Act and Paperwork Reduction Act Notice, see page 2. | Cat. No. 10220Q | Form **W-4** (2015)

FIGURE 56-12 Employee's Withholding Allowance Certificate (W-4) is completed upon hire and updated annually.

---

paycheck. These include additional federal withholding taxes, contributions to a 401(k) retirement plan, and payments to a company health insurance plan. Employees who want additional federal taxes taken out of their paycheck will indicate this deduction on their W-4 form.

Gross Earnings

Gross earnings refers to the total amount of income earned before deductions, and this figure must be calculated for each employee as a first step in the payroll process.

Calculating Gross Earnings For every payroll period, use data from the payroll information sheet to compute each employee's gross earnings. For an hourly employee, use this equation:

$$\text{Hourly Wage} \times \text{Hours Worked} = \text{Gross Earnings}$$

An employee who earns $12.50 per hour and works 35 hours, for example, has gross earnings of $437.50 ($12.50 × 35 hours) per week.

For a salaried employee, use the salary amount as the gross earnings for the pay period, no matter how many hours the employee worked. An employee who earns a weekly salary of $500, for example, receives that amount whether she worked 30, 40, or 50 hours during that week.

Fair Labor Standards Act The Fair Labor Standards Act primarily affects employees who earn hourly wages. It limits the number of hours they may work, sets their minimum wage, and regulates their overtime pay. It also requires the employer to record the number of hours they work, usually on a time card or in a time book.

For hourly employees, this act mandates payment of

- Time and a half (1½ times the normal hourly wage) for all hours worked beyond the normal 8 in a regular workday.
- Time and a half for all hours worked on the sixth consecutive day of the workweek.
- Twice the normal wage (double time) for all hours worked on the seventh consecutive workday.
- Double time, plus normal holiday pay, for all hours worked on a company-approved holiday.

The Fair Labor Standards Act also requires overtime payments for part-time hourly employees for every hour worked beyond the normal 8 in a day or 40 in a week.

Making Deductions

The law requires all employers to withhold money from employees' gross earnings to pay federal, state, and local (if any) income taxes and certain other taxes. In addition, employees may wish you to make certain voluntary deductions. For example, you might be asked to deduct an amount for child care, if the practice or hospital provides onsite child care. You also might deduct employee contributions to health insurance premiums.

You must deposit all employee deductions and employer payments into separate accounts, one for each deduction type. Accounts are typically set up for each type of deduction. The most common are **tax liability accounts** which are used to pay taxes to appropriate government agencies.

Income Taxes Enough money must be withheld to cover the employee's federal income tax for the pay period. You can determine this amount by finding the employee's number of exemptions (from Form W-4) and referring to the tax tables in *Circular E, Employer's Tax Guide,* published by the IRS. Consult the state and local tax tables for other income taxes.

FICA Taxes For **Federal Insurance Contributions Act (FICA)** tax, withhold from the employee's check half of the tax owed for the pay period. Pay the other half from the practice's accounts. The amount of FICA tax that funds Social Security differs from the amount that funds Medicare. Report these two amounts separately. Check IRS *Circular E* for the latest FICA tax percentages and level of taxable earnings.

Unemployment Taxes Federal unemployment tax is not a deduction from the employees' paychecks but rather is based on their earnings and paid by the employer. The **Federal Unemployment Tax Act (FUTA)** requires employers to pay a percentage of each employee's income, up to a certain dollar amount. The percentage may be reduced if the employer also pays state unemployment taxes.

States calculate unemployment taxes differently. Some states tax employers and employees; others tax only employers. State unemployment tax usually varies with the employer's past employment record. Employers with few layoffs, such as physicians, have lower tax rates than those with many layoffs. To compute state unemployment tax, apply the assigned tax rate to each employee's earnings, up to a maximum for the calendar year. For details, consult your state unemployment insurance department.

Workers' Compensation Some states require employers to insure their employees against possible loss of income resulting from work-related injury, disability, or disease. Although state laws vary, they typically require doctors to carry this insurance with a state insurance fund or state-authorized private insurer. Usually, a medical practice's insurance agent will audit the payroll books annually and then issue a bill for the workers' compensation premium due.

Calculating Net Earnings

Add each employee's required and voluntary deductions together to determine the total deductions. Then, subtract the total deductions from the gross earnings to get the employee's **net earnings,** or take-home pay. Use the following equation:

$$\text{Gross earnings} - \text{Total deductions} = \text{Net earnings}$$

The exception to this rule is contributions the employee makes to the employer retirement plan, if available. When sponsored by an employer, as with a 401(k) account, these deductions are often taken before taxes are calculated, reducing the employee's taxable income, which encourages the employee to take part in these plans.

Preparing Paychecks

The way you prepare the practice's payroll will depend on the system the practice uses. In a small practice, you may write paychecks manually. In this case, write the check amount for the employee's net earnings and deduct the check amount from the office checkbook. Payroll also may be handled through electronic banking; see the *Points on Practice* feature.

If the practice uses a payroll service, you may supply time cards or payroll data to the service by mail or electronically. The service calculates all the deductions, prepares paychecks, and mails them to the practice for distribution.

No matter how paychecks are prepared, they should include information about how the check amount was determined. This information usually appears on the check stub. It should match the information on the employee earnings records and payroll register. Procedure 56-4, at the end of the chapter, explains the process for generating payroll.

Maintaining Employee Earnings Records

You need to keep an employee earnings record for each employee (Figure 56-13). When creating the record, list the employee's name, address, phone number, Social Security

POINTS ON PRACTICE

Handling Payroll Through Electronic Banking

An electronic funds transfer system (EFTS) enables you to handle the practice's payroll without generating payroll checks manually. The practice must sign up for EFTS with the practice's bank and employees must supply their bank account numbers to the employer. Then, the bank electronically deposits employees' paychecks into their bank accounts, as directed.

Most employees like to have their paychecks deposited automatically. The money is available on the day of deposit and no one has to worry about losing a paycheck, getting to the bank before it closes, or carrying a paycheck around. Also, employees still receive a check stub along with a notification of deposit, so they can track their earnings and deductions. Contact your bank for more information and specific procedures for setting up EFTS and electronic payroll.

number, birth date, spouse's name, number of dependents, job title, employment start date, pay rate, and voluntary deductions.

Then, for each pay period, record the employee's gross earnings, individual deductions, net earnings, and related information. Properly completed earnings records show each employee's earning history.

Maintaining a Payroll Register

A payroll register summarizes vital information about all employees and their earnings (Figure 56-14). At the end of each pay period, record each employee's earnings to date, hourly rate, hours worked, overtime hours, overtime earnings, and total gross earnings. Also, list the gross earnings subject to unemployment taxes and FICA, all required and voluntary deductions, net earnings, and the paycheck number. Refer to Procedure 56-4, at the end of this chapter, for an example of how to prepare and complete the payroll procedure and register.

Handling Payroll Electronically

Manual payroll preparation and related tasks may take an hour per week for each employee. To save time and provide

Name ______________________ Soc. Sec. No. ______________________ Dependents ____________ Year ________

Address ______________________ Birth Date ______________________ Deductions ______________________

______________________ Job Title ______________________

______________________ Employed on ______________________ Pay Rate

Spouse ______________________ Terminated on ______________________ Record of Changes

Phone ______________________ Reason ______________________

Date	Rate

Check Number	Period Number	Earnings: Regular	Earnings: OT	Earnings: Total	Deductions: FICA	Deductions: Fed. Tax	Deductions: State	Deductions: SUI	Deductions: SDI	Net Pay	Cumulative FICA
1st Quarter Total											
2nd Quarter Total											

FIGURE 56-13 Earnings records show the earning history of each employee at the practice.

Emp. No.	Name	Earnings to Date	Hrly. Rate	Reg. Hrs.	OT Hrs.	OT Earnings	TOTAL GROSS	Earnings Subject to Unemp.	Earnings Subject to FICA	Social Security (FICA)	Medicare	Federal W/H	State W/H	Health Ins.	Net Pay	Check No.
0010	Scott, B.	9,823.14	14.00	70.00			980.00	980.00	980.00	60.50	14.10	147.92	15.10	25.00	717.38	11747
0020	Wilson, J.	14,290.38	17.00	70.00	6.50	165.75	1,355.75	1,355.75	1,355.75	83.26	19.47	160.45	15.85	67.50	1,009.22	11748
0030	Diaz, J.	2,750.26	5.50	46.25			254.37	254.37	254.37	15.77	3.68	38.20	3.75		192.97	11749
0040	Ling, W.	2,240.57	6.80	30.00			204.00	204.00	204.00	12.66	2.96	26.02	3.12		159.54	11750
0050	Harris, E.	2,600.98	10.00	23.50			235.00	235.00	235.00	14.57	3.41	33.52	3.36		180.14	11751

FIGURE 56-14   The payroll register is designed to summarize information about all employees and their earnings.

employees the convenience of having their paychecks automatically deposited, some practices handle payroll tasks electronically.

If you work in a relatively small practice, you may handle all payroll tasks in the office, using accounting or payroll software. If you work in a large practice, you may prepare payroll information on the computer and transmit it to an outside payroll service for processing. Depending on which system and software the practice has, you may use the computer to

- Create, update, and delete employee payroll information files.
- Prepare employee paychecks, stubs, and W-2 forms.
- Update and print employee earnings records.
- Update all appropriate bookkeeping records, such as the payroll ledger and general ledger, with payroll data.

To perform these payroll functions electronically, follow the specific instructions in the software manual or get instructions from the payroll service. Generally, you would follow these steps:

1. Select an option from the "Payroll" menu. Wait for the prompt and select the appropriate employee from the employee list.
2. Create a new employee file:
   a. Enter employee name, address, SSN, marital status, pay schedule, number of dependents, payroll type, and voluntary deductions.
   b. Print two copies—one for the employee and one for the personnel file.
3. Update employee payroll information after a life change such as change in marital status, birth of a child, change of address, or voluntary change in deductions:
   a. Select "Update Employee File."
   b. Make required changes.
   c. Print the form for the employee signature after he confirms information is correct.
   d. Print two signed copies—one for the employee and one for the personnel file.

   e. Payroll information must be correct and current. It should be updated yearly for each employee.
4. Delete an employee from payroll:
   a. Select "Terminate Employee."
   b. Print a copy of the file before deleting it, as the employer is required to keep employee payroll records for 4 years.
5. Generate paychecks and paystubs:
   a. Select the employee from the employee list.
   b. Choose the "Print Paycheck" option.
   c. Answer each prompt displayed (for example, hours worked).
   d. From the payroll information entered previously, the program calculates the employee's net earnings, generates a paycheck, and prints a pay stub with the appropriate information.
6. Create an employee earnings record:

   a. Select "Creating Employee Earnings Record."
   b. Follow the prompts to enter the required information.
   c. Depending on the software program used, this information may be updated automatically with each paycheck generated.

   Select an option from the "Payroll" menu. Wait for the prompt; then select the appropriate employee from a list of employees.

Calculating and Filing Taxes   LO 56.7

In many practices, administrative medical assistants set up tax liability accounts for money withheld from paychecks. These accounts are used to submit this money to appropriate agencies. Visit http://www.irs.gov for further information.

Setting Up Tax Liability Accounts

It is important to hold the money deducted from paychecks until it can be sent to the appropriate government agencies. Deductions from employees' paychecks for federal, state, and local income taxes and FICA taxes, as well as employer payments based on payroll, such as federal and state unemployment taxes, must be deposited until payment is due. For these accounts, choose a bank authorized by the IRS to accept federal tax deposits. If the practice makes other paycheck deductions, such as for workers' compensation or a 401(k) plan, other accounts are created and accurate records for this money must be maintained.

Each time you prepare paychecks, deposit the withheld money into the proper account as dictated by your practice. Record the deposited amounts as debits in the practice's checking account.

Understanding Federal Tax Deposit Schedules

You will probably deposit federal income taxes and FICA taxes (which together are known as employment taxes) on a quarterly, monthly, or biweekly (every-other-week) schedule. Every November, IRS personnel decide which deposit schedule your office should use for the next year.

If the IRS does not notify you about this matter, determine your deposit schedule based on the total employment taxes your office reported on the previous year's Employer's Quarterly Federal Tax Returns (Form 941). For example, if your office reported $50,000 or less in employment taxes during the past year, you would make monthly employment tax deposits the present year. If your office reported more than $50,000 during the past year, you would make semimonthly tax deposits.

Exceptions to the monthly or semimonthly tax deposit schedules are the $500 rule and the $100,000 rule. The $500 rule applies to employers who owe less than $500 in employment taxes during a tax period (such as a quarter). These employers do not have to make a deposit for that period. The $100,000 rule applies to employers who owe $100,000 or more in employment taxes on any one day during a tax period. These employers must deposit the tax by the next banking day after the day that ceiling is reached.

Submitting Federal Income Taxes and FICA Taxes

Since January 1, 2011, businesses must submit federal income taxes and FICA taxes to the IRS by electronic funds transfer (EFT), known as TAXLINK. If for any reason a check must be mailed, such as the office EFT process having not yet been completed, make the check payable to "Financial Agent." Put the practice EIN in the check's memo section and mail it to Financial Agent, Federal Tax Deposit Processing Center, in St. Louis, Missouri. If your office does not have electronic fund transfer capabilities, contact the office accountant or financial institution, who may be able to submit your tax liabilities for you (a fee is usually charged for this service).

If you work in a practice with a large payroll, you may need to make deposits every few days. In most practices, however, you will probably make deposits once a month. Then, every 3 months, a more complete accounting is required on a quarterly basis, which will be discussed in more detail a bit later in this chapter.

Submitting Federal Unemployment Tax Act (FUTA) and State Unemployment Tax Act (SUTA) Taxes

FUTA taxes provide money to workers who are unemployed. If the practice owes more than $100 in federal unemployment tax at the end of the quarter, deposit the tax amount with an FTD Coupon (Form 8109). At the end of the year, file an Employer's Annual Federal Unemployment (FUTA) Tax Return (Form 940) with any final taxes owed (Figure 56-15).

Generally, an employer must pay FUTA taxes if employees' wages total more than $1,500 in any quarter (3-month period) and if those employees are not seasonal or household workers. The FUTA tax, which is 6.2%, is applied to the first $7,000 of income for a year.

Some states are also governed by a State Unemployment Tax Act (SUTA). These taxes are filed along with FUTA taxes. Make sure you know the laws governing unemployment taxes in your state.

Filing an Employer's Quarterly Federal Tax Return

Each quarter, file an Employer's Quarterly Federal Tax Return (Form 941) with the IRS (Figure 56-16). This tax return summarizes the federal income and FICA taxes (employment taxes) withheld from employees' paychecks.

As a general rule, you should file Form 941 at the nearest IRS office by the last day of the first month after the quarter ends. If the practice has deposited all taxes on time, you have an additional 10 days after the due date to file.

Handling State and Local Income Taxes

Send withheld state and local income taxes to the proper agencies, using their forms, procedures, and schedules. If required, prepare quarterly or other tax forms for your state or local agency. If you are unsure of how often to submit these forms and taxes, you can visit your state website or the IRS website at http://www.irs.gov.

Filing Wage and Tax Statements

After the end of each year, file a Wage and Tax Statement (**Form W-2**) with the appropriate federal, state, and local government agencies for each employee who had federal income and FICA taxes withheld during the previous year (Figure 56-17). Also, supply copies of Form W-2 to each employee.

Form W-2 shows the employee's total taxable income for the previous year. It also shows the exact amount of federal income taxes and FICA taxes (for Social Security and Medicare) withheld, along with the amounts of state and local taxes withheld (if any).

Along with the W-2 forms, submit Form W-3, a Transmittal of Wage and Tax Statements (Figure 56-18). This form lists the employer's name, address, and EIN and summarizes the amount of all employees' earnings and the federal income taxes and FICA taxes withheld.

Form **940** for 2014: Employer's Annual Federal Unemployment (FUTA) Tax Return

Department of the Treasury — Internal Revenue Service

850113

OMB No. 1545-0028

Employer identification number (EIN)

Name (not your trade name)

Trade name (if any)

Address

Number   Street   Suite or room number

City   State   ZIP code

Foreign country name   Foreign province/county   Foreign postal code

Type of Return
(Check all that apply.)

☐ a. Amended

☐ b. Successor employer

☐ c. No payments to employees in 2014

☐ d. Final: Business closed or stopped paying wages

Instructions and prior-year forms are available at *www.irs.gov/form940*.

Read the separate instructions before you complete this form. Please type or print within the boxes.

Part 1: Tell us about your return. If any line does NOT apply, leave it blank.

1a If you had to pay state unemployment tax in one state only, enter the state abbreviation . **1a**

1b If you had to pay state unemployment tax in more than one state, you are a multi-state employer . . . . **1b** ☐ Check here. Complete Schedule A (Form 940).

2 If you paid wages in a state that is subject to CREDIT REDUCTION . . . . **2** ☐ Check here. Complete Schedule A (Form 940).

Part 2: Determine your FUTA tax before adjustments for 2014. If any line does NOT apply, leave it blank.

3 Total payments to all employees **3**

4 Payments exempt from FUTA tax **4**

Check all that apply: **4a** ☐ Fringe benefits   **4c** ☐ Retirement/Pension   **4e** ☐ Other
4b ☐ Group-term life insurance   **4d** ☐ Dependent care

5 Total of payments made to each employee in excess of $7,000 . . . . **5**

6 Subtotal (line 4 + line 5 = line 6) **6**

7 Total taxable FUTA wages (line 3 – line 6 = line 7) (see instructions) **7**

8 FUTA tax before adjustments (line 7 x .006 = line 8) **8**

Part 3: Determine your adjustments. If any line does NOT apply, leave it blank.

9 If ALL of the taxable FUTA wages you paid were excluded from state unemployment tax, multiply line 7 by .054 (line 7 × .054 = line 9). Go to line 12 . . . . . . **9**

10 If SOME of the taxable FUTA wages you paid were excluded from state unemployment tax, OR you paid ANY state unemployment tax late (after the due date for filing Form 940), complete the worksheet in the instructions. Enter the amount from line 7 of the worksheet . . **10**

11 If credit reduction applies, enter the total from Schedule A (Form 940) **11**

Part 4: Determine your FUTA tax and balance due or overpayment for 2014. If any line does NOT apply, leave it blank.

12 Total FUTA tax after adjustments (lines 8 + 9 + 10 + 11 = line 12) **12**

13 FUTA tax deposited for the year, including any overpayment applied from a prior year . **13**

14 Balance due (If line 12 is more than line 13, enter the excess on line 14.)
- If line 14 is more than $500, you must deposit your tax.
- If line 14 is $500 or less, you may pay with this return. (see instructions) **14**

15 Overpayment (If line 13 is more than line 12, enter the excess on line 15 and check a box below.) **15**

▶ You **MUST** complete both pages of this form and **SIGN** it.   Check one: ☐ Apply to next return. ☐ Send a refund.

Next ▶

For Privacy Act and Paperwork Reduction Act Notice, see the back of Form 940-V, Payment Voucher.   Cat. No. 11234O   Form **940** (2014)

FIGURE 56-15 Tax dollars filed with FUTA returns (Form 940) provide income to temporarily unemployed workers.

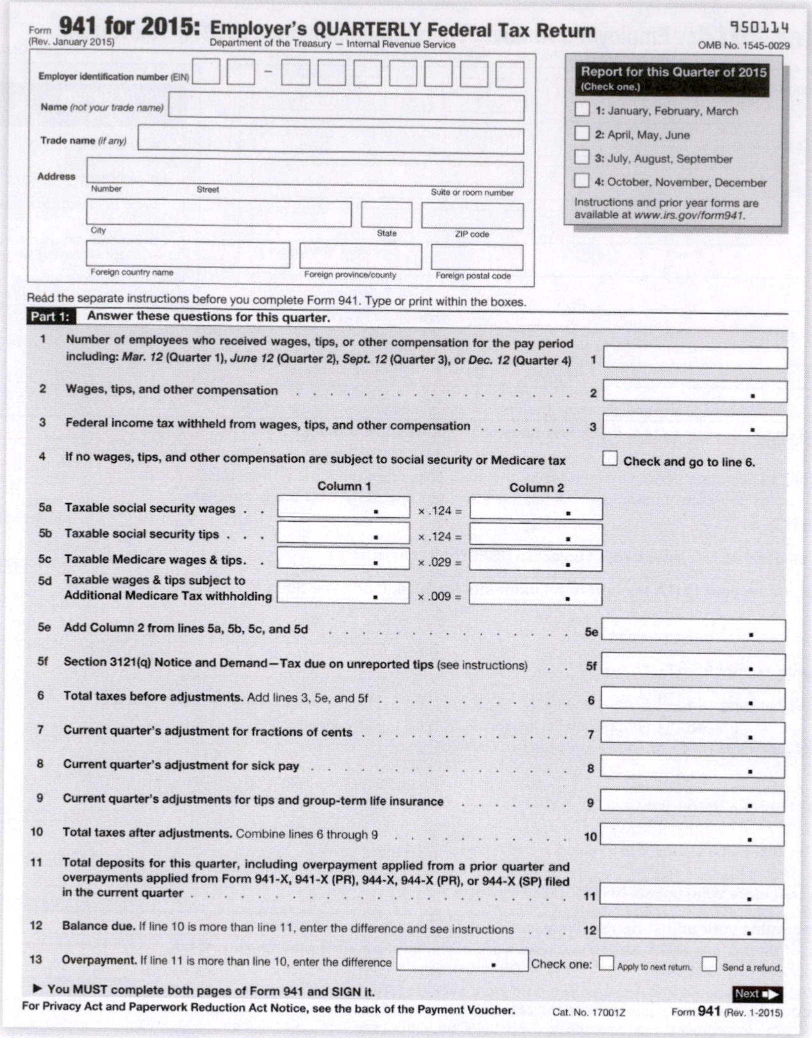

FIGURE 56-16 Most practices make tax deposits monthly and then make a more complete accounting quarterly on the Employer's Quarterly Federal Tax Return (Form 941), the first page of which is shown here.

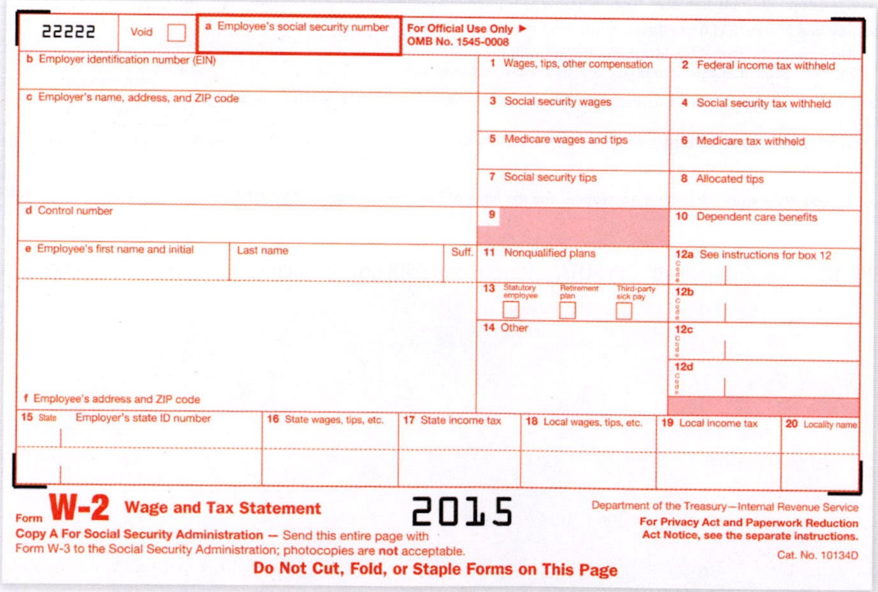

FIGURE 56-17 A Wage and Tax Statement (Form W-2) records the total amount of taxes withheld during the previous year for each employee.

Form W-3 (2015)

DO NOT STAPLE				
a Control number 33333		For Official Use Only ▶ OMB No. 1545-0008		

| **b** Kind of Payer (Check one) | 941 ☐ Military ☐ 943 ☐ 944 ☐ CT-1 ☐ Hshld. emp. ☐ Medicare govt. emp. ☐ | **Kind of Employer** (Check one) | None apply ☐ 501c non-govt. ☐ State/local non-501c ☐ State/local 501c ☐ Federal govt. ☐ | Third-party sick pay ☐ (Check if applicable) |

c Total number of Forms W-2	**d** Establishment number	**1** Wages, tips, other compensation	**2** Federal income tax withheld
e Employer identification number (EIN)		**3** Social security wages	**4** Social security tax withheld
f Employer's name		**5** Medicare wages and tips	**6** Medicare tax withheld
		7 Social security tips	**8** Allocated tips
		9	**10** Dependent care benefits
		11 Nonqualified plans	**12a** Deferred compensation
g Employer's address and ZIP code			
h Other EIN used this year		**13** For third-party sick pay use only	**12b**
15 State Employer's state ID number		**14** Income tax withheld by payer of third-party sick pay	
16 State wages, tips, etc.	**17** State income tax	**18** Local wages, tips, etc.	**19** Local income tax
Employer's contact person		Employer's telephone number	For Official Use Only
Employer's fax number		Employer's email address	

Under penalties of perjury, I declare that I have examined this return and accompanying documents and, to the best of my knowledge and belief, they are true, correct, and complete.

Signature ▶   Title ▶   Date ▶

Form W-3 Transmittal of Wage and Tax Statements   2015

Department of the Treasury
Internal Revenue Service

Send this entire page with the entire Copy A page of Form(s) W-2 to the Social Security Administration (SSA).
Photocopies are not acceptable. Do not send Form W-3 if you filed electronically with the SSA.
Do not send any payment (cash, checks, money orders, etc.) with Forms W-2 and W-3.

Reminder

Separate instructions. See the 2015 General Instructions for Forms W-2 and W-3 for information on completing this form. Do not file Form W-3 for Form(s) W-2 that were submitted electronically to the SSA.

Purpose of Form

A Form W-3 Transmittal is completed only when paper Copy A of Form(s) W-2, Wage and Tax Statement, is being filed. Do not file Form W-3 alone. All paper forms **must** comply with IRS standards and be machine readable. Photocopies are **not** acceptable. Use a Form W-3 even if only one paper Form W-2 is being filed. Make sure both the Form W-3 and Form(s) W-2 show the correct tax year and Employer Identification Number (EIN). Make a copy of this form and keep it with Copy D (For Employer) of Form(s) W-2 for your records. The IRS recommends retaining copies of these forms for four years.

E-Filing

The SSA strongly suggests employers report Form W-3 and Forms W-2 Copy A electronically instead of on paper. The SSA provides two free e-filing options on its Business Services Online (BSO) website:

• **W-2 Online.** Use fill-in forms to create, save, print, and submit up to 50 Forms W-2 at a time to the SSA.

• **File Upload.** Upload wage files to the SSA you have created using payroll or tax software that formats the files according to the SSA's *Specifications for Filing Forms W-2 Electronically (EFW2)*.

W-2 Online fill-in forms or file uploads will be on time if submitted by March 31, 2016. For more information, go to *www.socialsecurity.gov/employer*. First time filers select "*Go to Register*"; returning filers select "*Go To Log In*."

When To File

Mail Form W-3 with Copy A of Form(s) W-2 by February 29, 2016.

Where To File Paper Forms

Send this entire page with the entire Copy A page of Form(s) W-2 to:

Social Security Administration
Data Operations Center
Wilkes-Barre, PA 18769-0001

Note. If you use "Certified Mail" to file, change the ZIP code to "18769-0002." If you use an IRS-approved private delivery service, add "ATTN: W-2 Process, 1150 E. Mountain Dr." to the address and change the ZIP code to "18702-7997." See Publication 15 (Circular E), Employer's Tax Guide, for a list of IRS-approved private delivery services.

For Privacy Act and Paperwork Reduction Act Notice, see the separate instructions.

Cat. No. 10159Y

FIGURE 56-18 Submit the Transmittal of Wage and Tax Statements (Form W-3) with the W-2 forms.

PROCEDURE 56-1   Preparing a Travel Expense Report

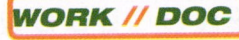

(Imagine that you have just attended the latest AAMA or AMT annual conference. Research the price of airfare from your locale to the city of the conference. Determine registration and other costs. Use these figures to perform the procedure.)

Procedure Goal: To obtain reimbursement or account for pre-approved travel funds and to provide documentation of expenses for the medical office

OSHA Guidelines: This procedure does not involve exposure to blood, body fluids, or tissues.

Materials: Travel expense report form, pen, receipts, conference web information, and a calculator

Method:

1. Ensure that your travel received prior approval.

RATIONALE: *Without prior approval, your expenses may be denied.*

2. Save receipts from the event.
3. Complete the personal identifying information on the form.
4. Insert the purpose of the travel, location, dates, and number of days.
5. Place the amounts as labeled in the expense table.
6. Total the amounts.
7. Check the appropriate box to indicate if you missed work and the dates and total number of days.
8. Sign and date the form.
9. Attach receipts (generally, original receipts are submitted; keep copies for your own records).
   RATIONALE: *Without receipts, the expenses will not be reimbursed.*
10. Submit the completed form and receipts.

PROCEDURE 56-2 Preparing an Agenda

Procedure Goal: To facilitate a meeting's organization and focus by providing a list of meeting topics, the name of the person reporting, and the order in which each topic will be addressed

OSHA Guidelines: This procedure does not involve exposure to blood, body fluids, or tissues.

Materials: Paper and pen or computer, copy machine, and minutes from last meeting

Method:

1. Approximately 1 week before the meeting, e-mail or post a memo to staff, offering them an opportunity to add items to the agenda. This is referred to as a *Call for Agenda Items.*
   RATIONALE: *Allows an opportunity for all staff members to suggest items for discussion.*
2. Place the following on top of the form used to create the agenda:
   - Name of the practice
   - Site name, if the practice has more than one location
   - Title: *Staff Meeting Agenda*
   - Date and time the meeting is scheduled to begin and end
3. Many offices have standing topics that go on the agenda every month; examples are
   - Introduction of new staff members.
   - Approval of minutes, if formal minutes are kept.
   - Staff news (promotions, birthdays, weddings, births, and so on).
   - Quality assurance report.
   - Policy and procedure updates.
   - Committee reports.
   - Report from individuals who have attended a conference.
   RATIONALE: *Consistency in meeting format ensures that items are not forgotten.*
4. Review the minutes from the previous meeting to determine any topics that required action with the person responsible. List these on the agenda under *Old Business.*
5. Add topics obtained from the *Call for Agenda Items* and any new topics the manager wishes to discuss. List these under *New Business.*
6. Add *Other* on the agenda to allow announcements or other brief information.
7. Place the date and time of the next meeting at the end of the agenda.
   RATIONALE: *Advance notice allows staff members to plan other meetings and events around previously scheduled items.*
8. At least 1 week prior to the meeting, inform and verify persons on the agenda who will present a topic at the meeting.
   RATIONALE: *Advance notice ensures that those presenting topics will be prepared.*
9. Send agenda to staff members prior to the meeting.
10. Make copies available at the staff meeting.

PROCEDURE 56-3 Completing an Incident Report

Procedure Goal: To provide documentation of an adverse incident or potential risk in order to facilitate investigation, correction, and avoidance of future occurrences

OSHA Guidelines: This procedure does not involve exposure to blood, body fluids, or tissues.

Materials: Paper, a pen, and an incident report form

Method:

1. If anyone is injured, make sure initial first aid and appropriate steps are taken to help the injured person.
   RATIONALE: *The injured person must be taken care of prior to completing any paperwork.*

2. Interview the person to whom the incident occurred, gathering the facts required for the incident report, including contact information.

RATIONALE: *The injured person's statement should be in her own words, clarifying information as needed.*

3. Interview witnesses, gathering the facts required for the incident report, including contact information.

RATIONALE: *Witnesses can add information to the injured person's statement of how the incident occurred.*

4. Ensure that the information is complete.
5. Transfer the information to the incident report form.
6. Review the form for accuracy and clarity.
7. Submit the form to the appropriate supervisor.

PROCEDURE 56-4 Generating Payroll

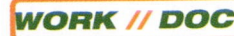

Procedure Goal: To handle the practice's payroll efficiently and accurately for each pay period

OSHA Guidelines: This procedure does not involve exposure to blood, body fluids, or tissues.

Materials: Employees' time cards, employees' earnings records, payroll register, IRS tax tables, and check register

Method:

1. Calculate the total regular and overtime hours worked, based on the employee's time card. Enter those totals under the appropriate headings on the payroll register.

2. Check the pay rate on the employee earnings record. Multiply the hours worked (including any paid vacation or paid holidays, if applicable) by the rates for regular time and overtime (time and a half or double time). This yields gross earnings.

3. Enter the gross earnings under the appropriate heading on the payroll register. Subtract any nontaxable benefits, such as healthcare or retirement programs.

4. Using IRS tax tables and data on the employee earnings record, determine the amount of federal income tax to withhold based on the employee's marital status and number of exemptions. Also, compute the amount of FICA tax to withhold for Social Security (6.2%) and Medicare (1.45%).

5. Following state and local procedures, determine the amount of state and local income taxes (if any) to withhold based on the employee's marital status and number of exemptions.

6. Calculate the employer's contributions to FUTA and to the state unemployment fund, if any. Post these amounts to the employer's account.

7. Enter any other required or voluntary deductions, such as health insurance or contributions to a 401(k) fund.

8. Subtract all deductions from the gross earnings to get the employee's net earnings.

9. Enter the total amount withheld from all employees for FICA under the headings for Social Security and Medicare. Remember that the employer must match these amounts. Enter other employer contributions, such as for federal and state unemployment taxes, under the appropriate headings.

10. Fill out the check stub, including the employee's name, the date, the pay period, gross earnings, all deductions, and net earnings. Make out the paycheck for the net earnings.

11. Deposit each deduction in a tax liability account.

SUMMARY OF LEARNING OUTCOMES

LEARNING OUTCOMES	KEY POINTS
56.1 **Explain the basic organizational designs of the medical office and the relationship of the physician and the medical assistant with the practice manager and direct supervisors.**	In a physician-owned medical practice, the medical assistant will often report directly to the practice manager. In a company-owned practice, the medical assistant will often report to the medical director. Regardless of the practice's organizational design, the medical assistant should always know the office chain of command and who her direct supervisor is and should consistently follow the chain of command as outlined in the organizational chart and the office policies and procedures manual.

LEARNING OUTCOMES	KEY POINTS
56.2 Describe the responsibilities of the practice manager.	The practice manager's job description may change from practice to practice, but common responsibilities include creating, updating, and maintaining the office policies and procedures manual; making sure all licenses and certifications necessary for all healthcare providers are up-to-date; and ensuring that all necessary contracts with payers and other providers are current. The practice manager is also in charge of the practice's finances and budget, including overseeing the office petty cash fund. Exceptional communication and interpersonal skills are required. On any given day, the manager may be communicating with staff, patients, healthcare providers, hospitals, insurers, vendors, contractors, government agencies, bankers, other employers, educators, attorneys, and community organizations. The manager also evaluates and purchases equipment and systems that fit the practice's needs and budget, facilitates the installation and staff training, and then oversees the ongoing operations. Other managerial functions include ensuring the availability of mailing and shipping services, inventory and supply purchases, and appropriate market and public relation strategies, which may include websites, brochures, and community event sponsorship.
56.3 Summarize the basic human resources functions in practice management.	The *human resources role* refers to how the practice manages employees and deals with elements of hiring, orienting, and training employees and terminating employees when necessary. Understanding the laws, acts, and regulations surrounding employment is also a large part of the human resources aspect of the practice manager's role.
56.4 Distinguish four of the possible traits of someone with leadership skills and the importance of these skills to the healthcare team.	Any of the following traits may be attributable to a leader: a desire to achieve both personal and organizational goals; confidence that is based on a good understanding of the situation at hand; the ability to be a team member and influence other members of the team to accomplish stated goals; excellent communication skills; the ability and willingness to accommodate change; integrity; the willingness to accept responsibility; the realization that goals are achieved best through the efforts of many; and the giving of genuine recognition to others who assist in achieving goals. All of these items and the ability to be a leader are important in a medical assistant as a healthcare team member because, when the office members work together with the common goal of caring for their patients, the result is excellent patient care.
56.5 Compare risk management and quality assurance in a medical facility.	The term *risk management* (RM) is defined as a plan and processes that continually identify, assess, correct, and monitor functions of the medical office to prevent negative outcomes and minimize risk exposure and consequent liability. When an incident does occur, an incident report is completed to track the cause of the incident to minimize future risk. *Quality assurance* (QA) consists of procedures that ensure that the services provided in the medical practice meet or exceed the requirements and standards.

LEARNING OUTCOMES	KEY POINTS
56.6 Calculate an employee's gross earnings, deductions, and net earnings for a pay period.	To calculate an employee's gross earnings, multiply the hours worked by the hourly rate. Using state, local, and federal tax guidelines, calculate the employee's tax deductions. Add to these any voluntary deductions and subtract the total deductions to obtain the employee's net earnings. Using the employee payroll record containing the employee's name, address, SSN, and number of exemptions, record the employee's gross earnings, deductions (including mandatory and voluntary deductions), and net paycheck.
56.7 Describe tax forms commonly used in the medical office and the purpose of the office tax liability account.	Tax forms used in a medical practice include, but are not limited to, W-2, W-3, and W-4 forms; NHR forms; I-9s; quarterly federal tax forms; wage and tax statements; and FUTA and SUTA forms. The practice liability account is set up to hold the money deducted from employees' paychecks until the funds can be appropriately disbursed to government agencies. There may be separate accounts for federal and state taxes as well as unemployment and retirement funds. Record the tax amounts deposited in the liability account as debits in the practice's checking account.

C A S E   S T U D Y   C R I T I C A L   T H I N K I N G

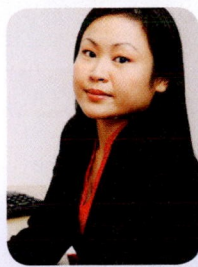

© Red Chopsticks/Getty Images RF

Recall Cindy Chen from the beginning of the chapter. Now that you have completed the chapter, answer the following questions regarding her case.

1. What questions would be appropriate to ask Cindy when interviewing her for the position?

2. If she is hired, other staff members may also know her medical status. How should this be best handled by the practice? By Cindy?

E X A M   P R E P A R A T I O N   Q U E S T I O N S

1. (LO 56.1) In most medical practices, the medical assistant will work under the supervision of
   a. The physician
   b. The physician assistant
   c. The nurse practitioner
   d. The staff nurse
   e. Any of these, depending on the practice structure

2. (LO 56.2) The document that is the backbone of the medical practice is its
   a. HIPAA manual
   b. Employee manual
   c. Policies and procedures manual
   d. SDS binder
   e. OSHA guidelines

3. (LO 56.2) The practice manager is responsible for which of the following tasks?
   a. Licenses, certifications, and contract updates
   b. Budgets and financial planning
   c. Petty cash management
   d. Schedule and travel for physicians and employees
   e. All of these

4. (LO 56.3) Which act does *not* come under the heading of human resources?
   a. EEOC
   b. ADA
   c. FMLA
   d. ECOA
   e. Fair Labor Standards Act

5. (LO 56.3) Which of the following questions cannot be asked during an interview?
   a. Do you have reliable transportation?
   b. Do you have small children at home?
   c. Are you capable of performing the duties listed on the job description?
   d. We require a certification for our medical assistants; are you certified?
   e. Our hours are 8:00 a.m.–4:30 p.m. and one Saturday a month from 8:00 a.m.–1:00 p.m. on a rotating schedule; can you be available for this schedule?

6. (LO 56.4) Why are goals important in building a team?
   a. Goals keep team members busy
   b. Goals keep each person focused solely on his or her own job
   c. Creating goals keeps supervisors busy
   d. Goals increase understanding of expectations
   e. None of these

7. (LO 56.5) There are five steps to the improvement process. Which one implements the plan?
   a. Identification
   b. Assessment
   c. Correction
   d. Monitoring
   e. Reevaluation

8. (LO 56.5) When is an incident report required?
   a. Only if an employee is injured while working
   b. Only if a patient is hurt because of employee error
   c. Only if a patient is hurt through no fault of the office staff
   d. For any adverse incident with risk of liability
   e. For any adverse incident with no risk of liability

9. (LO 56.6) Which tax form is more commonly known as the I-9?
   a. Form NHR
   b. Employment Eligibility and Verification
   c. Employee's Withholding Allowance Certificate
   d. Transmittal of Wage and Tax Statements
   e. Employee Wage and Tax Statement

10. (LO 56.7) Which tax provides for unemployment benefits?
   a. FUTA
   b. SUTA
   c. FICA
   d. State and local tax
   e. EFT

SOFT SKILLS SUCCESS

Recall Cindy Chen from the case study at the beginning of the chapter.

1. As an intern, Cindy went through a "mini" employee orientation. Malik explained to her that if she is hired, she will report directly to him. She will be expected to complete a 90-day probationary period, during which she will be expected to follow all office protocol and continue her learning process. Additionally, during this time, either the office or she can part ways if the employment does not appear to be a good fit for either party. He also explained that all employees are expected to cross-train to allow coverage for all positions during illness or vacation. Although Cindy loves the clinical aspect of the office, she understands she should take advantage of any learning opportunities that come her way. How do you think she should respond?

2. Malik asks Cindy if she understands the concept of the office petty cash fund, and Cindy states, "Yes"; she used it during her externship to purchase some tissues for the office when they ran out. Malik then asks her what she would do if she realized the petty cash fund appeared to be "short."

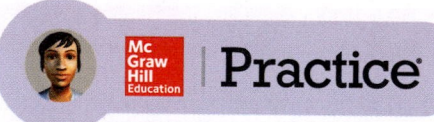

Go to PRACTICE MEDICAL OFFICE and complete the module Admin: Check Out—Privacy and Liability.

Emergency Preparedness

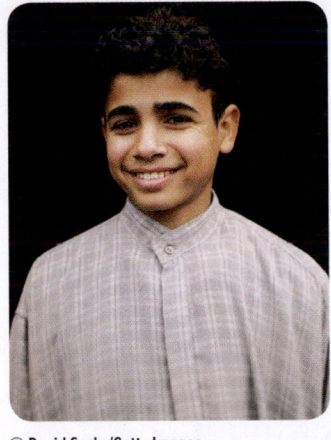
LEARNING OUTCOMES

After completing Chapter 57, you will be able to:

57.1 Discuss the importance of first aid during a medical emergency.

57.2 Identify items found on a crash cart.

57.3 Recognize various accidental emergencies and how to deal with them.

57.4 List common illnesses that can result in medical emergencies.

57.5 Identify less common illnesses that can result in medical emergencies.

57.6 Discuss your role in caring for people with psychosocial emergencies.

57.7 Carry out the procedure for calming a patient who is under extreme stress.

57.8 Discuss ways to educate patients about how to prevent and respond to emergencies.

57.9 Illustrate your role in responding to natural disasters and pandemic illness.

57.10 Discuss your role in responding to acts of bioterrorism.

KEY TERMS

automated external defibrillator (AED)

bioterrorism

cerebrovascular accident (CVA)

concussion

contusion

crash cart

dehydration

epistaxis

hematemesis

hematoma

hyperglycemia

hypoglycemia

hypovolemic shock

palpitations

septic shock

shelter-in-place

splint

sprain

strain

ventricular fibrillation (VF)

I.C.13	List principles and steps of professional/provider CPR
I.C.14	Describe basic principles of first aid as they pertain to the ambulatory healthcare setting
I.P.13	Perform first aid procedures for:
	(a) bleeding
	(b) diabetic coma or insulin shock
	(c) fractures
	(d) seizures
	(e) shock
	(f) syncope
I.A.1	Incorporate critical thinking skills when performing patient assessment
I.A.2	Incorporate critical thinking skills when performing patient care
III.P.2	Select appropriate barrier/personal protective equipment (PPE)
III.P.8	Perform wound care
III.P.9	Perform dressing change
X.C.7	Define:
	(d) Good Samaritan Act(s)
X.C.13	Define the following medical legal terms:
	(n) Good Samaritan laws
XII.C.6	Discuss protocols for disposal of biological chemical materials
XII.C.8	Identify critical elements of an emergency plan for response to a natural disaster or other emergency
XII.P.4	Participate in a mock exposure event with documentation of specific steps
XII.A.1	Recognize the physical and emotional effects on persons involved in an emergency situation
XII.A.2	Demonstrate self-awareness in responding to an emergency situation

2. Anatomy and Physiology

   c. Identify diagnostic and treatment modalities as they relate to each body system

9. Clinical Procedures

   b. Obtain vital signs, obtain patient history, and formulate chief complaint

   g. Recognize and respond to medical office emergencies

   j. Make adaptations with patients with special needs

▶ Introduction

Emergencies of all types can occur when you are working as a medical assistant. Patients may come to your facility with an acute illness or injury. You may have to handle phone calls from patients with urgent physical or psychological problems. You might even experience a disaster—from a simple office fire to a bomb threat or bioterrorism. As a medical assistant, you must be prepared to determine the level of urgency and handle any emergency that arises. Remember to stay calm and think through each situation in order to respond appropriately and create the best outcome.

▶ Understanding Medical Emergencies   LO 57.1

A medical emergency is any situation in which a person suddenly becomes ill or sustains an injury that requires immediate

help by a healthcare professional. Your prompt action in a medical emergency could prevent permanent disability or even death.

As a medical assistant, you may see life-threatening medical emergencies in the healthcare setting. For example, a patient in the waiting room may have chest pains that could indicate a heart attack is imminent. You also may see emergencies that are not life-threatening, such as a coworker sustaining a minor injury on the job. And you could encounter emergencies outside the office. For example, a family member might cut a finger while using a kitchen knife or a restaurant patron might choke on a piece of food. Your quick response is vital in all of these situations.

In or out of the office, a medical emergency may require you to perform first aid. First aid is the immediate care given to someone who is injured or suddenly becomes ill, before complete medical care can be obtained. Prompt and appropriate first aid can

- Save a life.
- Reduce pain.

- Prevent further injury.
- Reduce the risk of permanent disability.
- Increase the chance of early recovery.

Because most emergencies do not occur in a medical office, your role in patient education is critical. The more you teach patients about first aid and the proper way to respond to emergencies, the better equipped they will be to handle accidental injuries and illnesses. You also should make patients aware of Good Samaritan laws. These laws protect people who respond, in good faith, to medical emergencies but have no medical training. Every state in the United States has Good Samaritan laws or regulations.

▶ Preparing for Medical Emergencies
LO 57.2

How prepared you are for an emergency can mean the difference between life and death for a patient. You must be able to perform procedures quickly and correctly. Keeping your skills up-to-date will enable you to handle medical emergencies effectively.

Just as important is your ability to ensure that the medical office where you work is ready to handle whatever emergencies arise. This preparedness will depend on your own organizational skills and knowledge of community resources.

Preparing the Office
First, establish with the doctor which duties are expected of you and of other office personnel in case of an emergency and determine the available resources. One of your most important allies will be the local emergency medical services (EMS) system. An EMS system is a network of qualified emergency services personnel who use community resources and equipment to provide emergency care to victims of injury or sudden illness.

Posting Emergency Telephone Numbers Although the local EMS system's telephone number is 911 in most parts of the country, some areas may not have 911 service. Post the area's EMS system telephone number at every telephone and on the **crash cart** (the rolling cart of emergency supplies and equipment) or first-aid tray. Every office employee should know this number. If the community has no EMS system, post the telephone number of the local ambulance or rescue squad. You also should post the telephone numbers of the nearest fire company, police station, poison control center, women's shelter, rape hotline, and drug and alcohol center.

When you call EMS for medical assistance and transport, speak clearly and calmly to the dispatcher and be prepared to provide the following information:

- Your name, telephone number, and location
- Nature of the emergency
- Number of people in need of help
- Condition of the injured or ill patient(s)
- Summary of the first aid that has been given
- Directions on how to reach the location of the emergency

Do not hang up until the dispatcher gives you permission to do so.

Common Emergency and First-Aid Supplies
The crash cart or tray contains basic drugs, supplies, and equipment for medical emergencies. Most crash carts also contain a first-aid kit with supplies for managing minor injuries and ailments. Table 57-1 lists the usual items in a first-aid kit. The actual contents of the crash cart may vary slightly from practice to practice. Become familiar with these contents and know where they are located in the office. Procedure 57-1, at the end of this chapter, describes how to check and restock essential crash cart items.

TABLE 57-1 Contents of a First-Aid Kit
Absorbent compress bandages (sterile)
Adhesive bandages (assorted sizes)
Adhesive tape
Airway or breathing barrier
Analgesics, such as acetaminophen
Antiseptic solution or spray
Antiseptic wipes
Aspirin (81 mg)
Calamine lotion
Chemical cold packs
Diphenhydramine (Benadryl®)
Disposable gloves
Elastic bandages in various sizes
Emergency blanket
First-aid book or information card
Gauze pads (sterile)
Glucose tablets or sugar source
Hand sanitizer
Personal protective equipment (PPE): gloves, mask, and goggles or face shield, gown, shower cap, booties, pocket mask, or mouth shield
Plastic bags
Premoistened towelettes or hand cleaner
Roller bandages
Scissors
Splints in various sizes
Sterile gauze pads in various sizes
Sterile rolls of gauze
Sterile saline solution
Sunscreen
Thermometer (with extra batteries if digital)
Triangular bandage
Tweezers
Waterproof flashlight with extra batteries

Guidelines for Handling Emergencies

A medical emergency requires you to take certain steps. You are not responsible for diagnosing or providing medical care other than first aid. You are expected, however, to note the presence of serious conditions that threaten the patient's life and to take appropriate action, performing only those procedures you have been trained to perform.

Patient Emergencies Assess the situation and surroundings to determine whether it is safe for you to assist. If safe, don the appropriate PPE, such as gloves. Next, do an initial assessment to detect and immediately correct any life-threatening circulation, airway, and breathing problems. Correcting life-threatening problems is essential to survival. The initial assessment has six steps:

1. Form a general impression of the patient.
2. Determine the patient's level of responsiveness.
3. Assess the circulation (compressions or the need for them if no pulse detected), airway, and breathing status of the patient, sometimes referred to as the CABs.
4. Determine the priority or urgency of the patient's condition.
5. Conduct a focused exam.
6. Document a history.

Procedure 57-2, at the end of this chapter, provides guidelines for performing these six steps.

Telephone Emergencies Sometimes, a patient or a patient's family member calls the medical office with an emergency. If you are responsible for handling telephone calls, be prepared to triage the injuries by phone. Triaging is the classification of injuries according to severity, urgency of treatment, and place for treatment.

To handle emergency calls, follow the practice's telephone triage protocols. For example, if a parent calls to say her daughter has broken her arm and the child's bone is visible, tell her to call the local EMS system for immediate care and transport to the hospital. If, however, a parent calls to say her son swallowed half a bottle of baby bath, tell her to remain calm and give her the telephone number of the poison control center. Depending on circumstances, you may offer to make the necessary phone call yourself.

Adhere to the following general guidelines in any emergency situation:

- Stay calm.
- Reassure the patient.
- Act in a confident, organized manner.

Personal Protection Whenever you administer first aid and emergency treatment, try to reduce or eliminate the risk of exposing yourself and others to infection. Follow standard precautions and assume that all blood and other body fluids are infected with bloodborne pathogens. To protect yourself and others, take the following basic precautions.

- Include PPE in all first-aid kits (gloves, goggles, mask, gown, cap, and booties).
- Include a pocket mask or mouth shield for rescue breathing.
- Use PPE appropriate to the patient's condition. (See Table 57-2 for examples of PPE to use in various emergency situations.)
- Wear gloves if you expect hand contact with blood, other body fluids, or mucous membranes.
- If you have any cuts or lesions, wear PPE over the affected area.
- When in doubt, wear more PPE than you may think is called for.
- If blood or other body fluids splash into your eyes, nose, or mouth, flush the area with water as soon as possible.
- Wash your hands thoroughly with soap and water after removing the gloves.
- Wash other skin surfaces that have come in contact with blood or other body fluids.
- Do not touch your mouth, nose, or eyes and do not eat or drink after providing emergency care until you have washed your hands thoroughly.
- If you have been exposed to blood or other body fluids, be sure to tell your supervisor or healthcare practitioner. You may need postexposure treatment.

Documentation Properly document all office emergencies in the patient's chart. Be sure to include your assessment, the treatment given, and the patient's response. If the patient was transported to another facility, record the location.

TABLE 57-2	Personal Protective Equipment for Emergencies	
Equipment	**Conditions for Use**	**Sample Emergencies Requiring Equipment**
Gloves	Chance of contact with blood or other body secretion or excretion during emergency	Open wound, eye trauma
Goggles and mask or face shield and possible head cover	Chance of blood or other body secretion or excretion being splattered, coughed, or sprayed onto the mucus membranes of the eyes, mouth, or nose	Bleeding, vomiting, most emergency care for small children (because of squirming)
Gown and possibly booties	Chance of contact with excessive bleeding or secretion and excretion	Childbirth, severe nosebleed
Pocket mask or mouth shield	Needed for CPR or rescue breathing	Heart attack (MI), respiratory arrest

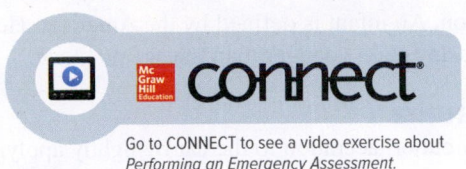
▶ Accidental Injuries   LO 57.3

No matter where you encounter an emergency, your knowledge and certifications should enable you to provide first aid for the patient until a physician or EMT arrives. To help you become familiar with how to handle various emergency situations, the following sections present accidental injuries, common illnesses, and less common illnesses.

Bites and Stings

Dog and cat bites and bee, wasp, and hornet stings are fairly common. Less common are snakebites and spider bites, which you are more likely to encounter in certain parts of the country, such as Florida or the Southwest, than in other areas.

Animal Bites An animal bite may bruise the skin, tear it, or leave a puncture wound. A wound that breaks the skin should be seen by a doctor and will need to be reported to the police, animal control officer, and local health department. If the animal can be found, it should be checked for rabies. Then, depending on the animal's rabies vaccination status, the animal may need to be quarantined. If the animal is a probable carrier of rabies and cannot be found, depending on the extent of the injury, the doctor may administer rabies immunoglobulin and rabies vaccination to the patient as a precaution.

Dogs, cats, skunks, squirrels, raccoons, bats, and foxes are more likely to carry rabies than are other animals. Hamsters, gerbils, guinea pigs, and mice are rarely infected by the rabies virus.

Human bites can raise concerns about transmitting the human immunodeficiency virus (HIV) or hepatitis B virus. HIV can be transmitted only if the bite breaks the skin and if the biter has bleeding gums. Hepatitis B virus may be transmitted by a human bite that punctures the skin. In this case, a series of three injections is required to immunize against hepatitis B.

Immediate care for bites calls for washing the area thoroughly with antiseptic soap and water. Apply a dry, sterile dressing. If the wound is bleeding profusely or spurting blood, apply pressure to the wound and seek medical attention. The healthcare practitioner will treat the wound and administer tetanus toxoid if the patient has not received it in the last 5 to 10 years.

Insect Stings Insect stings are merely a nuisance to most patients. The site of the sting can become red, swollen, itchy, and painful. If the patient was stung by a honeybee, you must first remove the stinger because it still has the ability to release venom. Remove the stinger by scraping the skin with a credit card or other flat, hard, sharp object. Be careful not to release more venom. Avoid using your fingers or tweezers because squeezing the stinger may force more venom into the wound.

(If you cannot remove the stinger, call the physician.) Wash the skin with soap and water. After the stinger is removed, apply ice to the site, 10 minutes on and 10 minutes off, to reduce the pain and swelling.

A sting can be deadly to a patient who is allergic to the insect venom because anaphylaxis can develop. The symptoms of and treatment for anaphylaxis are described later in this chapter.

Snakebites Poisonous snakes in the United States include rattlesnakes, water moccasins (or cottonmouths), copperheads, and coral snakes. Because snakes are cold-blooded, they often lie on rocks to warm themselves. Most bites occur when a person steps onto, sits down on, or reaches over or between rocks where a snake is sunning itself.

The bites of most poisonous snakes produce similar symptoms: one or two puncture marks, pain, and swelling at the site; rapid pulse; nausea; vomiting; and sometimes unconsciousness and seizures. If possible, get a description of the snake so that the EMS team or the hospital can procure the proper antivenin (a substance that counteracts the snake poison) ahead of time. Snakebites are dangerous, but with proper intervention, they rarely lead to death.

If a patient has been bitten by a potentially poisonous snake, call a doctor or the EMS system. If the patient must walk, have him walk slowly to prevent dispersion (spreading) of the poison through the circulation. To care for a poisonous snakebite while you await help, keep the patient calm and remove rings, watches, or tight clothing in the area. If possible, immobilize the injured part and position it below heart level. Do not apply ice or a tourniquet and do not cut or suction the wound.

Spider Bites Only two types of spiders in the United States are a serious threat to health: the black widow and the brown recluse.

- The black widow has a red hourglass mark on its abdomen. The bite causes swelling and pain at the site as well as nausea, vomiting, rigid abdomen, fever, rash, and difficulty breathing or swallowing.
- The brown recluse has a violin-shaped mark on its head. The bite causes severe swelling and tenderness and, eventually, ulceration, which enlarges around the location of the bite.

You are not expected to classify spiders and their bites accurately, so any patient bitten by a spider must be seen by a physician. To care for a patient with a spider bite, wash the area thoroughly with soap and water. Apply a cold compress to the area to reduce swelling and pain. If possible, elevate the area to slow the poison's spreading. Healing of the bite can sometimes take several months.

Burns

Burns involve tissue injury that occurs from heat, chemicals, electricity, or radiation. Be sure to teach patients about emergency treatment for burns and any follow-up care prescribed by the physician.

Types of Burns

Thermal Burns Thermal burns can be caused by contact with hot liquids, steam, flames, radiation, and excessive heat from fires or hot objects. If the burn is on the hands, face, or feet and is larger than 3 inches in diameter, call the EMS team immediately. If the burn is minor and less than 3 inches in diameter, stop the burning process by using water to cool the burn. If the victim's clothes or skin are on fire, use a wet cloth or blanket to put out the fire.

Chemical Burns Chemical burns are more likely to affect workers at chemical or industrial facilities than individuals in the home. To treat this type of burn, first remove the cause of the burn. Take care not to come in contact with the chemical. Brush off any excess dry chemical and remove any clothing contaminated with the chemical. If the Safety Data Sheet is available and it is indicated on the sheet, gently flood the area with cool water for at least 15 minutes. Cover the area with a dry, sterile dressing. If the burn is severe, call EMS to transport the patient to the hospital. Monitor the patient carefully for signs of shock.

Electrical Burns Electrical burns are injuries from exposure to electric currents, including lightning. These burns occur at the site where the electricity enters the body and where the current exits the body and enters the ground. Along the current's pathway, extensive tissue damage can occur from heat followed by chemical changes to nerve, muscle, and heart tissue. Call the EMS team immediately for these types of injuries.

Classifications of Burns The severity of a burn is determined by the following factors:

- The depth and extent of the burn area
- The source of the burn
- The age of the patient
- The body regions burned
- The patient's general health and condition

For more information about classifying and estimating the extent of burns, see the chapter *The Integumentary System*.

Choking

Choking occurs when food or a foreign object blocks a person's trachea, or windpipe. The main symptom of a choking emergency is the inability to speak. A choking person who cannot talk may give the universal sign of choking—a hand up to the throat and a fearful look. If you see someone giving the universal sign, be prepared to act promptly.

Procedure 57-3, at the end of this chapter, provides guidelines for assisting an adult or a child who is responsive and choking. The American Heart Association generally considers anyone between the ages of 1 and 8 years old a child. Procedure 57-4, at the end of this chapter, provides the guidelines for assisting an infant who is responsive and has a foreign body airway obstruction. An infant is defined by the American Heart Association as any child younger than the age of 1 year.

Ear Trauma

Treat any cut or laceration to the ear by lightly applying a bandage, with even pressure, over the injury. It may be possible to reattach a severed ear surgically. Carefully wrap the severed ear in a sterile dressing secured with a self-adherent gauze bandage. Then wrap the ear in plastic, label it, and place it in an ice chest or over an ice pack so that it is kept chilled but is not in direct contact with the ice. Send it with the patient to the hospital.

Eye Trauma

Depending on its severity, eye trauma may require no more than an ice pack or a cold compress, or it may require hospital care. Eye trauma may result from a fall, a blow to the eye, or a wound from a pointed object. Whatever the cause, carefully examine the eye to the best of your ability and notify the physician of the patient's condition.

Eye injuries are commonly caused by foreign objects in the eye. Tiny specks cause tearing and can be painful. To remove them, use moistened sterile gauze or a tissue. Do not use a cotton ball because it may leave behind eye-irritating cotton wisps. If an object has penetrated the eye, do not try to remove it. Seek medical attention immediately.

Falls

If a patient falls and cannot get up, you will need to call for help. Do not move the patient on your own; wait until the physician or an EMT examines him. Instruct the patient not to move his head, neck, or back if injuries to those areas are suspected. When this type of injury is suspected, have someone hold the patient's neck to stabilize it until the physician or EMT arrives. Move the patient only in a life-threatening situation, such as if the building is on fire. Arrange for transport to the hospital and document the fall and injury in the patient's chart.

If the fall results in only a bump, apply ice if ordered by the healthcare practitioner and observe for bruises and swelling. Give the patient time to collect himself. Be sure to notify the doctor, who should examine the patient. Then document the fall, the injury, and the treatment in the patient's chart.

Fractures, Dislocations, Sprains, and Strains

Fractures, sprains, and other musculoskeletal injuries can result from falls and slips in the medical office. As a medical assistant, you must be able to recognize the symptoms of a fracture, dislocation, sprain, or strain and provide immediate first aid. Table 57-3 summarizes the types of fractures. Additional information about fractures and dislocations can be found in the chapter *The Skeletal System*. For more information on muscle strains and sprains, see the chapter *The Muscular System*.

Fracture and dislocation treatment depends on factors such as the nature of the injury and the patient's age and physical condition. The basic emergency steps are:

1. Keep the person calm and limit his movement.
2. Assess him for any other injuries.

TABLE 57-3	Summary of Fracture Types and Their Symptoms
Fracture	**Symptoms**
Complete	The fracture extends across the bone, snapping it into two pieces.
Incomplete	The bone is cracked but not broken into two pieces.
Closed	The skin in the area of the fracture is not broken.
Open (compound)	The skin is broken by the bone fragments or the skin is broken during the course of the fracture.
Greenstick	The bone is cracked on one side and bent on the other. This is a common fracture in children.
Comminuted	The bone is broken into three or more pieces.

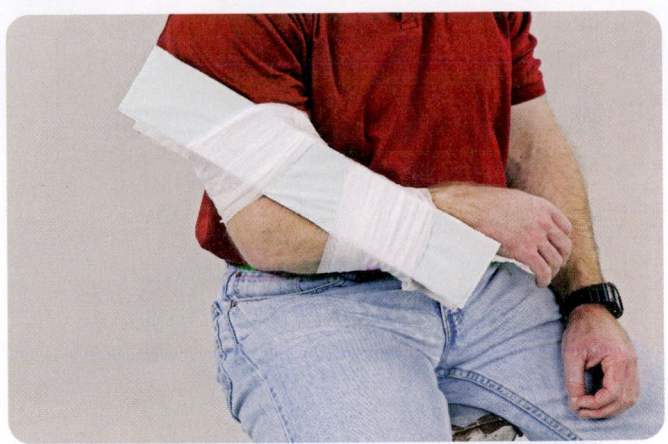

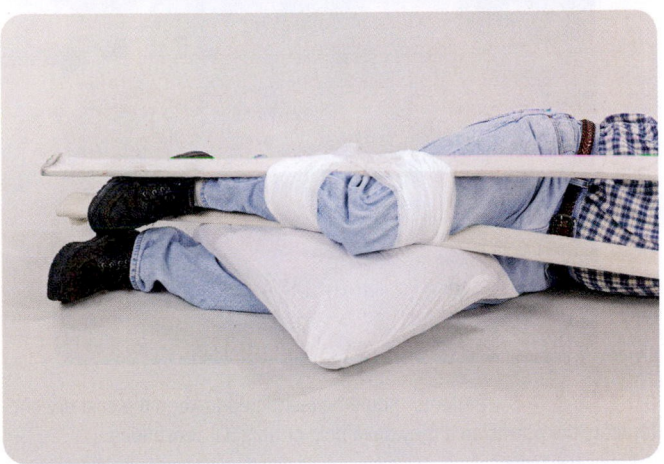

FIGURE 57-1   When using a splint, make sure you immobilize above and below the injured joint.

© National Safety Council/Rick Brady, photographer

3. Notify the doctor or call EMS if needed.
   - Do not try to move the person until the doctor or EMS arrives.
4. If the skin is broken, cover with a sterile dressing.
5. Immobilize the extremity with a splint or sling (Figure 57-1).
   - Use rolled-up newspaper, strips of wood, or the like.
   - Immobilize the joint above and below the injury.
   - Immobilize the bone in the position it is found.
   - Do not try to put the bone back in place.
6. Place an ice pack on the affected area.
7. Monitor him for signs of shock.
8. Assess for signs of lack of circulation in the injured limb, including pale or blue skin, loss of feeling, and tingling in the area.

Immobilization is sometimes provided by the application of a splint or cast. The purpose of both splints and casts is to keep an injured body part in place and protect it as it heals. A **splint** is an appliance used for conditions that do not require rigid immobilization or, as a temporary measure, for those in which swelling is anticipated. A *cast* is a rigid, external dressing, usually made of plaster or fiberglass, that is molded to the contours of the body part to which it is applied. You may assist the physician with the application of a cast (Figure 57-2). You also may educate the patient about these basic elements of cast care:

- Report any of the following to the physician immediately: pain, swelling, discoloration of exposed portions, lack of pulsation and warmth, or the inability to move exposed parts.
- Keep the casted extremity elevated for the first day.
- Avoid indenting the cast until it is completely dry.
- Check the movement and sensation of the visible extremities frequently.
- Restrict strenuous activities for the first few days.
- Avoid allowing the affected limb to hang down for any length of time.

- Do not put anything inside the cast.
- Keep the cast dry.
- Follow the physician's orders regarding activity restrictions.

Sprains and strains often result from sports injuries and accidents. A **sprain** is an injury characterized by partial tearing of a ligament that supports a joint, such as the ankle. A sprain also may involve injuries to tendons, muscles, and local blood vessels and contusions of the surrounding soft tissue. A **strain** is a muscle injury that results from overexertion. For example, back strain may occur when a person carries a heavy load.

Symptoms of a sprain include swelling, tenderness, pain during movement, and local discoloration. If you suspect a sprain, splint the joint, apply ice, and call the EMS system if needed. Inform the patient that an X-ray may be required to confirm there is no fracture. A strain causes pain on motion. In most cases, it should be examined by a physician, who may prescribe rest, application of heat, and a muscle relaxant.

Head Injuries

Head injuries include concussions; severe head injuries such as contusions, fractures, and intracranial bleeding; and scalp

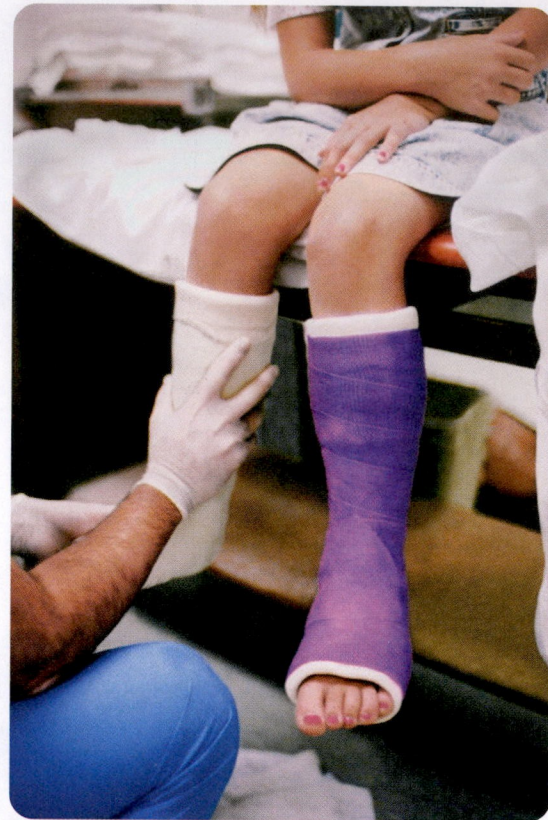

FIGURE 57-2 Patients should be instructed to keep the cast dry and to notify the physician if they have pain or unusual sensations.
© Royalty-Free/Corbis

hematomas and lacerations. Some head injuries are life-threatening and require immediate medical attention.

Concussion A **concussion** is a jarring injury to the brain. It is the most common type of head injury. Someone who has a concussion may lose consciousness. Temporary loss of vision, pallor (paleness), listlessness, memory loss, or vomiting also can occur. Symptoms may disappear rapidly or last up to 24 hours. A concussion may produce slow intracranial bleeding. Teach the patient and the patient's family basic precautions after this type of injury. See the *Educating the Patient* feature for more information on concussions.

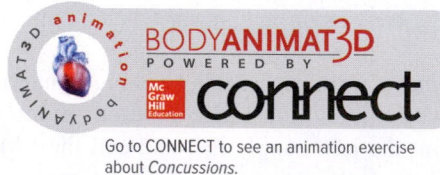

Go to CONNECT to see an animation exercise about *Concussions*.

Severe Head Injuries Contusions (bruises), fractures, and intracranial bleeding cause symptoms similar to, but more profound than, the symptoms of concussions. Signs and symptoms of severe head injuries include the following:

- Leakage of clear or bloody fluid from the ears or nose
- Seizures
- Respiratory arrest

A patient with a severe head injury requires immediate hospitalization. Your priority is to monitor the patient's CABs and to begin CPR if needed.

Scalp Hematomas and Lacerations A **hematoma** is a swelling caused by blood under the skin. A scalp hematoma causes a bump on the head. This swelling can be reduced by applying ice immediately after the injury. Because blood vessels in the scalp are close to the skin, scalp lacerations often bleed profusely and look worse than they really are. Apply direct pressure to stop bleeding from a scalp laceration, wash the area with soap and water, and apply a dry, sterile dressing over the area.

Hemorrhaging

Hemorrhaging (heavy or uncontrollable bleeding) is generally the result of an injury. It also may be caused by an illness. The first-aid treatment remains the same in both cases. Bleeding can be internal or external. When administering first aid to a patient who may have internal bleeding, cover the patient with a blanket for warmth, keep the patient quiet and calm, and get medical help immediately.

Control external bleeding to prevent rapid blood loss and shock. Use direct pressure, apply additional dressings as needed, elevate the bleeding body part, and put pressure over a pressure point, as described in Procedure 57-5 at the end of this chapter. Then transport the patient to an emergency care facility.

As a last resort, if medical help is more than an hour away, you may need to use a tourniquet (Figure 57-3) to save a person's life. You apply a tourniquet over the main pressure point above the wound and tighten the tourniquet until the bleeding stops. For upper limb injuries, place the tourniquet as high as possible and tighten as much as possible. If you apply a tourniquet, make sure you write the application time on the tourniquet or the patient's forehead. New research shows that with better trauma surgery techniques, a tourniquet may be used to stop life-threatening hemorrhage without loss of the affected limb.

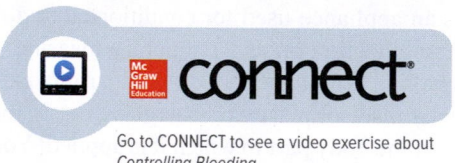

Go to CONNECT to see a video exercise about *Controlling Bleeding*.

Multiple Injuries

Sometimes, a patient sustains more than one type of injury—for example, an arm fracture, a head injury, lacerations, and internal bleeding. Multiple injuries often result from a car accident or a fall. If you need to assist a patient with multiple injuries, assess the CABs, call EMS (or have someone else call), and perform CPR if needed. Once you have ensured that the patient has a pulse and an open airway and is breathing on his own, perform first aid for the most life-threatening injuries first.

Poisoning

A poison is a substance that produces harmful effects if it enters the body. Poisoning is serious and can result in death or permanent injury if immediate medical care is not provided.

Concussion

Because a concussion can cause intracranial bleeding, handle gently a patient who is being treated for this type of injury. If bleeding is slow, it might take up to 24 hours to produce symptoms. Because intracranial bleeding may require brain surgery, use the following patient education guidelines to help ensure patient safety after a concussion:

- Inform the patient that the first 24 hours after the injury are the most critical.
- Tell the patient to refrain from strenuous activity, to rest, and to return to regular activity gradually. Instruct the patient to avoid using pain medicines other than acetaminophen, unless the drugs are approved by the physician.
- Advise the patient to eat lightly, especially if nausea and vomiting occur.
- Tell a family member to check on the patient every few hours. The family member should make sure the patient knows her own name, her location, and the name of the family member.

- Instruct the family member to call for medical assistance immediately if the patient exhibits any of these warning signs:

  - Any symptom that is getting worse, such as headaches, sleepiness, or nausea, including nausea that does not go away
  - Changes in behavior, such as irritability or confusion
  - Dilated pupils (pupils that are bigger than normal) or pupils of different sizes
  - Trouble walking or speaking
  - Drainage of bloody or clear fluids from ears or nose
  - Vomiting
  - Seizures
  - Weakness or numbness in the arms or legs
  - A less serious head injury in a patient taking blood thinners or who has a bleeding disorder such as hemophilia

---

In addition to being able to handle a poisoning emergency, you need to educate patients in how to do the same. Teach them about the symptoms of and treatment for the different types of poisoning and provide them with pamphlets that

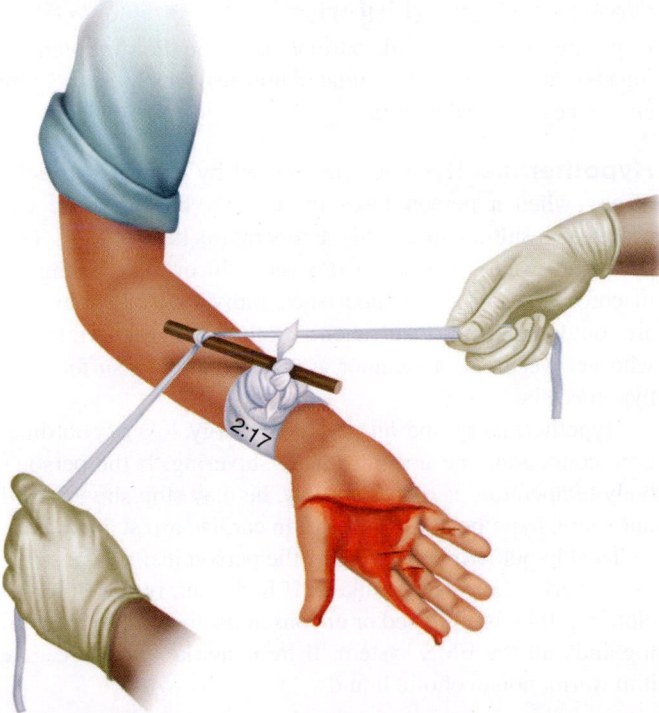

FIGURE 57-3 Apply a tourniquet as a last resort—if the bleeding cannot be stopped and medical help is more than an hour away. Record the time applied on the tourniquet or the patient's forehead.

describe the procedures to follow and stickers with the telephone number of the regional poison control center.

The majority of accidental poisonings happen to children younger than the age of 5. Young children are not necessarily put off by strong smells or burning sensations when they swallow something. Common causes of poisoning in children are household cleaning products, household plants, and medications. Poisons also can be caused by improperly prepared or contaminated food. These types of poisons are ingested or swallowed.

Poisoning that results from coming in contact with plants (called absorbed poisoning), such as poison ivy, poison sumac, and poison oak, is common and generally fairly minor. It can be serious, however, if the poisoning occurs over a large body surface.

Poisons also can be inhaled. This situation occurs when a person inhales a poisonous gas such as carbon monoxide or the fumes from burning poisonous plants.

Ingested Poisons Symptoms of ingested poisoning include abdominal pain and cramping; nausea; vomiting; diarrhea; odor, stains, or burns around or in the mouth; drowsiness; and unconsciousness. You also should suspect poisoning if packages containing poisonous substances are near a person who has one or more of these symptoms. Swallowed poison remains in the stomach only a short time. Most of it is absorbed while in the small intestine.

It is crucial to call a poison control center (1-800-222-1222), hospital emergency room, doctor, or the EMS system for instructions if you think a patient has swallowed a poison. When you call, you will need to know

- The patient's age.
- The name of the poison.
- The amount of poison swallowed.
- When the poison was swallowed.
- Whether or not the person has vomited.
- How much time it will take to get the patient to a medical facility.

Poisons vary in their toxicity. Some cause damage right away; others cause damage several hours later. If the patient is alert and not having convulsions, follow these steps:

1. Call the regional poison control center.
2. Seek immediate medical attention.
3. Monitor the patient's vital signs.
4. Watch for increasing nausea and vomiting.

Do not induce vomiting unless directed by a medical authority. The patient may have ingested a strong acid, alkali, or petroleum product, such as chlorine bleach or gasoline. These products may cause further damage to the throat and esophagus during vomiting. If you do not know what the patient ingested, never induce vomiting.

Turn the patient on her left side. This position delays stomach emptying by several hours and prevents aspiration if the patient vomits. Take both the poison container and vomited material to the hospital for inspection.

Food poisoning, another type of ingested poisoning, can occur when bacteria produce toxins in food. Botulism, for example, results from eating improperly canned or preserved foods contaminated with the bacterium *Clostridium botulinum*. Symptoms appear within 12 to 36 hours after eating contaminated food. Initial symptoms include dry mouth, sore throat, weakness, vomiting, and diarrhea.

Food poisoning is often difficult to detect because the signs and symptoms vary greatly. A patient with food poisoning usually has abdominal pain, nausea, vomiting, gas, frequent bowel sounds, and diarrhea. Chills, joint pain, and excessive sweating also may occur. If you suspect that a patient has food poisoning, call the poison control center and arrange for immediate transport to the hospital.

Absorbed Poisons Most people have had the red, itchy rash that results from contact with poison ivy, poison sumac, or poison oak. In some people, however, the rash may be accompanied by a generalized swelling, burning eyes, headache, fever, and abnormal pulse or respirations.

To treat a patient who has come in contact with an absorbed poison, call the regional poison control center. Have the patient immediately remove all contaminated clothing. Then wash the affected skin thoroughly with soap and water, drench it with alcohol, and rinse well. To help relieve symptoms, apply wet compresses soaked with calamine lotion. Also, suggest baths in colloidal oatmeal or applications of a paste made from 3 teaspoons baking soda and 1 teaspoon water to soothe the itching. If the rash is severe, the doctor may prescribe a corticosteroid ointment. Tell the patient to seek medical assistance if a fever or swelling develops.

Inhaled Poisons A patient may inhale poisons by breathing air contaminated by chemicals in the workplace or by a malfunctioning stove or furnace in the home. The patient may not realize she has been exposed to a poisonous gas until symptoms arise. Even then, she may merely suspect the flu because some symptoms of inhalation poisoning mimic those of influenza. Common symptoms include headache, tinnitus (ringing in the ears), angina (chest pain), shortness of breath, muscle weakness, nausea, vomiting, confusion, and dizziness, followed by blurred or double vision, difficulty breathing, unconsciousness, and cardiac arrest. Also, a patient who has facial burns may have sustained an inhalation injury.

To treat poisoning by inhalation, first get the patient into fresh air. Have someone call the EMS system or the regional poison control center. Loosen tight-fitting clothing and wrap the patient in a blanket to prevent shock. Check the patient's CABs and begin CPR if needed.

Carbon monoxide is a major cause of inhalation poisoning in the home. It is a colorless and odorless natural gas produced by incomplete combustion of organic fuels, such as coal, wood, or gasoline. Carbon monoxide is especially dangerous in closed spaces because, when inhaled, it replaces oxygen in the blood. If you suspect carbon monoxide poisoning, look for clues in the environment such as a malfunctioning furnace or a car engine left running in a closed space such as a garage.

Mild carbon monoxide poisoning can cause headache and flu-like symptoms without fever. Moderate poisoning may cause tinnitus, drowsiness, severe seizures, coma, and cardiopulmonary problems. Because the gas is odorless, people are often unaware they are being poisoned. They may fall asleep, lapse into unconsciousness, and die.

Weather-Related Injuries

Exposure to extreme cold, extreme heat, and the sun's damaging rays can cause weather-related injuries, which may require emergency medical attention.

Hypothermia Hypothermia, caused by exposure to cold, occurs when a person loses more body heat than he can produce, resulting in a body temperature below 95°F. This condition usually occurs in the very old or very young, or in chronically ill or malnourished individuals. People who are outdoors with insufficient clothing in the winter or who get wet in cold weather are more likely to suffer from hypothermia.

Hypothermia symptoms include lethargy, loss of coordination, confusion, and uncontrollable shivering. If the person's body temperature is extremely low, he may stop shivering. If untreated, hypothermia can result in cardiac arrest and coma.

Treat hypothermia by moving the person inside if possible and covering him with blankets. If he is wet, remove his wet clothing. If he is confused or unconscious, monitor his breathing and call the EMS system. If he is awake and alert, give him warm, nonalcoholic liquids.

Frostbite When body tissues are exposed to below-freezing temperatures, frostbite can occur. Frostbite causes ice crystals to form between tissue cells, and these crystals enlarge as they extract water from the cells. Frostbite also causes obstruction to the blood supply in the form of blood clots. This aspect of frostbite prevents blood from flowing to the tissues and causes additional, severe damage to cells.

Frostbite symptoms include white, waxy, or grayish yellow skin. The affected body part feels cold, tingling, and painful. The skin surface may feel crusty and the underlying tissue soft in comparison. If the frostbite is deep, the body part may feel cold and hard and not be sensitive to pain. Blisters may appear after rewarming.

Treat frostbite by wrapping warm clothing or blankets around the affected body part or placing it in contact with a warm body part. Do not rub or massage the affected area, or you may cause further damage to the frozen tissue. Call for medical assistance. If you are in a remote area, use the wet rapid rewarming method. This method involves placing the affected part in warm (100°F to 104°F) water. Hot water should be added at regular intervals to keep the temperature of the bath stable. As an alternative method, you can heat the affected area with warm compresses. Continue rewarming for 20 to 40 minutes. After the affected area becomes soft, place dry, sterile gauze between skin surfaces, such as between the toes or the fingers or between the ear and the side of the head. Do not massage the skin or break blisters.

Heatstroke Heatstroke is an overheating of the body, which results from prolonged exposure to high temperatures and humidity. This condition may lead to excessive loss of fluids (dehydration) and insufficient blood in the circulatory system (hypovolemic shock). High body temperature (over 104°F) can damage tissues and organs throughout the body. If untreated, the patient will die. People most susceptible to heatstroke are those who have previously had heatstroke, children, the elderly, athletes, and patients who are obese or have circulatory problems or other chronic illnesses.

Symptoms of heatstroke include the following:

- Hot, dry skin (lack of sweating)
- High body temperature
- Altered mental state
- Rapid pulse
- Rapid breathing
- Dizziness
- Headache
- Nausea and vomiting
- Weakness

If you suspect that a patient has heatstroke, check the patient's CABs and call the EMS system. Move the patient to a cool place and remove outer clothing unless it is made of light cotton or other light fabric. Also, cool the patient with any means available, such as gentle spraying with a hose. Move the patient to an air-conditioned place if available, fan vigorously, or apply a wet sheet. If the humidity is above 75%, place ice packs on the patient's groin and armpits. Stop cooling when the patient's mental state improves. Keep the patient's head and shoulders slightly elevated.

Sunburn Do not dismiss a sunburn as trivial. It is a burn that can cause redness, tenderness, pain, swelling, blisters, and peeling skin and may lead to skin damage or cancer later in life.

Soak sunburned skin in cool water to help reduce the heat. Apply cold compresses, and later calamine lotion, to relieve the burning sensation. Have the patient elevate the legs and arms to prevent swelling. The patient also should drink plenty of water and take a pain reliever.

Educate the patient about the importance of using sunscreen and reapplying it every 2 to 3 hours when outdoors. Advise the patient to stay out of direct sunlight between 10:00 a.m. and 2:00 p.m. because the sun's rays are strongest during that period.

Wounds

A wound is an injury in which the skin or tissues under the skin are damaged. Wounds can be either open or closed. Figure 57-4 shows the various types of wounds.

Open Wounds An open wound is a break in the skin or mucous membrane. Types of open wounds include incisions, lacerations, amputations, abrasions, and punctures.

Incisions and Lacerations An incision is a clean and smooth cut, like that from a kitchen knife. A laceration has jagged edges, as may result when a child steps on a piece of broken glass in the sand at the beach. Care of minor incisions and lacerations involves controlling bleeding by covering the wound with a clean or sterile dressing and applying direct pressure. After the bleeding stops, clean and dress the wound. Procedure 57-6, at the end of this chapter, explains how to clean minor wounds. Teach the patient the importance of keeping the wound clean and checking for signs of infection, such as heat, redness, pain, and swelling.

If the wound is deep and involves muscle, tendons, the face, the genitals, the mouth, or the tongue, control the bleeding with direct pressure to the wound (with a sterile dressing or clean cloth held against its surface), elevation, and use of pressure points. Contact the doctor and, if necessary, the EMS system.

Amputations If a fingertip or toe is completely or nearly severed, quick action may increase the likelihood that it can be saved. Elevate the injured extremity, cover the digit with a dry dressing, and immobilize the hand or foot. Retrieve the severed digit, wrap it in gauze, put it in a plastic bag, put the bag on ice (making sure the digit does not come in direct contact with the ice), and send the part with the patient to the hospital.

Abrasions An abrasion is a scraping of the skin, as when someone slides across rough dirt during a softball game. Abrasions require washing with soap and water. Be sure to remove all the dirt and debris to prevent tattooing (dark discoloration under the skin). Minor abrasions do not need a dressing or bandage, but large ones do. Various types of bandaging are shown in Figure 57-5. As with any wound, teach the patient to watch for signs of infection.

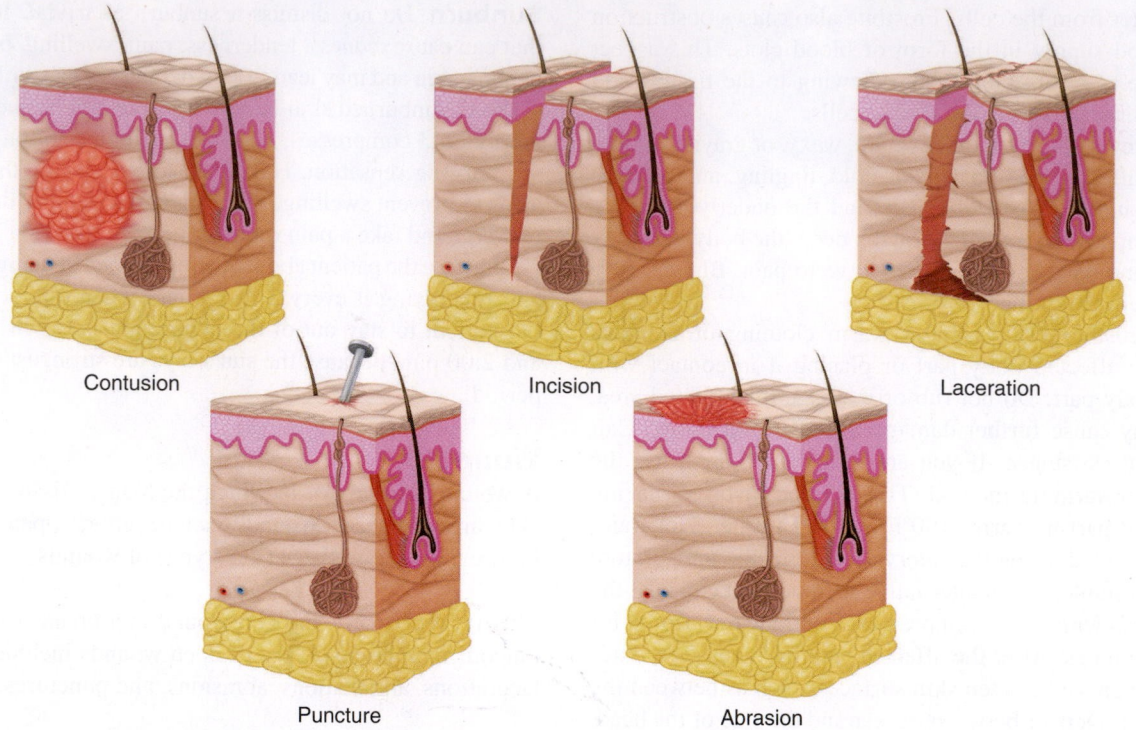

FIGURE 57-4 Different types of wounds produce different degrees of tissue damage.

Contusion

Incision

Laceration

Puncture

Abrasion

Punctures A puncture wound is a small hole created by a piercing object, such as a bullet, a knife, a nail, or an animal tooth. Rinse the wound under running water for 15 minutes. Then clean the wound with soap and water and apply a dry, sterile dressing. Puncture wounds are a potential breeding ground for tetanus bacteria because the bacteria can live and thrive in the absence of oxygen. If the patient has not had a tetanus toxoid immunization in the past 7 to 10 years, inform the physician so that one can be ordered.

Closed Wounds A closed wound is an injury that occurs inside the body without breaking the skin. Closed wounds, often called contusions, are caused by a blunt object striking the tissue. This action produces broken blood vessels and internal, localized bleeding (hematoma) below the area that has been struck. Treat such a wound with cold compresses to reduce swelling. The affected area will turn from black and blue to green to yellow as blood pigments oxidize. Inform the patient that these color changes are part of the normal healing process.

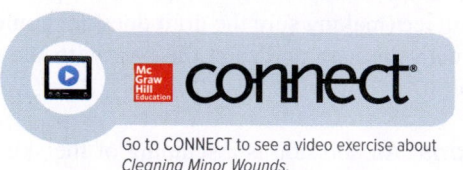

Go to CONNECT to see a video exercise about *Cleaning Minor Wounds.*

▶ Common Disorders   LO 57.4

A variety of common disorders frequently require emergency medical intervention. As a patient educator, you can help ensure that patients recognize the symptoms of illnesses and know when to call for medical assistance. Teaching patients

the importance of following the physician's orders for follow-up care is also your responsibility. Common disorders include the following:

- Abdominal pain
- Asthma
- Dehydration
- Diarrhea
- Fainting
- Fever
- Hyperventilation
- Nosebleed
- Tachycardia
- Vomiting

Abdominal Pain

Sudden, acute abdominal pain accompanied by fever may indicate an emergency that requires surgery. The patient may complain of spasmodic contractions and knife-like or dull pain. Ask the patient if the pain is localized or radiating. The pain's location gives clues to its cause. Right upper quadrant pain, for example, may signal a gallbladder attack. Right lower quadrant pain may indicate appendicitis. The following are other causes of abdominal pain:

- Internal hemorrhage
- Intestinal perforation
- Intestinal obstruction
- Peptic ulcer
- Hernia

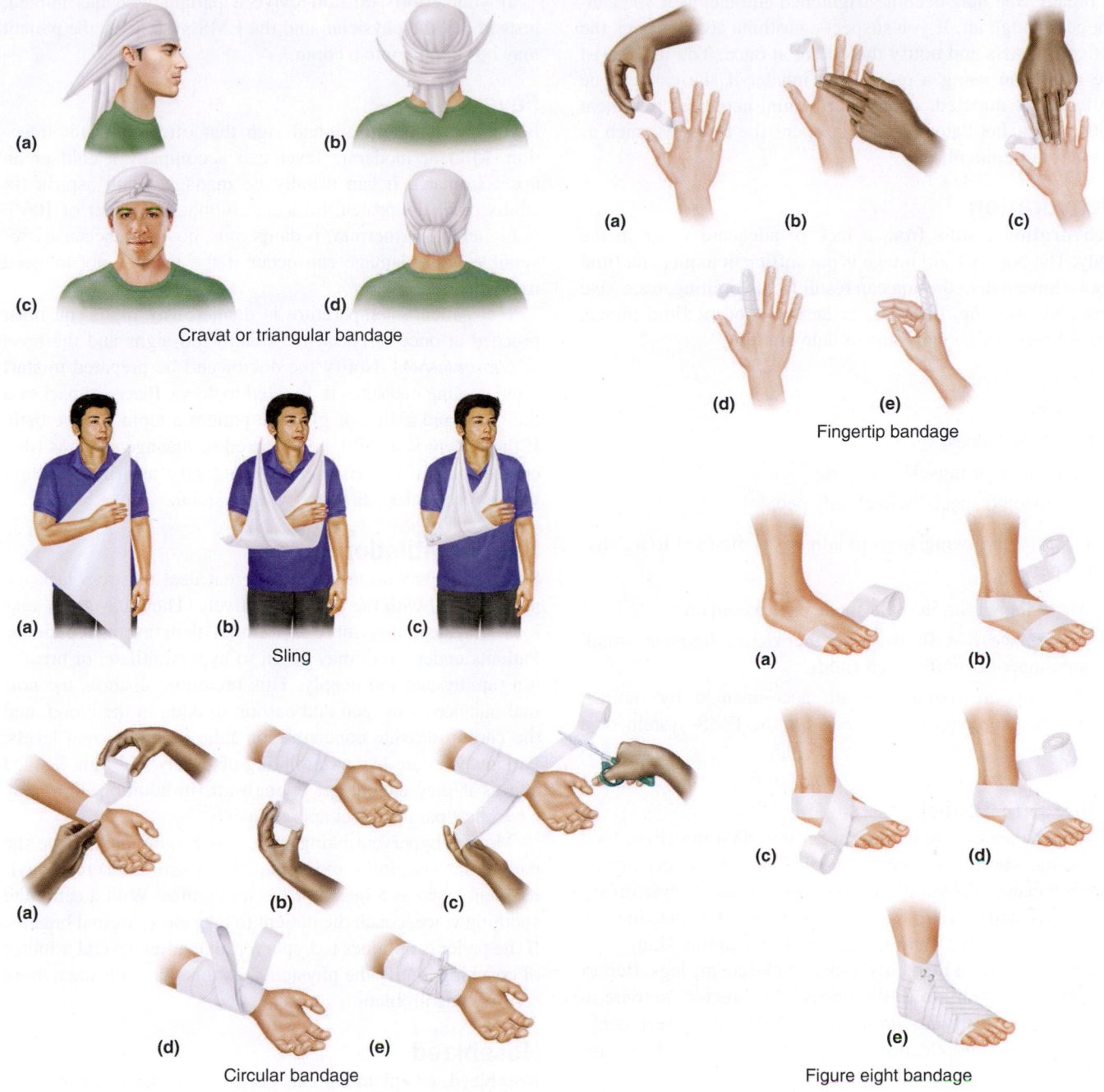

FIGURE 57-5 Apply a bandage, as needed, to a wound or an injury.

(a) (b) (c) (d)
Cravat or triangular bandage

(a) (b) (c) (d) (e)
Fingertip bandage

(a) (b) (c)
Sling

(a) (b) (c) (d) (e)
Circular bandage

(a) (b) (c) (d) (e)
Figure eight bandage

- Abdominal aortic aneurysm
- Ectopic pregnancy
- Kidney stones
- Trauma to the area (wounds or blows)

While waiting for patient transport, have the patient lie on his back with his knees flexed (unless there is a wound or swelling in the abdomen). This position lets the abdominal muscles relax. Keep the patient quiet and warm, and stay calm and attentive. Do not give anything by mouth, and keep an emesis (vomiting) basin handy in case the patient vomits. Do not apply heat to the abdomen, as heat may exacerbate inflammation. Monitor the patient's pulse and consciousness and check for signs of shock.

Asthma

Asthma is a common disorder caused by spasmodic narrowing of the bronchi. It is often an inherited tendency, and several members of one family may suffer from it. A patient who is having an acute attack wheezes, coughs, and is short of breath. She may become frightened and feel as if she cannot get enough air. If you suspect an asthma attack, check the patient's CABs and notify the doctor at once. You may assist the patient in using a respiratory inhaler if she carries one with her. If directed, administer a mini-nebulizer treatment with a bronchodilator (drug that opens the bronchi), such as albuterol or epinephrine.

Dehydration

Dehydration results from a lack of adequate water in the body. The body's fluid intake is not sufficient to meet its fluid needs. Severe dehydration can result from vomiting, excessive heat and sweating, diarrhea, or lack of food or fluid intake. The following are symptoms of dehydration:

- Extreme thirst
- Tiredness
- Light-headedness
- Abdominal or muscle cramping
- Confusion (especially in elderly people)

Perform the following steps to administer first aid to a dehydrated person:

1. Move the victim into the shade or to a cool area.
2. To replace lost fluids, give the victim frequent, small amounts of decaffeinated fluids.
3. If symptoms persist or are accompanied by nausea, diarrhea, or convulsions, call for the EMS system or a physician.

Diarrhea (Acute)

Acute diarrhea can be caused by an intestinal infection, food poisoning, a bowel disorder, or medication side effects. Severe diarrhea causes dehydration and dangerous electrolyte imbalances that can lead to shock. Symptoms of shock include rapid pulse, low blood pressure, and pale, clammy skin.

Help the patient lie on his back and elevate his legs. Report the patient's condition to the doctor. As directed, prepare to assist in administering intravenous fluids to correct dehydration and restore electrolytes, as well as to draw blood for testing.

Fainting (Syncope)

Fainting, or syncope, is a partial or complete loss of consciousness, which usually follows a decrease in blood flow to the brain. Before fainting, patients may feel weak, dizzy, cold, or nauseated. They may perspire or look pale and anxious.

If you are with a patient who feels as if she is going to faint, tell her to lower her head between her legs and to breathe deeply. Stay with her until the feeling passes. If the patient is having difficulty breathing or faints, lay her flat on her back with her feet slightly elevated. Loosen tight clothing and apply a cold cloth to her face. Observe the patient carefully, monitoring her breathing and level of consciousness. Observe for weakness in her arms and legs. Let her rest for at least 10 minutes after she regains full consciousness. Notify the physician that the patient fainted.

If your efforts do not revive a patient who has fainted, instead call the physician and the EMS system, as the patient may be slipping into a coma.

Fever

Fever is a common clinical sign that often indicates infection. Mild or moderate fever can accompany a cold or an upset stomach. It can usually be managed with aspirin (in adults only), ibuprofen, or acetaminophen. A fever of 106°F or higher (hyperthermia) is dangerous, however, because irreversible brain damage can occur if the fever is not lowered immediately.

If a patient's temperature is dangerously high, you must proceed at once to check the other vital signs and the level of consciousness. Notify the doctor and be prepared to start rapid cooling measures if directed to do so. Place ice packs on the groin and axilla, or give the patient a tepid sponge bath. If the patient is a child, be prepared to manage seizures (discussed later in this chapter). Do not give aspirin to a child with a fever unless directed by a physician.

Hyperventilation

Some patients who are under a great deal of stress lack the skills to deal with the stress effectively. They may seem anxious, frazzled, and more emotional than average patients. Patients under stress may begin to hyperventilate, or breathe too rapidly and too deeply. This breathing disturbs the normal balance of oxygen and carbon dioxide in the blood, and the carbon dioxide concentration falls below normal levels. Patients who are hyperventilating also may feel light-headed and as if they cannot get enough air. In addition, they may have chest pain and feel apprehensive.

Move a hyperventilating patient to a quiet area. Have the patient sit peacefully and visualize a calm and serene environment, such as a beach or the mountains. With a calm and soothing voice, coach the patient to take slow, normal breaths. If the patient continues to hyperventilate after several minutes of coaching, notify the physician, as this may indicate a more serious lung problem.

Nosebleed

Nosebleed, or **epistaxis,** can occur for a variety of reasons: blowing the nose too hard, local irritation or dryness, frequent sneezing, fragile or superficial blood vessels, high blood pressure, a blow to the nose, and a foreign body in the nose. Nosebleeds are common in children, especially at night.

Treat a nosebleed by having the patient sit up with the head tilted forward to prevent blood from running down the back of the throat. Next, have the patient gently pinch the nostrils shut at the bottom for at least 5 minutes. If that does not stop the bleeding, continue to pinch the nostrils for an additional 5 minutes. If the bleeding cannot be controlled within 10 minutes, alert the physician.

Tachycardia

Tachycardia is a rapid heart rate, generally in excess of 100 beats per minute. A patient with tachycardia may report having **palpitations,** unusually rapid, strong, or irregular pulsations of the heart. He may feel as if his heart is pounding. Help the patient lie down, take his vital signs, and, if instructed, obtain an electrocardiogram (ECG). (Electrocardiography is discussed in the *Electrocardiography and Pulmonary Function Testing* chapter.) If tachycardia is accompanied by low blood pressure and light-headedness, notify the physician immediately. These symptoms indicate the patient could faint or go into shock. Remain with the patient and keep him calm.

Vomiting

Vomiting is a symptom common to many disorders, ranging from food poisoning to various infections. When severe, it can lead to dehydration and dangerous changes in electrolyte levels, especially in patients who are very young, very old, or diabetic or who also have diarrhea. Because these problems can be severe, notify the doctor and provide appropriate care. Procedure 57-7, at the end of this chapter, describes how to provide emergency care for a patient who is vomiting.

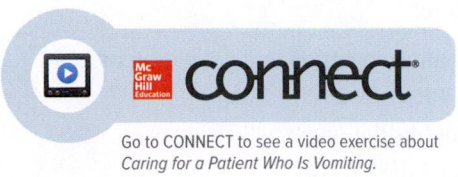

Go to CONNECT to see a video exercise about
Caring for a Patient Who Is Vomiting.

▶ Less Common Disorders LO 57.5

Even though some disorders are less common than those previously discussed, you should still be familiar enough with them to handle them effectively if a physician or an EMT is not immediately available. Educate patients about symptoms they may encounter that require emergency medical intervention and about the importance of follow-up care when recovering from such illnesses or disorders. Less common disorders that may require emergency medical intervention include the following:

- Anaphylaxis
- Bacterial meningitis
- Diabetic emergencies
- Gallbladder attack
- Heart attack (myocardial infarction)
- **Hematemesis** (the vomiting of blood)
- Obstetric emergencies
- Respiratory arrest
- Seizures
- Shock
- Stroke
- Toxic shock syndrome
- Viral encephalitis

Anaphylaxis

Anaphylaxis, or anaphylactic shock, is a severe, often life-threatening allergic reaction. The reaction can be immediate or delayed up to 2 hours or more. It happens to people who have become sensitized to certain substances. For example, it can result from eating certain foods, being stung by an insect, or taking a particular type of medication, such as penicillin.

Initial signs of anaphylaxis include itchy, red, hot skin. Swelling occurs in the face, mouth, and throat. The patient may have trouble breathing and swallowing and feels as if he has a "lump in the throat." Other symptoms include pallor, perspiration, abdominal pain or nausea, and a weak, rapid, irregular pulse. If you detect these symptoms or if the patient becomes restless, has a headache, or says his throat feels as if it is closing up, take the following steps immediately.

Check the patient's CABs and then notify the healthcare practitioner. As directed, administer epinephrine, oral antihistamines, and oxygen and help the patient into semi-Fowler's position. After the patient receives epinephrine, monitor his vital signs every 2 to 3 minutes. Note skin color and monitor the airway. If he does not recover quickly, arrange for immediate transport to the hospital.

When severely allergic patients stabilize, the practitioner prescribes an epinephrine autoinjector for patients to carry with them. You are responsible for teaching patients how to use this device. See the *Assisting in Other Medical Specialties* chapter for more information about using an autoinjector.

Because of the possibility of anaphylaxis, a patient who has just received any type of injection should routinely be kept in the office for 20 to 30 minutes of observation. This procedure reduces the possibility that an allergic reaction to the medication will occur while the patient is unattended.

Bacterial Meningitis

Bacterial meningitis is almost always a complication of another bacterial infection, such as otitis media (middle ear infection) or pneumonia. So first find out whether the patient currently has or recently has had a bacterial infection. The signs of bacterial meningitis are fever, chills, headache, neck stiffness, and vomiting. If the patient has these signs and then develops a fever of 102°F, becomes less alert, has altered respirations, or experiences seizures, the infection has progressed to a dangerous state.

If these signs are present, assess the patient's CABs and notify the physician of the change in the patient's condition. Expect to arrange for transport to the hospital, where the patient will be treated with intravenous antibiotics.

Diabetic Emergencies

Patients who have diabetes or prediabetes must maintain healthy blood glucose levels. It is important that they know the signs of both low and high blood sugar. Symptoms of **hypoglycemia** (low blood sugar) include the following:

- Dizziness
- Headache
- Confusion
- Hunger
- Weakness
- Shaking/trembling
- Full, rapid pulse
- Pallor

Symptoms of **hyperglycemia** (high blood sugar) include the following:

- Dry mouth
- Intense thirst
- Frequent urination
- Muscle weakness
- Blurred vision

You also should be familiar with the signs and symptoms of the two most common diabetic emergencies you will encounter: insulin shock and diabetic coma.

Insulin Shock Insulin shock is basically very severe hypoglycemia, in which a patient has too little sugar in the blood. Insulin shock occurs when insulin levels are so high that they move too much sugar from the blood into cells. Symptoms include rapid pulse; shallow respiration; hunger; profuse sweating; pale, cool, clammy skin; double vision; tremors; restlessness; confusion; numbness and tingling in the hands and feet; and possibly fainting. Insulin shock can usually be corrected with administration of some form of sugar (candy, juice, or regular soda for a conscious patient). If the cause of a diabetic emergency is unknown, give sugar if the patient is conscious. Patients will improve quickly if the cause is insulin shock and will not be harmed if the cause is diabetic coma, provided they are then transported to the hospital.

Diabetic Coma Diabetic coma is the end result of severe hyperglycemia. It occurs when insulin levels are insufficient to move blood sugar into body cells. Its symptoms include rapid, deep, gulping breaths; flushed, warm, dry skin; thirst; acetone breath (a sweet or fruity odor from the mouth); drowsiness, disorientation, or confusion; and gradual loss of consciousness. If you suspect diabetic coma, notify the doctor at once and expect to arrange transport to the hospital.

Gallbladder Attack (Acute)

A classic acute gallbladder attack occurs after a person eats a high-fat meal rich in cholesterol. The patient may wake up in the night with acute abdominal pain (gallbladder colic) in the right upper quadrant. The pain is caused by inflammation of the gallbladder, usually related to gallstones obstructing the cystic duct. This duct carries bile from the gallbladder to the hepatic duct, delivering bile to the duodenum. The pain may radiate to the back between the shoulder blades or be localized in the epigastric region (the upper central region of the abdomen) and the front chest area. The attack may be accompanied by nausea and vomiting. The pain is usually so severe that the patient seeks medical attention; many patients think they are having a heart attack.

Gallbladder attacks caused by gallstones are more common among women who are older than age 40 and obese, and the frequency of attacks increases with age (especially after age 65). Diagnosis is usually made with the help of ultrasonography. The patient may require surgery to remove the gallbladder.

Heart Attack

A heart attack, or myocardial infarction (MI), occurs when the blood flow to the heart is reduced as a result of blockage in the coronary arteries or their branches. Chest pain is the cardinal symptom of a myocardial infarction. The patient may describe the pain as crushing, burning, heavy, aching, or like that of indigestion. The pain may radiate down the left arm or into the jaw, throat, or both shoulders. It may be accompanied by shortness of breath, sweating, nausea, and vomiting. The patient may be pale and have a feeling of doom. If you cannot easily detect pallor (paleness) because the patient has dark skin, check the patient's inner lip for paleness. Elderly patients may experience atypical symptoms of a myocardial infarction, such as jaw pain, because responses to pain diminish during the aging process. The pain of a myocardial infarction is not relieved by nitroglycerin.

If you think a patient is having a myocardial infarction, follow the American Heart Association's "Chain of Survival," outlined here:

- Immediate recognition and activation of EMS
- Early CPR
- Rapid defibrillation
- Advanced life support
- Post-cardiac arrest care

Do not let the patient walk. Loosen tight clothing and have the patient sit up to aid breathing. The physician may order you to administer oxygen at 4 to 6 liters per minute; make sure no one in the area is smoking. Stay with the patient, observe the CABs, and begin CPR if required. If directed, obtain an ECG. Take apical and radial pulses, as instructed by the physician. Be prepared to obtain medication from the crash cart or use a defibrillator if required. The American Heart Association guidelines for CPR key components are found in Table 57-4.

Ventricular fibrillation (VF)—the most common cause of cardiac arrest—is an abnormal heart rhythm. During VF, the heart's rhythm becomes chaotic and the heart does not pump blood. VF treatment is defibrillation using a medical device called a defibrillator, which works by delivering an electric shock to the heart to interrupt the chaotic rhythm. Defibrillators are effective only if used within minutes of the patient's collapse. An **automated external defibrillator (AED)** is a computerized defibrillator programmed to recognize VF and other lethal heart rhythms (Figure 57-6). These devices are found in many public places, including airports, but also may be used at the clinic where you are employed.

To use an AED, attach the adhesive electrode pads to the client's chest in a specific arrangement as determined by the manufacturer. Look at the illustration on the electrode's packing or machine. Activate the AED and it will analyze the heart's rhythm and determine if a shock is required. Pressing the "Shock" button will deliver an electrical charge to the patient's heart by way of the AED's electrode wires attached to the chest.

In order to use an AED, you must be properly trained. Training is included as part of the CPR courses of the American Red Cross and the American Heart Association.

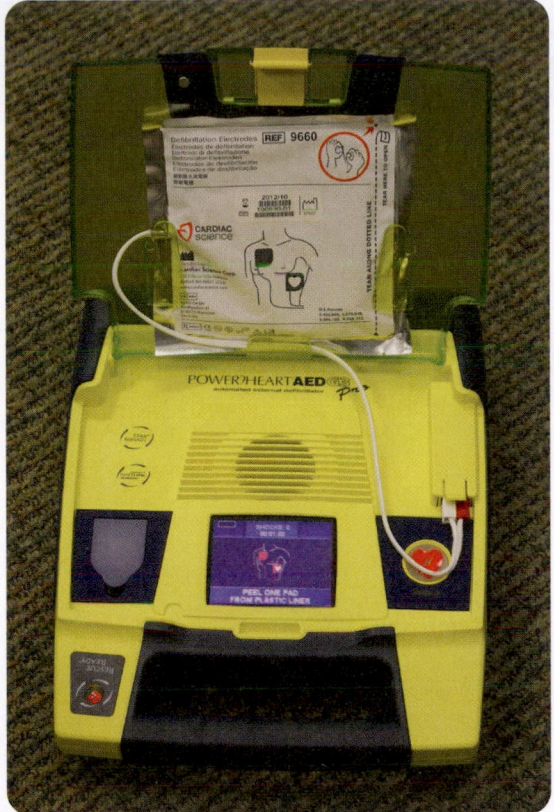

FIGURE 57-6 An automated external defibrillator delivers an electric current to the heart to stop a chaotic rhythm such as ventricular fibrillation.

© McGraw-Hill Education

Obtaining CPR and first-aid certification will be an asset to you as a medical assistant and is necessary to receive medical assisting certification by some agencies.

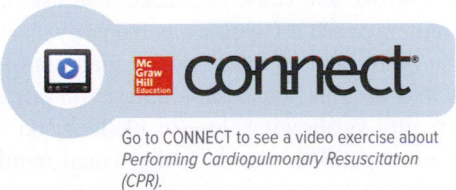

Go to CONNECT to see a video exercise about *Performing Cardiopulmonary Resuscitation (CPR)*.

Hematemesis

Hematemesis is the vomiting of blood. A patient who vomits bright red blood may have a gastrointestinal disorder, such as a bleeding ulcer. A patient who vomits blood that looks like coffee grounds may have slow bleeding into the stomach.

Quickly check the vital signs of a patient with hematemesis. If pulse and breathing are rapid and blood pressure is low, the patient may be going into shock. Notify the doctor immediately and get the crash cart to help the doctor start an intravenous line to replace lost fluid. Then call the EMS system.

Obstetric Emergencies

If you work in an obstetric practice, you may see emergencies unique to this specialty. Although the physician handles most obstetric emergencies, you can assist by asking the patient specific questions about her problem so that the physician can decide what treatment is necessary.

Set up written protocols to handle these situations. For example, if the patient calls from home and reports gushing vaginal bleeding, your protocol may be to call the EMS system for her and tell her to lie down with her feet elevated. If the patient has a miscarriage, have her bring the expelled tissue with her to the office or hospital. (See the *Assisting in Reproductive and Urinary Specialties* chapter for more information.)

Respiratory Arrest

Respiratory arrest, or lack of breathing, is usually preceded by respiratory distress symptoms, which include difficulty breathing, rapid breathing, palpitations, racing pulse, high or low blood pressure, sweating, pale or bluish skin, and decreasing level of consciousness. If a patient shows these symptoms, notify the doctor right away. If the patient develops respiratory arrest, have someone call the doctor and the EMS system while you perform CPR.

Seizures

A seizure, or convulsion, is a series of violent and involuntary muscle contractions caused by abnormal electrical activity in the brain. Seizures are usually related to brain malfunctions that can result from diseased or injured brain tissues. A seizure may be caused by high fever, epilepsy (a brain disorder that causes seizures with varying severity), meningitis, diabetic states, and many other medical problems.

Follow this emergency care for seizure patients:

1. Remove objects that may cause injury.
2. Place the patient on the floor or the ground. If possible, position him on his side with his head turned to the side to help keep the airway open and unobstructed by the tongue. This position is especially important if the patient vomits, to prevent aspiration of vomitus into the lungs.
3. Loosen restrictive clothing and never place anything in the patient's mouth.
4. Protect the patient from injury, but do not try to hold him still during convulsions.
5. After convulsions end, keep the patient at rest, positioned for drainage from the mouth.
6. Make sure the patient is breathing. If he is not, begin rescue breathing or CPR.
7. Take vital signs and monitor respirations closely.
8. Move the patient to an exam room or have him taken to a medical facility.

Shock

Generally speaking, shock is a life-threatening state associated with cardiovascular system failure. It can bring to a stop all normal metabolic functions. This condition prevents the vital organs from receiving blood.

Early symptoms of shock include restlessness; irritability; fear; rapid pulse; pale, cool skin; and increased respiratory rate. Treat a patient in shock by elevating the feet

TABLE 57-4	Key Components of Basic Life Support		
	Recommendations		
Component	**Adults**	**Children**	**Infants**
Recognition	Unresponsive, all ages		
	No breathing or abnormal breathing like gasping		
	No pulse palpated within 10 seconds (healthcare professionals)		
CPR sequence	CAB	CAB	CAB
Compression rate	At least 100/min		
Compression depth	At least 2 inches	2 inches or ⅓ anteroposterior chest circumference	1½ inches or ⅓ anteroposterior chest circumference
Chest wall recoil	Complete recoil between compressions		
Compression interruptions	Limit chest compression interruptions to less than 10 seconds if at all		
Airway	Head tilt–chin lift		
	Healthcare professionals only—jaw thrust if indicated by trauma		
Compression to ventilation ratio	30:2 (1 or 2 rescuers)	30:2 (single rescuer) 15:2 (2 healthcare professional rescuers)	30:2 (single rescuer) 15:2 (2 healthcare professional rescuers)
Ventilations for untrained rescuer	Compressions only		
Defibrillation	Use AED as soon as possible. Minimize interruptions in chest compressions before and after shock. Resume compressions immediately after each shock.		

Adapted from *2010 American Heart Association Guidelines for Cardiopulmonary Resuscitation and Emergency Cardiovascular Care Service*, Pt. 4, tab. 1.

8 to 12 inches. If you suspect a head injury, however, keep the patient flat. Monitor the patient's CABs and take steps to control bleeding. Keep the patient warm and loosen any tight clothing. Notify the physician and call the EMS system.

Several types of shock are possible. Anaphylactic shock, or anaphylaxis, is usually associated with an allergic reaction, as previously discussed. Hypovolemic shock and septic shock are two other types of shock.

Hypovolemic Shock **Hypovolemic shock** results from insufficient blood volume in the circulatory system. It occurs after an injury that causes major fluid loss, such as hemorrhage or burns. Patients with hypovolemic shock must be transported to an emergency facility immediately.

Septic Shock **Septic shock** results from massive, widespread infection that affects the ability of the blood vessels to circulate blood. Common causes are urinary tract infection (UTI) (especially in older adults), postpartum infection, and a variety of infections in patients with immunosuppression (as caused by chemotherapy or acquired immunodeficiency syndrome [AIDS]).

Stroke

A stroke, or **cerebrovascular accident** (**CVA**), occurs when the blood supply to the brain is impaired. This impairment may cause temporary or permanent damage, depending on how long the brain cells are deprived of oxygen.

A minor stroke can cause headache, confusion, dizziness, tinnitus, minor speech difficulties, personality changes, weakness of the limbs, and memory loss. A major stroke typically produces loss of consciousness, paralysis on one side of the body, difficulty swallowing, loss of bladder and bowel control, slurred or garbled speech, and unequal pupil size. The American Stroke Association recommends using the acronym FAST to assess if someone is having a stroke.

- F—facial drooping; ask the patient to smile, do both sides of the mouth raise?
- A—arm weakness; have the patient raise both arms, do both arms stay up?
- S—speech difficulty; have the patient repeat a simple sentence, is it correct?
- T—time to call 911; don't delay, even if the patient seems to be getting better.

If a patient has a stroke in the office, notify the physician at once and call the EMS system. Maintain the patient's airway by turning the head toward the affected side to allow secretions to drain out rather than be aspirated. Loosen tight clothing. If directed by the physician, monitor vital signs and administer oxygen.

Toxic Shock Syndrome

Toxic shock syndrome (TSS) is an acute infection most often caused by the bacterium *Staphylococcus aureus.* The toxin produced by bacterial overgrowth can act as a poison, causing severe, life-threatening symptoms. Although the infection is most common in menstruating women who are using tampons at the time of onset, the link between tampon use and TSS is unclear.

TSS symptoms include high fever, intense muscle aches, vomiting, diarrhea, headache, bouts of violent shivering, vaginal discharge, red eyes, and a decreased level of consciousness. A sign specific to TSS is a deep red rash on the palms of the hands and the soles of the feet. This skin then sloughs off. A menstruating patient with these symptoms should be instructed to remove the tampon immediately and replace it with a sanitary napkin.

TSS is treated with intravenous antibiotics and fluids. The patient will require hospitalization.

Viral Encephalitis

Viral encephalitis is a severe brain inflammation caused directly by a virus or secondary to a complication resulting from a viral infection. Viral encephalitis may result from an epidemic or may arise sporadically. This condition requires accurate identification and prompt treatment. Symptoms develop suddenly, beginning with fever, headache, and vomiting. They quickly progress to stiff neck and back, decreased level of consciousness (from drowsiness to coma), and paralysis and seizures.

The level of consciousness must be monitored frequently in a patient with viral encephalitis. Prepare the patient for treatment with antiviral drugs and arrange for transport to a hospital for a lumbar puncture and other diagnostic tests.

▶ Common Psychosocial Emergencies   LO 57.6

You will probably encounter psychosocial emergencies in the medical office at some point. These may result from drug or alcohol abuse, spousal abuse, child abuse, or elder abuse. Handle these situations as directed in the *Patient Interview and History* chapter. If you encounter patients who have overdosed on drugs, exhibit violent behavior, mention suicide, or have been raped, follow the specific clinical responsibilities described in this section.

You also may be responsible for referring patients with psychosocial emergencies to resources in the community. Some of these resources are listed in Table 57-5.

A patient who is overdosing on drugs can suffer serious medical problems and can even die. If a patient who has taken an overdose is brought to the medical office, call the EMS system immediately and arrange for transport to the hospital.

Patients on drugs may become violent during withdrawal from the substance or while under the influence. If, at any time, a patient becomes aggressive or threatening, follow office protocol for handling violent behavior. The protocol should state when to call the police, how to document the incident, and when to notify the insurance carrier.

TABLE 57-5   Resources for Patient Assistance
Resource
Al-Anon Family Groups
Alcoholics Anonymous
Mothers Against Drunk Driving (MADD)
Narcotics Anonymous
National Child Abuse Hotline
National Coalition Against Domestic Violence
National Council on Child Abuse and Family Violence
National Domestic Violence Hotline
National Institute for Alcohol Abuse and Alcoholism (NIAAA)
National Institute on Drug Abuse
National Organization for Victim Assistance
Students Against Destructive Decisions

During a psychosocial emergency, a patient may tell you he is so depressed that he has thought about killing himself. Allow the patient to talk freely. Listen carefully without interrupting. Whenever a patient mentions suicide or talks about life in ways that make you suspect suicidal tendencies, discuss your suspicions with the physician. Take comments on suicide seriously, no matter how casual they may seem.

Victims of rape may be of any age and either gender, but more than 90% are women. If a patient says she has been raped, provide privacy. Limit the number of people who ask her questions. She may feel traumatized, embarrassed, and fearful. Do not make her go through the office routine at this time.

If the physician asks you to speak to the patient, explain to her that you are legally required to contact the police so that they can file a report. The patient can decide later whether she wishes to press charges.

Contact the local rape hotline and request that a rape counselor come to the office to stay with the patient during the exam and police report procedures. The physician should be familiar with state laws for collecting specimens and the protocol for caring for a rape victim.

The procedure of ensuring that a specimen is obtained from the victim and is correctly identified, that the specimen is under the uninterrupted control of authorized personnel, and that the specimen has not been altered or replaced is called *establishing chain of custody.* This procedure is required for medicolegal issues such as evidence of rape and for tests for illicit drug use. If the chain between the victim and the specimen cannot be proved to have remained unbroken, the specimen must be considered invalid. The steps for establishing a chain of custody are outlined in the *Collecting, Processing, and Testing Urine and Stool Specimens* chapter and are essentially the same for any specimen with a medicolegal purpose. These general steps help maintain an intact chain of custody. Always refer to your office's procedures to make sure you are meeting all relevant requirements.

The Patient Under Stress   LO 57.7

In emergency situations, patients and family members are under a great deal of stress. You must realize that people react differently to emergency situations. You can learn how to detect signs of extreme stress by being alert for patients whose behavior varies from that previously observed or who cannot focus or follow directions.

Your role during many emergency situations may be to keep victims and their families and friends calm. You can promote calmness by listening carefully and giving your full attention. Your first priority, at all times, is the victim's well-being. If he is very distraught, for example, hold his hand while the doctor examines him. If one of his relatives is crying and causing him to become emotional, suggest that the relative do something to help—for example, fill out paperwork in another room.

You may face special challenges when communicating with victims during emergencies. Victims may not speak your language, or they may have a visual or hearing impairment. In such instances, follow these guidelines:

- Use gestures throughout the process for non-English-speaking victims. Continue to speak, however, because they may be able to understand some English.
- Tell patients who have visual impairments what you are going to do before you do it, and maintain voice and touch contact while caring for them.
- Ask patients who have hearing impairments whether they can read lips. If they can, speak slowly to them and never turn away while you are speaking. If they cannot read lips, communicate by writing and using gestures. At all times, try to remain face to face and keep direct physical contact.

Educating the Patient   LO 57.8

During minor medical emergencies, after major emergencies have been resolved, and during routine office visits, you can educate patients about ways to prevent and handle various medical emergencies. For example, you might tell them how to contact the local American Red Cross office, post notices of upcoming classes the Red Cross offers, and encourage patients and family members to learn basic first aid. You also might develop a first-aid kit checklist and make it available to patients and families.

Make sure all family members, including children, are familiar with the local EMS system and know how to contact it in an emergency. Suggest that families keep emergency numbers by the telephone. In addition, teach parents how to childproof their home for children of various ages. Remember, childproofing differs for different children—for example, for children who can crawl as opposed to children who can walk.

Provide brief, easy-to-read handouts to reinforce the information you present to patients. Prepare handouts in multiple languages if you provide care for non-English-speaking patients. Find and use patient education resources for the types of patients seen by the practice. For example, if you

work in an obstetric office, obtain educational materials for pregnant and postpartum patients from companies that provide pregnancy-related products. Ask company representatives what materials are available. Many companies provide free videos and booklets.

Disasters and Pandemics   LO 57.9

Your skills in dealing with emergencies, including first-aid and CPR training, will be an enormous help to your community in the event of a disaster or pandemic illness. To be fully effective, you also must be familiar with standard protocols for responding to disasters and pandemic illness. Table 57-6 shows ways you can help in certain types of disasters. You may even want to participate in fire or other disaster drills to familiarize yourself with emergency procedures.

Evacuation and Shelter-in-Place Plans

Every office should have evacuation and shelter-in-place plans in the event of an emergency. **Shelter-in-place** refers to an interior room or rooms within your medical facility that has few or no windows and is a place to take refuge. Plans should include means of communication for employees during and after the emergency. Maps of the facility with escape routes clearly marked should be posted. These plans should be in writing and there should be periodic practice drills. Employees should be trained in shelter-in-place procedures and their roles in implementing them. If a shelter-in-place option is a part of your emergency plan, be sure to implement a means of alerting your employees to shelter-in-place that is easy to distinguish from alerts used to signal an evacuation.

Pandemic Illness

A rapidly spreading influenza outbreak can overwhelm your office's resources very quickly. The influenza virus is capable of mutating, creating novel strains. Since the population has never been exposed to a novel influenza strain, no one has immunity to the new strain and the virus can spread quickly throughout the world. You must plan for pandemic illness before it occurs. Your office should have a written plan that includes

- Identification and isolation of patients with potential influenza.
- Communication and reporting.
- Occupational health.
- Education and training of patients and staff.
- Respiratory hygiene.

In the most serious scenario, a worldwide influenza outbreak may last 12 to 24 months. There may be waves of illness that come and go every 6 to 8 weeks. Vaccines may be unavailable at first and antivirals will likely be in short supply. To reduce confusion, essential personnel and their roles should be clearly defined. The practice's plan should be flexible, as it is likely the situation will rapidly change. Having a flexible plan will more easily accommodate an evolving pandemic. For more information, see the *Caution: Handle with Care* feature.

TABLE 57-6   Assisting in a Disaster

Type of Disaster	Action to Take
Weather disaster, such as a flood or hurricane	• Report to the community command post. • Have your credentials with you. • Receive an identifying tag or vest and assignment. • Accept only an assignment that is appropriate for your abilities. • Expect to be part of a team. • Document what medical care each victim receives on each person's disaster tag.
Office fire	• Activate the alarm system. • Use a fire extinguisher if the fire is confined to a small container, such as a trash can. • Turn off oxygen. • Shut windows and doors. • Seal doors with wet cloths to prevent smoke from entering. • If evacuation is necessary, proceed quietly and calmly. Direct ambulatory patients and family members to the appropriate exit route. Assist patients who need help leaving the building.
Bioterrorist attack	• Be alert for rapidly increasing incidence of disease in a healthy population (clusters). • Take appropriate isolation precautions. • Use standard precautions when cleaning/decontaminating patient rooms and equipment. • Inform local health departments of suspected bioterrorism agent.
Chemical emergency	• Don appropriate PPE to avoid secondary contamination. • Identify the chemical if possible and report to the local authorities. • Determine if there is a protocol for the specific chemical, if known. • Assist with patient decontamination. • Monitor patient's CABs and vital signs if indicated. • Document what medical care each victim receives. • Arrange for patient transport if possible.
Radiation emergencies	• Assess for contamination (contact with radioisotope released in liquid or power form) or exposure from an external source (for example, from a nuclear power plant accident). • If victim is contaminated, use PPE appropriate for radiation protection, assess for amount of contamination, and decontaminate victim following approved decontamination procedures. • If victim is exposed, look for signs of acute radiation syndrome (ARS) and assist physician in management of multisystem ARS symptoms.
Mass casualties	• Assess the situation for safety. • If there is an explosion, do not go toward the explosion. • Report to the community command post. • Triage victims as necessary. • Render first aid as required. • Document what medical care each victim receives.

Chemical Release Disasters

Whether a chemical release is the result of an industrial or transportation accident or an intentional release during a terrorist event, the results can quickly overwhelm emergency services and medical facilities. As a medical assistant, you may be asked to assist in treating and decontaminating patients exposed to chemicals released into the atmosphere. There are numerous chemicals that, when released into the atmosphere, can cause serious health concerns. Initial decontamination and assessment will most likely occur at the site of the release. Ambulatory patients who may need further decontamination and supportive care may be transferred to your medical facility. It is important that you use appropriate PPE and follow specific instructions based on the chemical that is released. Decontamination is often the same for most chemicals. Removing contaminated clothing and washing the area with soap and water or flooding with water for various periods of time are standard procedure. Procedure 57-8, at the end of this chapter, outlines the steps for assisting during a chemical release emergency.

▶ Bioterrorism   LO 57.10

Bioterrorism is the intentional release of a biologic agent with the intent to harm individuals. The Centers for Disease Control and Prevention (CDC) defines a biologic agent as a weapon when it is easy to disseminate, has a high potential for mortality, can cause a public panic or social disruption, and requires public health preparedness. Numerous biologic agents are identified as weapons, including anthrax, tularemia, smallpox, plague, and botulism. The CDC maintains an Internet site with current information about identified biologic agents at http://www.bt.cdc.gov.

Physicians' offices will be on the front lines if a biologic agent is intentionally released. It will be up to physicians and their staff to sound the alarm to public officials that something may be amiss. Physicians and medical assistants should be vigilant about cases that present themselves, as well as common trends in syndromes. Be on the lookout for unusual patterns in affected patients. Indications of a bioterrorist attack might include many patients having been in the same place at the same time or an unusual distribution for common illnesses, such as an increase in chickenpox-like illness in adults that might be smallpox.

If you suspect that bioterrorism is responsible for an illness, report your suspicions to the physician. It is the responsibility of your facility to immediately contact the local public

health department. The information about the patient should be recorded and appropriate tests should be performed. The laboratory should be notified of the potential for bioterrorism. Additionally, consultations with specialists and discussions of all findings are necessary when bioterrorism is suspected. The following is a list of clues of a bioterroristic attack, as defined by the American College of Physicians–American Society of Internal Medicine (Source: Epidemiological Clues of a Bioterroristic Attack: Clinical Information, Bioterrorism and Disaster Preparedness. Pocket Guide. Used with permission from American College of Physicians. ©American College of Physicians--American Society of Internal Medicine.):

- Unusual temporal or geographic clustering of illness
- Unusual age distribution of common disease, such as an illness that appears to be chickenpox in adults but is really smallpox
- A large epidemic with greater caseloads than expected, especially in a discrete population
- More severe disease than expected

- Unusual route of exposure
- A disease that is outside its normal transmission season or is impossible to transmit naturally in the absence of its normal vector
- Multiple simultaneous epidemics of different diseases
- A disease outbreak with health consequences to humans and animals
- Unusual strains or variants of organisms or antimicrobial resistance patterns

During a disaster, you may be asked to assist with various tasks. It is essential that you remain calm and follow instructions from your healthcare practitioner and local emergency personnel. Always protect yourself from injury during a disaster by assessing the situation, wearing appropriate PPE, and following OSHA guidelines at all times. You will be of no help in an emergency if you become a victim of the disaster by not following standard safety procedures.

PROCEDURE 57-1 Stocking the Crash Cart

Procedure Goal: To ensure that the crash cart includes all appropriate drugs, supplies, and equipment needed for emergencies

OSHA Guidelines: This procedure does not involve exposure to blood, body fluids, or tissues.

Materials: Protocol for or list of crash cart items, crash cart

Method:

1. Review the office protocol for or list of items that should be on the crash cart.
2. Verify each drug on the crash cart and check the amount against the office protocol or list. Restock those that were used and replace those that have passed their expiration date.
   RATIONALE: *Drugs on the crash cart should be available in quantities sufficient for use during an emergency. An out-of-date drug is of no use in an emergency.*
   Some typical crash cart drugs are listed here:
   - Activated charcoal
   - Adenosine
   - Atropine
   - Calcium
   - Dexamethasone
   - Dextrose 50%
   - Diazepam (Valium®)
   - Digoxin (Lanoxin®)
   - Diphenhydramine hydrochloride (Benadryl®)
   - Epinephrine, injectable
   - Furosemide (Lasix®)
   - Glucagon
   - Glucose paste or tablets
   - Insulin (regular or a variety)
   - Intravenous dextrose in saline and intravenous dextrose in water
   - Isoproterenol hydrochloride (Isuprel), aerosol inhaler and injectable
   - Lactated Ringer's solution
   - Lidocaine (Xylocaine®), injectable
   - Methylprednisolone tablets

- Narcan®
- Nitroglycerin tablets
- Phenobarbital, injectable
- Phenytoin (Dilantin®)
- Saline solution, isotonic (0.9%)
- Sodium bicarbonate, injectable
- Sterile water for injection

3. Check the supplies on the crash cart against the list. Restock items that were used and make sure the packaging of supplies on the cart has not been opened.
   RATIONALE: *Items on the cart must be available and ready for use at the time of an emergency.*
   Some typical crash cart supplies are listed here:
   - Adhesive tape
   - Constricting band or tourniquet
   - Dressing supplies (alcohol wipes, rolls of gauze, bandage strips, bandage scissors)
   - Intravenous tubing, venipuncture devices, and butterfly needles
   - Personal protective equipment
   - Syringes and needles in various sizes

4. Check the equipment on the crash cart against the list and examine it to make sure it is in working order. Restock missing or broken equipment.
   RATIONALE: *There is no time during an emergency to make sure equipment works.*
   Some typical crash cart equipment is listed here:
   - Airways in assorted sizes
   - Ambu-bag, a breathing bag used to assist respiratory ventilation
   - Automated external defibrillator (electrical device that shocks the heart to restore normal beating)
   - Endotracheal tubes in various sizes
   - Oxygen tank with oxygen mask and cannula

5. Check miscellaneous items on the crash cart against the list and restock as needed. Two typical crash cart items are listed here:
   - Orange juice
   - Sugar packets

PROCEDURE 57-2 Performing an Emergency Assessment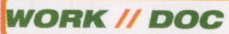

Procedure Goal: To assess a medical emergency quickly and accurately

OSHA Guidelines:

Materials:
Patient's chart/progress note, pen, gloves, and other PPE appropriate to the situation

Method:

1. Put on gloves.
2. Form a general impression of the patient, including his level of responsiveness, level of distress, facial expressions, age, ability to talk, and skin color.
3. If the patient can communicate clearly, ask what happened. If not, ask someone who observed the accident or injury.
4. Assess an unresponsive patient by tapping on his shoulder and asking, "Are you OK?" If there is no response, proceed to the next step.
   RATIONALE: *You must know if a patient is unresponsive before proceeding. The patient's responsiveness will determine if you need to assess his circulation, airway, and breathing.*
5. Assess the patient's circulation, airway, and breathing. Perform CPR as needed.
6. Is there any serious external bleeding? Control any significant bleeding.
7. If all life-threatening problems have been identified and treated, perform a focused exam. Start at the head and perform the following steps rapidly, taking about 90 seconds.
   a. Head: Check for deformities, bruises, open wounds, tenderness, depressions, and swelling. Check the ears, nose, and mouth for fluid, blood, or foreign bodies.
   b. Eyes: Open the eyes and compare the pupils. They should be the same size.
   c. Neck: Look and feel for deformities, bruises, depressions, open wounds, tenderness, and swelling. Check for a medical alert bracelet or necklace.
   d. Chest: Look and feel for deformities, bruises, open wounds, tenderness, depressions, and swelling.
   e. Abdomen: Look and feel for deformities, bruises, open wounds, tenderness, depressions, and swelling.
   f. Pelvis: Look and feel for deformities, bruises, open wounds, tenderness, depressions, and swelling.
   g. Arms: Look and feel for deformities, bruises, open wounds, depressions, tenderness, and swelling. Compare the arms for any differences in size, color, or temperature.
   h. Legs: Look and feel for deformities, bruises, open wounds, depressions, tenderness, and swelling. Compare the legs for any differences in size, color, or temperature.
   i. Back: Look and feel for deformities, bruises, open wounds, depressions, tenderness, and swelling. Feel under the patient for pools of blood.
   RATIONALE: *Pools of blood indicate rapid hemorrhage.*
8. Check vital signs and observe the patient for pallor (paleness) or cyanosis (a bluish tint). If the patient is dark-skinned, observe for pallor or cyanosis on the inside of the lips and mouth.
   RATIONALE: *A patient's status may change quickly. Checking vital signs often will alert you to any changes in the patient's condition.*
9. Document your findings and report them to the doctor or emergency medical technician (EMT).
10. Assist the doctor or EMT as requested.
11. Dispose of biohazardous waste according to OSHA guidelines.
12. Remove your gloves and wash your hands.

PROCEDURE 57-3 Foreign Body Airway Obstruction in a Responsive Adult or Child

Procedure Goal: To correctly relieve a foreign body from the airway of an adult or a child

OSHA Guidelines: This procedure does not involve exposure to blood, body fluids, or tissues.

Materials: Choking adult or child patient. *Caution: Never perform this procedure on someone who is not choking.*

Method:

1. Ask, "Are you choking?" If the answer is "Yes," indicated by a nod of the head or some other sign, tell the patient you can help.
   A choking person cannot speak, cough, or breathe and exhibits the universal sign of choking. If the patient is coughing, observe her closely to see if she clears the object. If she is not coughing or stops coughing, use abdominal thrusts.

2. Position yourself behind the patient. Place your fist against the abdomen just above the navel and below the xiphoid process.

3. Grasp your fist with your other hand and provide quick inward and upward thrusts into the patient's abdomen.

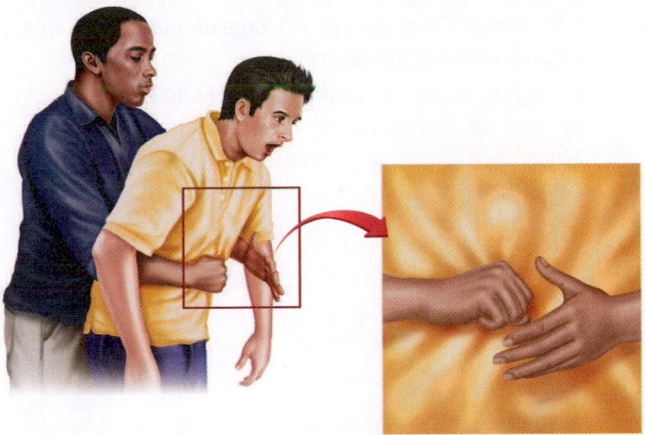

FIGURE Procedure 57-3 Step 3 Perform abdominal thrusts on a conscious choking victim.

RATIONALE: *The thrust should be sufficient to move enough air from the lungs so that the object can be displaced from the airway.*

Note: If a pregnant or obese person is choking, you will need to place your arms around the chest and perform thrusts over the center of the breastbone.

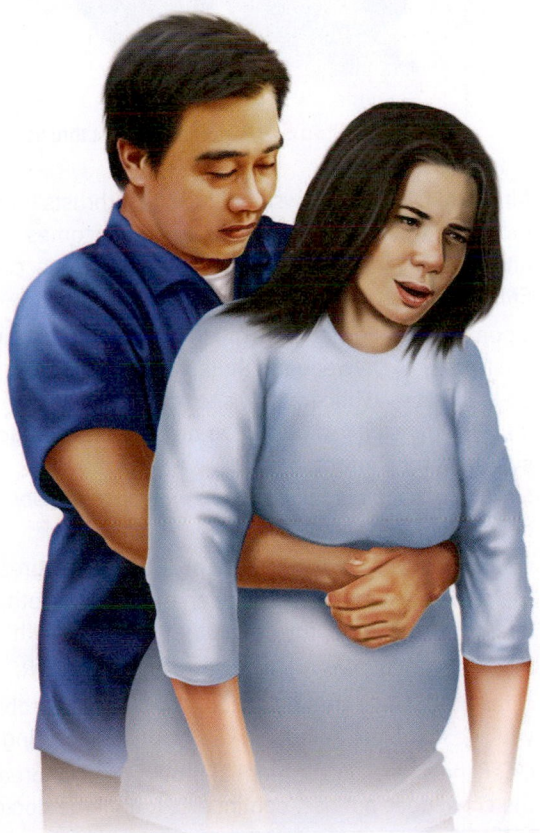

FIGURE Procedure 57-3 Step 3 Use a chest thrust for a choking victim who is pregnant or obese.

4. Continue the thrusts until the object is expelled or the patient becomes unresponsive.

5. If the patient becomes unresponsive, call EMS and position the patient on her back and begin chest compressions without a pulse check.
   RATIONALE: *A patient who becomes unresponsive is most likely not getting the necessary amount of oxygen to the brain.*

6. Use the head tilt–chin lift to open the patient's airway.

7. Look into the mouth. If you see the foreign body, remove it using your index finger. **Do not perform any blind finger sweeps.**
   RATIONALE: *Blind finger sweeps can result in pushing the foreign body further into the airway and may cause pharyngeal trauma.*

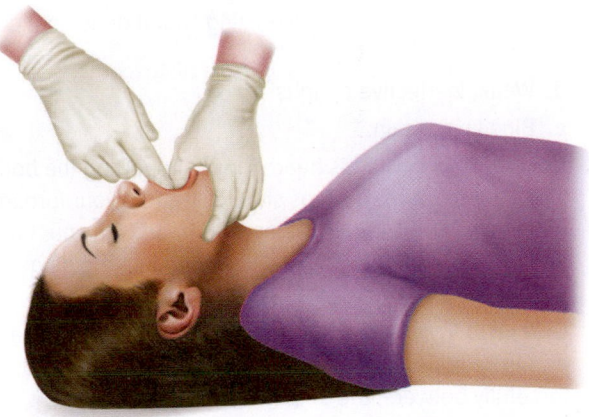

FIGURE Procedure 57-3 Step 7 If you see the foreign body, use your index finger to remove it from the mouth. Do not perform a blind finger sweep.

8. Open the airway. If the patient is not breathing, attempt a rescue breath. Observe the chest. If it does not rise with the breath, reposition the airway and administer another rescue breath. If the chest does not rise after the second attempt, assume the airway is still blocked and continue CPR.

PROCEDURE 57-4 Foreign Body Airway Obstruction in a Responsive Infant

Procedure Goal: To correctly relieve a foreign body from the airway of an infant

OSHA Guidelines: This procedure does not involve exposure to blood, body fluids, or tissues.

Materials: Choking infant. *Caution: Never perform this procedure on an infant who is not choking.*

Method:

1. Assess the infant for signs of severe or complete airway obstruction, which include
   a. Sudden onset of difficulty in breathing.
   b. Inability to speak, make sounds, or cry.
   c. A high-pitched, noisy, wheezing sound or no sounds while inhaling.
   d. Weak, ineffective coughs.
   e. Blue lips or skin.

2. Hold the infant with his head down, supporting the body with your forearm. His legs should straddle your forearm and you should support his jaw and head with your hand and fingers. This is best done in a sitting or kneeling position.

3. Give up to five back blows with the heel of your free hand, as shown in the figure below. Strike the infant's back forcefully between the shoulder blades. At any point, if the object is expelled, discontinue the back blows.
   RATIONALE: *Effective back blows may successfully dislodge the object. Having the infant's head down will allow the object to fall out.*

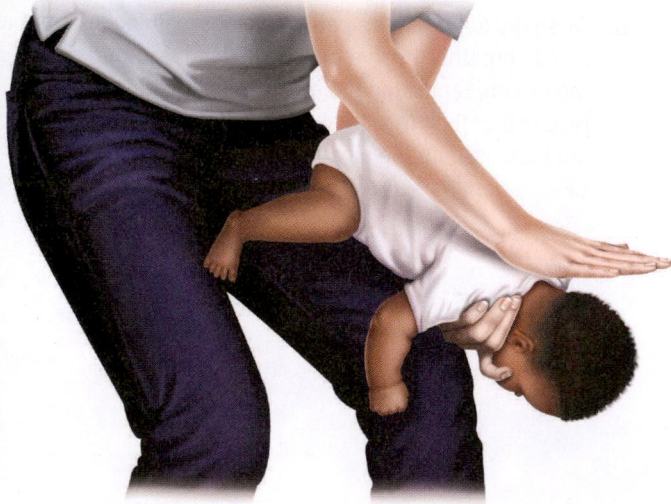

FIGURE Procedure 57-4 Step 3   Use back blows for a choking infant.

4. If the obstruction is not cleared, turn the infant over as a unit, supporting the head with your hands and the body between your forearms.

5. Keep the head lower than the chest and perform five chest thrusts.
   RATIONALE: *Chest thrusts will force air out of the lungs, helping dislodge the object.*
   Place two fingers over the breastbone (sternum), above the xiphoid. Give five quick chest thrusts about ½ to 1 inch deep. Stop the compressions if the object is expelled.

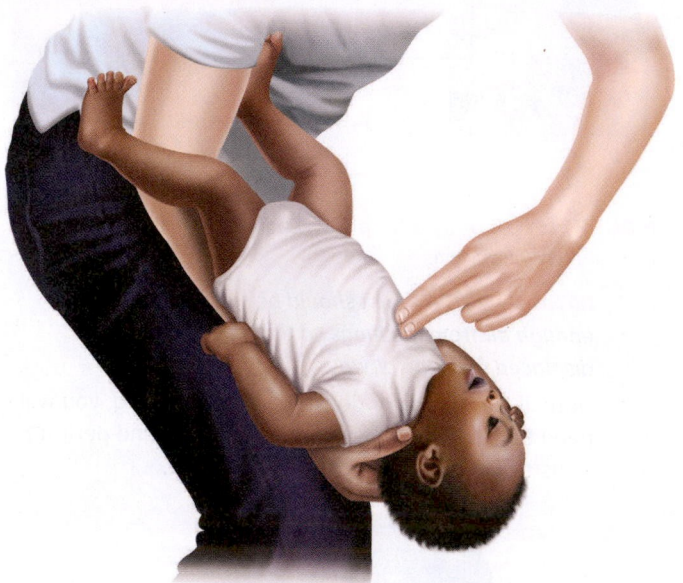

FIGURE Procedure 57-4 Step 5   Perform five chest thrusts.

6. Alternate five back blows and five chest thrusts until the object is expelled or until the infant becomes unconscious. If the infant becomes unconscious, call EMS or have someone do it for you.

7. Open the infant's mouth by grasping both the tongue and the lower jaw between the thumb and fingers, and pull up the lower jawbone. *If you see the object, remove it using your smallest finger.* **Do not use blind finger sweeps on an infant.**
   RATIONALE: *A blind finger sweep may push the object deeper into the airway.*

8. Open the airway and attempt to provide rescue breaths. If the chest does not rise, reposition the airway (both head and chin) and try to provide another rescue breath.

9. If the rescue breaths are unsuccessful, begin CPR.

10. Open the infant's mouth and look for the foreign object. If you see an object, remove it with your smallest finger.

11. Open the airway and attempt to provide rescue breaths. If the chest does not rise, continue CPR until the doctor or EMS arrives.

PROCEDURE 57-5 Controlling Bleeding

Procedure Goal: To control bleeding and minimize blood loss

OSHA Guidelines:

   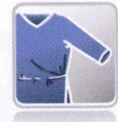 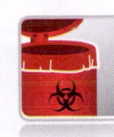

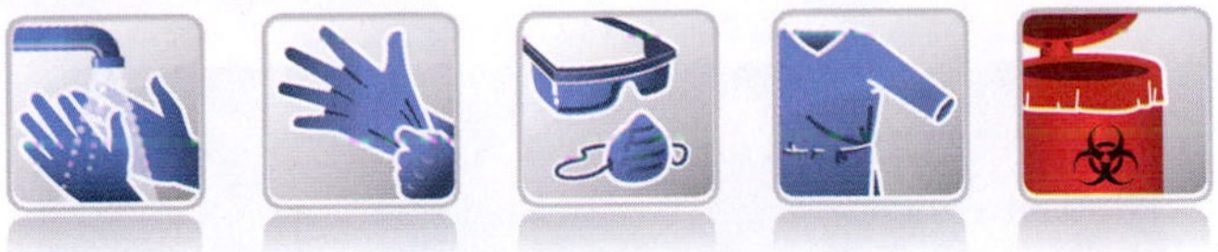

Materials: Patient chart/progress note, clean or sterile dressings

Method:

1. If you have time, wash your hands and don exam gloves, face protection, and a gown.
   RATIONALE: *To protect yourself from splatters, splashes, and sprays.*

2. Using a clean or sterile dressing, apply direct pressure over the wound.

3. If blood soaks through the dressing, do not remove it. Apply an additional dressing over the original one.
   RATIONALE: *Removing the dressing may dislodge a clot and cause more bleeding.*

4. If possible, elevate the bleeding body part.

5. If direct pressure and elevation do not stop the bleeding, apply pressure over the nearest pressure point between the bleeding and the heart. For example, if the wound is on the lower arm, apply pressure on the brachial artery. For a lower-leg wound, apply pressure on the femoral artery in the groin.

6. When the doctor or EMT arrives, assist as requested.

7. After the patient has been transferred to a hospital, properly dispose of contaminated materials.

8. Remove the gloves and wash your hands.

9. Document your care in the patient's chart.

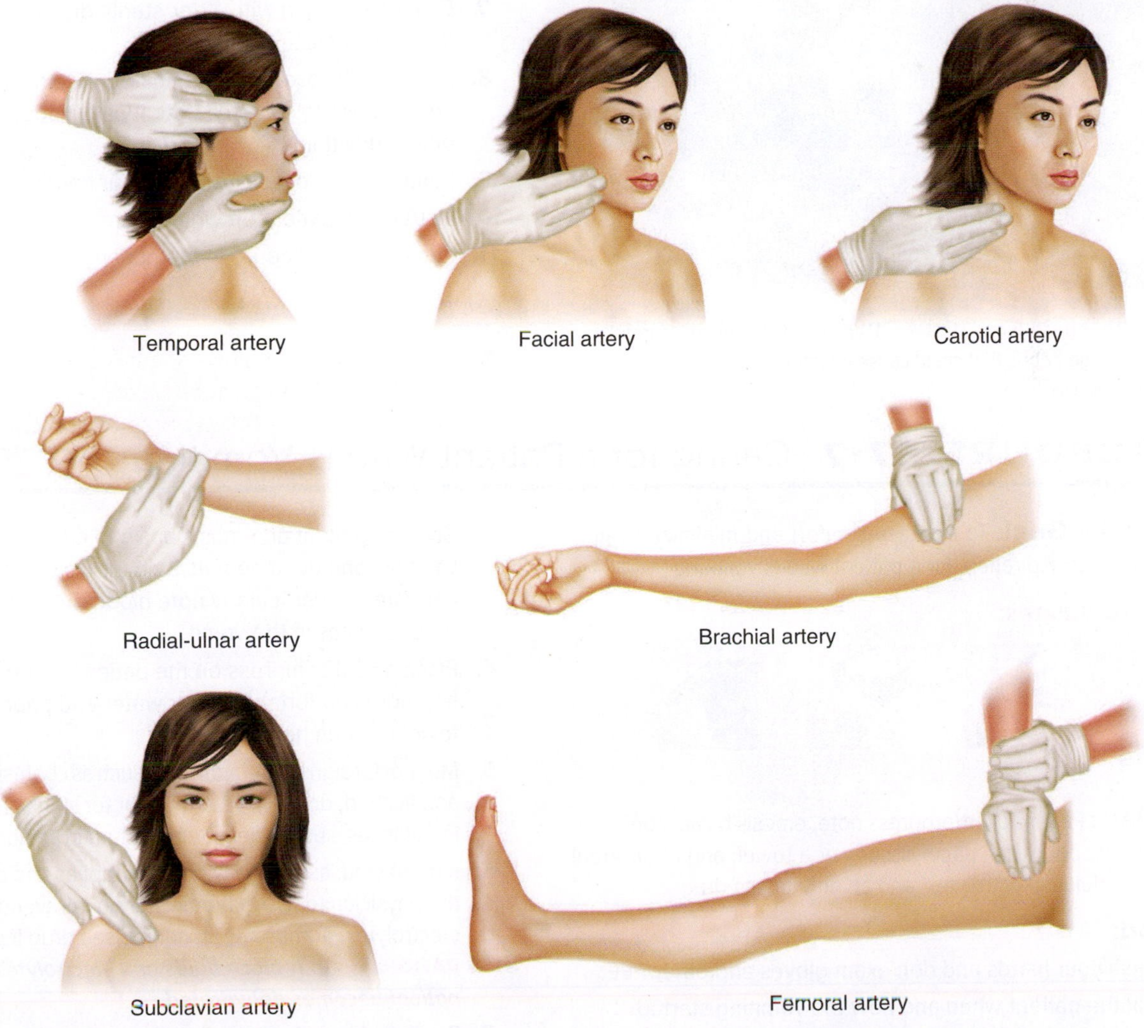

Temporal artery

Facial artery

Carotid artery

Radial-ulnar artery

Brachial artery

Subclavian artery

Femoral artery

FIGURE Procedure 57-5 Step 5 Apply pressure on these pressure points to stop bleeding.

PROCEDURE 57-6 Cleaning Minor Wounds

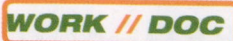

Procedure Goal: To clean and dress minor wounds

OSHA Guidelines:

Materials: Patient chart/progress note, sterile gauze squares, basin, antiseptic soap, warm water, and sterile dressing

Method:

1. Wash your hands and don exam gloves.

2. Dip several gauze squares in a basin of warm, soapy water.

3. Wash the wound from the center outward, using a new gauze square for each cleansing motion.
   RATIONALE: *To avoid bringing contaminants from the surrounding skin into the wound.*

4. As you wash, remove debris that could cause infection.

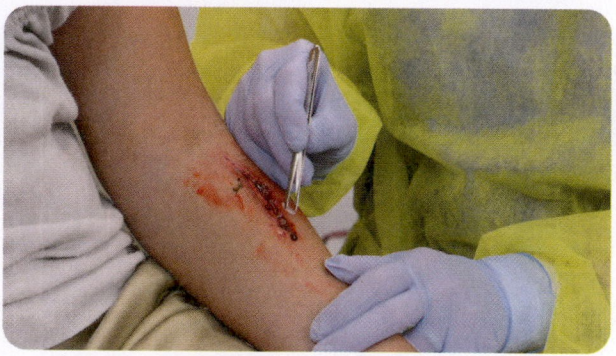

FIGURE Procedure 57-6 Step 4   Using a pair of forceps, carefully remove any large debris that could cause infection.
© McGraw-Hill Education

5. Rinse the area thoroughly, preferably by placing the wound under warm, running water.
   RATIONALE: *Running water will wash away debris.*

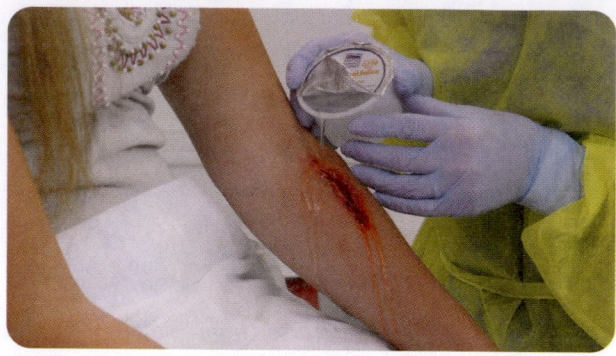

FIGURE Procedure 57-6 Step 5   Rinsing the area with water or sterile saline washes debris from the wound.
© McGraw-Hill Education

6. Pat the wound dry with sterile gauze squares.

7. Cover the wound with a dry, sterile dressing. Bandage the dressing in place.

8. Properly dispose of contaminated materials and decontaminate surfaces potentially exposed to blood or other body fluid.

9. Remove the gloves and wash your hands.

10. Instruct the patient on wound care.

11. Record the procedure in the patient's chart.

PROCEDURE 57-7 Caring for a Patient Who Is Vomiting

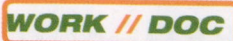

Procedure Goal: To increase comfort and minimize complications, such as aspiration, for a patient who is vomiting

OSHA Guidelines:

   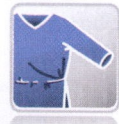

Materials: Patient chart/progress note, emesis basin, cool compress, cup of cool water, paper tissues or a towel, and (if ordered) intravenous fluids, electrolytes, and an antinausea drug

Method:

1. Wash your hands and don exam gloves and other PPE.

2. Ask the patient when and how the vomiting started and how frequently it occurs. Find out whether she is nauseated or in pain.

3. Give the patient an emesis basin to collect vomit. Observe and document its amount, color, odor, and consistency. Particularly note blood, bile, undigested food, or feces in the vomit.

4. Place a cool compress on the patient's forehead to make her more comfortable. Offer water and paper tissues or a towel to clean her mouth.

5. Monitor for signs of dehydration, such as confusion, irritability, and flushed, dry skin. Also monitor for signs of electrolyte imbalances, such as leg cramps or an irregular pulse.

6. If requested, assist by laying out supplies and equipment for the physician to use in administering intravenous fluids and electrolytes. Administer an antinausea drug if prescribed.
   RATIONALE: *To replace fluids and electrolytes if the patient becomes dehydrated.*

7. Prepare the patient for diagnostic tests if instructed.

8. Remove the gloves and wash your hands.

PROCEDURE 57-8 Assisting During a Chemical Disaster

Procedure Goal: To assist during a chemical disaster

OSHA Guidelines:

  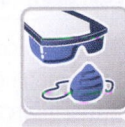 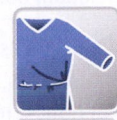

Materials: Soap, water, containment materials such as tubs or plastic covers, biohazard bags and boxes, watch with a second hand

Method:

1. Wash your hands and don exam gloves, moisture barrier gown, and other PPE appropriate for chemical released. **RATIONALE:** *To reduce the possibility that you are exposed to the chemical.*

2. Assess the victim for consciousness and respiratory distress.

3. Monitor the victim's vital signs.

4. Assess the victim for chemical contamination. Look for unusual powder or stains on skin or clothing.

5. Remove the victim's contaminated clothing. **RATIONALE:** *Removing the patient's clothing decreases the likelihood of further exposure to the chemical.*

6. Carefully place the clothes in a biohazard bag and seal the bag. Place the bag in a secondary box or container according to OSHA standards and label the box for disposal. Local authorities may provide labels with detailed information about the chemical.

7. Carefully brush any powder on the victim's skin off into a bag or other container, being careful not to disperse the powder into the air.

8. If you are directed to wash the affected area, place the affected body part over a tub, container, or other containment device.

9. Wash the exposed area with a surfactant detergent and large amounts of water.

10. Continue to flush the area with large amounts of water for at least 15 minutes.

11. Continue monitoring the victim's vital signs. If the victim develops difficulty breathing, alert the healthcare practitioner and place the patient in semi-Fowler's position.

12. Be prepared to arrange for transport if the victim requires additional care and facilities are available.

13. Carefully remove PPE and dispose of it properly, in accordance with OSHA standards.

14. Wash your hands and any other skin that may have been exposed to the chemical with soap and water. You may need to shower after decontaminating the victim if heavy contamination existed. **RATIONALE:** *Showering removes any chemical that may have been transferred from the victim to you and reduces the possibility of your being exposed to the chemical after removing PPE.*

15. Consult with local authorities regarding disposal of waste water and the victim's clothing.

SUMMARY OF LEARNING OUTCOMES

LEARNING OUTCOMES	KEY POINTS
57.1 Discuss the importance of first aid during a medical emergency.	Prompt and appropriate first aid can save a life, reduce pain, prevent further injury, reduce the risk of permanent disability, and increase the chance of early recovery.
57.2 Identify items found on a crash cart.	The crash cart should include all appropriate drugs, supplies, and equipment needed for emergencies. These include but are not limited to activated charcoal, atropine, dextrose 50%, epinephrine, lactated Ringer's solution, nitroglycerin tablets, and sodium bicarbonate.
57.3 Recognize various accidental emergencies and how to deal with them.	Accidental injuries you may encounter include bites and stings; burns; choking; ear trauma; eye trauma; falls; fractures, dislocations, sprains, and strains; head injuries; hemorrhaging; multiple injuries; poisoning; weather-related injuries; and wounds.

LEARNING OUTCOMES	KEY POINTS
57.4 **List common illnesses that can result in medical emergencies.**	Common illnesses that may cause a medical emergency include abdominal pain, asthma, dehydration, diarrhea, fainting, fever, hyperventilation, nosebleed, tachycardia, and vomiting.
57.5 **Identify less common illnesses that can result in medical emergencies.**	Less common illnesses you may encounter in a medical office include anaphylaxis, bacterial meningitis, diabetic emergencies, gallbladder attack, myocardial infarction, hematemesis, obstetric emergencies, respiratory arrest, seizures, shock, stroke, toxic shock syndrome, and viral encephalitis.
57.6 **Discuss your role in caring for people with psychosocial emergencies.**	Psychosocial emergencies in the medical office include drug or alcohol abuse, spousal abuse, child abuse, elder abuse, and rape. As a medical assistant, you may be involved in the direct care of someone suffering a psychosocial emergency, or you may arrange for his or her care at an outside agency.
57.7 **Carry out the procedure for calming a patient who is under extreme stress.**	A medical assistant can help calm a patient under stress by listening carefully and giving her or his full attention.
57.8 **Discuss ways to educate patients about how to prevent and respond to emergencies.**	Medical assistants should educate patients about ways to prevent and handle various medical emergencies by providing brief, easy-to-read handouts containing local emergency contact numbers and a first-aid kit checklist. The handouts should be prepared in multiple languages if the practice provides care for non-English-speaking patients.
57.9 **Illustrate your role in responding to natural disasters and pandemic illness.**	During a disaster, a medical assistant's first-aid and CPR training will be of enormous help. A medical assistant also must be familiar with standard protocols for responding to disasters and pandemic illness.
57.10 **Discuss your role in responding to acts of bioterrorism.**	Physicians' offices will be on the front lines if a biologic agent is intentionally released as an act of terror. You should be aware of unusual patterns of disease in patients being seen at your office. Indications of a bioterrorist attack might include many patients having been in the same place at the same time or an unusual distribution for common illnesses, such as an increase in chickenpox-like illness in adults that might be smallpox.

CASE STUDY CRITICAL THINKING

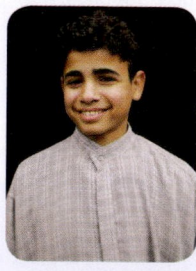

© David Sacks/Getty Images

Recall Mohammad Nassar from the beginning of the chapter. Now that you have completed the chapter, answer the following questions regarding his case.

1. What action should you take to keep Mohammad from exposing the other patients in the reception area?

2. What precautions should his mother take?

3. Mohammad tells you he feels like he is going to vomit. How should you care for Mohammad?

4. Dr. Williams tells you the office needs to implement the preparedness plan for pandemic illness. What steps should you take?

1. (LO 57.3) What is the first action you should take when administering first aid for an animal bite?
   a. Check to see if the animal has had a rabies vaccination
   b. Clean the wound with soap and water
   c. Call animal control
   d. Administer tetanus toxoid
   e. Put antibiotic ointment on the wound

2. (LO 57.3) A displacement of a bone end from the joint is a(n)
   a. Fracture
   b. Sprain
   c. Dislocation
   d. Impaction
   e. Greenstick

3. (LO 57.3) Which of the following is a jarring injury to the brain?
   a. Concussion
   b. Stroke
   c. Seizure
   d. TIA
   e. Aneurysm

4. (LO 57.3) When should you apply a tourniquet to a wound?
   a. To save the limb
   b. If medical help is less than an hour away
   c. Only if the patient is alert
   d. As a last resort, if bleeding cannot be stopped
   e. Before putting pressure on a wound

5. (LO 57.5) Severe hypoglycemia is known as
   a. Insulin shock
   b. Diabetic coma
   c. High blood sugar
   d. Diabetes mellitus
   e. Diabetes insipidus

6. (LO 57.4) The medical term for fainting is
   a. Hypoglycemia
   b. Epistaxis
   c. Shock
   d. Stroke
   e. Syncope

7. (LO 57.5) A severe, often life-threatening allergic reaction is known as
   a. Anaphylaxis
   b. Bee sting
   c. Hives
   d. Toxic shock syndrome
   e. CVA

8. (LO 57.10) The intentional release of a biologic agent with the intent to harm individuals is known as
   a. Pandemic illness
   b. Natural disaster
   c. Mass casualties
   d. Bioterrorism
   e. Radiation contamination

9. (LO 57.6) Drug abuse, attempted suicide, rape, child abuse, and alcohol abuse are examples of
   a. Common illnesses
   b. Psychosocial emergencies
   c. Stress-related diseases
   d. Psychiatric diseases
   e. Medical emergencies

10. (LO 57.3) An injury characterized by a clean, smooth cut through the skin is a(n)
    a. Puncture
    b. Contusion
    c. Laceration
    d. Abrasion
    e. Incision

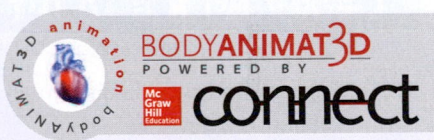

Go to CONNECT to see an animation exercise about *Burns*.

You arrive at the office the morning after a large accidental chemical release at the local fertilizer plant. Your office was utilized by emergency personnel as a decontamination station for victims with mild to moderate exposure. As you are checking the exam rooms, you notice that one of the rooms still has contaminated clothing from a victim of the chemical accident. The clothes are in the corner of the room and are not contained. What should you do?

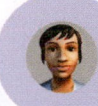 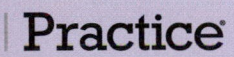

Go to PRACTICE MEDICAL OFFICE and complete the module Clinical - Privacy and Liability.

Preparing for the World of Work

CASE STUDY

	Employee Name	Position	Credentials
EMPLOYEE INFORMATION	Reagan Patrick	Student	In training
	Supervisor	**DOB**	**Other Information**
	Malik Katahri, CMM	09/07/19XX	Applying for a position that is opening where she is finishing her applied training.

Reagan Patrick, a 25-year-old-female, is just finishing her applied training and is beginning her job search. Her applied training included venipuncture, ECG, urinalysis, assisting with exams and procedures, patient reception, insurance claim form completion, patient scheduling, and many other clinical and administrative skills. She lives in a small town

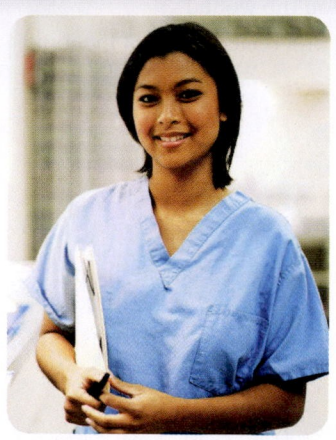

© Ablestock.com/Getty Images

but is willing to relocate. She is excited about her new career in healthcare because it is so different from her current job working as a teller at a bank.

Keep Reagan in mind as you study this chapter. There will be questions at the end of the chapter based on the case study. The information in the chapter will help you answer these questions.

LEARNING OUTCOMES

After completing Chapter 58, you will be able to:

58.1 Carry out professionalism in all applied training scenarios.

58.2 Summarize the steps necessary for obtaining professional certification.

58.3 Describe an appropriate strategy for finding a position.

58.4 Explain key factors for a successful interview.

58.5 Describe ways of becoming a successful employee.

KEY TERMS

affiliation agreement

applied training

applied training coordinator

chronological résumé

clinical preceptor

constructive criticism

functional résumé

networking

portfolio

professional objective

reference

targeted résumé

V.P.8 Compose professional correspondence utilizing electronic technology

1. General Orientation

  c. Describe medical assistant credentialing requirements and the process to obtain the credential. Comprehend the importance of credentialing

  d. List the general responsibilities & skills of the medical assistant

4. Medical Law and Ethics

  f. Comply with federal, state, and local health laws and regulations as they relate to healthcare settings

11. Career Development

  a. Perform the essential requirements for employment, such as résumé writing, effective interviewing, dressing professionally, and following up appropriately

  b. Demonstrate professional behavior

▶ Introduction

After completing a medical assisting program, you may be both excited and apprehensive about beginning your new career. Such a reaction is perfectly normal. In this chapter, you will learn how to maximize your applied training experience and gain the hands-on experience you need for securing a position in medical assisting. Your applied training is an opportunity for you to explore the different responsibilities required of a medical assistant. After completing this chapter, you will understand the process for becoming a nationally certified medical assistant. You also will know how to effectively begin searching for a position in medical assisting—which includes completing a résumé, cover letter, and thank-you letter—and how to form a strategic plan to secure this position. And as you explore this chapter, you will gain valuable interviewing techniques for successfully competing in the modern healthcare world.

▶ Training in Action   LO 58.1

An **applied training** experience is an opportunity to work in a medical facility to gain essential on-the-job experience for beginning your new career. Some schools call this training an externship, while others call it a practicum. Whether it is called an externship or a practicum, it is an opportunity to apply—in an actual medical environment—the knowledge and skills you have learned.

    Most applied training is measured by hours attended, usually a minimum of 160 hours. Applied training is a mandatory requirement of fulfilling a medical assisting program in educational institutions that are accredited by the Accrediting Bureau of Health Education Schools (ABHES) and the Commission on Accreditation of Allied Health Education Programs (CAAHEP). Some of the applied training is completed after the didactic, or academic, portion of the curriculum (for example, during the last module or semester) and some is completed during the last semester. Medical assisting applied training may be performed at physician offices, laboratories, hospitals, administrative billing offices, and clinics.

The Applied Training Process

To make the applied training process possible, the educational institution where the medical assisting student is enrolled partners with local medical facilities throughout the area. Most schools have an **applied training coordinator,** who is familiar with medical assisting and the medical community. The applied training coordinator procures applied training sites and qualifies, or assesses, them to make certain that they provide a thorough educational experience. The applied training coordinator is the liaison between the applied training site and the educational institution. A checklist is often designed to ensure that students are given a well-rounded, safe experience (Figure 58-1). Although student applied training experiences are unpaid, the student should be positive about the experience and appreciate the opportunity to train with the facility.

Applied Training Requirements Applied training sites are required to review and sign an **affiliation agreement.** The affiliation agreement states the expectations of the facility and the expectations of the student. Some examples of the expectations of the applied training site include

CLINICAL SITE ASSESSMENT

Name of Site _____

Address _____

Specialty _____ Supervisor _____

Telephone # _____ Fax # _____

Number of Staff _____

Administrative/clinical experience available to students
(check all that apply)

_____ Front office skills

_____ Word processing skills

_____ Measure/record vital signs

_____ Blood drawing (venipuncture, fingersticks)

_____ Injections

_____ Electrocardiograms

_____ Specimen collection/diagnostic procedures
(urinalysis, blood sugar, cholesterol, etc.)

_____ Assisting with minor surgical procedures

I have determined that this site meets the needs of the students in the medical assisting program.

Print name of evaluator _____

Signature of evaluator _____ Date _____

FIGURE 58-1 A form such as this clinical site assessment is often used by the applied training coordinator to determine if a clinical site will be appropriate for medical assisting applied training.

- Providing reasonable opportunities for clinical instruction by qualified facility personnel for students participating in the program.
- Supervising students in a manner that will provide safe practice and meaningful clinical education.

In addition, the expectations of the educational institution include

- Reinforcing patient confidentiality by having the student sign a statement of confidentiality.
- Providing professional liability insurance for the student, the educational institution, and the faculty.
- Ensuring that the student is medically able to perform the assigned duties of the applied training facility by providing proof of immunizations and health physicals.

Screening The applied training coordinator places students in applied training clinical sites. It is not uncommon for the clinical site to screen students prior to their applied training. This screening can include

- Interviewing students.
- Asking students to provide a urine or hair sample for drug screening.
- Asking students to consent to a criminal background check. Some medical facilities check only for felony convictions, and others check for misdemeanors and felonies. Honesty is the best policy for criminal background checks. Some institutions will waive some convictions as long as the student is honest and truthful about the conviction early in the process.

Time Sheets Students receive time sheets to be completed on a daily basis and faxed to the educational facility at the end of every week. The **clinical preceptor** (person at the clinical site who serves as an instructor but is an employee of the site) and the student both sign the time sheet (Figure 58-2). Weekly telephone calls and site visits may be performed by the clinical coordinator or a medical assisting instructor for each student. Some schools require weekly progress reports from each student, outlining the procedures and duties the student performed during the week. Figure 58-3 provides an example of

Clinical Training Time Sheet
Medical Assistant Program

Instructions:

Students are expected to attend their clinical site for a minimum of 32 hours per week and will not receive credit for more than 10 hours per day. **For shifts greater than 4 hours, you must include a 30-minute meal break.**

_____ Complete the log daily and fax or scan it weekly to the school no later than 5 p.m. Friday.

_____ For each day attended, please include a brief description of the duties performed.

_____ The time sheet must be signed and dated by both the student and the clinical site supervisor.

Student Information

Name:_____

Program:_____

Home Phone:_____

Alt. Phone:_____

Clinical Site Information

Name:_____

Phone:_____

Rotation:_____

Assignment Dates:_____

Site Supervisor's Name:_____

	Date	Time In	Time Out	Total Hours	General Duties Performed*
Monday					
Tuesday					
Wednesday					
Thursday					
Friday					
Saturday					
TOTAL HOURS					

*Examples of general duties include billing, vital signs, lab work, filing, charting.

Student Signature: _____

Date: _____

Supervisor: _____

Supervisor Signature: _____

Date: _____

FIGURE 58-2 Students participating in applied training complete a weekly time sheet.

this report. When students finish their applied training, the preceptors will complete a final evaluation, and the students will be graded on their performance.

Expectations of Applied Training Candidates

While in an applied training program, you are expected to be and look professional, report to the applied training site as scheduled, and display initiative and a willingness to learn.

Professionalism You are expected to conduct yourself in a professional manner at all times while attending your applied training. During this experience, you may often feel that you are being criticized by the site preceptor, but this is a normal part of learning, called **constructive criticism.** Constructive criticism is aimed at giving you feedback about your performance in order to improve that performance. You are not expected to know everything during your applied training, but you are expected to be open to suggestions and ideas.

STUDENT WEEKLY PROGRESS REPORT

This form needs to be completed and signed each week. It must be faxed or scanned with the time sheet on Friday afternoon. It is designed to help you maximize your clinical training experience. Having recognizable goals is the surest way to succeed!

Name: _____ Date: _____

Class Code: _____

Clinical Site: _____

Supervisor Signature: _____

Student Signature: _____

I.   Goals for next week:

           1. _____

           2. _____

           3. _____

II.   Personal assessment of progress this week:

           _____

           _____

           _____

III.   Supervisor's assessment of progress this week:

           _____

           _____

           _____

IV.   Identify one task/item/event you are most proud of that occurred this week:

           _____

           _____

V.   Did you meet your goals for this week? Why or why not?

           _____

           _____

FIGURE 58-3   A weekly progress report is a helpful way for students to track their applied training goals and achievements.

Asking questions during your applied training is expected, but you should not question why a procedure is done a certain way or why you are asked to do something. Do not argue with preceptors about their skills, and know that you may be exposed to some procedures that are not performed exactly as you were taught. After all, there is usually more than one way to get the desired result in patient care. Everything you do during your applied training is a learning experience and should be treated as such.

Your behavior at your applied training site is expected to be as professional as if you were an employee there. Foul language and inappropriate conversation are not tolerated in any workplace. You are expected to be professional with the patients under all circumstances. Medical facilities expect you to demonstrate empathy and compassion to every patient. Proper verbal skills and grammar are expected at all times. Do not use slang when communicating with office staff and patients.

Personal phone calls should not be made or accepted during working hours. Turn off your cell phone while at work and do not use the facility phone for personal calls. Park your car in the designated employee parking area, not in places reserved for patients. Many patients are older and have difficulty walking long distances. It is a professional courtesy and good customer practice to allow the patients to use the parking spots closest to the entrances.

Attendance You are expected to report to your applied training *every day* that you are assigned to a schedule. It is your responsibility to have several alternatives for babysitting and transportation. Employers are seeking dependable and punctual medical staff and do not tolerate attendance problems with their own staff, nor do they expect it from their applied training students. Chronic attendance and punctuality issues can be grounds for termination of your applied training. In the event of an emergency, you are expected to call the medical facility and the school 2 hours before the beginning of your shift, as would any other employee.

As a medical assisting student doing your applied training, also be sure to adhere to the facility's policy regarding breaks. Take breaks only when it is appropriate to do so. If you smoke, refrain from smoking during work hours, smoking only in designated areas if allowed. Many medical facilities are now considered no-smoking zones and smoking is prohibited on the grounds. Lunch breaks are permitted under facility policies. Be sure to adhere to break and lunch time frames, returning back to work on time.

Professional Appearance Medical facilities expect you to appear as a medical professional. Most facilities require a uniform that consists of a scrub top and bottom and a lab jacket. Your scrubs should be clean, pressed, and well fitting. Shoes should be clean, white, and in good repair. Your name tag or badge should always be worn and visible to patients. Nails should be trimmed and clean. Many medical facilities will not accept students with artificial nails. Facial and tongue piercings are not acceptable when working with patients, and visible tattoos must be covered. Your hair should be a natural color and pulled back from your face and off your collar. Makeup should be conservative and in good taste. Perfumes, colognes, scented shampoos, hair gels, and hairsprays should not be used because patients with respiratory conditions or allergies may not be able to tolerate them.

Remember that as a medical assisting student conducting your applied training, you represent several things:

- The school you attend. It is important to maintain a good reputation in the medical community. You will depend on the school's reputation to obtain a job.
- The profession of medical assisting. Participating in a medical assisting applied training program gives you an opportunity to represent the profession of medical assisting to patients and the community.
- Yourself. First impressions are lasting impressions. Make your first impression to the medical community an outstanding one. Even if you are not offered a position there, or if the site is not one where you would like a permanent position, the office will be able to give you your first professional reference and may be key to your obtaining your first position as a medical assistant.

Initiative and Willingness to Learn During your applied training, accept all assignments with enthusiasm and grace, no matter how mundane. These tasks are often a test of how well you accept assignments and work within a medical team. Ask for additional work if you are idle and look for tasks that need to be done. Keep a notebook and record the office policies and procedures. Be prepared to observe and participate in all office policies and procedures.

Make a Good Impression Often, a shy and passive medical assisting student in applied training will appear to the preceptor and facility as unmotivated or lacking initiative. It is important to be assertive and confident when working in

healthcare. Remember: Every day on your applied training is "show time"! You may have to step out of your comfort zone to make a good impression.

▶ Obtaining Professional Certification LO 58.2

Once you complete your education, you may be eligible to take a national certification exam. Some employers require—and many prefer—a medical assistant who is certified. Holding a medical assisting credential can make you more desirable in a competitive job market and enhance the possibilities of career advancement once you are hired. There are two major credentialing agencies: the American Association of Medical Assistants (AAMA) and the American Medical Technologists (AMT). The CMA (AAMA) exam is offered by the Certifying Board of the AAMA and the RMA exam is offered by the AMT. Each of these agencies has its own specific exam eligibility requirements.

Certification Qualifications

In order to sit for a national certification exam, you must meet certain criteria. Both agencies require that you be of good character, including having no felony convictions or guilty pleas to felonies. Other eligibility requirements include

- AAMA—graduation from a CAAHEP- or ABHES-accredited medical assisting program. If you are a student in a program accredited by either of these agencies, you may take the test up to 30 days prior to graduation or within 12 months after graduation.
- AMT—graduation from an ABHES- or CAAHEP-accredited medical assisting program or from a program at a college with regional accreditation and at least 720 clock hours of medical assisting skills training. If you have formal US Armed Forces medical services training, you are also eligible to take the RMA exam. In addition, someone with at least 5 years of experience working as a medical assistant may take the RMA exam.

Applying for the Exam

Once you determine that you are eligible for national certification, you must apply to take the exam. There are required fees for each exam and both require completion of an application form. The following are the steps for applying:

1. Request an application from the appropriate agency.
2. Gather required documents.
3. Review all exam policies and procedures in the examination handbooks.
4. Complete the application and submit it to the appropriate agency.
5. Schedule an exam time.

Be sure to provide all the required information when completing the application. Submitting an incomplete application will delay your taking the exam, which could affect the timing of your job search.

Preparing to Take the Exam

Taking the time to prepare will increase your chances of successfully completing the exam, so never try to take the exam without knowing the following:

- Test format. The CMA (AAMA) exam is a computer-based test. The RMA is either computer-based or paper-and-pencil.
- Content areas. This gives you general information about the material covered on the test.

General Content Areas When you begin studying for the exam, a good starting point is to know the content it covers. The areas of knowledge you should be familiar with for either exam are general medical, which includes medical terminology, anatomy and physiology, medical ethics and law, and human behavior; administrative; clinical; and laboratory. These general areas are expanded further in the content outlines available from the AAMA or AMT. Use the expanded content outlines as a study guide, making sure you review materials from each specific content area.

Study Tips At first, studying for a national exam can seem like an impossible task. You may feel overwhelmed, with no idea where to start or what to do. Do not panic. Instead, break it down. You cannot study everything at once, so you must find a way to make it manageable. If you are served a 12-ounce steak, you would not put the entire steak in your mouth and try to chew it. What would you do? Cut it into pieces. That is exactly what you need to do when studying for the certification exam. Study a piece at a time.

Start by taking a practice exam that covers all the content areas of the real exam. This will reveal your areas of weakness. Use this information to focus your studies on what you do not know. Students often make the mistake of studying what they do know because it feels good, but this will not help you in the long run. If you study what you do not know, you will ultimately spend less time studying. Once you have studied the content in your areas of weakness, take another practice test. You will most likely score higher on the second practice test. Identify the areas you are still having trouble with and study the content in those areas. You will soon feel comfortable with the information in all areas.

During your study process, follow these general guidelines:

- Start early; do not wait until a few days before the exam. Cramming does not work.
- Study some every day.
- Create a study schedule and follow it.
- Study in a quiet place free of distractions. Turn off your phone while you are studying; most calls can wait until you are finished.
- Make flash cards with terms, definitions, and concepts.
- Use mnemonic devices to help you remember difficult material. For example, if you are learning the stages of mitosis, in order, remember the first letter of each phase: IPMAT—interphase, prophase, metaphase, anaphase, telophase.

The Day of the Test This is the time to show your knowledge. You have followed your study plan and you are ready. Now, make the best of all that studying by getting a good start on the day. To prepare for test day,

- Get a good night's sleep the night before the test. Remember, do not cram—it does not work and just tires out your brain.
- Eat a balanced breakfast. Your brain, like your car, needs fuel.
- Take a short walk if you can. Exercise helps your brain as well as your body.
- Give yourself enough time to get to the testing site and make sure you know exactly where it is. Use a map if necessary.
- Take all necessary documents to the testing site. Do not forget your photo ID. You will have to identify yourself.
- If you are taking a paper-and-pencil test, take more than one pencil with you.
- Tell yourself that you are prepared. Believing in yourself is essential.

▶ Preparing to Find a Position   LO 58.3

The next phase of beginning your new career is seeking a position as a medical assistant. Most accredited schools have a career services department. Its primary focus is job placement after graduation. The department's counselors will assist you in writing your résumé, improving your interviewing skills, and learning about positions in your field. Many employers will contact a school's career services department to recruit medical personnel.

Seeking Employment

In addition to working with a career services department, you can take advantage of a number of other resources in seeking employment within the medical assisting field. These resources include Internet sites, classified ads, employment services, and networking with classmates and others.

Internet Sites and Classified Ads Many prospective employers use employment websites and classified advertisements in area newspapers to alert potential applicants to a career opportunity with their organization. The job listing or advertisement usually describes the position's duties and responsibilities as well as the type of education and experience preferred.

When you are first beginning to seek a medical assisting position, do not become discouraged if you see advertisements asking for a specified amount of experience, such as 2 years. You must realize that employers place ads seeking an experienced candidate, but many will consider a new graduate because experienced candidates are not always available. Becoming credentialed will help you bridge this experience gap. A local newspaper's classified advertisements and corresponding website are often a good place to start your search. You also might check for a medical practice network website in your area. These often have lists of local medical practices along with job postings for these practices. They may allow you to submit online job applications.

It is important to explore all the possibilities when seeking employment opportunities. A medical assistant is qualified for a number of positions. For example, new graduates can apply for the following positions:

- Unit secretary in hospitals
- Phlebotomist in labs
- Patient care associate or patient care technician in hospitals
- Entry-level medical coder and biller
- Customer service representative in medical-related companies
- Clinical or administrative positions in physician offices and clinics

The Internet is another useful tool when seeking employment. Websites for job seekers are becoming more and more popular, as they allow job seekers to post résumés online and to respond to advertisements that are posted by employers locally or statewide. Many hospitals and larger companies will not accept paper or faxed résumés; instead, they require all applicants to fill out an electronic application and post résumés on the facility website. Newly graduated medical assistants should post their résumé and cover letter on all local hospital and physician network websites and on local employment websites during their applied training to start circulating their résumés.

Employment Services Employment and temporary agencies provide assistance in locating a specific job. Both types of agencies have a variety of job openings on file. You should call to make an appointment with an employment counselor. Agencies usually require you to fill out an application, take a basic healthcare knowledge test, and provide a résumé. If the agency has positions that match your skills, it contacts the employer. If the service has no appropriate listings, it will place your résumé on file.

Employment services are an excellent way to gain experience and select a position. You are given an opportunity to try out the office or facility with little commitment on your part. Many permanent opportunities can result from a temporary job assignment.

Networking Networking involves making contacts with relatives, friends, and acquaintances who may have information about how to find a job in your field. People in your network may be able to give you job leads or tell you about openings. Word-of-mouth referrals—finding job information by talking with other people—can be very helpful. Other people may be able to introduce you to others who work in, or know people who work in, your field. You also may find opportunities at your applied training site. Although there might not be a position available directly within your site, the practice manager may know someone who is looking for a medical assistant. Networking is a valuable tool. It can advance your career even while you are employed.

Joining a medical assisting organization and attending conferences are the easiest ways to network. Attend an organization's local chapter meetings, such as the AAMA county or state chapters, and talk with as many people as possible. Always take along a pen and a notebook. Be prepared to exchange information with other attendees. Remember, networking is an exchange of information—it is not one-sided. What you learn through networking may enable you to provide others with information to help their job search or further their career.

Your classmates are often a good source of networking. It is important to build lasting friendships with your classmates and keep in touch after graduation. Oftentimes, they will know of positions as they gain employment. Networking begins in the classroom.

Creating a Résumé

Your résumé is a vital part of the employment process. It provides potential employers with information about your educational and work history and other aspects of your background.

Components of a Résumé In order to create a well-rounded, informative résumé, you need to include a wide variety of information about your background.

Personal Information Include your name, address, telephone number, cell phone number, and e-mail address. Do not include your marital status or the number of children you have. You should not include your height, weight, interests, or hobbies unless you think they are relevant to the position.

Professional Objective A **professional objective** is a brief, general statement that demonstrates a career goal. An example of an effective, professional objective is the following: "To work as a medical assistant, applying skills in patient relations and laboratory work while gaining increasing responsibility." If you want to list a specific career objective, such as applying your medical assisting skills in a pediatric medical facility, it would be best to mention it in the cover letter and not on your résumé.

Employment Experience List the title of your most recent or last job first, the dates you were employed there, and a brief description of your duties. Choose jobs that have been the most beneficial to your working career. Do not clutter your résumé with needless details or irrelevant jobs. You can elaborate on specific duties in your cover letter and in the interview. Only include jobs you have held for a longer period of time, such as 6 months to a year.

Educational Background In providing your educational history, list your highest degree first, the school attended, the dates, and the major field of study. Include educational experience that may be relevant to the job, such as certification, licensing, advanced training, and intensive seminars. Do not list individual classes on your résumé. However, do list the skills you acquired during your training, such as phlebotomy, CPT, and coding skills. If you have taken classes that relate directly to the job you are seeking, list them in your cover letter.

Awards and Honors List the awards and honors related to your career or that indicate excellence. Perfect attendance, academic honors, and student-of-the-month are excellent traits that employers are seeking. Highlight this information prominently rather than writing it as an afterthought. You can make the most impact by displaying your best qualities at the beginning of this section.

Campus and Community Activities List activities that show leadership abilities and a willingness to contribute. Include any volunteer work.

Professional Memberships and Activities List any career-related professional memberships. Student memberships are available through the American Medical Technologists (AMT) and the American Association of Medical Assistants (AAMA). You can contact the AMT and request a copy of the student by-laws and directions on how to form a student membership in your school. The AAMA provides continuing education through its local chapters and sponsors local meetings periodically throughout the year. Employers like medical professionals who are involved in their disciplines. It demonstrates a commitment and dedication to their chosen field.

Summary of Skills As you learn clinical and administrative skills, be sure to list them on your résumé. Under headings such as "Clinical Skills" or "Administrative Skills," list the skills you acquired in school and during your applied training. The following are some examples of clinical skills:

- ECG
- Venipuncture
- Urinalysis
- Parenteral injections
- Aseptic technique and bloodborne pathogens
- First aid and bandaging
- CPR
- Triage and vital statistics
- Spirometry

Some examples of administrative work include

- CPT, HCPCS, and ICD-10 coding.
- Insurance claim form completion and reimbursement posting.
- MediSoft® billing and reimbursement software (or any software you have experience with).
- Medical office accounting practices.
- Keyboarding speed.
- Microsoft Office® (list the software you are proficient with).

Choosing a Résumé Style Three résumé styles have been developed: functional, chronological, and targeted. Each has specific advantages and disadvantages. You will want to choose a style or combination of styles that best describes your strengths and skills.

Functional Résumé A **functional résumé** highlights specialty areas of your accomplishments, strengths, knowledge, and skills. You can organize these in an order that supports your objective. Functional résumés are useful when you change careers, reenter the job market after an absence, or have had a variety of unconnected work experiences. A sample of a functional résumé is shown in Figure 58-4.

Chronological Résumé Individuals who have a strong work history use a **chronological résumé.** List your most recent job first and end with your first job. Chronological résumés are best when you stay in the same field and when your employment history shows growth and development. Do not use a chronological résumé if you have gaps in your work history, if you have changed careers, if you have been in the same job for many years, or if you are looking for your first job. Figure 58-5 illustrates a chronological résumé.

Targeted Résumé A **targeted résumé** is best if you are focused on a specific job target. The résumé should contain a clear, concise objective about what you are looking for (targeting). This résumé should tailor your descriptions of your skills, academic achievements, student honors, and other pertinent information to the job you are seeking. This approach adds substance to your résumé when you have just graduated and do not have relevant job experience. Because the targeted résumé is an academic-type résumé, your skills, achievements, and community and volunteer work—your most significant assets—should be listed first. A sample of a targeted résumé is shown in Figure 58-6.

Writing the Résumé

One of the most daunting tasks of completing the résumé process is writing the résumé. Résumé writing is different from any other form of writing. The language you use in your résumé will affect its success, so it is important to be careful and conscientious when choosing your words.

You should use a direct, functional writing style that focuses on the use of verbs and other words that imply action on your part. Translate the facts of your academic and employment history into an active and precise résumé that will keep the reader's interest and highlight your major accomplishments in a concise, effective manner.

Writing with action words and strong verbs portrays you as an energetic, active person who is able to achieve results in your work. Choose words that display your strengths and demonstrate your initiative. Table 58-1 provides a list of commonly used verbs that help create a strong, active résumé.

The following are two writing samples that differ only in their style. The first example is ineffective because it does not use action words to accent the applicant's work experiences.

Example #1
WORK EXPERIENCE

Medical Assistant
Manager of eight medical assistants from three offices. Office manager of three offices located east and west sides. In charge of the daily operations of the medical office. Trainer of all new medical assistants.

Donna Turner-Smith
18 Kingsley Road
Olmsted Falls, OH 44138
(440) 555-4279

PUBLIC HEALTH EDUCATION:
> Instructed community groups on HIV awareness
> Instructed volunteers on how to set up community programs on domestic violence
> Facilitated workshops for parents of teenagers
> Provided in-services for public school teachers on signs and symptoms of substance abuse

COUNSELING:
> Consulted with social workers on individual cases for suspected child abuse
> Worked with parents from abused homes
> Counseled individual abused children

ORGANIZATIONAL:
> Wrote grants for federal funds for HIV awareness programs
> Served as a liaison for transitional shelters for victims of domestic violence
> Served as a liaison between community health agencies and public schools

PROFESSIONAL WORK HISTORY:

> 2006–2011   Project SAFE, Plymouth, Michigan
> HIV Public Health Instructor

> 2011–2012   Department of Child Health and Safety, Cleveland, Ohio
> Public Health Educator

EDUCATION:
> 2006 BS Sociology, Eastern Michigan University, Ypsilanti, Michigan

References available upon request

FIGURE 58-4   A functional résumé is often used by people who are reentering the job market.

Special Projects:	Coordinator and secretary for Cuyahoga County Chapter of the American Association of Medical Assistants.
Accomplishments:	Daily patient census went up 25% by implementing the "Patient First" customer service program. Patient-facility relations improved.

In the second example, the first paragraph has been rewritten. Notice how the tone has changed. The paragraph now makes the applicant sound stronger and more active. This person accomplished goals.

Example #2
WORK EXPERIENCE

Medical Assistant
Managed eight medical assistants from three different offices. Oversaw three offices in the Greater Cleveland area. Directed the daily operations of the medical offices. Coordinated events and served as secretary for the Cuyahoga County Chapter of the American Association of Medical Assistants. Increased daily patient census by 25% due to the success of a customer service model, "Patient First," which improved patient-facility relations during my tenure.

WORK EXPERIENCE:

September 2010–Present   NORTH BERGEN CLINIC FOUNDATION

Lead medical assistant for cardiology practice
Patient preparation
EKG and Holter monitor
Assist with stress testing
Patient follow-up

June 2002–August 2010   ST. JOSEPH HOSPITAL

Phlebotomist—inpatient and outpatient

March 2002–June 2002   ST. JOSEPH HOSPITAL

Medical assisting externship
Administrative and clinical responsibilities utilizing all
medical assisting skills in the emergency department

- Patient triage
- Foley catheters
- ECG
- Specimen collection
- Patient intake
- Insurance verification

EDUCATION AND CERTIFICATIONS:

Associate of Applied Science Degree, June 2008, Bergen Community College,
Paramus, New Jersey, 07645

Certified Medical Assistant, August 2002

References available upon request

FIGURE 58-5   A chronological résumé lists a person's job history in chronological order.

Résumé Writing Tips

Pay close attention to detail as you create your résumé:

- Organize your information by using a worksheet (Figure 58-7). List all the addresses, dates, phone numbers, and supervisors of previous positions you have held. Write down brief descriptions of all the responsibilities and duties of your positions.
- List your educational institutions and their addresses, your dates of attendance, and the type of diploma or degree, including your major.
- Choose a résumé format that best describes your experience, education, and achievements.
- Use a word processing program and save your résumé so that you can update it as needed.
- Proofread all spelling and grammar. Your completed résumé should be perfect. Do not rely on the spell-checking feature of your computer. Proofread your résumé line by line and request that someone else also proofread your résumé.
- Select a high-quality, standard-size (8½ × 11) résumé paper with a weight between 20 and 25 pounds. Use ivory or white paper with matching envelopes.

Kelly Adamson
220 Terrace Avenue
Mooresburg, TN 37811
(423) 555-2657

CAREER OBJECTIVE:

To obtain a challenging position as a medical assistant in a growth-oriented ambulatory care facility

ACHIEVEMENTS:

Registered Medical Assistant
Certified Phlebotomy Technician
Registered Medical Office Specialist
Graduate of an Accredited Medical Assistant Program
OSHA Compliance Officer
American Heart BLS Instructor

SKILLS AND CAPABILITIES:

Front Office and Clinical Medical Assistant Patient Triage
Specimen Collection Venipuncture
ECG and Holter Monitor Parenteral Injections
ICD-9 and CPT Coding Medical Billing

PROFESSIONAL EXPERIENCE:

September 2011–Present Affiliated Physician Network, Mooresburg, Tennessee
    Medical Assistant/Office Coordinator
June 2001–September 2011 Partners in Internal Medicine, Mooresburg,
    Tennessee Medical Assistant

EDUCATION:

Sanford Brown Institute, Diploma, Medical Assisting 2006

AFFILIATIONS:

American Medical Technologists

References available upon request

FIGURE 58-6 A targeted résumé is often used by a person who is focusing on a specific job target.

- Use clear and concise statements and sentences. Your writing should reflect a positive and confident tone. For example, if you are describing your duties as a food service worker, use sentences that focus on customer service, cash management, and the training and development of new food service workers. Avoid using the word "I" because the reader already knows that the résumé is referring to you.

- Be truthful about your strengths and abilities. Do not mislead or exaggerate any skills, talents, or experience.

Procedure 58-1, at the end of this chapter, provides information on how to write a résumé.

Writing a Cover Letter

A cover letter is an introduction to your résumé. It is a tool that markets your résumé as well as your skills and abilities. Your cover letter is just as important as your résumé in your job search. An effective cover letter motivates an employer to review your résumé and perhaps grant you a job interview.

Your cover letter should be direct and to the point. It should be no longer than one page and typed on paper that matches your résumé. If possible, your cover letter should be addressed to a specific person in the organization. You can call the facility and ask to whom you should address the letter.

TABLE 58-1 Effective Résumé Verbs

administered	inspected
advised	introduced
analyzed	maintained
billed	managed
carried out	motivated
compiled	negotiated
completed	operated
conducted	ordered
contacted	organized
coordinated	oversaw
counseled	performed
designed	planned
developed	prepared
directed	presented
distributed	produced
established	reviewed
functioned as	supervised
implemented	taught
improved	trained

If a name is not available, it is acceptable to address the letter to "Human Resources Manager" or "Recruitment Manager." Research the facility prior to writing the letter. This information can help you tailor your letter to show how your qualifications and interests directly relate to the needs of the company or medical facility. Make sure the description of your qualifications and interests reflects the words the company used in its advertisement. Always be truthful about the information in the cover letter; employers often verify all facts presented in your résumé and cover letter. Check each cover letter for errors in spelling, grammar, and punctuation. The format for a cover letter is shown in Figure 58-8.

Sending a Résumé
When mailing a résumé, make sure you have the correct name, address, and zip code of the facility. This information should be typed on a matching envelope. Many software programs have an envelope template feature that allows you to print an envelope using the address in your cover letter. Do not handwrite envelopes; professionally appearing mail is often opened first. Make sure that you attach sufficient postage.

If you fax a résumé, verify the fax number and person or department you are faxing to. Make sure your name is on all the faxed pages. If your fax machine provides a completion printout, save it to verify that the fax was delivered.

Some classified ads request that you send your résumé via e-mail. In order to send your résumé in electronic form, you must first have an account with an Internet service provider (ISP). You will be asked by the ISP to select a login or screen name. Do not use a casual name for your login; prospective

employers will see your login name in their inbox. Instead, choose a name that is conservative and professional. Verify that your e-mail was sent by checking your sent items.

Post your résumé and cover letter on the Internet by using a career job search site. Most job sites have local employers posting positions daily. A job search site will provide clear directions on how to post your résumé and cover letter. Some school career services departments host online job fairs and will assist you in posting your résumé.

Obtaining a Reference
Prior to the end of your applied training, meet with your preceptor and ask for a **reference,** a recommendation for employment from the facility and the preceptor. A reference can be in the form of a letter from the facility, preceptor, or physician or it can be a request to include these people on your reference list. It is professional to always ask before you list someone as a reference. References are important to career building because employers often like to inquire about a person prior to offering him or her employment. Your first references in medical assisting are your instructors and then the applied training facility.

You will want three to five references, including employment, academic, and character references. Ask instructors for a general letter before you finish your program. Fellow members of professional associations or your classmates can provide character references and your applied training facility can provide an employment reference. Make sure that you ask your references for permission to use their names and phone numbers. Do not print your references on the bottom of your résumé. List them on a separate sheet of paper so that you can provide them upon request, and update the list as needed.

Preparing a Portfolio
Prior to the interviewing phase, you should organize all your employment documentation into a portfolio. A **portfolio** is a collection of documents and may include your résumé; cover letter; reference list or reference letters; awards for volunteer service in a health-related field; and student recognition certificates for student-of-the-year or month, perfect attendance, or academic honors. Include a copy of your transcript, diploma or degree, and medical assisting credentials such as your CMA (AAMA) or RMA (AMT). You also can include any other certifications you hold, such as a CPR card or phlebotomy certification. Some employers request proof of immunizations, so include that in your portfolio. Give your portfolio a professional presentation by printing your documents on a high-quality printer and organizing them in a nice binder. A professional portfolio can help you obtain employment. If needed, look for a service that specializes in creating professional portfolios.

▶ Interviewing LO 58.4

Preparation for your interview begins long before the interview itself. After you send your cover letters and résumés, you must make sure that prospective employers can reach you by telephone. You must practice how you are going to handle

EMPLOYMENT WORKSHEET

Job Title _____

Dates _____

Employer _____

City, State _____

Major Duties _____

_____

_____

_____

_____

Special Projects _____

_____

_____

Accomplishments _____

_____

_____

_____

_____

FIGURE 58-7   An employment worksheet can be a useful tool in drafting a résumé.

your interview, and you must plan what to wear and how to present yourself in the most professional way.

Before starting your job search, invest in an answering machine or set up your voicemail to receive calls when you are not available. Be sure the outgoing message is clear, concise, and professional. Avoid cute messages and background music. An appropriate message would be "I'm unable to take your call at the moment, but your call is important to me. Please leave your name and number, the time you called, and a brief message after the tone and I will call you back as soon as I can. Thank you." Also, make sure all household members who answer the phone (especially children) know proper phone etiquette and how to take a written message. When a prospective employer calls with an interview invitation, write down the interviewer's name and the company or practice name, day, time, and location of the interview.

Interview Planning and Strategies

Just as the résumé is important for opening the door to opportunity, the job interview is critical in allowing you to present yourself professionally and to clearly articulate why you are the best person for the job. As you learned in the *Interpersonal Communication* chapter, being successful in a medical assisting career is centered on communication—both verbal and nonverbal. These communication skills will be assets during your job interviews. The following list provides some strategies that will help you improve your interviewing skills:

- Practice interviewing. Rehearse possible questions and be prepared to answer them directly. Have a friend or family member interview you as you sit in front of a mirror and observe your body language. Your college career center may help you prepare by offering mock interviews.

Your Street Address
City, State, Zip Code

Date

Name of person to whom you are writing
Title
Company or Organization
Street Address
City, State, Zip Code

Dear Dr., Mr., Mrs., Miss, or Ms. _____,

1st Paragraph: Tell why you are writing. Name the position or general area of work that interests you. Mention how you learned about the job opening. State why you are interested in the job.

2nd Paragraph: Refer to the enclosed résumé and give some background information. Indicate why you should be considered as a candidate, focusing on how your skills can fulfill the needs of the company. Relate your experiences to the company's needs and mention results/achievements. Do not restate what is said on your résumé—pull together all the information and tell how your background fits the position.

3rd Paragraph: Close by making a specific request for an interview. Say that you will follow up with a phone call to arrange a mutually convenient interview time. Offer to provide any additional information that may be needed. Thank the employer for his/her time and consideration.

Sincerely,

(your handwritten signature)

Type your name

Enclosure

FIGURE 58-8   The object of a cover letter is to convince the recipient to read your résumé.

- Anticipate question types. Expect open-ended questions such as the following: "What are your strengths?" "What are your weaknesses?" "Tell me about your best work experience." "Can you give me an example how you have worked with others to solve a problem?" Decide in advance what information and skills are pertinent to the position and reveal your strengths. For example, you could say, "While I was at school, I learned to get along with a diverse group of people."
- Learn about the company. Be prepared; research the company or medical facility. What is the type of specialty? How many physicians are there?

- Dress appropriately. Because much communication is nonverbal, dressing appropriately for the interview is important. In most situations, you will be safe if you wear clean, pressed, conservative business clothes in neutral colors. Do not wear current fashions or fad clothing to an interview. Pay special attention to grooming. Keep makeup light, and wear little jewelry. Make sure that your hair and nails are clean and styled conservatively. Do not carry a large purse, backpack, books, coat, or hat. Leave extra clothing in an outside office and simply carry a pen, your portfolio with extra copies of your résumé, and a small pad for taking notes. Turn cell phones and pagers off during the interview or leave them in your vehicle.

- Be punctual. A good first impression is important and can be lasting. If you arrive late for the interview, a prospective employer may conclude that you will be late in arriving to work. Make certain you know the location and the time of the interview. Allow time for traffic, parking, and other preliminaries.

- Be professional. Being too familiar in your manner can be a barrier to a professional interview. Never call anyone by his or her first name unless you are asked to.

- Know the interviewer's title and the pronunciation of his or her name. Do not sit down until the interviewer does.

- Exhibit appropriate interview behavior. Always greet the interviewer with a smile. The interview is an opportunity to sell yourself to the employer. Offer your hand for a firm, confident handshake and be alert to the interviewer's body language. The flow of conversation during an interview should be natural. Maintain eye contact, pay attention to the interviewer, and show interest. Ask intelligent questions that you prepared before the interview. Remember, the interview is an opportunity for both the prospective employer and the prospective employee to gather information and make a good impression. In addition to reviewing the experience listed on your résumé, the interviewer will evaluate your personality and behavior. At the same time, you will be observing the office and learning more about the position. Try to be aware of the office's atmosphere, its equipment and supplies, and the attitudes of the staff. Does it seem like a pleasant, professional place to work? Request a tour of the facility and ask yourself if you would be happy in that work environment.

- Be poised and relaxed. Avoid nervous habits like tapping your pencil, playing with your hair, or covering your mouth with your hand. Watch language such as "you know," "ah," and "stuff like that." Use proper grammar and pronunciation as you talk with the interviewer—do not use slang. Do not smoke beforehand (you will smell like smoke), chew gum, fidget, or bite your nails.

- Maintain comfortable eye contact. Look the interviewer in the eye and speak with confidence. Your eyes reveal much about you; use them to show interest, confidence, poise, and sincerity. Use other nonverbal techniques like a firm handshake to reinforce your confidence.

- Relate your experience to the job. Use every question as an opportunity to show how your skills relate to the job. Use examples taken from school, previous jobs, your applied training, volunteer work, leadership in student organizations, and personal experience to indicate that you have the personal qualities, aptitude, and skills needed for this job.

- Be honest. While it is important to be confident and stress your strengths, it is equally important to your sense of integrity to be honest. Dishonesty always catches up to you sooner or later. Someone will verify your background, so do not exaggerate your accomplishments, grade point average, or experience.

- Focus on how you can benefit the company. Do not ask about benefits, salary, or vacations until you are offered the job. During a first interview, try to show how you can contribute to the organization. Do not appear to be too eager to move up through the company or suggest that you are more interested in gaining experience than in contributing to the company.

- Close the interview on a positive note. Thank the interviewer for his or her time, shake hands, and say that you are looking forward to hearing from him or her. On the way out of the office, thank the staff members involved in the interview. Ask for a business card from anyone to whom you think you might want to send a thank-you note. After leaving the interview, write down any additional information you want to remember. Every interview provides you with information about the medical assisting profession. Even if an interview does not result in a job, you will have met new people, developed a larger network of professional contacts, and gained valuable interviewing experience.

- Follow up with a letter within 2 days of the interview. After an interview, it is professional to send a thank-you letter to the person or persons from the company who conducted your interview. Your letter may be brief, but it should express your appreciation for the opportunity to have met with the interviewer, reaffirm your interest in the organization, and state your desire to remain a part of the selection process. By sending a thank-you letter, you display common business courtesy, which can make a difference in the employer's hiring decision. Even if you are not interested in continuing the interview and selection process, you should thank the employer for holding the interview.

- Complete an application. Some employers ask you to complete an employment application at an interview even when you provide a résumé. You can use your résumé to help you complete the application. Fill out the application neatly. Spell all words correctly and read and follow the instructions on the form carefully. Your application represents you; it must make a good first impression. Fill in all sections of the application—do not write "see résumé." Because an application is signed, it is a legal document and, as such, referring to your résumé, even though the information is there, is not allowed.

- Comply with other aspects of the application process. As part of the application process, employers are required by federal law to request documents that prove your identity and eligibility to work in the United States. To maintain the safety and confidentiality of the medical office, hospital, or laboratory, employers may also check your police record, credit rating, and history of chemical or alcohol abuse. A drug screen may be requested. You may be asked to provide the needed documents or to give the employer authorization to obtain them.

- Do not excessively contact the interviewer by telephone or e-mail after the interview. Prior to leaving the interview, it is acceptable to ask the interviewer when a decision will be made and if the interviewer will call to let you know whether an offer of employment will be made. It is acceptable to ask permission to contact the interviewer to follow up on the position.

Interview Questions

In order to prepare for your interview, you can anticipate that you may be asked any of the following questions:

- I see from your résumé that you graduated from ABC School. What did that school have to offer you that others did not?
- What is your 5-year goal?
- Tell me about yourself.
- What do you consider to be your greatest strengths and weaknesses?
- How would your instructors describe you?
- What qualifications do you have that make you a good candidate for this position?
- How could you make a contribution to this facility?
- How well do you work with others?
- What is your concept of a team environment?
- How well do you work under pressure?
- Will you be able to work overtime?
- Do you have the flexibility to work various shifts?
- What has been your major accomplishment to date?
- Why did you choose medical assisting as your career?
- Do you have any questions that you would like to ask?

It is also helpful to be prepared with any questions that you may have for the interviewer about the position or the facility. Remember, however, that questions about salary and benefits are not appropriate in a first interview.

An interviewer may ask you questions that you are not obligated to answer. These questions refer to age, race, sexual orientation, marital status, or number of children. Even if the questions sound harmless or the interviewer seems nonjudgmental, these questions have nothing to do with your skills or abilities. If the interviewer asks even one of these questions, you should reconsider whether you want to work for the organization.

If you are asked an inappropriate question during an interview, be polite and remain professional in declining to answer. You may simply state that you do not believe the requested information is necessary for the employer to evaluate your qualifications for the job. Try to move the discussion on to a more relevant topic.

Reasons for Not Being Hired

Employers in business were asked to list reasons for not hiring a job candidate. Some of the biggest complaints included

1. Poor appearance, not being dressed properly, and being poorly groomed.
2. Acting like a know-it-all.
3. Not communicating clearly, as well as poor voice, diction, and grammar.
4. Lack of planning for the interview, with no purpose or goals communicated.
5. Lack of confidence or poise.
6. No interest in or enthusiasm for the job.

7. Objectionable content on personal social networking pages.
8. Being interested only in the best salary offer.
9. Inappropriate voicemail greeting.
10. Unwillingness to begin in an entry-level position.
11. Making excuses about an unfavorable record.
12. No tact.
13. No maturity.
14. No curiosity about the job.
15. Being critical of past employers.

Salary Negotiations

Medical assisting salaries are varied and differ by geographic area. When you are a new graduate, you will begin your career as an entry-level medical assistant. As you gain experience, your compensation will reflect that. Salary ranges are determined by geographic location, medical specialty, years of experience, credentialing, and the job description.

The first step in determining your compensation needs is to know how much income is required to meet your living expenses. You will need to prepare a budget. Keep track of your overall expenditures and living expenses. Itemizing your basic living expenses can help you to prepare a budget.

Establishing a budget will give you an idea of the amount of income you may need. Once your budget is established, you have a negotiating benchmark. Employers will often ask you what you are looking for with regard to salary. If you answer directly, you may risk either quoting yourself out of a job or leaving money on the table. The best response to this question is to ask the employer the range of the position. Most positions have a low-to-high range. For example, the range for a specific position might be between $23,000 and $32,000 annually. Once you know the range, quote a little higher than what your budgetary amount is, which will give the employer room to negotiate down if necessary. Allow the employer to bring up salary first.

▶ On the Job

Once you have a job, you must learn how to be an effective employee. There are many ways that your initiative enables the medical team in the office, hospital, clinic, or laboratory to function effectively. You must identify the important skills in your daily duties, stay competitive and marketable through continuing education, and integrate constructive criticism from your employee evaluations into your daily work and annual goals.

Job Description

During the initial paperwork process when you begin as a new employee, you may be asked to read and sign a job description for the position for which you have been hired. The purpose of a job description is to provide the standard benchmarks of your position. It will list and describe the position's expectations and the duties to be performed. A job description includes detailed information, such as

- Essential duties and responsibilities.
- Qualifications.

- Education and experience.
- Certificates, licenses, and registrations.
- Physical demands.
- Description of the work environment.

Employee Evaluations

Employee evaluations are usually held annually. An initial employment review generally occurs after a 90-day probationary period. Evaluations describe an employee's performance and, in most situations, the employee and the employer meet to discuss this. The purpose of an annual evaluation should be to check the goals and values of both the employer and the employee to make sure they support each other.

An employee evaluation form typically outlines the most important qualities and abilities needed for the job. It evaluates the employee's strengths and weaknesses. This form also may help determine whether an employee is worthy of a merit raise, which is a raise based on performance (as opposed to a cost-of-living raise). The quantity and quality of work are assessed on this form, as are initiative, judgment, and cooperation. A completed evaluation is placed in an official record of employment.

Continuing Education

After completing a medical assisting program, you should continue your education, setting specific educational advancement goals on a yearly basis. For example, you may decide to obtain further education to learn more about the medical specialty in which you work. Once you obtain your certification as a medical assistant, you will be required to obtain a specific number of continuing education units (CEUs) yearly to maintain your certification credential.

As medical research expands its discoveries and as new technologies emerge, the necessity for self-education increases. You must read to stay abreast of updates in medicine. The need for more highly specialized training presents you with an opportunity for growth in your education and career. Medical publications are the best source for the latest medical information. Local and state medical assisting meetings also provide information about advances in the field. And, of course, the Internet is a valuable source for staying current about today's technological advances.

Self-education is an important skill for the medical assistant. It helps you to stay up-to-date in topics about medicine, healthcare, wellness, insurance products, and pharmaceuticals. Patients may ask questions about information they have read or about the effectiveness of certain new treatments and having this knowledge will enable you to better discuss this information and to refer patients' questions to their physician for more details.

PROCEDURE 58-1 Résumé Writing

Procedure Goal: To develop a résumé that defines your career objective and highlights your skills

OSHA Guidelines: This procedure does not involve exposure to blood, body fluids, or tissues.

Materials: Paper, pen, dictionary, thesaurus, and computer

Method:

1. Type your full name, address (temporary and permanent, if you have both), telephone number with area code, and e-mail address (if you have one).

2. List your general career objective. You also may choose to summarize your skills. If you want to phrase your objective to fit a specific position, you should include that information in a cover letter to accompany the résumé.

3. List the highest level of education or the most recently obtained degree first. Include the school name, degree earned, and date of graduation. Be sure to list any special projects, courses, or participation in overseas study programs.

4. Summarize your work experience. List your most recent or most relevant employment first. Describe your responsibilities and list job titles, company names, and dates of employment. Summer employment, volunteer work, and student applied training also may be included. Use short sentences with strong action words such

as *directed, designed, developed,* and *organized.* For example, condense a responsibility into "Handled insurance and billing" or "Drafted correspondence as requested."
   RATIONALE: *Action verbs give the impression that you are an energetic and results-oriented employee.*

5. List any memberships and affiliations with professional organizations alphabetically or by order of importance.

6. Do not list references on your résumé.
   RATIONALE: *It is easier to update your reference list if you maintain it in a separate file.*

7. Do not list the salary you wish to receive in a medical assisting position. Salary requirements should not be discussed until a job offer is received. If the ad you are answering requests that you include a required salary, it is best to state a range (no broader than $5,000 from lowest to highest point in the range for an annual salary).

8. Print your résumé on an 8½ × 11-inch sheet of high-quality white or off-white bond paper. Carefully check your résumé for spelling, punctuation, and grammatical errors. Have someone else double-check your résumé if possible.
   RATIONALE: *Your résumé is a printed reflection of you, so ensuring its accuracy and completeness is essential.*

SUMMARY OF LEARNING OUTCOMES

LEARNING OUTCOMES	KEY POINTS
58.1 Carry out professionalism in all applied training scenarios.	Students' weekly progress sheets should reveal new goals each week and progress on previous weeks' goals. Their assessment and the preceptor's assessments should be similar and show professionalism, willingness to learn, and continual progress throughout the applied training.
58.2 Summarize the steps necessary for obtaining professional certification.	When seeking national certification, students should determine if they are eligible to take the certification exam, gather necessary documents, apply for the exam, and study and prepare to take the exam.
58.3 Describe an appropriate strategy for finding a position.	Students should be able to list classified advertisements available in local papers, employment websites, networking, and employment agencies where employment assistance is available and should provide a workable, professional résumé that can be used to begin the employment search.
58.4 Explain key factors for a successful interview.	Students should be able to list key factors, such as portraying confidence, smiling, looking the interviewer in the eye, having questions ready for the interviewer about the position, and practicing answers to common interviewing questions. If possible, participation in a mock interview should be considered.
58.5 Describe ways of becoming a successful employee.	The keys to becoming a successful employee include using the job description to provide benchmarks for performance standards, using employee evaluations to improve performance, and continuing self-education throughout your career.

CASE STUDY CRITICAL THINKING

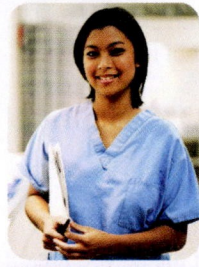

© Ablestock.com/
Getty Images

Recall Reagan from the beginning of the chapter. Now that you have completed the chapter, answer the following questions regarding her case.

1. What should be Reagan's first steps in seeking employment?

2. What style of résumé should she choose?

3. What advantages might Reagan have if she applies for a position at the practice where she is finishing her applied training?

4. You are Reagan's instructor; she tells you that she is only going to apply for the position at the office where she is completing her applied training. What should you tell her?

1. (LO 58.1) The document that states the expectations of the facility and student for the applied training site is a(n)
   a. Time sheet
   b. Affiliation agreement
   c. Progress report
   d. Applied training plan
   e. Job description

2. (LO 58.1) Feedback given in order to improve performance is
   a. Affiliation
   b. Benchmarking
   c. Training agreement
   d. Constructive criticism
   e. Negotiation

3. (LO 58.1) Which of the following personality types are generally the best for medical assisting students involved in applied training?
   a. Quiet/passive
   b. Aggressive/know-it-all
   c. Assertive/confident
   d. Shy/timid
   e. Tentative/unbending

4. (LO 58.3) Which résumé style generally works best for new medical assisting graduates seeking employment?
   a. Targeted résumé
   b. Chronological résumé
   c. Functional résumé
   d. Curriculum vitae
   e. Simple résumé

5. (LO 58.3) A reference is a recommendation for a position. Which of the following persons might you consider asking for a reference?
   a. Former supervisor
   b. Applied training supervisor/preceptor
   c. Medical assisting instructor
   d. Applied training coordinator
   e. All of these

6. (LO 58.1) If you are unable to attend your applied training due to an emergency, you should
   a. Call your instructor and ask that he or she call the applied training site
   b. Call the applied training site and the school 2 hours before you are to arrive
   c. E-mail the applied training site that you will not be in
   d. E-mail your instructor that you will be absent
   e. Call the applied training site when it opens

7. (LO 58.5) Employee evaluations are usually held
   a. Each month
   b. Yearly
   c. Every 90 days
   d. At the employee's request
   e. Only if there is an issue with an employee

8. (LO 58.2) Which of the following is a certification eligibility requirement of the AAMA?
   a. Graduation from a CAAHEP- or ABHES-accredited school
   b. US Armed Forces medical services training
   c. Working as a medical assistant for 5 years
   d. Teaching in a medical assisting program
   e. Attending a medical assisting program that has 720 hours of training

9. (LO 58.3) A chronological résumé is used most often when
   a. A person has gaps in his or her work history
   b. Someone has job experience
   c. A person is changing jobs
   d. A person is looking for a specific job
   e. A person has just graduated

10. (LO 58.3) A collection of documents you can take to a job interview is a(n)
    a. Affiliation
    b. Application
    c. Portfolio
    d. Reference
    e. Résumé

SOFT SKILLS SUCCESS

Recall Reagan Patrick from the case study at the beginning of the chapter. You are working with Reagan Patrick today in the administrative area of the office. Your duties include checking patients out after seeing the healthcare practitioner and calling to schedule any outside appointments they need. Reagan has been checking patients out with your assistance all day and is doing an excellent job. When Mrs. Lemmonds checks out, you see that she has a note on her encounter form that she needs to be scheduled for bone densitometry. You ask Reagan to perform this duty and notice that Reagan is slightly hesitant. How can you help Reagan maintain a professional demeanor even though she is unsure of her ability to schedule the appointment for Mrs. Lemmonds?

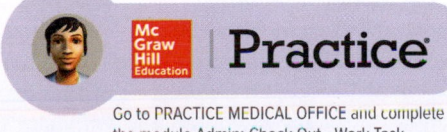

Go to PRACTICE MEDICAL OFFICE and complete the module Admin: Check Out—Work Task Proficiencies

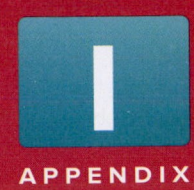
NOTE: When referencing this appendix, note that some word parts are used in more than one way. For example, "cyt" serves as a word root in "cytology" but as a suffix in "astrocyte." If you do not initially find the word part you are looking for, check the other sections of this appendix to see if it is listed as another type of word part.

Prefixes

a-, an- without, not
ab- from, away
acr-, acro- extremity, topmost
ad- to, toward
ambi-, amph-, amphi- both, on both sides, around
ante- before
antero- in front of
anti- against, opposing
aque- water
astro- star-like
auto- self
bi- twice, double
brachy- short
brady- slow
carboxy- containing carbon and oxygen or a carboxyl group
cata- down, lower, under
centi- hundred
cephal- head
chol-, chole-, cholo- gall
chromo- color
circum- around
co-, com-, con- together, with
contra- against
cryo- cold
crypt-, crypto- hidden
cyan-, cyano- blue
de- down, from
deca- ten
deci- tenth
demi- half
dextro- to the right
di- double, twice
dia- through, apart, between
dipla-, diplo- double, twin
dis- apart, away from
dys- difficult, painful, bad, abnormal
e-, ec-, ecto- away, from, without, outside
echo- sound, sound wave
electro- electric
em-, en- in, into, inside
endo- within, inside
ento- within, inner
epi- on, above
erythro- red
eu- good
ex-, exo- outside of, beyond, without
excori- scratch or abrasion, loss of skin

extra- outside of, beyond, in addition
fore- before, in front of
glauc- glauco- gray
gyn-, gyno-, gyne-, gyneco- woman, female
hemi- half
hetero- other, unlike
homeo-, homo- same, like
hyper- above, over, increased, excessive
hypo- below, under, decreased
idio- personal, self-produced
im-, in-, ir- not
in- in, into
inferi- below
infra- beneath
inter- between, among
intra-, intro- into, within, during
juxta- near, nearby
kata-, kath- down, lower, under
kineto- motion
leuco-, leuko- white
levo- to the left
macro- large, long
mal- bad
mega-, megalo- large, great
meio- contraction
melan-, melano- black
membran- pertaining to a membrane
mes-, meso- middle
metr-, metro- pertaining to the uterus
meta- beyond
micro- small
mid- middle
mio- smaller, less
mono- single, one
multi- many
neo- new
non-, not- no
nulli- none
ob- against
olig-, oligo- few, less than normal
ortho- straight
oxy- sharp, acid
pachy- thick
pan- all, every
par-, para- alongside of, with; woman who has given birth
per- through, excessive
peri- around
pes- foot

pluri- more, several
pneo- breathing
poly- many, much
post-, posteri- after, behind
pre-, pro- before, in front of
presby-, presbyo- old age
primi- first
pseudo- false
quadri- four
re- back, again
retro- backward, behind
semi- half
steno- contracted, narrow
stereo- firm, solid, three-dimensional
sub- under
super-, supra- above, upon, excess
sym-, syn- with, together
tachy- fast
tele- distant, far
tetra- four
tomo- incision, section
trans- across
tri- three
tropho- nutrition, growth
ultra- beyond, excess
uni- one
veni- vein
xanth-, xantho- yellow

Suffixes

-ad to, toward
-aesthesia, -esthesia sensation
-al characterized by, pertaining to
-algia pain
-ase enzyme
-asthenia weakness
-cele swelling, tumor
-centesis puncture, tapping
-ceps heads
-cidal killing
-cide causing death
-cise cut
-clast to break
-coele cavity
-crine to excrete
-cyst bladder, bag
-cyte cell, cellular
-duction to pull or move
-dynia pain
-ectomy cutting out, surgical removal

-edema   fluid buildup
-emesis   vomiting
-emia   blood
-esthesia   sensation
-extension   increasing the angle of a joint
-flexion   bending
-form   shape
-fuge   driving away
-gen, -genesis, -gon   born, produced
-gene, -genic, -genetic, -genesis, -genous   arising from, origin, formation
-glia   pertaining to glial cells
-globin, -globulin   protein
-gram   recorded information
-graph   instrument for recording
-graphy   the process of recording
-ia   condition
-iasis   condition of
-ic, -ical   pertaining to
-ician   specialist in a field
-id   having the characteristics of
-ism   condition, process, theory
-itis   inflammation of
-ium   membrane
-ive   with the properties of
-ize   to cause to be, to become, to treat by special method
-kinesis, -kinetic   motion
-lepsis, -lepsy   seizure, convulsion
-lith   stone
-logy   science of, study of
-lysis   setting free, disintegration, decomposition
-malacia   abnormal softening
-mania   insanity, abnormal desire
-megaly   enlargement
-meter   measure
-metrist   one who measures
-metry   process of measuring
-motor   movement
-odynia   pain
-oid   resembling
-ole   small, little
-oma   tumor
-opia   vision
-opsy   to view
-osis   disease, condition of
-or   relating to
-ostomy   to make a mouth, opening
-otomy   incision, surgical cutting
-ous   having
-pathy   disease, suffering
-pelvic   pelvis
-penia   too few, lack, decreased
-pexy   surgical fixation
-phagia, -phage   eating, consuming, swallowing
-phobia   fear, abnormal fear
-phylaxis   protection
-plasia   formation or development
-plastic   molded

-plasty   operation to reconstruct, surgical repair
-plegia   paralysis
-pnea   breathing
-poiesis   to make or produce
-ptysis   spitting
-receptor   cell that can send a signal to the brain
-rrhage, -rrhagia   abnormal or excessive discharge, hemorrhage, flow
-rrhaphy   suture of
-rrhea   flow, discharge
-sarcoma   malignant tumor
-sclerosis   hardening
-scope   instrument used to examine
-scopy   examining
-sepsis   poisoning, infection
-spasm   cramp or twitching
-stalsis   contraction
-stasis   stoppage
-stomy   opening
-thalamus   pertaining to the thalamus
-therapy   treatment
-thermy   heat
-thorax   chest
-tome   cutting instrument
-tomy   incision, section
-tory   pertaining to
-toxic   poison
-tripsy   surgical crushing
-trophy   turning, tendency
-tropic   in response to a stimulus
-tropy   turning, tendency
-ula, -ule   little
-uretic   pertaining to urine
-uria   urine
-verse, -version   turned or directed

Word Roots

abdomino-   abdomen
adeno-   gland, glandular
adipo-   fat
adreno-   adrenal glands
aero-   air
andr-, andro-   man, male
ambly-   dull, dim
angio-   blood vessel
ano-   anus
anthrac-, anthraco-   coal, carbon
arterio-   artery
arthro-   joint
athero-   soft, fatty deposit
atrio-   pertaining to the atria of the heart
audi-   hearing
baro-   weight, pressure
bili-   bile
bio-   life
blasto-, blast-   developing stage, bud, immature
bracheo-   arm
broncho-   bronchial (windpipe)
burs-   bursa
carcino-   cancer

cardio-   heart
caud-   tail
cellul-   cells
cephalo-   head
cerebr-, cerebro-   brain
cervico-   neck
chondro-   cartilage
chromo-   color
colo-   colon
colp-, colpo-   vagina
conjunctiv-   conjunctiva
coro-   body
cortico-   cortex
cost-, costo-   rib
cox-   hip
crani-, cranio-   skull
cusp-   projection
cysto-   bladder, bag
cyto-   cell, cellular
dacry-, dacryo-   tears, lacrimal apparatus
dactyl-, dactylo-   finger, toe
dent-, denti-, dento-   teeth
derma-, dermat-, dermato-   skin
dist-   farthest from the point of attachment
diverticul-   diverticula
dorsi-, dorso-   back
dur-, dura-   pertaining to the dura mater of the brain
encephalo-   brain
entero-   intestine
episi-, episio   pertaining to the pubic region
esophag-   esophagus
esthesio-   sensation
femor-   femur
fibro-   connective tissue
follicul-   follicle
front-   forehead
galact-, galacto-   milk
gastr-, gastro-   stomach
gingiv-   gums
glomerulo-   glomerulus
glosso-   tongue
gluco-, glyco-   sugar, sweet
granulo-   granules
gravid-   pregnant female
haemo-, hemato-, hem-, hemo-   blood
hepa-, hepar-, hepato-   liver
herni-   rupture
hidro-   sweat (perspiration)
histo-   tissue
hydra-, hydro-   water
hyster-, hystero-   uterus
ictero-   jaundice
ileo-   ileum
immuno-   pertaining to the immune system
interstit-   interstices
karyo-   nucleus, nut
kera-, kerato-   horn, hardness, cornea
keratino-   keratin
labyrinth-   pertaining to the labyrinth of the ears

lacrim-, lacrimo-   tears
lact-, lactifer-   milk
laparo-   abdomen
laryngo-   pertaining to the larynx
later-, latero-   side
linguo-   tongue
lipo-   fat
lith-   stone
lobo-   lobe
lun-, luna-   moon
lymph-, lympho-   lymphatic, spring water
mast-, masto-   breast
med-, medi-   middle
mening-   meninges (covers the brain)
metacarpo-   pertaining to the metacarpal bones
metatarso-   pertaining to the metatarsal bones
metro-, metra-   uterus
my-, myo-   muscle
myel-, myelo-   marrow
narco-   sleep
nas-, naso-   nose
nat-, nato-   born
natri-   sodium
necro-   dead
nephr-, nephro-   kidney
neu-, neuro-   nerve
niter-, nitro-   nitrogen
nucleo-   nucleus
oculo-   eye
odont-   tooth
omphalo-   navel, umbilicus
onco-   tumor
onych-, onycho-   pertaining to the nail of a finger or toe
oo-   ovum, egg
oophor-   ovary
ophthalmo-   eye
opt-, opto-   vision
or-, oro-   pertaining to the mouth

orchid-   testicle
os-   mouth, opening
oste-, osteo-   bone
oto-   ear
ov-, ovi-, ovo-   pertaining to an ovum or egg
paedo-, pedo-   child
palpebro-   eyelid
pancrea-   pancreas
path-, patho-   disease, suffering
pedicul-   lice
pepso-   digestion
peptid-   pertaining to a peptide
phag-, phago-   eating, consuming, swallowing
phalang-   pertaining to the phalanges
pharyng-, pharyngo-   throat, pharynx
phlebo-   vein
photo-   pertaining to light
pleuro-   side, rib
pneumo-   air, lungs
pod-   foot
procto-   rectum
proxim-   close to the point of attachment
psych-   the mind
pulmon-, pulmono-   lung
pyelo-   pelvis (renal)
pylor-   pylorus (part of the stomach)
pyo-, pus-   pus
pyro-   fever, heat
refract-   refraction, refractive
reni-, reno-   kidney
retino-   retina
rhabdo-   rod-shaped
rhino-   nose
sacchar-   sugar
sacro-   sacrum
sagitt-   dividing into left and right
salpingo-   tube, fallopian tube
sarco-   flesh
sclero-   hard, sclera

scolio-   lateral curvature
sebace-   oil
sensori-   the senses
septi-, septic-, septico-   poison, infection
sigmo-   S-shaped
som-, soma-   body
sperma-, spermato-   semen, spermatozoa
spleno-   spleen
steroid-   steroid (lipid-soluble substance)
stomato-   mouth
synapt-   pertaining to a synapse
synov-   synovium
sudorifer-   sweat
superfic-   near the surface
superi-   above
tempor-   pertaining to the temple
teno-, tenoto-, tendon-   tendon
thermo-   heat
thio-   sulfa
thoraco-   chest
thrombo-   blood clot
thymo-   thymus
thyro-   thyroid gland
tricho-   hair
tubulo-   tube, tubule
tympan-   eardrum
ureth-   urethra
urino-, uro-   urine, urinary organs
utero-   uterus, uterine
uvulo-   uvula
vagin-   vagina
vaso-, vasculo-   vessel
ventr-   front
ventricul-, ventriculo-   pertaining to the ventricles of the heart
ventri-, ventro-   abdomen
vesico-   blister
vulvo-   pertaining to the vulva

Abbreviations

a   before
āā, ĀĀ   of each
ABGs   arterial blood gases
a.c.   before meals
ADD   attention deficit disorder
ADL   activities of daily living
ad lib   as desired
ADT   admission, discharge, transfer
AIDS   acquired immunodeficiency syndrome
AKA   above knee amputation
a.m.a.   against medical advice
AMA   American Medical Association
amp.   ampule
amt   amount
aq., AQ   water; aqueous
ASHD   atherosclerotic heart disease
ausc.   auscultation
ax   axis
Bib, bib   drink
b.i.d., bid, BID   twice a day
BKA   below knee amputation
BM   bowel movement
BP, B/P   blood pressure
BPC   blood pressure check
BPH   benign prostatic hypertrophy
bpm   beats per minute
BSA   body surface area
c̄   with
Ca, CA   calcium; cancer
CABG   coronary artery bypass graft
cap, caps   capsules
CBC   complete blood (cell) count
C.C., CC   chief complaint
CDC   Centers for Disease Control and Prevention
CHF   congestive heart failure
chr   chronic
cm   centimeter
CNS   central nervous system
Comp, comp   compound
COPD   chronic obstructive pulmonary disease
CP   chest pain
CPE   complete physical examination
CPR   cardiopulmonary resuscitation
CSF   cerebrospinal fluid
CT   computed tomography
CV   cardiovascular
CVA   cerebrovascular accident
CXR   chest X-ray
d   day
D&C   dilation and curettage

DEA   Drug Enforcement Administration
Dil, dil   dilute
DM   diabetes mellitus
DNR   do not resuscitate
DOB   date of birth
Dr.   doctor
DTaP   diphtheria-tetanus-acellular pertussis vaccine
DTs   delirium tremens
DVT   deep venous thrombosis
D/W   dextrose in water
Dx, dx   diagnosis
ECG, EKG   electrocardiogram
ED   emergency department
EEG   electroencephalogram
EENT   eyes, ears, nose, and throat
EP   established patient
ER   emergency room
ESR   erythrocyte sedimentation rate
FBS   fasting blood sugar
FDA   Food and Drug Administration
FH   family history
Fl, fl , fld   fluid
fl oz   fluid ounce
F/u, F/U, f/u   follow-up
FUO   fever of unknown origin
Fx   fracture
g   gram
GBS   gallbladder series
GI   gastrointestinal
Gm, gm   gram
gr   grain
gt, gtt   drop, drops
GTT   glucose tolerance test
GU   genitourinary
GYN   gynecology
HA   headache
HB, Hgb   hemoglobin
hct   hematocrit
HEENT   head, eyes, ears, nose, throat
HIV   human immunodeficiency virus
HO   history of
HPI   history of present illness
HPV   human papillomavirus
Hx   history
ICU   intensive care unit
I&D   incision and drainage
I&O   intake and output
IDDM   insulin-dependent diabetes
IIHI   individually identifiable health information
IM   intramuscular
inf.   infusion; inferior
inj   injection

IT   inhalation therapy
IUD   intrauterine device
IV   intravenous
KUB   kidneys, ureters, bladder
L   liter
L1, L2, etc.   lumbar vertebrae
lab   laboratory
lb   pound
liq   liquid
LLE   left lower extremity (left leg)
LLL   left lower lobe
LLQ   left lower quadrant
LMP   last menstrual period
LUE   left upper extremity (left arm)
LUQ   left upper quadrant
m   meter
M   mix (Latin *misce*)
mcg   microgram
mg   milligram
MI   myocardial infarction
mL   milliliter
mm   millimeter
MM   mucous membrane
mmHg   millimeters of mercury
MRI   magnetic resonance imaging
MS   multiple sclerosis
NB   newborn
NED   no evidence of disease
NIDDM   noninsulin-dependent diabetes mellitus
NKA   no known allergies
no, #   number
noc, noct   night
npo, NPO   nothing by mouth
NPT   new patient
NS   normal saline
NSAID   nonsteroidal anti-inflammatory drug
NTP   normal temperature and pressure
N&V, N/V   nausea and vomiting
NYD   not yet diagnosed
OB   obstetrics
OC   oral contraceptive
oint   ointment
OOB   out of bed
OPD   outpatient department
OPS   outpatient services
OR   operating room
OT   occupational therapy
OTC   over-the-counter
oz   ounce
p̄   after
P&P   Pap smear (Papanicolaou smear) and pelvic exam

PA posteroanterior
Pap Pap smear
Path pathology
p.c., pc after meals
PE physical examination
per by, with
PH past history
PHI protected health information
PID pelvic inflammatory disease
PMFSH past medical, family, social history
PMS premenstrual syndrome
po by mouth
p/o postoperative
POMR problem-oriented medical record
p.r.n., prn, PRN whenever necessary
pt pint
Pt patient
PT physical therapy
PTA prior to admission
pulv powder
PVC premature ventricular contraction
q. every
q2, q2h every 2 hours
q.a.m., qam every morning
q.h., qh every hour
qns, QNS quantity not sufficient
qs, QS quantity sufficient
qt quart
RA rheumatoid arthritis; right atrium
RBC red blood cells; red blood (cell) count
RDA recommended dietary allowance; recommended daily allowance
REM rapid eye movement
RF rheumatoid factor
RLE right lower extremity (right leg)
RLL right lower lobe
RLQ right lower quadrant
R/O rule out
ROM range of motion
ROS/SR review of systems/systems review
RUE right upper extremity (right arm)
RUQ right upper quadrant
RV right ventricle
Rx prescription; take
s̄ without
SAD seasonal affective disorder
SIDS sudden infant death syndrome
sig sigmoidoscopy
Sig directions
SL sublingual
SOAP subjective, objective, assessment, plan
SOB shortness of breath

sol solution
SOMR source-oriented medical record
S/R suture removal
Staph staphylococcus
stat, STAT immediately
STI sexually transmitted infection
Strep streptococcus
subcu, subcut subcutaneous
subling sublingual
surg surgery
S/W saline in water
SX symptoms
T1, T2, etc. thoracic vertebrae
T&A tonsillectomy and adenoidectomy
tab tablet
TB tuberculosis
tbs, tbsp tablespoon
TIA transient ischemic attack
t.i.d., tid, TID three times a day
tinc, tinct, tr tincture
TMJ temporomandibular joint
top topically
TPR temperature, pulse, and respiration
TSH thyroid-stimulating hormone
tsp teaspoon
Tx treatment
U unit
UA urinalysis
UCHD usual childhood diseases
UGI upper gastrointestinal
ung, ungt ointment
URI upper respiratory infection
US ultrasound
UTI urinary tract infection
VA visual acuity
VD venereal disease
VF visual field
VS vital signs
WBC white blood cells; white blood (cell) count
WNL within normal limits
wt weight
y/o year old

Symbols

Weights and Measures

pounds
° degrees
′ foot; minute
″ inch; second
mEq milliequivalent
mL milliliter
dL deciliter
mg% milligrams percent; milligrams per 100 mL

Mathematical Functions and Terms

number
+ plus; positive; acid reaction
− minus; negative; alkaline reaction
± plus or minus; either positive or negative; indefinite
× multiply; magnification; crossed with, hybrid
÷ , / divided by
= equal to
≈ approximately equal to
> greater than; from which is derived
< less than; derived from
≮ not less than
≯ not greater than
≤ equal to or less than
≥ equal to or greater than
≠ not equal to
√ square root
³√ cube root
∞ infinity
: ratio; "is to"
∴ therefore
% percent
π pi (3.14159)—the ratio of circumference of a circle to its diameter

Chemical Notations

Δ change; heat
⇌ reversible reaction
↑ increase
↓ decrease

Warnings

Ⓒ Schedule I controlled substance
Ⓒ Schedule II controlled substance
Ⓒ Schedule III controlled substance
Ⓒ Schedule IV controlled substance
Ⓒ Schedule V controlled substance
☠ poison
☢ radiation
☣ biohazard

Others

℞ prescription; take
□, ♂ male
○, ♀ female
† one
†† two
††† three

Infectious Diseases Caused by Bacteria

NAME	DESCRIPTION
Boil	Localized skin infection usually caused by staphylococcus bactera.
Botulism	Type of food poisoning caused by a toxin produced by the bacterium *Clostridium botulinum*.
Chlamydia	Sexually transmitted infection caused by the bacterium *Chlamydia trachomatis*.
Conjunctivitis	Commonly called pink eye, this condition is highly contagious when the cause is bacterial. Can also be caused by viruses and allergies.
Gonorrhea	Highly contagious condition transmitted by sexual intercourse and caused by gonococcus bacteria.
Haemophilus influenzae serotype b (Hib) disease	Transferred by respiratory droplets. Can cause difficulty breathing through either epiglottitis and a sore throat or pneumonia with a fever.
Impetigo	A *Staphylococcus* or *Streptococcus* infection commonly found in children that causes lesions on the face or lower leg. Impetigo is highly contagious when contact is made with the lesions. This condition is treated with antibiotics.
Legionnaire's disease	Acute type of bacterial pneumonia caused by *Legionnaire* bacillus, a gram-negative organism. It grows in standing water such as that found in commercial air conditioners, humidifiers, water heaters, and evaporative condensers.
Lyme disease	Arthropod-borne disease caused by the spirochete *Borrelia burgdorferi*. The disease is transmitted by deer ticks. The signs and symptoms include skin lesions, central nervous system and cardiac involvement, and arthritis.
Meningitis	Inflammation of the meninges. Causes include bacterial, viral, and fungal infections.
Methicillin-resistant *Staphylococcus aureus*	Infection that causes red, swollen, painful pustules and is not responsive to methicillin and similar antibiotics.
Peptic ulcer	Gastrointestinal infection that causes gnawing or burning stomach pain; caused by the bacterium *Helicobacter pylori*.
Pertussis	Also called whooping cough. Caused by bacillus bacteria.
Pneumonia	Respiratory condition in which lung tissue is inflamed, usually causing difficulty breathing and a cough. Can also be caused by fungus or chemicals.
Rheumatic fever	Febrile (characterized by fever) disease, usually occurring after a streptococcal infection.
Strep throat	Inflammation and infection of the throat caused by streptococcus bacteria.
Syphilis	Infectious venereal disease, usually transmitted by sexual contact. Caused by a spirochete bacterium.
Tetanus	Infectious disease produced by the toxins from the tetanus bacillus. The first sign is stiffness of the jaw, hence the common name "lockjaw."
Tuberculosis (TB)	Disease that primarily affects the lungs but can spread to other parts of the body. Caused by various strains of the bacterium *Mycobacterium tuberculosis*.

Infectious Diseases Caused by Fungi

NAME	DESCRIPTION
Tinea (ringworm)	Fungal skin infection that gets its name because it appears serpentine like a worm. *Tinea corporis* means the location is on the trunk or body, *tinea capitis* affects the scalp, and *tinea pedis* refers to the feet and is commonly known as athlete's foot.
Candidiasis	Commonly called a "yeast infection," this disease can be caused by one of several bacteria in the Candida family but is most commonly caused by *Candida albicans*. It may be oropharyngeal (thrush), vaginal, or invasive.
Pneumocystis pneumonia (PCP)	Infection that causes fever, dry cough, shortness of breath, and fatigue. Caused by *Pneumocystis jirovecii.*

Infectious Diseases Caused by Parasites and Protozoans

NAME	DESCRIPTION
Amebic dysentery	Condition characterized by loose stools; causes inflammation of the intestines.
Giardiasis	Disease transmitted by the oral-fecal route and through untreated water. Causes diarrhea.
Lice	Can affect the head or the pubic area. Transmitted by contact with personal items used by someone who is infected. Lice and their eggs cause itching in the affected area.
Malaria	Disease transmitted to humans from the bite of an infected anopheles mosquito. Protozoan parasites invade the red blood cells and create symptoms such as high fever and chills.
Pinworm	Transmitted by oral-fecal route. This disease is common in children and causes anal itching and nighttime restlessness from eggs that are deposited around the anus.
Scabies	A highly contagious skin condition that results from a mite that burrows beneath the skin, leaving its feces behind. The feces leave red lines of inflammation on the skin.
Trichomoniasis	Condition that affects the reproductive organs and can be transmitted through sexual intercourse.

Infectious Diseases Caused by Viruses

NAME	DESCRIPTION
Acquired immune deficiency syndrome (AIDS)	Syndrome caused by HIV (human immunodeficiency virus), resulting in decreased resistance to infections. Transmitted by blood and body fluids.
Chickenpox	Highly contagious disease caused by the varicella-zoster virus. Also called varicella, it is characterized by the presence of skin lesions. Shingles is also caused by varicella and is seen in patients who have previously had chickenpox.
Hepatitis	Hepatitis types A, B, C, D, and E are all caused by a virus. This disease affects the liver and can cause mild to moderate symptoms or chronic illness, and possibly death. Healthcare workers are encouraged to be vaccinated for hepatitis B because they are at risk for contact with client blood and body fluids.
Herpes simplex virus types 1 and 2 (HSV-1, HSV-2)	Typically, HSV-1 causes cold sores, is very contagious, and is spread through contact with infected saliva. HSV-2, known as genital herpes, is sexually transmitted. However, it should be noted that there can be crossing over, with HSV-1 infecting the genitals and HSV-2 infecting the mouth.
Human immunodeficiency virus (HIV)	Virus that destroys the immune system and can result in AIDS (acquired immune deficiency syndrome).
Human papillomavirus (HPV)	The most common sexually transmitted infection. Some strains of HPV cause harmless verrucae (warts); other strains are the greatest single risk factor for cervical cancer and may cause other, less common cancers such as cancer of the vagina, penis, and oropharynx.
Influenza	Commonly called "the flu"; an infection of both the upper and lower respiratory tracts.
Mononucleosis	Highly contagious viral infection spread through the saliva of the infected person. Caused by either the Epstein-Barr virus or the cytomegalovirus (CMV).

Infectious Diseases Caused by Viruses *(concluded)*

NAME	DESCRIPTION
Norovirus	Most common cause of foodborne illness in the United States. Causes diarrhea, nausea, stomach pain, vomiting, fever, headache, and body aches.
Respiratory syncytial virus (RSV)	Infection that causes cough, sneezing, runny nose, fever, loss of appetite, wheezing, and dyspnea.
Severe acute respiratory syndrome (SARS)	Highly contagious disease that causes severe flu-like symptoms.
Upper respiratory (tract) infection (URI)	The common cold, including pharyngitis (sore throat). Caused by the rhinovirus.

Genetic Diseases

DISEASE	DESCRIPTION
Albinism	Genetic condition in which a person is born with little or no pigmentation in the skin, eyes, or hair.
Cystic fibrosis	Life-threatening disease that affects the lungs and pancreas. It is one of the most common inherited life-threatening disorders among Caucasians in the United States.
Down syndrome	Abnormal cell division involving chromosome 21 that results in physical abnormalities and some form of mental disability. It is the single most common type of birth defect.
Fragile X syndrome	Most common inherited cause of learning disability, caused by a defect on one of the genes on the X chromosome. It affects boys more severely than girls.
Hemophilia	Inheritable bleeding disorder in which an essential clotting factor is low or missing, primarily affecting males.
Klinefelter's syndrome	Disorder in which males have an extra X chromosome, resulting in tall stature, pear-shaped fat distribution, small testes, sparse body hair, infertility, and slightly lower intelligence.
Muscular dystrophy	Group of genetic disorders that affect the muscular and nervous systems, most often affecting males.
Phenylketonuria (PKU)	Genetic disorder in which the body is unable to properly eliminate phenylalanine, which is an essential amino acid. Organ damage, mental disability, and even death are possible.
Turner's syndrome	Disorder that results when females have a single X chromosome. Symptoms include a webbed neck, broad chest, short stature, and infertility. Intelligence is normal.

Common Diseases and Disorders in the United States*

DISEASE	EXAMPLES	SCREENING AND PREVENTION
Heart disease	Coronary artery disease, atherosclerosis, congestive heart failure	Monitor blood pressure and cholesterol and triglyceride levels, and have routine electrocardiograms (ECG).
Cancer	Skin, lung, breast, prostate, blood, colorectal, gynecologic, HPV-related	Have routine breast or prostate exam, Pap smear, and colonoscopy. Monitor size and shape of skin lesions. Maintain healthy eating habits and a good body weight, exercise, do not use tobacco products, and limit alcohol consumption.
Chronic lower respiratory diseases	Asthma, COPD, bronchitis	Do not use tobacco products, avoid irritants and allergens, and monitor air quality. Have routine screening tests (TB skin test) and vaccinations.
Cerebrovascular diseases	Stroke, deep vein thrombosis, aneurysm, embolism	Maintain healthy eating habits and a good body weight, exercise, do not use tobacco products, and limit alcohol consumption. Have routine screening tests and physical exams.

*Entries ordered from most to least common.

Common Diseases and Disorders in the United States* (concluded)

DISEASE	EXAMPLES	SCREENING AND PREVENTION
Alzheimer's disease		Maintain a healthy lifestyle and have a regular physical examination.
Diabetes mellitus	Type 1, Type 2, gestational	Have blood glucose tests, including fasting blood sugar, and hemoglobin A1c blood test. Maintain healthy eating habits and a good body weight, exercise, and limit alcohol and sugar consumption.
Influenza, pneumonia		Maintain a healthy lifestyle and obtain yearly flu and pneumonia vaccinations.
Nephritis/nephrosis	Chronic renal disease (CRD), end-stage renal disease (ESRD)	Have routine urinalysis. Maintain healthy eating habits and a good body weight, exercise, do not use tobacco products, and limit alcohol consumption.

*Entries ordered from most to least common.

Skin Lesions

NAME AND EXAMPLE	DESCRIPTION
Bulla	A large blister or cluster of blisters.
Cherry angioma	A common, noncancerous skin growth made up of blood.
Crust	Dried blood or pus on the skin.
Ecchymosis	A black-and-blue mark, or bruise.
Erosion	A shallow area of skin worn away by friction or pressure.

NAME AND EXAMPLE	DESCRIPTION
Excoriation	A scratch; may be covered with dried blood.
Fissure	A crack in the skin's surface.
Keloid	An overgrowth of scar tissue.
Macule	A flat skin discoloration, such as a freckle or a flat mole.
Nodule	A large pimple or small node (larger than 1 cm).
Papule	An elevated mass similar to but smaller than a nodule.
Patch color	A spot on the skin that is lighter or darker than regular skin.
Petechiae	Pinpoint skin hemorrhages that result from bleeding disorders.

Skin Lesions *(concluded)*

NAME AND EXAMPLE	DESCRIPTION
Plaque	A small, flat, scaly area of the skin.
Purpura	Purple-red bruises; usually the result of clotting abnormalities.
Pustule	An elevated (infected) lesion containing pus.
Scale	A thin plaque of epithelial tissue on the skin's surface.
Telangiesctasia	Widely open (dilated) blood vessels in the outer layer of the skin.
Tumor	A swelling of abnormal tissue growth.
Ulcer	A wound that results from tissue loss.
Vesicle	A blister.
Wheal	A hive.

Classifications of Fractures

NAME AND EXAMPLE	DESCRIPTION
Closed fracture (simple fracture)	Fracture in which the skin remains intact.
Comminuted fracture	Fracture in which the bone has broken into several fragments.
Complete fracture	Fracture that goes across the entire bone.

Classifications of Fractures *(continued)*

NAME AND EXAMPLE	DESCRIPTION
Greenstick fracture	Fracture commonly seen in children; occurs in bones that are not completely ossified, so there is a bending and only one side of the bone is fractured, rather than a complete breaking of bone.
Impacted fracture	Fracture in which one end of the fractured bone is driven into the interior of the other.
Incomplete fracture	Fracture that goes through only part of the bone.

Classifications of Fractures *(concluded)*

NAME AND EXAMPLE		DESCRIPTION
	Open fracture (compound fracture)	Fracture in which the skin is broken.

Bone Disorders

NAME	DESCRIPTION
Bursitis	Inflammation of a bursa, which is the fluid-filled sac that cushions tendons. (Tendons attach muscles to bone.)
Carpal tunnel syndrome (CTS)	Occurs when the median nerve in the wrist is excessively compressed by an inflamed tendon (the flexor retinaculum).
Fractures	Cracks, breaks, or splintering of a bone.
Gout (gouty arthritis)	A type of arthritis associated with high uric acid levels in the blood with crystalline deposits in the joints, kidneys, and various soft tissues.
Kyphosis	An abnormal, exaggerated curvature of the spine, most often at the thoracic level. This condition is often referred to as humpback.
Lordosis	An exaggerated inward (convex) curvature of the lumbar spine. The condition is sometimes called swayback.
Osteoarthritis (OA)	Also known as degenerative joint disease (DJD) or wear-and-tear arthritis.
Osteogenesis imperfecta (brittle bone disease)	People with brittle bone disease have decreased amounts of collagen in their bones, which leads to very fragile bones.
Osteoporosis	A condition in which bones become thin (more porous) over time.
Osteosarcoma	A type of bone cancer that originates from osteoblasts, the cells that make bone tissue. It is most often seen in children, teens, and young adults and occurs more often in males than females.
Paget's disease	Causes bones to enlarge and become deformed and weak. It usually affects people older than 40 years of age.
Rheumatoid arthritis (RA)	A chronic, systemic inflammatory disease that attacks the smaller joints such as those in the hands and feet.
Scoliosis	An abnormal, S-shaped lateral curvature of the thoracic or lumbar spine.

Classifications of Burns

NAME	DESCRIPTION
First-degree © Sheila Terry/Science Source	A superficial burn that causes pain and makes the surrounding skin turn red.
Second-degree © Dr. P. Marazzi/Science Source	A partial-thickness burn that extends deeper into the skin than first-degree burns; causes blistering along with pain and redness.
Third-degree © John Radcliffe Hospital/Science Source	A full-thickness burn that involves all layers of the skin and requires immediate medical assistance.

Diseases and Disorders of the Integumentary System

NAME	DESCRIPTION
Acne vulgaris	An inflammatory condition of the skin follicles and sebaceous glands.
Alopecia	The absence or loss of hair, especially of the head (baldness).
Basal cell carcinoma	Skin cancer that originates from the basal layer of the epidermis and rarely metastasizes (spreads).
Cellulitis	An inflammation of the connective tissue in skin that is most often seen on the face and legs. A bacterial infection by *Staphylococcus aureus* or *Streptococcus* is the most common cause.
Comedos	Commonly known as blackheads; collections of bacteria, dead epithelial cells, and dried sebum.
Dermatitis	A general term describing any inflammation of the skin; can be caused by a wide range of disorders.
Eczema	A common chronic dermatitis that often has acute phases or flareups followed by periods of remission. The rash of eczema can appear anywhere on the body and appears as a red, scaly, pruritic (itchy) rash that may be painful.

Diseases and Disorders of the Integumentary System *(concluded)*

NAME	DESCRIPTION
Folliculitis	Inflammation of hair follicles. When it involves a single hair follicle, the condition is called a furuncle. When more than one hair follicle is involved, it is a carbuncle.
Herpes simplex types 1 and 2	Type 1 causes cold sores and is very contagious. Type 2, which is genital herpes, is sexually transmitted.
Jaundice	A yellow cast to the skin that often occurs with liver disease.
Lentigos	Commonly called liver spots or age spots; these are not caused by the liver but are the result of excessive melanin production due to overexposure to sunlight (UV rays).
Malignant melanoma	Skin cancer that arises from melanocytes and often metastasizes (spreads).
Psoriasis	A common chronic inflammatory skin condition that has an autoimmune basis.
Rosacea	A skin disorder that commonly appears as facial redness, predominantly over the cheeks and nose.
Squamous cell carcinoma	Skin cancer that arises from the upper cells of the epidermis and often metastasizes (spreads).

Diseases and Disorders of the Muscular System

NAME	DESCRIPTION
Fibromyalgia	A fairly common condition that results in chronic pain primarily in joints, muscles, and tendons. It most commonly affects women between the ages of 20 and 50.
Muscular dystrophy (MD)	A group of inherited disorders characterized by muscle weakness and a loss of muscle tissue.
Myasthenia gravis	A condition in which affected persons experience muscle weakness. In this autoimmune condition, a person produces antibodies that prevent muscles from receiving neurotransmitters from neurons.
Sprains	Injuries that excessively stretch or tear ligaments at a joint.
Strains	Caused by stretching or tearing of muscles or tendons.
Tendonitis	Painful inflammation of a tendon as well as of the tendon–muscle attachment to a bone.
Tetanus	A condition caused by a toxin produced by the bacterium *Clostridium tetani*. It has a high mortality rate but is completely preventable through regular vaccinations.
Torticollis	Also known as wry neck. This condition is due to abnormally contracted neck muscles. The head typically bends toward the side of the contracted muscle and the chin rotates to the opposite side.

Diseases and Disorders of the Blood and Circulatory System

NAME	DESCRIPTION
Anemia	A symptom of an underlying disease process. Anemia occurs when the blood has less than its normal oxygen-carrying capacity. Anemia is the most common blood disorder in the United States and occurs more often in women than in men.
Aneurysm	A ballooned, weakened arterial wall. The most common locations of aneurysms are the aorta and the arteries in the brain, legs, intestines, and spleen. An aortic aneurysm is a bulge in the wall of the aorta.
Leukemia	A neoplastic condition in which the bone marrow produces a large number of WBCs that are not normal.
Thrombocythemia	A condition in which there is an increase in the platelet count. This condition is the opposite of thrombocytopenia.
Thrombocytopenia	A condition in which there are too few platelets, causing abnormal bleeding. This can be caused by a variety of situations, such as leukemia, certain medications, or idiopathic (unknown) reasons. The bleeding may be mild or life threatening.
Thrombophlebitis	A condition in which a thrombus and inflammation develop in a vein. It most commonly occurs in the deeper veins of the legs.
Varicose veins (varices or varicosities)	Tortuous or twisted, dilated veins that are usually seen in the legs. They affect women more often than men.

Diseases and Disorders of the Cardiovascular System

NAME	DESCRIPTION
Congenital heart disease	A problem with the heart's structure and function due to abnormal heart development before birth.
Congestive heart failure (CHF)	Failure of the heart to pump effectively. The heart weakens over time and loses its ability to supply blood to the body.
Coronary artery disease (CAD), atherosclerosis	A condition involving partial or complete blockage of major coronary arteries that supply blood to the heart.
Dysrhythmias	Also known as arrhythmias; abnormal heart rhythms and/or rates.
Endocarditis	An inflammation of the innermost lining of the heart and heart valves, usually caused by bacterial infections.
Murmurs	Abnormal heart sounds. Not all murmurs indicate a heart disorder. Murmurs are graded from 1 to 6, with 6 being quite loud and the most serious.
Myocardial infarction (MI, heart attack)	Death of heart tissue due to deprivation of oxygen. The cardiac muscle sustains damage because of ischemia.
Myocarditis	An inflammation of the muscular layer of the heart caused by a viral infection. It leads to weakening of the heart wall.
Pericarditis	An inflammation of the pericardium, usually caused by complications of viral or bacterial infections, MIs, or chest injuries.

Diseases and Disorders of the Lymphatic and Immune Systems

NAME	DESCRIPTION
Allergies	Excessive immune responses to stimuli that would not ordinarily cause a reaction.
Autoimmune disease	A disease in which the immune system targets itself.
Chronic fatigue syndrome (CFS)	Causes a person to feel severe tiredness; possibly caused by the Epstein-Barr virus (EBV).
HIV/AIDS	A viral disease spread through blood and body fluids. AIDS is caused by the human immunodeficiency virus (HIV). HIV attacks T lymphocytes.
Lymphadenitis	Inflammation of lymph nodes; can be viral or bacterial.
Lymphadenopathy	Any disease involving the lymph nodes; causes can be autoimmune disease or malignancy.
Lymphedema	Blockage of lymphatic vessels; can be caused by genetics, parasitic infections, trauma to the vessels, tumors, radiation therapy, cellulitis, and surgeries.
Systemic lupus erythematosus (SLE)	An autoimmune disorder that affects women more often than men. Affects many organ systems of the body and has numerous symptoms, usually including joint pain and swelling.

Diseases and Disorders of the Respiratory System

NAME	DESCRIPTION
Allergic rhinitis	A hypersensitivity reaction to various airborne allergens.
Asthma	Hyperactivity of the bronchioles; an inflammatory response with excess mucus production.
Atelectasis	Commonly called collapsed lung; may occur after surgery or due to pleural effusion.
Bronchitis	Inflammation of the bronchi; can be acute or chronic. Often follows a cold. One common cause of chronic bronchitis is cigarette smoking.
Chronic obstructive pulmonary disease (COPD)	A group of lung disorders in which obstruction limits airflow to the lungs. COPD includes chronic bronchitis and emphysema.

Diseases and Disorders of the Respiratory System (concluded)

NAME	DESCRIPTION
Emphysema	A lung disease in which the alveolar walls are destroyed; often caused by cigarette smoking.
Laryngitis	An acute inflammation of the larynx; caused by viruses, bacteria, polyp formation, excessive use due to talking and singing, allergies, smoking, heartburn, alcohol use, nerve damage, or stroke.
Lung cancer	The leading cancer-related cause of death in the United States. Caused by smoking or exposure to radon, asbestos, and industrial carcinogens. The three types are small cell lung cancer, squamous cell lung cancer, and adenocarcinoma.
Mesothelioma	A type of cancer that affects the pleura and is a result of asbestos exposure.
Pleuritis or pleurisy	A condition in which the pleura become inflamed.
Pneumonia (pneumonitis)	An inflammation of the lungs caused by a bacterial, viral, or fungal infection.
Pneumonoconiosis	Lung diseases that result from years of exposure to different environmental or occupational types of dust.
Pulmonary edema	A condition in which fluids fill the alveoli of the lungs, most commonly occurring with left heart failure.
Pulmonary embolism	A blocked artery in the lungs, usually caused by a blood clot.
Respiratory distress syndrome (RDS)	Kills apparently healthy infants; the cause is unknown.
Severe acute respiratory syndrome (SARS)	A viral disease that is highly contagious and sometimes fatal.
Sinusitis	An inflammation of the membranes lining the sinuses. It can be acute or chronic.
Sudden infant death syndrome (SIDS)	The sudden and unexpected death of an infant under 1 year of age. There is no explainable cause of death.

Diseases and Disorders of the Nervous System

NAME	DESCRIPTION
Alzheimer's disease	A progressive, degenerative disease of the gray matter of the brain that causes dementia.
Amyotrophic lateral sclerosis (ALS)	Commonly known as Lou Gehrig's disease; a fatal disorder characterized by the degeneration of neurons in the spinal cord and brain.
Bell's palsy	A disorder in which facial muscles are very weak or temporarily totally paralyzed. Results from damage to the facial nerve; causes are unknown.
Brain tumors and cancers	Abnormal growths in the brain. Malignant tumors that start in brain tissue are called primary brain cancers. Those that start elsewhere and metastasize to the brain are classified as secondary brain cancers.
Epilepsy	A condition in which the brain experiences repeated spontaneous seizures due to abnormal electrical activity of the brain.
Guillain-Barré syndrome	A disorder in which the body's immune system attacks part of the peripheral nervous system. It has a sudden and unexpected onset.
Headaches	Caused by a variety of factors. Include episodic tension headaches, chronic tension headaches, migraines, and cluster headaches.
Meningitis	An inflammation of the meninges.
Multiple sclerosis (MS)	A chronic disease of the central nervous system in which myelin is destroyed. Some known causes are viruses, genetic factors, and immune system abnormalities.

Diseases and Disorders of the Nervous System (concluded)

NAME	DESCRIPTION
Neuralgia	A group of disorders commonly referred to as nerve pain; most frequently occur in the nerves of the face.
Parkinson's disease	A nervous system disorder that is slowly progressive and degenerative.
Sciatica	A condition in which the sciatic nerve is damaged, commonly due to excessive pressure on the nerve from prolonged sitting.
Stroke or cerebrovascular accident (CVA)	Occurs when brain cells die because of inadequate blood perfusion of the brain.

Diseases and Disorders of the Urinary System

NAME	DESCRIPTION
Acute kidney (renal) failure (ARF)	A sudden loss of kidney function due to burns, dehydration, low blood pressure, hemorrhage, allergic reactions, obstructions, poisons, alcohol abuse, or trauma.
Chronic kidney (renal) failure (CRF)	A condition in which the kidneys slowly lose their ability to function due to diabetes, hypertension, kidney disease, or heart failure.
Cystitis	A urinary bladder infection caused by different types of bacteria.
Glomerulonephritis	An inflammation of the glomeruli of the kidney, caused by bacterial infections, renal diseases, and immune disorders.
Incontinence	A condition in which an adult cannot control urination. Can be temporary or long lasting; caused by various medications, UTIs, nervous system disorders, cancers, surgery, trauma, or pregnancy.
Polycystic kidney disease (PKD)	A disorder in which the kidneys enlarge because of the presence of many cysts within them. The cause is hereditary.
Pyelonephritis	A type of complicated UTI that begins as a bladder infection and spreads up one or both ureters into the kidneys.
Renal calculi (kidney stones)	Solid masses of crystals that obstruct the ducts within the kidneys or ureters. Painful condition caused by gouty arthritis, ureter defects, overly concentrated urine, or UTIs.

Diseases and Disorders of the Male Reproductive System

NAME	DESCRIPTION
Benign prostatic hypertrophy (BPH)	The nonmalignant enlargement of the prostate gland.
Epididymitis	An inflammation of the epididymis. Most cases start as an infection of the urinary tract.
Impotence, or erectile dysfunction (ED)	A disorder in which a male cannot achieve or maintain an erection to complete sexual intercourse. Can be caused by many physical or psychological conditions.
Prostate cancer	One of the most common cancers in men older than 40. A high-fat diet, increased age, and genetic predisposition all increase the risk.
Prostatitis	An inflammation of the prostate gland; can be acute or chronic. May be caused by bacterial infections, catheterization, trauma, excessive alcohol consumption, or scarring.
Testicular cancer	A malignant growth in one or both testicles. Occurs more commonly in males 15 to 30 years of age and is very aggressive.

Diseases and Disorders of the Female Reproductive System

NAME	DESCRIPTION
Breast cancer	One of the most common cancers in females. Evaluated and graded based on tumor size and how far cells have traveled from the site of origin.
Cervical cancer	This type of cancer usually develops slowly, and with early detection by a yearly Pap smear, treatment is often successful.
Cervicitis	Inflammation of the cervix, caused by an infection.
Dysmenorrhea	Condition of experiencing severe menstrual cramps that limit normal daily activities.
Endometriosis	A condition in which tissues that make up the lining of the uterus grow outside the uterus.
Fibrocystic breast change	A common condition consisting of abnormal but usually benign cysts in the breasts that vary in size related to the menstrual cycle.
Fibroids	Benign tumors that grow in the uterine wall.
Infertility	The inability to conceive a child due to scarring of the fallopian tubes, STIs, PID, endometriosis, or hormone imbalance.
Ovarian cancer	Considered more deadly than the other types of gynecologic cancers because its symptoms are mild and indistinct.
Pelvic inflammatory disease (PID)	An acute or chronic infection of the reproductive tract caused by untreated STIs or bacteria.
Premenstrual syndrome (PMS)	A collection of symptoms that occur just before the menstrual period. Symptoms include anxiety, depression, irritability, bloating, and diarrhea.
Uterine (endometrial) cancer	Most common in postmenopausal women. It may be related to increased levels of estrogen.
Vaginitis	An inflammation of the vagina, associated with abnormal vaginal discharge.
Vulvovaginitis	An inflammation of the vulva and vagina.

Diseases and Disorders of the Digestive System

NAME	DESCRIPTION
Appendicitis	An inflammation of the appendix. If not treated promptly, it can be life threatening.
Cholelithiasis (gallstones)	Hardened deposits of bile that can form in the gallbladder. Two types of calculi are cholesterol and pigment stones.
Cirrhosis	A chronic liver disease in which normal liver tissue is replaced with nonfunctional scar tissue.
Colitis	An inflammation of the large intestine. This condition can be chronic or short-lived, depending on the cause.
Colorectal cancer	Usually arises from the lining of the rectum or colon. This type of cancer is curable if diagnosed and treated early. It is the third most common cause of death due to cancer in both men and women.
Constipation	The condition of difficult defecation or elimination of feces.
Crohn's disease	A type of inflammatory bowel disease. It can affect any region of the digestive tract from the mouth to the anus, but most often affects the ileum (lower part of the small intestine).
Diarrhea	The condition of watery and frequent feces. Many cases of diarrhea do not require treatment because they are usually self-limiting and stop within a day or two.
Diverticulitis	An inflammation of diverticuli in the intestine. Diverticuli are abnormal dilations or pouches in the intestinal wall. When the diverticuli are not inflamed, the condition is known as *diverticulosis*.
Gastric, or stomach, ulcers	Occur when the lining of the stomach breaks down.

Diseases and Disorders of the Digestive System *(concluded)*

NAME	DESCRIPTION
Gastritis	An inflammation of the stomach lining; often referred to as an upset stomach.
Gastroesophageal reflux disorder (GERD)	This occurs when stomach acids are pushed into the esophagus (also called heartburn). If not treated, GERD can cause erosion of the esophagus and even esophageal cancer.
Helicobacter pylori (H. pylori)	Organism implicated as being responsible for many diseases and disorders, including gastric ulcers.
Hemorrhoids	Varicosities (varicose veins) of the rectum or anus.
Hepatitis	An inflammation of the liver. There are many different types of hepatitis, but they all involve inflammation of the liver. Many signs and symptoms are shared, regardless of the cause of the inflammation.
Hiatal hernias	Occur when a portion of the stomach protrudes into the thoracic cavity through an opening (esophageal hiatus) in the diaphragm.
Inguinal hernias	Occur when a portion of the large intestine protrudes into the inguinal canal, which is located where the thigh and the body trunk meet. In males, the hernia can also protrude into the scrotum.
Oral cancer	Usually involves the lips or tongue but can occur anywhere in the mouth. This type of cancer tends to spread rapidly to other organs because of the high vascularity of this area.
Pancreatic cancer	The fourth leading cause of cancer death in the United States. The poor prognosis and 5-year survival rate of only 5% is due to the late diagnosis in many cases.
Stomach cancer	Most commonly occurs in the uppermost (cardiac) portion of the stomach. It appears to occur more frequently in Japan, Chile, and Iceland than in the United States. This may be due to diets high in nitrates that are known to be carcinogenic.
Stomach ulcer	A condition in which the lining of the stomach breaks down.

Diseases and Disorders of Metabolism and Nutrition

NAME	DESCRIPTION
Anorexia nervosa	An eating disorder in which individuals have a perception of being overweight regardless of their actual weight.
Bulimia nervosa	An eating disorder in which the person may be of normal weight and may eat normal or even excessive amounts of food but then vomits to rid himself or herself of the calories. Also called binge-and-purge eating.
Celiac disease	An immune reaction to eating gluten that causes the individual's body to attack the small intestinal mucosa. In a similar disorder, known as non-celiac gluten sensitivity, patients cannot tolerate gluten and have similar symptoms, with the addition of headache, joint pain, and numbness in the extremities.
Hypercholesterolemia	An excess of cholesterol in the blood.
Kwashiorkor	A type of starvation in which there is too little protein in the diet.
Malnutrition	Inadequate or excessive caloric intake.
Marasmus	A type of starvation that entails both protein and calorie insufficiency.
Metabolic syndrome	A group of symptoms such as hypertension, hyperinsulinism, excess body fat around the waist, and hypercholesterolemia. Lifestyle changes, medication, and regular appointments with a healthcare provider are essential.
Obesity	A body weight greater than 20% above the standard is considered obesity, and 50% over the standard is considered morbid obesity.
Starvation	A type of malnutrition resulting from inadequate caloric intake, inadequate resources, dietary imbalances, illness, or self-imposed starvation.

Diseases and Disorders of the Endocrine System

NAME	DESCRIPTION
Acromegaly	A condition caused by the secretion of too much growth hormone after puberty that causes the hands, feet, and face to take on unusual enlargement.
Addison's syndrome	Hyposecretion of ACTH in which patients experience anorexia, fatigue, weight loss, GI problems, and bronzing of the skin.
Diabetes insipidus	Hyposecretion of ADH. Symptoms include excessive urination, thirst, and dehydration.
Diabetes mellitus	Hyposecretion of insulin, categorized into Type 1 (insulin dependent) and Type 2 (non-insulin dependent).
Dwarfism (achondroplasia)	Abnormal underdevelopment of the body due to hyposecretion of growth hormone (GH). Adult height is 4 feet 10 inches or less.
Epinephrine and norepinephrine imbalances	Cause increase in blood pressure, tachycardia, and tachypnea.
Estrogen imbalances	Hyposecretion before or during menopause results in hot flashes, vaginal dryness, mood changes, depression, and loss of bone density.
Gigantism	An abnormal increase in the length of long bones due to hypersecretion of growth hormone during childhood.
Hypercalcemia	An increase in blood calcium levels, resulting in more calcium going into bone.
Hyperthyroidism	Excess secretion of thyroid hormone (TSH). Also called Grave's disease, it causes an overall increase in metabolism.
Hypocalcemia	A condition in which there is too little calcium in the blood.
Hypoglycemia	A low level of glucose in the blood.
Hypothyroidism	Too little TSH is secreted, resulting in slowing of metabolism.
Melatonin imbalances	Hyposecretion disturbs the sleep cycle and contributes to depression.
Pancreatic tumors	Malignant tumors have a poor prognosis due to difficulty in diagnosing.
Pheochromocytoma	A benign tumor of the adrenal medulla that can cause an increase in blood pressure.
Thymosin imbalances	Hyposecretion results in lack of mature T lymphocytes and a decrease in immunity.
Thyroid tumor	An abnormal growth on the thyroid gland. May be benign or malignant.

Diseases and Disorders of the Special Senses—the Eye

NAME	DESCRIPTION
Amblyopia	Commonly called lazy eye; occurs when a child does not use one eye regularly.
Astigmatism	Occurs when the cornea or lens has an abnormal shape, which causes blurred images in near or distant vision.
Blepharitis	An inflammation of the eyelid, as well as corneal abrasions (scratching of the cornea).
Cataracts	Opaque structures within the lens that prevent light from going through the lens. Over time, images begin to look fuzzy; if left untreated, cataracts may cause blindness.
Color blindness	The inability to see certain colors. May be inherited; occurs more commonly in males.
Dry eye syndrome (xerophthalmia)	One of the most common eye problems treated by physicians. This syndrome results from a decreased production of the oil within tears, which normally occurs with age.
Ectropion	Eversion of the lower eyelid.
Entropion	Inversion of the lower eyelid.

Diseases and Disorders of the Special Senses—the Eye *(concluded)*

NAME	DESCRIPTION
Glaucoma	Indicated by an increase in intraocular pressure, caused by a buildup of aqueous humor in the anterior chamber. If untreated, this excess pressure can lead to permanent damage of the optic nerve that can result in blindness.
Hyperopia	Farsightedness.
Macular degeneration	A progressive disease that usually affects people over the age of 50. It occurs when the retina no longer receives an adequate blood supply. It is the most common cause of vision loss in the United States.
Myopia	Nearsightedness.
Nystagmus	Rapid, involuntary eye movements. The movements may be horizontal or vertical.
Presbyopia	A common eye disorder that results in the loss of lens elasticity. It develops with age and causes a person to have difficulty seeing objects that are close up.
Retinal detachment	Occurs when the layers of the retina separate. It is considered a medical emergency and if not treated right away leads to permanent vision loss.
Strabismus	A misalignment of the eyes. Convergent strabismus is commonly referred to as crossed eyes.

Diseases and Disorders of the Special Senses—the Ear

NAME	DESCRIPTION
Cerumen impaction	A buildup of ear wax within the external auditory canal.
Menière's disease	A disturbance in the equilibrium characterized by *vertigo* (dizziness), ringing in the ears, nausea, and progressive hearing loss.
Otitis externa	An inflammation of the outer ear.
Otitis media	An inflammation of the middle ear.
Otosclerosis	The immobilization of the stapes within the middle ear; a common cause of conductive hearing loss.
Presbycusis	Hearing loss because of the aging process.
Tinnitus	Ringing in the ears.
Vertigo	Dizziness.

10× lens (ten lenz) A magnifying lens in the ocular of a microscope that magnifies an image ten times.

24-hour urine specimen (Twen′t ē fŭr owr′ yŭr′in spes′i-mĕn) A urine specimen collected over a 24-hour period and used to complete a quantitative and qualitative analysis of one or more substances, such as sodium, chloride, and calcium.

AAMA See **American Association of Medical Assistants.**

abandonment (ă-ban′dŏn-mĕnt) A situation in which a healthcare professional stops caring for a patient without arranging for care by an equally qualified substitute.

ABA number (nŭm′bĕr) A fraction appearing in the upper-right corner of all printed checks that identifies the geographic area and specific bank on which the check is drawn.

abduction (ab-dŭk′shŭn) Movement away from the body.

ABHES See **Accrediting Bureau of Health Education Schools.**

abscess (ab′ses) A collection of pus (white blood cells, bacteria, and dead skin cells) that forms as a result of infection.

absorption (ăb-sōrp′shŭn) The process by which one substance is absorbed, or taken in and incorporated, into another, as when the body converts food or drugs into a form it can use.

abuse (ă-byūs′) A practice or behavior that is not indicative of or in line with sound medical or fiscal activity.

access (ak′ses) The way patients enter and exit a medical office.

accessibility (ak-ses′ă-bil′i-tē) The ease with which people can move into and out of a space.

accommodation (ă-kom′ŏ-dā′shŭn) The ability of the lens to change shape, allowing the eye to focus images of objects that are near or far away.

accounting (ă-kownt-ing) The process of communicating the income and expenses of a business and its financial health.

accounts payable (A/P) (ă-kownts′ pā′ŭ-bĕl) Money owed by a business; the practice's expenses.

accounts receivable (A/R) (ă-kownts′ rĕ-sē′vă-bĕl) Income or money owed to a business.

accreditation (ă-kred′i-tā′shŭn) The documentation of official authorization or approval of a program.

Accrediting Bureau of Health Education Schools (ABHES) (ă′kre-dăt-ing byoor-oh helth ed′yū-kā′shŭn skulz) An accrediting body that accredits private postsecondary institutions and programs that prepare individuals for entry into the medical assisting profession.

acetabulum (as-ĕ-tab′yū-lŭm) The hip socket.

acetylcholine (as′ĕ-til-kō′lēn) A neurotransmitter released by the parasympathetic nerves onto organs and glands for resting and digesting.

acetylcholinesterase (as′ĕ-til-kō′lin-es′tĕr-ās) An enzyme within the nervous system that hydrolyzes acetylcholine to acetate and choline.

acid-fast stain (as′id-fast stān) A staining procedure for identifying bacteria that have a waxy cell wall.

acids (as′idz) Electrolytes that release hydrogen ions in water.

acinar cells (as′i-năr selz) Cells in the pancreas that produce pancreatic juice.

acquired immunodeficiency syndrome (AIDS) (ă-kwīrd′ im′yū-nō-dĕ-fish′ĕn-sē sin′drōm) The most advanced stage of HIV infection; it severely weakens the body's immune system.

acromegaly (ak′rō-meg′ă-lē) A disorder in which too much growth hormone is produced in adults.

acrosome (ak′rō-sōm) An enzyme-filled sac covering the head of a sperm that aids in the penetration of the egg during fertilization.

ACTH See **adrenocorticotropic hormone.**

action potential (ak′shŭn pŏ-ten′shăl) The flow of electrical current along the axon membrane.

active file (ăk′tĭv fīl) A file used on a consistent basis.

active listening (ak′tiv lis′ĕn-ing) Part of two-way communication, such as offering feedback or asking questions; contrast with **passive listening.**

active transport (ak′-tiv trans′pōrt) The movement of a substance across a cell membrane from an area of low concentration to an area of high concentration.

acupressure (ak′yū-presh-ŭr) Pressure applied by hands to various areas of the body to restore balance in the body's energy flow.

acupuncture (ak′yū-pŭngk′shŭr) The practice of inserting needles into various areas of the body to restore balance in the body's energy flow.

acupuncturist (ak′yū-pŭngk′shŭr-ist) A practitioner of acupuncture. The acupuncturist uses hollow needles inserted into the patient's skin to treat pain, discomfort, or systemic imbalances.

acute (ă-kyūt′) Having a rapid onset and progress, as acute appendicitis.

ADA See **Americans with Disabilities Act.**

ADA Amendments Act of 2008 (ADAAA) (ă-mend′mĕnts akt) A 2008 amendment to the ADA that broadens the definition of disability, making it easier for individuals who seek ADA protection to establish that they have a disability.

addiction (ă-dik′shŭn) A physical or psychological dependence on a substance, usually involving a pattern of behavior that includes obsessive or compulsive preoccupation with the substance and the security of its supply, as well as a high rate of relapse after withdrawal.

Addison's disease (ad′i-sŏns di-zēz) A condition in which the adrenal glands fail to produce enough corticosteroids.

add-on code (ad′on′ kōd) A code indicating procedures that are usually carried out in addition to another procedure. Add-on codes are used together with the primary code.

add-on safety features (ad′on saf′tē fē′chūrz) Features on injection, phlebotomy, and winged steel needles that provide protection from needlestick injury. They consist of a hinged or sliding sheath attached to the needle that can be activated with one hand, keeping the user's hands behind the needle.

adduction (ă-dŭk′shŭn) Movement toward the body.

adenoids (ad′ĕ-noydz) See **pharyngeal tonsils.**

ADH See **antidiuretic hormone.**

adjustment (ă-jŭst′mĕnt) Manual treatment given by a chiropractor that moves the joints of the spine and other joints into proper alignment. Also, an amount taken off a bill which is the difference between the fees charged for a service and the fees allowed by insurance. Also known as a write-off.

administer (ad-min′i-stir) To give a drug directly by injection, by mouth, or by any other route that introduces the drug into the body.

adrenocorticotropic hormone (ACTH) (ă-drē′nō-kōr′ti-kō-trō′fik hor′mōn) Hormone that stimulates the adrenal cortex to release its hormones.

advance scheduling (ad-vans′ sked′jūl-ing) Booking an appointment several weeks or even months in advance.

adverse effect (ad-vĕrs′ e-fekt′) An unintended negative reaction to a medication or treatment. Adverse effects are potentially more harmful than side effects, but are less common.

AED See **automated external defibrillator.**

aerobes (âr′ōbz) Bacteria that grow best in the presence of oxygen.

aerobic respiration (ār-ō′bik res′pir-ā′shŭn) A process that requires large amounts of oxygen and uses glucose to make ATP.

afebrile (ā-feb′ril) Having a body temperature within one's normal range.

afferent arterioles (af′ĕr-ĕnt ahr-tēr′ē-ōls) Structures that deliver blood to the glomeruli of the kidneys.

afferent nerves (af′ĕr-ĕnt nĕrvs) Sensory nerves that are responsible for detecting sensory information from the environment or even from inside the body and taking it to the CNS for interpretation.

affiliation agreement (ă-fili′ā-shŭn ă-grē′mĕnt) An agreement that applied training participants must sign that states the expectations of the facility and the expectations of the student.

agar (ā′gahr) A gelatin-like substance derived from seaweed that gives a culture medium its semisolid consistency.

age analysis (āj ă-nal′i-sis) The process of clarifying and reviewing past-due accounts by age from the first date of billing.

agenda (ă′jĕn-dă) The list of topics discussed or presented at a meeting, in order of presentation.

agent (ā′jĕnt) (legal) A person who acts on a physician's behalf while performing professional tasks; (clinical) an active principal or entity that produces a certain effect, for example, an infectious agent.

agglutination (ă-glū-ti-nā′shŭn) The clumping of red blood cells following a blood transfusion.

aggressive (ă-gres′iv) Imposing one's position on others or trying to manipulate them.

agonist (ag′ŏn-ist) See **antagonist.**

agranular leukocyte (ă-gran′yū-lăr lū′kō-sīt) A type of leukocyte (white blood cell) with a solid nucleus and clear cytoplasm; includes lymphocytes and monocytes.

agranulocyte (ā-grăn′ŭ-lō-sīt) See **agranular leukocyte.**

AIDS See **Acquired Immune Deficiency Syndrome.**

albumins (al-bū′mins) The smallest of the plasma proteins. Albumins are important for pulling water into the bloodstream to help maintain blood pressure.

alcohol-based hand disinfectants (AHD) (al′kŏ-hol băsd hand dis-infek′tănts) Gels, foams, or liquids with an alcohol content of 60% to 95% that are used for hand disinfection.

aldosterone (al-dos′tĕr-ōn) A hormone produced in the adrenal glands that acts on the kidney. It causes the body to retain sodium and excrete potassium. Its role is to maintain blood volume and pressure.

alimentary canal (al′i-men′tăr-ē kă-nal′) The organs of the digestive system that extend from the mouth to the anus.

allele (ă-lēl′) Any one of a pair or series of **genes** that occupy a specific position on a specific **chromosome.**

allergen (al′ĕr-jĕn) An antigen that induces an allergic reaction.

allergic rhinitis (ă-lĕr′jik rī-nī′tis) A hypersensitivity reaction to various airborne allergens.

allergist (al′ĕr-jist) A specialist who diagnoses and treats physical reactions to substances including mold, dust, fur, pollen, foods, drugs, and chemicals.

allopathy (al-op′ă-thē) The usual medical practice of physicians and other health professionals; also known as conventional medicine.

allowed charge (ă-low′d chahrj) The amount that is the most the payer will pay any provider for each procedure or service.

alopecia (al-ō-pē′shē-ă) The clinical term for baldness.

alphabetic filing system (ăl′fă-bĕt′ĭk fī′lĭng sis′tăm) A filing system in which the files are arranged in alphabetical order, with the patient's last name first, followed by the first name and middle initial.

Alphabetic Index (al′fă′bet-ik in′deks) One of two ways diagnoses are listed in the ICD manual. They appear in alphabetical order with their corresponding diagnosis codes.

alternative medicine (awl-tĕr′nă-tiv med′i-sin) The type of medicine used in place of conventional medicine to promote health and treat disease.

alveolar glands (al-vē′ŏ-lăr glands) Glands that make milk under the influence of the hormone **prolactin.**

alveoli (al-vē′ŏ-lī) Clusters of air sacs in which the exchange of gases between air and blood takes place; located in the lungs.

amblyopia (am′blē-ō′pē-ă) Poor vision in one eye without a detectable cause.

amenorrhea (ā-men′ŏ-rē′ă) Absence or abnormal cessation of the menses.

American Association of Medical Assistants (AAMA) (ă-mer′i-kăn ă-sō′sē-ā′shŭn med′i-kăl ă-sis′tănts) The professional organization that certifies medical assistants and works to maintain professional standards in the medical assisting profession.

American Medical Technologists (AMT) (ă-mer′i-kăn med′i-kăl tek-nol′ŏ-jists) The registering organization for medical assistants that provides online continuing education, certification information, and member news.

Americans with Disabilities Act (ADA) (ă-mer′i-kănz dis′ă-bil′i-tēz akt) A US civil rights act forbidding discrimination against people because of a physical or mental handicap.

amino acid (ă-mē′nō as′id) Natural organic compound found in plant and animal foods and used by the body to create protein.

amnion (am′nē-on) The innermost membrane enveloping the embryo and containing amniotic fluid.

amount to administer *(A)* **(ă-mownt ad-min′ĭ-stĭr′)** The amount of medication the patient will receive.

AMT See American Medical Technologists.

anabolism (ă-nab′ŏ-lizm) The stage of metabolism in which substances such as nutrients are changed into more complex substances and used to build body tissues.

anaerobe (an′ār-ōb) A bacterium that grows best in the absence of oxygen.

anal canal (ā′năl kă-nal′) The last few centimeters of the rectum.

anaphase (an′ă-fāz) The period of mitosis when the centromeres divide and pull the chromosomes (formerly chromatids) toward the centrioles at opposite sides of the cell.

anaphylactic shock (an′ă-fi-lak′tik shok) A severe, often fatal form of shock characterized by smooth muscle contraction and capillary dilation initiated by cytotropic (IgE class) antibodies.

anaphylaxis (an′ă-fī-lak′sis) A severe allergic reaction with symptoms that include respiratory distress, difficulty in swallowing, pallor, and a drastic drop in blood pressure that can lead to circulatory collapse.

anatomical position (an-ă-tom′i-kăl pŏ-zish′ŏn) When the body is standing upright and facing forward with the arms at the side and the palms of the hands facing forward.

anatomy (ă-nat′ŏ-mē) The scientific term for the study of body structure.

anemia (ă-nē′mē-ă) A condition characterized by low red blood cell count. This condition decreases the ability to transport oxygen throughout the body.

anergic reaction (an-er′jik rē-ăk′shən) A lack of response to skin testing that indicates the body's inability to mount a normal response to invasion by a pathogen.

anesthesia (an′es-thē′zē-ă) A loss of sensation, particularly the feeling of pain.

anesthetic (an′es-thet′ik) A medication that causes anesthesia.

anesthetist (ă-nes′thĕ-tist) A specialist who uses medications to cause patients to lose sensation or feeling during surgery.

aneurysm (an′yūr-izm) A serious and potentially life-threatening bulge in the wall of a blood vessel.

angiography (an-jē-og′ră-fē) An X-ray examination of a blood vessel, performed after the injection of a contrast medium, that evaluates the function and structure of one or more arteries or veins.

annotate (an′ō-tāt′) To underline or highlight key points of a document or to write reminders, make comments, and suggest actions in the margins.

anorexia nervosa (an′ŏ-rek′sē-ă nĕr-vō′să) An eating disorder in which people starve themselves because they fear that if they lose control of eating they will become grossly overweight.

antagonist (an-tag′ŏ-nist) A muscle that produces the opposite movement of the **prime mover.**

antecubital space (an-te-kyū′bi-tăl spās) The inner side or bend of the elbow; the site at which the brachial artery is felt or heard when a pulse or blood pressure is taken.

anterior (an-tēr′ē-ŏr) Anatomical term meaning toward the front of the body; also called ventral.

anthracosis (an′thră-kō′sis) Chronic lung disease caused by the inhalation of coal deposits; also known as black lung disease.

antibodies (ăn′ti-bod′ēs) Highly specific proteins that attach themselves to foreign substances in an initial step in destroying such substances, as part of the body's defenses.

antibody-mediated response (an′ti-bod-ē mē′dē-ăt-ed rĕ-spons′) The part of our body's immune response that occurs when B cells respond to antigens by becoming plasma cells, which make antibodies that attach to antigens.

anticoagulants (an′tē-kō-ag′yŭ-lăntz) Substances that prevent clotting.

antidiuretic hormone (ADH) (an′tē-dī-yŭr-et′ik hōr′mōn) A hormone that increases water reabsorption, which decreases urine production and helps to maintain blood pressure.

antigens (an′ti-jenz) Foreign substances that stimulate white blood cells to create antibodies when they enter the body.

antihistamines (an′tē-his′tă-mēnz) Medications used to treat allergies.

antimicrobial (an′tē-mī-krō′bē-ăl) An agent that kills microorganisms or suppresses their growth.

antioxidant (an′tē-ok′si-dănt) Chemical agent that fights cell-destroying chemical substances called free radicals.

antiseptic (an′ti-sep′tik) A cleaning product used on human tissue as an anti-infection agent.

antivirus software (an′tē-vī′rŭs sahft′wēr) Software that prevents and removes computer viruses. Such programs may also detect and remove adware and spyware.

anuria (an-yū′rē-ă) The absence of urine production.

aortic semilunar valve (ā-ōr′tik sem′ē-lū′năr valv) Heart valve that is a semilunar valve and that is situated between the left ventricle and the aorta.

apex (ā′peks) The left lower corner of the heart, where the strongest heart sounds can be heard.

APGAR (ap′gar) A test performed 1 minute and 5 minutes after a baby is born to determine how well the baby is breathing and how well the heart is working. Its five categories are respiratory effort, heart rate, skin color, reflexes, and muscle tone.

apical (ap′i-kăl) Located at the **apex** of the heart.

apnea (ap′nē-ă) The absence of respiration.

apocrine gland (ap′ō-krin glănd) A type of sweat gland. It produces a thicker type of sweat than other sweat glands and contains more proteins.

aponeurosis (ap′ō-nū-rō′sis) A tough, sheet-like structure that is made of fibrous connective tissue. It typically attaches muscles to other muscles.

apothecary system (ă-poth′ĕ-kār-ē sis′tĕm) An older system of measurement that includes units such as fluid ounces, fluid drams, pints, and quarts.

appendicitis (ă-pen′di-sī′tis) Inflammation of the appendix.

appendicular (ap′en-dik′yū-lăr) The division of the skeletal system that consists of the bones of the arms, legs, pectoral girdle, and pelvic girdle.

applied training (ă-plīd trān′ing) An opportunity to work in a medical facility to gain the essential on-the-job experience for beginning your new career, sometimes known as an externship or practicum.

applied training coordinator (ă-plīd trān′ing kō-ōr′di-nā-tōr) A professional who procures applied training sites and qualifies, or assesses, them to make certain that they provide a thorough educational experience. May also be known as a clinical coordinator.

approximate (a-prŏks′i māt) To bring the edges of a wound together so that the tissue surfaces are close in order to protect the area from further contamination and to minimize scar and scab formation.

aqueous humor (ā′kwē-ŭs hyū′mŏr) A liquid produced by the eye's ciliary body that fills the space between the cornea and the lens.

arbitration (ahr′bi-trā′shŭn) A process in which opposing sides choose a person or persons outside the court system, often someone with special knowledge in the field, to hear and decide a dispute.

areflexia (ā-rē-flek′sē-ă) The absence of reflexes.

areola (ă-rē′ō-lă) The pigmented area that surrounds the nipple.

aromatherapy (ă-rō′mă-thār′ă-pē) The use of essential oil extracts or essences from flowers, herbs, and trees to promote health and well-being.

arrector pili (ă-rek′tōr pī′lī) Muscles attached to most hair follicles and found in the dermis.

arrhythmia (ā-ridh′mē-ă) Irregularity in heart rhythm.

arterial blood gases (ahr-tēr′ē-ăl blŭd găs′sez) A test that measures the amount of gases, such as oxygen and carbon dioxide, dissolved in arterial blood.

arthritis (ahr-thrī′tis) A general term meaning joint inflammation.

arthrography (ahr-throg′ră-fē) A radiologic procedure performed by a radiologist, who uses a contrast medium and fluoroscopy to help diagnose abnormalities or injuries in the cartilage, tendons, or ligaments of the joints—usually the knee or shoulder.

arthroscopy (ahr-thros′kŏ-pē) A procedure in which an orthopedist examines a joint, usually the knee or shoulder, with a tubular instrument called an arthroscope; also used to guide surgical procedures.

articular cartilage (ahr-tik′yū-lăr kahr′ti-lăj) The cartilage that covers the **epiphysis** of long bones.

articulations (ahr-tik′yū-lā′shŭnz) The areas where bones are joined together; joints.

artifact (ahr′ti-fakt) Any irrelevant object or mark observed when examining specimens or graphic records that is not related to the object being examined—for example, a foreign object visible through a microscope or an erroneous mark on an ECG strip.

asbestosis (as-bes-tō′sis) Chronic lung disease caused by the inhalation of asbestos fibers.

ascending colon (ă-send′ing kō′lŏn) The segment of the large intestine that runs up the right side of the abdominal cavity.

ascending tracts (ă-send′ing trakts) The tracts of the spinal cord that carry sensory information to the brain.

asepsis (ā-sep′sis) The condition in which pathogens are absent or controlled.

assault (ă-sawlt) The open threat of bodily harm to another.

assertive (ă-sĕr′tiv) Being firm and standing up for oneself while showing respect for others.

asset (as′-ĕt) An item owned by the practice that has a dollar value, such as the medical practice building, office equipment, or accounts receivable.

assignment of benefits (ă-sīn′mĕnt ben′ĕ-fits) An authorization for an insurance carrier to pay a physician or practice directly.

asthma (az′mă) A condition in which the tubes of the bronchial tree become obstructed due to inflammation.

astigmatism (ă-stig′mă-tizm) A condition in which the cornea has an abnormal shape, which causes blurred images during near or distant vision.

astrocytes (ăs′trō-sīts) Star-shaped cells within the nervous system that anchor blood vessels to the nerve cells.

atelectasis (at′ĕ-lek′tă-sis) The collapse of a lung because of fluid, air, pus, or blood.

atherosclerosis (ath′ĕr-ō-skler-ō′sis) The accumulation of fatty deposits along the inner walls of arteries.

atlas (at′lăs) The first cervical vertebra.

atoms (at′ŏmz) The simplest units of all matter.

atria (ā′trē-ă) [*Singular:* **atrium**] Chambers of the heart that receive blood from the veins and circulate it to the ventricles.

atrial natriuretic peptide (ā′trē-ăl nā′trēyū-ret′ik pep′tīd) A hormone secreted by the heart that regulates blood pressure.

atrioventricular bundle (ā′trē-ō-ventrik′yū-lar bŭn′dĕl) A structure that is located between the ventricles of the heart and that sends the electrical impulse to the Purkinje fibers.

atrioventricular node (AV node) (ā′trē-ō-ventrik′yū-lar nōd) A node that is located between the atria of the heart. After the electrical impulse reaches the atrioventricular node, the atria contract and the impulse is sent to the ventricles.

atrioventricular septum (ā′trē-ō-ventrik′yū-lar sep′tŭm) The wall separating the upper atrial chambers from the lower ventricular chambers of the heart.

attitude (at′i-tūd) A disposition to act in a certain way.

audiologist (aw-dē-ol′ōjist) A healthcare specialist who focuses on evaluating and correcting hearing problems.

audiometer (aw-dē-om′ĕ-ter) An electronic device that measures hearing acuity by producing sounds in specific frequencies and intensities.

audit (aw′dit) To examine and review a group of patient records for completeness and accuracy—particularly as related to their ability to back up the charges sent to health insurance carriers for reimbursement.

auricle (awr′i-kĕl) The outside part of the ear, made of cartilage and covered with skin.

auscultated blood pressure (aws′kŭl-tāt-ĕd blŭd presh′ŭr) Blood pressure as measured by listening with a stethoscope.

auscultation (aws′kŭl-tā′shŭn) The process of listening to body sounds.

authorization (aw′thŏr-ī-zā′shŭn) A form that explains in detail the standards for the use and disclosure of patient information for purposes other than treatment, payment, or healthcare operations.

autoclave (aw′tō-klāv) A device that uses pressurized steam to sterilize instruments and equipment.

autoimmune disease (aw′tō-i-myūn′ di-zēz′) Any condition in which the body attacks its own antigens, causing illness to the patient.

automated external defibrillator (AED) (aw′tō-mā-tĕd eks-tĕr′năl dē-fib′ri-lā-tŏr) A computerized defibrillator programmed to recognize lethal heart rhythms and deliver an electric shock to restore a normal rhythm.

automated voice response unit (aw′tō-mā′tĕd voys rĕ-spons′ yū′nit) Automated answering unit with a recorded voice that offers the caller various options for routing the call.

automatic puncturing devices (aw′tō-mat′ik pungk′shŭr-ing dĕ-vīs′iz) A type of lancet that is spring loaded, is self-contained, and has a mechanically controlled skin puncture depth.

autonomic (aw′tō-nom′ik) A division of the peripheral nervous system that connects the central nervous system to viscera such as the heart, stomach, intestines, glands, blood vessels, and bladder.

autonomic nervous system (aw′tō-nom′ik nĕr′vŭs sis′tĕm) A system that is in charge of the body's automatic functions, such as the respiratory and gastrointestinal systems.

autopsy (aw′top-sē) The examination of a cadaver to determine or confirm the cause of death.

autosome (aw′tō-sōm) A chromosome that is not a sex chromosome.

axial (ak′sē-ăl) The division of the skeletal system that consists of the skull, vertebral column, and rib cage.

axilla (ak-sil′ă) Armpit; one of the four locations for temperature readings.

axis (ak′-sis) The second vertebra of the neck on which the head turns.

axon (ak′son) A type of nerve fiber that is typically long and branches far from the cell body. Its function is to send information away from the cell body.

Ayurveda (ī′yŭr-vā′d′ă) A form of medicine, originated in India, that uses herbal preparations, dietary changes, exercises, and meditation to restore health and promote well-being.

bacillus (bă-sil′ŭs) A rod-shaped bacterium.

bacterial spore (bak-tēr′ē-ăl spōr) A primitive, thick-walled reproductive body capable of developing into a new individual; resistant to killing through disinfection.

balance billing (bal′ăns bil′ing) Billing a patient for the difference between a higher usual fee and a lower allowed charge.

balloon angioplasty (bă-lūn′ an′jē-ō-plas′tē) A procedure using a slender, hollow tube passed through a coronary artery to compress a blockage in the artery.

bandwidth (bānd′wĭdth) A measurement, calculated in bits or bytes, of how much information can be sent or processed with one single instruction.

barium enema (bar′ē-ŭm en′ĕ-mă) A radiologic procedure performed by a radiologist who administers barium sulfate through the anus, into the rectum, and then into the colon to help diagnose and evaluate obstructions, ulcers, polyps, diverticuloses, tumors, or motility problems of the colon or rectum; also called a lower GI (gastrointestinal) series.

barium swallow (bar′ē-ŭm swahl′ō) A radiologic procedure that involves oral administration of a barium sulfate drink to help diagnose and evaluate obstructions, ulcers, polyps, diverticuloses, tumors, or motility problems of the esophagus, stomach, duodenum, and small intestine; also called an upper GI (gastrointestinal) series.

baroreceptors (bar′ō-rē-sep′terz) Structures, located in the aorta and carotid arteries, that help regulate blood pressure.

Bartholin's glands (bahr′tō-lĭn glandz) Glands lateral to the vagina that produce mucus for lubrication of the vagina.

bases (bā′sēz) Electrolytes that release hydroxyl ions in water.

basophil (bā′sō-fil) A type of granular leukocyte that produces the chemical histamine, which aids the body in controlling allergic reactions and other exaggerated immunologic responses.

battery (bat′ĕr-ē) An action that causes bodily harm to another.

behavior modification (bē-hāv′yŏr mod′i-fi-kā′shŭn) The altering of personal habits to promote a healthier lifestyle.

benefits (ben′ĕ-fits) Payments for medical services.

benign (bē-nīn′) A noncancerous or non-malignant growth or condition.

benign prostatic hypertrophy (bē-nīn′ pros-tat′ik hī-pĕr′trŏ-fē) A noncancerous enlargement of the prostate gland.

bicarbonate ions (bī-kahr′bŏn-āt ī′onz) Elements formed when carbon dioxide gets into the bloodstream and reacts with water. In the alimentary canal, these ions neutralize acidic chyme arriving from the stomach.

bicuspids (bī-kŭs′pidz) Teeth with two cusps. There are two in front of each set of molars.

bicuspid valve (bī-kŭs′pid valv) Heart valve that has two cusps and that is located between the left atrium and the left ventricle. Also known as the mitral valve.

bile (bīl) A substance created in the liver and stored in the gallbladder. Bile is a bitter, yellow-green fluid that is used in the digestion of fats.

bilirubin (bil′i-rū′bin) A bile pigment formed by the breakdown of hemoglobin in the liver.

bilirubinuria (bil′i-rū-bi-nyūr′ē-ă) The presence of bilirubin in the urine; one of the first signs of liver disease or conditions that involve the liver.

biliverdin (bil′i-vĕr-din) A pigment released when a red blood cell is destroyed.

biochemistry (bī′ō-kem′is-trē) The study of matter and chemical reactions in the body.

bioelectromagnetic-based therapies (bī′ō-ĕ-lek′trō-mag′nĕt-ik bās-ĕd thār′ă-pēz) The use of measurable energy fields in such things as magnetic therapy, millimeter wave therapy, sound energy therapy, and light therapy.

bioethics (bī-ō-ĕth′ĭks) Principles of right and wrong in issues that arise from medical advances.

biofeedback (bī-ō-fēd′bak) A type of therapy in which an individual learns how to control involuntary body responses in order to promote health and treat disease.

biofield therapies (bī′ō-fēld thār′ă-pēz) Treatments that affect the energy fields that surround and penetrate the human body in order to promote health and well-being.

biohazardous materials (bī′ō-haz′ărd-ŭs mă-tēr′ē-ălz) Biologic agents that can spread disease to living things.

biohazardous waste container (bī′ō-haz′ărd-ŭs wāst kŏn-tā′nĕr) A leakproof, puncture-resistant container, color-coded red or labeled with a biohazard symbol, that is used to store and dispose of contaminated supplies and equipment.

biohazard symbol (bī′ō-haz′ărd sim′bŏl)   A symbol that must appear on all containers used to store waste products, blood, blood products, or other specimens that may be infectious.

biological indicator (bī′ŏ-loj′i-kălin′di-kā-tŏr)   An indicator consisting of bacterial spores that is used as a quality control method in autoclaves to confirm that sterilization has occurred.

biopsy (bī-op′-sē)   The removal and examination of a sample of tissue from a living body for diagnostic purposes.

biopsy specimen (bī′ŏp′sē spes′i-měn)   A small amount of tissue removed from the body for examination under a microscope to diagnose an illness.

bioterrorism (bī′o-ter′ŏr-izm)   The intentional release of a biologic agent with the intent to harm individuals.

birthday rule (bĭrth′dā rūl)   A rule that states that the insurance policy of a policyholder whose birthday comes first in the year is the primary payer for all dependents.

blastocyst (blas′tō-sist)   A morula that travels down the uterine tube to the uterus and is invaded with fluid. It then implants into the wall of the uterus.

bloodborne pathogen (blŭd′bōrn path′ŏ-jĕn)   A disease-causing microorganism carried in a host's blood and transmitted through contact with infected blood, tissue, or body fluids.

blood-brain barrier (blŭd brān bar′ē-ĕr)   A structure that is formed from tight capillaries to protect the tissues of the central nervous system from certain substances.

B lymphocyte (bē lim′fŏ-sīt)   A type of nongranular leukocyte that produces antibodies to combat specific pathogens.

board-certified physician (bōrd sěr′ti-fīd fi-zish′ŭn)   A licensed practitioner who has obtained education and licensing for 9 to 12 years and taken multiple tests known as board tests.

body (bod′ē)   Single-spaced lines of text that are the content of a business letter.

body language (bod′ē lang′gwăj)   Nonverbal communication, including facial expressions, eye contact, posture, touch, and attention to personal space.

body mass index (BMI) (bod′ē mas in′deks)   A reliable indicator of healthy weight that is calculated based on height and weight.

body mechanics (bod′ē mě-kan′iks)   The application of physical principles to achieve maximum efficiency and to limit risk of physical stress or injury to the practitioner of physical therapy, massage therapy, or chiropractic or osteopathic manipulation.

body surface area (BSA) (bod′ē sŭr′făs ār′ē-ă)   The area of the external surface of the body, expressed in square meters (m^2); used to calculate metabolic, electrolyte, and nutritional requirements; drug dosage; and expected pulmonary function measurements.

bolus (bō′lŭs)   The mass created when food is combined with saliva and mucus.

bone conduction (bōn kŏn-dŭk′shŭn)   The process by which sound waves pass through the bones of the skull directly to the inner ear, bypassing the outer and middle ears.

bookkeeping (buk kēp′ing)   The systematic recording of business transactions.

botulism (boch′ŭ-lizm)   A life-threatening type of food poisoning that results from eating improperly canned or preserved foods that have been contaminated with the bacterium *Clostridium botulinum*.

boundaries (bown′dăr-ēz)   A physical or psychological space that indicates the limit of appropriate versus inappropriate behavior.

Bowman's capsule (bō′mănz kap′sŭl)   A capsule that surrounds the **glomerulus** of the kidney.

brachial artery (brā′kē-ăl ahr′těr-ē)   An artery that provides a palpable pulse and audible vascular sounds in the antecubital space (the bend of the elbow).

brachytherapy (brak-ē-thār′ă-pe′)   A radiation therapy technique in which a radiologist places temporary radioactive implants close to or directly into cancerous tissue; used for treating localized cancers.

bradycardia (brad′ē-kahr′dē-ă)   A slow heart rate; usually less than 60 beats per minute.

brain stem (brān stem)   A structure that connects the cerebrum to the spinal cord.

breach of contract (brēch kon′trakt)   The violation of or failure to live up to a contract's terms.

bronchi (brong′kī)   The two branches of the trachea that enter the lungs.

bronchial tree (brong′kē-al trē)   A series of tubes that begins where the distal end of the trachea branches.

bronchioles (brong′kē-ōlz)   A part of the respiratory tract that branches from the tertiary bronchi.

buccal (bŭk′ăl)   Between the cheek and gum.

budget (bŭj′ět)   The total sum of money allocated for a particular purpose or period of time.

buffy coat (buf′ē kōt)   The layer between the packed red blood cells and plasma in a centrifuged blood sample; this layer contains the white blood cells and platelets.

bulbourethral glands (bŭl′bō-yū-rē′thrăl glăndz)   Glands that lie beneath the prostate and empty their fluid into the urethra. Their fluid aids in sperm movement.

bulimia nervosa (bŭ-lĭm′ē-ă něr-vō′să)   An eating disorder in which people eat a large quantity of food in a short period of time (bingeing) and then attempt to counter the effects of bingeing by self-induced vomiting, use of laxatives or diuretics, and/or excessive exercise.

bundled codes (bŭn′děld kōds)   When healthcare services that are usually separate are considered as a single entity for purposes of classification and payment.

bundle of His (bŭn′děl hiss)   Also known as the AV bundle, this is the node located between the ventricles of the heart that carries the electrical impulse from the AV node to the bundle branches.

burnout (bŭrn′owt)   The end result of prolonged periods of stress without relief. Burnout is an energy-depleting condition that can affect one's health and career. It can be common for those who work in healthcare.

bursitis (bŭr-sī′tis)   Inflammation of a bursa.

butterfly system (bŭt′ěr-flī sis′těm)   A type of needle used to draw blood from patients with small or fragile veins. Sometimes called a winged infusion set, it has flexible wings attached to the needle and a length of flexible tubing.

CABG   See **coronary artery bypass graft**.

calcaneus (kal-kā′nē-ŭs)   The largest tarsal bone; also called the heel bone.

calcitonin (kal-si-tō′nin)   A hormone produced by the thyroid gland that lowers blood calcium levels by activating osteoblasts.

calibrate (kal′i-brāt) To determine the caliber of; to standardize a measuring instrument.

calibrated spoon (kal′i-brā-tĕd spūn) A spoon that has special markings, or calibrations, that allow you to measure a dose of liquid medication.

calibration syringe (kal′i-brā′shun sir-inj′) A standardized measuring instrument used to check and adjust the volume indicator on a spirometer.

calorie (kal′ŏr-ē) A unit used to measure the amount of energy food produces; the amount of energy needed to raise the temperature of 1 kg of water by 1°C.

calyces (kal′ih-sēz) Small cavities of the renal pelvis of the kidney.

CAM (kam) The acronym for complementary and alternative medicine. Complementary medicine is used with conventional medicine. Alternative medicine is used in place of conventional medicine.

canaliculi (kan-ă-lik′yū-lī) Tiny canals that connect lacunae to each other.

cancellous (kan-sĕl′ŭs) Bone also known as spongy bone. It contains spaces within it containing the red bone marrow.

capillary (kap′i-lar-ē) Branches of arterioles and the smallest type of blood vessel.

capillary puncture (kap′i-lar-ē pungk′shŭr) A blood-drawing technique that requires a superficial puncture of the skin with a sharp point.

capitation (kap′i-tā′shŭn) A payment structure in which a health maintenance organization prepays an annual set fee per patient to a physician.

carboxyhemoglobin (kahr-bok′sē-hē′mŏ-glō′bin) The term used when the hemoglobin of red blood cells is carrying carbon dioxide.

carboxypeptidase (kahr-bok′sē-pep′ti-dās) A pancreatic enzyme that digests proteins.

carcinogen (kahr-sin′ŏ-jen) A factor that is known to cause the formation of cancer.

cardiac catheterization (kahr′dē-ak kath′ĕ-tĕr-ī-zā′shŭn) A diagnostic method in which a catheter is inserted into a vein or an artery in the arm or leg and passed through blood vessels into the heart.

cardiac cycle (kahr′dē-ak sī′kĕl) The sequence of contraction and relaxation that makes up a complete heartbeat.

cardiac output (kahr′dē-ak owt′put) The product of heart rate and stroke volume, measured in liters per minute; the amount of blood that is pumped by the heart in 1 minute.

cardiac rehabilitation (kahr′dē-ak rē′hă-bil′i-tā′shŭn) A systematic program of exercise and nutritional, behavioral, and vocational counseling to optimize the recovery and physiologic capacity of the patient with cardiovascular disease.

cardiac sphincter (kahr′dē-ak sfingk′tĕr) The valve-like structure composed of a circular band of muscle at the juncture of the esophagus and stomach. Also known as the esophageal sphincter.

cardiologist (kahr′dē-ol′ŏ-jist) A specialist who diagnoses and treats diseases of the heart and blood vessels (cardiovascular diseases).

carditis (kahr-dī′tis) Inflammation of the heart.

carpal (kahr′păl) Bone of the wrist.

carpal tunnel syndrome (kahr′păl tŭn′ĕl sin′drōm) A painful disorder caused by compression of the median nerve in the carpal tunnel of the wrist.

carrier (kar′ē-ĕr) A reservoir host who is unaware of the presence of a pathogen and so spreads the disease while exhibiting no symptoms of infection.

cash flow statement (kash flō stāt′mĕnt) A statement that shows the cash on hand at the beginning of a period, the income and disbursements made during the period, and the new amount of cash on hand at the end of the period.

cashier's check (ka-shērz chek) A bank check issued by a bank on bank paper and signed by a bank representative; usually purchased by individuals who do not have checking accounts.

cast (kast) Cylinder-shaped elements with flat or rounded ends, differing in composition and size, that form when protein from the breakdown of cells accumulates and precipitates in the kidney tubules and is washed into the urine. A rigid, external dressing, usually made of plaster or fiberglass, that is molded to the contours of the body part to which it is applied; used to immobilize a fractured or dislocated bone.

catabolism (kă-tab′ō-lizm) The stage of metabolism in which complex substances, including nutrients and body tissues, are broken down into simpler substances and converted into energy.

cataracts (kat′ăr-akt) Cloudy areas that form in the lens of the eye that prevent light from reaching visual receptors.

category (kat′ĕ-gōr′ē) In both ICD-9 and ICD-10, the first three digits of the diagnosis code.

catheter-associated urinary tract infection (CAUTI) (kath′ĕ-tĕr ă-sō′sē-āt-ĕd yūr′i-nar-ē trakt infek′shŭn) A urinary tract infection that may be caused by long-term use of urinary catheters; the longer the catheter is in place, the greater the chance of infection.

catheterization (kath′ĕ-ter-ī-ză′shun) The procedure during which a catheter is inserted into a vessel, an organ, or a body cavity.

caudal (kaw′dăl) See **inferior.**

CD-ROM (sē′dē′rŏm′) A compact disc that contains software programs; an abbreviation for "compact disc—read-only memory."

cecum (sē′kŭm) The first section of the large intestine.

celiac disease (sē′lē-ak di-zēz′) An intolerance to gluten that causes an immune response in the body and reduces the absorption of nutrients in the small intestine.

cell body (sel bŏd′ē) The portion of the neuron that contains the nucleus and organelles.

cell-mediated response (sel mē′dē-āt-id rĕ-spons′) The part of our body's immune response that occurs when T cells bind to antigens on cells and attack the antigens directly.

cell membrane (sel mem′brān) The outer limit of a cell that is thin and selectively permeable. It controls the movement of substances into and out of the cell.

cells (selz) The smallest living units of structure and function.

cellulitis (sel-yū-lī′tis) Inflammation of cellular or connective tissue.

cellulose (sel′yū-lōs) A type of carbohydrate that is found in vegetables and cannot be digested by humans; commonly called fiber.

Celsius (centigrade) (sel′sē-ŭs) One of two common scales for measuring temperature; measured in degrees Celsius, or °C.

Centers for Medicare and Medicaid Services (CMS) (sen′tĕrs med′i-kār medi-kād sĕr′vis-ez) A congressional agency designed to handle Medicare and Medicaid insurance claims. It was formerly known as the Health Care Financing Administration.

central line (sen′trăl līn) A catheter placed in a large vein, usually in the neck, chest, or groin, that is used to give fluids or medications.

central line–associated bloodstream infections (CLABSI) (sen′trăl līn ă-sō′sē-āt-ĕd blŭd′strēm in-fek′shŭnz) Bloodstream infections caused by the entry of infectious microorganisms into the bloodstream through a central line.

central nervous system (CNS) (sen′trăl nĕr′vŭs sis′tĕm) A system that consists of the brain and the spinal cord.

central processing unit (CPU) (sen′trăl pros′es-ing yū′nit) A microprocessor, the primary computer chip responsible for interpreting and executing programs.

centrifuge (sen′tri-fyūzh) A device used to spin a specimen at high speed until it separates into its component parts.

centrioles (sen′trē ōlz) Two cylinder-shaped organs near the cell nucleus that are essential for cell division, by equally dividing chromosomes to the daughter cells.

cerebellum (ser′ĕ-bel′ŭm) An area of the brain inferior to the cerebrum that coordinates complex skeletal muscle coordination.

cerebrospinal fluid (CSF) (ser′ĕ-brō-spī′năl flūo′ĭd) The fluid in the subarachnoid space of the meninges and the central canal of the spinal cord.

cerebrovascular accident (ser′ĕ-brō-vas′kyū-lăr ak′si-dĕnt) A stroke; caused by a hemorrhage in the brain or more often by a clot lodged in a cerebral artery.

cerebrum (ser′ĕ-brŭm) The largest part of the brain; it mainly includes the cerebral hemispheres.

Certificate of Waiver tests (sĕr′ti-fi-kŭt wāv′ĕr tests) Laboratory tests that pose an insignificant risk to the patient if they are performed or interpreted incorrectly, are simple and accurate to such a degree that the risk of obtaining incorrect results is minimal, and have been approved by the Food and Drug Administration for use by patients at home; laboratories performing only Certificate of Waiver tests must meet less stringent standards than laboratories that perform tests in other categories.

certification (sĕr′ti-fi-kā′shŭn) The attainment of board approval and credentialing in a specialty.

certified check (sĕr′ti-fid chek) A payer's check written and signed by the payer, which is stamped "certified" by the bank. The bank has already drawn money from the payer's account to guarantee that the check will be paid.

Certified Medical Assistant (CMA) (sĕr′ti-fid med′i-kăl ă-sis′tănt) A medical assistant whose knowledge about the skills of medical assistants, as summarized by the 2003 AAMA Role Delineation Study areas of competence, has been certified by the Certifying Board of the American Association of Medical Assistants (AAMA).

cerumen (sĕ-rū′mĕn) A wax-like substance produced by glands in the ear canal; also called earwax.

cervical enlargement (sĕr′vi-kăl en-lahrj′mĕnt) The thickening of the spinal cord in the neck region.

cervical orifice (sĕr′vi-kăl ōr′i-fis) The opening of the uterus through the cervix into the vagina.

cervicitis (ser-vi-sī′tis) Inflammation of the cervix.

cervix (sĕr′viks) The lowest portion of the uterus that extends into the vagina.

cesarean section (se-zār′ē-ăn sek′shŭn) A surgical incision of the abdomen and uterus to deliver a baby transabdominally.

chain of command (chān kŏ-mand′) A command hierarchy where a group of people are committed to carrying out orders from the highest authority.

chain of custody (chān kŭs′tŏ-dē) A procedure for ensuring that a specimen is obtained from a specified individual, is correctly identified, is under the uninterrupted control of authorized personnel, and has not been altered or replaced.

CHAMPVA (Civilian Health and Medical Program of the Veterans Administration) (si-vil′yăn helth med′i-kăl prō′gram) A type of health insurance that covers the expenses of families (dependent spouses and children) of veterans with total, permanent, and service-connected disabilities. It also covers the surviving families of veterans who die in the line of duty or as a result of service-connected disabilities.

chancre (shang′ker) A painless ulcer that may appear on the tongue, the lips, the genitalia, the rectum, or elsewhere.

chapters (chap-tĕrz) The breakdown of diagnosis codes by body system or disease. There are 17 chapters in ICD-9 and 21 in ICD-10.

charge slip (chahrj slip) The original record of services performed for a patient and the charges for those services.

check (chek) A bank draft or order written by a payer that directs the bank to pay a sum of money on demand to the payee.

CHEDDAR (ched′er) C: Chief complaint. H: History. E: Examination. D: Details of problem and complaints. D: Drugs and dosage. A: Assessment. R: Return visit information or referral, if applicable.

chemical digestion (kem′i-kăl di-jes′chŭn) The breaking down of food for use by the body caused by enzymes in the body such as amylase.

chemistry (kem′is-trē) The study of the composition of matter and how matter changes.

chemoreceptor (kē′mō-rĕ-sep′tŏr) Any cell that is activated by a change in chemical concentration and results in a nerve impulse. The olfactory, or smell, receptors in the nose are an example of a chemoreceptor.

Cheyne-Stokes respirations (chān stōks res′pir-ā′shŭnz) A pattern of breathing that gradually alternates between deep and shallow breaths with a period of apnea or no breathing that can last from 5 to 40 seconds.

chief cells (chēf sĕlz) Cells in the lining of the stomach that secrete pepsinogen.

chief complaint (CC) (chēf kōm-plānt) The patient's main issue of pain or ailment.

chiropractor (kī′rō-prak′tŏr) A licensed practitioner who uses a system of therapy, including manipulation of the spine, to treat illness or pain. This treatment is done without drugs or surgery.

chlamydia (klă-mid′ē-ă) A common bacterial STI caused by bacterium *Chlamydia trachomatis* that can lead to PID in women.

cholangiography (kō-lan-jē-og′ră-fē) A test that evaluates the function of the bile ducts by injection of a contrast medium directly into the common bile duct (during gallbladder surgery) or through a T-tube (after gallbladder surgery or during radiologic testing) and taking an X-ray.

cholecystography (kō-lē-sis-tog′ră-fē) A gallbladder function test performed by X-ray after the patient ingests an oral contrast agent; used to detect gallstones and bile duct obstruction.

cholesterol (kŏ-les′tĕr-ol) A fat-related substance that the body produces in the liver and obtains from dietary sources; needed in small amounts to carry out several vital functions. High levels of cholesterol in the blood increase the risk of heart and artery disease.

chordae tendineae (kōr′dē ten-din′ē-ē) Cord-like structures that attach the cusps of the heart valves to the papillary muscles in the ventricles.

choroid (kōr′oyd) The middle layer of the eye, which contains the iris, the ciliary body, and most of the eye's blood vessels.

chromosome (krō′mə-sōm′) Thread-like structure composed of DNA.

chronic (kron′ik) Lasting a long time or recurring frequently, as in chronic osteoarthritis.

chronic obstructive pulmonary disease (COPD) (kron′ik ŏb-strŭk′tiv pul′mŏ-nar-ē di-zēz′) A disease characterized by the presence of airflow obstruction as a result of chronic bronchitis or emphysema. It is typically progressive. Cigarette smoking is the leading cause.

chronological résumé (kron′ŏ-loj′ik′ĕl res-yūm′ā) The type of résumé used by individuals who have job experience. Jobs are listed according to date, with the most recent listed first.

chylomicron (kī-lō-mi′kron) The least dense of the lipoproteins; it functions in lipid transportation.

chyme (kīm) The mixture of food and gastric juice.

chymotrypsin (kī-mō-trip′sin) A pancreatic enzyme that digests proteins.

cilia (sil′ēa) Hair-like projections from the outside of the cell membrane on some cell types.

ciliary body (sil′ē-ar-ē bod′ē) A wedge-shaped thickening in the middle layer of the eyeball that contains the muscles that control the shape of the lens.

circumduction (ser-kŭm-dŭk′shŭn) Moving a body part in a circle; for example, tracing a circle with your arm.

cirrhosis (sĭr-ō′sis) A long-lasting liver disease in which normal liver tissue is replaced with nonfunctioning scar tissue.

Civilian Health and Medical Program of the Veterans Administration See CHAMPVA.

civil law (si′vĭl law) Involves crimes against persons. A person can sue another person, business, or the government. Judgments often require a payment of money.

clarification (klar′i-fi-kā′shŭn) Asking questions that provide an increased understanding of a problem.

clarity (klār′i-tē) Clearness in writing or stating a message.

class action lawsuit (klas ak′shŭn law′sŭt) A lawsuit in which one or more people sue a company or other legal entity that allegedly wronged all of them in the same way.

clavicle (klav′i-kĕl) A slender, curved long bone that connects the sternum and the scapula; also called the collar bone.

clean-catch mid-stream urine specimen (klēn kach mid-strēm yūr′in spes′i-mĕn) A type of urine specimen that requires special cleansing of the external genitalia to avoid contamination by organisms residing near the external opening of the urethra and is used to identify the number and types of pathogens present in urine; sometimes referred to as midvoid.

clearinghouse (klēr′ing-hows) A group that takes nonstandard medical billing software formats and translates them into the standard EDI formats.

cleavage (klēv′ăj) The rapid rate of mitosis of a zygote immediately following fertilization.

CLIA ′88 See **Clinical Laboratory Improvement Amendments of 1988.**

clinical diagnosis (klin′i-kăl dī-ăg-nō′sis) A diagnosis based on the signs and symptoms of a disease or condition.

clinical drug trial (klin′i-kăl drŭg trī′al) An internationally recognized research protocol designed to evaluate the efficacy or safety of drugs and to produce scientifically valid results.

Clinical Laboratory Improvement Amendments of 1988 (CLIA ′88) (klin′i-kăl la′bōr-ă-tōr′ē im-prūv′ment ă-mend′ments) A law enacted by Congress in 1988 that placed all laboratory facilities that conduct tests for diagnosing, preventing, or treating human disease or for assessing human health under federal regulations administered by the Health Care Financing Administration (HCFA) and the Centers for Disease Control and Prevention (CDC).

clinical preceptor (klin′i-kăl prē′sep-tŏr) The person at the clinical site who serves as an instructor, but is an employee of the site.

clitoris (klit′ŏr-is) Located anterior to the urethral opening in females. It contains erectile tissue and is rich in sensory nerves.

clock speed (klŏk spēd) A measurement of how many instructions per second that a CPU can process. Clock speed is measured in megahertz (MHz) or gigahertz (GHz).

closed file (klōzd fīl) A file for a patient who has died, has moved away, or for some other reason no longer consults the office for medical expertise.

closed posture (klōzd pŏs′chŭr) A position that conveys the feeling of not being totally receptive to what is being said; arms are often rigid or folded across the chest.

cluster scheduling (klŭs′tĕr sked′jūl-ing) The scheduling of similar appointments together at a certain time of the day or week.

CMA See **Certified Medical Assistant.**

CMS See **Centers for Medicare and Medicaid Services.**

CNS See **central nervous system.**

coagulation (kō-ag′yū-lā′shŭn) The process by which a clot forms in blood.

coccus (kŏk′ŭs) A spherical, round, or ovoid bacterium.

coccyx (kŏk′sĭks) A small, triangular-shaped bone consisting of three to five fused vertebrae.

cochlea (kok′lē-ă) A spiral-shaped canal in the inner ear that contains the hearing receptors.

cochlear implant (kok′lē-ăr im′plant) Amplification device surgically implanted with its stimulating electrodes inserted directly into the non-functioning cochlea.

code linkage (kōd lĭng′kĭj) Analysis of the connection between diagnostic and procedural information in order to evaluate the medical necessity of the reported charges. This analysis is performed by insurance company representatives.

coding (kōd′ing) Putting an identifying mark or phrase on a document to ensure that it is placed in the correct file folder.

coinsurance (kō-in-shŭr′ăns) A fixed percentage of covered charges paid by the insured person after a deductible has been met.

colitis (kō-lī′tis) Inflammation of the colon.

colonoscopy (kō-lon-os′kŏ-pē) A procedure used to determine the cause of diarrhea, constipation, bleeding, or lower abdominal pain by inserting a scope through the anus to provide direct visualization of the large intestine.

colony (kol′ŏ-nē) A distinct group of microorganisms, visible with the naked eye, on the surface of a culture medium.

color family (kŭl′ŏr fam′i-lē) A group of colors that share certain characteristics, such as warmth or coolness, allowing them to blend well together.

colposcopy (kol-pos′kŏ-pē) The examination of the vagina and cervix with an instrument called a colposcope to identify abnormal tissue, such as cancerous or precancerous cells.

combination code (kom′bi-nā′shŭn kōd′) An ICD code in which two diagnoses are included in one code.

combining vowel (kom′bīn-ing vow′ĕl) A vowel (often an *o*) that is placed between a word root and suffix to ease pronunciation.

Commission on Accreditation of Allied Health Education Programs (CAA-HEP) (kŏ-mish′ŭn ă-kred′i-tā′shŭn al′īd helth) A voluntary organization that accredits allied health education programs.

common bile duct (kom′ŏn bīl dŭkt) Duct that carries bile to the duodenum. It is formed from the merger of the cystic and hepatic ducts.

compactible file (kom-pakt′ăbl fīl) File kept on rolling shelves that slide along permanent tracks in the floor and stored close together or stacked when not in use.

complements (kom′plĕ-mĕnts) Proteins, present in serum, that are involved in specific defenses.

complementary medicine (kom′plĕ-men′tăr-ē med′i-sin) A type of medicine that is used with conventional medicine.

complete blood (cell) count (CBC) (kom-plēt′ blŭd kownt) A combination of the following determinations: red blood cell indices and count, white blood cell count, hematocrit, hemoglobin, platelets, and differential blood count.

complete proteins (kom-plēt′ prō′tēnz) Proteins that contain all nine essential amino acids.

complex carbohydrate (kom′pleks kahr′bō-hī′drāt) A long chain of sugar units; also known as a polysaccharide.

complex inheritance (kom′pleks in-her′i-tăns) The inheritance of traits determined by multiple genes.

compliance plan (kom-plī′ăns plan) A process for finding, correcting, and preventing illegal medical office practices.

complimentary closing (kom′plĕ-mĕnt-ăr-ē klōz′ing) The closing remark of a business letter found two spaces below the last line of the body of the letter.

compound (kom′pownd) A substance that is formed when two or more atoms of more than one element are chemically combined.

compound microscope (kom′pownd mī′krŏ-skōp) A microscope that uses two lenses to magnify the image created by condensed light focused through the object being examined.

comprehension (kom′prē-hen′shŭn) Knowledge or understanding of an object, a situation, an event, or a verbal statement.

computed tomography (kŏm-pyū′tĕd tŏ-mog′ră-fē) A radiographic examination that produces a three-dimensional, cross-sectional view of an area of the body; may be performed with or without a contrast medium.

concise (kon-sīs′) Brevity; the use of no unnecessary words.

concurrent care (kon-kŭr′ĕnt kār) Care being provided by more than one physician, such as with specialists.

concussion (kŏn-kŭsh′ŭn) A jarring injury to the brain; the most common type of head injury.

conditioning (kŏn-dish′ŭn-ing) Preparing documents for filing by removing paper clips or other fasteners from documents and mending any tears prior to filing. Also known as inspecting.

conductive hearing loss (kon-dŭk′tiv′hēr′ing laws) A type of hearing loss that occurs when sound waves cannot be conducted through the ear. Most types are temporary.

condyle (kon′dīl) Rounded articular surface on a bone.

cones (kōnz) Light-sensing nerve cells in the eye, at the posterior of the retina, that are sensitive to color, provide sharp images, and function only in bright light.

conflict (kon′flĭkt) An opposition of opinions or ideas.

conjunctiva (kon′jŭngk-tī′vă) The protective membrane that lines the eyelid and covers the anterior of the sclera, or the white of the eye.

conjunctivitis (kōn-jŭngk′ti-vī′tis) A contagious infection of the conjunctiva caused by bacteria, viruses, and allergies. The symptoms may include discharge, red eyes, itching, and swollen eyelids; also commonly called pinkeye.

connective tissue (kŏ-nek′tiv tish′ū) A tissue type that is the framework of the body.

consent (kon-sent′) A voluntary agreement that a patient gives to allow a medically trained person the permission to touch, examine, and perform a treatment.

constructive criticism (kon′strŭkt-iv krit′ĭ-sis′ŭm) A type of critique aimed at giving an individual feedback about his or her performance in order to improve that performance.

consultation (kon′sŭl-tā′shŭn) Meeting of two or more physicians or surgeons to evaluate the nature and progress of disease in a particular patient and to establish diagnosis, prognosis, and/or therapy.

consumable (kŏn-sum′ă-bĕl) Able to be emptied or used up, as with supplies.

consumer education (kŏn-sum′ĕr ed′yū-kā′shŭn) The process by which the average person learns to make informed decisions about goods and services, including healthcare.

contagious (kŏn-tā′jŭs) Having a disease that can easily be transmitted to others.

contaminated (kŏn-tam′i-nā-tĕd) Soiled or stained, particularly through contact with potentially infectious substances; no longer clean or sterile.

continuing education (kŏn-tin′yū-ing ed′yū-kā′shŭn) Systematic professional learning experiences designed to augment knowledge and skills of healthcare professionals; education completed after the initial educational program; required for relicensure in some fields.

contract (kon′trakt) A voluntary agreement between two parties in which specific promises are made.

contraindication (kon'tră-in-di-kā'shŭn) A symptom that renders use of a remedy or procedure inadvisable, usually because of risk.

contrast medium (kon'trast mē'dē-ŭm) A substance that makes internal organs denser and blocks the passage of X-rays to photographic film. Introducing a contrast medium into certain structures or areas of the body can provide a clear image of organs and tissues and highlight indications of how well they are functioning.

controlled substance (kŏn-trōld' sŭb'stăns) A drug or drug product that is categorized as potentially dangerous and addictive and is strictly regulated by federal laws.

control sample (kŏn-trŏl sam'pĕl) A specimen that has a known value; used as a comparison for test results on a patient sample.

contusion (kŏn-tū'zhŭn) A closed wound, or bruise.

conventional medicine (kŏn-vĕn'zhŭn-ĕl med'i-sin) The usual practice of physicians and other allied health professionals, such as physical therapists, psychologists, medical assistants, and registered nurses. Also known as allopathy.

conventions (kŏn-vĕn'zhŭnz) A list of abbreviations, punctuation, symbols, typefaces, and instructional notes appearing in the beginning of the ICD-9. The items provide guidelines for using the code set.

convolutions (kon-vŏ-lū'shŭnz) The ridges of brain matter between the sulci; also called gyri.

coordination of benefits (kō-ōr'di-nā'shŭn ben'ĕ-fits) A legal principle that limits payment by insurance companies to 100% of the cost of covered expenses.

copayment (kō'pā-mĕnt) A fixed or set amount paid for each healthcare or medical service; the remainder is paid by the health insurance plan. Also called a copay.

COPD See **chronic obstructive pulmonary disease.**

cornea (kōr'nē-ă) A transparent area on the front of the outer layer of the eye that acts as a window to let light into the eye.

coronary artery bypass graft (CABG) (kōr'ŏ-nār-ē ahr'tĕr-ē bī'pās graft) A surgery performed to bypass a blockage within a coronary artery with a vessel taken from another area.

coronary circulation (kōr'ŏ-nār-ē sĭr'kyū-lā'shŭn) The part of systemic circulation that provides the heart muscle with oxygen and nutrients and carries away waste products.

corporation (kōr'pŏ-rā'shŭn) A type of business group, such as a medical practice, that is established by law and managed by a board of directors.

corpus callosum (kōr'pŭs ka-lō'sŭm) A thick bundle of nerve fibers that connects the cerebral hemispheres.

corpus luteum (kôr'pŭs lū-tē'ŭm) A ruptured follicle cell in the ovary following ovulation.

cortex (kōr'teks) The outermost layer of the cerebrum.

cortisol (kōr'ti-sol) A steroid hormone that is released when a person is stressed. It decreases protein synthesis.

coryza (kō-rī'ză) Another name for an upper respiratory tract infection; the common cold.

costal (kos'tăl) Cartilage that attaches true ribs to the sternum.

counseling (kown'sĕl-ing) Provision of advice and instruction by a healthcare professional to patients.

counter check (kown'tĕr chek) A special bank check that allows a depositor to draw funds from his own account only, as when he has forgotten his checkbook.

courtesy title (kŭr'ti-sē tī'tl) A title used before a person's name, such as Dr., Mr., or Ms.

covered entity (kŭv'ĕrd en'ti-tē) Any organization that transmits health information in an electronic form that is related in any way with a HIPAA-covered business.

cover sheet (kŭv'ĕr shēt) A form sent with a fax that provides details about the transmission.

Cowper's glands (kow'pĕrz glandz) Bulbourethral glands.

coxal (koks'-al) Pertaining to the bones of the pelvic girdle. The coxa is composed of the ilium, ischium, and pubis. (24)

CPT See **Current Procedural Terminology.**

CPU See **central processing unit.**

cranial (krā'nē-ăl) See **superior.**

cranial nerves (krā'nē-ăl nĕrvs) Peripheral nerves that originate from the brain.

crash cart (krăsh kärt) A rolling cart of emergency supplies and equipment.

creatine phosphate (krē'ă-tēn fos'făt) A protein that stores extra phosphate groups.

credentialing (krĕ-den'shăl-ing) A formal review of the qualifications of a healthcare provider who has applied to participate in a healthcare system or plan.

credit (krĕd'ĭt) An extension of time to pay for services, which are provided on trust.

credit bureau (krĕd'ĭt būr-ō) A company that provides information about the creditworthiness of a person seeking credit.

cricoid cartilage (krī'koyd kahr'ti-lăj) A cartilage of the larynx that forms most of the posterior wall and a small part of the anterior wall.

crime (krīm) An offense against the state committed or omitted in violation of public law.

criminal law (krim'i-năl law) Involves crimes against the state. When a state or federal law is violated, the government brings criminal charges against the alleged offender.

critical care (krit'i-kăl kār) Care provided to unstable, critically ill patients. Constant bedside attention is needed in order to code critical care.

critical thinking (krit'i-kăl thingk'ing) The practice of considering all aspects of a situation when deciding what to believe or what to do.

cross-reference (kraws ref'rĕns) The notation within the ICD-9 of the word *see* after a main term in the index. The *see* reference means that the main term first checked is not correct. Another category must then be used.

cross-referenced (kraws ref'rĕns'd) Filed in two or more places, with each place noted in each file; the exact contents of the file may be duplicated, or a cross-reference form can be created, listing all the places to find the file.

cross-training (kraws trān'ing) The acquisition of training in a variety of tasks and skills.

cryosurgery (krī'ō-sŭr'jĕr-ē) The use of extreme cold to destroy unwanted tissue, such as skin lesions.

cryotherapy (krī'ō-thār'ă-pē) The application of cold to a patient's body for therapeutic reasons.

cryptorchidism (kript-ōr'ki-dizm) Congenital failure of the testes to descend into the scrotal sac.

crystal (kris'tăl) Naturally produced solid of definite form; commonly seen in urine specimens, especially those permitted to cool.

cultural diversity (kŭl′chŭr-ăl di-vĕr′si-tē) The inevitable variety in customs, attitudes, practices, and behavior that exists among groups of people from different ethnic, racial, or national backgrounds who come into contact.

culture (kŭl′chŭr) In the sociologic sense, a pattern of assumptions, beliefs, and practices that shape the way people think and act.

To place a sample of a specimen in or on a substance that allows microorganisms to grow in order to identify the microorganisms present.

culture and sensitivity (C&S) (kŭl′chŭr sen′si-tiv′i-tē) A procedure that involves culturing a specimen and then testing the isolated bacteria's susceptibility (sensitivity) to certain antibiotics to determine which antibiotics would be most effective in treating an infection.

culture medium (kŭl′chŭr mē′dē-ŭm) A substance containing all the nutrients a particular type of microorganism needs to grow.

Current Procedural Terminology (CPT) (kŭr′rĕnt prō-sē′jŭr-ăl tĕr-mi-nol′ŏ-jē) A book with the most commonly used system of procedure codes. It is the HIPAA-required code set for physicians' procedures.

cursor (kŭrs′ōr) A blinking line or cube on a computer screen that shows where the next character that is keyed will appear.

Cushing's disease (kush′ingz dĭ-zēz′) A condition in which a person produces too much cortisol or has used too many steroid hormones. Some of the signs and symptoms include buffalo hump, obesity, a moon face, and abdominal stretch marks; also called hypercortisolism.

cuspids (kŭs′pidz) The sharpest teeth; they tear food.

customized (kŭs′tŏm-īzd) Altering something to meet individual specifications such as when creating unique settings within an EHR software program to meet the needs of a specialty physician or medical office.

cyanosis (sī′ă-nō′sis) A bluish color of skin that results when the supply of oxygen is low in the blood.

cycle billing (sī′kĕl bil′ing) A system that sends invoices to groups of patients every few days, spreading the work of billing all patients over the month while billing each patient only once.

cystic duct (sis′tik dŭkt) The duct from the gallbladder that merges with the hepatic duct to form the common bile duct.

cystitis (sis-tī′tis) Inflammation of the urinary bladder caused by infection.

cytokines (sī′tō-kīnz) Chemicals secreted by T lymphocytes in response to an antigen. Cytokines increase T- and B-cell production, kill cells that have antigens, and stimulate red bone marrow to produce more white blood cells.

cytokinesis (sī′tō-ki-nē′sis) Splitting of the cytoplasm during cell division.

cytoplasm (sī′tō-plazm) The watery intracellular substance that consists mostly of water, proteins, ions, and nutrients.

damages (dam′ij-iz) Money paid as compensation for violating legal rights.

database (dā′tă-bās) A collection of records created and stored on a computer.

dateline (dāt′līn) The line at the top of a letter that contains the month, day, and year.

debridement (dā-brēd-mont′) The removal of debris or dead tissue from a wound to expose healthy tissue.

decibels (des′i-bĕlz) Units for measuring the relative intensity of sounds on a scale from 0 to 130.

deductible (dĕ-dŭk′ti-bĕl) A fixed dollar amount that must be paid by the insured before additional expenses are covered by an insurer.

deep (dēp) Anatomical term meaning closer to the inside of the body.

defamation (def′ĕ-mā′shŭn) Damaging a person's reputation by making public statements that are both false and malicious.

defecation reflex (def-ĕ-kā′shŭn rē′fleks′) The relaxation of the anal sphincters so that feces can move through the anus in the process of elimination.

deflection (dĕ-flek′shŭn) A peak or valley on an electrocardiogram.

dehydration (dē-hī-drā′shŭn) The condition that results from a lack of adequate water in the body.

dementia (dĕ-men′shē-ă) The deterioration of mental faculties from organic disease of the brain.

demographic (dĕ-mog′ră-fik) Statistical data relating to the population and particular groups within it.

dendrite (dĕn′drīt) A type of nerve fiber that is short and branches near the cell body. Its function is to receive information from the neuron.

deoxyhemoglobin (dē-oks′ē-hē′mō-glō-bin) A type of hemoglobin that is not carrying oxygen. It is darker red in color than hemoglobin.

dependent (dē-pen′dĕnt) A person who depends on another person for financial support.

depolarization (dē-pō′lăr-i-zā′shŭn) The loss of polarity, or opposite charges inside and outside; the electrical impulse that initiates a chain reaction resulting in contraction.

depolarized (dē-pō′lăr-īzd) A state in which sodium ions flow to the inside of the cell membrane, making the outside less positive. Depolarization occurs when a neuron responds to stimuli such as heat, pressure, or chemicals.

depression (dē-presh′ŭn) The lowering of a body part.

dermatitis (dĕr′mă-tī′tis) Inflammation of the skin.

dermatologist (dĕr′mă-tol′ŏ-jist) A specialist who diagnoses and treats diseases of the skin, hair, and nails.

dermatome (dĕr′mă-tōm) An area of skin innervated by a spinal nerve.

dermis (dĕr′mis) The middle layer of the skin, which contains connective tissue, nerve endings, hair follicles, sweat glands, and oil glands.

descending colon (dĕ-send′ing kō′lŏn) The segment of the large intestine after the transverse colon that descends the left side of the abdominal cavity.

descending tracts (dĕ-send′ing trakts) Tracts of the spinal cord that carry motor information from the brain to muscles and glands.

desired dose (D) (dez′ īrd dōs) The amount of medication the licensed practitioner has ordered the patient to take.

detrusor muscle (dĕ-trū′sŏr mŭs′ĕl) A smooth muscle that contracts to push urine from the bladder into the urethra.

diabetes insipidus (dī-ă-bē′tēz in-sip′i-dŭs) The condition of excessive thirst and excessive urination related to hyposecretion of ADH so that water is not retained by the kidney.

diabetes mellitus (dī-ă-bē′tēz me-lī′tŭs) Any of several related endocrine disorders characterized by an elevated level of glucose in the blood, caused by a deficiency of insulin or insulin resistance at the cellular level.

diagnosis (Dx) (dī-ăg-nō′sis) The primary condition for which a patient is receiving care.

diagnosis code (dī-ăg-nō′sis kōd) The way a diagnosis is communicated to the third-party payer on the healthcare claim.

diagnostic radiology (dī-ăg-nōs′tik rā′dē-ol′ŏ-jē) The use of X-ray technology to determine the cause of a patient's symptoms.

diapedesis (dī′ă-pĕ-dē′sis) The squeezing of a cell through a blood vessel wall.

diaphoresis (dī′ă-fŏr-ē′sis) Excessive sweating as a result of illness or injury.

diaphragm (dī′ă-fram) A muscle that separates the thoracic and abdominopelvic cavities.

diaphysis (dī′af′i-sis) The shaft of a long bone.

diastolic pressure (dī′ă-stol′ik presh′ŭr) The blood pressure measured when the heart relaxes.

diathermy (dī′ă-thĕr-mē) A type of heat therapy in which a machine produces high-frequency electromagnetic waves that achieve deep heat penetration in muscle tissue.

diencephalon (dī-en-sef′ă-lon) A structure that includes the thalamus and the hypothalamus. It is located between the cerebral hemispheres and is superior to the brain stem.

dietary supplements (dī′ĕ-tār-ē sŭp′lĕ-mĕnts) Vitamins, minerals, herbals, and other substances taken by mouth without a prescription to promote health and well-being.

differential diagnosis (dif′ĕr-en′shăl dī-ăg-nō′sis) The process of determining the correct diagnosis when two or more diagnoses are possible.

differently abled (dif′ĕr-ent′lē ā-bld) Having a condition that limits or changes a person's abilities and may require special accommodations.

diffusion (di-fyū′zhŭn) The movement of a substance from an area of high concentration to an area of low concentration.

digital examination (dij′i-tăl eg-zam′i-nā′shŭn) Part of a physical examination in which the physician inserts one or two fingers of one hand into the opening of a body canal such as the vagina or the rectum; used to palpate canal and related structures.

digital subscriber line (DSL) (dij′i-tăl sŭb-skrī′br līn) A type of modem that operates over telephone lines but uses a different frequency than a telephone, allowing a computer to access the Internet at the same time that a telephone is being used.

diluent (dil′yū-ĕnt) A liquid used to dissolve and dilute another substance, such as a drug.

disability insurance (dis′ă-bil′i-tē in-shŭr′ăns) Insurance that provides a monthly, prearranged payment to an individual who cannot work as the result of an injury or disability.

disaccharide (dī-sak′ă-rīd) A type of carbohydrate that is a simple sugar.

disbursement (dis-bĕrs′-mĕnt) Any payment of funds made by the physician's office for goods and services.

disclaimer (dis-clām′ĕr) A statement of denial of legal liability or that refutes the authenticity of a claim.

disclosure (dĭs-klō′zhŭr) The release of, the transfer of, the provision of access to, or the divulgence in any manner of patient information.

disclosure statement (dis-klō′zhŭr stāt′mĕnt) A written description of agreed terms of payment; also called a federal Truth in Lending Statement.

discrimination (dis-krim′i-nā′shŭn) Unequal and unfair treatment.

disinfectant (dis-in-fek′tănt) A cleaning product applied to instruments and equipment to reduce or eliminate infectious organisms; not used on human tissue.

disinfection (dis-in-fek′shŭn) Destruction of pathogenic microorganisms or their toxins or vectors by direct exposure to chemical or physical agents.

disk cleanup (dĭsk klēn-up) A computer maintenance untility designed to free up disk space on computer users' hard drive.

disk defragmentation (dĭsk dē-frag′mĕnt-tā′shŭn) A computer program designed to increase access speed by rearranging files stored on a disk to occupy contiguous storage locations, a technique commonly known as defragmenting.

dislocation (dis′lō-kā′shŭn) The displacement of a bone end from a joint.

dispense (dis-pens′) To distribute a drug, in a properly labeled container, to a patient who is to use it.

distal (dis′tăl) Anatomical term meaning farther away from a point of attachment or farther away from the trunk of the body.

distal convoluted tubule (dis′tăl kon′vŏ-lūt′ed tū′byūl) The last twisted section of the renal tubule; it is located after the loop of Henle. Several of these tubules merge together to form collecting ducts.

distribution (dis′tri-byū′shŭn) The biochemical process of transporting a drug from its administration site in the body to its site of action.

diversity (di-vĕr′si-tē) Differences among people in terms of identity, age, sex, race, physical ability, ethnicity, religious beliefs, values and mores, sexual orientation, and personality.

diverticula (dī′vĕr-tik′yū-lă) Pouches or sacs opening from a tubular or saccular organ, such as the gut or bladder. Plural of *diverticulum.*

diverticulitis (dī′vĕr-tik′yū-lī′tis) Inflammation of the diverticuli, which are abnormal dilations in the intestine.

diverticulosis (dī′vĕr-tik′ū-lō′sis) Abnormal outpouchings or dilations of the intestine.

DNA (dē′ĕn-ā′) A nucleic acid that contains the genetic information of cells.

doctor of osteopathy (dok′tŏr os′tē-op′ă-thē) A doctor who focuses on the musculoskeletal system and uses hands and eyes to identify and adjust structural problems, supporting the body's natural tendency toward health and self-healing.

doctrine of informed consent (dok′trin in-fōrmd′ kŏn-sent′) The legal basis for informed consent, usually outlined in a state's medical practice act.

doctrine of professional discretion (dok′trin prŏ-fesh′i-năl dis-krē′shŭn) A principle under which a physician can exercise judgment as to whether to show patients who are being treated for mental or emotional conditions their records.

documentation (dok′yū-mĕn-tā′shŭn) The recording of information in a patient's medical record; includes detailed notes about each contact with the patient and about the treatment plan, patient progress, and treatment outcomes.

dorsal (dōr′săl) See **posterior.**

dorsal root (dōr′săl rūt) A portion of a spinal nerve that contains axons of sensory neurons only.

dorsiflexion (dōr-si-flek′shŭn) Pointing the toes upward.

dosage (dō′săj) The size, frequency, and number of doses.

dose (dōs) The amount of a drug given or taken at one time.

dose on hand (*H*) (dōs hand) The amount of medication in each unit of the drug.

dot matrix printer (dŏt mā′trĭks prĭn′ter) An impact printer that creates characters by placing a series of tiny dots next to one another.

double-booking system (dŭb′ĕl buk′-ing sis′tĕm) A system of scheduling in which two or more patients are booked for the same appointment slot, with the assumption that both patients will be seen by the doctor within the scheduled period.

douche (dūsh) Vaginal irrigation, which can be used to administer vaginal medication in liquid form.

downcoding (down′kōd-ing) The insurance carrier bases reimbursement on a code level lower than the one submitted by the provider.

drainage catheter (drān′ăj kath′ĕ-ter) A type of catheter used to withdraw fluids.

dressing (drĕs′ĭng) A sterile material used to cover a surgical or other wound.

dual coverage (d′yū-ăl kŭv′ĕr-ăj) Term used when a patient is covered by Medicare and Medicaid.

dual-energy X-ray absorptiometry (DXA) (dū′ăl en′ĕr-jē x-rā ăb-sōrp′shē-om′ĕ-trē) A screening test that uses small doses of X-rays to determine the mineral density of a person's bones; also called *bone densitometry.*

ductus arteriosus (dŭk′tŭs ar-tēr′ē-ō′sus) The connection in the fetus between the pulmonary trunk and the aorta.

ductus venosus (duk′tŭs vē-nō′sŭs) A blood vessel that allows most of the blood to bypass the liver in the fetus.

duodenum (dū′ō-dē′nŭm) The first section of the small intestine.

durable item (dūr′ă-bĕl ĭ′tem) A piece of equipment that is used repeatedly, such

as a telephone, computer, or examination table; contrast with *expendable item.*

durable power of attorney (dūr′ă-bĕl pow′ĕr ă-tŏr′nē) A document naming the person who will make decisions regarding medical care on behalf of another person if that person becomes unable to do so.

dwarfism (dwōrf′ĭzm) A condition in which too little growth hormone is produced, resulting in an abnormally small stature.

dysmenorrhea (dis-men-ōr-ē′ă) Severe menstrual cramps that limit daily activity.

dysrhythmia (dis-ritĭh′mē-ă) An irregularity in heart rhythm; also called *arrhythmia.*

dyspnea (disp′-nēă) Difficult or painful breathing.

ear ossicles (ēr os′i-kĕlz) Three tiny bones called the malleus, the incus, and the stapes located in the middle ear cavity. They are the smallest bones of the body.

eccrine gland (ek′rin glănd) The most numerous type of sweat gland. Eccrine sweat glands produce a watery type of sweat and are activated primarily by heat.

ECG See **electrocardiogram.**

echocardiography (ek′ō-kahr-dē-og′ră-fē) A procedure that tests the structure and function of the heart through the use of reflected sound waves, or echoes.

E code (ē kōd) A type of code in the ICD-9. E codes identify the external causes of injuries and poisoning.

ectoderm (ek′tō-derm) The primary germ layer that gives rise to nervous tissue and some epithelial tissue.

ectropion (ek-trō′pē-ŭn) Eversion of the lower eyelid.

eczema (ek′sĕ-mă) Inflammatory condition of the skin.

edema (ĕ-dē′mă) An excessive buildup of fluid in body tissue.

EDI See **electronic data interchange.**

editing (ed′i-ting) The process of ensuring that a document is accurate, clear, and complete; free of grammatical errors; organized logically; and written in the appropriate style.

effacement (e-fās′mĕnt) Thinning of the cervix in preparation for childbirth.

effectors (e-fek′tŏrz) Muscles and glands that are stimulated by motor neurons in the peripheral nervous system.

efferent arterioles (ef′ĕr-ĕnt ahr-tēr′ē-ōlz) Structures that deliver blood to peritubular capillaries that are wrapped around the renal tubules of the nephron in the kidneys.

efferent nerves (ef′ĕr-ĕnt nĕrvz) Motor nerves that take information or impulses from the central nervous system to the peripheral nervous system to allow for the movement or action of a muscle or gland.

efficacy (ef′i-kă-sē) The therapeutic value of a procedure or therapy, such as a drug.

efficiency (ĕ-fish′ĕn-sē) The ability to produce a desired result with the least effort, expense, and waste.

EHR See **electronic health records.**

EIA See **enzyme immunoassay.**

elderly (el′dĕr-lē) Individuals over the age of 65.

elective procedure (ĕ-lek′tiv prŏ-sē′jŭr) A medical procedure that is not required to sustain life but is requested for payment to the third-party payer by the patient or physician. Some elective procedures are paid for by third-party payers, whereas others are not.

electrocardiogram (ECG) (ĕ-lek′trō-kahr′dē-ō-gram) The tracing made by an electrocardiograph.

electrocardiograph (ĕ-lek′trō-kahr′dē-ō-graf) An instrument that measures and displays the waves of electrical impulses responsible for the cardiac cycle.

electrocardiography (ĕ-lek′trō-kahr-dē-og′ră-fē) The process by which a graphic pattern is created to reflect the electrical impulses generated by the heart as it pumps.

electrocauterization (ĕ-lek′trō-kaw′tĕr-ī-zā′shŭn) The use of a needle, probe, or loop heated by electric current to remove growths such as warts, to stop bleeding, and to control nosebleeds that either will not subside or continually recur.

electrode (ĕ-lek′trōd) Sensor that detects electrical activity.

electroencephalography (ĕ-lek′trō-en-se-f′ă-log′ră-fē) A procedure that records the electrical activity of the brain as a tracing called an electroencephalogram, or EEG, on a strip of graph paper.

electrolytes (ĕ-lek′trō-līts) Substances that carry electrical current through the movement of ions.

electromyography (ĕ-lek′trō-mī-og′ră-fē) A procedure in which needle electrodes are inserted into some of the skeletal muscles and a monitor records the nerve impulses and measures conduction time; used to detect neuromuscular disorders or nerve damage.

electronic data interchange (EDI) (ĕ-lek-tron′ik dā′tă in′tĕr-chānj) Transmitting electronic medical insurance claims from providers to payers using the necessary information systems.

electronic health records (EHR) (ĕ-lek-tron′ik helth rek′ŏrdz) Patient health records created and stored on a computer or other electronic storage device. Also known as *electronic medical records.*

electronic mail (ĕ-lek-tron′ik māl) A method of sending and receiving messages through a computer network; commonly known as e-mail.

electronic media (ĕ-lek-tron′ik mē′dē-ă) Any transmissions that are physically moved from one location to another through the use of magnetic tape, disk, compact disk media, or any other form of digital or electronic technology.

electronic medical record (EMR) (ĕ-lek-tron′ik med′i-kăl rek′ŏrd) Patient medical record created and stored on a computer or other electronic storage device.

electronic transaction record (ĕ-lek-tron′ik tranz-ak′shŭn rek′ŏrd) The standardized codes and formats used for the exchange of medical data.

elevation (el′ĕ-vā′shŭn) The raising of a body part.

ELISA test See **enzyme-linked immuno-sorbent assay test.**

embolism (em′bŏ-lizm) An obstruction in a blood vessel.

embolus (em′bŏ-lŭs) A portion of a thrombus that breaks off and moves through the bloodstream.

embryo (em′brē-ō) A group of cells, called the *inner cell mass,* that develops from the blastocyst during the embryonic prenatal period to become the fetus.

embryonic period (em-brē-on′ik pēr′ē-ŏd) The second through eighth weeks of pregnancy.

E/M code (ē/ĕm kōd) Evaluation and management codes that are often considered the most important of all CPT codes. The E/M section guidelines explain how to code different levels of services.

empathy (ĕm′pă-thē) Identification with or sensitivity to another person's feelings and problems.

emphysema (em′fi-sē′mă) A chronic lung condition consisting of damage to the alveoli of the lungs. It is heavily associated with smoking, which causes stretching of the spaces between the alveoli and paralyzes the cilia of the respiratory system.

employee handbook (em-ploy′ē hand′-buk) A synopsis of human resources policies and procedures.

employment contract (em-ploy′mĕnt kon′trakt) A written agreement of employment terms between employer and employee that describes the employee's duties and the considerations (money, benefits, and so on) to be given by the employer in exchange.

empyema (em′pī-ē′mă) A collection of pus in the pleural cavity.

EMR See **electronic medical record.**

enclosures (en-klō′zhŭrz) Materials that are included in the same envelope as the primary letter.

encounter form (en-kown′tĕr fōrm) A form that combines the charges for services rendered, an invoice for payment or insurance copayment, and all the information for submitting an insurance claim; also known as a superbill.

endocardium (en′dō-kahr′dē-ŭm) The innermost layer of the heart.

endochondral (en′dō-kon′drăl) A type of ossification in which bones start out as cartilage models.

endocrine gland (en′dō-krin gland) A gland that secretes its products directly into tissue, fluid, or blood.

endocrinologist (en′dō-kri-nol′ŏ-jist) A specialist who diagnoses and treats disorders of the endocrine system, which regulates many body functions by circulating hormones that are secreted by glands throughout the body.

endoderm (ĕn′dō-derm) The primary germ layer that gives rise to epithelial tissues only.

endogenous infection (en-doj′ĕ-nŭs in-fek′shŭn) An infection in which an abnormality or a malfunction in routine body processes causes normally beneficial or harmless microorganisms to become pathogenic.

endolymph (ĕn′dō-limf) A fluid in the inner ear. When this fluid moves, it activates hearing and equilibrium receptors.

endometriosis (en′dō-mē-trē-ō′sis) A condition in which tissues that make up the lining of the uterus grow outside the uterus.

endometrium (en′dō-mē′trē-ŭm) The innermost layer of the uterus. It undergoes significant changes during the menstrual cycle.

endomysium (en′dō-miz′ē-ŭm) A connective tissue covering that surrounds individual muscle cells.

endoplasmic reticulum (en′dō-plas′mik rĕ-tik′yū-lŭm) The organelles of the endoplasmic reticulum are composed of both smooth and rough types. The rough type contains ribosomes on its surface. The smooth type has no ribosomes. Both types create a network of passageways throughout the cytoplasm.

endorse (en-dōrs′) To sign or stamp the back of a check with the proper identification of the person or organization to whom the check is made out, to prevent the check from being cashed if it is stolen or lost.

endorsement (en-dōrs′-mĕnt) Signature on the back of a check with the terms for accepting the check as payment.

endoscopy (en-dos′kŏ-pē) Any procedure in which a scope is used to visually inspect a canal or cavity within the body.

endosteum (en-dos′tē-ŭm) A membrane that lines the medullary cavity and the holes of spongy bone.

engineered safety devices (en′jin-ērd sāf′tē dĕ-vīs′) Devices specifically designed to isolate or remove a hazard. These include needles with safety shields and self-shielding needles.

entropion (en-trō′pē-on) Inversion of the lower eyelid.

enunciation (ē-nŭn-sī-ā′shŭn) Clear and distinct speaking.

enuresis (en-yūr-ē′sis) Bed wetting.

enzyme immunoassay (EIA) (ĕn′zīm im′yū-nō-as′ā) The detection of substances by immunologic methods. This method involves an antigen, an antibody specific for the antigen, and a second antibody conjugated to an enzyme.

enzyme-linked immunosorbent assay (ELISA) test (ĕn′zīm-lĭngkt im′yū-nō-sōr′bent ăs′ā tĕst) A blood test that confirms the presence of antibodies developed by the body's immune system in response to an initial HIV infection.

EOB See **explanation of benefits.**

eosinophil (ē-ō-sin′ō-fil)   A type of granular leukocyte that captures invading bacteria and antigen-antibody complexes through phagocytosis.

epicardium (ep-i-kar′dē-ŭm)   The outermost layer of the wall of the heart. Also known as the **visceral pericardium**.

epidermis (ep′i-děr′mis)   The most superficial layer of the skin.

epididymis (ep-i-did′i-mis)   An elongated structure attached to the back of the testes and in which sperm cells mature.

epididymitis (ep-i-did-i-mī′tis)   Inflammation of an **epididymis**. Most cases result from infection.

epiglottic cartilage (ep-i-glot′ik kahr′ti-lăj)   A cartilage of the larynx that forms the framework of the epiglottis.

epiglottis (ep-i-glot′is)   The flap-like structure that closes off the larynx during swallowing.

epilepsy (ep′i-lep′sē)   A condition that occurs when parts of the brain receive a burst of electrical signals that disrupt normal brain function; also called seizures.

epimysium (ep′i-mis′ē-ŭm)   A thin covering that is just deep to the fascia of a muscle. It surrounds the entire muscle.

epinephrine (ep′i-nef′rin)   An injectable medication used to treat anaphylaxis by causing vasoconstriction to increase blood pressure. Also, a hormone secreted from the adrenal glands. It increases heart rate, breathing rate, and blood pressure.

epiphyseal disk (ep-i-fiz′ē-ăl dĭsk)   A plate of cartilage between the **epiphysis** and the **diaphysis**.

epiphysis (e-pif′i-sis)   The expanded end of a long bone.

episiotomy (e-piz′ē-ot′ŏ-mē)   A surgical incision of the female perineum to enlarge the vaginal opening for delivery.

epistaxis (ĕp′i-stak′sis)   Nosebleed.

epithelial tissue (ep′i-thē′lē-ăl tish′ū)   A tissue type that lines the tubes, hollow organs, and cavities of the body.

e-prescribing (ē-prĕ-skrĭb′ing)   Prescriptions are entered electronically and transmitted directly to the pharmacy.

erectile tissue (ĕ-rek′tĭl tish′ū)   A highly specialized tissue located in the shaft of the penis. It fills with blood to achieve an erection.

ergonomics (ĕr′gŏ-nom′iks)   The science of workplace, tools, and equipment designed to reduce worker discomfort, strain, and fatigue and to prevent work-related injuries.

erythema (er-i-thē′mă)   Redness of the skin.

erythroblastosis fetalis (ĕ-rith′rō-blas-tō′sis fē-tā′lis)   A serious anemia that develops in a fetus with Rh-positive blood as a result of antibodies in an Rh-negative mother's body.

erythrocyte (ĕ-rith′rŏ-sīt)   Red blood cell.

erythrocyte sedimentation rate (ESR) (ĕ-rith′rŏ-sīt sed′i-měn-tā′shŭn rāt)   The rate at which red blood cells, the heaviest blood component, settle to the bottom of a blood sample.

erythropoietin (ĕ-rith′rō-poy′ĕ-tin)   A hormone secreted by the kidney and responsible for regulating the production of red blood cells.

esophageal hiatus (ĕ-sof′ă-jē′ăl hī-ā′tŭs)   Hole in the diaphragm through which the esophagus passes.

ESR   See erythrocyte sedimentation rate.

established patient (es-tab′lisht pā′shěnt)   A patient who has seen the physician within the past 3 years. This determination is important when using E/M codes.

estrogen (es′trŏ-jen)   A female sex hormone; when produced during ovulation, estrogen causes a buildup of the lining of the uterus (womb) to prepare it for a possible pregnancy.

ethics (ĕth′ĭks)   General principles of right and wrong, as opposed to requirements of law.

ethmoid (ĕth′moyd)   Bones located between the sphenoid and nasal bone that form part of the floor of the cranium.

ethylenediaminetetraacetic acid (EDTA) (eth′i-lĕn-dī′ă-mēn-tet′ră-ă-sē′tik as′id)   A chelating agent and anticoagulant; added to blood specimens for hematologic and other tests.

etiologic agent (ē′tē-ə-lŏj′ĭk ā′jənt)   A living microorganism or its toxin that may cause human disease.

etiology (ē′tē-ol′ŏ-jē)   The science and study of the causes of disease and their mode of operation.

etiquette (ĕt′ĭ-ket′)   Good manners.

eustachian tube (yū-stā′-shē-an tūb)   An opening in the middle ear, leading to the back of the throat, that helps equalize air pressure on both sides of the eardrum.

eversion (ē-ver′zhŭn)   Turning the sole of the foot laterally.

exclusion (eks-klū′zhŭn)   An expense that is not covered by a particular insurance policy, such as an eye examination or dental care.

excretion (eks-krē′shŭn)   The elimination of waste by a discharge; in drug metabolism, the manner in which a drug is eliminated from the body.

exocrine gland (ek′sō-krin gland)   A gland that secretes its product into a duct.

exogenous infection (eks-oj′ĕ-nŭs in-fek′shŭn)   An infection that is caused by the introduction of a pathogen from outside the body.

exophthalmos (eks′of-thal′mos)   Bulging of the eyeballs, often related to hyperthyroidism.

expendable item (eks-pen′dă-běl ī′tem)   An item that is used and must then be restocked; also known collectively as supplies. Contrast with *durable item.*

expiration (eks-pir-ā′shŭn)   The process of breathing out; also called exhalation.

explanation of benefits (EOB) (eks′plă-nā′shŭn ben′ĕ-fits)   Information that explains the medical claim in detail; also called **remittance advice (RA).**

explanation of payment (EOP) (eks′plă-nā′shŭn pā′měnt)   Document sent by an insurance carrier when payment is made describing the terms of the payments. Also known as **explanation of benefits (EOB)** or **remittance advice (RA).**

exposure control plan (eks-pō′zhŭr kŏn-trōl′ plan)   A written document of practices and procedures, required equipment, and facilities designed to minimize employee exposure to infectious agents or biohazardous materials.

expressed contract (eks-prest′ kon′trakt)   A contract clearly stated in written or spoken words.

extension (eks-ten′shŭn)   An unbending or straightening movement of the two elements of a jointed body part.

external auditory canal (eks-těr′năl aw′di-tōr-ē kă-nal′)   Canal that carries sound waves to the tympanic membrane; commonly called the ear canal.

extrinsic eye muscles (eks-trin′zik ī mŭs′ělz)   The skeletal muscles that move the eyeball.

face page (fās pāj′)   A screen that provides an overview or "snapshot" of the patient demographic information in an EHR system.

face sheet (fās shēt) A screen that provides an overview or "snapshot" of the patient demographic information in an EHR system.

facsimile machine (fak-si′milē mă-shēn′) A piece of office equipment used to send a facsimile, or fax, over telephone lines from one modem to another; more commonly called a fax machine.

factual teaching (fak′chū-ăl tēch′ing) Method of teaching that provides the patient with details of the information that is being taught.

facultative (fak′ŭl-tā-tiv) Able to adapt to different conditions; in microbiology, able to grow in environments either with or without oxygen.

Fahrenheit (far′ĕn-hīt) One of two common scales used for measuring temperature; measured in degrees Fahrenheit, or °F.

fallopian tubes (fă-lō′pē-ăn tūbz) Tubes that extend from the uterus on each side and that open near an ovary.

family practitioner (făm′i-lē prăk-tĭsh′i-ner) A physician who does not specialize in a branch of medicine but treats all types and ages of patients; also called a general practitioner.

fascia (fash′e-ă) A structure that covers entire skeletal muscles and separates them from each other.

fascicle (fas′i-kĕl) Sections of a muscle divided by connective tissue called perimysium.

febrile (feb′ril) Having a body temperature above one's normal range.

fecal occult blood test (FOBT) (fē′kăl ŏ-kŭlt′ blŭd test) A test to find hidden blood in the stool.

feces (fē′sēz) Material found in the large intestine and made from leftover chyme. Feces are eventually eliminated through the anus.

Federal Insurance Contributions Act (FICA) (fed′ĕr′ăl in-shŭr′ăns kon′tri-byū-shunz akt) A law that requires employers to deduct a certain amount from each employee's paycheck to fund Social Security and Medicare.

Federal Unemployment Tax Act (FUTA) (fĕd′ĕr-al em-ploy′mĕnt taks akt) This act requires employers to pay a percentage of each employee's income up to a certain dollar amount.

feedback (fēd′băk) Verbal and nonverbal evidence that a message was received and understood.

feedback loop (fēd′băk lūp) A mechanism to control hormone levels. The two types are positive and negative feedback loops.

fee-for-service (fē sĕr′vis) A major type of health plan. It repays policyholders for the costs of healthcare that are due to illness and accidents.

fee schedule (fē sked′jūl) A list of the costs of common services and procedures performed by a physician.

felony (fel′ŏnē) A serious crime, such as murder or rape, that is punishable by imprisonment. In certain crimes, a felony is punishable by death.

femoral (fem′ŏ-răl) Relating to the femur or thigh.

femur (fē′mŭr) The bone in the upper leg; commonly called the thigh bone.

fenestrated drape (fen′ĕs-trāt-ĕd drāp) A drape that has a round or slit-like opening that provides access to the surgical site.

fertilization (fĕr′til-i-zā′shŭn) The process in which an egg unites with a sperm.

fetal period (fē′tăl pēr′ē-ŏd) A period that begins at week nine of pregnancy and continues through delivery of the offspring.

fetus (fē′tŭs) The product of conception from the end of the eighth week to the moment of birth.

fiber (fī′bĕr) The tough, stringy part of vegetables and grains, which is not absorbed by the body but aids in a variety of bodily functions.

fibrinogen (fī-brin′ō-jen) A protein found in plasma that is important for blood clotting.

fibroid (fī′broyd) A benign tumor in the uterus composed of fibrous tissue.

fibromyalgia (fī-brō-mī-al′jē-ă) A condition that exhibits chronic pain primarily in joints, muscles, and tendons.

fibula (fib′yū-lă) The lateral bone of the lower leg.

file guide (fīl gīd) A heavy cardboard or plastic insert used to identify a group of file folders in a file drawer.

filtration (fil-trā′shŭn) A process that separates substances into solutions by forcing them across a membrane.

fimbriae (fi′m-brē-ē) Fringe-like structures that border the entrances of the fallopian tubes.

firewall (fīr′wawl) A system that protects a computer network from unauthorized access by users on its own network or another network such as the Internet.

first morning urine specimen (first mōr′ning yūr′in spes′i-mĕn) A urine specimen that is collected after a night's sleep; contains greater concentrations of substances that collect over time than specimens taken during the day.

fixative (fik′să-tiv) A solution sprayed on a slide immediately after the specimen is applied. It is used to preserve and hold the cells in place until a microscopic examination is performed.

flaccid (fla′sid) Weak, soft; not erect.

flagellum (flă-jel′ŭm) The "tail-like" structure on some cell membranes that provides cell movement.

flexion (flek′shŭn) A bending movement of the two elements of a jointed body part.

floater (flōt′ĕr) A nonsterile assistant who is free to move about the room during surgery and attend to unsterile needs.

fluidotherapy (flū′id-ō-thār′ă-pē) A technique for stimulating healing, particularly in the hands and feet, by placing the affected body part in a container of glass beads that are heated and agitated with hot air.

follicle (fol′i-kĕl) An accessory organ of the skin that is found in the dermis and the sites at which hairs emerge.

follicle-stimulating hormone (FSH) (fol′i-kĕl stim′yū-lāt-ing hōr′mōn) A hormone that in females stimulates the production of estrogen by the ovaries; in males, it stimulates sperm production.

follicular cells (fŏ-lik′yū-lăr selz) Small cells contained in the primordial follicle along with a large cell called a primary oocyte.

folliculitis (fŏ-lik-yū-lī′tis) Inflammation of the hair follicle.

fomite (fō′mīt) An inanimate object, such as clothing, body fluids, water, or food, that may be contaminated with infectious organisms and thus transmit disease.

fontanels (fon′tă-nelz′) Soft spots in an infant's skull that consist of tough membranes that connect to incompletely developed bone.

food exchange (fūd eks-chānj′) A unit of food in a particular food category that provides the same amounts of protein, fat, and carbohydrates as all other units of food in that category.

foramen magnum (fōr-ā′měn mag′nŭm) The large hole in the occipital bone that allows the brain to connect to the spinal cord.

foramen ovale (fōr-ā′měn ō-va′lē) A hole in the fetal heart between the right atrium and the left atrium.

forced vital capacity (FVC) (fōrst vī′tăl kă-pas′i-tē) The greatest volume of air that a person is able to expel when performing rapid, forced expiration.

formalin (fōr′mă-lin) A dilute solution of formaldehyde used to preserve biological specimens.

formed elements (fōrmd el′ě-měnts) Red blood cells, white blood cells, and platelets; compose 45% of blood volume.

Form I-9 A federal form for verifying that an employee is a US citizen, a legally admitted alien, or an alien authorized to work in the United States.

formula method (fōrm′yū-lă meth′ŏd) A basic formula to calculate dosage. D/H × Q, where D: desired dose, H: dose on hand, Q: quantity of the dose.

formulary (fōrm′yū-lar-ē) An insurance plan's list of approved prescription medications.

Form W-2 The tax form that an employer must send to an employee and the IRS at the end of the year. It reports an employee's annual wages and the amount of taxes withheld from his or her paycheck.

Form W-4 A tax form completed by an employee to indicate his or her tax situation, such as exemptions and status, to the employer.

fracture (frak′shŭr) Any break in a bone.

fraud (frawd) An act of deception that is used to take advantage of another person or entity.

frequency (frē′kwěn-sē) The number of complete fluctuations of energy per second in the form of waves.

frontal (frŏn′tăl) Anatomical term that refers to the plane that divides the body into anterior and posterior portions. Also called coronal.

FSH See **follicle-stimulating hormone.**

fulgurated (ful′gŭr-āt-ed) The use of heat or laser to burn or destroy tissue.

full-block letter style (ful′ blok let′ěr stīl) A letter format in which all lines begin flush left; also called block style.

functional résumé (fŭngk′shŭn-ăl rez′ŭm-ā) A résumé that highlights specialty areas of a person's accomplishments and strengths.

fundus (fun′dŭs) The upper, domed portion of an organ.

fungus (fŭng′gŭs) A eukaryotic organism that has a rigid cell wall at some stage in the life cycle.

FUTA See **Federal Unemployment Tax Act.**

FVC See **forced vital capacity.**

gait (gāt) The way a person walks, consisting of two phases: stance and swing.

ganglia (gang′glē-ă) Collections of neuron cell bodies outside the central nervous system.

gastric juice (găs′trĭk jūs) Secretions from the stomach lining that begin the process of digesting protein.

gastritis (gă-strī′tĭs) Inflammation of the stomach lining.

gastroenterologist (găs′trō-ěn-ter-ol′ō-jist) A specialist who diagnoses and treats disorders of the entire gastrointestinal tract, including the stomach, intestines, and associated digestive organs.

gastroesophageal reflux disease (GERD) (gas′trō-ě-sof′ă-jē′ăl rē′flŭks di-zēz) A condition that occurs when stomach acids are pushed into the esophagus and cause heartburn.

gene (jēn) A segment of DNA that determines a body trait.

general duty clause (jen′ěr-ăl dū′tē klawz) An OSHA clause that requires an employer to maintain a workplace free from hazards that are recognized as likely to cause death or serious injury.

general physical examination (jen′ěr-ăl fiz′i-kăl eg-zam′i-nā′shŭn) An examination performed by a physician to confirm a patient's health or to diagnose a medical problem.

generic name (jě-ner′ik năm) A drug's official name.

geriatrician (jer′ē-at′-trish′ăn) A specialist who cares for elderly individuals, usually those over the age of 65.

gerontologist (jer′ŏn-tol′ŏ-jist) A specialist who studies the aging process.

GH See **growth hormone.**

gigantism (jī-gan′tizm) A condition in which too much growth hormone is produced in childhood, resulting in an abnormally increased stature.

glans penis (glanz pē′nĭs) A cone-shaped structure at the end of the penis.

glaucoma (glaw-kō′mă) A condition in which too much pressure is created in the eye by excessive aqueous humor. This excess pressure can lead to permanent damage of the optic nerves, resulting in blindness.

Globally Harmonized System of Classification and Labeling of Chemicals (GHS) (glō′băl-lē har′-mŏn-izd sis′těm klas′i-fi-kā′shŭn lā′běl-ing kem′i-kălz) A system for standardizing the classification and labeling of chemicals developed by the United Nations as a guide for regulatory systems around the world. In the United States, OSHA's Hazard Communication Standard is now aligned with the GHS.

global period (glō′băl pěr′ē-ŏd) The period of time that is covered for follow-up care of a procedure or surgical service.

globulins (glob′yū-linz) Plasma proteins that transport lipids and some vitamins.

glomerular filtrate (glō-mer′yū-lăr fil′trāt) The fluid remaining in the glomerular capsule after glomerular filtration.

glomerular filtration (glō-mer′yū-lăr fil′trā-shŭn) The process by which urine forms in the kidneys as blood moves through a tight ball of capillaries called the glomerulus.

glomerulonephritis (glō-mer′yū-lō-ně-frī′tis) An inflammation of the glomeruli of the kidney.

glomerulus (glō-mer′yū-lŭs) A group of capillaries in the renal corpuscle.

glottis (glot′is) The opening between the vocal cords.

glucagon (glū′kă-gon) A hormone that increases glucose concentrations in the bloodstream and slows down protein synthesis.

gluten (glū′těn) The insoluble protein (prolamines) constituent of wheat and other grains; a mixture of gliadin, glutenin, and other proteins; believed to be an agent in celiac disease.

glycogen (glī′kō-jen) An excess of glucose that is stored in the liver and in skeletal muscle.

glycosuria (glī′kō-syūr′ē-ă) The presence of significant levels of glucose in the urine.

goiter (goy′těr) Enlargement of the thyroid gland, which causes swelling of the neck, often related to iodine insufficiency in the diet.

Golgi apparatus (gol′jē ap′ă-rat′ŭs) The cell's Golgi apparatus synthesizes carbohydrates and appears to prepare and store secretions for discharge from the cell.

gonadotropin-releasing hormone (GnRH) (gō-nad′ō-trō′pin-rĕ-lēs′ing hōr′mōn) Hormone that stimulates the anterior pituitary gland to release follicle-stimulating hormone (FSH).

gonads (gō′nădz) The reproductive organs: namely, in women the ovaries, and in men the testes.

goniometer (gō′nē-om′ĕ-tĕr) A protractor device that measures range of motion.

gout (gowt) A medical condition characterized by an elevated uric acid level and recurrent acute arthritis.

G-protein (jē-prō′tēn) A substance that causes enzymes in the cell to activate following the activation of the hormone-receptor complex in the cell membrane.

Gram-negative (gram′ nĕg′ă-tĭv) Referring to bacteria that lose their purple color when a decolorizer has been added during a Gram stain.

Gram-positive (gram′ pŏz′ĭ-tĭv) Referring to bacteria that retain their purple color after a decolorizer has been added during a Gram stain.

Gram stain (gram stān) A method of staining that differentiates bacteria according to the chemical composition of their cell walls.

granular leukocyte (gran′yū-lăr lū′kō-sīt) A type of leukocyte (white blood cell) with a segmented nucleus and granulated cytoplasm; also known as a polymorphonuclear leukocyte.

granulocyte (gran′yū-lō-sīt) See **granular leukocyte.**

Graves' disease (grāvz dĭ-zēz′) A disorder in which a person develops antibodies that attack the thyroid gland.

gray matter (grā măt′ər) The inner tissue of the brain and the spinal cord that is darker in color than white matter. It contains all the bodies and dendrites of nerve cells.

grievance process (grē-văns pros′es) A mediation process through the human resources department utilized when an employee or employees feel they are treated unjustly.

gross earnings (grōs ĕrn′ingz) The total amount an employee earns before deductions.

group practice (grūp prak′tis) A medical management system in which a group of three or more licensed physicians share their collective income, expenses, facilities, equipment, records, and personnel.

growth chart (grōth chahrt) A chart consisting of percentile curves that are used to determine a child's growth in relation to average rates.

growth hormone (GH) (grōth hôr′mōn′) A hormone that stimulates an increase in the size of the muscles and bones of the body.

growth plate (grōth plāt) A shaft of cartilage between the epiphysis and the diaphysis; also known as the *epiphyseal disk.*

guarantor (gar′ăn-tōr) The patient, caregiver, or entity responsible for payment of the healthcare bill.

gustatory cortex (gŭs′tă-tōr-ē kōr′teks) An area of the brain that is responsible for interpreting taste sensations by integrating information from the taste cells with other information to provide a more complete interpretation.

gustatory receptors (gŭs′tă-tōr-ē rĕ-sep′tŏrz) Taste receptors that are found on taste buds.

gynecologist (gīnĕ-kol′ō-jist) A specialist who performs routine physical care and examinations of the female reproductive system.

gyri (jī′rī) The ridges of brain matter between the sulci; also called **convolutions.**

hairy leukoplakia (hār′ē lū′kō-plā′kē-ă) A white lesion on the tongue associated with AIDS.

hapten (hap′tĕn) Foreign substances in the body too small to start an immune response by themselves.

hard copy (hahrd kŏp′ē) A readable paper copy or printout of information.

hard skills (hahrd skilz) Specific technical and operational proficiencies.

hardware (hahrd′wār) The physical components of a computer system, including the monitor, keyboard, and printer.

Hazard Communication Standard (HCS) (haz′ărd kŏ-myūn′i-kā′shŭn stan′dărd) OSHA's standard for worker safety when working with hazardous chemicals. In 2012, the standard was updated to align with the Globally Harmonized System of Classification and Labeling of Chemicals (GHS).

hazard label (haz′ărd lā′bĕl) A shortened version of the Safety Data Sheet; permanently affixed to a hazardous substance container.

HCG See **human chorionic gonadotropin.**

HCPCS See **Healthcare Common Procedure Coding System.**

HCPCS Level II codes (hik-piks lĕv′ĕl tū kōdz) Codes that cover many supplies such as sterile trays, drugs, and durable medical equipment; also referred to as national codes. They also cover services and procedures not included in the CPT.

healthcare-associated infections (HAI) (helth kār ă-sō′sē-ăt-ed in-fek′shŭns) Infections acquired by a patient in a healthcare facility.

Healthcare Common Procedure Coding System (HCPCS) (helth′kār kom′ŏn prŏ-sē′jŭr kōd′ing sis′tĕm) A coding system developed by the Centers for Medicare and Medicaid Services that is used in coding services for Medicare patients.

health fraud (helth frawd) A deception or trickery related to health prevention or care for profit.

Health Insurance Portability and Accountability Act See **HIPAA.**

Health Information Technology for Economics and Clinical Health See **HITECH.**

health maintenance organization (HMO) (helth mān′tĕn-ăns ōr′găn-ī-zā′shŭn) A healthcare organization that provides specific services to individuals and their dependents who are enrolled in the plan. Doctors who enroll in an HMO agree to provide certain services in exchange for a prepaid fee.

helper T-cells (hel′pĕr selz) White blood cells that are a key component of the body's immune system and that work in coordination with other white blood cells to combat infection.

hematemesis (hē′-mă-tem′ĕ-sis) The vomiting of blood.

hematocrit (Hct) (hē-mat′ō-krit) The percentage of the volume of a sample made up of red blood cells after the sample has been spun in a centrifuge.

hematology (hē′mă-tol′ō-jē) The study of blood.

hematoma (hē′mă-tō′mă) A swelling caused by blood under the skin.

hematopoiesis (hē′mă-tō-poy-ē′sis) The process of new blood cell formation in the red bone marrow of cancellous bone.

hematuria (hē′mă-tyūr′ē-ă) The presence of blood in the urine.

hemocytoblast (hē′mō-sī′tō-blast) Cells of the red bone marrow that produce most red blood cells.

hemoglobin (Hgb) (hē′mō-glō′bin) A protein that contains iron and bonds with and carries oxygen to cells; the main component of erythrocytes.

hemoglobinuria (hē′mō-glō′bi-nyūr′ē-ă) The presence of free hemoglobin in the urine; a rare condition caused by transfusion reactions, malaria, drug reactions, snake bites, or severe burns.

hemolysis (hē-mol′ĭ-sis) The rupturing of red blood cells, which releases hemoglobin.

hemolytic anemias (hē′mō-lit′ik ă-nē′mē-ăz) Types of anemia that cause red blood cells to be destroyed faster than they can be made.

hemoptysis (hē-mop′ti-sis) The spitting up of blood from the respiratory tract.

hemorrhoids (hem′ŏr-oydz) Varicose veins of the rectum or anus.

hemostasis (hē′mō-stā′sis) The stoppage of bleeding.

hemothorax (hē′mō-thōr′aks) Blood collection in the pleural cavity, causing collapse of the lung.

hepatic duct (hĕ-pat′ik dŭkt) A duct that leaves the liver carrying bile and merges with the cystic duct to form the common bile duct.

hepatic lobule (hĕ-pat′ik lob′yūl) Smaller division within the lobes of the liver.

hepatic portal system (hĕ-pat′ik pōr′tăl sis′tĕm) The collection of veins carrying blood to the liver.

hepatic portal vein (hĕ-pat′ik pōr′tăl vān) A blood vessel that carries blood from the other digestive organs to the **hepatic lobules.**

hepatitis (hep′ă-tī′tis) Inflammation of the liver usually caused by viruses or toxins.

hepatocytes (hepă′-tō-sītz) The cells within the lobules of the liver. Hepatocytes process nutrients in the blood and make bile.

hernia (hĕr′nē-ă) The protrusion of an organ through the wall that usually contains it, such as a hiatal or inguinal hernia.

herpes simplex (her′pēz sim′plĕks) A medical condition characterized by an eruption of one or more groups of vesicles on the lips or genitalia.

herpes zoster (her′pēz zos′ter) A medical condition characterized by an eruption of a group of vesicles on one side of the body following a nerve root.

hierarchy (hī′ĕr-ahr-kē) A term that pertains to Abraham Maslow's hierarchy of needs. This hierarchy states that human beings are motivated by unsatisfied needs and that certain lower needs must be satisfied before higher needs can be met.

hilum (hī′lŭm) The indented side of a lymph node. Also, the entrance of the renal sinus that contains the renal artery, renal vein, and ureter.

HIPAA (Health Insurance Portability and Accountability Act) (hĭp-uh) A set of regulations whose goals include the following: (1) improving the portability and continuity of healthcare coverage in group and individual markets; (2) combating waste, fraud, and abuse in healthcare insurance and healthcare delivery; (3) promoting the use of a medical savings account; (4) improving access to long-term care services and coverage; and (5) simplifying the administration of health insurance.

HITECH (Health Information Technology for Economics and Clinical Health) (hī-tek′) The expansion of HIPAA coverage through increased regulations and enforcement penalties related to EHR and practice management systems.

HIV See **human immunodeficiency virus.**

HMO See **health maintenance organization.**

Holter monitor (hōl′tĕr mon′i-tŏr) An electrocardiography device that includes a microchip or a small cassette recorder worn around a patient's waist or on a shoulder strap to record the heart's electrical activity.

homeopathic medicine (hō-mē-ō-păth′ĭk med′i-sin) A system of medicine that uses remedies in an attempt to stimulate the body to recover itself.

homeostasis (hō′mē-ō-stā′sĭs) A balanced, stable state within the body.

homologous chromosomes (hŏ-mol′ŏ-gŭs krō′mŏ-sōmz) Members in each pair of chromosomes.

hormone (hōr′mōn′) A chemical secreted by a cell that affects the functions of other cells.

hospice (hŏs′pĭs) Volunteers who work with terminally ill patients and their families.

household system (hows′hōld sis′tĕm) A system of measurement that includes drops, teaspoons, tablespoons, ounces, cups, pints, quarts, and gallons.

human chorionic gonadotropin (HCG) (hyū′măn kōr′ē-on′ik gō-nad′ō-trō′pin) A hormone secreted by cells of the embryo after implantation. It maintains the corpus luteum in the ovary so that it will continue to secrete estrogen and progesterone.

human immunodeficiency virus (HIV) (hyū′măn im′yū-nō-dĕ-fish′ĕn-sē vī′rŭs) A retrovirus that gradually destroys the body's immune system and causes AIDS.

humerus (hyū′mĕr-ŭs) The bone of the upper arm.

humors (hyū′mŏrz) Fluids of the body.

hydrotherapy (hī′drō-thār′ă-pē) The therapeutic use of water to treat physical problems.

hydrothorax (hī′drō-thōr′aks) Fluid collection in the pleural cavity causing collapse of the lung.

hyoid (hī′ŏid) The bone that anchors the tongue.

hyperextension (hī′pĕr-eks-ten′shŭn) Extension of a body part past the normal anatomical position.

hyperglycemia (hī′pĕr-glī-sē′mē-ă) High blood sugar.

hyperopia (hī′pĕr-ō′pē-ă) A condition that occurs when light entering the eye is focused behind the retina; commonly called farsightedness.

hyperpnea (hī′pĕrp-nē′ă) Abnormally deep, rapid breathing.

hyperpyrexia (hī′pĕr-pī-rek′sē-ă) An exceptionally high fever.

hyperreflexia (hī′pĕr-rē-flek′sē-ă) Reflexes that are stronger than normal reflexes.

hypertension (hī′pĕr-ten′shŭn) High blood pressure.

hyperventilation (hī′pĕr-ven′ti-lā′shŭn) The condition of breathing rapidly and deeply. Hyperventilating decreases the amount of carbon dioxide in the blood.

hypnosis (hĭp-nō′sĭs) A trance-like state usually induced by another person to access the subconscious mind and promote healing.

hypodermis (hī′pō-dĕr′mis) The subcutaneous layer of the skin that is largely made of adipose tissue.

hypoglycemia (hī′pō-glī-sē′mē-ă) Low blood sugar.

hyporeflexia (hī′pō-rē-flek′sē-ă) A condition of decreased reflexes.

hypotension (hī′pō-tĕn′shŭn) Low blood pressure.

hypothalamus (hī′pō-thal′ă-mŭs) A region of the diencephalon. It maintains homeostasis by regulating many vital activities such as heart rate, blood pressure, and breathing rate.

hypovolemic shock (hī′pō-vŏ-lē′mik shok) A state of shock resulting from insufficient blood volume in the circulatory system.

hypoxemia (hī′pok-sē′mē-ă) Subnormal oxygenation of arterial blood, short of anoxia.

hypoxia (hī-pok′sē-ă) Inadequate oxygenation of the cells of the body.

hysterectomy (his′tĕr-ek′tŏ-mē) Surgical removal of the uterus.

ICD-10 See *International Classification of Diseases, Tenth Revision.*

icons (ī′konz′) Pictorial images; on a computer screen, graphic symbols that identify menu choices.

identification line (ī-den′ti-fi-kā′shŭn līn) A line at the bottom of a letter containing the letter writer's initials and the typist's initials.

idiopathic (ĭd-ē-ō-path′ik) A disease or condition of unknown cause.

IFFA See **immunofluorescent antibody test.**

ileocecal sphincter (il′ē-ō-sē′kăl sfingk′tĕr) A structure that controls the movement of chime from the ileum to the cecum.

ileum (ĭl′ē-əm) The last portion of the small intestine. It is directly attached to the large intestine.

ilium (il′ē-ŭm) The most superior part of the hip bone. It is broad and flaring.

immunity (i-myū′ni-tē) The condition of being resistant or not susceptible to pathogens and the diseases they cause.

immunizations (im′yū-nī-zā-shŭnz) Administration of a vaccine to protect susceptible individuals from communicable diseases.

immunocompromised (im′yū-nō-kom′pro-mīzd) Having an impaired or weakened immune system.

immunofluorescent antibody (IFFA) test (im′yū-nō-flōr-es′ent an′ti-bod-ē test) A blood test used to confirm enzyme-linked immunosorbent assay (ELISA) test results for HIV infection.

immunoglobulins (im′yū-nō-glob′yū-linz) A class of structurally related proteins that include IgG, IgA, IgM, and IgE; also called **antibodies.**

impetigo (im′pě-tī′gō) A contagious skin infection usually caused by germs commonly called staph and strep.

implied consent (im-plīd′ kŏn-sent′) A form of consent that is not expressly granted by a person, but rather inferred from a person's actions and the facts and circumstances of a particular situation (or in some cases by a person's silence or inaction).

implied contract (ĭm-plīd′ kon′trakt) A contract that is created by the acceptance or conduct of the parties rather than the written word.

impotence (ĭm′pŏ-tĕns) A disorder in which a male cannot maintain an erect penis to complete sexual intercourse; also called erectile dysfunction.

inactive file (in-ak′tiv fīl) A file used infrequently.

incident report (in′si-dĕnt rē-pōrt′) A report required by a facility when an adverse incident with risk of liability occurs.

incision (in-sizh′ŭn) A surgical wound made by cutting into body tissue.

incisors (in-sī′zŏrz) The most medial teeth. They act as chisels to bite off food.

incomplete proteins (in′kŏm-plēt′ prō′tēnz) Proteins that lack one or more of the essential amino acids.

incontinence (in-kon′ti-nens) The involuntary leakage of urine.

incus (ĭng′kŭs) A small bone in the middle ear, located between the malleus and the stapes; also called the anvil.

indexing (in′dĕks′ ing) The naming of a file.

indexing rules (in′dĕks′ing rūlz) Rules used as guidelines for the sequencing of files based on current business practice.

indication (in′di-kā′shŭn) The purpose or reason for using a drug, as approved by the FDA.

indirect filing system (in′dir-ekt′ fīl-ing sis′tĕm) A numeric filing system, which organizes files by numbers instead of by names.

individual identifiable health information (IIHI) (in′di-vij′yū-ăl ī-den′ti-fī′ă-bĕl helth in′fŏr-mā′shun) Any part of an individual's health information, including demographic information, collected from an individual that is received by a covered entity (e.g., a healthcare provider).

induction (in-dŭk′shŭn) The pregnant patient is admitted to the delivering healthcare facility, then given medication to start uterine contractions.

induration (in′dūr-ā′shŭn) The process of hardening or of becoming hard.

infection (in-fek′shŭn) The presence of a pathogen in or on the body.

infectious waste (in-fek′shŭs wāst) Waste that can be dangerous to those who handle it or to the environment; includes human waste, human tissue, and body fluids as well as potentially hazardous waste, such as used needles, scalpels, and dressings, and cultures of human cells.

inferior (in-fēr′ē-ŏr) Anatomical term meaning below or closer to the feet; also called caudal.

infertility (in′fĕr-til′i-tē) Diminished ability to produce offspring; does not imply sterility.

inflammation (in′flă-mā′shŭn) The body's reaction when tissue becomes injured or infected. The four cardinal signs are redness, heat, pain, and swelling.

inflammatory phase (in-flam′ă-tōr-ē fāz) The initial phase of wound healing in which bleeding is reduced as blood vessels in the affected area constrict.

informed consent (in-fōrmd′ kŏn-sent′) The patient's right to receive all information relative to his or her condition and then make a decision regarding treatment based upon that knowledge.

informed consent form (in-fōrmd′ kŏn-sent′ fōrm) A form that verifies that a patient understands the offered treatment and its possible outcomes or side effects.

infundibulum (in-fŭn-dib′yū-lŭm) The funnel-like end of the uterine tube near an ovary. It catches the secondary oocyte as it leaves the ovary.

infusion (in-fyū′zhŭn) A slow drip, as of an intravenous solution into a vein.

ink-jet printer (ĭngk′jĕt′ prĭn′tĕr) A nonimpact printer that forms characters by using a series of dots created by tiny drops of ink.

innate immunity (i-nāt′ i-myū′ni-tē) The body's mechanisms to protect itself against pathogens in general; also called nonspecific defenses.

inner cell mass (in′ĕr sel mas) A group of cells in a blastocyte that gives rise to an embryo.

inorganic (in′ŏr-gan′ik) Matter that generally does not contain carbon and hydrogen.

insertion (in-sĕr′shŭn) An attachment site of a skeletal muscle that moves when a muscle contracts.

inside address (ĭn-sīd′ ă-dres′) The name and address of the person to whom the letter is being sent. It appears on a business letter two to four spaces down from the date. It should be two, three, or four lines in length.

inspecting (conditioning) (in-spek′t-ing (kuhn-dih′shun-ing)) The process of making sure an item is ready for filing, including removing paper clips and stapling related documents together.

inspection (ĭn-spĕk′shŭn) The visual examination of the patient's entire body and overall appearance.

inspiration (in′spir-ă′shŭn) The act of breathing in; also called inhalation.

instruction set (in-strŭkt′shŭn set) Includes the groups of instructions from installed programming that a CPU can implement.

insulin (in′sŭ-lin) A hormone that regulates the amount of sugar in the blood by facilitating its entry into the cells.

integrative medicine (in′tĕ-grā-tiv med′i-sin) The combination of components of conventional medicine with complementary and alternative medicine modalities.

integrity (in-teg′ri-tē) Adhering to the appropriate code of law and ethics and being honest and trustworthy.

interactive pager (in′tĕr-ak′tiv pāj′ĕr) A pager designed for two-way communication. The pager screen displays a printed message and allows the physician to respond by way of a mini-keyboard.

interatrial septum (in′tĕr-ā′trē-ăl sep′tŭm) The wall separating the right and left atria from each other.

intercalated disc (in-ter′kă-lā-ted disk) A disk that connects groups of cardiac muscles. This disc allows the fibers in that group to contract and relax together.

interferon (in-tĕr-fēr′on) A protein that blocks viruses from infecting cells.

interim room (ĭn′tĕr-ĭm rūm) A room off the patient reception area and away from the examination rooms for occasions when patients require privacy.

International Classification of Diseases (in′tĕr-nash′ŭn-ăl klas′i-fi-kā′shŭn di-zēz′ĕz) Code set that is based on a system maintained by the World Health Organization of the United Nations. The use of the ICD-10 codes in the healthcare industry is mandated by HIPAA for reporting patients' diseases, conditions, and signs and symptoms. ICD-10 codes, adopted 10/1/15, allow for more specificity and accuracy when coding.

Internet (ĭn′tĕr-net) A global network of computers.

interneurons (in′tĕr-nū′ronz) Structures found only in the central nervous system that link sensory and motor neurons together.

internist (ĭn-tĕr′nĭst) A doctor who specializes in diagnosing and treating problems related to the internal organs.

interpersonal skills (in′tĕr-pĕr′sŏn-ăl skĭlz) Attitudes, qualities, and abilities that influence the level of success and satisfaction achieved in interacting with other people.

interphalangeal (in′tĕr-fă-lan′jē-ăl) Pertaining to the joints between the phalangeal bones.

interphase (in′ter-fāz) The state of a cell carrying out its normal daily functions and not dividing.

interstitial cell (in′tĕr-stish′ăl sel) A cell located between the seminiferous tubules that is responsible for making testosterone.

interstitial fluid (in′tĕr-stish′ăl flū′id) Fluid found between tissue cells that is absorbed by lymphatic capillaries to become lymph.

interventricular septum (in′tĕr-ven-trik′yū-lăr sep′tŭm) The wall separating the right and left ventricles from each other.

intestinal lipase (in-tes′ti-năl liīp′ās) An enzyme that digests fat.

intradermal (ID) (in′tră-der′măl) Within the upper layers of the skin.

intradermal test (in′tră-dĕr′măl tĕst) An allergy test in which dilute solutions of allergens are introduced into the skin of the inner forearm or upper back with a fine-gauge needle.

intramembranous (in′tră-mem′bră-nŭs) A type of ossification in which bones begin as tough, fibrous membranes.

intramuscular (IM) (in′tră-mŭs′kyū-lăr) Within muscle; an IM injection allows administration of a larger amount of a drug than a subcutaneous injection allows.

intraoperative (in′tră-op′ĕr-ă-tiv) Taking place during surgery.

intravenous (IV) (in′tră-vē′nŭs) Injected directly into a vein.

intravenous pyelography (IVP) (in′tră-vē′nŭs pī′ĕ-log′ră-fē) A radiologic procedure in which the doctor injects a contrast medium into a vein and takes a series of X-rays of the kidneys, ureters, and bladder to evaluate urinary system abnormalities or trauma to the urinary system; also known as excretory urography.

intrinsic factor (ĭn-trĭn′zĭk făk′tŏr) A substance secreted by parietal cells in the lining of the stomach. It is necessary for vitamin B_{12} absorption.

invasive (ĭn-vā′sĭv) Referring to a procedure in which a catheter, wire, or other foreign object is introduced into a blood vessel or organ through the skin or a body orifice. Surgical asepsis is required during all invasive tests.

invasive procedure (in-vā′siv prŏ-sē′jŭr) Any procedure that requires entry into a body cavity or cutting into skin or mucous membranes.

inventory (in′vĕn-tōr-ē) A list of supplies used regularly and the quantities in stock.

inversion (in-vĕr′zhŭn) Turning the sole of the foot medially.

invoice (ĭn′vois) A listing of products or services rendered that is used when billing for that product or service..

ions (ī′onz) Positively or negatively charged particles.

iris (ī′rĭs) The colored part of the eye, made of muscular tissue that contracts and relaxes, altering the size of the pupil.

ischium (is′kē-ŭm) A structure that forms the lower part of the hip bone.

islets of Langerhans (ī'lĕts lahng'er-hahnz) Structures in the pancreas that secrete insulin and glucagon into the bloodstream.

itinerary (ī-tĭn'ĕ-rar'ē) A detailed travel plan listing dates and times for specific transportation arrangements and events, the location of meetings and lodgings, and phone numbers.

IV See **intravenous.**

IVP See **intravenous pyelography.**

jaundice (jawn'dis) A condition characterized by yellowness of the skin, eyes, mucous membranes, and excretions; occurs during the second stage of hepatitis infection.

jejunum (je-jū'nŭm) The mid-portion and the majority of the small intestine.

journalizing (jûr'nă-līz'ĭng) The process of logging charges and receipts in a chronological list each day; used in the single-entry system of bookkeeping.

juxtaglomerular apparatus (jŭks'tă-glō-mer'yū-lăr ap-ă-rat'ŭs) A structure contained in the nephron and made up of the macula densa and juxtaglomerular cells.

juxtaglomerular cells (jŭks'tă-glō-mer'yū-lăr sĕlz) Enlarged smooth muscle cells in the walls of either the afferent or efferent arterioles.

Kaposi's sarcoma (kap'ŏ-shē sahr-kō'mă) Abnormal tissue occurring in the skin, and sometimes in the lymph nodes and organs, manifested by reddish-purple to dark blue patches or spots on the skin.

keratin (kĕr'ă-tĭn) A tough, hard protein contained in skin, hair, and nails.

keratinocyte (kĕ-rat'i-nō-sīt) The most common cell type in the epidermis of the skin.

key (kē) The act of inputting or entering information into a computer.

KOH mount (kā'ō-āch mownt) A type of mount used when a physician suspects a patient has a fungal infection of the skin, nails, or hair and to which potassium hydroxide is added to dissolve the keratin in cell walls.

Krebs cycle (krĕbz sī'kĕl) Also called the citric acid cycle. This cycle generates ATP for muscle cells.

KUB radiography (kā'ȳoo-bē rā'dē-og'ră-fē) The process of X-raying the abdomen to help assess the size, shape, and position of the urinary organs; evaluate urinary system diseases or disorders; or determine the presence of kidney stones. It can also be helpful in determining the position of an intrauterine device (IUD) or in locating foreign bodies in the digestive tract; also called a flat plate of the abdomen.

kyphosis (kī-fō'sis) A deformity of the spine characterized by a bent-over position; more commonly called humpback.

labeling (lā'bĕl-ing) Information provided with a drug, including FDA-approved indications and the form of the drug.

labia majora (lā'bē-ă mă'jôr-ă) The rounded folds of adipose tissue and skin that protect the other female reproductive organs.

labia minora (lā'bē-ă mĭ'nôr-ă) The folds of skin between the labia majora.

labor relations (lā'bŏr rĕ-lā'shŭnz) An HR role that refers to issues that arise between employees and management.

labyrinth (lab'i-rinth) The inner ear.

laceration (las'ĕr-ā'shŭn) A jagged, open wound in the skin that can extend down into the underlying tissue.

lacrimal apparatus (lak'ri-măl ap'ă-rat'ŭs) A structure that consists of the lacrimal glands and nasolacrimal ducts.

lacrimal gland (lak'ri-măl gland) A gland in the eye that produces tears.

lactase (lăk'tās) An enzyme that digests sugars.

lactic acid (lăk'tĭk ăs'ĭd) A waste product that must be released from the cell. It is produced when a cell is low on oxygen and converts pyruvic acid.

lactiferous (lak-tif'ĭr-ŭs) Pertaining to producing milk.

lactogen (lak'tō-jen) Substance secreted by the placenta that stimulates the enlargement of the mammary glands.

lacunae (lă-kū'nē) Holes in the matrix of bone that hold osteocytes.

lamella (lă-mel'ă) Layer of bone surrounding the canals of osteons.

LAN (local area network) (lăn) See **local area network.**

lancet (lăn'sĭt) A small, disposable instrument with a sharp point used to puncture the skin and make a shallow incision; used for capillary puncture.

laryngopharynx (lă-ring'gō-făr-ingks) The portion of the pharynx behind the larynx.

larynx (lăr'ĭngks) The part of the respiratory tract between the pharynx and the trachea that is responsible for voice production; also called the voice box.

laser printer (lā'zĕr prĭn'tĕr) A high-resolution printer that uses a technology similar to that of a photocopier. It is the fastest type of computer printer and produces the highest-quality output.

last menstrual period (LMP) (lăst men'strū-ăl pēr'ē-ŏd) The date of the first day of the last menstruation; used to determine an estimated expected delivery date for a pregnant patient.

lateral (lat'ĕr-ăl) A directional term that means farther away from the midline of the body.

lateral file (lat'ĕr-ăl fīl) A horizontal filing cabinet that features doors that flip up and a pull-out drawer, where files are arranged with sides facing out.

laterality (lat'ĕr-al'i-tē) In ICD-10, the side of the body affected by the diagnosis.

law (lô) A rule of conduct established and enforced by an authority or governing body, such as the federal government.

law of agency (law ā'jĕn-sē) A law stating that an employee is considered to be acting on the physician's behalf while performing professional duties.

lead (lēd) A view of a specific area of the heart on an electrocardiogram.

lease (lēs) To rent an item or piece of equipment.

legal custody (lā-gal' kŭs'tŏ-dē) The court-decreed right to have control over a child's upbringing and to take responsibility for the child's care, including healthcare.

lens (lenz) A clear, circular disc located in the eye, just posterior to the iris, that can change shape to help the eye focus images of objects that are near or far away.

lentigos (len-tī'gōz) Brown macules resembling a freckle except that the border is usually regular and microscopic proliferation of rete ridges is present; scattered melanocytes are seen in the basal cell layer. They are usually caused by sun exposure in someone of middle age or older.

letterhead (lĕt′ĕr-hĕd′) Formal business stationery, with the doctor's (or office's) name and address printed at the top, used for correspondence with patients, colleagues, and vendors.

leukemia (lū-kē′mē-ă) A medical condition in which bone marrow produces a large number of white blood cells that are not normal.

leukocyte (lū′kō-sīt) White blood cell.

leukocytosis (lū′kō-sī-tō′sis) A white blood cell count that is above normal.

leukopenia (lū′kō-pē′nē-ă) A white blood cell count that is below normal.

LH See **luteinizing hormone.**

liability insurance (lī′ă-bil′ī′-tē in-shūr′ents) A type of insurance that covers injuries caused by the insured or injuries that occurred on the insured's property.

liable (lī′ă-bĕl) Legally responsible.

libel (lī′bĕl) A false publication, as in writing, print, signs, or pictures, that damages a person's reputation.

licensed practitioner (lī′sĕnst prak′ti′shŭn-ĕr) A healthcare provider who has obtained the necessary education and skills and is licensed to provide specified healthcare to patients.

lifetime maximum benefit (līf′tīm′ mak′si-mŭm ben′ĕ-fit) The total sum that a health plan will pay out over the patient's life.

ligament (lig′ă-mĕnt) A tough, fibrous band of tissue that connects bone to bone.

ligature (lig′ă-chŭr) Suture material.

limbus (lim′bŭs) The corneal-scleral junction, which is the area where the sclera (the white of the eye) gives way to the clear covering of the iris (cornea).

limited check (lim′ĭ-ted chek) A check that is void after a certain time limit; commonly used for payroll.

lingual frenulum (ling′gwăl fren′yŭlŭm) A flap of mucosa that holds the body of the tongue to the floor of the oral cavity.

lingual tonsils (ling′gwăl ton′silz) Two lumps of lymphatic tissue at the back of the tongue that destroy bacteria and viruses.

linoleic acid (lin-ō-lē′ik as′id) An essential fatty acid found in corn and sunflower oils.

lipid (lip′id) "Fat-soluble," an operational term describing a solubility characteristic, not a chemical substance, denoting substances extracted from animal or vegetable cells by nonpolar solvents; included in the heterogeneous collection of materials thus extractable are fatty acids, glycerides, glyceryl ethers, phospholipids, sphingolipids, long-chain alcohols, waxes, terpenes, steroids, and "fat-soluble" vitamins such as A, D, and E.

lipoproteins (lip-ō-prō′tēnz) Large molecules that are fat-soluble on the inside and water-soluble on the outside and carry lipids such as cholesterol and triglycerides through the bloodstream.

lithotripsy (lith′ō-trip-sē) The crushing of a stone in the renal pelvis, ureter, or bladder by mechanical force or sound waves.

living will (liv′ing wil) A legal document addressed to a patient's family and healthcare providers stating what type of treatment the patient wishes or does not wish to receive if terminally ill, unconscious, or permanently comatose; sometimes called an advance directive.

lobe (lōb) The frontal, parietal, temporal, or occipital region of the cerebral hemisphere.

local area network (LAN) (lō′kăl ār′ē-ă net′wŏrk) A network that connects computers in one building or a group of buildings.

locum tenens **(lō′kum ten′enz)** A substitute physician hired to see patients while the regular physician is away from the office.

loop electrosurgical excision procedure (LEEP) (lūp ĕ-lek′trō-sŭr′jik-ăl ek-sizh′ŭn prŏ-sē′jŭr) A diagnostic and therapeutic gynecologic surgical technique for removing dysplastic cells from the cervix with a small wire loop.

loop of Henle (lūp hen′lē) The portion of the renal tubule that curves back toward the renal corpuscle and twists again to become the distal convoluted tubule.

lubricant (lū′bri-kănt) A water-soluble gel used during examination of the rectum or vaginal cavity.

lumbar enlargement (lŭm′bahr en-lahrj′mĕnt) The thickening of the spinal cord in the low back region.

lunula (lūn′yŭ-lă) The white, half-moon-shaped area at the base of a nail.

luteinizing hormone (LH) (lū′tē-in-ī′zing hōr′mōn) Hormone that in females stimulates ovulation and the production of estrogen; in males, it stimulates the production of testosterone.

lymph (limf) The fluid inside lymphatic vessels.

lymphedema (limf′ĕ-dē′mă) The blockage of lymphatic vessels that results in the swelling of tissue from the accumulation of lymphatic fluid.

lymph nodes (limf nōdz) Very small, glandular structures that filter pathogens from lymph and generate lymphocytes.

lymphocytes (lim′fō-sīts) Granular leukocytes formed in lymphoid tissue. Lymphocytes are generally small. See *T lymphocyte* and *B lymphocyte.*

lymphokines (limf′ō-kĭnz) A type of cytokine secreted by T cells that increases T-cell production and directly kills cells with antigens.

lysosomes (lī′sō-sōmz) Structures that are known to perform the digestive function of the cells.

lysozyme (lī′sō-zīm) An enzyme in tears that destroys pathogens on the surface of the eye.

macrophages (mak′rō-fāj-ez) A type of phagocytic cell found in the liver, spleen, lungs, bone marrow, and connective tissue. Macrophages play several roles in humoral and cell-mediated immunity, including presenting the antigens to the lymphocytes involved in these defenses; also known as monocytes while in the bloodstream.

macula densa (mak′yū-lă den′sa) An area of the distal convoluted tubule that touches afferent and efferent arterioles.

macular degeneration (mak′yū-lahr dĕ-jen′ĕr-ā′shŭn) A progressive disease that usually affects people older than the age of 50. It occurs when the retina no longer receives an adequate blood supply.

magnetic resonance imaging (MRI) (mag-net′ik rez′ō-năns im′ăj-ing) A viewing technique that uses a powerful magnetic field to produce an image of internal body structures.

magnetic therapy (măg-nĕt′ĭk thār′ă-pē) A type of therapy in which magnets are placed on the body to penetrate and correct the body's energy fields.

maintenance contract (mān′tĕ-năns kon′trakt) A contract that specifies when a piece of equipment will be cleaned, checked for worn parts, and repaired.

major histocompatibility complex (MHC) (mā′jŏr his′tō-kŏm-pat′i-bil′i-tē kom′pleks) A large protein complex that plays a role in T-cell activation.

malignant (mă-lig′nănt) A type of tumor or neoplasm that is invasive and destructive and that tends to metastasize; it is commonly known as cancerous.

malleus (măl′ē-ŭs) A small bone in the middle ear that is attached to the eardrum; also called the hammer.

malpractice claim (mal-prak′tis clăm) A lawsuit brought by a patient against a physician for errors in diagnosis or treatment.

maltase (mawl′tās) An enzyme that digests sugars.

mammary glands (mam′ă-rē glăndz) Accessory organs of the female reproductive system that secrete milk after pregnancy.

mammography (mă-mog′ră-fē) X-ray examination of the breasts.

managed care organization (MCO) (man′ăjd kār ōr′găn-ī-zā′shŭn) A healthcare business that, through mergers and buyouts, can deliver healthcare more cost-effectively.

mandible (man′di-běl) A bone that forms the lower portion of the jaw.

manipulation (mă-nip′yū-lā′shŭn) The systematic movement of a patient's body parts.

margin (mahr′jin) The space or measurement around the edges of a form or letter that is left blank.

marrow (ma′rō) A substance that is contained in the medullary cavity. In adults, it consists primarily of fat.

massage (mă-sahzh′) The use of pressure, kneading, stroking, and the human touch to alleviate pain and promote healing through relaxation.

massage therapist (mă-sahzh′ thār′ă-pist) An individual who is trained to use pressure, kneading, and stroking to promote muscle and full-body relaxation.

mastoid process (mas′toyd pros′es) A large bump on each temporal bone just behind each ear. It resembles a nipple, hence the name mastoid.

matrix (mā′trĭks) The basic format of an appointment book, established by blocking off times on the schedule during which the doctor is able to see patients. Also, the material between the cells of connective tissue.

matter (măt′er) Anything that takes up space and has weight. Liquids, solids, and gases are matter.

maturation phase (mach′ūr-ā′shŭn fāz) The third phase of wound healing, in which scar tissue forms.

maxilla (mak-sil′ă) A bone that forms the upper portion of the jaw.

Mayo stand (mā′ō stănd) A movable stainless steel instrument tray on a stand.

MCO See **managed care organization.**

meaningful use (mēn′ing-ful yüs) The use of certified electronic health record technology to improve quality, safety, and efficiency, and reduce health disparities; to engage patients and family; to improve care coordination, and population and public health; and to maintain privacy and security of patient health information.

mechanical digestion (mě-kan′i-kăl dī-jes′chŭn) The breaking down of food for use by the body by a physical method such as chewing.

medial (mē′dē-ăl) A directional term that describes areas closer to the midline of the body.

mediation (mē′dē-ā′-shun) Intervention in a dispute in order to resolve it.

Medicaid (med′i-kād) A federally funded health cost–assistance program for low-income, blind, and disabled patients; families receiving aid to dependent children; foster children; and children with birth defects.

medical asepsis (med′i-kăl ā-sep′sis) Measures taken to reduce the number of microorganisms, such as handwashing and wearing examination gloves, that do not necessarily eliminate microorganisms; also called clean technique.

medical identity theft (med′i-kăl ī-den′ti-tē theft) Using another person's name or insurance to seek healthcare.

medical practice act (med′i-kăl prak′tis akt) A law that defines the exact duties that physicians and other healthcare personnel may perform.

Medicare (med′i-kār) A national health insurance program for Americans aged 65 and older.

Medicare Choice Plan (med′i-kār choys plan) Medicare benefit in which beneficiaries can choose to enroll in one of three major types of plans instead of the Original Medicare Plan.

Medigap (med′i-gap) Private insurance that Medicare recipients can purchase to reduce the gap in coverage—the amount they would have to pay from their own pockets after receiving Medicare benefits.

meditation (měd′ĭ-tā′shŭn) A state in which the body is consciously relaxed and the mind becomes calm and focused.

medullary cavity (med′ŭ-lar′ē kav′i-tē) The canal that runs through the center of the diaphysis.

megakaryocytes (meg-ă-kar′ē-ō-sīts) Cells within red blood marrow that give rise to platelets.

meiosis (mī-ō′sis) A type of cell division in which each new cell contains only one member of each chromosome pair.

melanin (mel′ă-nĭn) A pigment that is deposited throughout the layers of the epidermis.

melanocyte (mel′ă-nō-sīt) A cell type within the epidermis that makes the pigment **melanin.**

melanocyte-stimulating hormone (MSH) (mel′ă-nō-sīt stim′yū-lā-ting hōr′mōn) A hormone released from the anterior pituitary to stimulate melanin production in the skin's epidermal cells.

melatonin (měl′ă-tō′nĭn) A hormone that helps to regulate circadian rhythms.

membrane potential (mem′brăn pŏ-ten′shăl) The potential inside a cell relative to the fluid outside the cell.

menarche (men′-ahrkē) The first menstrual period.

Ménière's disease (me-nērz′ di-zēz′) An inner-ear disease characterized by attacks of vertigo, tinnitus, and nausea. Permanent hearing loss may result.

meninges (mě-nin′jēz) Membranes that protect the brain and spinal cord.

meningitis (měn′ĭn-jī′tĭs) An inflammation of the meninges.

meniscus (mě-nis′kŭs) The curve in the air-to-liquid surface of a liquid specimen in a container.

menopause (men′ŏ-pawz) The termination of the menstrual cycle due to the normal aging of the ovaries.

menorrhagia (men′ŏ-rā′jē-ă) Excessively prolonged or profuse menses.

menses (měn′sēz) The clinical term for menstrual flow.

menstrual cycle (men′strū-ăl sī′kĕl) The female reproductive cycle. It consists of regular changes in the uterine lining that lead to monthly bleeding.

menstruation (men′strū-ā′shŭn) Cyclic endometrial shedding and discharge of a bloody fluid from the uterus during the menstrual cycle.

mensuration (men′sŭr-ā′shŭn) The process of measuring.

meridians (měr-id′ē-anz) Pathways of energetic flow that are distributed symmetrically throughout the body. These pathways are used in acupuncture, traditional Chinese medicine, and Ayurveda.

mesentery (mes′ĕn-ter-ē) The fan-like tissue that attaches the jejunum and ileum to the posterior abdominal wall.

mesoderm (mez′ō-derm) The primary germ layer that gives rise to connective tissue and some epithelial tissue.

metabolic wastes (met′ă-bol′ik wāsts) Substances produced during the normal operation of the kidneys and excreted through the urine.

metabolism (mě-tab′ě-lizm) The overall chemical functioning of the body, including all body processes that build small molecules into large ones (anabolism) and break down large molecules into small ones (catabolism).

metacarpal (met′ă-kahr′păl) One of the bones that form the palms of the hand.

metacarpophalangeal (met′ă-kahr′pō-fă-lan′jē-ăl) Pertaining to the joints that join the phalanges to the metacarpals.

metaphase (met′ăfāz) Period of mitosis when the chromosomes line up on the spindle fibers created by the centrioles during prophase.

metastasis (mě-tas′tă-sis) The transfer of abnormal cells to body sites far removed from the original tumor; the spread of tumor cells.

metatarsal (met′ă-tahr′săl) One of the bones that form the front of the foot.

metatarsophalangeal (met′ă-tahr′sō-fă-lan′jē-ăl) Pertaining to the joints that join the phalanges to the metatarsals.

metric system (met′rik sis′tĕm) A system of measurement based on multiples of 10.

metrorrhagia (mī′krō-bī-ol′ŏ-jē) Any irregular, acyclic bleeding from the uterus between periods.

MHC See **major histocompatibility complex.**

microbiology (mī′krō-bī-ŏl′ŏ-jē) The study of microorganisms.

microfiche (mī′krō-fēsh′) Microfilm in rectangular sheets.

microfilm (mī′krō-film) A roll of film stored on a reel and imprinted with information on a reduced scale to minimize storage space requirements.

microglia (mī-krŏg′lēa) Small cells within the nervous system that act as phagocytes, watching for and engulfing invaders.

microorganism (mī′krō-ōr′găn-izm) A simple form of life, commonly made up of a single cell and so small that it can be seen only with a microscope.

micropipette (mī′krō-pĭ-pet′) A small pipette that holds a small, precise volume of fluid; used to collect capillary blood.

microvilli (mī′krō-vil′ī) Structures found in the lining of the small intestine. They greatly increase the surface area of the small intestine so that it can absorb many nutrients.

micturition (mik-chŭr-ish′ŭn) The process of urination.

middle digit (mid′ĕl dij′it) A small group of two to three numbers in the middle of a patient number that is used as an identifying unit in a filing system.

midlevel provider (mid-lev′ĕl prō-vī′dĕr) Physician assistant or nurse practitioner who provides patient care under the supervision of a physician.

midsagittal (mid′saj′i-tăl) Anatomical term that refers to the plane that runs lengthwise down the midline of the body, dividing it into equal left and right halves.

mineral (min′ĕr-ăl) Natural, inorganic substance the body needs to help build and maintain body tissues and carry on life functions.

minor (mī′nŏr) Anyone under the age of majority—18 in most states, 21 in some jurisdictions.

minutes (min′ŭtz) A report of what happened and what was discussed and decided at a meeting.

mirroring (mir′ŏr-ing) Restating in your own words what a person is saying.

misdemeanor (mis′di-mēn-ŏr) A less serious crime such as theft under a certain dollar amount or disturbing the peace. A misdemeanor is punishable by fines or imprisonment.

mitochondria (mi′tō-kon′drē-ă) Structures that provide energy for cells and are the respiratory centers for the cell.

mitosis (mī-tō′sĭs) A type of cell division that produces ordinary body, or somatic, cells; each new cell receives a complete set of paired chromosomes.

mitral valve (mī′trăl vălv) See **bicuspid valve.**

mobility aid (mō-bil′i-tē ād) Device that improves one's ability to move from one place to another; also called mobility assistive device.

modeling (mod′ĕl-ing) The process of teaching the patient a new skill by having the patient observe and imitate it.

modem (mō′dĕm) A device used to transfer information from one computer to another through telephone lines.

modified-block letter style (mod′i-fīd blok let′ĕr stīl) A letter format similar to full-block style, except that the dateline, complimentary closing, signature block, and notations are aligned and begin at the center of the page or slightly to the right of center.

modified-wave scheduling (mod′i-fīd wāv sked′jūl-ing) A scheduling system similar to the wave system, with patients arriving at planned intervals during the hour, allowing time to catch up before the next hour begins.

modifier (mod′i-fī′ĕr) One or more 2-digit codes assigned to the 5-digit main code to show that some special circumstance applied to the service or procedure that the physician performed.

molars (mō′lărz) Back teeth that are flat and are designed to grind food.

mold (mōld) Fungi that grow into large, fuzzy, multicelled organisms that produce spores.

molecule (mol′ě-kyūl) The smallest unit into which an element can be divided and still retain its properties; it is formed when atoms bond together.

money order (mŭn′ē ôr′dĕr) A certificate of guaranteed payment, which may be purchased from a bank, a post office, or some convenience stores.

monocyte (mon′o-sīt) A type of phagocyte that is formed in bone marrow and circulates throughout the blood for a very short period of time. It then migrates to specific tissues and is called a macrophage.

monokines (mon′ō kīnz) A type of cytokine secreted by lymphocytes and macrophages that assists in regulating the immune response by increasing B-cell production and stimulating red bone marrow to produce more white blood cells.

mononucleosis (mon′ō-nū-klē-ō′sis) A highly contagious viral infection caused by the Epstein-Barr virus (EBV).

monosaccharide (mon-ō-sak′ă-rīd) A type of carbohydrate that is a simple sugar.

mons pubis (monz pyū′bis) A fatty area that overlies the public bone.

moral values (mōr′ăl val′yūz) Values or types of behavior that serve as a basis for ethical conduct and are formed through the influence of the family, culture, or society.

morbidity (mōr-bid′i-tē) The frequency of the appearance of complications following a surgical procedure or other treatment.

mordant (mōr′dănt) A substance, such as iodine, that can intensify or deepen the response a specimen has to a stain.

moro reflex (mō′rō rē′fleks) A reflex in which an infant's arms spread out and then back in, often with crying, because the infant feels as if she is falling. The moro reflex is a result of the infant's immature nervous system.

morphology (mōr-fol′ŏ-jē) The study of the shape or form of objects.

mortality (mōr-tal′i-tē) A fatal outcome.

morula (mōr′yū-lă) A zygote that has undergone cleavage and results in a ball of cells.

motherboard (mŏth′ĕr-bōrd) The main circuit board of a computer that controls the other components in the system.

motility (mō-til′i-tē) To be capable of movement.

motor (mō′tŏr) Efferent neurons that carry information from the central nervous system to the effectors.

motor nerve (mō′tŏr nĕrv) An efferent nerve conveying an impulse that excites muscular contraction; motor nerves in the autonomic nervous system also elicit secretions from glandular epithelia.

mouse (mous) A pointing device that can be added to a computer that directs activity on the computer screen by positioning a pointer, or cursor, on the screen. It can be directly attached to the computer or can be wireless.

moxibustion (mok′sē-bŭs′chŭn) The application of heat at the points where the needles are inserted during acupuncture.

MRI See **magnetic resonance imaging.**

MSH See **melanocyte-stimulating hormone.**

mucocutaneous exposure (myū′kō-kyū-tā′nē-ŭs eks-pō′zhŭr) Exposure to a pathogen through mucous membranes.

mucosa (myū-kō′să) The innermost layer of the wall of the alimentary canal.

mucous cells (myū′kŭs selz) Cells that are found in the salivary glands and the lining of the stomach and that secrete mucous.

MUGA scan (nuclear ventriculography) (mŭg′ă skan [nōōklē-ĕr ven-trĭ-kyōō-log′ră-fē]) A radiologic procedure that evaluates the condition of the heart's myocardium; it involves injection of radioisotopes that concentrate in the myocardium, followed by the use of a gamma camera to measure ventricular contractions to evaluate the patient's heart wall.

multimedia (mŭl′tē-mē′dē-ă) More than one medium, such as in graphics, sound, and text, used to convey information.

multiskilled healthcare professional (MSHP) (mŭl′tē skild helth′kār prŏ-fesh′i-năl) A healthcare team member who has been cross-trained to handle many different duties.

multi-unit smooth muscle (mŭl′tē yū′nit smūth mŭs′ĕl) A type of smooth muscle that is found in the iris of the eye and in the walls of blood vessels.

murmur (mŭr′mŭr) An abnormal heart sound heard when the ventricles contract and blood leaks back into the atria.

muscle fatigue (mus′ĕl fă-tēg′) A condition caused by a buildup of lactic acid.

muscle fibers (mŭs′ĕl fī′bĕrz) Muscle cells that are called fibers because of their long lengths.

muscle tissue (mŭs′ĕl tish′ū) A tissue type that is specialized to shorten and elongate.

muscular dystrophy (mŭs′kyū-lăr dis′trŏ-fē) A group of inherited disorders characterized by a loss of muscle tissue and by muscle weakness.

mutation (myū-tā′shŭn) An error that sometimes occurs when DNA is duplicated. When it occurs, it is passed to descendent cells and may or may not affect them in harmful ways.

myasthenia gravis (mī-as-thē′nē-ă grăv′is) An autoimmune disorder that is characterized by muscle weakness.

myelin (mī′ĕ-lin) A fatty substance that insulates the axon and allows it to send nerve impulses quickly.

myelin sheath (mī′ĕ-lin shēth) Insulation around some nerve cell axons that allows nerve impulses to move more quickly through the axons.

myelography (mī′ĕ-log′ră-fē) An X-ray visualization of the spinal cord after the injection of a radioactive contrast medium or air into the spinal subarachnoid space (between the second and innermost of three membranes that cover the spinal cord). This test can reveal tumors, cysts, spinal stenosis, or herniated disks.

myocardial infarction (mī′ō-kahr′dē-ăl in-fahrk′shŭn) A heart attack that occurs when the blood flow to the heart is reduced as a result of blockage in the coronary arteries or their branches.

myocardium (mī′ō-kahr′dē-ŭm) The middle and thickest layer of the heart. It is made primarily of cardiac muscle.

myocytes (mī′ō-sīts) Muscle cells; also called muscle fibers.

myofibrils (mī-ō-fī′brils) Long structures that fill the sarcoplasm of a muscle fiber.

myoglobin (mī′ō-glō′bin) A pigment contained in muscle cells that stores extra oxygen.

myoglobinuria (mī′ō-glō-bi-nyūr′ē-ă) The presence of myoglobin in the urine; can be caused by injured or damaged muscle tissue.

myometrium (mī′ō-mē′trē-ŭm) The middle, thick, muscular layer of the uterus.

myopia (mī-ō′pē-ă) A condition that occurs when light entering the eye is focused in front of the retina; commonly called nearsightedness.

myxedema (mik-se-dē′mă) A severe type of hypothyroidism that is most common in women older than 50.

nail bed (nāl bĕd) The layer beneath each nail.

narcotic (nahr-kot′ik) A popular term for an opioid and term of choice in government agencies; see **opioid.**

nares (nā′-rēz) The openings of the nose, or nostrils.

nasal (nā′zăl) Relating to the nose. The nasal bones fuse to form the bridge of the nose.

nasal conchae (nā′zăl kon′kē) Structures that extend from the lateral walls of the nasal cavity.

nasal mucosa (nā′zăl myū-kō′să) The lining of the nose.

nasal septum (nā′zăl sĕp′tŭm) A structure that divides the nasal cavity into a left and right portion.

nasolacrimal duct (nā′zō-lak′ri-măl dŭkt) A structure located on the medial aspect of each eyeball. These ducts drain tears into the nose.

nasopharynx (nā′zō-far′ingks) The portion of the pharynx behind the nasal cavity.

National Center for Complementary and Alternative Medicine (NCCAM) (nash′ŏ-năl sen′tĕr kom′plĕ-ment′ă-rē awl-tĕr′nă-tiv med′i-sin) National organization that conducts and supports CAM research and provides CAM information to healthcare providers and the public.

natural killer (NK) cells (na′chŭr-ăl kil′ĕr selz) Non-B and non-T lymphocytes. NK cells kill cancer cells and virus-infected cells without previous exposure to the antigen.

naturopathic medicine (nā′chŭr-ō-path′ik mĕd-i-sin) A system of medicine that relies on the healing power of the body and supports that power through various healthcare practices, such as nutritional counseling, lifestyle counseling, and exercise.

needle biopsy (nē′dĕl bī′op-sē) A procedure in which a needle and syringe are used to aspirate (withdraw by suction) fluid or tissue cells.

negligence (nĕg′li-jĕns) A medical professional's failure to perform an essential action or performance of an improper action that directly results in the harm of a patient.

negotiable (nĭ-gō′shē-ă-bəl) Legally transferable from one person to another.

neonatal period (nē′ō-nā′tăl pēr′e-ŏd) The first 4 weeks of the postnatal period of an offspring.

neonate (nē′ō-nāt′) An infant during the first 4 weeks of life.

nephrologist (ne-frol′ō-jĭst) A specialist who studies, diagnoses, and manages diseases of the kidney.

nephrons (nef′ronz) Microscopic structures in the kidneys that filter blood and form urine.

nerve fiber (nĕrv fī′bĕr) A structure that extends from the cell body. It consists of two types: axons and dendrites.

nerve impulse (nĕrv im′pŭls) Electrochemical messages transmitted from neurons to other neurons and effectors.

nervous tissue (nĕr′vŭs tish′ū) A tissue type located in the brain, spinal cord, and peripheral nerves.

netbook (net-buk) A small, portable laptop computer designed for wireless communication and access to the Internet.

net earnings (net ûr′nĭngz) Take-home pay, calculated by subtracting total deductions from gross earnings.

network (net′wŏrk) A system that links several computers together.

networking (nĕt′wŏrk-ĭng) Making contacts with relatives, friends, and acquaintances who may have information about how to find a job in your field.

neuralgia (nūr-al′jē-ă) A medical condition characterized by severe pain along the distribution of a nerve.

neuroglia (nūr-ŏg′lēă) Structures that function as support cells for other neurons, including astrocytes, microglia, and oligodendrocytes; also called *neuroglial cells.*

neurologist (nūr-ol′ŏ-jist) A specialist who diagnoses and treats disorders and diseases of the nervous system, including the brain, spinal cord, and nerves.

neuron (nūr′on) A nerve cell; it carries nerve impulses between the brain or spinal cord and other parts of the body.

neurotransmitter (nūr′ō-trans′mit-ĕr) A chemical within the vesicles of the synaptic knob that is released into the postsynaptic structures when a nerve impulse reaches the synaptic knob.

neutrophil (nū′trō-fil) A type of granular leukocyte that aids in phagocytosis by attacking bacterial invaders; also responsible for the release of pyrogens.

new patient (nū pā′shĕnt) Patient that, for CPT reporting purposes, has not received professional services from the physician within the past 3 years.

NK cells See **natural killer cells.**

nocturia (nok-tyūr′ē-ă) Excessive nighttime urination.

nomogram (nō′mō-gram) A form of line chart showing scales for the variables involved in a particular formula in such a way that corresponding values for each variable lie in a straight line intersecting all the scales.

noncompliant (non-kŏm-plī′ănt) The term used to describe a patient who does not follow the medical advice given.

noninvasive (non-in-vā′siv) Referring to procedures that do not require inserting devices, breaking the skin, or monitoring to the degree needed with invasive procedures.

nonsteroidal hormone (non′ster-oy′dăl hŏr′mōn) A type of hormone made of amino acids and proteins.

norepinephrine (nor-ep′i-nef′rin) A neurotransmitter released by sympathetic neurons onto organs and glands for fight-or-flight (stressful) situations.

no-show (nō shō) A patient who does not call to cancel and does not come to an appointment.

nosocomial infection (nō′zō-kō′mē-ăl in-fek′shŭn) An infection contracted in a hospital.

notations (nō-tā′shŭnz) Information found at the end of a business letter indicating enclosures included with the letter and the names of other people who will be receiving copies of the letter.

Notice of Privacy Practices (NPP) (nō′tis prī′vă-sē prak′tis-ĕz) A document that informs patients of their rights as outlined under **HIPAA.**

NPP See **Notice of Privacy Practices.**

nuclear medicine (nū′klē-ăr med′i-sin) The use of radionuclides, or radioisotopes (radioactive elements or their compounds), to evaluate the bone, brain, lungs, kidneys, liver, pancreas, thyroid, and spleen; also known as radionuclide imaging.

nucleases (nū′klē-ās-ez) Pancreatic enzymes that digest nucleic acids.

nucleus (nū′klē-ŭs) The control center of a cell; contains the chromosomes that direct cellular processes.

numeric filing system (nū-mer′ik fīl′-ing sis′tĕm) A filing system that organizes files by numbers instead of names. Each patient is assigned a number in the order in which she joins the practice.

nutrient (nū′trē-ĕnt) A constituent of food necessary for normal physiologic function.

nystagmus (nis-tag′mŭs) Rapid, involuntary eye movements that may be the result of drug or alcohol use, brain injury or lesion, or cerebrovascular accident (CVA).

O&P specimen (ō and pē spes′i-mĕn)   An ova and parasites specimen, or a stool sample, that is examined for the presence of certain forms of protozoans or parasites, including their eggs (ova).

objective (ŏb-jek′tĭv)   Pertaining to data that are readily apparent and measurable, such as vital signs, test results, or physical examination findings.

objective data (ŏb-jek′tĭv dā′tă)   Information about the patient's condition that is readily apparent or measurable.

objectives (ob-jek′tĭvs)   The set of magnifying lenses contained in the nosepiece of a compound microscope.

occipital (ok-sip′i-tăl)   Relating to the back of the head. The occipital bone forms the back of the skull.

occult blood (ŏ-kŭlt′ blŭd)   Blood contained in some other substance, not visible to the naked eye.

Occupational Safety and Health Administration (OSHA)   See **OSHA.**

Occupational Safety and Health Act. (ok′yū-pā′shŭn-ăl sāf′tē helth akt)   A set of regulations designed to save lives, prevent injuries, and protect the health of workers in the United States.

OCR   See **optical character recognition.**

ocular (ok′yū-lăr)   An eyepiece of a microscope.

oil-immersion objective (oyl i-mĕr′zhŭn ŏb-jek′tiv)   A microscope objective that is designed to be lowered into a drop of immersion oil placed directly above the prepared specimen under examination, eliminating the air space between the microscope slide and the objective and producing a much sharper, brighter image.

ointment (oynt′mĕnt)   A form of topical drug; also known as a salve.

Older Americans Act of 1965 (ōl′dĕr ă-mĕr′ĭ-kăns akt)   A US law that guarantees certain benefits to elderly citizens, including healthcare, retirement income, and protection against abuse.

olfactory (ōl-fak′tŏr-ē)   Relating to the sense of smell.

oligodendrocytes (ol′i-gō-den′drō-sīts)   Specialized neuroglial cells that assist in the production of the myelin sheath.

oliguria (ol′i-gyūr′ē-ă)   Insufficient production (or volume) of urine.

OMM   See **osteopathic manipulative medicine.**

oncologist (on-kol′ŏ-jist)   A specialist who identifies tumors and treats patients who have cancer.

onychectomy (ŏn-i-kek′tŏ-mē)   The removal of a fingernail or toenail.

oocyte (ō′ŏ-sīt)   The immature egg.

oogenesis (ō-ŏ-jen′ĭ-sis)   The process of egg cell formation.

open-book account (ō′pĕn buk ă-kownt′)   An account that is open to charges made occasionally as needed.

open-hours scheduling (ō′pĕn owrz sked′jūl-ing)   A system of scheduling in which patients arrive at the doctor's office at their convenience and are seen on a first-come, first-served basis.

open posture (ō′pĕn pos′chŭr)   A position that conveys a feeling of receptiveness and friendliness; facing another person with arms comfortably at the sides or in the lap.

ophthalmologist (of′thăl-mol′ŏ-jist)   A medical doctor who is an eye specialist.

ophthalmoscope (of-thal′mō-skōp)   A hand-held instrument with a light; used to view inner eye structures.

opioid (ō′-pē-oyd)   A natural or synthetic drug that produces opium-like effects.

opportunistic infection (op′ŏr-tū-nis′tik in-fek′shŭn)   Infection by microorganisms that can cause disease only when a host's resistance is low.

optical character reader (OCR) (op′ti-kăl kar′ăk-tĕr rēd′ĕr)   An electronic scanner that can "read" typed letters.

optical character recognition (OCR) (op′ti-kăl kar′ăk-tĕr rek′ŏg-nish′ŭn)   The process or technology of reading data in printed form by a device that scans and identifies characters.

optical microscope (op′ti-kăl mī′krŏ-skōp)   A microscope that uses light, concentrated through a condenser and focused through the object being examined, to project an image.

optic chiasm (ŏp′tĭk kī′azm)   A structure located at the base of the brain where parts of the optic nerves cross. It carries visual information to the brain.

optician (op-tish′ăn)   An eye professional who fills prescriptions for eyeglasses and contact lenses.

optometrist (op-tom′ĕ-trist)   A trained and licensed vision specialist who is not a physician.

orbicularis oculi (ōr-bik′yū-lā′ris ok′yū-lī)   The muscle in the eyelid responsible for blinking.

orbit (ōr′bit)   The eye socket, which forms a protective shell around the eye.

organ (ōr′găn)   Structure formed by the organization of two or more different tissue types that carries out specific functions.

organ of Corti (ōr′găn kōr′tē)   The organ of hearing, located within the cochlea of the inner ear.

organelle (ōr′gă-nel′)   A structure within a cell that performs a specific function.

organic (ōr-gan′ik)   Pertaining to matter that contains carbon and hydrogen.

organism (ōr′gă-nizm)   A whole living being that is formed from organ systems.

organization (ōr′găn-ī-zā′shŭn)   A facility or set of coordinated facilities that provide health care.

organizational chart (ōr′găn-ī-zā′shŭn-ăl chahrt)   A formal drawing of the supervisory structure and reporting relationships of an organization such as a medical facility.

organ system (ōr′găn sis′tĕm)   A system that consists of organs that join together to carry out vital functions.

orifice (ōr′i-fis)   An opening.

origin (ōr′i-jin)   An attachment site of a skeletal muscle that does not move when a muscle contracts.

Original Medicare Plan (ōr′i-jin′ăl med′i-kār plan)   The Medicare fee-for-service plan that allows the beneficiary to choose any licensed physician certified by Medicare.

oropharynx (ōr′ō-far′ingks)   The portion of the pharynx behind the oral cavity.

orthopedist (ōr′thŏ-pē′dist)   A specialist who diagnoses and treats diseases and disorders of the muscles and bones.

orthopnea (ōr-thop′nē′ă)   Condition of difficulty breathing except while in an upright position.

orthostatic hypotension (ōr-thō-stat′ik hī′pō-ten′shŭn)   A situation in which blood pressure becomes low and the pulse increases when a patient is moved from a lying to standing position; also known as postural hypotension.

OSHA (ō′shuh)   A federal organization (part of the Department of Labor) that ensures safe and healthy working conditions for Americans by enforcing standards and providing workplace safety training.

osmosis (ŏz-mō′sĭs) The diffusion of water across a semipermeable membrane such as a cell membrane.

ossicles (os′i-kĕls) Small bones; specifically, one of the bones of the tympanic cavity or middle ear.

ossification (os′i-fi-kā′shŭn) The process of bone growth.

osteoarthritis (os′tē-ō-ahr-thrī′tis) Arthritis characterized by erosion of articular cartilage, which becomes soft, frayed, and thinned with eburnation of subchondral bone and outgrowths of marginal osteophytes; pain and loss of function result; mainly affects weight-bearing joints and is more common in women, the overweight, and older people.

osteoblasts (os′tē-ō-blasts) Bone-forming cells that turn membrane into bone. They use excess blood calcium to build new bone.

osteoclast (os′tē-ō-klast) Bone-dissolving cell. When bone is dissolved, calcium is released into the bloodstream.

osteocyte (os′tē-ō-sĭt A cell of osseous tissue; also called a bone cell.

osteon (os′tē-on) Elongated cylinders that run up and down the long axis of bone.

osteopathic manipulative medicine (OMM) (ŏs′tē-ō-păth′ĭk mă-nip′yū-lă-tiv med′i-sin) A system of hands-on techniques that help relieve pain, restore motion, support the body's natural functions, and influence the body's structure. Osteopathic physicians study OMM in addition to medical courses.

osteoporosis (os′tē-ō-pŏr-ō′sis) An endocrine and metabolic disorder of the musculoskeletal system, more common in women than in men, characterized by hunched-over posture.

osteosarcoma (os′tē-ō-sahr-kō′mă) A type of bone cancer that originates from osteoblasts, the cells that make bony tissue.

OT See **oxytocin.**

otologist (ō-tol′ŏ-jist) A medical doctor who specializes in the health of the ear.

otorhinolaryngologist (ō-tō-rī′nō-lar-ing-gol′ŏ-jist) A specialist who diagnoses and treats diseases of the ear, nose, and throat.

otosclerosis (ō′tō-skle-rō′sis) Hardening or immobilization of the stapes within the inner ear.

out guide (owt gīd) A marker made of stiff material and used as a placeholder when a file is taken out of a filing system.

ova (ōva) Eggs.

oval window (ō′văl win′dō) The beginning of the inner ear.

overbooking (ō′vĕr-buk′ing) Scheduling appointments for more patients than can reasonably be seen in the time allowed.

oviduct (ō′vi-dŭkt) A fallopian tube.

ovulation (ov′yū-lā′shŭn) The process by which the ovaries release one ovum (egg) approximately every 28 days.

ovum (ō′vŭm) One egg. The female "egg" that unites with the male sperm to begin reproduction.

oxygenated (ok′si-jĕ-nāt-ĕd) *Oxygenated blood* refers to blood that has been to the lungs and is carrying oxygen in the hemoglobin.

oxygen debt (ok′sĭ-jĕn det) A condition that develops when skeletal muscles are used strenuously for a minute or two.

oxyhemoglobin (ok′sē-hē′mŏ-glō′bin) Hemoglobin that is bound to oxygen. It is bright red in color.

oxytocin (OT) (ok-sē-tō′sin) A hormone that causes contraction of the uterus during childbirth and the ejection of milk from mammary glands during breast-feeding. (32)

package insert (pak′ăj in′sĕrt) A manufacturer's printed guideline for the use and dosing of a drug; includes the pharmacokinetics, dosage forms, and other relevant information about a drug.

packed red blood cells (păkt rĕd blud sĕlz) Red blood cells that collect at the bottom of a centrifuged blood sample.

palate (pal′ăt) The roof of the mouth.

palatine (pal′ă-tīn) Bones that form the anterior portion of the roof of the mouth and the palate.

palatine tonsils (pal′ă-tīn tŏn′silz) Two masses of lymphatic tissue located at the back of the throat.

palpation (pal-pā′shŭn) A type of touch used by healthcare providers to determine characteristics such as texture, temperature, shape, and the presence of movement.

palpatory method (pal′pă-tōr′ē meth′ŏd) Systolic blood pressure measured by using the sense of touch. This measurement provides a necessary preliminary approximation of the systolic blood pressure to ensure an adequate level of inflation when the actual auscultatory measurement is made.

palpitations (pal′pi-tā′shŭn) Unusually rapid, strong, or irregular pulsations of the heart.

pancreatic amylase (pan-krē-at′ik am′il-ās) An enzyme that digests carbohydrates.

pancreatic lipase (pan-krē-at′ik lip′ās) An enzyme that digests lipids.

panel (păn′el) Tests frequently ordered together that are organ or disease oriented.

papillae (pă-pĭl′ē) The "bumps" of the tongue in which the taste buds are found. (35)

paranasal sinuses (par′ă-nā′zăl sī′nŭs-ĕz) Air-filled spaces within skull bones that open into the nasal cavity.

parasite (păr′ă-sīt′) An organism that lives on or in another organism and relies on it for nourishment or some other advantage to the detriment of the host organism.

parasympathetic branch (par′ă-sim′pă-thet′ik branch) A branch of the autonomic nervous system that prepares the body for rest and digestion.

parathyroid glands (par′ă-thī′royd glăndz) Four small glands embedded in the posterior thyroid gland that secrete parathyroid hormone (PTH), also known as parathormone.

parathyroid hormone (PH) (par′ă-thī′royd hôr′mōn′) A hormone that helps regulate calcium levels in the bloodstream. It increases blood calcium by decreasing bone calcium.

parenteral nutrition (pă-ren′tĕr-ăl nū-trish′ŭn) Nutrition obtained when specially prepared nutrients are injected directly into patients' veins rather than taken by mouth.

paresthesia (par′es-thē′zē-ă) Abnormal sensations ranging from burning to tingling.

parietal (pă-rī′ĕ-tăl) Bones that form most of the top and sides of the skull.

parietal cells (pă-rī′ĕ-tăl selz) Stomach cells that secrete hydrochloric acid, which is necessary to convert pepsinogen to pepsin. Parietal cells also secrete intrinsic factor, which is necessary for vitamin B_{12} absorption.

parietal pericardium (pă-rī′ĕ-tăl per-i-kar′dē-ŭm) The layer on top of the visceral pericardium.

parietal peritoneum (pă-rī′ĕ-tăl per′i-tŏ-nē′ŭm) The lining of the abdominal cavity.

parotid glands (pă-rot′id glandz) The largest of the salivary glands. The parotid glands are located beneath the skin just in front of the ears.

participating physicians (pahr-tis′i-pāt-ing fi-zish′ŭnz) Physicians who enroll in managed care plans. They have contracts with MCOs that stipulate their fees.

participatory teaching (pahr-tis′i-pă-to′rē tēch′ing) Method of teaching that includes demonstrations of techniques that may be necessary to show that something has been learned.

partnership (pahrt′nĕr-ship) A form of medical practice management in which two or more parties practice together under a written agreement, specifying the rights, obligations, and responsibilities of each partner.

parturition (pahr′chŭr-ish′ŭn) The act of giving birth.

passive listening (păs′ĭv lĭs′ĕn-ĭng) Hearing what a person has to say without responding in any way; contrast with **active listening.**

patch test (pach test) An allergy test in which a gauze patch soaked with a suspected allergen is taped onto the skin with nonallergenic tape; used to discover the cause of contact dermatitis.

patella (pă-tel′ă) The bone commonly referred to as the kneecap.

pathogen (path′ŏ-jĕn) A microorganism capable of causing disease.

pathologist (pă-thol′ŏ-jist) A medical doctor who studies the changes a disease produces in the cells, fluids, and processes of the entire body.

patient advocacy (pā′shĕnt ad′vŏ-kă-sē) The act of speaking and acting on behalf of the patient's needs and well-being.

patient-centered medical home (PCMH) (pā′shĕnt-sen′tĕrd med′i-kăl hōm) A healthcare model designed to change the organization and delivery of primary care in the United States. Primary functions include comprehensive, patient-centered, coordinated care that is accessible and ensures the quality and safety of healthcare provided.

patient compliance (pā′shĕnt kŏm-plī′ăns) Obedience in terms of following a physician's orders.

patient ledger card (pā′shĕnt lej′ĕr kahrd) A card containing information needed for insurance purposes, including the patient's name, address, telephone number, Social Security number, insurance information, employer's name, and any special billing instructions. It also includes the name of the person who is responsible for charges if this is anyone other than the patient.

patient navigator (pā′shĕnt nav′i-gā′tŏr) A healthcare professional who helps patients find their way through the sometimes complex healthcare system, helping them overcome any barriers they encounter to ensure that they get the diagnosis and treatment they need in a timely manner.

patient record/chart (pā′shĕnt rĕk′ŏrd/ chärt) A compilation of important information about a patient's medical history and present condition.

payee (pā-ē′) A person who receives a payment.

payer (pā′ĕr) A person who pays a bill or writes a check.

pay schedule (pā sked′jūl) A list showing how often an employee is paid, such as weekly, biweekly, or monthly.

peak expiratory flow rate (PEFR) (pēk ek-spīr′ă-tōr-ē flō rāt) A measurement taken, usually with a peak flow meter, to determine the amount of air that can be forced quickly from the lungs.

pectoral girdle (pek′tŏr-ăl gĭr′dĕl) The structure that attaches the arms to the axial skeleton.

pediatrician (pē′dē-ă-trish′ăn) A specialist who diagnoses and treats childhood diseases and teaches parents skills for keeping their children healthy.

pediculosis (pĕ-dik′yū-lō′sis) The medical term for lice.

pegboard system (peg′bōrd sis′tĕm) A bookkeeping system that uses a lightweight board with pegs on which forms can be stacked, allowing each transaction to be entered and recorded on four different bookkeeping forms at once; also called the one-write system.

pelvic girdle (pel′vik gĭr′dĕl) The strcture that attaches the legs to the axial skeleton.

pepsin (pep′sin) An enzyme that allows the body to digest proteins.

pepsinogen (pep-sin′ō-jen) Substance that is secreted by the chief cells in the lining of the stomach and becomes pepsin in the presence of acid.

peptidases (pep′ti-dās-ez) Enzymes that digest proteins.

percussion (pĕr-kŭsh′ŭn) Tapping or striking the body to hear sounds or feel vibration.

percutaneous exposure (pĕr′kyū-tā′nē-ŭs eks-pō′zhŭr) Exposure to a pathogen through a puncture wound or needlestick.

pericardium (pĕr-i-kahr′dē-ŭm) A membrane that covers the heart and large blood vessels attached to it.

perilymph (per′i-limf) A fluid in the inner ear. When this fluid moves, it activates hearing and equilibrium receptors.

perimetrium (peri-mē′trē-ŭm) The thin layer that covers the myometrium of the uterus.

perimysium (per′i-mis′ē-ŭm) The connective tissue that divides a muscle into sections called fascicles.

perineum (per′i-nē′ŭm) In the male, the area between the scrotum and anus; in the female, the area between the vagina and rectum.

periosteum (per′ē-os′tē-ŭm) The membrane that surrounds the **diaphysis** of a bone.

peripheral nervous system (PNS) (pĕr-if′ĕr-ăl nĕr′vŭs sis′tĕm) A system that consists of nerves that branch off the central nervous system.

peristalsis (per′i-stal′sis) The rhythmic muscular contractions that move a substance through a tract, such as food through the digestive tract and the ovum through the fallopian tube.

peritoneum (per′i-tŏ-nē′ŭm) The double-walled, outermost layer of the alimentary canal; also called the *serosa*.

persistence (pĕr-sis′tĕns) Survival despite opposition or adverse environmental conditions.

personal health record (PHR) (pĕr′sŏn-ăl helth rek′ŏrd) A health record that provides a summary of medical information, maintained in electronic or other format by an individual, that can be shared with anyone of the patient's choosing.

personal protective equipment (PPE) (pĕr′sŏn-ăl prŏ-tek′tiv ĕ-kwip′mĕnt) Any type of protective gear worn to guard against physical hazards.

personal space (pĕr′sŏn-ăl spās) A certain area that surrounds an individual and within which another person's physical presence is felt as an intrusion.

PET See **positron emission tomography.** (42, 50)

petty cash fund (pĕt′ē-kăsh fŭnd) Cash kept on hand in the office for small purchases.

PH See **parathyroid hormone.**

phagocyte (fag′ō-sīt) A specialized white blood cell that engulfs and digests pathogens.

phagocytosis (fag′ō-sī-tō′sis) The process by which white blood cells defend the body against infection by engulfing invading pathogens.

phalanges (fă-lan′jēz) The bones of the fingers.

pharmaceutical (fahr′mă-sū′ti-kăl) Pertaining to medicinal drugs.

pharmacodynamics (far′mă-kō-dī-nam′iks) The study of what drugs do to the body: the mechanism of action, or how they work to produce a therapeutic effect.

pharmacognosy (far-mă-kog′nō-sē) The study of characteristics of natural drugs and their sources.

pharmacokinetics (far′mă-kō-ki-net′iks) The study of what the body does to drugs: how the body absorbs, metabolizes, distributes, and excretes the drugs.

pharmacology (fär′ma-kŏl′ŏ-jē) The study of drugs.

pharmacotherapeutics (far′mă-kō-thār′ă-pyū′tiks) The study of how drugs are used to treat disease; also called clinical pharmacology.

pharyngeal tonsils (fă-rin′jē-ăl tŏn′sils) Two masses of lymphatic tissue located above the palatine tonsils; also called adenoids.

pharynx (făr′ĭngks) Structure below the mouth and nasal cavities that is an organ of the respiratory system as well as the digestive system.

phenylketonuria (PKU) (fen′il-kē′tō-nyūr′ē-ă) A genetically inherited disorder in which the body cannot properly metabolize the nutrient phenylalanine, resulting in the buildup of phenylketones in the blood and their presence in the urine. The accumulation of phenylketones results in mental retardation.

PHI See **protected health information.**

philosophy (fĭ-lŏs′ĕ-fē) The system of values and principles an office has adopted in its everyday practice.

phlebotomy (fle-bot′ŏ-mē) The insertion of a needle or cannula (small tube) into a vein for the purpose of withdrawing blood.

photometer (fō-tom′ĕ-tĕr) An instrument that measures light intensity.

PHR See **personal health record.**

physiatrist (fiz-i-a′-trist) A physical medicine specialist, who diagnoses and treats diseases and disorders with physical therapy.

physical therapy (fiz′i-kăl thār′ă-pē) A medical specialty that uses cold, heat, water, exercise, massage, traction, and other physical means to treat musculoskeletal, nervous, and cardiopulmonary disorders.

physician assistant (PA) (fi-zish′ŭn ă-sis′tănt) A healthcare provider who practices medicine under the supervision of a physician.

physician's office laboratory (POL) (fi-zish′ŭnz aw′fis lă′brūh-tō-rē) A laboratory contained in a physician's office; processing tests in the POL produces quick turnaround and eliminates the need for patients to travel to other test locations.

physiology (fĭz′ē-ŏl″ŏ-jē) The science of the study of the body's functions.

pineal body (pin′ē-ăl bŏd′ē) A small gland located between the cerebral hemispheres that secretes melatonin.

pitch (pĭch) The high or low quality in the sound of a person's speaking voice.

PKU See **phenylketonuria.**

placebo effect (plă-sē′bō e-fekt′) The belief that a medication or treatment works even though it is not scientifically substantiated. In research, a placebo is an inactive substance or preparation used as a control to determine the effectiveness of a medicinal drug.

placenta (plă-sen′tă) An organ located between the mother and the fetus. It permits the absorption of nutrients and oxygen. In some cases, harmful substances such as viruses are absorbed through the placenta.

plantar flexion (plan′tăr flek′shŭn) Pointing the toes downward.

plasma (plăz′mă) The fluid component of blood, in which formed elements are suspended; makes up 55% of blood volume.

plastic surgeon (plăs′tĭk sûr′jĕn) A specialist who reconstructs, corrects, or improves body structures.

platelets (plāt′lĕt) Fragments of cytoplasm in the blood that are crucial to clot formation; also called thrombocytes.

pleura (plūr′ă) The membranes that surround the lungs.

pleural effusion (plūr′ăl ĕ-fyū′zhŭn) A buildup of fluid within the pleural cavity.

pleurisy (plūr′i-sē) Also known as pleuritis; this is an inflammation of the parietal pleura of the lungs.

pleuritis (plūr-ī′tis) A condition in which the pleura become inflamed, which causes them to stick together. It can also cause an excess amount of fluid to form between the membranes.

plexus (plĕk′sŭs) A structure that is formed when spinal nerves fuse together. It includes the cervical, brachial, and lumbosacral nerves.

PMS See **premenstrual syndrome.**

pneumoconiosis (nŭ-mŏ-kō-nē-ō′sis) Lung diseases that result from years of exposure to different environmental or occupational types of dust.

pneumothorax (nū-mō-thōr′aks) The presence of air or gas in the pleural cavity. The lung typically collapses with pneumothorax.

PNS See **peripheral nervous system.**

podiatrist (pŏ-dī′ă-trist) Physician who specializes in the study and treatment of the foot and ankle.

POL See **physician's office laboratory.**

polar body (pō′lăr bod′ē) A nonfunctional cell that is one of two small cells formed during the division of an oocyte.

polarity (pō-lăr′ĭ-tē) The condition of having two separate poles, one of which is positive and the other negative.

polarized (pō′lăr-īzd′) The state in which the outside of a cell membrane is positively charged and the inside is negatively charged. Polarization occurs when a neuron is at rest.

policies and procedures (P&P) manual (pol′i-sēz prŏ-sē′jŭrz) A key written communication tool in the medical office that covers all office policies for administrative and clinical procedures.

polypharmacy (pol′ē-fahr′mă-sē) The administration of many drugs at the same time.

polysaccharide (pol-ē-sak′ă-rīd) A type of carbohydrate that is a starch.

POMR The problem-oriented medical record system for keeping patients' charts. Information in a POMR includes the database of information about the patient and the patient's condition, the problem list, the diagnostic and treatment plan, and progress notes.

portfolio (pôrt-fō′lē-ō′) A collection of an applicant's résumé, reference letters, and other documents of interest to a potential employer.

positive tilt test (pŏz′ĭ-tĭv tĭlt tĕst) When the pulse rate increases more than 10 beats per minute (bpm) and the blood pressure drops more than 20 points while taking vital signs in the lying, sitting, and standing positions.

positron emission tomography (PET) (pŏz′ĭ-tron ĕ-mish′ŭn tŏ-mog′rǎ-fē) A radiologic procedure that entails injecting isotopes combined with other substances involved in metabolic activity, such as glucose. These isotopes emit positrons, which a computer processes and displays on a screen.

postcoital (pōst-kō′ĭ-tǎl) After sexual union.

posterior (pos-tēr′ē-ŏr) Anatomical term meaning toward the back of the body. Also called dorsal.

postnatal period (pōst-nā′tǎl pēr′ē-ŏd) The period following childbirth.

postoperative (pōst-op′ĕr-ǎ-tiv) Taking place after a surgical procedure.

postural hypotension (pŏs-chŭr′-ǎl hī-pō-tĕn-shŭn) A situation in which blood pressure becomes low and the pulse increases when a patient is moved from a lying to a standing position; also known as orthostatic hypotension.

posture (pŏs′chŭr) Body position and alignment.

power of attorney (pow′ĕr ǎ-tŏr′nē) The legal right to act as the attorney or agent of another person, including handling that person's financial matters.

PPE See **personal protective equipment.**

PPO See **preferred provider organization.**

practitioner (prak-tish′ŭn-ĕr) One who practices a profession.

practice management system (prak′tis man′ǎj-mĕnt sis′tĕm) Multi-functional electronic health system programs which, in addition to medical records management, provide other functionalities including, but not limited to electronic scheduler, billing and accounts receivable capability, report writer, insurance eligibility and referral management system and billing and coding software.

preauthorization (prē′awth′ŏr-ĭ-zā′shun) Authorization or approval for payment from a third-party payer requested in advance of a specific procedure.

pre-certification (prē′sĕr-ti-fi-kā′shŭn) A determination of the amount of money that will be paid by a third-party payer for a specific procedure before the procedure is conducted.

preferred provider organization (PPO) (prĕ-fĕrd′ prŏ-vī′dĕr ōr′gǎ-nī-zā′shun) A managed care plan that establishes a network of providers to perform services for plan members.

prefix (prē′fĭks) A word part that comes at the beginning of a medical term that alters the meaning of the term.

premenstrual syndrome (PMS) (prē-men′strū-ǎl sin′drōm) A collection of symptoms that occur just before the menstrual period.

premium (prē′mē-ŭm) The basic annual cost of healthcare insurance.

prenatal period (prē-nā′tǎl pîr′ē-ŏd) The period that includes the embryonic and fetal periods until the delivery of the offspring.

preoperative (prē-op′ĕr-ǎ-tiv) Taking place prior to surgery.

prepuce (prē′pyŭs) A piece of skin in the uncircumcized male that covers the glans penis.

presbyopia (prez-bē-ō′pē-ǎ) A common eye disorder that results in the loss of lens elasticity. Presbyopia develops with age and causes a person to have difficulty seeing objects close up.

prescribe (prĕ-skrīb′) To give a patient a prescription to be filled by a pharmacy.

prescription (prĕ-skrip′shŭn) A physician's written order for medication.

prescription drug (prĕ-skrip′shŭn drŭg) A drug that can be legally used only by order of a physician and must be administered or dispensed by a licensed healthcare professional.

preventive care (prĕ-ven′tiv kār) Screening tests and drugs to prevent disease.

preventive medicine (prĕ-ven′tiv med′i-sin) The branch of medical science concerned with the prevention of disease and with promotion of physical and mental health, through study of the etiology and epidemiology of disease processes.

primary care physician (PCP) (prī′mar-ē kār fi-zish′ǎn) A physician who provides routine medical care and referrals to specialists.

primary diagnosis (prī′mar-ē dī-ǎg-nō′sis) The diagnosis given as the primary reason for the patient seeking care.

primary germ layer (prī′mar-ē jĕrm lā′ĕr) An inner cell mass that organizes into layers: the ectoderm, mesoderm, and endoderm.

prime mover (prīm mū′vĕr) The muscle responsible for most of the movement when a body movement is produced by a group of muscles.

primordial follicle (prī-mōr′dē-ǎl fol′i-kĕl) A structure that develops in the ovarian cortex of a female infant before she is born.

principal diagnosis (prin′si-pǎl dī′ǎg-nō′sis) The diagnosis that is found, after testing and study, to be the main reason for the patient's need for health-care services.

prioritizing (prī-ôr′-ĭ-tīz-ing) Sorting and dealing with matters in the order of urgency and importance.

Privacy Rule (prī′vǎ-sē rūl) Common name for the HIPAA Standard for Privacy of Individually Identifiable Health Information, which provides the first comprehensive federal protection for the privacy of health information. The Privacy Rule creates national standards to protect individuals' medical records and other personal health information.

PRL See **prolactin.**

probationary period (prō-bā-shŭn-ār-ē pĕr′ē-ŏd) A trial period during which the employer may terminate the new employee without cause.

problem solving (prob′lĕm sŏlv-ing) A step-by-step approach that uses critical thinking and good judgment to deal with situations or occurrences that need resolution.

procedure code (prŏ-sē′jĕr kōd) Code that represents a medical procedure, such as surgery and diagnostic tests, and medical services, such as an examination to evaluate a patient's condition.

proctologist (prok-tol′ŏ-jist) Physician who diagnoses and treats disorders of the anus, rectum, and intestines.

proctoscopy (prok-tos′kō-pē) An examination of the lower rectum and anal canal with a 3-inch instrument called a proctoscope to detect hemorrhoids, polyps, fissures, fistulas, and abscesses.

professional development (prŏ-fesh'ŭn-ăl dĕ-vel'ŏp-mĕnt) The skills and knowledge attained for both personal development and career advancement.

professional objective (prŏ-fesh'un-ăl ŏb-jek'tiv) A brief, general statement that demonstrates a career goal.

proficiency testing program (prō-fish'ĕn-sē test'ing prō'grăm) A required set of tests for clinical laboratories; the tests measure the accuracy of the laboratory's test results and adherence to standard operating procedures.

progesterone (prŏ-jes'tĕr-ōn) A female steroid hormone primarily produced by the ovary.

prognosis (prŏg-nō'sĭs) A prediction of the probable course of a disease in an individual and the chances of recovery.

prolactin (PRL) (prō-lak'tin) A hormone that stimulates milk production in the mammary glands.

prolapse (prō'laps) A sinking of an organ or other part, especially its appearance at a natural or artificial orifice.

proliferation phase (prŏ-lif'ĕr-ā'shŭn fāz) The second phase of wound healing, in which new tissue forms, closing off the wound.

pronation (prō-nā'shŭn) Turning the palms of the hand downward.

pronunciation (prō-nun'cē-ā'shŭn) The sounding out of words.

proofreading (prūf'rēd-ing) Checking a document for formatting, data, and mechanical errors.

prophase (prō'faz) Movement of the replicated centrioles to the opposite ends of the cell, creating spindle-like fibers during mitosis.

proportion (prŏ-pōr'shŭn) Two fractions that are equal to each other. When three of the four values are known, the fourth value can be calculated by cross-multiplying and solving for the unknown value.

proportion method (prō-pōr'shŭn meth'ŏd) A fraction formula based on ratios and proportions that is used to calculate dosage.

prostaglandins (pros-tă-glan'dinz) Local hormones derived from lipid molecules. Prostaglandins typically do not travel in the bloodstream to find their target cells because their targets are close by. These hormones have numerous effects, including uterine stimulation during childbirth.

prostate gland (prŏs'tāt glănd) A chestnut-shaped gland that surrounds the beginning of the urethra in the male.

prostatitis (pros-tă-tī'tis) Inflammation of the prostate gland, which can be acute or chronic.

protected health information (PHI) (prŏ-tek'tĕd helth in'fŏr-mā'shŭn) Individually identifiable health information that is transmitted or maintained by electronic or other media, such as computer storage devices. The core of the HIPAA Privacy Rule is the protection, use, and disclosure of protected health information.

protein (prō'tēn) Macromolecules consisting of long sequences of α-amino acids [H_2N-CHR-COOH] in peptide (amide) linkage (elimination of H_2O between the α-NH_2 and α-COOH of successive residues). Protein is three-fourths of the dry weight of most cell matter and is involved in structures, hormones, enzymes, muscle contraction, immunologic response, and essential life functions. The amino acids involved are generally the 20 α-amino acids (glycine, l-alanine) recognized by the genetic code. Cross-links yielding globular forms of protein are often effected through the 2SH groups of two sulfur-containing l-cysteinyl residues, as well as by noncovalent forces (such as hydrogen bonds, lipophilic attractions).

proteinuria (prō'tē-nyūr'ē-ă) An excess of protein in the urine.

protozoan (prō'tō-zō'ăn) A single-celled eukaryotic organism much larger than a bacterium; some protozoans can cause disease in humans.

protraction (prō-trăk'shŭn) Moving a body part anteriorly.

proximal (prok'si-măl) Anatomical term meaning closer to a point of attachment or closer to the trunk of the body.

proximal convoluted tubule (prok'simăl kon'vō-lūt'ed tū'byūl) The portion of the renal tubule that is directly attached to the glomerular capsule and becomes the loop of Henle.

psoriasis (sōr-ī'ă-sis) A common skin condition characterized by reddish-silver, scaly lesions most often found on the elbows, knees, scalp, and trunk.

puberty (pyu'bĕr-tē) The period of adolescence when a person begins to develop secondary sexual traits and reproductive functions.

pubis (pyu'bis) The area that forms the front of a hip bone.

pulmonary circuit (pul'mŏ-nār-ē sĭr'kŭt) The route that blood takes from the heart to the lungs and back to the heart again.

pulmonary circulation (pul'mŏ-nar-ē sĭr'kyū-lā'shŭn) The passage of blood from the right ventricle through the pulmonary artery to the lungs and back through the pulmonary veins to the left atrium.

pulmonary function test (pul'mŏ-nār-ē fŭngk'shŭn test) A test that evaluates a patient's lung volume and capacity; used to detect and diagnose pulmonary problems or to monitor certain respiratory disorders and evaluate the effectiveness of treatment.

pulmonary semilunar valve (pul'mŏ-nār-ē sem'ē-lū'năr valv) A heart valve that is a semilunar valve. It is situated between the right ventricle and the pulmonary trunk.

pulmonary trunk (pul'mŏ-nār-ē trŭngk) A large artery that branches into the pulmonary arteries and carries blood to the lungs.

punctuality (pŭngk'chū'ăl'i-tē) Showing up on appointed dates and at appointed times.

puncture wound (pungk'shŭr wūnd) A deep wound caused by a sharp, pointed object.

punitive damages (pyū'ni-tiv dam'ij'iz) Money paid as punishment for intentionally breaking the law.

pupil (pyū'pil) The opening at the center of the iris, which grows smaller or larger as the iris contracts or relaxes, respectively; it regulates the amount of light that enters the eye.

purchase order (pŭr'chăs ōr'dĕr) A form that authorizes a purchase for the practice.

purchasing groups (pur'chăs-ĭng grūps) Groups of medical offices associated with a nearby hospital that order supplies through the hospital to obtain a quantity discount.

Purkinje fibers (pŭr-kin'jē fī'bĕrz) Cardiac fibers located in the lateral walls of the ventricles.

pyelonephritis (pī'ĕ-lō-ne-frī'-tis) A urinary tract infection that involves one or both of the kidneys.

pyloric sphincter (pī-lōr′ik sfingk′tĕr) The valve-like structure composed of a circular band of muscle at the juncture of the stomach and small intestine.

pyothorax (pī′ō-thōr′aks) Pus or infected fluid in the pleural cavity, causing collapse of the lung.

pyrogens (pī′rō-jenz) Fever-producing substances released by neutrophils.

QC See **quality control.**

qi (chē) According to traditional Chinese medicine, a vital energy that flows throughout the body.

quadrant (kwahd′rănt) One of four equal sections, such as those into which the abdomen is figuratively divided during an examination.

qualitative analysis (kwahl′i-tā′tiv ă-nal′i-sis) In microbiology, identification of bacteria present in a specimen by the appearance of colonies grown on a culture plate.

qualitative test response (kwahl′i-tā′tiv test rĕ-spons′) A test result that indicates the substance tested for is either present or absent.

quality assurance (kwahl′i-tē ă-shŭr′ăns) Procedures that ensure that the services provided in the medical practice meet or exceed requirements and standards.

quality assurance program (kwahl′i-tē ă-shŭr′ăns prō′gram) A required program for clinical laboratories designed to monitor the quality of patient care, including quality control, instrument and equipment maintenance, proficiency testing, training and continuing education, and standard operating procedures documentation.

quality control (QC) (kwahl′i-tē kŏn-trōl′) An ongoing system, required in every physician's office, to evaluate the quality of medical care provided.

quality control program (kwahl′i-tē kŏn-trōl′ prō′gram) A component of a quality assurance program that focuses on ensuring accuracy in laboratory test results through careful monitoring of test procedures.

quantitative analysis (kwahn′ti-tā′tiv ă-nal′i-sis) In microbiology, a determination of the number of bacteria present in a specimen by direct count of colonies grown on a culture plate.

quantitative test results (kwahn′ti-tā′tiv test rĕ-sŭlt) The concentration of a test substance in a specimen.

quantity (Q) (kwahn′ti-tē) Amount of a medication on hand; for example, a pill or an amount of liquid.

quarterly return (kwahr′tĕr-lē rē-tŭrn′) The Employer's Quarterly Federal Tax Return, a form submitted to the IRS every 3 months that summarizes the federal income and employment taxes withheld from employees' paychecks.

qui tam (kwē tahm) Latin, meaning "to bring action for the king and for one's self."

RA See **explanation of benefits, remittance advice.**

radial artery (rā′dē-ăl ahr′tĕr-ē) An artery located in the groove on the thumb side of the inner wrist, where the pulse is taken on adults.

radiation therapy (rā′dē-ā′shŭn thār′ă-pē) The use of X-rays and radioactive substances to treat cancer.

radiography (rā′dē-og′ră-fē) Examination of any part of the body for diagnostic purposes by means of X-rays, with the record of the findings usually impressed on a photographic film.

radiologist (rā′dē-ol′ŏ-jist) A physician who specializes in taking and reading X-rays.

radius (rā′dē-ŭs) The lateral bone of the forearm.

rales (rahlz) Noisy respirations usually due to blockage of the bronchial tubes.

RAM See **random-access memory.**

random-access memory (RAM) (ran′dŏm ak′ses mem′ŏ-rē) The temporary, or programmable, memory in a computer.

random urine specimen (ran′dŏm yūr′in spes′i-mĕn) A single urine specimen taken at any time of the day; the most common type of sample collected.

range of motion (ROM) (rānj mō′shŭn) The degree to which a joint is able to move.

rapport (ră-pôr′) A harmonious, positive relationship.

RBRVS See **resource-based relative value scale.**

read-only memory (ROM) (rēd ōn′lē mem′ŏ-rē) A computer's permanent memory, which can be read by the computer but not changed. It provides the computer with the basic operating instructions it needs to function.

reagent (rē-ā′jĕnt) A chemical or chemically treated substance used in test procedures and formulated to react in specific ways when exposed under specific conditions.

reconciliation (rē-kon-sil′ē-ā′shŭn) A comparison of the office's financial records with bank records to ensure that they are consistent and accurate; usually done when the monthly checking account statement is received from the bank.

records management system (rĕ-kôrdz man′ăj-mĕnt sis′tĕm) How patient records are created, filed, and maintained.

recovery position (rē-kŏv′ĕr-ē pŏ-zish′ŏn) The position a person is placed in after receiving first aid for choking or cardiopulmonary resuscitation.

rectum (rĕk′tŭm) The last section of the sigmoid colon that straightens out and becomes the anal canal.

Red Flags Rule (rĕd flăgz rūl) A law requiring certain businesses, including most medical offices and other healthcare facilities, to develop written programs to detect the warning signs, or red flags, of identity theft.

reference (refer-′rĕns) A recommendation for employment from a facility or a preceptor.

reference laboratory (ref′er-rĕns lă′brŭh-tō-rē) A laboratory owned and operated by an organization outside the physician's practice.

referral (rĕ-fĕr′ăl) An authorization from a medical practice for a patient to have specialized services performed by another practice; often required for insurance purposes.

reflection (rĕ-flek′shŭn) When a thought, an idea, or an opinion is formed as a result of deeper thought.

reflex (rē′fleks) A predictable automatic response to stimuli.

reflexology (rē′flek-sol′ŏ-jē) Manual therapy to the foot and/or hand in which pressure is applied to "reflex" points mapped out on the feet or hands.

refraction (rē-frak′shŭn) The bending of light by the cornea, lens, and eye fluids to focus light onto the retina.

refraction examination (rē-frak′shŭn eg-zam′i-nā′shŭn) An eye examination in which the patient looks through a succession of different lenses to find out which ones create the clearest image.

refractometer (rē-frak-tom′ĕ-ter) An optical instrument that measures the refraction, or bending, of light as it passes through a liquid.

Registered Medical Assistant (RMA) (rej′i-stĕrd med′i-kăl ă-sis′tănt) A medical assistant who has met the educational requirements and taken and passed the certification examination for medical assisting given by the American Medical Technologists (AMT).

registration (rej′is-trā′shŭn) The recording of information (e.g., licensure, birth or death date).

Reiki (rā′kē) The use of visualization and touch to balance energy flow and bring healthy energy to affected body parts.

relaxin (rē-lak′sin) A hormone that comes from the corpus luteum. It inhibits uterine contractions and relaxes the ligaments of the pelvis in preparation for childbirth.

releasing (rĕ-lēs′ing) Placing a mark or stamp on an item that indicates that the responsible licensed practitioner has seen the document and is giving permission to file it in the patient's medical record.

remedy (rem′ĕ-dē) A treatment prescribed by a homeopath in small amounts that in large doses would produce the same symptoms seen in the patient.

remittance advice (RA) (rē-mit′ăns ad-vīs′) A form that the patient and the practice receive for each encounter that outlines the amount billed by the practice, the amount allowed, the amount of subscriber liability, the amount paid, and notations of any service not covered, including an explanation of why that service is not covered; also called an explanation of benefits.

renal calculi (rē′năl kal′kyū-lī) Kidney stones.

renal column (rē′năl kol′ŭm) The portion of the renal cortex between the renal pyramids.

renal corpuscle (rē′năl kōr′pŭs-ĕl) Corpuscle that is composed of the glomerulus and the glomerular capsule. The filtration of blood occurs here.

renal cortex (rē′năl kōr′teks) The outermost layer of the kidney.

renal medulla (rē′năl mĕ-dŭl′ă) The middle portion of the kidney.

renal pelvis (rē′năl pel′vis) The internal structure of the kidney. Urine flows from the renal pelvis down the ureter.

renal pyramids (rē′năl pir′ă-midz) Triangular-shaped areas in the medulla of the kidney.

renal sinus (rē′năl sī′nŭs) The medial depression of a kidney.

renal tubule (rē′năl tū′byūl) Structure that extends from the glomerular capsule of a nephron and is composed of the proximal convoluted tubule, the loop of Henle, and the distal convoluted tubule.

renin (rē′nin) A hormone secreted by the kidney that helps to regulate blood pressure.

repolarization (rē-pō′lăr-i-zā′shŭn) The process of returning to the original polar (resting) state.

reputable (rĕp′yū-ti-bĕl) Having a good reputation.

requisition (rĕk′wĭ-zĭsh′ŭn) A formal request from a staff member or doctor for the purchase of equipment or supplies.

reservoir host (rĕz′er-vwahr′ hōst) An animal, an insect, or a human whose body is susceptible to growth of a pathogen.

re-sheathing scalpel (rĕ-sheth′ing skalp′ĕl) A single-use, disposable scalpel that has a sheath that can be slid over the blade and locked in position after use.

resident normal flora (rez′i-dĕnt nōr′ măl flōr′ă) Bacteria, fungi, and protozoa that have taken up residence either in or on the human body. Some of these organisms neither help nor harm the host and some are beneficial, creating a barrier against pathogens.

res ipsa loquitur **(res ip′să lō′ kwi-tŭr)** Latin, meaning "the thing speaks for itself," which is also known as the doctrine of common knowledge.

resource-based relative value scale (RBRVS) (rē′sōrs-băst rel′ă-tiv val′yū skāl) The payment system used by Medicare. It establishes the relative value units for services, replacing the providers' consensus on usual fees.

respiratory capacity (res′pir-ă-tōr-ē kă-pas′i-tē) The amount of air the lungs can hold; calculated by adding certain respiratory volumes together.

respiratory distress syndrome (res′pir-ă-tōr-ē dis-tres′ sin′drōm) Condition found usually in premature babies, who lack the substance surfactant in their lungs, causing the lungs to collapse on expiration.

respiratory hygiene/cough etiquette (res′pir-ă-tōr-ē hī′jēn kawf e-ti′ket) Infection control guideline that includes teaching the patient to cover his or her mouth/nose when coughing and dispose of tissues in the proper receptacle.

respiratory volume (res′pir-ă-tōr-ē vol′yūm) The different volumes of air that move into and out of the lungs during different intensities of breathing. These volumes can be measured to assess the healthiness of the respiratory system.

respondeat superior **(rē-spon′dē-ăt sŭ-pēr′e-ŏr)** Latin, meaning "let the master answer," a doctrine under which an employer is legally liable for the acts of his or her employees, if such acts were performed within the scope of the employee's duties.

restatement (rē-stāt′ment) Repeating what a patient says in your own words back to the patient.

résumé (rē-zūm-ā′) A document summarizing one's employment and educational history.

retention schedule (rĭ-ten′shŭn sked′jūl) A schedule that details how long to keep different types of patient records in the office after they have become inactive or closed and how long the records should be stored.

retina (ret′i-nă) The inner layer of the eye; contains light-sensing nerve cells.

retractable needle (rē-trak′tă-bĕl nē′dĕl) A needle that retracts inside the barrel of a syringe after it is activated.

retraction (rē-trăk′shŭn) Moving a body part posteriorly.

retrograde pyelography (ret′rō-grād pī′ĕ-log′ră-fē) A radiologic procedure in which the doctor injects a contrast medium through a urethral catheter and takes a series of X-rays to evaluate function of the ureters, bladder, and urethra.

retroperitoneal (ret′rō-per′i-tŏ-nē′ăl) An anatomical term that means behind the peritoneal cavity. It is where the kidneys lie.

return demonstration (rē-tŭrn′ dem′on-strā′shŭn) Participatory teaching method in which the technique is first described to the patient and then demonstrated to the patient; the patient is then asked to repeat the demonstration.

reverse chronological order (rĕ-vĕrs′ kron′ŏ-loj′ik ĕl ōr′dĕr) A filing system in which the most recent files (by date) are inserted so they are on top of documents with earlier dates in the file folder.

review of symptoms (rē-vū′ simp′tŏmz) A process of gathering information about a patient's health history regardless of apparent relevance to the chief complaint.

rhabdomyolysis (rab′dō-mī-ol′i-sis) A condition in which the kidneys have been damaged due to toxins released from muscle cells.

rhonchi (rong′kī) Deep snoring or rattling sounds during breathing; associated with asthma, acute bronchitis, or any condition involving partial obstruction of the lung's airway.

Rh antigen (an′ti-jen) A protein first discovered on the red blood cells of rhesus monkeys, hence the name Rh.

RhoGAM (rō′găm) A medication that prevents an Rh-negative mother from making antibodies against the Rh antigen.

rhythm strip (rith′ŭm strip) An ECG tracing obtained using an electrocardiograph machine.

ribosomes (rī′bŏ-sōmz) The organelle within the cytoplasm responsible for protein synthesis.

risk management (RM) (risk man′ăj-mĕnt) Plans and processes that continually identify, assess, correct, and monitor functions of the medical office to prevent negative outcomes and minimize exposure to risk and consequent liability.

RMA See **Registered Medical Assistant.**

RNA A nucleic acid used to make protein.

rods (rŏdz) Light-sensing nerve cells in the eye, at the posterior of the retina, that function in dim light but do not provide sharp images or detect color.

ROM See **read-only memory.**

rosacea (rō-zā′shē-ă) A condition characterized by chronic redness and acne over the nose and cheeks.

rotation (rō-tā′shŭn) Twisting a body part.

route (rūt) The way a drug is introduced into the body.

rubrics (rū′briks) Three-character ICD categories used to specify diseases, injuries, and symptoms.

rugae (rū′jē) The expandable folds of an organ. The folds of the stomach lining.

sacrum (sā′krŭm) A triangular-shaped bone that consists of five fused vertebra.

Safety Data Sheet (SDS) (sāf′tē dā′tă shēt) A form that is required for all hazardous chemicals or other substances used in the laboratory and that contains information about the product's name, ingredients, chemical characteristics, physical and health hazards, guidelines for safe handling, and procedures to be followed in the event of exposure.

sagittal (saj′i-tăl) An anatomical term that refers to the plane that divides the body into left and right portions.

salutation (sal′yū-tā′shŭn) A written greeting, such as "Dear," used at the beginning of a letter.

sanitization (san′i-tī-zā′shŭn) A reduction of the number of microorganisms on an object or a surface to a fairly safe level.

sarcolemma (sahr′kō-lem′ă) The cell membrane of a muscle fiber.

sarcoplasm (sahr′kō-plazm) The cytoplasm of a muscle fiber.

sarcoplasmic reticulum (sahr′kō-plaz′mik rĕ-tik′yū-lŭm) The endoplasmic reticulum of a muscle fiber.

SARS (severe acute respiratory syndrome) (sārz) A severe and acute respiratory illness characterized by fever and a nonproductive cough that progresses to the point at which insufficient oxygen is present in the blood.

saturated fat (sach′ūr-āt′ĕd fat) Fat, derived primarily from animal sources, that is usually solid at room temperature and that tends to raise blood cholesterol levels.

scabies (skā′bēz) Skin lesions that are very itchy and caused by a burrowing mite. Scabies is most commonly found between the fingers and on the genitalia.

scanner (skan′er) An optical device that converts printed matter into a format that can be read by the computer and inputs the converted information.

scapula (skap′yū-lă) Thin, triangular-shaped, flat bone located on the dorsal surface of the rib cage; also called shoulder blade.

Schwann cells (shwahn sĕlz) Neuroglial cells whose cell membrane coats the axons.

sciatica (sī-ăt′i-kă) Pain in the low back and hip radiating down the back of the leg along the sciatic nerve.

sclera (skler′ă) The tough, outermost layer, or "white," of the eye, through which light cannot pass; covers all except the front of the eye.

scoliosis (skō′lē-ō′sis) A lateral curvature of the spine, which is normally straight when viewed from behind.

scope of practice (skōp prak′tis) The procedures, processes, and actions a healthcare worker is allowed to perform under the terms of his or her professional license.

scored (skōrd) An indented line on a tablet where the medication can be broken into pieces.

scratch test (skrăch tĕst) An allergy test in which extracts of suspected allergens are applied to the patient's skin and the skin is then scratched to allow the extracts to penetrate.

screening (skrēn′ĭng) Performing a diagnostic test on a person who is typically free of symptoms.

screen saver (skrēn sāv′er) A program that automatically changes the monitor display at short intervals or constantly shows moving images to prevent burn-in of images on the computer screen.

scrotum (skrō′tŭm) In a male, the sac of skin below the pelvic cavity that contains the testes.

sebaceous (sĕ-bā′shŭs) A type of oil gland found in the dermis.

sebum (sē′bŭm) An oily substance produced by sebaceous glands.

secondary diagnosis (sek′ŏn-dār-ē dī-ăg-nō′sis) Diagnosis other than the primary diagnosis for other conditions that are also affecting the patient at the time of the visit.

Security Rule (sĕ-kyūr′i-tē rūl) The technical safeguards that protect the confidentiality, integrity, and availability of health information covered by HIPAA. The Security Rule specifies how patient information is protected on computer networks, the Internet, disks, and other storage media.

seizure (sē′zhŭr) A series of violent and involuntary contractions of the muscles; also called a convulsion.

self-blunting/blunt tip blood drawing needle (self blŭnt′ing) A blood-drawing needle that has a blunt tip that slides forward through the needle past the sharp point to protect the user from needlestick injury.

self-confidence (self-kŏn′fĭ-dĕns) Believing in oneself; assured.

self-sheathing needle (self-shēth´ing) A needle that has a sheath over the barrel of the syringe. After injecting the medication, the user slides the sheath forward over the needle and locks it in place to prevent needlestick injuries.

sella turcica (sel´ă tŭr´sē-kă) A deep depression in the sphenoid bone where the pituitary gland sits.

semen (sē´měn) Sperm and the various substances that nourish and transport them.

semicircular canals (sem´ē-sĭr´kyū-lăr kă-nalz´) Structures in the inner ear that help a person maintain balance; each of the three canals is positioned at right angles to the other two.

seminal vesicles (sem´i-năl ves´i-kĕlz) A pair of convoluted tubes that lie behind the bladder. These tubes secrete a fluid that provides nutrition for the sperm.

seminiferous tubules (sem´i-nif´er-ŭs tū´byūlz) These tubes contain spermatogenic cells and are located in the lobules of the testes.

sensorineural hearing loss (sen´sĕr-ē-nūr´ăl hēr´ing laws) Hearing loss that occurs when neural structures associated with the ear are damaged. Neural structures include hearing receptors and the auditory nerve.

sensory (sen´sŏr-ē) Afferent neurons that carry sensory information from the periphery to the central nervous system.

sensory adaptation (sen´sŏr-ē ad´ap-tā´shŭn) A process in which the same chemical can stimulate receptors only for a limited amount of time until the receptors eventually no longer respond to the chemical.

sensory teaching (sen´sŏr-ē tēch´ing) Method of teaching that provides a patient with a description of the physical sensations he or she may have as part of the learning or the procedure involved.

septic shock (sĕp´tĭk shŏk) A state of shock resulting from massive, widespread infection that affects the blood vessels' ability to circulate blood.

sequential order (sē-kwen´shăl ōr´dĕr) One after another in a predictable pattern or sequence.

serosa (se-rō´să) The outermost layer of the alimentary canal; also known as the visceral peritoneum.

serous cells (sēr´ŭs sĕlz) One of two types of cells that make up the salivary glands.

These cells secrete a watery fluid that contains amylase.

serum (sēr´ŭm) The liquid portion of blood (plasma) when all of the clotting factors have been removed.

serum separators (sēr´ŭm sep´ăr-ā´tŏrz) A type of blood collection tube with an additive that, when spun, forms a gel-like barrier between serum and the clot in a coagulated blood sample.

service contract (sĕr´vis kŏn´-trakt) A contract that covers services for equipment that are not included in a standard maintenance contract.

severe acute respiratory syndrome See **SARS.**

sex chromosome (seks krō´mŏ-sōm) Chromosome of the 23rd pair.

sex-linked trait (seks´linkt trāt) Trait carried on the sex chromosomes, or X and Y chromosomes.

sexual harassment (sek´shū-ăl hăr-ăs´-ment) Unwelcome verbal, visual, or physical conduct of a sexual nature that is severe or pervasive and affects working conditions or creates a hostile work environment.

shelter-in-place (shel´tĕr in plas) An interior room or rooms with few or no windows that form a place to take refuge in case of an emergency or a disaster.

side effects (sīd e-fekts´) Unintended, but fairly mild and common, effects of a medication.

sigmoid colon (sig´moyd kō´lŏn) An S-shaped tube that lies between the **descending colon** and the **rectum.**

sigmoidoscopy (sig´moy-dos´kŏ-pē) A procedure in which the interior of the sigmoid area of the large intestine, between the descending colon and the rectum, is examined with a sigmoidoscope, a lighted instrument with a magnifying lens.

sign (sīn) An objective, or external, factor, such as blood pressure, rash, or swelling, that can be seen or felt by the physician or measured by an instrument.

signature block (sig´nă-chŭr blok) The writer's name and business title found four lines below the complimentary closing in a business letter.

silicosis (sil´i-kō´sis) Chronic lung disease caused by the inhalation of silica dust.

simplified letter style (sim´pli-fīd let´ĕr stīl) A modification of the full-block style in which the salutation and complimentary closing are omitted and a subject line typed in all capital letters is

placed between the address and the body of the letter.

single-entry account (sing´gĕl en´trē ă-kownt) An account that has only one charge, usually for a small amount, for a patient who does not come in regularly.

sinoatrial node (SA node) (sī´nō-ā´trē-ăl nōd) A small bundle of heart muscle tissue in the superior wall of the right atrium that sets the rhythm (pattern) of the heart's contractions; also called sinus node or pacemaker.

sinusitis (sī´nŭ-sī´tis) Inflammation of the lining of a sinus.

skinfold test (skĭn´fōld tĕst) A method of measuring fat as a percentage of body weight by measuring the thickness of a fold of skin with a caliper.

skip (skĭp) A patient who has moved without leaving a forwarding address and his bill is unpaid.

slander (slăn´dĕr) The speaking of defamatory words intended to prejudice others against an individual in a manner that jeopardizes his or her reputation or means of livelihood.

SLE See **systemic lupus erythematosus.**

sleep apnea (slēp ap´nē-ă) A condition characterized by pauses in breathing during sleep.

slit lamp (slit lămp) An instrument composed of a magnifying lens combined with a light source; used to provide a minute examination of the eye's anatomy.

smear (smēr) A specimen spread thinly and unevenly across a slide.

SOAP (sōp) An approach to medical records documentation that documents information in the following order: S (subjective data), O (objective data), A (assessment), P (plan of action).

soft skills (sawft skilz) Personal attributes that enhance an individual's interactions, job performance, and career prospects.

software (soft´wār) A program, or set of instructions, that tells a computer what to do.

sole proprietorship (sōl prŏ-prī´ĕ-tŏr-ship) A form of medical practice management in which a physician practices alone, assuming all benefits and liabilities for the business.

solution (sŏ-lū´shŭn) A homogeneous mixture of a solid, liquid, or gaseous substance in a liquid, such as a dissolved drug in liquid form.

somatic (sō-măt′ĭk) A division of the peripheral nervous system that connects the central nervous system to skin and skeletal muscle.

somatic nervous system (sō-măt′ĭk něr′vŭs sis′tĕm) A system that governs the body's skeletal, or voluntary, muscles.

SOMR Source-oriented medical record.

SPECT (spĕkt) Single photon emission computed tomography; a radiologic procedure in which a gamma camera detects signals induced by gamma radiation and a computer converts these signals into two- or three-dimensional images that are displayed on a screen.

speculum (spek′yŭ-lŭm) An instrument that expands the vaginal opening to permit viewing of the vagina and cervix.

spermatids (sper′mă-tidz) Immature sperm before they develop their flagella (tails).

spermatocytes (sper-mătō′-sīts) The cells that result when spermatogonia undergo mitosis.

spermatogenesis (sper′mă-t′ō-jen′ĕ-sis) The process of sperm cell formation.

spermatogenic cells (sper′mă-tō-jen′ik sĕlz) The cells that give rise to sperm cells.

spermatogonia (sper′mă-tō-gō′nē-ă) The earliest cell in the process of spermatogenesis.

sphenoid (sfē′noyd) A bone that forms part of the floor of the cranium.

sphincter (sfĭngk′tĕr) A valve-like structure formed from circular bands of muscle. Sphincters are located around various body openings and passages.

sphygmomanometer (sfig′mō-mă-nom′ĕ-ter) An instrument for measuring blood pressure; consists of an inflatable cuff, a pressure bulb used to inflate the cuff, and a device to read the pressure.

spinal nerves (spī′năl něrvs) Peripheral nerves that originate from the spinal cord.

spirillum (spī-ril′ŭm) A spiral-shaped bacterium.

spirometer (spī-rom′ĕ-ter) An instrument that measures the air taken in and expelled from the lungs.

spirometry (spī-rom′ĕ-trē) A test used to measure breathing capacity.

spleen (splēn) An abdominal organ that assists in the production and removal of blood cells.

splenectomy (sple-nek′tŏ-mē) Surgical removal of the spleen.

splint (splĭnt) A device used to immobilize and protect a body part.

splinting catheter (splĭnt′ĭng kath′ĕ-tĕr) A type of catheter inserted after plastic repair of the ureter; it must remain in place for at least a week after surgery.

spores (spōrz) A resistant form of certain species of bacteria.

sprain (sprān) An injury characterized by partial tearing of a ligament that supports a joint, such as the ankle. A sprain may also involve injuries to tendons, muscles, and local blood vessels and contusions of the surrounding soft tissue.

stain (stān) In microbiology, a solution of a dye or group of dyes that imparts a color to microorganisms.

standard (stan′dărd) A specimen for which test values are already known; used to calibrate test equipment.

standardization (stan′dărd-ī-zā′shŭn) The consistency of the active ingredient(s) in a supplement from batch to batch and from manufacturer to manufacturer.

standard of care (stan′dărd kār) A legal term that refers to the care that would ordinarily be provided by an average, prudent healthcare provider in a given situation.

standard precautions (stan′dărd prĕ-kaw′shŭnz) A combination of Universal Precautions and Body Substance Isolation guidelines; used in hospitals for the care of all patients.

stapes (stā′pēz) A small bone in the middle ear that is attached to the inner ear; also called the stirrup.

statement (stāt′mĕnt) Similar to an invoice; a summary of total amounts owed, including outstanding charges as well as payments received for services provided by the office.

State Unemployment Tax Act (SUTA) (stāt un-em-ploy′mĕnt taks akt) Some states are also governed by this act; these taxes are filed along with FUTA taxes.

statute of limitations (stach′yū′t lim′i-tā′shŭnz) A state law that sets a time limit on when a collection suit on a past-due account can legally be filed.

stenosis (stĕ-nō′sis) An abnormal narrowing of a body passage.

stent (stĕnt) A metal mesh tube used to hold a vessel open.

stereoscopy (ster-ē-os′kŏ-pē) An X-ray procedure that uses a specially designed microscope (stereoscopic, or Greenough, microscope) with double eyepieces and objectives to take films at different angles and produce three-dimensional images; used primarily to study the skull.

sterile field (ster′il fēld) An area free of microorganisms used as a work area during a surgical procedure.

sterile scrub assistant (ster′il skrŭb ă-sis′tănt) An assistant who handles sterile equipment during a surgical procedure.

sterilization (ster′i-lī-zā′shŭn) The destruction of all microorganisms, including bacterial spores, by specific means.

sterilization indicator (ster′i-lī-zā′shŭn in′di-kā-tŏr) A tag, insert, tape, tube, or strip that confirms that the items in an autoclave have been exposed to the correct volume of steam at the correct temperature for the correct amount of time.

sternum (stĕr′nŭm) A bone that forms the front and middle portion of the rib cage; also called the breastbone or breast plate.

steroidal hormone (ster-oy′dăl hŏr′mōn) A hormone derived from steroids that are soluble in lipids and can cross cell membranes very easily.

stethoscope (stĕth′ĕ-skōp) An instrument that amplifies body sounds.

strabismus (stră-biz′mŭs) A condition that results in a lack of parallel visual axes of the eyes; commonly called crossed eyes.

strain (strān) A muscle injury that results from overexertion or overstretching.

stratum basale (strat′ŭm bā-sā′lē) The deepest layer of the epidermis of the skin.

stratum corneum (strat′ŭm kŏr′nē-ŭm) The most superficial layer of the epidermis of the skin.

stratum germinativum (strā′tŭm jer-mi-nā- tī′vŭm) The deepest layer of the epidermis; also known as stratum basale.

stressor (stres′or) Any stimulus that produces stress.

stress test (stres tĕst) A procedure that involves recording an electrocardiogram while the patient is exercising on a stationary bicycle, treadmill, or stair-stepping ergometer, which measures work performed.

striations (strī-ā′shŭns) Bands produced from the arrangement of filaments in myofibrils in skeletal and cardiac muscle cells.

stroke (strōk) A condition that occurs when the blood supply to the brain is impaired. It may cause temporary or permanent damage.

stylus (stī′lŭs) A pen-like instrument that records electrical impulses on ECG paper.

subarachnoid space (sŭb-ă-rak′noyd spās) An area between the arachnoid mater and the pia mater.

subcategory (sŭb-kăt′ĭ-gôr′ē) The fourth digit added to many ICD-9 codes giving further specificity to the diagnosis.

subclinical case (sŭb-klin′i-kăl kās) An infection in which the host experiences only some of the symptoms of the infection or milder symptoms than in a full case.

subcutaneous (subcut) (sŭb′kyŭ-tā′nē-ŭs) Under the skin.

subjective (sŭb-jĕk′tĭv) Pertaining to data that are obtained from conversation with a person or patient.

subjective data (sŭb-jĕk′tĭv dā′tă) Information about the patient's condition that includes thoughts, feelings, and perceptions.

subject line (sŭb′jekt līn) Optional line of two to three words that appears three lines below the inside address of a business letter.

sublingual (sŭb-ling′gwăl) Under the tongue.

sublingual gland (sŭb-ling′gwăl glănd) The smallest of the salivary glands.

submandibular gland (sŭb-man-dib′yu-lăr glănd) The gland that is located in the floor of the mouth.

submucosa (sŭb′myū-kō′să) The layer of the alimentary canal located between the mucosa and the muscular layer.

subpoena (sŭ-pē′nă) A written court order that is addressed to a specific person and requires that person's presence in court on a specific date at a specific time.

subpoena duces tecum (sŭ-pē′nă dŭ′sēz tē′kum) Latin; a legal document that requires the recipient to bring certain written records to court to be used as evidence in a lawsuit.

substance abuse (sŭb′stăns ă-byŭs′) The use of a substance in a way that is not medically approved, such as using diet pills to stay awake or consuming large quantities of cough syrup that contains codeine. Substance abusers are not necessarily addicts.

sucrase (sū′krās) An enzyme that digests sugars.

sudoriferous (sŭ′dŏr-if′ĕr-ŭs) The sweat glands.

suffix (sŭ-fiks) A word part that comes at the end of a medical term that alters the meaning of the term.

sulci (sŭl′si) The grooves on the surface of the cerebrum.

superbill (sū′pĕr-bil) A form that combines the charges for services rendered, an invoice for payment or insurance copayment, and all the information for submitting an insurance claim; also known as an encounter form.

superficial (sŭ′pĕr-fish′ăl) Anatomical term meaning closer to the surface of the body.

superior (sŭ-pēr′ē-ŏr) Anatomical term meaning above or closer to the head; also called cranial.

supernatant (sū-per-nā′tănt) The liquid portion of a substance from which solids have settled to the bottom, as with a urine specimen after centrifugation.

supination (sū′pi-nā′shŭn) Turning the palm of the hand upward.

surfactant (sŭr-fak′tănt) Fatty substance secreted by some alveolar cells that helps maintain the inflation of the alveoli so that they do not collapse in on themselves between inspirations.

surgeon (sûr′jŏn) A physician who uses hands and medical instruments to diagnose and correct deformities and treat external and internal injuries or disease.

surgical asepsis (sûr′ji-kăl ā-sep′sis) The elimination of all microorganisms from objects or working areas; also called sterile technique.

surgical site infection (SSI) (sûr′ji-kăl sīt in-fek′shŭn) An infection that occurs after a surgical procedure at the site of surgery.

susceptible host (sŭ-sep′ti-bĕl hōst) An individual who has little or no immunity to infection by a particular organism.

SUTA See **State Unemployment Tax Act.**

suture (sŭ′chŭr) Fibrous joint in the skull. Also, a surgical stitch made to close a wound.

swaged needle (swājd nē′dĕl) A suturing needle that has the suture material permanently attached to the needle.

symmetry (sim′ĕ-trē) The degree to which one side of the body is the same as the other.

sympathetic branch (sim′pă-thet′ik branch) A branch of the autonomic nervous system that prepares organs for fight-or-flight (stressful) situations.

symptom (simp′tŏm) A subjective, or internal, condition felt by a patient, such as pain, headache, or nausea, or another indication that generally cannot be seen or felt by the doctor or measured by instruments.

synaptic knob (si-nap′tik nŏb) The end of the axon branch.

synaptic space (si-nap-′tik spās) The space between the axon of one neuron and the dendrite of the next.

synergist (sĭn′ər-jist) Muscle that helps the prime mover by stabilizing joints.

synovial (sin-ō′vē-ăl) A type of joint, such as the elbow or knee, that is freely moveable.

systemic circuit (sis-tem′ik sĭr′kŭt) The route that blood takes from the heart through the body and back to the heart.

systemic circulation (sis-tem′ik sĭr′kyū-lā′shŭn) The circulation of blood through the arteries, capillaries, and veins of the general system, from the left ventricle to the right atrium.

systemic lupus erythematosus (SLE) (sis-tem′ik lū′pŭs ĕr-ith′ĕ-mă-tō′sŭs) An autoimmune disorder in which a person produces antibodies that target the person's own cells and tissues.

systolic pressure (sis-tol′ik presh′ŭr) The blood pressure measured when the left ventricle of the heart contracts.

tab (tăb) A tapered rectangular or rounded extension at the top of a file folder.

Tabular List (tab′yŭ-lăr list) One of two ways that diagnoses are listed in the ICD-10. In the Tabular List, the diagnosis codes are listed in numeric order with additional instructions.

tachycardia (tak′i-kahr′dē-ă) Rapid heart rate, generally in excess of 100 beats per minute.

tachypnea (tăk′ĕp-nē′ă) Abnormally rapid breathing.

targeted résumé (tahr′gĕt-ed rē′zŭm-ā) A résumé that is focused on a specific job target.

tarsals (tahr′sălz) Bones of the ankle.

taste bud (tāst bŭd) A structure that is made of taste cells (a type of chemoreceptor) and supporting cells.

tax liability account (taks lī′ă-bil′ĭ-tē ă-kownt′) Money withheld from employees' paychecks and held in a separate account that must be used to pay taxes to appropriate government agencies.

teamwork (tēm′-wŏrk) Working with others in the best interest of completing the job.

telecommunications device for the deaf (TDD) (tel′ĕ-kŏ-myū′ni-kā′shŭns dĕ-vīs′ def) Telephone accessory that transmits and receives text over standard telephone lines.

telephone triage (tĕl′ĕ-fōn′trē′ahzh) A process of determining the level of urgency of each incoming telephone call and how it should be handled.

teletherapy (tel-ĕ-thăr′ă-pē) A radiation therapy technique that allows deeper penetration than brachytherapy; used primarily for deep tumors.

teletype (TTY) device (tĕl′ĕ-tīp) A specially designed telephone that looks very much like a laptop computer with a cradle for the receiver of a traditional telephone. It is used by the hearing impaired to type communications onto a keyboard.

telophase (tel′ō-fāz) The final stage of mitosis; chromosomes reach the centrioles and the division creating two cells, each with a complete set of chromosomes, is completed.

template (tem′plăt) A guide that ensures consistency and accuracy.

temporal (tem′pŏr-ăl) Bones that form the lower sides of the skull.

temporal mandibular joint (TMJ) (tem′pŏr-ăl man-dib′yū-lăr joynt) The location where the mandible attaches to the temporal bone.

temporal scanner (tem′pŏr-ăl skan′ĕr) An instrument used to measure the body temperature by scanning the temporal artery in the forehead.

tendon (ten′dŏn) A cord-like, fibrous tissue that connects muscle to bone.

tendonitis (ten′dŏ-nī′tis) Inflammation of a tendon.

terminal (tĕr′mi-năl) Fatal.

terminal digit (tĕr′mi-năl dij′it) A small group of two to three numbers at the end of a patient number that is used as an identifying unit in a filing system.

testes (tĕs′tēz) The primary organs of the male reproductive system. Testes produce the hormone **testosterone.**

testosterone (tĕs-tŏs′tĕ-rōn) A hormone produced by the testes that maintains the male reproductive structures and male characteristics such as deep voice, body hair, and muscle mass.

tetanus (tet′ă-nŭs) A disease caused by *Clostridium tetani* living in the soil and water; more commonly called lockjaw.

thalamus (thal′ă-mŭs) Structure that acts as a relay station for sensory information heading to the cerebral cortex for interpretation; a subdivision of the diencephalon.

thalassemia (thal′ă-sē′mē-ă) An inherited form of anemia with a defective hemoglobin chain causing micocytic (small), hypochromic (pale), and short-lived red blood cells.

therapeutic team (thăr′ă-pyū′tik tēm) A group of physicians, nurses, medical assistants, and other specialists who work with patients dealing with chronic illness or recovery from major injuries.

therapeutic touch (thăr′ă-pyū′tik tŭch) The use of touch to detect and correct a person's energy fields, thus promoting healing and health.

thermography (ther-mog′ră-fē) A radiologic procedure in which an infrared camera is used to take photographs that record variations in skin temperature as dark (cool areas), light (warm areas), or shades of gray (areas with temperatures between cool and warm); used to diagnose breast tumors, breast abscesses, and fibrocystic breast disease.

thermometer (ther-mom′ĕ-ter) An instrument, either electronic or disposable, that is used to measure body temperature.

thermotherapy (ther′mō-thăr′ă-pē) The application of heat to the body to treat a disorder or injury.

third-party check (thĭrd-pahr′tē chek) A check made out to one recipient and given in payment to another, as with one made out to a patient rather than the medical practice.

third-party payer (thĭrd-pahr′tē pā′ĕr) A health plan that agrees to carry the risk of paying for patient services.

thoracocentesis (thōr′ă-kō-sen-tē′sis) Medical procedure where a sterile needle is introduced into the chest to remove fluid and pus.

thoracostomy (thōr′ă-kos′tŏ-mē) The surgical insertion of a chest tube to provide continuous drainage of the thoracic (chest) cavity.

thorax (thō′raks) The chest cavity.

thrombocytes (throm′bō-sīts) See **platelets.**

thrombophlebitis (thrŏm′bō-flĕ-bī′tis) A medical condition that most commonly occurs in leg veins when a blood clot and inflammation develop.

thrombus (thrŏm′bŭs) A blood clot that forms on the inside of an injured blood vessel wall.

thymosin (thī′mō-sin) A hormone that promotes the production of certain lymphocytes.

thymus (thī′mŭs) A gland that lies between the lungs. It secretes a hormone called thymosin.

thyroid cartilage (thī′royd kahr′ti-lăj) The largest cartilage in the larynx. It forms the anterior wall of the larynx.

thyroid gland (thī′royd gland) An endocrine gland, consisting of irregularly spheroid follicles, lying in front and to the sides of the upper part of the trachea, in a horseshoe shape, with two lateral lobes connected by a narrow central portion, the isthmus; occasionally an elongated offshoot, the pyramidal lobe, passes upward from the isthmus in front of the trachea. It is supplied by branches from the external carotid and subclavian arteries, and its nerves are derived from the middle cervical and cervicothoracic ganglia of the sympathetic system. It secretes thyroid hormone and calcitonin.

thyroid hormone (thī′royd hōr′mōn) A hormone produced by the thyroid gland that increases energy production, stimulates protein synthesis, and speeds up the repair of damaged tissue.

thyroid-stimulating hormone (TSH) (thī′royd-stim′yū-lāt-ing hōr′mōn) A hormone that stimulates the thyroid gland to release its hormone.

tibia (ti′bē-ă) The medial bone of the lower leg; commonly called the shin bone.

tickler file (tĭk′lĕr fīl) A reminder file for keeping track of time-sensitive obligations.

timed urine specimen (tīmd yūr′in spes′i-mĕn) A specimen of a patient's urine collected over a specific time period.

time management (tīm man′ăj-mĕnt) Utilizing time in an effective manner to accomplish the desired results.

time-specified scheduling (tīm spĕs'i-fīd sked'jūl-ing) A system of scheduling where patients arrive at regular, specified intervals, assuring the practice a steady stream of patients throughout the day.

tinea (tin'ē-ă) A fungal infection.

tinnitus (tin'i-tŭs) An abnormal ringing in the ear.

tissue (tish'ū) A structure that is formed when cells of the same type organize together.

T lymphocyte (tē lim'fŏ-sīt) A type of nongranular leukocyte that regulates immunologic response; includes helper T cells and suppressor T cells.

tonsils (ton'silz) Sets of lymphoid tissue in and around the oral cavity. The three sets are the pharyngeal tonsils (adenoids), palatine tonsils, and lingual tonsils.

tonometer (tō-nom'ĕ-tĕr) An instrument for determining pressure or tension, especially determining ocular tension.

topical (tŏp'ĭ-kăl) Applied to the skin.

tort (tōrt) In civil law, a breach of some obligation that causes harm or injury to someone.

torticollis (tōr'ti-kol'is) A muscular disease causing a cervical deformity in which the head bends toward the affected side while the chin rotates to the opposite side.

touchpad (tŭch păd) A type of pointing device common to laptop and notebook computers that directs activity on the computer screen by positioning a pointer or cursor on the screen. It is a small, flat device or surface that is highly sensitive to touch.

touch screen (tŭch skrēn) A type of computer monitor that acts as an intake device, receiving information through the touch of a pen, wand, or hand directly to the screen.

tourniquet (tŭr'ni-kĕt) An instrument for temporarily arresting the flow of blood to or from a distal part by pressure applied with an encircling device.

tower case (tou'ĕr kās) A vertical housing for the system unit of a personal computer.

toxicology (tŏk'sĭ-kŏl'ŏ-jē) The study of poisons or poisonous effects of drugs.

TPO See **treatment, payments, and operations.**

trachea (trā'kē-ă) The part of the respiratory tract between the larynx and the bronchial tree that is tubular and made of rings of cartilage and smooth muscle; also called the windpipe.

trackball (trăk-bawl) A pointing device with a ball that is rolled to position a pointer or cursor on a computer screen. It can be directly attached to the computer or can be wireless.

tracking (trăk'ĭng) Watching for changes in spending so as to help control expenses.

traction (trak'shŭn) The pulling or stretching of the musculoskeletal system to treat dislocated joints, joints afflicted by arthritis or other diseases, and fractured bones.

trade name (trād nām) A drug's brand, or proprietary, name.

traditional Chinese medicine (TCM) (tră-di'shŭn-ăl chī-nēz' med'i-sin) An ancient system of medicine originating in China that involves herbal and animal source preparations to treat illness. TCM includes various treatments such as acupuncture and acupressure.

transcription (trăn-skrĭp'shŭn) The transforming of spoken notes into accurate written form.

transcutaneous absorption (tranz'kyū-tā'nē-ŭs ăb-sōrp'shŭn) Entry (as of a pathogen) through a cut or crack in the skin.

transdermal (trans-der'măl) A type of topical drug administration that slowly and evenly releases a systemic drug through the skin directly into the bloodstream; a transdermal unit is also called a patch.

transfer (trăns'fĕr) To give something, such as information, to another party outside the doctor's office.

transmission-based precautions (trans-mish'ŭn-bāsd prē-kaw'shŭnz) CDC guidelines that supplement standard precautions when caring for patients with suspected or confirmed infection. The three types of transmission-based precautions are contact, droplet, and airborne precautions.

transurethral resection of prostate (trans'yŭr-ē'thrăl rē-sek'shŭn pros'tāt) Removal of the prostate through the urethra.

transverse (trans-vĕrs') Anatomical term that refers to the plane that divides the body into superior and inferior portions.

transverse colon (trans-vĕrs' kō'lŏn) The segment of the large intestine that crosses the upper abdominal cavity between the ascending and descending colon.

traveler's check (trăv'ĕl-rz chĕk) A check purchased and signed at a bank and later signed over to a payee.

treatment, payments, and operations (TPO) (trēt'mĕnt pā-mĕnt op-ĕr-ā'shŭns) The portion of **HIPAA** that allows the provider to use and share patient healthcare information for treatment, payment, and operations (such as quality improvement).

triage (trē'ahzh) To assess the urgency and types of conditions patients present as well as their immediate medical needs.

TRICARE (trī'kār) A program that provides healthcare benefits for families of military personnel and military retirees.

trichinosis (trik-i-nō'sis) A disease caused by a worm that is usually ingested from undercooked meat.

tricuspid valve (trī-kŭs'pid vălv) A heart valve that has three cusps and is situated between the right atrium and the right ventricle.

triglycerides (trī-glis'ĕr-īdz) Simple lipids consisting of glycerol (an alcohol) and three fatty acids.

trigone (trī'gōn) The triangle formed by the openings of the two ureters and the urethra in the internal floor of the bladder.

triple check (trip'ĕl chek) The process of checking a medication three times before administering it. First check is when you take it from the storage container and match it to the MAR; second check is when you prepare the medication; third check is before you close the container or just before you administer the medication.

troubleshooting (trŭb'ĕl-shū'tĭng) Trying to determine and correct a problem without having to call a service supplier.

Truth in Lending Statement (trūth lending stāt'mĕnt) A written description of the agreed terms of payment between the patient and medical practice when payment will be made in more than four installments.

trypsin (trip'sin) A pancreatic enzyme that digests proteins.

TSH See **thyroid-stimulating hormone.**

TTY device   See **teletype device.**

tubular reabsorption (tū′byū-lăr re-ab-sôrp′shŭn)   The second process of urine formation in which the glomerular filtrate flows into the proximal convoluted tubule.

tubular secretion (tū′byū-lăr sĭ-krē′shŭn)   The third process of urine formation in which substances move out of the blood in the peritubular capillaries into renal tubules.

tutorial (tūt-or′rē-ĕl)   A small program included in a software package designed to give users an overall picture of the product and its functions.

tympanic membrane (tim-păn′ik mĕm′brān)   A fibrous partition located at the inner end of the ear canal and separating the outer ear from the middle ear; also called the eardrum.

tympanic thermometer (tim-pan′ik ther-mom′ĕ-ter)   A type of electronic thermometer that measures infrared energy emitted from the tympanic membrane.

ulna (ŭl′nă)   The medial bone of the lower arm.

ultrasonic cleaning (ŭl′tră-sŏn′ĭk klēn′ĭng)   A method of sanitization that involves placing instruments in a cleaning solution in a receptacle that generates sound waves through the cleaning solution, loosening contaminants. Ultrasonic cleaning is safe for even very fragile instruments.

ultrasound (ŭl′tră-sownd)   The noninvasive therapeutic or diagnostic use of very high frequency sound waves for examination of internal body structures.

umami (ū-mom′ē)   Savory taste produced by glutamic acid (monosodium glutamate), recognized as the fifth taste sensation.

umbilical cord (ŭm-bil′i-kăl kōrd)   The rope-like connection between the fetus and the placenta. It contains the umbilical blood vessels.

unbundling (ŭn-bŭnd′ling)   Use of several *Current Procedural Terminology* codes for a service when one inclusive code is available.

underbooking (ŭn′dĕr buk′ing)   Leaving large, unused gaps in the doctor's schedule; this approach does not make the best use of the doctor's time.

uniform donor card (yū′ni-fŏrm dō′nŏr kahr′d)   A legal document that states a person's wish to make a gift upon death of one or more organs for medical research, organ transplants, or placement in a tissue bank.

unit (yū′nit)   A part of an individual's name or title, described in indexing rules.

unit price (yū′nit prīs)   The total price of a package divided by the number of items that comprise the package.

universal precautions (yū′ni-vĕr′săl prē-kaw′shŭnz)   Specific precautions required by the Centers for Disease Control and Prevention (CDC) to prevent healthcare workers from exposing themselves and others to infection by bloodborne pathogens.

unsaturated fats (ŭn-săch′ŭr-āt-ĕd fats)   Fats, including most vegetable oils, that is usually liquid at room temperature and tends to lower blood cholesterol.

upcoding (ŭp′kōd-ing)   Coding to a higher level of service than that provided to obtain higher reimbursements.

upper respiratory (tract) infection (ŭp′ĕr res′pir-ă-tōr-ē trakt in-fek′shŭn)   The common cold. (29)

urea (yūr-ē′ă)   Waste product formed by the breakdown of proteins and nucleic acids.

ureters (yŭr′ĕ-tĕrz)   Long, slender, muscular tubes that carry urine from the kidneys to the urinary bladder.

urethra (yūr-ē′thră)   The tube that conveys urine from the bladder during urination.

uric acid (yūr′ik as′id)   Waste product formed by the breakdown of proteins and nucleic acids.

urinalysis (yūr′in-al′i-sis)   The physical, chemical, and microscopic evaluation of urine to obtain information about body health and disease.

urinary catheter (yūr′i-nar-ē kath′ĕ-tĕr)   A sterile plastic tube inserted to provide urinary drainage.

urinary pH (yūr′i-nar-ē)   A measure of the degree of acidity or alkalinity of urine.

urine culture (yūr′in kŭl′chŭr)   A laboratory test in which urine is placed on a growth medium and bacteria are allowed to grow for 24 to 48 hours. Any large growths of bacteria are then identified. Urine cultures are often followed by a sensitivity or susceptibility test to determine which antibiotic will be most effective against the bacteria.

urine specific gravity (yūr′in spĕ-sif′ik grav′i-tē)   A measure of the concentration or amount (total weight) of substances dissolved in urine.

urobilinogen (yūr-ō-bī-lin′ō-jen)   A colorless compound formed by the breakdown of hemoglobin in the intestines. Elevated levels in urine may indicate increased red blood cell destruction or liver disease, whereas lack of urobilinogen in the urine may suggest total bile duct obstruction.

urologist (yŭr-ol′ŏ-jist)   A specialist who diagnoses and treats diseases of the kidney, bladder, and urinary system.

use (ūs)   The sharing, employing, applying, utilizing, examining, or analyzing of individually identifiable health information by employees or other members of an organization's workforce.

uterus (yū′tĕr-ŭs)   A hollow, muscular organ that functions to receive an embryo and sustain its development; also called the womb.

utilization review (UR) (yū′ti-lī-zā′shŭn rē-vyū′)   The process of reviewing medical care in individual cases to be sure that all services provided were medically necessary and that there was appropriate use of medical resources; performed by medical peers and used as a cost control measure by managed care organizations.

uvula (ū′vyū-lă)   The part of the soft palate that hangs down in the back of the throat.

uvulotomy (ū′vyū-lot′ŏ-mē)   Surgical procedure removing all or part of the uvula of the soft palate.

vaccine (văk-sēn′)   A preparation made from microorganisms and administered to a person to produce reduced sensitivity to or increased immunity to, an infectious disease.

vagina (vă-jī′nă)   A tubular organ that extends from the uterus to the labia.

vaginal introitus (vaj′i-năl in-trō′i-tŭs)   The vaginal os, or orifice. The opening of the vagina to the outside of the body.

vaginitis (vaj-i-nī′tis)   Inflammation of the vagina characterized by an abnormal vaginal discharge.

varicose veins (vār′i-kōs vānz)   Distended veins that result when vein valves are destroyed and blood pools in the veins, causing these veins to dilate.

vas deferens (vas def′ĕr-enz)   A tube that connects the epididymis with the urethra and that carries sperm.

vasectomy (vas-ek′tŏ-mē) A male steril-ization procedure in which a section of each vas deferens is removed.

vasoconstriction (vā′sō-kŏn-strik′shŭn) The constriction of the muscular wall of an artery to increase blood pressure.

vasodilation (vā-sō-dī-lā′shŭn) The wid-ening of the muscular wall of an artery to decrease blood pressure.

V code (vē kōd) A code used to identify encounters for reasons other than ill-ness or injury, such as annual checkups, immunizations, and normal childbirth.

vector (vek′tŏr) A living organism, such as an insect, that carries microorgan-isms from an infected person to another person.

venipuncture (ven′i-pŭngk′shŭr) The puncture of a vein, usually with a needle, for the purpose of drawing blood.

venoscope (vē′no-skōp) An instrument that helps visualize a vein; LED lights illuminate the subcutaneous tissue to highlight the veins.

ventilation (ven′ti-lā′shŭn) Moving air into and out of the lungs; also called breathing.

ventral (vĕn′trăl) See **anterior**.

ventral root (ven′trăl rūt) A portion of the spinal nerve that contains axons of motor neurons only.

ventricle (ven′tri-kĕl) Interconnected cavities in the brain filled with cerebro-spinal fluid.

ventricular fibrillation (VF) (ven-trik′yū-lăr fib′ri-lā′shŭn) An abnormal heart rhythm that is the most common cause of cardiac arrest.

verbalizing (vûr′bă-līz′ĭng) Stating what you believe the patient is suggesting or implying.

vermiform appendix (vĕr′mi-fōrm ă-pen′diks) A structure made mostly of lymphoid tissue and projecting off the cecum. It is commonly referred to as simply the appendix.

vertical file (vĕr′ti-kăl) A filing cabinet featuring pull-out drawers that usually contain a metal frame or bar equipped to handle letter- or legal-sized documents in hanging file folders.

vertigo (vĕr′ti-gō) Dizziness.

vesicles (vĕs′ĭ-kĕlz) Small sacs within the synaptic knobs that contain chemicals called neurotransmitters.

vestibule (ves′ti-byūl) The area in the inner ear between the semicircular canals and the cochlea.

VF See **ventricular fibrillation**.

vial (vī′ăl) A small glass bottle with a self-sealing rubber stopper.

vibrio (vib′rē-ō) A comma-shaped bacterium.

virtual private network (VPN) (vir′chū-ăl prī′văt net′wŏrk) These are used to connect two or more computer systems.

virulence (vir′yū-lĕns) A microorgan-ism's disease-producing power.

virus (vī′rŭs) One of the smallest known infectious agents, consisting only of nucleic acid surrounded by a protein coat; can live and grow only within the living cells of other organisms.

visceral pericardium (vis′er-ăl per-i-kahr′dē-ŭm) The innermost layer of the pericardium that lies directly on top of the heart; also known as the epicardium.

visceral peritoneum (vis′ĕr-ăl per-i-tō-nē′ŭm) Also known as the serosa, the outermost layer of the abdominal organs that secretes serous fluid to keep the organs from sticking to each other.

visceral smooth muscle (vis′ĕr-ăl smūth mŭs′ĕl) A type of smooth muscle containing sheets of muscle that closely contact each other. It is found in the walls of hollow organs such as the stomach, intestines, bladder, and uterus.

viscosity (vis-kos′i-tē) Thickness.

vitamin (vīt′ă-min) Organic substance that is essential for normal body growth and maintenance and resistance to infection.

vitreous humor (vit′rē-ŭs hyū′mŏr) A jelly-like substance that fills the part of the eye behind the lens and helps the eye keep its shape.

voice mail (voys māl) An advanced form of answering machine that allows a caller to leave a message when the phone line is busy.

void (voyd) A term used to describe some-thing that is not legally enforceable.

volume (vol′yūm) The amount of space an object, such as a drug, occupies.

vomer (vō′mĕr) A thin bone that divides the nasal cavity.

voucher check (vow′chĕr chĕk) A busi-ness check with an attached stub, which is kept as a receipt.

VPN See **virtual private network**.

vulva (vŭl′vă) External female genitalia.

vulvovaginitis (vul-vō-vaj′i-nī′tis) Inflammation of the external female genitalia and vagina.

walk-in (wôk′in) A patient who arrives without an appointment.

WAN (wăn) See **wide-area network**.

warranty (wōr′ăn-tē) A contract that specifies free service and replacement of parts for a piece of equipment during a certain period, usually a year.

warts (wōrts) Flesh-colored skin lesions with distinct, round borders that are raised and often have small, finger-like projections; also called verruca.

wave scheduling (wāv sked′jūl-ing) A system of scheduling in which the num-ber of patients seen each hour is deter-mined by dividing the hour by the length of the average visit and then giving that number of patients appointments with the doctor at the beginning of each hour.

weight (wāt) The product of the force of gravity, defined internationally as 9.81 (m/sec)/sec, × the mass of the body.

wellness (wĕl′nĕs) A philosophy of life and personal hygiene that views health as not merely the absence of illness but the fullest realization of one's physical and mental potential, as achieved through positive attitudes, fitness training, a diet low in fat and high in fiber, and the avoidance of unhealthful practices.

Western blot test (wes′tĕrn blŏt tĕst) A blood test used to confirm enzyme-linked immunosorbent assay (ELISA) test results for HIV infection.

wet mount (wĕt mount) A preparation of a specimen in a liquid that allows the organisms to remain alive and mobile while they are being identified.

white matter (hwīt măt′ĕr) The outer tissue of the spinal cord that is lighter in color than gray matter. It contains myelinated axons.

whole blood (hōl blŭd) The total volume of plasma and formed elements, or blood in which the elements have not been sep-arated by coagulation or centrifugation.

whole-body skin examination (hōl-bŏd′ē skĭn eg-zam′i-nā′shŭn) An examina-tion of the visible top layer of the entire surface of the skin, including the scalp, genital area, and areas between the toes, to look for lesions, especially suspicious moles or precancerous growths.

whole foods (hōl fūdz) Foods that have little or no processing before they are eaten.

wide-area network (WAN) (wīd ār′ē-ă net′wŏrk) A computer network in which the computers connected may be far apart, generally having a radius of half a mile or more.

Wood's light examination (wudz līt eg-zam′i-nā′shŭn) A type of dermatologic examination in which a physician inspects the patient's skin under an ultraviolet lamp in a darkened room.

word root (wŏrd rūt) The base meaning of a medical term.

work ethic (wŏrk eth′ik) A set of values of hard work held by employees.

work practice controls (wŏrk prak′tis kŏn-trōzl′) Controlling workplace injuries by altering the way a task is performed.

work quality (wŏrk kwahl′i-tē) Striving for excellence in doing the job; pride in one's performance.

World Health Organization (WHO) (wŏrld helth ōr′găn-ĭ-zā′shŭn) A unit of the United Nations devoted to international health problems.

write-it-once (pegboard) system (rīt it wŭns pĕg-bōrd′ sis′tĕm) A manual bookkeeping system where the daily log has prepunched holes on the right or left side of the log. Prepunched charge sheets (of NCR paper) are placed in designated areas on top of the day sheet, which has been placed on the pegboard. The patient ledger card is placed between the day sheet and the charge sheet and an entry is made; it appears on all three documents at the same time.

written-contract account (rĕ′ten kŏn′trăkt ă-kownt) An agreement between the physician and patient stating that the patient will pay a bill in more than four installments.

X12 837 Health Care Claim (hĕlth kār klăm) An electronic claim transaction that is the HIPAA Health Care Claim or Equivalent Encounter Information ("HIPAA claim").

xeroradiography (zē′rō-rā′dē-og′ră-fē) A radiologic procedure in which X-rays are developed with a powder toner, similar to the toner in photocopiers, and the X-ray image is processed on specially treated xerographic paper; used to diagnose breast cancer, abscesses, lesions, or calcifications.

xiphoid process (zī′foyd pros′es) The lower extension of the breastbone; the cartilaginous tip of the sternum.

yeast (yēst) A fungus that grows mainly as a single-celled organism and reproduces by budding.

yoga (yō′gă) A series of poses and breathing exercises that provide awareness of the unity of the whole being. The practice of yoga also increases flexibility and strength.

yolk sac (yōk săk) The sac that holds the materials for the nutrition of the embryo.

Zip drive (zip drīv) A high-capacity disk drive developed by Iomega®. Zip drives can hold 100 to 750 MB of data. They are durable and relatively inexpensive. They may be used for backing up hard disks and transporting large files.

zona pellucida (zō′nă pe-lū′sid-ă) A layer that surrounds the cell membrane of an egg.

Z-track method (zē′trăk mĕth′ŏd) A technique used when injecting an intramuscular (IM) drug that can irritate subcutaneous tissue; involves pulling the skin and subcutaneous tissue to the side before inserting the needle at the site, creating a zigzag path in the tissue layers that prevents the drug from leaking into the subcutaneous tissue and causing irritation.

zygomatic (zī′gō-mat′ik) The bones that form the prominence of the cheeks.

zygote (zī′gōt) The cell that is formed from the union of the egg and sperm.

Index

Page numbers in **boldface** indicate figures. Page numbers followed by b indicate box features, p procedures, and t tables, respectively.

A

AAMA. *See* American Association of Medical Assistants

AAPC (American Academy of Professional Coders), 22t

AAPC (American Association of Professional Coders), 24t

ABA (American Banking Association), 453

Abandonment of patients, 68, 69–70, 73

ABA numbers, **452,** 453

Abbreviations
  in appointment scheduling, 325, 326t
  for blood tests, 1004–1005t
  in charting, 727, 727–728t
  for laboratory measurements, 936, 938t
  in medical notation, 1285–1286
  in prescriptions, 1099, 1101t
  in transcription, 235
  for urine analysis and stool testing, 974, 975t

Abdomen
  examination of, 765–766
  flat plate of, 1074
  pain and emergency intervention, 1242–1243
  quadrants of, 766

Abdominal girth, 749

Abdominal lining, 650

Abdominal muscles, **531,** 533, **534**

Abdominopelvic cavity, 479, **481**

Abducens nerves, 606, **607**

Abduction, 529, **529, 1156–1157**

ABHES (Accrediting Bureau of Health Education Schools), 6, 7, 1263

ABMS (American Board of Medical Specialties), 15

ABN (Advance Beneficiary Notice of Noncoverage), 358–359, **359**

ABO blood types, 563, 563t, **564**

Abrasions, 869, 1241, **1242**

Abscesses, 759t, 897

Absorbed poisons, 1240

Absorption
  of drugs, 1088
  of nutrients in digestive system, 657–658, 658t

Abuse. *See also* Substance abuse
  of children, 721–722, 820
  of elderly, 722, 839
  of healthcare system, 65, 77
  in Medicare program, 354
  physical, 720–721

psychological, 720–721

ACA (Affordable Care Act of 2010), 14, 247, 348

Academy of Nutrition and Dietetics, 306t

ACAP (Alliance of Claims Assistance Professionals), 22t

Acceptance
  in stages of dying, **55**
  in therapeutic communication, 50

Accepting assignment, 353, 355

Accessibility
  to electronic health records, 253
  exam room guidelines for, 177
  to healthcare, 14, 350
  of medical offices, **125–126,** 125–128
  to medical records, 269

Accessory nerves, 607, **607**

Accidental injuries, 1235–1242

Accident reporting, for laboratories, 928, **929**

Accommodation, 681, 872

Account cards. *See* Patient ledger cards

Accounting. *See also* Banking; Billing; Bookkeeping; Collections; Payments; Payroll
  accuracy in, 433
  attaching superbills to patient charts, 438
  defined, 433
  disbursement records, 435–436, **437,** 459
  electronic bookkeeping, 434
  end of day tasks, 445
  manual, 434–437
  methods for, 433–437
  patient check out and, 438
  payment collection, 128, 438–440, 444
  procedures for, 433
  software for, 144
  start of business day tasks, 438

Accounts. *See also* Accounts payable; Accounts receivable
  age analysis of, **445,** 445–446, 462–463p
  checking, 454
  open-book, 443
  past-due, 443
  single-entry, 443
  uncollectable, 445
  written-contract, 443

Accounts payable
  as bookkeeping record, 435
  categories of, 458
  disbursement management, 459

financial summaries, 460
  report generators for, 252
  writing checks for, 459

Accounts receivable
  as bookkeeping record, 435
  daily logs for tracking, 435
  insuring, 448
  report generators for, 252

Accreditation, 4, 7

Accrediting Bureau of Health Education Schools (ABHES), 6, 7, 1263

Accuracy
  in accounting, 433
  of electronic health records, 253
  of medical records, 235
  of telephone messages, 291

ACE (angiotensin-converting enzyme), 1013t

Acetabulum, 516

Acetaminophen, 1136

Acetylcholine, 526, 527, 608–609

Acetylcholinesterase, 526

Acetyl coenzyme A, 528

Acid-fast stains, 950

Acidosis, 981t

Acids, 179, 179t, 481–482, **482**

Acinar cells, 656

Acne vulgaris, **500,** 500–501b, 852t, 1296

ACOG (American College of Obstetricians and Gynecologists), 777, 777t

Acoustic neuroma, 688b

ACP (American College of Physicians), 24, 24t, 1252

Acromegaly, 670–671b, 670t, **671,** 1303

Acrosome, 627, **631**

ACTH (adrenocorticotropic hormone), **666,** 667t, 668, 670t

Active files, 270

Active immunity, 577

Active listening, 49, **49,** 718

Active mechanisms, 484

Active mobility exercises, 1161

Active resistance exercises, 1162

Active transport, 484

Active voice, 193

Activity-monitoring systems, 148–149

Acupuncture, 1102

Acupuncturists, 18

Acute conditions, 389

Acute drug therapy, 1089

Acute kidney failure, 623b, 1300

ADA. *See* Americans with Disabilities Act of 1990

ADA Amendments Act of 2008 (ADAAA), 177

Adam's apple, 586

Addiction
  in adolescents, 721b, 820–821, 821b
  defined, 721b, 821b

Adding machines, 151–152

Addison's disease, 670t, **671,** 671b, 1303

Add-on codes, **411,** 411–412

Add-on safety features, for needles, 699, **700**

Addresses
  format for, 209, 209t
  inside, 195, **196**
  patient address change and relocation, 451–452
  placement of, 208–209, **208–209**

Address labels, 192

Adduction, 529, **529, 1156–1157**

Adductor longus, **531,** 533

Adductor magnus, **531,** 533

Adenohypophysis, 667–668

Adenoids, 651

Adenosine triphosphate (ATP), 527–528, 657

Adenovirus, 947t

ADH. *See* Antidiuretic hormone

ADHD (attention deficit hyperactivity disorder), 817

Adipocytes, 472, 473

Adipose (fat) tissue, 473, **474,** 493, **493**

Adjectives, 193t

Adjustments
  billing, 357
  chiropractic, 18
  posting, 460p

Administration of drugs. *See* Drug administration

Administrative medical assistants
  legal considerations for, 73–76
  preoperative duties of, 907
  responsibilities of, 2, 3t
  specialty careers for, 21, 22t

Administrative office equipment, 149–154

Administrative office supplies, 157, 158t, 159

Administrative simplification, 83

ADNs (associate degrees in nursing), 21

Adolescents. *See also* Children; Pediatrics
  depression, substance abuse and addiction in, 721b, 820–821, 821b
  developmental stages of, **46**

Induction of labor, 782
Induration, 1131
Industry vs. inferiority stage, **46**
Indwelling catheters, 977, **977**
Infants. *See also* Breast-feeding;
    Children; Pediatrics
  aspects of care for, 802, 802t
  body measurements of, 747, 814,
    814, 822–823p
  bottle feeding, 782
  capillary puncture in, 1011, **1012**
  choking, 1236, 1256p
  developmental stages of, **46**
  head circumference of, 814, **814,**
    822–823p
  hearing problems in, 688
  intellectual-cognitive
    development of, 802
  neonates, 641, 800–801, **800–801**
  physical development of,
    801–802, **802**
  postnatal period, 641–642
  psycho-emotional development
    of, 802
  respiratory distress syndrome in,
    588, 595b
  safety tips for, 805b
  skull bones, 511
  social development of, 802
  transmission of bloodborne
    infections during
    childbirth, 96
Infection-control techniques
  Bloodborne Pathogens Protection
    Standard, 76–77, 98–99,
    99t, 103
  disinfection, 178–180, 179t
  for examination rooms, 180–182,
    181b
  for exposure incidents, 102–103
  hand hygiene, 97–98, **98,**
    105–106p, 180, 180t
  HBV vaccine for healthcare
    workers, 99, 103, 696
  for medical equipment, 701
  in Needlestick Safety and
    Prevention Act, 103
  OSHA guidelines for, 94–95,
    98–99
  personal protective equipment,
    99, 102
  respiratory hygiene and cough
    etiquette, 96b
  sanitization, 177–178
  for spirometers, 1055
  transmission-based precautions,
    103–104
  Universal Precautions, 99, 101
  written exposure plans, 102
Infections, 93–108. *See also*
    Diseases; Infection-control
    techniques
  breaking cycle of, 97
  congenital, 96
  cycle of, **95,** 95–98
  defenses against, 574–576, 575t,
    577
  defined, 575
  diagnosis of, 957, **958**
  of ears, 688–689b
  endogenous, 95, 701

environmental factors in
  transmission of, 97
exogenous, 95, 701
exposure incidents, 102–103
healthcare-associated infections,
  105, 693–695, **694**
means of entrance, **95,** 97
means of exit, 95, **95**
means of transmission, **95,** 95–97
opportunistic, 948
reservoir hosts for, 95, **95**
superficial, 701
surgical site infections, 701–702
susceptible hosts for, **95,** 97
as venipuncture complication,
  1013
wound healing and, 898b
Infectious diseases
  conjunctivitis, 818t
  examination of patients with, 758
  ICD-10-CM coding guidelines
    for, 398
  reporting guidelines for, 706,
    706–707t, 710–712p
  transmission by airborne droplets,
    758, 758t
  urinalysis for, 981t
Infectious waste, 125. *See also*
    Biohazardous waste
Inferior (caudal), 477, 477t, 478,
    478–479
Inferior vena cava, 547, **548**
Infertility, 644, 787, 1301
Infestations, 955
Inflammation
  of heart tissue, 851t
  as nonspecific defense, 575, 575t
  signs of, 575
Inflammatory bowel disease. *See*
    Crohn's disease
Inflammatory phase, of wound
    healing, 897
Inflation reflex, 589
Influenza
  droplet precautions for, 104
  in elderly patients, 838
  ICD-10-CM coding guidelines
    for, 400, **400**
  immunization for, **811, 1103**
  pathophysiology of, 592b
  personal protective equipment
    for, 759t
  prevention of, 1290
  transmission of, 96, 699
  viral pathogens causing, **946,**
    947t, 1288
Information. *See* Patient
    information; Protected health
    information (PHI)
Information packets. *See* Patient
    information packets
Information sheets, patient, 303,
    303–304
Informed consent
  defined, 66–67
  for immunizations, 810, **812**
  in medical records, 225–226,
    228, 724
  of minors, 67
  in physician-patient contracts,
    66–67

surgical, 312, **313,** 907
  for treatment, 311, **312**
Infrared rays, 1159
Infraspinatus, **531,** 533
Infundibulum, 633, **634**
Infusion, for IV injections, 1133
Ingested poisons, 1239–1240
Inguinal hernias, 661b, 1302
Inhalants, 722t
Inhalation therapy, 1126t, 1134,
    1146p
Inhaled poisons, 1240
Inhalers, 1134, 1146p
Inheritance, 486
Initialing, of medical records, 227,
    232, 233
Initiative vs. guilt stage, **46**
Injections
  advantages and disadvantages
    of, 1129
  of anesthetics, 909, **909**
  for children, 1135–1136
  intradermal, 1126t, 1129, **1130,**
    1131, 1131t, 1143–1144p
  intramuscular, 1126t, 1129, **1130,**
    1131t, 1132, **1133,** 1135,
    1145–1146p
  intravenous, 1126t, 1129, **1130,**
    1132–1133
  methods of, 1131–1133, **1133**
  needles and syringes for, 1129,
    1130–1132, 1131t
  packaging of, 1129–1130, **1132**
  reconstituting and drawing drugs
    for, 1142–1143p
  safe practices for, 698–699,
    699–700
  sites for, 1123, 1135
  subcutaneous, 1127t, 1129, **1130,**
    1131t, 1132, 1144–1145p
Injuries. *See also* Medical
    emergencies
  accidental, 1235–1242
  to brain and spinal cord, 606b
  ICD-10-CM coding guidelines
    for, 401–402
  multiple, 1238
  needlestick, 699
  prevention of, 307–308, 307b
  strains and sprains, 534b, 855t,
    1297
Ink-jet printers, 143
Innate (nonspecific) immunity,
    574–575, 575t
Inner cell mass, 639
Inner ear, 686, **686–687,** 878
Inoculation of culture plates,
    963–964, 963–965
In-office transactions, 437–441
Inorganic matter, 482
Input devices, for computers, 141
INR (International Normalized
    Ratio), 1021
Insects
  bites and stings from, 1235
  in infection transmission, 96–97
  parasitic, **956,** 956–957
Insertions, in muscle attachment
    sites, 528, **528**
Inside address, of business letters,
    195, **196**

Inspection
  of examination room instruments,
    183
  in filing process, 267
  in general physical examinations,
    762
Inspiration, **588,** 588–589
Institute for Safe Medication
    Practice (ISMP), 727
In-store clinics, 88
Instruments
  adding sterile instruments to
    sterile field, 906
  arranging, 183
  cleaning, 184, 185t
  for cutting and dissecting,
    900–901, **900–901**
  in examination rooms, 183–184,
    184, 185t
  for general physical examinations,
    183–184, **184,** 185t, 763,
    763t, **764**
  for grasping and clamping, 901,
    902
  handling by sterile scrub
    assistants, 911, **911**
  inspecting and maintaining, 183
  for minor surgery, 900–904,
    900–904
  preparing, 184
  for retracting, dilating, and
    probing, 901, **902**
  sanitizing, disinfecting, and
    sterilizing, 177–178, 907
  for suturing, 901, **903,** 903–904
  trays and packs of, 904, **904**
Insulin
  chemical development of, 1087
  diseases and disorders involving,
    670t
  function of, **666,** 667t, 669–670
  negative feedback loop and, 666
  normal ranges for, 1018t
Insulin-dependent diabetes mellitus,
    578b
Insulin shock, 1246
Insurance, 346–357. *See also*
    Medicaid; Medicare
  for accounts receivable, 448
  Affordable Care Act and, 348
  coinsurance, 347
  commercial carriers, 350
  copayments, 347
  deductibles, 347, 348
  disability, 350
  fee-for-service plans, 348
  fraud, 425
  government plans, 351–357
  information packets on, 311
  liability, 71–72, 350
  malpractice, 71–72
  managed care organizations, 239,
    348–350, **349**
  for military personnel, 355–356,
    356
  patient centered medical homes,
    350–351
  portability of coverage, 77
  premiums, 347
  private health plans, 347–351,
    349